ICD•9•CM

Professional for Physicians
Volumes 1 and 2

International Classification of Diseases
9th Revision
Clinical Modification

Sixth Edition

Effective October 1, 2002–September 30, 2003

Edited by:
Anita C. Hart, RHIA, CCS, CCS-P
Catherine A. Hopkins, CPC

ingenix®
St. Anthony Publishing/Medicode

Copyright © 2002 Ingenix, Inc.

All Rights Reserved

First Printing — August 2002

This book, or parts hereof, may not be reproduced in any form without permission.

Additional copies may be ordered from:

Your local bookstore
or
1-800-INGENIX (464-3649)

IPPC ISBN 1-56329-873-2

DISCLAIMER

All the codes, indexes and other material in the ICD-9-CM are compiled from official ICD-9-CM codes and instructions as well as the Medicare regulations and manuals issued or authorized by the Centers for Medicare and Medicaid Services. The code book is designed to provide accurate and authoritative information in regard to the subject covered, and every reasonable effort has been made to ensure the accuracy of the information within these pages. However, the ultimate responsibility for correct coding lies with the provider of services.

Ingenix, Inc., its employees, agents and staff make no representation, warranty or guarantee that this compilation of codes and narratives is error-free or that the use of this code book will prevent differences of opinion or disputes with Medicare or other third-party payers as to the codes that are accepted or the amounts that will be paid to providers of services, and will bear no responsibility or liability for the results or consequences of the use of this code book.

American Academy of Professional Coders (AAPC)
Continuing Education Units Credits: 5 CEUs
Contact AAPC directly for credits: 1.800.626.CODE

St. Anthony Publishing/Medicode

2525 Lake Park Boulevard • Salt Lake City, UT 84120
11410 Isaac Newton Square • Reston, VA 20190

St. Anthony Publishing/Medicode

September 2002

Dear Ingenix Customer:

St. Anthony Publishing and Medicode joined their expertise and after intense research involving real-world coders developed a new and innovative code book. Your *2003 ICD-9-CM Professional for Physicians, Volumes 1 & 2*, is the result of this effort. Designed by coders for coders, we are certain you will find the new page design and intuitive symbols will improve coding accuracy and efficiency.

The codes contained in this book are the official code set issued by the U.S. Department of Health and Human Services, effective October 1, 2002 through September 30, 2003.

Your new *2003 ICD-9-CM Professional for Physicians, Volumes 1 and 2*, features:

- New! ICD-9-CM convention — Code, if applicable any causal condition first
- fiscal year 2003 official ICD-9-CM codes
- summary of code changes for 2003
- symbols indicating code changes and pages are dated to indicate when the changes occurred
- clinically-oriented illustrations and comprehensive definitions
- check fourth- and fifth-digit symbols in the index and tabular sections
- age and sex edit symbols

.......PLUS the accuracy and quality you expect from the leaders!

> **Note: The ICD-9-CM Coordination and Maintenance Committee has undertaken the task of completely revising the official coding guidelines. At the time of press the guidelines had not yet been finalized. The new guidelines build upon the current set and therefore, the guidance provided by the current set is still valid. Release of the revised guidelines is expected before the effective date of October 1, 2002. We have created a web site specifically to provide you with the revised guidelines once they are released. You will be able to log on to www.ingenixonline.com/I9guidelines toward the end of September to view and print the new ICD-9-CM official coding guidelines.**

We appreciate your choosing Ingenix/St. Anthony Publishing/Medicode/ to meet your coding needs. If you have any questions or comments concerning your *2003 ICD-9-CM Professional for Physicians, Volumes 1 and 2*, please do not hesitate to call our customer service department. The toll free number is 1.800.INGENIX (464-3649).

Cordially,

Elizabeth Boudrie

Elizabeth Boudrie
Vice President, Regulatory Services

IPPC/10/02

Preface

ICD-9-CM for Physicians has been designed with the physician office coder in mind. The most recent official government versions of volumes 1 and 2 have been combined to provide physicians and their office staff with an ICD-9-CM book that is easy to use.

In addition, our technical experts have drawn upon their extensive hands-on experience to enhance the government's official version with valuable features essential to correct coding and reimbursement. With these enhancements, physician office coders will increase the efficiency and timeliness of claim submission for both Medicare and other third-party payers.

As you review the content, you'll find the following:

- All the official ICD-9-CM codes, indexes, notes, footnotes and symbols
- Complete official coding guidelines
- Our exclusive color coding, symbols, and footnotes that alert coders to coding and reimbursement issues. Medicare outpatient code edits, such as invalid fourth or fifth digit for diagnosis codes and circumstances under which Medicare may be secondary payer (MSP), are identified.
- Illustrations and clinically oriented definitions to aid in correct code assignment
- Symbols identifying new codes and text revisions; pages are dated to indicate when the changes were made
- Exclusive QuickFlip Color Tabs for quick, easy location of terms and codes in the index and tabular list

USE OF OFFICIAL SOURCES

This *ICD-9-CM for Physicians* contains the official U.S. Department of Health and Human Services, ICD-9-CM codes, effective for the current year.

The color coding, footnotes and symbols, which identify coding and reimbursement issues, are derived from official federal government sources, including the Medicare Outpatient Code Editor as well as the knowledge of our technical experts.

In addition to the editors, the following people have contributed to this book:

Kerrie Hornsby, Desktop Publishing Manger
Stacy Perry, Desktop Publishing Manager
Paul Driscoll, Illustrator
Sheri Bernard, Director of Essential Regulatory Products
Lynn Speirs, Managing Editor

TECHNICAL EDITORS
Anita C. Hart, RHIA, CCS, CCS-P
Product Manager, Ingenix, Inc., Reston, VA
Ms. Hart's experience includes fifteen years conducting and publishing research in clinical medicine and human genetics for Yale University, Massachusetts General Hospital, and Massachusetts Institute of Technology. In addition, Ms. Hart has supervised medical records management, health information management, coding and reimbursement, and worker's compensation issues as the office manager for a physical therapy rehabilitation clinic. Ms. Hart is an expert in physician and facility coding, reimbursement systems, and compliance issues. Ms. Hart developed the *Complete Coding Tutor*, an advanced self-study guide for ICD-9-CM, CPT, and HCPCS Level II coding and served as technical consultant for numerous other publications for hospital and physician practices. Currrently, Ms. Hart is the Product Manager for the ICD-9-CM and DRG product lines.

Catherine A. Hopkins, CPC
Technical Consultant, Ingenix, Inc., Reston, VA
Ms. Hopkins has 17 years of experience in the healthcare field. Her experience includes six years as office manager and senior coding specialist for a large multi-specialty practice. Ms. Hopkins has written several coding manuals and newsletters and has taught seminars on CPT, HCPCS, and ICD-9-CM coding. She also serves as technical support for various software products.

WHAT TO DO IF YOU HAVE QUESTIONS
If you have any questions about your subscription, call our customer service department toll free at (800) INGENIX (464.3649).

If you have comments on the content of the code book, please address them in writing to:

> Product Manager, Ingenix, Inc.
> 11410 Isaac Newton Square, Reston, VA 20190
> Tel no.: (800) INGENIX (464.3649)
> Fax no.: (801) 982-4033

ADDITIONAL COPIES
Contact the customer service order department toll free at (800) INGENIX (464-3649).

Introduction

HISTORY AND FUTURE OF ICD•9

The International Classification of Diseases, Ninth Revision, Clinical Modification (ICD-9-CM) is based on the official version of the World Health Organization's Ninth Revision, International Classification of Diseases (ICD-9). ICD-9-CM classifies morbidity and mortality information for statistical purposes, indexing of hospital records by disease and operations, data storage, and retrieval.

This modification of ICD-9 supplants the Eighth Revision International Classification of Diseases, Adapted for Use in the United States (ICDA-8) and the Hospital Adaptation of ICDA (H-ICDA).

The concept of extending the International Classification of Diseases for use in hospital indexing was originally developed in response to a need for a more efficient basis for storage and retrieval of diagnostic data. In 1950, the U.S. Public Health Service and the Veterans Administration began independent tests of the International Classification of Diseases for hospital indexing purposes. The following year, the Columbia Presbyterian Medical Center in New York City adopted the International Classification of Diseases, Sixth Revision, with some modifications for use in its medical record department. A few years later, the Commission on Professional and Hospital Activities (CPHA) in Ann Arbor, Mich., adopted the International Classification of Diseases with similar modifications for use in hospitals participating in the Professional Activity Study.

The problem of adapting ICD for indexing hospital records was addressed by the U.S. National Committee on Vital and Health Statistics through its subcommittee on hospital statistics. The subcommittee reviewed the modifications made by the various users of ICD and proposed that uniform changes be made. This was done by a small working party.

In view of the growing interest in the use of the International Classification of Diseases for hospital indexing, a study was undertaken in 1956 by the American Hospital Association and the American Medical Record Association (then the American Association of Medical Record Librarians) of the relative efficiencies of coding systems for diagnostic indexing. This study indicated the International Classification of Diseases provided a suitable and efficient framework for indexing hospital records. The major users of the International Classification of Diseases for hospital indexing purposes then consolidated their experiences, and an adaptation was first published in December 1959. A revision was issued in 1962 and the first "Classification of Operations and Treatments" was included.

In 1966, the international conference for revising the International Classification of Diseases noted the eighth revision of ICD had been constructed with hospital indexing in mind and considered the revised classification suitable, in itself, for hospital use in some countries. However, it was recognized that the basic classification might provide inadequate detail for diagnostic indexing in other countries. A group of consultants was asked to study the eighth revision of ICD (ICD-8) for applicability to various users in the United States. This group recommended that further detail be provided for coding of hospital and morbidity data. The American Hospital Association was requested to develop the needed adaptation proposals. This was done by an advisory committee (the Advisory Committee to the Central Office on ICDA). In 1968 the United States Public Health Service published the product, Eighth Revision International Classification of Diseases, Adapted for Use in the United States. This became commonly known as ICDA-8, and beginning in 1968 it served as the basis for coding diagnostic data for both official morbidity and mortality statistics in the United States.

In 1968, the CPHA published the Hospital Adaptation of ICDA (H-ICDA) based on both the original ICD-8 and ICDA-8. In 1973, CPHA published a revision of H-ICDA, referred to as H-ICDA-2. Hospitals throughout the United States were divided in their use of these classifications until January 1979, when ICD-9-CM was made the single classification intended primarily for use in the United States, replacing these earlier related, but somewhat dissimilar, classifications.

Physicians have been required by law to submit diagnosis codes for Medicare reimbursement since the passage of the Medicare Catastrophic Coverage Act of 1988. This act requires physician offices to include the appropriate diagnosis codes when billing for services provided to Medicare beneficiaries on or after April 1, 1989. The Health Care Financing Administration designated ICD-9-CM as the coding system physicians must use.

In 1993 the World Health Organization published the newest version of International Classification of Diseases, Tenth Revision, ICD-10. This version contains the greatest number of changes in the history of ICD. There are more codes (5,500 more than ICD-9) to allow more specific reporting of diseases and newly recognized conditions. ICD-10 consists of three volumes; tabular list (volume I), instructions (volume 2) and the alphabetic index (volume 3). It contains 21 chapters including two supplementary ones. The codes are alphanumeric (A00–T98, V01–Y98 and Z00–Z99). Currently ICD-10 is being used in some European countries with implementation expected after the year 2000 in the United States.

ICD-9-CM BACKGROUND

In February 1977, a steering committee was convened by the National Center for Health Statistics to provide advice and counsel in developing a clinical modification of ICD-9. The organizations represented on the steering committee included the following:

- American Association of Health Data Systems
- American Hospital Association
- American Medical Record Association
- Association for Health Records
- Council on Clinical Classifications
- Centers for Medicare and Medicaid (formerly known as Health Care Financing Administration), Department of Health and Human Services
- WHO Center for Classification of Diseases for North America, sponsored by the National Center for Health Statistics, Department of Health and Human Services

The Council on Clinical Classifications was sponsored by the following:

- American Academy of Pediatrics
- American College of Obstetricians and Gynecologists
- American College of Physicians

- American College of Surgeons
- American Psychiatric Association
- Commission on Professional and Hospital Activities

The steering committee met periodically in 1977. Clinical guidance and technical input were provided by task forces on classification from the Council on Clinical Classification's sponsoring organizations.

ICD-9-CM is a clinical modification of the World Health Organization's ICD-9. The term "clinical" is used to emphasize the modification's intent: to serve as a useful tool to classify morbidity data for indexing medical records, medical care review, and ambulatory and other medical care programs, as well as for basic health statistics. To describe the clinical picture of the patient, the codes must be more precise than those needed only for statistical groupings and trend analysis.

CHARACTERISTICS OF ICD-9-CM

ICD-9-CM far exceeds its predecessors in the number of codes provided. The disease classification has been expanded to include health-related conditions and to provide greater specificity at the fifth-digit level of detail. These fifth digits are not optional; they are intended for use in recording the information substantiated in the clinical record.

Volume I (tabular list) of ICD-9-CM contains five appendices:

Appendix A: Morphology of Neoplasms
Appendix B: Glossary of Mental Disorders
Appendix C: Classification of Drugs by American Hospital Formulary Service List Number and Their ICD-9-CM Equivalents
Appendix D: Classification of Industrial Accidents According to Agency
Appendix E: List of Three-Digit Categories

These appendices are included as a reference to provide further information about the patient's clinical picture, to further define a diagnostic statement, to aid in classifying new drugs or to reference three-digit categories.

Volume 2 (alphabetic index) of ICD-9-CM contains many diagnostic terms that do not appear in volume I since the index includes most diagnostic terms currently in use.

THE DISEASE CLASSIFICATION

ICD-9-CM is totally compatible with its parent system, ICD-9, thus meeting the need for comparability of morbidity and mortality statistics at the international level. A few fourth-digit codes were created in existing three-digit rubrics only when the necessary detail could not be accommodated by the use of a fifth-digit subclassification. To ensure that each rubric of ICD-9-CM collapses back to its ICD-9 counterpart the following specifications governed the ICD-9-CM disease classification:

Specifications for the tabular list:

1. Three-digit rubrics and their contents are unchanged from ICD-9.
2. The sequence of three-digit rubrics is unchanged from ICD-9.
3. Three-digit rubrics are not added to the main body of the classification.
4. Unsubdivided three-digit rubrics are subdivided where necessary to

- add clinical detail
- isolate terms for clinical accuracy

5. The modification in ICD-9-CM is accomplished by adding a fifth digit to existing ICD-9 rubrics, except as noted under #7 below.
6. The optional dual classification in ICD-9 is modified.
    - Duplicate rubrics are deleted:
        - four-digit manifestation categories duplicating etiology entries
        - manifestation inclusion terms duplicating etiology entries
    - Manifestations of disease are identified, to the extent possible, by creating five-digit codes in the etiology rubrics.
    - When the manifestation of a disease cannot be included in the etiology rubrics, provision for its identification is made by retaining the ICD-9 rubrics used for classifying manifestations of disease.
7. The format of ICD-9-CM is revised from that used in ICD-9.
    - American spelling of medical terms is used.
    - Inclusion terms are indented beneath the titles of codes.
    - Codes not to be used for primary tabulation of disease are printed in italics with the notation, "code first underlying disease."

Specifications for the alphabetic index:

1. The format of the alphabetic index follows that of ICD-9.
2. When two codes are required to indicate etiology and manifestation, the manifestation code appears in brackets (e.g., diabetic cataract 250.5 [*366.41*]).

How to Use the ICD•9•CM for Physicians (Volumes 1 & 2)

This *ICD-9-CM for Physicians* is based on the official version of the International Classification of Diseases, Ninth Revision, Clinical Modification, Sixth Edition, issued by the U.S. Department of Health and Human Services. Annual code changes are implemented by the government and are effective Oct. 1 and valid through Sept. 30 of the following year.

To accommodate the coder's approach to coding, the alphabetic index (Volume 2) has been placed before the tabular list (Volume 1). This allows the user to locate the term in the index, then confirm the accuracy of the code in the tabular list.

10 STEPS TO CORRECT CODING

To code accurately, it is necessary to have a working knowledge of medical terminology and to understand the characteristics, terminology and conventions of ICD-9-CM. Transforming descriptions of diseases, injuries, conditions and procedures into numerical designations (coding) is a complex activity and should not be undertaken without proper training.

Originally, coding allowed retrieval of medical information by diagnoses and operations for medical research, education and administration. Coding today is used to describe the medical necessity of a procedure which then facilitates payment of health services, to evaluate utilization patterns and to study the appropriateness of health care costs. Coding provides the basis for epidemiological studies and research into the quality of health care. Incorrect or inaccurate coding can lead to investigations of fraud and abuse. Therefore, coding must be performed correctly and consistently to produce meaningful statistics to aid in planning for the health needs of the nation.

Follow the steps below to code correctly:

Step 1: Identify the reason for the visit (e.g., sign, symptom, diagnosis, condition to be coded).
Physicians describe the patient's condition using terminology that includes specific diagnoses as well as symptoms, problems or reasons for the encounter. If symptoms are present but a definitive diagnosis has not yet been determined, code the symptoms. Do not code conditions that are referred to as "rule out," "suspected," "probable" or "questionable."

Step 2: Always consult the Alphabetic Index, Volume 2, before turning to the tabular list.
The most critical rule is to begin a code search in the index. Never turn first to the Tabular List (Volume 1), as this will lead to coding errors and less specificity in code

assignments. To prevent coding errors, use both the Alphabetic Index and the tabular list when locating and assigning a code.

Step 3: Locate the main entry term.
The Alphabetic Index is arranged by condition. Conditions may be expressed as nouns, adjectives and eponyms. Some conditions have multiple entries under their synonyms. Main terms are identified using boldface type.

Step 4: Read and interpret any notes listed with the main term
Notes are identified using italicized type.

Step 5: Review entries for modifiers
Nonessential modifiers are in parentheses. These parenthetical terms are supplementary words or explanatory information that may either be present or absent in the diagnostic statement and do not affect code assignment.

Step 6: Interpret abbreviations, cross-references, symbols and brackets
Cross-references used are "*see*," "*see* category" or "*see* also." The abbreviation NEC may follow main terms or subterms. NEC (not elsewhere classified) indicates that there is no specific code for the condition even though the medical documentation may be very specific. The ✓5ᵗʰ box indicates the code requires a fifth digit. If the appropriate fifth digits are not found in the index, in a box beneath the main term, you MUST refer to the tabular list. Italicized brackets [ ], are used to enclose a second code number that must be used with the code immediately preceding it and in that sequence.

Step 7: Choose a tentative code and locate it in the tabular list.
Be guided by any inclusion or exclusion terms, notes or other instructions, such as "*code first*" and "use additional code," that would direct the use of a different or additional code from that selected in the index for a particular diagnosis, condition or disease.

Step 8: Determine whether the code is at the highest level of specificity.
Assign three-digit codes (category codes) if there are no four-digit codes within the code category. Assign four-digit codes (subcategory codes) if there are no five-digit codes for that category. Assign five-digit codes (fifth-digit subclassification codes) for those categories where they are available.

Step 9: Consult the color coding and reimburse-ment prompts, including the age, sex and Medicare as secondary payer edits. Refer to the key at the bottom of the page for definitions of colors and symbols.

Step 10: Assign the code.

ORGANIZATION

Introduction
The introductory material in this book includes the history and future of ICD-9-CM as well as an overview of the classification system

Official ICD-9-CM Conventions
This section provides a full explanation of all the official footnotes, symbols, instructional notes, and conventions found in the official government version

Additional Conventions
Exclusive color-coding, symbols, and notations have been included in the *ICD-9-CM for Physicians, Volumes 1 and 2,* to alert coders to important coding and reimbursement issues. This section provides a full explanation of the additional conventions used throughout this book.

Synopsis of Code Changes
This section includes a complete listing of all code changes for the current year.

Coding Guidelines
Included in this book are the official ICD-9-CM coding guidelines as approved by the four cooperating parties of the ICD-9-CM Coordination and Maintenance Committee. Failure to comply with these official coding guidelines may result in denied or delayed claims.

Disease Classification: Alphabetic Index to Diseases
The Alphabetic Index to Diseases is separated by tabs labeled with the letters of the alphabet, contains diagnostic terms for illnesses, injuries and reasons for encounters with health care professionals. Both the Table of Drugs and Chemicals and the Alphabetic Index to External Causes of Injury and Poisoning are easily located with the tabs in this section.

Disease Classification: Tabular List of Diseases
The Tabular List of Diseases arranges the ICD-9-CM codes and descriptors numerically. Tabs divide this section into chapters, identified by the code range on the tab.

The tabular list includes two supplementary classifications:

- V Codes—Supplementary Classification of Factors Influencing Health Status and Contact with Health Services (V01–V83)
- E Codes—Supplementary Classification of External Causes of Injury and Poisoning (E800–E999)

ICD-9-CM includes five official appendixes.

- Appendix A   Morphology of Neoplasms
- Appendix B   Glossary of Mental Disorders
- Appendix C   Classification of Drugs by AHFS List
- Appendix D   Classification of Industrial Accidents According to Agency
- Appendix E   List of Three-digit Categories

ICD-9-CM Official Conventions

ICD-9-CM FOOTNOTES, SYMBOLS, INSTRUCTIONAL NOTES AND CONVENTIONS

This *ICD-9-CM for Physicians* preserves all the footnotes, symbols, instructional notes and conventions found in the government's official version. Accurate coding depends upon understanding the meaning of these elements.

The following appear in the disease tabular list, unless otherwise noted.

OFFICIAL GOVERNMENT SYMBOLS

§   The section mark preceding a code denotes a footnote on the page. This symbol is used only in the Tabular List of Diseases.

ICD-9-CM CONVENTIONS USED IN THE TABULAR LIST

In addition to the symbols and footnotes above, the ICD-9-CM disease tabular has certain abbreviations, punctuation, symbols and other conventions. Our *ICD-9-CM for Physicians* preserves these conventions. Proper use of the conventions will lead to efficient and accurate coding.

Abbreviations

NEC   Not elsewhere classifiable

This abbreviation is used when the ICD-9-CM system does not provide a code specific for the patient's condition.

NOS   Not otherwise specified

This abbreviation is the equivalent of 'unspecified' and is used only when the coder lacks the information necessary to code to a more specific four-digit subcategory.

[ ]   Brackets enclose synonyms, alternative terminology or explanatory phrases:

482.2 Pneumonia due to Hemophilus influenzae [H. influenzae]

Brackets that appear beneath a code indicate the fifth digits that are considered valid fifth digits for the code. This convention is applied for those instances in ICD-9-CM where not all common fifth digits are considered valid for each subcategory within a category.

715.0 Osteoarthrosis, generalized
[0,4,9]

Generalized arthrosis can only be assigned in cases for which the degenerative joint disease involves multiple joints. Therefore, this code is considered for arthrosis in the sites described as unspecified, hand (which consists of multiple joints), or multiple sites. Therefore, only fifth digits 0, 4, and 9 are valid with subcategory 715.0.

( )   Parentheses enclose supplementary words, called nonessential modifiers, that may be present in the narrative description of a disease without affecting the code assignment:

       198.4 Other parts of nervous system
          Meninges (cerebral) (spinal)

:   Colons are used in the tabular list after an incomplete term that needs one or more of the modifiers that follow in order to make it assignable to a given category:

       021.1 Enteric tularemia
          Tularemia:
             cryptogenic
             intestinal
             typhoidal

}   Braces enclose a series of terms, each of which is modified by the statement appearing to the right of the brace:

       560.2 Volvulus
          Knotting
          Strangulation   } of intestine, bowel, or
          Torsion   colon
          Twist

OTHER CONVENTIONS

Boldface   Boldface type is used for all codes and titles in the tabular list.

Italicized   Italicized type is used for all exclusion notes and to identify codes that should not be used for describing the primary diagnosis.

INSTRUCTIONAL NOTES

These notes appear only in the Tabular List of Diseases

Includes   An includes note further defines or clarifies the content of the chapter, subchapter, category, subcategory or subclassification. The includes note in the example below applies only to category 461.

Excludes   Terms following the word "*Excludes*" are not classified to the chapter, subchapter, category, subcategory or specific subclassification code under which it is found. The note also may provide the location of the excluded diagnosis. Excludes notes are italicized.

       461 Acute sinusitis

          INCLUDES   abscess
                         empyema   } acute, of sinus
                         infection   (accessory)
                         inflammation   (nasal)
                         suppuration

          EXCLUDES   *chronic or unspecified sinusitis (473.0-473.9)*

Use additional code:
       This instruction signals the coder that an additional code should be used if the information is available to provide a more complete picture of that diagnosis.

       330 Cerebral degenerations usually manifest in childhood
          Use additional code to identify
             associated mental retardation

Code first underlying disease:
>This instruction is used in those categories not intended for primary tabulation of disease. These codes, called manifestation codes, may never be used alone or indicated as the primary diagnosis (i.e., sequenced first). They must always be preceded by another code.
>
>The code and its descriptor appear in italics in the tabular list. The instruction "*Code first underlying disease*" is usually followed by the code or codes for the most common underlying disease (etiology). Record the code for the etiology or origin of the disease, and then record the italicized manifestation code in the next position.
>
>**590.81 Pyelitis or pyelonephritis in diseases classified elsewhere**
>>*Code first underlying disease as:*
>>tuberculosis (016.0)

Code, if applicable, any causal condition first:
>A code with this note may be principal if no causal condition is applicable or known.
>
>**590.0 Chronic pyelonephritis**
>>Chronic pyelitis
>>Chronic pyonephrosis
>>Code, if applicable, any causal condition first

Omit code
>"*Omit code*" is used to instruct the coder that no code is to be assigned. When this instruction is found in the Alphabetic Index to Diseases the medical term should not be coded as a diagnosis.
>>**Metaplasia**
>>>cervix—*omit code*

Additional Conventions

SYMBOLS AND NOTATIONS

New and Revised Text Symbols
- • A bullet at a code or line of text indicates that that the entry is new.
- ▲ A triangle in the Tabular List indicates that the code title is revised. In the Alphabetic Index the triangle indicates that a code has changed.
- ►◄ These symbols appear at the beginning and at the end of a section of new or revised text.

When these symbols appear on a page there will be a date on the lower outside corner of the page indicating the date of the change, (e.g., October 2002).

Additional Digits Required
✓4th This symbol indicates that the code requires a fourth digit.

✓5th This symbol indicates that a code requires a fifth digit.

Age and Sex Edit Symbols
The age edits below address OCE edits and are used to detect inconsistencies between the patient's age and diagnosis. They appear in the Tabular List of Diseases to the right of the code description.

Newborn Age: 0

These diagnoses are intended for newborns and neonates and the patient's age must be 0 years

Pediatric Age: 0-17

These diagnoses are intended for children and the patient's age must between 0 and 17 years

Maternity Age: 12-55

These diagnoses are intended for the patients between the age of 12 and 55 years

Adult Age 15-124

These diagnoses are intended for the patients between the age of 15 and 124 years.

The sex symbols below address OCE edits and are used to detect inconsistencies between the patient's sex and diagnosis. They appear in the Tabular List of Diseases to the right of the code description:

♂ **Male diagnosis only**

This symbol appears to the right of the code description. This reference appears in the disease tabular list.

♀ **Female diagnosis only**
> This symbol appears to the right of the code description. This reference appears in the disease tabular list.

COLOR CODING

To alert the coder to Medicare outpatient code edits and other important reimbursement issues, color bars have been added over the code descriptors in the tabular list. Some codes carry more than one color.

Carriers use the Medicare Outpatient Code Editor (OCE) to examine claims for coding and billing accuracy and completeness. Color codes in this book signify Medicare code edits for E codes and manifestation codes as a primary diagnosis, Medicare secondary payer alerts and when a more specific diagnosis or code should be used.

Manifestation Code
> These codes will appear in italic type as well as with a blue color bar over the code title. A manifestation code is not allowed to be reported as a primary diagnosis because each describes a manifestation of some other underlying disease, not the disease itself. This is also referred to as mandatory multiple coding. Code the underlying disease first. A *'Code first underlying disease'* instructional note will appear with underlying disease codes identified. In the Alphabetic Index these codes are listed as the secondary code in slanted bracket with the code for the underlying disease listed first.

Other Specified Code
> These codes will appear with a gray color bar over the code title. Use these codes when the documentation indicates a specified diagnosis, but the ICD-9-CM system does not have a specific code that describes the diagnosis. These codes are may be stated as "Other" or "Not elsewhere classified (NEC)."

Unspecified Code
> These codes will have a yellow color bar over the code title. Use these codes when the neither the diagnostic statement nor the documentation provides enough information to assign a more specified diagnosis code. These codes may be stated as "Unspecified" or "Not otherwise specified (NOS)." Note: Do not assign these codes when a more specific diagnosis has been determined.

OTHER NOTATIONS

DEF: This symbol indicates a definition of disease or procedure term. The definition will appear in blue type in the Disease Tabular Lists.

MSP This identifies specific trauma codes that alert the carrier that another carrier should be billed first and Medicare billed second if payment from the first payer does not equal or exceed the amount Medicare would pay.

PDx This symbol identifies a V code that can only be used as a primary diagnosis

SDx This symbol identifies a V code that can only be used as a secondary diagnosis

Note: A V code without a symbol may be used as either a primary or secondary diagnosis

Summary of Code Changes

DISEASE TABULAR LIST (VOLUME 1)

038	Excludes term added
● 040.82	Toxic shock syndrome Use additional code note added
062.8	Excludes note added
066.3	Includes term deleted
● 066.4	West Nile fever Includes notes added
256.2	Use additional code note added Excludes term deleted
256.3	Use additional code note revised
277.00	Includes note added
● 277.02	Cystic fibrosis with pulmonary manifestations Includes note added Use additional code note added
● 277.03	Cystic fibrosis with gastrointestinal manifestations Excludes note added
● 277.09	Cystic fibrosis with other manifestations
277.7	Use additional code note revised
337.3	Use additional code note revised
357.8	Includes note deleted
● 357.81	Chronic inflammatory demyelinating polyneuritis
● 357.82	Critical illness polyneuropathy Includes note added
● 357.89	Other inflammatory and toxic neuropathy
● 359.81	Critical illness myopathy Includes note added
● 359.89	Other myopathies
● 365.83	Aqueous misdirection Includes note added
368.6	Includes term deleted
402	Use additional code note added
▲ 402.00	Hypertensive heart disease, malignant, without congestive heart failure
▲ 402.01	Hypertensive heart disease, malignant, with ~~congestive~~ heart failure
▲ 402.10	Hypertensive heart disease, benign, without ~~congestive~~ heart failure
▲ 402.11	Hypertensive heart disease, benign, with ~~congestive~~ heart failure
▲ 402.90	Hypertensive heart disease, unspecified, without ~~congestive~~ heart failure
▲ 402.91	Hypertensive heart disease, unspecified, with ~~congestive~~ heart failure
404	Use additional code note added Fifth-digit code definitions revised 0 without mention of ~~congestive~~ heart failure or renal failure 1 with ~~congestive~~ heart failure 2 with ~~congestive~~ heart failure and renal failure
▲ 404.00	Hypertensive heart and renal disease, malignant, without mention of ~~congestive~~ heart failure or renal failure
▲ 404.01	Hypertensive heart and renal disease, malignant, with ~~congestive~~ heart failure
▲ 404.03	Hypertensive heart and renal disease, malignant, with ~~congestive~~ heart failure and renal failure
▲ 404.10	Hypertensive heart and renal disease, benign, without mention of ~~congestive~~ heart failure or renal failure
▲ 404.11	Hypertensive heart and renal disease, benign, with ~~congestive~~ heart failure
▲ 404.13	Hypertensive heart and renal disease, benign, with ~~congestive~~ heart failure and renal failure
▲ 404.90	Hypertensive heart and renal disease, unspecified, without mention of ~~congestive~~ heart failure or renal failure
▲ 404.91	Hypertensive heart and renal disease, unspecified, with ~~congestive~~ heart failure
▲ 404.93	Hypertensive heart and renal disease, unspecified, with ~~congestive~~ heart failure and renal failure
411.81	Excludes terms revised
● 414.06	Coronary atherosclerosis of coronary artery of transplanted heart
▲ 414.1	Aneurysm ▶and dissection◀ of heart

▲ 414.10	▶Aneurysm◀ of heart (wall)	● 443.22	Dissection of iliac artery
▲ 414.11	▶Aneurysm◀ of coronary vessels	● 443.23	Dissection of renal artery
● 414.12	Dissection of coronary artery	● 443.24	Dissection of vertebral artery
▲ 414.19	Other ▶aneurysm of heart◀	● 443.29	Dissection of other artery
427.89	Excludes terms added	444	Excludes term added
428	Excludes term deleted Code, if applicable, note added	● 445	Atheroembolism Includes note added
▲ 428.0	Congestive heart failure, ▶unspecified◀ Excludes note added	● 445.0	Atheroembolism, of extremities
		● 445.01	Atheroembolism, upper extermity
		● 445.02	Atheroembolism, lower extremity
● 428.2	Systolic heart failure Excludes note added	● 445.8	Atheroembolism, of other sites
		● 445.81	Atheroembolism, kidney Use additional code note added
● 428.20	Systolic heart failure, unspecified		
● 428.21	Systolic heart failure, acute	● 445.89	Atheroembolism, other site
● 428.22	Systolic heart failure, chronic	447.6	Excludes term revised
● 428.23	Systolic heart failure, acute on chronic	● 454.8	Varicose veins of the lower extremities, with other complications Includes note added
● 428.3	Diastolic heart failure Excludes note added		
● 428.30	Diastolic heart failure, unspecified	▲ 454.9	Varicose veins of lower extremities, ~~without mention of ulcer or inflammation~~ ▶asmyptomatic varicose veins◀ Includes term added
● 428.31	Diastolic heart failure, acute		
● 428.32	Diastolic heart failure, chronic		
● 428.33	Diastolic heart failure, acute on chronic		
		459.1	Includes note added Excludes note added
● 428.4	Combined systolic and diastolic heart failure		
● 428.40	Combined systolic and diastolic heart failure, unspecified	● 459.10	Postphlebetic syndrome without complications Includes note added
● 428.41	Combined systolic and diastolic heart failure, acute	● 459.11	Postphlebetic syndrome with ulcer
		● 459.12	Postphlebetic syndrome with inflammation
● 428.42	Combined systolic and diastolic heart failure, chronic		
● 428.43	Combined systolic and diastolic heart failure, acute on chronic	● 459.13	Postphlebetic syndrome with ulcer and inflammation
		● 459.19	Postphlebetic syndrome with other complication
(430-438)	Cerebrovascular Disease section Excludes term added		
436	Excludes term added	● 459.3	Chronic venous hypertension (idiopathic) Includes note added Excludes note added
● 438.6	Late effects of cerebrovascular disease, alterations of sensations Use additional code note added		
		● 459.30	Chronic venous hypertension without complications Includes note added
● 438.7	Late effects of cerebrovascular disease, disturbances of vision Use additional code note added		
		● 459.31	Chronic venous hypertension with ulcer
● 438.83	Other late effects of cerebrovascular disease, facial weakness Includes term added	● 459.32	Chronic venous hypertension with inflammation
		● 459.33	Chronic venous hypertension with ulcer and inflammation
● 438.84	Other late effects of cerebrovascular disease, ataxia		
● 438.85	Other late effects of cerebrovascular disease, vertigo	● 459.39	Chronic venous hypertension with other complication
440	Excludes term added	491.2	Includes term deleted
440.8	Excludes term revised	491.20	Includes term deleted
441.0	Includes note deleted	491.21	Includes term deleted
● 443.2	Other arterial dissection Excludes note added	493.2	Includes term added Excludes term deleted
● 443.21	Dissection of carotid artery	518.81	Excludes term revised

	518.82	Excludes term revised		Fifth-digit subclassification instructions revised
●	537.84	Dieulafoy lesion (hemorrhagic) of stomach and duodenum	▲ 765	Disorders relating to short gestation and low birthweight
●	569.86	Dieulafoy lesion (hemorrhagic) of intestine	765.0	Instructional note revised Use additional code note added
	577.8	Excludes term revised	765.1	Instrucitonal note revised Use additional code note added
	590.0	Code first note deleted Code, if applicable, note added	● 765.2	Disorders relating to short gestation and low birthweight, weeks of gestation
	593.7	Use additional code note deleted		
	599.0	Excludes term added	● 765.20	Unspecified weeks of gestation
	602.3	Includes terms revised Excludes terms revised	● 765.21	Less than 24 completed weeks of gestation
	622.1	Includes terms added	● 765.22	24 completed weeks of gestation
▲	627.2	►Symptomatic◄ menopausal or female climacteric states	● 765.23	25-26 completed weeks of gestation
▲	627.4	►Symptomatic◄ states associated with artificial menopause	● 765.24	27-28 completed weeks of gestation
			● 765.25	29-30 completed weeks of gestation
	629.0	Excludes term revised	● 765.26	31-32 completed weeks of gestation
●	633.00	Abdominal pregnancy without intrauterine pregnancy	● 765.27	33-34 completed weeks of gestation
●	633.01	Abdominal pregnancy with intrauterine pregnancy	● 765.28	35-36 completed weeks of gestation
●	633.10	Tubal pregnancy without intrauterine pregnancy	● 765.29	37 or more completed weeks of gestation
			770.8	Includes note deleted
●	633.11	Tubal pregnancy with intrauterine pregnancy	● 770.81	Primary apnea of newborn Includes note added
●	633.20	Ovarian pregnancy without intrauterine pregnancy	● 770.82	Other apnea of newborn Includes note added
●	633.21	Ovarian pregnancy with intrauterine pregnancy	● 770.83	Cyanotic attacks of newborn
●	633.80	Other ectopic pregnancy without intrauterine pregnancy	● 770.84	Respiratory failure of newborn Excludes note added
●	633.81	Other ectopic pregnancy with intrauterine pregnancy	● 770.89	Other respiratory problems after birth
●	633.90	Unspecified ectopic pregnancy without intrauterine pregnancy	771.8	Includes note deleted Use additional code note added
			● 771.81	Septicemia [sepsis] of newborn
●	633.91	Unspecified ectopic pregnancy with intrauterine pregnancy	● 771.82	Urinary tract infection of newborn
			● 771.83	Bacteremia of newborn
	646.6	Includes term revised	● 771.89	Other infections specific to the perinatal period Includes note added
	647.1	Excludes note added		
	707.1	Code first note revised Code, if applicable, terms added	774.5	Code first term revised
	710	Use additional code note deleted	● 779.81	Neonatal bradycardia Excludes note added
	710.1	Use additional code note added	● 779.82	Neonatal tachycardia Excludes note added
	718.7	Excludes terms deleted Excludes terms added	● 779.89	Other specified conditions originating in the perinatal period
	723.5	Excludes term added		
	730.1	Includes term deleted	780.9	Includes note deleted
	733.4	Excludes term deleted	● 780.91	Fussy infant (baby)
●	747.83	Persistent fetal circulation Includes note added	● 780.92	Excessive crying of infant (baby)
			● 780.99	Other general symptoms Includes note added
	751.7	Excludes term revised		
	753.0	Code first note deleted	● 781.93	Ocular torticollis
	753.15	Code first note deleted	782.5	Excludes note revised
	(764-779)	Other conditions originating in the perinatal period section	785.0	Excludes note added
			786.03	Excludes term added

Code	Change
786.09	Excludes terms revised
788.3	Code first note deleted
	Code, if applicable, note added
790.7	Excludes term added
795.0	Includes note deleted
	Excludes note added
● 795.00	Nonspecific abnormal Papanicolaou smear of cervix, unspecified
● 795.01	Atypical squamous cell changes of undetermined significance favor benign (ASCUS favor benign) Includes note added
● 795.02	Atypical squamous cell changes of undetermined significance favor dysplasia (ASCUS favor dysplasia) Includes note added
● 795.09	Other nonspecific abnormal Papanicolaou smear of cervix Includes note added
● 795.31	Nonspecific positive findings for anthrax Includes term added
● 795.39	Other nonspecific positive culture findings
799.1	Excludes terms revised
(800-829)	Fractures section Instructional note revised
● 813.45	Torus fracture of radius
● 823.4	Fracture of tibia and fibula, torus fracture
959.01	Excludes term added
991.6	Excludes term revised
995.0	Code first note deleted
● 995.9	Systemic inflammatory response syndrome (SIRS)
● 995.90	Systemic inflammatory response syndrome, unspecified Includes note added
● 995.91	Systemic inflammatory response syndrome due to infectious process without organ dysfunction
● 995.92	Systemic inflammatory response syndrome due to infectious process with organ dysfunction Includes note added Use additional code note added
● 995.93	Systemic inflammatory response syndrome due to non-infectious process without organ dysfunction
● 995.94	Systemic inflammatory response syndrome due to non-infectious process with organ dysfunction Use additional code note added
996.72	Excludes note revised
● 998.31	Disruption of internal operation wound
● 998.32	Disruption of external operation wound Includes note added
● V01.81	Contact with or exposure to anthrax
● V01.89	Contact with or exposure to other communicable diseases
● V13.21	Personal history of pre-term labor Excludes note added
● V13.29	Personal history of other genital system and obstetric disorders
● V23.41	Pregnancy with history of pre-term labor
● V23.49	Pregnancy with other poor obstetric history
● V46.2	Other dependence on machines, supplemental oxygen Includes note added
▲ V49.81	▶Asymptomatic◀ postmenopausal status (age-related) (natural)
V54.0	Excludes term revised
● V54.1	Aftercare for healing traumatic fracture
● V54.10	Aftercare for healing traumatic fracture of arm, unspecified
● V54.11	Aftercare for healing traumatic fracture of upper arm
● V54.12	Aftercare for healing traumatic fracture of lower arm
● V54.13	Aftercare for healing traumatic fracture of hip
● V54.14	Aftercare for healing traumatic fracture of leg, unspecified
● V54.15	Aftercare for healing traumatic fracture of upper leg Excludes note added
● V54.16	Aftercare for healing traumatic fracture of lower leg
● V54.17	Aftercare for healing traumatic fracture of vertebrae
● V54.19	Aftercare for healing traumatic fracture of other bone
● V54.2	Aftercare for healing pathologic fracture
● V54.20	Aftercare for healing pathologic fracture of arm, unspecified
● V54.21	Aftercare for healing pathologic fracture of upper arm
● V54.22	Aftercare for healing pathologic fracture of lower arm
● V54.23	Aftercare for healing pathologic fracture of hip
● V54.24	Aftercare for healing pathologic fracture of leg, unspecified
● V54.25	Aftercare for healing pathologic fracture of upper leg Excludes note added
● V54.26	Aftercare for healing pathologic fracture of lower leg
● V54.27	Aftercare for healing pathologic fracture of vertebrae

• V54.29	Aftercare for healing pathologic fracture of other bone		• V83.89	Other genetic carrier status	
V54.8	Includes note deleted		• E885.0	Fall from (nonmotorized) scooter	
• V54.81	Aftercare following joint replacement Use additional code note added		• E922.5	Accident caused by firearm, and air gun missle, paintball gun	
• V54.89	Other orthopedic aftercare Includes note added		• E955.7	Suicide and self-inflicted injury by firearms, air guns and explosives, paintball gun	
V58.4	Instructional note added		E960-E969	Homicide and injury purposely inflicted by other persons section Excludes term added	
• V58.42	Aftercare following surgery for neoplasm Includes note added		• (E979)	Terrorism (E979) new section	
• V58.43	Aftercare following surgery for injury and trauma Includes note added Excludes note added		• E979	Terrorism Instructional note added	
			• E979.0	Terrorism involving explosion of marine weapons Includes note added	
• V58.7	Aftercare following surgery to specified body systems, not elsewhere classified Instructional note added		• E979.1	Terrorism involving destruction of aircraft Includes note added	
• V58.71	Aftercare following surgery of the sense organs, NEC Includes note added		• E979.2	Terrorism involving other explosions and fragments Includes note added	
• V58.72	Aftercare following surgery of the nervous system, NEC Includes note added Excludes note added		• E979.3	Terrorism involving fires, conflagration and hot substances Includes note added	
			• E979.4	Terrorism involving firearms Includes note added	
• V58.73	Aftercare following surgery of the circulatory system, NEC Includes note added		• E979.5	Terrorism involving nuclear weapons Includes note added	
• V58.74	Aftercare following surgery of the respiratory system, NEC Includes note added		• E979.6	Terrorism involving biological weapons Includes note added	
• V58.75	Aftercare following surgery of the teeth, oral cavity and digestive system, NEC Includes note added		• E979.7	Terrorism involving chemical weapons Includes note added	
			• E979.8	Terrorism involving other means Includes note added	
• V58.76	Aftercare following surgery of the genitourinary system, NEC Includes note added Excludes note added		• E979.9	Terrorism, secondary effects Instructional note added Excludes note added	
• V58.77	Aftercare following surgery of the skin and subcutaneous tissue, NEC Includes note added		• E985.7	Injury by paintball gun, undetermined whether accidentally or purposely inflicted	
• V58.78	Aftercare following surgery of the musculoskeletal system, NEC Includes note added		▲ E999	Late effect of injury due to war operations wand terrorismx Instructional note revised	
V58.83	Use additional code note added		• E999.0	Late effect of injury due to war operations	
▲ V71.8	Observation ▶and evaluation◀ for other specified suspected conditions		• E999.1	Late effect of injury due to terrorism	
• V71.82	Observation and evaluation for suspected exposure to anthrax				
• V71.83	Observation and evaluation for suspected exposure to other biological agent				
• V83.8	Other genetic carrier status				
• V83.81	Cystic fibrosis gene carrier				

Coding Guidelines

OFFICIAL ICD-9-CM GUIDELINES FOR CODING AND REPORTING

The Public Health Service and the Centers for Medicare and Medicaid (formerly know as Health Care Financing Administration) of the U.S. Department of Health and Human Services present the following guidelines for coding and reporting using the International Classification of Diseases, 9th Revision, Clinical Modification (ICD-9-CM). These guidelines should be used as a companion document to the official versions of the ICD-9-CM.

These guidelines for coding and reporting have been developed and approved by the cooperating parties for ICD-9-CM: American Hospital Association, American Health Information Management Association, Center for Medicare and Medicaid Services and the National Center for Health Statistics. These guidelines previously appeared in the Coding Clinic for ICD-9-CM, published by the American Hospital Association.

These guidelines have been developed to assist the user in coding and reporting in situations where the ICD-9-CM manual does not provide direction. Coding and sequencing instructions in the three ICD-9-CM manuals take precedence over any guidelines.

These guidelines are not exhaustive. The cooperating parties are continuing to conduct review of these guidelines and develop new guidelines as needed. Users of the ICD-9-CM should be aware that only guidelines approved by the cooperating parties are official. Revision of these guidelines and new guidelines will be published by the U.S. Department of Health and Human Services when they are approved by the cooperating parties.

OUTPATIENT SERVICES

(Hospital-Based and Physician Office)

Table of Contents

Introduction
Code Range . . . . A
Accurate Reporting . . . . B
Code Selection C
Symptoms, Signs and Ill-defined Conditions . . . . D
Circumstances other than Disease or Injury . . . . E
Code Specificity . . . . F
Code Sequence . . . . G
Uncertain Diagnosis . . . . H
Chronic Disease I
Coexisting Conditions . . . . J
Ancillary Diagnostic Services . . . . K
Ancillary Therapeutic Services L
Preoperative Evaluations . . . . N
Ambulatory Surgery . . . . O

INPATIENT SERVICES

Table of Contents

Adverse Effects and Poisoning 9
   Adverse Effect 9.1
   Poisoning 9.2
External Causes of Diseases and Injuries 11
   Child and Adult Abuse 11.5
   General Coding guidelines 11.1
   Late effects 11.8

Misadventures and complications of care	11.9
Multiple external causes	11.4
Place of occurrence	11.2
Poisonings and adverse effects of drugs	11.3
Undetermined cause	11.7
Unknown intent	11.6
General Inpatient Coding Guidelines	1
Acute and Chronic Conditions	1.4; 2.3
Combination Code	1.5
Impending or Threatened Condition	1.9
Late Effect	1.7
Level of Specificity in Coding	1.2
Multiple Coding of Diagnoses	1.6
Other and Unspecified (NOS) Code Titles	1.3
Uncertain Diagnosis	1.8
Use of Alphabetic Index and Tabular List	1.1
Human Immunodeficiency Virus (HIV) Infections	10
Asymptomatic HIV Infection	10.6
Confirmed Cases of HIV Infection/Illness	10.1
HIV Infection in Pregnancy, Childbirth and the Puerperium	10.5
Inconclusive Lab Test for HIV	10.7
Previously Diagnosed HIV-related Illness	10.3
Selection of HIV Code	10.2
Sequencing	10.4
Testing for HIV	10.8
Hypertension	4
Controlled Hypertension	4.9
Elevated Blood Pressure	4.11
Essential Hypertension	4.1
Hypertension with Heart Disease	4.2
Hypertensive Cardiovascular Disease	4.5
Hypertensive Heart and Renal Disease	4.4
Hypertensive Renal Disease with Chronic Renal Failure	4.3
Hypertensive Retinopathy	4.6
Secondary Hypertension	4.7
Transient Hypertension	4.8
Uncontrolled Hypertension	4.10
Newborn Coding	6
Category V29	6.3
Congenital Anomalies	6.5
Maternal Causes of Perinatal Morbidity	6.4
Newborn Transfers	6.2
Other (Additional) Diagnoses	6.6
Prematurity and Fetal Growth Retardation	6.7
Use of Codes V30-V39	6.1
Obstetrics	5
General Rules	5.1
Selection of Principal Diagnosis	5.2
Chapter 11 Fifth-digits	5.3
Fetal Conditions Affecting Managment of Mother	5.4
Normal Delivery 650	5.5
Procedure Codes	5.6
Postpartum Period	5.7
Abortions	5.8
Late Effects of Complications of Pregnancy, Childbirth and the Puerperium	5.9
Reporting Other (Additional) Diagnoses	3
Abnormal Findings	3.5
Conditions Integral to a Disease Process	3.3

Conditions Not Integral to a Disease Process 3.4
Diagnoses Not Listed in Final Diagnostic Statement 3.2
Previous Conditions 3.1
Selection of Principal Diagnosis 2
   Acute and Chronic Conditions 2.3; 1.4
   Codes from V71.0-V71.9, Observation and Evaluation for Suspected Conditions,
      not found 2.8
   Complications of Pregnancy. 2.16
   Complications of Surgery and Other Medical Care 2.15
   Codes in Brackets in the Alphabetic Index 2.2
   Multiple Burns. 2.11; 8.3
   Multiple Injuries 2.12
   Neoplasms 2.13
   Original Treatment Plan Not Carried Out 2.9
   Poisoning 2.14
   Residual Condition or Nature of Late Effect 2.10
   Symptoms, Signs, and Ill-defined Conditions 2.1
   Symptom Followed by Contrasting/Comparative Diagnoses 2.7
   Two or More Interrelated Conditions 2.4
   Two or More Equally Meet Definition 2.5
   Two or More Comparative or Contrasting
      Conditions 2.6
Septicemia and Shock 7
Trauma 8
   Current Burns and Encounters for Late Effectsof Burns 8.3
   Debridement of Wound, Infection or Burn 8.4
   Multiple Fractures 8.2
   Multiple Injuries 8.1

OFFICIAL GUIDELINES FOR CODING AND REPORTING OUTPATIENT SERVICES (HOSPITAL-BASED AND PHYSICIAN OFFICE)

Introduction

These revised coding guidelines for outpatient diagnoses have been approved for use by hospitals/physicians in coding and reporting hospital-based outpatient services and physician office visits.

The terms encounter and visit are often used interchangeably in describing outpatient service contacts and, therefore, appear together in these guidelines without distinguishing one from the other.

Coding guidelines for outpatient and physician reporting of diagnoses will vary in a number of instances from those for inpatient diagnoses, recognizing that:

The Uniform Hospital Discharge Data Set (UHDDS) definition of principal diagnosis applies only to inpatients in acute, short-term, general hospitals.

Coding guidelines for inconclusive diagnoses (probable, suspected, rule out, etc.) were developed for inpatient reporting and do not apply to outpatients.

Diagnoses often are not established at the time of the initial encounter/visit. It may take two or more visits before the diagnosis is confirmed.

The most critical rule involves beginning the search for the correct code assignment through the Alphabetic Index. Never begin searching initially in the Tabular List as this will lead to coding errors.

Basic Coding Guidelines for Outpatient Services

A. Code Range

The appropriate code or codes from 001.0 through V82.9 must be used to identify diagnoses, symptoms, conditions, problems, complaints, or other reason(s) for the encounter/visit.

B. Accurate Reporting

For accurate reporting of ICD-9-CM diagnosis codes, the documentation should describe the patient's condition, using terminology which includes specific diagnoses as well as symptoms, problems, or reasons for the encounter. There are ICD-9-CM codes to describe all of these.

C. Code Selection

The selection of codes 001.0 through 999.9 will frequently be used to describe the reason for the encounter. These codes are from the section of ICD-9-CM for the classification of diseases and injuries (e.g. infectious and parasitic diseases; neoplasms; symptoms, signs, and ill-defined conditions, etc.).

D. Symptoms, Signs and Ill-defined Conditions

Codes that describe symptoms and signs, as opposed to diagnoses, are acceptable for reporting purposes when an established diagnosis has not been diagnosed (confirmed) by the physician. Chapter 16 of ICD-9-CM, Symptoms, Signs, and Ill-defined conditions (codes 780.0 - 799.9) contain many, but not all codes for symptoms.

E. Circumstances other than Disease or Injury

ICD-9-CM provides codes to deal with encounters for circumstances other than a disease or injury. The Supplementary Classification of factors Influencing Health Status and Contact with Health Services (V01.0- V82.9) is provided to deal with occasions when circumstances other than a disease or injury are recorded as diagnosis or problems. The V codes should be used for encounters of this type. For example, the correct code for a cancer patient who is seen solely for radiotherapy is V58.0, radiotherapy session.

Example:

Discharge diagnosis: Open-angle glaucoma

Reason for visit code: 365.10

Discharge diagnosis: Follow-up examination after surgery

Reason for visit code: V67.0

F. Code Specificity

ICD-9-CM is composed of codes with either 3, 4, or 5 digits. Codes with 3 digits are included in ICD-9-CM as the heading of a category of codes that may be further subdivided by the use of fourth and/or fifth digits which provide greater specificity. A code is invalid if it has not been coded to the full number of digits required for that code.

- Assign three-digit codes only if there are no four-digit codes within that code category.
- Assign four-digit codes only if there is no fifth-digit subclassification for that subcategory.
- Assign the fifth-digit subclassification code for those subcategories where it exists

Example:

Diagnosis: Acute tonsillitis

Correct code: 463

Diagnosis: Benign neoplasm of colon

Incorrect code: 211

Correct code: 211.3

G. Code Sequence

List first the ICD-9-CM code for the diagnosis, condition, problem, or other reason for encounter/visit shown in the medical record to be chiefly responsible for the services provided. List additional codes that describe any coexisting conditions.

H. Uncertain Diagnosis

Do not code diagnoses documented as "probable", "suspected," "questionable," "rule out," or working diagnosis. Rather, code the condition(s) to the highest degree of certainty for that encounter/visit, such as symptoms, signs, abnormal test results, or other reason for the visit.

Coders should be aware that this is contrary to the coding practices used by health information management departments for coding the diagnoses of hospital inpatients. For inpatient coding, all discharge diagnoses listed as "probable," "suspected," "questionable" or "rule out" would be coded as if the condition existed. Further, coding symptoms for inpatients is generally unacceptable, particularly when there is an established diagnosis. A requirement that conditions listed as "probable," "suspected," "questionable" or "rule out" be coded in the outpatient setting as if the condition existed would lead to significant over-reporting of conditions. Therefore codes for symptoms and signs are appropriate and acceptable for hospital outpatient reporting.

Example:

Reason for visit: Chest pain, code 786.50

Discharge diagnosis: Rule out angina, code 413.9

Correct code: 786.50

Comment: Do not code angina as if it were established; code the reason for the visit.

I. Chronic Disease

Chronic diseases treated on an ongoing basis may be coded and reported as many times as the patient receives treatment and care for the condition(s).

Example:

History of illness: Patient is seen for monthly lumbar epidural block with steroid injection.

Discharge diagnosis: Chronic low back pain, code 724.2

Comment: Report code 724.2, low back pain, for each visit during which the patient receives lumbar-block treatment, regardless of the number or frequency of visits.

J. Coexisting Conditions

Code all documented conditions that coexist at the time of the encounter/visit, and require or affect patient care treatment or management. Do not code conditions that were previously treated and no longer exist. However, history codes (V10- V19) may be used as secondary codes if the historical condition or family history has an impact on current care or influences treatment.

Coders are advised to exercise care in identifying (a) conditions presently existing, (b) conditions no longer existing, (c) residuals (late effects) of conditions no longer existing, and (d) certain postoperative status conditions that require consideration in managing patient care and that warrant coding. Some physicians add to the list of conditions currently being treated any previous surgery or conditions that no longer exist to provide easy reference of the patient's history for recapitulation in the ongoing care of the patient. These conditions should not be coded unless they require or affect patient care treatment or management.

Example:

Chief complaint: Uncontrolled diabetes mellitus, 250.02

Review of systems: Patient has congestive heart failure (428.0) and is curently on Lasix.

Medical history: Patient is status three months post right inguinal herniorrherapy for incarcerated inguinal hernia.

Comment: First code "uncontrolled diabetes mellitus" as the reason for the visit, followed by "congestive heart failure" as a coexisting condition. Do not code the incarcerated inguinal hernia; it was treated successfully.

Code sequence: 250.02, 428.0

K. Ancillary Diagnostic Services

For patients receiving diagnostic services only during an encounter/visit, sequence first the diagnosis, condition, problem, or other reason for encounter/visit shown in the medical record to be chiefly responsible for the outpatient services provided during the encounter/visit. Codes for other diagnoses (e.g., chronic conditions) may be sequenced as additional diagnoses.

Example:

Chief complaint: Hematuria, code 599.7

Laboratory studies: Intravenous pyelogram, code V72.5

History of illness: Patient was referred to hospital outpatient clinic for intravenous pyelogram only. Will provide patient's physician with the results.

Code sequence: 599.7

L. Ancillary Therapeutic Services

For patients receiving therapeutic services only during an encounter/visit, sequence first the diagnosis, condition, problem, or other reason for encounter/visit shown in the medical record to be chiefly responsible for the outpatient services provided during the encounter/visit. Codes for other diagnoses (e.g., chronic conditions) may be sequenced as additional diagnoses.

Example:

Chief complaint: Chronic renal failure, code 585

Procedure performed: Hemodialysis, code V56.0

History of illness: Patient is being seen for hemodialysis treatment.

Code sequence: 585

NOTE: The appropriate V code can be listed first for patients receiving the following (the diagnosis or problem for which the service is being performed should be listed second):

- chemotherapy
- radiation therapy
- rehabilitation.

Example:

Chief complaint: Trigone bladder cancer, code 188.0

Procedure performed: Chemotherapy infusion, code V58.1

History of illness: Patient is being seen for second course of five chemotherapy infusions.

Code sequence: V58.1, 188.0

M. [Guideline M-deleted in the official guidelines]

N. Preoperative Evaluations

For patient's receiving preoperative evaluations only, sequence a code from category V72.8, Other specified examinations, to describe the pre-op consultations. Assign a code for the condition to describe the reason for the surgery as an additional diagnosis. Code also any findings related to the pre-op evaluation.

Example:

Chief complaint: Rhegmatogenous retinal detachment in left eye, code 361.00

Procedure performed: Preoperative cardiovascular examination, V72.81

History of illness: Patient is being seen for preoperative cardiovascular examination, due to history of myocardial infarction 1 year ago. Patient is scheduled for a repair of his retinal detachment next week.

Code sequence: V72.81, 361.00

O. Ambulatory Surgery

For ambulatory surgery, code the diagnosis for which the surgery was performed. If the postoperative diagnosis is known to be different from the preoperative diagnosis at the time the diagnosis is confirmed, select the postoperative diagnosis for coding, since it is the most definitive.

Example:

Preoperative diagnosis: Breast mass, code 611.72

Postoperative diagnosis: Fibrocystic breast disease, code 610.3

Comment: Code 610.3 as the reason for the visit because it is the postoperative diagnosis.

OFFICIAL GUIDELINES FOR CODING AND REPORTING INPATIENT SERVICES

1. GENERAL INPATIENT CODING GUIDELINES

   1.1. Use of Both Alphabetic Index and Tabular List

   A. Use both the Alphabetic Index and the Tabular List when locating and assigning a code. Reliance on only the Alphabetic Index or the Tabular List leads to errors in code assignments and less specificity in code selection.

   B. Locate each term in the Alphabetic Index and verify the code selected in the Tabular List. Read and be guided by instructional notations that appear in both the Alphabetic Index and the Tabular List.

   1.2. Level of Specificity in Coding

   Diagnostic and procedure codes are to be used at their highest level of specificity:

   - Assign three-digit codes only if there are no four-digit codes within that code category.
   - Assign four-digit codes only if there is no fifth-digit subclassification for that category.
   - Assign the fifth-digit subclassification code for those categories where it exists.

   1.3. Other (NEC) and Unspecified (NOS) Code Titles

   Codes labeled "other specified" (NEC—not elsewhere classified) or "unspecified" (NOS—not otherwise specified) are used only when neither the diagnostic statement nor a thorough review of the medical record provides adequate information to permit assignment of a more specific code.

   - Use the code assignment for "other" or NEC when the information at hand specifies a condition but no separate code for that condition is provided.
   - Use "unspecified" (NOS) when the information at hand does not permit either a more specific or "other" code assignment.
   - When the Alphabetic Index assigns a code to a category labeled "other (NEC)" or to a category labeled "unspecified (NOS)", refer to the Tabular List and review the titles and inclusion terms in the subdivisions under that particular three-digit category (or subdivision under the four-digit code) to determine if the information at hand can be appropriately assigned to a more specific code.

   1.4. Acute and Chronic Conditions

   If the same condition is described as both acute (subacute) and chronic and separate subentries exist in the Alphabetic Index at the same indentation level, code both and sequence the acute (subacute) code first.

   1.5. Combination Code

   A single code used to classify two diagnoses or a diagnosis with an associated secondary process (manifestation) or an associated complication is called a combination code. Combination codes are identified by referring to subterm entries in the Alphabetic Index and by reading the inclusion and exclusion notes in the Tabular List.

   Assign only the combination code when that code fully identifies the diagnostic conditions involved or when the Alphabetic Index so directs.

Multiple coding should not be used when the classification provides a combination code that clearly identifies all of the elements documented in the diagnosis. When the combination code lacks necessary specificity in describing the manifestation or complication, an additional code may be used as a secondary code.

1.6. Multiple Coding of Diagnoses

Multiple coding is required for certain conditions not subject to the rules for combination codes.

Instruction for conditions that require multiple coding appear in the Alphabetic Index and the Tabular List.

A. Alphabetic Index: Codes for both etiology and manifestation of a disease appear following the subentry term, with the second code in brackets. Assign both codes in the same sequence in which they appear in the Alphabetic Index.

B. Tabular List: Instructional terms, such as "Code first...," "Use additional code for any...," and "Note...," indicate when to use more than one code.

- "Code first underlying disease" - Assign the codes for both the manifestation and underlying cause. The codes for manifestations cannot be used (designated) as principal diagnosis.
- "Use additional code, to identify manifestation, as ..." - Assign also the code that identifies the manifestation, such as, but not limited to, the examples listed. The codes for manifestations cannot be used (designated) as principal diagnosis.

C. Apply multiple coding instructions throughout the classification where appropriate, whether or not multiple coding directions appear in the Alphabetic Index or the Tabular List. Avoid indiscriminate multiple coding or irrelevant information, such as symptoms or signs characteristic of the diagnosis.

1.7. Late Effect

A late effect is the residual effect (condition produced) after the acute phase of an illness or injury has terminated. There is no time limit on when a late effect code can be used. The residual may be apparent early, such as in cerebrovascular accident cases, or it may occur months or years later, such as that due to a previous injury.

Coding of late effects requires two codes:

- The residual condition or nature of the late effect
- The cause of the late effect

The residual condition or nature of the late effect is sequenced first, followed by the cause of the late effect, except in those few instances where the code for late effect is followed by a manifestation code identified in the Tabular List and title or the late effect code has been expanded (at the fourth and fifth-digit levels) to include the manifestation(s).

The code for the acute phase of an illness or injury that led to the late effect is never used with a code for the cause of the late effect.

A. Late Effects of Cerebrovascular Disease

Category 438 is used to indicate conditions classifiable to categories 430-437 as the causes of late effects (neurologic deficits), themselves classified elsewhere. These "late effects" include neurologic deficits that persist after initial onset of conditions classifiable to 430-437. The neurologic deficits caused by cerebrovascular disease may be present from the onset or may arise at any time after the onset of the condition classifiable to 430–437.

- Codes from category 438 may be assigned on a health care record with codes from 430–437, if the patient has a current CVA and deficits from an old CVA.
- Assign code V12.59 (and not a code from category 438) as an additional code for history of cerebrovascular disease when no neurologic deficits are present.

1.8. Uncertain Diagnosis

If the diagnosis documented at the time of discharge is qualified as "probable", "suspected", "likely", "questionable", "possible", or "still to be ruled out", code the condition as if it existed or was established. The bases for this guidelines are the diagnostic workup, arrangements for further workup or observation, and initial therapeutic approach that correspond most closely with the established diagnosis.

1.9. Impending or Threatened Condition

Code any condition described at the time of discharge as "impending" or "threatened" as follows:

If it did occur, code as confirmed diagnosis.

If it did not occur, reference the Alphabetic Index to determine if the condition has a subentry term for "impending" or "threatened" and also reference main term entries for Impending and for Threatened.

- If the subterms are listed, assign the given code.
- If the subterms are not listed, code the existing forerunner condition(s) and not the condition described as impending or threatened.

2. SELECTION OF PRINCIPAL DIAGNOSIS

The circumstances of inpatient admission always govern the selection of principal diagnosis. The principal diagnosis is defined in the Uniform Hospital Discharge Data Set (UHDDS) as "that condition established after study to be chiefly responsible for occasioning the admission of the patient to the hospital for care".

In determining principal diagnosis the coding directives in the ICD-9-CM manuals, Volumes I, II, and III, take precedence over all other guidelines.

The importance of consistent, complete documentation in the medical record cannot be overemphasized. Without such documentation the application of all coding guidelines is a difficult, if not impossible, task.

2.1. Codes for symptoms, signs, and ill-defined conditions

Codes for symptoms, signs, and ill-defined conditions from Chapter 16 are not to be used as principal diagnosis when a related definitive diagnosis has been established.

2.2. Codes in brackets

Codes in brackets in the Alphabetic Index can never be sequenced as principal diagnosis. Coding directives require that the codes in brackets be sequenced in the order as they appear in the Alphabetic Index.

2.3. Acute and chronic conditions

If the same condition is described as both acute (subacute) and chronic and separate subentries exist in the Alphabetic Index at the same indentation level, code both and sequence the acute (subacute) code first.

2.4. Two or more interrelated conditions, each potentially meeting the definition for principal diagnosis

When there are two or more interrelated conditions (such as diseases in the same ICD-9-CM chapter or manifestations characteristically associated with a certain disease) potentially meeting the definition of principal diagnosis, either condition may be sequenced first, unless the circumstances of the admission, the therapy provided, the Tabular List, or the Alphabetic Index indicate otherwise.

2.5. Two or more diagnoses that equally meet the definition for principal diagnosis

In the unusual instance when two or more diagnoses equally meet the criteria for principal diagnosis as determined by the circumstances of admission, diagnostic workup and/or therapy provided, and the Alphabetic Index, Tabular List, or another coding guidelines does not provide sequencing direction, any one of the diagnoses may be sequenced first.

2.6. Two or more comparative or contrasting conditions

In those rare instances when two or more contrasting or comparative diagnoses are documented as "either/or" (or similar terminology), they are coded as if the diagnoses were confirmed and the diagnoses are sequenced according to the circumstances of the admission. If no further determination can be made as to which diagnosis should be principal, either diagnosis may be sequenced first.

2.7. A symptom(s) followed by contrasting/comparative diagnoses

When a symptom(s) is followed by contrasting/comparative diagnoses, the symptom code is sequenced first. All the contrasting/comparative diagnoses should be coded as suspected conditions.

2.8. Codes from the V71.0-V71.9 series, Observation and evaluation for suspected conditions

Codes from the V71.0-V71.9 series are assigned as principal diagnoses for encounters or admissions to evaluate the patient's condition when there is some evidence to suggest the existence of an abnormal condition or following an accident or other incident that ordinarily results in a health problem, and where no supporting evidence for the suspected condition is found and no treatment is currently required. The fact that the patient may be scheduled for continuing observation in the office/clinic setting following discharge does not limit the use of this category.

2.9. Original treatment plan not carried out

Sequence as the principal diagnosis the condition which after study occasioned the admission to the hospital, even though treatment may not have been carried out due to unforeseen circumstances.

2.10. Residual condition or nature of late effect

The residual condition or nature of the late effect is sequenced first, followed by the late effect code for the cause of the residual condition, except in a few instances where the Alphabetic Index or Tabular List directs otherwise.

2.11. Multiple burns

Sequence first the code that reflects the highest degree of burn when more than one burn is present. (See also Burns guideline 8.3)

2.12. Multiple injuries

When multiple injuries exist, the code for the most severe injury as determined by the attending physician is sequenced first.

2.13. Neoplasms

A. If the treatment is directed at the malignancy, designate the malignancy as the principal diagnosis, except when the purpose of the encounter or hospital admission is for radiotherapy session(s), V58.0, or for chemotherapy session(s), V58.1, in which instance the malignancy is coded and sequenced second.

B. When a patient is admitted for the purpose of radiotherapy or chemotherapy and develops complications such as uncontrolled nausea and vomiting or dehydration, the principal diagnosis is Encounter for radiotherapy, V58.0, or Encounter for chemotherapy, V58.1.

C. When an episode of inpatient care involves surgical removal of a primary site or secondary site malignancy followed by adjunct chemotherapy or radiotherapy, code the malignancy as the principal diagnosis, using codes in the 140-198 series or where appropriate in the 200-203 series.

D. When the reason for admission is to determine the extent of the malignancy, or for a procedure such as paracentesis or thoracentesis, the primary malignancy or appropriate metastatic site is designated as the principal diagnosis, even though chemotherapy or radiotherapy is administered.

E. When the primary malignancy has been previously excised or eradicated from its site and there is not adjunct treatment directed to that site and no evidence of any remaining malignancy at the primary site, use the appropriate code from the V10 series to indicate the former site of primary malignancy. Any mention of extension, invasion, or metastasis to a nearby structure or organ or to a distant site is coded as a secondary malignant neoplasm to that site and may be the principal diagnosis in the absence of the primary site.

F. When a patient is admitted because of a primary neoplasm with metastasis and treatment is directed toward the secondary site only, the secondary neoplasm is designated as the principal diagnosis even though the primary malignancy is still present.

G. Symptoms, signs, and ill-defined conditions listed in Chapter 16 characteristic of, or associated with, an existing primary or secondary site malignancy cannot be used to replace the malignancy as principal diagnosis, regardless of the number of admissions or encounters for treatment and care of the neoplasm.

H. Coding and sequencing of complications associated with the malignant neoplasm or with the therapy thereof are subject to the following guidelines:

- When admission is for management of an anemia associated with the malignancy, and the treatment is only for anemia, the anemia is designated at the principal diagnosis and is followed by the appropriate code(s) for the malignancy.
- When the admission is for management of an anemia associated with chemotherapy or radiotherapy and the only treatment is for the anemia, the anemia is designated as the principal diagnosis followed by the appropriate code(s) for the malignancy.
- When the admission is for management of dehydration due to the malignancy or the therapy, or a combination of both, and only the dehydration is being treated (intravenous rehydration), the dehydration is designated as the principal diagnosis, followed by the code(s) for the malignancy.
- When the admission is for treatment of a complication resulting from a surgical procedure performed for the

treatment of an intestinal malignancy, designate the complication as the principal diagnosis if treatment is directed at resolving the complication.

2.14. Poisoning

When coding a poisoning or reaction to the improper use of a medication (e.g., wrong dose, wrong substance, wrong route of administration) the poisoning code is sequenced first, followed by a code for the manifestation. If there is also a diagnosis of drug abuse or dependence to the substance, the abuse or dependence is coded as an additional code.

2.15. Complications of surgery and other medical care

When the admission is for treatment of a complication resulting from surgery or other medical care, the complication code is sequenced as the principal diagnosis. If the complication is classified to the 996-999 series, an additional code for the specific complication may be assigned.

2.16. Complication of pregnancy

When a patient is admitted because of a condition that is either a complication pregnancy or that is complicating the pregnancy, the code for the obstetric complication is the principal diagnosis. An additional code may be assigned as needed to provide specificity.

3. REPORTING OTHER (ADDITIONAL) DIAGNOSES

A joint effort between the attending physician and coder is essential to achieve complete and accurate documentation, code assignment, and reporting of diagnoses and procedures.

These guidelines have been developed and approved by the Cooperating Parties to assure both the physician and the coder in identifying those diagnoses that are to be reported in addition to the principal diagnosis. Hospitals may record other diagnoses as needed for internal data use.

The UHDDS definitions are used by acute care short-term hospitals to report inpatient data elements in a standardized manner. These data elements and their definitions can be found in the July 31, 1985, Federal Register (Vol. 50, No, 147), pp. 31038-40.

The UHDDS item #11-b defines Other Diagnoses as "all conditions that coexist at the time of admission, that develop subsequently, or that affect the treatment received and/or the length of stay. Diagnoses that relate to an earlier episode which have no bearing on the current hospital stay are to be excluded".

General Rule

For reporting purposes the definition for "other diagnoses" is interpreted as additional conditions that affect patient care in terms of requiring:

- clinical evaluation; or
- therapeutic treatment; or
- diagnostic procedures; or
- extended length of hospital stay; or
- increased nursing care and/or monitoring.

The following guidelines are to be applied in designating "other diagnoses" when neither the Alphabetic Index nor the Tabular List in ICD-9-CM provide direction.

The listing of the diagnoses on the attestation statement is the responsibility of the attending physician.

3.1. Previous conditions

If the physician has included a diagnosis in the final diagnostic statement, such as the discharge summary or the face sheet, it should ordinarily be coded. Some physicians include in the diagnostic statement resolved conditions or diagnoses and status-post procedures from previous admission that have no bearing on the current stay. Such conditions are not to be reported and are coded only if required by hospital policy.

However, history codes (V10-V19) may be used as secondary codes if the historical condition or family history has an impact on current care or influences treatment.

3.2. Diagnoses not listed in the final diagnostic statement

When the physician has documented what appears to be a current diagnosis in the body of the record, but has not included the diagnosis in the final diagnostic statement, the physician should be asked whether the diagnosis should be added.

3.3. Conditions that are an integral part of a disease process

Conditions that are integral to the disease process should not be assigned as additional codes.

3.4. Conditions that are not an integral part of a disease process

Additional conditions that may not be associated routinely with a disease process should be coded when present.

3.5. Abnormal findings

Abnormal findings (laboratory, x-ray, pathologic, and other diagnostic results) are not coded and reported unless the physician indicates their clinical significance. If the findings are outside the normal range and the physician has ordered other tests to evaluate the condition or prescribed treatment, it is appropriate to ask the physician whether the diagnosis should be added.

4. HYPERTENSION

4.1. Hypertension, Essential, or NOS

Assign hypertension (arterial) (essential) (primary) (systemic) (NOS) to category code 401 with the appropriate fourth digit to indicate malignant (.0), benign (.1), or unspecified (.9). Do not use either .0 malignant or .1 benign unless medical record documentation supports such a designation.

4.2. Hypertension with Heart Disease

Certain heart conditions (425.8, 428, 429.0-429.3, 429.8, 429.9) are assigned to a code from category 402 when a causal relationship is stated (due to hypertension) or implied (hypertensive). Use only the code from category 402.

The same heart conditions (425.8, 428, 429.0-429.3, 429.8, 429.9) with hypertension, but without a stated casual relationship, are coded separately. Sequence according to the circumstances of the admission.

4.3. Hypertensive Renal Disease with Chronic Renal Failure

Assign codes from category 403, Hypertensive renal disease, when conditions classified to categories 585-587 are present. Unlike hypertension with heart disease, ICD-9-CM presumes a cause-and-effect relationship and classifies renal failure with hypertension as hypertensive renal disease.

4.4. Hypertensive Heart and Renal Disease

Assign codes from combination category 404, Hypertensive heart and renal disease, when both hypertensive renal disease and hypertensive heart disease are stated in the diagnosis. Assume a relationship between the hypertension and the renal disease, whether or not the condition is so designated.

4.5. Hypertensive Cerebrovascular Disease.

First assign codes from 430-438, Cerebrovascular disease, then the appropriate hypertension code from categories 401-405.

4.6. Hypertensive Retinopathy

Two codes are necessary to identify the condition. First assign the code from subcategory 362.11, Hypertensive retinopathy, then the appropriate code from categories 401-405 to indicate the type of hypertension.

4.7. Hypertension, Secondary

Two codes are required: one to identify the underlying condition and one from category 405 to identify the hypertension. Sequencing of codes is determined by the reason for admission to the hospital.

4.8. Hypertension, Transient

Assign code 796.2, Elevated blood pressure reading without diagnosis of hypertension, unless patient has an established diagnosis of hypertension. Assign code 642.3x for transient hypertension of pregnancy.

4.9. Hypertension, Controlled

Assign appropriate code from categories 401-405. This diagnostic statement usually refers to an existing state of hypertension under control by therapy.

4.10. Hypertension, Uncontrolled

Uncontrolled hypertension may refer to untreated hypertension or hypertension not responding to current therapeutic regimen. In either case. assign the appropriate code from categories 401-405 to designate the stage and type of hypertension. Code to the type of hypertension.

4.11. Elevated Blood Pressure

For a statement of elevated blood pressure without further specificity, assign code 796.2, Elevated blood pressure reading without diagnosis of hypertension, rather than a code from category 401.

5. OBSTETRICS

Introduction

These guidelines have been developed and approved by the Cooperating Parties in conjunction with the Editorial Advisory Board of Coding Clinic and the American College of Obstetricians and Gynecologists, to assist the coder in coding and reporting obstetric cases. Where feasible, previously published advice has been incorporated. Some advice in these new guidelines may supersede previous advice. The guidelines are provided for reporting purposes. Health care facilities may record additional diagnoses as needed for internal data needs.

5.1. General Rules

A. Obstetric cases require codes from chapter 11, codes in the range 630-677, Complications of Pregnancy, Childbirth, and the Puerperium. Should the physician document that the pregnancy is incidental to the encounter then code V22.2 should be used in place of any chapter 11 codes. It is the physician's responsibility to state that the condition being treated is not affecting the pregnancy.

B. Chapter 11 codes have sequencing priority over codes from other chapters. Additional codes from other chapters may be used in conjunction with chapter 11 codes to further specify conditions.

C. Chapter 11 codes are to be used only on the maternal record, never on the record of the newborn.

D. An outcome of delivery code, V27.0-V27.9, should be included on every maternal record when a delivery has occurred. These codes are not to be used on subsequent records or on the newborn record.

5.2. Selection of Principal Diagnosis

A. The circumstances of the encounter govern the selection of the principal diagnosis.

B. In episodes when no delivery occurs the principal diagnosis should correspond to the principal complication of the pregnancy which necessitated the encounter. Should more than one complication exist, all of which are treated or monitored, any of the complications codes may be sequenced first.

C. When a delivery occurs the principal diagnosis should correspond to the main circumstances or complication of the delivery. In cases of cesarean deliveries, the principal diagnosis should correspond to the reason the cesarean was performed, unless the reason for admission was unrelated to the condition resulting in the cesarean delivery.

D. For routine prenatal visits when no complications are present codes V22.0, Supervision of normal first pregnancy, and V22.1, Supervision of other normal pregnancy, should be used as principal diagnoses. These codes should not be used in conjunction with chapter 11 codes.

E. For prenatal outpatient visits for patients with high-risk pregnancies, a code from category V23, Supervision of high-risk pregnancy, should be used as the principal diagnosis. Secondary chapter 11 codes may be used in conjunction with these codes if appropriate. A thorough review of any pertinent excludes note is necessary to be certain that these V codes are being used properly.

5.3. Chapter 11 Fifth-digits

A. Categories 640-648, 651-676 have required fifth-digits which indicate whether the encounter is antepartum, postpartum and whether a delivery has also occurred.

B. The fifth-digits which are appropriate for each code number are listed in brackets under each code. The fifth-digits on each code should all be consistent with each other. That is, should a delivery occur all of the fifth-digits should indicate the delivery.

5.4. Fetal Conditions Affecting the Management of the Mother.

Codes from category 655, Known or suspected fetal abnormality affecting management of the mother, and category 656, Other fetal and placental problems affecting the management of the mother, are assigned only when the fetal condition is actually responsible for modifying the management of the mother, i.e., by requiring diagnostic studies, additional observation, special care, or termination of pregnancy. The fact that the fetal condition exists does not justify assigning a code from this series to the mother's record.

5.5. Normal Delivery, 650

A. Code 650 is for use in cases when a woman is admitted for a full-term normal delivery and delivers a single, healthy infant without any complications antepartum, during the delivery, or postpartum during the delivery episode.

B. 650 may be used if the patient had a complications at some point during her pregnancy but the complication is not present at the time of the admission for delivery.

- C. Code 650 is always a principal diagnosis. It is not to be used if any other code from chapter 11 is needed to describe a current complication of the antenatal, delivery, or perinatal period. Additional codes from other chapters may be used with code 650 if they are not related to or are in any way complicating the pregnancy.
- D. V27.0, Single liveborn, is the only outcome of delivery code appropriate for use with 650.

5.6. Procedure Codes
- A. In cases of cesarean delivery, the selection of the principal diagnosis should correspond to the reason the cesarean delivery was performed unless the reason for admission was unrelated to the condition resulting in the cesarean delivery.
- B. A delivery procedure code should not be used for a woman who has delivered prior to admission to the hospital. Any postpartum repairs should be coded.

5.7. The Postpartum Period
- A. The postpartum period begins immediately after delivery and continues for 6 weeks following delivery.
- B. A postpartum complication is any complication occurring within the 6 week period.
- C. Chapter 11 codes may also be used to describe pregnancy-related complications after the 6 week period should the physician document that a condition is pregnancy related.
- D. Postpartum complications that occur during the same admission as the delivery are identified with a fifth digit of "2". Subsequent admissions for postpartum complications should identified with a fifth digit of "4".
- E. When the mother delivers outside the hospital prior to admission and is admitted for routine postpartum care and no complications are noted, code V24.0, Postpartum care and examination immediately after delivery, should be assigned as the principal diagnosis.

5.8. Abortions
- A. Fifth-digits are required for abortion categories 634-637. Fifth-digit 1, incomplete, indicates that all of the products of conception have not been expelled from the uterus. Fifth-digit 2, complete, indicates that all products of conception have been expelled from the uterus prior to the episode of care.
- B. A code from categories 640-648 and 651-657 may be used as additional codes with an abortion code to indicate the complication leading to the abortion.

    Fifth digit 3 is assigned with codes from these categories when used with an abortion code because the other fifth digits will not apply. Codes from the 660-669 series are not to be used for complications of abortion.
- C. Code 639 is to be used for all complications following abortion. Code 639 cannot be assigned with codes from categories 634-638.
- D. Abortion with Liveborn Fetus. When an attempted termination of pregnancy results in a liveborn fetus assign code 644.21, Early onset of delivery, with an appropriate code from category V27,

Outcome of Delivery. The procedure code for the attempted termination of pregnancy should also be assigned.

E. Retained Products of Conception following an abortion. Subsequent admissions for retained products of conception following a spontaneous or legally induced abortion are assigned the appropriate code from category 634, Spontaneous abortion, or legally induced abortion, with a fifth digit of "1" (incomplete). This advice is appropriate even when the patient was discharged previously with a discharge diagnosis of complete abortion.

5.9. Code 677, Late effect of complication of pregnancy, childbirth, and the puerperium

A. Code 677, Late effect of complication of pregnancy, childbirth, and the puerperium is for use in those cases when an initial complication of a pregnancy develops a sequelae requiring care or treatment at a future date.

B. This code may be used at any time after the initial postpartum period.

C. This code, like all late effect codes, is to be sequenced following the code describing the sequelae of the complication.

6. NEWBORN GUIDELINES

Definition

The newborn period is defined as beginning at birth and lasting through the 28th day following birth.

The following guidelines are provided for reporting purposes. Hospitals may record other diagnoses as needed for internal data use.

General Rule

All clinically significant conditions noted on routine newborn examination should be coded. A condition is clinically significant if it requires:

- clinical evaluation; or
- therapeutic treatment; or
- diagnostic procedures; or
- extended length of hospital stay; or
- increased nursing care and/or monitoring; or
- has implications for future health care needs.

Note: The newborn guidelines listed above are the same as the general coding guidelines for "other diagnoses," except for the final bullet regarding implications for future health care needs. Whether or not a condition is clinically significant can only be determined by the physician.

6.1. Use of Codes V30-V39

When coding the birth of an infant, assign a code from categories V30-V39, according to the type of birth. A code from this series is assigned as a principal diagnosis, and assigned only once to a newborn at the time of birth.

6.2. Newborn Transfers

If the newborn is transferred to another institution, the V30 series is not used.

6.3. Use of Category V29

A. Assign a code from category V29, Observation and evaluation of newborns and infants for suspected conditions not found, to identify those instances when a healthy newborn is evaluated for a suspected condition that is determined after study not to be present. Do not use a code from category V29 when the patient has identified signs or symptoms of a suspected problem; in such cases, code the sign or symptom.

B. A V29 code is to be used as a secondary code after the V30, Outcome of delivery, code. It may also be assigned as a principal code for readmissions or encounters when the V30 code no longer applies. It is for use only for healthy newborns and infants for which no condition after study is found to be present.

6.4. Maternal Causes of Perinatal Morbidity

Codes from categories 760-763, Maternal causes of perinatal morbidity and mortality, are assigned only when the maternal condition has actually affected the fetus or newborn. The fact that the mother has an associated medical condition or experiences some complication of pregnancy, labor or delivery does not justify the routine assignment of codes from these categories to the newborn record.

6.5. Congenital Anomalies

Assign an appropriate code from categories 740-759, Congenital Anomalies, when a specific abnormality is diagnosed for an infant. Such abnormalities may occur as a set of symptoms or multiple malformations. A code should be assigned for each presenting manifestation of the syndrome if the syndrome is not specifically indexed in ICD-9-CM.

6.6. Coding of Other (Additional) Diagnoses

A. Assign codes for conditions that require treatment or further investigation, prolong the length of stay, or require resource utilization.

B. Assign codes for conditions that have been specified by the physician as having implications for future health care needs.

NOTE: This guideline should not be used for adult patients.

C. Assign a code for Newborn conditions originating in the perinatal period (categories 760-779), as well as complications arising during the current episode of care classified in other chapters, only if the diagnoses have been documented by the responsible physician at the time of transfer or discharge as having affected the fetus or newborn.

D. Insignificant conditions or signs or symptoms that resolve without treatment are not coded.

6.7. Prematurity and Fetal Growth Retardation

Codes from categories 764 and 765 should not be assigned based solely on recorded birthweight or estimated gestational age, but upon the attending physician's clinical assessment of maturity of the infant.

NOTE: Since physicians may utilize different criteria in determining prematurity, do not code the diagnosis of prematurity unless the physician documents this condition.

7. SEPTICEMIA AND SEPTIC SHOCK

When the diagnosis of septicemia with shock or the diagnosis of general sepsis with septic shock is documented, code and list the septicemia first and report the septic shock code as a secondary condition. The septicemia code assignment should identify the type of bacteria if it is known.

Sepsis and septic shock associated with abortion, ectopic pregnancy, and molar pregnancy are classified to category codes in Chapter 11 (630-639).

Negative or inconclusive blood cultures do not preclude a diagnosis of septicemia in patients with clinical evidence of the condition.

8. TRAUMA

8.1. Coding for Multiple Injuries

When coding multiple injuries such as fracture of tibia and fibula, assign separate codes for each injury unless a combination code is provided, in which case the combination code is assigned. Multiple injury codes are provided in ICD-9-CM, but should not be assigned unless information for a more specific code is not available.

A. The code for the most serious injury, as determined by the physician, is sequenced first.

B. Superficial injuries such as abrasions or contusions are not coded when associated with more severe injuries of the same site.

C. When a primary injury results in minor damage to peripheral nerves or blood vessels, the primary injury is sequenced first with additional code(s) from categories 950-957, Injury to nerves and spinal cord, and/or 900-904, Injury to blood vessels. When the primary injury is to the blood vessels or nerves, that injury should be sequenced first.

8.2. Coding for Multiple Fractures

The principle of multiple coding of injuries should be followed in coding multiple fractures. Multiple fractures of specified sites are coded individually by site in accordance with both the provisions within categories 800-829 and the level of detail furnished by medical record content. Combination categories for multiple fractures are provided for use when there is insufficient detail in the medical record (such as trauma cases transferred to another hospital), when the reporting form limits the number of codes that can be used in reporting pertinent clinical data, or when there is insufficient specificity at the fourth-digit or fifth-digit level. More specific guidelines are as follows:

A. Multiple fractures of same limb classifiable to the same three-digit or four-digit category are coded to that category.

B. Multiple unilateral or bilateral fractures of same bone(s) but classified to different fourth-digit subdivisions (bone part) within the same three-digit category are coded individually by site.

C. Multiple fracture categories 819 and 828 classify bilateral fractures of both upper limbs (819) and both lower limbs (828), but without any detail at the fourth-digit level other than open and closed type of fractures.

D. Multiple fractures are sequenced in accordance with the severity of the fracture and the physician should be asked to list the fracture diagnoses in the order of severity.

8.3. Current Burns and Encounters for Late Effects of Burns

Current burns (940-948) are classified by depth, extent and, if desired, by agent (E code). By depth burns are classified as first degree (erythema), second degree (blistering), and third degree (full-thickness involvement).

A. All burns are coded with the highest degree of burn sequenced first.

B. Classify burns of the same local site (three-digit category level, (940-947) but of different degrees to the subcategory identifying the highest degree recorded in the diagnosis.

C. Non-healing burns are coded as acute burns. Necrosis of burned skin should be coded as a non-healed burn.

    D.   Assign code 958.3, Posttraumatic wound infection, not elsewhere classified, as an additional code for any documented infected burn site.

    E.   When coding multiple burns, assign separate codes for each burn site. Category 946 Burns of Multiple specified sites, should only be used if the location of the burns are not documented. Category 949, Burn, unspecified, is extremely vague and should rarely be used.

    F.   Assign codes from category 948, Burns classified according to extent of body surface involved, when the site of the burn is not specified or when there is a need for additional data. It is advisable to use category 948 as additional coding when needed to provide data for evaluating burn mortality, such as that needed by burn units. It is also advisable to use category 948 as an additional code for reporting purposes when there is mention of a third-degree burn involving 20 percent or more of the body surface. In assigning a code from category 948:

- Four-digit codes are used to identify the percentage of total body surface involved in a burn (all degree).
- Fifth-digits are assigned to identify the percentage of body surface involved in third-degree burn.
- Fifth-digit zero (0) is assigned when less than 10 percent or when no body surface is involved in a third-degree burn.

Category 948 is based on the classic "rule of nines" in estimating body surface involved: head and neck are assigned nine percent, each arm nine percent, each leg 18 percent, the anterior trunk 18 percent, posterior trunk 18 percent, and genitalia one percent. Physicians may change these percentage assignments where necessary to accommodate infants and children who have proportionately larger heads than adults and patients who have large buttocks, thighs, or abdomen that involve burns.

    G.   Encounters for the treatment of the late effects of burns (i.e., scars or joint contractures) should be coded to the residual condition (sequelae) followed by the appropriate late effect code (906.5-906.9). A late effect E code may also be used, if desired.

    H.   When appropriate, both a sequelae with a late effect code, and a current burn code may be assigned on the same record.

8.4. Debridement of Wound, Infection, or Burn

    A.   For coding purposes, excisional debridement, 86.22, is assigned only when the procedure is performed by a physician.

    B.   For coding purposes, nonexcisional debridement performed by the physician or nonphysician health care professional is assigned to 86.28. Any "excisional" type procedure performed by a nonphysician is assigned to 86.28.

9. ADVERSE EFFECTS AND POISONING

The properties of certain drugs, medicinal and biological substances or combinations of such substances, may cause toxic reactions. The occurrence of drug toxicity is classified in ICD-9-CM as follows:

9.1. Adverse Effect

When the drug was correctly prescribed and properly administered, code the reaction plus the appropriate code from the E930-E949 series.

Adverse effects of therapeutic substances correctly prescribed and properly administered (toxicity, synergistic reaction, side effect, and idiosyncratic reaction) may be due to (1) differences among patients, such as age, sex, disease, and genetic factors, and (2) drug-related factors, such as type of drug, route of administration, duration of therapy, dosage, and bioavailability.

Codes from the E930-E949 series must be used to identify the causative substance for an adverse effect of drug, medicinal and biological substances, correctly prescribed and properly administered. The effect, such as tachycardia, delirium, gastrointestinal hemorrhaging, vomiting, hypokalemia, hepatitis, renal failure, or respiratory failure, is coded and followed by the appropriate code from the E930-E949 series.

9.2. Poisoning

Poisoning when an error was made in drug prescription or in the administration of the drug by physician, nurse, patient, or other person, use the appropriate code from the 960-979 series. If an overdose of a drug was intentionally taken or administered and resulted in drug toxicity, it would be coded as a poisoning (960-979 series). If a nonprescribed drug or medicinal agent was taken in combination with a correctly prescribed and properly administered drug, any drug toxicity or other reaction resulting from the interaction of the two drugs would be classified as a poisoning.

10. HUMAN IMMUNODEFICIENCY VIRUS (HIV) INFECTIONS

10.1. Code only confirmed cases of HIV infection/illness.

This is an exception to guideline 1.8 which states "If the diagnosis documented at the time of discharge is qualified as 'probable,' 'suspected,' 'likely,' 'questionable,' 'possible,' or 'still to be ruled out,' code the condition as if it existed or was established..."

In this context, "confirmation" does not require documentation of positive serology or culture for HIV; the physician's diagnostic statement that the patient is HIV positive, or has an HIV-related illness is sufficient.

10.2. Selection of HIV code

042   Human Immunodeficiency Virus [HIV] Disease

Patients with an HIV-related illness should be coded to 042, Human Immunodeficiency Virus [HIV] Disease.

V08   Asymptomatic Human Immunodeficiency Virus [HIV] Infection

Patients with physician-documented asymptomatic HIV infections who have never had an HIV-related illness should be coded to V08, Asymptomatic Human Immunodeficiency Virus [HIV] Infection.

795.71   Nonspecific Serologic Evidence of Human Immunodeficiency Virus [HIV]

Code 795.71, Nonspecific serologic evidence of human immunodeficiency virus [HIV], should be used for patients (including infants) with inconclusive HIV test results.

10.3. Previously diagnosed HIV-related illness

Patients with any known prior diagnosis of an HIV-related illness should be coded to 042. Once a patient had developed an HIV-related illness, the patient should always be assigned code 042 on every subsequent admission. Patients previously diagnosed with any HIV illness (042) should never be assigned to 795.71 or V08.

10.4. Sequencing

The sequencing of diagnoses for patients with HIV-related illnesses follows guideline 2 for selection of principal diagnosis. That is, the circumstances of admission govern the selection of principal diagnosis, "that condition established after study to be chiefly responsible for occasioning the admission of the patient to the hospital for care."

Patients who are admitted for an HIV-related illness should be assigned a minimum of two codes: first assign code 042 to identify the HIV disease and then sequence additional codes to identify the other diagnoses. If a patient is admitted for an HIV-related condition, the principal diagnosis should be 042, followed by additional diagnosis codes for all reported HIV-related conditions.

If a patient with HIV disease is admitted for an unrelated condition (such as a traumatic injury), the code for the unrelated condition (e.g., the nature of injury code) should be the principal diagnosis. Other diagnoses would be 042 followed by additional diagnosis codes for all reported HIV-related conditions.

Whether the patient is newly diagnosed or has had previous admissions for HIV conditions (or has expired) is irrelevant to the sequencing decision.

10.5. HIV Infection in Pregnancy, Childbirth and the Puerperium

During pregnancy, childbirth or the puerperium, a patient admitted because of an HIV-related illness should receive a principal diagnosis of 647.6X, Other specified infectious and parasitic diseases in the mother classifiable elsewhere, but complicating the pregnancy, childbirth or the puerperium, followed by 042 and the code(s) for the HIV-related illness(es). This is an exception to the sequencing rule found in 10.4 above.

Patients with asymptomatic HIV infection status admitted during pregnancy, childbirth, or the puerperium should receive codes of 647.6X and V08.

10.6. Asymptomatic HIV Infection

V08 Asymptomatic human immunodeficiency virus [HIV] infection, is to be applied when the patient without any documentation of symptoms is listed as being "HIV positive," "known HIV," "HIV test positive," or similar terminology. Do not use this code if the term "AIDS" is used or if the patient is treated for any HIV-related illness or is described as having any condition(s) resulting from his/her HIV positive status; use 042 in these cases.

10.7. Inconclusive Laboratory Test for HIV

Patients with inconclusive HIV serology, but no definitive diagnosis or manifestations of the illness may be assigned code 795.71.Inconclusive serologic test for Human Immunodeficiency Virus [HIV]

10.8. Testing for HIV

If the patient is asymptomatic but wishes to know his/her HIV status, use code V73.89, Screening for other specified viral disease. Use code V69.8, Other problems related to lifestyle, as a secondary code if an asymptomatic patient is in a known high-risk group for HIV. Should a patient with signs or symptoms or illness, or a confirmed HIV related diagnosis be tested for HIV code the signs and symptoms or the diagnosis. An additional counseling code V65.44 may be used if counseling is provided during the encounter for the test.

When the patient returns to be informed of his/her HIV test results use code V65.44, HIV counseling, if the results of the test are negative. If the results are positive but the patient is asymptomatic use code V08, Asymptomatic HIV infection. If the results are positive and the patient is symptomatic use code 042, HIV infection, with codes for the HIV related symptoms or diagnosis. The HIV counseling code may also be used if counseling is provided for patients with positive test results.

11. GUIDELINES FOR CODING EXTERNAL CAUSES OF INJURIES, POISONINGS AND ADVERSE EFFECTS OF DRUGS (E Codes)

Introduction

These guidelines are provided for those who are currently collecting E codes in order that there will be standardization in the process. If your institution plans to begin collecting E codes, these guidelines are to be applied. The use of E codes are supplemental to the application of basic ICD-9-CM codes. E codes are never to be recorded as principal diagnosis (first listed in the outpatient setting) and are not required for reporting to the Health Care Financing Administration.

Injuries are a major cause of mortality, morbidity and disability. In the United States, the care of patients who suffer intentional and unintentional injuries and poisonings contributes significantly to the increase in medical care costs. External causes of injury and poisoning codes (E codes) are intended to provide data for injury research and evaluation of injury prevention strategies. E codes capture how the injury or poisoning happened (cause), the intent (unintentional or accidental; or intentional, such as suicide or assault), and the place where the event occurred. Some major categories of E codes include:

- transport accidents
- poisoning and adverse effects of drugs, medicinal substances and biologicals
- accidental falls
- accidents caused by fire and flames
- accidents due to natural and environmental factors
- late effects of accidents, assaults or self injury
- assaults or purposely inflicted injury
- suicide or self inflicted injury

These guidelines apply for the coding and collection of E code from records in hospitals, outpatient clinics, emergency departments, other ambulatory care settings and physician offices except when other specific guidelines apply. (See Reporting Diagnostic Guidelines for Hospital-based Outpatient Services/Reporting Requirements for Physician Billing.)

11.1. General E Code Coding Guidelines

A. An E code may be used with any code in the range of 001-V82.9 which indicates an injury, poisoning, or adverse effect due to an external cause.

B. Assign the appropriate E-code for all initial treatments of an injury, poisoning, or adverse effect of drugs.

C. Use a late effect E code for subsequent visits when a late effect of the initial injury or poisoning is being treated. There is no late effect E code for adverse effects of drugs.

D. Use the full range of E codes to completely describe the cause, the intent and the place of occurrence, if applicable, for all injuries, poisonings, and adverse effects of drugs.

E. Assign as many E codes as necessary to fully explain each cause. If only one E code can be recorded, assign the E code most related to the principal diagnosis.

F. The selection of the appropriate E code is guided by the Index to External Causes which is located after the alphabetical index to diseases and by Inclusion and Exclusion notes in the Tabular List.

G. An E code can never be a principal (first listed) diagnosis.

11.2. Place of Occurrence Guideline

Use an additional code from category E849 to indicate the Place of Occurrence for injuries and poisonings. The Place of Occurrence describes the place where the event occurred and not the patient's activity at the time of the event.

Do not use E849.9 if the place of occurrence is not stated.

11.3. Poisonings and Adverse Effects of Drugs, Medicinal and Biological Substances Guidelines

    A. Do not code directly from the Table of Drugs and Chemicals. Always refer back to the Tabular List.

    B. Use as many codes as necessary to describe completely all drugs, medicinal or biological substances.

    C. If the same E code would describe the causative agent for more than one adverse reaction, assign the code only once.

    D. If two or more drugs, medicinal or biological substances are reported, code each individually unless the combination code is listed in the Table of Drugs and Chemicals. In that case, assign the E code for the combination.

    E. When a reaction results from the interaction of a drug(s) and alcohol, use poisoning codes and E codes for both.

    F. If the reporting format limits the number of E codes that can be used in reporting clinical data, code the one most related to the principal diagnosis. Include at least one from each category (cause, intent, place) if possible.

- If there are different fourth digit codes in the same three digit category, use the code for "Other specified" of that category. If there is no "Other specified" code in that category, use the appropriate "Unspecified" code in that category.
- If the codes are in different three digit categories, assign the appropriate E code for other multiple drugs and medicinal substances.

11.4. Multiple Cause E Code Coding Guidelines

If two or more events cause separate injuries, an E code should be assigned for each cause. The first listed E code will be selected in the following order:

- E codes for child and adult abuse take priority over all other E code—see Child and Adult abuse guidelines
- E codes for cataclysmic events take priority over all other E codes except child and adult abuse
- E codes for transport accidents take priority over all other E codes except cataclysmic events and child and adult abuse

The first listed E code should correspond to the cause of the most serious diagnosis due to an assault, accident, or self-harm, following the order of hierarchy listed above.

11.5. Child and Adult Abuse Guideline

    A. When the cause of an injury or neglect is intentional child or adult abuse, the first listed E code should be assigned from categories E960-E968, Homicide and injury purposely inflicted by other persons, (except category E967). An E code from category E967, Child and adult battering and other maltreatment, should be added as an additional code to identify the perpetrator, if known.

    B. In cases of neglect when the intent is determined to be accidental E code E904.0, Abandonment or neglect of infant and helpless person, should be the first listed E code.

11.6. Unknown or Suspected Intent Guideline

    A. If the intent (accident, self-harm, assault) of the cause of an injury or poisoning is unknown or unspecified, code the intent as undetermined E980-E989.

    B. If the intent (accident, self-harm, assault) of the cause of an injury or poisoning is questionable, probable or suspected, code the intent as undetermined E980-E989.

11.7. Undetermined Cause

When the intent of an injury or poisoning is known, but the cause is unknown, use codes: E928.9, Unspecified accident, E958.9, Suicide and self-inflicted injury by unspecified means, and E968.9, Assault by unspecified means.

These E codes should rarely be used as the documentation in the medical record, in both the inpatient and outpatient settings, should normally provide sufficient detail to determine the cause of the injury.

11.8. Late Effects of External Cause Guidelines

    A. Late effect E codes exist for injuries and poisonings but not for adverse effects of drugs, misadventures and surgical complications.

    B. A late effect E code (E929, E959, E969, E977, E989, or E999) should be used with any report of a late effect or sequela resulting from a previous injury or poisoning (905-909).

    C. A late effect E code should never be used with a related current nature of injury code.

11.9. Misadventures and Complications of Care Guidelines

    A. Assign a code in the range of E870-E876 if misadventures are stated by the physician.

    B. Assign a code in the range of E878-E879 if the physician attributes an abnormal reaction or later complication to a surgical or medical procedure, but does not mention misadventure at the time of the procedure as the cause of the reaction.

A

AAV (disease) (illness) (infection) — see Human immunodeficiency virus (disease) (illness) (infection)
Abactio — see Abortion, induced
Abactus venter — see Abortion, induced
Abarognosis 781.99
Abasia (-astasia) 307.9
    atactica 781.3
    choreic 781.3
    hysterical 300.11
    paroxysmal trepidant 781.3
    spastic 781.3
    trembling 781.3
    trepidans 781.3
Abderhalden-Kaufmann-Lignac syndrome (cystinosis) 270.0
Abdomen, abdominal — see also condition
    accordion 306.4
    acute 789.0 ✓5ᵗʰ
    angina 557.1
    burst 868.00
    convulsive equivalent (see also Epilepsy) 345.5 ✓5ᵗʰ
    heart 746.87
    muscle deficiency syndrome 756.79
    obstipum 756.79
Abdominalgia 789.0 ✓5ᵗʰ
    periodic 277.3
Abduction contracture, hip or other joint — see Contraction, joint
Abercrombie's syndrome (amyloid degeneration) 277.3
Aberrant (congenital) — see also Malposition, congenital
    adrenal gland 759.1
    blood vessel NEC 747.60
        arteriovenous NEC 747.60
        cerebrovascular 747.81
        gastrointestinal 747.61
        lower limb 747.64
        renal 747.62
        spinal 747.82
        upper limb 747.63
    breast 757.6
    endocrine gland NEC 759.2
    gastrointestinal vessel (peripheral) 747.61
    hepatic duct 751.69
    lower limb vessel (peripheral) 747.64
    pancreas 751.7
    parathyroid gland 759.2
    peripheral vascular vessel NEC 747.60
    pituitary gland (pharyngeal) 759.2
    renal blood vessel 747.62
    sebaceous glands, mucous membrane, mouth 750.26
    spinal vessel 747.82
    spleen 759.0
    testis (descent) 752.51
    thymus gland 759.2
    thyroid gland 759.2
    upper limb vessel (perpipheral) 747.63
Aberratio
    lactis 757.6
    testis 752.51
Aberration — see also Anomaly
    chromosome — see Anomaly, chromosome(s)
    distantial 368.9

Aberration — continued
    mental (see also Disorder, mental, nonpsychotic) 300.9
Abetalipoproteinemia 272.5
Abionarce 780.79
Abiotrophy 799.8
Ablatio
    placentae — see Placenta, ablatio
    retinae (see also Detachment, retina) 361.9
Ablation
    pituitary (gland) (with hypofunction) 253.7
    placenta — see Placenta, ablatio
    uterus 621.8
Ablepharia, ablepharon, ablephary 743.62
Ablepsia — see Blindness
Ablepsy — see Blindness
Ablutomania 300.3
Abnormal, abnormality, abnormalities — see also Anomaly
    acid-base balance 276.4
        fetus or newborn — see Distress, fetal
    adaptation curve, dark 368.63
    alveolar ridge 525.9
    amnion 658.9 ✓5ᵗʰ
        affecting fetus or newborn 762.9
    anatomical relationship NEC 759.9
    apertures, congenital, diaphragm 756.6
    auditory perception NEC 388.40
    autosomes NEC 758.5
        13 758.1
        18 758.2
        21 or 22 758.0
        D₁ 758.1
        E₃ 758.2
        G 758.0
    ballistocardiogram 794.39
    basal metabolic rate (BMR) 794.7
    biosynthesis, testicular androgen 257.2
    blood level (of)
        cobalt 790.6
        copper 790.6
        iron 790.6
        lithium 790.6
        magnesium 790.6
        mineral 790.6
        zinc 790.6
    blood pressure
        elevated (without diagnosis of hypertension) 796.2
        low (see also Hypotension) 458.9
            reading (incidental) (isolated) (nonspecific) 796.3
    bowel sounds 787.5
    breathing behavior — see Respiration
    caloric test 794.19
    cervix (acquired) NEC 622.9
        congenital 752.40
        in pregnancy or childbirth 654.6 ✓5ᵗʰ
            causing obstructed labor 660.2 ✓5ᵗʰ
                affecting fetus or newborn 763.1
    chemistry, blood NEC 790.6
    chest sounds 786.7
    chorion 658.9 ✓5ᵗʰ
        affecting fetus or newborn 762.9
    chromosomal NEC 758.89
        analysis, nonspecific result 795.2
        autosomes (see also Abnormal, autosomes NEC) 758.5
        fetal, (suspected) affecting management of pregnancy 655.1 ✓5ᵗʰ

Abnormal, abnormality, abnormalities —
continued
  chromosomal NEC — *continued*
    sex 758.81
  clinical findings NEC 796.4
  communication — *see* Fistula
  configuration of pupils 379.49
  coronary
    artery 746.85
    vein 746.9
  cortisol-binding globulin 255.8
  course, Eustachian tube 744.24
  dentofacial NEC 524.9
    functional 524.5
    specified type NEC 524.8
  development, developmental NEC 759.9
    bone 756.9
    central nervous system 742.9
  direction, teeth 524.3
  Dynia (*see also* Defect, coagulation) 286.9
  Ebstein 746.2
  echocardiogram 793.2
  echoencephalogram 794.01
  echogram NEC — *see* Findings, abnormal, structure
  electrocardiogram (ECG) (EKG) 794.31
  electroencephalogram (EEG) 794.02
  electromyogram (EMG) 794.17
    ocular 794.14
  electro-oculogram (EOG) 794.12
  electroretinogram (ERG) 794.11
  erythrocytes 289.9
    congenital, with perinatal jaundice 282.9 [774.0]
  Eustachian valve 746.9
  excitability under minor stress 301.9
  fat distribution 782.9
  feces 787.7
  fetal heart rate — *see* Distress, fetal
  fetus NEC
    affecting management of pregnancy — *see* Pregnancy, management affected by, fetal
    causing disproportion 653.7
      affecting fetus or newborn 763.1
      causing obstructed labor 660.1
        affecting fetus or newborn 763.1
  findings without manifest disease — *see* Findings, abnormal
  fluid
    amniotic 792.3
    cerebrospinal 792.0
    peritoneal 792.9
    pleural 792.9
    synovial 792.9
    vaginal 792.9
  forces of labor NEC 661.9
    affecting fetus or newborn 763.7
  form, teeth 520.2
  function studies
    auditory 794.15
    bladder 794.9
    brain 794.00
    cardiovascular 794.30
    endocrine NEC 794.6
    kidney 794.4
    liver 794.8
    nervous system
      central 794.00
      peripheral 794.19
    oculomotor 794.14

Abnormal, abnormality, abnormalities —
continued
  function studies — *continued*
    pancreas 794.9
    placenta 794.9
    pulmonary 794.2
    retina 794.11
    special senses 794.19
    spleen 794.9
    thyroid 794.5
    vestibular 794.16
  gait 781.2
    hysterical 300.11
  gastrin secretion 251.5
  globulin
    cortisol-binding 255.8
    thyroid-binding 246.8
  glucagon secretion 251.4
  glucose tolerance test 790.2
    in pregnancy, childbirth, or puerperium 648.8
    fetus or newborn 775.0
  gravitational (G) forces or states 994.9
  hair NEC 704.2
  hard tissue formation in pulp 522.3
  head movement 781.0
  heart
    rate
      fetus, affecting liveborn infant
        before the onset of labor 763.81
        during labor 763.82
        unspecified as to time of onset 763.83
      intrauterine
        before the onset of labor 763.81
        during labor 763.82
        unspecified as to time of onset 763.83
      newborn
        before the onset of labor 763.81
        during labor 763.82
        unspecified as to time of onset 763.83
    shadow 793.2
    sounds NEC 785.3
  hemoglobin (*see also* Disease, hemoglobin) 282.7
    trait — *see* Trait, hemoglobin, abnormal
  hemorrhage, uterus — *see* Hemorrhage, uterus
  histology NEC 795.4
  increase
    in
      appetite 783.6
      development 783.9
  involuntary movement 781.0
  jaw closure 524.5
  karyotype 795.2
  knee jerk 796.1
  labor NEC 661.9
    affecting fetus or newborn 763.7
  laboratory findings — *see* Findings, abnormal
  length, organ or site, congenital — *see* Distortion
  loss of height 781.91
  loss of weight 783.21
  lung shadow 793.1
  mammogram 793.80
    microcalcification 793.81
  Mantoux test 795.5
  membranes (fetal)
    affecting fetus or newborn 762.9
    complicating pregnancy 658.8
  menstruation — *see* Menstruation

Index to Diseases

Abnormal, abnormality, abnormalities — *continued*
- metabolism (*see also* condition) 783.9
- movement 781.0
    - disorder NEC 333.90
        - specified NEC 333.99
    - head 781.0
    - involuntary 781.0
    - specified type NEC 333.99
- muscle contraction, localized 728.85
- myoglobin (Aberdeen) (Annapolis) 289.9
- narrowness, eyelid 743.62
- optokinetic response 379.57
- organs or tissues of pelvis NEC
    - in pregnancy or childbirth 654.9 ✓5ᵗʰ
        - affecting fetus or newborn 763.89
        - causing obstructed labor 660.2 ✓5ᵗʰ
            - affecting fetus or newborn 763.1
- origin — *see* Malposition, congenital
- palmar creases 757.2
- Papanicolaou (smear)
    - cervix 795.00 ▲
        - atypical squamous cell changes of ●
            - undetermined significance ●
            - favor benign (ASCUS favor benign) ●
                - 795.01
            - favor dysplasia (ASCUS favor ●
                - dysplasia) 795.02
            - nonspecific finding NEC 795.09 ●
    - other site 795.1
- parturition
    - affecting fetus or newborn 763.9
    - mother — *see* Delivery, complicated
- pelvis (bony) — *see* Deformity, pelvis
- percussion, chest 786.7
- periods (grossly) (*see also* Menstruation) 626.9
- phonocardiogram 794.39
- placenta — *see* Placenta, abnormal
- plantar reflex 796.1
- plasma protein — *see* Deficiency, plasma, protein
- pleural folds 748.8
- position — *see also* Malposition
    - gravid uterus 654.4 ✓5ᵗʰ
        - causing obstructed labor 660.2 ✓5ᵗʰ
            - affecting fetus or newborn 763.1
- posture NEC 781.92
- presentation (fetus) — *see* Presentation, fetus, abnormal
- product of conception NEC 631
- puberty — *see* Puberty
- pulmonary
    - artery 747.3
    - function, newborn 770.89 ▲
    - test results 794.2
    - ventilation, newborn 770.89 ▲
        - hyperventilation 786.01
- pulsations in neck 785.1
- pupil reflexes 379.40
- quality of milk 676.8 ✓5ᵗʰ
- radiological examination 793.9
    - abdomen NEC 793.6
    - biliary tract 793.3
    - breast 793.89
        - mammogram NOS 793.80
        - mammographic microcalcification 793.81
    - gastrointestinal tract 793.4
    - genitourinary organs 793.5
    - head 793.0
    - intrathoracic organ NEC 793.2

Abnormal, abnormality, abnormalities — *continued*
- radiological examination — *continued*
    - lung (field) 793.1
    - musculoskeletal system 793.7
    - retroperitoneum 793.6
    - skin and subcutaneous tissue 793.9
    - skull 793.0
- red blood cells 790.09
    - morphology 790.09
    - volume 790.09
- reflex NEC 796.1
- renal function test 794.4
- respiration signs — *see* Respiration
- response to nerve stimulation 794.10
- retinal correspondence 368.34
- rhythm, heart — *see also* Arrhythmia
    - fetus — *see* Distress, fetal
- saliva 792.4
- scan
    - brain 794.09
    - kidney 794.4
    - liver 794.8
    - lung 794.2
    - thyroid 794.5
- secretion
    - gastrin 251.5
    - glucagon 251.4
- semen 792.2
- serum level (of)
    - acid phosphatase 790.5
    - alkaline phosphatase 790.5
    - amylase 790.5
    - enzymes NEC 790.5
    - lipase 790.5
- shape
    - cornea 743.41
    - gallbladder 751.69
    - gravid uterus 654.4 ✓5ᵗʰ
        - affecting fetus or newborn 763.89
        - causing obstructed labor 660.2 ✓5ᵗʰ
            - affecting fetus or newborn 763.1
    - head (*see also* Anomaly, skull) 756.0
    - organ or site, congenital NEC — *see* Distortion
- sinus venosus 747.40
- size
    - fetus, complicating delivery 653.5 ✓5ᵗʰ
        - causing obstructed labor 660.1 ✓5ᵗʰ
    - gallbladder 751.69
    - head (*see also* Anomaly, skull) 756.0
    - organ or site, congenital NEC — *see* Distortion
    - teeth 520.2
- skin and appendages, congenital NEC 757.9
- soft parts of pelvis — *see* Abnormal, organs or tissues of pelvis
- spermatozoa 792.2
- sputum (amount) (color) (excessive) (odor) (purulent) 786.4
- stool NEC 787.7
    - bloody 578.1
        - occult 792.1
    - bulky 787.7
    - color (dark) (light) 792.1
    - content (fat) (mucus) (pus) 792.1
    - occult blood 792.1
- synchondrosis 756.9
- test results without manifest disease — *see* Findings, abnormal
- thebesian valve 746.9

Abnormal, abnormality, abnormalities —
  continued
  thermography — *see* Findings, abnormal,
    structure
  threshold, cones or rods (eye) 368.63
  thyroid-binding globulin 246.8
  thyroid product 246.8
  toxicology (findings) NEC 796.0
  tracheal cartilage (congenital) 748.3
  transport protein 273.8
  ultrasound results — *see* Findings, abnormal,
    structure
  umbilical cord
    affecting fetus or newborn 762.6
    complicating delivery 663.9 ✓5ᵗʰ
    specified NEC 663.8 ✓5ᵗʰ
  union
    cricoid cartilage and thyroid cartilage 748.3
    larynx and trachea 748.3
    thyroid cartilage and hyoid bone 748.3
  urination NEC 788.69
    psychogenic 306.53
    stream
      intermittent 788.61
      slowing 788.62
      splitting 788.61
      weak 788.62
  urine (constituents) NEC 791.9
  uterine hemorrhage (*see also* Hemorrhage,
      uterus) 626.9
    climacteric 627.0
    postmenopausal 627.1
  vagina (acquired) (congenital)
    in pregnancy or childbirth 654.7 ✓5ᵗʰ
      affecting fetus or newborn 763.89
      causing obstructed labor 660.2 ✓5ᵗʰ
        affecting fetus or newborn 763.1
  vascular sounds 785.9
  vectorcardiogram 794.39
  visually evoked potential (VEP) 794.13
  vulva (acquired) (congenital)
    in pregnancy or childbirth 654.8 ✓5ᵗʰ
      affecting fetus or newborn 763.89
      causing obstructed labor 660.2 ✓5ᵗʰ
        affecting fetus or newborn 763.1
  weight
    gain 783.1
      of pregnancy 646.1 ✓5ᵗʰ
        with hypertension — *see* Toxemia, of
            pregnancy
    loss 783.21
  x-ray examination — *see* Abnormal,
      radiological examination
Abnormally formed uterus — *see* Anomaly,
    uterus
Abnormity (any organ or part) — *see* Anomaly
ABO
  hemolytic disease 773.1
  incompatibility reaction 999.6
Abocclusion 524.2
Abolition, language 784.69
Aborter, habitual or recurrent NEC
  without current pregnancy 629.9
  current abortion (*see also* Abortion,
      spontaneous) 634.9 ✓5ᵗʰ
    affecting fetus or newborn 761.8
  observation in current pregnancy 646.3 ✓5ᵗʰ

Abortion (complete) (incomplete) (inevitable) (with
    retained products of conception) 637.9 ✓5ᵗʰ

> Note — Use the following fifth-digit
> subclassification with categories 634–637:
>
> 0   unspecified
> 1   incomplete
> 2   complete

  with
    complication(s) (any) following previous
        abortion — *see* category 639 ✓4ᵗʰ
    damage to pelvic organ (laceration)
        (rupture) (tear) 637.2 ✓5ᵗʰ
    embolism (air) (amniotic fluid) (blood clot)
        (pulmonary) (pyemic) (septic) (soap)
        637.6 ✓5ᵗʰ
    genital tract and pelvic infection 637.0 ✓5ᵗʰ
    hemorrhage, delayed or excessive 637.1 ✓5ᵗʰ
    metabolic disorder 637.4 ✓5ᵗʰ
    renal failure (acute) 637.3 ✓5ᵗʰ
    sepsis (genital tract) (pelvic organ)
        637.0 ✓5ᵗʰ
      urinary tract 637.7 ✓5ᵗʰ
    shock (postoperative) (septic) 637.5 ✓5ᵗʰ
    specified complication NEC 637.7 ✓5ᵗʰ
    toxemia 637.3 ✓5ᵗʰ
    unspecified complication(s) 637.8 ✓5ᵗʰ
    urinary tract infection 637.7 ✓5ᵗʰ
  accidental — *see* Abortion, spontaneous
  artificial — *see* Abortion, induced
  attempted (failed) — *see* Abortion, failed
  criminal — *see* Abortion, illegal
  early — *see* Abortion, spontaneous
  elective — *see* Abortion, legal
  failed (legal) 638.9
    with
      damage to pelvic organ (laceration)
          (rupture) (tear) 638.2
      embolism (air) (amniotic fluid) (blood
          clot) (pulmonary) (pyemic) (septic)
          (soap) 638.6
      genital tract and pelvic infection 638.0
      hemorrhage, delayed or excessive 638.1
      metabolic disorder 638.4
      renal failure (acute) 638.3
      sepsis (genital tract) (pelvic organ) 638.0
        urinary tract 638.7
      shock (postoperative) (septic) 638.5
      specified complication NEC 638.7
      toxemia 638.3
      unspecified complication(s) 638.8
      urinary tract infection 638.7
  fetal indication — *see* Abortion, legal
  fetus 779.6
  following threatened abortion — *see* Abortion,
      by type
  habitual or recurrent (care during pregnancy)
      646.3 ✓5ᵗʰ
    with current abortion (*see also* Abortion,
        spontaneous) 634.9 ✓5ᵗʰ
      affecting fetus or newborn 761.8
    without current pregnancy 629.9
  homicidal — *see* Abortion, illegal
  illegal 636.9 ✓5ᵗʰ
    with
      damage to pelvic organ (laceration)
          (rupture) (tear) 636.2 ✓5ᵗʰ
      embolism (air) (amniotic fluid) (blood
          clot) (pulmonary) (pyemic) (septic)
          (soap) 636.6 ✓5ᵗʰ

Abortion — continued
  illegal — continued
    with — continued
      genital tract and pelvic infection 636.0 ✓5ᵗʰ
      hemorrhage, delayed or excessive 636.1 ✓5ᵗʰ
      metabolic disorder 636.4 ✓5ᵗʰ
      renal failure 636.3 ✓5ᵗʰ
      sepsis (genital tract) (pelvic organ) 636.0 ✓5ᵗʰ
        urinary tract 636.7 ✓5ᵗʰ
      shock (postoperative) (septic) 636.5 ✓5ᵗʰ
      specified complication NEC 636.7 ✓5ᵗʰ
      toxemia 636.3 ✓5ᵗʰ
      unspecified complication(s) 636.8 ✓5ᵗʰ
      urinary tract infection 636.7 ✓5ᵗʰ
    fetus 779.6
  induced 637.9 ✓5ᵗʰ
    illegal — see Abortion, illegal
    legal indications — see Abortion, legal
    medical indications — see Abortion, legal
    therapeutic — see Abortion, legal
  late — see Abortion, spontaneous
  legal (legal indication) (medical indication) (under medical supervision) 635.9 ✓5ᵗʰ
    with
      damage to pelvic organ (laceration) (rupture) (tear) 635.2 ✓5ᵗʰ
      embolism (air) (amniotic fluid) (blood clot) (pulmonary) (pyemic) (septic) (soap) 635.6 ✓5ᵗʰ
      genital tract and pelvic infection 635.0 ✓5ᵗʰ
      hemorrhage, delayed or excessive 635.1 ✓5ᵗʰ
      metabolic disorder 635.4 ✓5ᵗʰ
      renal failure (acute) 635.3 ✓5ᵗʰ
      sepsis (genital tract) (pelvic organ) 635.0 ✓5ᵗʰ
        urinary tract 635.7 ✓5ᵗʰ
      shock (postoperative) (septic) 635.5 ✓5ᵗʰ
      specified complication NEC 635.7 ✓5ᵗʰ
      toxemia 635.3 ✓5ᵗʰ
      unspecified complication(s) 635.8 ✓5ᵗʰ
      urinary tract infection 635.7 ✓5ᵗʰ
    fetus 779.6
  medical indication — see Abortion, legal
  mental hygiene problem — see Abortion, legal
  missed 632
  operative — see Abortion, legal
  psychiatric indication — see Abortion, legal
  recurrent — see Abortion, spontaneous
  self-induced — see Abortion, illegal
  septic — see Abortion, by type, with sepsis
  spontaneous 634.9 ✓5ᵗʰ
    with
      damage to pelvic organ (laceration) (rupture) (tear) 634.2 ✓5ᵗʰ
      embolism (air) (amniotic fluid) (blood clot) (pulmonary) (pyemic) (septic) (soap) 634.6 ✓5ᵗʰ
      genital tract and pelvic infection 634.0 ✓5ᵗʰ
      hemorrhage, delayed or excessive 634.1 ✓5ᵗʰ
      metabolic disorder 634.4 ✓5ᵗʰ
      renal failure 634.3 ✓5ᵗʰ
      sepsis (genital tract) (pelvic organ) 634.0 ✓5ᵗʰ
        urinary tract 634.7 ✓5ᵗʰ

Abortion — continued
  spontaneous — continued
    with — continued
      shock (postoperative) (septic) 634.5 ✓5ᵗʰ
      specified complication NEC 634.7 ✓5ᵗʰ
      toxemia 634.3 ✓5ᵗʰ
      unspecified complication(s) 634.8 ✓5ᵗʰ
      urinary tract infection 634.7 ✓5ᵗʰ
    fetus 761.8
    threatened 640.0 ✓5ᵗʰ
      affecting fetus or newborn 762.1
  surgical — see Abortion, legal
  therapeutic — see Abortion, legal
  threatened 640.0 ✓5ᵗʰ
    affecting fetus or newborn 762.1
  tubal — see Pregnancy, tubal
  voluntary — see Abortion, legal

Abortus fever 023.9

Aboulomania 301.6

Abrachia 755.20

Abrachiatism 755.20

Abrachiocephalia 759.89

Abrachiocephalus 759.89

Abrami's disease (acquired hemolytic jaundice) 283.9

Abramov-Fiedler myocarditis (acute isolated myocarditis) 422.91

Abrasion — see also Injury, superficial, by site
  cornea 918.1
  dental 521.2
  teeth, tooth (dentifrice) (habitual) (hard tissues) (occupational) (ritual) (traditional) (wedge defect) 521.2

Abrikossov's tumor (M9580/0) — see also Neoplasm, connective tissue, benign
  malignant (M9580/3) — see Neoplasm, connective tissue, malignant

Abrism 988.8

Abruption, placenta — see Placenta, abruptio

Abruptio placentae — see Placenta, abruptio

Abscess (acute) (chronic) (infectional) (lymphangitic) (metastatic) (multiple) (pyogenic) (septic) (with lymphangitis) (see also Cellulitis) 682.9
  abdomen, abdominal
    cavity — see Abscess, peritoneum
    wall 682.2
  abdominopelvic — see Abscess, peritoneum
  accessory sinus (chronic) (see also Sinusitis) 473.9
  adrenal (capsule) (gland) 255.8
  alveolar 522.5
    with sinus 522.7
  amebic 006.3
    bladder 006.8
    brain (with liver or lung abscess) 006.5
    liver (without mention of brain or lung abscess) 006.3
      with
        brain abscess (and lung abscess) 006.5
        lung abscess 006.4
    lung (with liver abscess) 006.4
      with brain abscess 006.5
    seminal vesicle 006.8
    specified site NEC 006.8
    spleen 006.8
  anaerobic 040.0
  ankle 682.6

Abscess — *continued*
- anorectal 566
- antecubital space 682.3
- antrum (chronic) (Highmore) (*see also* Sinusitis, maxillary) 473.0
- anus 566
- apical (tooth) 522.5
  - with sinus (alveolar) 522.7
- appendix 540.1
- areola (acute) (chronic) (nonpuerperal) 611.0
  - puerperal, postpartum 675.1 ✓5ᵗʰ
- arm (any part, above wrist) 682.3
- artery (wall) 447.2
- atheromatous 447.2
- auditory canal (external) 380.10
- auricle (ear) (staphylococcal) (streptococcal) 380.10
- axilla, axillary (region) 682.3
  - lymph gland or node 683
- back (any part) 682.2
- Bartholin's gland 616.3
  - with
    - abortion — *see* Abortion, by type, with sepsis
    - ectopic pregnancy (*see also* categories 633.0-633.9) 639.0
    - molar pregnancy (*see also* categories 630-632) 639.0
    - complicating pregnancy or puerperium 646.6 ✓5ᵗʰ
  - following
    - abortion 639.0
    - ectopic or molar pregnancy 639.0
- bartholinian 616.3
- Bezold's 383.01
- bile, biliary, duct or tract (*see also* Cholecystitis) 576.8
- bilharziasis 120.1
- bladder (wall) 595.89
  - amebic 006.8
- bone (subperiosteal) (*see also* Osteomyelitis) 730.0 ✓5ᵗʰ
  - accessory sinus (chronic) (*see also* Sinusitis) 473.9
  - acute 730.0 ✓5ᵗʰ
  - chronic or old 730.1 ✓5ᵗʰ
  - jaw (lower) (upper) 526.4
  - mastoid — *see* Mastoiditis, acute
  - petrous (*see also* Petrositis) 383.20
  - spinal (tuberculous) (*see also* Tuberculosis) 015.0 ✓5ᵗʰ [730.88]
    - nontuberculous 730.08
- bowel 569.5
- brain (any part) 324.0
  - amebic (with liver or lung abscess) 006.5
  - cystic 324.0
  - late effect — *see* category 326
  - otogenic 324.0
  - tuberculous (*see also* Tuberculosis) 013.3 ✓5ᵗʰ
- breast (acute) (chronic) (nonpuerperal) 611.0
  - newborn 771.5
  - puerperal, postpartum 675.1 ✓5ᵗʰ
  - tuberculous (*see also* Tuberculosis) 017.9 ✓5ᵗʰ
- broad ligament (chronic) (*see also* Disease, pelvis, inflammatory) 614.4
  - acute 614.3
- Brodie's (chronic) (localized) (*see also* Osteomyelitis) 730.1 ✓5ᵗʰ
- bronchus 519.1

Abscess — *continued*
- buccal cavity 528.3
- bulbourethral gland 597.0
- bursa 727.89
  - pharyngeal 478.29
- buttock 682.5
- canaliculus, breast 611.0
- canthus 372.20
- cartilage 733.99
- cecum 569.5 ▲●
  - with appendicitis 540.1
- cerebellum, cerebellar 324.0
  - late effect — *see* category 326
- cerebral (embolic) 324.0
  - late effect — *see* category 326
- cervical (neck region) 682.1
  - lymph gland or node 683
  - stump (*see also* Cervicitis) 616.0
- cervix (stump) (uteri) (*see also* Cervicitis) 616.0
- cheek, external 682.0
  - inner 528.3
- chest 510.9
  - with fistula 510.0
  - wall 682.2
- chin 682.0
- choroid 363.00
- ciliary body 364.3
- circumtonsillar 475
- cold (tuberculous) — *see also* Tuberculosis, abscess
  - articular — *see* Tuberculosis, joint
- colon (wall) 569.5
- colostomy or enterostomy 569.61
- conjunctiva 372.00
- connective tissue NEC 682.9
- cornea 370.55
  - with ulcer 370.00
- corpus
  - cavernosum 607.2
  - luteum (*see also* Salpingo-oophoritis) 614.2
- Cowper's gland 597.0
- cranium 324.0
- cul-de-sac (Douglas') (posterior) (*see also* Disease, pelvis, inflammatory) 614.4
  - acute 614.3
- dental 522.5
  - with sinus (alveolar) 522.7
- dentoalveolar 522.5
  - with sinus (alveolar) 522.7
- diaphragm, diaphragmatic — *see* Abscess, peritoneum
- digit NEC 681.9
- Douglas' cul-de-sac or pouch (*see also* Disease, pelvis, inflammatory) 614.4
- Douglas' cul-de-sac or pouch — *continued*
  - acute 614.3
- Dubois' 090.5
- ductless gland 259.8
- ear
  - acute 382.00
  - external 380.10
  - inner 386.30
  - middle — *see* Otitis media
- elbow 682.3
- endamebic — *see* Abscess, amebic
- entamebic — *see* Abscess, amebic
- enterostomy 569.61
- epididymis 604.0
- epidural 324.9
  - brain 324.0

Abscess — continued
  epidural — continued
    late effect — see category 326
      spinal cord 324.1
  epiglottis 478.79
  epiploon, epiploic — see Abscess, peritoneum
  erysipelatous (see also Erysipelas) 035
  esophagus 530.19
  ethmoid (bone) (chronic) (sinus) (see also Sinusitis, ethmoidal) 473.2
  external auditory canal 380.10
  extradural 324.9
    brain 324.0
    late effect — see category 326
      spinal cord 324.1
  extraperitoneal — see Abscess, peritoneum
  eye 360.00
  eyelid 373.13
  face (any part, except eye) 682.0
  fallopian tube (see also Salpingo-oophoritis) 614.2
  fascia 728.89
  fauces 478.29
  fecal 569.5
  femoral (region) 682.6
  filaria, filarial (see also Infestation, filarial) 125.9
  finger (any) (intrathecal) (periosteal) (subcutaneous) (subcuticular) 681.00
  fistulous NEC 682.9
  flank 682.2
  foot (except toe) 682.7
  forearm 682.3
  forehead 682.0
  frontal (sinus) (chronic) (see also Sinusitis, frontal) 473.1
  gallbladder (see also Cholecystitis, acute) 575.0
  gastric 535.0 ✓5ᵗʰ
  genital organ or tract NEC
    female 616.9
      with
        abortion — see Abortion, by type, with sepsis
        ectopic pregnancy (see also categories 633.0-633.9) 639.0
        molar pregnancy (see also categories 630-632) 639.0
      following
        abortion 639.0
        ectopic or molar pregnancy 639.0
      puerperal, postpartum, childbirth 670 ✓4ᵗʰ
    male 608.4
  genitourinary system, tuberculous (see also Tuberculosis) 016.9 ✓5ᵗʰ
  gingival 523.3
  gland, glandular (lymph) (acute) NEC 683
  glottis 478.79
  gluteal (region) 682.5
  gonorrheal NEC (see also Gonococcus) 098.0
  groin 682.2
  gum 523.3
  hand (except finger or thumb) 682.4
  head (except face) 682.8
  heart 429.89
  heel 682.7
  helminthic (see also Infestation, by specific parasite) 128.9

Abscess — continued
  hepatic 572.0
    amebic (see also Abscess, liver, amebic) 006.3
    duct 576.8
  hip 682.6
    tuberculous (active) (see also Tuberculosis) 015.1 ✓5ᵗʰ
  ileocecal 540.1
  ileostomy (bud) 569.61
  iliac (region) 682.2
    fossa 540.1
  iliopsoas (tuberculous) (see also Tuberculosis) 015.0 ✓5ᵗʰ [730.88]
    nontuberculous 728.89
  infraclavicular (fossa) 682.3
  inguinal (region) 682.2
    lymph gland or node 683
  intersphincteric (anus) 566
  intestine, intestinal 569.5
    rectal 566
  intra-abdominal (see also Abscess, peritoneum) 567.2
    postoperative 998.59
  intracranial 324.0
    late effect — see category 326
  intramammary — see Abscess, breast
  intramastoid (see also Mastoiditis, acute) 383.00
  intraorbital 376.01
  intraperitoneal — see Abscess, peritoneum
  intraspinal 324.1
    late effect — see category 326
  intratonsillar 475
  iris 364.3
  ischiorectal 566
  jaw (bone) (lower) (upper) 526.4
    skin 682.0
  joint (see also Arthritis, pyogenic) 711.0 ✓5ᵗʰ
    vertebral (tuberculous) (see also Tuberculosis) 015.0 ✓5ᵗʰ [730.88]
    nontuberculous 724.8
  kidney 590.2
    with
      abortion — see Abortion, by type, with urinary tract infection
      calculus 592.0
      ectopic pregnancy (see also categories 633.0-633.9) 639.8
      molar pregnancy (see also categories 630-632) 639.8
      complicating pregnancy or puerperium 646.6 ✓5ᵗʰ
        affecting fetus or newborn 760.1
      following
        abortion 639.8
        ectopic or molar pregnancy 639.8
  knee 682.6
    joint 711.06
    tuberculous (active) (see also Tuberculosis) 015.2 ✓5ᵗʰ
  labium (majus) (minus) 616.4
    complicating pregnancy, childbirth, or puerperium 646.6 ✓5ᵗʰ
  lacrimal (passages) (sac) (see also Dacryocystitis) 375.30
    caruncle 375.30
    gland (see also Dacryoadenitis) 375.00
  lacunar 597.0
  larynx 478.79

Abscess

Abscess — *continued*
- lateral (alveolar) 522.5
  - with sinus 522.7
- leg, except foot 682.6
- lens 360.00
- lid 373.13
- lingual 529.0
  - tonsil 475
- lip 528.5
- Littre's gland 597.0
- liver 572.0
  - amebic 006.3
    - with
      - brain abscess (and lung abscess) 006.5
      - lung abscess 006.4
    - due to Entamoeba histolytica 006.3
  - dysenteric (*see also* Abscess, liver, amebic) 006.3
  - pyogenic 572.0
  - tropical (*see also* Abscess, liver, amebic) 006.3
- loin (region) 682.2
- lumbar (tuberculous) (*see also* Tuberculosis) 015.0 ✓5ᵗʰ [730.88]
  - nontuberculous 682.2
- lung (miliary) (putrid) 513.0
  - amebic (with liver abscess) 006.4
    - with brain abscess 006.5
- lymph, lymphatic, gland or node (acute) 683
  - any site, except mesenteric 683
  - mesentery 289.2
- lymphangitic, acute — *see* Cellulitis
- malar 526.4
- mammary gland — *see* Abscess, breast
- marginal (anus) 566
- mastoid (process) (*see also* Mastoiditis, acute) 383.00
  - subperiosteal 383.01
- maxilla, maxillary 526.4
  - molar (tooth) 522.5
    - with sinus 522.7
  - premolar 522.5
  - sinus (chronic) (*see also* Sinusitis, maxillary) 473.0
- mediastinum 513.1
- meibomian gland 373.12
- meninges (*see also* Meningitis) 320.9
- mesentery, mesenteric — *see* Abscess, peritoneum
- mesosalpinx (*see also* Salpingo-oophoritis) 614.2
- milk 675.1 ✓5ᵗʰ
- Monro's (psoriasis) 696.1
- mons pubis 682.2
- mouth (floor) 528.3
- multiple sites NEC 682.9
- mural 682.2
- muscle 728.89
- myocardium 422.92
- nabothian (follicle) (*see also* Cervicitis) 616.0
- nail (chronic) (with lymphangitis) 681.9
  - finger 681.02
  - toe 681.11
- nasal (fossa) (septum) 478.1
  - sinus (chronic) (*see also* Sinusitis) 473.9
- nasopharyngeal 478.29
- nates 682.5
- navel 682.2
  - newborn NEC 771.4

Abscess — *continued*
- neck (region) 682.1
  - lymph gland or node 683
- nephritic (*see also* Abscess, kidney) 590.2
- nipple 611.0
  - puerperal, postpartum 675.0 ✓5ᵗʰ
- nose (septum) 478.1
  - external 682.0
- omentum — *see* Abscess, peritoneum
- operative wound 998.59
- orbit, orbital 376.01
- ossifluent — *see* Abscess, bone
- ovary, ovarian (corpus luteum) (*see also* Salpingo-oophoritis) 614.2
- oviduct (*see also* Salpingo-oophoritis) 614.2
- palate (soft) 528.3
  - hard 526.4
- palmar (space) 682.4
- pancreas (duct) 577.0
- paradontal 523.3
- parafrenal 607.2
- parametric, parametrium (chronic) (*see also* Disease, pelvis, inflammatory) 614.4
  - acute 614.3
- paranephric 590.2
- parapancreatic 577.0
- parapharyngeal 478.22
- pararectal 566
- parasinus (*see also* Sinusitis) 473.9
- parauterine (*see also* Disease, pelvis, inflammatory) 614.4
  - acute 614.3
- paravaginal (*see also* Vaginitis) 616.10
- parietal region 682.8
- parodontal 523.3
- parotid (duct) (gland) 527.3
  - region 528.3
- parumbilical 682.2
  - newborn 771.4
- pectoral (region) 682.2
- pelvirectal — *see* Abscess, peritoneum
- pelvis, pelvic
  - female (chronic) (*see also* Disease, pelvis, inflammatory) 614.4
    - acute 614.3
  - male, peritoneal (cellular tissue) — *see* Abscess, peritoneum
  - tuberculous (*see also* Tuberculosis) 016.9 ✓5ᵗʰ
- penis 607.2
  - gonococcal (acute) 098.0
    - chronic or duration of 2 months or over 098.2
- perianal 566
- periapical 522.5
  - with sinus (alveolar) 522.7
- periappendiceal 540.1
- pericardial 420.99
- pericecal 540.1
- pericemental 523.3
- pericholecystic (*see also* Cholecystitis, acute) 575.0
- pericoronal 523.3
- peridental 523.3
- perigastric 535.0 ✓5ᵗʰ
- perimetric (*see also* Disease, pelvis, inflammatory) 614.4
  - acute 614.3
- perinephric, perinephritic (*see also* Abscess, kidney) 590.2

Abscess — *continued*
  perineum, perineal (superficial) 682.2
    deep (with urethral involvement) 597.0
    urethra 597.0
  periodontal (parietal) 523.3
    apical 522.5
  periosteum, periosteal (*see also* Periostitis) 730.3 ✓5ᵗʰ
    with osteomyelitis (*see also* Osteomyelitis) 730.2 ✓5ᵗʰ
      acute or subacute 730.0 ✓5ᵗʰ
      chronic or old 730.1 ✓5ᵗʰ
  peripleuritic 510.9
    with fistula 510.0
  periproctic 566
  periprostatic 601.2
  perirectal (staphylococcal) 566
  perirenal (tissue) (*see also* Abscess, kidney) 590.2
  perisinuous (nose) (*see also* Sinusitis) 473.9
  peritoneum, peritoneal (perforated) (ruptured) 567.2
    with
      abortion — *see* Abortion, by type, with sepsis
      appendicitis 540.1
      ectopic pregnancy (*see also* categories 633.0-633.9) 639.0
      molar pregnancy (*see also* categories 630-632) 639.0
      following
        abortion 639.0
        ectopic or molar pregnancy 639.0
      pelvic, female (*see also* Disease, pelvis, inflammatory) 614.4
        acute 614.3
      postoperative 998.59
      puerperal, postpartum, childbirth 670 ✓4ᵗʰ
      tuberculous (*see also* Tuberculosis) 014.0 ✓5ᵗʰ
  peritonsillar 475
  perityphlic 540.1
  periureteral 593.89
  periurethral 597.0
    gonococcal (acute) 098.0
      chronic or duration of 2 months or over 098.2
  periuterine (*see also* Disease, pelvis, inflammatory) 614.4
    acute 614.3
  perivesical 595.89
  pernicious NEC 682.9
  petrous bone — *see* Petrositis
  phagedenic NEC 682.9
    chancroid 099.0
  pharynx, pharyngeal (lateral) 478.29
  phlegmonous NEC 682.9
  pilonidal 685.0
  pituitary (gland) 253.8
  pleura 510.9
    with fistula 510.0
  popliteal 682.6
  postanal 566
  postcecal 540.1
  postlaryngeal 478.79
  postnasal 478.1
  postpharyngeal 478.24
  posttonsillar 475
  posttyphoid 002.0
  Pott's (*see also* Tuberculosis) 015.0 ✓5ᵗʰ [730.88]

Abscess — *continued*
  pouch of Douglas (chronic) (*see also* Disease, pelvis, inflammatory) 614.4
  premammary — *see* Abscess, breast
  prepatellar 682.6
  prostate (*see also* Prostatitis) 601.2
    gonococcal (acute) 098.12
      chronic or duration of 2 months or over 098.32
  psoas (tuberculous) (*see also* Tuberculosis) 015.0 ✓5ᵗʰ [730.88]
    nontuberculous 728.89
  pterygopalatine fossa 682.8
  pubis 682.2
  puerperal — Puerperal, abseess, by site
  pulmonary — *see* Abscess, lung
  pulp, pulpal (dental) 522.0
    finger 681.01
    toe 681.10
  pyemic — *see* Septicemia
  pyloric valve 535.0 ✓5ᵗʰ
  rectovaginal septum 569.5
  rectovesical 595.89
  rectum 566
  regional NEC 682.9
  renal (*see also* Abscess, kidney) 590.2
  retina 363.00
  retrobulbar 376.01
  retrocecal — *see* Abscess, peritoneum
  retrolaryngeal 478.79
  retromammary — *see* Abscess, breast
  retroperineal 682.2
  retroperitoneal — *see* Abscess, peritoneum
  retropharyngeal 478.24
    tuberculous (*see also* Tuberculosis) 012.8 ✓5ᵗʰ
  retrorectal 566
  retrouterine (*see also* Disease, pelvis, inflammatory) 614.4
    acute 614.3
  retrovesical 595.89
  root, tooth 522.5
    with sinus (alveolar) 522.7
  round ligament (*see also* Disease, pelvis, inflammatory) 614.4
    acute 614.3
  rupture (spontaneous) NEC 682.9
  sacrum (tuberculous) (*see also* Tuberculosis) 015.0 ✓5ᵗʰ [730.88]
    nontuberculous 730.08
  salivary duct or gland 527.3
  scalp (any part) 682.8
  scapular 730.01
  sclera 379.09
  scrofulous (*see also* Tuberculosis) 017.2 ✓5ᵗʰ
  scrotum 608.4
  seminal vesicle 608.0
    amebic 006.8
  septal, dental 522.5
    with sinus (alveolar) 522.7
  septum (nasal) 478.1
  serous (*see also* Periostitis) 730.3 ✓5ᵗʰ
  shoulder 682.3
  side 682.2
  sigmoid 569.5
  sinus (accessory) (chronic) (nasal) (*see also* Sinusitis) 473.9
    intracranial venous (any) 324.0
    late effect — *see* category 326
  Skene's duct or gland 597.0

Abscess

Abscess — *continued*
  skin NEC 682.9
    tuberculous (primary) (*see also* Tuberculosis) 017.0 ✓5ᵗʰ
  sloughing NEC 682.9
  specified site NEC 682.8
    amebic 006.8
  spermatic cord 608.4
  sphenoidal (sinus) (*see also* Sinusitis, sphenoidal) 473.3
  spinal
    cord (any part) (staphylococcal) 324.1
      tuberculous (*see also* Tuberculosis) 013.5 ✓5ᵗʰ
    epidural 324.1
  spine (column) (tuberculous) (*see also* Tuberculosis) 015.0 ✓5ᵗʰ [730.88]
    nontuberculous 730.08
  spleen 289.59
    amebic 006.8
  staphylococcal NEC 682.9
  stitch 998.59
  stomach (wall) 535.0 ✓5ᵗʰ
  strumous (tuberculous) (*see also* Tuberculosis) 017.2 ✓5ᵗʰ
  subarachnoid 324.9
    brain 324.0
    cerebral 324.0
    late effect — *see* category 326
    spinal cord 324.1
  subareolar — *see also* Abscess, breast
    puerperal, postpartum 675.1 ✓5ᵗʰ
  subcecal 540.1
  subcutaneous NEC 682.9
  subdiaphragmatic — *see* Abscess, peritoneum
  subdorsal 682.2
  subdural 324.9
    brain 324.0
    late effect — *see* category 326
    spinal cord 324.1
  subgaleal 682.8
  subhepatic — *see* Abscess, peritoneum
  sublingual 528.3
    gland 527.3
  submammary — *see* Abscess, breast
  submandibular (region) (space) (triangle) 682.0
    gland 527.3
  submaxillary (region) 682.0
    gland 527.3
  submental (pyogenic) 682.0
    gland 527.3
  subpectoral 682.2
  subperiosteal — *see* Abscess, bone
  subperitoneal — *see* Abscess, peritoneum
  subphrenic — *see also* Abscess, peritoneum
    postoperative 998.59
  subscapular 682.2
  subungual 681.9
  suburethral 597.0
  sudoriparous 705.89
  suppurative NEC 682.9
  supraclavicular (fossa) 682.3
  suprahepatic — *see* Abscess, peritoneum
  suprapelvic (*see also* Disease, pelvis, inflammatory) 614.4
    acute 614.3
  suprapubic 682.2
  suprarenal (capsule) (gland) 255.8
  sweat gland 705.89
  syphilitic 095.8
  teeth, tooth (root) 522.5
    with sinus (alveolar) 522.7

Abscess — *continued*
  teeth, tooth — *continued*
    supporting structures NEC 523.3
  temple 682.0
  temporal region 682.0
  temporosphenoidal 324.0
    late effect — *see* category 326
  tendon (sheath) 727.89
  testicle — *see* Orchitis
  thecal 728.89
  thigh (acquired) 682.6
  thorax 510.9
    with fistula 510.0
  throat 478.29
  thumb (intrathecal) (periosteal) (subcutaneous) (subcuticular) 681.00
  thymus (gland) 254.1
  thyroid (gland) 245.0
  toe (any) (intrathecal) (periosteal) (subcutaneous) (subcuticular) 681.10
  tongue (staphylococcal) 529.0
  tonsil(s) (lingual) 475
  tonsillopharyngeal 475
  tooth, teeth (root) 522.5
    with sinus (alveolar) 522.7
    supporting structure NEC 523.3
  trachea 478.9
  trunk 682.2
  tubal (*see also* Salpingo-oophoritis) 614.2
  tuberculous — *see* Tuberculosis, abscess
  tubo-ovarian (*see also* Salpingo-oophoritis) 614.2
  tunica vaginalis 608.4
  umbilicus NEC 682.2
    newborn 771.4
  upper arm 682.3
  upper respiratory 478.9
  urachus 682.2
  urethra (gland) 597.0
  urinary 597.0
  uterus, uterine (wall) (*see also* Endometritis) 615.9
    ligament (*see also* Disease, pelvis, inflammatory) 614.4
      acute 614.3
    neck (*see also* Cervicitis) 616.0
  uvula 528.3
  vagina (wall) (*see also* Vaginitis) 616.10
  vaginorectal (*see also* Vaginitis) 616.10
  vas deferens 608.4
  vermiform appendix 540.1
  vertebra (column) (tuberculous) (*see also* Tuberculosis) 015.0 ✓5ᵗʰ [730.88]
    nontuberculous 730.0 ✓5ᵗʰ
  vesical 595.89
  vesicouterine pouch (*see also* Disease, pelvis, inflammatory) 614.4
  vitreous (humor) (pneumococcal) 360.04
  vocal cord 478.5
  von Bezold's 383.01
  vulva 616.4
    complicating pregnancy, childbirth, or puerperium 646.6 ✓5ᵗʰ
  vulvovaginal gland (*see also* Vaginitis) 616.3
  web-space 682.4
  wrist 682.4

Absence (organ or part) (complete or partial)
  acoustic nerve 742.8
  adrenal (gland) (congenital) 759.1
    acquired V45.79
  albumin (blood) 273.8

Index to Diseases

Absence — *continued*
  alimentary tract (complete) (congenital) (partial) 751.8
    lower 751.5
    upper 750.8
  alpha-fucosidase 271.8
  alveolar process (acquired) 525.8
    congenital 750.26
  anus, anal (canal) (congenital) 751.2
  aorta (congenital) 747.22
  aortic valve (congenital) 746.89
  appendix, congenital 751.2
  arm (acquired) V49.60
    above elbow V49.66
    below elbow V49.65
    congenital (*see also* Deformity, reduction, upper limb) 755.20
      lower — *see* Absence, forearm, congenital
      upper (complete) (partial) (with absence of distal elements, incomplete) 755.24
        with
          complete absence of distal elements 755.21
          forearm (incomplete) 755.23
  artery (congenital) (peripheral) NEC (*see also* Anomaly, peripheral vascular system) 747.60
    brain 747.81
    cerebral 747.81
    coronary 746.85
    pulmonary 747.3
    umbilical 747.5
  atrial septum 745.69
  auditory canal (congenital) (external) 744.01
  auricle (ear) (with stenosis or atresia of auditory canal), congenital 744.01
  bile, biliary duct (common) or passage (congenital) 751.61
  bladder (acquired) V45.74
    congenital 753.8
  bone (congenital) NEC 756.9
    marrow 284.9
      acquired (secondary) 284.8
      congenital 284.0
      hereditary 284.0
      idiopathic 284.9
    skull 756.0
  bowel sounds 787.5
  brain 740.0
    specified part 742.2
  breast(s) (acquired) V45.71
    congenital 757.6
  broad ligament (congenital) 752.19
  bronchus (congenital) 748.3
  calvarium, calvaria (skull) 756.0
  canaliculus lacrimalis, congenital 743.65
  carpal(s) (congenital) (complete) (partial) (with absence of distal elements, incomplete) (*see also* Deformity, reduction, upper limb) 755.28
    with complete absence of distal elements 755.21
  cartilage 756.9
  caudal spine 756.13
  cecum (acquired) (postoperative) (posttraumatic) V45.72
    congenital 751.2
  cementum 520.4
  cerebellum (congenital) (vermis) 742.2

Absence — *continued*
  cervix (acquired) (uteri) V45.77
    congenital 752.49
  chin, congenital 744.89
  cilia (congenital) 743.63
    acquired 374.89
  circulatory system, part NEC 747.89
  clavicle 755.51
  clitoris (congenital) 752.49
  coccyx, congenital 756.13
  cold sense (*see also* Disturbance, sensation) 782.0
  colon (acquired) (postoperative) V45.72
    congenital 751.2
  congenital
    lumen — *see* Atresia
    organ or site NEC — *see* Agenesis
    septum — *see* Imperfect, closure
  corpus callosum (congenital) 742.2
  cricoid cartilage 748.3
  diaphragm (congenital) (with hernia) 756.6
    with obstruction 756.6
  digestive organ(s) or tract, congenital (complete) (partial) 751.8
    acquired V45.79
    lower 751.5
    upper 750.8
  ductus arteriosus 747.89
  duodenum (acquired) (postoperative) V45.72
    congenital 751.1
  ear, congenital 744.09
    acquired V45.79
    auricle 744.01
    external 744.01
    inner 744.05
    lobe, lobule 744.21
    middle, except ossicles 744.03
      ossicles 744.04
    ossicles 744.04
  ejaculatory duct (congenital) 752.8
  endocrine gland NEC (congenital) 759.2
  epididymis (congenital) 752.8
    acquired V45.77
  epiglottis, congenital 748.3
  epileptic (atonic) (typical) (*see also* Epilepsy) 345.0 ✓5ᵗʰ
  erythrocyte 284.9
  erythropoiesis 284.9
    congenital 284.0
  esophagus (congenital) 750.3
  Eustachian tube (congenital) 744.24
  extremity (acquired)
    congenital (*see also* Deformity, reduction) 755.4
    lower V49.70
    upper V49.60
  extrinsic muscle, eye 743.69
  eye (acquired) V45.78
    adnexa (congenital) 743.69
    congenital 743.00
    muscle (congenital) 743.69
  eyelid (fold), congenital 743.62
    acquired 374.89
  face
    bones NEC 756.0
    specified part NEC 744.89
  fallopian tube(s) (acquired) V45.77
    congenital 752.19

Absence — *continued*
  femur, congenital (complete) (partial) (with
      absence of distal elements, incomplete)
      (*see also* Deformity, reduction, lower
      limb) 755.34
    with
      complete absence of distal elements
          755.31
      tibia and fibula (incomplete) 755.33
  fibrin 790.92
  fibrinogen (congenital) 286.3
    acquired 286.6
  fibula, congenital (complete) (partial) (with
      absence of distal elements, incomplete)
      (*see also* Deformity, reduction, lower
      limb) 755.37
    with
      complete absence of distal elements
          755.31
      tibia 755.35
        with
          complete absence of distal
              elements 755.31
          femur (incomplete) 755.33
            with complete absence of distal
                elements 755.31
  finger (acquired) V49.62
    congenital (complete) (partial) (*see also*
        Deformity, reduction, upper limb)
        755.29
      meaning all fingers (complete) (partial)
          755.21
      transverse 755.21
  fissures of lungs (congenital) 748.5
  foot (acquired) V49.73
    congenital (complete) 755.31
  forearm (acquired) V49.65
    congenital (complete) (partial) (with absence
        of distal elements, incomplete) (*see
        also* Deformity, reduction, upper
        limb) 755.25
      with
        complete absence of distal elements
            (hand and fingers) 755.21
        humerus (incomplete) 755.23
  fovea centralis 743.55
  fucosidase 271.8
  gallbladder (acquired) V45.79
    congenital 751.69
  gamma globulin (blood) 279.00
  genital organs
    acquired V45.77
    congenital
      female 752.8
        external 752.49
        internal NEC 752.8
      male 752.8
        penis 752.69
  genitourinary organs, congenital NEC 752.8
  glottis 748.3
  gonadal, congenital NEC 758.6
  hair (congenital) 757.4
    acquired — *see* Alopecia
  hand (acquired) V49.63
    congenital (complete) (*see also* Deformity,
        reduction, upper limb) 755.21
  heart (congenital) 759.89
    acquired — *see* Status, organ replacement
  heat sense (*see also* Disturbance, sensation)
      782.0

Absence — *continued*
  humerus, congenital (complete) (partial) (with
      absence of distal elements, incomplete)
      (*see also* Deformity, reduction, upper
      limb) 755.24
    with
      complete absence of distal elements
          755.21
      radius and ulna (incomplete) 755.23
  hymen (congenital) 752.49
  ileum (acquired) (postoperative)
      (posttraumatic) V45.72
    congenital 751.1
  immunoglobulin, isolated NEC 279.03
    IgA 279.01
    IgG 279.03
    IgM 279.02
  incus (acquired) 385.24
    congenital 744.04
  internal ear (congenital) 744.05
  intestine (acquired) (small) V45.72
    congenital 751.1
    large 751.2
    large V45.72
      congenital 751.2
  iris (congenital) 743.45
  jaw — *see* Absence, mandible
  jejunum (acquired) V45.72
    congenital 751.1
  joint, congenital NEC 755.8
  kidney(s) (acquired) V45.73
    congenital 753.0
  labium (congenital) (majus) (minus) 752.49
  labyrinth, membranous 744.05
  lacrimal apparatus (congenital) 743.65
  larynx (congenital) 748.3
  leg (acquired) V49.70
    above knee V49.76
    below knee V49.75
    congenital (partial) (unilateral) (*see also*
        Deformity, reduction, lower limb)
        755.31
      lower (complete) (partial) (with absence
          of distal elements, incomplete)
          755.35
        with
          complete absence of distal
              elements (foot and toes)
              755.31
          thigh (incomplete) 755.33
            with complete absence of distal
                elements 755.31
      upper — *see* Absence, femur
  lens (congenital) 743.35
    acquired 379.31
  ligament, broad (congenital) 752.19
  limb (acquired)
    congenital (complete) (partial) (*see also*
        Deformity, reduction) 755.4
      lower 755.30
        complete 755.31
        incomplete 755.32
        longitudinal — *see* Deficiency, lower
            limb, longitudinal
        transverse 755.31
      upper 755.20
        complete 755.21
        incomplete 755.22
        longitudinal — *see* Deficiency, upper
            limb, longitudinal
        transverse 755.21

Index to Diseases

Absence — *continued*
  limb — *continued*
    lower NEC V49.70
    upper NEC V49.60
  lip 750.26
  liver (congenital) (lobe) 751.69
  lumbar (congenital) (vertebra) 756.13
    isthmus 756.11
    pars articularis 756.11
  lumen — *see* Atresia
  lung (bilateral) (congenital) (fissure) (lobe) (unilateral) 748.5
    acquired (any part) V45.76
  mandible (congenital) 524.09
  maxilla (congenital) 524.09
  menstruation 626.0
  metacarpal(s), congenital (complete) (partial) (with absence of distal elements, incomplete) (*see also* Deformity, reduction, upper limb) 755.28
    with all fingers, complete 755.21
  metatarsal(s), congenital (complete) (partial) (with absence of distal elements, incomplete) (*see also* Deformity, reduction, lower limb) 755.38
    with complete absence of distal elements 755.31
  muscle (congenital) (pectoral) 756.81
    ocular 743.69
  musculoskeletal system (congenital) NEC 756.9
  nail(s) (congenital) 757.5
  neck, part 744.89
  nerve 742.8
  nervous system, part NEC 742.8
  neutrophil 288.0
  nipple (congenital) 757.6
  nose (congenital) 748.1
    acquired 738.0
  nuclear 742.8
  ocular muscle (congenital) 743.69
  organ
    of Corti (congenital) 744.05
    or site
      acquired V45.79
      congenital NEC 759.89
  osseous meatus (ear) 744.03
  ovary (acquired) V45.77
    congenital 752.0
  oviduct (acquired) V45.77
    congenital 752.19
  pancreas (congenital) 751.7
    acquired (postoperative) (posttraumatic) V45.79
  parathyroid gland (congenital) 759.2
  parotid gland(s) (congenital) 750.21
  patella, congenital 755.64
  pelvic girdle (congenital) 755.69
  penis (congenital) 752.69
    acquired V45.77
  pericardium (congenital) 746.89
  perineal body (congenital) 756.81
  phalange(s), congenital 755.4
    lower limb (complete) (intercalary) (partial) (terminal) (*see also* Deformity, reduction, lower limb) 755.39
      meaning all toes (complete) (partial) 755.31
      transverse 755.31

Absence — *continued*
  phalange(s), congenital — *continued*
    upper limb (complete) (intercalary) (partial) (terminal) (*see also* Deformity, reduction, upper limb) 755.29
      meaning all digits (complete) (partial) 755.21
      transverse 755.21
  pituitary gland (congenital) 759.2
  postoperative — *see* Absence, by site, acquired
  prostate (congenital) 752.8
    acquired V45.77
  pulmonary
    artery 747.3
    trunk 747.3
    valve (congenital) 746.01
    vein 747.49
  punctum lacrimale (congenital) 743.65
  radius, congenital (complete) (partial) (with absence of distal elements, incomplete) 755.26
    with
      complete absence of distal elements 755.21
      ulna 755.25
        with
          complete absence of distal elements 755.21
          humerus (incomplete) 755.23
  ray, congenital 755.4
    lower limb (complete) (partial) (*see also* Deformity, reduction, lower limb) 755.38
      meaning all rays 755.31
      transverse 755.31
    upper limb (complete) (partial) (*see also* Deformity, reduction, upper limb) 755.28
      meaning all rays 755.21
      transverse 755.21
  rectum (congenital) 751.2
    acquired V45.79
  red cell 284.9
    acquired (secondary) 284.8
    congenital 284.0
    hereditary 284.0
    idiopathic 284.9
  respiratory organ (congenital) NEC 748.9
  rib (acquired) 738.3
    congenital 756.3
  roof of orbit (congenital) 742.0
  round ligament (congenital) 752.8
  sacrum, congenital 756.13
  salivary gland(s) (congenital) 750.21
  scapula 755.59
  scrotum, congenital 752.8
  seminal tract or duct (congenital) 752.8
    acquired V45.77
  septum (congenital) — *see also* Imperfect, closure, septum
    atrial 745.69
      and ventricular 745.7
    between aorta and pulmonary artery 745.0
    ventricular 745.3
      and atrial 745.7
  sex chromosomes 758.81
  shoulder girdle, congenital (complete) (partial) 755.59
  skin (congenital) 757.39

Absence — *continued*
  skull bone 756.0
    with
      anencephalus 740.0
      encephalocele 742.0
      hydrocephalus 742.3
        with spina bifida (*see also* Spina bifida) 741.0 ✓5ᵗʰ
      microcephalus 742.1
  spermatic cord (congenital) 752.8
  spinal cord 742.59
  spine, congenital 756.13
  spleen (congenital) 759.0
    acquired V45.79
  sternum, congenital 756.3
  stomach (acquired) (partial) (postoperative) V45.75
    with postgastric surgery syndrome 564.2
    congenital 750.7
  submaxillary gland(s) (congenital) 750.21
  superior vena cava (congenital) 747.49
  tarsal(s), congenital (complete) (partial) (with absence of distal elements, incomplete) (*see also* Deformity, reduction, lower limb) 755.38
  teeth, tooth (congenital) 520.0
    with abnormal spacing 524.3
    acquired 525.10
      with malocclusion 524.3
      due to
        caries 525.13
        extraction 525.10
        periodontal disease 525.12
        trauma 525.11
  tendon (congenital) 756.81
  testis (congenital) 752.8
    acquired V45.77
  thigh (acquired) 736.89
  thumb (acquired) V49.61
    congenital 755.29
  thymus gland (congenital) 759.2
  thyroid (gland) (surgical) 246.8
    with hypothyroidism 244.0
    cartilage, congenital 748.3
    congenital 243
  tibia, congenital (complete) (partial) (with absence of distal elements, incomplete) (*see also* Deformity, reduction, lower limb) 755.36
    with
      complete absence of distal elements 755.31
      fibula 755.35
        with
          complete absence of distal elements 755.31
          femur (incomplete) 755.33
            with complete absence of distal elements 755.31
  toe (acquired) V49.72
    congenital (complete) (partial) 755.39
      meaning all toes 755.31
      transverse 755.31
      great V49.71
  tongue (congenital) 750.11
  tooth, teeth (congenital) 520.0
    with abnormal spacing 524.3
    acquired 525.10
      with malocclusion 524.3
      due to
        caries 525.13

Absence — *continued*
  tooth, teeth — *continued*
    acquired — *continued*
      due to — *continued*
        extraction 525.10
        periodontal disease 525.12
        trauma 525.11
  trachea (cartilage) (congenital) (rings) 748.3
  transverse aortic arch (congenital) 747.21
  tricuspid valve 746.1
  ulna, congenital (complete) (partial) (with absence of distal elements, incomplete) (*see also* Deformity, reduction, upper limb) 755.27
    with
      complete absence of distal elements 755.21
      radius 755.25
        with
          complete absence of distal elements 755.21
          humerus (incomplete) 755.23
  umbilical artery (congenital) 747.5
  ureter (congenital) 753.4
    acquired V45.74
  urethra, congenital 753.8
    acquired V45.74
  urinary system, part NEC, congenital 753.8
    acquired V45.74
  uterus (acquired) V45.77
    congenital 752.3
  uvula (congenital) 750.26
  vagina, congenital 752.49
    acquired V45.77
  vas deferens (congenital) 752.8
    acquired V45.77
  vein (congenital) (peripheral) NEC (*see also* Anomaly, peripheral vascular system) 747.60
    brain 747.81
    great 747.49
    portal 747.49
    pulmonary 747.49
    vena cava (congenital) (inferior) (superior) 747.49
  ventral horn cell 742.59
  ventricular septum 745.3
  vermis of cerebellum 742.2
  vertebra, congenital 756.13
  vulva, congenital 752.49
Absentia epileptica (*see also* Epilepsy) 345.0 ✓5ᵗʰ
Absinthemia (*see also* Dependence) 304.6 ✓5ᵗʰ
Absinthism (*see also* Dependence) 304.6 ✓5ᵗʰ
Absorbent system disease 459.89
Absorption
  alcohol, through placenta or breast milk 760.71
  antibiotics, through placenta or breast milk 760.74
  anti-infective, through placenta or breast milk 760.74
  chemical NEC 989.9
    specified chemical or substance — *see* Table of Drugs and Chemicals
    through placenta or breast milk (fetus or newborn) 760.70
      alcohol 760.71
      anti-infective agents 760.74
      cocaine 760.75
      "crack" 760.75
      diethylstilbestrol [DES] 760.76

Index to Diseases

Absorption — *continued*
  chemical NEC — *continued*
    through placenta or breast milk —
      continued
      hallucinogenic agents 760.73
      medicinal agents NEC 760.79
      narcotics 760.72
      obstetric anesthetic or analgesic drug 763.5
      specified agent NEC 760.79
      suspected, affecting management of pregnancy 655.5 ✓5ᵗʰ
  cocaine, through placenta or breast milk 760.75
  drug NEC (*see also* Reaction, drug)
    through placenta or breast milk (fetus or newborn) 760.70
      alcohol 760.71
      anti-infective agents 760.74
      cocaine 760.75
      "crack" 760.75
      diethylstilbestrol [DES] 760.76
      hallucinogenic agents 760.73
      medicinal agents NEC 760.79
      narcotics 760.72
      obstetric anesthetic or analgesic drug 763.5
      specified agent NEC 760.79
      suspected, affecting management of pregnancy 655.5 ✓5ᵗʰ
  fat, disturbance 579.8
  hallucinogenic agents, through placenta or breast milk 760.73
  immune sera, through placenta or breast milk 760.79
  lactose defect 271.3
  medicinal agents NEC, through placenta or breast milk 760.79
  narcotics, through placenta or breast milk 760.72
  noxious substance, — *see* Absorption, chemical
  protein, disturbance 579.8
  pus or septic, general — *see* Septicemia
  quinine, through placenta or breast milk 760.74
  toxic substance, — *see* Absorption, chemical
  uremic — *see* Uremia

Abstinence symptoms or syndrome
  alcohol 291.81
  drug 292.0

Abt-Letterer-Siwe syndrome (acute histiocytosis X) (M9722/3) 202.5 ✓5ᵗʰ

Abulia 799.8

Abulomania 301.6

Abuse
  adult 995.80
    emotional 995.82
    multiple forms 995.85
    neglect (nutritional) 995.84
    physical 995.81
    psychological 995.82
    sexual 995.83
  alcohol (*see also* Alcoholism) 305.0 ✓5ᵗʰ
    dependent 303.9 ✓5ᵗʰ
    non-dependent 305.0 ✓5ᵗʰ
  child 995.50
    counseling
      perpetrator
        non-parent V62.83
        parent V61.22

Abuse — *continued*
  child — *continued*
    counseling — *continued*
      victim V61.21
    emotional 995.51
    multiple forms 995.59
    neglect (nutritional) 995.52
    psychological 995.51
    physical 995.54
      shaken infant syndrome 995.55
    sexual 995.53
  drugs, nondependent 305.9 ✓5ᵗʰ

> **Note** — Use the following *fifth-digit* subclassification with the following codes: 305.0, 305.2-305.9:
>
> 0 unspecified   2 episodic
> 1 continuous   3 in remission

    amphetamine type 305.7 ✓5ᵗʰ
    antidepressants 305.8 ✓5ᵗʰ
    barbiturates 305.4 ✓5ᵗʰ
    caffeine 305.9 ✓5ᵗʰ
    cannabis 305.2 ✓5ᵗʰ
    cocaine type 305.6 ✓5ᵗʰ
    hallucinogens 305.3 ✓5ᵗʰ
    hashish 305.2 ✓5ᵗʰ
    LSD 305.3 ✓5ᵗʰ
    marijuana 305.2 ✓5ᵗʰ
    mixed 305.9 ✓5ᵗʰ
    morphine type 305.5 ✓5ᵗʰ
    opioid type 305.5 ✓5ᵗʰ
    phencyclidine (PCP) 305.9 ✓5ᵗʰ
    specified NEC 305.9 ✓5ᵗʰ
    tranquilizers 305.4 ✓5ᵗʰ
  spouse 995.80
  tobacco 305.1

Acalcerosis 275.40

Acalcicosis 275.40

Acalculia 784.69
  developmental 315.1

Acanthocheilonemiasis 125.4

Acanthocytosis 272.5

Acanthokeratodermia 701.1

Acantholysis 701.8
  bullosa 757.39

Acanthoma (benign) (M8070/0) — *see also* Neoplasm, by site, benign
  malignant (M8070/3) — *see* Neoplasm, by site, malignant

Acanthosis (acquired) (nigricans) 701.2
  adult 701.2
  benign (congenital) 757.39
  congenital 757.39
  glycogenic
    esophagus 530.89
  juvenile 701.2
  tongue 529.8

Acanthrocytosis 272.5

Acapnia 276.3

Acarbia 276.2

Acardia 759.89

Acardiacus amorphus 759.89

Acardiotrophia 429.1

Acardius 759.89

Acariasis 133.9
  sarcoptic 133.0

Acaridiasis 133.9

Acarinosis 133.9
Acariosis 133.9
Acarodermatitis 133.9
　urticarioides 133.9
Acarophobia 300.29
Acatalasemia 277.8
Acatalasia 277.8
Acatamathesia 784.69
Acataphasia 784.5
Acathisia 781.0
　due to drugs 333.99
Acceleration, accelerated
　atrioventricular conduction 426.7
　idioventricular rhythm 427.89
Accessory (congenital)
　adrenal gland 759.1
　anus 751.5
　appendix 751.5
　atrioventricular conduction 426.7
　auditory ossicles 744.04
　auricle (ear) 744.1
　autosome(s) NEC 758.5
　　21 or 22 758.0
　biliary duct or passage 751.69
　bladder 753.8
　blood vessels (peripheral) (congenital) NEC
　　(see also Anomaly, peripheral vascular
　　system) 747.60
　　cerebral 747.81
　　coronary 746.85
　bone NEC 756.9
　　foot 755.67
　breast tissue, axilla 757.6
　carpal bones 755.56
　cecum 751.5
　cervix 752.49
　chromosome(s) NEC 758.5
　　13-15 758.1
　　16-18 758.2
　　21 or 22 758.0
　　autosome(s) NEC 758.5
　　D_1 758.1
　　E_3 758.2
　　G 758.0
　　sex 758.81
　coronary artery 746.85
　cusp(s), heart valve NEC 746.89
　　pulmonary 746.09
　cystic duct 751.69
　digits 755.00
　ear (auricle) (lobe) 744.1
　endocrine gland NEC 759.2
　external os 752.49
　eyelid 743.62
　eye muscle 743.69
　face bone(s) 756.0
　fallopian tube (fimbria) (ostium) 752.19
　fingers 755.01
　foreskin 605
　frontonasal process 756.0
　gallbladder 751.69
　genital organ(s)
　　female 752.8
　　　external 752.49
　　　internal NEC 752.8
　　male NEC 752.8
　　　penis 752.69
　genitourinary organs NEC 752.8

Accessory — continued
　heart 746.89
　　valve NEC 746.89
　　　pulmonary 746.09
　hepatic ducts 751.69
　hymen 752.49
　intestine (large) (small) 751.5
　kidney 753.3
　lacrimal canal 743.65
　leaflet, heart valve NEC 746.89
　　pulmonary 746.09
　ligament, broad 752.19
　liver (duct) 751.69
　lobule (ear) 744.1
　lung (lobe) 748.69
　muscle 756.82
　navicular of carpus 755.56
　nervous system, part NEC 742.8
　nipple 757.6
　nose 748.1
　organ or site NEC — see Anomaly, specified
　　type NEC
　ovary 752.0
　oviduct 752.19
　pancreas 751.7
　parathyroid gland 759.2
　parotid gland (and duct) 750.22
　pituitary gland 759.2
　placental lobe — see Placenta, abnormal
　preauricular appendage 744.1
　prepuce 605
　renal arteries (multiple) 747.62
　rib 756.3
　　cervical 756.2
　roots (teeth) 520.2
　salivary gland 750.22
　sesamoids 755.8
　sinus — see condition
　skin tags 757.39
　spleen 759.0
　sternum 756.3
　submaxillary gland 750.22
　tarsal bones 755.67
　teeth, tooth 520.1
　　causing crowding 524.3
　tendon 756.89
　thumb 755.01
　thymus gland 759.2
　thyroid gland 759.2
　toes 755.02
　tongue 750.13
　tragus 744.1
　ureter 753.4
　urethra 753.8
　urinary organ or tract NEC 753.8
　uterus 752.2
　vagina 752.49
　valve, heart NEC 746.89
　　pulmonary 746.09
　vertebra 756.19
　vocal cords 748.3
　vulva 752.49
Accident, accidental — see also condition
　birth NEC 767.9
　cardiovascular (see also Disease,
　　cardiovascular) 429.2
　cerebral (see also Disease, cerebrovascular,
　　acute) 436
　cerebrovascular (current) (CVA) (see also
　　Disease, cerebrovascular, acute) 436
　　healed or old V12.59
　　impending 435.9

Index to Diseases

Accident, accidental — *continued*
  cerebrovascular — *continued*
    late effect — *see* Late effect(s) (of) cerebrovascular disease
    postoperative 997.02
  coronary (*see also* Infarct, myocardium) 410.9 ✓5ᵗʰ
  craniovascular (*see also* Disease, cerebrovascular, acute) 436
  during pregnancy, to mother affecting fetus or newborn 760.5
  heart, cardiac (*see also* Infarct, myocardium) 410.9 ✓5ᵗʰ
  intrauterine 779.89
  vascular — *see* Disease, cerebrovascular, acute
Accommodation
  disorder of 367.51
    drug-induced 367.89
    toxic 367.89
  insufficiency of 367.4
  paralysis of 367.51
    hysterical 300.11
  spasm of 367.53
Accouchement — *see* Delivery
Accreta placenta (without hemorrhage) 667.0 ✓5ᵗʰ
  with hemorrhage 666.0 ✓5ᵗʰ
Accretio cordis (nonrheumatic) 423.1
Accretions on teeth 523.6
Accumulation secretion, prostate 602.8
Acephalia, acephalism, acephaly 740.0
Acephalic 740.0
Acephalobrachia 759.89
Acephalocardia 759.89
Acephalocardius 759.89
Acephalochiria 759.89
Acephalochirus 759.89
Acephalogaster 759.89
Acephalostomus 759.89
Acephalothorax 759.89
Acephalus 740.0
Acetonemia 790.6
  diabetic 250.1 ✓5ᵗʰ
Acetonglycosuria 982.8
Acetonuria 791.6
Achalasia 530.0
  cardia 530.0
  digestive organs congenital NEC 751.8
  esophagus 530.0
  pelvirectal 751.3
  psychogenic 306.4
  pylorus 750.5
  sphincteral NEC 564.89
Achard-Thiers syndrome (adrenogenital) 255.2
Ache(s) — *see* Pain
Acheilia 750.26
Acheiria 755.21
Achillobursitis 726.71
Achillodynia 726.71
Achlorhydria, achlorhydric 536.0
  anemia 280.9
  diarrhea 536.0
  neurogenic 536.0
  postvagotomy 564.2
  psychogenic 306.4
  secondary to vagotomy 564.2

Achloroblepsia 368.52
Achloropsia 368.52
Acholia 575.8
Acholuric jaundice (familial) (splenomegalic) (*see also* Spherocytosis) 282.0
  acquired 283.9
Achondroplasia 756.4
Achrestic anemia 281.8
Achroacytosis, lacrimal gland 375.00
  tuberculous (*see also* Tuberculosis) 017.3 ✓5ᵗʰ
Achroma, cutis 709.00
Achromate (congenital) 368.54
Achromatopia 368.54
Achromatopsia (congenital) 368.54
Achromia
  congenital 270.2
  parasitica 111.0
  unguium 703.8
Achylia
  gastrica 536.8
    neurogenic 536.3
    psychogenic 306.4
  pancreatica 577.1
Achylosis 536.8
Acid
  burn — *see also* Burn, by site
    from swallowing acid — *see* Burn, internal organs
  deficiency
    amide nicotinic 265.2
    amino 270.9
    ascorbic 267
    folic 266.2
    nicotinic (amide) 265.2
    pantothenic 266.2
  intoxication 276.2
  peptic disease 536.8
  stomach 536.8
    psychogenic 306.4
Acidemia 276.2
  arginosuccinic 270.6
  fetal
    affecting management of pregnancy 656.3 ✓5ᵗʰ
    before onset of labor, in liveborn infant 768.2
    during labor, in liveborn infant 768.3
    intrauterine — *see* Distress, fetal 656.3 ✓5ᵗʰ
    unspecified as to time of onset, in liveborn infant 768.4
  pipecolic 270.7
Acidity, gastric (high) (low) 536.8
  psychogenic 306.4
Acidocytopenia 288.0
Acidocytosis 288.3
Acidopenia 288.0
Acidosis 276.2
  diabetic 250.1 ✓5ᵗʰ
  fetal, affecting management of pregnancy 656.8 ✓5ᵗʰ
  fetal, affecting newborn 768.9
  kidney tubular 588.8
  lactic 276.2
  metabolic NEC 276.2
    with respiratory acidosis 276.4
    late, of newborn 775.7
  renal
    hyperchloremic 588.8

✓4ᵗʰ Fourth-digit Required   ✓5ᵗʰ Fifth-digit Required

Acidosis — continued
  renal — continued
    tubular (distal) (proximal) 588.8
  respiratory 276.2
    complicated by
      metabolic acidosis 276.4
      metabolic alkalosis 276.4
Aciduria 791.9
  arginosuccinic 270.6
  beta-aminoisobutyric (BAIB) 277.2
  glycolic 271.8
  methylmalonic 270.3
    with glycinemia 270.7
  organic 270.9
  orotic (congenital) (hereditary) (pyrimidine deficiency) 281.4
Acladiosis 111.8
  skin 111.8
Aclasis
  diaphyseal 756.4
  tarsoepiphyseal 756.59
Acleistocardia 745.5
Aclusion 524.4
Acmesthesia 782.0
Acne (pustular) (vulgaris) 706.1
  agminata (*see also* Tuberculosis) 017.0 ✓5ᵗʰ
  artificialis 706.1
  atrophica 706.0
  cachecticorum (Hebra) 706.1
  conglobata 706.1
  conjunctiva 706.1
  cystic 706.1
  decalvans 704.09
  erythematosa 695.3
  eyelid 706.1
  frontalis 706.0
  indurata 706.1
  keloid 706.1
  lupoid 706.0
  necrotic, necrotica 706.0
    miliaris 704.8
  nodular 706.1
  occupational 706.1
  papulosa 706.1
  rodens 706.0
  rosacea 695.3
  scorbutica 267
  scrofulosorum (Bazin) (*see also* Tuberculosis) 017.0 ✓5ᵗʰ
  summer 692.72
  tropical 706.1
  varioliformis 706.0
Acneiform drug eruptions 692.3
Acnitis (primary) (*see also* Tuberculosis) 017.0 ✓5ᵗʰ
Acomia 704.00
Acontractile bladder 344.61
Aconuresis (*see also* Incontinence) 788.30
Acosta's disease 993.2
Acousma 780.1
Acoustic — *see* condition
Acousticophobia 300.29
Acquired — *see* condition
Acquired immune deficiency syndrome — *see* Human immunodeficiency virus (disease) (illness) (infection)

Acquired immunodeficiency syndrome — *see* Human immunodeficiency virus (disease) (illness) (infection)
Acragnosis 781.99
Acrania 740.0
Acroagnosis 781.99
Acroasphyxia, chronic 443.89
Acrobrachycephaly 756.0
Acrobystiolith 608.89
Acrobystitis 607.2
Acrocephalopolysyndactyly 755.55
Acrocephalosyndactyly 755.55
Acrocephaly 756.0
Acrochondrohyperplasia 759.82
Acrocyanosis 443.89
  newborn 770.83 ▲
Acrodermatitis 686.8
  atrophicans (chronica) 701.8
  continua (Hallopeau) 696.1
  enteropathica 686.8
  Hallopeau's 696.1
  perstans 696.1
  pustulosa continua 696.1
  recalcitrant pustular 696.1
Acrodynia 985.0
Acrodysplasia 755.55
Acrohyperhidrosis 780.8
Acrokeratosis verruciformis 757.39
Acromastitis 611.0
Acromegaly, acromegalia (skin) 253.0
Acromelalgia 443.89
Acromicria acromikria 756.59
Acronyx 703.0
Acropachy, thyroid (*see also* Thyrotoxicosis) 242.9 ✓5ᵗʰ
Acropachyderma 757.39
Acroparesthesia 443.89
  simple (Schultz's type) 443.89
  vasomotor (Nothnagel's type) 443.89
Acropathy thyroid (*see also* Thyrotoxicosis) 242.9 ✓5ᵗʰ
Acrophobia 300.29
Acroposthitis 607.2
Acroscleriasis (*see also* Scleroderma) 710.1
Acroscleroderma (*see also* Scleroderma) 710.1
Acrosclerosis (*see also* Scleroderma) 710.1
Acrosphacelus 785.4
Acrosphenosyndactylia 755.55
Acrospiroma, eccrine (M8402/0) — *see* Neoplasm, skin, benign
Acrostealgia 732.9
Acrosyndactyly (*see also* Syndactylism) 755.10
Acrotrophodynia 991.4
Actinic — *see also* condition
  cheilitis (due to sun) 692.72
    chronic NEC 692.74
    due to radiation, except from sun 692.82
  conjunctivitis 370.24
  dermatitis (due to sun) (*see also* Dermatitis, actinic 692.70
    due to
      roentgen rays or radioactive substance 692.82

Index to Diseases

Actinic — *continued*
  dermatitis — *continued*
    due to — *continued*
      ultraviolet radiation, except from sun 692.82
        sun NEC 692.70
    elastosis solare 692.74
    granuloma 692.73
    keratitis 370.24
    ophthalmia 370.24
    reticuloid 692.73
Actinobacillosis, general 027.8
Actinobacillus
  lignieresii 027.8
  mallei 024
  muris 026.1
Actinocutitis NEC (*see also* Dermatitis, actinic) 692.70
Actinodermatitis NEC (*see also* Dermatitis, actinic) 692.70
Actinomyces
  israelii (infection) — *see* Actinomycosis
  muris-ratti (infection) 026.1
Actinomycosis, actinomycotic 039.9
  with
    pneumonia 039.1
    abdominal 039.2
    cervicofacial 039.3
    cutaneous 039.0
    pulmonary 039.1
    specified site NEC 039.8
    thoracic 039.1
Actinoneuritis 357.89 ▲
Action, heart
  disorder 427.9
    postoperative 997.1
  irregular 427.9
    postoperative 997.1
    psychogenic 306.2
Active — *see* condition
Activity decrease, functional 780.99 ▲
Acute — *see also* condition
  abdomen NEC 789.0 ✓5ᵗʰ
  gallbladder (*see also* Cholecystitis, acute) 575.0
Acyanoblepsia 368.53
Acyanopsia 368.53
Acystia 753.8
Acystinervia — *see* Neurogenic, bladder
Acystineuria — *see* Neurogenic, bladder
Adactylia, adactyly (congenital) 755.4
  lower limb (complete) (intercalary) (partial) (terminal) (*see also* Deformity, reduction, lower limb) 755.39
    meaning all digits (complete) (partial) 755.31
    transverse (complete) (partial) 755.31
  upper limb (complete) (intercalary) (partial) (terminal) (*see also* Deformity, reduction, upper limb) 755.29
    meaning all digits (complete) (partial) 755.21
    transverse (complete) (partial) 755.21
Adair-Dighton syndrome (brittle bones and blue sclera, deafness) 756.51
Adamantinoblastoma (M9310/0) — *see* Ameloblastoma

Adamantinoma (M9310/0) — *see* Ameloblastoma
Adamantoblastoma (M9310/0) — *see* Ameloblastoma
Adams-Stokes (-Morgagni) disease or syndrome (syncope with heart block) 426.9
Adaptation reaction (*see also* Reaction, adjustment) 309.9
Addiction — *see also* Dependence
  absinthe 304.6 ✓5ᵗʰ
  alcoholic (ethyl) (methyl) (wood) 303.9 ✓5ᵗʰ
    complicating pregnancy, childbirth, or puerperium 648.4 ✓5ᵗʰ
      affecting fetus or newborn 760.71
    suspected damage to fetus affecting management of pregnancy 655.4 ✓5ᵗʰ
  drug (*see also* Dependence) 304.9 ✓5ᵗʰ
  ethyl alcohol 303.9 ✓5ᵗʰ
  heroin 304.0 ✓5ᵗʰ
  hospital 301.51
  methyl alcohol 303.9 ✓5ᵗʰ
  methylated spirit 303.9 ✓5ᵗʰ
  morphine (-like substances) 304.0 ✓5ᵗʰ
  nicotine 305.1
  opium 304.0 ✓5ᵗʰ
  tobacco 305.1
  wine 303.9 ✓5ᵗʰ
Addison's
  anemia (pernicious) 281.0
  disease (bronze) (primary adrenal insufficiency) 255.4
    tuberculous (*see also* Tuberculosis) 017.6 ✓5ᵗʰ
  keloid (morphea) 701.0
  melanoderma (adrenal cortical hypofunction) 255.4
Addison-Biermer anemia (pernicious) 281.0
Addison-Gull disease — *see* Xanthoma
Addisonian crisis or melanosis (acute adrenocortical insufficiency) 255.4
Additional — *see also* Accessory
  chromosome(s) 758.5
    13-15 758.1
    16-18 758.2
    21 758.0
  autosome(s) NEC 758.5
  sex 758.81
Adduction contracture, hip or other joint — *see* Contraction, joint
Adenasthenia gastrica 536.0
Aden fever 061
Adenitis (*see also* Lymphadenitis) 289.3
  acute, unspecified site 683
    epidemic infectious 075
  axillary 289.3
    acute 683
    chronic or subacute 289.1
  Bartholin's gland 616.8
  bulbourethral gland (*see also* Urethritis) 597.89
  cervical 289.3
    acute 683
    chronic or subacute 289.1
  chancroid (Ducrey's bacillus) 099.0
  chronic (any lymph node, except mesenteric) 289.1
    mesenteric 289.2
  Cowper's gland (*see also* Urethritis) 597.89
  epidemic, acute 075

✓4ᵗʰ Fourth-digit Required
✓5ᵗʰ Fifth-digit Required

Adenitis — continued
- gangrenous 683
- gonorrheal NEC 098.89
- groin 289.3
  - acute 683
  - chronic or subacute 289.1
- infectious 075
- inguinal (region) 289.3
  - acute 683
  - chronic or subacute 289.1
- lymph gland or node, except mesenteric 289.3
  - acute 683
  - chronic or subacute 289.1
- mesenteric (acute) (chronic) (nonspecific) (subacute) 289.2
- mesenteric (acute) (chronic) (nonspecific) (subacute) 289.2
  - due to Pasteurella multocida (P. septica) 027.2
- parotid gland (suppurative) 527.2
- phlegmonous 683
- salivary duct or gland (any) (recurring) (suppurative) 527.2
- scrofulous (*see also* Tuberculosis) 017.2 ✓5ᵗʰ
- septic 289.3
- Skene's duct or gland (*see also* Urethritis) 597.89
- strumous, tuberculous (*see also* Tuberculosis) 017.2 ✓5ᵗʰ
- subacute, unspecified site 289.1
- sublingual gland (suppurative) 527.2
- submandibular gland (suppurative) 527.2
- submaxillary gland (suppurative) 527.2
- suppurative 683
- tuberculous — *see* Tuberculosis, lymph gland
- urethral gland (*see also* Urethritis) 597.89
- venereal NEC 099.8
- Wharton's duct (suppurative) 527.2

Adenoacanthoma (M8570/3) — *see* Neoplasm, by site, malignant

Adenoameloblastoma (M9300/0) 213.1
- upper jaw (bone) 213.0

Adenocarcinoma (M8140/3) — *see also* Neoplasm, by site, malignant

> Note — The following list of adjectival modifiers is not exhaustive. A description of adenocarcinoma that does not appear in this list should be coded in the same manner as carcinoma with that description. Thus, "mixed acidophil-basophil adenocarcinoma," should be coded in the same manner as "mixed acidophil-basophil carcinoma," which appears in the list under "Carcinoma."
>
> Except where otherwise indicated, the morphological varieties of adenocarcinoma in the list should be coded by site as for "Neoplasm, malignant."

- with
  - apocrine metaplasia (M8573/3)
  - cartilaginous (and osseous) metaplasia (M8571/3)
  - osseous (and cartilaginous) metaplasia (M8571/3)
  - spindle cell metaplasia (M8572/3)
  - squamous metaplasia (M8570/3)
- acidophil (M8280/3)
  - specified site — *see* Neoplasm, by site, malignant
  - unspecified site 194.3

Adenocarcinoma — continued
- acinar (M8550/3)
- acinic cell (M8550/3)
- adrenal cortical (M8370/3) 194.0
- alveolar (M8251/3)
- and
  - epidermoid carcinoma, mixed (M8560/3)
  - squamous cell carcinoma, mixed (M8560/3)
- apocrine (M8401/3)
  - breast — *see* Neoplasm, breast, malignant
  - specified site NEC — *see* Neoplasm, skin, malignant
  - unspecified site 173.9
- basophil (M8300/3)
  - specified site — *see* Neoplasm, by site, malignant
  - unspecified site 194.3
- bile duct type (M8160/3)
  - liver 155.1
  - specified site NEC — *see* Neoplasm, by site, malignant
  - unspecified site 155.1
- bronchiolar (M8250/3) — *see* Neoplasm, lung, malignant
- ceruminous (M8420/3) 173.2
- chromophobe (M8270/3)
  - specified site — *see* Neoplasm, by site, malignant
  - unspecified site 194.3
- clear cell (mesonephroid type) (M8310/3)
- colloid (M8480/3)
- cylindroid type (M8200/3)
- diffuse type (M8145/3)
  - specified site — *see* Neoplasm, by site, malignant
  - unspecified site 151.9
- duct (infiltrating) (M8500/3)
  - with Paget's disease (M8541/3) — *see* Neoplasm, breast, malignant
  - specified site — *see* Neoplasm, by site, malignant
  - unspecified site 174.9
- embryonal (M9070/3)
- endometrioid (M8380/3) — *see* Neoplasm, by site, malignant
- eosinophil (M8280/3)
  - specified site — *see* Neoplasm, by site malignant
  - unspecified site 194.3
- follicular (M8330/3)
  - and papillary (M8340/3) 193
  - moderately differentiated type (M8332/3) 193
  - pure follicle type (M8331/3) 193
  - specified site — *see* Neoplasm, by site, malignant
  - trabecular type (M8332/3) 193
  - unspecified type 193
  - well differentiated type (M8331/3) 193
- gelatinous (M8480/3)
- granular cell (M8320/3)
- Hürthle cell (M8290/3) 193
- in
  - adenomatous
    - polyp (M8210/3)
    - polyposis coli (M8220/3) 153.9
  - polypoid adenoma (M8210/3)
  - tubular adenoma (M8210/3)
  - villous adenoma (M8261/3)

Adenocarcinoma — *continued*
  infiltrating duct (M8500/3)
    with Paget's disease (M8541/3) — *see*
      Neoplasm, breast, malignant
    specified site — *see* Neoplasm, by site,
      malignant
    unspecified site 174.9
  inflammatory (M8530/3)
    specified site — *see* Neoplasm, by site,
      malignant
    unspecified site 174.9
  in situ (M8140/2) — *see* Neoplasm, by site, in
    situ
  intestinal type (M8144/3)
    specified site — *see* Neoplasm, by site,
      malignant
    unspecified site 151.9
  intraductal (noninfiltrating) (M8500/2)
    papillary (M8503/2)
      specified site — *see* Neoplasm, by site,
        in situ
      unspecified site 233.0
    specified site — *see* Neoplasm, by site, in
      situ
    unspecified site 233.0
  islet cell (M8150/3)
    and exocrine, mixed (M8154/3)
      specified site — *see* Neoplasm, by site,
        malignant
      unspecified site 157.9
    pancreas 157.4
    specified site NEC — *see* Neoplasm, by site,
      malignant
    unspecified site 157.4
  lobular (M8520/3)
    specified site — *see* Neoplasm, by site,
      malignant
    unspecified site 174.9
  medullary (M8510/3)
  mesonephric (M9110/3)
  mixed cell (M8323/3)
  mucinous (M8480/3)
  mucin-producing (M8481/3)
  mucoid (M8480/3) — *see also* Neoplasm, by
    site, malignant
    cell (M8300/3)
      specified site — *see* Neoplasm, by site,
        malignant
      unspecified site 194.3
  nonencapsulated sclerosing (M8350/3) 193
  oncocytic (M8290/3)
  oxyphilic (M8290/3)
  papillary (M8260/3)
    and follicular (M8340/3) 193
    intraductal (noninfiltrating) (M8503/2)
      specified site — *see* Neoplasm, by site,
        in situ
      unspecified site 233.0
    serous (M8460/3)
      specified site — *see* Neoplasm, by site,
        malignant
      unspecified site 183.0
    papillocystic (M8450/3)
      specified site — *see* Neoplasm, by site,
        malignant
      unspecified site 183.0
  pseudomucinous (M8470/3)
    specified site — *see* Neoplasm, by site,
      malignant
    unspecified site 183.0
  renal cell (M8312/3) 189.0

Adenocarcinoma — *continued*
  sebaceous (M8410/3)
  serous (M8441/3) — *see also* Neoplasm, by
    site, malignant
    papillary
      specified site — *see* Neoplasm, by site
        malignant
      unspecified site 183.0
  signet ring cell (M8490/3)
  superficial spreading (M8143/3)
  sweat gland (M8400/3) — *see* Neoplasm, skin,
    malignant
  trabecular (M8190/3)
  tubular (M8211/3)
  villous (M8262/3)
  water-clear cell (M8322/3) 194.1
Adenofibroma (M9013/0)
  clear cell (M8313/0) — *see* Neoplasm, by site,
    benign
  endometrioid (M8381/0) 220
    borderline malignancy (M8381/1) 236.2
    malignant (M8381/3) 183.0
  mucinous (M9015/0)
    specified site — *see* Neoplasm, by site,
      benign
    unspecified site 220
  prostate 600.2
  serous (M9014/0)
    specified site — *see* Neoplasm, by site,
      benign
    unspecified site 220
  specified site — *see* Neoplasm, by site, benign
  unspecified site 220
Adenofibrosis
  breast 610.2
  endometrioid 617.0
Adenoiditis 474.01
  acute 463
  chronic 474.01
    with chronic tonsillitis 474.02
Adenoids (congenital) (of nasal fossa) 474.9
  hypertrophy 474.12
  vegetations 474.2
Adenolipomatosis (symmetrical) 272.8
Adenolymphoma (M8561/0)
  specified site — *see* Neoplasm, by site, benign
  unspecified 210.2
Adenoma (sessile) (M8140/0) — *see also*
  Neoplasm, by site, benign

> Note — Except where otherwise indicated,
> the morphological varieties of adenoma in the
> list below should be coded by site as for
> "Neoplasm, benign."

  acidophil (M8280/0)
    specified site — *see* Neoplasm, by site,
      benign
    unspecified site 227.3
  acinar (cell) (M8550/0)
  acinic cell (M8550/0)
  adrenal (cortex) (cortical) (functioning)
    (M8370/0) 227.0
    clear cell type (M8373/0) 227.0
    compact cell type (M8371/0) 227.0
    glomerulosa cell type (M8374/0) 227.0
    heavily pigmented variant (M8372/0) 227.0
    mixed cell type (M8375/0) 227.0
  alpha cell (M8152/0)
    pancreas 211.7

Adenoma — *continued*
  alpha cell — *continued*
    specified site NEC — *see* Neoplasm, by site, benign
    unspecified site 211.7
  alveolar (M8251/0)
  apocrine (M8401/0)
    breast 217
    specified site NEC — *see* Neoplasm, skin, benign
    unspecified site 216.9
  basal cell (M8147/0)
  basophil (M8300/0)
    specified site — *see* Neoplasm, by site, benign
    unspecified site 227.3
  beta cell (M8151/0)
    pancreas 211.7
    specified site NEC — *see* Neoplasm, by site, benign
    unspecified site 211.7
  bile duct (M8160/0) 211.5
  black (M8372/0) 227.0
  bronchial (M8140/1) 235.7
    carcinoid type (M8240/3) — *see* Neoplasm, lung, malignant
    cylindroid type (M8200/3) — *see* Neoplasm, lung, malignant
  ceruminous (M8420/0) 216.2
  chief cell (M8321/0) 227.1
  chromophobe (M8270/0)
    specified site — *see* Neoplasm, by site, benign
    unspecified site 227.3
  clear cell (M8310/0)
  colloid (M8334/0)
    specified site — *see* Neoplasm, by site, benign
    unspecified site 226
  cylindroid type, bronchus (M8200/3) — *see* Neoplasm, lung, malignant
  duct (M8503/0)
  embryonal (M8191/0)
  endocrine, multiple (M8360/1)
    single specified site — *see* Neoplasm, by site, uncertain behavior
    two or more specified sites 237.4
    unspecified site 237.4
  endometrioid (M8380/0) — *see also* Neoplasm, by site, benign
    borderline malignancy (M8380/1) — *see* Neoplasm, by site, uncertain behavior
  eosinophil (M8280/0)
    specified site — *see* Neoplasm, by site, benign
    unspecified site 227.3
  fetal (M8333/0)
    specified site — *see* Neoplasm, by site, benign
    unspecified site 226
  follicular (M8330/0)
    specified site — *see* Neoplasm, by site, benign
    unspecified site 226
  hepatocellular (M8170/0) 211.5
  Hürthle cell (M8290/0) 226
  intracystic papillary (M8504/0)
  islet cell (functioning) (M8150/0)
    pancreas 211.7
    specified site NEC — *see* Neoplasm, by site, benign

Adenoma — *continued*
  islet cell — *continued*
    unspecified site 211.7
  liver cell (M8170/0) 211.5
  macrofollicular (M8334/0)
    specified site NEC — *see* Neoplasm, by site, benign
    unspecified site 226
  malignant, malignum (M8140/3) — *see* Neoplasm, by site, malignant
  mesonephric (M9110/0)
  microfollicular (M8333/0)
    specified site — *see* Neoplasm, by site, benign
    unspecified site 226
  mixed cell (M8323/0)
  monomorphic (M8146/0)
  mucinous (M8480/0)
  mucoid cell (M8300/0)
    specified site — *see* Neoplasm, by site, benign
    unspecified site 227.3
  multiple endocrine (M8360/1)
    single specified site — *see* Neoplasm, by site, uncertain behavior
    two or more specified sites 237.4
    unspecified site 237.4
  nipple (M8506/0) 217
  oncocytic (M8290/0)
  oxyphilic (M8290/0)
  papillary (M8260/0) — *see also* Neoplasm, by site, benign
    intracystic (M8504/0)
  papillotubular (M8263/0)
  Pick's tubular (M8640/0)
    specified site — *see* Neoplasm, by site, benign
    unspecified site
      female 220
      male 222.0
  pleomorphic (M8940/0)
  polypoid (M8210/0)
  prostate (benign) 600.2
  rete cell 222.0
  sebaceous, sebaceum (gland) (senile) (M8410/0) — *see also* Neoplasm, skin, benign
    disseminata 759.5
  Sertoli cell (M8640/0)
    specified site — *see* Neoplasm, by site, benign
    unspecified site
      female 220
      male 222.0
  skin appendage (M8390/0) — *see* Neoplasm, skin, benign
  sudoriferous gland (M8400/0) — *see* Neoplasm, skin, benign
  sweat gland or duct (M8400/0) — *see* Neoplasm, skin, benign
  testicular (M8640/0)
    specified site — *see* Neoplasm, by site, benign
    unspecified site
      female 220
      male 222.0
  thyroid 226
  trabecular (M8190/0)
  tubular (M8211/0) — *see also* Neoplasm, by site, benign
    papillary (M8460/3)

Adenoma — continued
  tubular — continued
    Pick's (M8640/0)
      specified site — see Neoplasm, by site, benign
      unspecified site
        female 220
        male 222.0
  tubulovillous (M8263/0)
  villoglandular (M8263/0)
  villous (M8261/1) — see Neoplasm, by site, uncertain behavior
  water-clear cell (M8322/0) 227.1
  wolffian duct (M9110/0)
Adenomatosis (M8220/0)
  endocrine (multiple) (M8360/1)
    single specified site — see Neoplasm, by site, uncertain behavior
    two or more specified sites 237.4
    unspecified site 237.4
  erosive of nipple (M8506/0) 217
  pluriendocrine — see Adenomatosis, endocrine
  pulmonary (M8250/1) 235.7
    malignant (M8250/3) — see Neoplasm, lung, malignant
    specified site — see Neoplasm, by site, benign
    unspecified site 211.3
Adenomatous
  cyst, thyroid (gland) — see Goiter, nodular
  goiter (nontoxic) (see also Goiter, nodular) 241.9
    toxic or with hyperthyroidism 242.3 ✓5ᵗʰ
Adenomyoma (M8932/0) — see also Neoplasm, by site, benign
  prostate 600.2
Adenomyometritis 617.0
Adenomyosis (uterus) (internal) 617.0
Adenopathy (lymph gland) 785.6
  inguinal 785.6
  mediastinal 785.6
  mesentery 785.6
  syphilitic (secondary) 091.4
  tracheobronchial 785.6
    tuberculous (see also Tuberculosis) 012.1 ✓5ᵗʰ
      primary, progressive 010.8 ✓5ᵗʰ
  tuberculous (see also Tuberculosis, lymph gland) 017.2 ✓5ᵗʰ
    tracheobronchial 012.1 ✓5ᵗʰ
      primary, progressive 010.8 ✓5ᵗʰ
Adenopharyngitis 462
Adenophlegmon 683
Adenosalpingitis 614.1
Adenosarcoma (M8960/3) 189.0
Adenosclerosis 289.3
Adenosis
  breast (sclerosing) 610.2
  vagina, congenital 752.49
Adentia (complete) (partial) (see also Absence, teeth) 520.0
Adherent
  labium (minus) 624.4
  pericardium (nonrheumatic) 423.1
    rheumatic 393
  placenta 667.0 ✓5ᵗʰ
    with hemorrhage 666.0 ✓5ᵗʰ
  prepuce 605
  scar (skin) NEC 709.2
  tendon in scar 709.2

Adhesion(s), adhesive (postinfectional) (postoperative)
  abdominal (wall) (see also Adhesions, peritoneum) 568.0
  amnion to fetus 658.8 ✓5ᵗʰ
    affecting fetus or newborn 762.8
  appendix 543.9
  arachnoiditis — see Meningitis
  auditory tube (Eustachian) 381.89
  bands — see Adhesions, peritoneum
    cervix 622.3
    uterus 621.5
  bile duct (any) 576.8
  bladder (sphincter) 596.8
  bowel (see also Adhesions, peritoneum) 568.0
  cardiac 423.1
    rheumatic 398.99
  cecum (see also Adhesions, peritoneum) 568.0
  cervicovaginal 622.3
    congenital 752.49
    postpartal 674.8 ✓5ᵗʰ
    old 622.3
  cervix 622.3
  clitoris 624.4
  colon (see also Adhesions, peritoneum) 568.0
  common duct 576.8
  congenital — see also Anomaly, specified type NEC
    fingers (see also Syndactylism, fingers) 755.11
    labium (majus) (minus) 752.49
    omental, anomalous 751.4
    ovary 752.0
    peritoneal 751.4
    toes (see also Syndactylism, toes) 755.13
    tongue (to gum or roof of mouth) 750.12
  conjunctiva (acquired) (localized) 372.62
    congenital 743.63
    extensive 372.63
  cornea — see Opacity, cornea
  cystic duct 575.8
  diaphragm (see also Adhesions, peritoneum) 568.0
  due to foreign body — see Foreign body
  duodenum (see also Adhesions, peritoneum) 568.0
    with obstruction 537.3
  ear, middle — see Adhesions, middle ear
  epididymis 608.89
  epidural — see Adhesions, meninges
  epiglottis 478.79
  Eustachian tube 381.89
  eyelid 374.46
    postoperative 997.99
      surgically created V45.69
  gallbladder (see also Disease, gallbladder) 575.8
  globe 360.89
  heart 423.1
    rheumatic 398.99
  ileocecal (coil) (see also Adhesions, peritoneum) 568.0
  ileum (see also Adhesions, peritoneum) 568.0
  intestine (postoperative) (see also Adhesions, peritoneum) 568.0
    with obstruction 560.81
      with hernia — see also Hernia, by site, with obstruction
      gangrenous — see Hernia, by site, with gangrene

Adhesion(s), adhesive — *continued*
  intra-abdominal (*see also* Adhesions,
      peritoneum) 568.0
  iris 364.70
    to corneal graft 996.79
  joint (*see also* Ankylosis) 718.5 ✓5ᵗʰ
  kidney 593.89
  labium (majus) (minus), congenital 752.49
  liver 572.8
  lung 511.0
  mediastinum 519.3
  meninges 349.2
    cerebral (any) 349.2
      congenital 742.4
    congenital 742.8
    spinal (any) 349.2
      congenital 742.59
    tuberculous (cerebral) (spinal) (*see also*
        Tuberculosis, meninges) 013.0 ✓5ᵗʰ
  mesenteric (*see also* Adhesions, peritoneum)
      568.0
  middle ear (fibrous) 385.10
    drum head 385.19
      to
        incus 385.11
        promontorium 385.13
        stapes 385.12
    specified NEC 385.19
  nasal (septum) (to turbinates) 478.1
  nerve NEC 355.9
    spinal 355.9
      root 724.9
        cervical NEC 723.4
        lumbar NEC 724.4
        lumbosacral 724.4
        thoracic 724.4
  ocular muscle 378.60
  omentum (*see also* Adhesions, peritoneum)
      568.0
  organ or site, congenital NEC — *see* Anomaly,
      specified type NEC
  ovary 614.6
    congenital (to cecum, kidney, or omentum)
        752.0
  parauterine 614.6
  parovarian 614.6
  pelvic (peritoneal)
    female (postoperative) (postinfection) 614.6
    male (postoperative) (postinfection) (*see also*
        Adhesions, peritoneum) 568.0
    postpartal (old) 614.6
    tuberculous (*see also* Tuberculosis)
        016.9 ✓5ᵗʰ
  penis to scrotum (congenital) 752.69
  periappendiceal (*see also* Adhesions,
      peritoneum) 568.0
  pericardium (nonrheumatic) 423.1
    rheumatic 393
    tuberculous (*see also* Tuberculosis)
        017.9 ✓5ᵗʰ [420.0]
  pericholecystic 575.8
  perigastric (*see also* Adhesions, peritoneum)
      568.0
  periovarian 614.6
  periprostatic 602.8
  perirectal (*see also* Adhesions, peritoneum)
      568.0
  perirenal 593.89
  peritoneum, peritoneal (fibrous) (postoperative)
      568.0

Adhesion(s), adhesive — *continued*
  peritoneum, peritoneal — *continued*
    with obstruction (intestinal) 560.81
      with hernia — *see also* Hernia, by site,
          with obstruction
        gangrenous — *see* Hernia, by site,
            with gangrene
      duodenum 537.3
      congenital 751.4
      female (postoperative) (postinfective) 614.6
      pelvic, female 614.6
      pelvic, male 568.0
      postpartal, pelvic 614.6
      to uterus 614.6
  peritubal 614.6
  periureteral 593.89
  periuterine 621.5
  perivesical 596.8
  perivesicular (seminal vesicle) 608.89
  pleura, pleuritic 511.0
    tuberculous (*see also* Tuberculosis, pleura)
        012.0 ✓5ᵗʰ
  pleuropericardial 511.0
  postoperative (gastrointestinal tract) (*see also*
      Adhesions, peritoneum) 568.0
    eyelid 997.99
      surgically created V45.69
    pelvic female 614.9
    pelvic male 568.0
    urethra 598.2
  postpartal, old 624.4
  preputial, prepuce 605
  pulmonary 511.0
  pylorus (*see also* Adhesions, peritoneum)
      568.0
  Rosenmüller's fossa 478.29
  sciatic nerve 355.0
  seminal vesicle 608.89
  shoulder (joint) 726.0
  sigmoid flexure (*see also* Adhesions,
      peritoneum) 568.0
  spermatic cord (acquired) 608.89
    congenital 752.8
  spinal canal 349.2
    nerve 355.9
      root 724.9
        cervical NEC 723.4
        lumbar NEC 724.4
        lumbosacral 724.4
        thoracic 724.4
  stomach (*see also* Adhesions, peritoneum)
      568.0
  subscapular 726.2
  tendonitis 726.90
    shoulder 726.0
  testicle 608.89
  tongue (congenital) (to gum or roof of mouth)
      750.12
    acquired 529.8
  trachea 519.1
  tubo-ovarian 614.6
  tunica vaginalis 608.89
  ureter 593.89
  uterus 621.5
    to abdominal wall 614.6
    in pregnancy or childbirth 654.4 ✓5ᵗʰ
      affecting fetus or newborn 763.89
  vagina (chronic) (postoperative) (postradiation)
      623.2
  vaginitis (congenital) 752.49
  vesical 596.8
  vitreous 379.29

Index to Diseases

Adie (-Holmes) syndrome (tonic pupillary reaction) 379.46
Adiponecrosis neonatorum 778.1
Adiposa dolorosa 272.8
Adiposalgia 272.8
Adiposis 278.0 ✓5ᵗʰ
  cerebralis 253.8
  dolorosa 272.8
  tuberosa simplex 272.8
Adiposity 278.00
  heart (see also Degeneration, myocardial) 429.1
  localized 278.1
Adiposogenital dystrophy 253.8
Adjustment
  prosthesis or other device — see Fitting of
  reaction — see Reaction, adjustment
Administration, prophylactic
  antibiotics V07.39
  antitoxin, any V07.2
  antivenin V07.2
  chemotherapeutic agent NEC V07.39
  chemotherapy V07.39
  diphtheria antitoxin V07.2
  fluoride V07.31
  gamma globulin V07.2
  immune sera (gamma globulin) V07.2
  passive immunization agent V07.2
  RhoGAM V07.2
Admission (encounter)
  as organ donor — see Donor
  by mistake V68.9
  for
    adequacy testing (for)
      hemodialysis V56.31
      peritoneal dialysis V56.32
    adjustment (of)
      artificial
        arm (complete) (partial) V52.0
        eye V52.2
        leg (complete) (partial) V52.1
      brain neuropacemaker V53.02
      breast
        implant V52.4
        prosthesis V52.4
      cardiac device V53.39
        defibrillator, automatic implantable V53.32
        pacemaker V53.31
          carotid sinus V53.39
      catheter
        non-vascular V58.82
        vascular V58.81
      cerebral ventricle (communicating) shunt V53.01
      colostomy belt V55.3
      contact lenses V53.1
      cystostomy device V55.3
      dental prosthesis V52.3
      device NEC V53.9
        abdominal V53.5
        cardiac V53.39
          defibrillator, automatic implantable V53.32
          pacemaker V53.31
            carotid sinus V53.39
        cerebral ventricle (communicating) shunt V53.01
        intrauterine contraceptive V25.1
        nervous system V53.09

Admission — continued
  for — continued
    adjustment (of) — continued
      device NEC — continued
        orthodontic V53.4
        prosthetic V52.9
          breast V52.4
          dental V52.3
          eye V52.2
          specified type NEC V52.8
        special senses V53.09
        substitution
          auditory V53.09
          nervous system V53.09
          visual V53.09
        urinary V53.6
      dialysis catheter
        extracorporeal V56.1
        peritoneal V56.2
      diaphragm (contraceptive) V25.02
      hearing aid V53.2
      ileostomy device V55.2
      intestinal appliance or device NEC V53.5
      intrauterine contraceptive device V25.1
      neuropacemaker (brain) (peripheral nerve) (spinal cord) V53.02
      orthodontic device V53.4
      orthopedic (device) V53.7
        brace V53.7
        cast V53.7
        shoes V53.7
      pacemaker
        brain V53.02
        cardiac V53.31
        carotid sinus V53.39
        peripheral nerve V53.02
        spinal cord V53.02
      prosthesis V52.9
        arm (complete) (partial) V52.0
        breast V52.4
        dental V52.3
        eye V52.2
        leg (complete) (partial) V52.1
        specified type NEC V52.8
      spectacles V53.1
      wheelchair V53.8
    adoption referral or proceedings V68.89
    aftercare (see also Aftercare) V58.9
      cardiac pacemaker V53.31
      chemotherapy V58.1
      dialysis
        extracorporeal (renal) V56.0
        peritoneal V56.8
        renal V56.0
      fracture (see also Aftercare, fracture) V54.9
      medical NEC V58.89
      orthopedic V54.9
        specified care NEC V54.89 ▲
      pacemaker device
        brain V53.02
        cardiac V53.31
        carotid sinus V53.39
        nervous system V53.02
        spinal cord V53.02
      postoperative NEC V58.49
        wound closure, planned V58.41
      postpartum
        immediately after delivery V24.0
        routine follow-up V24.2
      postradiation V58.0

Admission — Index to Diseases

Admission — *continued*
  for — *continued*
    aftercare — *continued*
      radiation therapy V58.0
      removal of
        non-vascular catheter V58.82
        vascular catheter V58.81
      specified NEC V58.89
      surgical NEC V58.49
      wound closure, planned V58.41
    artificial insemination V26.1
    attention to artificial opening (of) V55.9
      artificial vagina V55.7
      colostomy V55.3
      cystostomy V55.5
      enterostomy V55.4
      gastrostomy V55.1
      ileostomy V55.2
      jejunostomy V55.4
      nephrostomy V55.6
      specified site NEC V55.8
        intestinal tract V55.4
        urinary tract V55.6
      tracheostomy V55.0
      ureterostomy V55.6
      urethrostomy V55.6
    battery replacement
      cardiac pacemaker V53.31
    boarding V65.0
    breast
      augmentation or reduction V50.1
      removal, prophylactic V50.41
    change of
      cardiac pacemaker (battery) V53.31
      carotid sinus pacemaker V53.39
      catheter in artificial opening — *see*
        Attention to, artificial, opening
      dressing V58.3
      fixation device
        external V54.89 ▲
        internal V54.0
      Kirschner wire V54.89 ▲
      neuropacemaker device (brain)
        (peripheral nerve) (spinal cord)
        V53.02
      pacemaker device
        brain V53.02
        cardiac V53.31
        carotid sinus V53.39
        nervous system V53.02
      plaster cast V54.89 ▲
      splint, external V54.89 ▲
      Steinmann pin V54.89 ▲
      surgical dressing V58.3
      traction device V54.89 ▲
    checkup only V70.0
    chemotherapy V58.1
    circumcision, ritual or routine (in absence
      of medical indication) V50.2
    clinical research investigation (control)
      (normal comparison) (participant)
      V70.7
    closure of artificial opening — *see* Attention
      to, artificial, opening
    contraceptive
      counseling V25.09
      management V25.9
        specified type NEC V25.8
    convalescence following V66.9
      chemotherapy V66.2
      psychotherapy V66.3

Admission — *continued*
  for — *continued*
    convalescence following — *continued*
      radiotherapy V66.1
      surgery V66.0
      treatment (for) V66.5
        combined V66.6
        fracture V66.4
        mental disorder NEC V66.3
        specified condition NEC V66.5
    cosmetic surgery NEC V50.1
      following healed injury or operation V51
    counseling (*see also* Counseling) V65.40
      without complaint or sickness V65.49
      contraceptive management V25.09
      dietary V65.3
      exercise V65.41
      for
        nonattending third party V65.1
        victim of abuse
          child V61.21
          partner or spouse V61.11
      genetic V26.3
      gonorrhea V65.45
      HIV V65.44
      human immunodeficiency virus V65.44
      injury prevention V65.43
      procreative management V26.4
      sexually transmitted disease NEC
        V65.45
        HIV V65.44
      specified reason NEC V65.49
      substance use and abuse V65.42
      syphilis V65.45
      victim of abuse
        child V61.21
        partner or spouse V61.11
    desensitization to allergens V07.1
    dialysis V56.0
      catheter
        fitting and adjustment
          extracorporeal V56.1
          peritoneal V56.2
        removal or replacement
          extracorporeal V56.1
          peritoneal V56.2
      extracorporeal (renal) V56.0
      peritoneal V56.8
      renal V56.0
    dietary surveillance and counseling V65.3
    drug monitoring, therapeutic V58.83
    ear piercing V50.3
    elective surgery V50.9
      breast
        augmentation or reduction V50.1
        removal, prophylactic V50.41
      circumcision, ritual or routine (in
        absence of medical indication)
        V50.2
      cosmetic NEC V50.1
        following healed injury or operation
          V51
      ear piercing V50.3
      face-lift V50.1
      hair transplant V50.0
      plastic
        cosmetic NEC V50.1
        following healed injury or operation
          V51
      prophylactic organ removal V50.49
        breast V50.41
        ovary V50.42

Admission — *continued*
  for — *continued*
    elective surgery — *continued*
      repair of scarred tissue (following healed injury or operation) V51
      specified type NEC V50.8
    end-of-life care V66.7
    examination (*see also* Examination) V70.9
      administrative purpose NEC V70.3
      adoption V70.3
      allergy V72.7
      at health care facility V70.0
      athletic team V70.3
      camp V70.3
      cardiovascular, preoperative V72.81
      clinical research investigation (control) (participant) V70.7
      dental V72.2
      developmental testing (child) (infant) V20.2
      donor (potential) V70.8
      driver's license V70.3
      ear V72.1
      employment V70.5
      eye V72.0
      follow-up (routine) — *see* Examination, follow-up
      for admission to
        old age home V70.3
        school V70.3
      general V70.9
        specified reason NEC V70.8
      gynecological V72.3
      health supervision (child) (infant) V20.2
      hearing V72.1
      immigration V70.3
      insurance certification V70.3
      laboratory V72.6
      marriage license V70.3
      medical (general) (*see also* Examination, medical) V70.9
      medicolegal reasons V70.4
      naturalization V70.3
      pelvic (annual) (periodic) V72.3
      postpartum checkup V24.2
      pregnancy (possible) (unconfirmed) V72.4
      preoperative V72.84
        cardiovascular V72.81
        respiratory V72.82
        specified NEC V72.83
      prison V70.3
      psychiatric (general) V70.2
        requested by authority V70.1
      radiological NEC V72.5
      respiratory, preoperative V72.82
      school V70.3
      screening — *see* Screening
      skin hypersensitivity V72.7
      specified type NEC V72.85
      sport competition V70.3
      vision V72.0
      well baby and child care V20.2
    exercise therapy V57.1
    face-lift, cosmetic reason V50.1
    fitting (of)
      artificial
        arm (complete) (partial) V52.0
        eye V52.2
        leg (complete) (partial) V52.1
      biliary drainage tube V58.82

Admission — *continued*
  for — *continued*
    fitting (of) — *continued*
      brain neuropacemaker V53.02
      breast V52.4
        implant V52.4
        prosthesis V52.4
      cardiac pacemaker V53.31
      catheter
        non-vascular V58.82
        vascular V58.81
      cerebral ventricle (communicating) shunt V53.01
      chest tube V58.82
      colostomy belt V55.2
      contact lenses V53.1
      cystostomy device V53.6
      dental prosthesis V52.3
      device NEC V53.9
        abdominal V53.5
        cerebral ventricle (communicating) shunt V53.01
        intrauterine contraceptive V25.1
        nervous system V53.09
        orthodontic V53.4
        prosthetic V52.9
          breast V52.4
          dental V52.3
          eye V52.2
        special senses V53.09
        substitution
          auditory V53.09
          nervous system V53.09
          visual V53.09
      diaphragm (contraceptive) V25.02
      fistula (sinus tract) drainage tube V58.82
      hearing aid V53.2
      ileostomy device V55.2
      intestinal appliance or device NEC V53.5
      intrauterine contraceptive device V25.1
      neuropacemaker (brain) (peripheral nerve) (spinal cord) V53.02
      orthodontic device V53.4
      orthopedic (device) V53.7
        brace V53.7
        cast V53.7
        shoes V53.7
      pacemaker
        brain V53.02
        cardiac V53.31
        carotid sinus V53.39
        spinal cord V53.02
      pleural drainage tube V58.82
      prosthesis V52.9
        arm (complete) (partial) V52.0
        breast V52.4
        dental V52.3
        eye V52.2
        leg (complete) (partial) V52.1
        specified type NEC V52.8
      spectacles V53.1
      wheelchair V53.8
    follow-up examination (routine) (following) V67.9
      cancer chemotherapy V67.2
      chemotherapy V67.2
      high-risk medication NEC V67.51
      injury NEC V67.59
      psychiatric V67.3
      psychotherapy V67.3

Admission — continued
for — continued
    follow-up examination — continued
        radiotherapy V67.1
        specified surgery NEC V67.09
        surgery V67.00
            vaginal pap smear V67.01
        treatment (for) V67.9
            combined V67.6
            fracture V67.4
            involving high-risk medication NEC
                V67.51
            mental disorder V67.3
            specified NEC V67.59
    hair transplant, for cosmetic reason V50.0
    health advice, education, or instruction
        V65.4
    hospice care V66.7
    insertion (of)
        subdermal implantable contraceptive
            V25.5
        intrauterine device
            insertion V25.1
            management V25.42
    investigation to determine further
        disposition V63.8
    isolation V07.0
    issue of
        medical certificate NEC V68.0
        repeat prescription NEC V68.1
            contraceptive device NEC V25.49
    kidney dialysis V56.0
    mental health evaluation V70.2
        requested by authority V70.1
    nonmedical reason NEC V68.89
    nursing care evaluation V63.8
    observation (without need for further
        medical care) (see also Observation)
        V71.9
        accident V71.4
        alleged rape or seduction V71.5
        criminal assault V71.6
        following accident V71.4
            at work V71.3
        foreign body ingestion V71.89
        growth and development variations,
            childhood V21.0
        inflicted injury NEC V71.6
        ingestion of deleterious agent or foreign
            body V71.89
        injury V71.6
        malignant neoplasm V71.1
        mental disorder V71.09
        newborn — see Observation, suspected,
            condition, newborn
        rape V71.5
        specified NEC V71.89
        suspected disorder V71.9
            abuse V71.81
            accident V71.4
                at work V71.3
            benign neoplasm V71.89
            cardiovascular V71.7
            exposure
                anthrax V71.82
                biological agent NEC V71.83
            heart V71.7
            inflicted injury NEC V71.6
            malignant neoplasm V71.1
            mental NEC V71.09
            neglect V71.81

Admission — continued
for — continued
    observation — continued
        suspected disorder — continued
            specified condition NEC V71.89
            tuberculosis V71.2
        tuberculosis V71.2
    occupational therapy V57.21
    organ transplant, donor — see Donor
    ovary, ovarian removal, prophylactic
        V50.42
    palliative care V66.7
    Papanicolaou smear
        cervix V76.2
            for suspected malignant neoplasm
                V76.2
            no disease found V71.1
            routine, as part of gynecological
                examination V72.3
        vaginal V76.47
            following hysterectomy for malignant
                condition V67.01
    passage of sounds or bougie in artificial
        opening — see Attention to, artificial,
        opening
    paternity testing V70.4
    peritoneal dialysis V56.32
    physical therapy NEC V57.1
    plastic surgery
        cosmetic NEC V50.1
        following healed injury or operation V51
    postmenopausal hormone replacement
        therapy V07.4
    postpartum observation
        immediately after delivery V24.0
        routine follow-up V24.2
    poststerilization (for restoration) V26.0
    procreative management V26.9
        specified type NEC V26.8
    prophylactic
        administration of
            antibiotics V07.39
            antitoxin, any V07.2
            antivenin V07.2
            chemotherapeutic agent NEC V07.39
            chemotherapy NEC V07.39
            diphtheria antitoxin V07.2
            fluoride V07.31
            gamma globulin V07.2
            immune sera (gamma globulin) V07.2
            RhoGAM V07.2
            tetanus antitoxin V07.2
        breathing exercises V57.0
        chemotherapy NEC V07.39
            fluoride V07.31
        measure V07.9
            specified type NEC V07.8
        organ removal V50.49
            breast V50.41
            ovary V50.42
    psychiatric examination (general) V70.2
        requested by authority V70.1
    radiation management V58.0
    radiotherapy V58.0
    reforming of artificial opening — see
        Attention to, artificial, opening
    rehabilitation V57.9
        multiple types V57.89
        occupational V57.21
        orthoptic V57.4
        orthotic V57.81
        physical NEC V57.1

Index to Diseases — Admission

Admission — continued
  for — continued
    rehabilitation — continued
      specified type NEC V57.89
      speech V57.3
      vocational V57.22
    removal of
      cardiac pacemaker V53.31
      cast (plaster) V54.89 ▲
      catheter from artificial opening — see Attention to, artificial, opening
      cerebral ventricle (communicating) shunt V53.01
      cystostomy catheter V55.5
      device
        cerebral ventricle (communicating) shunt V53.01
        fixation
          external V54.89 ▲
          internal V54.0
        intrauterine contraceptive V25.42
        traction, external V54.89 ▲
      dressing V58.3
      fixation device
        external V54.89 ▲
        internal V54.0
      intrauterine contraceptive device V25.42
      Kirschner wire V54.89 ▲
      neuropacemaker (brain) (peripheral nerve) (spinal cord) V53.02
      orthopedic fixation device
        external V54.89 ▲
        internal V54.0
      pacemaker device
        brain V53.02
        cardiac V53.31
        carotid sinus V53.39
        nervous system V53.02
      plaster cast V54.89 ▲
      plate (fracture) V54.0
      rod V54.0
      screw (fracture) V54.0
      splint, traction V54.89 ▲
      Steinmann pin V54.89 ▲
      subdermal implantable contraceptive V25.43
      surgical dressing V58.3
      sutures V58.3
      traction device, external V54.89 ▲
      ureteral stent V53.6
    repair of scarred tissue (following healed injury or operation) V51
    reprogramming of cardiac pacemaker V53.31
    restoration of organ continuity (poststerilization) (tuboplasty) (vasoplasty) V26.0
    sensitivity test — see also Test, skin
      allergy NEC V72.7
      bacterial disease NEC V74.9
      Dick V74.8
      Kveim V82.89
      Mantoux V74.1
      mycotic infection NEC V75.4
      parasitic disease NEC V75.8
      Schick V74.3
      Schultz-Charlton V74.8
    social service (agency) referral or evaluation V63.8
    speech therapy V57.3
    sterilization V25.2

Admission — continued
  for — continued
    suspected disorder (ruled out) (without need for further care) — see Observation
    terminal care V66.7
    tests only — see Test
    therapeutic drug monitoring V58.83
    therapy
      blood transfusion, without reported diagnosis V58.2
      breathing exercises V57.0
      chemotherapy V58.1
        prophylactic NEC V07.39
          fluoride V07.31
      dialysis (intermittent) (treatment)
        extracorporeal V56.0
        peritoneal V56.8
        renal V56.0
        specified type NEC V56.8
      exercise (remedial) NEC V57.1
        breathing V57.0
      long-term (current) drug use NEC V58.69
        antibiotics V58.62
        anticoagulant V58.61
      occupational V57.21
      orthoptic V57.4
      physical NEC V57.1
      radiation V58.0
      speech V57.3
      vocational V57.22
    toilet or cleaning
      of artificial opening — see Attention to, artificial, opening
      of non-vascular catheter V58.82
      of vascular catheter V58.81
    tubal ligation V25.2
    tuboplasty for previous sterilization V26.0
    vaccination, prophylactic (against)
      arthropod-borne virus, viral NEC V05.1
        disease NEC V05.1
        encephalitis V05.0
      Bacille Calmette Guérin (BCG) V03.2
      BCG V03.2
      chickenpox V05.4
      cholera alone V03.0
        with typhoid-paratyphoid (cholera + TAB) V06.0
      common cold V04.7
      dengue V05.1
      diphtheria alone V03.5
      diphtheria-tetanus [Td] without pertussis V06.5
      diphtheria-tetanus-pertussis (DTP) V06.1
        with
          poliomyelitis (DTP + polio) V06.3
          typhoid-paratyphoid (DTP + TAB) V06.2
      disease (single) NEC V05.9
        bacterial NEC V03.9
          specified type NEC V03.89
        combinations NEC V06.9
          specified type NEC V06.8
        specified type NEC V05.8
      encephalitis, viral, arthropod-borne V05.0
      Hemophilus infuenzae, type B [Hib] V03.81
      hepatitis, viral V05.3

Admission — *continued*
  for — *continued*
    vaccination, prophylactic — *continued*
      immune sera (gamma globulin) V07.2
      influenza V04.8
        with
          Streptococcus pneumoniae [pneumococcus] V06.6
      Leishmaniasis V05.2
      measles alone V04.2
      measles-mumps-rubella (MMR) V06.4
      mumps alone V04.6
        with measles and rubella (MMR) V06.4
      not done because of contraindication V64.0
      pertussis alone V03.6
      plague V03.3
      pneumonia V03.82
      poliomyelitis V04.0
        with diphtheria-tetanus-pertussis (DTP+ polio) V06.3
      rabies V04.5
      rubella alone V04.3
        with measles and mumps (MMR) V06.4
      smallpox V04.1
      specified type NEC V05.8
      Streptococcus pneumoniae [pneumococcus] V03.82
        with
          influenza V06.6
      tetanus toxoid alone V03.7
        with diphtheria [Td] V06.5
          and pertussis (DTP) V06.1
      tuberculosis (BCG) V03.2
      tularemia V03.4
      typhoid alone V03.1
        with diphtheria-tetanus-pertussis (TAB + DTP) V06.2
      typhoid-paratyphoid alone (TAB) V03.1
      typhus V05.8
      varicella (chicken pox) V05.4
      viral encephalitis, arthropod-borne V05.0
      viral hepatitis V05.3
      yellow fever V04.4
    vasectomy V25.2
    vasoplasty for previous sterilization V26.0
    vision examination V72.0
    vocational therapy V57.22
    waiting period for admission to other facility V63.2
      undergoing social agency investigation V63.8
    well baby and child care V20.2
    x-ray of chest
      for suspected tuberculosis V71.2
      routine V72.5
Adnexitis (suppurative) (*see also* Salpingo-oophoritis) 614.2
Adolescence NEC V21.2
Adoption
  agency referral V68.89
  examination V70.3
  held for V68.89
Adrenal gland — *see* condition
Adrenalism 255.9
  tuberculous (*see also* Tuberculosis) 017.6 ✓5th

Adrenalitis, adrenitis 255.8
  meningococcal hemorrhagic 036.3
Adrenarche, precocious 259.1
Adrenocortical syndrome 255.2
Adrenogenital syndrome (acquired) (congenital) 255.2
  iatrogenic, fetus or newborn 760.79
Adventitious bursa — *see* Bursitis
Adynamia (episodica) (hereditary) (periodic) 359.3
Adynamic
  ileus or intestine (*see also* Ileus) 560.1
  ureter 753.22
Aeration lung, imperfect, newborn 770.5
Aerobullosis 993.3
Aerocele — *see* Embolism, air
Aerodermectasia
  subcutaneous (traumatic) 958.7
    surgical 998.81
  surgical 998.81
Aerodontalgia 993.2
Aeroembolism 993.3
Aerogenes capsulatus infection (*see also* Gangrene, gas) 040.0
Aero-otitis media 993.0
Aerophagy, aerophagia 306.4
  psychogenic 306.4
Aerosinusitis 993.1
Aerotitis 993.0
Affection, affections — *see also* Disease
  sacroiliac (joint), old 724.6
  shoulder region NEC 726.2
Afibrinogenemia 286.3
  acquired 286.6
  congenital 286.3
  postpartum 666.3 ✓5th
African
  sleeping sickness 086.5
  tick fever 087.1
  trypanosomiasis 086.5
    Gambian 086.3
    Rhodesian 086.4
Aftercare V58.9
  artificial openings — *see* Attention to, artificial, opening
  blood transfusion without reported diagnosis V58.2
  breathing exercise V57.0
  cardiac device V53.39
    defibrillator, automatic implantable V53.32
    pacemaker V53.31
      carotid sinus V53.39
  carotid sinus pacemaker V53.39
  cerebral ventricle (communicating) shunt V53.01
  chemotherapy session (adjunctive) (maintenance) V58.1
  defibrillator, automatic implantable cardiac V53.32
  exercise (remedial) (therapeutic) V57.1
    breathing V57.0
  extracorporeal dialysis (intermittent) (treatment) V56.0
  following surgery NEC V58.49
    for
      injury V58.43
      neoplasm V58.42
      trauma V58.43

Index to Diseases

Aftercare — *continued*
  following surgery NEC — *continued*
    joint replacement V54.81
    of
      circulatory system V58.73
      digestive system V58.75
      genital organs V58.76
      genitourinary system V58.76
      musculoskeletal system V58.78
      nervous system V58.72
      oral cavity V58.75
      respiratory system V58.74
      sense organs V58.71
      skin V58.77
      subcutaneous tissue V58.77
      teeth V58.75
      urinary system V58.76
    wound closure, planned V58.41
  fracture V54.9
    healing V54.89
      pathologic
        arm V54.20
          lower V54.22
          upper V54.21
        hip V54.23
        leg V54.24
          lower V54.26
          upper V54.25
        specified site NEC V54.29
        vertebrae V54.27
      traumatic
        arm V54.10
          lower V54.12
          upper V54.11
        hip V54.13
        leg V54.14
          lower V54.16
          upper V54.15
        specified site NEC V54.19
        vertebrae V54.17
    removal of
      external fixation device V54.89
      internal fixation device V54.0
    specified care NEC V54.89
  gait training V57.1
    for use of artificial limb(s) V57.81
  involving
    dialysis (intermittent) (treatment)
      extracorporeal V56.0
      peritoneal V56.8
      renal V56.0
    gait training V57.1
      for use of artificial limb(s) V57.81
    orthoptic training V57.4
    orthotic training V57.81
    radiotherapy session V58.0
    removal of
      dressings V58.3
      fixation device
        external V54.89
        internal V54.0
      fracture plate V54.0
      pins V54.0
      plaster cast V54.89
      rods V54.0
      screws V54.0
      surgical dressings V58.3
      sutures V58.3
      traction device, external V54.89
  neuropacemaker (brain) (peripheral nerve)
    (spinal cord) V53.02

Aftercare — *continued*
  occupational therapy V57.21
  orthodontic V58.5
  orthopedic V54.9
    change of external fixation or traction
      device V54.89
    following joint replacement V54.81
    removal of fixation device
      external V54.89
      internal V54.0
    specified care NEC V54.89
  orthoptic training V57.4
  orthotic training V57.81
  pacemaker
    brain V53.02
    cardiac V53.31
    carotid sinus V53.39
    peripheral nerve V53.02
    spinal cord V53.02
  peritoneal dialysis (intermittent) (treatment)
    V56.8
  physical therapy NEC V57.1
    breathing exercises V57.0
  radiotherapy session V58.0
  rehabilitation procedure V57.9
    breathing exercises V57.0
    multiple types V57.89
    occupational V57.21
    orthoptic V57.4
    orthotic V57.81
    physical therapy NEC V57.1
    remedial exercises V57.1
    specified type NEC V57.89
    speech V57.3
    therapeutic exercises V57.1
    vocational V57.22
  renal dialysis (intermittent) (treatment) V56.0
  specified type NEC V58.89
    removal of non-vascular catheter V58.82
    removal of vascular catheter V58.81
  speech therapy V57.3
  vocational rehabilitation V57.22
After-cataract 366.50
  obscuring vision 366.53
  specified type, not obscuring vision 366.52
Agalactia 676.4
Agammaglobulinemia 279.00
  with lymphopenia 279.2
  acquired (primary) (secondary) 279.06
  Bruton's X-linked 279.04
  infantile sex-linked (Bruton's) (congenital)
    279.04
  Swiss-type 279.2
Aganglionosis (bowel) (colon) 751.3
AGCUS (atypical glandular cell changes of
  undetermined significance)
  favor benign 795.01
  favor dysplasia 795.02
Age (old) (*see also* Senile) 797
Agenesis — *see also* Absence, by site, congenital
  acoustic nerve 742.8
  adrenal (gland) 759.1
  alimentary tract (complete) (partial) NEC 751.8
    lower 751.2
    upper 750.8
  anus, anal (canal) 751.2
  aorta 747.22
  appendix 751.2
  arm (complete) (partial) (*see also* Deformity,
    reduction, upper limb) 755.20

Agenesis — *continued*
  artery (peripheral) NEC (*see also* Anomaly,
    peripheral vascular system) 747.60
    brain 747.81
    coronary 746.85
    pulmonary 747.3
    umbilical 747.5
  auditory (canal) (external) 744.01
  auricle (ear) 744.01
  bile, biliary duct or passage 751.61
  bone NEC 756.9
  brain 740.0
    specified part 742.2
  breast 757.6
  bronchus 748.3
  canaliculus lacrimalis 743.65
  carpus NEC (*see also* Deformity, reduction,
    upper limb) 755.28
  cartilage 756.9
  cecum 751.2
  cerebellum 742.2
  cervix 752.49
  chin 744.89
  cilia 743.63
  circulatory system, part NEC 747.89
  clavicle 755.51
  clitoris 752.49
  coccyx 756.13
  colon 751.2
  corpus callosum 742.2
  cricoid cartilage 748.3
  diaphragm (with hernia) 756.6
  digestive organ(s), or tract (complete) (partial)
    NEC 751.8
    lower 751.2
    upper 750.8
  ductus arteriosus 747.89
  duodenum 751.1
  ear NEC 744.09
    auricle 744.01
    lobe 744.21
  ejaculatory duct 752.8
  endocrine (gland) NEC 759.2
  epiglottis 748.3
  esophagus 750.3
  Eustachian tube 744.24
  extrinsic muscle, eye 743.69
  eye 743.00
    adnexa 743.69
  eyelid (fold) 743.62
  face
    bones NEC 756.0
    specified part NEC 744.89
  fallopian tube 752.19
  femur NEC (*see also* Absence, femur,
    congenital) 755.34
  fibula NEC (*see also* Absence, fibula,
    congenital) 755.37
  finger NEC (*see also* Absence, finger,
    congenital) 755.29
  foot (complete) (*see also* Deformity, reduction,
    lower limb) 755.31
  gallbladder 751.69
  gastric 750.8
  genitalia, genital (organ)
    female 752.8
      external 752.49
      internal NEC 752.8
    male 752.8
      penis 752.69
  glottis 748.3

Agenesis — *continued*
  gonadal 758.6
  hair 757.4
  hand (complete) (*see also* Deformity,
    reduction, upper limb) 755.21
  heart 746.89
    valve NEC 746.89
      aortic 746.89
      mitral 746.89
      pulmonary 746.01
  hepatic 751.69
  humerus NEC (*see also* Absence, humerus,
    congenital) 755.24
  hymen 752.49
  ileum 751.1
  incus 744.04
  intestine (small) 751.1
    large 751.2
  iris (dilator fibers) 743.45
  jaw 524.09
  jejunum 751.1
  kidney(s) (partial) (unilateral) 753.0
  labium (majus) (minus) 752.49
  labyrinth, membranous 744.05
  lacrimal apparatus (congenital) 743.65
  larynx 748.3
  leg NEC (*see also* Deformity, reduction, lower
    limb) 755.30
  lens 743.35
  limb (complete) (partial) (*see also* Deformity,
    reduction) 755.4
    lower NEC 755.30
    upper 755.20
  lip 750.26
  liver 751.69
  lung (bilateral) (fissures) (lobe) (unilateral)
    748.5
  mandible 524.09
  maxilla 524.09
  metacarpus NEC 755.28
  metatarsus NEC 755.38
  muscle (any) 756.81
  musculoskeletal system NEC 756.9
  nail(s) 757.5
  neck, part 744.89
  nerve 742.8
  nervous system, part NEC 742.8
  nipple 757.6
  nose 748.1
  nuclear 742.8
  organ
    of Corti 744.05
    or site not listed — *see* Anomaly, specified
      type NEC
  osseous meatus (ear) 744.03
  ovary 752.0
  oviduct 752.19
  pancreas 751.7
  parathyroid (gland) 759.2
  patella 755.64
  pelvic girdle (complete) (partial) 755.69
  penis 752.69
  pericardium 746.89
  perineal body 756.81
  pituitary (gland) 759.2
  prostate 752.8
  pulmonary
    artery 747.3
    trunk 747.3
    vein 747.49
  punctum lacrimale 743.65

Agenesis — *continued*
  radioulnar NEC (*see also* Absence, forearm, congenital) 755.25
  radius NEC (*see also* Absence, radius, congenital) 755.26
  rectum 751.2
  renal 753.0
  respiratory organ NEC 748.9
  rib 756.3
  roof of orbit 742.0
  round ligament 752.8
  sacrum 756.13
  salivary gland 750.21
  scapula 755.59
  scrotum 752.8
  seminal duct or tract 752.8
  septum
    atrial 745.69
    between aorta and pulmonary artery 745.0
    ventricular 745.3
  shoulder girdle (complete) (partial) 755.59
  skull (bone) 756.0
    with
      anencephalus 740.0
      encephalocele 742.0
      hydrocephalus 742.3
        with spina bifida (*see also* Spina bifida) 741.0 ✓5ᵗʰ
      microcephalus 742.1
  spermatic cord 752.8
  spinal cord 742.59
  spine 756.13
    lumbar 756.13
      isthmus 756.11
      pars articularis 756.11
  spleen 759.0
  sternum 756.3
  stomach 750.7
  tarsus NEC 755.38
  tendon 756.81
  testicular 752.8
  testis 752.8
  thymus (gland) 759.2
  thyroid (gland) 243
    cartilage 748.3
  tibia NEC (*see also* Absence, tibia, congenital) 755.36
  tibiofibular NEC 755.35
  toe (complete) (partial) (*see also* Absence, toe, congenital) 755.39
  tongue 750.11
  trachea (cartilage) 748.3
  ulna NEC (*see also* Absence, ulna, congenital) 755.27
  ureter 753.4
  urethra 753.8
  urinary tract NEC 753.8
  uterus 752.3
  uvula 750.26
  vagina 752.49
  vas deferens 752.8
  vein(s) (peripheral) NEC (*see also* Anomaly, peripheral vascular system) 747.60
    brain 747.81
    great 747.49
    portal 747.49
    pulmonary 747.49
  vena cava (inferior) (superior) 747.49
  vermis of cerebellum 742.2

Agenesis — *continued*
  vertebra 756.13
    lumbar 756.13
      isthmus 756.11
      pars articularis 756.11
    vulva 752.49
Ageusia (*see also* Disturbance, sensation) 781.1
Aggressiveness 301.3
Aggressive outburst (*see also* Disturbance, conduct) 312.0 ✓5ᵗʰ
  in children and adolescents 313.9
Aging skin 701.8
Agitated — *see* condition
Agitation 307.9
  catatonic (*see also* Schizophrenia) 295.2 ✓5ᵗʰ
Aglossia (congenital) 750.11
Aglycogenosis 271.0
Agnail (finger) (with lymphangitis) 681.02
Agnosia (body image) (tactile) 784.69
  verbal 784.69
    auditory 784.69
      secondary to organic lesion 784.69
    developmental 315.8
    secondary to organic lesion 784.69
  visual 784.69
    developmental 315.8
    secondary to organic lesion 784.69
  visual 368.16
    developmental 315.31
Agoraphobia 300.22
  with panic attacks 300.21
Agrammatism 784.69
Agranulocytopenia 288.0
Agranulocytosis (angina) (chronic) (cyclical) (genetic) (infantile) (periodic) (pernicious) 288.0
Agraphia (absolute) 784.69
  with alexia 784.61
  developmental 315.39
Agrypnia (*see also* Insomnia) 780.52
Ague (*see also* Malaria) 084.6
  brass-founders' 985.8
  dumb 084.6
  tertian 084.1
Agyria 742.2
Ahumada-del Castillo syndrome (nonpuerperal galactorrhea and amenorrhea) 253.1
AIDS 042
AIDS-associated retrovirus (disease) (illness) 042
  infection — *see* Human immunodeficiency virus, infection
AIDS-associated virus (disease) (illness) 042
  infection — *see* Human immunodeficiency virus, infection
AIDS-like disease (illness) (syndrome) 042
AIDS-related complex 042
AIDS-related conditions 042
AIDS-related virus (disease) (illness) 042
  infection — *see* Human immunodeficiency virus, infection
AIDS virus (disease) (illness) 042
  infection — *see* Human immunodeficiency virus, infection
Ailment, heart — *see* Disease, heart
Ailurophobia 300.29

Ainhum (disease) 136.0
Air
 anterior mediastinum 518.1
 compressed, disease 993.3
 embolism (any site) (artery) (cerebral) 958.0
  with
   abortion — see Abortion, by type, with embolism
   ectopic pregnancy (see also categories 633.0-633.9) 639.6
   molar pregnancy (see also categories 630-632) 639.6
  due to implanted device — see Complications, due to (presence of) any device, implant, or graft classified to 996.0-996.5 NEC
  following
   abortion 639.6
   ectopic or molar pregnancy 639.6
   infusion, perfusion, or transfusion 999.1
  in pregnancy, childbirth, or puerperium 673.0
  traumatic 958.0
 hunger 786.09
  psychogenic 306.1
 leak (lung) (pulmonary) (thorax) 512.8
  iatrogenic 512.1
  postoperative 512.1
 rarefied, effects of — see Effect, adverse, high altitude
 sickness 994.6
Airplane sickness 994.6
Akathisia, acathisia 781.0
 due to drugs 333.99
Akinesia algera 352.6
Akiyami 100.89
Akureyri disease (epidemic neuromyasthenia) 049.8
Alacrima (congenital) 743.65
Alactasia (hereditary) 271.3
Alalia 784.3
 developmental 315.31
  receptive-expressive 315.32
 secondary to organic lesion 784.3
Alaninemia 270.8
Alastrim 050.1
Albarrán's disease (colibacilluria) 791.9
Albers-Schönberg's disease (marble bones) 756.52
Albert's disease 726.71
Albinism, albino (choroid) (cutaneous) (eye) (generalized) (isolated) (ocular) (oculocutaneous) (partial) 270.2
Albinismus 270.2
Albright (-Martin) (-Bantam) disease (pseudohypoparathyroidism) 275.49
Albright (-McCune) (-Sternberg) syndrome (osteitis fibrosa disseminata) 756.59
Albuminous — see condition
Albuminuria, albuminuric (acute) (chronic) (subacute) 791.0
 Bence-Jones 791.0
 cardiac 785.9
 complicating pregnancy, childbirth, or puerperium 646.2
  with hypertension — see Toxemia, of pregnancy
 affecting fetus or newborn 760.1

Albuminuria, albuminuric — continued
 cyclic 593.6
 gestational 646.2
 gravidarum 646.2
  with hypertension — see Toxemia, of pregnancy
  affecting fetus or newborn 760.1
 heart 785.9
 idiopathic 593.6
 orthostatic 593.6
 postural 593.6
 pre-eclamptic (mild) 642.4
  affecting fetus or newborn 760.0
  severe 642.5
   affecting fetus or newborn 760.0
 recurrent physiologic 593.6
 scarlatinal 034.1
Albumosuria 791.0
 Bence-Jones 791.0
 myelopathic (M9730/3) 203.0
Alcaptonuria 270.2
Alcohol, alcoholic
 abstinence 291.81
 acute intoxication 305.0
  with dependence 303.0
 addiction (see also Alcoholism) 303.9
  maternal
   with suspected fetal damage affecting management of pregnancy 655.4
   affecting fetus or newborn 760.71
 amnestic disorder, persisting 291.1
 anxiety 291.89
 brain syndrome, chronic 291.2
 cardiopathy 425.5
 chronic (see also Alcoholism) 303.9
 cirrhosis (liver) 571.2
 delirium 291.0
  acute 291.0
  chronic 291.1
  tremens 291.0
  withdrawal 291.0
 dementia NEC 291.2
 deterioration 291.2
 drunkenness (simple) 305.0
 hallucinosis (acute) 291.3
 insanity 291.9
 intoxication (acute) 305.0
  with dependence 303.0
  pathological 291.4
 jealousy 291.5
 Korsakoff's, Korsakov's, Korsakow's 291.1
 liver NEC 571.3
  acute 571.1
  chronic 571.2
 mania (acute) (chronic) 291.9
 mood 291.89
 paranoia 291.5
 paranoid (type) psychosis 291.5
 pellagra 265.2
 poisoning, accidental (acute) NEC 980.9
  specified type of alcohol — see Table of Drugs and Chemicals
 psychosis (see also Psychosis, alcoholic) 291.9
  Korsakoff's, Korsakov's, Korsakow's 291.1
 polyneuritic 291.1
  with
   delusions 291.5
   hallucinations 291.3

Index to Diseases

Alcohol, alcoholic — *continued*
  withdrawal symptoms, syndrome NEC 291.81
    delirium 291.0
    hallucinosis 291.3
Alcoholism 303.9 ✓5ᵗʰ

> Note — *Use the following fifth-digit subclassification with category 303:*
>
> 0   unspecified
> 1   continuous
> 2   episodic
> 3   in remission

  with psychosis (*see also* Psychosis, alcoholic) 291.9
  acute 303.0 ✓5ᵗʰ
  chronic 303.9 ✓5ᵗʰ
    with psychosis 291.9
  complicating pregnancy, childbirth, or puerperium 648.4 ✓5ᵗʰ
    affecting fetus or newborn 760.71
  history V11.3
  Korsakoff's, Korsakov's, Korsakow's 291.1
  suspected damage to fetus affecting management of pregnancy 655.4 ✓5ᵗʰ
Alder's anomaly or syndrome (leukocyte granulation anomaly) 288.2
Alder-Reilly anomaly (leukocyte granulation) 288.2
Aldosteronism (primary) (secondary) 255.1
  congenital 255.1
Aldosteronoma (M8370/1) 237.2
Aldrich (-Wiskott) syndrome (eczema-thrombocytopenia) 279.12
Aleppo boil 085.1
Aleukemic — *see* condition
Aleukia
  congenital 288.0
  hemorrhagica 284.9
    acquired (secondary) 284.8
    congenital 284.0
    idiopathic 284.9
  splenica 289.4
Alexia (congenital) (developmental) 315.01
  secondary to organic lesion 784.61
Algoneurodystrophy 733.7
Algophobia 300.29
Alibert's disease (mycosis fungoides) (M9700/3) 202.1 ✓5ᵗʰ
Alibert-Bazin disease (M9700/3) 202.1 ✓5ᵗʰ
Alice in Wonderland syndrome 293.89
Alienation, mental (*see also* Psychosis) 298.9
Alkalemia 276.3
Alkalosis 276.3
  metabolic 276.3
    with respiratory acidosis 276.4
  respiratory 276.3
Alkaptonuria 270.2
Allen-Masters syndrome 620.6
Allergic bronchopulmonary aspergillosis 518.6
Allergy, allergic (reaction) 995.3
  air-borne substance (*see also* Fever, hay) 477.9
    specified allergen NEC 477.8
  alveolitis (extrinsic) 495.9
    due to
      Aspergillus clavatus 495.4
      cryptostroma corticale 495.6

Allergy, allergic — *continued*
  alveolitis — *continued*
    due to — *continued*
      organisms (fungal, thermophilic actinomycete, other) growing in ventilation (air conditioning systems) 495.7
    specified type NEC 495.8
  anaphylactic shock 999.4
    due to food — *see* Anaphylactic shock, due to, food
  angioneurotic edema 995.1
  animal (dander) (epidermal) (hair) 477.8
  arthritis (*see also* Arthritis, allergic) 716.2 ✓5ᵗʰ
  asthma — *see* Asthma
  bee sting (anaphylactic shock) 989.5
  biological — *see* Allergy, drug
  bronchial asthma — *see* Asthma
  conjunctivitis (eczematous) 372.14
  dander (animal) 477.8
  dandruff 477.8
  dermatitis (venenata) — *see* Dermatitis
  diathesis V15.09
  drug, medicinal substance, and biological (any) (correct medicinal substance properly administered) (external) (internal) 995.2
    wrong substance given or taken NEC 977.9
      specified drug or substance — *see* Table of Drugs and Chemicals
  dust (house) (stock) 477.8
  eczema — *see* Eczema
  endophthalmitis 360.19
  epidermal (animal) 477.8
  feathers 477.8
  food (any) (ingested) 693.1
    atopic 691.8
    in contact with skin 692.5
  gastritis 535.4 ✓5ᵗʰ
  gastroenteritis 558.3
  gastrointestinal 558.3
  grain 477.0
  grass (pollen) 477.0
    asthma (*see also* Asthma) 493.0 ✓5ᵗʰ
    hay fever 477.0
  hair (animal) 477.8
  hay fever (grass) (pollen) (ragweed) (tree) (*see also* Fever, hay) 477.9
  history (of) V15.09
    to
      eggs V15.03
      food additives V15.05
      insect bite V15.06
      latex V15.07
      milk products V15.02
      nuts V15.05
        peanuts V15.01
      radiographic dye V15.08
      seafood V15.04
      specified food NEC V15.05
      spider bite V15.06
  horse serum — *see* Allergy, serum
  inhalant 477.9
    dust 477.8
    pollen 477.0
    specified allergen other than pollen 477.8
  kapok 477.8
  medicine — *see* Allergy, drug
  migraine 346.2 ✓5ᵗʰ
  pannus 370.62
  pneumonia 518.3

Allergy, allergic — continued
  pollen (any) (hay fever) 477.0
    asthma (see also Asthma) 493.0 ✓5ᵗʰ
  primrose 477.0
  primula 477.0
  purpura 287.0
  ragweed (pollen) (Senecio jacobaea) 477.0
    asthma (see also Asthma) 493.0 ✓5ᵗʰ
    hay fever 477.0
  respiratory (see also Allergy, inhalant) 477.9
    due to
      drug — see Allergy, drug
      food — see Allergy, food
  rhinitis (see also Fever, hay) 477.9
    due to food 477.1
  rose 477.0
  Senecio jacobae 477.0
  serum (prophylactic) (therapeutic) 999.5
    anaphylactic shock 999.4
  shock (anaphylactic) (due to adverse effect of correct medicinal substance properly administered) 995.0
    food — (see Anaphylactic shock, due to, food
    from serum or immunization 999.5
      anaphylactic 999.4
  sinusitis (see also Fever, hay) 477.9
  skin reaction 692.9
    specified substance — see Dermatitis, due to
  tree (any) (hay fever) (pollen) 477.0
    asthma (see also Asthma) 493.0 ✓5ᵗʰ
  upper respiratory (see also Fever, hay) 477.9
  urethritis 597.89
  urticaria 708.0
  vaccine — see Allergy, serum
Allescheriosis 117.6
Alligator skin disease (ichthyosis congenita) 757.1
  acquired 701.1
Allocheiria, allochiria (see also Disturbance, sensation) 782.0
Almeida's disease (Brazilian blastomycosis) 116.1
Alopecia (atrophicans) (pregnancy) (premature) (senile) 704.00
  adnata 757.4
  areata 704.01
  celsi 704.01
  cicatrisata 704.09
  circumscripta 704.01
  congenital, congenitalis 757.4
  disseminata 704.01
  effluvium (telogen) 704.02
  febrile 704.09
  generalisata 704.09
  hereditaria 704.09
  marginalis 704.01
  mucinosa 704.09
  postinfectional 704.09
  seborrheica 704.09
  specific 091.82
  syphilitic (secondary) 091.82
  telogen effluvium 704.02
  totalis 704.09
  toxica 704.09
  universalis 704.09
  x-ray 704.09
Alpers' disease 330.8
Alpha-lipoproteinemia 272.4

Alpha thalassemia 282.4
Alphos 696.1
Alpine sickness 993.2
Alport's syndrome (hereditary hematurianephropathy-deafness) 759.89
Alteration (of), altered
  awareness 780.09
    transient 780.02
  consciousness 780.09
    persistent vegetative state 780.03
    transient 780.02
  mental status 780.99 ▲
Alternaria (infection) 118
Alternating — see condition
Altitude, high (effects) — see Effect, adverse, high altitude
Aluminosis (of lung) 503
Alvarez syndrome (transient cerebral ischemia) 435.9
Alveolar capillary block syndrome 516.3
Alveolitis
  allergic (extrinsic) 495.9
    due to organisms (fungal, thermophilic actinomycete, other) growing in ventilation (air conditioning systems) 495.7
    specified type NEC 495.8
  due to
    Aspergillus clavatus 495.4
    Cryptostroma corticale 495.6
  fibrosing (chronic) (cryptogenic) (lung) 516.3
    idiopathic 516.3
    rheumatoid 714.81
  jaw 526.5
  sicca dolorosa 526.5
Alveolus, alveolar — see condition
Alymphocytosis (pure) 279.2
Alymphoplasia, thymic 279.2
Alzheimer's
  dementia (senile)
    with behavioral disturbance 331.0 [294.11]
    without behavioral disturbance 331.0 [294.10]
  disease or sclerosis 331.0
    with dementia — see Alzheimer's, dementia
Amastia (see also Absence, breast) 611.8
Amaurosis (acquired) (congenital) (see also Blindness) 369.00
  fugax 362.34
  hysterical 300.11
  Leber's (congenital) 362.76
  tobacco 377.34
  uremic — see Uremia
Amaurotic familial idiocy (infantile) (juvenile) (late) 330.1
Ambisexual 752.7
Amblyopia (acquired) (congenital) (partial) 368.00
  color 368.59
    acquired 368.55
  deprivation 368.02
  ex anopsia 368.00
  hysterical 300.11
  nocturnal 368.60
    vitamin A deficiency 264.5
  refractive 368.03
  strabismic 368.01
  suppression 368.01

Amblyopia — *continued*
  tobacco 377.34
  toxic NEC 377.34
  uremic — *see* Uremia
Ameba, amebic (histolytica) — *see also* Amebiasis
  abscess 006.3
    bladder 006.8
    brain (with liver and lung abscess) 006.5
    liver 006.3
      with
        brain abscess (and lung abscess) 006.5
        lung abscess 006.4
      lung (with liver abscess) 006.4
        with brain abscess 006.5
      seminal vesicle 006.8
      spleen 006.8
  carrier (suspected of) V02.2
  meningoencephalitis
    due to Naegleria (gruberi) 136.2
    primary 136.2
Amebiasis NEC 006.9
  with
    brain abscess (with liver or lung abscess) 006.5
    liver abscess (without mention of brain or lung abscess) 006.3
    lung abscess (with liver abscess) 006.4
      with brain abscess 006.5
  acute 006.0
  bladder 006.8
  chronic 006.1
  cutaneous 006.6
  cutis 006.6
  due to organism other than Entamoeba histolytica 007.8
  hepatic (*see also* Abscess, liver, amebic) 006.3
  nondysenteric 006.2
  seminal vesicle 006.8
  specified
    organism NEC 007.8
    site NEC 006.8
Ameboma 006.8
Amelia 755.4
  lower limb 755.31
  upper limb 755.21
Ameloblastoma (M9310/0) 213.1
  jaw (bone) (lower) 213.1
    upper 213.0
  long bones (M9261/3) — *see* Neoplasm, bone, malignant
  malignant (M9310/3) 170.1
    jaw (bone) (lower) 170.1
      upper 170.0
  mandible 213.1
  tibial (M9261/3) 170.7
Amelogenesis imperfecta 520.5
  nonhereditaria (segmentalis) 520.4
Amenorrhea (primary) (secondary) 626.0
  due to ovarian dysfunction 256.2
  hyperhormonal 256.8
Amentia (*see also* Retardation, mental) 319
  Meynert's (nonalcoholic) 294.0
    alcoholic 291.1
  nevoid 759.6
American
  leishmaniasis 085.5
  mountain tick fever 066.1

American — *continued*
  trypanosomiasis — *see* Trypanosomiasis, American
Ametropia (*see also* Disorder, accommodation) 367.9
Amianthosis 501
Amimia 784.69
Amino acid
  deficiency 270.9
    anemia 281.4
  metabolic disorder (*see also* Disorder, amino acid) 270.9
Aminoaciduria 270.9
  imidazole 270.5
Amnesia (retrograde) 780.99
  auditory 784.69
    developmental 315.31
    secondary to organic lesion 784.69
  hysterical or dissociative type 300.12
  psychogenic 300.12
  transient global 437.7
Amnestic (confabulatory) syndrome 294.0
  alcohol induced 291.1
  drug-induced 292.83
  posttraumatic 294.0
Amniocentesis screening (for) V28.2
  alphafetoprotein level, raised V28.1
  chromosomal anomalies V28.0
Amnion, amniotic — *see also* condition
  nodosum 658.8
Amnionitis (complicating pregnancy) 658.4
  affecting fetus or newborn 762.7
Amoral trends 301.7
Amotio retinae (*see also* Detachment, retina) 361.9
Ampulla
  lower esophagus 530.89
  phrenic 530.89
Amputation
  any part of fetus, to facilitate delivery 763.89
  cervix (supravaginal) (uteri) 622.8
    in pregnancy or childbirth 654.6
      affecting fetus or newborn 763.89
  clitoris — *see* Wound, open, clitoris
  congenital
    lower limb 755.31
    upper limb 755.21
  neuroma (traumatic) — *see also* Injury, nerve, by site
  surgical complication (late) 997.61
  penis — *see* Amputation, traumatic, penis
  status (without complication) — *see* Absence, by site, acquired
  stump (surgical) (posttraumatic)
    abnormal, painful, or with complication (late) 997.60
    healed or old NEC — *see also* Absence, by site, acquired
      lower V49.70
      upper V49.60
  traumatic (complete) (partial)

Note — "Complicated" includes traumatic amputation with delayed healing, delayed treatment, foreign body, or infection.

    arm 887.4
      at or above elbow 887.2
        complicated 887.3

Amputation — *continued*
  traumatic — *continued*
    arm — *continued*
      below elbow 887.0
        complicated 887.1
      both (bilateral) (any level(s)) 887.6
        complicated 887.7
      complicated 887.5
      finger(s) (one or both hands) 886.0
        with thumb(s) 885.0
          complicated 885.1
        complicated 886.1
    foot (except toe(s) only) 896.0
      and other leg 897.6
        complicated 897.7
      both (bilateral) 896.2
        complicated 896.3
      complicated 896.1
      toe(s) only (one or both feet) 895.0
        complicated 895.1
    genital organ(s) (external) NEC 878.8
      complicated 878.9
    hand (except finger(s) only) 887.0
      and other arm 887.6
        complicated 887.7
      both (bilateral) 887.6
        complicated 887.7
      complicated 887.1
      finger(s) (one or both hands) 886.0
        with thumb(s) 885.0
          complicated 885.1
        complicated 886.1
      thumb(s) (with fingers of either hand) 885.0
        complicated 885.1
    head 874.9
    late effect — *see* Late, effects (of), amputation
    leg 897.4
      and other foot 897.6
        complicated 897.7
      at or above knee 897.2
        complicated 897.3
      below knee 897.0
        complicated 897.1
      both (bilateral) 897.6
        complicated 897.7
      complicated 897.5
    lower limb(s) except toe(s) — *see* Amputation, traumatic, leg
    nose — *see* Wound, open, nose
    penis 878.0
      complicated 878.1
    sites other than limbs — *see* Wound, open, by site
    thumb(s) (with finger(s) of either hand) 885.0
      complicated 885.1
    toe(s) (one or both feet) 895.0
      complicated 895.1
    upper limb(s) — *see* Amputation, traumatic, arm

Amputee (bilateral) (old) — *see also* Absence, by site, acquired V49.70

Amusia 784.69
  developmental 315.39
  secondary to organic lesion 784.69

Amyelencephalus 740.0

Amyelia 742.59

Amygdalitis — *see* Tonsillitis

Amygdalolith 474.8

Amyloid disease or degeneration 277.3
  heart 277.3 *[425.7]*

Amyloidosis (familial) (general) (generalized) (genetic) (primary) (secondary) 277.3
  with lung involvement 277.3 *[517.8]*
  heart 277.3 *[425.7]*
  nephropathic 277.3 *[583.81]*
  neuropathic (Portuguese) (Swiss) 277.3 *[357.4]*
  pulmonary 277.3 *[517.8]*
  systemic, inherited 277.3

Amylopectinosis (brancher enzyme deficiency) 271.0

Amylophagia 307.52

Amyoplasia, congenita 756.89

Amyotonia 728.2
  congenita 358.8

Amyotrophia, amyotrophy, amyotrophic 728.2
  congenita 756.89
  diabetic 250.6 ✓5ᵗʰ *[358.1]*
  lateral sclerosis (syndrome) 335.20
  neuralgic 353.5
  sclerosis (lateral) 335.20
  spinal progressive 335.21

Anacidity, gastric 536.0
  psychogenic 306.4

Anaerosis of newborn 768.9 ▲

Analbuminemia 273.8

Analgesia (*see also* Anesthesia) 782.0

Analphalipoproteinemia 272.5

Anaphylactic shock or reaction (correct substance properly administered) 995.0
  due to
    food 995.60
      additives 995.66
      crustaceans 995.62
      eggs 995.68
      fish 995.65
      fruits 995.63
      milk products 995.67
      nuts (tree) 995.64
      peanuts 995.61
      seeds 995.64
      specified NEC 995.69
      tree nuts 995.64
      vegetables 995.63
    immunization 999.4
    overdose or wrong substance given or taken 977.9
      specified drug — *see* Table of Drugs and Chemicals
    serum 999.4
  following sting(s) 989.5
  purpura 287.0
  serum 999.4

Anaphylactoid shock or reaction — *see* Anaphylactic shock

Anaphylaxis — *see* Anaphylactic shock

Anaplasia, cervix 622.1

Anarthria 784.5

Anarthritic rheumatoid disease 446.5

Anasarca 782.3
  cardiac (*see also* Failure, heart) 428.0
  fetus or newborn 778.0
  lung 514
  nutritional 262
  pulmonary 514
  renal (*see also* Nephrosis) 581.9

Anaspadias 752.62

Anastomosis
  aneurysmal — see Aneurysm
  arteriovenous, congenital NEC (see also
      Anomaly, arteriovenous) 747.60
    ruptured, of brain (see also Hemorrhage,
        subarachnoid) 430
    intestinal 569.89
      complicated NEC 997.4
        involving urinary tract 997.5
    retinal and choroidal vessels 743.58
      acquired 362.17
Anatomical narrow angle (glaucoma) 365.02
Ancylostoma (infection) (infestation) 126.9
  americanus 126.1
  braziliense 126.2
  caninum 126.8
  ceylanicum 126.3
  duodenale 126.0
  Necator americanus 126.1
Ancylostomiasis (intestinal) 126.9
  Ancylostoma
    americanus 126.1
    caninum 126.8
    ceylanicum 126.3
    duodenale 126.0
  braziliense 126.2
  Necator americanus 126.1
Anders' disease or syndrome (adiposis tuberosa simplex) 272.8
Andersen's glycogen storage disease 271.0
Anderson's disease 272.7
Andes disease 993.2
Andrews' disease (bacterid) 686.8
Androblastoma (M8630/1)
  benign (M8630/0)
    specified site — see Neoplasm, by site, benign
    unspecified site
      female 220
      male 222.0
  malignant (M8630/3)
    specified site — see Neoplasm, by site, malignant
    unspecified site
      female 183.0
      male 186.9
  specified site — see Neoplasm, by site, uncertain behavior
  tubular (M8640/0)
    with lipid storage (M8641/0)
      specified site — see Neoplasm, by site, benign
      unspecified site
        female 220
        male 222.0
    specified site — see Neoplasm, by site, benign
    unspecified site
      female 220
      male 222.0
  unspecified site
    female 236.2
    male 236.4
Android pelvis 755.69
  with disproportion (fetopelvic) 653.3 ✓5ᵗʰ
    affecting fetus or newborn 763.1
    causing obstructed labor 660.1 ✓5ᵗʰ
      affecting fetus or newborn 763.1
Anectasis, pulmonary (newborn or fetus) 770.5

Anemia 285.9
  with
    disorder of
      anaerobic glycolysis 282.3
      pentose phosphate pathway 282.2
    koilonychia 280.9
  6-phosphogluconic dehydrogenase deficiency 282.2
  achlorhydric 280.9
  achrestic 281.8
  Addison's (pernicious) 281.0
  Addison-Biermer (pernicious) 281.0
  agranulocytic 288.0
  amino acid deficiency 281.4
  aplastic 284.9
    acquired (secondary) 284.8
    congenital 284.0
    constitutional 284.0
    due to
      chronic systemic disease 284.8
      drugs 284.8
      infection 284.8
      radiation 284.8
    idiopathic 284.9
    myxedema 244.9
    of or complicating pregnancy 648.2 ✓5ᵗʰ
    red cell (acquired) (pure) (with thymoma) 284.8
      congenital 284.0
    specified type NEC 284.8
    toxic (paralytic) 284.8
  aregenerative 284.9
    congenital 284.0
  asiderotic 280.9
  atypical (primary) 285.9
  autohemolysis of Selwyn and Dacie (type I) 282.2
  autoimmune hemolytic 283.0
  Baghdad Spring 282.2
  Balantidium coli 007.0
  Biermer's (pernicious) 281.0
  blood loss (chronic) 280.0
    acute 285.1
  bothriocephalus 123.4
  brickmakers' (see also Ancylostomiasis) 126.9
  cerebral 437.8
  childhood 285.9
  chlorotic 280.9
  chronica congenita aregenerativa 284.0
  chronic simple 281.9
  combined system disease NEC 281.0 [336.2]
    due to dietary deficiency 281.1 [336.2]
  complicating pregnancy or childbirth 648.2 ✓5ᵗʰ
  congenital (following fetal blood loss) 776.5
    aplastic 284.0
    due to isoimmunization NEC 773.2
    Heinz-body 282.7
    hereditary hemolytic NEC 282.9
    nonspherocytic
      Type I 282.2
      Type II 282.3
    pernicious 281.0
    spherocytic (see also Spherocytosis) 282.0
  Cooley's (erythroblastic) 282.4
  crescent — see Disease, sickle-cell
  cytogenic 281.0
  Dacie's (nonspherocytic)
    type I 282.2
    type II 282.3
  Davidson's (refractory) 284.9

Anemia — continued
  deficiency 281.9
    2, 3 diphosphoglycerate mutase 282.3
    2, 3 PG 282.3
    6-PGD 282.2
    6-phosphogluronic dehydrogenase 282.2
    amino acid 281.4
    combined B_{12} and folate 281.3
    enzyme, drug-induced (hemolytic) 282.2
    erythrocytic glutathione 282.2
    folate 281.2
      dietary 281.2
      drug-induced 281.2
    folic acid 281.2
      dietary 281.2
      drug-induced 281.2
    G-6-PD 282.2
    GGS-R 282.2
    glucose-6-phosphate dehydrogenase (G-6-PD) 282.2
    glucose-phosphate isomerase 282.3
    glutathione peroxidase 282.2
    glutathione reductase 282.2
    glyceraldehyde phosphate dehydrogenase 282.3
    GPI 282.3
    G SH 282.2
    hexokinase 282.3
    iron (Fe) 280.9
      specified NEC 280.8
    nutritional 281.9
      with
        poor iron absorption 280.9
        specified deficiency NEC 281.8
      due to inadequate dietary iron intake 280.1
      specified type NEC 281.8
    of or complicating pregnancy 648.2 ✓5ᵗʰ
    pentose phosphate pathway 282.2
    PFK 282.3
    phosphofructo-aldolase 282.3
    phosphofructokinase 282.3
    phosphoglycerate kinase 282.3
    PK 282.3
    protein 281.4
    pyruvate kinase (PK) 282.3
    TPI 282.3
    triosephosphate isomerase 282.3
    vitamin B_{12} NEC 281.1
      dietary 281.1
      pernicious 281.0
  Diamond-Blackfan (congenital hypoplastic) 284.0
  dibothriocephalus 123.4
  dimorphic 281.9
  diphasic 281.8
  diphtheritic 032.89
  Diphyllobothrium 123.4
  drepanocytic (see also Disease, sickle-cell) 282.60
  due to
    blood loss (chronic) 280.0
      acute 285.1
    defect of Embden-Meyerhof pathway glycolysis 282.3
    disorder of glutathione metabolism 282.2
    fetal blood loss 776.5
    fish tapeworm (D. latum) infestation 123.4
    glutathione metabolism disorder 282.2
    hemorrhage (chronic) 280.0
      acute 285.1

Anemia — continued
  due to — continued
    hexose monophosphate (HMP) shunt deficiency 282.2
    impaired absorption 280.9
    loss of blood (chronic) 280.0
      acute 285.1
    myxedema 244.9
    Necator americanus 126.1
    prematurity 776.6
    selective vitamin B_{12} malabsorption with proteinuria 281.1
  Dyke-Young type (secondary) (symptomatic) 283.9
  dyserythropoietic (congenital) (types I, II, III) 285.8
  dyshemopoietic (congenital) 285.8
  Egypt (see also Ancylostomiasis) 126.9
  elliptocytosis (see also Elliptocytosis) 282.1
  enzyme deficiency, drug-induced 282.2
  epidemic (see also Ancylostomiasis) 126.9
  erythroblastic
    familial 282.4
    fetus or newborn (see also Disease, hemolytic) 773.2
      late 773.5
  erythrocytic glutathione deficiency 282.2
  essential 285.9
  Faber's (achlorhydric anemia) 280.9
  factitious (self-induced blood letting) 280.0
  familial erythroblastic (microcytic) 282.4
  Fanconi's (congenital pancytopenia) 284.0
  favism 282.2
  fetal, following blood loss 776.5
  fetus or newborn
    due to
      ABO
        antibodies 773.1
        incompatibility, maternal/fetal 773.1
        isoimmunization 773.1
      Rh
        antibodies 773.0
        incompatibility, maternal/fetal 773.0
        isoimmunization 773.0
    following fetal blood loss 776.5
  fish tapeworm (D. latum) infestation 123.4
  folate (folic acid) deficiency 281.2
    dietary 281.2
    drug-induced 281.2
  folate malabsorption, congenital 281.2
  folic acid deficiency 281.2
    dietary 281.2
    drug-induced 281.2
  G-6-PD 282.2
  general 285.9
  glucose-6-phosphate dehydrogenase deficiency 282.2
  glutathione-reductase deficiency 282.2
  goat's milk 281.2
  granulocytic 288.0
  Heinz-body, congenital 282.7
  hemoglobin deficiency 285.9
  hemolytic 283.9
    acquired 283.9
      with hemoglobinuria NEC 283.2
      autoimmune (cold type) (idiopathic) (primary) (secondary) (symptomatic) (warm type) 283.0
      due to
        cold reactive antibodies 283.0
        drug exposure 283.0

Index to Diseases — Anemia

Anemia — *continued*
  hemolytic — *continued*
    acquired — *continued*
      due to — *continued*
        warm reactive antibodies 283.0
        fragmentation 283.19
        idiopathic (chronic) 283.9
        infectious 283.19
          autoimmune 283.0
        non-autoimmune NEC 283.10
        toxic 283.19
        traumatic cardiac 283.19
      acute 283.9
        due to enzyme deficiency NEC 282.3
        fetus or newborn (*see also* Disease, hemolytic) 773.2
          late 773.5
        Lederer's (acquired infectious hemolytic anemia) 283.19
      autoimmune (acquired) 283.0
      chronic 282.9
        idiopathic 283.9
      cold type (secondary) (symptomatic) 283.0
      congenital (spherocytic) (*see also* Spherocytosis) 282.0
        nonspherocytic — *see* Anemia, hemolytic, nonspherocytic, congenital
      drug-induced 283.0
        enzyme deficiency 282.2
      due to
        cardiac conditions 283.19
        drugs 283.0
        enzyme deficiency NEC 282.3
          drug-induced 282.2
        presence of shunt or other internal prosthetic device 283.19
        thrombotic thrombocytopenic purpura 446.6
      elliptocytotic (*see also* Elliptocytosis) 282.1
      familial 282.9
      hereditary 282.9
        due to enzyme deficiency NEC 282.3
        specified NEC 282.8
      idiopathic (chronic) 283.9
      infectious (acquired) 283.19
      mechanical 283.19
      microangiopathic 283.19
      non-autoimmune NEC 283.10
      nonspherocytic
        congenital or hereditary NEC 282.3
          glucose-6-phosphate dehydrogenase deficiency 282.2
          pyruvate kinase (PK) deficiency 282.3
            type I 282.2
            type II 282.3
        type I 282.2
        type II 282.3
      of or complicating pregnancy 648.2 ✓5ᵗʰ
      resulting from presence of shunt or other internal prosthetic device 283.19
      secondary 283.19
        autoimmune 283.0
      sickle-cell — *see* Disease, sickle-cell
      Stransky-Regala type (Hb-E) (*see also* Disease, hemoglobin) 282.7
      symptomatic 283.19
        autoimmune 283.0
      toxic (acquired) 283.19
      uremic (adult) (child) 283.11
      warm type (secondary) (symptomatic) 283.0
  hemorrhagic (chronic) 280.0
    acute 285.1
  HEMPAS 285.8
  hereditary erythroblast multinuclearity-positive acidified serum test 285.8
  Herrick's (hemoglobin S disease) 282.61
  hexokinase deficiency 282.3
  high A_2 282.4
  hookworm (*see also* Ancylostomiasis) 126.9
  hypochromic (idiopathic) (microcytic) (normoblastic) 280.9
    with iron loading 285.0
    due to blood loss (chronic) 280.0
      acute 285.1
    familial sex linked 285.0
    pyridoxine-responsive 285.0
  hypoplasia, red blood cells 284.8
    congenital or familial 284.0
  hypoplastic (idiopathic) 284.9
    congenital 284.0
    familial 284.0
    of childhood 284.0
  idiopathic 285.9
    hemolytic, chronic 283.9
  in
    chronic illness NEC 285.29
    end-stage renal disease 285.21
    neoplastic disease 285.22
  infantile 285.9
  infective, infectional 285.9
  intertropical (*see also* Ancylostomiasis) 126.9
  iron (Fe) deficiency 280.9
    due to blood loss (chronic) 280.0
      acute 285.1
    of or complicating pregnancy 648.2 ✓5ᵗʰ
    specified NEC 280.8
  Jaksch's (pseudoleukemia infantum) 285.8
  Joseph-Diamond-Blackfan (congenital hypoplastic) 284.0
  labyrinth 386.50
  Lederer's (acquired infectious hemolytic anemia) 283.19
  leptocytosis (hereditary) 282.4
  leukoerythroblastic 285.8
  macrocytic 281.9
    nutritional 281.2
    of or complicating pregnancy 648.2 ✓5ᵗʰ
    tropical 281.2
  malabsorption (familial), selective B_{12} with proteinuria 281.1
  malarial (*see also* Malaria) 084.6
  malignant (progressive) 281.0
  malnutrition 281.9
  marsh (*see also* Malaria) 084.6
  Mediterranean (with hemoglobinopathy) 282.4
  megaloblastic 281.9
    combined B_{12} and folate deficiency 281.3
    nutritional (of infancy) 281.2
    of infancy 281.2
    of or complicating pregnancy 648.2 ✓5ᵗʰ
    refractory 281.3
    specified NEC 281.3
  megalocytic 281.9
  microangiopathic hemolytic 283.19
  microcytic (hypochromic) 280.9
    due to blood loss (chronic) 280.0
      acute 285.1
    familial 282.4
    hypochromic 280.9
  microdrepanocytosis 282.4

Anemia — continued
- miners' (see also Ancylostomiasis) 126.9
- myelopathic 285.8
- myelophthisic (normocytic) 285.8
- newborn (see also Disease, hemolytic) 773.2
    - due to isoimmunization (see also Disease, hemolytic) 773.2
    - late, due to isoimmunization 773.5
    - posthemorrhagic 776.5
- nonregenerative 284.9
- nonspherocytic hemolytic — see Anemia, hemolytic, nonspherocytic
- normocytic (infectional) (not due to blood loss) 285.9
    - due to blood loss (chronic) 280.0
        - acute 285.1
    - myelophthisic 284.8
- nutritional (deficiency) 281.9
    - with
        - poor iron absorption 280.9
        - specified deficiency NEC 281.8
    - due to inadequate dietary iron intake 280.1
    - megaloblastic (of infancy) 281.2
- of childhood (see also Thalassemia) 282.4
- of chronic illness NEC 285.29
- of or complicating pregnancy 648.2 ✓5ᵗʰ
    - affecting fetus or newborn 760.8
- of prematurity 776.6
- orotic aciduric (congenital) (hereditary) 281.4
- osteosclerotic 289.8
- ovalocytosis (hereditary) (see also Elliptocytosis) 282.1
- paludal (see also Malaria) 084.6
- pentose phosphate pathway deficiency 282.2
- pernicious (combined system disease) (congenital) (dorsolateral spinal degeneration) (juvenile) (myelopathy) (neuropathy) (posterior sclerosis) (primary) (progressive) (spleen) 281.0
    - of or complicating pregnancy 648.2 ✓5ᵗʰ
- pleochromic 285.9
    - of sprue 281.8
- portal 285.8
- posthemorrhagic (chronic) 280.0
    - acute 285.1
    - newborn 776.5
- pressure 285.9
- primary 285.9
- profound 285.9
- progressive 285.9
    - malignant 281.0
    - pernicious 281.0
- protein-deficiency 281.4
- pseudoleukemica infantum 285.8
- puerperal 648.2 ✓5ᵗʰ
- pure red cell 284.8
    - congenital 284.0
- pyridoxine-responsive (hypochromic) 285.0
- pyruvate kinase (PK) deficiency 282.3
- refractoria sideroblastica 285.0
- refractory (primary) 284.9
    - with hemochromatosis 285.0
    - megaloblastic 281.3
    - sideroblastic 285.0
    - sideropenic 280.9
- Rietti-Greppi-Micheli (thalassemia minor) 282.4
- scorbutic 281.8
- secondary (to) 285.9
    - blood loss (chronic) 280.0
        - acute 285.1

Anemia — continued
- secondary — continued
    - hemorrhage 280.0
        - acute 285.1
    - inadequate dietary iron intake 280.1
- semiplastic 284.9
- septic 285.9
- sickle-cell (see also Disease, sickle-cell) 282.60
- sideroachrestic 285.0
- sideroblastic (acquired) (any type) (congenital) (drug-induced) (due to disease) (hereditary) (primary) (refractory) (secondary) (sex-linked hypochromic) (vitamin B_6 responsive) 285.0
- sideropenic (refractory) 280.9
    - due to blood loss (chronic) 280.0
        - acute 285.1
- simple chronic 281.9
- specified type NEC 285.8
- spherocytic (hereditary) (see also Spherocytosis) 282.0
- splenic 285.8
    - familial (Gaucher's) 272.7
- splenomegalic 285.8
- stomatocytosis 282.8
- syphilitic 095.8
- target cell (oval) 282.4
- thalassemia 282.4
- thrombocytopenic (see also Thrombocytopenia) 287.5
- toxic 284.8
- triosephosphate isomerase deficiency 282.3
- tropical, macrocytic 281.2
- tuberculous (see also Tuberculosis) 017.9 ✓5ᵗʰ
- vegan's 281.1
- vitamin
    - B_6-responsive 285.0
    - B_{12} deficiency (dietary) 281.1
        - pernicious 281.0
- von Jaksch's (pseudoleukemia infantum) 285.8
- Witts' (achlorhydric anemia) 280.9
- Zuelzer (-Ogden) (nutritional megaloblastic anemia) 281.2

Anencephalus, anencephaly 740.0
- fetal, affecting management of pregnancy 655.0 ✓5ᵗʰ

Anergasia (see also Psychosis, organic) 294.9
- senile 290.0

Anesthesia, anesthetic 782.0
- complication or reaction NEC 995.2
    - due to
        - correct substance properly administered 995.2
        - overdose or wrong substance given 968.4
        - specified anesthetic — see Table of Drugs and Chemicals
- cornea 371.81
- death from
    - correct substance properly administered 995.4
    - during delivery 668.9 ✓5ᵗʰ
    - overdose or wrong substance given 968.4
    - specified anesthetic — see Table of Drugs and Chemicals
- eye 371.81
- functional 300.11
- hyperesthetic, thalamic 348.8
- hysterical 300.11
- local skin lesion 782.0

Index to Diseases — Aneurysm

Anesthesia, anesthetic — *continued*
  olfactory 781.1
  sexual (psychogenic) 302.72
  shock
    due to
      correct substance properly administered 995.4
      overdose or wrong substance given 968.4
      specified anesthetic — *see* Table of Drugs and Chemicals
  skin 782.0
  tactile 782.0
  testicular 608.9
  thermal 782.0
Anetoderma (maculosum) 701.3
Aneuploidy NEC 758.5
Aneurin deficiency 265.1
Aneurysm (anastomotic) (artery) (cirsoid) (diffuse) (false) (fusiform) (multiple) (ruptured) (saccular) (varicose) 442.9
  abdominal (aorta) 441.4
    ruptured 441.3
    syphilitic 093.0
  aorta, aortic (nonsyphilitic) 441.9
    abdominal 441.4
      dissecting 441.02
      ruptured 441.3
      syphilitic 093.0
    arch 441.2
      ruptured 441.1
    arteriosclerotic NEC 441.9
      ruptured 441.5
    ascending 441.2
      ruptured 441.1
    congenital 747.29
    descending 441.9
      abdominal 441.4
        ruptured 441.3
        ruptured 441.5
      thoracic 441.2
        ruptured 441.1
    dissecting 441.00
      abdominal 441.02
      thoracic 441.01
      thoracoabdominal 441.03
    due to coarctation (aorta) 747.10
    ruptured 441.5
    sinus, right 747.29
    syphilitic 093.0
    thoracoabdominal 441.7
      ruptured 441.6
    thorax, thoracic (arch) (nonsyphilitic) 441.2
      dissecting 441.01
      ruptured 441.1
      syphilitic 093.0
    transverse 441.2
      ruptured 441.1
    valve (heart) (*see also* Endocarditis, aortic) 424.1
  arteriosclerotic NEC 442.9
    cerebral 437.3
      ruptured (*see also* Hemorrhage, subarachnoid) 430
  arteriovenous (congenital) (peripheral) NEC (*see also* Anomaly, arteriovenous) 747.60
    acquired NEC 447.0
      brain 437.3
        ruptured (*see also* Hemorrhage, subarachnoid) 430
      coronary 414.11

Aneurysm — *continued*
  arteriovenous — *continued*
    acquired NEC — *continued*
      pulmonary 417.0
    brain (cerebral) 747.81
      ruptured (*see also* Hemorrhage, subarachnoid) 430
    coronary 746.85
    pulmonary 747.3
    retina 743.58
    specified site NEC 747.89
      acquired 447.0
    traumatic (*see also* Injury, blood vessel, by site) 904.9
  basal — *see* Aneurysm, brain
  berry (congenital) (ruptured) (*see also* Hemorrhage, subarachnoid) 430
  brain 437.3
    arteriosclerotic 437.3
      ruptured (*see also* Hemorrhage, subarachnoid) 430
    arteriovenous 747.81
      acquired 437.3
        ruptured (*see also* Hemorrhage, subarachnoid) 430
      ruptured (*see also* Hemorrhage, subarachnoid) 430
    berry (congenital) (ruptured) (*see also* Hemorrhage, subarachnoid) 430
    congenital 747.81
      ruptured (*see also* Hemorrhage, subarachnoid) 430
    meninges 437.3
      ruptured (*see also* Hemorrhage, subarachnoid) 430
    miliary (congenital) (ruptured) (*see also* Hemorrhage, subarachnoid) 430
    mycotic 421.0
      ruptured (*see also* Hemorrhage, subarachnoid) 430
    nonruptured 437.3
    ruptured (*See also* Hemorrhage, subarachnoid) 430
    syphilitic 094.87
    syphilitic (hemorrhage) 094.87
    traumatic — *see* Injury, intracranial
  cardiac (false) (*see also* Aneurysm, heart) 414.10
  carotid artery (common) (external) 442.81
    internal (intracranial portion) 437.3
      extracranial portion 442.81
      ruptured into brain (*see also* Hemorrhage, subarachnoid) 430
    syphilitic 093.89
      intracranial 094.87
  cavernous sinus (*see also* Aneurysm, brain) 437.3
    arteriovenous 747.81
      ruptured (*see also* Hemorrhage, subarachnoid) 430
    congenital 747.81
      ruptured (*see also* Hemorrhage, subarachnoid) 430
  celiac 442.84
  central nervous system, syphilitic 094.89
  cerebral — *see* Aneurysm, brain
  chest — *see* Aneurysm, thorax
  circle of Willis (*see also* Aneurysm, brain) 437.3
    congenital 747.81

Aneurysm — *continued*
  circle of Willis — *continued*
    congenital — *continued*
      ruptured (*see also* Hemorrhage,
        subarachnoid) 430
    ruptured (*see also* Hemorrhage,
      subarachnoid) 430
  common iliac artery 442.2
  congenital (peripheral) NEC 747.60
    brain 747.81
      ruptured (*see also* Hemorrhage,
        subarachnoid) 430
    cerebral — *see* Aneurysm, brain, congenital
    coronary 746.85
    gastrointestinal 747.61
    lower limb 747.64
    pulmonary 747.3
    renal 747.62
    retina 743.58
    specified site NEC 747.89
    spinal 747.82
    upper limb 747.63
  conjunctiva 372.74
  conus arteriosus (*see also* Aneurysm, heart)
    414.10
  coronary (arteriosclerotic) (artery) (vein) (*see
    also* Aneurysm, heart) 414.11
    arteriovenous 746.85
    congenital 746.85
    syphilitic 093.89
  cylindrical 441.9
    ruptured 441.5
    syphilitic 093.9
  dissecting 442.9
    aorta (any part) 441.00
      abdominal 441.02
      thoracic 441.01
      thoracoabdominal 441.03
    syphilitic 093.9
  ductus arteriosus 747.0
  embolic — *see* Embolism, artery
  endocardial, infective (any valve) 421.0
  femoral 442.3
  gastroduodenal 442.84
  gastroepiploic 442.84
  heart (chronic or with a stated duration of
    over 8 weeks) (infectional) (wall) 414.10
    acute or with a stated duration of 8 weeks
      or less (*see also* Infarct, myocardium)
      410.9 ✓5ᵗʰ
    congenital 746.89
    valve — *see* Endocarditis
  hepatic 442.84
  iliac (common) 442.2
  infective (any valve) 421.0
  innominate (nonsyphilitic) 442.89
    syphilitic 093.89
  interauricular septum (*see also* Aneurysm,
    heart) 414.10
  interventricular septum (*see also* Aneurysm,
    heart) 414.10
  intracranial — *see* Aneurysm, brain
  intrathoracic (nonsyphilitic) 441.2
    ruptured 441.1
    syphilitic 093.0
  jugular vein 453.8
  lower extremity 442.3
  lung (pulmonary artery) 417.1
  malignant 093.9
  mediastinal (nonsyphilitic) 442.89
    syphilitic 093.89

Aneurysm — *continued*
  miliary (congenital) (ruptured) (*see also*
    Hemorrhage, subarachnoid) 430
  mitral (heart) (valve) 424.0
  mural (arteriovenous) (heart) (*see also*
    Aneurysm, heart) 414.10
  mycotic, any site 421.0
    ruptured, brain (*see also* Hemorrhage,
      subarachnoid) 430
  myocardium (*see also* Aneurysm, heart)
    414.10
  neck 442.81
  pancreaticoduodenal 442.84
  patent ductus arteriosus 747.0
  peripheral NEC 442.89
    congenital NEC (*see also* Aneurysm,
      congenital) 747.60
  popliteal 442.3
  pulmonary 417.1
    arteriovenous 747.3
      acquired 417.0
    syphilitic 093.89
    valve (heart) (*see also* Endocarditis,
      pulmonary) 424.3
  racemose 442.9
    congenital (peripheral) NEC 747.60
  radial 442.0
  Rasmussen's (*see also* Tuberculosis) 011.2 ✓5ᵗʰ
  renal 442.1
  retinal (acquired) 362.17
    congenital 743.58
    diabetic 250.5 ✓5ᵗʰ *[362.01]*
  sinus, aortic (of Valsalva) 747.29
  specified site NEC 442.89
  spinal (cord) 442.89
    congenital 747.82
    syphilitic (hemorrhage) 094.89
  spleen, splenic 442.83
  subclavian 442.82
    syphilitic 093.89
  superior mesenteric 442.84
  syphilitic 093.9
    aorta 093.0
    central nervous system 094.89
    congenital 090.5
    spine, spinal 094.89
  thoracoabdominal 441.7
    ruptured 441.6
  thorax, thoracic (arch) (nonsyphilitic) 441.2
    dissecting 441.0 ✓5ᵗʰ
    ruptured 441.1
    syphilitic 093.0
  traumatic (complication) (early) — *see* Injury,
    blood vessel, by site
  tricuspid (heart) (valve) — *see* Endocarditis,
    tricuspid
  ulnar 442.0
  upper extremity 442.0
  valve, valvular — *see* Endocarditis
  venous 456.8
    congenital NEC (*see also* Aneurysm,
      congenital) 747.60
  ventricle (arteriovenous) (*see also* Aneurysm,
    heart) 414.10
  visceral artery NEC 442.84
Angiectasis 459.89
Angiectopia 459.9
Angiitis 447.6
  allergic granulomatous 446.4
  hypersensitivity 446.20
    Goodpasture's syndrome 446.21

Angiitis — continued
  hypersensitivity — continued
    specified NEC 446.29
  necrotizing 446.0
  Wegener's (necrotizing respiratory
    granulomatosis) 446.4
Angina (attack) (cardiac) (chest) (effort) (heart)
    (pectoris) (syndrome) (vasomotor) 413.9
  abdominal 557.1
  agranulocytic 288.0
  aphthous 074.0
  catarrhal 462
  crescendo 411.1
  croupous 464.4
  cruris 443.9
    due to atherosclerosis NEC (see also
      Arteriosclerosis, extremities) 440.20
  decubitus 413.0
  diphtheritic (membranous) 032.0
  erysipelatous 034.0
  erythematous 462
  exudative, chronic 476.0
  faucium 478.29
  gangrenous 462
    diphtheritic 032.0
  infectious 462
  initial 411.1
  intestinal 557.1
  ludovici 528.3
  Ludwig's 528.3
  malignant 462
    diphtheritic 032.0
  membranous 464.4
    diphtheritic 032.0
  mesenteric 557.1
  monocytic 075
  nocturnal 413.0
  phlegmonous 475
    diphtheritic 032.0
  preinfarctional 411.1
  Prinzmetal's 413.1
  progressive 411.1
  pseudomembranous 101
  psychogenic 306.2
  pultaceous, diphtheritic 032.0
  scarlatinal 034.1
  septic 034.0
  simple 462
  stable NEC 413.9
  staphylococcal 462
  streptococcal 034.0
  stridulous, diphtheritic 032.3
  syphilitic 093.9
    congenital 090.5
  tonsil 475
  trachealis 464.4
  unstable 411.1
  variant 413.1
  Vincent's 101
Angioblastoma (M9161/1) — see Neoplasm,
  connective tissue, uncertain behavior
Angiocholecystitis (see also Cholecystitis, acute)
  575.0
Angiocholitis (see also Cholecystitis, acute)
  576.1
Angiodysgensis spinalis 336.1
Angiodysplasia (intestinalis) (intestine) 569.84
  with hemorrhage 569.85
  duodenum 537.82
    with hemorrhage 537.83

Angiodysplasia — continued
  stomach 537.82
    with hemorrhage 537.83
Angioedema (allergic) (any site) (with urticaria)
  995.1
  hereditary 277.6
Angioendothelioma (M9130/1) — see also
    Neoplasm, by site, uncertain behavior
  benign (M9130/0) (see also Hemangioma, by
    site) 228.00
  bone (M9260/3) — see Neoplasm, bone,
    malignant
  Ewing's (M9260/3) — see Neoplasm, bone,
    malignant
  nervous system (M9130/0) 228.09
Angiofibroma (M9160/0) — see also Neoplasm,
    by site, benign
  juvenile (M9160/0) 210.7
  specified site — see Neoplasm, by site,
    benign
  unspecified site 210.7
Angiohemophilia (A) (B) 286.4
Angioid streaks (choroid) (retina) 363.43
Angiokeratoma (M9141/0) — see also Neoplasm,
    skin, benign
  corporis diffusum 272.7
Angiokeratosis
  diffuse 272.7
Angioleiomyoma (M8894/0) — see Neoplasm,
    connective tissue, benign
Angioleucitis 683
Angiolipoma (M8861/0) (see also Lipoma, by
    site) 214.9
  infiltrating (M8861/1) — see Neoplasm,
    connective tissue, uncertain behavior
Angioma (M9120/0) (see also Hemangioma, by
    site) 228.00
  capillary 448.1
  hemorrhagicum hereditaria 448.0
  malignant (M9120/3) — see Neoplasm,
    connective tissue, malignant
  pigmentosum et atrophicum 757.33
  placenta — see Placenta, abnormal
  plexiform (M9131/0) — see Hemangioma, by
    site
  senile 448.1
  serpiginosum 709.1
  spider 448.1
  stellate 448.1
Angiomatosis 757.32
  bacillary 083.8
  corporis diffusum universale 272.7
  cutaneocerebral 759.6
  encephalocutaneous 759.6
  encephalofacial 759.6
  encephalotrigeminal 759.6
  hemorrhagic familial 448.0
  hereditary familial 448.0
  heredofamilial 448.0
  meningo-oculofacial 759.6
  multiple sites 228.09
  neuro-oculocutaneous 759.6
  retina (Hippel's disease) 759.6
  retinocerebellosa 759.6
  retinocerebral 759.6
  systemic 228.09
Angiomyolipoma (M8860/0)
  specified site — see Neoplasm, connective
    tissue, benign
  unspecified site 223.0

Angiomyoliposarcoma (M8860/3) — see Neoplasm, connective tissue, malignant
Angiomyoma (M8894/0) — see Neoplasm, connective tissue, benign
Angiomyosarcoma (M8894/3) — see Neoplasm, connective tissue, malignant
Angioneurosis 306.2
Angioneurotic edema (allergic) (any site) (with urticaria) 995.1
  hereditary 277.6
Angiopathia, angiopathy 459.9
  diabetic (peripheral) 250.7 ✓5ᵗʰ *[443.81]*
  peripheral 443.9
    diabetic 250.7 ✓5ᵗʰ *[443.81]*
    specified type NEC 443.89
  xretinae syphilitica 093.89
  retinalis (juvenilis) 362.18
    background 362.10
    diabetic 250.5 ✓5ᵗʰ *[362.01]*
    proliferative 362.29
    tuberculous (see also Tuberculosis) 017.3 ✓5ᵗʰ *[362.18]*
Angiosarcoma (M9120/3) — see Neoplasm, connective tissue, malignant
Angiosclerosis — see Arteriosclerosis
Angioscotoma, enlarged 368.42
Angiospasm 443.9
  brachial plexus 353.0
  cerebral 435.9
  cervical plexus 353.2
  nerve
    arm 354.9
      axillary 353.0
      median 354.1
      ulnar 354.2
    autonomic (see also Neuropathy, peripheral, autonomic) 337.9
      axillary 353.0
      leg 355.8
        plantar 355.6
      lower extremity — see Angiospasm, nerve, leg
      median 354.1
    peripheral NEC 355.9
    spinal NEC 355.9
    sympathetic (see also Neuropathy, peripheral, autonomic) 337.9
    ulnar 354.2
    upper extremity — see Angiospasm, nerve, arm
  peripheral NEC 443.9
  traumatic 443.9
    foot 443.9
    leg 443.9
  vessel 443.9
Angiospastic disease or edema 443.9
Anguillulosis 127.2
Angulation
  cecum (see also Obstruction, intestine) 560.9
  coccyx (acquired) 738.6
    congenital 756.19
  femur (acquired) 736.39
    congenital 755.69
  intestine (large) (small) (see also Obstruction, intestine) 560.9
  sacrum (acquired) 738.5
    congenital 756.19
  sigmoid (flexure) (see also Obstruction, intestine) 560.9

Angulation — *continued*
  spine (see also Curvature, spine) 737.9
  tibia (acquired) 736.89
    congenital 755.69
  ureter 593.3
  wrist (acquired) 736.09
    congenital 755.59
Angulus infectiosus 686.8
Anhedonia 302.72
Anhidrosis (lid) (neurogenic) (thermogenic) 705.0
Anhydration 276.5
  with
    hypernatremia 276.0
    hyponatremia 276.1
Anhydremia 276.5
  with
    hypernatremia 276.0
    hyponatremia 276.1
Anidrosis 705.0
Aniridia (congenital) 743.45
Anisakiasis (infection) (infestation) 127.1
Anisakis larva infestation 127.1
Aniseikonia 367.32
Anisocoria (pupil) 379.41
  congenital 743.46
Anisocytosis 790.09
Anisometropia (congenital) 367.31
Ankle — see condition
Ankyloblepharon (acquired) (eyelid) 374.46
  filiforme (adnatum) (congenital) 743.62
  total 743.62
Ankylodactly (see also Syndactylism) 755.10
Ankyloglossia 750.0
Ankylosis (fibrous) (osseous) 718.50
  ankle 718.57
  any joint, produced by surgical fusion V45.4
  cricoarytenoid (cartilage) (joint) (larynx) 478.79
  dental 521.6
  ear ossicle NEC 385.22
    malleus 385.21
  elbow 718.52
  finger 718.54
  hip 718.55
  incostapedial joint (infectional) 385.22
  joint, produced by surgical fusion NEC V45.4
  knee 718.56
  lumbosacral (joint) 724.6
  malleus 385.21
  multiple sites 718.59
  postoperative (status) V45.4
  sacroiliac (joint) 724.6
  shoulder 718.51
  specified site NEC 718.58
  spine NEC 724.9
  surgical V45.4
  teeth, tooth (hard tissues) 521.6
  temporomandibular joint 524.61
  wrist 718.53
Ankylostoma — see Ancylostoma
Ankylostomiasis (intestinal) — see Ancylostomiasis
Ankylurethria (see also Stricture, urethra) 598.9
Annular — see also condition
  detachment, cervix 622.8
  organ or site, congenital NEC — see Distortion
  pancreas (congenital) 751.7

Index to Diseases

Anodontia (complete) (partial) (vera) 520.0
  with abnormal spacing 524.3
  acquired 525.10
    causing malocclusion 524.3
    due to
      caries 525.13
      extraction 525.10
      periodontal disease 525.12
      trauma 525.11
Anomaly, anomalous (congenital) (unspecified type) 759.9
  abdomen 759.9
  abdominal wall 756.70
  acoustic nerve 742.9
  adrenal (gland) 759.1
  Alder (-Reilly) (leukocyte granulation) 288.2
  alimentary tract 751.9
    lower 751.5
    specified type NEC 751.8
    upper (any part, except tongue) 750.9
      tongue 750.10
        specified type NEC 750.19
  alveolar ridge (process) 525.8
  ankle (joint) 755.69
  anus, anal (canal) 751.5
  aorta, aortic 747.20
    arch 747.21
    coarctation (postductal) (preductal) 747.10
    cusp or valve NEC 746.9
    septum 745.0
    specified type NEC 747.29
  aorticopulmonary septum 745.0
  apertures, diaphragm 756.6
  appendix 751.5
  aqueduct of Sylvius 742.3
    with spina bifida (*see also* Spina bifida) 741.0 ✓5ᵗʰ
  arm 755.50
    reduction (*see also* Deformity, reduction, upper limb) 755.20
  arteriovenous (congenital) (peripheral) NEC 747.60
    brain 747.81
    cerebral 747.81
    coronary 746.85
    gastrointestinal 747.61
    lower limb 747.64
    renal 747.62
    specified site NEC 747.69
    spinal 747.82
    upper limb 747.63
  artery (*see also* Anomaly, peripheral vascular system) NEC 747.60
    brain 747.81
    cerebral 747.81
    coronary 746.85
    eye 743.9
    pulmonary 747.3
    renal 747.62
    retina 743.9
    umbilical 747.5
  arytenoepiglottic folds 748.3
  atrial
    bands 746.9
    folds 746.9
    septa 745.5
  atrioventricular
    canal 745.69
    common 745.69
    conduction 426.7
    excitation 426.7

Anomaly, anomalous — *continued*
  atrioventricular — *continued*
    septum 745.4
  atrium — *see* Anomaly, atrial
  auditory canal 744.3
    specified type NEC 744.29
      with hearing impairment 744.02
  auricle
    ear 744.3
      causing impairment of hearing 744.02
    heart 746.9
      septum 745.5
  autosomes, autosomal NEC 758.5
  Axenfeld's 743.44
  back 759.9
  band
    atrial 746.9
    heart 746.9
    ventricular 746.9
  Bartholin's duct 750.9
  biliary duct or passage 751.60
    atresia 751.61
  bladder (neck) (sphincter) (trigone) 753.9
    specified type NEC 753.8
  blood vessel 747.9
    artery — *see* Anomaly, artery
    peripheral vascular — *see* Anomaly, peripheral vascular system
    vein — *see* Anomaly, vein
  bone NEC 756.9
    ankle 755.69
    arm 755.50
    chest 756.3
    cranium 756.0
    face 756.0
    finger 755.50
    foot 755.67
    forearm 755.50
    frontal 756.0
    head 756.0
    hip 755.63
    leg 755.60
    lumbosacral 756.10
    nose 748.1
    pelvic girdle 755.60
    rachitic 756.4
    rib 756.3
    shoulder girdle 755.50
    skull 756.0
      with
        anencephalus 740.0
        encephalocele 742.0
        hydrocephalus 742.3
          with spina bifida (*see also* Spina bifida) 741.0 ✓5ᵗʰ
        microcephalus 742.1
    toe 755.66
  brain 742.9
    multiple 742.4
    reduction 742.2
    specified type NEC 742.4
    vessel 747.81
  branchial cleft NEC 744.49
    cyst 744.42
    fistula 744.41
    persistent 744.41
    sinus (external) (internal) 744.41
  breast 757.9
  broad ligament 752.10
    specified type NEC 752.19
  bronchus 748.3

Anomaly, anomalous — *continued*
  bulbar septum 745.0
  bulbus cordis 745.9
    persistent (in left ventricle) 745.8
  bursa 756.9
  canal of Nuck 752.9
  canthus 743.9
  capillary NEC (*see also* Anomaly, peripheral vascular system) 747.60
  cardiac 746.9
    septal closure 745.9
      acquired 429.71
    valve NEC 746.9
      pulmonary 746.00
      specified type NEC 746.89
  cardiovascular system 746.9
    complicating pregnancy, childbirth, or puerperium 648.5
  carpus 755.50
  cartilage, trachea 748.3
  cartilaginous 756.9
  caruncle, lacrimal, lachrymal 743.9
  cascade stomach 750.7
  cauda equina 742.59
  cecum 751.5
  cerebral — *see also* Anomaly, brain vessels 747.81
  cerebrovascular system 747.81
  cervix (uterus) 752.40
    with doubling of vagina and uterus 752.2
    in pregnancy or childbirth 654.6
      affecting fetus or newborn 763.89
      causing obstructed labor 660.2
        affecting fetus or newborn 763.1
  Chédiak-Higashi (-Steinbrinck) (congenital gigantism of peroxidase granules) 288.2
  cheek 744.9
  chest (wall) 756.3
  chin 744.9
    specified type NEC 744.89
  chordae tendineae 746.9
  choroid 743.9
    plexus 742.9
  chromosomes, chromosomal 758.9
    13 (13-15) 758.1
    18 (16-18) 758.2
    21 or 22 758.0
    autosomes NEC (*see also* Abnormality, autosomes) 758.5
      deletion 758.3
      Christchurch 758.3
    D_1 758.1
    E_3 758.2
    G 758.0
    mitochondrial 758.9
    mosaics 758.89
    sex 758.81
      complement, XO 758.6
      complement, XXX 758.81
      complement, XXY 758.7
      complement, XYY 758.81
      gonadal dysgenesis 758.6
      Klinefelter's 758.7
      Turner's 758.6
    trisomy 21 758.0
  cilia 743.9
  circulatory system 747.9
    specified type NEC 747.89
  clavicle 755.51
  clitoris 752.40
  coccyx 756.10

Anomaly, anomalous — *continued*
  colon 751.5
  common duct 751.60
  communication
    coronary artery 746.85
    left ventricle with right atrium 745.4
  concha (ear) 744.3
  connection
    renal vessels with kidney 747.62
    total pulmonary venous 747.41
  connective tissue 756.9
    specified type NEC 756.89
  cornea 743.9
    shape 743.41
    size 743.41
    specified type NEC 743.49
  coronary
    artery 746.85
    vein 746.89
  cranium — *see* Anomaly, skull
  cricoid cartilage 748.3
  cushion, endocardial 745.60
    specified type NEC 745.69
  cystic duct 751.60
  dental arch relationship 524.2
  dentition 520.6
  dentofacial NEC 524.9
    functional 524.5
    specified type NEC 524.8
  dermatoglyphic 757.2
  Descemet's membrane 743.9
    specified type NEC 743.49
  development
    cervix 752.40
    vagina 752.40
    vulva 752.40
  diaphragm, diaphragmatic (apertures) NEC 756.6
  digestive organ(s) or system 751.9
    lower 751.5
    specified type NEC 751.8
    upper 750.9
  distribution, coronary artery 746.85
  ductus
    arteriosus 747.0
    Botalli 747.0
  duodenum 751.5
  dura 742.9
    brain 742.4
    spinal cord 742.59
  ear 744.3
    causing impairment of hearing 744.00
      specified type NEC 744.09
    external 744.3
      causing impairment of hearing 744.02
      specified type NEC 744.29
    inner (causing impairment of hearing) 744.05
    middle, except ossicles (causing impairment of hearing) 744.03
      ossicles 744.04
    ossicles 744.04
    prominent auricle 744.29
    specified type NEC 744.29
      with hearing impairment 744.09
  Ebstein's (heart) 746.2
    tricuspid valve 746.2
  ectodermal 757.9
  Eisenmenger's (ventricular septal defect) 745.4
  ejaculatory duct 752.9
    specified type NEC 752.8

Anomaly, anomalous — *continued*
  elbow (joint) 755.50
  endocardial cushion 745.60
    specified type NEC 745.69
  endocrine gland NEC 759.2
  epididymis 752.9
  epiglottis 748.3
  esophagus 750.9
    specified type NEC 750.4
  Eustachian tube 744.3
    specified type NEC 744.24
  eye (any part) 743.9
    adnexa 743.9
      specified type NEC 743.69
    anophthalmos 743.00
    anterior
      chamber and related structures 743.9
      angle 743.9
        specified type NEC 743.44
      specified type NEC 743.44
      segment 743.9
        combined 743.48
        multiple 743.48
        specified type NEC 743.49
    cataract (*see also* Cataract) 743.30
    glaucoma (*see also* Buphthalmia) 743.20
    lid 743.9
      specified type NEC 743.63
    microphthalmos (*see also* Microphthalmos) 743.10
    posterior segment 743.9
      specified type NEC 743.59
      vascular 743.58
      vitreous 743.9
        specified type NEC 743.51
    ptosis (eyelid) 743.61
    retina 743.9
      specified type NEC 743.59
    sclera 743.9
      specified type NEC 743.47
    specified type NEC 743.8
  eyebrow 744.89
  eyelid 743.9
    specified type NEC 743.63
  face (any part) 744.9
    bone(s) 756.0
    specified type NEC 744.89
  fallopian tube 752.10
    specified type NEC 752.19
  fascia 756.9
    specified type NEC 756.89
  femur 755.60
  fibula 755.60
  finger 755.50
    supernumerary 755.01
    webbed (*see also* Syndactylism, fingers) 755.11
  fixation, intestine 751.4
  flexion (joint) 755.9
    hip or thigh (*see also* Dislocation, hip, congenital) 754.30
  folds, heart 746.9
  foot 755.67
  foramen
    Botalli 745.5
    ovale 745.5
  forearm 755.60
  forehead (*see also* Anomaly, skull) 756.0
  form, teeth 520.2
  fovea centralis 743.9
  frontal bone (*see also* Anomaly, skull) 756.0

Anomaly, anomalous — *continued*
  gallbladder 751.60
  Gartner's duct 752.11
  gastrointestinal tract 751.9
    specified type NEC 751.8
    vessel 747.61
  genitalia, genital organ(s) or system
    female 752.9
      external 752.40
        specified type NEC 752.49
      internal NEC 752.9
    male (external and internal) 752.9
      epispadias 752.62
      hidden penis 752.65
      hydrocele, congenital 778.6
      hypospadias 752.61
      micropenis 752.64
      testis, undescended 752.51
        retractile 752.52
    specified type NEC 752.8
  genitourinary NEC 752.9
  Gerbode 745.4
  globe (eye) 743.9
  glottis 748.3
  granulation or granulocyte, genetic 288.2
    constitutional 288.2
    leukocyte 288.2
  gum 750.9
  gyri 742.9
  hair 757.9
    specified type NEC 757.4
  hand 755.50
  hard tissue formation in pulp 522.3
  head (*see also* Anomaly, skull) 756.0
  heart 746.9
    auricle 746.9
    bands 746.9
    fibroelastosis cordis 425.3
    folds 746.9
    malposition 746.87
    maternal, affecting fetus or newborn 760.3
    obstructive NEC 746.84
    patent ductus arteriosus (Botalli) 747.0
    septum 745.9
      acquired 429.71
      aortic 745.0
      aorticopulmonary 745.0
      atrial 745.5
      auricular 745.5
      between aorta and pulmonary artery 745.0
      endocardial cushion type 745.60
        specified type NEC 745.69
      interatrial 745.5
      interventricular 745.4
        with pulmonary stenosis or atresia, dextraposition of aorta, and hypertrophy of right ventricle 745.2
        acquired 429.71
      specified type NEC 745.8
      ventricular 745.4
        with pulmonary stenosis or atresia, dextraposition of aorta, and hypertrophy of right ventricle 745.2
        acquired 429.71
    specified type NEC 746.89
    tetralogy of Fallot 745.2

Anomaly, anomalous — continued
- heart — continued
  - valve NEC 746.9
    - aortic 746.9
      - atresia 746.89
      - bicuspid valve 746.4
      - insufficiency 746.4
      - specified type NEC 746.89
      - stenosis 746.3
        - subaortic 746.81
        - supravalvular 747.22
    - mitral 746.9
      - atresia 746.89
      - insufficiency 746.6
      - specified type NEC 746.89
      - stenosis 746.5
    - pulmonary 746.00
      - atresia 746.01
      - insufficiency 746.09
      - stenosis 746.02
        - infundibular 746.83
        - subvalvular 746.83
    - tricuspid 746.9
      - atresia 746.1
      - stenosis 746.1
  - ventricle 746.9
- heel 755.67
- Hegglin's 288.2
- hemianencephaly 740.0
- hemicephaly 740.0
- hemicrania 740.0
- hepatic duct 751.60
- hip (joint) 755.63
- hourglass
  - bladder 753.8
  - gallbladder 751.69
  - stomach 750.7
- humerus 755.50
- hymen 752.40
- hypersegmentation of neutrophils, hereditary 288.2
- hypophyseal 759.2
- ileocecal (coil) (valve) 751.5
- ileum (intestine) 751.5
- ilium 755.60
- integument 757.9
  - specified type NEC 757.8
- intervertebral cartilage or disc 756.10
- intestine (large) (small) 751.5
  - fixational type 751.4
- iris 743.9
  - specified type NEC 743.46
- ischium 755.60
- jaw NEC 524.9
  - closure 524.5
  - size (major) NEC 524.00
  - specified type NEC 524.8
- jaw-cranial base relationship 524.10
  - specified NEC 524.19
- jejunum 751.5
- joint 755.9
  - hip
    - dislocation (see also Dislocation, hip, congenital) 754.30
    - predislocation (see also Subluxation, congenital, hip) 754.32
    - preluxation (see also Subluxation, congenital, hip) 754.32
    - subluxation (see also Subluxation, congenital, hip) 754.32

Anomaly, anomalous — continued
- joint — continued
  - lumbosacral 756.10
    - spondylolisthesis 756.12
    - spondylosis 756.11
  - multiple arthrogryposis 754.89
  - sacroiliac 755.69
- Jordan's 288.2
- kidney(s) (calyx) (pelvis) 753.9
  - vessel 747.62
- Klippel-Feil (brevicollis) 756.16
- knee (joint) 755.64
- labium (majus) (minus) 752.40
- labyrinth, membranous (causing impairment of hearing) 744.05
- lacrimal
  - apparatus, duct or passage 743.9
    - specified type NEC 743.65
  - gland 743.9
    - specified type NEC 743.64
- Langdon Down (mongolism) 758.0
- larynx, laryngeal (muscle) 748.3
  - web, webbed 748.2
- leg (lower) (upper) 755.60
  - reduction NEC (see also Deformity, reduction, lower limb) 755.30
- lens 743.9
  - shape 743.36
  - specified type NEC 743.39
- leukocytes, genetic 288.2
  - granulation (constitutional) 288.2
- lid (fold) 743.9
- ligament 756.9
  - broad 752.10
  - round 752.9
- limb, except reduction deformity 755.9
  - lower 755.60
    - reduction deformity (see also Deformity, reduction, lower limb) 755.30
    - specified type NEC 755.69
  - upper 755.50
    - reduction deformity (see also Deformity, reduction, upper limb) 755.20
    - specified type NEC 755.59
- lip 750.9
  - harelip (see also Cleft, lip) 749.10
  - specified type NEC 750.26
- liver (duct) 751.60
  - atresia 751.69
- lower extremity 755.60
  - vessel 747.64
- lumbosacral (joint) (region) 756.10
- lung (fissure) (lobe) NEC 748.60
  - agenesis 748.5
  - specified type NEC 748.69
- lymphatic system 759.9
- Madelung's (radius) 755.54
- mandible 524.9
  - size NEC 524.00
- maxilla 524.9
  - size NEC 524.00
- May (-Hegglin) 288.2
- meatus urinarius 753.9
  - specified type NEC 753.8
- meningeal bands or folds, constriction of 742.8
- meninges 742.9
  - brain 742.4
  - spinal 742.59
- meningocele (see also Spina bifida) 741.9
- mesentery 751.9

Index to Diseases

Anomaly, anomalous — *continued*
  metacarpus 755.50
  metatarsus 755.67
  middle ear, except ossicles (causing
      impairment of hearing) 744.03
    ossicles 744.04
  mitral (leaflets) (valve) 746.9
    atresia 746.89
    insufficiency 746.6
    specified type NEC 746.89
    stenosis 746.5
  mouth 750.9
    specified type NEC 750.26
  multiple NEC 759.7
    specified type NEC 759.89
  muscle 756.9
    eye 743.9
      specified type NEC 743.69
    specified type NEC 756.89
  musculoskeletal system, except limbs 756.9
    specified type NEC 756.9
  nail 757.9
    specified type NEC 757.5
  narrowness, eyelid 743.62
  nasal sinus or septum 748.1
  neck (any part) 744.9
    specified type NEC 744.89
  nerve 742.9
    acoustic 742.9
      specified type NEC 742.8
    optic 742.9
      specified type NEC 742.8
    specified type NEC 742.8
  nervous system NEC 742.9
    brain 742.9
      specified type NEC 742.4
    specified type NEC 742.8
  neurological 742.9
  nipple 757.9
  nonteratogenic NEC 754.89
  nose, nasal (bone) (cartilage) (septum) (sinus) 748.1
  ocular muscle 743.9
  omphalomesenteric duct 751.0
  opening, pulmonary veins 747.49
  optic
    disc 743.9
      specified type NEC 743.57
    nerve 742.9
  opticociliary vessels 743.9
  orbit (eye) 743.9
    specified type NEC 743.66
  organ
    of Corti (causing impairment of hearing) 744.05
    or site 759.9
      specified type NEC 759.89
  origin
    both great arteries from same ventricle 745.11
    coronary artery 746.85
    innominate artery 747.69
    left coronary artery from pulmonary artery 746.85
    pulmonary artery 747.3
    renal vessels 747.62
    subclavian artery (left) (right) 747.21
  osseous meatus (ear) 744.03
  ovary 752.0
  oviduct 752.10

Anomaly, anomalous — *continued*
  palate (hard) (soft) 750.9
    cleft (*see also* Cleft, palate) 749.00
  pancreas (duct) 751.7
  papillary muscles 746.9
  parathyroid gland 759.2
  paraurethral ducts 753.9
  parotid (gland) 750.9
  patella 755.64
  Pelger-Huët (hereditary hyposegmentation) 288.2
  pelvic girdle 755.60
    specified type NEC 755.69
  pelvis (bony) 755.60
    complicating delivery 653.0 ✓5ᵗʰ
    rachitic 268.1
      fetal 756.4
  penis (glans) 752.69
  pericardium 746.89
  peripheral vascular system NEC 747.60
    gastrointestinal 747.61
    lower limb 747.64
    renal 747.62
    specified site NEC 747.69
    spinal 747.82
    upper limb 747.63
  Peter's 743.44
  pharynx 750.9
    branchial cleft 744.41
    specified type NEC 750.29
  Pierre Robin 756.0
  pigmentation NEC 709.00
    congenital 757.33
  pituitary (gland) 759.2
  pleural folds 748.8
  portal vein 747.40
  position tooth, teeth 524.3
  preauricular sinus 744.46
  prepuce 752.9
  prostate 752.9
  pulmonary 748.60
    artery 747.3
    circulation 747.3
    specified type NEC 748.69
    valve 746.00
      atresia 746.01
      insufficiency 746.09
      specified type NEC 746.09
      stenosis 746.02
        infundibular 746.83
        subvalvular 746.83
    vein 747.40
    venous
      connection 747.49
        partial 747.42
        total 747.41
      return 747.49
        partial 747.42
        total (TAPVR) (complete) (subdiaphragmatic) (supradiaphrag-matic) 747.41
  pupil 743.9
  pylorus 750.9
    hypertrophy 750.5
    stenosis 750.5
  rachitic, fetal 756.4
  radius 755.50
  rectovaginal (septum) 752.40
  rectum 751.5
  refraction 367.9

Anomaly, anomalous

Anomaly, anomalous — *continued*
  renal 753.9
    vessel 747.62
  respiratory system 748.9
    specified type NEC 748.8
  rib 756.3
    cervical 756.2
  Rieger's 743.44
  rings, trachea 748.3
  rotation — *see also* Malrotation
    hip or thigh (*see also* Subluxation, congenital, hip) 754.32
  round ligament 752.9
  sacroiliac (joint) 755.69
  sacrum 756.10
  saddle
    back 754.2
    nose 754.0
      syphilitic 090.5
  salivary gland or duct 750.9
    specified type NEC 750.26
  scapula 755.50
  sclera 743.9
    specified type NEC 743.47
  scrotum 752.9
  sebaceous gland 757.9
  seminal duct or tract 752.9
  sense organs 742.9
    specified type NEC 742.8
  septum
    heart — *see* Anomaly, heart, septum
    nasal 748.1
  sex chromosomes NEC (*see also* Anomaly, chromosomes) 758.81
  shoulder (girdle) (joint) 755.50
    specified type NEC 755.59
  sigmoid (flexure) 751.5
  sinus of Valsalva 747.29
  site NEC 759.9
  skeleton generalized NEC 756.50
  skin (appendage) 757.9
    specified type NEC 757.39
  skull (bone) 756.0
    with
      anencephalus 740.0
      encephalocele 742.0
      hydrocephalus 742.3
        with spina bifida (*see also* Spina bifida) 741.0 ✓5ᵗʰ
      microcephalus 742.1
  specified type NEC
    adrenal (gland) 759.1
    alimentary tract (complete) (partial) 751.8
      lower 751.5
      upper 750.8
    ankle 755.69
    anus, anal (canal) 751.5
    aorta, aortic 747.29
      arch 747.21
    appendix 751.5
    arm 755.59
    artery (peripheral) NEC (*see also* Anomaly, peripheral vascular system) 747.60
      brain 747.81
      coronary 746.85
      eye 743.58
      pulmonary 747.3
      retinal 743.58
      umbilical 747.5
    auditory canal 744.29
      causing impairment of hearing 744.02

Anomaly, anomalous — *continued*
  specified type NEC — *continued*
    bile duct or passage 751.69
    bladder 753.8
      neck 753.8
    bone(s) 756.9
      arm 755.59
      face 756.0
      leg 755.69
      pelvic girdle 755.69
      shoulder girdle 755.59
      skull 756.0
        with
          anencephalus 740.0
          encephalocele 742.0
          hydrocephalus 742.3
            with spina bifida (*see also* Spina bifida) 741.0 ✓5ᵗʰ
          microcephalus 742.1
    brain 742.4
    breast 757.6
    broad ligament 752.19
    bronchus 748.3
    canal of Nuck 752.8
    cardiac septal closure 745.8
    carpus 755.59
    cartilaginous 756.9
    cecum 751.5
    cervix 752.49
    chest (wall) 756.3
    chin 744.89
    ciliary body 743.46
    circulatory system 747.89
    clavicle 755.51
    clitoris 752.49
    coccyx 756.19
    colon 751.5
    common duct 751.69
    connective tissue 756.89
    cricoid cartilage 748.3
    cystic duct 751.69
    diaphragm 756.6
    digestive organ(s) or tract 751.8
      lower 751.5
      upper 750.8
    duodenum 751.5
    ear 744.29
      auricle 744.29
        causing impairment of hearing 744.02
      causing impairment of hearing 744.09
      inner (causing impairment of hearing) 744.05
      middle, except ossicles 744.03
        ossicles 744.04
    ejaculatory duct 752.8
    endocrine 759.2
    epiglottis 748.3
    esophagus 750.4
    Eustachian tube 744.24
    eye 743.8
      lid 743.63
      muscle 743.69
    face 744.89
      bone(s) 756.0
    fallopian tube 752.19
    fascia 756.89
    femur 755.69
    fibula 755.69
    finger 755.59
    foot 755.67

Index to Diseases **Anomaly, anomalous**

Anomaly, anomalous — *continued*
  specified type NEC — *continued*
    fovea centralis 743.55
    gallbladder 751.69
    Gartner's duct 752.8
    gastrointestinal tract 751.8
    genitalia, genital organ(s)
      female 752.8
        external 752.49
        internal NEC 752.8
      male 752.8
        penis 752.69
    genitourinary tract NEC 752.8
    glottis 748.3
    hair 757.4
    hand 755.59
    heart 746.89
      valve NEC 746.89
        pulmonary 746.09
    hepatic duct 751.69
    hydatid of Morgagni 752.8
    hymen 752.49
    integument 757.8
    intestine (large) (small) 751.5
      fixational type 751.4
    iris 743.46
    jejunum 751.5
    joint 755.8
    kidney 753.3
    knee 755.64
    labium (majus) (minus) 752.49
    labyrinth, membranous 744.05
    larynx 748.3
    leg 755.69
    lens 743.39
    limb, except reduction deformity 755.8
      lower 755.69
        reduction deformity (*see also*
          Deformity, reduction, lower
          limb) 755.30
      upper 755.59
        reduction deformity (*see also*
          Deformity, reduction, upper
          limb) 755.20
    lip 750.26
    liver 751.69
    lung (fissure) (lobe) 748.69
    meatus urinarius 753.8
    metacarpus 755.59
    mouth 750.26
    muscle 756.89
      eye 743.69
    musculoskeletal system, except limbs 756.9
    nail 757.5
    neck 744.89
    nerve 742.8
      acoustic 742.8
      optic 742.8
    nervous system 742.8
    nipple 757.6
    nose 748.1
    organ NEC 759.89
      of Corti 744.05
    osseous meatus (ear) 744.03
    ovary 752.0
    oviduct 752.19
    pancreas 751.7
    parathyroid 759.2
    patella 755.64
    pelvic girdle 755.69
    penis 752.69

Anomaly, anomalous — *continued*
  specified type NEC — *continued*
    pericardium 746.89
    peripheral vascular system NEC (*see also*
      Anomaly, peripheral vascular system)
      747.60
    pharynx 750.29
    pituitary 759.2
    prostate 752.8
    radius 755.59
    rectum 751.5
    respiratory system 748.8
    rib 756.3
    round ligament 752.8
    sacrum 756.19
    salivary duct or gland 750.26
    scapula 755.59
    sclera 743.47
    scrotum 752.8
    seminal duct or tract 752.8
    shoulder girdle 755.59
    site NEC 759.89
    skin 757.39
    skull (bone(s)) 756.0
      with
        anencephalus 740.0
        encephalocele 742.0
        hydrocephalus 742.3
          with spina bifida (*see also* Spina
            bifida) 741.0 ✓5
        microcephalus 742.1
    specified organ or site NEC 759.89
    spermatic cord 752.8
    spinal cord 742.59
    spine 756.19
    spleen 759.0
    sternum 756.3
    stomach 750.7
    tarsus 755.67
    tendon 756.89
    testis 752.8
    thorax (wall) 756.3
    thymus 759.2
    thyroid (gland) 759.2
      cartilage 748.3
    tibia 755.69
    toe 755.66
    tongue 750.19
    trachea (cartilage) 748.3
    ulna 755.59
    urachus 753.7
    ureter 753.4
      obstructive 753.29
    urethra 753.8
      obstructive 753.6
    urinary tract 753.8
    uterus 752.3
    uvula 750.26
    vagina 752.49
    vascular NEC (*see also* Anomaly, peripheral
      vascular system) 747.60
      brain 747.81
    vas deferens 752.8
    vein(s) (peripheral) NEC (*see also* Anomaly,
      peripheral vascular system) 747.60
      brain 747.81
      great 747.49
      portal 747.49
      pulmonary 747.49
    vena cava (inferior) (superior) 747.49
    vertebra 756.19

Anomaly, anomalous

Anomaly, anomalous — *continued*
  specified type NEC — *continued*
    vulva 752.49
  spermatic cord 752.9
  spine, spinal 756.10
    column 756.10
    cord 742.9
      meningocele (*see also* Spina bifida) 741.9 ✓5ᵗʰ
      specified type NEC 742.59
      spina bifida (*see also* Spina bifida) 741.9 ✓5ᵗʰ
      vessel 747.82
    meninges 742.59
    nerve root 742.9
  spleen 759.0
  Sprengel's 755.52
  sternum 756.3
  stomach 750.9
    specified type NEC 750.7
  submaxillary gland 750.9
  superior vena cava 747.40
  talipes — *see* Talipes
  tarsus 755.67
    with complete absence of distal elements 755.31
  teeth, tooth NEC 520.9
    position 524.3
    spacing 524.3
  tendon 756.9
    specified type NEC 756.89
  termination
    coronary artery 746.85
  testis 752.9
  thebesian valve 746.9
  thigh 755.60
    flexion (*see also* Subluxation, congenital, hip) 754.32
  thorax (wall) 756.3
  throat 750.9
  thumb 755.50
    supernumerary 755.01
  thymus gland 759.2
  thyroid (gland) 759.2
    cartilage 748.3
  tibia 755.60
    saber 090.5
  toe 755.66
    supernumerary 755.02
    webbed (*see also* Syndactylism, toes) 755.13
  tongue 750.10
    specified type NEC 750.19
  trachea, tracheal 748.3
    cartilage 748.3
    rings 748.3
  tragus 744.3
  transverse aortic arch 747.21
  trichromata 368.59
  trichromatopsia 368.59
  tricuspid (leaflet) (valve) 746.9
    atresia 746.1
    Ebstein's 746.2
    specified type NEC 746.89
    stenosis 746.1
  trunk 759.9
  Uhl's (hypoplasia of myocardium, right ventricle) 746.84
  ulna 755.50
  umbilicus 759.9
    artery 747.5

Anomaly, anomalous — *continued*
  union, trachea with larynx 748.3
  unspecified site 759.9
  upper extremity 755.50
    vessel 747.63
  urachus 753.7
    specified type NEC 753.7
  ureter 753.9
    obstructive 753.20
    specified type NEC 753.4
      obstructive 753.29
  urethra (valve) 753.9
    obstructive 753.6
    specified type NEC 753.8
  urinary tract or system (any part, except urachus) 753.9
    specified type NEC 753.8
    urachus 753.7
  uterus 752.3
    with only one functioning horn 752.3
    in pregnancy or childbirth 654.0 ✓5ᵗʰ
      affecting fetus or newborn 763.89
    causing obstructed labor 660.2 ✓5ᵗʰ
      affecting fetus or newborn 763.1
  uvula 750.9
  vagina 752.40
  valleculae 748.3
  valve (heart) NEC 746.9
    formation, ureter 753.29
    pulmonary 746.00
    specified type NEC 746.89
  vascular NEC (*see also* Anomaly, peripheral vascular system) 747.60
    ring 747.21
  vas deferens 752.9
  vein(s) (peripheral) NEC (*see also* Anomaly, peripheral vascular system) 747.60
    brain 747.81
    cerebral 747.81
    coronary 746.89
    great 747.40
      specified type NEC 747.49
    portal 747.40
    pulmonary 747.40
    retina 743.9
  vena cava (inferior) (superior) 747.40
  venous return (pulmonary) 747.49
    partial 747.42
    total 747.41
  ventricle, ventricular (heart) 746.9
    bands 746.9
    folds 746.9
    septa 745.4
  vertebra 756.10
  vesicourethral orifice 753.9
  vessels NEC (*see also* Anomaly, peripheral vascular system) 747.60
    optic papilla 743.9
  vitelline duct 751.0
  vitreous humor 743.9
    specified type NEC 743.51
  vulva 752.40
  wrist (joint) 755.50

Anomia 784.69

Anonychia 757.5
  acquired 703.8

Anophthalmos, anophthalmus (clinical) (congenital) (globe) 743.00
  acquired V45.78

Anopsia (altitudinal) (quadrant) 368.46

Anorchia 752.8

Anorchism, anorchidism 752.8
Anorexia 783.0
  hysterical 300.11
  nervosa 307.1
Anosmia (see also Disturbance, sensation) 781.1
  hysterical 300.11
  postinfectional 478.9
  psychogenic 306.7
  traumatic 951.8
Anosognosia 780.99
Anosphrasia 781.1
Anosteoplasia 756.50
Anotia 744.09
Anovulatory cycle 628.0
Anoxemia 799.0
  newborn 768.9
Anoxia 799.0
  altitude 993.2
  cerebral 348.1
    with
      abortion — see Abortion, by type, with specified complication NEC
      ectopic pregnancy (see also categories 633.0-633.9) 639.8
      molar pregnancy (see also categories 630-632) 639.8
    complicating
      delivery (cesarean) (instrumental) 669.4
      ectopic or molar pregnancy 639.8
      obstetric anesthesia or sedation 668.2
      during or resulting from a procedure 997.01
    following
      abortion 639.8
      ectopic or molar pregnancy 639.8
    newborn (see also Distress, fetal, liveborn infant) 768.9
  due to drowning 994.1
  fetal, affecting newborn 768.9
  heart — see Insufficiency, coronary
  high altitude 993.2
  intrauterine
    fetal death (before onset of labor) 768.0
      during labor 768.1
    liveborn infant — see Distress, fetal, liveborn infant
  myocardial — see Insufficiency, coronary
  newborn 768.9
    mild or moderate 768.6
    severe 768.5
  pathological 799.0
Anteflexion — see Anteversion
Antenatal
  care, normal pregnancy V22.1
    first V22.0
  screening (for) V28.9
    based on amniocentesis NEC V28.2
      chromosomal anomalies V28.0
      raised alphafetoprotein levels V28.1
    chromosomal anomalies V28.0
    fetal growth retardation using ultrasonics V28.4
    isoimmunization V28.5
    malformations using ultrasonics V28.3
    raised alphafetoprotein levels in amniotic fluid V28.1

Antenatal — continued
  screening — continued
    specified condition NEC V28.8
    Streptococcus B V28.6
Antepartum — see condition
Anterior — see also condition
  spinal artery compression syndrome 721.1
Antero-occlusion 524.2
Anteversion
  cervix (see also Anteversion, uterus) 621.6
  femur (neck), congenital 755.63
  uterus, uterine (cervix) (postinfectional) (postpartal, old) 621.6
    congenital 752.3
    in pregnancy or childbirth 654.4
      affecting fetus or newborn 763.89
      causing obstructed labor 660.2
        affecting fetus or newborn 763.1
Anthracosilicosis (occupational) 500
Anthracosis (lung) (occupational) 500
  lingua 529.3
Anthrax 022.9
  with pneumonia 022.1 [484.5]
  colitis 022.2
  cutaneous 022.0
  gastrointestinal 022.2
  intestinal 022.2
  pulmonary 022.1
  respiratory 022.1
  septicemia 022.3
  specified manifestation NEC 022.8
Anthropoid pelvis 755.69
  with disproportion (fetopelvic) 653.2
    affecting fetus or newborn 763.1
    causing obstructed labor 660.1
      affecting fetus or newborn 763.1
Anthropophobia 300.29
Antibioma, breast 611.0
Antibodies
  maternal (blood group) (see also Incompatibility) 656.2
    anti-D, cord blood 656.1
  fetus or newborn 773.0
Antibody deficiency syndrome
  agammaglobulinemic 279.00
  congenital 279.04
  hypogammaglobulinemic 279.00
Anticoagulant, circulating (see also Circulating anticoagulants) 286.5
Antimongolism syndrome 758.3
Antimonial cholera 985.4
Antisocial personality 301.7
Antithrombinemia (see also Circulating anticoagulants) 286.5
Antithromboplastinemia (see also Circulating anticoagulants) 286.5
Antithromboplastinogenemia (see also Circulating anticoagulants) 286.5
Antitoxin complication or reaction — see Complications, vaccination
Anton (-Babinski) syndrome (hemiasomatognosia) 307.9
Antritis (chronic) 473.0
  acute 461.0
Antrum, antral — see condition

Anuria 788.5
　with
　　abortion — see Abortion, by type, with renal failure
　　ectopic pregnancy (see also categories 633.0-633.9) 639.3
　　molar pregnancy (see also categories 630-632) 639.3
　calculus (impacted) (recurrent) 592.9
　　kidney 592.0
　　ureter 592.1
　congenital 753.3
　due to a procedure 997.5
　following
　　abortion 639.3
　　ectopic or molar pregnancy 639.3
　newborn 753.3
　postrenal 593.4
　puerperal, postpartum, childbirth 669.3 ✓5ᵗʰ
　specified as due to a procedure 997.5
　sulfonamide
　　correct substance properly administered 788.5
　　overdose or wrong substance given or taken 961.0
　traumatic (following crushing) 958.5
Anus, anal — see condition
Anusitis 569.49
Anxiety (neurosis) (reaction) (state) 300.00
　alcohol-induced 291.89
　depression 300.4
　drug-induced 292.89
　due to or associated with physical condition 293.84
　generalized 300.02
　hysteria 300.20
　in
　　acute stress reaction 308.0
　　transient adjustment reaction 309.24
　panic type 300.01
　separation, abnormal 309.21
　syndrome (organic) (transient) 293.84
Aorta, aortic — see condition
Aortectasia 441.9
Aortitis (nonsyphilitic) 447.6
　arteriosclerotic 440.0
　calcific 447.6
　Döhle-Heller 093.1
　luetic 093.1
　rheumatic (see also Endocarditis, acute, rheumatic) 391.1
　rheumatoid — see Arthritis, rheumatoid
　specific 093.1
　syphilitic 093.1
　　congenital 090.5
Apethetic thyroid storm (see also Thyrotoxicosis) 242.9 ✓5ᵗʰ
Apepsia 536.8
　achlorhydric 536.0
　psychogenic 306.4
Aperistalsis, esophagus 530.0
Apert's syndrome (acrocephalosyndactyly) 755.55
Apert-Gallais syndrome (adrenogenital) 255.2
Apertognathia 524.2
Aphagia 787.2
　psychogenic 307.1

Aphakia (acquired) (bilateral) (postoperative) (unilateral) 379.31
　congenital 743.35
Aphalangia (congenital) 755.4
　lower limb (complete) (intercalary) (partial) (terminal) 755.39
　　meaning all digits (complete) (partial) 755.31
　　transverse 755.31
　upper limb (complete) (intercalary) (partial) (terminal) 755.29
　　meaning all digits (complete) (partial) 755.21
　　transverse 755.21
Aphasia (amnestic) (ataxic) (auditory) (Broca's) (choreatic) (classic) (expressive) (global) (ideational) (ideokinetic) (ideomotor) (jargon) (motor) (nominal) (receptive) (semantic) (sensory) (syntactic) (verbal) (visual) (Wernicke's) 784.3
　developmental 315.31
　syphilis, tertiary 094.89
　uremic — see Uremia
Aphemia 784.3
　uremic — see Uremia
Aphonia 784.41
　clericorum 784.49
　hysterical 300.11
　organic 784.41
　psychogenic 306.1
Aphthae, aphthous — see also condition
　Bednar's 528.2
　cachectic 529.0
　epizootic 078.4
　fever 078.4
　oral 528.2
　stomatitis 528.2
　thrush 112.0
　ulcer (oral) (recurrent) 528.2
　　genital organ(s) NEC
　　　female 629.8
　　　male 608.89
　larynx 478.79
Apical — see condition
Aplasia — see also Agenesis
　alveolar process (acquired) 525.8
　　congenital 750.26
　aorta (congenital) 747.22
　aortic valve (congenital) 746.89
　axialis excorticalis (congenital) 330.0
　bone marrow (myeloid) 284.9
　　acquired (secondary) 284.8
　　congenital 284.0
　　idiopathic 284.9
　brain 740.0
　　specified part 742.2
　breast 757.6
　bronchus 748.3
　cementum 520.4
　cerebellar 742.2
　congenital pure red cell 284.0
　corpus callosum 742.2
　erythrocyte 284.8
　　congenital 284.0
　extracortical axial 330.0
　eye (congenital) 743.00
　fovea centralis (congenital) 743.55
　germinal (cell) 606.0
　iris 743.45
　labyrinth, membranous 744.05

Aplasia — continued
　limb (congenital) 755.4
　　lower NEC 755.30
　　upper NEC 755.20
　lung (bilateral) (congenital) (unilateral) 748.5
　nervous system NEC 742.8
　nuclear 742.8
　ovary 752.0
　Pelizaeus-Merzbacher 330.0
　prostate (congenital) 752.8
　red cell (pure) (with thymoma) 284.8
　　acquired (secondary) 284.8
　　congenital 284.0
　　hereditary 284.0
　　of infants 284.0
　　primary 284.0
　round ligament (congenital) 752.8
　salivary gland 750.21
　skin (congenital) 757.39
　spinal cord 742.59
　spleen 759.0
　testis (congenital) 752.8
　thymic, with immunodeficiency 279.2
　thyroid 243
　uterus 752.3
　ventral horn cell 742.59

Apleuria 756.3

Apnea, apneic (spells) 786.03
　newborn, neonatorum 770.81
　　essential 770.81
　　obstructive 770.82
　　primary 770.81
　　sleep 770.81
　　specified NEC 770.82
　psychogenic 306.1
　sleep NEC 780.57
　　with
　　　hypersomnia 780.53
　　　hyposomnia 780.51
　　　insomnia 780.51
　　　sleep disturbance NEC 780.57

Apneumatosis newborn 770.4

Apodia 755.31

Apophysitis (bone) (see also Osteochondrosis) 732.9
　calcaneus 732.5
　juvenile 732.6

Apoplectiform convulsions (see also Disease, cerebrovascular, acute) 436

Apoplexia, apoplexy, apoplectic (see also Disease, cerebrovascular, acute) 436
　abdominal 569.89
　adrenal 036.3
　attack 436
　basilar (see also Disease, cerebrovascular, acute) 436
　brain (see also Disease, cerebrovascular, acute) 436
　bulbar (see also Disease, cerebrovascular, acute) 436
　capillary (see also Disease, cerebrovascular, acute) 436
　cardiac (see also Infarct, myocardium) 410.9
　cerebral (see also Disease, cerebrovascular, acute) 436
　chorea (see also Disease, cerebrovascular, acute) 436
　congestive (see also Disease, cerebrovascular, acute) 436

Apoplexia, apoplexy, apoplectic — continued
　congestive — continued
　　newborn 767.4
　embolic (see also Embolism, brain) 434.1
　fetus 767.0
　fit (see also Disease, cerebrovascular, acute) 436
　healed or old V12.59
　heart (auricle) (ventricle) (see also Infarct, myocardium) 410.9
　heat 992.0
　hemiplegia (see also Disease, cerebrovascular, acute) 436
　hemorrhagic (stroke) (see also Hemorrhage, brain) 432.9
　ingravescent (see also Disease, cerebrovascular, acute) 436
　late effect — see Late effect(s) (of) cerebrovascular disease
　lung — see Embolism, pulmonary
　meninges, hemorrhagic (see also Hemorrhage subarachnoid) 430
　neonatorum 767.0
　newborn 767.0
　pancreatitis 577.0
　placenta 641.2
　progressive (see also Disease, cerebrovascular, acute) 436
　pulmonary (artery) (vein) — see Embolism, pulmonary
　sanguineous (see also Disease, cerebrovascular, acute) 436
　seizure (see also Disease, cerebrovascular, acute) 436
　serous (see also Disease, cerebrovascular, acute) 436
　spleen 289.59
　stroke (see also Disease, cerebrovascular, acute) 436
　thrombotic (see also Thrombosis, brain) 434.0
　uremic — see Uremia
　uteroplacental 641.2

Appendage
　fallopian tube (cyst of Morgagni) 752.11
　intestine (epiploic) 751.5
　preauricular 744.1
　testicular (organ of Morgagni) 752.8

Appendicitis 541
　with
　　perforation, peritonitis (generalized), or rupture 540.0
　　　with peritoneal abscess 540.1
　　peritoneal abscess 540.1
　acute (catarrhal) (fulminating) (gangrenous) (inflammatory) (obstructive) (retrocecal) (suppurative) 540.9
　　with
　　　perforation, peritonitis, or rupture 540.0
　　　　with peritoneal abscess 540.1
　　　peritoneal abscess 540.1
　amebic 006.8
　chronic (recurrent) 542
　exacerbation — see Appendicitis, acute
　fulminating — see Appendicitis, acute
　gangrenous — see Appendicitis, acute
　healed (obliterative) 542
　interval 542
　neurogenic 542
　obstructive 542
　pneumococcal 541
　recurrent 542

Appendicitis — continued
  relapsing 542
  retrocecal 541
  subacute (adhesive) 542
  subsiding 542
  suppurative — *see* Appendicitis, acute
  tuberculous (*see also* Tuberculosis) 014.8 ✓5ᵗʰ
Appendiclausis 543.9
Appendicolithiasis 543.9
Appendicopathia oxyurica 127.4
Appendix, appendicular — *see also* condition
  Morgagni (male) 752.8
    fallopian tube 752.11
Appetite
  depraved 307.52
  excessive 783.6
    psychogenic 307.51
  lack or loss (*see also* Anorexia) 783.0
    nonorganic origin 307.59
  perverted 307.52
    hysterical 300.11
Apprehension, apprehensiveness (abnormal) (state) 300.00
  specified type NEC 300.09
Approximal wear 521.1
Apraxia (classic) (ideational) (ideokinetic) (ideomotor) (motor) 784.69
  oculomotor, congenital 379.51
  verbal 784.69
Aptyalism 527.7
Aqueous misdirection 365.83
Arabicum elephantiasis (*see also* Infestation, filarial) 125.9
Arachnidism 989.5
Arachnitis — *see* Meningitis
Arachnodactyly 759.82
Arachnoidism 989.5
Arachnoiditis (acute) (adhesive) (basic) (brain) (cerebrospinal) (chiasmal) (chronic) (spinal) (*see also* Meningitis) 322.9
  meningococcal (chronic) 036.0
  syphilitic 094.2
  tuberculous (*see also* Tuberculosis meninges) 013.0 ✓5ᵗʰ
Araneism 989.5
Arboencephalitis, Australian 062.4
Arborization block (heart) 426.6
Arbor virus, arbovirus (infection) NEC 066.9
ARC 042
Arches — *see* condition
Arcuatus uterus 752.3
Arcus (cornea)
  juvenilis 743.43
    interfering with vision 743.42
  senilis 371.41
Arc-welders' lung 503
Arc-welders' syndrome (photokeratitis) 370.24
Areflexia 796.1
Areola — *see* condition
Argentaffinoma (M8241/1) — *see also* Neoplasm, by site, uncertain behavior
  benign (M8241/0) — *see* Neoplasm, by site, benign
  malignant (M8241/3) — *see* Neoplasm, by site, malignant
  syndrome 259.2

Argentinian hemorrhagic fever 078.7
Arginosuccinicaciduria 270.6
Argonz-Del Castillo syndrome (nonpuerperal galactorrhea and amenorrhea) 253.1
Argyll-Robertson phenomenon, pupil, or syndrome (syphilitic) 094.89
  atypical 379.45
  nonluetic 379.45
  nonsyphilitic 379.45
  reversed 379.45
Argyria, argyriasis NEC 985.8
  conjunctiva 372.55
  cornea 371.16
  from drug or medicinal agent
    correct substance properly administered 709.09
    overdose or wrong substance given or taken 961.2
Arhinencephaly 742.2
Arias-Stella phenomenon 621.3
Ariboflavinosis 266.0
Arizona enteritis 008.1
Arm — *see* condition
Armenian disease 277.3
Arnold-Chiari obstruction or syndrome (*see also* Spina bifida) 741.0 ✓5ᵗʰ
  type I 348.4
  type II (*see also* Spina bifida) 741.0 ✓5ᵗʰ
  type III 742.0
  type IV 742.2
Arrest, arrested
  active phase of labor 661.1 ✓5ᵗʰ
    affecting fetus or newborn 763.7
  any plane in pelvis
    complicating delivery 660.1 ✓5ᵗʰ
      affecting fetus or newborn 763.1
  bone marrow (*see also* Anemia, aplastic) 284.9
  cardiac 427.5
    with
      abortion — *see* Abortion, by type, with specified complication NEC
      ectopic pregnancy (*see also* categories 633.0-633.9) 639.8
      molar pregnancy (*see also* categories 630-632) 639.8
    complicating
      anesthesia
        correct substance properly administered 427.5
        obstetric 668.1 ✓5ᵗʰ
        overdose or wrong substance given 968.4
        specified anesthetic — *see* Table of Drugs and Chemicals
      delivery (cesarean) (instrumental) 669.4 ✓5ᵗʰ
      ectopic or molar pregnancy 639.8
      surgery (nontherapeutic) (therapeutic) 997.1
    fetus or newborn 779.89 ▲
    following
      abortion 639.8
      ectopic or molar pregnancy 639.8
    postoperative (immediate) 997.1
      long-term effect of cardiac surgery 429.4
    cardiorespiratory (*see also* Arrest, cardiac) 427.5
  deep transverse 660.3 ✓5ᵗʰ
    affecting fetus or newborn 763.1

Index to Diseases

Arrest, arrested — *continued*
  development or growth
    bone 733.91
    child 783.40
    fetus 764.9 ✓5ᵗʰ
      affecting management of pregnancy 656.5 ✓5ᵗʰ
    tracheal rings 748.3
  epiphyseal 733.91
  granulopoiesis 288.0
  heart — *see* Arrest, cardiac
  respiratory 799.1
    newborn 770.89
  sinus 426.6
  transverse (deep) 660.3 ✓5ᵗʰ
    affecting fetus or newborn 763.1
Arrhenoblastoma (M8630/1)
  benign (M8630/0)
    specified site — *see* Neoplasm, by site, benign
    unspecified site
      female 220
      male 222.0
  malignant (M8630/3)
    specified site — *see* Neoplasm, by site, malignant
    unspecified site
      female 183.0
      male 186.9
  specified site — *see* Neoplasm, by site, uncertain behavior
  unspecified site
    female 236.2
    male 236.4
Arrhinencephaly 742.2
  due to
    trisomy 13 (13-15) 758.1
    trisomy 18 (16-18) 758.2
Arrhythmia (auricle) (cardiac) (cordis) (gallop rhythm) (juvenile) (nodal) (reflex) (sinus) (supraventricular) (transitory) (ventricle) 427.9
  bigeminal rhythm 427.89
  block 426.9
  bradycardia 427.89
  contractions, premature 427.60
  coronary sinus 427.89
  ectopic 427.89
  extrasystolic 427.60
  postoperative 997.1
  psychogenic 306.2
  vagal 780.2
Arrillaga-Ayerza syndrome (pulmonary artery sclerosis with pulmonary hypertension) 416.0
Arsenical
  dermatitis 692.4
  keratosis 692.4
  pigmentation 985.1
    from drug or medicinal agent
      correct substance properly administered 709.09
      overdose or wrong substance given or taken 961.1
Arsenism 985.1
  from drug or medicinal agent
    correct substance properly administered 692.4
    overdose or wrong substance given or taken 961.1

Arterial — *see* condition
Arteriectasis 447.8
Arteriofibrosis — *see* Arteriosclerosis
Arteriolar sclerosis — *see* Arteriosclerosis
Arteriolith — *see* Arteriosclerosis
Arteriolitis 447.6
  necrotizing, kidney 447.5
  renal — *see* Hypertension, kidney
Arteriolosclerosis — *see* Arteriosclerosis
Arterionephrosclerosis (*see also* Hypertension, kidney) 403.90
Arteriopathy 447.9
Arteriosclerosis, arteriosclerotic (artery) (deformans) (diffuse) (disease) (endarteritis) (general) (obliterans) (obliterative) (occlusive) (senile) (with calcification) 440.9
  with
    gangrene 440.24
    psychosis (*see also* Psychosis, arteriosclerotic) 290.40
    ulceration 440.23
  aorta 440.0
  arteries of extremities — *see* Arteriosclerosis, extremities
  basilar (artery) (*see also* Occlusion, artery, basilar) 433.0 ✓5ᵗʰ
  brain 437.0
  bypass graft
    coronary artery 414.05
      autologous artery (gastroepiploic) (internal mammary) 414.04
      autologous vein 414.02
      nonautologous biological 414.03
    extremity 440.30
      autologous vein 440.31
      nonautologous biological 440.32
  cardiac — *see* Arteriosclerosis, coronary
  cardiopathy — *see* Arteriosclerosis, coronary
  cardiorenal (*see also* Hypertension, cardiorenal) 404.90
  cardiovascular (*see also* Disease, cardiovascular) 429.2
  carotid (artery) (common) (internal) (*see also* Occlusion, artery, carotid) 433.1 ✓5ᵗʰ
  central nervous system 437.0
  cerebral 437.0
    late effect — *see* Late effect(s) (of) cerebrovascular disease
  cerebrospinal 437.0
  cerebrovascular 437.0
  coronary (artery) 414.00
    graft — *see* Arteriosclerosis, bypass graft
    native artery 414.01
    of transplanted heart 414.06
  extremities (native artery) NEC 440.20
    bypass graft 440.30
      autologous vein 440.31
      nonautologous biological 440.32
    claudication (intermittent) 440.21
    and
      gangrene 440.24
      rest pain 440.22
      and
        gangrene 440.24
        ulceration 440.23
          and gangrene 440.24
      ulceration 440.23
        and gangrene 440.24
    gangrene 440.24

Arteriosclerosis, arteriosclerotic

Arteriosclerosis, arteriosclerotic — continued
  extremities — continued
    rest pain 440.22
    and
      gangrene 440.24
      ulceration 440.23
        and gangrene 440.24
    specified site NEC 440.29
    ulceration 440.23
      and gangrene 440.24
  heart (disease) — see also Arteriosclerosis, coronary
    valve 424.99
      aortic 424.1
      mitral 424.0
      pulmonary 424.3
      tricuspid 424.2
  kidney (see also Hypertension, kidney) 403.90
  labyrinth, labyrinthine 388.00
  medial NEC 440.20
  mesentery (artery) 557.1
  Mönckeberg's 440.20
  myocarditis 429.0
  nephrosclerosis (see also Hypertension, kidney) 403.90
  peripheral (of extremities) — see Arteriosclerosis, extremities
  precerebral 433.9 ✓5ᵗʰ
    specified artery NEC 433.8 ✓5ᵗʰ
  pulmonary (idiopathic) 416.0
  renal (see also Hypertension, kidney) 403.90
    arterioles (see also Hypertension, kidney) 403.90
    artery 440.1
  retinal (vascular) 440.8 [362.13]
  specified artery NEC 440.8
    with gangrene 440.8 [785.4]
  spinal (cord) 437.0
  vertebral (artery) (see also Occlusion, artery, vertebral) 433.2 ✓5ᵗʰ
Arteriospasm 443.9
Arteriovenous — see condition
Arteritis 447.6
  allergic (see also Angiitis, hypersensitivity) 446.20
  aorta (nonsyphilitic) 447.6
    syphilitic 093.1
  aortic arch 446.7
  brachiocephalica 446.7
  brain 437.4
    syphilitic 094.89
  branchial 446.7
  cerebral 437.4
    late effect — see Late effect(s) (of) cerebrovascular disease
    syphilitic 094.89
  coronary (artery) — see also Arteriosclerosis, coronary
    rheumatic 391.9
      chronic 398.99
    syphilitic 093.89
  cranial (left) (right) 446.5
  deformans — see Arteriosclerosis
  giant cell 446.5
  necrosing or necrotizing 446.0
  nodosa 446.0
  obliterans — see also Arteriosclerosis
    subclaviocarotica 446.7
  pulmonary 417.8
  retina 362.18
  rheumatic — see Fever, rheumatic

Arteritis — continued
  senile — see Arteriosclerosis
  suppurative 447.2
  syphilitic (general) 093.89
    brain 094.89
    coronary 093.89
    spinal 094.89
    temporal 446.5
  young female, syndrome 446.7
Artery, arterial — see condition
Arthralgia (see also Pain, joint) 719.4 ✓5ᵗʰ
  allergic (see also Pain, joint) 719.4 ✓5ᵗʰ
  in caisson disease 993.3
  psychogenic 307.89
  rubella 056.71
  Salmonella 003.23
  temporomandibular joint 524.62
Arthritis, arthritic (acute) (chronic) (subacute) 716.9 ✓5ᵗʰ
  meaning Osteoarthritis — see Osteoarthrosis

Note — Use the following fifth-digit subclassification with categories 711-712, 715-716:

0	site unspecified
1	shoulder region
2	upper arm
3	forearm
4	hand
5	pelvic region and thigh
6	lower leg
7	ankle and foot
8	other specified sites
9	multiple sites

  allergic 716.2 ✓5ᵗʰ
  ankylosing (crippling) (spine) 720.0
    sites other than spine 716.9 ✓5ᵗʰ
  atrophic 714.0
    spine 720.9
  back (see also Arthritis, spine) 721.90
  Bechterew's (ankylosing spondylitis) 720.0
  blennorrhagic 098.50
  cervical, cervicodorsal (see also Spondylosis, cervical) 721.0
  Charcôt's 094.0 [713.5]
    diabetic 250.6 ✓5ᵗʰ [713.5]
    syringomyelic 336.0 [713.5]
    tabetic 094.0 [713.5]
  chylous (see also Filariasis) 125.9 [711.7] ✓5ᵗʰ
  climacteric NEC 716.3 ✓5ᵗʰ
  coccyx 721.8
  cricoarytenoid 478.79
  crystal (-induced) — see Arthritis, due to crystals
  deformans (see also Osteoarthrosis) 715.9 ✓5ᵗʰ
    spine 721.90
      with myelopathy 721.91
  degenerative (see also Osteoarthrosis) 715.9 ✓5ᵗʰ
    idiopathic 715.09
    polyarticular 715.09
    spine 721.90
      with myelopathy 721.91
  dermatoarthritis, lipoid 272.8 [713.0]
  due to or associated with
    acromegaly 253.0 [713.0]
    actinomycosis 039.8 [711.4] ✓5ᵗʰ
    amyloidosis 277.3 [713.7]

Arthritis, arthritic — *continued*
  due to or associated with — *continued*
    bacterial disease NEC 040.89 *[711.4]* ✓5
    Behçet's syndrome 136.1 *[711.2]* ✓5
    blastomycosis 116.0 *[711.6]* ✓5
    brucellosis (*see also* Brucellosis) 023.9 *[711.4]* ✓5
    caisson disease 993.3
    coccidioidomycosis 114.3 *[711.6]* ✓5
    coliform (Escherichia coli) 711.0 ✓5
    colitis, ulcerative (*see also* Colitis, ulcerative) 556.9 *[713.1]*
    cowpox 051.0 *[711.5]* ✓5
    crystals — *see also* Gout
      dicalcium phosphate 275.49 *[712.1]*
      pyrophosphate 275.49 *[712.2]*
      specified NEC 275.49 *[712.8]*
    dermatoarthritis, lipoid 272.8 *[713.0]*
    dermatological disorder NEC 709.9 *[713.3]*
    diabetes 250.6 ✓5 *[713.5]*
    diphtheria 032.89 *[711.4]* ✓5
    dracontiasis 125.7 *[711.7]* ✓5
    dysentery 009.0 *[711.3]* ✓5
    endocrine disorder NEC 259.9 *[713.0]*
    enteritis NEC 009.1 *[711.3]* ✓5
      infectious (*see also* Enteritis, infectious) 009.0 *[711.3]* ✓5
        specified organism NEC 008.8 *[711.3]* ✓5
      regional (*see also* Enteritis, regional) 555.9 *[713.1]*
      specified organism NEC 008.8 *[711.3]* ✓5
    epiphyseal slip, nontraumatic (old) 716.8 ✓5
    erysipelas 035 *[711.4]* ✓5
    erythema
      epidemic 026.1
      multiforme 695.1 *[713.3]*
      nodosum 695.2 *[713.3]*
    Escherichia coli 711.0 ✓5
    filariasis NEC 125.9 *[711.7]* ✓5
    gastrointestinal condition NEC 569.9 *[713.1]*
    glanders 024 *[711.4]* ✓5
    Gonococcus 098.50
    gout 274.0
    H. influenzae 711.0 ✓5
    helminthiasis NEC 128.9 *[711.7]* ✓5
    hematological disorder NEC 289.9 *[713.2]*
    hemochromatosis 275.0 *[713.0]*
    hemoglobinopathy NEC (*see also* Disease, hemoglobin) 282.7 *[713.2]*
    hemophilia (*see also* Hemophilia) 286.0 *[713.2]*
    Hemophilus influenzae (H. influenzae) 711.0 ✓5
    Henoch (-Schönlein) purpura 287.0 *[713.6]*
    histoplasmosis NEC (*see also* Histoplasmosis) 115.99 *[711.6]* ✓5
    hyperparathyroidism 252.0 *[713.0]*
    hypersensitivity reaction NEC 995.3 *[713.6]*
    hypogammaglobulinemia (*see also* Hypogamma-globulinemia) 279.00 *[713.0]*
    hypothyroidism NEC 244.9 *[713.0]*
    infection (*see also* Arthritis, infectious) 711.9 ✓5
    infectious disease NEC 136.9 *[711.8]* ✓5
    leprosy (*see also* Leprosy) 030.9 *[711.4]* ✓5
    leukemia NEC (M9800/3) 208.9 ✓5 *[713.2]*
    lipoid dermatoarthritis 272.8 *[713.0]*

Arthritis, arthritic — *continued*
  due to or associated with — *continued*
    Lyme disease 088.81 *[711.8]* ✓5
    Mediterranean fever, familial 277.3 *[713.7]*
    meningococcal infection 036.82
    metabolic disorder NEC 277.9 *[713.0]*
    multiple myelomatosis (M9730/3) 203.0 ✓5 *[713.2]*
    mumps 072.79 *[711.5]* ✓5
    mycobacteria 031.8 *[711.4]* ✓5
    mycosis NEC 117.9 *[711.6]* ✓5
    neurological disorder NEC 349.9 *[713.5]*
    ochronosis 270.2 *[713.0]*
    O'Nyong Nyong 066.3 *[711.5]* ✓5
    parasitic disease NEC 136.9 *[711.8]* ✓5
    paratyphoid fever (*see also* Fever, paratyphoid) 002.9 *[711.3]* ✓5
    Pneumococcus 711.0 ✓5
    poliomyelitis (*see also* Poliomyelitis) 045.9 ✓5 *[711.5]* ✓5
    Pseudomonas 711.0 ✓5
    psoriasis 696.0
    pyogenic organism (E. coli) (H. influenzae) (Pseudomonas) (Streptococcus) 711.0 ✓5
    rat-bite fever 026.1 *[711.4]* ✓5
    regional enteritis (*see also* Enteritis, regional) 555.9 *[713.1]*
    Reiter's disease 099.3 *[711.1]* ✓5
    respiratory disorder NEC 519.9 *[713.4]*
    reticulosis, malignant (M9720/3) 202.3 ✓5 *[713.2]*
    rubella 056.71
    salmonellosis 003.23
    sarcoidosis 135 *[713.7]*
    serum sickness 999.5 *[713.6]*
    Staphylococcus 711.0 ✓5
    Streptococcus 711.0 ✓5
    syphilis (*see also* Syphilis) 094.0 *[711.4]* ✓5
    syringomyelia 336.0 *[713.5]*
    thalassemia 282.4 *[713.2]*
    tuberculosis (*see also* Tuberculosis, arthritis) 015.9 ✓5 *[711.4]* ✓5
    typhoid fever 002.0 *[711.3]* ✓5
    ulcerative colitis (*see also* Colitis, ulcerative) 556.9 *[713.1]*
    urethritis
      nongonococcal (*see also* Urethritis, nongonococcal) 099.40 *[711.1]* ✓5
      nonspecific (*see also* Urethritis, nongonococcal) 099.40 *[711.1]* ✓5
      Reiter's 099.3 *[711.1]* ✓5
    viral disease NEC 079.99 *[711.5]* ✓5
  erythema epidemic 026.1
  gonococcal 098.50
  gouty (acute) 274.0
  hypertrophic (*see also* Osteoarthrosis) 715.9 ✓5
    spine 721.90
      with myelopathy 721.91
  idiopathic, blennorrheal 099.3
  in caisson disease 993.3 *[713.8]*
  infectious or infective (acute) (chronic) (subacute) NEC 711.9 ✓5
    nonpyogenic 711.9 ✓5
    spine 720.9
  inflammatory NEC 714.9
  juvenile rheumatoid (chronic) (polyarticular) 714.30
    acute 714.31
    monoarticular 714.33

Arthritis, arthritic — *continued*
  juvenile rheumatoid — *continued*
    pauciarticular 714.32
  lumbar (*see also* Spondylosis, lumbar) 721.3
  meningococcal 036.82
  menopausal NEC 716.3 ✓5ᵗʰ
  migratory — *see* Fever, rheumatic
  neuropathic (Charcôt's) 094.0 *[713.5]*
    diabetic 250.6 ✓5ᵗʰ *[713.5]*
    nonsyphilitic NEC 349.9 *[713.5]*
    syringomyelic 336.0 *[713.5]*
    tabetic 094.0 *[713.5]*
  nodosa (*see also* Osteoarthrosis) 715.9 ✓5ᵗʰ
    spine 721.90
      with myelopathy 721.91
  nonpyogenic NEC 716.9 ✓5ᵗʰ
    spine 721.90
      with myelopathy 721.91
  ochronotic 270.2 *[713.0]*
  palindromic (see also Rheumatism, palindromic) 719.3 ✓5ᵗʰ
  pneumococcal 711.0 ✓5ᵗʰ
  postdysenteric 009.0 *[711.3]* ✓5ᵗʰ
  postrheumatic, chronic (Jaccoud's) 714.4
  primary progressive 714.0
    spine 720.9
  proliferative 714.0
    spine 720.0
  psoriatic 696.0
  purulent 711.0 ✓5ᵗʰ
  pyogenic or pyemic 711.0 ✓5ᵗʰ
  rheumatoid 714.0
    acute or subacute — *see* Fever, rheumatic
    chronic 714.0
    spine 720.0
  rheumatoid (nodular) 714.0
    with
      splenoadenomegaly and leukopenia 714.1
      visceral or systemic involvement 714.2
    aortitis 714.89
    carditis 714.2
    heart disease 714.2
    juvenile (chronic) (polyarticular) 714.30
      acute 714.31
      monoarticular 714.33
      pauciarticular 714.32
      spine 720.0
  rubella 056.71
  sacral, sacroiliac, sacrococcygeal (*see also* Spondylosis, sacral) 721.3
  scorbutic 267
  senile or senescent (*see also* Osteoarthrosis) 715.9 ✓5ᵗʰ
    spine 721.90
      with myelopathy 721.91
  septic 711.0 ✓5ᵗʰ
  serum (nontherapeutic) (therapeutic) 999.5 *[713.6]*
  specified form NEC 716.8 ✓5ᵗʰ
  spine 721.90
    with myelopathy 721.91
    atrophic 720.9
    degenerative 721.90
      with myelopathy 721.91
    hypertrophic (with deformity) 721.90
      with myelopathy 721.91
    infectious or infective NEC 720.9
    Marie-Strümpell 720.0
    nonpyogenic 721.90
      with myelopathy 721.91

Arthritis, arthritic — *continued*
  spine — *continued*
    pyogenic 720.9
    rheumatoid 720.0
    traumatic (old) 721.7
    tuberculous (*see also* Tuberculosis) 015.0 ✓5ᵗʰ *[720.81]*
  staphylococcal 711.0 ✓5ᵗʰ
  streptococcal 711.0 ✓5ᵗʰ
  suppurative 711.0 ✓5ᵗʰ
  syphilitic 094.0 *[713.5]*
    congenital 090.49 *[713.5]*
  syphilitica deformans (Charcôt) 094.0 *[713.5]*
  temporomandibular joint 524.69
  thoracic (*see also* Spondylosis, thoracic) 721.2
  toxic of menopause 716.3 ✓5ᵗʰ
  transient 716.4 ✓5ᵗʰ
  traumatic (chronic) (old) (post) 716.1 ✓5ᵗʰ
    current injury — *see* nature of injury
    tuberculous (*see also* Tuberculosis, arthritis) 015.9 ✓5ᵗʰ *[711.4]* ✓5ᵗʰ
  urethritica 099.3 *[711.1]* ✓5ᵗʰ
  urica, uratic 274.0
  venereal 099.3 *[711.1]* ✓5ᵗʰ
  vertebral (*see also* Arthritis, spine) 721.90
  villous 716.8 ✓5ᵗʰ
  von Bechterew's 720.0
Arthrocele (*see also* Effusion, joint) 719.0 ✓5ᵗʰ
Arthrochondritis — *see* Arthritis
Arthrodesis status V45.4
Arthrodynia (*see also* Pain, joint) 719.4 ✓5ᵗʰ
  psychogenic 307.89
Arthrodysplasia 755.9
Arthrofibrosis, joint (*see also* Ankylosis) 718.5 ✓5ᵗʰ
Arthrogryposis 728.3
  multiplex, congenita 754.89
Arthrokatadysis 715.35
Arthrolithiasis 274.0
Arthro-onychodysplasia 756.89
Arthro-osteo-onychodysplasia 756.89
Arthropathy (*see also* Arthritis) 716.9 ✓5ᵗʰ

Note — *Use the following fifth-digit subclassification with categories 711-712, 716:*	
0	site unspecified
1	shoulder region
2	upper arm
3	forearm
4	hand
5	pelvic region and thigh
6	lower leg
7	ankle and foot
8	other specified sites
9	multiple sites

  Behçets 136.1 *[711.2]* ✓5ᵗʰ
  Charcôt's 094.0 *[713.5]*
    diabetic 250.6 ✓5ᵗʰ *[713.5]*
    syringomyelic 336.0 *[713.5]*
    tabetic 094.0 *[713.5]*
  crystal (-induced) — *see* Arthritis, due to crystals
  gouty 274.0
  neurogenic, neuropathic (Charcôt's) (tabetic) 094.0 *[713.5]*

Arthropathy — continued
  neurogenic, neuropathic — continued
    diabetic 250.6 ✓5ᵗʰ [713.5]
    nonsyphilitic NEC 349.9 [713.5]
    syringomyelic 336.0 [713.5]
  postdysenteric NEC 009.0 [711.3] ✓5ᵗʰ
  postrheumatic, chronic (Jaccoud's) 714.4
  psoriatic 696.0
  pulmonary 731.2
  specified NEC 716.8 ✓5ᵗʰ
  syringomyelia 336.0 [713.5]
  tabes dorsalis 094.0 [713.5]
  tabetic 094.0 [713.5]
  transient 716.4 ✓5ᵗʰ
  traumatic 716.1 ✓5ᵗʰ
  uric acid 274.0
Arthophyte (see also Loose, body, joint) 718.1 ✓5ᵗʰ
Arthrophytis 719.80
  ankle 719.87
  elbow 719.82
  foot 719.87
  hand 719.84
  hip 719.85
  knee 719.86
  multiple sites 719.89
  pelvic region 719.85
  shoulder (region) 719.81
  specified site NEC 719.88
  wrist 719.83
Arthropyosis (see also Arthritis, pyogenic) 711.0 ✓5ᵗʰ
Arthrosis (deformans) (degenerative) (see also Osteoarthrosis) 715.9 ✓5ᵗʰ
  Charcôt's 094.0 [713.5]
  polyarticular 715.09
  spine (see also Spondylosis) 721.90
Arthus' phenomenon 995.2
  due to
    correct substance properly administered 995.2
    overdose or wrong substance given or taken 977.9
      specified drug — see Table of Drugs and Chemicals
    serum 999.5
Articular — see also condition
  disc disorder (reducing or non-reducing) 524.63
  spondylolisthesis 756.12
Artificial
  device (prosthetic) — see Fitting, device
  insemination V26.1
  menopause (states) (symptoms) (syndrome) 627.4
  opening status (functioning) (without complication) V44.9
    anus (colostomy) V44.3
    colostomy V44.3
    cystostomy V44.50
      appendico-vesicostomy V44.52
      cutaneous-vesicostomy V44.51
      specified type NEC V44.59
    enterostomy V44.4
    gastrostomy V44.1
    ileostomy V44.2
    intestinal tract NEC V44.4
    jejunostomy V44.4
    nephrostomy V44.6
    specified site NEC V44.8

Artificial — continued
  opening status — continued
    tracheostomy V44.0
    ureterostomy V44.6
    urethrostomy V44.6
    urinary tract NEC V44.6
    vagina V44.7
    vagina status V44.7
ARV (disease) (illness) (infection) — see Human immunodeficiency virus (disease) (illness) (infection)
Arytenoid — see condition
Asbestosis (occupational) 501
Asboe-Hansen's disease (incontinentia pigmenti) 757.33
Ascariasis (intestinal) (lung) 127.0
Ascaridiasis 127.0
Ascaris 127.0
  lumbricoides (infestation) 127.0
  pneumonia 127.0
Ascending — see condition
Aschoff's bodies (see also Myocarditis, rheumatic) 398.0
Ascites 789.5
  abdominal NEC 789.5
  cancerous (M8000/6) 197.6
  cardiac 428.0
  chylous (nonfilarial) 457.8
    filarial (see also Infestation, filarial) 125.9
  congenital 778.0
  due to S. japonicum 120.2
  fetal, causing fetopelvic disproportion 653.7 ✓5ᵗʰ
  heart 428.0
  joint (see also Effusion, joint) 719.0 ✓5ᵗʰ
  malignant (M8000/6) 197.6
  pseudochylous 789.5
  syphilitic 095.2
  tuberculous (see also Tuberculosis) 014.0 ✓5ᵗʰ
Ascorbic acid (vitamin C) deficiency (scurvy) 267
ASCUS (atypical squamous cell changes of undetermined significance)
  favor benign 795.01
  favor dysplasia 795.02
ASCVD (arteriosclerotic cardiovascular disease) 429.2
Aseptic — see condition
Asherman's syndrome 621.5
Asialia 527.7
Asiatic cholera (see also Cholera) 001.9
Asocial personality or trends 301.7
Asomatognosia 781.8
Aspergillosis 117.3
  with pneumonia 117.3 [484.6]
  allergic bronchopulmonary 518.6
  nonsyphilitic NEC 117.3
Aspergillus (flavus) (fumigatus) (infection) (terreus) 117.3
Aspermatogenesis 606.0
Aspermia (testis) 606.0
Asphyxia, asphyxiation (by) 799.0
  antenatal — see Distress, fetal
  bedclothes 994.7
  birth (see also Ashpyxia, newborn) 768.9
  bunny bag 994.7
  carbon monoxide 986

Asphyxia, asphyxiation — continued
- caul (see also Asphyxia, newborn)
- cave-in 994.7
  - crushing — see Injury, internal, intrathoracic organs
- constriction 994.7
- crushing — see Injury, internal, intrathoracic organs
- drowning 994.1
- fetal, affecting newborn 768.9 ▲
- food or foreign body (in larynx) 933.1
  - bronchioles 934.8
  - bronchus (main) 934.1
  - lung 934.8
  - nasopharynx 933.0
  - nose, nasal passages 932
  - pharynx 933.0
  - respiratory tract 934.9
    - specified part NEC 934.8
  - throat 933.0
  - trachea 934.0
- gas, fumes, or vapor NEC 987.9
  - specified — see Table of Drugs and Chemicals
- gravitational changes 994.7
- hanging 994.7
- inhalation — see Inhalation
- intrauterine
  - fetal death (before onset of labor) 768.0
    - during labor 768.1
  - liveborn infant — see Distress, fetal, liveborn infant
- local 443.0
- mechanical 994.7
  - during birth (see also Distress, fetal) 768.9 ▲
- mucus 933.1
  - bronchus (main) 934.1
  - larynx 933.1
  - lung 934.8
  - nasal passages 932
  - newborn 770.1
  - pharynx 933.0
  - respiratory tract 934.9
    - specfied part NEC 934.8
  - throat 933.0
  - trachea 934.0
  - vaginal (fetus or newborn) 770.1
- newborn 768.9
  - blue 768.6
  - livida 768.6
  - mild or moderate 768.6
  - pallida 768.5
  - severe 768.5
  - white 768.5
- pathological 799.0
- plastic bag 994.7
- postnatal (see also Asphyxia, newborn) 768.9
  - mechanical 994.7
- pressure 994.7
- reticularis 782.61
- strangulation 994.7
- submersion 994.1
- traumatic NEC — see Injury, internal, intrathoracic organs
- vomiting, vomitus — see Asphyxia, food or foreign body

Aspiration
- acid pulmonary (syndrome) 997.3
  - obstetric 668.0 ✓5ᵗʰ
- amniotic fluid 770.1

Aspiration — continued
- bronchitis 507.0
- contents of birth canal 770.1
- fetal pneumonitis 770.1
- food, foreign body, or gasoline (with asphyxiation) — see Asphyxia, food or foreign body
- meconium 770.1
- mucus 933.1
  - into
    - bronchus (main) 934.1
    - lung 934.8
    - respiratory tract 934.9
      - specified part NEC 934.8
    - trachea 934.0
  - newborn 770.1
  - vaginal (fetus or newborn) 770.1
- newborn 770.1
- pneumonia 507.0
- pneumonitis 507.0
  - fetus or newborn 770.1
  - obstetric 668.0 ✓5ᵗʰ
- syndrome of newborn (massive) (meconium) 770.1
- vernix caseosa 770.1

Asplenia 759.0
- with mesocardia 746.87

Assam fever 085.0

Assimilation, pelvis
- with disproportion 653.2 ✓5ᵗʰ
  - affecting fetus or newborn 763.1
  - causing obstructed labor 660.1 ✓5ᵗʰ
    - affecting fetus or newborn 763.1

Assmann's focus (see also Tuberculosis) 011.0 ✓5ᵗʰ

Astasia (-asbasia) 307.9
- hysterical 300.11

Asteatosis 706.8
- cutis 706.8

Astereognosis 780.99 ▲

Asterixis 781.3
- in liver disease 572.8

Asteroid hyalitis 379.22

Asthenia, asthenic 780.79
- cardiac (see also Failure, heart) 428.9
  - psychogenic 306.2
- cardiovascular (see also Failure, heart) 428.9
  - psychogenic 306.2
- heart (see also Failure, heart) 428.9
  - psychogenic 306.2
- hysterical 300.11
- myocardial (see also Failure, heart) 428.9
  - psychogenic 306.2
- nervous 300.5
- neurocirculatory 306.2
- neurotic 300.5
- psychogenic 300.5
- psychoneurotic 300.5
- psychophysiologic 300.5
- reaction, psychoneurotic 300.5
- senile 797
- Stiller's 780.79
- tropical anhidrotic 705.1

Asthenopia 368.13
- accommodative 367.4
- hysterical (muscular) 300.11
- psychogenic 306.7

Asthenospermia 792.2

Index to Diseases

Asthma, asthmatic (bronchial) (catarrh) (spasmodic) 493.9 ✓5ᵗʰ

> Note — Use the following fifth-digit subclassification with category 493:
>
> 0   without mention of status asthmaticus or acute exacerbation or unspecified
> 1   with status asthmaticus
> 2   with acute exacerbation

   with
      chronic obstructive pulmonary disease (COPD) 493.2 ✓5ᵗʰ
      hay fever 493.0 ✓5ᵗʰ
      rhinitis, allergic 493.0 ✓5ᵗʰ
   allergic 493.9 ✓5ᵗʰ
      stated cause (external allergen) 493.0 ✓5ᵗʰ
   atopic 493.0 ✓5ᵗʰ
   cardiac (see also Failure, ventricular, left) 428.1
   cardiobronchial (see also Failure, ventricular, left) 428.1
   cardiorenal (see also Hypertension, cardiorenal) 404.90
   childhood 493.0 ✓5ᵗʰ
   colliers' 500
   croup 493.9 ✓5ᵗʰ
   detergent 507.8
   due to
      detergent 507.8
      inhalation of fumes 506.3
      internal immunological process 493.0 ✓5ᵗʰ
   endogenous (intrinsic) 493.1 ✓5ᵗʰ
   eosinophilic 518.3
   exogenous (cosmetics) (dander or dust) (drugs) (dust) (feathers) (food) (hay) (platinum) (pollen) 493.0 ✓5ᵗʰ
   extrinsic 493.0 ✓5ᵗʰ
   grinders' 502
   hay 493.0 ✓5ᵗʰ
   heart (see also Failure, ventricular, left) 428.1
   IgE 493.0 ✓5ᵗʰ
   infective 493.1 ✓5ᵗʰ
   intrinsic 493.1 ✓5ᵗʰ
   Kopp's 254.8
   late-onset 493.1 ✓5ᵗʰ
   meat-wrappers' 506.9
   Millar's (laryngismus stridulus) 478.75
   millstone makers' 502
   miners' 500
   Monday morning 504
   New Orleans (epidemic) 493.0 ✓5ᵗʰ
   platinum 493.0 ✓5ᵗʰ
   pneumoconiotic (occupational) NEC 505
   potters' 502
   psychogenic 316 [493.9] ✓5ᵗʰ
   pulmonary eosinophilic 518.3
   red cedar 495.8
   Rostan's (see also Failure, ventricular, left) 428.1
   sandblasters' 502
   sequoiosis 495.8
   stonemasons' 502
   thymic 254.8
   tuberculous (see also Tuberculosis, pulmonary) 011.9 ✓5ᵗʰ
   Wichmann's (laryngismus stridulus) 478.75
   wood 495.8
Astigmatism (compound) (congenital) 367.20
   irregular 367.22

Astigmatism — continued
   regular 367.21
Astroblastoma (M9430/3)
   nose 748.1
   specified site — see Neoplasm, by site, malignant
   unspecified site 191.9
Astrocytoma (cystic) (M9400/3)
   anaplastic type (M9401/3)
      specified site — see Neoplasm, by site, malignant
      unspecified site 191.9
   fibrillary (M9420/3)
      specified site — see Neoplasm, by site, malignant
      unspecified site 191.9
   fibrous (M9420/3)
      specified site — see Neoplasm, by site, malignant
      unspecified site 191.9
   gemistocytic (M9411/3)
      specified site — see Neoplasm, by site, malignant
      unspecified site 191.9
   juvenile (M9421/3)
      specified site — see Neoplasm, by site, malignant
      unspecified site 191.9
   nose 748.1
   pilocytic (M9421/3)
      specified site — see Neoplasm, by site, malignant
      unspecified site 191.9
   piloid (M9421/3)
      specified site — see Neoplasm, by site, malignant
      unspecified site 191.9
   protoplasmic (M9410/3)
      specified site — see Neoplasm, by site, malignant
      unspecified site 191.9
   specified site — see Neoplasm, by site, malignant
   subependymal (M9383/1) 237.5
      giant cell (M9384/1) 237.5
   unspecified site 191.9
Astroglioma (M9400/3)
   nose 748.1
   specified site — see Neoplasm, by site, malignant
   unspecified site 191.9
Asymbolia 784.60
Asymmetrical breathing 786.09
Asymmetry — see also Distortion
   chest 786.9
   face 754.0
   jaw NEC 524.12
      maxillary 524.11
   pelvis with disproportion 653.0 ✓5ᵗʰ
      affecting fetus or newborn 763.1
      causing obstructed labor 660.1 ✓5ᵗʰ
         affecting fetus or newborn 763.1
Asynergia 781.3
Asynergy 781.3
   ventricular 429.89
Asystole (heart) (see also Arrest, cardiac) 427.5
Ataxia, ataxy, ataxic 781.3
   acute 781.3
   brain 331.89

Ataxia, ataxy, ataxic — *continued*
    cerebellar 334.3
        hereditary (Marie's) 334.2
        in
            alcoholism 303.9 ✓5ᵗʰ *[334.4]*
            myxedema (*see also* Myxedema) 244.9
                [334.4]
            neoplastic disease NEC 239.9 *[334.4]*
    cerebral 331.89
    family, familial 334.2
        cerebral (Marie's) 334.2
        spinal (Friedreich's) 334.0
    Friedreich's (heredofamilial) (spinal) 334.0
    frontal lobe 781.3
    gait 781.2
        hysterical 300.11
    general 781.3
    hereditary NEC 334.2
        cerebellar 334.2
        spastic 334.1
        spinal 334.0
    heredofamilial (Marie's) 334.2
    hysterical 300.11
    locomotor (progressive) 094.0
        diabetic 250.6 ✓5ᵗʰ *[337.1]*
    Marie's (cerebellar) (heredofamilial) 334.2
    nonorganic origin 307.9
    partial 094.0
    postchickenpox 052.7
    progressive locomotor 094.0
    psychogenic 307.9
    Sanger-Brown's 334.2
    spastic 094.0
        hereditary 334.1
        syphilitic 094.0
    spinal
        hereditary 334.0
        progressive locomotor 094.0
    telangiectasia 334.8
Ataxia-telangiectasia 334.8
Atelectasis (absorption collapse) (complete)
    (compression) (massive) (partial)
    (postinfective) (pressure collapse)
    (pulmonary) (relaxation) 518.0
    newborn (congenital) (partial) 770.5
        primary 770.4
    primary 770.4
    tuberculous (*see also* Tuberculosis,
        pulmonary) 011.9 ✓5ᵗʰ
Ateleiosis, ateliosis 253.3
Atelia — *see* Distortion
Ateliosis 253.3
Atelocardia 746.9
Atelomyelia 742.59
Athelia 757.6
Atheroembolism
    extremity
        lower 445.02
        upper 445.01
    kidney 445.81
    specified site NEC 445.89
Atheroma, atheromatous (*see also*
        Arteriosclerosis) 440.9
    aorta, aortic 440.0
        valve (*see also* Endocarditis, aortic) 424.1
    artery — *see* Arteriosclerosis
    basilar (artery) (*see also* Occlusion, artery,
        basilar) 433.0 ✓5ᵗʰ
    carotid (artery) (common) (internal) (*see also*
        Occlusion, artery, carotid) 433.1 ✓5ᵗʰ

Atheroma, atheromatous — *continued*
    cerebral (arteries) 437.0
    coronary (artery) — *see* Arteriosclerosis,
        coronary
    degeneration — *see* Arteriosclerosis
    heart, cardiac — *see* Arteriosclerosis, coronary
    mitral (valve) 424.0
    myocardium, myocardial — *see*
        Arteriosclerosis, coronary
    pulmonary valve (heart) (*see also* Endocarditis,
        pulmonary) 424.3
    skin 706.2
    tricuspid (heart) (valve) 424.2
    valve, valvular — *see* Endocarditis
    vertebral (artery) (*see also* Occlusion, artery,
        vertebral) 433.2 ✓5ᵗʰ
Atheromatosis — *see also* Arteriosclerosis
    arterial, congenital 272.8
Atherosclerosis — *see* Arteriosclerosis
Athetosis (acquired) 781.0
    bilateral 333.7
    congenital (bilateral) 333.7
    double 333.7
    unilateral 781.0
Athlete's
    foot 110.4
    heart 429.3
Athletic team examination V70.3
Athrepsia 261
Athyrea (acquired) (*see also* Hypothyroidism)
        244.9
    congenital 243
Athyreosis (congenital) 243
    acquired — *see* Hypothyroidism
Athyroidism (acquired) (*see also*
        Hypothyroidism) 244.9
    congenital 243
Atmospheric pyrexia 992.0
Atonia, atony, atonic
    abdominal wall 728.2
    bladder (sphincter) 596.4
        neurogenic NEC 596.54
            with cauda equina syndrome 344.61
    capillary 448.9
    cecum 564.89
        psychogenic 306.4
    colon 564.89
        psychogenic 306.4
    congenital 779.89
    dyspepsia 536.3
        psychogenic 306.4
    intestine 564.89
        psychogenic 306.4
    stomach 536.3
        neurotic or psychogenic 306.4
        psychogenic 306.4
    uterus 666.1 ✓5ᵗʰ
        affecting fetus or newborn 763.7
    vesical 596.4
Atopy NEC V15.09
Atransferrinemia, congenital 273.8
Atresia, atretic (congenital) 759.89
    alimentary organ or tract NEC 751.8
        lower 751.2
        upper 750.8
    ani, anus, anal (canal) 751.2

Atresia, atretic — *continued*
  aorta 747.22
    with hypoplasia of ascending aorta and
        defective development of left ventricle
        (with mitral valve atresia) 746.7
    arch 747.11
    ring 747.21
  aortic (orifice) (valve) 746.89
    arch 747.11
  aqueduct of Sylvius 742.3
    with spina bifida (*see also* Spina bifida)
        741.0 ✓5ᵗʰ
  artery NEC (*see also* Atresia, blood vessel)
    747.60
    cerebral 747.81
    coronary 746.85
    eye 743.58
    pulmonary 747.3
    umbilical 747.5
  auditory canal (external) 744.02
  bile, biliary duct (common) or passage 751.61
    acquired (*see also* Obstruction, biliary)
        576.2
  bladder (neck) 753.6
  blood vessel (peripheral) NEC 747.60
    cerebral 747.81
    gastrointestinal 747.61
    lower limb 747.64
    pulmonary artery 747.3
    renal 747.62
    spinal 747.82
    upper limb 747.63
  bronchus 748.3
  canal, ear 744.02
  cardiac
    valve 746.89
      aortic 746.89
      mitral 746.89
      pulmonary 746.01
      tricuspid 746.1
  cecum 751.2
  cervix (acquired) 622.4
    congenital 752.49
    in pregnancy or childbirth 654.6 ✓5ᵗʰ
      affecting fetus or newborn 763.89
      causing obstructed labor 660.2 ✓5ᵗʰ
        affecting fetus or newborn 763.1
  choana 748.0
  colon 751.2
  cystic duct 751.61
    acquired 575.8
      with obstruction (*see also* Obstruction,
        gallbladder) 575.2
  digestive organs NEC 751.8
  duodenum 751.1
  ear canal 744.02
  ejaculatory duct 752.8
  epiglottis 748.3
  esophagus 750.3
  Eustachian tube 744.24
  fallopian tube (acquired) 628.2
    congenital 752.19
  follicular cyst 620.0
  foramen of
    Luschka 742.3
      with spina bifida (*see also* Spina bifida)
        741.0 ✓5ᵗʰ
    Magendie 742.3
      with spina bifida (*see also* Spina bifida)
        741.0 ✓5ᵗʰ
  gallbladder 751.69

Atresia, atretic — *continued*
  genital organ
    external
      female 752.49
      male NEC 752.8
        penis 752.69
    internal
      female 752.8
      male 752.8
  glottis 748.3
  gullet 750.3
  heart
    valve NEC 746.89
      aortic 746.89
      mitral 746.89
      pulmonary 746.01
      tricuspid 746.1
  hymen 752.42
    acquired 623.3
    postinfective 623.3
  ileum 751.1
  intestine (small) 751.1
    large 751.2
  iris, filtration angle (*see also* Buphthalmia)
    743.20
  jejunum 751.1
  kidney 753.3
  lacrimal, apparatus 743.65
    acquired — *see* Stenosis, lacrimal
  larynx 748.3
  ligament, broad 752.19
  lung 748.5
  meatus urinarius 753.6
  mitral valve 746.89
    with atresia or hypoplasia of aortic orifice
        or valve, with hypoplasia of ascending
        aorta and defective development of
        left ventricle 746.7
  nares (anterior) (posterior) 748.0
  nasolacrimal duct 743.65
  nasopharynx 748.8
  nose, nostril 748.0
    acquired 738.0
  organ or site NEC — *see* Anomaly, specified
    type NEC
  osseous meatus (ear) 744.03
  oviduct (acquired) 628.2
    congenital 752.19
  parotid duct 750.23
    acquired 527.8
  pulmonary (artery) 747.3
    valve 746.01
    vein 747.49
  pulmonic 746.01
  pupil 743.46
  rectum 751.2
  salivary duct or gland 750.23
    acquired 527.8
  sublingual duct 750.23
    acquired 527.8
  submaxillary duct or gland 750.23
    acquired 527.8
  trachea 748.3
  tricuspid valve 746.1
  ureter 753.29
  ureteropelvic junction 753.21
  ureterovesical orifice 753.22
  urethra (valvular) 753.6
  urinary tract NEC 753.29
  uterus 752.3
    acquired 621.8

Atresia, atretic — *continued*
  vagina (acquired) 623.2
    congenital 752.49
    postgonococcal (old) 098.2
    postinfectional 623.2
    senile 623.2
  vascular NEC (*see also* Atresia, blood vessel) 747.60
    cerebral 747.81
  vas deferens 752.8
  vein NEC (*see also* Atresia, blood vessel) 747.60
    cardiac 746.89
    great 747.49
    portal 747.49
    pulmonary 747.49
  vena cava (inferior) (superior) 747.49
  vesicourethral orifice 753.6
  vulva 752.49
    acquired 624.8

Atrichia, atrichosis 704.00
  congenital (universal) 757.4

Atrioventricularis commune 745.69

Atrophia — *see also* Atrophy
  alba 709.09
  cutis 701.8
    idiopathica progressiva 701.8
    senilis 701.8
  dermatological, diffuse (idiopathic) 701.8
  flava hepatis (acuta) (subacuta) (*see also* Necrosis, liver) 570
  gyrata of choroid and retina (central) 363.54
    generalized 363.57
  senilis 797
    dermatological 701.8
  unguium 703.8
    congenita 757.5

Atrophoderma, atrophodermia 701.9
  diffusum (idiopathic) 701.8
  maculatum 701.3
    et striatum 701.3
      due to syphilis 095.8
    syphilitic 091.3
  neuriticum 701.8
  pigmentosum 757.33
  reticulatum symmetricum faciei 701.8
  senile 701.8
  symmetrical 701.8
  vermiculata 701.8

Atrophy, atrophic
  adrenal (autoimmune) (capsule) (cortex) (gland) 255.4
    with hypofunction 255.4
  alveolar process or ridge (edentulous) 525.2
  appendix 543.9
  Aran-Duchenne muscular 335.21
  arm 728.2
  arteriosclerotic — *see* Arteriosclerosis
  arthritis 714.0
    spine 720.9
  bile duct (any) 576.8
  bladder 596.8
  blanche (of Milian) 701.3
  bone (senile) 733.99
    due to
      disuse 733.7
      infection 733.99
      tabes dorsalis (neurogenic) 094.0
    posttraumatic 733.99
  brain (cortex) (progressive) 331.9
    with dementia 290.10

Atrophy, atrophic — *continued*
  brain — *continued*
    Alzheimer's 331.0
      with dementia — *see* Alzheimer's, dementia
    circumscribed (Pick's) 331.1
      with dementia
        with behavioral disturbance 331.1 [294.11]
        without behavioral disturbance 331.1 [294.10]
    congenital 742.4
    hereditary 331.9
    senile 331.2
  breast 611.4
    puerperal, postpartum 676.3
  buccal cavity 528.9
  cardiac (brown) (senile) (*see also* Degeneration, myocardial) 429.1
  cartilage (infectional) (joint) 733.99
  cast, plaster of Paris 728.2
  cerebellar — *see* Atrophy, brain
  cerebral — *see* Atrophy, brain
  cervix (endometrium) (mucosa) (myometrium) (senile) (uteri) 622.8
    menopausal 627.8
  Charcôt-Marie-Tooth 356.1
  choroid 363.40
    diffuse secondary 363.42
    hereditary (*see also* Dystrophy, choroid) 363.50
      gyrate
        central 363.54
        diffuse 363.57
        generalized 363.57
    senile 363.41
  ciliary body 364.57
  colloid, degenerative 701.3
  conjunctiva (senile) 372.89
  corpus cavernosum 607.89
  cortical (*see also* Atrophy, brain) 331.9
  Cruveilhier's 335.21
  cystic duct 576.8
  dacryosialadenopathy 710.2
  degenerative
    colloid 701.3
    senile 701.3
  Déjérine-Thomas 333.0
  diffuse idiopathic, dermatological 701.8
  disuse
    bone 733.7
    muscle 728.2
  Duchenne-Aran 335.21
  ear 388.9
  edentulous alveolar ridge 525.2
  emphysema, lung 492.8
  endometrium (senile) 621.8
    cervix 622.8
  enteric 569.89
  epididymis 608.3
  eyeball, cause unknown 360.41
  eyelid (senile) 374.50
  facial (skin) 701.9
  facioscapulohumeral (Landouzy-Déjérine) 359.1
  fallopian tube (senile), acquired 620.3
  fatty, thymus (gland) 254.8
  gallbladder 575.8
  gastric 537.89
  gastritis (chronic) 535.1
  gastrointestinal 569.89

Atrophy, atrophic — *continued*
  genital organ, male 608.89
  glandular 289.3
  globe (phthisis bulbi) 360.41
  gum 523.2
  hair 704.2
  heart (brown) (senile) (*see also* Degeneration, myocardial) 429.1
  hemifacial 754.0
    Romberg 349.89
  hydronephrosis 591
  infantile 261
    paralysis, acute (*see also* Poliomyelits, with paralysis) 045.1 ✓5ᵗʰ
  intestine 569.89
  iris (generalized) (postinfectional) (sector shaped) 364.59
    essential 364.51
    progressive 364.51
    sphincter 364.54
  kidney (senile) (*see also* Sclerosis, renal) 587
    with hypertension (*see also* Hypertension, kidney) 403.90
    congenital 753.0
    hydronephrotic 591
    infantile 753.0
  lacrimal apparatus (primary) 375.13
    secondary 375.14
  Landouzy-Déjérine 359.1
  laryngitis, infection 476.0
  larynx 478.79
  Leber's optic 377.16
  lip 528.5
  liver (acute) (subacute) (*see also* Necrosis, liver) 570
    chronic (yellow) 571.8
    yellow (congenital) 570
      with
        abortion — *see* Abortion, by type, with specified complication NEC
        ectopic pregnancy (*see also* categories 633.0-633.9) 639.8
        molar pregnancy (*see also* categories 630-632) 639.8
      chronic 571.8
      complicating pregnancy 646.7 ✓5ᵗʰ
      following
        abortion 639.8
        ectopic or molar pregnancy 639.8
      from injection, inoculation or transfusion (onset within 8 months after administration) — *see* Hepatitis, viral
      healed 571.5
      obstetric 646.7 ✓5ᵗʰ
      postabortal 639.8
      postimmunization — *see* Hepatitis, viral
      posttransfusion — *see* Hepatitis, viral
      puerperal, postpartum 674.8 ✓5ᵗʰ
  lung (senile) 518.89
    congenital 748.69
  macular (dermatological) 701.3
    syphilitic, skin 091.3
      striated 095.8
  muscle, muscular 728.2
    disuse 728.2
    Duchenne-Aran 335.21
    extremity (lower) (upper) 728.2
    familial spinal 335.11
    general 728.2
    idiopathic 728.2

Atrophy, atrophic — *continued*
  muscle, muscular — *continued*
    infantile spinal 335.0
    myelopathic (progressive) 335.10
    myotonic 359.2
    neuritic 356.1
    neuropathic (peroneal) (progressive) 356.1
    peroneal 356.1
    primary (idiopathic) 728.2
    progressive (familial) (hereditary) (pure) 335.21
      adult (spinal) 335.19
      infantile (spinal) 335.0
      juvenile (spinal) 335.11
      spinal 335.10
        adult 335.19
        Aran-Duchenne 335.10
        hereditary or familial 335.11
        infantile 335.0
    pseudohypertrophic 359.1
    spinal (progressive) 335.10
      adult 335.19
      Aran-Duchenne 335.21
      familial 335.11
      hereditary 335.11
      infantile 335.0
      juvenile 335.11
    syphilitic 095.6
  myocardium (*see also* Degeneration, myocardial) 429.1
  myometrium (senile) 621.8
    cervix 622.8
  myotatic 728.2
  myotonia 359.2
  nail 703.8
    congenital 757.5
  nasopharynx 472.2
  nerve — *see also* Disorder, nerve
    abducens 378.54
    accessory 352.4
    acoustic or auditory 388.5
    cranial 352.9
      first (olfactory) 352.0
      second (optic) (*see also* Atrophy, optic nerve) 377.10
      third (oculomotor)(partial) 378.51
        total 378.52
      fourth (trochlear) 378.53
      fifth (trigeminal) 350.8
      sixth (abducens) 378.54
      seventh (facial) 351.8
      eighth (auditory) 388.5
      ninth (glossopharyngeal) 352.2
      tenth (pneumogastric) (vagus) 352.3
      eleventh (accessory) 352.4
      twelfth (hypoglossal) 352.5
    facial 351.8
    glossopharyngeal 352.2
    hypoglossal 352.5
    oculomotor (partial) 378.51
      total 378.52
    olfactory 352.0
    peripheral 355.9
    pneumogastric 352.3
    trigeminal 350.8
    trochlear 378.53
    vagus (pneumogastric) 352.3
  nervous system, congenital 742.8
  neuritic (*see also* Disorder, nerve) 355.9

Atrophy, atrophic — continued
  neurogenic NEC 355.9
    bone
      tabetic 094.0
  nutritional 261
  old age 797
  olivopontocerebellar 333.0
  optic nerve (ascending) (descending)
      (infectional) (nonfamilial) (papillomacular
      bundle) (postretinal) (secondary NEC)
      (simple) 377.10
    associated with retinal dystrophy 377.13
    dominant hereditary 377.16
    glaucomatous 377.14
    hereditary (dominant) (Leber's) 377.16
    Leber's (hereditary) 377.16
    partial 377.15
    postinflammatory 377.12
    primary 377.11
    syphilitic 094.84
      congenital 090.49
      tabes dorsalis 094.0
  orbit 376.45
  ovary (senile), acquired 620.3
  oviduct (senile), acquired 620.3
  palsy, diffuse 335.20
  pancreas (duct) (senile) 577.8
  papillary muscle 429.81
  paralysis 355.9
  parotid gland 527.0
  patches skin 701.3
    senile 701.8
  penis 607.89
  pharyngitis 472.1
  pharynx 478.29
  pluriglandular 258.8
  polyarthritis 714.0
  prostate 602.2
  pseudohypertrophic 359.1
  renal (see also Sclerosis, renal) 587
  reticulata 701.8
  retina (see also Degeneration, retina) 362.60
    hereditary (see also Dystrophy, retina)
        362.70
  rhinitis 472.0
  salivary duct or gland 527.0
  scar NEC 709.2
  sclerosis, lobar (of brain) 331.0
    with dementia
      with behavioral disturbance 331.1
          [294.11]
      without behavioral disturbance 331.1
          [294.10]
  scrotum 608.89
  seminal vesicle 608.89
  senile 797
    degenerative, of skin 701.3
  skin (patches) (senile) 701.8
  spermatic cord 608.89
  spinal (cord) 336.8
    acute 336.8
    muscular (chronic) 335.10
      adult 335.19
      familial 335.11
      juvenile 335.10
    paralysis 335.10
      acute (see also Poliomyelitis, with
          paralysis) 045.1
  spine (column) 733.99
  spleen (senile) 289.59

Atrophy, atrophic — continued
  spots (skin) 701.3
    senile 701.8
  stomach 537.89
  striate and macular 701.3
    syphilitic 095.8
  subcutaneous 701.9
    due to injection 999.9
  sublingual gland 527.0
  submaxillary gland 527.0
  Sudeck's 733.7
  suprarenal (autoimmune) (capsule) (gland)
      255.4
    with hypofunction 255.4
  tarso-orbital fascia, congenital 743.66
  testis 608.3
  thenar, partial 354.0
  throat 478.29
  thymus (fat) 254.8
  thyroid (gland) 246.8
    with
      cretinism 243
      myxedema 244.9
    congenital 243
  tongue (senile) 529.8
    papillae 529.4
    smooth 529.4
  trachea 519.1
  tunica vaginalis 608.89
  turbinate 733.99
  tympanic membrane (nonflaccid) 384.82
    flaccid 384.81
  ulcer (see also Ulcer, skin) 707.9
  upper respiratory tract 478.9
  uterus, uterine (acquired) (senile) 621.8
    cervix 622.8
    due to radiation (intended effect) 621.8
  vagina (senile) 627.3
  vascular 459.89
  vas deferens 608.89
  vertebra (senile) 733.99
  vulva (primary) (senile) 624.1
  Werdnig-Hoffmann 335.0
  yellow (acute) (congenital) (liver) (subacute)
      (see also Necrosis, liver) 570
    chronic 571.8
    resulting from administration of blood,
        plasma, serum, or other biological
        substance (within 8 months of
        administration) — see Hepatitis, viral

Attack
  akinetic (see also Epilepsy) 345.0
  angina — see Angina
  apoplectic (see also Disease, cerebrovascular,
      acute) 436
  benign shuddering 333.93
  bilious — see Vomiting
  cataleptic 300.11
  cerebral (see also Disease, cerebrovascular,
      acute) 436
  coronary (see also Infarct, myocardium)
      410.9
  cyanotic, newborn 770.83
  epileptic (see also Epilepsy) 345.9
  epileptiform 780.39
  heart (see also Infarct, myocardium) 410.9
  hemiplegia (see also Disease, cerebrovascular,
      acute) 436
  hysterical 300.11
  jacksonian (see also Epilepsy) 345.5

Index to Diseases

Attack — *continued*
- myocardium, myocardial (*see also* Infarct, myocardium) 410.9 ✓5ᵗʰ
- myoclonic (*see also* Epilepsy) 345.1 ✓5ᵗʰ
- panic 300.01
- paralysis (*see also* Disease, cerebrovascular, acute) 436
- paroxysmal 780.39
- psychomotor (*see also* Epilepsy) 345.4 ✓5ᵗʰ
- salaam (*see also* Epilepsy) 345.6 ✓5ᵗʰ
- schizophreniform (*see also* Schizophrenia) 295.4 ✓5ᵗʰ
- sensory and motor 780.39
- syncope 780.2
- toxic, cerebral 780.39
- transient ischemic (TIA) 435.9
- unconsciousness 780.2
  - hysterical 300.11
- vasomotor 780.2
- vasovagal (idiopathic) (paroxysmal) 780.2

Attention to
- artificial opening (of) V55.9
  - digestive tract NEC V55.4
  - specified site NEC V55.8
  - urinary tract NEC V55.6
  - vagina V55.7
- colostomy V55.3
- cystostomy V55.5
- gastrostomy V55.1
- ileostomy V55.2
- jejunostomy V55.4
- nephrostomy V55.6
- surgical dressings V58.3
- sutures V58.3
- tracheostomy V55.0
- ureterostomy V55.6
- urethrostomy V55.6

Attrition
- gum 523.2
- teeth (excessive) (hard tissues) 521.1

Atypical — *see also* condition
- distribution, vessel (congenital) (peripheral) NEC 747.60
- endometrium 621.9
- glandular cell changes of undetermined significance •
  - favor benign (AGCUS favor benign) 795.01 •
  - favor dysplasia (AGCUS favor dysplasia) 795.02 •
- kidney 593.89
- squamous cell changes of undetermined significance •
  - favor benign (ASCUS favor benign) 795.01 •
  - favor dysplasia (ASCUS favor dysplasia) 795.02 •

Atypism, cervix 622.1
Audible tinnitus (*see also* Tinnitus) 388.30
Auditory — *see* condition
Audry's syndrome (acropachyderma) 757.39
Aujeszky's disease 078.89
Aura, jacksonian (*see also* Epilepsy) 345.5 ✓5ᵗʰ
Aurantiasis, cutis 278.3
Auricle, auricular — *see* condition
Auriculotemporal syndrome 350.8
Australian
- Q fever 083.0
- X disease 062.4

Autism, autistic (child) (infantile) 299.0 ✓5ᵗʰ
Autodigestion 799.8
Autoerythrocyte sensitization 287.2
Autographism 708.3
Autoimmune
- cold sensitivity 283.0
- disease NEC 279.4
- hemolytic anemia 283.0
- thyroiditis 245.2

Autoinfection, septic — *see* Septicemia
Autointoxication 799.8
Automatism 348.8
- epileptic (*see also* Epilepsy) 345.4 ✓5ᵗʰ
- paroxysmal, idiopathic (*see also* Epilepsy) 345.4 ✓5ᵗʰ

Autonomic, autonomous
- bladder 596.54
  - neurogenic NEC 596.54
    - with cauda equina 344.61
- dysreflexia 337.3
- faciocephalalgia (*see also* Neuropathy, peripheral, autonomic) 337.9
- hysterical seizure 300.11
- imbalance (*see also* Neuropathy, peripheral, autonomic) 337.9

Autophony 388.40
Autosensitivity, erythrocyte 287.2
Autotopagnosia 780.99
Autotoxemia 799.8
Autumn — *see* condition
Avellis' syndrome 344.89
Aviators
- disease or sickness (*see also* Effect, adverse, high altitude) 993.2
- ear 993.0
- effort syndrome 306.2

Avitaminosis (multiple NEC) (*see also* Deficiency, vitamin) 269.2
- A 264.9
- B 266.9
  - with
    - beriberi 265.0
    - pellagra 265.2
- B_1 265.1
- B_2 266.0
- B_6 266.1
- B_{12} 266.2
- C (with scurvy) 267
- D 268.9
  - with
    - osteomalacia 268.2
    - rickets 268.0
- E 269.1
- G 266.0
- H 269.1
- K 269.0
- multiple 269.2
- nicotinic acid 265.2
- P 269.1

Avulsion (traumatic) 879.8
- blood vessel — *see* Injury, blood vessel, by site
- cartilage — *see also* Dislocation, by site
- knee, current (*see also* Tear, meniscus) 836.2
- symphyseal (inner), complicating delivery 665.6 ✓5ᵗʰ
- complicated 879.9
- diaphragm — *see* Injury, internal, diaphragm

Avulsion — *continued*
 ear — *see* Wound, open, ear
 epiphysis of bone — *see* Fracture, by site
 external site other than limb — *see* Wound, open, by site
 eye 871.3
 fingernail — *see* Wound, open, finger
 fracture — *see* Fracture, by site
 genital organs, external — *see* Wound, open, genital organs
 head (intracranial) NEC — *see also* Injury, intracranial, with open intracranial wound
  complete 874.9
  external site NEC 873.8
   complicated 873.9
 internal organ or site — *see* Injury, internal, by site
 joint — *see also* Dislocation, by site
  capsule — *see* Sprain, by site
 ligament — *see* Sprain, by site
 limb — *see also* Amputation, traumatic, by site
 skin and subcutaneous tissue — *see* Wound, open, by site
 muscle — *see* Sprain, by site
 nerve (root) — *see* Injury, nerve, by site
 scalp — *see* Wound, open, scalp
 skin and subcutaneous tissue — *see* Wound, open, by site
 symphyseal cartilage (inner), complicating delivery 665.6
 tendon — *see also* Sprain, by site
  with open wound — *see* Wound, open, by site
 toenail — *see* Wound, open, toe(s)
 tooth 873.63
  complicated 873.73
Awareness of heart beat 785.1
Axe grinders' disease 502
Axenfeld's anomaly or syndrome 743.44
Axilla, axillary — *see also* condition
 breast 757.2
Axonotmesis — *see* Injury, nerve, by site
Ayala's disease 756.89
Ayerza's disease or syndrome (pulmonary artery sclerosis with pulmonary hypertension) 416.0
Azoospermia 606.0
Azotemia 790.6
 meaning uremia (*see also* Uremia) 586
Aztec ear 744.29
Azorean disease (of the nervous system) 334.8
Azygos lobe, lung (fissure) 748.69

B

Baader's syndrome (erythema multiforme exudativum) 695.1
Baastrup's syndrome 721.5
Babesiasis 088.82
Babesiosis 088.82
Babington's disease (familial hemorrhagic telangiectasia) 448.0
Babinski's syndrome (cardiovascular syphilis) 093.89
Babinski-Fröhlich syndrome (adiposogenital dystrophy) 253.8

Babinski-Nageotte syndrome 344.89
Bacillary — *see* condition
Bacilluria 791.9
 asymptomatic, in pregnancy or puerperium 646.5
 tuberculous (*see also* Tuberculosis) 016.9
Bacillus — *see also* Infection, bacillus
 abortus infection 023.1
 anthracis infection 022.9
 coli
  infection 041.4
   generalized 038.42
   intestinal 008.00
  pyemia 038.42
  septicemia 038.42
 Flexner's 004.1
 fusiformis infestation 101
 mallei infection 024
 Shiga's 004.0
 suipestifer infection (*see also* Infection, Salmonella) 003.9
Back — *see* condition
Backache (postural) 724.5
 psychogenic 307.89
 sacroiliac 724.6
Backflow (pyelovenous) (*see also* Disease, renal) 593.9
Backknee (*see also* Genu, recurvatum) 736.5
Bacteremia 790.7
 with
  sepsis — *see* Septicemia
 during
  labor 659.3
  pregnancy 647.8
 newborn 771.83
Bacteria
 in blood (*see also* Bacteremia) 790.7
 in urine (*see also* Bacteriuria) 599.0
Bacterial — *see* condition
Bactericholia (*see also* Cholecystitis, acute) 575.0
Bacterid, bacteride (Andrews' pustular) 686.8
Bacteriuria, bacteruria 791.9
 with
  urinary tract infection 599.0
 asymptomatic 791.9
  in pregnancy or puerperium 646.5
   affecting fetus or newborn 760.1
Bad
 breath 784.9
 heart — *see* Disease, heart
 trip (*see also* Abuse, drugs, nondependent) 305.3
Baehr-Schiffrin disease (thrombotic thrombocytopenic purpura) 446.6
Baelz's disease (cheilitis glandularis apostematosa) 528.5
Baerensprung's disease (eczema marginatum) 110.3
Bagassosis (occupational) 495.1
Baghdad boil 085.1
Bagratuni's syndrome (temporal arteritis) 446.5
Baker's
 cyst (knee) 727.51
  tuberculous (*see also* Tuberculosis) 015.2
 itch 692.82

Index to Diseases

Bakwin-Krida syndrome (craniometaphyseal dysplasia) 756.89
Balanitis (circinata) (gangraenosa) (infectious) (vulgaris) 607.1
  amebic 006.8
  candidal 112.2
  chlamydial 099.53
  due to Ducrey's bacillus 099.0
  erosiva circinata et gangraenosa 607.1
  gangrenous 607.1
  gonococcal (acute) 098.0
    chronic or duration of 2 months or over 098.2
  nongonococcal 607.1
  phagedenic 607.1
  venereal NEC 099.8
  xerotica obliterans 607.81
Balanoposthitis 607.1
  chlamydial 099.53
  gonococcal (acute) 098.0
    chronic or duration of 2 months or over 098.2
  ulcerative NEC 099.8
Balanorrhagia — see Balanitis
Balantidiasis 007.0
Balantidiosis 007.0
Balbuties, balbutio 307.0
Bald
  patches on scalp 704.00
  tongue 529.4
Baldness (see also Alopecia) 704.00
Balfour's disease (chloroma) 205.3 ✓5ᵗʰ
Balint's syndrome (psychic paralysis of visual fixation) 368.16
Balkan grippe 083.0
Ball
  food 938
  hair 938
Ballantyne (-Runge) syndrome (postmaturity) 766.2
Balloon disease (see also Effect, adverse, high altitude) 993.2
Ballooning posterior leaflet syndrome 424.0
Baló's disease or concentric sclerosis 341.1
Bamberger's disease (hypertrophic pulmonary osteoarthropathy) 731.2
Bamberger-Marie disease (hypertrophic pulmonary osteoarthropathy) 731.2
Bamboo spine 720.0
Bancroft's filariasis 125.0
Band(s)
  adhesive (see also Adhesions, peritoneum) 568.0
  amniotic 658.8 ✓5ᵗʰ
    affecting fetus or newborn 762.8
  anomalous or congenital — see also Anomaly, specified type NEC
    atrial 746.9
    heart 746.9
    intestine 751.4
    omentum 751.4
    ventricular 746.9
  cervix 622.3
  gallbladder (congenital) 751.69
  intestinal (adhesive) (see also Adhesions, peritoneum) 568.0
    congenital 751.4

Band(s) — continued
  obstructive (see also Obstruction, intestine) 560.81
  periappendiceal (congenital) 751.4
  peritoneal (adhesive) (see also Adhesions, peritoneum) 568.0
    with intestinal obstruction 560.81
    congenital 751.4
  uterus 621.5
  vagina 623.2
Bandl's ring (contraction)
  complicating delivery 661.4 ✓5ᵗʰ
    affecting fetus or newborn 763.7
Bang's disease (Brucella abortus) 023.1
Bangkok hemorrhagic fever 065.4
Bannister's disease 995.1
Bantam-Albright-Martin disease (pseudohypoparathyroidism) 275.49
Banti's disease or syndrome (with cirrhosis) (with portal hypertension) — see Cirrhosis, liver
Bar
  calcaneocuboid 755.67
  calcaneonavicular 755.67
  cubonavicular 755.67
  prostate 600.9
  talocalcaneal 755.67
Baragnosis 780.99
Barasheh, barashek 266.2
Barcoo disease or rot (see also Ulcer, skin) 707.9
Bard-Pic syndrome (carcinoma, head of pancreas) 157.0
Bärensprung's disease (eczema marginatum) 110.3
Baritosis 503
Barium lung disease 503
Barlow's syndrome (meaning mitral valve prolapse) 424.0
Barlow (-Möller) disease or syndrome (meaning infantile scurvy) 267
Barodontalgia 993.2
Baron Münchausen syndrome 301.51
Barosinusitis 993.1
Barotitis 993.0
Barotrauma 993.2
  odontalgia 993.2
  otitic 993.0
  sinus 993.1
Barraquer's disease or syndrome (progressive lipodystrophy) 272.6
Barré-Guillain syndrome 357.0
Barré-Liéou syndrome (posterior cervical sympathetic) 723.2
Barrel chest 738.3
Barrett's syndrome or ulcer (chronic peptic ulcer of esophagus) 530.2
Bársony-Polgár syndrome (corkscrew esophagus) 530.5
Bársony-Teschendorf syndrome (corkscrew esophagus) 530.5
Bartholin's
  adenitis (see also Bartholinitis) 616.8
  gland — see condition

Bartholinitis (suppurating) 616.8
  gonococcal (acute) 098.0
    chronic or duration of 2 months or over 098.2
Bartonellosis 088.0
Bartter's syndrome (secondary hyperaldosteronism with juxtaglomerular hyperplasia) 255.1
Basal — see condition
Basan's (hidrotic) ectodermal dysplasia 757.31
Baseball finger 842.13
Basedow's disease or syndrome (exophthalmic goiter) 242.0
Basic — see condition
Basilar — see condition
Bason's (hidrotic) ectodermal dysplasia 757.31
Basopenia 288.0
Basophilia 288.8
Basophilism (corticoadrenal) (Cushing's) (pituitary) (thymic) 255.0
Bassen-Kornzweig syndrome (abetalipoproteinemia) 272.5
Bat ear 744.29
Bateman's
  disease 078.0
  purpura (senile) 287.2
Bathing cramp 994.1
Bathophobia 300.23
Batten's disease, retina 330.1 [362.71]
Batten-Mayou disease 330.1 [362.71]
Batten-Steinert syndrome 359.2
Battered
  adult (syndrome) 995.81
  baby or child (syndrome) 995.54
  spouse (syndrome) 995.81
Battey mycobacterium infection 031.0
Battledore placenta — see Placenta, abnormal
Battle exhaustion (see also Reaction, stress, acute) 308.9
Baumgarten-Cruveilhier (cirrhosis) disease, or syndrome 571.5
Bauxite
  fibrosis (of lung) 503
  workers' disease 503
Bayle's disease (dementia paralytica) 094.1
Bazin's disease (primary) (see also Tuberculosis) 017.1
Beach ear 380.12
Beaded hair (congenital) 757.4
Beard's disease (neurasthenia) 300.5
Bearn-Kunkel (-Slater) syndrome (lupoid hepatitis) 571.49
Beat
  elbow 727.2
  hand 727.2
  knee 727.2
Beats
  ectopic 427.60
  escaped, heart 427.60
    postoperative 997.1
  premature (nodal) 427.60
    atrial 427.61
    auricular 427.61
    postoperative 997.1
    specified type NEC 427.69

Beats — continued
  premature — continued
    supraventricular 427.61
    ventricular 427.69
Beau's
  disease or syndrome (see also Degeneration, myocardial) 429.1
  lines (transverse furrows on fingernails) 703.8
Bechterew's disease (ankylosing spondylitis) 720.0
Bechterew-Strümpell-Marie syndrome (ankylosing spondylitis) 720.0
Beck's syndrome (anterior spinal artery occlusion) 433.8
Becker's
  disease (idiopathic mural endomyocardial disease) 425.2
  dystrophy 359.1
Beckwith (-Wiedemann) syndrome 759.89
Bedclothes, asphyxiation or suffocation by 994.7
Bednar's aphthae 528.2
Bedsore 707.0
  with gangrene 707.0 [785.4]
Bedwetting (see also Enuresis) 788.36
Beer-drinkers' heart (disease) 425.5
Bee sting (with allergic or anaphylactic shock) 989.5
Begbie's disease (exophthalmic goiter) 242.0
Behavior disorder, disturbance — see also Disturbance, conduct
  antisocial, without manifest psychiatric disorder
    adolescent V71.02
    adult V71.01
    child V71.02
  dyssocial, without manifest psychiatric disorder
    adolescent V71.02
    adult V71.01
    child V71.02
  high risk — see Problem
Behçet's syndrome 136.1
Behr's disease 362.50
Beigel's disease or morbus (white piedra) 111.2
Bejel 104.0
Bekhterev's disease (ankylosing spondylitis) 720.0
Bekhterev-Strümpell-Marie syndrome (ankylosing spondylitis) 720.0
Belching (see also Eructation) 787.3
Bell's
  disease (see also Psychosis, affective) 296.0
  mania (see also Psychosis, affective) 296.0
  palsy, paralysis 351.0
    infant 767.5
    newborn 767.5
    syphilitic 094.89
  spasm 351.0
Bence-Jones albuminuria, albuminosuria, or proteinuria 791.0
Bends 993.3
Benedikt's syndrome (paralysis) 344.89
Benign — see also condition
  cellular changes, cervix 795.09

Index to Diseases

Benign — *continued*
  prostate
    hyperplasia 600.0
    neoplasm 222.2
Bennett's
  disease (leukemia) 208.9 ✓5ᵗʰ
  fracture (closed) 815.01
    open 815.11
Benson's disease 379.22
Bent
  back (hysterical) 300.11
  nose 738.0
    congenital 754.0
Bereavement V62.82
  as adjustment reaction 309.0
Berger's paresthesia (lower limb) 782.0
Bergeron's disease (hysteroepilepsy) 300.11
Beriberi (acute) (atrophic) (chronic) (dry) (subacute) (wet) 265.0
  with polyneuropathy 265.0 *[357.4]*
  heart (disease) 265.0 *[425.7]*
  leprosy 030.1
  neuritis 265.0 *[357.4]*
Berlin's disease or edema (traumatic) 921.3
Berloque dermatitis 692.72
Bernard-Horner syndrome (*see also* Neuropathy, peripheral, autonomic) 337.9
Bernard-Sergent syndrome (acute adrenocortical insufficiency) 255.4
Bernard-Soulier disease or thrombopathy 287.1
Bernhardt's disease or paresthesia 355.1
Bernhardt-Roth disease or syndrome (paresthesia) 355.1
Bernheim's syndrome (*see also* Failure, heart) 428.0
Bertielliasis 123.8
Bertolotti's syndrome (sacralization of fifth lumbar vertebra) 756.15
Berylliosis (acute) (chronic) (lung) (occupational) 503
Besnier's
  lupus pernio 135
  prurigo (atopic dermatitis) (infantile eczema) 691.8
Besnier-Boeck disease or sarcoid 135
Besnier-Boeck-Schaumann disease (sarcoidosis) 135
Best's disease 362.76
Bestiality 302.1
Beta-adrenergic hyperdynamic circulatory state 429.82
Beta-aminoisobutyric aciduria 277.2
Beta-mercaptolactate-cysteine disulfiduria 270.0
Beta thalassemia (major) (minor) (mixed) 282.4
Beurmann's disease (sporotrichosis) 117.1
Bezoar 938
  intestine 936
  stomach 935.2
Bezold's abscess (*see also* Mastoiditis) 383.01
Bianchi's syndrome (aphasia-apraxia-alexia) 784.69

Bicornuate or bicornis uterus 752.3
  in pregnancy or childbirth 654.0 ✓5ᵗʰ
    with obstructed labor 660.2 ✓5ᵗʰ
      affecting fetus or newborn 763.1
    affecting fetus or newborn 763.89
Bicuspid aortic valve 746.4
Biedl-Bardet syndrome 759.89
Bielschowsky's disease 330.1
Bielschowsky-Jansky
  amaurotic familial idiocy 330.1
  disease 330.1
Biemond's syndrome (obesity, polydactyly, and mental retardation) 759.89
Biermer's anemia or disease (pernicious anemia) 281.0
Biett's disease 695.4
Bifid (congenital) — *see also* Imperfect, closure
  apex, heart 746.89
  clitoris 752.49
  epiglottis 748.3
  kidney 753.3
  nose 748.1
  patella 755.64
  scrotum 752.8
  toe 755.66
  tongue 750.13
  ureter 753.4
  uterus 752.3
  uvula 749.02
    with cleft lip (*see also* Cleft, palate, with cleft lip) 749.20
Biforis uterus (suprasimplex) 752.3
Bifurcation (congenital) — *see also* Imperfect, closure
  gallbladder 751.69
  kidney pelvis 753.3
  renal pelvis 753.3
  rib 756.3
  tongue 750.13
  trachea 748.3
  ureter 753.4
  urethra 753.8
  uvula 749.02
    with cleft lip (*see also* Cleft, palate, with cleft lip) 749.20
  vertebra 756.19
Bigeminal pulse 427.89
Bigeminy 427.89
Big spleen syndrome 289.4
Bilateral — *see* condition
Bile duct — *see* condition
Bile pigments in urine 791.4
Bilharziasis (*see also* Schistosomiasis) 120.9
  chyluria 120.0
  cutaneous 120.3
  galacturia 120.0
  hematochyluria 120.0
  intestinal 120.1
  lipemia 120.9
  lipuria 120.0
  Oriental 120.2
  piarhemia 120.9
  pulmonary 120.2
  tropical hematuria 120.0
  vesical 120.0
Biliary — *see* condition
Bilious (attack) — *see also* Vomiting
  fever, hemoglobinuric 084.8

Bilirubinuria 791.4
Biliuria 791.4
Billroth's disease
 meningocele (*see also* Spina bifida) 741.9
Bilobate placenta — *see* Placenta, abnormal
Bilocular
 heart 745.7
 stomach 536.8
Bing-Horton syndrome (histamine cephalgia) 346.2
Binswanger's disease or dementia 290.12
Biörck (-Thorson) syndrome (malignant carcinoid) 259.2
Biparta, bipartite — *see also* Imperfect, closure
 carpal scaphoid 755.59
 patella 755.64
 placenta — *see* Placenta, abnormal
 vagina 752.49
Bird
 face 756.0
 fanciers' lung or disease 495.7
Bird's disease (oxaluria) 271.8
Birth
 abnormal fetus or newborn 763.9
 accident, fetus or newborn — *see* Birth, injury
 complications in mother — *see* Delivery, complicated
 compression during NEC 767.9
 defect — *see* Anomaly
 delayed, fetus 763.9
 difficult NEC, affecting fetus or newborn 763.9
 dry, affecting fetus or newborn 761.1
 forced, NEC, affecting fetus or newborn 763.89
 forceps, affecting fetus or newborn 763.2
 hematoma of sternomastoid 767.8
 immature 765.1
  extremely 765.0
 inattention, after or at 995.52
 induced, affecting fetus or newborn 763.89
 infant — *see* Newborn
 injury NEC 767.9
  adrenal gland 767.8
  basal ganglia 767.0
  brachial plexus (paralysis) 767.6
  brain (compression) (pressure) 767.0
  cerebellum 767.0
  cerebral hemorrhage 767.0
  conjunctiva 767.8
  eye 767.8
  fracture
   bone, any except clavicle or spine 767.3
   clavicle 767.2
   femur 767.3
   humerus 767.3
   long bone 767.3
   radius and ulna 767.3
   skeleton NEC 767.3
   skull 767.3
   spine 767.4
   tibia and fibula 767.3
  hematoma 767.8
   liver (subcapsular) 767.8
   mastoid 767.8
   skull 767.1
   sternomastoid 767.8
   testes 767.8
   vulva 767.8
  intracranial (edema) 767.0

Birth — *continued*
 injury NEC — *continued*
  laceration
   brain 767.0
   by scalpel 767.8
   peripheral nerve 767.7
  liver 767.8
  meninges
   brain 767.0
   spinal cord 767.4
  nerves (cranial, peripheral) 767.7
   brachial plexus 767.6
   facial 767.5
  paralysis 767.7
   brachial plexus 767.6
   Erb (-Duchenne) 767.6
   facial nerve 767.5
   Klumpke (-Déjérine) 767.6
   radial nerve 767.6
   spinal (cord) (hemorrhage) (laceration) (rupture) 767.4
  rupture
   intracranial 767.0
   liver 767.8
   spinal cord 767.4
   spleen 767.8
   viscera 767.8
  scalp 767.1
  scalpel wound 767.8
  skeleton NEC 767.3
  specified NEC 767.8
  spinal cord 767.4
  spleen 767.8
  subdural hemorrhage 767.0
  tentorial, tear 767.0
  testes 767.8
  vulva 767.8
 instrumental, NEC, affecting fetus or newborn 763.2
 lack of care, after or at 995.52
 multiple
  affected by maternal complications of pregnancy 761.5
  healthy liveborn — *see* Newborn, multiple
 neglect, after or at 995.52
 newborn — *see* Newborn
 palsy or paralysis NEC 767.7
 precipitate, fetus or newborn 763.6
 premature (infant) 765.1
 prolonged, affecting fetus or newborn 763.9
 retarded, fetus or newborn 763.9
 shock, newborn 779.89 ▲
 strangulation or suffocation due to aspiration of amniotic fluid 770.1
  mechanical 767.8
 trauma NEC 767.9
 triplet
  affected by maternal complications of pregnancy 761.5
  healthy liveborn — *see* Newborn, multiple
 twin
  affected by maternal complications of pregnancy 761.5
  healthy liveborn — *see* Newborn, twin
 ventouse, affecting fetus or newborn 763.3
Birthmark 757.32
Bisalbuminemia 273.8
Biskra button 085.1
Bite(s)
 with intact skin surface — *see* Contusion

Bite(s) — *continued*
  animal — *see* Wound, open, by site
    intact skin surface — *see* Contusion
  centipede 989.5
  chigger 133.8
  fire ant 989.5
  flea — *see* Injury, superficial, by site
  human (open wound) — *see also* Wound, open, by site
    intact skin surface — *see* Contusion
  insect
    nonvenomous — *see* Injury, superficial, by site
    venomous 989.5
  mad dog (death from) 071
  poisonous 989.5
  red bug 133.8
  reptile 989.5
    nonvenomous — *see* Wound, open, by site
  snake 989.5
    nonvenomous — *see* Wound, open, by site
  spider (venomous) 989.5
    nonvenomous — *see* Injury, superficial, by site
    venomous 989.5
Biting
  cheek or lip 528.9
  nail 307.9
Black
  death 020.9
  eye NEC 921.0
  hairy tongue 529.3
  lung disease 500
Blackfan-Diamond anemia or syndrome (congenital hypoplastic anemia) 284.0
Blackhead 706.1
Blackout 780.2
Blackwater fever 084.8
Bladder — *see* condition
Blast
  blindness 921.3
  concussion — *see* Blast, injury
  injury 869.0
    with open wound into cavity 869.1
    abdomen or thorax — *see* Injury, internal, by site
    brain (*see also* Concussion, brain) 850.9
      with skull fracture — *see* Fracture, skull
    ear (acoustic nerve trauma) 951.5
      with perforation, tympanic membrane — *see* Wound, open, ear, drum
    lung (*see also* Injury, internal, lung) 861.20
    otitic (explosive) 388.11
Blastomycosis, blastomycotic (chronic) (cutaneous) (disseminated) (lung) (pulmonary) (systemic) 116.0
  Brazilian 116.1
  European 117.5
  keloidal 116.2
  North American 116.0
  primary pulmonary 116.0
  South American 116.1
Bleb(s) 709.8
  emphysematous (bullous) (diffuse) (lung) (ruptured) (solitary) 492.0
  filtering, eye (postglaucoma) (status) V45.69
    with complication 997.99
      postcataract extraction (complication) 997.99

Bleb(s) — *continued*
  lung (ruptured) 492.0
  congenital 770.5
  subpleural (emphysematous) 492.0
Bleeder (familial) (hereditary) (*see also* Defect, coagulation) 286.9
  nonfamilial 286.9
Bleeding (*see also* Hemorrhage) 459.0
  anal 569.3
  anovulatory 628.0
  atonic, following delivery 666.1 ✓5ᵗʰ
  capillary 448.9
  due to subinvolution 621.1
    puerperal 666.2 ✓5ᵗʰ
  ear 388.69
  excessive, associated with menopausal onset 627.0
  familial (*see also* Defect, coagulation) 286.9
  following intercourse 626.7
  gastrointestinal 578.9
  gums 523.8
  hemorrhoids — *see* Hemorrhoids, bleeding
  intermenstrual
    irregular 626.6
    regular 626.5
  intraoperative 998.11
  irregular NEC 626.4
  menopausal 627.0
  mouth 528.9
  nipple 611.79
  nose 784.7
  ovulation 626.5
  postclimacteric 627.1
  postcoital 626.7
  postmenopausal 627.1
    following induced menopause 627.4
  postoperative 998.11
  preclimacteric 627.0
  puberty 626.3
    excessive, with onset of menstrual periods 626.3
  rectum, rectal 569.3
  tendencies (*see also* Defect, coagulation) 286.9
  throat 784.8
  umbilical stump 772.3
  umbilicus 789.9
  unrelated to menstrual cycle 626.6
  uterus, uterine 626.9
    climacteric 627.0
    dysfunctional 626.8
    functional 626.8
    unrelated to menstrual cycle 626.6
  vagina, vaginal 623.8
    functional 626.8
  vicarious 625.8
Blennorrhagia, blennorrhagic — *see* Blennorrhea
Blennorrhea (acute) 098.0
  adultorum 098.40
  alveolaris 523.4
  chronic or duration of 2 months or over 098.2
  gonococcal (neonatorum) 098.40
  inclusion (neonatal) (newborn) 771.6
  neonatorum 098.40
Blepharelosis (*see also* Entropion) 374.00
Blepharitis (eyelid) 373.00
  angularis 373.01
  ciliaris 373.00
    with ulcer 373.01

Blepharitis — continued
  marginal 373.00
    with ulcer 373.01
    scrofulous (see also Tuberculosis) 017.3 [5]
      [373.00]
    squamous 373.02
    ulcerative 373.01
Blepharochalasis 374.34
  congenital 743.62
Blepharoclonus 333.81
Blepharoconjunctivitis (see also Conjunctivitis) 372.20
  angular 372.21
  contact 372.22
Blepharophimosis (eyelid) 374.46
  congenital 743.62
Blepharoplegia 374.89
Blepharoptosis 374.30
  congenital 743.61
Blepharopyorrhea 098.49
Blepharospasm 333.81
Blessig's cyst 362.62
Blighted ovum 631
Blind
  bronchus (congenital) 748.3
  eye — see also Blindness
    hypertensive 360.42
    hypotensive 360.41
  loop syndrome (postoperative) 579.2
  sac, fallopian tube (congenital) 752.19
  spot, enlarged 368.42
  tract or tube (congenital) NEC — see Atresia
Blindness (acquired) (congenital) (both eyes) 369.00
  blast 921.3
    with nerve injury — see Injury, nerve, optic
  Bright's — see Uremia
  color (congenital) 368.59
    acquired 368.55
    blue 368.53
    green 368.52
    red 368.51
    total 368.54
  concussion 950.9
  cortical 377.75
  day 368.10
    acquired 368.10 ▲
    congenital 368.10 ▲
    hereditary 368.10 ▲
    specified type NEC 368.10 ▲
  due to
    injury NEC 950.9
    refractive error — see Error, refractive
  eclipse (total) 363.31
  emotional 300.11
  hysterical 300.11
  legal (both eyes) (USA definition) 369.4
    with impairment of better (less impaired) eye
      near-total 369.02
        with
          lesser eye impairment 369.02
            near-total 369.04
            total 369.03
      profound 369.05
        with
          lesser eye impairment 369.05
            near-total 369.07

Blindness — continued
  legal — continued
    with impairment of better (less impaired) eye — continued
      profound — continued
        with — continued
          lesser eye impairment — continued
            profound 369.08
            total 369.06
      severe 369.21
        with
          lesser eye impairment 369.21
            blind 369.11
            near-total 369.13
            profound 369.14
            severe 369.22
            total 369.12
      total
        with lesser eye impairment
          total 369.01
  mind 784.69
  moderate
    both eyes 369.25
      with impairment of lesser eye (specified as)
        blind, not further specified 369.15
        low vision, not further specified 369.23
        near-total 369.17
        profound 369.18
        severe 369.24
        total 369.16
    one eye 369.74
      with vision of other eye (specified as)
        near-normal 369.75
        normal 369.76
  near-total
    both eyes 369.04
      with impairment of lesser eye (specified as)
        blind, not further specified 369.02
        total 369.03
    one eye 369.64
      with vision of other eye (specified as)
        near-normal 369.65
        normal 369.66
  night 368.60
    acquired 368.62
    congenital (Japanese) 368.61
    hereditary 368.61
    specified type NEC 368.69
    vitamin A deficiency 264.5
  nocturnal — see Blindness, night
  one eye 369.60
    with low vision of other eye 369.10
  profound
    both eyes 369.08
      with impairment of lesser eye (specified as)
        blind, not further specified 369.05
        near-total 369.07
        total 369.06
    one eye 369.67
      with vision of other eye (specified as)
        near-normal 369.68
        normal 369.69
  psychic 784.69
  severe
    both eyes 369.22
      with impairment of lesser eye (specified as)

Index to Diseases

Blindness — *continued*
- severe — *continued*
  - both eyes — *continued*
    - with impairment of lesser eye (specified as) — *continued*
      - blind, not further specified 369.11
      - low vision, not further specified 369.21
      - near-total 369.13
      - profound 369.14
      - total 369.12
  - one eye 369.71
    - with vision of other eye (specified as)
      - near-normal 369.72
      - normal 369.73
- snow 370.24
- sun 363.31
- temporary 368.12
- total
  - both eyes 369.01
  - one eye 369.61
    - with vision of other eye (specified as)
      - near-normal 369.62
      - normal 369.63
- transient 368.12
- traumatic NEC 950.9
- word (developmental) 315.01
  - acquired 784.61
  - secondary to organic lesion 784.61

Blister — *see also* Injury, superficial, by site
- beetle dermatitis 692.89
- due to burn — *see* Burn, by site, second degree
- fever 054.9
- multiple, skin, nontraumatic 709.8

Bloating 787.3

Bloch-Siemens syndrome (incontinentia pigmenti) 757.33

Bloch-Stauffer dyshormonal dermatosis 757.33

Bloch-Sulzberger disease or syndrome (incontinentia pigmenti) (melanoblastosis) 757.33

Block
- alveolar capillary 516.3
- arborization (heart) 426.6
- arrhythmic 426.9
- atrioventricular (AV) (incomplete) (partial) 426.10
  - with
    - 2:1 atrioventricular response block 426.13
    - atrioventricular dissociation 426.0
  - first degree (incomplete) 426.11
  - second degree (Mobitz type I) 426.13
    - Mobitz (type) II 426.12
  - third degree 426.0
  - complete 426.0
    - congenital 746.86
  - congenital 746.86
  - Mobitz (incomplete)
    - type I (Wenckebach's) 426.13
    - type II 426.12
  - partial 426.13
- auriculoventricular (*see also* Block, atrioventricular) 426.10
  - complete 426.0
    - congenital 746.86
  - congenital 746.86
- bifascicular (cardiac) 426.53

Block — *continued*
- bundle branch (complete) (false) (incomplete) 426.50
  - bilateral 426.53
  - left (complete) (main stem) 426.3
    - with right bundle branch block 426.53
    - anterior fascicular 426.2
      - with
        - posterior fascicular block 426.3
        - right bundle branch block 426.52
    - hemiblock 426.2
    - incomplete 426.2
      - with right bundle branch block 426.53
    - posterior fascicular 426.2
      - with
        - anterior fascicular block 426.3
        - right bundle branch block 426.51
  - right 426.4
    - with
      - left bundle branch block (incomplete) (main stem) 426.53
      - left fascicular block 426.53
        - anterior 426.52
        - posterior 426.51
  - Wilson's type 426.4
- cardiac 426.9
- conduction 426.9
- complete 426.0
- Eustachian tube (*see also* Obstruction, Eustachian tube) 381.60
- fascicular (left anterior) (left posterior) 426.2
- foramen Magendie (acquired) 331.3
  - congenital 742.3
    - with spina bifida (*see also* Spina bifida) 741.0
- heart 426.9
  - first degree (atrioventricular) 426.11
  - second degree (atrioventricular) 426.13
  - third degree (atrioventricular) 426.0
  - bundle branch (complete) (false) (incomplete) 426.50
    - bilateral 426.53
    - left (*see also* Block, bundle branch, left) 426.3
    - right (*see also* Block, bundle branch, right) 426.4
  - complete (atrioventricular) 426.0
  - congenital 746.86
  - incomplete 426.13
  - intra-atrial 426.6
  - intraventricular NEC 426.6
  - sinoatrial 426.6
  - specified type NEC 426.6
- hepatic vein 453.0
- intraventricular (diffuse) (myofibrillar) 426.6
  - bundle branch (complete) (false) (incomplete) 426.50
    - bilateral 426.53
    - left (*see also* Block, bundle branch, left) 426.3
    - right (*see also* Block, bundle branch, right) 426.4
- kidney (*see also* Disease, renal) 593.9
  - postcystoscopic 997.5
- myocardial (*see also* Block, heart) 426.9
- nodal 426.10
- optic nerve 377.49
- organ or site (congenital) NEC — *see* Atresia
- parietal 426.6
- peri-infarction 426.6

Block — *continued*
  portal (vein) 452
  sinoatrial 426.6
  sinoauricular 426.6
  spinal cord 336.9
  trifascicular 426.54
  tubal 628.2
  vein NEC 453.9
Blocq's disease or syndrome (astasia-abasia) 307.9
Blood
  constituents, abnormal NEC 790.6
  disease 289.9
    specified NEC 289.8
  donor V59.01
    other blood components V59.09
    stem cells V59.02
    whole blood V59.01
  dyscrasia 289.9
    with
      abortion — *see* Abortion, by type, with hemorrhage, delayed or excessive
      ectopic pregnancy (*see also* categories 633.0-633.9) 639.1
      molar pregnancy (*see also* categories 630-632) 639.1
    fetus or newborn NEC 776.9
    following
      abortion 639.1
      ectopic or molar pregnancy 639.1
    puerperal, postpartum 666.3 ✓5ᵗʰ
  flukes NEC (*see also* Infestation, Schistosoma) 120.9
  in
    feces (*see also* Melena) 578.1
      occult 792.1
    urine (*see also* Hematuria) 599.7
  mole 631
  occult 792.1
  poisoning (*see also* Septicemia) 038.9
  pressure
    decreased, due to shock following injury 958.4
    fluctuating 796.4
    high (*see also* Hypertension) 401.9
      incidental reading (isolated) (nonspecific), without diagnosis of hypertension 796.2
    low (*see also* Hypotension) 458.9
      incidental reading (isolated) (nonspecific), without diagnosis of hypotension 796.3
  spitting (*see also* Hemoptysis) 786.3
  staining cornea 371.12
  transfusion
    without reported diagnosis V58.2
    donor V59.01
      stem cells V59.02
    reaction or complication — *see* Complications, transfusion
  tumor — *see* Hematoma
  vessel rupture — *see* Hemorrhage
  vomiting (*see also* Hematemesis) 578.0
Blood-forming organ disease 289.9
Bloodgood's disease 610.1
Bloodshot eye 379.93
Bloom (-Machacek) (-Torre) syndrome 757.39
Blotch, palpebral 372.55
Blount's disease (tibia vara) 732.4
Blount-Barber syndrome (tibia vara) 732.4

Blue
  baby 746.9
  bloater 491.20
    with acute bronchitis or exacerbation 491.21
  diaper syndrome 270.0
  disease 746.9
  dome cyst 610.0
  drum syndrome 381.02
  sclera 743.47
    with fragility of bone and deafness 756.51
  toe syndrome — *see* Atherosclerosis
Blueness (*see also* Cyanosis) 782.5
Blurring, visual 368.8
Blushing (abnormal) (excessive) 782.62
Boarder, hospital V65.0
  infant V65.0
Bockhart's impetigo (superficial folliculitis) 704.8
Bodechtel-Guttmann disease (subacute sclerosing panencephalitis) 046.2
Boder-Sedgwick syndrome (ataxia-telangiectasia) 334.8
Body, bodies
  Aschoff (*see also* Myocarditis, rheumatic) 398.0
  asteroid, vitreous 379.22
  choroid, colloid (degenerative) 362.57
    hereditary 362.77
  cytoid (retina) 362.82
  drusen (retina) (*see also* Drusen) 362.57
    optic disc 377.21
  fibrin, pleura 511.0
  foreign — *see* Foreign body
  Hassall-Henle 371.41
  loose
    joint (*see also* Loose, body, joint) 718.1 ✓5ᵗʰ
      knee 717.6
    knee 717.6
    sheath, tendon 727.82
  Mallory's 034.1
  Mooser 081.0
  Negri 071
  rice (joint) (*see also* Loose, body, joint) 718.1 ✓5ᵗʰ
    knee 717.6
  rocking 307.3
Boeck's
  disease (sarcoidosis) 135
  lupoid (miliary) 135
  sarcoid 135
Boerhaave's syndrome (spontaneous esophageal rupture) 530.4
Boggy
  cervix 622.8
  uterus 621.8
Boil (*see also* Carbuncle) 680.9
  abdominal wall 680.2
  Aleppo 085.1
  ankle 680.6
  anus 680.5
  arm (any part, above wrist) 680.3
  auditory canal, external 680.0
  axilla 680.3
  back (any part) 680.2
  Baghdad 085.1
  breast 680.2
  buttock 680.5
  chest wall 680.2
  corpus cavernosum 607.2

Boil — continued
  Delhi 085.1
  ear (any part) 680.0
  eyelid 373.13
  face (any part, except eye) 680.0
  finger (any) 680.4
  flank 680.2
  foot (any part) 680.7
  forearm 680.3
  Gafsa 085.1
  genital organ, male 608.4
  gluteal (region) 680.5
  groin 680.2
  hand (any part) 680.4
  head (any part, except face) 680.8
  heel 680.7
  hip 680.6
  knee 680.6
  labia 616.4
  lacrimal (see also Dacryocystitis) 375.30
    gland (see also Dacryoadenitis) 375.00
    passages (duct) (sac) (see also Dacryocystitis) 375.30
  leg, any part except foot 680.6
  multiple sites 680.9
  natal 085.1
  neck 680.1
  nose (external) (septum) 680.0
  orbit, orbital 376.01
  partes posteriores 680.5
  pectoral region 680.2
  penis 607.2
  perineum 680.2
  pinna 680.0
  scalp (any part) 680.8
  scrotum 608.4
  seminal vesicle 608.0
  shoulder 680.3
  skin NEC 680.9
  specified site NEC 680.8
  spermatic cord 608.4
  temple (region) 680.0
  testis 608.4
  thigh 680.6
  thumb 680.4
  toe (any) 680.7
  tropical 085.1
  trunk 680.2
  tunica vaginalis 608.4
  umbilicus 680.2
  upper arm 680.3
  vas deferens 608.4
  vulva 616.4
  wrist 680.4
Bold hives (see also Urticaria) 708.9
Bolivian hemorrhagic fever 078.7
Bombé, iris 364.74
Bomford-Rhoads anemia (refractory) 284.9
Bone — see condition
Bonnevie-Ullrich syndrome 758.6
Bonnier's syndrome 386.19
Bonvale Dam fever 780.79
Bony block of joint 718.80
  ankle 718.87
  elbow 718.82
  foot 718.87
  hand 718.84
  hip 718.85
  knee 718.86
  multiple sites 718.89
  pelvic region 718.85

Bony block of joint — continued
  shoulder (region) 718.81
  specified site NEC 718.88
  wrist 718.83
Borderline
  intellectual functioning V62.89
  pelvis 653.1
    with obstruction during labor 660.1
    affecting fetus or newborn 763.1
  psychosis (see also Schizophrenia) 295.5
    of childhood (see also Psychosis, childhood) 299.8
  schizophrenia (see also Schizophrenia) 295.5
Borna disease 062.9
Bornholm disease (epidemic pleurodynia) 074.1
Borrelia vincentii (mouth) (pharynx) (tonsils) 101
Bostock's catarrh (see also Fever, hay) 477.9
Boston exanthem 048
Botalli, ductus (patent) (persistent) 747.0
Bothriocephalus latus infestation 123.4
Botulism 005.1
Bouba (see also Yaws) 102.9
Bouffée délirante 298.3
Bouillaud's disease or syndrome (rheumatic heart disease) 391.9
Bourneville's disease (tuberous sclerosis) 759.5
Boutonneuse fever 082.1
Boutonniere
  deformity (finger) 736.21
  hand (intrinsic) 736.21
Bouveret (-Hoffmann) disease or syndrome (paroxysmal tachycardia) 427.2
Bovine heart — see Hypertrophy, cardiac
Bowel — see condition
Bowen's
  dermatosis (precancerous) (M8081/2) — see Neoplasm, skin, in situ
  disease (M8081/2) — see Neoplasm, skin, in situ
  epithelioma (M8081/2) — see Neoplasm, skin, in situ
  type
    epidermoid carcinoma in situ (M8081/2) — see Neoplasm, skin, in situ
    intraepidermal squamous cell carcinoma (M8081/2) — see Neoplasm, skin, in situ
Bowing
  femur 736.89
    congenital 754.42
  fibula 736.89
    congenital 754.43
  forearm 736.09
    away from midline (cubitus valgus) 736.01
    toward midline (cubitus varus) 736.02
  leg(s), long bones, congenital 754.44
  radius 736.09
    away from midline (cubitus valgus) 736.01
    toward midline (cubitus varus) 736.02
  tibia 736.89
    congenital 754.43
Bowleg(s) 736.42
  congenital 754.44
  rachitic 268.1
Boyd's dysentery 004.2

Brachial — see condition
Brachman-de Lange syndrome (Amsterdam dwarf, mental retardation, and brachycephaly) 759.89
Brachycardia 427.89
Brachycephaly 756.0
Brachymorphism and ectopia lentis 759.89
Bradley's disease (epidemic vomiting) 078.82
Bradycardia 427.89
   chronic (sinus) 427.81
   newborn 779.81
   nodal 427.89
   postoperative 997.1
   reflex 337.0
   sinoatrial 427.89
      with paroxysmal tachyarrhythmia or tachycardia 427.81
         chronic 427.81
   sinus 427.89
      with paroxysmal tachyarrhythmia or tachycardia 427.81
         chronic 427.81
      persistent 427.81
      severe 427.81
   tachycardia syndrome 427.81
   vagal 427.89
Bradypnea 786.09
Brailsford's disease 732.3
   radial head 732.3
   tarsal scaphoid 732.5
Brailsford-Morquio disease or syndrome (mucopolysac-charidosis IV) 277.5
Brain — see also condition
   death 348.8
   syndrome (acute) (chronic) (nonpsychotic) (organic) (with neurotic reaction) (with behavioral reaction) (*see also* Syndrome, brain) 310.9
      with
         presenile brain disease 290.10
         psychosis, psychotic reaction (*see also* Psychosis, organic) 294.9
      congenital (*see also* Retardation, mental) 319
Branched-chain amino-acid disease 270.3
Branchial — see condition
Branchopulmonitis — see Pneumonia, broncho-
Brandt's syndrome (acrodermatitis enteropathica) 686.8
Brash (water) 787.1
Brass-founders', ague 985.8
Bravais-Jacksonian epilepsy (*see also* Epilepsy) 345.5
Braxton Hicks contractions 644.1
Braziers' disease 985.8
Brazilian
   blastomycosis 116.1
   leishmaniasis 085.5
Break
   cardiorenal — see Hypertension, cardiorenal
   retina (*see also* Defect, retina) 361.30
Breakbone fever 061
Breakdown
   device, implant, or graft — see Complications, mechanical
   nervous (*see also* Disorder, mental, nonpsychotic) 300.9

Breakdown — *continued*
   perineum 674.2
Breast — see condition
Breast feeding difficulties 676.8
Breath
   foul 784.9
   holder, child 312.81
   holding spells 786.9
   shortness 786.05
Breathing
   asymmetrical 786.09
   bronchial 786.09
   exercises V57.0
   labored 786.09
   mouth 784.9
   periodic 786.09
   tic 307.20
Breathlessness 786.09
Breda's disease (*see also* Yaws) 102.9
Breech
   delivery, affecting fetus or newborn 763.0
   extraction, affecting fetus or newborn 763.0
   presentation (buttocks) (complete) (frank) 652.2
      with successful version 652.1
      before labor, affecting fetus or newborn 761.7
      during labor, affecting fetus or newborn 763.0
Breisky's disease (kraurosis vulvae) 624.0
Brennemann's syndrome (acute mesenteric lymphadenitis) 289.2
Brenner's
   tumor (benign) (M9000/0) 220
   borderline malignancy (M9000/1) 236.2
   malignant (M9000/3) 183.0
   proliferating (M9000/1) 236.2
Bretonneau's disease (diphtheritic malignant angina) 032.0
Breus' mole 631
Brevicollis 756.16
Bricklayers' itch 692.89
Brickmakers' anemia 126.9
Bridge
   myocardial 746.85
Bright's
   blindness — see Uremia
   disease (*see also* Nephritis) 583.9
      arteriosclerotic (*see also* Hypertension, kidney) 403.90
Brill's disease (recrudescent typhus) 081.1
   flea-borne 081.0
   louse-borne 081.1
Brill-Symmers disease (follicular lymphoma) (M9690/3) 202.0
Brill-Zinsser disease (recrudescent typhus) 081.1
Brinton's disease (linitis plastica) (M8142/3) 151.9
Brion-Kayser disease (*see also* Fever, paratyphoid) 002.9
Briquet's disorder or syndrome 300.81
Brissaud's
   infantilism (infantile myxedema) 244.9
   motor-verbal tic 307.23
Brissaud-Meige syndrome (infantile myxedema) 244.9

Brittle
  bones (congenital) 756.51
  nails 703.8
    congenital 757.5
Broad — *see also* condition
  beta disease 272.2
  ligament laceration syndrome 620.6
Brock's syndrome (atelectasis due to enlarged lymph nodes) 518.0
Brocq's disease 691.8
  atopic (diffuse) neurodermatitis 691.8
  lichen simplex chronicus 698.3
  parakeratosis psoriasiformis 696.2
  parapsoriasis 696.2
Brocq-Duhring disease (dermatitis herpetiformis) 694.0
Brodie's
  abscess (localized) (chronic) (*see also* Osteomyelitis) 730.1 ✓5ᵗʰ
  disease (joint) (*see also* Osteomyelitis) 730.1 ✓5ᵗʰ
Broken
  arches 734
    congenital 755.67
  back — *see* Fracture, vertebra, by site
  bone — *see* Fracture, by site
  compensation — *see* Disease, heart
  implant or internal device — *see* listing under Complications, mechanical
  neck — *see* Fracture, vertebra, cervical
  nose 802.0
    open 802.1
  tooth, teeth 873.63
    complicated 873.73
Bromhidrosis 705.89
Bromidism, bromism
  acute 967.3
    correct substance properly administered 349.82
    overdose or wrong substance given or taken 967.3
  chronic (*see also* Dependence) 304.1 ✓5ᵗʰ
Bromidrosiphobia 300.23
Bromidrosis 705.89
Bronchi, bronchial — *see* condition
Bronchiectasis (cylindrical) (diffuse) (fusiform) (localized) (moniliform) (postinfectious) (recurrent) (saccular) 494.0
  with acute exacerbation 494.1
  congenital 748.61
  tuberculosis (*see also* Tuberculosis) 011.5 ✓5ᵗʰ
Bronchiolectasis — *see* Bronchiectasis
Bronchiolitis (acute) (infectious) (subacute) 466.19
  with
    bronchospasm or obstruction 466.19
    influenza, flu, or grippe 487.1
  catarrhal (acute) (subacute) 466.19
  chemical 506.0
    chronic 506.4
  chronic (obliterative) 491.8
  due to external agent — *see* Bronchitis, acute, due to
  fibrosa obliterans 491.8
  influenzal 487.1
  obliterans 491.8
    with organizing pneumonia (B.O.O.P.) 516.8
    status post lung transplant 996.84

Bronchiolitis — *continued*
  obliterative (chronic) (diffuse) (subacute) 491.8
    due to fumes or vapors 506.4
  respiratory syncytial virus 466.11
  vesicular — *see* Pneumonia, broncho-
Bronchitis (diffuse) (hypostatic) (infectious) (inflammatory) (simple) 490
  with
    emphysema — *see* Emphysema
    influenza, flu, or grippe 487.1
    obstruction airway, chronic 491.20
      with acute exacerbation 491.21
    tracheitis 490
      acute or subacute 466.0
        with bronchospasm or obstruction 466.0
      chronic 491.8
  acute or subacute 466.0
    with
      bronchospasm 466.0
      chronic
        bronchitis (obstructive) 491.21
        obstructive pulmonary disease (COPD) 491.21
      obstruction 466.0
      tracheitis 466.0
    chemical (due to fumes or vapors) 506.0
    due to
      fumes or vapors 506.0
      radiation 508.8
  allergic (acute) (*see also* Asthma) 493.9 ✓5ᵗʰ
  arachidic 934.1
  aspiration 507.0
    due to fumes or vapors 506.0
  asthmatic (acute) 493.90
    with
      acute exacerbation 493.92
      status asthmaticus 493.91
    chronic 493.2 ✓5ᵗʰ ▲
  capillary 466.19
    with bronchospasm or obstruction 466.19
    chronic 491.8
  caseous (*see also* Tuberculosis) 011.3 ✓5ᵗʰ
  Castellani's 104.8
  catarrhal 490
    acute — *see* Bronchitis, acute
    chronic 491.0
  chemical (acute) (subacute) 506.0
    chronic 506.4
    due to fumes or vapors (acute) (subacute) 506.0
      chronic 506.4
  chronic 491.9
    with
      tracheitis (chronic) 491.8
    asthmatic 493.2 ✓5ᵗʰ ▲
    catarrhal 491.0
    chemical (due to fumes and vapors) 506.4
    due to
      fumes or vapors (chemical) (inhalation) 506.4
      radiation 508.8
      tobacco smoking 491.0
    mucopurulent 491.1
    obstructive 491.20
      with acute bronchitis or acute exacerbation 491.21
    purulent 491.1
    simple 491.0
    specified type NEC 491.8
  croupous 466.0
    with bronchospasm or obstruction 466.0

Bronchitis — continued
  croupous — continued
    due to fumes or vapors 506.0
  emphysematous 491.20
    with acute bronchitis or acute exacerbation 491.21
  exudative 466.0
  fetid (chronic) (recurrent) 491.1
  fibrinous, acute or subacute 466.0
    with bronchospasm or obstruction 466.0
  grippal 487.1
  influenzal 487.1
  membranous, acute or subacute 466.0
    with bronchospasm or obstruction 466.0
  moulders' 502
  mucopurulent (chronic) (recurrent) 491.1
    acute or subacute 466.0
  non-obstructive 491.0
  obliterans 491.8
  obstructive (chronic) 491.20
    with acute bronchitis or acute exacerbation 491.21
  pituitous 491.1
  plastic (inflammatory) 466.0
  pneumococcal, acute or subacute 466.0
    with bronchospasm or obstruction 466.0
  pseudomembranous 466.0
  purulent (chronic) (recurrent) 491.1
    acute or subacute 466.0
      with bronchospasm or obstruction 466.0
  putrid 491.1
  scrofulous (see also Tuberculosis) 011.3
  senile 491.9
  septic, acute or subacute 466.0
    with bronchospasm or obstruction 466.0
  smokers' 491.0
  spirochetal 104.8
  suffocative, acute or subacute 466.0
  summer (see also Asthma) 493.9
  suppurative (chronic) 491.1
    acute or subacute 466.0
  tuberculous (see also Tuberculosis) 011.3
  ulcerative 491.8
    Vincent's 101
  Vincent's 101
  viral, acute or subacute 466.0
Bronchoalveolitis 485
Bronchoaspergillosis 117.3
Bronchocele
  meaning
    dilatation of bronchus 519.1
    goiter 240.9
Bronchogenic carcinoma 162.9
Bronchohemisporosis 117.9
Broncholithiasis 518.89
  tuberculous (see also Tuberculosis) 011.3
Bronchomalacia 748.3
Bronchomoniliasis 112.89
Bronchomycosis 112.89
Bronchonocardiosis 039.1
Bronchopleuropneumonia — see Pneumonia, broncho-
Bronchopneumonia — see Pneumonia, broncho-
Bronchopneumonitis — see Pneumonia, broncho-
Bronchopulmonary — see condition
Bronchorrhagia 786.3
  newborn 770.3
  tuberculous (see also Tuberculosis) 011.3

Bronchorrhea (chronic) (purulent) 491.0
  acute 466.0
Bronchospasm 519.1
  with
    asthma — see Asthma
    bronchiolitis
      due to respiratory syncytial virus 466.11
    bronchitis — see Bronchitis
    chronic obstructive pulmonary disease (COPD) 496
    emphysema — see Emphysema
    due to external agent — see Condition, respiratory, acute, due to
Bronchospirochetosis 104.8
Bronchostenosis 519.1
Bronchus — see condition
Bronze, bronzed
  diabetes 275.0
  disease (Addison's) (skin) 255.4
    tuberculous (see also Tuberculosis) 017.6
Brooke's disease or tumor (M8100/0) — see Neoplasm, skin, benign
Brown's tendon sheath syndrome 378.61
Brown enamel of teeth (hereditary) 520.5
Brown-Séquard's paralysis (syndrome) 344.89
Brow presentation complicating delivery 652.4
Brucella, brucellosis (infection) 023.9
  abortus 023.1
  canis 023.3
  dermatitis, skin 023.9
  melitensis 023.0
  mixed 023.8
  suis 023.2
Bruck's disease 733.99
Bruck-de Lange disease or syndrome (Amsterdam dwarf, mental retardation, and brachycephaly) 759.89
Brugada syndrome 746.89
Brugsch's syndrome (acropachyderma) 757.39
Brug's filariasis 125.1
Bruhl's disease (splenic anemia with fever) 285.8
Bruise (skin surface intact) — see also Contusion
  with
    fracture — see Fracture, by site
    open wound — see Wound, open, by site
    internal organ (abdomen, chest, or pelvis) — see Injury, internal, by site
  umbilical cord 663.6
    affecting fetus or newborn 762.6
Bruit 785.9
  arterial (abdominal) (carotid) 785.9
  supraclavicular 785.9
Brushburn — see Injury, superficial, by site
Bruton's X-linked agammaglobulinemia 279.04
Bruxism 306.8
Bubbly lung syndrome 770.7
Bubo 289.3
  blennorrhagic 098.89
  chancroidal 099.0
  climatic 099.1
  due to Hemophilus ducreyi 099.0
  gonococcal 098.89
  indolent NEC 099.8
  inguinal NEC 099.8
    chancroidal 099.0

Bubo — continued
  inguinal NEC — continued
    climatic 099.1
    due to H. ducreyi 099.0
    scrofulous (see also Tuberculosis) 017.2 ✓5ᵗʰ
    soft chancre 099.0
    suppurating 683
    syphilitic 091.0
      congenital 090.0
    tropical 099.1
    venereal NEC 099.8
    virulent 099.0
Bubonic plague 020.0
Bubonocele — see Hernia, inguinal
Buccal — see condition
Buchanan's disease (juvenile osteochondrosis of iliac crest) 732.1
Buchem's syndrome (hyperostosis corticalis) 733.3
Buchman's disease (osteochondrosis, juvenile) 732.1
Bucket handle fracture (semilunar cartilage) (see also Tear, meniscus) 836.2
Budd-Chiari syndrome (hepatic vein thrombosis) 453.0
Budgerigar-fanciers' disease or lung 495.2
Büdinger-Ludloff-Läwen disease 717.89
Buerger's disease (thromboangiitis obliterans) 443.1
Bulbar — see condition
Bulbus cordis 745.9
  persistent (in left ventricle) 745.8
Bulging fontanels (congenital) 756.0
Bulimia 783.6
  nonorganic origin 307.51
Bulky uterus 621.2
Bulla(e) 709.8
  lung (emphysematous) (solitary) 492.0
Bullet wound — see also Wound, open, by site
  fracture — see Fracture, by site, open
  internal organ (abdomen, chest, or pelvis) — see Injury, internal, by site, with open wound
  intracranial — see Laceration, brain, with open wound
Bullis fever 082.8
Bullying (see also Disturbance, conduct) 312.0 ✓5ᵗʰ
Bundle
  branch block (complete) (false) (incomplete) 426.50
    bilateral 426.53
    left (see also Block, bundle branch, left) 426.3
      hemiblock 426.2
    right (see also Block, bundle branch, right) 426.4
  of His — see condition
  of Kent syndrome (anomalous atrioventricular excitation) 426.7
Bungpagga 040.81
Bunion 727.1
Bunionette 727.1
Bunyamwera fever 066.3
Buphthalmia, buphthalmos (congenital) 743.20
  associated with
    keratoglobus, congenital 743.22

Buphthalmia, buphthalmos — continued
  associated with — continued
    megalocornea 743.22
    ocular anomalies NEC 743.22
  isolated 743.21
  simple 743.21
Bürger-Grütz disease or syndrome (essential familial hyperlipemia) 272.3
Buried roots 525.3
Burke's syndrome 577.8
Burkitt's
  tumor (M9750/3) 200.2 ✓5ᵗʰ
  type malignant, lymphoma, lymphoblastic, or undifferentiated (M9750/3) 200.2 ✓5ᵗʰ
Burn (acid) (cathode ray) (caustic) (chemical) (electric heating appliance) (electricity) (fire) (flame) (hot liquid or object) (irradiation) (lime) (radiation) (steam) (thermal) (x-ray) 949.0

> Note — Use the following fifth-digit subclassification with category 948 to indicate the percent of body surface with third degree burn:
>
> 0 Less than 10% or unspecified
> 1 10–19%
> 2 20–29%
> 3 30–39%
> 4 40–49%
> 5 50–59%
> 6 60–69%
> 7 70–79%
> 8 80–89%
> 9 90% or more of body surface

with
  blisters — see Burn, by site, second degree
  erythema — see Burn, by site, first degree
  skin loss (epidermal) — see also Burn, by site, second degree
    full thickness — see also Burn, by site, third degree
      with necrosis of underlying tissues — see Burn, by site, third degree, deep
  first degree — see Burn, by site, first degree
  second degree — see Burn, by site, second degree
  third degree — see Burn, by site, third degree
    deep — see Burn, by site, third degree, deep
abdomen, abdominal (muscle) (wall) 942.03
  with
    trunk — see Burn, trunk, multiple sites
  first degree 942.13
  second degree 942.23
  third degree 942.33
    deep 942.43
      with loss of body part 942.53
ankle 945.03
  with
    lower limb(s) — see Burn, leg, multiple sites
  first degree 945.13
  second degree 945.23
  third degree 945.33
    deep 945.43
      with loss of body part 945.53

Burn — *continued*
  anus — *see* Burn, trunk, specified site NEC
  arm(s) 943.00
    first degree 943.10
    second degree 943.20
    third degree 943.30
      deep 943.40
        with loss of body part 943.50
    lower — *see* Burn, forearm(s)
    multiple sites, except hand(s) or wrist(s) 943.09
      first degree 943.19
      second degree 943.29
      third degree 943.39
        deep 943.49
          with loss of body part 943.59
    upper 943.03
      first degree 943.13
      second degree 943.23
      third degree 943.33
        deep 943.43
          with loss of body part 943.53
  auditory canal (external) — *see* Burn, ear
  auricle (ear) — *see* Burn, ear
  axilla 943.04
    with
      upper limb(s) except hand(s) or wrist(s) — *see* Burn, arm(s), multiple sites
    first degree 943.14
    second degree 943.24
    third degree 943.34
      deep 943.44
        with loss of body part 943.54
  back 942.04
    with
      trunk — *see* Burn, trunk, multiple sites
    first degree 942.14
    second degree 942.24
    third degree 942.34
      deep 942.44
        with loss of body part 942.54
  biceps
    brachii — *see* Burn, arm(s), upper
    femoris — *see* Burn, thigh
  breast(s) 942.01
    with
      trunk — *see* Burn, trunk, multiple sites
    first degree 942.11
    second degree 942.21
    third degree 942.31
      deep 942.41
        with loss of body part 942.51
  brow — *see* Burn, forehead
  buttock(s) — *see* Burn, back
  canthus (eye) 940.1
    chemical 940.0
  cervix (uteri) 947.4
  cheek (cutaneous) 941.07
    with
      face or head — *see* Burn, head, multiple sites
    first degree 941.17
    second degree 941.27
    third degree 941.37
      deep 941.47
        with loss of body part 941.57
  chest wall (anterior) 942.02
    with
      trunk — *see* Burn, trunk, multiple sites
    first degree 942.12
    second degree 942.22

Burn — *continued*
  chest wall — *continued*
    third degree 942.32
      deep 942.42
        with loss of body part 942.52
  chin 941.04
    with
      face or head — *see* Burn, head, multiple sites
    first degree 941.14
    second degree 941.24
    third degree 941.34
      deep 941.44
        with loss of body part 941.54
  clitoris — *see* Burn, genitourinary organs, external
  colon 947.3
  conjunctiva (and cornea) 940.4
    chemical
      acid 940.3
      alkaline 940.2
  cornea (and conjunctiva) 940.4
    chemical
      acid 940.3
      alkaline 940.2
  costal region — *see* Burn, chest wall
  due to ingested chemical agent — *see* Burn, internal organs
  ear (auricle) (canal) (drum) (external) 941.01
    with
      face or head — *see* Burn, head, multiple sites
    first degree 941.11
    second degree 941.21
    third degree 941.31
      deep 941.41
        with loss of a body part 941.51
  elbow 943.02
    with
      hand(s) and wrist(s) — *see* Burn, multiple specified sites
      upper limb(s) except hand(s) or wrist(s) — *see also* Burn, arm(s), multiple sites
    first degree 943.12
    second degree 943.22
    third degree 943.32
      deep 943.42
        with loss of body part 943.52
  electricity, electric current — *See* Burn, by site
  entire body — *see* Burn, multiple, specified sites
  epididymis — *see* Burn, genitourinary organs, external
  epigastric region — *see* Burn, abdomen
  epiglottis 947.1
  esophagus 947.2
  extent (percent of body surface)
    less than 10 percent 948.0
    10-19 percent 948.1
    20-29 percent 948.2
    30-39 percent 948.3
    40-49 percent 948.4
    50-59 percent 948.5
    60-69 percent 948.6
    70-79 percent 948.7
    80-89 percent 948.8
    90 percent or more 948.9
  extremity
    lower — *see* Burn, leg
    upper — *see* Burn, arm(s)

Index to Diseases — Burn

Burn — *continued*
  eye(s) (and adnexa) (only) 940.9
    with
      face, head, or neck 941.02
        first degree 941.12
        second degree 941.22
        third degree 941.32
          deep 941.42
            with loss of body part 941.52
      other sites (classifiable to more than one category in 940-945) — *see* Burn, multiple, specified sites
      resulting rupture and destruction of eyeball 940.5
      specified part — *see* Burn, by site
  eyeball — *see also* Burn, eye with resulting rupture and destruction of eyeball 940.5
  eyelid(s) 940.1
    chemical 940.0
  face — *see* Burn, head
  finger (nail) (subungual) 944.01
    with
      hand(s) — *see* Burn, hand(s), multiple sites
      other sites — *see* Burn, multiple, specified sites
      thumb 944.04
        first degree 944.14
        second degree 944.24
        third degree 944.34
          deep 944.44
            with loss of body part 944.54
    first degree 944.11
    second degree 944.21
    third degree 944.31
      deep 944.41
        with loss of body part 944.51
    multiple (digits) 944.03
      with thumb — *see* Burn, finger, with thumb
      first degree 944.13
      second degree 944.23
      third degree 944.33
        deep 944.43
          with loss of body part 944.53
  flank — *see* Burn, abdomen
  foot 945.02
    with
      lower limb(s) — *see* Burn, leg, multiple sites
    first degree 945.12
    second degree 945.22
    third degree 945.32
      deep 945.42
        with loss of body part 945.52
  forearm(s) 943.01
    with
      upper limb(s) except hand(s) or wrist(s) — *see* Burn, arm(s), multiple sites
    first degree 943.11
    second degree 943.21
    third degree 943.31
      deep 943.41
        with loss of body part 943.51
  forehead 941.07
    with
      face or head — *see* Burn, head, multiple sites
    first degree 941.17
    second degree 941.27

Burn — *continued*
  forehead — *continued*
    third degree 941.37
      deep 941.47
        with loss of body part 941.57
  fourth degree — *see* Burn, by site, third degree, deep
  friction — *see* Injury, superficial, by site
  from swallowing caustic or corrosive substance NEC — *see* Burn, internal organs
  full thickness — *see* Burn, by site, third degree
  gastrointestinal tract 947.3
  genitourinary organs
    external 942.05
      with
        trunk — *see* Burn, trunk, multiple sites
      first degree 942.15
      second degree 942.25
      third degree 942.35
        deep 942.45
          with loss of body part 942.55
    internal 947.8
  globe (eye) — *see* Burn, eyeball
  groin — *see* Burn, abdomen
  gum 947.0
  hand(s) (phalanges) (and wrist) 944.00
    first degree 944.10
    second degree 944.20
    third degree 944.30
      deep 944.40
        with loss of body part 944.50
    back (dorsal surface) 944.06
      first degree 944.16
      second degree 944.26
      third degree 944.36
        deep 944.46
          with loss of body part 944.56
    multiple sites 944.08
      first degree 944.18
      second degree 944.28
      third degree 944.38
        deep 944.48
          with loss of body part 944.58
  head (and face) 941.00
    eye(s) only 940.9
    specified part — *see* Burn, by site
    first degree 941.10
    second degree 941.20
    third degree 941.30
      deep 941.40
        with loss of body part 941.50
    multiple sites 941.09
      with eyes — *see* Burn, eyes, with face, head, or neck
      first degree 941.19
      second degree 941.29
      third degree 941.39
        deep 941.49
          with loss of body part 941.59
  heel — *see* Burn, foot
  hip — *see* Burn, trunk, specified site NEC
  iliac region — *see* Burn, trunk, specified site NEC
  infected 958.3
  inhalation (*see also* Burn, internal organs) 947.9

Burn

Burn — *continued*
- internal organs 947.9
  - from caustic or corrosive substance (swallowing) NEC 947.9
  - specified NEC (*see also* Burn, by site) 947.8
- interscapular region — *see* Burn, back
- intestine (large) (small) 947.3
- iris — *see* Burn, eyeball
- knee 945.05
  - with
    - lower limb(s) — *see* Burn, leg, multiple sites
  - first degree 945.15
  - second degree 945.25
  - third degree 945.35
    - deep 945.45
      - with loss of body part 945.55
- labium (majorus) (minus) — *see* Burn, genitourinary organs, external
- lacrimal apparatus, duct, gland, or sac 940.1
  - chemical 940.0
- larynx 947.1
- late effect — *see* Late, effects (of), burn
- leg 945.00
  - first degree 945.10
  - second degree 945.20
  - third degree 945.30
    - deep 945.40
      - with loss of body part 945.50
  - lower 945.04
    - with other part(s) of lower limb(s) — *see* Burn, leg, multiple sites
    - first degree 945.14
    - second degree 945.24
    - third degree 945.34
      - deep 945.44
        - with loss of body part 945.54
  - multiple sites 945.09
    - first degree 945.19
    - second degree 945.29
    - third degree 945.39
      - deep 945.49
        - with loss of body part 945.59
  - upper — *see* Burn, thigh
- lightning — *see* Burn, by site
- limb(s)
  - lower (including foot or toe(s)) — *see* Burn, leg
  - upper (except wrist and hand) — *see* Burn, arm(s)
- lip(s) 941.03
  - with
    - face or head — *see* Burn, head, multiple sites
  - first degree 941.13
  - second degree 941.23
  - third degree 941.33
    - deep 941.43
      - with loss of body part 941.53
- lumbar region — *see* Burn, back
- lung 947.1
- malar region — *see* Burn, cheek
- mastoid region — *see* Burn, scalp
- membrane, tympanic — *see* Burn, ear
- midthoracic region — *see* Burn, chest wall
- mouth 947.0
- multiple (*see also* Burn, unspecified) 949.0
  - specified sites classifiable to more than one category in 940-945 946.0
    - first degree 946.1
    - second degree 946.2

Burn — *continued*
- multiple — *continued*
  - specified sites classifiable to more than one category in 940-945 946.0 — *continued*
    - third degree 946.3
      - deep 946.4
        - with loss of body part 946.5
- muscle, abdominal — *see* Burn, abdomen
- nasal (septum) — *see* Burn, nose
- neck 941.08
  - with
    - face or head — *see* Burn, head, multiple sites
  - first degree 941.18
  - second degree 941.28
  - third degree 941.38
    - deep 941.48
      - with loss of body part 941.58
- nose (septum) 941.05
  - with
    - face or head — *see* Burn, head, multiple sites
  - first degree 941.15
  - second degree 941.25
  - third degree 941.35
    - deep 941.45
      - with loss of body part 941.55
- occipital region — *see* Burn, scalp
- orbit region 940.1
  - chemical 940.0
- oronasopharynx 947.0
- palate 947.0
- palm(s) 944.05
  - with
    - hand(s) and wrist(s) — *see* Burn, hand(s), multiple sites
  - first degree 944.15
  - second degree 944.25
  - third degree 944.35
    - deep 944.45
      - with loss of a body part 944.55
- parietal region — *see* Burn, scalp
- penis — *see* Burn, genitourinary organs, external
- perineum — *see* Burn, genitourinary organs, external
- periocular area 940.1
  - chemical 940.0
- pharynx 947.0
- pleura 947.1
- popliteal space — *see* Burn, knee
- prepuce — *see* Burn, genitourinary organs, external
- pubic region — *see* Burn, genitourinary organs, external
- pudenda — *see* Burn, genitourinary organs, external
- rectum 947.3
- sac, lacrimal 940.1
  - chemical 940.0
- sacral region — *see* Burn, back
- salivary (ducts) (glands) 947.0
- scalp 941.06
  - with
    - face or neck — *see* Burn, head, multiple sites
  - first degree 941.16
  - second degree 941.26

Index to Diseases

Burn — *continued*
  scalp — *continued*
    third degree 941.36
      deep 941.46
        with loss of body part 941.56
  scapular region 943.06
    with
      upper limb(s), except hand(s) or wrist(s) — *see* Burn, arm(s), multiple sites
    first degree 943.16
    second degree 943.26
    third degree 943.36
      deep 943.46
        with loss of body part 943.56
  sclera — *see* Burn, eyeball
  scrotum — *see* Burn, genitourinary organs, external
  septum, nasal — *see* Burn, nose
  shoulder(s) 943.05
    with
      hand(s) and wrist(s) — *see* Burn, multiple, specified sites
      upper limb(s), except hand(s) or wrist(s) — *see* Burn, arm(s), multiple sites
    first degree 943.15
    second degree 943.25
    third degree 943.35
      deep 943.45
        with loss of body part 943.55
  skin NEC (*see also* Burn, unspecified) 949.0
  skull — *see* Burn, head
  small intestine 947.3
  sternal region — *see* Burn, chest wall
  stomach 947.3
  subconjunctival — *see* Burn, conjunctiva
  subcutaneous — *see* Burn, by site, third degree
  submaxillary region — *see* Burn, head
  submental region — *see* Burn, chin
  sun — *see* Sunburn
  supraclavicular fossa — *see* Burn, neck
  supraorbital — *see* Burn, forehead
  temple — *see* Burn, scalp
  temporal region — *see* Burn, scalp
  testicle — *see* Burn, genitourinary organs, external
  testis — *see* Burn, genitourinary organs, external
  thigh 945.06
    with
      lower limb(s) — *see* Burn, leg, multiple sites
    first degree 945.16
    second degree 945.26
    third degree 945.36
      deep 945.46
        with loss of body part 945.56
  thorax (external) — *see* Burn, chest wall
  throat 947.0
  thumb(s) (nail) (subungual) 944.02
    with
      finger(s) — *see* Burn, finger, with other sites, thumb
      hand(s) and wrist(s) — *see* Burn, hand(s), multiple sites
    first degree 944.12
    second degree 944.22
    third degree 944.32
      deep 944.42
        with loss of body part 944.52

Burn — *continued*
  toe (nail) (subungual) 945.01
    with
      lower limb(s) — *see* Burn, leg, multiple sites
    first degree 945.11
    second degree 945.21
    third degree 945.31
      deep 945.41
        with loss of body part 945.51
  tongue 947.0
  tonsil 947.0
  trachea 947.1
  trunk 942.00
    first degree 942.10
    second degree 942.20
    third degree 942.30
      deep 942.40
        with loss of body part 942.50
    multiple sites 942.09
      first degree 942.19
      second degree 942.29
      third degree 942.39
        deep 942.49
          with loss of body part 942.59
    specified site NEC 942.09
      first degree 942.19
      second degree 942.29
      third degree 942.39
        deep 942.49
          with loss of body part 942.59
  tunica vaginalis — *see* Burn, genitourinary organs, external
  tympanic membrane — *see* Burn, ear
  tympanum — *see* Burn, ear
  ultraviolet 692.82
  unspecified site (multiple) 949.0
    with extent of body surface involved specified
      less than 10 percent 948.0 ✓5ᵗʰ
      10-19 percent 948.1 ✓5ᵗʰ
      20-29 percent 948.2 ✓5ᵗʰ
      30-39 percent 948.3 ✓5ᵗʰ
      40-49 percent 948.4 ✓5ᵗʰ
      50-59 percent 948.5 ✓5ᵗʰ
      60-69 percent 948.6 ✓5ᵗʰ
      70-79 percent 948.7 ✓5ᵗʰ
      80-89 percent 948.8 ✓5ᵗʰ
      90 percent or more 948.9 ✓5ᵗʰ
    first degree 949.1
    second degree 949.2
    third degree 949.3
      deep 949.4
        with loss of body part 949.5
  uterus 947.4
  uvula 947.0
  vagina 947.4
  vulva — *see* Burn, genitourinary organs, external
  wrist(s) 944.07
    with
      hand(s) — *see* Burn, hand(s), multiple sites
    first degree 944.17
    second degree 944.27
    third degree 944.37
      deep 944.47
        with loss of body part 944.57
Burnett's syndrome (milk-alkali) 999.9
Burnier's syndrome (hypophyseal dwarfism) 253.3

✓4ᵗʰ Fourth-digit Required   ✓5ᵗʰ Fifth-digit Required

Burning

feet syndrome 266.2
sensation (see also Disturbance, sensation) 782.0
tongue 529.6

Burns' disease (osteochondrosis, lower ulna) 732.3

Bursa — see also condition
pharynx 478.29

Bursitis NEC 727.3
Achilles tendon 726.71
adhesive 726.90
   shoulder 726.0
ankle 726.79
buttock 726.5
calcaneal 726.79
collateral ligament
   fibular 726.63
   tibial 726.62
Duplay's 726.2
elbow 726.33
finger 726.8
foot 726.79
gonococcal 098.52
hand 726.4
hip 726.5
infrapatellar 726.69
ischiogluteal 726.5
knee 726.60
occupational NEC 727.2
olecranon 726.33
pes anserinus 726.61
pharyngeal 478.29
popliteal 727.51
prepatellar 726.65
radiohumeral 727.3
scapulohumeral 726.19
   adhesive 726.0
shoulder 726.10
   adhesive 726.0
subacromial 726.19
   adhesive 726.0
subcoracoid 726.19
subdeltoid 726.19
   adhesive 726.0
subpatellar 726.69
syphilitic 095.7
Thornwaldt's, Tornwaldt's (pharyngeal) 478.29
toe 726.79
trochanteric area 726.5
wrist 726.4

Burst stitches or sutures (complication of surgery) ▶(external)◀ 998.32
internal 998.31

Buruli ulcer 031.1

Bury's disease (erythema elevatum diutinum) 695.89

Buschke's disease or scleredema (adultorum) 710.1

Busquet's disease (osteoperiostitis) (see also Osteomyelitis) 730.1

Busse-Buschke disease (cryptococcosis) 117.5

Buttock — see condition

Button
Biskra 085.1
Delhi 085.1
oriental 085.1

Buttonhole hand (intrinsic) 736.21

Bwamba fever (encephalitis) 066.3

Byssinosis (occupational) 504

Bywaters' syndrome 958.5

C

Cacergasia 300.9

Cachexia 799.4
cancerous (M8000/3) 199.1
cardiac — see Disease, heart
dehydration 276.5
   with
      hypernatremia 276.0
      hyponatremia 276.1
due to malnutrition 261
exophthalmic 242.0
heart — see Disease, heart
hypophyseal 253.2
hypopituitary 253.2
lead 984.9
   specified type of lead — see Table of Drugs and Chemicals
malaria 084.9
malignant (M8000/3) 199.1
marsh 084.9
nervous 300.5
old age 797
pachydermic — see Hypothyroidism
paludal 084.9
pituitary (postpartum) 253.2
renal (see also Disease, renal) 593.9
saturnine 984.9
   specified type of lead — see Table of Drugs and Chemicals
senile 797
Simmonds' (pituitary cachexia) 253.2
splenica 289.59
strumipriva (see also Hypothyroidism) 244.9
tuberculous NEC (see also Tuberculosis) 011.9

Café au lait spots 709.09

Caffey's disease or syndrome (infantile cortical hyperostosis) 756.59

Caisson disease 993.3

Caked breast (puerperal, postpartum) 676.2

Cake kidney 753.3

Calabar swelling 125.2

Calcaneal spur 726.73

Calcaneoapophysitis 732.5

Calcaneonavicular bar 755.67

Calcareous — see condition

Calcicosis (occupational) 502

Calciferol (vitamin D) deficiency 268.9
with
   osteomalacia 268.2
   rickets (see also Rickets) 268.0

Calcification
adrenal (capsule) (gland) 255.4
   tuberculous (see also Tuberculosis) 017.6
aorta 440.0
artery (annular) — see Arteriosclerosis
auricle (ear) 380.89
bladder 596.8
   due to S. hematobium 120.0
brain (cortex) — see Calcification, cerebral
bronchus 519.1
bursa 727.82

Calcification — *continued*
    cardiac (*see also* Degeneration, myocardial) 429.1
    cartilage (postinfectional) 733.99
    cerebral (cortex) 348.8
        artery 437.0
    cervix (uteri) 622.8
    choroid plexus 349.2
    conjunctiva 372.54
    corpora cavernosa (penis) 607.89
    cortex (brain) — *see* Calcification, cerebral
    dental pulp (nodular) 522.2
    dentinal papilla 520.4
    disc, intervertebral 722.90
        cervical, cervicothoracic 722.91
        lumbar, lumbosacral 722.93
        thoracic, thoracolumbar 722.92
    fallopian tube 620.8
    falx cerebri — *see* Calcification, cerebral
    fascia 728.89
    gallbladder 575.8
    general 275.40
    heart (*see also* Degeneration, myocardial) 429.1
        valve — *see* Endocarditis
    intervertebral cartilage or disc (postinfectional) 722.90
        cervical, cervicothoracic 722.91
        lumbar, lumbosacral 722.93
        thoracic, thoracolumbar 722.92
    intracranial — *see* Calcification, cerebral
    intraspinal ligament 728.89
    joint 719.80
        ankle 719.87
        elbow 719.82
        foot 719.87
        hand 719.84
        hip 719.85
        knee 719.86
        multiple sites 719.89
        pelvic region 719.85
        shoulder (region) 719.81
        specified site NEC 719.88
        wrist 719.83
    kidney 593.89
        tuberculous (*see also* Tuberculosis) 016.0 ✓5
    larynx (senile) 478.79
    lens 366.8
    ligament 728.89
        intraspinal 728.89
        knee (medial collateral) 717.89
    lung 518.89
        active 518.89
        postinfectional 518.89
        tuberculous (*see also* Tuberculosis, pulmonary) 011.9 ✓5
    lymph gland or node (postinfectional) 289.3
        tuberculous (*see also* Tuberculosis, lymph gland) 017.2 ✓5
    massive (paraplegic) 728.10
    medial NEC (*see also* Arteriosclerosis, extremities) 440.20
    meninges (cerebral) 349.2
    metastatic 275.40
    Mönckeberg's — *see* Arteriosclerosis
    muscle 728.10
        heterotopic, postoperative 728.13
    myocardium, myocardial (*see also* Degeneration, myocardial) 429.1
    ovary 620.8

Calcification — *continued*
    pancreas 577.8
    penis 607.89
    periarticular 728.89
    pericardium (*see also* Pericarditis) 423.8
    pineal gland 259.8
    pleura 511.0
        postinfectional 518.89
        tuberculous (*see also* Tuberculosis, pleura) 012.0 ✓5
    pulp (dental) (nodular) 522.2
    renal 593.89
    Rider's bone 733.99
    sclera 379.16
    semilunar cartilage 717.89
    spleen 289.59
    subcutaneous 709.3
    suprarenal (capsule) (gland) 255.4
    tendon (sheath) 727.82
        with bursitis, synovitis or tenosynovitis 727.82
    trachea 519.1
    ureter 593.89
    uterus 621.8
    vitreous 379.29
Calcified — *see also* Calcification
    hematoma NEC 959.9
Calcinosis (generalized) (interstitial) (tumoral) (universalis) 275.49
    circumscripta 709.3
    cutis 709.3
    intervertebralis 275.49 [722.90]
    Raynaud's phenomenonsclerodactylytelangiectasis (CRST) 710.1
Calcium
    blood
        high (*see also* Hypercalcemia) 275.42
        low (*see also* Hypocalcemia) 275.41
    deposits — *see also* Calcification, by site
        in bursa 727.82
        in tendon (sheath) 727.82
            with bursitis, synovitis or tenosynovitis 727.82
    salts or soaps in vitreous 379.22
Calciuria 791.9
Calculi — *see* Calculus
Calculosis, intrahepatic — *see* Choledocholithiasis
Calculus, calculi, calculous 592.9
    ampulla of Vater — *see* Choledocholithiasis
    anuria (impacted) (recurrent) 592.0
    appendix 543.9
    bile duct (any) — *see* Choledocholithiasis
    biliary — *see* Cholelithiasis
    bilirubin, multiple — *see* Cholelithiasis
    bladder (encysted) (impacted) (urinary) 594.1
        diverticulum 594.0
    bronchus 518.89
    calyx (kidney) (renal) 592.0
        congenital 753.3
    cholesterol (pure) (solitary) — *see* Cholelithiasis
    common duct (bile) — *see* Choledocholithiasis
    conjunctiva 372.54
    cystic 594.1
        duct — *see* Cholelithiasis
    dental 523.6
        subgingival 523.6
        supragingival 523.6

Calculus, calculi, calculous

Calculus, calculi, calculous — continued
  epididymis 608.89
  gallbladder — see also Cholelithiasis
    congenital 751.69
  hepatic (duct) — see Choledocholithiasis
  intestine (impaction) (obstruction) 560.39
  kidney (impacted) (multiple) (pelvis) (recurrent)
    (staghorn) 592.0
    congenital 753.3
  lacrimal (passages) 375.57
  liver (impacted) — see Choledocholithiasis
  lung 518.89
  nephritic (impacted) (recurrent) 592.0
  nose 478.1
  pancreas (duct) 577.8
  parotid gland 527.5
  pelvis, encysted 592.0
  prostate 602.0
  pulmonary 518.89
  renal (impacted) (recurrent) 592.0
    congenital 753.3
  salivary (duct) (gland) 527.5
  seminal vesicle 608.89
  staghorn 592.0
  Stensen's duct 527.5
  sublingual duct or gland 527.5
    congenital 750.26
  submaxillary duct, gland, or region 527.5
  suburethral 594.8
  tonsil 474.8
  tooth, teeth 523.6
  tunica vaginalis 608.89
  ureter (impacted) (recurrent) 592.1
  urethra (impacted) 594.2
  urinary (duct) (impacted) (passage) (tract)
    592.9
    lower tract NEC 594.9
      specified site 594.8
  vagina 623.8
  vesical (impacted) 594.1
  Wharton's duct 527.5
Caliectasis 593.89
California
  disease 114.0
  encephalitis 062.5
Caligo cornea 371.03
Callositas, callosity (infected) 700
Callus (infected) 700
  bone 726.91
  excessive, following fracture — see also Late, effect (of), fracture
Calvé (-Perthes) disease (osteochondrosis, femoral capital) 732.1
Calvities (see also Alopecia) 704.00
Cameroon fever (see also Malaria) 084.6
Camptocormia 300.11
Camptodactyly (congenital) 755.59
Camurati-Engelmann disease (diaphyseal sclerosis) 756.59
Canal — see condition
Canaliculitis (lacrimal) (acute) 375.31
  Actinomyces 039.8
  chronic 375.41
Canavan's disease 330.0

Cancer (M8000/3) — see also Neoplasm, by site, malignant

> Note — The term "cancer" when modified by an adjective or adjectival phrase indicating a morphological type should be coded in the same manner as "carcinoma" with that adjective or phrase. Thus, "squamous-cell cancer" should be coded in the same manner as "squamous-cell carcinoma," which appears in the list under "Carcinoma."

  bile duct type (M8160/3), liver 155.1
  hepatocellular (M8170/3) 155.0
Cancerous (M8000/3) — see Neoplasm, by site, malignant
Cancerphobia 300.29
Cancrum oris 528.1
Candidiasis, candidal 112.9
  with pneumonia 112.4
  balanitis 112.2
  congenital 771.7
  disseminated 112.5
  endocarditis 112.81
  esophagus 112.84
  intertrigo 112.3
  intestine 112.85
  lung 112.4
  meningitis 112.83
  mouth 112.0
  nails 112.3
  neonatal 771.7
  onychia 112.3
  otitis externa 112.82
  otomycosis 112.82
  paronychia 112.3
  perionyxis 112.3
  pneumonia 112.4
  pneumonitis 112.4
  skin 112.3
  specified site NEC 112.89
  systemic 112.5
  urogenital site NEC 112.2
  vagina 112.1
  vulva 112.1
  vulvovaginitis 112.1
Candidiosis — see Candidiasis
Candiru infection or infestation 136.8
Canities (premature) 704.3
  congenital 757.4
Canker (mouth) (sore) 528.2
  rash 034.1
Cannabinosis 504
Canton fever 081.9
Cap
  cradle 690.11
Capillariasis 127.5
Capillary — see condition
Caplan's syndrome 714.81
Caplan-Colinet syndrome 714.81
Capsule — see condition
Capsulitis (joint) 726.90
  adhesive (shoulder) 726.0
  hip 726.5
  knee 726.60
  labyrinthine 387.8
  thyroid 245.9
  wrist 726.4

Index to Diseases

Caput
 crepitus 756.0
 medusae 456.8
 succedaneum 767.1
Carapata disease 087.1
Carate — *see* Pinta
Carboxyhemoglobinemia 986
Carbuncle 680.9
 abdominal wall 680.2
 ankle 680.6
 anus 680.5
 arm (any part, above wrist) 680.3
 auditory canal, external 680.0
 axilla 680.3
 back (any part) 680.2
 breast 680.2
 buttock 680.5
 chest wall 680.2
 corpus cavernosum 607.2
 ear (any part) (external) 680.0
 eyelid 373.13
 face (any part except eye) 680.0
 finger (any) 680.4
 flank 680.2
 foot (any part) 680.7
 forearm 680.3
 genital organ (male) 608.4
 gluteal (region) 680.5
 groin 680.2
 hand (any part) 680.4
 head (any part except face) 680.8
 heel 680.7
 hip 680.6
 kidney (*see also* Abscess, kidney) 590.2
 knee 680.6
 labia 616.4
 lacrimal
   gland (*see also* Dacryoadenitis) 375.00
   passages (duct) (sac) (*see also*
    Dacryocystitis) 375.30
 leg, any part except foot 680.6
 lower extremity, any part except foot 680.6
 malignant 022.0
 multiple sites 680.9
 neck 680.1
 nose (external) (septum) 680.0
 orbit, orbital 376.01
 partes posteriores 680.5
 pectoral region 680.2
 penis 607.2
 perineum 680.2
 pinna 680.0
 scalp (any part) 680.8
 scrotum 608.4
 seminal vesicle 608.0
 shoulder 680.3
 skin NEC 680.9
 specified site NEC 680.8
 spermatic cord 608.4
 temple (region) 680.0
 testis 608.4
 thigh 680.6
 thumb 680.4
 toe (any) 680.7
 trunk 680.2
 tunica vaginalis 608.4
 umbilicus 680.2
 upper arm 680.3
 urethra 597.0

Carcinoma

Carbuncle — *continued*
 vas deferens 608.4
 vulva 616.4
 wrist 680.4
Carbunculus (*see also* Carbuncle) 680.9
Carcinoid (tumor) (M8240/1) — *see also*
  Neoplasm, by site, uncertain behavior
  and struma ovarii (M9091/1) 236.2
 argentaffin (M8241/1) — *see* Neoplasm, by
   site, uncertain behavior
   malignant (M8241/3) — *see* Neoplasm, by
    site, malignant
 benign (M9091/0) 220
 composite (M8244/3) — *see* Neoplasm, by
   site, malignant
 goblet cell (M8243/3) — *see* Neoplasm, by
   site, malignant
 malignant (M8240/3) — *see* Neoplasm, by
   site, malignant
 nonargentaffin (M8242/1) — *see also*
   Neoplasm, by site, uncertain behavior
   malignant (M8242/3) — *see* Neoplasm, by
    site, malignant
 strumal (M9091/1) 236.2
 syndrome (intestinal) (metastatic) 259.2
 type bronchial adenoma (M8240/3) — *see*
   Neoplasm, lung, malignant
Carcinoidosis 259.2
Carcinoma (M8010/3) — *see also* Neoplasm, by
  site, malignant

> Note — Except where otherwise indicated,
> the morphological varieties of carcinoma in
> the list below should be coded by site as for
> "Neoplasm, malignant."

 with
   apocrine metaplasia (M8573/3)
   cartilaginous (and osseous) metaplasia
    (M8571/3)
   osseous (and cartilaginous) metaplasia
    (M8571/3)
   productive fibrosis (M8141/3)
   spindle cell metaplasia (M8572/3)
   squamous metaplasia (M8570/3)
 acidophil (M8280/3)
   specified site — *see* Neoplasm, by site,
    malignant
   unspecified site 194.3
 acidophil-basophil, mixed (M8281/3)
   specified site — *see* Neoplasm, by site,
    malignant
   unspecified site 194.3
 acinar (cell) (M8550/3)
 acinic cell (M8550/3)
 adenocystic (M8200/3)
 adenoid
   cystic (M8200/3)
   squamous cell (M8075/3)
 adenosquamous (M8560/3)
 adnexal (skin) (M8390/3) — *see* Neoplasm,
   skin, malignant
 adrenal cortical (M8370/3) 194.0
 alveolar (M8251/3)
   cell (M8250/3) — *see* Neoplasm, lung,
    malignant
 anaplastic type (M8021/3)
 apocrine (M8401/3)
   breast — *see* Neoplasm, breast, malignant
   specified site NEC — *see* Neoplasm, skin,
    malignant

Carcinoma — *continued*
  apocrine — *continued*
    unspecified site 173.9
  basal cell (pigmented) (M8090/3) — *see also* Neoplasm, skin, malignant
    fibro-epithelial type (M8093/3) — *see* Neoplasm, skin, malignant
    morphea type (M8092/3) — *see* Neoplasm, skin, malignant
    multicentric (M8091/3) — *see* Neoplasm, skin, malignant
  basaloid (M8123/3)
  basal-squamous cell, mixed (M8094/3) — *see* Neoplasm, skin, malignant
  basophil (M8300/3)
    specified site — *see* Neoplasm, by site, malignant
    unspecified site 194.3
  basophil-acidophil, mixed (M8281/3)
    specified site — *see* Neoplasm, by site, malignant
    unspecified site 194.3
  basosquamous (M8094/3) — *see* Neoplasm, skin, malignant
  bile duct type (M8160/3)
    and hepatocellular, mixed (M8180/3) 155.0
    liver 155.1
    specified site NEC — *see* Neoplasm, by site, malignant
    unspecified site 155.1
  branchial or branchiogenic 146.8
  bronchial or bronchogenic — *see* Neoplasm, lung, malignant
  bronchiolar (terminal) (M8250/3) — *see* Neoplasm, lung, malignant
  bronchiolo-alveolar (M8250/3) — *see* Neoplasm, lung, malignant
  bronchogenic (epidermoid) 162.9
  C cell (M8510/3)
    specified site — *see* Neoplasm, by site, mailignant
    unspecified site 193
  ceruminous (M8420/3) 173.2
  chorionic (M9100/3)
    specified site — *see* Neoplasm, by site, malignant
    unspecified site
      female 181
      male 186.9
  chromophobe (M8270/3)
    specified site — *see* Neoplasm, by site, malignant
    unspecified site 194.3
  clear cell (mesonephroid type) (M8310/3)
  cloacogenic (M8124/3)
    specified site — *see* Neoplasm, by site, malignant
    unspecified site 154.8
  colloid (M8480/3)
  cribriform (M8201/3)
  cylindroid type (M8200/3)
  diffuse type (M8145/3)
    specified site — *see* Neoplasm, by site, malignant
    unspecified site 151.9
  duct (cell) (M8500/3)
    with Paget's disease (M8541/3) — *see* Neoplasm, breast, malignant
    infiltrating (M8500/3)
      specified site — *see* Neoplasm, by site, malignant

Carcinoma — *continued*
  duct — *continued*
    infiltrating — *continued*
      unspecified site 174.9
  ductal (M8500/3)
  ductular, infiltrating (M8521/3)
  embryonal (M9070/3)
    and teratoma, mixed (M9081/3)
    combined with choriocarcinoma (M9101/3) — *see* Neoplasm, by site, malignant
    infantile type (M9071/3)
    liver 155.0
    polyembryonal type (M9072/3)
  endometrioid (M8380/3)
  eosinophil (M8280/3)
    specified site — *see* Neoplasm, by site, malignant
    unspecified site 194.3
  epidermoid (M8070/3) — *see also* Carcinoma, squamous cell
    and adenocarcinoma, mixed (M8560/3)
    in situ, Bowen's type (M8081/2) — *see* Neoplasm, skin, in situ
    intradermal — *see* Neoplasm, skin, in situ
  fibroepithelial type basal cell (M8093/3) — *see* Neoplasm, skin, malignant
  follicular (M8330/3)
    and papillary (mixed) (M8340/3) 193
    moderately differentiated type (M8332/3) 193
    pure follicle type (M8331/3) 193
    specified site — *see* Neoplasm, by site, malignant
    trabecular type (M8332/3) 193
    unspecified site 193
    well differentiated type (M8331/3) 193
  gelatinous (M8480/3)
  giant cell (M8031/3)
    and spindle cell (M8030/3)
  granular cell (M8320/3)
  granulosa cell (M8620/3) 183.0
  hepatic cell (M8170/3) 155.0
  hepatocellular (M8170/3) 155.0
    and bile duct, mixed (M8180/3) 155.0
  hepatocholangiolitic (M8180/3) 155.0
  Hürthle cell (thyroid) 193
  hypernephroid (M8311/3)
  in
    adenomatous
      polyp (M8210/3)
      polyposis coli (M8220/3) 153.9
    pleomorphic adenoma (M8940/3)
    polypoid adenoma (M8210/3)
    situ (M8010/3) — *see* Carcinoma, in situ
    tubular adenoma (M8210/3)
    villous adenoma (M8261/3)
  infiltrating duct (M8500/3)
    with Paget's disease (M8541/3) — *see* Neoplasm, breast, malignant
    specified site — *see* Neoplasm, by site, malignant
    unspecified site 174.9
  inflammatory (M8530/3)
    specified site — *see* Neoplasm, by site, malignant
    unspecified site 174.9
  in situ (M8010/2) — *see also* Neoplasm, by site, in situ
    epidermoid (M8070/2) — *see also* Neoplasm, by site, in situ

Index to Diseases   **Carcinoma**

Carcinoma — *continued*
  in situ — *continued*
    epidermoid — *continued*
      with questionable stromal invasion (M8076/2)
        specified site — *see* Neoplasm, by site, in situ
        unspecified site 233.1
      Bowen's type (M8081/2) — *see* Neoplasm, skin, in situ
    intraductal (M8500/2)
      specified site — *see* Neoplasm, by site, in situ
      unspecified site 233.0
    lobular (M8520/2)
      specified site — *see* Neoplasm, by site, in situ
      unspecified site 233.0
    papillary (M8050/2) — *see* Neoplasm, by site, in situ
    squamous cell (M8070/2) — *see also* Neoplasm, by site, in situ
      with questionable stromal invasion (M8076/2)
        specified site — *see* Neoplasm, by site, in situ
        unspecified site 233.1
    transitional cell (M8120/2) — *see* Neoplasm, by site, in situ
  intestinal type (M8144/3)
    specified site — *see* Neoplasm, by site, malignant
    unspecified site 151.9
  intraductal (noninfiltrating) (M8500/2)
    papillary (M8503/2)
      specified site — *see* Neoplasm, by site, in situ
      unspecified site 233.0
    specified site — *see* Neoplasm, by site, in situ
    unspecified site 233.0
  intraepidermal (M8070/2) — *see also* Neoplasm, skin, in situ
    squamous cell, Bowen's type (M8081/2) — *see* Neoplasm, skin, in situ
  intraepithelial (M8010/2) — *see also* Neoplasm, by site, in situ
    squamous cell (M8072/2) — *see* Neoplasm, by site, in situ
  intraosseous (M9270/3) 170.1
    upper jaw (bone) 170.0
  islet cell (M8150/3)
    and exocrine, mixed (M8154/3)
      specified site — *see* Neoplasm, by site, malignant
      unspecified site 157.9
    pancreas 157.4
    specified site NEC — *see* Neoplasm, by site, malignant
    unspecified site 157.4
  juvenile, breast (M8502/3) — *see* Neoplasm, breast, malignant
  Kulchitsky's cell (carcinoid tumor of intestine) 259.2
  large cell (M8012/3)
    squamous cell, nonkeratinizing type (M8072/3)
  Leydig cell (testis) (M8650/3)
    specified site — *see* Neoplasm, by site, malignant

Carcinoma — *continued*
  Leydig cell — *continued*
    unspecified site 186.9
      female 183.0
      male 186.9
  liver cell (M8170/3) 155.0
  lobular (infiltrating) (M8520/3)
    non-infiltrating (M8520/3)
      specified site — *see* Neoplasm, by site, in situ
      unspecified site 233.0
    specified site — *see* Neoplasm, by site, malignant
    unspecified site 174.9
  lymphoepithelial (M8082/3)
  medullary (M8510/3)
    with
      amyloid stroma (M8511/3)
        specified site — *see* Neoplasm, by site, malignant
        unspecified site 193
      lymphoid stroma (M8512/3)
        specified site — *see* Neoplasm, by site, malignant
        unspecified site 174.9
  mesometanephric (M9110/3)
  mesonephric (M9110/3)
  metastatic (M8010/6) — *see* Metastasis, cancer
  metatypical (M8095/3) — *see* Neoplasm, skin, malignant
  morphea type basal cell (M8092/3) — *see* Neoplasm, skin, malignant
  mucinous (M8480/3)
  mucin-producing (M8481/3)
  mucin-secreting (M8481/3)
  mucoepidermoid (M8430/3)
  mucoid (M8480/3)
    cell (M8300/3)
      specified site — *see* Neoplasm, by site, malignant
      unspecified site 194.3
  mucous (M8480/3)
  nonencapsulated sclerosing (M8350/3) 193
  noninfiltrating
    intracystic (M8504/2) — *see* Neoplasm, by site, in situ
    intraductal (M8500/2)
      papillary (M8503/2)
        specified site — *see* Neoplasm, by site, in situ
        unspecified site 233.0
      specified site — *see* Neoplasm, by site, in situ
      unspecified site 233.0
    lobular (M8520/2)
      specified site — *see* Neoplasm, by site, in situ
      unspecified site 233.0
  oat cell (M8042/3)
    specified site — *see* Neoplasm, by site, malignant
    unspecified site 162.9
  odontogenic (M9270/3) 170.1
    upper jaw (bone) 170.0
  onocytic (M8290/3)
  oxyphilic (M8290/3)
  papillary (M8050/3)
    and follicular (mixed) (M8340/3) 193
    epidermoid (M8052/3)

Carcinoma — *continued*
  papillary — *continued*
    intraductal (noninfiltrating) (M8503/2)
      specified site — *see* Neoplasm, by site, in situ
      unspecified site 233.0
    serous (M8460/3)
      specified site — *see* Neoplasm, by site, malignant
      surface (M8461/3)
        specified site — *see* Neoplasm, by site, malignant
        unspecified site 183.0
      unspecified site 183.0
    squamous cell (M8052/3)
    transitional cell (M8130/3)
  papillocystic (M8450/3)
    specified site — *see* Neoplasm, by site, malignant
    unspecified site 183.0
  parafollicular cell (M8510/3)
    specified site — *see* Neoplasm, by site, malignant
    unspecified site 193
  pleomorphic (M8022/3)
  polygonal cell (M8034/3)
  prickle cell (M8070/3)
  pseudoglandular, squamous cell (M8075/3)
  pseudomucinous (M8470/3)
    specified site — *see* Neoplasm, by site, malignant
    unspecified site 183.0
  pseudosarcomatous (M8033/3)
  regaud type (M8082/3) — *see* Neoplasm, nasopharynx, malignant
  renal cell (M8312/3) 189.0
  reserve cell (M8041/3)
  round cell (M8041/3)
  Schmincke (M8082/3) — *see* Neoplasm, nasopharynx, malignant
  Schneiderian (M8121/3)
    specified site — *see* Neoplasm, by site, malignant
    unspecified site 160.0
  scirrhous (M8141/3)
  sebaceous (M8410/3) — *see* Neoplasm, skin, malignant
  secondary (M8010/6) — *see* Neoplasm, by site, malignant, secondary
  secretory, breast (M8502/3) — *see* Neoplasm, breast, malignant
  serous (M8441/3)
    papillary (M8460/3)
      specified site — *see* Neoplasm, by site, malignant
      unspecified site 183.0
    surface, papillary (M8461/3)
      specified site — *see* Neoplasm, by site, malignant
      unspecified site 183.0
  Sertoli cell (M8640/3)
    specified site — *see* Neoplasm, by site, malignant
    unspecified site 186.9
  signet ring cell (M8490/3)
    metastatic (M8490/6) — *see* Neoplasm, by site, secondary
  simplex (M8231/3)
  skin appendage (M8390/3) — *see* Neoplasm, skin, malignant

Carcinoma — *continued*
  small cell (M8041/3)
    fusiform cell type (M8043/3)
    squamous cell, non-keratinizing type (M8073/3)
  solid (M8230/3)
    with amyloid stroma (M8511/3)
      specified site — *see* Neoplasm, by site, malignant
      unspecified site 193
  spheroidal cell (M8035/3)
  spindle cell (M8032/3)
    and giant cell (M8030/3)
  spinous cell (M8070/3)
  squamous (cell) (M8070/3)
    adenoid type (M8075/3)
    and adenocarcinoma, mixed (M8560/3)
    intraepidermal, Bowen's type — *see* Neoplasm, skin, in situ
    keratinizing type (large cell) (M8071/3)
    large cell, non-keratinizing type (M8072/3)
    microinvasive (M8076/3)
      specified site — *see* Neoplasm, by site, malignant
      unspecified site 180.9
    non-keratinizing type (M8072/3)
    papillary (M8052/3)
    pseudoglandular (M8075/3)
    small cell, non-keratinizing type (M8073/3)
    spindle cell type (M8074/3)
    verrucous (M8051/3)
  superficial spreading (M8143/3)
  sweat gland (M8400/3) — *see* Neoplasm, skin, malignant
  theca cell (M8600/3) 183.0
  thymic (M8580/3) 164.0
  trabecular (M8190/3)
  transitional (cell) (M8120/3)
    papillary (M8130/3)
    spindle cell type (M8122/3)
  tubular (M8211/3)
  undifferentiated type (M8020/3)
  urothelial (M8120/3)
  ventriculi 151.9
  verrucous (epidermoid) (squamous cell) (M8051/3)
  villous (M8262/3)
  water-clear cell (M8322/3) 194.1
  wolffian duct (M9110/3)

Carcinomaphobia 300.29

Carcinomatosis
  peritonei (M8010/6) 197.6
  specified site NEC (M8010/3) — *see* Neoplasm, by site, malignant
  unspecified site (M8010/6) 199.0

Carcinosarcoma (M8980/3) — *see also* Neoplasm, by site, malignant
  embryonal type (M8981/3) — *see* Neoplasm, by site, malignant

Cardia, cardial — *see* condition

Cardiac — *see also* condition
  death — *see* Disease, heart
  device
    defibrillator, automatic implantable V45.02
    in situ NEC V45.00
    pacemaker
      cardiac
        fitting or adjustment V53.31
        in situ V45.01

Cardiac — *continued*
  device — *continued*
    pacemaker — *continued*
      carotid sinus
        fitting or adjustment V53.39
        in situ V45.09
    pacemaker — *see* Cardiac, device, pacemaker
  tamponade 423.9
Cardialgia (*see also* Pain, precordial) 786.51
Cardiectasis — *see* Hypertrophy, cardiac
Cardiochalasia 530.81
Cardiomalacia (*see also* Degeneration, myocardial) 429.1
Cardiomegalia glycogenica diffusa 271.0
Cardiomegaly (*see also* Hypertrophy, cardiac) 429.3
  congenital 746.89
  glycogen 271.0
  hypertensive (*see also* Hypertension, heart) 402.90
  idiopathic 429.3
Cardiomyoliposis (*see also* Degeneration, myocardial) 429.1
Cardiomyopathy (congestive) (constrictive) (familial) (infiltrative) (obstructive) (restrictive) (sporadic) 425.4
  alcoholic 425.5
  amyloid 277.3 *[425.7]*
  beriberi 265.0 *[425.7]*
  cobalt-beer 425.5
  congenital 425.3
  due to
    amyloidosis 277.3 *[425.7]*
    beriberi 265.0 *[425.7]*
    cardiac glycogenosis 271.0 *[425.7]*
    Chagas' disease 086.0
    Friedreich's ataxia 334.0 *[425.8]*
    hypertension —*see* Hypertension, with, heart involvement
    mucopolysaccharidosis 277.5 *[425.7]*
    myotonia atrophica 359.2 *[425.8]*
    progressive muscular dystrophy 359.1 *[425.8]*
    sarcoidosis 135 *[425.8]*
  glycogen storage 271.0 *[425.7]*
  hypertensive — *see* Hypertension, with, heart involvement
  hypertrophic
    nonobstructive 425.4
    obstructive 425.1
      congenital 746.84
  idiopathic (concentric) 425.4
  in
    Chagas' disease 086.0
    sarcoidosis 135 *[425.8]*
  ischemic 414.8
  metabolic NEC 277.9 *[425.7]*
    amyloid 277.3 *[425.7]*
    thyrotoxic (*see also* Thyrotoxicosis) 242.9 ✓5ᵗʰ *[425.7]*
    thyrotoxicosis (*see also* Thyrotoxicosis) 242.9 ✓5ᵗʰ *[425.7]*
  nutritional 269.9 *[425.7]*
    beriberi 265.0 *[425.7]*
  obscure of Africa 425.2
  postpartum 674.8 ✓5ᵗʰ
  primary 425.4
  secondary 425.9
  thyrotoxic (*see also* Thyrotoxicosis) 242.9 ✓5ᵗʰ *[425.7]*

Cardiomyopathy — *continued*
  toxic NEC 425.9
  tuberculous (*see also* Tuberculosis) 017.9 ✓5ᵗʰ *[425.8]*
Cardionephritis — *see* Hypertension, cardiorenal
Cardionephropathy — *see* Hypertension, cardiorenal
Cardionephrosis — *see* Hypertension, cardiorenal
Cardioneurosis 306.2
Cardiopathia nigra 416.0
Cardiopathy (*see also* Disease, heart) 429.9
  hypertensive (*see also* Hypertension, heart) 402.90
  idiopathic 425.4
  mucopolysaccharidosis 277.5 *[425.7]*
Cardiopericarditis (*see also* Pericarditis) 423.9
Cardiophobia 300.29
Cardioptosis 746.87
Cardiorenal — *see* condition
Cardiorrhexis (*see also* Infarct, myocardium) 410.9 ✓5ᵗʰ
Cardiosclerosis — *see* Arteriosclerosis, coronary
Cardiosis — *see* Disease, heart
Cardiospasm (esophageal) (reflex) (stomach) 530.0
  congenital 750.7
Cardiostenosis — *see* Disease, heart
Cardiosymphysis 423.1
Cardiothyrotoxicosis — *see* Hyperthyroidism
Cardiovascular — *see* condition
Carditis (acute) (bacterial) (chronic) (subacute) 429.89
  Coxsackie 074.20
  hypertensive (*see also* Hypertension, heart) 402.90
  meningococcal 036.40
  rheumatic — *see* Disease, heart, rheumatic
  rheumatoid 714.2
Care (of)
  child (routine) V20.1
  convalescent following V66.9
    chemotherapy V66.2
    medical NEC V66.5
    psychotherapy V66.3
    radiotherapy V66.1
    surgery V66.0
    surgical NEC V66.0
    treatment (for) V66.5
      combined V66.6
      fracture V66.4
      mental disorder NEC V66.3
      specified type NEC V66.5
  end-of-life V66.7
  family member (handicapped) (sick)
    creating problem for family V61.49
    provided away from home for holiday relief V60.5
    unavailable, due to
      absence (person rendering care) (sufferer) V60.4
      inability (any reason) of person rendering care V60.4
  holiday relief V60.5
  hospice V66.7
  lack of (at or after birth) (infant) (child) 995.52
    adult 995.84
  lactation of mother V24.1

Care (of) — *continued*
  palliative V66.7
  postpartum
    immediately after delivery V24.0
    routine follow-up V24.2
  prenatal V22.1
    first pregnancy V22.0
    high risk pregnancy V23.9
      specified problem NEC V23.89
  terminal V66.7
  unavailable, due to
    absence of person rendering care V60.4
    inability (any reason) of person rendering care V60.4
  well baby V20.1

Caries (bone) (*see also* Tuberculosis, bone) 015.9 [5] *[730.8]* [5]
  arrested 521.04
  cementum 521.03
  cerebrospinal (tuberculous) 015.0 [5] *[730.88]*
  dental (acute) (chronic) (incipient) (infected) 521.09
    with pulp exposure 521.03
    extending to
      dentine 521.02
      pulp 521.03
    other specified NEC 521.09
  dentin (acute) (chronic) 521.02
  enamel (acute) (chronic) (incipient) 521.01
  external meatus 380.89
  hip (*see also* Tuberculosis) 015.1 [5] *[730.85]*
  knee 015.2 [5] *[730.86]*
  labyrinth 386.8
  limb NEC 015.7 [5] *[730.88]*
  mastoid (chronic) (process) 383.1
  middle ear 385.89
  nose 015.7 [5] *[730.88]*
  orbit 015.7 [5] *[730.88]*
  ossicle 385.24
  petrous bone 383.20
  sacrum (tuberculous) 015.0 [5] *[730.88]*
  spine, spinal (column) (tuberculous) 015.0 [5] *[730.88]*
  syphilitic 095.5
    congenital 090.0 *[730.8]* [5]
  teeth (internal) 521.00
    initial 521.01
  vertebra (column) (tuberculous) 015.0 [5] *[730.88]*

Carini's syndrome (ichthyosis congenita) 757.1
Carious teeth 521.00
Carneous mole 631
Carnosinemia 270.5
Carotid body or sinus syndrome 337.0
Carotidynia 337.0
Carotinemia (dietary) 278.3
Carotinosis (cutis) (skin) 278.3
Carpal tunnel syndrome 354.0
Carpenter's syndrome 759.89
Carpopedal spasm (*see also* Tetany) 781.7
Carpoptosis 736.05
Carrier (suspected) of
  amebiasis V02.2
  bacterial disease (meningococcal, staphylococcal, streptococcal) NEC V02.59
  cholera V02.0
  cystic fibrosis gene V83.81 ●
  defective gene V83.89 ▲

Carrier — *continued*
  diphtheria V02.4
  dysentery (bacillary) V02.3
    amebic V02.2
  Endamoeba histolytica V02.2
  gastrointestinal pathogens NEC V02.3
  genetic defect V83.89 ▲
  gonorrhea V02.7
  group B streptococcus V02.51
  HAA (hepatitis Australian-antigen) V02.61
  hemophilia A (asymptomatic) V83.01
    symptomatic V83.02
  hepatitis V02.60
    Australian-antigen (HAA) V02.61
    B V02.61
    C V02.62
    serum V02.61
    specified type NEC V02.69
    viral V02.60
  infective organism NEC V02.9
  malaria V02.9
  paratyphoid V02.3
  Salmonella V02.3
    typhosa V02.1
  serum hepatitis V02.61
  Shigella V02.3
  Staphylococcus NEC V02.59
  Streptococcus NEC V02.52
    group B V02.51
  typhoid V02.1
  venereal disease NEC V02.8

Carrión's disease (Bartonellosis) 088.0
Car sickness 994.6
Carter's
  relapsing fever (Asiatic) 087.0
Cartilage — *see* condition
Caruncle (inflamed)
  abscess, lacrimal (*see also* Dacryocystitis) 375.30
  conjunctiva 372.00
    acute 372.00
  eyelid 373.00
  labium (majus) (minus) 616.8
  lacrimal 375.30
  urethra (benign) 599.3
  vagina (wall) 616.8
Cascade stomach 537.6
Caseation lymphatic gland (*see also* Tuberculosis) 017.2 [5]
Caseous
  bronchitis — *see* Tuberculosis, pulmonary
  meningitis 013.0 [5]
  pneumonia — *see* Tuberculosis, pulmonary
Cassidy (-Scholte) syndrome (malignant carcinoid) 259.2
Castellani's bronchitis 104.8
Castleman's tumor or lymphoma (mediastinal lymph node hyperplasia) 785.6
Castration, traumatic 878.2
  complicated 878.3
Casts in urine 791.7
Cat's ear 744.29
Catalepsy 300.11
  catatonic (acute) (*see also* Schizophrenia) 295.2 [5]
  hysterical 300.11
  schizophrenic (*see also* Schizophrenia) 295.2 [5]
Cataphasia 307.0

Cataplexy (idiopathic) 347
Cataract (anterior cortical) (anterior polar) (black) (capsular) (central) (cortical) (hypermature) (immature) (incipient) (mature) 366.9
  anterior
    and posterior axial embryonal 743.33
    pyramidal 743.31
    subcapsular polar
      infantile, juvenile, or presenile 366.01
      senile 366.13
  associated with
    calcinosis 275.40 *[366.42]*
    craniofacial dysostosis 756.0 *[366.44]*
    galactosemia 271.1 *[366.44]*
    hypoparathyroidism 252.1 *[366.42]*
    myotonic disorders 359.2 *[366.43]*
    neovascularization 366.33
  blue dot 743.39
  cerulean 743.39
  complicated NEC 366.30
  congenital 743.30
    capsular or subcapsular 743.31
    cortical 743.32
    nuclear 743.33
    specified type NEC 743.39
    total or subtotal 743.34
    zonular 743.32
  coronary (congenital) 743.39
  acquired 366.12
  cupuliform 366.14
  diabetic 250.5 ✓5ᵗʰ *[366.41]*
  drug-induced 366.45
  due to
    chalcosis 360.24 *[366.34]*
    chronic choroiditis (*see also* Choroiditis) 363.20 *[366.32]*
    degenerative myopia 360.21 *[366.34]*
    glaucoma (*see also* Glaucoma) 365.9 *[366.31]*
    infection, intraocular NEC 366.32
    inflammatory ocular disorder NEC 366.32
    iridocyclitis, chronic 364.10 *[366.33]*
    pigmentary retinal dystrophy 362.74 *[366.34]*
    radiation 366.46
  electric 366.46
  glassblowers' 366.46
  heat ray 366.46
  heterochromic 366.33
  in eye disease NEC 366.30
  infantile (*see also* Cataract, juvenile) 366.00
  intumescent 366.12
  irradiational 366.46
  juvenile 366.00
    anterior subcapsular polar 366.01
    combined forms 366.09
    cortical 366.03
    lamellar 366.03
    nuclear 366.04
    posterior subcapsular polar 366.02
    specified NEC 366.09
    zonular 366.03
  lamellar 743.32
    infantile, juvenile, or presenile 366.03
  morgagnian 366.18
  myotonic 359.2 *[366.43]*
  myxedema 244.9 *[366.44]*
  nuclear 366.16
  posterior, polar (capsular) 743.31
    infantile, juvenile, or presenile 366.02
    senile 366.14

Cataract — *continued*
  presenile (*see also* Cataract, juvenile) 366.00
  punctate
    acquired 366.12
    congenital 743.39
  secondary (membrane) 366.50
    obscuring vision 366.53
    specified type, not obscuring vision 366.52
  senile 366.10
    anterior subcapsular polar 366.13
    combined forms 366.19
    cortical 366.15
    hypermature 366.18
    immature 366.12
    incipient 366.12
    mature 366.17
    nuclear 366.16
    posterior subcapsular polar 366.14
    specified NEC 366.19
    total or subtotal 366.17
  snowflake 250.5 ✓5ᵗʰ *[366.41]*
  specified NEC 366.8
  subtotal (senile) 366.17
    congenital 743.34
  sunflower 360.24 *[366.34]*
  tetanic NEC 252.1 *[366.42]*
  total (mature) (senile) 366.17
    congenital 743.34
    localized 366.21
    traumatic 366.22
  toxic 366.45
  traumatic 366.20
    partially resolved 366.23
    total 366.22
  zonular (perinuclear) 743.32
    infantile, juvenile, or presenile 366.03
Cataracta 366.10
  brunescens 366.16
  cerulea 743.39
  complicata 366.30
  congenita 743.30
  coralliformis 743.39
  coronaria (congenital) 743.39
    acquired 366.12
  diabetic 250.5 ✓5ᵗʰ *[366.41]*
  floriformis 360.24 *[366.34]*
  membranacea
    accreta 366.50
    congenita 743.39
  nigra 366.16
Catarrh, catarrhal (inflammation) (*see also* condition) 460
  acute 460
  asthma, asthmatic (*see also* Asthma) 493.9 ✓5ᵗʰ
  Bostock's (*see also* Fever, hay) 477.9
  bowel — *see* Enteritis
  bronchial 490
    acute 466.0
    chronic 491.0
    subacute 466.0
  cervix, cervical (canal) (uteri) — *see* Cervicitis
  chest (*see also* Bronchitis) 490
  chronic 472.0
  congestion 472.0
  conjunctivitis 372.03
  due to syphilis 095.9
    congenital 090.0
  enteric — *see* Enteritis
  epidemic 487.1
  Eustachian 381.50

Catarrh, catarrhal — *continued*
  eye (acute) (vernal) 372.03
  fauces (*see also* Pharyngitis) 462
  febrile 460
  fibrinous acute 466.0
  gastroenteric — *see* Enteritis
  gastrointestinal — *see* Enteritis
  gingivitis 523.0
  hay (*see also* Fever, hay) 477.9
  infectious 460
  intestinal — *see* Enteritis
  larynx (*see also* Laryngitis, chronic) 476.0
  liver 070.1
    with hepatic coma 070.0
  lung (*see also* Bronchitis) 490
    acute 466.0
    chronic 491.0
  middle ear (chronic) — *see* Otitis media, chronic
  mouth 528.0
  nasal (chronic) (*see also* Rhinitis) 472.0
    acute 460
  nasobronchial 472.2
  nasopharyngeal (chronic) 472.2
    acute 460
  nose — *see* Catarrh, nasal
  ophthalmia 372.03
  pneumococcal, acute 466.0
  pulmonary (*see also* Bronchitis) 490
    acute 466.0
    chronic 491.0
  spring (eye) 372.13
  suffocating (*see also* Asthma) 493.9 ✓5ᵗʰ
  summer (hay) (*see also* Fever, hay) 477.9
  throat 472.1
  tracheitis 464.10
    with obstruction 464.11
  tubotympanal 381.4
    acute (*see also* Otitis media, acute, nonsuppurative) 381.00
    chronic 381.10
  vasomotor (*see also* Fever, hay) 477.9
  vesical (bladder) — *see* Cystitis
Catarrhus aestivus (*see also* Fever, hay) 477.9
Catastrophe, cerebral (*see also* Disease, cerebrovascular, acute) 436
Catatonia, catatonic (acute) 781.99
  with
    affective psychosis — *see* Psychosis, affective
    agitation 295.2 ✓5ᵗʰ
    Churg-Strauss syndrome 446.4
    dementia (praecox) 295.2 ✓5ᵗʰ
    due to or associated with physical condition 293.89
    excitation 295.2 ✓5ᵗʰ
    excited type 295.2 ✓5ᵗʰ
    schizophrenia 295.2 ✓5ᵗʰ
    stupor 295.2 ✓5ᵗʰ
Cat-scratch — *see also* Injury, superficial
  disease or fever 078.3
Cauda equina — *see also* condition
  syndrome 344.60
Cauliflower ear 738.7
Caul over face 768.9
Causalgia 355.9
  lower limb 355.71
  upper limb 354.4
Cause
  external, general effects NEC 994.9

Cause — *continued*
  not stated 799.9
  unknown 799.9
Caustic burn — *see also* Burn, by site
  from swallowing caustic or corrosive substance — *see* Burn, internal organs
Cavare's disease (familial periodic paralysis) 359.3
Cave-in, injury
  crushing (severe) (*see also* Crush, by site) 869.1
  suffocation 994.7
Cavernitis (penis) 607.2
  lymph vessel — *see* Lymphangioma
Cavernositis 607.2
Cavernous — *see* condition
Cavitation of lung (*see also* Tuberculosis) 011.2 ✓5ᵗʰ
  nontuberculous 518.89
  primary, progressive 010.8 ✓5ᵗʰ
Cavity
  lung — *see* Cavitation of lung
  optic papilla 743.57
  pulmonary — *see* Cavitation of lung
  teeth 521.00
  vitreous (humor) 379.21
Cavovarus foot, congenital 754.59
Cavus foot (congenital) 754.71
  acquired 736.73
Cazenave's
  disease (pemphigus) NEC 694.4
  lupus (erythematosus) 695.4
Cecitis — *see* Appendicitis
Cecocele — *see* Hernia
Cecum — *see* condition
Celiac
  artery compression syndrome 447.4
  disease 579.0
  infantilism 579.0
Cell, cellular — *see also* condition
  anterior chamber (eye) (positive aqueous ray) 364.04
Cellulitis (diffuse) (with lymphangitis) (*see also* Abscess) 682.9
  abdominal wall 682.2
  anaerobic (*see also* Gas gangrene) 040.0
  ankle 682.6
  anus 566
  areola 611.0
  arm (any part, above wrist) 682.3
  auditory canal (external) 380.10
  axilla 682.3
  back (any part) 682.2
  breast 611.0
    postpartum 675.1 ✓5ᵗʰ
  broad ligament (*see also* Disease, pelvis, inflammatory) 614.4
    acute 614.3
  buttock 682.5
  cervical (neck region) 682.1
  cervix (uteri) (*see also* Cervicitis) 616.0
  cheek, external 682.0
    internal 528.3
  chest wall 682.2
  chronic NEC 682.9
  corpus cavernosum 607.2
  digit 681.9

Cellulitis — *continued*
  Douglas' cul-de-sac or pouch (chronic) (*see also* Disease, pelvis, inflammatory) 614.4
    acute 614.3
  drainage site (following operation) 998.59
  ear, external 380.10
  enterostomy 569.61
  erysipelar (*see also* Erysipelas) 035
  eyelid 373.13
  face (any part, except eye) 682.0
  finger (intrathecal) (periosteal) (subcutaneous) (subcuticular) 681.00
  flank 682.2
  foot (except toe) 682.7
  forearm 682.3
  gangrenous (*see also* Gangrene) 785.4
  genital organ NEC
    female — *see* Abscess, genital organ, female
    male 608.4
  glottis 478.71
  gluteal (region) 682.5
  gonococcal NEC 098.0
  groin 682.2
  hand (except finger or thumb) 682.4
  head (except face) NEC 682.8
  heel 682.7
  hip 682.6
  jaw (region) 682.0
  knee 682.6
  labium (majus) (minus) (*see also* Vulvitis) 616.10
  larynx 478.71
  leg, except foot 682.6
  lip 528.5
  mammary gland 611.0
  mouth (floor) 528.3
  multiple sites NEC 682.9
  nasopharynx 478.21
  navel 682.2
    newborn NEC 771.4
  neck (region) 682.1
  nipple 611.0
  nose 478.1
    external 682.0
  orbit, orbital 376.01
  palate (soft) 528.3
  pectoral (region) 682.2
  pelvis, pelvic
    with
      abortion — *see* Abortion, by type, with sepsis
      ectopic pregnancy (*see also* categories 633.0— 633.9) 639.0
      molar pregnancy (*see also* categories 630— 632) 639.0
    female (*see also* Disease, pelvis, inflammatory) 614.4
      acute 614.3
    following
      abortion 639.0
      ectopic or molar pregnancy 639.0
    male (*see also* Abscess, peritoneum) 567.2
    puerperal, postpartum, childbirth 670 ✓4ᵗʰ
  penis 607.2
  perineal, perineum 682.2
  perirectal 566
  peritonsillar 475
  periurethral 597.0
  periuterine (*see also* Disease, pelvis, inflammatory) 614.4
    acute 614.3

Cellulitis — *continued*
  pharynx 478.21
  phlegmonous NEC 682.9
  rectum 566
  retromammary 611.0
  retroperitoneal (*see also* Peritonitis) 567.2
  round ligament (*see also* Disease, pelvis, inflammatory) 614.4
    acute 614.3
  scalp (any part) 682.8
    dissecting 704.8
  scrotum 608.4
  seminal vesicle 608.0
  septic NEC 682.9
  shoulder 682.3
  specified sites NEC 682.8
  spermatic cord 608.4
  submandibular (region) (space) (triangle) 682.0
    gland 527.3
  submaxillary 528.3
    gland 527.3
  submental (pyogenic) 682.0
    gland 527.3
  suppurative NEC 682.9
  testis 608.4
  thigh 682.6
  thumb (intrathecal) (periosteal) (subcutaneous) (subcuticular) 681.00
  toe (intrathecal) (periosteal) (subcutaneous) (subcuticular) 681.10
  tonsil 475
  trunk 682.2
  tuberculous (primary) (*see also* Tuberculosis) 017.0 ✓5ᵗʰ
  tunica vaginalis 608.4
  umbilical 682.2
    newborn NEC 771.4
  vaccinal 999.3
  vagina — *see* Vaginitis
  vas deferens 608.4
  vocal cords 478.5
  vulva (*see also* Vulvitis) 616.10
  wrist 682.4

Cementoblastoma, benign (M9273/0) 213.1
  upper jaw (bone) 213.0
Cementoma (M9273/0) 213.1
  gigantiform (M9276/0) 213.1
    upper jaw (bone) 213.0
  upper jaw (bone) 213.0
Cementoperiostitis 523.4
Cephalgia, cephalagia (*see also* Headache) 784.0
  histamine 346.2 ✓5ᵗʰ
  nonorganic origin 307.81
  psychogenic 307.81
  tension 307.81
Cephalhematocele, cephalematocele
  due to birth injury 767.1
  fetus or newborn 767.1
  traumatic (*see also* Contusion, head) 920
Cephalhematoma, cephalematoma (calcified)
  due to birth injury 767.1
  fetus or newborn 767.1
  traumatic (*see also* Contusion, head) 920
Cephalic — *see* condition
Cephalitis — *see* Encephalitis
Cephalocele 742.0
Cephaloma — *see* Neoplasm, by site, malignant
Cephalomenia 625.8
Cephalopelvic — *see* condition

Cercomoniasis 007.3
Cerebellitis — see Encephalitis
Cerebellum (cerebellar) — see condition
Cerebral — see condition
Cerebritis — see Encephalitis
Cerebrohepatorenal syndrome 759.89
Cerebromacular degeneration 330.1
Cerebromalacia (see also Softening, brain) 434.9 ✓5th
Cerebrosidosis 272.7
Cerebrospasticity — see Palsy, cerebral
Cerebrospinal — see condition
Cerebrum — see condition
Ceroid storage disease 272.7
Cerumen (accumulation) (impacted) 380.4
Cervical — see also condition
   auricle 744.43
   rib 756.2
Cervicalgia 723.1
Cervicitis (acute) (chronic) (nonvenereal) (subacute) (with erosion or ectropion) 616.0
   with
     abortion — see Abortion, by type, with sepsis
     ectopic pregnancy (see also categories 633.0-633.9) 639.0
     molar pregnancy (see also categories 630-632) 639.0
     ulceration 616.0
   chlamydial 099.53
   complicating pregnancy or puerperium 646.6 ✓5th
     affecting fetus or newborn 760.8
   following
     abortion 639.0
     ectopic or molar pregnancy 639.0
   gonococcal (acute) 098.15
     chronic or duration of 2 months or more 098.35
   senile (atrophic) 616.0
   syphilitic 095.8
   trichomonal 131.09
   tuberculous (see also Tuberculosis) 016.7 ✓5th
Cervicoaural fistula 744.49
Cervicocolpitis (emphysematosa) (see also Cervicitis) 616.0
Cervix — see condition
Cesarean delivery, operation or section NEC 669.7 ✓5th
   affecting fetus or newborn 763.4
   post mortem, affecting fetus or newborn 761.6
   previous, affecting management of pregnancy 654.2 ✓5th
Céstan's syndrome 344.89
Céstan-Chenais paralysis 344.89
Céstan-Raymond syndrome 433.8 ✓5th
Cestode infestation NEC 123.9
   specified type NEC 123.8
Cestodiasis 123.9
Chabert's disease 022.9
Chacaleh 266.2
Chafing 709.8
Chagas' disease (see also Trypanosomiasis, American) 086.2
   with heart involvement 086.0
Chagres fever 084.0

Chalasia (cardiac sphincter) 530.81
Chalazion 373.2
Chalazoderma 757.39
Chalcosis 360.24
   cornea 371.15
   crystalline lens 360.24 [366.34]
   retina 360.24
Chalicosis (occupational) (pulmonum) 502
Chancre (any genital site) (hard) (indurated) (infecting) (primary) (recurrent) 091.0
   congenital 090.0
   conjunctiva 091.2
   Ducrey's 099.0
   extragenital 091.2
   eyelid 091.2
   Hunterian 091.0
   lip (syphilis) 091.2
   mixed 099.8
   nipple 091.2
   Nisbet's 099.0
   of
     carate 103.0
     pinta 103.0
     yaws 102.0
   palate, soft 091.2
   phagedenic 099.0
   Ricord's 091.0
   Rollet's (syphilitic) 091.0
   seronegative 091.0
   seropositive 091.0
   simple 099.0
   soft 099.0
     bubo 099.0
   urethra 091.0
   yaws 102.0
Chancriform syndrome 114.1
Chancroid 099.0
   anus 099.0
   penis (Ducrey's bacillus) 099.0
   perineum 099.0
   rectum 099.0
   scrotum 099.0
   urethra 099.0
   vulva 099.0
Chandipura fever 066.8
Chandler's disease (osteochondritis dissecans, hip) 732.7
Change(s) (of) — see also Removal of
   arteriosclerotic — see Arteriosclerosis
   battery
     cardiac pacemaker V53.31
   bone 733.90
     diabetic 250.8 ✓5th [731.8]
     in disease, unknown cause 733.90
   bowel habits 787.99
   cardiorenal (vascular) (see also Hypertension, cardiorenal) 404.90
   cardiovascular — see Disease, cardiovascular
   circulatory 459.9
   cognitive or personality change of other type, nonpsychotic 310.1
   color, teeth, tooth
     during formation 520.8
     posteruptive 521.7
   contraceptive device V25.42
   cornea, corneal
     degenerative NEC 371.40
     membrane NEC 371.30
     senile 371.41
   coronary (see also Ischemia, heart) 414.9

Change(s) (of) — *continued*
degenerative
　chamber angle (anterior) (iris) 364.56
　ciliary body 364.57
　spine or vertebra (*see also* Spondylosis) 721.90
dental pulp, regressive 522.2
dressing V58.3
fixation device V54.89 ▲
　external V54.89 ▲
　internal V54.0
heart — *see also* Disease, heart
hip joint 718.95
hyperplastic larynx 478.79
hypertrophic
　nasal sinus (*see also* Sinusitis) 473.9
　turbinate, nasal 478.0
　upper respiratory tract 478.9
inflammatory — *see* Inflammation
joint (*see also* Derangement, joint) 718.90
　sacroiliac 724.6
Kirschner wire V54.89 ▲
knee 717.9
macular, congenital 743.55
malignant (M—— /3) — *see also* Neoplasm, by site, malignant

> Note — for malignant change occurring in a neoplasm, use the appropriate M code with behavior digit /3 e.g., malignant change in uterine fibroid — M8890/3. For malignant change occurring in a nonneoplastic condition (e.g., gastric ulcer) use the M code M8000/3.

　mental (status) NEC 780.99 ▲
　　due to or associated with physical condition — *see* Syndrome, brain
　myocardium, myocardial — *see* Degeneration, myocardial
　of life (*see also* Menopause) 627.2
　pacemaker battery (cardiac) V53.31
　peripheral nerve 355.9
　personality (nonpsychotic) NEC 310.1
　plaster cast V54.89 ▲
　refractive, transient 367.81
　regressive, dental pulp 522.2
　retina 362.9
　　myopic (degenerative) (malignant) 360.21
　　vascular appearance 362.13
　sacroiliac joint 724.6
　scleral 379.19
　　degenerative 379.16
　senile (*see also* Senility) 797
　sensory (*see also* Disturbance, sensation) 782.0
　skin texture 782.8
　spinal cord 336.9
　splint, external V54.89 ▲
　subdermal implantable contraceptive V25.5
　suture V58.3
　traction device V54.89 ▲
　trophic 355.9
　　arm NEC 354.9
　　leg NEC 355.8
　　lower extremity NEC 355.8
　　upper extremity NEC 354.9
　vascular 459.9
　vasomotor 443.9
　voice 784.49
　　psychogenic 306.1

Changing sleep-work schedule, affecting sleep 307.45
Changuinola fever 066.0
Chapping skin 709.8
Character
　depressive 301.12
Charcôt's
　arthropathy 094.0 *[713.5]*
　cirrhosis — *see* Cirrhosis, biliary
　disease 094.0
　　spinal cord 094.0
　fever (biliary) (hepatic) (intermittent) — *see* Choledocholithiasis
　joint (disease) 094.0 *[713.5]*
　　diabetic 250.6 ✓5ᵗʰ *[713.5]*
　syringomyelic 336.0 *[713.5]*
　syndrome (intermittent claudication) 443.9
　　due to atherosclerosis 440.21
Charcôt-Marie-Tooth disease, paralysis, or syndrome 356.1
Charleyhorse (quadriceps) 843.8
　muscle, except quadriceps — *see* Sprain, by site
Charlouis' disease (*see also* Yaws) 102.9
Chauffeur's fracture — *see* Fracture, ulna, lower end
Cheadle (-Möller) (-Barlow) disease or syndrome (infantile scurvy) 267
Checking (of)
　contraceptive device (intrauterine) V25.42
　device
　　fixation V54.89 ▲
　　　external V54.89 ▲
　　　internal V54.0
　　traction V54.89 ▲
　　Kirschner wire V54.89 ▲
　　plaster cast V54.89 ▲
　　splint, external V54.89 ▲
Checkup
　following treatment — *see* Examination
　health V70.0
　infant (not sick) V20.2
　pregnancy (normal) V22.1
　　first V22.0
　　high risk pregnancy V23.9
　　specified problem NEC V23.89
Chédiak-Higashi (-Steinbrinck) anomaly, disease, or syndrome (congenital gigantism of peroxidase granules) 288.2
Cheek — *see also* condition
　biting 528.9
Cheese itch 133.8
Cheese washers' lung 495.8
Cheilitis 528.5
　actinic (due to sun) 692.72
　　chronic NEC 692.72
　　　due to radiation, except from sun 692.82
　　due to radiation, except from sun 692.82
　acute 528.5
　angular 528.5
　catarrhal 528.5
　chronic 528.5
　exfoliative 528.5
　gangrenous 528.5
　glandularis apostematosa 528.5
　granulomatosa 351.8
　infectional 528.5
　membranous 528.5
　Miescher's 351.8

Cheilitis — *continued*
  suppurative 528.5
  ulcerative 528.5
  vesicular 528.5
Cheilodynia 528.5
Cheilopalatoschisis (*see also* Cleft, palate, with cleft lip) 749.20
Cheilophagia 528.9
Cheiloschisis (*see also* Cleft, lip) 749.10
Cheilosis 528.5
  with pellagra 265.2
  angular 528.5
  due to
    dietary deficiency 266.0
    vitamin deficiency 266.0
Cheiromegaly 729.89
Cheiropompholyx 705.81
Cheloid (*see also* Keloid) 701.4
Chemical burn — *see also* Burn, by site
  from swallowing chemical — *see* Burn, internal organs
Chemodectoma (M8693/1) — *see* Paraganglioma, nonchromaffin
Chemoprophylaxis NEC V07.39
Chemosis, conjunctiva 372.73
Chemotherapy
  convalescence V66.2
  encounter (for) V58.1
  maintenance V58.1
  prophylactic NEC V07.39
    fluoride V07.31
Cherubism 526.89
Chest — *see* condition
Cheyne-Stokes respiration (periodic) 786.04
Chiari's
  disease or syndrome (hepatic vein thrombosis) 453.0
  malformation
    type I 348.4
    type II (*see also* Spina bifida) 741.0
    type III 742.0
    type IV 742.2
    network 746.89
Chiari-Frommel syndrome 676.6
Chicago disease (North American blastomycosis) 116.0
Chickenpox (*see also* Varicella) 052.9
  vaccination and inoculation (prophylactic) V05.4
Chiclero ulcer 085.4
Chiggers 133.8
Chignon 111.2
  fetus or newborn (from vacuum extraction) 767.1
Chigoe disease 134.1
Chikungunya fever 066.3
Chilaiditi's syndrome (subphrenic displacement, colon) 751.4
Chilblains 991.5
  lupus 991.5
Child
  behavior causing concern V61.20
Childbed fever 670
Childbirth — *see also* Delivery
  puerperal complications — *see* Puerperal
Childhood, period of rapid growth V21.0

Chill(s) 780.99
  with fever 780.6
  congestive 780.99
    in malarial regions 084.6
  septic — *see* Septicemia
  urethral 599.84
Chilomastigiasis 007.8
Chin — *see* condition
Chinese dysentery 004.9
Chiropractic dislocation (*see also* Lesion, nonallopathic, by site) 739.9
Chitral fever 066.0
Chlamydia, chlamydial — *see* condition
Chloasma 709.09
  cachecticorum 709.09
  eyelid 374.52
    congenital 757.33
    hyperthyroid 242.0
  gravidarum 646.8
  idiopathic 709.09
  skin 709.09
  symptomatic 709.09
Chloroma (M9930/3) 205.3
Chlorosis 280.9
  Egyptian (*see also* Ancylostomiasis) 126.9
  miners' (*see also* Ancylostomiasis) 126.9
Chlorotic anemia 280.9
Chocolate cyst (ovary) 617.1
Choked
  disk or disc — *see* Papilledema
  on food, phlegm, or vomitus NEC (*see also* Asphyxia, food) 933.1
  phlegm 933.1
  while vomiting NEC (*see also* Asphyxia, food) 933.1
Chokes (resulting from bends) 993.3
Choking sensation 784.9
Cholangiectasis (*see also* Disease, gallbladder) 575.8
Cholangiocarcinoma (M8160/3)
  and hepatocellular carcinoma, combined (M8180/3) 155.0
  liver 155.1
  specified site NEC — *see* Neoplasm, by site, malignant
  unspecified site 155.1
Cholangiohepatitis 575.8
  due to fluke infestation 121.1
Cholangiohepatoma (M8180/3) 155.0
Cholangiolitis (acute) (chronic) (extrahepatic) (gangrenous) 576.1
  intrahepatic 575.8
  paratyphoidal (*see also* Fever, paratyphoid) 002.9
  typhoidal 002.0
Cholangioma (M8160/0) 211.5
  malignant — *see* Cholangiocarcinoma
Cholangitis (acute) (ascending) (catarrhal) (chronic) (infective) (malignant) (primary) (recurrent) (sclerosing) (secondary) (stenosing) (suppurative) 576.1
  chronic nonsuppurative destructive 571.6
  nonsuppurative destructive (chronic) 571.6
Cholecystdocholithiasis — *see* Choledocholithiasis

Cholecystitis 575.10
 with
  calculus, stones in
   bile duct (common) (hepatic) — see
    Choledocholithiasis
   gallbladder — see Cholelithiasis
 acute 575.0
 acute and chronic 575.12
 chronic 575.11
 emphysematous (acute) (see also Cholecystitis,
   acute) 575.0
 gangrenous (see also Cholecystitis, acute)
   575.0
 paratyphoidal, current (see also Fever,
   paratyphoid) 002.9
 suppurative (see also Cholecystitis, acute)
   575.0
 typhoidal 002.0
Choledochitis (suppurative) 576.1
Choledocholith — see Choledocholithiasis
Choledocholithiasis 574.5 ✓5ᵗʰ

> Note — Use the following fifth-digit
> subclassification with category 574:
>
> 0   without mention of obstruction
> 1   with obstruction

 with
  cholecystitis 574.4 ✓5ᵗʰ
   acute 574.3 ✓5ᵗʰ
   chronic 574.4 ✓5ᵗʰ
  cholelithiasis 574.9 ✓5ᵗʰ
   with
    cholecystitis 574.7 ✓5ᵗʰ
     acute 574.6 ✓5ᵗʰ
      and chronic 574.8 ✓5ᵗʰ
     chronic 574.7 ✓5ᵗʰ
Cholelithiasis (impacted) (multiple) 574.2 ✓5ᵗʰ

> Note — Use the following fifth-digit
> subclassification with category 574:
>
> 0   without mention of obstruction
> 1   with obstruction

 with
  cholecystitis 574.1 ✓5ᵗʰ
   acute 574.0 ✓5ᵗʰ
   chronic 574.1 ✓5ᵗʰ
  choledocholithiasis 574.9 ✓5ᵗʰ
   with
    cholecystitis 574.7 ✓5ᵗʰ
     acute 574.6 ✓5ᵗʰ
      and chronic 574.8 ✓5ᵗʰ
     chronic cholecystitis 574.7 ✓5ᵗʰ
Cholemia (see also Jaundice) 782.4
 familial 277.4
 Gilbert's (familial nonhemolytic) 277.4
Cholemic gallstone — see Cholelithiasis
Choleperitoneum, choleperitonitis (see also
  Disease, gallbladder) 567.8
Cholera (algid) (Asiatic) (asphyctic) (epidemic)
  (gravis) (Indian) (malignant) (morbus)
  (pestilential) (spasmodic) 001.9
 antimonial 985.4
 carrier (suspected) of V02.0
 classical 001.0
 contact V01.0

Cholera — continued
 due to
  Vibrio
   cholerae (Inaba, Ogawa, Hikojima
    serotypes) 001.0
    El Tor 001.1
  El Tor 001.1
 exposure to V01.0
 vaccination, prophylactic (against) V03.0
Cholerine (see also Cholera) 001.9
Cholestasis 576.8
Cholesteatoma (ear) 385.30
 attic (primary) 385.31
 diffuse 385.35
 external ear (canal) 380.21
 marginal (middle ear) 385.32
  with involvement of mastoid cavity 385.33
  secondary (with middle ear involvement)
   385.33
 mastoid cavity 385.30
 middle ear (secondary) 385.32
  with involvement of mastoid cavity 385.33
 postmastoidectomy cavity (recurrent) 383.32
 primary 385.31
 recurrent, postmastoidectomy cavity 383.32
 secondary (middle ear) 385.32
  with involvement of mastoid cavity 385.33
Cholesteatosis (middle ear) (see also
  Cholesteatoma) 385.30
 diffuse 385.35
Cholesteremia 272.0
Cholesterin
 granuloma, middle ear 385.82
 in vitreous 379.22
Cholesterol
 deposit
  retina 362.82
  vitreous 379.22
 imbibition of gallbladder (see also Disease,
  gallbladder) 575.6
Cholesterolemia 272.0
 essential 272.0
 familial 272.0
 hereditary 272.0
Cholesterosis, cholesterolosis (gallbladder)
  575.6
 with
  cholecystitis — see Cholecystitis
  cholelithiasis — see Cholelithiasis
 middle ear (see also Cholesteatoma) 385.30
Cholocolic fistula (see also Fistula, gallbladder)
  575.6
Choluria 791.4
Chondritis (purulent) 733.99
 costal 733.6
  Tietze's 733.6
 patella, posttraumatic 717.7
 posttraumatica patellae 717.7
 tuberculous (active) (see also Tuberculosis)
  015.9 ✓5ᵗʰ
  intervertebral 015.0 ✓5ᵗʰ [730.88]
Chondroangiopathia calcarea seu punctate
  756.59
Chondroblastoma (M9230/0) — see also
  Neoplasm, bone, benign
 malignant (M9230/3) — see Neoplasm, bone,
  malignant

Chondrocalcinosis (articular) (crystal deposition) (dihydrate) (see also Arthritis, due to, crystals) 275.49 [712.3]
  due to
    calcium pyrophosphate 275.49 [712.2]
    dicalcium phosphate crystals 275.49 [712.1]
    pyrophosphate crystals 275.49 [712.2]
Chondrodermatitis nodularis helicis 380.00
Chondrodysplasia 756.4
  angiomatose 756.4
  calcificans congenita 756.59
  epiphysialis punctata 756.59
  hereditary deforming 756.4
Chondrodystrophia (fetalis) 756.4
  calcarea 756.4
  calcificans congenita 756.59
  fetalis hypoplastica 756.59
  hypoplastica calcinosa 756.59
  punctata 756.59
  tarda 277.5
Chondrodystrophy (familial) (hypoplastic) 756.4
Chondroectodermal dysplasia 756.55
Chondrolysis 733.99
Chondroma (M9220/0) — see also Neoplasm, cartilage, benign
  juxtacortical (M9221/0) — see Neoplasm, bone, benign
  periosteal (M9221/0) — see Neoplasm, bone, benign
Chondromalacia 733.92
  epiglottis (congenital) 748.3
  generalized 733.92
  knee 717.7
  larynx (congenital) 748.3
  localized, except patella 733.92
  patella, patellae 717.7
  systemic 733.92
  tibial plateau 733.92
  trachea (congenital) 748.3
Chondromatosis (M9220/1) — see Neoplasm, cartilage, uncertain behavior
Chondromyxosarcoma (M9220/3) — see Neoplasm, cartilage, malignant
Chondro-osteodysplasia (Morquio-Brailsford type) 277.5
Chondro-osteodystrophy 277.5
Chondro-osteoma (M9210/0) — see Neoplasm, bone, benign
Chondropathia tuberosa 733.6
Chondrosarcoma (M9220/3) — see also Neoplasm, cartilage, malignant
  juxtacortical (M9221/3) — see Neoplasm, bone, malignant
  mesenchymal (M9240/3) — see Neoplasm, connective tissue, malignant
Chordae tendineae rupture (chronic) 429.5
Chordee (nonvenereal) 607.89
  congenital 752.63
  gonococcal 098.2
Chorditis (fibrinous) (nodosa) (tuberosa) 478.5
Chordoma (M9370/3) — see Neoplasm, by site, malignant
Chorea (gravis) (minor) (spasmodic) 333.5
  with
    heart involvement — see Chorea with rheumatic heart disease

Chorea — continued
  with — continued
    rheumatic heart disease (chronic, inactive, or quiescent) (conditions classifiable to 393-398) — see also Rheumatic heart condition involved
      active or acute (conditions classifiable to 391) 392.0
  acute — see Chorea, Sydenham's
  apoplectic (see also Disease, cerebrovascular, acute) 436
  chronic 333.4
  electric 049.8
  gravidarum — see Eclampsia, pregnancy
  habit 307.22
  hereditary 333.4
  Huntington's 333.4
  posthemiplegic 344.89
  pregnancy — see Eclampsia, pregnancy
  progressive 333.4
    chronic 333.4
    hereditary 333.4
  rheumatic (chronic) 392.9
    with heart disease or involvement — see Chorea, with rheumatic heart disease
  senile 333.5
  Sydenham's 392.9
    with heart involvement — see Chorea, with rheumatic heart disease
    nonrheumatic 333.5
  variabilis 307.23
Choreoathetosis (paroxysmal) 333.5
Chorioadenoma (destruens) (M9100/1) 236.1
Chorioamnionitis 658.4
  affecting fetus or newborn 762.7
Chorioangioma (M9120/0) 219.8
Choriocarcinoma (M9100/3)
  combined with
    embryonal carcinoma (M9101/3) — see Neoplasm, by site, malignant
    teratoma (M9101/3) — see Neoplasm, by site, malignant
  specified site — see Neoplasm, by site, malignant
  unspecified site
    female 181
    male 186.9
Chorioencephalitis, lymphocytic (acute) (serous) 049.0
Chorioepithelioma (M9100/3) — see Choriocarcinoma
Choriomeningitis (acute) (benign) (lymphocytic) (serous) 049.0
Chorionepithelioma (M9100/3) — see Choriocarcinoma
Chorionitis (see also Scleroderma) 710.1
Chorioretinitis 363.20
  disseminated 363.10
  generalized 363.13
  in
    neurosyphilis 094.83
    secondary syphilis 091.51
  peripheral 363.12
  posterior pole 363.11
  tuberculous (see also Tuberculosis) 017.3 [363.13]
  due to
    histoplasmosis (see also Histoplasmosis) 115.92

Chorioretinitis — *continued*
  due to — *continued*
    toxoplasmosis (acquired) 130.2
      congenital (active) 771.2
  focal 363.00
    juxtapapillary 363.01
    peripheral 363.04
    posterior pole NEC 363.03
  juxtapapillaris, juxtapapillary 363.01
  progressive myopia (degeneration) 360.21
  syphilitic (secondary) 091.51
    congenital (early) 090.0 *[363.13]*
      late 090.5 *[363.13]*
      late 095.8 *[363.13]*
  tuberculous (*see also* Tuberculosis) 017.3 ✓5ᵗʰ *[363.13]*

Choristoma — *see* Neoplasm, by site, benign
Choroid — *see* condition
Choroideremia, choroidermia (initial stage) (late stage) (partial or total atrophy) 363.55
Choroiditis (*see also* Chorioretinitis) 363.20
  leprous 030.9 *[363.13]*
  senile guttate 363.41
  sympathetic 360.11
  syphilitic (secondary) 091.51
    congenital (early) 090.0 *[363.13]*
      late 090.5 *[363.13]*
      late 095.8 *[363.13]*
  Tay's 363.41
  tuberculous (*see also* Tuberculosis) 017.3 ✓5ᵗʰ *[363.13]*

Choroidopathy NEC 363.9
  degenerative (*see also* Degeneration, choroid) 363.40
  hereditary (*see also* Dystrophy, choroid) 363.50
  specified type NEC 363.8

Choroidoretinitis — *see* Chorioretinitis
Choroidosis, central serous 362.41
Choroidretinopathy, serous 362.41
Christian's syndrome (chronic histiocytosis X) 277.8
Christian-Weber disease (nodular nonsuppurative panniculitis) 729.30
Christmas disease 286.1
Chromaffinoma (M8700/0) — *see also* Neoplasm, by site, benign
  malignant (M8700/3) — *see* Neoplasm, by site, malignant
Chromatopsia 368.59
Chromhidrosis, chromidrosis 705.89
Chromoblastomycosis 117.2
Chromomycosis 117.2
Chromophytosis 111.0
Chromotrichomycosis 111.8
Chronic — *see* condition
Churg-Strauss syndrome 446.4
Chyle cyst, mesentery 457.8
Chylocele (nonfilarial) 457.8
  filarial (*see also* Infestation, filarial) 125.9
  tunica vaginalis (nonfilarial) 608.84
    filarial (*see also* Infestation, filarial) 125.9
Chylomicronemia (fasting) (with hyperprebetalipoproteinemia) 272.3
Chylopericardium (acute) 420.90
Chylothorax (nonfilarial) 457.8
  filarial (*see also* Infestation, filarial) 125.9

Chylous
  ascites 457.8
  cyst of peritoneum 457.8
  hydrocele 603.9
  hydrothorax (nonfilarial) 457.8
    filarial (*see also* Infestation, filarial) 125.9
Chyluria 791.1
  bilharziasis 120.0
  due to
    Brugia (malayi) 125.1
    Wuchereria (bancrofti) 125.0
      malayi 125.1
  filarial (*see also* Infestation, filarial) 125.9
  filariasis (*see also* Infestation, filarial) 125.9
  nonfilarial 791.1
Cicatricial (deformity) — *see* Cicatrix
Cicatrix (adherent) (contracted) (painful) (vicious) 709.2
  adenoid 474.8
  alveolar process 525.8
  anus 569.49
  auricle 380.89
  bile duct (*see also* Disease, biliary) 576.8
  bladder 596.8
  bone 733.99
  brain 348.8
  cervix (postoperative) (postpartal) 622.3
    in pregnancy or childbirth 654.6 ✓5ᵗʰ
      causing obstructed labor 660.2 ✓5ᵗʰ
  chorioretinal 363.30
    disseminated 363.35
    macular 363.32
    peripheral 363.34
    posterior pole NEC 363.33
  choroid — *see* Cicatrix, chorioretinal
  common duct (*see also* Disease, biliary) 576.8
  congenital 757.39
  conjunctiva 372.64
  cornea 371.00
    tuberculous (*see also* Tuberculosis) 017.3 ✓5ᵗʰ *[371.05]*
  duodenum (bulb) 537.3
  esophagus 530.3
  eyelid 374.46
    with
      ectropion — *see* Ectropion
      entropion — *see* Entropion
  hypopharynx 478.29
  knee, semilunar cartilage 717.5
  lacrimal
    canaliculi 375.53
    duct
      acquired 375.56
      neonatal 375.55
    punctum 375.52
    sac 375.54
  larynx 478.79
  limbus (cystoid) 372.64
  lung 518.89
  macular 363.32
    disseminated 363.35
    peripheral 363.34
  middle ear 385.89
  mouth 528.9
  muscle 728.89
  nasolacrimal duct
    acquired 375.56
    neonatal 375.55
  nasopharynx 478.29
  palate (soft) 528.9
  penis 607.89

Cicatrix — *continued*
 prostate 602.8
 rectum 569.49
 retina 363.30
  disseminated 363.35
  macular 363.32
  peripheral 363.34
  posterior pole NEC 363.33
 semilunar cartilage — *see* Derangement, meniscus
 seminal vesicle 608.89
 skin 709.2
  infected 686.8
  postinfectional 709.2
  tuberculous (*see also* Tuberculosis) 017.0 ✓5ᵗʰ
 specified site NEC 709.2
 throat 478.29
 tongue 529.8
 tonsil (and adenoid) 474.8
 trachea 478.9
 tuberculous NEC (*see also* Tuberculosis) 011.9 ✓5ᵗʰ
 ureter 593.89
 urethra 599.84
 uterus 621.8
 vagina 623.4
  in pregnancy or childbirth 654.7 ✓5ᵗʰ
   causing obstructed labor 660.2 ✓5ᵗʰ
 vocal cord 478.5
 wrist, constricting (annular) 709.2
CIN I [cervical intraepithelial neoplasia I] 622.1
CIN II [cervical intraepithelial neoplasia II] 622.1
CIN III [cervical intraepithelial neoplasia III] 233.1
Cinchonism
 correct substance properly administered 386.9
 overdose or wrong substance given or taken 961.4
Circine herpes 110.5
Circle of Willis — *see* condition
Circular — *see also* condition
 hymen 752.49
Circulating anticoagulants 286.5
 following childbirth 666.3 ✓5ᵗʰ
 postpartum 666.3 ✓5ᵗʰ
Circulation
 collateral (venous), any site 459.89
 defective 459.9
  congenital 747.9
  lower extremity 459.89
 embryonic 747.9
 failure 799.8
  fetus or newborn 779.89 ▲
  peripheral 785.59
 fetal, persistent 747.83 ▲
 heart, incomplete 747.9
Circulatory system — *see* condition
Circulus senilis 371.41
Circumcision
 in absence of medical indication V50.2
 ritual V50.2
 routine V50.2
Circumscribed — *see* condition
Circumvallata placenta — *see* Placenta, abnormal
Cirrhosis, cirrhotic 571.5
 with alcoholism 571.2
 alcoholic (liver) 571.2

Cirrhosis, cirrhotic — *continued*
 atrophic (of liver) — *see* Cirrhosis, portal
 Baumgarten-Cruveilhier 571.5
 biliary (cholangiolitic) (cholangitic) (cholestatic) (extrahepatic) (hypertrophic) (intrahepatic) (nonobstructive) (obstructive) (pericholangiolitic) (posthepatic) (primary) (secondary) (xanthomatous) 571.6
  due to
   clonorchiasis 121.1
   flukes 121.3
 brain 331.9
 capsular — *see* Cirrhosis, portal
 cardiac 571.5
  alcoholic 571.2
 central (liver) — *see* Cirrhosis, liver
 Charcôt's 571.6
 cholangiolitic — *see* Cirrhosis, biliary
 cholangitic — *see* Cirrhosis, biliary
 cholestatic — *see* Cirrhosis, biliary
 clitoris (hypertrophic) 624.2
 coarsely nodular 571.5
 congestive (liver) — *see* Cirrhosis, cardiac
 Cruveilhier-Baumgarten 571.5
 cryptogenic (of liver) 571.5
  alcoholic 571.2
 dietary (*see also* Cirrhosis, portal) 571.5
 due to
  bronzed diabetes 275.0
  congestive hepatomegaly — *see* Cirrhosis, cardiac
  cystic fibrosis 277.00
  hemochromatosis 275.0
  hepatolenticular degeneration 275.1
  passive congestion (chronic) — *see* Cirrhosis, cardiac
  Wilson's disease 275.1
  xanthomatosis 272.2
 extrahepatic (obstructive) — *see* Cirrhosis, biliary
 fatty 571.8
  alcoholic 571.0
 florid 571.2
 Glisson's — *see* Cirrhosis, portal
 Hanot's (hypertrophic) — *see* Cirrhosis, biliary
 hepatic — *see* Cirrhosis, liver
 hepatolienal — *see* Cirrhosis, liver
 hobnail — *see* Cirrhosis, portal
 hypertrophic — *see also* Cirrhosis, liver
  biliary — *see* Cirrhosis, biliary
  Hanot's — *see* Cirrhosis, biliary
 infectious NEC — *see* Cirrhosis, portal
 insular — *see* Cirrhosis, portal
 intrahepatic (obstructive) (primary) (secondary) — *see* Cirrhosis, biliary
 juvenile (*see also* Cirrhosis, portal) 571.5
 kidney (*see also* Sclerosis, renal) 587
 Laennec's (of liver) 571.2
  nonalcoholic 571.5
 liver (chronic) (hepatolienal) (hypertrophic) (nodular) (splenomegalic) (unilobar) 571.5
  with alcoholism 571.2
   alcoholic 571.2
  congenital (due to failure of obliteration of umbilical vein) 777.8
  cryptogenic 571.5
   alcoholic 571.2
  fatty 571.8
   alcoholic 571.0

Index to Diseases — Cleft

Cirrhosis, cirrhotic — *continued*
  liver — *continued*
    macronodular 571.5
      alcoholic 571.2
    micronodular 571.5
      alcoholic 571.2
    nodular, diffuse 571.5
      alcoholic 571.2
    pigmentary 275.0
    portal 571.5
      alcoholic 571.2
    postnecrotic 571.5
      alcoholic 571.2
    syphilitic 095.3
  lung (chronic) (*see also* Fibrosis, lung) 515
  macronodular (of liver) 571.5
    alcoholic 571.2
  malarial 084.9
  metabolic NEC 571.5
  micronodular (of liver) 571.5
    alcoholic 571.2
  monolobular — *see* Cirrhosis, portal
  multilobular — *see* Cirrhosis, portal
  nephritis (*see also* Sclerosis, renal) 587
  nodular — *see* Cirrhosis, liver
  nutritional (fatty) 571.5
  obstructive (biliary) (extrahepatic)
    (intrahepatic) — *see* Cirrhosis, biliary
  ovarian 620.8
  paludal 084.9
  pancreas (duct) 577.8
  pericholangiolitic — *see* Cirrhosis, biliary
  periportal — *see* Cirrhosis, portal
  pigment, pigmentary (of liver) 275.0
  portal (of liver) 571.5
    alcoholic 571.2
  posthepatitic (*see also* Cirrhosis, postnecrotic) 571.5
  postnecrotic (of liver) 571.5
    alcoholic 571.2
  primary (intrahepatic) — *see* Cirrhosis, biliary
  pulmonary (*see also* Fibrosis, lung) 515
  renal (*see also* Sclerosis, renal) 587
  septal (*see also* Cirrhosis, postnecrotic) 571.5
  spleen 289.51
  splenomegalic (of liver) — *see* Cirrhosis, liver
  stasis (liver) — *see* Cirrhosis, liver
  stomach 535.4 ✓5ᵗʰ
  Todd's (*see also* Cirrhosis, biliary) 571.6
  toxic (nodular) — *see* Cirrhosis, postnecrotic
  trabecular — *see* Cirrhosis, postnecrotic
  unilobar — *see* Cirrhosis, liver
  vascular (of liver) — *see* Cirrhosis, liver
  xanthomatous (biliary) (*see also* Cirrhosis, biliary) 571.6
    due to xanthomatosis (familial) (metabolic) (primary) 272.2
Cistern, subarachnoid 793.0
Citrullinemia 270.6
Citrullinuria 270.6
Ciuffini-Pancoast tumor (M8010/3) (carcinoma, pulmonary apex) 162.3
Civatte's disease or poikiloderma 709.09
Clam diggers' itch 120.3
Clap — *see* Gonorrhea
Clark's paralysis 343.9
Clarke-Hadfield syndrome (pancreatic infantilism) 577.8
Clastothrix 704.2

Claude's syndrome 352.6
Claude Bernard-Horner syndrome (*see also* Neuropathy, peripheral, autonomic) 337.9
Claudication, intermittent 443.9
  cerebral (artery) (*see also* Ischemia, cerebral, transient) 435.9
  due to atherosclerosis 440.21
  spinal cord (arteriosclerotic) 435.1
    syphilitic 094.89
  spinalis 435.1
  venous (axillary) 453.8
Claudicatio venosa intermittens 453.8
Claustrophobia 300.29
Clavus (infected) 700
Clawfoot (congenital) 754.71
  acquired 736.74
Clawhand (acquired) 736.06
  congenital 755.59
Clawtoe (congenital) 754.71
  acquired 735.5
Clay eating 307.52
Clay shovelers' fracture — *see* Fracture, vertebra, cervical
Cleansing of artificial opening (*see also* Attention to artificial opening) V55.9
Cleft (congenital) — *see also* Imperfect, closure
  alveolar process 525.8
  branchial (persistent) 744.41
    cyst 744.42
  clitoris 752.49
  cricoid cartilage, posterior 748.3
  facial (*see also* Cleft, lip) 749.10
  lip 749.10
    with cleft palate 749.20
      bilateral (lip and palate) 749.24
        with unilateral lip or palate 749.25
        complete 749.23
        incomplete 749.24
      unilateral (lip and palate) 749.22
        with bilateral lip or palate 749.25
        complete 749.21
        incomplete 749.22
    bilateral 749.14
      with cleft palate, unilateral 749.25
      complete 749.13
      incomplete 749.14
    unilateral 749.12
      with cleft palate, bilateral 749.25
      complete 749.11
      incomplete 749.12
  nose 748.1
  palate 749.00
    with cleft lip 749.20
      bilateral (lip and palate) 749.24
        with unilateral lip or palate 749.25
        complete 749.23
        incomplete 749.24
      unilateral (lip and palate) 749.22
        with bilateral lip or palate 749.25
        complete 749.21
        incomplete 749.22
    bilateral 749.04
      with cleft lip, unilateral 749.25
      complete 749.03
      incomplete 749.04
    unilateral 749.02
      with cleft lip, bilateral 749.25
      complete 749.01
      incomplete 749.02

Cleft — continued
  penis 752.69
  posterior, cricoid cartilage 748.3
  scrotum 752.8
  sternum (congenital) 756.3
  thyroid cartilage (congenital) 748.3
  tongue 750.13
  uvula 749.02
    with cleft lip (see also Cleft, lip, with cleft palate) 749.20
  water 366.12
Cleft hand (congenital) 755.58
Cleidocranial dysostosis 755.59
Cleidotomy, fetal 763.89
Cleptomania 312.32
Clérambault's syndrome 297.8
  erotomania 302.89
Clergyman's sore throat 784.49
Click, clicking
  systolic syndrome 785.2
Clifford's syndrome (postmaturity) 766.2
Climacteric (see also Menopause) 627.2
  arthritis NEC (see also Arthritis, climacteric) 716.3
  depression (see also Psychosis, affective) 296.2
  disease 627.2
    recurrent episode 296.3
    single episode 296.2
  female (symptoms) 627.2
  male (symptoms) (syndrome) 608.89
  melancholia (see also Psychosis, affective) 296.2
    recurrent episode 296.3
    single episode 296.2
  paranoid state 297.2
  paraphrenia 297.2
  polyarthritis NEC 716.39
    male 608.89
  symptoms (female) 627.2
Clinical research investigation (control) (participant) V70.7
Clinodactyly 755.59
Clitoris — see condition
Cloaca, persistent 751.5
Clonorchiasis 121.1
Clonorchiosis 121.1
Clonorchis infection, liver 121.1
Clonus 781.0
Closed bite 524.2
Closure
  artificial opening (see also Attention to artificial opening) V55.9
  congenital, nose 748.0
  cranial sutures, premature 756.0
  defective or imperfect NEC — see Imperfect, closure
  fistula, delayed — see Fistula
  fontanelle, delayed 756.0
  foramen ovale, imperfect 745.5
  hymen 623.3
  interauricular septum, defective 745.5
  interventricular septum, defective 745.4
  lacrimal duct 375.56
    congenital 743.65
    neonatal 375.55
  nose (congenital) 748.0
    acquired 738.0

Closure — continued
  vagina 623.2
  valve — see Endocarditis
  vulva 624.8
Clot (blood)
  artery (obstruction) (occlusion) (see also Embolism) 444.9
  bladder 596.7
  brain (extradural or intradural) (see also Thrombosis, brain) 434.0
    late effects — see Late effect(s) (of) cerebrovascular disease
  circulation 444.9
  heart (see also Infarct, myocardium) 410.9
  vein (see also Thrombosis) 453.9
Clotting defect NEC (see also Defect, coagulation) 286.9
Clouded state 780.09
  epileptic (see also Epilepsy) 345.9
  paroxysmal (idiopathic) (see also Epilepsy) 345.9
Clouding
  corneal graft 996.51
Cloudy
  antrum, antra 473.0
  dialysis effluent 792.5
Clouston's (hidrotic) ectodermal dysplasia 757.31
Clubbing of fingers 781.5
Clubfinger 736.29
  acquired 736.29
  congenital 754.89
Clubfoot (congenital) 754.70
  acquired 736.71
  equinovarus 754.51
  paralytic 736.71
Club hand (congenital) 754.89
  acquired 736.07
Clubnail (acquired) 703.8
  congenital 757.5
Clump kidney 753.3
Clumsiness 781.3
  syndrome 315.4
Cluttering 307.0
Clutton's joints 090.5
Coagulation, intravascular (diffuse) (disseminated) (see also Fibrinolysis) 286.6
  newborn 776.2
Coagulopathy (see also Defect, coagulation) 286.9
  consumption 286.6
  intravascular (disseminated) NEC 286.6
    newborn 776.2
Coalition
  calcaneoscaphoid 755.67
  calcaneus 755.67
  tarsal 755.67
Coal miners'
  elbow 727.2
  lung 500
Coal workers' lung or pneumoconiosis 500
Coarctation
  aorta (postductal) (preductal) 747.10
  pulmonary artery 747.3
Coated tongue 529.3
Coats' disease 362.12
Cocainism (see also Dependence) 304.2

Coccidioidal granuloma 114.3
Coccidioidomycosis 114.9
  with pneumonia 114.0
  cutaneous (primary) 114.1
  disseminated 114.3
  extrapulmonary (primary) 114.1
  lung 114.5
    acute 114.0
    chronic 114.4
    primary 114.0
  meninges 114.2
  primary (pulmonary) 114.0
    acute 114.0
  prostate 114.3
  pulmonary 114.5
    acute 114.0
    chronic 114.4
    primary 114.0
  specified site NEC 114.3
Coccidioidosis 114.9
  lung 114.5
    acute 114.0
    chronic 114.4
    primary 114.0
  meninges 114.2
Coccidiosis (colitis) (diarrhea) (dysentery) 007.2
Cocciuria 791.9
Coccus in urine 791.9
Coccydynia 724.79
Coccygodynia 724.79
Coccyx — *see* condition
Cochin-China
  diarrhea 579.1
    anguilluliasis 127.2
  ulcer 085.1
Cock's peculiar tumor 706.2
Cockayne's disease or syndrome (microcephaly and dwarfism) 759.89
Cockayne-Weber syndrome (epidermolysis bullosa) 757.39
Cocked-up toe 735.2
Codman's tumor (benign chondroblastoma) (M9230/0) — *see* Neoplasm, bone, benign
Coenurosis 123.8
Coffee workers' lung 495.8
Cogan's syndrome 370.52
  congenital oculomotor apraxia 379.51
  nonsyphilitic interstitial keratitis 370.52
Coiling, umbilical cord — *see* Complications, umbilical cord
Coitus, painful (female) 625.0
  male 608.89
  psychogenic 302.76
Cold 460
  with influenza, flu, or grippe 487.1
    abscess — *see also* Tuberculosis, abscess
  articular — *see* Tuberculosis, joint
  agglutinin
    disease (chronic) or syndrome 283.0
    hemoglobinuria 283.0
      paroxysmal (cold) (nocturnal) 283.2
  allergic (*see also* Fever, hay) 477.9
  bronchus or chest — *see* Bronchitis
    with grippe or influenza 487.1
  common (head) 460
    vaccination, prophylactic (against) V04.7
  deep 464.10

Cold — *continued*
  effects of 991.9
    specified effect NEC 991.8
  excessive 991.9
    specified effect NEC 991.8
  exhaustion from 991.8
  exposure to 991.9
    specified effect NEC 991.8
  grippy 487.1
  head 460
  injury syndrome (newborn) 778.2
  intolerance 780.99
  on lung — *see* Bronchitis
  rose 477.0
  sensitivity, autoimmune 283.0
  virus 460
Coldsore (*see also* Herpes, simplex) 054.9
Colibacillosis 041.4
  generalized 038.42
Colibacilluria 791.9
Colic (recurrent) 789.0
  abdomen 789.0
    psychogenic 307.89
  appendicular 543.9
  appendix 543.9
  bile duct — *see* Choledocholithiasis
  biliary — *see* Cholelithiasis
  bilious — *see* Cholelithiasis
  common duct — *see* Choledocholithiasis
  Devonshire NEC 984.9
    specified type of lead — *see* Table of Drugs and Chemicals
  flatulent 787.3
  gallbladder or gallstone — *see* Cholelithiasis
  gastric 536.8
  hepatic (duct) — *see* Choledocholithiasis
  hysterical 300.11
  infantile 789.0
  intestinal 789.0
  kidney 788.0
  lead NEC 984.9
    specified type of lead — *see* Table of Drugs and Chemicals
  liver (duct) — *see* Choledocholithiasis
  mucous 564.9
    psychogenic 316 [564.9]
  nephritic 788.0
  painter's NEC 984.9
  pancreas 577.8
  psychogenic 306.4
  renal 788.0
  saturnine NEC 984.9
    specified type of lead — *see* Table of Drugs and Chemicals
  spasmodic 789.0
  ureter 788.0
  urethral 599.84
    due to calculus 594.2
  uterus 625.8
    menstrual 625.3
  vermicular 543.9
  virus 460
  worm NEC 128.9
Colicystitis (*see also* Cystitis) 595.9
Colitis (acute) (catarrhal) (croupous) (cystica superficialis) (exudative) (hemorrhagic) (noninfectious) (phlegmonous) (presumed noninfectious) 558.9
  adaptive 564.9
  allergic 558.3

Colitis — continued
  amebic (see also Amebiasis) 006.9
    nondysenteric 006.2
  anthrax 022.2
  bacillary (see also Infection, Shigella) 004.9
  balantidial 007.0
  chronic 558.9
    ulcerative (see also Colitis, ulcerative) 556.9
  coccidial 007.2
  dietetic 558.9
  due to radiation 558.1
  functional 558.9
  gangrenous 009.0
  giardial 007.1
  granulomatous 555.1
  gravis (see also Colitis, ulcerative) 556.9
  infectious (see also Enteritis, due to, specific organism) 009.0
    presumed 009.1
  ischemic 557.9
    acute 557.0
    chronic 557.1
    due to mesenteric artery insufficiency 557.1
  membranous 564.9
    psychogenic 316 [564.9]
  mucous 564.9
    psychogenic 316 [564.9]
  necrotic 009.0
  polyposa (see also Colitis, ulcerative) 556.9
  protozoal NEC 007.9
  pseudomembranous 008.45
  pseudomucinous 564.9
  regional 555.1
  segmental 555.1
  septic (see also Enteritis, due to, specific organism) 009.0
  spastic 564.9
    psychogenic 316 [564.9]
  staphylococcus 008.41
    food 005.0
  thromboulcerative 557.0
  toxic 558.2
  transmural 555.1
  trichomonal 007.3
  tuberculous (ulcerative) 014.8 ✓5ᵗʰ
  ulcerative (chronic) (idiopathic) (nonspecific) 556.9
    entero- 556.0
    fulminant 557.0
    ileo- 556.1
    left-sided 556.5
    procto- 556.2
    proctosigmoid 556.3
    psychogenic 316 [556] ✓4ᵗʰ
    specified NEC 556.8
    universal 556.6
Collagen disease NEC 710.9
  nonvascular 710.9
  vascular (allergic) (see also Angiitis, hypersensitivity) 446.20
Collagenosis (see also Collagen disease) 710.9
  cardiovascular 425.4
  mediastinal 519.3
Collapse 780.2
  adrenal 255.8
  cardiorenal (see also Hypertension, cardiorenal) 404.90
  cardiorespiratory 785.51
    fetus or newborn 779.89 ▲

Collapse — continued
  cardiovascular (see also Disease, heart) 785.51
    fetus or newborn 779.89 ▲
  circulatory (peripheral) 785.59
    with
      abortion — see Abortion, by type, with shock
      ectopic pregnancy (see also categories 633.0-633.9) 639.5
      molar pregnancy (see also categories 630-632) 639.5
    during or after labor and delivery 669.1 ✓5ᵗʰ
    fetus or newborn 779.89 ▲
    following
      abortion 639.5
      ectopic or molar pregnancy 639.5
    during or after labor and delivery 669.1 ✓5ᵗʰ
    fetus or newborn 779.89 ▲
  external ear canal 380.50
    secondary to
      inflammation 380.53
      surgery 380.52
      trauma 380.51
  general 780.2
  heart — see Disease, heart
  heat 992.1
  hysterical 300.11
  labyrinth, membranous (congenital) 744.05
  lung (massive) (see also Atelectasis) 518.0
    pressure, during labor 668.0 ✓5ᵗʰ
  myocardial — see Disease, heart
  nervous (see also Disorder, mental, nonpsychotic) 300.9
  neurocirculatory 306.2
  nose 738.0
  postoperative (cardiovascular) 998.0
  pulmonary (see also Atelectasis) 518.0
    fetus or newborn 770.5
      partial 770.5
      primary 770.4
  thorax 512.8
    iatrogenic 512.1
    postoperative 512.1
  trachea 519.1
  valvular — see Endocarditis
  vascular (peripheral) 785.59
    with
      abortion — see Abortion, by type, with shock
      ectopic pregnancy (see also categories 633.0-633.9) 639.5
      molar pregnancy (see also categories 630-632) 639.5
      cerebral (see also Disease, cerebrovascular, acute) 436
    during or after labor and delivery 669.1 ✓5ᵗʰ
    fetus or newborn 779.89 ▲
    following
      abortion 639.5
      ectopic or molar pregnancy 639.5
  vasomotor 785.59
  vertebra 733.13
Collateral — see also condition
  circulation (venous) 459.89
  dilation, veins 459.89
Colles' fracture (closed) (reversed) (separation) 813.41
  open 813.51
Collet's syndrome 352.6
Collet-Sicard syndrome 352.6

Index to Diseases

Colliculitis urethralis (see also Urethritis) 597.89
Colliers'
  asthma 500
  lung 500
  phthisis (see also Tuberculosis) 011.4 ✓5ᵗʰ
Collodion baby (ichthyosis congenita) 757.1
Colloid milium 709.3
Coloboma NEC 743.49
  choroid 743.59
  fundus 743.52
  iris 743.46
  lens 743.36
  lids 743.62
  optic disc (congenital) 743.57
    acquired 377.23
  retina 743.56
  sclera 743.47
Coloenteritis — see Enteritis
Colon — see condition
Coloptosis 569.89
Color
  amblyopia NEC 368.59
    acquired 368.55
  blindness NEC (congenital) 368.59
    acquired 368.55
Colostomy
  attention to V55.3
  fitting or adjustment V53.5
  malfunctioning 569.62
  status V44.3
Colpitis (see also Vaginitis) 616.10
Colpocele 618.6
Colpocystitis (see also Vaginitis) 616.10
Colporrhexis 665.4 ✓5ᵗʰ
Colpospasm 625.1
Column, spinal, vertebral — see condition
Coma 780.01
  apoplectic (see also Disease, cerebrovascular, acute) 436
  diabetic (with ketoacidosis) 250.3 ✓5ᵗʰ
    hyperosmolar 250.2 ✓5ᵗʰ
  eclamptic (see also Eclampsia) 780.39
  epileptic 345.3
  hepatic 572.2
  hyperglycemic 250.2 ✓5ᵗʰ
  hyperosmolar (diabetic) (nonketotic) 250.2 ✓5ᵗʰ
  hypoglycemic 251.0
    diabetic 250.3 ✓5ᵗʰ
  insulin 250.3 ✓5ᵗʰ
    hyperosmolar 250.2 ✓5ᵗʰ
    non-diabetic 251.0
    organic hyperinsulinism 251.0
  Kussmaul's (diabetic) 250.3 ✓5ᵗʰ
  liver 572.2
  newborn 779.2
  prediabetic 250.2 ✓5ᵗʰ
  uremic — see Uremia
Combat fatigue (see also Reaction, stress, acute) 308.9
Combined — see condition
Comedo 706.1
Comedocarcinoma (M8501/3) — see also
  Neoplasm, breast, malignant
  noninfiltrating (M8501/2)
    specified site — see Neoplasm, by site, in situ
    unspecified site 233.0
Comedomastitis 610.4
Comedones 706.1
  lanugo 757.4
Comma bacillus, carrier (suspected) of V02.3
Comminuted fracture — see Fracture, by site
Common
  aortopulmonary trunk 745.0
  atrioventricular canal (defect) 745.69
  atrium 745.69
  cold (head) 460
    vaccination, prophylactic (against) V04.7
  truncus (arteriosus) 745.0
  ventricle 745.3
Commotio (current)
  cerebri (see also Concussion, brain) 850.9
    with skull fracture — see Fracture, skull, by site
  retinae 921.3
  spinalis — see Injury, spinal, by site
Commotion (current)
  brain (without skull fracture) (see also Concussion, brain) 850.9
    with skull fracture — see Fracture, skull, by site
  spinal cord — see Injury, spinal, by site
Communication
  abnormal — see also Fistula
    between
      base of aorta and pulmonary artery 745.0
      left ventricle and right atrium 745.4
      pericardial sac and pleural sac 748.8
      pulmonary artery and pulmonary vein 747.3
    congenital, between uterus and anterior abdominal wall 752.3
      bladder 752.3
      intestine 752.3
      rectum 752.3
  left ventricular— right atrial 745.4
  pulmonary artery— pulmonary vein 747.3
Compensation
  broken — see Failure, heart
  failure — see Failure, heart
  neurosis, psychoneurosis 300.11
Complaint — see also Disease
  bowel, functional 564.9
    psychogenic 306.4
  intestine, functional 564.9
    psychogenic 306.4
  kidney (see also Disease, renal) 593.9
  liver 573.9
  miners' 500
Complete — see condition
Complex
  cardiorenal (see also Hypertension, cardiorenal) 404.90
  castration 300.9
  Costen's 524.60
  ego-dystonic homosexuality 302.0
  Eisenmenger's (ventricular septal defect) 745.4
  homosexual, ego-dystonic 302.0
  hypersexual 302.89
  inferiority 301.9
  jumped process
    spine — see Dislocation, vertebra
  primary, tuberculosis (see also Tuberculosis) 010.0 ✓5ᵗʰ

Complex — *continued*
  Taussig-Bing (transposition, aorta and overriding pulmonary artery) 745.11
Complications
  abortion NEC — *see* categories 634-639
  accidental puncture or laceration during a procedure 998.2
  amputation stump (late) (surgical) 997.60
    traumatic — *see* Amputation, traumatic
  anastomosis (and bypass) NEC — *see also* Complications, due to (presence of) any device, implant, or graft classified to 996.0-996.5 NEC
    hemorrhage NEC 998.11
    intestinal (internal) NEC 997.4
      involving urinary tract 997.5
    mechanical — *see* Complications, mechanical, graft
    urinary tract (involving intestinal tract) 997.5
  anesthesia, anesthetic NEC (*see also* Anesthesia, complication) 995.2
    in labor and delivery 668.9 ✓5ᵗʰ
      affecting fetus or newborn 763.5
      cardiac 668.1 ✓5ᵗʰ
      central nervous system 668.2 ✓5ᵗʰ
      pulmonary 668.0 ✓5ᵗʰ
      specified type NEC 668.8 ✓5ᵗʰ
  aortocoronary (bypass) graft 996.03
    atherosclerosis — *see* Arteriosclerosis, coronary
    embolism 996.72
    occlusion NEC 996.72
    thrombus 996.72
  arthroplasty 996.4
  artificial opening
    cecostomy 569.60
    colostomy 569.60
    cystostomy 997.5
    enterostomy 569.60
    gastrostomy 536.40
    ileostomy 569.60
    jejunostomy 569.60
    nephrostomy 997.5
    tracheostomy 519.00
    ureterostomy 997.5
    urethrostomy 997.5
  bile duct implant (prosthetic) NEC 996.79
    infection or inflammation 996.69
    mechanical 996.59
  bleeding (intraoperative) (postoperative) 998.11
  blood vessel graft 996.1
    aortocoronary 996.03
      atherosclerosis — *see* Arteriosclerosis, coronary
      embolism 996.72
      occlusion NEC 996.72
      thrombus 996.72
    atherosclerosis — *see* Arteriosclerosis, extremities
    embolism 996.74
    occlusion NEC 996.74
    thrombus 996.74
  bone growth stimulator 996.78
    infection or inflammation 996.67
  bone marrow transplant 996.85
  breast implant (prosthetic) NEC 996.79
    infection or inflammation 996.69
    mechanical 996.54
  bypass — *see also* Complications, anastomosis

Complications — *continued*
  bypass — *continued*
    aortocoronary 996.03
      atherosclerosis — *see* Arteriosclerosis, coronary
      embolism 996.72
      occlusion NEC 996.72
      thrombus 996.72
    carotid artery 996.1
      atherosclerosis — *see* Arteriosclerosis, extremities
      embolism 996.74
      occulsion NEC 996.74
      thrombus 996.74
  cardiac (*see also* Disease, heart) 429.9
    device, implant, or graft NEC 996.72
      infection or inflammation 996.61
      long-term effect 429.4
      mechanical (*see also* Complications, mechanical, by type) 996.00
      valve prosthesis 996.71
        infection or inflammation 996.61
    postoperative NEC 997.1
      long-term effect 429.4
  cardiorenal (*see also* Hypertension, cardiorenal) 404.90
  carotid artery bypass graft 996.1
    atherosclerosis — *see* Arteriosclerosis, extremities
    embolism 996.74
    occlusion NEC 996.74
    thrombus 996.74
  cataract fragments in eye 998.82
  catheter device NEC — *see also* Complications, due to (presence of) any device, implant, or graft classified to 996.0-996.5 NEC
    mechanical — *see* Complications, mechanical, catheter
  cecostomy 569.60
  cesarean section wound 674.3 ✓5ᵗʰ
  chin implant (prosthetic) NEC 996.79
    infection or inflammation 996.69
    mechanical 996.59
  colostomy (enterostomy) 569.60
    specified type NEC 569.69
  contraceptive device, intrauterine NEC 996.76
    infection 996.65
    inflammation 996.65
    mechanical 996.32
  cord (umbilical) — *see* Complications, umbilical cord
  cornea
    due to
      contact lens 371.82
  coronary (artery) bypass (graft) NEC 996.03
    atherosclerosis — *see* Arterio-sclerosis, coronary
    embolism 996.72
    infection or inflammation 996.61
    mechanical 996.03
    occlusion NEC 996.72
    specified type NEC 996.72
    thrombus 996.72
  cystostomy 997.5
  delivery 669.9 ✓5ᵗʰ
    procedure (instrumental) (manual) (surgical) 669.4 ✓5ᵗʰ
    specified type NEC 669.8 ✓5ᵗʰ
  dialysis (hemodialysis) (peritoneal) (renal) NEC 999.9

Complications — *continued*
- dialysis — *continued*
  - catheter NEC — *see also* Complications, due to (presence of) any device, implant or graft classified to 996.0-996.5 NEC
    - infection or inflammation 996.62
      - peritoneal 996.68
    - mechanical 996.1
      - peritoneal 996.56
- due to (presence of) any device, implant, or graft classified to 996.0-996.5 NEC 996.70
  - with infection or inflammation — *see* Complications, infection or inflammation, due to (presence of) any device, implant, or graft classified to 996.0-996.5 NEC
  - arterial NEC 996.74
    - coronary NEC 996.03
      - atherosclerosis — *see* Arteriosclerosis, coronary
      - embolism 996.72
      - occlusion NEC 996.72
      - specified type NEC 996.72
      - thrombus 996.72
    - renal dialysis 996.73
  - arteriovenous fistula or shunt NEC 996.74
  - bone growth stimulator 996.78
  - breast NEC 996.70
  - cardiac NEC 996.72
    - defibrillator 996.72
    - pacemaker 996.72
    - valve prosthesis 996.71
  - catheter NEC 996.79
    - spinal 996.75
    - urinary, indwelling 996.76
    - vascular NEC 996.74
      - renal dialysis 996.73
      - ventricular shunt 996.75
  - coronary (artery) bypass (graft) NEC 996.03
    - atherosclerosis — *see* Arteriosclerosis, coronary
    - embolism 996.72
    - occlusion NEC 996.72
    - thrombus 996.72
  - electrodes
    - brain 996.75
    - heart 996.72
  - gastrointestinal NEC 996.79
  - genitourinary NEC 996.76
  - heart valve prosthesis NEC 996.71
  - infusion pump 996.74
  - internal
    - joint prosthesis 996.77
    - orthopedic NEC 996.78
    - specified type NEC 996.79
  - intrauterine contraceptive device NEC 996.76
  - joint prosthesis, internal NEC 996.77
  - mechanical — *see* Complications, mechanical
  - nervous system NEC 996.75
  - ocular lens NEC 996.79
  - orbital NEC 996.79
  - orthopedic NEC 996.78
    - joint, internal 996.77
  - renal dialysis 996.73
  - specified type NEC 996.79
  - urinary catheter, indwelling 996.76
  - vascular NEC 996.74

Complications — *continued*
- due to (presence of) any device, implant, or graft classified to 996.0-996.5 NEC — *continued*
  - ventricular shunt 996.75
- during dialysis NEC 999.9
- ectopic or molar pregnancy NEC 639.9
- electroshock therapy NEC 999.9
- enterostomy 569.60
  - specified type NEC 569.69
- external (fixation) device with internal component(s) NEC 996.78
  - infection or inflammation 996.67
  - mechanical 996.4
- extracorporeal circulation NEC 999.9
- eye implant (prosthetic) NEC 996.79
  - infection or inflammation 996.69
  - mechanical
    - ocular lens 996.53
    - orbital globe 996.59
- gastrointestinal, postoperative NEC (*see also* Complications, surgical procedures) 997.4
- gastrostomy 536.40
  - specified type NEC 536.49
- genitourinary device, implant or graft NEC 996.76
  - infection or inflammation 996.65
    - urinary catheter, indwelling 996.64
  - mechanical (*see also* Complications, mechanical, by type) 996.30
  - specified NEC 996.39
- graft (bypass) (patch) NEC — *see also* Complications, due to (presence of) any device, implant, or graft classified to 996.0-996.5 NEC
  - bone marrow 996.85
  - corneal NEC 996.79
    - infection or inflammation 996.69
    - rejection or reaction 996.51
  - mechanical — *see* Complications, mechanical, graft
  - organ (immune or nonimmune cause) (partial) (total) 996.80
    - bone marrow 996.85
    - heart 996.83
    - intestines 996.87
    - kidney 996.81
    - liver 996.82
    - lung 996.84
    - pancreas 996.86
    - specified NEC 996.89
  - skin NEC 996.79
    - infection or inflammation 996.69
    - rejection 996.52
      - artificial 996.55
      - decellularized allodermis 996.55
- heart — *see also* Disease, heart transplant (immune or nonimmune cause) 996.83
- hematoma (intraoperative) (postoperative) 998.12
- hemorrhage (intraoperative) (postoperative) 998.11
- hyperalimentation therapy NEC 999.9
- immunization (procedure) — *see* Complications, vaccination
- implant — *see also* Complications, due to (presence of) any device, implant, or graft classified to 996.0-996.5 NEC
  - mechanical — *see* Complications, mechanical, implant

Complications

Complications — *continued*
  infection and inflammation
    due to (presence of) any device, implant or graft classified to 996.0-996.5 NEC 996.60
      arterial NEC 996.62
        coronary 996.61
        renal dialysis 996.62
      arteriovenous fistula or shunt 996.62
      bone growth stimulator 996.67
      breast 996.69
      cardiac 996.61
      catheter NEC 996.69
        peritoneal 996.68
        spinal 996.63
        urinary, indwelling 996.64
        vascular NEC 996.62
        ventricular shunt 996.63
      coronary artery bypass 996.61
      electrodes
        brain 996.63
        heart 996.61
      gastrointestinal NEC 996.69
      genitourinary NEC 996.65
        indwelling urinary catheter 996.64
      heart valve 996.61
      infusion pump 996.62
      intrauterine contraceptive device 996.65
      joint prosthesis, internal 996.66
      ocular lens 996.69
      orbital (implant) 996.69
      orthopedic NEC 996.67
        joint, internal 996.66
      specified type NEC 996.69
      urinary catheter, indwelling 996.64
      ventricular shunt 996.63
  infusion (procedure) 999.9
    blood — *see* Complications, transfusion
    infection NEC 999.3
    sepsis NEC 999.3
  inhalation therapy NEC 999.9
  injection (procedure) 999.9
    drug reaction (*see also* Reaction, drug) 995.2
    infection NEC 999.3
    sepsis NEC 999.3
    serum (prophylactic) (therapeutic) — *see* Complications, vaccination
    vaccine (any) — *see* Complications, vaccination
  inoculation (any) — *see* Complications, vaccination
  internal device (catheter) (electronic) (fixation) (prosthetic) NEC — *see* Complications, due to (presence of) any device, implant, or graft classified to 996.0-996.5 NEC
    mechanical — *see* Complications, mechanical
  intestinal transplant (immune or nonimmune cause) 996.87
  intraoperative bleeding or hemorrhage 998.11
  intrauterine contraceptive device 996.76 — *see also* Complications, contraceptive device
    with fetal damage affecting management of pregnancy 655.8
    infection or inflammation 996.65
  jejunostomy 569.60
  kidney transplant (immune or nonimmune cause) 996.81

Complications — *continued*
  labor 669.9
    specified condition NEC 669.8
  liver transplant (immune or nonimmune cause) 996.82
  lumbar puncture 349.0
  mechanical
    anastomosis — *see* Complications, mechanical, graft
    bypass — *see* Complications, mechanical, graft
    catheter NEC 996.59
      cardiac 996.09
      cystostomy 996.39
      dialysis (hemodialysis) 996.1
        peritoneal 996.56
      during a procedure 998.2
      urethral, indwelling 996.31
    colostomy 569.62
    device NEC 996.59
      balloon (counterpulsation), intra-aortic 996.1
      cardiac 996.00
        automatic implantable defibrillator 996.04
        long-term effect 429.4
        specified NEC 996.09
      contraceptive, intrauterine 996.32
      counterpulsation, intra-aortic 996.1
      fixation, external, with internal components 996.4
      fixation, internal (nail, rod, plate) 996.4
      genitourinary 996.30
        specified NEC 996.39
      nervous system 996.2
      orthopedic, internal 996.4
      prosthetic NEC 996.59
      umbrella, vena cava 996.1
      vascular 996.1
    dorsal column stimulator 996.2
    electrode NEC 996.59
      brain 996.2
      cardiac 996.01
      spinal column 996.2
    enterostomy 569.62
    fistula, arteriovenous, surgically created 996.1
    gastrostomy 536.42
    graft NEC 996.52
      aortic (bifurcation) 996.1
      aortocoronary bypass 996.03
      blood vessel NEC 996.1
      bone 996.4
      cardiac 996.00
      carotid artery bypass 996.1
      cartilage 996.4
      corneal 996.51
      coronary bypass 996.03
      decellularized allodermis 996.55
      genitourinary 996.30
        specified NEC 996.39
      muscle 996.4
      nervous system 996.2
      organ (immune or nonimmune cause) 996.80
        heart 996.83
        intestines 996.87
        kidney 996.81
        liver 996.82
        lung 996.84
        pancreas 996.86

Index to Diseases — Complications

Complications — *continued*
  mechanical — *continued*
    graft NEC — *continued*
      organ — *continued*
        specified NEC 996.89
      orthopedic, internal 996.4
      peripheral nerve 996.2
      prosthetic NEC 996.59
      skin 996.52
        artificial 996.55
      specified NEC 996.59
      tendon 996.4
      tissue NEC 996.52
      tooth 996.59
      ureter, without mention of resection 996.39
      vascular 996.1
    heart valve prosthesis 996.02
      long-term effect 429.4
    implant NEC 996.59
      cardiac 996.00
        automatic implantable defibrillator 996.04
        long-term effect 429.4
        specified NEC 996.09
      electrode NEC 996.59
        brain 996.2
        cardiac 996.01
        spinal column 996.2
      genitourinary 996.30
      nervous system 996.2
      orthopedic, internal 996.4
      prosthetic NEC 996.59
        in
          bile duct 996.59
          breast 996.54
          chin 996.59
          eye
            ocular lens 996.53
            orbital globe 996.59
      vascular 996.1
    nonabsorbable surgical material 996.59
    pacemaker NEC 996.59
      brain 996.2
      cardiac 996.01
      nerve (phrenic) 996.2
    patch — *see* Complications, mechanical, graft
    prosthesis NEC 996.59
      bile duct 996.59
      breast 996.54
      chin 996.59
      ocular lens 996.53
      reconstruction, vas deferens 996.39
    reimplant NEC 996.59
      extremity (*see also* Complications, reattached, extremity) 996.90
      organ (*see also* Complications, transplant, organ, by site) 996.80
    repair — *see* Complications, mechanical, graft
    shunt NEC 996.59
      arteriovenous, surgically created 996.1
      ventricular (communicating) 996.2
    stent NEC 996.59
    tracheostomy 519.02
    vas deferens reconstruction 996.39
  medical care NEC 999.9
    cardiac NEC 997.1
    gastrointestinal NEC 997.4
    nervous system NEC 997.00

Complications — *continued*
  medical care NEC — *continued*
    peripheral vascular NEC 997.2
    respiratory NEC 997.3
    urinary NEC 997.5
    vascular
      mesenteric artery 997.71
      other vessels 997.79
      peripheral vessels 997.2
      renal artery 997.72
  nephrostomy 997.5
  nervous system
    device, implant, or graft NEC 349.1
      mechanical 996.2
    postoperative NEC 997.00
  obstetric 669.9
    procedure (instrumental) (manual) (surgical) 669.4
    specified NEC 669.8
    surgical wound 674.3
  ocular lens implant NEC 996.79
    infection or inflammation 996.69
    mechanical 996.53
  organ transplant — *see* Complications, transplant, organ, by site
  orthopedic device, implant, or graft
    internal (fixation) (nail) (plate) (rod) NEC 996.78
      infection or inflammation 996.67
    joint prosthesis 996.77
      infection or inflammation 996.66
    mechanical 996.4
  pacemaker (cardiac) 996.72
    infection or inflammation 996.61
    mechanical 996.01
  pancreas transplant (immune or nonimmune cause) 996.86
  perfusion NEC 999.9
  perineal repair (obstetrical) 674.3
    disruption 674.2
  pessary (uterus) (vagina) — *see* Complications, contraceptive device
  phototherapy 990
  postcystoscopic 997.5
  postmastoidectomy NEC 383.30
  postoperative — *see* Complications, surgical procedures
  pregnancy NEC 646.9
    affecting fetus or newborn 761.9
  prosthetic device, internal NEC — *see also* Complications, due to (presence of) any device, implant or graft classified to 996.0-996.5 NEC
    mechanical NEC (*see also* Complications, mechanical) 996.59
  puerperium NEC (*see also* Puerperal) 674.9
  puncture, spinal 349.0
  pyelogram 997.5
  radiation 990
  radiotherapy 990
  reattached
    body part, except extremity 996.99
    extremity (infection) (rejection) 996.90
      arm(s) 996.94
      digit(s) (hand) 996.93
        foot 996.95
      finger(s) 996.93
      foot 996.95
      forearm 996.91
      hand 996.92

Complications — *continued*
  reattached — *continued*
    extremity — *continued*
      leg 996.96
      lower NEC 996.96
      toe(s) 996.95
      upper NEC 996.94
    reimplant NEC — *see also* Complications, to (presence of) any device, implant, or graft classified to 996.0-996.5 NEC
  bone marrow 996.85
    extremity (*see also* Complications, reattached, extremity) 996.90
      due to infection 996.90
    mechanical — *see* Complications, mechanical, reimplant
    organ (immune or nonimmune cause) (partial) (total) (*see also* Complications, transplant, organ, by site) 996.80
  renal allograft 996.81
  renal dialysis — *see* Complications, dialysis
  respiratory 519.9
    device, implant or graft NEC 996.79
      infection or inflammation 996.69
      mechanical 996.59
    distress syndrome, adult, following trauma or surgery 518.5
    insufficiency, acute, postoperative 518.5
    postoperative NEC 997.3
    therapy NEC 999.9
  sedation during labor and delivery 668.9 ✓5ᵗʰ
    affecting fetus or newborn 763.5
    cardiac 668.1 ✓5ᵗʰ
    central nervous system 668.2 ✓5ᵗʰ
    pulmonary 668.0 ✓5ᵗʰ
    specified type NEC 668.8 ✓5ᵗʰ
  seroma (intraoperative) (postoperative) (noninfected) 998.13
    infected 998.51
  shunt NEC — *see also* Complications, due to (presence of) any device, implant, or graft classified to 996.0-996.5 NEC
    mechanical — *see* Complications, mechanical, shunt
  specified body system NEC
    device, implant, or graft NEC — *see* Complications, due to (presence of) any device, implant, or graft classified to 996.0-996.5 NEC
    postoperative NEC 997.99
  spinal puncture or tap 349.0
  stoma, external
    gastrointestinal tract
      colostomy 569.60
      enterostomy 569.60
      gastrostomy 536.40
    urinary tract 997.5
  surgical procedures 998.9
    accidental puncture or laceration 998.2
    amputation stump (late) 997.60
    anastomosis — *see* Complications, anastomosis
    burst stitches or sutures ▶(external)◀ 998.32 ▲
      internal 998.31 ●
    cardiac 997.1
      long-term effect following cardiac surgery 429.4
    cataract fragments in eye 998.82

Complications — *continued*
  surgical procedures — *continued*
    catheter device — *see* Complications, catheter device
    cecostomy malfunction 569.62
    colostomy malfunction 569.62
    cystostomy malfunction 997.5
    dehiscence (of incision) ▶(external)◀ 998.32 ▲
      internal 998.31 ●
    dialysis NEC (*see also* Complications, dialysis) 999.9
    disruption
      anastomosis (internal) — *see* Complications, mechanical, graft
      internal suture (line) 998.31 ▲
      wound ▶(external)◀ 998.32 ▲
        internal 998.31 ●
    dumping syndrome (postgastrectomy) 564.2
    elephantiasis or lymphedema 997.99
      postmastectomy 457.0
    emphysema (surgical) 998.81
    enterostomy malfunction 569.62
    evisceration 998.32 ▲
    fistula (persistent postoperative) 998.6
    foreign body inadvertently left in wound (sponge) (suture) (swab) 998.4
    from nonabsorbable surgical material (Dacron) (mesh) (permanent suture) (reinforcing) (Teflon) — *see* Complications, due to (presence of) any device, implant, or graft classified to 996.0-996.5 NEC
    gastrointestinal NEC 997.4
    gastrostomy malfunction 536.42
    hematoma 998.12
    hemorrhage 998.11
    ileostomy malfunction 569.62
    internal prosthetic device NEC (*see also* Complications, internal device) 996.70
      hemolytic anemia 283.19
      infection or inflammation 996.60
      malfunction — *see* Complications, mechanical
      mechanical complication — *see* Complications, mechanical
      thrombus 996.70
    jejunostomy malfunction 569.62
    nervous system NEC 997.00
    obstruction, internal anastomosis — *see* Complications, mechanical, graft
    other body system NEC 997.99
    peripheral vascular NEC 997.2
    postcardiotomy syndrome 429.4
    postcholecystectomy syndrome 576.0
    postcommissurotomy syndrome 429.4
    postgastrectomy dumping syndrome 564.2
    postmastectomy lymphedema syndrome 457.0
    postmastoidectomy 383.30
      cholesteatoma, recurrent 383.32
      cyst, mucosal 383.31
      granulation 383.33
      inflammation, chronic 383.33
    postvagotomy syndrome 564.2
    postvalvulotomy syndrome 429.4
    reattached extremity (infection) (rejection) (*see also* Complications, reattached, extremity) 996.90
    respiratory NEC 997.3

Complications — *continued*
  surgical procedures — *continued*
    seroma 998.13
    shock (endotoxic) (hypovolemic) (septic) 998.0
    shunt, prosthetic (thrombus) — *see also* Complications, due to (presence of) any device, implant, or graft classified to 996.0-996.5 NEC
      hemolytic anemia 283.19
    specified complication NEC 998.89
    stitch abscess 998.59
    transplant — *see* Complications, graft
    ureterostomy malfunction 997.5
    urethrostomy malfunction 997.5
    urinary NEC 997.5
    vascular
      mesenteric artery 997.71
      other vessels 997.79
      peripheral vessels 997.2
      renal artery 997.72
    wound infection 998.59
  therapeutic misadventure NEC 999.9
    surgical treatment 998.9
  tracheostomy 519.00
  transfusion (blood) (lymphocytes) (plasma) NEC 999.8
    atrophy, liver, yellow, subacute (within 8 months of administration) — *see* Hepatitis, viral
    bone marrow 996.85
    embolism
      air 999.1
      thrombus 999.2
    hemolysis NEC 999.8
      bone marrow 996.85
    hepatitis (serum) (type B) (within 8 months after administration) — *see* Hepatitis, viral
    incompatibility reaction (ABO) (blood group) 999.6
      Rh (factor) 999.7
    infection 999.3
    jaundice (serum) (within 8 months after administration) — *see* Hepatitis, viral
    sepsis 999.3
    shock or reaction NEC 999.8
      bone marrow 996.85
    subacute yellow atrophy of liver (within 8 months after administration) — *see* Hepatitis, viral
    thromboembolism 999.2
  transplant NEC — *see also* Complications, due to (presence of) any device, implant, or graft classified to 996.0-996.5 NEC
    bone marrow 996.85
    organ (immune or nonimmune cause) (partial) (total) 996.80
      bone marrow 996.85
      heart 996.83
      intestines 996.87
      kidney 996.81
      liver 996.82
      lung 996.84
      pancreas 996.86
      specified NEC 996.89
  trauma NEC (early) 958.8
  ultrasound therapy NEC 999.9
  umbilical cord
    affecting fetus or newborn 762.6
    complicating delivery 663.9

Complications — *continued*
  umbilical cord — *continued*
    complicating delivery — *continued*
      affecting fetus or newborn 762.6
      specified type NEC 663.8
  urethral catheter NEC 996.76
    infection or inflammation 996.64
    mechanical 996.31
  urinary, postoperative NEC 997.5
  vaccination 999.9
    anaphylaxis NEC 999.4
    cellulitis 999.3
    encephalitis or encephalomyelitis 323.5
    hepatitis (serum) (type B) (within 8 months after administration) — *see* Hepatitis, viral
    infection (general) (local) NEC 999.3
    jaundice (serum) (within 8 months after administration) — *see* Hepatitis, viral
    meningitis 997.09 *[321.8]*
    myelitis 323.5
    protein sickness 999.5
    reaction (allergic) 999.5
      Herxheimer's 995.0
      serum 999.5
    sepsis 999.3
    serum intoxication, sickness, rash, or other serum reaction NEC 999.5
    shock (allergic) (anaphylactic) 999.4
    subacute yellow atrophy of liver (within 8 months after administration) — *see* Hepatitis, viral
    vaccinia (generalized) 999.0
      localized 999.3
  vascular
    device, implant, or graft NEC 996.74
    infection or inflammation 996.62
    mechanical NEC 996.1
      cardiac (*see also* Complications, mechanical, by type) 996.00
    following infusion, perfusion, or transfusion 999.2
    postoperative NEC 997.2
      mesenteric artery 997.71
      other vessels 997.79
      peripheral vessels 997.2
      renal artery 997.72
  ventilation therapy NEC 999.9

Compound presentation, complicating delivery 652.8
  causing obstructed labor 660.0

Compressed air disease 993.3

Compression
  with injury — *see* specific injury
  arm NEC 354.9
  artery 447.1
    celiac, syndrome 447.4
  brachial plexus 353.0
  brain (stem) 348.4
    due to
      contusion, brain — *see* Contusion, brain
      injury NEC — *see also* Hemorrhage, brain, traumatic
      birth — *see* Birth, injury, brain
      laceration, brain — *see* Laceration, brain
    osteopathic 739.0
  bronchus 519.1
  by cicatrix — *see* Cicatrix
  cardiac 423.9
  cauda equina 344.60
    with neurogenic bladder 344.61

Compression — *continued*
  celiac (artery) (axis) 447.4
  cerebral — *see* Compression, brain
  cervical plexus 353.2
  cord (umbilical) — *see* Compression, umbilical
    cord
  cranial nerve 352.9
    second 377.49
    third (partial) 378.51
      total 378.52
    fourth 378.53
    fifth 350.8
    sixth 378.54
    seventh 351.8
  divers' squeeze 993.3
  duodenum (external) (*see also* Obstruction,
    duodenum) 537.3
  during birth 767.9
  esophagus 530.3
    congenital, external 750.3
  Eustachian tube 381.63
  facies (congenital) 754.0
  fracture — *see* Fracture, by site
  heart — *see* Disease, heart
  intestine (*see also* Obstruction, intestine)
    560.9
    with hernia — *see* Hernia, by site, with
      obstruction
  laryngeal nerve, recurrent 478.79
  leg NEC 355.8
  lower extremity NEC 355.8
  lumbosacral plexus 353.1
  lung 518.89
  lymphatic vessel 457.1
  medulla — *see* Compression, brain
  nerve NEC — *see also* Disorder, nerve
    arm NEC 354.9
    autonomic nervous system (*see also*
      Neuropathy, peripheral, autonomic)
      337.9
    axillary 353.0
    cranial NEC 352.9
    due to displacement of intervertebral disc
      722.2
      with myelopathy 722.70
      cervical 722.0
        with myelopathy 722.71
      lumbar, lumbosacral 722.10
        with myelopathy 722.73
      thoracic, thoracolumbar 722.11
        with myelopathy 722.72
    iliohypogastric 355.79
    ilioinguinal 355.79
    leg NEC 355.8
    lower extremity NEC 355.8
    median (in carpal tunnel) 354.0
    obturator 355.79
    optic 377.49
    plantar 355.6
    posterior tibial (in tarsal tunnel) 355.5
    root (by scar tissue) NEC 724.9
      cervical NEC 723.4
      lumbar NEC 724.4
      lumbosacral 724.4
      thoracic 724.4
    saphenous 355.79
    sciatic (acute) 355.0
    sympathetic 337.9
    traumatic — *see* Injury, nerve
    ulnar 354.2
    upper extremity NEC 354.9

Compression — *continued*
  peripheral — *see* Compression, nerve
  spinal (cord) (old or nontraumatic) 336.9
    by displacement of intervertebral disc —
      see Displacement, intervertebral disc
    nerve
      root NEC 724.9
        postoperative 722.80
          cervical region 722.81
          lumbar region 722.83
          thoracic region 722.82
        traumatic — *see* Injury, nerve, spinal
      traumatic — *see* Injury, nerve, spinal
    spondylogenic 721.91
      cervical 721.1
      lumbar, lumbosacral 721.42
      thoracic 721.41
    traumatic — *see also* Injury, spinal, by site
      with fracture, vertebra — *see* Fracture,
        vertebra, by site, with spinal cord
        injury
  spondylogenic — *see* Compression, spinal
    cord, spondylogenic
  subcostal nerve (syndrome) 354.8
  sympathetic nerve NEC 337.9
  syndrome 958.5
  thorax 512.8
    iatrogenic 512.1
    postoperative 512.1
  trachea 519.1
    congenital 748.3
  ulnar nerve (by scar tissue) 354.2
  umbilical cord
    affecting fetus or newborn 762.5
      cord prolapsed 762.4
    complicating delivery 663.2
      cord around neck 663.1
      cord prolapsed 663.0
  upper extremity NEC 354.9
  ureter 593.3
  urethra — *see* Stricture, urethra
  vein 459.2
  vena cava (inferior) (superior) 459.2
  vertebral NEC — *see* Compression, spinal
    (cord)

Compulsion, compulsive
  eating 307.51
  neurosis (obsessive) 300.3
  personality 301.4
  states (mixed) 300.3
  swearing 300.3
    in Gilles de la Tourette's syndrome 307.23
  tics and spasms 307.22
  water drinking NEC (syndrome) 307.9

Concato's disease (pericardial polyserositis)
  423.2
  peritoneal 568.82
  pleural — *see* Pleurisy

Concavity, chest wall 738.3

Concealed
  hemorrhage NEC 459.0
  penis 752.65

Concentric fading 368.12

Concern (normal) about sick person in family
  V61.49

Concrescence (teeth) 520.2

Concretio cordis 423.1
  rheumatic 393

Index to Diseases

Concretion — *see also* Calculus
  appendicular 543.9
  canaliculus 375.57
  clitoris 624.8
  conjunctiva 372.54
  eyelid 374.56
  intestine (impaction) (obstruction) 560.39
  lacrimal (passages) 375.57
  prepuce (male) 605
    female (clitoris) 624.8
  salivary gland (any) 527.5
  seminal vesicle 608.89
  stomach 537.89
  tonsil 474.8
Concussion (current) 850.9
  with
    loss of consciousness 850.5
      brief (less than one hour) 850.1
      moderate (1-24 hours) 850.2
      prolonged (more than 24 hours) (with complete recovery) (with return to pre-existing conscious level) 850.3
        without return to pre-existing conscious level 850.4
      mental confusion or disorientation (without loss of consciousness) 850.0
        with loss of consciousness — *see* Concussion, with, loss of consciousness
    without loss of consciousness 850.0
  blast (air) (hydraulic) (immersion) (underwater) 869.0
    with open wound into cavity 869.1
    abdomen or thorax — *see* Injury, internal, by site
    brain — *see* Concussion, brain
    ear (acoustic nerve trauma) 951.5
      with perforation, tympanic membrane — *see* Wound, open, ear drum
    thorax — *see* Injury, internal, intrathoracic organs NEC
  brain or cerebral (without skull fracture) 850.9
    with
      loss of consciousness 850.5
        brief (less than one hour) 850.1
        moderate (1-24 hours) 850.2
        prolonged (more than 24 hours) (with complete recovery) (with return to pre-existing conscious level) 850.3
          without return to pre-existing conscious level 850.4
        mental confusion or disorientation (without loss of consciousness) 850.0
          with loss of consciousness — *see* Concussion, brain, with, loss of consciousness
      skull fracture — *see* Fracture, skull, by site
    without loss of consciousness 850.0
  cauda equina 952.4
  cerebral — *see* Concussion, brain
  conus medullaris (spine) 952.4
  hydraulic — *see* Concussion, blast
  internal organs — *see* Injury, internal, by site
  labyrinth — *see* Injury, intracranial
  ocular 921.3
  osseous labyrinth — *see* Injury, intracranial

Concussion — *continued*
  spinal (cord) — *see also* Injury, spinal, by site
  due to
    broken
      back — *see* Fracture, vertebra, by site, with spinal cord injury
      neck — *see* Fracture, vertebra, cervical, with spinal cord injury
    fracture, fracture dislocation, or compression fracture of spine or vertebra — *see* Fracture, vertebra, by site, with spinal cord injury
  syndrome 310.2
  underwater blast — *see* Concussion, blast
Condition — *see also* Disease
  psychiatric 298.9
  respiratory NEC 519.9
    acute or subacute NEC 519.9
      due to
        external agent 508.9
          specified type NEC 508.8
        fumes or vapors (chemical) (inhalation) 506.3
        radiation 508.0
    chronic NEC 519.9
      due to
        external agent 508.9
          specified type NEC 508.8
        fumes or vapors (chemical) (inhalation) 506.4
        radiation 508.1
    due to
      external agent 508.9
        specified type NEC 508.8
      fumes or vapors (chemical) (inhalation) 506.9
Conduct disturbance (*see also* Disturbance, conduct) 312.9
  adjustment reaction 309.3
  hyperkinetic 314.2
Condyloma NEC 078.10
  acuminatum 078.11
  gonorrheal 098.0
  latum 091.3
  syphilitic 091.3
    congenital 090.0
  venereal, syphilitic 091.3
Confinement — *see* Delivery
Conflagration — *see also* Burn, by site
  asphyxia (by inhalation of smoke, gases, fumes, or vapors) 987.9
  specified agent — *see* Table of Drugs and Chemicals
Conflict
  family V61.9
    specified circumstance NEC V61.8
  interpersonal NEC V62.81
  marital V61.10
    involving divorce or estrangement V61.0
  parent-child V61.20
  partner V61.10
Confluent — *see* condition
Confusion, confused (mental) (state) (*see also* State, confusional) 298.9
  acute 293.0
  epileptic 293.0
  postoperative 293.9
  psychogenic 298.2
  reactive (from emotional stress, psychological trauma) 298.2
  subacute 293.1

Congelation 991.9
Congenital — *see also* condition
　aortic septum 747.29
　intrinsic factor deficiency 281.0
　malformation — *see* Anomaly
Congestion, congestive (chronic) (passive)
　asphyxia, newborn 768.9
　bladder 596.8
　bowel 569.89
　brain (*see also* Disease, cerebrovascular NEC) 437.8
　　malarial 084.9
　breast 611.79
　bronchi 519.1
　bronchial tube 519.1
　catarrhal 472.0
　cerebral — *see* Congestion, brain
　cerebrospinal — *see* Congestion, brain
　chest 514
　chill 780.99
　　malarial (*see also* Malaria) 084.6
　circulatory NEC 459.9
　conjunctiva 372.71
　due to disturbance of circulation 459.9
　duodenum 537.3
　enteritis — *see* Enteritis
　eye 372.71
　fibrosis syndrome (pelvic) 625.5
　gastroenteritis — *see* Enteritis
　general 799.8
　glottis 476.0
　heart (*see also* Failure, heart) 428.0
　hepatic 573.0
　hypostatic (lung) 514
　intestine 569.89
　intracranial — *see* Congestion, brain
　kidney 593.89
　labyrinth 386.50
　larynx 476.0
　liver 573.0
　lung 514
　　active or acute (*see also* Pneumonia) 486
　　　congenital 770.0
　　chronic 514
　　hypostatic 514
　　idiopathic, acute 518.5
　　passive 514
　malaria, malarial (brain) (fever) (*see also* Malaria) 084.6
　medulla — *see* Congestion, brain
　nasal 478.1
　orbit, orbital 376.33
　　inflammatory (chronic) 376.10
　　　acute 376.00
　ovary 620.8
　pancreas 577.8
　pelvic, female 625.5
　pleural 511.0
　prostate (active) 602.1
　pulmonary — *see* Congestion, lung
　renal 593.89
　retina 362.89
　seminal vesicle 608.89
　spinal cord 336.1
　spleen 289.51
　　chronic 289.51
　stomach 537.89
　trachea 464.11
　urethra 599.84

Congestion, congestive — *continued*
　uterus 625.5
　　with subinvolution 621.1
　viscera 799.8
Congestive — *see* Congestion
Conical
　cervix 622.6
　cornea 371.60
　teeth 520.2
Conjoined twins 759.4
　causing disproportion (fetopelvic) 653.7 ▲
Conjugal maladjustment V61.10
　involving divorce or estrangement V61.0
Conjunctiva — *see* condition
Conjunctivitis (exposure) (infectious) (nondiphtheritic) (pneumococcal) (pustular) (staphylococcal) (streptococcal) NEC 372.30
　actinic 370.24
　acute 372.00
　　atopic 372.05
　　contagious 372.03
　　follicular 372.02
　　hemorrhagic (viral) 077.4
　adenoviral (acute) 077.3
　allergic (chronic) 372.14
　　with hay fever 372.05
　anaphylactic 372.05
　angular 372.03
　Apollo (viral) 077.4
　atopic 372.05
　blennorrhagic (neonatorum) 098.40
　catarrhal 372.03
　chemical 372.05
　chlamydial 077.98
　　due to
　　　Chlamydia trachomatis — *see* Trachoma
　　paratrachoma 077.0
　chronic 372.10
　　allergic 372.14
　　follicular 372.12
　　simple 372.11
　　specified type NEC 372.14
　　vernal 372.13
　diphtheritic 032.81
　due to
　　dust 372.05
　　enterovirus type 70 077.4
　　erythema multiforme 695.1 *[372.33]*
　　filiariasis (*see also* Filiariasis) 125.9 *[372.15]*
　　mucocutaneous
　　　disease NEC 372.33
　　　leishmaniasis 085.5 *[372.15]*
　　Reiter's disease 099.3 *[372.33]*
　　syphilis 095.8 *[372.10]*
　　toxoplasmosis (acquired) 130.1
　　　congenital (active) 771.2
　　trachoma — *see* Trachoma
　dust 372.05
　eczematous 370.31
　epidemic 077.1
　　hemorrhagic 077.4
　follicular (acute) 372.02
　　adenoviral (acute) 077.3
　　chronic 372.12
　glare 370.24
　gonococcal (neonatorum) 098.40
　granular (trachomatous) 076.1
　　late effect 139.1
　hemorrhagic (acute) (epidemic) 077.4

Index to Diseases

Conjunctivitis — *continued*
  herpetic (simplex) 054.43
    zoster 053.21
  inclusion 077.0
  infantile 771.6
  influenzal 372.03
  Koch-Weeks 372.03
  light 372.05
  medicamentosa 372.05
  membranous 372.04
  meningococcic 036.89
  Morax-Axenfeld 372.02
  mucopurulent NEC 372.03
  neonatal 771.6
    gonococcal 098.40
  Newcastle's 077.8
  nodosa 360.14
  of Beal 077.3
  parasitic 372.15
    filariasis (*see also* Filariasis) 125.9
      [372.15]
    mucocutaneous leishmaniasis 085.5
      [372.15]
  Parinaud's 372.02
  petrificans 372.39
  phlyctenular 370.31
  pseudomembranous 372.04
    diphtheritic 032.81
  purulent 372.03
  Reiter's 099.3 [372.33]
  rosacea 695.3 [372.31]
  serous 372.01
    viral 077.99
  simple chronic 372.11
  specified NEC 372.39
  sunlamp 372.04
  swimming pool 077.0
  trachomatous (follicular) 076.1
    acute 076.0
    late effect 139.1
  traumatic NEC 372.39
  tuberculous (*see also* Tuberculosis) 017.3 ✓5ᵗʰ
    [370.31]
  tularemic 021.3
  tularensis 021.3
  vernal 372.13
    limbar 372.13 [370.32]
  viral 077.99
    acute hemorrhagic 077.4
    specified NEC 077.8
Conjunctivochalasis 372.81
Conjunctoblepharitis — *see* Conjunctivitis
Conn (-Louis) syndrome (primary aldosteronism) 255.1
Connective tissue — *see* condition
Conradi (-Hünermann) syndrome or disease
  (chondrodysplasia calcificans congenita) 756.59
Consanguinity V19.7
Consecutive — *see* condition
Consolidated lung (base) — *see* Pneumonia, lobar
Constipation 564.00
  atonic 564.09
  drug induced
    correct substance properly administered 564.09

Constipation — *continued*
  drug induced — *continued*
    overdose or wrong substance given or taken 977.9
    specified drug — *see* Table of Drugs and Chemicals
  neurogenic 564.09
  other specified NEC 564.09
  outlet dysfunction 564.02
  psychogenic 306.4
  simple 564.00
  slow transit 564.01
  spastic 564.09
Constitutional — *see also* condition
  arterial hypotension (*see also* Hypotension) 458.9
  obesity 278.00
    morbid 278.01
  psychopathic state 301.9
  short stature in childhood 783.43
  state, developmental V21.9
    specified development NEC V21.8
  substandard 301.6
Constitutionally substandard 301.6
Constriction
  anomalous, meningeal bands or folds 742.8
  aortic arch (congenital) 747.10
  asphyxiation or suffocation by 994.7
  bronchus 519.1
  canal, ear (*see also* Stricture, ear canal, acquired) 380.50
  duodenum 537.3
  gallbladder (*see also* Obstruction, gallbladder) 575.2
    congenital 751.69
  intestine (*see also* Obstruction, intestine) 560.9
  larynx 478.74
    congenital 748.3
  meningeal bands or folds, anomalous 742.8
  organ or site, congenital NEC — *see* Atresia
  prepuce (congenital) 605
  pylorus 537.0
    adult hypertrophic 537.0
    congenital or infantile 750.5
      newborn 750.5
  ring (uterus) 661.4 ✓5ᵗʰ
    affecting fetus or newborn 763.7
  spastic — *see also* Spasm
    ureter 593.3
    urethra — *see* Stricture, urethra
  stomach 537.89
  ureter 593.3
  urethra — *see* Stricture, urethra
  visual field (functional) (peripheral) 368.45
Constrictive — *see* condition
Consultation
  medical — *see also* Counseling, medical
    specified reason NEC V65.8
  without complaint or sickness V65.9
    feared complaint unfounded V65.5
    specified reason NEC V65.8
Consumption — *see* Tuberculosis
Contact
  with
    AIDS virus V01.7
    anthrax V01.81
    cholera V01.0
    communicable disease V01.9
      specified type NEC V01.89

Contact — continued
  with — continued
    communicable disease — continued
      viral NEC V01.7
      German measles V01.4
      gonorrhea V01.6
      HIV V01.7
      human immunodeficiency virus V01.7
      parasitic disease NEC V01.89 ▲
      poliomyelitis V01.2
      rabies V01.5
      rubella V01.4
      smallpox V01.3
      syphilis V01.6
      tuberculosis V01.1
      venereal disease V01.6
      viral disease NEC V01.7
    dermatitis — see Dermatitis

Contamination, food (see also Poisoning, food) 005.9

Contraception, contraceptive
  advice NEC V25.09
    family planning V25.09
    fitting of diaphragm V25.02
    prescribing or use of
      oral contraceptive agent V25.01
      specified agent NEC V25.02
  counseling NEC V25.09
    family planning V25.09
    fitting of diaphragm V25.02
    prescribing or use of
      oral contraceptive agent V25.01
      specified agent NEC V25.02
  device (in situ) V45.59
    causing menorrhagia 996.76
    checking V25.42
    complications 996.32
    insertion V25.1
    intrauterine V45.51
    reinsertion V25.42
    removal V25.42
    subdermal V45.52
  fitting of diaphragm V25.02
  insertion
    intrauterine contraceptive device V25.1
    subdermal implantable V25.5
  maintenance V25.40
    examination V25.40
      subdermal implantable V25.43
        intrauterine device V25.42
      oral contraceptive V25.41
      specified method NEC V25.49
    intrauterine device V25.42
    oral contraceptive V25.41
    specified method NEC V25.49
    subdermal implantable V25.43
  management NEC V25.49
  prescription
    oral contraceptive agent V25.01
      repeat V25.41
    specified agent NEC V25.02
      repeat V25.49
  sterilization V25.2
  surveillance V25.40
    intrauterine device V25.42
    oral contraceptive agent V25.41
      subdermal implantable V25.43
    specified method NEC V25.49

Contraction, contracture, contracted
  Achilles tendon (see also Short, tendon, Achilles) 727.81

Contraction, contracture, contracted — continued
  anus 564.89
  axilla 729.9
  bile duct (see also Disease, biliary) 576.8
  bladder 596.8
    neck or sphincter 596.0
  bowel (see also Obstruction, intestine) 560.9
  Braxton Hicks 644.1 ✓5ᵗʰ
  bronchus 519.1
  burn (old) — see Cicatrix
  cecum (see also Obstruction, intestine) 560.9
  cervix (see also Stricture, cervix) 622.4
    congenital 752.49
  cicatricial — see Cicatrix
  colon (see also Obstruction, intestine) 560.9
  conjunctiva trachomatous, active 076.1
    late effect 139.1
  Dupuytren's 728.6
  eyelid 374.41
  eye socket (after enucleation) 372.64
  face 729.9
  fascia (lata) (postural) 728.89
    Dupuytren's 728.6
    palmar 728.6
    plantar 728.71
  finger NEC 736.29
    congenital 755.59
    joint (see also Contraction, joint) 718.44
  flaccid, paralytic
    joint (see also Contraction, joint) 718.4 ✓5ᵗʰ
    muscle 728.85
    ocular 378.50
  gallbladder (see also Obstruction, gallbladder) 575.2
  hamstring 728.89
    tendon 727.81
  heart valve — see Endocarditis
  Hicks' 644.1 ✓5ᵗʰ
  hip (see also Contraction, joint) 718.4 ✓5ᵗʰ
  hourglass
    bladder 596.8
      congenital 753.8
    gallbladder (see also Obstruction, gallbladder) 575.2
      congenital 751.69
    stomach 536.8
      congenital 750.7
      psychogenic 306.4
    uterus 661.4 ✓5ᵗʰ
      affecting fetus or newborn 763.7
  hysterical 300.11
  infantile (see also Epilepsy) 345.6 ✓5ᵗʰ
  internal os (see also Stricture, cervix) 622.4
  intestine (see also Obstruction, intestine) 560.9
  joint (abduction) (acquired) (adduction) (flexion) (rotation) 718.40
    ankle 718.47
    congenital NEC 755.8
      generalized or multiple 754.89
        lower limb joints 754.89
          hip (see also Subluxation, congenital, hip) 754.32
        lower limb (including pelvic girdle) not involving hip 754.89
        upper limb (including shoulder girdle) 755.59
    elbow 718.42
    foot 718.47
    hand 718.44

Contraction, contracture, contracted — *continued*
  joint — *continued*
    hip 718.45
    hysterical 300.11
    knee 718.46
    multiple sites 718.49
    pelvic region 718.45
    shoulder (region) 718.41
    specified site NEC 718.48
    wrist 718.43
  kidney (granular) (secondary) (*see also* Sclerosis, renal) 587
    congenital 753.3
    hydronephritic 591
    pyelonephritic (*see also* Pyelitis, chronic) 590.00
    tuberculous (*see also* Tuberculosis) 016.0 ✓5ᵗʰ
  ligament 728.89
    congenital 756.89
  liver — *see* Cirrhosis, liver
  muscle (postinfectional) (postural) NEC 728.85
    congenital 756.89
      sternocleidomastoid 754.1
    extraocular 378.60
    eye (extrinsic) (*see also* Strabismus) 378.9
      paralytic (*see also* Strabismus, paralytic) 378.50
    flaccid 728.85
    hysterical 300.11
    ischemic (Volkmann's) 958.6
    paralytic 728.85
    posttraumatic 958.6
    psychogenic 306.0
    specified as conversion reaction 300.11
  myotonic 728.85
  neck (*see also* Torticollis) 723.5
    congenital 754.1
    psychogenic 306.0
  ocular muscle (*see also* Strabismus) 378.9
    paralytic (*see also* Strabismus, paralytic) 378.50
  organ or site, congenital NEC — *see* Atresia
  outlet (pelvis) — *see* Contraction, pelvis
  palmar fascia 728.6
  paralytic
    joint (*see also* Contraction, joint) 718.4 ✓5ᵗʰ
    muscle 728.85
      ocular (*see also* Strabismus, paralytic) 378.50
  pelvis (acquired) (general) 738.6
    affecting fetus or newborn 763.1
    complicating delivery 653.1 ✓5ᵗʰ
      causing obstructed labor 660.1 ✓5ᵗʰ
    generally contracted 653.1 ✓5ᵗʰ
      causing obstructed labor 660.1 ✓5ᵗʰ
    inlet 653.2 ✓5ᵗʰ
      causing obstructed labor 660.1 ✓5ᵗʰ
    midpelvic 653.8 ✓5ᵗʰ
      causing obstructed labor 660.1 ✓5ᵗʰ
    midplane 653.8 ✓5ᵗʰ
      causing obstructed labor 660.1 ✓5ᵗʰ
    outlet 653.3 ✓5ᵗʰ
      causing obstructed labor 660.1 ✓5ᵗʰ
  plantar fascia 728.71
  premature
    atrial 427.61
    auricular 427.61
    auriculoventricular 427.61
    heart (junctional) (nodal) 427.60

Contraction, contracture, contracted — *continued*
  premature — *continued*
    supraventricular 427.61
    ventricular 427.69
  prostate 602.8
  pylorus (*see also* Pylorospasm) 537.81
  rectosigmoid (*see also* Obstruction, intestine) 560.9
  rectum, rectal (sphincter) 564.89
    psychogenic 306.4
  ring (Bandl's) 661.4 ✓5ᵗʰ
    affecting fetus or newborn 763.7
  scar — *see* Cicatrix
  sigmoid (*see also* Obstruction, intestine) 560.9
  socket, eye 372.64
  spine (*see also* Curvature, spine) 737.9
  stomach 536.8
    hourglass 536.8
      congenital 750.7
      psychogenic 306.4
    psychogenic 306.4
  tendon (sheath) (*see also* Short, tendon) 727.81
  toe 735.8
  ureterovesical orifice (postinfectional) 593.3
  urethra 599.84
  uterus 621.8
    abnormal 661.9 ✓5ᵗʰ
      affecting fetus or newborn 763.7
    clonic, hourglass or tetanic 661.4 ✓5ᵗʰ
      affecting fetus or newborn 763.7
    dyscoordinate 661.4 ✓5ᵗʰ
      affecting fetus or newborn 763.7
    hourglass 661.4 ✓5ᵗʰ
      affecting fetus or newborn 763.7
    hypotonic NEC 661.2 ✓5ᵗʰ
      affecting fetus or newborn 763.7
    incoordinate 661.4 ✓5ᵗʰ
      affecting fetus or newborn 763.7
    inefficient or poor 661.2 ✓5ᵗʰ
      affecting fetus or newborn 763.7
    irregular 661.2 ✓5ᵗʰ
      affecting fetus or newborn 763.7
    tetanic 661.4 ✓5ᵗʰ
      affecting fetus or newborn 763.7
  vagina (outlet) 623.2
  vesical 596.8
    neck or urethral orifice 596.0
  visual field, generalized 368.45
  Volkmann's (ischemic) 958.6

Contusion (skin surface intact) 924.9
  with
    crush injury — *see* Crush
    dislocation — *see* Dislocation, by site
    fracture — *see* Fracture, by site
    internal injury — *see also* Injury, internal, by site
      heart — *see* Contusion, cardiac
      kidney — *see* Contusion, kidney
      liver — *see* Contusion, liver
      lung — *see* Contusion, lung
      spleen — *see* Contusion, spleen
    intracranial injury — *see* Injury, intracranial
    nerve injury — *see* Injury, nerve
    open wound — *see* Wound, open, by site
  abdomen, abdominal (muscle) (wall) 922.2
    organ(s) NEC 868.00
  adnexa, eye NEC 921.9

Contusion

Contusion — *continued*
- ankle 924.21
  - with other parts of foot 924.20
- arm 923.9
  - lower (with elbow) 923.10
  - upper 923.03
    - with shoulder or axillary region 923.09
- auditory canal (external) (meatus) (and other part(s) of neck, scalp, or face, except eye) 920
- auricle, ear (and other part(s) of neck, scalp, or face except eye) 920
- axilla 923.02
  - with shoulder or upper arm 923.09
- back 922.31
- bone NEC 924.9
- brain (cerebral) (membrane) (with hemorrhage) 851.8 ✓5ᵗʰ

Note — *Use the following fifth-digit subclassification with categories 851-854:*

0	unspecified state of consciousness
1	with no loss of consciousness
2	with brief [less than one hour] loss of consciousness
3	with moderate [1-24 hours] loss of consciousness
4	with prolonged [more than 24 hours] loss of consciousness and return to pre-existing conscious level
5	with prolonged [more than 24 hours] loss of consciousness, without return to pre-existing conscious level

Use fifth-digit to designate when a patient is unconscious and dies before regaining consciousness, regardless of the duration of the loss of consciousness

6	with loss of consciousness of unspecified duration
9	with concussion, unspecified

- with
  - open intracranial wound 851.9 ✓5ᵗʰ
  - skull fracture — *see* Fracture, skull, by site
- cerebellum 851.4 ✓5ᵗʰ
  - with open intracranial wound 851.5 ✓5ᵗʰ
- cortex 851.0 ✓5ᵗʰ
  - with open intracranial wound 851.1 ✓5ᵗʰ
- occipital lobe 851.4 ✓5ᵗʰ
  - with open intracranial wound 851.5 ✓5ᵗʰ
- stem 851.4 ✓5ᵗʰ
  - with open intracranial wound 851.5 ✓5ᵗʰ
- breast 922.0
- brow (and other part(s) of neck, scalp, or face, except eye) 920
- buttock 922.32
- canthus 921.1
- cardiac 861.01
  - with open wound into thorax 861.11
- cauda equina (spine) 952.4
- cerebellum — *see* Contusion, brain, cerebellum
- cerebral — *see* Contusion, brain
- cheek(s) (and other part(s) of neck, scalp, or face, except eye) 920
- chest (wall) 922.1

Contusion — *continued*
- chin (and other part(s) of neck, scalp, or face, except eye) 920
- clitoris 922.4
- conjunctiva 921.1
- conus medullaris (spine) 952.4
- cornea 921.3
- corpus cavernosum 922.4
- cortex (brain) (cerebral) — *see* Contusion, brain, cortex
- costal region 922.1
- ear (and other part(s) of neck, scalp, or face except eye) 920
- elbow 923.11
  - with forearm 923.10
- epididymis 922.4
- epigastric region 922.2
- eye NEC 921.9
- eyeball 921.3
- eyelid(s) (and periocular area) 921.1
- face (and neck, or scalp, any part except eye) 920
- femoral triangle 922.2
- fetus or newborn 772.6
- finger(s) (nail) (subungual) 923.3
- flank 922.2
- foot (with ankle) (excluding toe(s)) 924.20
- forearm (and elbow) 923.10
- forehead (and other part(s) of neck, scalp, or face, except eye) 920
- genital organs, external 922.4
- globe (eye) 921.3
- groin 922.2
- gum(s) (and other part(s) of neck, scalp, or face, except eye) 920
- hand(s) (except fingers alone) 923.20
- head (any part, except eye) (and face) (and neck) 920
- heart — *see* Contusion, cardiac
- heel 924.20
- hip 924.01
  - with thigh 924.00
- iliac region 922.2
- inguinal region 922.2
- internal organs (abdomen, chest, or pelvis) NEC — *see* Injury, internal, by site
- interscapular region 922.33
- iris (eye) 921.3
- kidney 866.01
  - with open wound into cavity 866.11
- knee 924.11
  - with lower leg 924.10
- labium (majus) (minus) 922.4
- lacrimal apparatus, gland, or sac 921.1
- larynx (and other part(s) of neck, scalp, or face, except eye) 920
- late effect — *see* Late, effects (of), contusion
- leg 924.5
  - lower (with knee) 924.10
- lens 921.3
- lingual (and other part(s) of neck, scalp, or face, except eye) 920
- lip(s) (and other part(s) of neck, scalp, or face, except eye) 920
- liver 864.01
  - with
    - laceration — *see* Laceration, liver
    - open wound into cavity 864.11
- lower extremity 924.5
  - multiple sites 924.4
- lumbar region 922.31

Contusion — *continued*
  lung 861.21
    with open wound into thorax 861.31
  malar region (and other part(s) of neck, scalp, or face, except eye) 920
  mandibular joint (and other part(s) of neck, scalp, or face, except eye) 920
  mastoid region (and other part(s) of neck, scalp, or face, except eye) 920
  membrane, brain — *see* Contusion, brain
  midthoracic region 922.1
  mouth (and other part(s) of neck, scalp, or face, except eye) 920
  multiple sites (not classifiable to same three-digit category) 924.8
    lower limb 924.4
    trunk 922.8
    upper limb 923.8
  muscle NEC 924.9
  myocardium — *see* Contusion, cardiac
  nasal (septum) (and other part(s) of neck, scalp, or face, except eye) 920
  neck (and scalp, or face any part, except eye) 920
  nerve — *see* Injury, nerve, by site
  nose (and other part(s) of neck, scalp, or face, except eye) 920
  occipital region (scalp) (and neck or face, except eye) 920
    lobe — *see* Contusion, brain, occipital lobe
  orbit (region) (tissues) 921.2
  palate (soft) (and other part(s) of neck, scalp, or face, except eye) 920
  parietal region (scalp) (and neck, or face, except eye) 920
    lobe — *see* Contusion, brain
  penis 922.4
  pericardium — *see* Contusion, cardiac
  perineum 922.4
  periocular area 921.1
  pharynx (and other part(s) of neck, scalp, or face, except eye) 920
  popliteal space (*see also* Contusion, knee) 924.11
  prepuce 922.4
  pubic region 922.4
  pudenda 922.4
  pulmonary — *see* Contusion, lung
  quadriceps femoralis 924.00
  rib cage 922.1
  sacral region 922.32
  salivary ducts or glands (and other part(s) of neck, scalp, or face, except eye) 920
  scalp (and neck, or face any part, except eye) 920
  scapular region 923.01
    with shoulder or upper arm 923.09
  sclera (eye) 921.3
  scrotum 922.4
  shoulder 923.00
    with upper arm or axillar regions 923.09
  skin NEC 924.9
  skull 920
  spermatic cord 922.4
  spinal cord — *see also* Injury, spinal, by site
    cauda equina 952.4
    conus medullaris 952.4
  spleen 865.01
    with open wound into cavity 865.11
  sternal region 922.1
  stomach — *see* Injury, internal, stomach

Contusion — *continued*
  subconjunctival 921.1
  subcutaneous NEC 924.9
  submaxillary region (and other part(s) of neck, scalp, or face, except eye) 920
  submental region (and other part(s) of neck, scalp, or face, except eye) 920
  subperiosteal NEC 924.9
  supraclavicular fossa (and other part(s) of neck, scalp, or face, except eye) 920
  supraorbital (and other part(s) of neck, scalp, or face, except eye) 920
  temple (region) (and other part(s) of neck, scalp, or face, except eye) 920
  testis 922.4
  thigh (and hip) 924.00
  thorax 922.1
    organ — *see* Injury, internal, intrathoracic
  throat (and other part(s) of neck, scalp, or face, except eye) 920
  thumb(s) (nail) (subungual) 923.3
  toe(s) (nail) (subungual) 924.3
  tongue (and other part(s) of neck, scalp, or face, except eye) 920
  trunk 922.9
    multiple sites 922.8
    specified site — *see* Contusion, by site
  tunica vaginalis 922.4
  tympanum (membrane) (and other part(s) of neck, scalp, or face, except eye) 920
  upper extremity 923.9
    multiple sites 923.8
  uvula (and other part(s) of neck, scalp, or face, except eye) 920
  vagina 922.4
  vocal cord(s) (and other part(s) of neck, scalp, or face, except eye) 920
  vulva 922.4
  wrist 923.21
    with hand(s), except finger(s) alone 923.20
Conus (any type) (congenital) 743.57
  acquired 371.60
  medullaris syndrome 336.8
Convalescence (following) V66.9
  chemotherapy V66.2
  medical NEC V66.5
  psychotherapy V66.3
  radiotherapy V66.1
  surgery NEC V66.0
  treatment (for) NEC V66.5
    combined V66.6
    fracture V66.4
    mental disorder NEC V66.3
    specified disorder NEC V66.5
Conversion
  hysteria, hysterical, any type 300.11
  laparoscopic surgical procedure to open procedure V64.4
  neurosis, any 300.11
  reaction, any 300.11
Converter, tuberculosis (test reaction) 795.5
Convulsions (idiopathic) 780.39
  apoplectiform (*see also* Disease, cerebrovascular, acute) 436
  brain 780.39
  cerebral 780.39
  cerebrospinal 780.39
  due to trauma NEC — *see* Injury, intracranial
  eclamptic (*see also* Eclampsia) 780.39
  epileptic (*see also* Epilepsy) 345.9 ✓5ᵗʰ

Convulsions — *continued*
  epileptiform (*see also* Seizure, epileptiform) 780.39
  epileptoid (*see also* Seizure, epileptiform) 780.39
  ether
    anesthetic
      correct substance properly administered 780.39
      overdose or wrong substance given 968.2
    other specified type — *see* Table of Drugs and Chemicals
  febrile 780.31
  generalized 780.39
  hysterical 300.11
  infantile 780.39
    epilepsy — *see* Epilepsy
  internal 780.39
  jacksonian (*see also* Epilepsy) 345.5
  myoclonic 333.2
  newborn 779.0
  paretic 094.1
  pregnancy (nephritic) (uremic) — *see* Eclampsia, pregnancy
  psychomotor (*see also* Epilepsy) 345.4
  puerperal, postpartum — *see* Eclampsia, pregnancy
  recurrent 780.39
    epileptic — *see* Epilepsy
  reflex 781.0
  repetitive 780.39
    epileptic — *see* Epilepsy
  salaam (*see also* Epilepsy) 345.6
  scarlatinal 034.1
  spasmodic 780.39
  tetanus, tetanic (*see also* Tetanus) 037
  thymic 254.8
  uncinate 780.39
  uremic 586

Convulsive — *see also* Convulsions
  disorder or state 780.39
    epileptic — *see* Epilepsy
  equivalent, abdominal (*see also* Epilepsy) 345.5

Cooke-Apert-Gallais syndrome (adrenogenital) 255.2

Cooley's anemia (erythroblastic) 282.4

Coolie itch 126.9

Cooper's
  disease 610.1
  hernia — *see* Hernia, Cooper's

Coordination disturbance 781.3

Copper wire arteries, retina 362.13

Copra itch 133.8

Coprolith 560.39

Coprophilia 302.89

Coproporphyria, hereditary 277.1

Coprostasis 560.39
  with hernia — *see also* Hernia, by site, with obstruction
    gangrenous — *see* Hernia, by site, with gangrene

Cor
  biloculare 745.7
  bovinum — *see* Hypertrophy, cardiac
  bovis — *see also* Hypertrophy, cardiac
  pulmonale (chronic) 416.9
    acute 415.0

Cor — *continued*
  triatriatum, triatrium 746.82
  triloculare 745.8
    biatriatum 745.3
    biventriculare 745.69

Corbus' disease 607.1

Cord — *see also* condition
  around neck (tightly) (with compression)
    affecting fetus or newborn 762.5
    complicating delivery 663.1
      without compression 663.3
        affecting fetus or newborn 762.6
  bladder NEC 344.61
    tabetic 094.0
  prolapse
    affecting fetus or newborn 762.4
    complicating delivery 663.0

Cord's angiopathy (*see also* Tuberculosis) 017.3 [362.18]

Cordis ectopia 746.87

Corditis (spermatic) 608.4

Corectopia 743.46

Cori type glycogen storage disease — *see* Disease, glycogen storage

Cork-handlers' disease or lung 495.3

Corkscrew esophagus 530.5

Corlett's pyosis (impetigo) 684

Corn (infected) 700

Cornea — *see also* condition
  donor V59.5
  guttata (dystrophy) 371.57
  plana 743.41

Cornelia de Lange's syndrome (Amsterdam dwarf, mental retardation, and brachycephaly) 759.89

Cornual gestation or pregnancy — *see* Pregnancy, cornual

Cornu cutaneum 702.8

Coronary (artery) — *see also* condition
  arising from aorta or pulmonary trunk 746.85

Corpora — *see also* condition
  amylacea (prostate) 602.8
  cavernosa — *see* condition

Corpulence (*see also* Obesity) 278.0

Corpus — *see* condition

Corrigan's disease — *see* Insufficiency, aortic

Corrosive burn — *see* Burn, by site

Corsican fever (*see also* Malaria) 084.6

Cortical — *see also* condition
  blindness 377.75
  necrosis, kidney (bilateral) 583.6

Corticoadrenal — *see* condition

Corticosexual syndrome 255.2

Coryza (acute) 460
  with grippe or influenza 487.1
  syphilitic 095.8
    congenital (chronic) 090.0

Costen's syndrome or complex 524.60

Costiveness (*see also* Constipation) 564.00

Costochondritis 733.6

Cotard's syndrome (paranoia) 297.1

Cot death 798.0

Cotungo's disease 724.3

Cough 786.2
  with hemorrhage (*see also* Hemoptysis) 786.3

Index to Diseases

Cough — *continued*
  affected 786.2
  bronchial 786.2
    with grippe or influenza 487.1
  chronic 786.2
  epidemic 786.2
  functional 306.1
  hemorrhagic 786.3
  hysterical 300.11
  laryngeal, spasmodic 786.2
  nervous 786.2
  psychogenic 306.1
  smokers' 491.0
  tea tasters' 112.89
Counseling NEC V65.40
  without complaint or sickness V65.49
  abuse victim NEC V62.89
    child V61.21
    partner V61.11
    spouse V61.11
  child abuse, maltreatment, or neglect V61.21
  contraceptive NEC V25.09
    device (intrauterine) V25.02
    maintenance V25.40
      intrauterine contraceptive device V25.42
      oral contraceptive (pill) V25.41
      specified type NEC V25.49
      subdermal implantable V25.43
    management NEC V25.9
    oral contraceptive (pill) V25.01
    prescription NEC V25.02
      oral contraceptive (pill) V25.01
      repeat prescription V25.41
      repeat prescription V25.40
      subdermal implantable V25.43
    surveillance NEC V25.40
  dietary V65.3
  excercise V65.41
  explanation of
    investigation finding NEC V65.49
    medication NEC V65.49
  family planning V25.09
  for nonattending third party V65.1
  genetic V26.3
  gonorrhea V65.45
  health (advice) (education) (instruction) NEC V65.49
  HIV V65.44
  human immunodeficiency virus V65.44
  injury prevention V65.43
  marital V61.10
  medical (for) V65.9
    boarding school resident V60.6
    condition not demonstrated V65.5
    feared complaint and no disease found V65.5
    institutional resident V60.6
    on behalf of another V65.1
    person living alone V60.3
  parent-child conflict V61.20
    specified problem NEC V61.29
  partner abuse
    perpetrator V61.12
    victim V61.11
  perpetrator of
    child abuse V62.83
      parental V61.22
    partner abuse V61.12
    spouse abuse V61.12
  procreative V65.49

Counseling NEC — *continued*
  sex NEC V65.49
    transmitted disease NEC V65.45
      HIV V65.44
  specified reason NEC V65.49
  spousal abuse
    perpetrator V61.12
    victim V61.11
  substance use and abuse V65.42
  syphilis V65.45
  victim (of)
    abuse NEC V62.89
    child abuse V61.21
    partner abuse V61.11
    spousal abuse V61.11
Coupled rhythm 427.89
Couvelaire uterus (complicating delivery) — *see* Placenta, separation
Cowper's gland — *see* condition
Cowperitis (*see also* Urethritis) 597.89
  gonorrheal (acute) 098.0
    chronic or duration of 2 months or over 098.2
Cowpox (abortive) 051.0
  due to vaccination 999.0
  eyelid 051.0 *[373.5]*
    postvaccination 999.0 *[373.5]*
Coxa
  plana 732.1
  valga (acquired) 736.31
    congenital 755.61
    late effect of rickets 268.1
  vara (acquired) 736.32
    congenital 755.62
    late effect of rickets 268.1
Coxae malum senilis 715.25
Coxalgia (nontuberculous) 719.45
  tuberculous (*see also* Tuberculosis) 015.1 ✓5ᵗʰ *[730.85]*
Coxalgic pelvis 736.30
Coxitis 716.65
Coxsackie (infection) (virus) 079.2
  central nervous system NEC 048
  endocarditis 074.22
  enteritis 008.67
  meningitis (aseptic) 047.0
  myocarditis 074.23
  pericarditis 074.21
  pharyngitis 074.0
  pleurodynia 074.1
  specific disease NEC 074.8
Crabs, meaning pubic lice 132.2
Crack baby 760.75
Cracked nipple 611.2
  puerperal, postpartum 676.1 ✓5ᵗʰ
Cradle cap 690.11
Craft neurosis 300.89
Craigiasis 007.8
Cramp(s) 729.82
  abdominal 789.0 ✓5ᵗʰ
  bathing 994.1
  colic 789.0 ✓5ᵗʰ
  psychogenic 306.4
  due to immersion 994.1
  extremity (lower) (upper) NEC 729.82
  fireman 992.2
  heat 992.2
  hysterical 300.11

Cramp(s) — continued
  immersion 994.1
  intestinal 789.0 ✓5ᵗʰ
    psychogenic 306.4
  linotypist's 300.89
    organic 333.84
  muscle (extremity) (general) 729.82
    due to immersion 994.1
    hysterical 300.11
  occupational (hand) 300.89
    organic 333.84
  psychogenic 307.89
  salt depletion 276.1
  stoker 992.2
  stomach 789.0 ✓5ᵗʰ
  telegraphers' 300.89
    organic 333.84
  typists' 300.89
    organic 333.84
  uterus 625.8
    menstrual 625.3
  writers' 333.84
    organic 333.84
    psychogenic 300.89
Cranial — see condition
Cranioclasis, fetal 763.89
Craniocleidodysostosis 755.59
Craniofenestria (skull) 756.0
Craniolacunia (skull) 756.0
Craniopagus 759.4
Craniopathy, metabolic 733.3
Craniopharyngeal — see condition
Craniopharyngioma (M9350/1) 237.0
Craniorachischisis (totalis) 740.1
Cranioschisis 756.0
Craniostenosis 756.0
Craniosynostosis 756.0
Craniotabes (cause unknown) 733.3
  rachitic 268.1
  syphilitic 090.5
Craniotomy, fetal 763.89
Cranium — see condition
Craw-craw 125.3
Creaking joint 719.60
  ankle 719.67
  elbow 719.62
  foot 719.67
  hand 719.64
  hip 719.65
  knee 719.66
  multiple sites 719.69
  pelvic region 719.65
  shoulder (region) 719.61
  specified site NEC 719.68
  wrist 719.63
Creeping
  eruption 126.9
  palsy 335.21
  paralysis 335.21
Crenated tongue 529.8
Creotoxism 005.9
Crepitus
  caput 756.0
  joint 719.60
    ankle 719.67
    elbow 719.62
    foot 719.67

Crepitus — continued
  joint — continued
    hand 719.64
    hip 719.65
    knee 719.66
    multiple sites 719.69
    pelvic region 719.65
    shoulder (region) 719.61
    specified site NEC 719.68
    wrist 719.63
Crescent or conus choroid, congenital 743.57
Cretin, cretinism (athyrotic) (congenital) (endemic) (metabolic) (nongoitrous) (sporadic) 243
  goitrous (sporadic) 246.1
  pelvis (dwarf type) (male type) 243
    with disproportion (fetopelvic) 653.1 ✓5ᵗʰ
      affecting fetus or newborn 763.1
      causing obstructed labor 660.1 ✓5ᵗʰ
        affecting fetus or newborn 763.1
  pituitary 253.3
Cretinoid degeneration 243
Creutzfeldt-Jakob disease (syndrome) 046.1
  with dementia
    with behavioral disturbance 046.1 [294.11]
    without behavioral disturbance 046.1 [294.10]
Crib death 798.0
Cribriform hymen 752.49
Cri-du-chat syndrome 758.3
Crigler-Najjar disease or syndrome (congenital hyperbilirubinemia) 277.4
Crimean hemorrhagic fever 065.0
Criminalism 301.7
Crisis
  abdomen 789.0 ✓5ᵗʰ
  addisonian (acute adrenocortical insufficiency) 255.4
  adrenal (cortical) 255.4
  asthmatic — see Asthma
  brain, cerebral (see also Disease, cerebrovascular, acute) 436
  celiac 579.0
  Dietl's 593.4
  emotional NEC 309.29
    acute reaction to stress 308.0
    adjustment reaction 309.9
    specific to childhood and adolescence 313.9
  gastric (tabetic) 094.0
  glaucomatocyclitic 364.22
  heart (see also Failure, heart) 428.9
  hypertensive — see Hypertension
  nitritoid
    correct substance properly administered 458.2
    overdose or wrong substance given or taken 961.1
  oculogyric 378.87
    psychogenic 306.7
  Pel's 094.0
  psychosexual identity 302.6
  rectum 094.0
  renal 593.81
  sickle cell 282.62
  stomach (tabetic) 094.0
  tabetic 094.0
  thyroid (see also Thyrotoxicosis) 242.9 ✓5ᵗʰ
  thyrotoxic (see also Thyrotoxicosis) 242.9 ✓5ᵗʰ

Crisis — continued
  vascular — see Disease, cerebrovascular, acute
Crocq's disease (acrocyanosis) 443.89
Crohn's disease (see also Enteritis, regional) 555.9
Cronkhite-Canada syndrome 211.3
Crooked septum, nasal 470
Cross
  birth (of fetus) complicating delivery 652.3 ✓5ᵗʰ
    with successful version 652.1 ✓5ᵗʰ
    causing obstructed labor 660.0 ✓5ᵗʰ
  bite, anterior or posterior 524.2
  eye (see also Esotropia) 378.00
Crossed ectopia of kidney 753.3
Crossfoot 754.50
Croup, croupous (acute) (angina) (catarrhal) (infective) (inflammatory) (laryngeal) (membranous) (nondiphtheritic) (pseudomembranous) 464.4
  asthmatic (see also Asthma) 493.9 ✓5ᵗʰ
  bronchial 466.0
  diphtheritic (membranous) 032.3
  false 478.75
  spasmodic 478.75
    diphtheritic 032.3
  stridulous 478.75
    diphtheritic 032.3
Crouzon's disease (craniofacial dysostosis) 756.0
Crowding, teeth 524.3
CRST syndrome (cutaneous systemic sclerosis) 710.1
Cruchet's disease (encephalitis lethargica) 049.8
Cruelty in children (see also Disturbance, conduct) 312.9
Crural ulcer (see also Ulcer, lower extremity) 707.10
Crush, crushed, crushing (injury) 929.9
  with
    fracture — see Fracture, by site
  abdomen 926.19
    internal — see Injury, internal, abdomen
  ankle 928.21
    with other parts of foot 928.20
  arm 927.9
    lower (and elbow) 927.10
    upper 927.03
      with shoulder or axillary region 927.09
  axilla 927.02
    with shoulder or upper arm 927.09
  back 926.11
  breast 926.19
  buttock 926.12
  cheek 925.1
  chest — see Injury, internal, chest
  ear 925.1
  elbow 927.11
    with forearm 927.10
  face 925.1
  finger(s) 927.3
    with hand(s) 927.20
      and wrist(s) 927.21
  flank 926.19
  foot, excluding toe(s) alone (with ankle) 928.20
  forearm (and elbow) 927.10
  genitalia, external (female) (male) 926.0
    internal — see Injury, internal, genital organ NEC
  hand, except finger(s) alone (and wrist) 927.20

Crush, crushed, crushing — continued
  head — see Fracture, skull, by site
  heel 928.20
  hip 928.01
    with thigh 928.00
  internal organ (abdomen, chest, or pelvis) — see Injury, internal, by site
  knee 928.11
    with leg, lower 928.10
  labium (majus) (minus) 926.0
  larynx 925.2
  late effect — see Late, effects (of), crushing
  leg 928.9
    lower 928.10
      and knee 928.11
    upper 928.00
  limb
    lower 928.9
      multiple sites 928.8
    upper 927.9
      multiple sites 927.8
  multiple sites NEC 929.0
  neck 925.2
  nerve — see Injury, nerve, by site
  nose 802.0
    open 802.1
  penis 926.0
  pharynx 925.2
  scalp 925.1
  scapular region 927.01
    with shoulder or upper arm 927.09
  scrotum 926.0
  shoulder 927.00
    with upper arm or axillary region 927.09
  skull or cranium — see Fracture, skull, by site
  spinal cord — see Injury, spinal, by site
  syndrome (complication of trauma) 958.5
  testis 926.0
  thigh (with hip) 928.00
  throat 925.2
  thumb(s) (and fingers) 927.3
  toe(s) 928.3
    with foot 928.20
      and ankle 928.21
  tonsil 925.2
  trunk 926.9
    chest — see Injury, internal, intrathoracic organs NEC
    internal organ — see Injury, internal, by site
    multiple sites 926.8
    specified site NEC 926.19
  vulva 926.0
  wrist 927.21
    with hand(s), except fingers alone 927.20
Crusta lactea 690.11
Crusts 782.8
Crutch paralysis 953.4
Cruveilhier's disease 335.21
Cruveilhier-Baumgarten cirrhosis, disease, or syndrome 571.5
Cruz-Chagas disease (see also Trypanosomiasis) 086.2
Cryoglobulinemia (mixed) 273.2
Crypt (anal) (rectal) 569.49
Cryptitis (anal) (rectal) 569.49
Cryptococcosis (European) (pulmonary) (systemic) 117.5

Cryptococcus 117.5
  epidermicus 117.5
  neoformans, infection by 117.5
Cryptopapillitis (anus) 569.49
Cryptophthalmos (eyelid) 743.06
Cryptorchid, cryptorchism, cryptorchidism 752.51
Cryptosporidiosis 007.4
Cryptotia 744.29
Crystallopathy
  calcium pyrophosphate (*see also* Arthritis) 275.49 *[712.2]*
  dicalcium phosphate (*see also* Arthritis) 275.49 *[712.1]*
  gouty 274.0
  pyrophosphate NEC (*see also* Arthritis) 275.49 *[712.2]*
  uric acid 274.0
Crystalluria 791.9
Csillag's disease (lichen sclerosus or atrophicus) 701.0
Cuban itch 050.1
Cubitus
  valgus (acquired) 736.01
    congenital 755.59
    late effect of rickets 268.1
  varus (acquired) 736.02
    congenital 755.59
    late effect of rickets 268.1
Cultural deprivation V62.4
Cupping of optic disc 377.14
Curling's ulcer — *see* Ulcer, duodenum
Curling esophagus 530.5
Curschmann (-Batten) (-Steinert) disease or syndrome 359.2
Curvature
  organ or site, congenital NEC — *see* Distortion
  penis (lateral) 752.69
  Pott's (spinal) (*see also* Tuberculosis) 015.0 ✓5ᵗʰ *[737.43]*
  radius, idiopathic, progressive (congenital) 755.54
  spine (acquired) (angular) (idiopathic) (incorrect) (postural) 737.9
    congenital 754.2
    due to or associated with
      Charcôt-Marie-Tooth disease 356.1 *[737.40]*
      mucopolysaccharidosis 277.5 *[737.40]*
      neurofibromatosis 237.71 *[737.40]*
      osteitis
        deformans 731.0 *[737.40]*
        fibrosa cystica 252.0 *[737.40]*
      osteoporosis (*see also* Osteoporosis) 733.00 *[737.40]*
      poliomyelitis (*see also* Poliomyelitis) 138 *[737.40]*
      tuberculosis (Pott's curvature) (*see also* Tuberculosis) 015.0 ✓5ᵗʰ *[737.43]*
    kyphoscoliotic (*see also* Kyphoscoliosis) 737.30
    kyphotic (*see also* Kyphosis) 737.10
    late effect of rickets 268.1 *[737.40]*
    Pott's 015.0 ✓5ᵗʰ *[737.40]*
    scoliotic (*see also* Scoliosis) 737.30
    specified NEC 737.8
    tuberculous 015.0 ✓5ᵗʰ *[737.40]*

Cushing's
  basophilism, disease, or syndrome (iatrogenic) (idiopathic) (pituitary basophilism) (pituitary dependent) 255.0
  ulcer — *see* Ulcer, peptic
Cushingoid due to steroid therapy
  correct substance properly administered 255.0
  overdose or wrong substance given or taken 962.0
Cut (external) — *see* Wound, open, by site
Cutaneous — *see also* condition
  hemorrahage 782.7
  horn (cheek) (eyelid) (mouth) 702.8
  larva migrans 126.9
Cutis — *see also* condition
  hyperelastic 756.83
    acquired 701.8
  laxa 756.83
    senilis 701.8
  marmorata 782.61
  osteosis 709.3
  pendula 756.83
    acquired 701.8
  rhomboidalis nuchae 701.8
  verticis gyrata 757.39
    acquired 701.8
Cyanopathy, newborn 770.83 ▲
Cyanosis 782.5
  autotoxic 289.7
  common atrioventricular canal 745.69 ▲
  congenital 770.83 ▲
  conjunctiva 372.71
  due to
    endocardial cushion defect 745.60
    nonclosure, foramen botalli 745.5
    patent foramen botalli 745.5
    persistent foramen ovale 745.5
  enterogenous 289.7
  fetus or newborn 770.83 ▲
  ostium primum defect 745.61
  paroxysmal digital 443.0
  retina, retinal 362.10
Cycle
  anovulatory 628.0
  menstrual, irregular 626.4
Cyclencephaly 759.89
Cyclical vomiting 536.2
  psychogenic 306.4
Cyclitic membrane 364.74
Cyclitis (*see also* Iridocyclitis) 364.3
  acute 364.00
    primary 364.01
    recurrent 364.02
  chronic 364.10
    in
      sarcoidosis 135 *[364.11]*
      tuberculosis (*see also* Tuberculosis) 017.3 ✓5ᵗʰ *[364.11]*
  Fuchs' heterochromic 364.21
  granulomatous 364.10
  lens induced 364.23
  nongranulomatous 364.00
  posterior 363.21
  primary 364.01
  recurrent 364.02
  secondary (noninfectious) 364.04
    infectious 364.03
  subacute 364.00
    primary 364.01

Index to Diseases

Cyclitis — continued
  subacute — continued
    recurrent 364.02
Cyclokeratitis — see Keratitis
Cyclophoria 378.44
Cyclopia, cyclops 759.89
Cycloplegia 367.51
Cyclospasm 367.53
Cyclosporiasis 007.5
Cyclothymia 301.13
Cyclothymic personality 301.13
Cyclotropia 378.33
Cyesis — see Pregnancy
Cylindroma (M8200/3) — see also Neoplasm, by site, malignant
  eccrine dermal (M8200/0) — see Neoplasm, skin, benign
  skin (M8200/0) — see Neoplasm, skin, benign
Cylindruria 791.7
Cyllosoma 759.89
Cynanche
  diphtheritic 032.3
  tonsillaris 475
Cynorexia 783.6
Cyphosis — see Kyphosis
Cyprus fever (see also Brucellosis) 023.9
Cyriax's syndrome (slipping rib) 733.99
Cyst (mucus) (retention) (serous) (simple)

> Note — In general, cysts are not neoplastic and are classified to the approriate category for disease of the specified anatomical site. This generalization does not apply to certain types of cysts which are neoplastic in nature, for example, dermoid, nor does it apply to cysts of certain structures, for example, branchial cleft, which are classified as developmental anomalies.
>
> The following listing includes some of the most frequently reported sites of cysts as well as qualifiers which indicate the type of cyst. The latter qualifiers usually are not repeated under the anatomical sites. Since the code assignment for a given site may vary depending upon the type of cyst, the coder should refer to the listings under the specified type of cyst before consideration is given to the site.

  accessory, fallopian tube 752.11
  adenoid (infected) 474.8
  adrenal gland 255.8
    congenital 759.1
  air, lung 518.89
  allantoic 753.7
  alveolar process (jaw bone) 526.2
  amnion, amniotic 658.8 ✓5ᵗʰ
  anterior chamber (eye) 364.60
    exudative 364.62
    implantation (surgical) (traumatic) 364.61
    parasitic 360.13
  anterior nasopalatine 526.1
  antrum 478.1
  anus 569.49
  apical (periodontal) (tooth) 522.8
  appendix 543.9
  arachnoid, brain 348.0
  arytenoid 478.79

Cyst — continued
  auricle 706.2
  Baker's (knee) 727.51
    tuberculous (see also Tuberculosis) 015.2 ✓5ᵗʰ
  Bartholin's gland or duct 616.2
  bile duct (see also Disease, biliary) 576.8
  bladder (multiple) (trigone) 596.8
  Blessig's 362.62
  blood, endocardial (see also Endocarditis) 424.90
  blue dome 610.0
  bone (local) 733.20
    aneurysmal 733.22
    jaw 526.2
      developmental (odontogenic) 526.0
      fissural 526.1
      latent 526.89
    solitary 733.21
    unicameral 733.21
  brain 348.0
    congenital 742.4
    hydatid (see also Echinococcus) 122.9
    third ventricle (colloid) 742.4
  branchial (cleft) 744.42
  branchiogenic 744.42
  breast (benign) (blue dome) (pedunculated) (solitary) (traumatic) 610.0
    involution 610.4
    sebaceous 610.8
  broad ligament (benign) 620.8
    embryonic 752.11
  bronchogenic (mediastinal) (sequestration) 518.89
    congenital 748.4
  buccal 528.4
  bulbourethral gland (Cowper's) 599.89
  bursa, bursal 727.49
    pharyngeal 478.26
  calcifying odontogenic (M9301/0) 213.1
    upper jaw (bone) 213.0
  canal of Nuck (acquired) (serous) 629.1
    congenital 752.41
  canthus 372.75
  carcinomatous (M8010/3) — see Neoplasm, by site, malignant
  cartilage (joint) — see Derangement, joint
  cauda equina 336.8
  cavum septi pellucidi NEC 348.0
  celomic (pericardium) 746.89
  cerebellopontine (angle) — see Cyst, brain
  cerebellum — see Cyst, brain
  cerebral — see Cyst, brain
  cervical lateral 744.42
  cervix 622.8
    embryonal 752.41
    nabothian (gland) 616.0
  chamber, anterior (eye) 364.60
    exudative 364.62
    implantation (surgical) (traumatic) 364.61
    parasitic 360.13
  chiasmal, optic NEC (see also Lesion, chiasmal) 377.54
  chocolate (ovary) 617.1
  choledochal (congenital) 751.69
    acquired 576.8
  choledochus 751.69
  chorion 658.8 ✓5ᵗʰ
  choroid plexus 348.0
  chyle, mesentery 457.8

✓4ᵗʰ Fourth-digit Required   ✓5ᵗʰ Fifth-digit Required

Cyst — *continued*
- ciliary body 364.60
  - exudative 364.64
  - implantation 364.61
  - primary 364.63
- clitoris 624.8
- coccyx (*see also* Cyst, bone) 733.20
- colloid
  - third ventricle (brain) 742.4
  - thyroid gland — *see* Goiter
- colon 569.89
- common (bile) duct (*see also* Disease, biliary) 576.8
- congenital NEC 759.89
  - adrenal glands 759.1
  - epiglottis 748.3
  - esophagus 750.4
  - fallopian tube 752.11
  - kidney 753.10
    - multiple 753.19
    - single 753.11
  - larynx 748.3
  - liver 751.62
  - lung 748.4
  - mediastinum 748.8
  - ovary 752.0
  - oviduct 752.11
  - pancreas 751.7
  - periurethral (tissue) 753.8
  - prepuce NEC 752.69
    - penis 752.69
  - sublingual 750.26
  - submaxillary gland 750.26
  - thymus (gland) 759.2
  - tongue 750.19
  - ureterovesical orifice 753.4
  - vulva 752.41
- conjunctiva 372.75
- cornea 371.23
- corpora quadrigemina 348.0
- corpus
  - albicans (ovary) 620.2
  - luteum (ruptured) 620.1
- Cowper's gland (benign) (infected) 599.89
- cranial meninges 348.0
- craniobuccal pouch 253.8
- craniopharyngeal pouch 253.8
- cystic duct (*see also* Disease, gallbladder) 575.8
- Cysticercus (any site) 123.1
- Dandy-Walker 742.3
  - with spina bifida (*see also* Spina bifida) 741.0 ◢5ᵗʰ
- dental 522.8
  - developmental 526.0
  - eruption 526.0
  - lateral periodontal 526.0
  - primordial (keratocyst) 526.0
  - root 522.8
- dentigerous 526.0
  - mandible 526.0
  - maxilla 526.0
- dermoid (M9084/0) — *see also* Neoplasm, by site, benign
  - with malignant transformation (M9084/3) 183.0
  - implantation
    - external area or site (skin) NEC 709.8
    - iris 364.61
    - skin 709.8
    - vagina 623.8

Cyst — *continued*
- dermoid — *continued*
  - implantation — *continued*
    - vulva 624.8
  - mouth 528.4
  - oral soft tissue 528.4
  - sacrococcygeal 685.1
    - with abscess 685.0
- developmental of ovary, ovarian 752.0
- dura (cerebral) 348.0
  - spinal 349.2
- ear (external) 706.2
- echinococcal (*see also* Echinococcus) 122.9
- embryonal
  - cervix uteri 752.41
  - genitalia, female external 752.41
  - uterus 752.3
  - vagina 752.41
- endometrial 621.8
  - ectopic 617.9
- endometrium (uterus) 621.8
  - ectopic — *see* Endometriosis
- enteric 751.5
- enterogenous 751.5
- epidermal (inclusion) (*see also* Cyst, skin) 706.2
- epidermoid (inclusion) (*see also* Cyst, skin) 706.2
  - mouth 528.4
  - not of skin — *see* Cyst, by site
  - oral soft tissue 528.4
- epididymis 608.89
- epiglottis 478.79
- epiphysis cerebri 259.8
- epithelial (inclusion) (*see also* Cyst, skin) 706.2
- epoophoron 752.11
- eruption 526.0
- esophagus 530.89
- ethmoid sinus 478.1
- eye (retention) 379.8
  - congenital 743.03
  - posterior segment, congenital 743.54
- eyebrow 706.2
- eyelid (sebaceous) 374.84
  - infected 373.13
  - sweat glands or ducts 374.84
- falciform ligament (inflammatory) 573.8
- fallopian tube 620.8
- female genital organs NEC 629.8
- fimbrial (congenital) 752.11
- fissural (oral region) 526.1
- follicle (atretic) (graafian) (ovarian) 620.0
  - nabothian (gland) 616.0
- follicular (atretic) (ovarian) 620.0
  - dentigerous 526.0
- frontal sinus 478.1
- gallbladder or duct 575.8
- ganglion 727.43
- Gartner's duct 752.11
- gas, of mesentery 568.89
- gingiva 523.8
- gland of moll 374.84
- globulomaxillary 526.1
- graafian follicle 620.0
- granulosal lutein 620.2
- hemangiomatous (M9121/0) (*see also* Hemangioma) 228.00
- hydatid (*see also* Echinococcus) 122.9
  - fallopian tube (Morgagni) 752.11
  - liver NEC 122.8

Index to Diseases — Cyst

Cyst — *continued*
- hydatid — *continued*
  - lung NEC 122.9
  - Morgagni 752.8
    - fallopian tube 752.11
  - specified site NEC 122.9
- hymen 623.8
  - embryonal 752.41
- hypopharynx 478.26
- hypophysis, hypophyseal (duct) (recurrent) 253.8
  - cerebri 253.8
- implantation (dermoid)
  - anterior chamber (eye) 364.61
  - external area or site (skin) NEC 709.8
  - iris 364.61
  - vagina 623.8
  - vulva 624.8
- incisor, incisive canal 526.1
- inclusion (epidermal) (epithelial) (epidermoid) (mucous) (squamous) (*see also* Cyst, skin) 706.2
  - not of skin — *see* Neoplasm, by site, benign
- intestine (large) (small) 569.89
- intracranial — *see* Cyst, brain
- intraligamentous 728.89
  - knee 717.89
- intrasellar 253.8
- iris (idiopathic) 364.60
  - exudative 364.62
  - implantation (surgical) (traumatic) 364.61
  - miotic pupillary 364.55
  - parasitic 360.13
- Iwanoff's 362.62
- jaw (bone) (aneurysmal) (extravasation) (hemorrhagic) (traumatic) 526.2
  - developmental (odontogenic) 526.0
  - fissural 526.1
- keratin 706.2
- kidney (congenital) 753.10
  - acquired 593.2
  - calyceal (*see also* Hydronephrosis) 591
  - multiple 753.19
  - pyelogenic (*see also* Hydronephrosis) 591
  - simple 593.2
  - single 753.11
  - solitary (not congenital) 593.2
- labium (majus) (minus) 624.8
  - sebaceous 624.8
- lacrimal
  - apparatus 375.43
  - gland or sac 375.12
- larynx 478.79
- lens 379.39
  - congenital 743.39
- lip (gland) 528.5
- liver 573.8
  - congenital 751.62
  - hydatid (*see also* Echinococcus) 122.8
    - granulosis 122.0
    - multilocularis 122.5
- lung 518.89
  - congenital 748.4
  - giant bullous 492.0
- lutein 620.1
- lymphangiomatous (M9173/0) 228.1
- lymphoepithelial
  - mouth 528.4
  - oral soft tissue 528.4
- macula 362.54

Cyst — *continued*
- malignant (M8000/3) — *see* Neoplasm, by site, malignant
- mammary gland (sweat gland) (*see also* Cyst, breast) 610.0
- mandible 526.2
  - dentigerous 526.0
  - radicular 522.8
- maxilla 526.2
  - dentigerous 526.0
  - radicular 522.8
- median
  - anterior maxillary 526.1
  - palatal 526.1
- mediastinum (congenital) 748.8
- meibomian (gland) (retention) 373.2
  - infected 373.12
- membrane, brain 348.0
- meninges (cerebral) 348.0
  - spinal 349.2
- meniscus knee 717.5
- mesentery, mesenteric (gas) 568.89
  - chyle 457.8
  - gas 568.89
- mesonephric duct 752.8
- mesothelial
  - peritoneum 568.89
  - pleura (peritoneal) 569.89
- milk 611.5
- miotic pupillary (iris) 364.55
- Morgagni (hydatid) 752.8
  - fallopian tube 752.11
- mouth 528.4
- mullerian duct 752.8
- multilocular (ovary) (M8000/1) 239.5
- myometrium 621.8
- nabothian (follicle) (ruptured) 616.0
- nasal sinus 478.1
- nasoalveolar 528.4
- nasolabial 528.4
- nasopalatine (duct) 526.1
  - anterior 526.1
- nasopharynx 478.26
- neoplastic (M8000/1) — *see also* Neoplasm, by site, unspecified nature
  - benign (M8000/0) — *see* Neoplasm, by site, benign
  - uterus 621.8
- nervous system — *see* Cyst, brain
- neuroenteric 742.59
- neuroepithelial ventricle 348.0
- nipple 610.0
- nose 478.1
  - skin of 706.2
- odontogenic, developmental 526.0
- omentum (lesser) 568.89
  - congenital 751.8
- oral soft tissue (dermoid) (epidermoid) (lymphoepithelial) 528.4
- ora serrata 361.19
- orbit 376.81
- ovary, ovarian (twisted) 620.2
  - adherent 620.2
  - chocolate 617.1
  - corpus
    - albicans 620.2
    - luteum 620.1
  - dermoid (M9084/0) 220
  - developmental 752.0
  - due to failure of involution NEC 620.2
  - endometrial 617.1

Cyst

Cyst — *continued*
  ovary, ovarian — *continued*
    follicular (atretic) (graafian) (hemorrhagic) 620.0
    hemorrhagic 620.2
    in pregnancy or childbirth 654.4 ✓5ᵗʰ
      affecting fetus or newborn 763.89
      causing obstructed labor 660.2 ✓5ᵗʰ
        affecting fetus or newborn 763.1
    multilocular (M8000/1) 239.5
    pseudomucinous (M8470/0) 220
    retention 620.2
    serous 620.2
    theca lutein 620.2
    tuberculous (*see also* Tuberculosis) 016.6 ✓5ᵗʰ
    unspecified 620.2
  oviduct 620.8
  palatal papilla (jaw) 526.1
  palate 526.1
    fissural 526.1
    median (fissural) 526.1
  palatine, of papilla 526.1
  pancreas, pancreatic 577.2
    congenital 751.7
    false 577.2
    hemorrhagic 577.2
    true 577.2
  paranephric 593.2
  para ovarian 752.11
  paraphysis, cerebri 742.4
  parasitic NEC 136.9
  parathyroid (gland) 252.8
  paratubal (fallopian) 620.8
  paraurethral duct 599.89
  paroophoron 752.11
  parotid gland 527.6
    mucous extravasation or retention 527.6
  parovarian 752.11
  pars planus 364.60
    exudative 364.64
    primary 364.63
  pelvis, female
    in pregnancy or childbirth 654.4 ✓5ᵗʰ
      affecting fetus or newborn 763.89
      causing obstructed labor 660.2 ✓5ᵗʰ
        affecting fetus or newborn 763.1
  penis (sebaceous) 607.89
  periapical 522.8
  pericardial (congenital) 746.89
    acquired (secondary) 423.8
  pericoronal 526.0
  perineural (Tarlov's) 355.9
  periodontal 522.8
    lateral 526.0
  peripancreatic 577.2
  peripelvic (lymphatic) 593.2
  peritoneum 568.89
    chylous 457.8
  pharynx (wall) 478.26
  pilonidal (infected) (rectum) 685.1
    with abscess 685.0
    malignant (M9084/3) 173.5
  pituitary (duct) (gland) 253.8
  placenta (amniotic) — *see* Placenta, abnormal
  pleura 519.8
  popliteal 727.51
  porencephalic 742.4
    acquired 348.0
  postanal (infected) 685.1
    with abscess 685.0

Cyst — *continued*
  posterior segment of eye, congenital 743.54
  postmastoidectomy cavity 383.31
  preauricular 744.47
  prepuce 607.89
    congenital 752.69
  primordial (jaw) 526.0
  prostate 600.3
  pseudomucinous (ovary) (M8470/0) 220
  pudenda (sweat glands) 624.8
  pupillary, miotic 364.55
    sebaceous 624.8
  radicular (residual) 522.8
  radiculodental 522.8
  ranular 527.6
  Rathke's pouch 253.8
  rectum (epithelium) (mucous) 569.49
  renal — *see* Cyst, kidney
  residual (radicular) 522.8
  retention (ovary) 620.2
  retina 361.19
    macular 362.54
    parasitic 360.13
    primary 361.13
    secondary 361.14
  retroperitoneal 568.89
  sacrococcygeal (dermoid) 685.1
    with abscess 685.0
  salivary gland or duct 527.6
    mucous extravasation or retention 527.6
  Sampson's 617.1
  sclera 379.19
  scrotum (sebaceous) 706.2
    sweat glands 706.2
  sebaceous (duct) (gland) 706.2
    breast 610.8
    eyelid 374.84
    genital organ NEC
      female 629.8
      male 608.89
    scrotum 706.2
  semilunar cartilage (knee) (multiple) 717.5
  seminal vesicle 608.89
  serous (ovary) 620.2
  sinus (antral) (ethmoidal) (frontal) (maxillary) (nasal) (sphenoidal) 478.1
  Skene's gland 599.89
  skin (epidermal) (epidermoid, inclusion) (epithelial) (inclusion) (retention) (sebaceous) 706.2
    breast 610.8
    eyelid 374.84
    genital organ NEC
      female 629.8
      male 608.89
    neoplastic 216.3
    scrotum 706.2
    sweat gland or duct 705.89
  solitary
    bone 733.21
    kidney 593.2
  spermatic cord 608.89
  sphenoid sinus 478.1
  spinal meninges 349.2
  spine (*see also* Cyst, bone) 733.20
  spleen NEC 289.59
    congenital 759.0
    hydatid (*see also* Echinococcus) 122.9
  spring water (pericardium) 746.89
  subarachnoid 348.0
    intrasellar 793.0

Index to Diseases

Cyst — continued
- subdural (cerebral) 348.0
    - spinal cord 349.2
- sublingual gland 527.6
    - mucous extravasation or retention 527.6
- submaxillary gland 527.6
    - mucous extravasation or retention 527.6
- suburethral 599.89
- suprarenal gland 255.8
- suprasellar — see Cyst, brain
- sweat gland or duct 705.89
- sympathetic nervous system 337.9
- synovial 727.40
    - popliteal space 727.51
- Tarlov's 355.9
- tarsal 373.2
- tendon (sheath) 727.42
- testis 608.89
- theca-lutein (ovary) 620.2
- Thornwaldt's, Tornwaldt's 478.26
- thymus (gland) 254.8
- thyroglossal (duct) (infected) (persistent) 759.2
- thyroid (gland) 246.2
    - adenomatous — see Goiter, nodular
    - colloid (see also Goiter) 240.9
- thyrolingual duct (infected) (persistent) 759.2
- tongue (mucous) 529.8
- tonsil 474.8
- tooth (dental root) 522.8
- tubo-ovarian 620.8
    - inflammatory 614.1
- tunica vaginalis 608.89
- turbinate (nose) (see also Cyst, bone) 733.20
- Tyson's gland (benign) (infected) 607.89
- umbilicus 759.89
- urachus 753.7
- ureter 593.89
- ureterovesical orifice 593.89
    - congenital 753.4
- urethra 599.84
- urethral gland (Cowper's) 599.89
- uterine
    - ligament 620.8
        - embryonic 752.11
    - tube 620.8
- uterus (body) (corpus) (recurrent) 621.8
    - embryonal 752.3
- utricle (ear) 386.8
    - prostatic 599.89
- utriculus masculinus 599.89
- vagina, vaginal (squamous cell) (wall) 623.8
    - embryonal 752.41
    - implantation 623.8
    - inclusion 623.8
- vallecula, vallecular 478.79
- ventricle, neuroepithelial 348.0
- verumontanum 599.89
- vesical (orifice) 596.8
- vitreous humor 379.29
- vulva (sweat glands) 624.8
    - congenital 752.41
    - implantation 624.8
    - inclusion 624.8
    - sebaceous gland 624.8
- vulvovaginal gland 624.8
- wolffian 752.8

Cystadenocarcinoma (M8440/3) — see also Neoplasm, by site, malignant
- bile duct type (M8161/3) 155.1
- endometrioid (M8380/3) — see Neoplasm, by site, malignant

Cystadenocarcinoma — continued
- mucinous (M8470/3)
    - papillary (M8471/3)
        - specified site — see Neoplasm, by site, malignant
        - unspecified site 183.0
    - specified site — see Neoplasm, by site, malignant
    - unspecified site 183.0
- papillary (M8450/3)
    - mucinous (M8471/3)
        - specified site — see Neoplasm, by site, malignant
        - unspecified site 183.0
    - pseudomucinous (M8471/3)
        - specified site — see Neoplasm, by site, malignant
        - unspecified site 183.0
    - serous (M8460/3)
        - specified site — see Neoplasm, by site, malignant
        - unspecified site 183.0
    - specified site — see Neoplasm, by site, malignant
    - unspecified site 183.0
- pseudomucinous (M8470/3)
    - papillary (M8471/3)
        - specified site — see Neoplasm, by site, malignant
        - unspecified site 183.0
    - specified site — see Neoplasm, by site, malignant
    - unspecified site 183.0
- serous (M8441/3)
    - papillary (M8460/3)
        - specified site — see Neoplasm, by site, malignant
        - unspecified site 183.0
    - specified site — see Neoplasm, by site, malignant
    - unspecified site 183.0

Cystadenofibroma (M9013/0)
- clear cell (M8313/0) — see Neoplasm, by site, benign
- endometrioid (M8381/0) 220
    - borderline malignancy (M8381/1) 236.2
    - malignant (M8381/3) 183.0
- mucinous (M9015/0)
    - specified site — see Neoplasm, by site, benign
    - unspecified site 220
- serous (M9014/0)
    - specified site — see Neoplasm, by site, benign
    - unspecified site 220
- specified site — see Neoplasm, by site, benign
- unspecified site 220

Cystadenoma (M8440/0) — see also Neoplasm, by site, benign
- bile duct (M8161/0) 211.5
- endometrioid (M8380/0) — see also Neoplasm, by site, benign
    - borderline malignancy (M8380/1) — see Neoplasm, by site, uncertain behavior
    - malignant (M8440/3) — see Neoplasm, by site, malignant
- mucinous (M8470/0)
    - borderline malignancy (M8470/1)
        - specified site — see Neoplasm, uncertain behavior
        - unspecified site 236.2

Cystadenoma — *continued*
  mucinous — *continued*
    papillary (M8471/0)
      borderline malignancy (M8471/1)
        specified site — *see* Neoplasm, by site, uncertain behavior
        unspecified site 236.2
      specified site — *see* Neoplasm, by site, benign
      unspecified site 220
    specified site — *see* Neoplasm, by site, benign
    unspecified site 220
  papillary (M8450/0)
    borderline malignancy (M8450/1)
      specified site — *see* Neoplasm, by site, uncertain behavior
      unspecified site 236.2
    lymphomatosum (M8561/0) 210.2
    mucinous (M8471/0)
      borderline malignancy (M8471/1)
        specified site — *see* Neoplasm, by site, uncertain behavior
        unspecified site 236.2
      specified site — *see* Neoplasm, by site, benign
      unspecified site 220
    pseudomucinous (M8471/0)
      borderline malignancy (M8471/1)
        specified site — *see* Neoplasm, by site, uncertain behavior
        unspecified site 236.2
      specified site — *see* Neoplasm, by site, benign
      unspecified site 220
    serous (M8460/0)
      borderline malignancy (M8460/1)
        specified site — *see* Neoplasm, by site, uncertain behavior
        unspecified site 236.2
      specified site — *see* Neoplasm, by site, benign
      unspecified site 220
    specified site — *see* Neoplasm, by site, benign
    unspecified site 220
  pseudomucinous (M8470/0)
    borderline malignancy (M8470/1)
      specified site — *see* Neoplasm, by site, uncertain behavior
      unspecified site 236.2
    papillary (M8471/0)
      borderline malignancy (M8471/1)
        specified site — *see* Neoplasm, by site, uncertain behavior
        unspecified site 236.2
      specified site — *see* Neoplasm, by site, benign
      unspecified site 220
    specified site — *see* Neoplasm, by site, benign
    unspecified site 220
  serous (M8441/0)
    borderline malignancy (M8441/1)
      specified site — *see* Neoplasm, by site, uncertain behavior
      unspecified site 236.2
    papillary (M8460/0)
      borderline malignancy (M8460/1)
        specified site — *see* Neoplasm, by site, uncertain behavior

Cystadenoma — *continued*
  serous — *continued*
    papillary — *continued*
      borderline malignancy — *continued*
        unspecified site 236.2
      specified site — *see* Neoplasm, by site, benign
      unspecified site 220
    specified site — *see* Neoplasm, by site, benign
    unspecified site 220
  thyroid 226
Cystathioninemia 270.4
Cystathioninuria 270.4
Cystic — *see also* condition
  breast, chronic 610.1
  corpora lutea 620.1
  degeneration, congenital
    brain 742.4
    kidney 753.10
  disease
    breast, chronic 610.1
    kidney, congenital 753.10
      medullary 753.16
      multiple 753.19
      polycystic — *see* Polycystic, kidney
      single 753.11
      specified NEC 753.19
    liver, congenital 751.62
    lung 518.89
      congenital 748.4
    pancreas, congenital 751.7
    semilunar cartilage 717.5
  duct — *see* condition
  eyeball, congenital 743.03
  fibrosis (pancreas) 277.00
    with
      manifestations
        gastrointestinal 277.03
        pulmonary 277.02
        specified NEC 277.09
      meconium ileus 277.01
      pulmonary exacerbation 277.02
  hygroma (M9173/0) 228.1
  kidney, congenital 753.10
    medullary 753.16
    multiple 753.19
    polycystic — *see* Polycystic, kidney
    single 753.11
    specified NEC 753.19
  liver, congenital 751.62
  lung 518.89
    congenital 748.4
  mass — *see* Cyst
  mastitis, chronic 610.1
  ovary 620.2
  pancreas, congenital 751.7
Cysticerciasis 123.1
Cysticercosis (mammary) (subretinal) 123.1
Cysticercus 123.1
  cellulosae infestation 123.1
Cystinosis (malignant) 270.0
Cystinuria 270.0
Cystitis (bacillary) (colli) (diffuse) (exudative) (hemorrhagic) (purulent) (recurrent) (septic) (suppurative) (ulcerative) 595.9
  with
    abortion — *see* Abortion, by type, with urinary tract infection

Cystitis — *continued*
 with — *continued*
  ectopic pregnancy (*see also* categories 633.0-633.9) 639.8
  fibrosis 595.1
  leukoplakia 595.1
  malakoplakia 595.1
  metaplasia 595.1
  molar pregnancy (*see also* categories 630-632) 639.8
 actinomycotic 039.8 *[595.4]*
 acute 595.0
  of trigone 595.3
 allergic 595.89
 amebic 006.8 *[595.4]*
 bilharzial 120.9 *[595.4]*
 blennorrhagic (acute) 098.11
  chronic or duration of 2 months or more 098.31
 bullous 595.89
 calculus 594.1
  chlamydial 099.53
 chronic 595.2
  interstitial 595.1
  of trigone 595.3
 complicating pregnancy, childbirth, or puerperium 646.6 ✓5ᵗʰ
  affecting fetus or newborn 760.1
 cystic(a) 595.81
 diphtheritic 032.84
 echinococcal
  granulosus 122.3 *[595.4]*
  multilocularis 122.6 *[595.4]*
 emphysematous 595.89
 encysted 595.81
 follicular 595.3
 following
  abortion 639.8
  ectopic or molar pregnancy 639.8
 gangrenous 595.89
 glandularis 595.89
 gonococcal (acute) 098.11
  chronic or duration of 2 months or more 098.31
 incrusted 595.89
 interstitial 595.1
 irradiation 595.82
 irritation 595.89
 malignant 595.89
 monilial 112.2
 of trigone 595.3
 panmural 595.1
 polyposa 595.89
 prostatic 601.3
 radiation 595.82
 Reiter's (abacterial) 099.3
 specified NEC 595.89
 subacute 595.2
 submucous 595.1
 syphilitic 095.8
 trichomoniasis 131.09
 tuberculous (*see also* Tuberculosis) 016.1 ✓5ᵗʰ
 ulcerative 595.1
Cystocele (-rectocele)
 female (without uterine prolapse) 618.0
  with uterine prolapse 618.4
   complete 618.3
   incomplete 618.2
 in pregnancy or childbirth 654.4 ✓5ᵗʰ
  affecting fetus or newborn 763.89

Cystocele — *continued*
 in pregnancy or childbirth — *continued*
  causing obstructed labor 660.2 ✓5ᵗʰ
   affecting fetus or newborn 763.1
 male 596.8
Cystoid
 cicatrix limbus 372.64
 degeneration macula 362.53
Cystolithiasis 594.1
Cystoma (M8440/0) — *see also* Neoplasm, by site, benign
 endometrial, ovary 617.1
 mucinous (M8470/0)
  specified site — *see* Neoplasm, by site, benign
  unspecified site 220
 serous (M8441/0)
  specified site — *see* Neoplasm, by site, benign
  unspecified site 220
 simple (ovary) 620.2
Cystoplegia 596.53
Cystoptosis 596.8
Cystopyelitis (*see also* Pyelitis) 590.80
Cystorrhagia 596.8
Cystosarcoma phyllodes (M9020/1) 238.3
 benign (M9020/0) 217
 malignant (M9020/3) — *see* Neoplasm, breast, malignant
Cystostomy status V44.50
 appendico-vesicostomy V44.52
 cutaneous-vesicostomy V44.51
 specified type NEC V44.59
 with complication 997.5
Cystourethritis (*see also* Urethritis) 597.89
Cystourethrocele (*see also* Cystocele)
 female (without uterine prolapse) 618.0
  with uterine prolapse 618.4
   complete 618.3
   incomplete 618.2
 male 596.8
Cytomegalic inclusion disease 078.5
 congenital 771.1
Cytomycosis, reticuloendothelial (*see also* Histoplasmosis, American) 115.00

D

Daae (-Finsen) disease (epidemic pleurodynia) 074.1
Dabney's grip 074.1
Da Costa's syndrome (neurocirculatory asthenia) 306.2
Dacryoadenitis, dacryadenitis 375.00
 acute 375.01
 chronic 375.02
Dacryocystitis 375.30
 acute 375.32
 chronic 375.42
 neonatal 771.6
 phlegmonous 375.33
 syphilitic 095.8
  congenital 090.0
 trachomatous, active 076.1
  late effect 139.1
 tuberculous (*see also* Tuberculosis) 017.3 ✓5ᵗʰ
Dacryocystoblenorrhea 375.42
Dacryocystocele 375.43
Dacryolith, dacryolithiasis 375.57
Dacryoma 375.43
Dacryopericystitis (acute) (subacute) 375.32
 chronic 375.42
Dacryops 375.11
Dacryosialadenopathy, atrophic 710.2
Dacryostenosis 375.56
 congenital 743.65
Dactylitis 686.9
 bone (*see also* Osteomyelitis) 730.2 ✓5ᵗʰ
 sickle cell 282.61
 syphilitic 095.5
 tuberculous (*see also* Tuberculosis) 015.5 ✓5ᵗʰ
Dactylolysis opontaned 136.0
Dactylosymphysis (*see also* Syndactylism) 755.10
Damage
 arteriosclerotic — *see* Arteriosclerosis
 brain 348.9
  anoxic, hypoxic 348.1
   during or resulting from a procedure 997.01
  child NEC 343.9
  due to birth injury 767.0
  minimal (child) (*see also* Hyperkinesia) 314.9
  newborn 767.0
 cardiac — *see also* Disease, heart
 cardiorenal (vascular) (*see also* Hypertension, cardiorenal) 404.90
 central nervous system — *see* Damage, brain
 cerebral NEC — *see* Damage, brain
 coccyx, complicating delivery 665.6 ✓5ᵗʰ
 coronary (*see also* Ischemia, heart) 414.9
 eye, birth injury 767.8
 heart — *see also* Disease, heart
  valve — *see* Endocarditis
 hypothalamus NEC 348.9
 liver 571.9
  alcoholic 571.3
 myocardium (*see also* Degeneration, myocardial) 429.1
 pelvic
  joint or ligament, during delivery 665.6 ✓5ᵗʰ

Damage — *continued*
 pelvic — *continued*
  organ NEC
   with
    abortion — *see* Abortion, by type, with damage to pelvic organs
    ectopic pregnancy (*see also* categories 633.0-633.9) 639.2
    molar pregnancy (*see also* categories 630-632) 639.2
   during delivery 665.5 ✓5ᵗʰ
   following
    abortion 639.2
    ectopic or molar pregnancy 639.2
 renal (*see also* Disease, renal) 593.9
 skin, solar 692.79
  acute 692.72
  chronic 692.74
 subendocardium, subendocardial (*see also* Degeneration, myocardial) 429.1
 vascular 459.9
Dameshek's syndrome (erythroblastic anemia) 282.4
Dana-Putnam syndrome (subacute combined sclerosis with pernicious anemia) 281.0 [336.2]
Danbolt (-Closs) syndrome (acrodermatitis enteropathica) 686.8
Dandruff 690.18
Dandy fever 061
Dandy-Walker deformity or syndrome (atresia, foramen of Magendie) 742.3
 with spina bifida (*see also* Spina bifida) 741.0 ✓5ᵗʰ
Dangle foot 736.79
Danielssen's disease (anesthetic leprosy) 030.1
Danlos' syndrome 756.83
Darier's disease (congenital) (keratosis follicularis) 757.39
 due to vitamin A deficiency 264.8
 meaning erythema annulare centrifugum 695.0
Darier-Roussy sarcoid 135
Darling's
 disease (*see also* Histoplasmosis, American) 115.00
 histoplasmosis (*see also* Histoplasmosis, American) 115.00
Dartre 054.9
Darwin's tubercle 744.29
Davidson's anemia (refractory) 284.9
Davies' disease 425.0
Davies-Colley syndrome (slipping rib) 733.99
Dawson's encephalitis 046.2
Day blindness (*see also* Blindness, day) 368.60
Dead
 fetus
  retained (in utero) 656.4 ✓5ᵗʰ
   early pregnancy (death before 22 completed weeks gestation) 632
   late (death after 22 completed weeks gestation) 656.4 ✓5ᵗʰ
  syndrome 641.3 ✓5ᵗʰ
 labyrinth 386.50
 ovum, retained 631
Deaf and dumb NEC 389.7

Deaf mutism (acquired) (congenital) NEC 389.7
  endemic 243
  hysterical 300.11
  syphilitic, congenital 090.0
Deafness (acquired) (bilateral) (both ears) (complete) (congenital) (hereditary) (middle ear) (partial) (unilateral) 389.9
  with blue sclera and fragility of bone 756.51
  auditory fatigue 389.9
  aviation 993.0
    nerve injury 951.5
  boilermakers' 951.5
  central 389.14
    with conductive hearing loss 389.2
  conductive (air) 389.00
    with sensorineural hearing loss 389.2
    combined types 389.08
    external ear 389.01
    inner ear 389.04
    middle ear 389.03
    multiple types 389.08
    tympanic membrane 389.02
  emotional (complete) 300.11
  functional (complete) 300.11
  high frequency 389.8
  hysterical (complete) 300.11
  injury 951.5
  low frequency 389.8
  mental 784.69
  mixed conductive and sensorineural 389.2
  nerve 389.12
    with conductive hearing loss 389.2
  neural 389.12
    with conductive hearing loss 389.2
  noise-induced 388.12
    nerve injury 951.5
  nonspeaking 389.7
  perceptive 389.10
    with conductive hearing loss 389.2
    central 389.14
    combined types 389.18
    multiple types 389.18
    neural 389.12
    sensory 389.11
  psychogenic (complete) 306.7
  sensorineural (see also Deafness, perceptive) 389.10
  sensory 389.11
    with conductive hearing loss 389.2
  specified type NEC 389.8
  sudden NEC 388.2
  syphilitic 094.89
  transient ischemic 388.02
  transmission — see Deafness, conductive
  traumatic 951.5
  word (secondary to organic lesion) 784.69
    developmental 315.31
Death
  after delivery (cause not stated) (sudden) 674.9
  anesthetic
    due to
      correct substance properly administered 995.4
      overdose or wrong substance given 968.4
      specified anesthetic — see Table of Drugs and Chemicals
    during delivery 668.9
  brain 348.8
  cardiac — see Disease, heart

Death — continued
  cause unknown 798.2
  cot (infant) 798.0
  crib (infant) 798.0
  fetus, fetal (cause not stated) (intrauterine) 779.9
    early, with retention (before 22 completed weeks gestation) 632
    from asphyxia or anoxia (before labor) 768.0
    during labor 768.1
    late, affecting management of pregnancy (after 22 completed weeks gestation) 656.4
  from pregnancy NEC 646.9
  instantaneous 798.1
  intrauterine (see also Death, fetus) 779.9
    complicating pregnancy 656.4
  maternal, affecting fetus or newborn 761.6
  neonatal NEC 779.9
  sudden (cause unknown) 798.1
    during delivery 669.9
      under anesthesia NEC 668.9
    infant, syndrome (SIDS) 798.0
    puerperal, during puerperium 674.9
  unattended (cause unknown) 798.9
  under anesthesia NEC
    due to
      correct substance properly administered 995.4
      overdose or wrong substance given 968.4
      specified anesthetic — see Table of Drugs and Chemicals
    during delivery 668.9
  violent 798.1
de Beurmann-Gougerot disease (sporotrichosis) 117.1
Debility (general) (infantile) (postinfectional) 799.3
  with nutritional difficulty 269.9
  congenital or neonatal NEC 779.9
  nervous 300.5
  old age 797
  senile 797
Débove's disease (splenomegaly) 789.2
Decalcification
  bone (see also Osteoporosis) 733.00
  teeth 521.8
Decapitation 874.9
  fetal (to facilitate delivery) 763.89
Decapsulation, kidney 593.89
Decay
  dental 521.00
  senile 797
  tooth, teeth 521.00
Decensus, uterus — see Prolapse, uterus
Deciduitis (acute)
  with
    abortion — see Abortion, by type, with sepsis
    ectopic pregnancy (see also categories 633.0-633.9) 639.0
    molar pregnancy (see also categories 630-632) 639.0
  affecting fetus or newborn 760.8
  following
    abortion 639.0
    ectopic or molar pregnancy 639.0

Deciduitis — continued
  in pregnancy 646.6 ✓5ᵗʰ
  puerperal, postpartum 670 ✓4ᵗʰ
Deciduoma malignum (M9100/3) 181
Deciduous tooth (retained) 520.6
Decline (general) (*see also* Debility) 799.3
Decompensation
  cardiac (acute) (chronic) (*see also* Disease, heart) 429.9
    failure — *see* Failure, heart
  cardiorenal (*see also* Hypertension, cardiorenal) 404.90
  cardiovascular (*see also* Disease, cardiovascular) 429.2
  heart (*see also* Disease, heart) 429.9
    failure — *see* Failure, heart
  hepatic 572.2
  myocardial (acute) (chronic) (*see also* Disease, heart) 429.9
    failure — *see* Failure, heart
  respiratory 519.9
Decompression sickness 993.3
Decrease, decreased
  blood
    platelets (*see also* Thrombocytopenia) 287.5
    pressure 796.3
      due to shock following
        injury 958.4
        operation 998.0
  cardiac reserve — *see* Disease, heart
  estrogen 256.39
    postablative 256.2
  fetal movements 655.7 ✓5ᵗʰ
  fragility of erythrocytes 289.8
  function
    adrenal (cortex) 255.4
      medulla 255.5
    ovary in hypopituitarism 253.4
    parenchyma of pancreas 577.8
    pituitary (gland) (lobe) (anterior) 253.2
      posterior (lobe) 253.8
  functional activity 780.99 ▲
  glucose 790.2
  haptoglobin (serum) NEC 273.8
  platelets (*see also* Thrombocytopenia) 287.5
  pulse pressure 785.9
  respiration due to shock following injury 958.4
  tear secretion NEC 375.15
  tolerance
    fat 579.8
    glucose 790.2
    salt and water 276.9
  vision NEC 369.9
Decubital gangrene 707.0 [785.4]
Decubiti (*see also* Decubitus) 707.0
Decubitus (ulcer) 707.0
  with gangrene 707.0 [785.4]
Deepening acetabulum 718.85
Defect, defective 759.9
  3-beta-hydroxysteroid dehydrogenase 255.2
  11-hydroxylase 255.2
  21-hydroxylase 255.2
  abdominal wall, congenital 756.70
  aorticopulmonary septum 745.0
  aortic septal 745.0
  atrial septal (ostium secundum type) 745.5
    acquired 429.71
    ostium primum type 745.61
    sinus venosus 745.8

Defect, defective — continued
  atrioventricular
    canal 745.69
    septum 745.4
      acquired 429.71
  atrium secundum 745.5
    acquired 429.71
  auricular septal 745.5
    acquired 429.71
  bilirubin excretion 277.4
  biosynthesis, testicular androgen 257.2
  bulbar septum 745.0
  butanol-insoluble iodide 246.1
  chromosome — *see* Anomaly, chromosome
  circulation (acquired) 459.9
    congenital 747.9
    newborn 747.9
  clotting NEC (*see also* Defect, coagulation) 286.9
  coagulation (factor) (*see also* Deficiency, coagulation factor) 286.9
    with
      abortion — *see* Abortion, by type, with hemorrhage
      ectopic pregnancy (*see also* categories 634-638) 639.1
      molar pregnancy (*see also* categories 630-632) 639.1
    acquired (any) 286.7
    antepartum or intrapartum 641.3 ✓5ᵗʰ
      affecting fetus or newborn 762.1
    causing hemorrhage of pregnancy or delivery 641.3 ✓5ᵗʰ
    due to
      liver disease 286.7
      vitamin K deficiency 286.7
    newborn, transient 776.3
    postpartum 666.3 ✓5ᵗʰ
    specified type NEC 286.3
  conduction (heart) 426.9
    bone (*see also* Deafness, conductive) 389.00
  congenital, organ or site NEC — *see also* Anomaly
    circulation 747.9
    Descemet's membrane 743.9
      specified type NEC 743.49
    diaphragm 756.6
    ectodermal 757.9
    esophagus 750.9
    pulmonic cusps — *see* Anomaly, heart valve
    respiratory system 748.9
      specified type NEC 748.8
  cushion endocardial 745.60
  dentin (hereditary) 520.5
  Descemet's membrane (congenital) 743.9
    acquired 371.30
    specific type NEC 743.49
  deutan 368.52
  developmental — *see also* Anomaly, by site
    cauda equina 742.59
    left ventricle 746.9
      with atresia or hypoplasia of aortic orifice or valve, with hypoplasia of ascending aorta 746.7
      in hypoplastic left heart syndrome 746.7
    testis 752.9
    vessel 747.9

Defect, defective — *continued*
  diaphragm
    with elevation, eventration, or hernia — *see* Hernia, diaphragm
    congenital 756.6
      with elevation, eventration, or hernia 756.6
        gross (with elevation, eventration, or hernia) 756.6
  ectodermal, congenital 757.9
  Eisenmenger's (ventricular septal defect) 745.4
  endocardial cushion 745.60
    specified type NEC 745.69
  esophagus, congenital 750.9
  extensor retinaculum 728.9
  fibrin polymerization (*see also* Defect, coagulation) 286.3
  filling
    biliary tract 793.3
    bladder 793.5
    gallbladder 793.3
    kidney 793.5
    stomach 793.4
    ureter 793.5
  fossa ovalis 745.5
  gene, carrier (suspected) of V83.89 ▲
  Gerbode 745.4
  glaucomatous, without elevated tension 365.89
  Hageman (factor) (*see also* Defect, coagulation) 286.3
  hearing (*see also* Deafness) 389.9
  high grade 317
  homogentisic acid 270.2
  interatrial septal 745.5
    acquired 429.71
  interauricular septal 745.5
    acquired 429.71
  interventricular septal 745.4
    with pulmonary stenosis or atresia, dextraposition of aorta, and hypertrophy of right ventricle 745.2
    acquired 429.71
    in tetralogy of Fallot 745.2
  iodide trapping 246.1
  iodotyrosine dehalogenase 246.1
  kynureninase 270.2
  learning, specific 315.2
  mental (*see also* Retardation, mental) 319
  osteochondral NEC 738.8
  ostium
    primum 745.61
    secundum 745.5
  pericardium 746.89
  peroxidase-binding 246.1
  placental blood supply — *see* Placenta, insufficiency
  platelet (qualitative) 287.1
    constitutional 286.4
  postural, spine 737.9
  protan 368.51
  pulmonic cusps, congenital 746.00
  renal pelvis 753.9
    obstructive 753.29
    specified type NEC 753.3
  respiratory system, congenital 748.9
    specified type NEC 748.8
  retina, retinal 361.30
    with detachment (*see also* Detachment, retina, with retinal defect) 361.00

Defect, defective — *continued*
  retina, retinal — *continued*
    multiple 361.33
      with detachment 361.02
    nerve fiber bundle 362.85
    single 361.30
      with detachment 361.01
  septal (closure) (heart) NEC 745.9
    acquired 429.71
    atrial 745.5
    specified type NEC 745.8
  speech NEC 784.5
    developmental 315.39
    secondary to organic lesion 784.5
  Taussig-Bing (transposition, aorta and overriding pulmonary artery) 745.11
  teeth, wedge 521.2
  thyroid hormone synthesis 246.1
  tritan 368.53
  ureter 753.9
    obstructive 753.29
  vascular (acquired) (local) 459.9
    congenital (peripheral) NEC 747.60
      gastrointestinal 747.61
      lower limb 747.64
      renal 747.62
      specified NEC 747.69
      spinal 747.82
      upper limb 747.63
  ventricular septal 745.4
    with pulmonary stenosis or atresia, dextraposition of aorta, and hypertrophy of right ventricle 745.2
    acquired 429.71
    atrioventricular canal type 745.69
    between infundibulum and anterior portion 745.4
    in tetralogy of Fallot 745.2
    isolated anterior 745.4
  vision NEC 369.9
  visual field 368.40
    arcuate 368.43
    heteronymous, bilateral 368.47
    homonymous, bilateral 368.46
    localized NEC 368.44
    nasal step 368.44
    peripheral 368.44
    sector 368.43
  voice 784.40
  wedge, teeth (abrasion) 521.2
Defeminization syndrome 255.2
Deferentitis 608.4
  gonorrheal (acute) 098.14
    chronic or duration of 2 months or over 098.34
Defibrination syndrome (*see also* Fibrinolysis) 286.6
Deficiency, deficient
  3-beta-hydroxysteroid dehydrogenase 255.2
  6-phosphogluconic dehydrogenase (anemia) 282.2
  11-beta-hydroxylase 255.2
  17-alpha-hydroxylase 255.2
  18-hydroxysteroid dehydrogenase 255.2
  20-alpha-hydroxylase 255.2
  21-hydroxylase 255.2
  abdominal muscle syndrome 756.79
  accelerator globulin (Ac G) (blood) (*see also* Defect, coagulation) 286.3

Deficiency, deficient — *continued*
- AC globulin (congenital) (*see also* Defect, coagulation) 286.3
  - acquired 286.7
- activating factor (blood) (*see also*, Defect, coagulation) 286.3
- adenohypophyseal 253.2
- adenosine deaminase 277.2
- aldolase (hereditary) 271.2
- alpha-1-antitrypsin 277.6
- alpha-1-trypsin inhibitor 277.6
- alpha-fucosidase 271.8
- alpha-lipoprotein 272.5
- alpha-mannosidase 271.8
- amino acid 270.9
- anemia — *see* Anemia, deficiency
- aneurin 265.1
  - with beriberi 265.0
- antibody NEC 279.00
- antidiuretic hormone 253.5
- antihemophilic
  - factor (A) 286.0
    - B 286.1
    - C 286.2
  - globulin (AHG) NEC 286.0
- antitrypsin 277.6
- argininosuccinate synthetase or lyase 270.6
- ascorbic acid (with scurvy) 267
- autoprothrombin
  - I (*see also* Defect, coagulation) 286.3
  - II 286.1
  - C (*see also* Defect, coagulation) 286.3
- bile salt 579.8
- biotin 266.2
- biotinidase 277.6
- bradykinase-1 277.6
- brancher enzyme (amylopectinosis) 271.0
- calciferol 268.9
  - with
    - osteomalacia 268.2
    - rickets (*see also* Rickets) 268.0
- calcium 275.40
  - dietary 269.3
- calorie, severe 261
- carbamyl phosphate synthetase 270.6
- cardiac (*see also* Insufficiency, myocardial) 428.0
- carnitine palmityl transferase 791.3
- carotene 264.9
- Carr factor (*see also* Defect, coagulation) 286.9
- central nervous system 349.9
- ceruloplasmin 275.1
- cevitamic acid (with scurvy) 267
- choline 266.2
- Christmas factor 286.1
- chromium 269.3
- citrin 269.1
- clotting (blood) (*see also* Defect, coagulation) 286.9
- coagulation factor NEC 286.9
  - with
    - abortion — *see* Abortion, by type, with hemorrhage
    - ectopic pregnancy (*see also* categories 634-638) 639.1
    - molar pregnancy (*see also* categories 630-632) 639.1
  - acquired (any) 286.7
  - antepartum or intrapartum 641.3 ✓5ᵗʰ
    - affecting fetus or newborn 762.1

Deficiency, deficient — *continued*
- coagulation factor NEC — *continued*
  - due to
    - liver disease 286.7
    - vitamin K deficiency 286.7
  - newborn, transient 776.3
  - postpartum 666.3 ✓5ᵗʰ
  - specified type NEC 286.3
- color vision (congenital) 368.59
  - acquired 368.55
- combined, two or more coagulation factors (*see also* Defect, coagulation) 286.9
- complement factor NEC 279.8
- contact factor (*see also* Defect, coagulation) 286.3
- copper NEC 275.1
- corticoadrenal 255.4
- craniofacial axis 756.0
- cyanocobalamin (vitamin B_{12}) 266.2
- debrancher enzyme (limit dextrinosis) 271.0
- desmolase 255.2
- diet 269.9
- dihydrofolate reductase 281.2
- dihydropteridine reductase 270.1
- disaccharidase (intestinal) 271.3
- disease NEC 269.9
- ear(s) V48.8
- edema 262
- endocrine 259.9
- enzymes, circulating NEC (*see also* Deficiency, by specific enzyme) 277.6
- ergosterol 268.9
  - with
    - osteomalacia 268.2
    - rickets (*see also* Rickets) 268.0
- erythrocytic glutathione (anemia) 282.2
- eyelid(s) V48.8
- factor (*See also* Defect, coagulation) 286.9
  - I (congenital) (fibrinogen) 286.3
    - antepartum or intrapartum 641.3 ✓5ᵗʰ
    - affecting fetus or newborn 762.1
    - newborn, transient 776.3
    - postpartum 666.3 ✓5ᵗʰ
  - II (congenital) (prothrombin) 286.3
  - V (congenital) (labile) 286.3
  - VII (congenital) (stable) 286.3
  - VIII (congenital) (functional) 286.0
    - with
      - functional defect 286.0
      - vascular defect 286.4
  - IX (Christmas) (congenital) (functional) 286.1
  - X (congenital) (Stuart-Prower) 286.3
  - XI (congenital) (plasma thromboplastin antecedent) 286.2
  - XII (congenital) (Hageman) 286.3
  - XIII (congenital) (fibrin stabilizing) 286.3
  - Hageman 286.3
  - multiple (congenital) 286.9
    - acquired 286.7
- fibrinase (*see also* Defect, coagulation) 286.3
- fibrinogen (congenital) (*see also* Defect, coagulation) 286.3
  - acquired 286.6
- fibrin-stabilizing factor (congenital) (*see also* Defect, coagulation) 286.3
- finger — *see* Absence, finger
- fletcher factor (*see also* Defect, coagulation) 286.9
- fluorine 269.3
- folate, anemia 281.2

Deficiency, deficient

Deficiency, deficient — *continued*
  folic acid (vitamin B$_6$) 266.2
    anemia 281.2
  fructokinase 271.2
  fructose-1, 6-diphosphate 271.2
  fructose-1-phosphate aldolase 271.2
  FSH (follicle-stimulating hormone) 253.4
  fucosidase 271.8
  galactokinase 271.1
  galactose-1-phosphate uridyl transferase 271.1
  gamma globulin in blood 279.00
  glass factor (*see also* Defect, coagulation) 286.3
  glucocorticoid 255.4
  glucose-6-phosphatase 271.0
  glucose-6-phosphate dehydrogenase anemia 282.2
  glucuronyl transferase 277.4
  glutathione-reductase (anemia) 282.2
  glycogen synthetase 271.0
  growth hormone 253.3
  Hageman factor (congenital) (*see also* Defect, coagulation) 286.3
  head V48.0
  hemoglobin (*see also* Anemia) 285.9
  hepatophosphorylase 271.0
  hexose monophosphate (HMP) shunt 282.2
  HGH (human growth hormone) 253.3
  HG-PRT 277.2
  homogentisic acid oxidase 270.2
  hormone — *see also* Deficiency, by specific hormone
    anterior pituitary (isolated) (partial) NEC 253.4
      growth (human) 253.3
      follicle-stimulating 253.4
      growth (human) (isolated) 253.3
      human growth 253.3
      interstitial cell-stimulating 253.4
      luteinizing 253.4
      melanocyte-stimulating 253.4
      testicular 257.2
    human growth hormone 253.3
    humoral 279.00
      with
        hyper-IgM 279.05
          autosomal recessive 279.05
          X-linked 279.05
        increased IgM 279.05
      congenital hypogammaglobulinemia 279.04
      non-sex-linked 279.06
      selective immunoglobulin NEC 279.03
        IgA 279.01
        IgG 279.03
        IgM 279.02
        increased 279.05
        specified NEC 279.09
    hydroxylase 255.2
    hypoxanthine-guanine phosphoribosyltransferase (HG-PRT) 277.2
    ICSH (interstitial cell-stimulating hormone) 253.4
    immunity NEC 279.3
      cell-mediated 279.10
        with
          hyperimmunoglob-ulinemia 279.2
          thrombocytopenia and eczema 279.12
        specified NEC 279.19
      combined (severe) 279.2
        syndrome 279.2

Deficiency, deficient — *continued*
  immunity NEC — *continued*
    common variable 279.06
    humoral NEC 279.00
    IgA (secretory) 279.01
    IgG 279.03
    IgM 279.02
  immunoglobulin, selective NEC 279.03
    IgA 279.01
    IgG 279.03
    IgM 279.02
  inositol (B complex) 266.2
  interferon 279.4
  internal organ V47.0
  interstitial cell-stimulating hormone (ICSH) 253.4
  intrinsic factor (Castle's) (congenital) 281.0
  intrinsic (urethral) sphincter (ISD) 599.82
  invertase 271.3
  iodine 269.3
  iron, anemia 280.9
  labile factor (congenital) (*see also* Defect, coagulation) 286.3
    acquired 286.7
  lacrimal fluid (acquired) 375.15
    congenital 743.64
  lactase 271.3
  Laki-Lorand factor (*see also* Defect, coagulation) 286.3
  lecithin-cholesterol acyltranferase 272.5
  LH (luteinizing hormone) 253.4
  limb V49.0
    lower V49.0
      congenital (*see also* Deficiency, lower limb, congenital) 755.30
    upper V49.0
      congenital (*see also* Deficiency, upper limb, congenital) 755.20
  lipocaic 577.8
  lipoid (high-density) 272.5
  lipoprotein (familial) (high density) 272.5
  liver phosphorylase 271.0
  lower limb V49.0
    congenital 755.30
      with complete absence of distal elements 755.31
      longitudinal (complete) (partial) (with distal deficiencies, incomplete) 755.32
        with complete absence of distal elements 755.31
        combined femoral, tibial, fibular (incomplete) 755.33
        femoral 755.34
        fibular 755.37
        metatarsal(s) 755.38
        phalange(s) 755.39
          meaning all digits 755.31
        tarsal(s) 755.38
        tibia 755.36
        tibiofibular 755.35
      transverse 755.31
  luteinizing hormone (LH) 253.4
  lysosomal alpha-1, 4 glucosidase 271.0
  magnesium 275.2
  mannosidase 271.8
  melanocyte-stimulating hormone (MSH) 253.4
  menadione (vitamin K) 269.0
    newborn 776.0
  mental (familial) (hereditary) (*see also* Retardation, mental) 319

Deficiency, deficient — continued
　mineral NEC 269.3
　molybdenum 269.3
　moral 301.7
　multiple, syndrome 260
　myocardial (see also Insufficiency myocardial)
　　428.0
　myophosphorylase 271.0
　NADH (DPNH)-methemoglobin-reductase
　　(congenital) 289.7
　NADH-diaphorase or reductase (congenital)
　　289.7
　neck V48.1
　niacin (amide) (-tryptophan) 265.2
　nicotinamide 265.2
　nicotinic acid (amide) 265.2
　nose V48.8
　number of teeth (see also Anodontia) 520.0
　nutrition, nutritional 269.9
　　specified NEC 269.8
　ornithine transcarbamylase 270.6
　ovarian 256.39
　oxygen (see also Anoxia) 799.0
　pantothenic acid 266.2
　parathyroid (gland) 252.1
　phenylalanine hydroxylase 270.1
　phosphofructokinase 271.2
　phosphoglucomutase 271.0
　phosphohexosisomerase 271.0
　phosphorylase kinase, liver 271.0
　pituitary (anterior) 253.2
　　posterior 253.5
　placenta — see Placenta, insufficiency
　plasma
　　cell 279.00
　　protein (paraproteinemia)
　　　(pyroglobulinemia) 273.8
　　　gamma globulin 279.00
　　thrombosplastin
　　　antecedent (PTA) 286.2
　　　component (PTC) 286.1
　platelet NEC 287.1
　　constitutional 286.4
　polyglandular 258.9
　potassium (K) 276.8
　proaccelerin (congenital) (see also Defect,
　　congenital) 286.3
　　acquired 286.7
　proconvertin factor (congenital) (see also
　　Defect, coagulation) 286.3
　　acquired 286.7
　prolactin 253.4
　protein 260
　　anemia 281.4
　　plasma — see Deficiency, plasma protein
　prothrombin (congenital) (see also Defect
　　coagulation) 286.3
　　acquired 286.7
　Prower factor (see also Defect, coagulation)
　　286.3
　PRT 277.2
　pseudocholinesterase 289.8
　psychobiological 301.6
　PTA 286.2
　PTC 286.1
　purine nucleoside phosphorylase 277.2
　pyracin (alpha) (Beta) 266.1
　pyridoxal 266.1
　pyridoxamine 266.1
　pyridoxine (derivatives) 266.1
　pyruvate kinase (PK) 282.3

Deficiency, deficient — continued
　riboflavin (vitamin B_2) 266.0
　saccadic eye movements 379.57
　salivation 527.7
　salt 276.1
　secretion
　　ovary 256.39
　　salivary gland (any) 527.7
　　urine 788.5
　selenium 269.3
　serum
　　antitrypsin, familial 277.6
　　protein (congenital) 273.8
　smooth pursuit movements (eye) 379.58
　sodium (Na) 276.1
　SPCA (see also Defect, coagulation) 286.3
　specified NEC 269.8
　stable factor (congenital) (see also Defect,
　　coagulation) 286.3
　　acquired 286.7
　Stuart (-Prower) factor (see also Defect,
　　coagulation) 286.3
　sucrase 271.3
　sucrase-isomaltase 271.3
　sulfite oxidase 270.0
　syndrome, multiple 260
　thiamine, thiaminic (chloride) 265.1
　thrombokinase (see also Defect, coagulation)
　　286.3
　　newborn 776.0
　thrombopoieten 287.3
　thymolymphatic 279.2
　thyroid (gland) 244.9
　tocopherol 269.1
　toe — see Absence, toe
　tooth bud (see also Anodontia) 520.0
　trunk V48.1
　UDPG-glycogen transferase 271.0
　upper limb V49.0
　　congenital 755.20
　　　with complete absence of distal elements
　　　　755.21
　　　longitudinal (complete) (partial) (with
　　　　distal deficiencies, incomplete)
　　　　755.22
　　　carpal(s) 755.28
　　　combined humeral, radial, ulnar
　　　　(incomplete) 755.23
　　　humeral 755.24
　　　metacarpal(s) 755.28
　　　phalange(s) 755.29
　　　　meaning all digits 755.21
　　　radial 755.26
　　　radioulnar 755.25
　　　ulnar 755.27
　　　transverse (complete) (partial) 755.21
　vascular 459.9
　vasopressin 253.5
　viosterol (see also Deficiency, calciferol) 268.9
　vitamin (multiple) NEC 269.2
　　A 264.9
　　with
　　　Bitôt's spot 264.1
　　　corneal 264.2
　　　　with corneal ulceration 264.3
　　　keratomalacia 264.4
　　　keratosis, follicular 264.8
　　　night blindness 264.5
　　　scar of cornea, xerophthalmic 264.6
　　　specified manifestation NEC 264.8
　　　ocular 264.7

Deficiency, deficient — *continued*
  vitamin — *continued*
    A — *continued*
      with — *continued*
        xeroderma 264.8
        xerophthalmia 264.7
        xerosis
          conjunctival 264.0
            with Bitôt's spot 264.1
          corneal 264.2
            with corneal ulceraton 264.3
    B (complex) NEC 266.9
      with
        beriberi 265.0
        pellagra 265.2
      specified type NEC 266.2
    B_1 NEC 265.1
      beriberi 265.0
    B_2 266.0
    B_6 266.1
    B_{12} 266.2
    B_9 (folic acid) 266.2
    C (ascorbic acid) (with scurvy) 267
    D (calciferol) (ergosterol) 268.9
      with
        osteomalacia 268.2
        rickets (*see also* Rickets) 268.0
    E 269.1
    folic acid 266.2
    G 266.0
    H 266.2
    K 269.0
      of newborn 776.0
    nicotinic acid 265.2
    P 269.1
    PP 265.2
    specified NEC 269.1
  zinc 269.3

Deficient — *see also* Deficiency
  blink reflex 374.45
  craniofacial axis 756.0
  number of teeth (*see also* Anodontia) 520.0
  secretion of urine 788.5

Deficit
  neurologic NEC 781.99
    due to
      cerebrovascular lesion (*see also* Disease, cerebrovascular, acute) 436
      late effect — *see* Late effect(s) (of) cerebrovascular disease
      transient ischemic attack 435.9
  oxygen 799.0

Deflection
  radius 736.09
  septum (acquired) (nasal) (nose) 470
  spine — *see* Curvature, spine
  turbinate (nose) 470

Defluvium
  capillorum (*see also* Alopecia) 704.00
  ciliorum 374.55
  unguium 703.8

Deformity 738.9
  abdomen, congenital 759.9
  abdominal wall
    acquired 738.8
    congenital 756.70
    muscle deficiency syndrome 756.79
  acquired (unspecified site) 738.9
    specified site NEC 738.8
  adrenal gland (congenital) 759.1

Deformity — *continued*
  alimentary tract, congenital 751.9
    lower 751.5
    specified type NEC 751.8
    upper (any part, except tongue) 750.9
      specified type NEC 750.8
      tongue 750.10
        specified type NEC 750.19
  ankle (joint) (acquired) 736.70
    abduction 718.47
    congenital 755.69
    contraction 718.47
    specified NEC 736.79
  anus (congenital) 751.5
    acquired 569.49
  aorta (congenital) 747.20
    acquired 447.8
    arch 747.21
      acquired 447.8
    coarctation 747.10
  aortic
    arch 747.21
      acquired 447.8
    cusp or valve (congenital) 746.9
      acquired (*see also* Endocarditis, aortic) 424.1
    ring 747.21
  appendix 751.5
  arm (acquired) 736.89
    congenital 755.50
  arteriovenous (congenital) (peripheral) NEC 747.60
    gastrointestinal 747.61
    lower limb 747.64
    renal 747.62
    specified NEC 747.69
    spinal 747.82
    upper limb 747.63
  artery (congenital) (peripheral) NEC (*see also* Deformity, vascular) 747.60
    acquired 447.8
    cerebral 747.81
    coronary (congenital) 746.85
      acquired (*see also* Ischemia, heart) 414.9
    retinal 743.9
    umbilical 747.5
  atrial septal (congenital) (heart) 745.5
  auditory canal (congenital) (external) (*see also* Deformity, ear) 744.3
    acquired 380.50
  auricle
    ear (congenital) (*see also* Deformity, ear) 744.3
      acquired 380.32
    heart (congenital) 746.9
  back (acquired) — *see* Deformity, spine
  Bartholin's duct (congenital) 750.9
  bile duct (congenital) 751.60
    acquired 576.8
      with calculus, choledocholithiasis, or stones — *see* Choledocholithiasis
  biliary duct or passage (congenital) 751.60
    acquired 576.8
      with calculus, choledocholithiasis, or stones — *see* Choledocholithiasis
  bladder (neck) (spincter) (trigone) (acquired) 596.8
    congenital 753.9
  bone (acquired) NEC 738.9
    congenital 756.9
    turbinate 738.0

Deformity — *continued*
  boutonniere (finger) 736.21
  brain (congenital) 742.9
    acquired 348.8
    multiple 742.4
    reduction 742.2
    vessel (congenital) 747.81
  breast (acquired) 611.8
    congenital 757.9
  bronchus (congenital) 748.3
    acquired 519.1
  bursa, congenital 756.9
  canal of Nuck 752.9
  canthus (congenital) 743.9
    acquired 374.89
  capillary (acquired) 448.9
    congenital NEC (*see also* Deformity, vascular) 747.60
  cardiac — *see* Deformity, heart
  cardiovascular system (congenital) 746.9
  caruncle, lacrimal (congenital) 743.9
    acquired 375.69
  cascade, stomach 537.6
  cecum (congenital) 751.5
    acquired 569.89
  cerebral (congenital) 742.9
    acquired 348.8
  cervix (acquired) (uterus) 622.8
    congenital 752.40
  cheek (acquired) 738.19
    congenital 744.9
  chest (wall) (acquired) 738.3
    congenital 754.89
    late effect of rickets 268.1
  chin (acquired) 738.19
    congenital 744.9
  choroid (congenital) 743.9
    acquired 363.8
    plexus (congenital) 742.9
      acquired 349.2
  cicatricial — *see* Cicatrix
  cilia (congenital) 743.9
    acquired 374.89
  circulatory system (congenital) 747.9
  clavicle (acquired) 738.8
    congenital 755.51
  clitoris (congenital) 752.40
    acquired 624.8
  clubfoot — *see* Clubfoot
  coccyx (acquired) 738.6
    congenital 756.10
  colon (congenital) 751.5
    acquired 569.89
  concha (ear) (congenital) (*see also* Deformity, ear) 744.3
    acquired 380.32
  congenital, organ or site not listed (*see also* Anomaly) 759.9
  cornea (congenital) 743.9
    acquired 371.70
  coronary artery (congenital) 746.85
    acquired (*see also* Ischemia, heart) 414.9
  cranium (acquired) 738.19
    congenital (*see also* Deformity, skull, congenital) 756.0
  cricoid cartilage (congenital) 748.3
    acquired 478.79
  cystic duct (congenital) 751.60
    acquired 575.8

Deformity — *continued*
  Dandy-Walker 742.3
    with spina bifida (*see also* Spina bifida) 741.0 ✓5ᵗʰ
  diaphragm (congenital) 756.6
    acquired 738.8
  digestive organ(s) or system (congenital) NEC 751.9
    specified type NEC 751.8
  ductus arteriosus 747.0
  duodenal bulb 537.89
  duodenum (congenital) 751.5
    acquired 537.89
  dura (congenital) 742.9
    brain 742.4
      acquired 349.2
    spinal 742.59
      acquired 349.2
  ear (congenital) 744.3
    acquired 380.32
    auricle 744.3
      causing impairment of hearing 744.02
    causing impairment of hearing 744.00
    external 744.3
      causing impairment of hearing 744.02
    internal 744.05
    lobule 744.3
    middle 744.03
      ossicles 744.04
    ossicles 744.04
  ectodermal (congenital) NEC 757.9
    specified type NEC 757.8
  ejaculatory duct (congenital) 752.9
    acquired 608.89
  elbow (joint) (acquired) 736.00
    congenital 755.50
    contraction 718.42
  endocrine gland NEC 759.2
  epididymis (congenital) 752.9
    acquired 608.89
    torsion 608.2
  epiglottis (congenital) 748.3
    acquired 478.79
  esophagus (congenital) 750.9
    acquired 530.89
  Eustachian tube (congenital) NEC 744.3
    specified type NEC 744.24
  extremity (acquired) 736.9
    congenital, except reduction deformity 755.9
      lower 755.60
      upper 755.50
    reduction — *see* Deformity, reduction
  eye (congenital) 743.9
    acquired 379.8
    muscle 743.9
  eyebrow (congenital) 744.89
  eyelid (congenital) 743.9
    acquired 374.89
    specified type NEC 743.62
  face (acquired) 738.19
    congenital (any part) 744.9
      due to intrauterine malposition and pressure 754.0
  fallopian tube (congenital) 752.10
    acquired 620.8
  femur (acquired) 736.89
    congenital 755.60
  fetal
    with fetopelvic disproportion 653.7 ✓5ᵗʰ
      affecting fetus or newborn 763.1

Deformity — *continued*
  fetal — *continued*
    causing obstructed labor 660.1 ✓5ᵗʰ
      affecting fetus or newborn 763.1
    known or suspected, affecting management
      of pregnancy 655.9 ✓5ᵗʰ
  finger (acquired) 736.20
    boutonniere type 736.21
    congenital 755.50
    flexion contracture 718.44
    swan neck 736.22
  flexion (joint) (acquired) 736.9
    congenital NEC 755.9
    hip or thigh (acquired) 736.39
      congenital (*see also* Subluxation,
        congenital, hip) 754.32
  foot (acquired) 736.70
    cavovarus 736.75
      congenital 754.59
    congenital NEC 754.70
      specified type NEC 754.79
    valgus (acquired) 736.79
      congenital 754.60
        specified type NEC 754.69
    varus (acquired) 736.79
      congenital 754.50
        specified type NEC 754.59
  forearm (acquired) 736.00
    congenital 755.50
  forehead (acquired) 738.19
    congenital (*see also* Deformity, skull,
      congenital) 756.0
  frontal bone (acquired) 738.19
    congenital (*see also* Deformity, skull,
      congenital) 756.0
  gallbladder (congenital) 751.60
    acquired 575.8
  gastrointestinal tract (congenital) NEC 751.9
    acquired 569.89
    specified type NEC 751.8
  genitalia, genital organ(s) or system NEC
    congenital 752.9
    female (congenital) 752.9
      acquired 629.8
      external 752.40
      internal 752.9
    male (congenital) 752.9
      acquired 608.89
  globe (eye) (congenital) 743.9
    acquired 360.89
  gum (congenital) 750.9
    acquired 523.9
  gunstock 736.02
  hand (acquired) 736.00
    claw 736.06
    congenital 755.50
    minus (and plus) (intrinsic) 736.09
    pill roller (intrinsic) 736.09
    plus (and minus) (intrinsic) 736.09
    swan neck (intrinsic) 736.09
  head (acquired) 738.10
    congenital (*see also* Deformity, skull
      congenital) 756.0
    specified NEC 738.19
  heart (congenital) 746.9
    auricle (congenital) 746.9
    septum 745.9
      auricular 745.5
      specified type NEC 745.8
      ventricular 745.4

Deformity — *continued*
  heart — *continued*
    valve (congenital) NEC 746.9
      acquired — *see* Endocarditis
      pulmonary (congenital) 746.00
      specified type NEC 746.89
    ventricle (congenital) 746.9
  heel (acquired) 736.76
    congenital 755.67
  hepatic duct (congenital) 751.60
    acquired 576.8
    with calculus, choledocholithiasis, or
      stones — *see* Choledocholithiasis
  hip (joint) (acquired) 736.30
    congenital NEC 755.63
    flexion 718.45
      congenital (*see also* Subluxation,
        congenital, hip) 754.32
  hourglass — *see* Contraction, hourglass
  humerus (acquired) 736.89
    congenital 755.50
  hymen (congenital) 752.40
  hypophyseal (congenital) 759.2
  ileocecal (coil) (valve) (congenital) 751.5
    acquired 569.89
  ileum (intestine) (congenital) 751.5
    acquired 569.89
  ilium (acquired) 738.6
    congenital 755.60
  integument (congenital) 757.9
  intervertebral cartilage or disc (acquired) —
    see also Displacement, intervertebral
    disc
    congenital 756.10
  intestine (large) (small) (congenital) 751.5
    acquired 569.89
  iris (acquired) 364.75
    congenital 743.9
    prolapse 364.8
  ischium (acquired) 738.6
    congenital 755.60
  jaw (acquired) (congenital) NEC 524.9
    due to intrauterine malposition and
      pressure 754.0
  joint (acquired) NEC 738.8
    congenital 755.9
    contraction (abduction) (adduction)
      (extension) (flexion) — *see*
      Contraction, joint
  kidney(s) (calyx) (pelvis) (congenital) 753.9
    acquired 593.89
    vessel 747.62
      acquired 459.9
  Klippel-Feil (brevicollis) 756.16
  knee (acquired) NEC 736.6
    congenital 755.64
  labium (majus) (minus) (congenital) 752.40
    acquired 624.8
  lacrimal apparatus or duct (congenital) 743.9
    acquired 375.69
  larynx (muscle) (congenital) 748.3
    acquired 478.79
    web (glottic) (subglottic) 748.2
  leg (lower) (upper) (acquired) NEC 736.89
    congenital 755.60
      reduction — *see* Deformity, reduction,
        lower limb
  lens (congenital) 743.9
    acquired 379.39
  lid (fold) (congenital) 743.9
    acquired 374.89

Deformity — *continued*
  ligament (acquired) 728.9
    congenital 756.9
  limb (acquired) 736.9
    congenital, except reduction deformity 755.9
      lower 755.60
        reduction (*see also* Deformity, reduction, lower limb) 755.30
      upper 755.50
        reduction (*see also* Deformity, reduction, upper limb) 755.20
    specified NEC 736.89
  lip (congenital) NEC 750.9
    acquired 528.5
    specified type NEC 750.26
  liver (congenital) 751.60
    acquired 573.8
    duct (congenital) 751.60
      acquired 576.8
        with calculus, choledocholithiasis, or stones — *see* Choledocholithiasis
  lower extremity — *see* Deformity, leg
  lumbosacral (joint) (region) (congenital) 756.10
    acquired 738.5
  lung (congenital) 748.60
    acquired 518.89
    specified type NEC 748.69
  lymphatic system, congenital 759.9
  Madelung's (radius) 755.54
  maxilla (acquired) (congenital) 524.9
  meninges or membrane (congenital) 742.9
    brain 742.4
      acquired 349.2
    spinal (cord) 742.59
      acquired 349.2
  mesentery (congenitial) 751.9
    acquired 568.89
  metacarpus (acquired) 736.00
    congenital 755.50
  metatarsus (acquired) 736.70
    congenital 754.70
  middle ear, except ossicles (congenital) 744.03
    ossicles 744.04
  mitral (leaflets) (valve) (congenital) 746.9
    acquired — *see* Endocarditis, mitral
    Ebstein's 746.89
    parachute 746.5
    specified type NEC 746.89
    stenosis, congenital 746.5
  mouth (acquired) 528.9
    congenital NEC 750.9
      specified type NEC 750.26
  multiple, congenital NEC 759.7
    specified type NEC 759.89
  muscle (acquired) 728.9
    congenital 756.9
      specified type NEC 756.89
        sternocleidomastoid (due to intrauterine malposition and pressure) 754.1
  musculoskeletal system, congenital NEC 756.9
    specified type NEC 756.9
  nail (acquired) 703.9
    congenital 757.9
  nasal — *see* Deformity, nose
  neck (acquired) NEC 738.2
    congenital (any part) 744.9
    sternocleidomastoid 754.1
  nervous system (congenital) 742.9

Deformity — *continued*
  nipple (congenital) 757.9
    acquired 611.8
  nose, nasal (cartilage) (acquired) 738.0
    bone (turbinate) 738.0
    congenital 748.1
      bent 754.0
      squashed 754.0
    saddle 738.0
      syphilitic 090.5
    septum 470
      congenital 748.1
    sinus (wall) (congenital) 748.1
      acquired 738.0
    syphilitic (congenital) 090.5
      late 095.8
  ocular muscle (congenital) 743.9
    acquired 378.60
  opticociliary vessels (congenital) 743.9
  orbit (congenital) (eye) 743.9
    acquired NEC 376.40
      associated with craniofacial deformities 376.44
      due to
        bone disease 376.43
        surgery 376.47
        trauma 376.47
  organ of Corti (congenital) 744.05
  ovary (congenital) 752.0
    acquired 620.8
  oviduct (congenital) 752.10
    acquired 620.8
  palate (congenital) 750.9
    acquired 526.89
    cleft (congenital) (*see also* Cleft, palate) 749.00
    hard, acquired 526.89
    soft, acquired 528.9
  pancreas (congenital) 751.7
    acquired 577.8
  parachute, mitral valve 746.5
  parathyroid (gland) 759.2
  parotid (gland) (congenital) 750.9
    acquired 527.8
  patella (acquired) 736.6
    congenital 755.64
  pelvis, pelvic (acquired) (bony) 738.6
    with disproportion (fetopelvic) 653.0 ✓5ᵗʰ
      affecting fetus or newborn 763.1
      causing obstructed labor 660.1 ✓5ᵗʰ
        affecting fetus or newborn 763.1
    congenital 755.60
    rachitic (late effect) 268.1
  penis (glans) (congenital) 752.9
    acquired 607.89
  pericardium (congenital) 746.9
    acquired — *see* Pericarditis
  pharynx (congenital) 750.9
    acquired 478.29
  Pierre Robin (congenital) 756.0
  pinna (acquired) 380.32
    congenital 744.3
  pituitary (congenital) 759.2
  pleural folds (congenital) 748.8
  portal vein (congenital) 747.40
  posture *see* Curvature, spine
  prepuce (congenital) 752.9
    acquired 607.89
  prostate (congenital) 752.9
    acquired 602.8

Index to Diseases

Deformity — *continued*
  pulmonary valve — *see* Endocarditis, pulmonary
  pupil (congenital) 743.9
    acquired 364.75
  pylorus (congenital) 750.9
    acquired 537.89
  rachitic (acquired), healed or old 268.1
  radius (acquired) 736.00
    congenital 755.50
      reduction — *see* Deformity, reduction, upper limb
  rectovaginal septum (congenital) 752.40
    acquired 623.8
  rectum (congenital) 751.5
    acquired 569.49
  reduction (extremity) (limb) 755.4
    brain 742.2
    lower limb 755.30
      with complete absence of distal elements 755.31
      longitudinal (complete) (partial) (with distal deficiencies, incomplete) 755.32
        with complete absence of distal elements 755.31
        combined femoral, tibial, fibular (incomplete) 755.33
        femoral 755.34
        fibular 755.37
        metatarsal(s) 755.38
        phalange(s) 755.39
          meaning all digits 755.31
        tarsal(s) 755.38
        tibia 755.36
        tibiofibular 755.35
      transverse 755.31
    upper limb 755.20
      with complete absence of distal elements 755.21
      longitudinal (complete) (partial) (with distal deficiencies, incomplete) 755.22
        with complete absence of distal elements 755.21
        carpal(s) 755.28
        combined humeral, radial, ulnar (incomplete) 755.23
        humeral 755.24
        metacarpal(s) 755.28
        phalange(s) 755.29
          meaning all digits 755.21
        radial 755.26
        radioulnar 755.25
        ulnar 755.27
      transverse (complete) (partial) 755.21
  renal — *see* Deformity, kidney
  respiratory system (congenital) 748.9
    specified type NEC 748.8
  rib (acquired) 738.3
    congenital 756.3
      cervical 756.2
  rotation (joint) (acquired) 736.9
    congenital 755.9
    hip or thigh 736.39
      congenital (*see also* Subluxation, congenital, hip) 754.32
  sacroiliac joint (congenital) 755.69
    acquired 738.5
  sacrum (acquired) 738.5
    congenital 756.10

Deformity — *continued*
  saddle
    back 737.8
    nose 738.0
      syphilitic 090.5
  salivary gland or duct (congenital) 750.9
    acquired 527.8
  scapula (acquired) 736.89
    congenital 755.50
  scrotum (congenital) 752.9
    acquired 608.89
  sebaceous gland, acquired 706.8
  seminal tract or duct (congenital) 752.9
    acquired 608.89
  septum (nasal) (acquired) 470
    congenital 748.1
  shoulder (joint) (acquired) 736.89
    congenital 755.50
      specified type NEC 755.59
    contraction 718.41
  sigmoid (flexure) (congenital) 751.5
    acquired 569.89
  sinus of Valsalva 747.29
  skin (congenital) 757.9
    acquired NEC 709.8
  skull (acquired) 738.19
    congenital 756.0
      with
        anencephalus 740.0
        encephalocele 742.0
        hydrocephalus 742.3
          with spina bifida (*see also* Spina bifida) 741.0 ✓5ᵗʰ
        microcephalus 742.1
    due to intrauterine malposition and pressure 754.0
  soft parts, organs or tissues (of pelvis)
    in pregnancy or childbirth NEC 654.9 ✓5ᵗʰ
      affecting fetus or newborn 763.89
      causing obstructed labor 660.2 ✓5ᵗʰ
        affecting fetus or newborn 763.1
  spermatic cord (congenital) 752.9
    acquired 608.89
    torsion 608.2
  spinal
    column — *see* Deformity, spine
    cord (congenital) 742.9
      acquired 336.8
      vessel (congenital) 747.82
    nerve root (congenital) 742.9
      acquired 724.9
  spine (acquired) NEC 738.5
    congenital 756.10
      due to intrauterine malposition and pressure 754.2
    kyphoscoliotic (*see also* Kyphoscoliosis) 737.30
    kyphotic (*see also* Kyphosis) 737.10
    lordotic (*see also* Lordosis) 737.20
    rachitic 268.1
    scoliotic (*see also* Scoliosis) 737.30
  spleen
    acquired 289.59
    congenital 759.0
  Sprengel's (congenital) 755.52
  sternum (acquired) 738.3
    congenital 756.3
  stomach (congenital) 750.9
    acquired 537.89
  submaxillary gland (congenital) 750.9
    acquired 527.8

Deformity — *continued*
  swan neck (acquired)
    finger 736.22
    hand 736.09
  talipes — *see* Talipes
  teeth, tooth NEC 520.9
  testis (congenital) 752.9
    acquired 608.89
      torsion 608.2
  thigh (acquired) 736.89
    congenital 755.60
  thorax (acquired) (wall) 738.3
    congenital 754.89
    late effect of rickets 268.1
  thumb (acquired) 736.20
    congenital 755.50
  thymus (tissue) (congenital) 759.2
  thyroid (gland) (congenital) 759.2
    cartilage 748.3
      acquired 478.79
  tibia (acquired) 736.89
    congenital 755.60
    saber 090.5
  toe (acquired) 735.9
    congenital 755.66
    specified NEC 735.8
  tongue (congenital) 750.10
    acquired 529.8
  tooth, teeth NEC 520.9
  trachea (rings) (congenital) 748.3
    acquired 519.1
  transverse aortic arch (congenital) 747.21
  tricuspid (leaflets) (valve) (congenital) 746.9
    acquired — *see* Endocarditis, tricuspid
    atresia or stenosis 746.1
    specified type NEC 746.89
  trunk (acquired) 738.3
    congenital 759.9
  ulna (acquired) 736.00
    congenital 755.50
  upper extremity — *see* Deformity, arm
  urachus (congenital) 753.7
  ureter (opening) (congenital) 753.9
    acquired 593.89
  urethra (valve) (congenital) 753.9
    acquired 599.84
  urinary tract or system (congenital) 753.9
    urachus 753.7
  uterus (congenital) 752.3
    acquired 621.8
  uvula (congenital) 750.9
    acquired 528.9
  vagina (congenital) 752.40
    acquired 623.8
  valve, valvular (heart) (congenital) 746.9
    acquired — *see* Endocarditis
    pulmonary 746.00
    specified type NEC 746.89
  vascular (congenital) (peripheral) NEC 747.60
    acquired 459.9
  vas deferens (congenital) 752.9
    acquired 608.89
  vein (congenital) NEC (*see also* Deformity, vascular) 747.60
    brain 747.81
    coronary 746.9
    great 747.40
  vena cava (inferior) (superior) (congenital) 747.40
  vertebra — *see* Deformity, spine

Deformity — *continued*
  vesicourethral orifice (acquired) 596.8
    congenital NEC 753.9
      specified type NEC 753.8
  vessels of optic papilla (congenital) 743.9
  visual field (contraction) 368.45
  vitreous humor (congenital) 743.9
    acquired 379.29
  vulva (congenital) 752.40
    acquired 624.8
  wrist (joint) (acquired) 736.00
    congenital 755.50
    contraction 718.43
    valgus 736.03
      congenital 755.59
    varus 736.04
      congenital 755.59
Degeneration, degenerative
  adrenal (capsule) (gland) 255.8
    with hypofunction 255.4
    fatty 255.8
    hyaline 255.8
    infectional 255.8
    lardaceous 277.3
  amyloid (any site) (general) 277.3
  anterior cornua, spinal cord 336.8
  aorta, aortic 440.0
    fatty 447.8
    valve (heart) (*see also* Endocarditis, aortic) 424.1
  arteriovascular — *see* Arteriosclerosis
  artery, arterial (atheromatous) (calcareous) — *see also* Arteriosclerosis
    amyloid 277.3
    lardaceous 277.3
    medial NEC (*see also* Arteriosclerosis, extremities) 440.20
  articular cartilage NEC (*see also* Disorder, cartilage, articular) 718.0 ▲5ᵗʰ
    elbow 718.02
    knee 717.5
    patella 717.7
    shoulder 718.01
    spine (*see also* Spondylosis) 721.90
  atheromatous — *see* Arteriosclerosis
  bacony (any site) 277.3
  basal nuclei or ganglia NEC 333.0
  bone 733.90
  brachial plexus 353.0
  brain (cortical) (progressive) 331.9
    arteriosclerotic 437.0
    childhood 330.9
      specified type NEC 330.8
    congenital 742.4
    cystic 348.0
      congenital 742.4
    familial NEC 331.89
    grey matter 330.8
    heredofamilial NEC 331.89
    in
      alcoholism 303.9 ▲5ᵗʰ [331.7]
      beriberi 265.0 [331.7]
      cerebrovascular disease 437.9 [331.7]
      congenital hydrocephalus 742.3 [331.7]
        with spina bifida (*see also* Spina bifida) 741.0 ▲5ᵗʰ [331.7]
      Fabry's disease 272.7 [330.2]
      Gaucher's disease 272.7 [330.2]
      Hunter's disease or syndrome 277.5 [330.3]

Degeneration, degenerative — *continued*
  brain — *continued*
    in — *continued*
      lipidosis
        cerebral 330.1
          generalized 272.7 *[330.2]*
        mucopolysaccharidosis 277.5 *[330.3]*
        myxedema (*see also* Myxedema) 244.9
          [331.7]
        neoplastic disease NEC (M8000/1) 239.9
          [331.7]
        Niemann-Pick disease 272.7 *[330.2]*
        sphingolipidosis 272.7 *[330.2]*
        vitamin B₁₂ deficiency 266.2 *[331.7]*
    motor centers 331.89
    senile 331.2
    specified type NEC 331.89
  breast — *see* Disease, breast
  Bruch's membrane 363.40
  bundle of His 426.50
    left 426.3
    right 426.4
  calcareous NEC 275.49
  capillaries 448.9
    amyloid 277.3
    fatty 448.9
    lardaceous 277.3
  cardiac (brown) (calcareous) (fatty) (fibrous)
    (hyaline) (mural) (muscular) (pigmentary)
    (senile) (with arteriosclerosis) (*see also*
    Degeneration, myocardial) 429.1
    valve, valvular — *see* Endocarditis
  cardiorenal (*see also* Hypertension,
    cardiorenal) 404.90
  cardiovascular (*see also* Disease,
    cardiovascular) 429.2
    renal (*see also* Hypertension, cardiorenal)
      404.90
  cartilage (joint) — *see* Derangement, joint
  cerebellar NEC 334.9
    primary (hereditary) (sporadic) 334.2
  cerebral — *see* Degeneration, brain
  cerebromacular 330.1
  cerebrovascular 437.1
    due to hypertension 437.2
    late effect — *see* Late effect(s) (of)
      cerbrovascular disease
  cervical plexus 353.2
  cervix 622.8
    due to radiation (intended effect) 622.8
      adverse effect or misadventure 622.8
  changes, spine or vertebra (*see also*
    Spondylosis) 721.90
  chitinous 277.3
  chorioretinal 363.40
    congenital 743.53
    hereditary 363.50
  choroid (colloid) (drusen) 363.40
    hereditary 363.50
    senile 363.41
      diffuse secondary 363.42
  cochlear 386.8
  collateral ligament (knee) (medial) 717.82
    lateral 717.81
  combined (spinal cord) (subacute) 266.2
    [336.2]
    with anemia (pernicious) 281.0 *[336.2]*
      due to dietary deficiency 281.1 *[336.2]*
      due to vitamin B₁₂ deficiency anemia
        (dietary) 281.1 *[336.2]*

Degeneration, degenerative — *continued*
  conjunctiva 372.50
    amyloid 277.3 *[372.50]*
  cornea 371.40
    calcerous 371.44
    familial (hereditary) (*see also* Dystrophy,
      cornea) 371.50
      macular 371.55
      reticular 371.54
    hyaline (of old scars) 371.41
    marginal (Terrien's) 371.48
    mosaic (shagreen) 371.41
    nodular 371.46
    peripheral 371.48
    senile 371.41
  cortical (cerebellar) (parenchymatous) 334.2
    alcoholic 303.9 ✓5ᵗʰ *[334.4]*
    diffuse, due to arteriopathy 437.0
  corticostriatal-spinal 334.8
  cretinoid 243
  cruciate ligament (knee) (posterior) 717.84
    anterior 717.83
  cutis 709.3
    amyloid 277.3
  dental pulp 522.2
  disc disease — *see* Degeneration,
    intervertebral disc
  dorsolateral (spinal cord) — *see* Degeration,
    combined
  endocardial 424.90
  extrapyramidal NEC 333.90
  eye NEC 360.40
    macular (*see also* Degeneration, macula)
      362.50
      congenital 362.75
      hereditary 362.76
  fatty (diffuse) (general) 272.8
    liver 571.8
      alcoholic 571.0
    localized site — *see* Degeneration, by site,
      fatty
    placenta — *see* Placenta, abnormal
  globe (eye) NEC 360.40
    macular — *see* Degeneration, macula
  grey matter 330.8
  heart (brown) (calcareous) (fatty) (fibrous)
    (hyaline) (mural) (muscular) (pigmentary)
    (senile) (with arteriosclerosis) (*see also*
    Degeneration, myocardial) 429.1
    amyloid 277.3 *[425.7]*
    atheromatous —*see* Arteriosclerosis,
      coronary
    gouty 274.82
    hypertensive (*see also* Hypertension, heart)
      402.90
    ischemic 414.9
    valve, valvular — *see* Endocarditis
  hepatolenticular (Wilson's) 275.1
  hepatorenal 572.4
  heredofamilial
    brain NEC 331.89
    spinal cord NEC 336.8
  hyaline (diffuse) (generalized) 728.9
    localized — *see also* Degeneration, by site
      cornea 371.41
      keratitis 371.41
  hypertensive vascular — *see* Hypertension
  infrapatellar fat pad 729.31
  internal semilunar cartilage 717.3
  intervertebral disc 722.6
    with myelopathy 722.70

Degeneration, degenerative — *continued*
 intervertebral disc — *continued*
  cervical, cervicothoracic 722.4
   with myelopathy 722.71
  lumbar, lumbosacral 722.52
   with myelopathy 722.73
  thoracic, thoracolumbar 722.51
   with myelopathy 722.72
 intestine 569.89
  amyloid 277.3
  lardaceous 277.3
 iris (generalized) (*see also* Atrophy, iris) 364.59
  pigmentary 364.53
  pupillary margin 364.54
 ischemic — *see* Ischemia
 joint disease (*see also* Osteoarthrosis) 715.9 ✓5ᵗʰ
  multiple sites 715.09
  spine (*see also* Spondylosis) 721.90
 kidney (*see also* Sclerosis, renal 587
  amyloid 277.3 *[583.81]*
  cyst, cystic (multiple) (solitary) 593.2
   congenital (*see also* Cystic, disease, kidney) 753.10
  fatty 593.89
  fibrocystic (congenital) 753.19
  lardaceous 277.3 *[583.81]*
  polycystic (congenital) 753.12
   adult type (APKD) 753.13
   autosomal dominant 753.13
   autosomal recessive 753.14
   childhood type (CPKD) 753.14
   infantile type 753.14
  waxy 277.3 *[583.81]*
 Kuhnt-Junius (retina) 362.52
 labyrinth, osseous 386.8
 lacrimal passages, cystic 375.12
 lardaceous (any site) 277.3
 lateral column (posterior), spinal cord (*see also* Degeneration, combined) 266.2 *[336.2]*
 lattice 362.63
 lens 366.9
  infantile, juvenile, or presenile 366.00
  senile 366.10
 lenticular (familial) (progressive) (Wilson's) (with cirrhosis of liver) 275.1
  striate artery 437.0
 lethal ball, prosthetic heart valve 996.02
 ligament
  collateral (knee) (medial) 717.82
   lateral 717.81
  cruciate (knee) (posterior) 717.84
   anterior 717.83
 liver (diffuse) 572.8
  amyloid 277.3
  congenital (cystic) 751.62
  cystic 572.8
   congenital 751.62
  fatty 571.8
   alcoholic 571.0
  hypertrophic 572.8
  lardaceous 277.3
  parenchymatous, acute or subacute (*see also* Necrosis, liver) 570
  pigmentary 572.8
  toxic (acute) 573.8
  waxy 277.3
 lung 518.89
 lymph gland 289.3
  hyaline 289.3
  lardaceous 277.3

Degeneration, degenerative — *continued*
 macula (acquired) (senile) 362.50
  atrophic 362.51
  Best's 362.76
  congenital 362.75
  cystic 362.54
  cystoid 362.53
  disciform 362.52
  dry 362.51
  exudative 362.52
  familial pseudoinflammatory 362.77
  hereditary 362.76
  hole 362.54
  juvenile (Stargardt's) 362.75
  nonexudative 362.51
  pseudohole 362.54
  wet 362.52
 medullary — *see* Degeneration, brain
 membranous labyrinth, congenital (causing impairment of hearing) 744.05
 meniscus — *see* Derangement, joint
 microcystoid 362.62
 mitral — *see* Insufficiency, mitral
 Mönckeberg's (*see also* Arteriosclerosis, extremities) 440.20
 moral 301.7
 motor centers, senile 331.2
 mural (*see also* Degeneration, myocardial) 429.1
  heart, cardiac (*see also* Degeneration, myocardial) 429.1
  myocardium, myocardial (*see also* Degeneration, myocardial) 429.1
 muscle 728.9
  fatty 728.9
  fibrous 728.9
  heart (*see also* Degeneration, myocardial) 429.1
  hyaline 728.9
 muscular progressive 728.2
 myelin, central nervous system NEC 341.9
 myocardium, myocardial (brown) (calcareous) (fatty) (fibrous) (hyaline) (mural) (muscular) (pigmentary) (senile) (with arteriosclerosis) 429.1
  with rheumatic fever (conditions classifiable to 390) 398.0
   active, acute, or subacute 391.2
    with chorea 392.0
   inactive or quiescent (with chorea) 398.0
  amyloid 277.3 *[425.7]*
  congenital 746.89
  fetus or newborn 779.89 ▲
  gouty 274.82
  hypertensive (*see also* Hypertension, heart) 402.90
  ischemic 414.8
  rheumatic (*see also* Degeneration, myocardium, with rheumatic fever) 398.0
  syphilitic 093.82
 nasal sinus (mucosa) (*see also* Sinusitis) 473.9
  frontal 473.1
  maxillary 473.0
 nerve — *see* Disorder, nerve
 nervous system 349.89
  amyloid 277.3 *[357.4]*
  autonomic (*see also* Neuropathy, peripheral, autonomic) 337.9
  fatty 349.89

Index to Diseases

Degeneration, degenerative — *continued*
nervous system — *continued*
  peripheral autonomic NEC (*see also*
    Neuropathy, peripheral, autonomic)
    337.9
nipple 611.9
nose 478.1
oculoacousticocerebral, congenital
  (progressive) 743.8
olivopontocerebellar (familial) (hereditary)
  333.0
osseous labyrinth 386.8
ovary 620.8
  cystic 620.2
  microcystic 620.2
pallidal, pigmentary (progressive) 333.0
pancreas 577.8
  tuberculous (*see also* Tuberculosis)
    017.9 ✓5ᵗʰ
papillary muscle 429.81
paving stone 362.61
penis 607.89
peritoneum 568.89
pigmentary (diffuse) (general)
  localized — *see* Degeneration, by site
  pallidal (progressive) 333.0
  secondary 362.65
pineal gland 259.8
pituitary (gland) 253.8
placenta (fatty) (fibrinoid) (fibroid) — *see*
  Placenta, abnormal
popliteal fat pad 729.31
posterolateral (spinal cord) (*see also*
  Degeneration, combined) 266.2 *[336.2]*
pulmonary valve (heart) (*see also* Endocarditis,
  pulmonary) 424.3
pulp (tooth) 522.2
pupillary margin 364.54
renal (*see also* Sclerosis, renal) 587
  fibrocystic 753.19
  polycystic 753.12
    adult type (APKD) 753.13
    autosomal dominant 753.13
    autosomal recessive 753.14
    childhood type (CPKD) 753.14
    infantile type 753.14
reticuloendothelial system 289.8
retina (peripheral) 362.60
  with retinal defect (*see also* Detachment,
    retina, with retinal defect) 361.00
  cystic (senile) 362.50
  cystoid 362.53
  hereditary (*see also* Dystrophy, retina)
    362.70
    cerebroretinal 362.71
    congenital 362.75
    juvenile (Stargardt's) 362.75
    macula 362.76
  Kuhnt-Junius 362.52
  lattice 362.63
  macular (*see also* Degeneration, macula)
    362.50
  microcystoid 362.62
  palisade 362.63
  paving stone 362.61
  pigmentary (primary) 362.74
    secondary 362.65
  posterior pole (*see also* Degeneration,
    macula) 362.50
  secondary 362.66

Degeneration, degenerative — *continued*
retina — *continued*
  senile 362.60
    cystic 362.53
    reticular 362.64
saccule, congenital (causing impairment of
  hearing) 744.05
sacculocochlear 386.8
senile 797
  brain 331.2
  cardiac, heart, or myocardium (*see also*
    Degeneration, myocardial) 429.1
  motor centers 331.2
  reticule 362.64
  retina, cystic 362.50
  vascular — *see* Arteriosclerosis
silicone rubber poppet (prosthetic valve)
  996.02
sinus (cystic) (*see also* Sinusitis) 473.9
  polypoid 471.1
skin 709.3
  amyloid 277.3
  colloid 709.3
spinal (cord) 336.8
  amyloid 277.3
  column 733.90
  combined (subacute) (*see also*
    Degeneration, combined) 266.2
    [336.2]
    with anemia (pernicious) 281.0 *[336.2]*
  dorsolateral (*see also* Degeneration,
    combined) 266.2 *[336.2]*
  familial NEC 336.8
  fatty 336.8
  funicular (*see also* Degeneration, combined)
    266.2 *[336.2]*
  heredofamilial NEC 336.8
  posterolateral (*see also* Degeneration,
    combined) 266.2 *[336.2]*
  subacute combined — *see* Degeneration,
    combined
  tuberculous (*see also* Tuberculosis)
    013.8 ✓5ᵗʰ
spine 733.90
spleen 289.59
  amyloid 277.3
  lardaceous 277.3
stomach 537.89
  lardaceous 277.3
strionigral 333.0
sudoriparous (cystic) 705.89
suprarenal (capsule) (gland) 255.8
  with hypofunction 255.4
sweat gland 705.89
synovial membrane (pulpy) 727.9
tapetoretinal 362.74
  adult or presenile form 362.50
testis (postinfectional) 608.89
thymus (gland) 254.8
  fatty 254.8
  lardaceous 277.3
thyroid (gland) 246.8
tricuspid (heart) (valve) *see* Endocarditis,
  tricuspid
tuberculous NEC (*see also* Tuberculosis)
  011.9 ✓5ᵗʰ
turbinate 733.90
uterus 621.8
  cystic 621.8
vascular (senile) — *see also* Arteriosclerosis
  hypertensive — *see* Hypertension

✓4ᵗʰ Fourth-digit Required   ✓5ᵗʰ Fifth-digit Required

Degeneration, degenerative — continued
  vitreoretinal (primary) 362.73
    secondary 362.66
  vitreous humor (with infiltration) 379.21
  wallerian NEC — see Disorder, nerve
  waxy (any site) 277.3
  Wilson's hepatolenticular 275.1
Deglutition
  paralysis 784.9
    hysterical 300.11
  pneumonia 507.0
Degos' disease or syndrome 447.8
Degradation disorder, branched-chain amino acid 270.3
Dehiscence
  anastomosis — see Complications, anastomosis
  cesarean wound 674.1 ✓5ᵗʰ
  episiotomy 674.2 ✓5ᵗʰ
  operation wound 998.32
    internal 998.31
  perineal wound (postpartum) 674.2 ✓5ᵗʰ
  postoperative 998.32
    abdomen 998.32
      internal 998.31
    internal 998.31
  uterine wound 674.1 ✓5ᵗʰ
Dehydration (cachexia) 276.5
  with
    hypernatremia 276.0
    hyponatremia 276.1
  newborn 775.5
Deiters' nucleus syndrome 386.19
Déjérine's disease 356.0
Déjérine-Klumpke paralysis 767.6
Déjérine-Roussy syndrome 348.8
Déjérine-Sottas disease or neuropathy (hypertrophic) 356.0
Déjérine-Thomas atrophy or syndrome 333.0
de Lange's syndrome (Amsterdam dwarf, mental retardation, and brachycephaly) 759.89
Delay, delayed
  adaptation, cones or rods 368.63
  any plane in pelvis
    affecting fetus or newborn 763.1
    complicating delivery 660.1 ✓5ᵗʰ
  birth or delivery NEC 662.1 ✓5ᵗʰ
    affecting fetus or newborn 763.89
    second twin, triplet, or multiple mate 662.3 ✓5ᵗʰ
  closure — see also Fistula
    cranial suture 756.0
    fontanel 756.0
  coagulation NEC 790.92
  conduction (cardiac) (ventricular) 426.9
  delivery NEC 662.1 ✓5ᵗʰ
    second twin, triplet, etc. 662.3 ✓5ᵗʰ
      affecting fetus or newborn 763.89
  development
    in childhood 783.40
      physiological 783.40
    intellectual NEC 315.9
    learning NEC 315.2
    reading 315.00
    sexual 259.0
    speech 315.39
      associated with hyperkinesis 314.1
    spelling 315.09
  gastric emptying 536.8

Delay, delayed — continued
  menarche 256.39
    due to pituitary hypofunction 253.4
  menstruation (cause unknown) 626.8
  milestone in childhood 783.42
  motility — see Hypomotility
  passage of meconium (newborn) 777.1
  primary respiration 768.9
  puberty 259.0
  sexual maturation, female 259.0
Del Castillo's syndrome (germinal aplasia) 606.0
Déleage's disease 359.89 ▲
Delhi (boil) (button) (sore) 085.1
Delinquency (juvenile) 312.9
  group (see also Disturbance, conduct) 312.2 ✓5ᵗʰ
  neurotic 312.4
Delirium, delirious 780.09
  acute (psychotic) 293.0
  alcoholic 291.0
    acute 291.0
    chronic 291.1
  alcoholicum 291.0
  chronic (see also Psychosis) 293.89
    due to or associated with physical condition — see Psychosis, organic
  drug-induced 292.81
  eclamptic (see also Eclampsia) 780.39
  exhaustion (see also Reaction, stress, acute) 308.9
  hysterical 300.11
  in
    presenile dementia 290.11
    senile dementia 290.3
  induced by drug 292.81
  manic, maniacal (acute) (see also Psychosis, affective) 296.0 ✓5ᵗʰ
    recurrent episode 296.1 ✓5ᵗʰ
    single episode 296.0 ✓5ᵗʰ
  puerperal 293.9
  senile 290.3
  subacute (psychotic) 293.1
  thyroid (see also Thyrotoxicosis) 242.9 ✓5ᵗʰ
  traumatic — see also Injury, intracranial
    with
      lesion, spinal cord — see Injury, spinal, by site
      shock, spinal — see Injury, spinal, by site
  tremens (impending) 291.0
  uremic — see Uremia
  withdrawal
    alcoholic (acute) 291.0
      chronic 291.1
    drug 292.0

Delivery

Note — Use the following fifth-digit subclassification with categories 640-648, 651-676:

0	unspecified as to episode of care
1	delivered, with or without mention of antepartum condition
2	delivered, with mention of postpartum complication
3	antepartum condition or complication
4	postpartum condition or complication

Index to Diseases

Delivery

Delivery — *continued*
  breech (assisted) (spontaneous) 652.2 ✓5th
    affecting fetus or newborn 763.0
    extraction NEC 669.6 ✓5th
  cesarean (for) 669.7 ✓5th
    abnormal
      cervix 654.6 ✓5th
      pelvic organs or tissues 654.9 ✓5th
      pelvis (bony) (major) NEC 653.0 ✓5th
      presentation or position 652.9 ✓5th
        in multiple gestation 652.6 ✓5th
      size, fetus 653.5 ✓5th
      soft parts (of pelvis) 654.9 ✓5th
      uterus, congenital 654.0 ✓5th
      vagina 654.7 ✓5th
      vulva 654.8 ✓5th
    abruptio placentae 641.2 ✓5th
    acromion presentation 652.8 ✓5th
    affecting fetus or newborn 763.4
    anteversion, cervix or uterus 654.4 ✓5th
    atony, uterus 666.1 ✓5th
    bicornis or bicornuate uterus 654.0 ✓5th
    breech presentation 652.2 ✓5th
    brow presentation 652.4 ✓5th
    cephalopelvic disproportion (normally
        formed fetus) 653.4 ✓5th
    chin presentation 652.4 ✓5th
    cicatrix of cervix 654.6 ✓5th
    contracted pelvis (general) 653.1 ✓5th
      inlet 653.2 ✓5th
      outlet 653.3 ✓5th
    cord presentation or prolapse 663.0 ✓5th
    cystocele 654.4 ✓5th
    deformity (acquired) (congenital)
      pelvic organs or tissues NEC 654.9 ✓5th
      pelvis (bony) NEC 653.0 ✓5th
    displacement, uterus NEC 654.4 ✓5th
    disproportion NEC 653.9 ✓5th
    distress
      fetal 656.8 ✓5th
      maternal 669.0 ✓5th
    eclampsia 642.6 ✓5th
    face presentation 652.4 ✓5th
    failed
      forceps 660.7 ✓5th
      trial of labor NEC 660.6 ✓5th
      vacuum extraction 660.7 ✓5th
      ventouse 660.7 ✓5th
    fetal deformity 653.7 ✓5th
    fetal-maternal hemorrhage 656.0 ✓5th
    fetus, fetal
      distress 656.8 ✓5th
      prematurity 656.8 ✓5th
    fibroid (tumor) (uterus) 654.1 ✓5th
    footling 652.8 ✓5th
      with successful version 652.1 ✓5th
    hemorrhage (antepartum) (intrapartum)
        NEC 641.9 ✓5th
    hydrocephalic fetus 653.6 ✓5th
    incarceration of uterus 654.3 ✓5th
    incoordinate uterine action 661.4 ✓5th
    inertia, uterus 661.2 ✓5th
      primary 661.0 ✓5th
      secondary 661.1 ✓5th
    lateroversion, uterus or cervix 654.4 ✓5th
    mal lie 652.9 ✓5th
    malposition
      fetus 652.9 ✓5th
        in multiple gestation 652.6 ✓5th
      pelvic organs or tissues NEC 654.9 ✓5th
      uterus NEC or cervix 654.4 ✓5th

Delivery — *continued*
  cesarean — *continued*
    malpresentation NEC 652.9 ✓5th
      in multiple gestation 652.6 ✓5th
    maternal
      diabetes mellitus 648.0 ✓5th
      heart disease NEC 648.6 ✓5th
    meconium in liquor 656.8 ✓5th
      staining only 792.3
    oblique presentation 652.3 ✓5th
    oversize fetus 653.5 ✓5th
    pelvic tumor NEC 654.9 ✓5th
    placental insufficiency 656.5 ✓5th
    placenta previa 641.0 ✓5th
      with hemorrhage 641.1 ✓5th
    poor dilation, cervix 661.0 ✓5th
    preeclampsia 642.4 ✓5th
      severe 642.5 ✓5th
    previous
      cesarean delivery 654.2 ✓5th
      surgery (to)
        cervix 654.6 ✓5th
        gynecological NEC 654.9 ✓5th
        uterus NEC 654.9 ✓5th
          previous cesarean delivery
            654.2 ✓5th
        vagina 654.7 ✓5th
    prolapse
      arm or hand 652.7 ✓5th
      uterus 654.4 ✓5th
    prolonged labor 662.1 ✓5th
    rectocele 654.4 ✓5th
    retroversion, uterus or cervix 654.3 ✓5th
    rigid
      cervix 654.6 ✓5th
      pelvic floor 654.4 ✓5th
      perineum 654.8 ✓5th
      vagina 654.7 ✓5th
      vulva 654.8 ✓5th
    sacculation, pregnant uterus 654.4 ✓5th
    scar(s)
      cervix 654.6 ✓5th
      cesarean delivery 654.2 ✓5th
      uterus NEC 654.9 ✓5th
        due to previous cesarean delivery
          654.2 ✓5th
    Shirodkar suture in situ 654.5 ✓5th
    shoulder presentation 652.8 ✓5th
    stenosis or stricture, cervix 654.6 ✓5th
    transverse presentation or lie 652.3 ✓5th
    tumor, pelvic organs or tissues NEC
        654.4 ✓5th
    umbilical cord presentation or prolapse
        663.0 ✓5th
  completely normal case — *see* category 650
  complicated (by) NEC 669.9 ✓5th
    abdominal tumor, fetal 653.7 ✓5th
      causing obstructed labor 660.1 ✓5th
    abnormal, abnormality of
      cervix 654.6 ✓5th
        causing obstructed labor 660.2 ✓5th
      forces of labor 661.9 ✓5th
      formation of uterus 654.0 ✓5th
      pelvic organs or tissues 654.9 ✓5th
        causing obstructed labor 660.2 ✓5th
      pelvis (bony) (major) NEC 653.0 ✓5th
        causing obstructed labor 660.1 ✓5th
      presentation or position NEC 652.9 ✓5th
        causing obstructed labor 660.0 ✓5th
      size, fetus 653.5 ✓5th
        causing obstructed labor 660.1 ✓5th

Delivery — *continued*
  complicated — *continued*
    abnormal, abnormality of — *continued*
      soft parts (of pelvis) 654.9
        causing obstructed labor 660.2
      uterine contractions NEC 661.9
      uterus (formation) 654.0
        causing obstructed labor 660.2
      vagina 654.7
        causing obstructed labor 660.2
    abnormally formed uterus (any type) (congenital) 654.0
      causing obstructed labor 660.2
    acromion presentation 652.8
      causing obstructed labor 660.0
    adherent placenta 667.0
      with hemorrhage 666.0
    adhesions, uterus (to abdominal wall) 654.4
    advanced maternal age NEC 659.6
      multigravida 659.6
      primigravida 659.5
    air embolism 673.0
    amnionitis 658.4
    amniotic fluid embolism 673.1
    anesthetic death 668.9
    annular detachment, cervix 665.3
    antepartum hemorrhage — *see* Delivery, complicated, hemorrhage
    anteversion, cervix or uterus 654.4
      causing obstructed labor 660.2
    apoplexy 674.0
      placenta 641.2
    arrested active phase 661.1
    asymmetrical pelvis bone 653.0
      causing obstructed labor 660.1
    atony, uterus (hypotonic) (inertia) 666.1
      hypertonic 661.4
    Bandl's ring 661.4
    battledore placenta — *see* Placenta, abnormal
    bicornis or bicornuate uterus 654.0
      causing obstructed labor 660.2
    birth injury to mother NEC 665.9
    bleeding (*see also* Delivery, complicated, hemorrhage) 641.9
    breech presentation (assisted) (buttocks) (complete) (frank) (spontaneous) 652.2
      with successful version 652.1
    brow presentation 652.4
    cephalopelvic disproportion (normally formed fetus) 653.4
      causing obstructed labor 660.1
    cerebral hemorrhage 674.0
    cervical dystocia 661.0
    chin presentation 652.4
      causing obstructed labor 660.0
    cicatrix
      cervix 654.6
        causing obstructed labor 660.2
      vagina 654.7
        causing obstructed labor 660.2
    colporrhexis 665.4
      with perineal laceration 664.0
    compound presentation 652.8
      causing obstructed labor 660.0
    compression of cord (umbilical) 663.2
      around neck 663.1
      cord prolapsed 663.0

Delivery — *continued*
  complicated — *continued*
    contraction, contracted pelvis 653.1
      causing obstructed labor 660.1
      general 653.1
        causing obstructed labor 660.1
      inlet 653.2
        causing obstructed labor 660.1
      midpelvic 653.8
        causing obstructed labor 660.1
      midplane 653.8
        causing obstructed labor 660.1
      outlet 653.3
        causing obstructed labor 660.1
    contraction ring 661.4
    cord (umbilical) 663.9
      around neck, tightly or with compression 663.1
        without compression 663.3
      bruising 663.6
      complication NEC 663.9
        specified type NEC 663.8
      compression NEC 663.2
      entanglement NEC 663.3
        with compression 663.2
      forelying 663.0
      hematoma 663.6
      marginal attachment 663.8
      presentation 663.0
      prolapse (complete) (occult) (partial) 663.0
      short 663.4
      specified complication NEC 663.8
      thrombosis (vessels) 663.6
      vascular lesion 663.6
      velamentous insertion 663.8
    Couvelaire uterus 641.2
    cretin pelvis (dwarf type) (male type) 653.1
      causing obstructed labor 660.1
    crossbirth 652.3
      with successful version 652.1
      causing obstructed labor 660.0
    cyst (Gartner's duct) 654.7
    cystocele 654.4
      causing obstructed labor 660.2
    death of fetus (near term) 656.4
      early (before 22 completed weeks gestation) 632
    deformity (acquired) (congenital)
      fetus 653.7
        causing obstructed labor 660.1
      pelvic organs or tissues NEC 654.9
        causing obstructed labor 660.2
      pelvis (bony) NEC 653.0
        causing obstructed labor 660.1
    delay, delayed
      delivery in multiple pregnancy 662.3
        due to locked mates 660.5
      following rupture of membranes (spontaneous) 658.2
        artificial 658.3
    depressed fetal heart tones 659.7
    diastasis recti 665.8
    dilation
      bladder 654.4
        causing obstructed labor 660.2
      cervix, incomplete, poor or slow 661.0
    diseased placenta 656.7

Index to Diseases — Delivery

Delivery — *continued*
- complicated — *continued*
    - displacement uterus NEC 654.4
        - causing obstructed labor 660.2
    - disproportion NEC 653.9
        - causing obstructed labor 660.1
    - disruptio uteri — *see* Delivery, complicated, rupture, uterus
    - distress
        - fetal 656.8
        - maternal 669.0
    - double uterus (congenital) 654.0
        - causing obstructed labor 660.2
    - dropsy amnion 657
    - dysfunction, uterus 661.9
        - hypertonic 661.4
        - hypotonic 661.2
            - primary 661.0
            - secondary 661.1
        - incoordinate 661.4
    - dystocia
        - cervical 661.0
        - fetal — *see* Delivery, complicated, abnormal presentation
        - maternal — *see* Delivery, complicated, prolonged labor
        - pelvic — *see* Delivery, complicated, contraction pelvis
        - positional 652.8
        - shoulder girdle 660.4
    - eclampsia 642.6
    - ectopic kidney 654.4
        - causing obstructed labor 660.2
    - edema, cervix 654.6
        - causing obstructed labor 660.2
    - effusion, amniotic fluid 658.1
    - elderly multigravida 659.6
    - elderly primigravida 659.5
    - embolism (pulmonary) 673.2
        - air 673.0
        - amniotic fluid 673.1
        - blood clot 673.2
        - cerebral 674.0
        - fat 673.8
        - pyemic 673.3
        - septic 673.3
    - entanglement, umbilical cord 663.3
        - with compression 663.2
            - around neck (with compression) 663.1
    - eversion, cervix or uterus 665.2
    - excessive
        - fetal growth 653.5
            - causing obstructed labor 660.1
        - size of fetus 653.5
            - causing obstructed labor 660.1
    - face presentation 652.4
        - causing obstructed labor 660.0
        - to pubes 660.3
    - failure, fetal head to enter pelvic brim 652.5
        - causing obstructed labor 660.0
    - fetal
        - acid-base balance 656.8
        - death (near term) NEC 656.4
            - early (before 22 completed weeks gestation) 632
        - deformity 653.7
            - causing obstructed labor 660.1
        - distress 656.8
        - heart rate or rhythm 659.7

Delivery — *continued*
- complicated — *continued*
    - fetopelvic disproportion 653.4
        - causing obstructed labor 660.1
    - fever during labor 659.2
    - fibroid (tumor) (uterus) 654.1
        - causing obstructed labor 660.2
    - fibromyomata 654.1
        - causing obstructed labor 660.2
    - forelying umbilical cord 663.0
    - fracture of coccyx 665.6
    - hematoma 664.5
        - broad ligament 665.7
        - ischial spine 665.7
        - pelvic 665.7
        - perineum 664.5
        - soft tissues 665.7
        - subdural 674.0
        - umbilical cord 663.6
        - vagina 665.7
        - vulva or perineum 664.5
    - hemorrhage (uterine) (antepartum) (intrapartum) (pregnancy) 641.9
        - accidental 641.2
        - associated with
            - afibrinogenemia 641.3
            - coagulation defect 641.3
            - hyperfibrinolysis 641.3
            - hypofibrinogenemia 641.3
        - cerebral 674.0
        - due to
            - low-lying placenta 641.1
            - placenta previa 641.1
            - premature separation of placenta (normally implanted) 641.2
            - retained placenta 666.0
            - trauma 641.8
            - uterine leiomyoma 641.8
        - marginal sinus rupture 641.2
        - placenta NEC 641.9
        - postpartum (atonic) (immediate) (within 24 hours) 666.1
            - with retained or trapped placenta 666.0
            - delayed 666.2
            - secondary 666.2
            - third stage 666.0
    - hourglass contraction, uterus 661.4
    - hydramnios 657
    - hydrocephalic fetus 653.6
        - causing obstructed labor 660.1
    - hydrops fetalis 653.7
        - causing obstructed labor 660.1
    - hypertension — *see* Hypertension, complicating pregnancy
    - hypertonic uterine dysfunction 661.4
    - hypotonic uterine dysfunction 661.2
    - impacted shoulders 660.4
    - incarceration, uterus 654.3
        - causing obstructed labor 660.2
    - incomplete dilation (cervix) 661.0
    - incoordinate uterus 661.4
    - indication NEC 659.9
        - specified type 659.8
    - inertia, uterus 661.2
        - hypertonic 661.4
        - hypotonic 661.2
            - primary 661.0
            - secondary 661.1

Delivery — continued
  complicated — continued
    infantile
      genitalia 654.4
        causing obstructed labor 660.2
      uterus (os) 654.4
        causing obstructed labor 660.2
    injury (to mother) NEC 665.9
    intrauterine fetal death (near term) NEC 656.4
      early (before 22 completed weeks gestation) 632
    inversion, uterus 665.2
    kidney, ectopic 654.4
      causing obstructed labor 660.2
    knot (true), umbilical cord 663.2
    labor, premature (before 37 completed weeks gestation) 644.2
    laceration 664.9
      anus (spincter) 664.2
        with mucosa 664.3
      bladder (urinary) 665.5
      bowel 665.5
      central 664.4
      cervix (uteri) 665.3
      fourchette 664.0
      hymen 664.0
      labia (majora) (minora) 664.0
      pelvic
        floor 664.1
        organ NEC 665.5
      perineum, perineal 664.4
        first degree 664.0
        second degree 664.1
        third degree 664.2
        fourth degree 664.3
        central 664.4
        extensive NEC 664.4
        muscles 664.1
        skin 664.0
        slight 664.0
      peritoneum 665.5
      periurethral tissue 665.5
      rectovaginal (septum) (without perineal laceration) 665.4
        with perineum 664.2
          with anal rectal mucosa 664.3
      skin (perineum) 664.0
      specified site or type NEC 664.8
      sphincter ani 664.2
        with mucosa 664.3
      urethra 665.5
      uterus 665.1
        before labor 665.0
      vagina, vaginal (deep) (high) (sulcus) (wall) (without perineal laceration) 665.4
        with perineum 664.0
        muscles, with perineum 664.1
      vulva 664.0
    lateroversion, uterus or cervix 654.4
      causing obstructed labor 660.2
    locked mates 660.5
    low implantation of placenta — see Delivery, complicated, placenta, previa
    mal lie 652.9
    malposition
      fetus NEC 652.9
        causing obstructed labor 660.0

Delivery — continued
  complicated — continued
    malposition — continued
      pelvic organs or tissues NEC 654.9
        causing obstructed labor 660.2
      placenta 641.1
        without hemorrhage 641.0
      uterus NEC or cervix 654.4
        causing obstructed labor 660.2
    malpresentation 652.9
      causing obstructed labor 660.0
    marginal sinus (bleeding) (rupture) 641.2
    maternal hypotension syndrome 669.2
    meconium in liquor 656.8
    membranes, retained — see Delivery, complicated, placenta, retained
    mentum presentation 652.4
      causing obstructed labor 660.0
    metrorrhagia (myopathia) — see Delivery, complicated, hemorrhage
    metrorrhexis — see Delivery, complicated, rupture, uterus
    multiparity (grand) 659.4
    myelomeningocele, fetus 653.7
      causing obstructed labor 660.1
    Nägele's pelvis 653.0
      causing obstructed labor 660.1
    nonengagement, fetal head 652.5
      causing obstructed labor 660.0
    oblique presentation 652.3
      causing obstructed labor 660.0
    obstetric
      shock 669.1
      trauma NEC 665.9
    obstructed labor 660.9
      due to
        abnormality pelvic organs or tissues (conditions classifiable to 654.0-654.9) 660.2
        deep transverse arrest 660.3
        impacted shoulders 660.4
        locked twins 660.5
        malposition and malpresentation of fetus (conditions classifiable to 652.0-652.9) 660.0
        persistent occipitoposterior 660.3
        shoulder dystocia 660.4
    occult prolapse of umbilical cord 663.0
    oversize fetus 653.5
      causing obstructed labor 660.1
    pathological retraction ring, uterus 661.4
    pelvic
      arrest (deep) (high) (of fetal head) (transverse) 660.3
      deformity (bone) — see also Deformity, pelvis, with disproportion
        soft tissue 654.9
          causing obstructed labor 660.2
        tumor NEC 654.9
          causing obstructed labor 660.2
    penetration, pregnant uterus by instrument 665.1
    perforation — see Delivery, complicated, laceration
    persistent
      hymen 654.8
        causing obstructed labor 660.2
      occipitoposterior 660.3

Index to Diseases

Delivery — *continued*
  complicated — *continued*
    placenta, placental
      ablatio 641.2 ✓5
      abnormality 656.7 ✓5
        with hemorrhage 641.2 ✓5
      abruptio 641.2 ✓5
      accreta 667.0 ✓5
        with hemorrhage 666.0 ✓5
      adherent (without hemorrhage)
          667.0 ✓5
        with hemorrhage 666.0 ✓5
      apoplexy 641.2 ✓5
      battledore placenta — see Placenta,
          abnormal 663.8 ✓5
      detachment (premature) 641.2 ✓5
      disease 656.7 ✓5
      hemorrhage NEC 641.9 ✓5
      increta (without hemorrhage) 667.0 ✓5
        with hemorrhage 666.0 ✓5
      low (implantation) 641.0 ✓5
        without hemorrhage 641.0 ✓5
      malformation 656.7 ✓5
        with hemorrhage 641.2 ✓5
      malposition 641.1 ✓5
        without hemorrhage 641.0 ✓5
      marginal sinus rupture 641.2 ✓5
      percreta 667.0 ✓5
        with hemorrhage 666.0 ✓5
      premature separation 641.2 ✓5
      previa (central) (lateral) (marginal)
          partial) 641.1 ✓5
        without hemorrhage 641.0 ✓5
      retained (with hemorrhage) 666.0 ✓5
        without hemorrhage 667.0 ✓5
      rupture of marginal sinus 641.2 ✓5
      separation (premature) 641.2 ✓5
      trapped 666.0 ✓5
        without hemorrhage 667.0 ✓5
      vicious insertion 641.1 ✓5
    polyhydramnios 657 ✓4
    polyp, cervix 654.6 ✓5
      causing obstructed labor 660.2 ✓5
    precipitate labor 661.3 ✓5
    premature
      labor (before 37 completed weeks
          gestation) 644.2 ✓5
      rupture, membranes 658.1 ✓5
        delayed delivery following 658.2 ✓5
    presenting umbilical cord 663.0 ✓5
    previous
      cesarean delivery 654.2 ✓5
      surgery
        cervix 654.6 ✓5
          causing obstructed labor 660.2 ✓5
        gynecological NEC 654.9 ✓5
          causing obstructed labor 660.2 ✓5
        perineum 654.8 ✓5
        uterus NEC 654.9 ✓5
          due to previous cesarean delivery
              654.2 ✓5
        vagina 654.7 ✓5
          causing obstructed labor 660.2 ✓5
        vulva 654.8 ✓5
    primary uterine inertia 661.0 ✓5
    primipara, elderly or old 659.5 ✓5
    prolapse
      arm or hand 652.7 ✓5
        causing obstructed labor 660.0 ✓5
      cord (umbilical) 663.0 ✓5
      fetal extremity 652.8 ✓5

Delivery — *continued*
  complicated — *continued*
    prolapse — *continued*
      foot or leg 652.8 ✓5
        causing obstructed labor 660.0 ✓5
      umbilical cord (complete) (occult)
          (partial) 663.0 ✓5
      uterus 654.4 ✓5
        causing obstructed labor 660.2 ✓5
    prolonged labor 662.1 ✓5
      first stage 662.0 ✓5
      second stage 662.2 ✓5
      active phase 661.2 ✓5
      due to
        cervical dystocia 661.0 ✓5
        contraction ring 661.4 ✓5
        tetanic uterus 661.4 ✓5
        uterine inertia 661.2 ✓5
          primary 661.0 ✓5
          secondary 661.1 ✓5
      latent phase 661.0 ✓5
    pyrexia during labor 659.2 ✓5
    rachitic pelvis 653.2 ✓5
      causing obstructed labor 660.1 ✓5
    rectocele 654.4 ✓5
      causing obstructed labor 660.2 ✓5
    retained membranes or portions of placenta
        666.2 ✓5
      without hemorrhage 667.1 ✓5
    retarded (prolonged) birth 662.1 ✓5
    retention secundines (with hemorrhage)
        666.2 ✓5
      without hemorrhage 667.1 ✓5
    retroversion, uterus or cervix 654.3 ✓5
      causing obstructed labor 660.2 ✓5
    rigid
      cervix 654.6 ✓5
        causing obstructed labor 660.2 ✓5
      pelvic floor 654.4 ✓5
        causing obstructed labor 660.2 ✓5
      perineum or vulva 654.8 ✓5
        causing obstructed labor 660.2 ✓5
      vagina 654.7 ✓5
        causing obstructed labor 660.2 ✓5
    Robert's pelvis 653.0 ✓5
      causing obstructed labor 660.1 ✓5
    rupture — see also Delivery, complicated,
        laceration
      bladder (urinary) 665.5 ✓5
      cervix 665.3 ✓5
      marginal sinus 641.2 ✓5
      membranes, premature 658.1 ✓5
      pelvic organ NEC 665.5 ✓5
      perineum (without mention of other
          laceration) — see Delivery,
          complicated, laceration, perineum
      peritoneum 665.5 ✓5
      urethra 665.5 ✓5
      uterus (during labor) 665.1 ✓5
        before labor 665.0 ✓5
    sacculation, pregnant uterus 654.4 ✓5
    sacral teratomas, fetal 653.7 ✓5
      causing obstructed labor 660.1 ✓5
    scar(s)
      cervix 654.6 ✓5
        causing obstructed labor 660.2 ✓5
      cesarean delivery 654.2 ✓5
        causing obstructed labor 660.2 ✓5
      perineum 654.8 ✓5
        causing obstructed labor 660.2 ✓5

Delivery

Delivery — *continued*
  complicated — *continued*
    scar(s) — *continued*
      uterus NEC 654.9 ✓5ᵗʰ
        causing obstructed labor 660.2 ✓5ᵗʰ
        due to previous cesarean delivery 654.2 ✓5ᵗʰ
      vagina 654.7 ✓5ᵗʰ
        causing obstructed labor 660.2 ✓5ᵗʰ
      vulva 654.8 ✓5ᵗʰ
        causing obstructed labor 660.2 ✓5ᵗʰ
    scoliotic pelvis 653.0 ✓5ᵗʰ
      causing obstructed labor 660.1 ✓5ᵗʰ
    secondary uterine inertia 661.1 ✓5ᵗʰ
    secundines, retained — *see* Delivery, complicated, placenta, retained
    separation
      placenta (premature) 641.2 ✓5ᵗʰ
      pubic bone 665.6 ✓5ᵗʰ
      symphysis pubis 665.6 ✓5ᵗʰ
    septate vagina 654.7 ✓5ᵗʰ
      causing obstructed labor 660.2 ✓5ᵗʰ
    shock (birth) (obstetric) (puerperal) 669.1 ✓5ᵗʰ
    short cord syndrome 663.4 ✓5ᵗʰ
    shoulder
      girdle dystocia 660.4 ✓5ᵗʰ
      presentation 652.8 ✓5ᵗʰ
        causing obstructed labor 660.0 ✓5ᵗʰ
    Siamese twins 653.7 ✓5ᵗʰ
      causing obstructed labor 660.1 ✓5ᵗʰ
    slow slope active phase 661.2 ✓5ᵗʰ
    spasm
      cervix 661.4 ✓5ᵗʰ
      uterus 661.4 ✓5ᵗʰ
    spondylolisthesis, pelvis 653.3 ✓5ᵗʰ
      causing obstructed labor 660.1 ✓5ᵗʰ
    spondylolysis (lumbosacral) 653.3 ✓5ᵗʰ
      causing obstructed labor 660.1 ✓5ᵗʰ
    spondylosis 653.0 ✓5ᵗʰ
      causing obstructed labor 660.1 ✓5ᵗʰ
    stenosis or stricture
      cervix 654.6 ✓5ᵗʰ
        causing obstructed labor 660.2 ✓5ᵗʰ
      vagina 654.7 ✓5ᵗʰ
        causing obstructed labor 660.2 ✓5ᵗʰ
    sudden death, unknown cause 669.9 ✓5ᵗʰ
    tear (pelvic organ) (*see also* Delivery, complicated, laceration) 664.9 ✓5ᵗʰ
    teratomas, sacral, fetal 653.7 ✓5ᵗʰ
      causing obstructed labor 660.1 ✓5ᵗʰ
    tetanic uterus 661.4 ✓5ᵗʰ
    tipping pelvis 653.0 ✓5ᵗʰ
      causing obstructed labor 660.1 ✓5ᵗʰ
    transverse
      arrest (deep) 660.3 ✓5ᵗʰ
      presentation or lie 652.3 ✓5ᵗʰ
        with successful version 652.1 ✓5ᵗʰ
        causing obstructed labor 660.0 ✓5ᵗʰ
    trauma (obstetrical) NEC 665.9 ✓5ᵗʰ
    tumor
      abdominal, fetal 653.7 ✓5ᵗʰ
        causing obstructed labor 660.1 ✓5ᵗʰ
      pelvic organs or tissues NEC 654.9 ✓5ᵗʰ
        causing obstructed labor 660.2 ✓5ᵗʰ
    umbilical cord (*see also* Delivery, complicated, cord) 663.9 ✓5ᵗʰ
      around neck tightly, or with compression 663.1 ✓5ᵗʰ
      entanglement NEC 663.3 ✓5ᵗʰ
        with compression 663.2 ✓5ᵗʰ

Delivery — *continued*
  complicated — *continued*
    umbilical cord — *continued*
      prolapse (complete) (occult) (partial) 663.0 ✓5ᵗʰ
      unstable lie 652.0 ✓5ᵗʰ
        causing obstructed labor 660.0 ✓5ᵗʰ
      uterine
        inertia (*see also* Delivery, complicated, inertia, uterus) 661.2 ✓5ᵗʰ
        spasm 661.4 ✓5ᵗʰ
      vasa previa 663.5 ✓5ᵗʰ
      velamentous insertion of cord 663.8 ✓5ᵗʰ
      young maternal age 659.8 ✓5ᵗʰ
    delayed NEC 662.1 ✓5ᵗʰ
      following rupture of membranes
        (spontaneous) 658.2 ✓5ᵗʰ
        artificial 658.3 ✓5ᵗʰ
      second twin, triplet, etc. 662.3 ✓5ᵗʰ
    difficult NEC 669.9 ✓5ᵗʰ
      previous, affecting management of pregnancy or childbirth V23.49 ▲
      specified type NEC 669.8 ✓5ᵗʰ
    early onset (spontaneous) 644.2 ✓5ᵗʰ
    footling 652.8 ✓5ᵗʰ
      with successful version 652.1 ✓5ᵗʰ
    forceps NEC 669.5 ✓5ᵗʰ
      affecting fetus or newborn 763.2
    missed (at or near term) 656.4 ✓5ᵗʰ
    multiple gestation NEC 651.9 ✓5ᵗʰ
      with fetal loss and retention of one or more fetus(es) 651.6 ✓5ᵗʰ
      specified type NEC 651.8 ✓5ᵗʰ
        with fetal loss and retention of one or more fetus(es) 651.6 ✓5ᵗʰ
    nonviable infant 656.4 ✓5ᵗʰ
    normal — *see* category 650
    precipitate 661.3 ✓5ᵗʰ
      affecting fetus or newborn 763.6
    premature NEC (before 37 completed weeks gestation) 644.2 ✓5ᵗʰ
      previous, affecting management of pregnancy V23.41 ▲
    quadruplet NEC 651.2 ✓5ᵗʰ
      with fetal loss and retention of one or more fetus(es) 651.5 ✓5ᵗʰ
    quintuplet NEC 651.8 ✓5ᵗʰ
      with fetal loss and retention of one or more fetus(es) 651.6 ✓5ᵗʰ
    sextuplet NEC 651.8 ✓5ᵗʰ
      with fetal loss and retention of one or more fetus(es) 651.6 ✓5ᵗʰ
    specified complication NEC 669.8 ✓5ᵗʰ
    stillbirth (near term) NEC 656.4 ✓5ᵗʰ
      early (before 22 completed weeks gestation) 632
    term pregnancy (live birth) NEC — *see* category 650
    stillbirth NEC 656.4 ✓5ᵗʰ
    threatened premature 644.2 ✓5ᵗʰ
    triplets NEC 651.1 ✓5ᵗʰ
      with fetal loss and retention of one or more fetus(es) 651.4 ✓5ᵗʰ
      delayed delivery (one or more mates) 662.3 ✓5ᵗʰ
      locked mates 660.5 ✓5ᵗʰ
    twins NEC 651.0 ✓5ᵗʰ
      with fetal loss and retention of one fetus 651.3 ✓5ᵗʰ
      delayed delivery (one or more mates) 662.3 ✓5ᵗʰ

Delivery — continued
  twins NEC — continued
    locked mates 660.5 ✓5ᵗʰ
  uncomplicated — see category 650
  vacuum extractor NEC 669.5 ✓5ᵗʰ
    affecting fetus or newborn 763.3
  ventouse NEC 669.5 ✓5ᵗʰ
    affecting fetus or newborn 763.3
Dellen, cornea 371.41
Delusions (paranoid) 297.9
  grandiose 297.1
  parasitosis 300.29
  systematized 297.1
Dementia 294.8
  alcoholic (see also Psychosis, alcoholic) 291.2
  Alzheimer's — see Alzheimer's dementia
  arteriosclerotic (simple type) (uncomplicated) 290.40
    with
      acute confusional state 290.41
      delirium 290.41
      delusional features 290.42
      depressive features 290.43
    depressed type 290.43
    paranoid type 290.42
  Binswanger's 290.12
  catatonic (acute) (see also Schizophrenia) 295.2 ✓5ᵗʰ
  congenital (see also Retardation, mental) 319
  degenerative 290.9
    presenile-onset — see Dementia, presenile
    senile-onset — see Dementia, senile
  developmental (see also Schizophrenia) 295.9 ✓5ᵗʰ
  dialysis 294.8
    transient 293.9
  due to or associated with condition(s) classified elsewhere
    Alzheimer's
      with behavioral disturbance 331.0 [294.11]
      without behavioral disturbance 331.0 [294.10]
    cerebral lipidoses
      with behavioral disturbance 330.1 [294.11]
      without behavioral disturbance 330.1 [294.10]
    epilepsy
      with behavioral disturbance 345.9 ✓5ᵗʰ [294.11]
      without behavioral disturbance 345.9 ✓5ᵗʰ [294.10]
    hepatolenticular degeneration
      with behavioral disturbance 275.1 [294.11]
      without behavioral disturbance 275.1 [294.10]
    HIV
      with behavioral disturbance 042 [294.11]
      without behavioral disturbance 042 [294.10]
    Huntington's chorea
      with behavioral disturbance 333.4 [294.11]
      without behavioral disturbance 333.4 [294.10]
    Jakob-Cruetzfeldt disease
      with behavioral disturbance 046.1 [294.11]

Dementia — continued
  due to or associated with condition(s) classified elsewhere — continued
    Jakob-Cruetzfeldt disease — continued
      without behavioral disturbance 046.1 [294.10]
    multiple sclerosis
      with behavioral disturbance 340 [294.11]
      without behavioral disturbance 340 [294.10]
    neurosyphilis
      with behavioral disturbance 094.9 [294.11]
      without behavioral disturbance 094.9 [294.10]
    Pelizaeus-Merzbacher disease
      with behavioral disturbance 333.0 [294.11]
      without behavioral disturbance 333.0 [294.10]
    Pick's disease
      with behavioral disturbance 331.1 [294.11]
      without behavioral disturbance 331.1 [294.10]
    polyarteritis nodosa
      with behavioral disturbance 446.0 [294.11]
      without behavioral disturbance 446.0 [294.10]
    syphilis
      with behavioral disturbance 094.1 [294.11]
      without behavioral disturbance 094.1 [294.10]
    Wilson's disease
      with behavioral disturbance 275.1 [294.11]
      without behavioral disturbance 275.1 [294.10]
  hebephrenic (acute) 295.1 ✓5ᵗʰ
  Heller's (infantile psychosis) (see also Psychosis, childhood) 299.1 ✓5ᵗʰ
  idiopathic 290.9
    presenile-onset — see Dementia, presenile
    senile-onset — see Dementia, senile
  in
    arteriosclerotic brain disease 290.40
    senility 290.0
  induced by drug 292.82
  infantile, infantilia (see also Psychosis, childhood) 299.0 ✓5ᵗʰ
  multi-infarct (cerebrovascular) (see also Dementia, arteriosclerotic) 290.40
  old age 290.0
  paralytica, paralytic 094.1
    juvenilis 090.40
    syphilitic 094.1
      congenital 090.40
    tabetic form 094.1
  paranoid (see also Schizophrenia) 295.3 ✓5ᵗʰ
  paraphrenic (see also Schizophrenia) 295.3 ✓5ᵗʰ
  paretic 094.1
  praecox (see also Schizophrenia) 295.9 ✓5ᵗʰ
  presenile 290.10
    with
      acute confusional state 290.11
      delirium 290.11
      delusional features 290.12
      depressive features 290.13

Dementia — *continued*
  presenile — *continued*
    depressed type 290.13
    paranoid type 290.12
    simple type 290.10
    uncomplicated 290.10
  primary (acute) (*see also* Schizophrenia) 295.0
  progressive, syphilitic 094.1
  puerperal — *see* Psychosis, puerperal
  schizophrenic (*see also* Schizophrenia) 295.9
  senile 290.0
    with
      acute confusional state 290.3
      delirium 290.3
      delusional features 290.20
      depressive features 290.21
    depressed type 290.21
    exhaustion 290.0
    paranoid type 290.20
  simple type (acute) (*see also* Schizophrenia) 295.0
  simplex (acute) (*see also* Schizophrenia) 295.0
  syphilitic 094.1
  uremic — *see* Uremia
  vascular 290.40

Demerol dependence (*see also* Dependence) 304.0

Demineralization, ankle (*see also* Osteoporosis) 733.00

Demodex folliculorum (infestation) 133.8

de Morgan's spots (senile angiomas) 448.1

Demyelinating
  polyneuritis, chronic inflammatory 357.81 ▲

Demyelination, demyelinization
  central nervous system 341.9
    specified NEC 341.8
  corpus callosum (central) 341.8
  global 340

Dengue (fever) 061
  sandfly 061
  vaccination, prophylactic (against) V05.1
  virus hemorrhagic fever 065.4

Dens
  evaginatus 520.2
  in dente 520.2
  invaginatus 520.2

Density
  increased, bone (disseminated) (generalized) (spotted) 733.99
  lung (nodular) 518.89

Dental — *see also* condition
  examination only V72.2

Dentia praecox 520.6

Denticles (in pulp) 522.2

Dentigerous cyst 526.0

Dentin
  irregular (in pulp) 522.3
  opalescent 520.5
  secondary (in pulp) 522.3
  sensitive 521.8

Dentinogenesis imperfecta 520.5

Dentinoma (M9271/0) 213.1
  upper jaw (bone) 213.0

Dentition 520.7
  abnormal 520.6

Dentition — *continued*
  anomaly 520.6
  delayed 520.6
  difficult 520.7
  disorder of 520.6
  precocious 520.6
  retarded 520.6

Denture sore (mouth) 528.9

Dependence

> Note — Use the following fifth-digit subclassification with category 304:
>
> 0   unspecified
> 1   continuous
> 2   episodic
> 3   in remission

  with
    withdrawal symptoms
      alcohol 291.81
      drug 292.0
  14-hydroxy-dihydromorphinone 304.0
  absinthe 304.6
  acemorphan 304.0
  acetanilid(e) 304.6
  acetophenetidin 304.6
  acetorphine 304.0
  acetyldihydrocodeine 304.0
  acetyldihydrocodeinone 304.0
  Adalin 304.1
  Afghanistan black 304.3
  agrypnal 304.1
  alcohol, alcoholic (ethyl) (methyl) (wood) 303.9
    maternal, with suspected fetal damage affecting management of pregnancy 655.4
  allobarbitone 304.1
  allonal 304.1
  allylisopropylacetylurea 304.1
  alphaprodine (hydrochloride) 304.0
  Alurate 304.1
  Alvodine 304.0
  amethocaine 304.6
  amidone 304.0
  amidopyrine 304.6
  aminopyrine 304.6
  amobarbital 304.1
  amphetamine(s) (type) (drugs classifiable to 969.7) 304.4
  amylene hydrate 304.6
  amylobarbitone 304.1
  amylocaine 304.6
  Amytal (sodium) 304.1
  analgesic (drug) NEC 304.6
    synthetic with morphine-like effect 304.0
  anesthetic (agent) (drug) (gas) (general) (local) NEC 304.6
  Angel dust 304.6
  anileridine 304.0
  antipyrine 304.6
  aprobarbital 304.1
  aprobarbitone 304.1
  atropine 304.6
  Avertin (bromide) 304.6
  barbenyl 304.1
  barbital(s) 304.1
  barbitone 304.1

Index to Diseases

Dependence

Dependence — *continued*
- barbiturate(s) (compounds) (drugs classifiable to 967.0) 304.1 ✓5ᵗʰ
- barbituric acid (and compounds) 304.1 ✓5ᵗʰ
- benzedrine 304.4 ✓5ᵗʰ
- benzylmorphine 304.0 ✓5ᵗʰ
- Beta-chlor 304.1 ✓5ᵗʰ
- bhang 304.3 ✓5ᵗʰ
- blue velvet 304.0 ✓5ᵗʰ
- Brevital 304.1 ✓5ᵗʰ
- bromal (hydrate) 304.1 ✓5ᵗʰ
- bromide(s) NEC 304.1 ✓5ᵗʰ
- bromine compounds NEC 304.1 ✓5ᵗʰ
- bromisovalum 304.1 ✓5ᵗʰ
- bromoform 304.1 ✓5ᵗʰ
- Bromo-seltzer 304.1 ✓5ᵗʰ
- bromural 304.1 ✓5ᵗʰ
- butabarbital (sodium) 304.1 ✓5ᵗʰ
- butabarpal 304.1 ✓5ᵗʰ
- butallylonal 304.1 ✓5ᵗʰ
- butethal 304.1 ✓5ᵗʰ
- buthalitone (sodium) 304.1 ✓5ᵗʰ
- Butisol 304.1 ✓5ᵗʰ
- butobarbitone 304.1 ✓5ᵗʰ
- butyl chloral (hydrate) 304.1 ✓5ᵗʰ
- caffeine 304.4 ✓5ᵗʰ
- cannabis (indica) (sativa) (resin) (derivatives) (type) 304.3 ✓5ᵗʰ
- carbamazepine 304.6 ✓5ᵗʰ
- Carbrital 304.1 ✓5ᵗʰ
- carbromal 304.1 ✓5ᵗʰ
- carisoprodol 304.6 ✓5ᵗʰ
- Catha (edulis) 304.4 ✓5ᵗʰ
- chloral (betaine) (hydrate) 304.1 ✓5ᵗʰ
- chloralamide 304.1 ✓5ᵗʰ
- chloralformamide 304.1 ✓5ᵗʰ
- chloralose 304.1 ✓5ᵗʰ
- chlordiazepoxide 304.1 ✓5ᵗʰ
- Chloretone 304.1 ✓5ᵗʰ
- chlorobutanol 304.1 ✓5ᵗʰ
- chlorodyne 304.1 ✓5ᵗʰ
- chloroform 304.6 ✓5ᵗʰ
- Cliradon 304.0 ✓5ᵗʰ
- coca (leaf) and derivatives 304.2 ✓5ᵗʰ
- cocaine 304.2 ✓5ᵗʰ
  - hydrochloride 304.2 ✓5ᵗʰ
  - salt (any) 304.2 ✓5ᵗʰ
- codeine 304.0 ✓5ᵗʰ
- combination of drugs (excluding morphine or opioid type drug) NEC 304.8 ✓5ᵗʰ
  - morphine or opioid type drug with any other drug 304.7 ✓5ᵗʰ
- croton-chloral 304.1 ✓5ᵗʰ
- cyclobarbital 304.1 ✓5ᵗʰ
- cyclobarbitone 304.1 ✓5ᵗʰ
- dagga 304.3 ✓5ᵗʰ
- Delvinal 304.1 ✓5ᵗʰ
- Demerol 304.0 ✓5ᵗʰ
- desocodeine 304.0 ✓5ᵗʰ
- desomorphine 304.0 ✓5ᵗʰ
- desoxyephedrine 304.4 ✓5ᵗʰ
- DET 304.5 ✓5ᵗʰ
- dexamphetamine 304.4 ✓5ᵗʰ
- dexedrine 304.4 ✓5ᵗʰ
- dextromethorphan 304.0 ✓5ᵗʰ
- dextromoramide 304.0 ✓5ᵗʰ
- dextronorpseudoephedrine 304.4 ✓5ᵗʰ
- dextrorphan 304.0 ✓5ᵗʰ
- diacetylmorphine 304.0 ✓5ᵗʰ
- Dial 304.1 ✓5ᵗʰ
- diallylbarbituric acid 304.1 ✓5ᵗʰ

Dependence — *continued*
- diamorphine 304.0 ✓5ᵗʰ
- diazepam 304.1 ✓5ᵗʰ
- dibucaine 304.6 ✓5ᵗʰ
- dichloroethane 304.6 ✓5ᵗʰ
- diethyl barbituric acid 304.1 ✓5ᵗʰ
- diethylsulfone-diethylmethane 304.1 ✓5ᵗʰ
- difencloxazine 304.0 ✓5ᵗʰ
- dihydrocodeine 304.0 ✓5ᵗʰ
- dihydrocodeinone 304.0 ✓5ᵗʰ
- dihydrohydroxycodeinone 304.0 ✓5ᵗʰ
- dihydroisocodeine 304.0 ✓5ᵗʰ
- dihydromorphine 304.0 ✓5ᵗʰ
- dihydromorphinone 304.0 ✓5ᵗʰ
- dihydroxcodeinone 304.0 ✓5ᵗʰ
- Dilaudid 304.0 ✓5ᵗʰ
- dimenhydrinate 304.6 ✓5ᵗʰ
- dimethylmeperidine 304.0 ✓5ᵗʰ
- dimethyltriptamine 304.5 ✓5ᵗʰ
- Dionin 304.0 ✓5ᵗʰ
- diphenoxylate 304.6 ✓5ᵗʰ
- dipipanone 304.0 ✓5ᵗʰ
- d-lysergic acid diethylamide 304.5 ✓5ᵗʰ
- DMT 304.5 ✓5ᵗʰ
- Dolophine 304.0 ✓5ᵗʰ
- DOM 304.2 ✓5ᵗʰ
- Doriden 304.1 ✓5ᵗʰ
- dormiral 304.1 ✓5ᵗʰ
- Dormison 304.1 ✓5ᵗʰ
- Dromoran 304.0 ✓5ᵗʰ
- drug NEC 304.9 ✓5ᵗʰ
  - analgesic NEC 304.6 ✓5ᵗʰ
  - combination (excluding morphine or opioid type drug) NEC 304.8 ✓5ᵗʰ
    - morphine or opioid type drug with any other drug 304.7 ✓5ᵗʰ
  - complicating pregnancy, childbirth, or puerperium 648.3 ✓5ᵗʰ
    - affecting fetus or newborn 779.5
  - hallucinogenic 304.5 ✓5ᵗʰ
  - hypnotic NEC 304.1 ✓5ᵗʰ
  - narcotic NEC 304.9 ✓5ᵗʰ
  - psychostimulant NEC 304.4 ✓5ᵗʰ
  - sedative 304.1 ✓5ᵗʰ
  - soporific NEC 304.1 ✓5ᵗʰ
  - specified type NEC 304.6 ✓5ᵗʰ
  - suspected damage to fetus affecting management of pregnancy 655.5 ✓5ᵗʰ
  - synthetic, with morphine-like effect 304.0 ✓5ᵗʰ
  - tranquilizing 304.1 ✓5ᵗʰ
- duboisine 304.6 ✓5ᵗʰ
- ectylurea 304.1 ✓5ᵗʰ
- Endocaine 304.6 ✓5ᵗʰ
- Equanil 304.1 ✓5ᵗʰ
- Eskabarb 304.1 ✓5ᵗʰ
- ethchlorvynol 304.1 ✓5ᵗʰ
- ether (ethyl) (liquid) (vapor) (vinyl) 304.6 ✓5ᵗʰ
- ethidene 304.6 ✓5ᵗʰ
- ethinamate 304.1 ✓5ᵗʰ
- ethoheptazine 304.6 ✓5ᵗʰ
- ethyl
  - alcohol 303.9 ✓5ᵗʰ
  - bromide 304.6 ✓5ᵗʰ
  - carbamate 304.6 ✓5ᵗʰ
  - chloride 304.6 ✓5ᵗʰ
  - morphine 304.0 ✓5ᵗʰ
- ethylene (gas) 304.6 ✓5ᵗʰ
  - dichloride 304.6 ✓5ᵗʰ
- ethylidene chloride 304.6 ✓5ᵗʰ
- etilfen 304.1 ✓5ᵗʰ

Dependence — *continued*
- etorphine 304.0
- etoval 304.1
- eucodal 304.0
- euneryl 304.1
- Evipal 304.1
- Evipan 304.1
- fentanyl 304.0
- ganja 304.3
- gardenal 304.1
- gardenpanyl 304.1
- gelsemine 304.6
- Gelsemium 304.6
- Gemonil 304.1
- glucochloral 304.1
- glue (airplane) (sniffing) 304.6
- glutethimide 304.1
- hallucinogenics 304.5
- hashish 304.3
- headache powder NEC 304.6
- Heavenly Blue 304.5
- hedonal 304.1
- hemp 304.3
- heptabarbital 304.1
- Heptalgin 304.0
- heptobarbitone 304.1
- heroin 304.0
  - salt (any) 304.0
- hexethal (sodium) 304.1
- hexobarbital 304.1
- Hycodan 304.0
- hydrocodone 304.0
- hydromorphinol 304.0
- hydromorphinone 304.0
- hydromorphone 304.0
- hydroxycodeine 304.0
- hypnotic NEC 304.1
- Indian hemp 304.3
- intranarcon 304.1
- Kemithal 304.1
- ketobemidone 304.0
- khat 304.4
- kif 304.3
- Lactuca (virosa) extract 304.1
- lactucarium 304.1
- laudanum 304.0
- Lebanese red 304.3
- Leritine 304.0
- lettuce opium 304.1
- Levanil 304.1
- Levo-Dromoran 304.0
- levo-iso-methadone 304.0
- levorphanol 304.0
- Librium 304.1
- Lomotil 304.6
- Lotusate 304.1
- LSD (-25) (and derivatives) 304.5
- Luminal 304.1
- lysergic acid 304.5
  - amide 304.5
- maconha 304.3
- magic mushroom 304.5
- marihuana 304.3
- MDA (methylene dioxyamphetamine) 304.4
- Mebaral 304.1
- Medinal 304.1
- Medomin 304.1
- megahallucinogenics 304.5
- meperidine 304.0
- mephobarbital 304.1

Dependence — *continued*
- meprobamate 304.1
- mescaline 304.5
- methadone 304.0
- methamphetamine(s) 304.4
- methaqualone 304.1
- metharbital 304.1
- methitural 304.1
- methobarbitone 304.1
- methohexital 304.1
- methopholine 304.6
- methyl
  - alcohol 303.9
  - bromide 304.6
  - morphine 304.0
  - sulfonal 304.1
- methylated spirit 303.9
- methylbutinol 304.6
- methyldihydromorphinone 304.0
- methylene
  - chloride 304.6
  - dichloride 304.6
  - dioxyamphetamine (MDA) 304.4
- methylaparafynol 304.1
- methylphenidate 304.4
- methyprylone 304.1
- metopon 304.0
- Miltown 304.1
- morning glory *seed*s 304.5
- morphinan(s) 304.0
- morphine (sulfate) (sulfite) (type) (drugs classifiable to 965.00-965.09) 304.0
- morphine or opioid type drug (drugs classifiable to 965.00-965.09) with any other drug 304.7
- morphinol(s) 304.0
- morphinon 304.0
- morpholinylethylmorphine 304.0
- mylomid 304.1
- myristicin 304.5
- narcotic (drug) NEC 304.9
- nealbarbital 304.1
- nealbarbitone 304.1
- Nembutal 304.1
- Neonal 304.1
- Neraval 304.1
- Neravan 304.1
- neurobarb 304.1
- nicotine 305.1
- Nisentil 304.0
- nitrous oxide 304.6
- Noctec 304.1
- Noludar 304.1
- nonbarbiturate sedatives and tranquilizers with similar effect 304.1
- noptil 304.1
- normorphine 304.0
- noscapine 304.0
- Novocaine 304.6
- Numorphan 304.0
- nunol 304.1
- Nupercaine 304.6
- Oblivon 304.1
- on
  - aspirator V46.0
  - hyperbaric chamber V46.8
  - iron lung V46.1
  - machine (enabling) V46.9
    - specified type NEC V46.8
  - Possum (Patient-Operated-Selector-Mechanism) V46.8

Dependence — *continued*
on — *continued*
renal dialysis machine V45.1
respirator V46.1
supplemental oxygen V46.2
opiate 304.0 ✓5ᵗʰ
opioids 304.0 ✓5ᵗʰ
opioid type drug 304.0 ✓5ᵗʰ
with any other drug 304.7 ✓5ᵗʰ
opium (alkaloids) (derivatives) (tincture) 304.0 ✓5ᵗʰ
ortal 304.1 ✓5ᵗʰ
Oxazepam 304.1 ✓5ᵗʰ
oxycodone 304.0 ✓5ᵗʰ
oxymorphone 304.0 ✓5ᵗʰ
Palfium 304.0 ✓5ᵗʰ
Panadol 304.6 ✓5ᵗʰ
pantopium 304.0 ✓5ᵗʰ
pantopon 304.0 ✓5ᵗʰ
papaverine 304.0 ✓5ᵗʰ
paracetamol 304.6 ✓5ᵗʰ
paracodin 304.0 ✓5ᵗʰ
paraldehyde 304.1 ✓5ᵗʰ
paregoric 304.0 ✓5ᵗʰ
Parzone 304.0 ✓5ᵗʰ
PCP (phencyclidine) 304.6 ✓5ᵗʰ
Pearly Gates 304.5 ✓5ᵗʰ
pentazocine 304.0 ✓5ᵗʰ
pentobarbital 304.1 ✓5ᵗʰ
pentobarbitone (sodium) 304.1 ✓5ᵗʰ
Pentothal 304.1 ✓5ᵗʰ
Percaine 304.6 ✓5ᵗʰ
Percodan 304.0 ✓5ᵗʰ
Perichlor 304.1 ✓5ᵗʰ
Pernocton 304.1 ✓5ᵗʰ
Pernoston 304.1 ✓5ᵗʰ
peronine 304.0 ✓5ᵗʰ
pethidine (hydrochloride) 304.0 ✓5ᵗʰ
petrichloral 304.1 ✓5ᵗʰ
peyote 304.5 ✓5ᵗʰ
Phanodron 304.1 ✓5ᵗʰ
phenacetin 304.6 ✓5ᵗʰ
phenadoxone 304.0 ✓5ᵗʰ
phenaglycodol 304.1 ✓5ᵗʰ
phenazocine 304.0 ✓5ᵗʰ
phencyclidine 304.6 ✓5ᵗʰ
phenmetrazine 304.4 ✓5ᵗʰ
phenobal 304.1 ✓5ᵗʰ
phenobarbital 304.1 ✓5ᵗʰ
phenobarbitone 304.1 ✓5ᵗʰ
phenomorphan 304.0 ✓5ᵗʰ
phenonyl 304.1 ✓5ᵗʰ
phenoperidine 304.0 ✓5ᵗʰ
pholcodine 304.0 ✓5ᵗʰ
piminodine 304.0 ✓5ᵗʰ
Pipadone 304.0 ✓5ᵗʰ
Pitkin's solution 304.6 ✓5ᵗʰ
Placidyl 304.1 ✓5ᵗʰ
polysubstance 304.8 ✓5ᵗʰ
Pontocaine 304.6 ✓5ᵗʰ
pot 304.3 ✓5ᵗʰ
potassium bromide 304.1 ✓5ᵗʰ
Preludin 304.4 ✓5ᵗʰ
Prinadol 304.0 ✓5ᵗʰ
probarbital 304.1 ✓5ᵗʰ
procaine 304.6 ✓5ᵗʰ
propanal 304.1 ✓5ᵗʰ
propoxyphene 304.6 ✓5ᵗʰ
psilocibin 304.5 ✓5ᵗʰ
psilocin 304.5 ✓5ᵗʰ
psilocybin 304.5 ✓5ᵗʰ

Dependence — *continued*
psilocyline 304.5 ✓5ᵗʰ
psilocyn 304.5 ✓5ᵗʰ
psychedelic agents 304.5 ✓5ᵗʰ
psychostimulant NEC 304.4 ✓5ᵗʰ
psychotomimetic agents 304.5 ✓5ᵗʰ
pyrahexyl 304.3 ✓5ᵗʰ
Pyramidon 304.6 ✓5ᵗʰ
quinalbarbitone 304.1 ✓5ᵗʰ
racemoramide 304.0 ✓5ᵗʰ
racemorphan 304.0 ✓5ᵗʰ
Rela 304.6 ✓5ᵗʰ
scopolamine 304.6 ✓5ᵗʰ
secobarbital 304.1 ✓5ᵗʰ
Seconal 304.1 ✓5ᵗʰ
sedative NEC 304.1 ✓5ᵗʰ
nonbarbiturate with barbiturate effect 304.1 ✓5ᵗʰ
Sedormid 304.1 ✓5ᵗʰ
sernyl 304.1 ✓5ᵗʰ
sodium bromide 304.1 ✓5ᵗʰ
Soma 304.6 ✓5ᵗʰ
Somnal 304.1 ✓5ᵗʰ
Somnos 304.1 ✓5ᵗʰ
Soneryl 304.1 ✓5ᵗʰ
soporific (drug) NEC 304.1 ✓5ᵗʰ
specified drug NEC 304.6 ✓5ᵗʰ
speed 304.4 ✓5ᵗʰ
spinocaine 304.6 ✓5ᵗʰ
Stovaine 304.6 ✓5ᵗʰ
STP 304.5 ✓5ᵗʰ
stramonium 304.6 ✓5ᵗʰ
Sulfonal 304.1 ✓5ᵗʰ
sulfonethylmethane 304.1 ✓5ᵗʰ
sulfonmethane 304.1 ✓5ᵗʰ
Surital 304.1 ✓5ᵗʰ
synthetic drug with morphine-like effect 304.0 ✓5ᵗʰ
talbutal 304.1 ✓5ᵗʰ
tetracaine 304.6 ✓5ᵗʰ
tetrahydrocannabinol 304.3 ✓5ᵗʰ
tetronal 304.1 ✓5ᵗʰ
THC 304.3 ✓5ᵗʰ
thebacon 304.0 ✓5ᵗʰ
thebaine 304.0 ✓5ᵗʰ
thiamil 304.1 ✓5ᵗʰ
thiamylal 304.1 ✓5ᵗʰ
thiopental 304.1 ✓5ᵗʰ
tobacco 305.1
toluene, toluol 304.6 ✓5ᵗʰ
tranquilizer NEC 304.1 ✓5ᵗʰ
nonbarbiturate with barbiturate effect 304.1 ✓5ᵗʰ
tribromacetaldehyde 304.6 ✓5ᵗʰ
tribromethanol 304.6 ✓5ᵗʰ
tribromomethane 304.6 ✓5ᵗʰ
trichloroethanol 304.6 ✓5ᵗʰ
trichoroethyl phosphate 304.1 ✓5ᵗʰ
triclofos 304.1 ✓5ᵗʰ
Trional 304.1 ✓5ᵗʰ
Tuinal 304.1 ✓5ᵗʰ
Turkish Green 304.3 ✓5ᵗʰ
urethan(e) 304.6 ✓5ᵗʰ
Valium 304.1 ✓5ᵗʰ
Valmid 304.1 ✓5ᵗʰ
veganin 304.0 ✓5ᵗʰ
veramon 304.1 ✓5ᵗʰ
Veronal 304.1 ✓5ᵗʰ
versidyne 304.6 ✓5ᵗʰ
vinbarbital 304.1 ✓5ᵗʰ
vinbarbitone 304.1 ✓5ᵗʰ

Dependence — *continued*
    vinyl bitone 304.1
    vitamin B₆ 266.1
    wine 303.9
    Zactane 304.6

Dependency
    passive 301.6
    reactions 301.6

Depersonalization (episode, in neurotic state) (neurotic) (syndrome) 300.6

Depletion
    carbohydrates 271.9
    complement factor 279.8
    extracellular fluid 276.5
    plasma 276.5
    potassium 276.8
        nephropathy 588.8
    salt or sodium 276.1
        causing heat exhaustion or prostration 992.4
        nephropathy 593.9
    volume 276.5
        extracellular fluid 276.5
        plasma 276.5

Deposit
    argentous, cornea 371.16
    bone, in Boeck's sarcoid 135
    calcareous, calcium — *see* Calcification
    cholesterol
        retina 362.82
        skin 709.3
        vitreous (humor) 379.22
    conjunctival 372.56
    cornea, corneal NEC 371.10
        argentous 371.16
        in
            cystinosis 270.0 *[371.15]*
            mucopolysaccharidosis 277.5 *[371.15]*
    crystalline, vitreous (humor) 379.22
    hemosiderin, in old scars of cornea 371.11
    metallic, in lens 366.45
    skin 709.3
    teeth, tooth (betel) (black) (green) (materia alba) (orange) (soft) (tobacco) 523.6
    urate, in kidney (*see also* Disease, renal) 593.9

Depraved appetite 307.52

Depression 311
    acute (*see also* Psychosis, affective) 296.2
        recurrent episode 296.3
        single episode 296.2
    agitated (*see also* Psychosis, affective) 296.2
        recurrent episode 296.3
        single episode 296.2
    anaclitic 309.21
    anxiety 300.4
    arches 734
        congenital 754.61
    autogenous (*see also* Psychosis, affective) 296.2
        recurrent episode 296.3
        single episode 296.2
    basal metabolic rate (BMR) 794.7
    bone marrow 289.9
    central nervous system 799.1
        newborn 779.2
    cerebral 331.9
        newborn 779.2

Depression — *continued*
    cerebrovascular 437.8
        newborn 779.2
    chest wall 738.3
    endogenous (*see also* Psychosis, affective) 296.2
        recurrent episode 296.3
        single episode 296.2
    functional activity 780.99 ▲
    hysterical 300.11
    involutional, climacteric, or menopausal (*see also* Psychosis, affective) 296.2
        recurrent episode 296.3
        single episode 296.2
    manic (*see also* Psychosis, affective) 296.80
    medullary 348.8
        newborn 779.2
    mental 300.4
    metatarsal heads — *see* Depression, arches
    metatarsus — *see* Depression, arches
    monopolar (*see also* Psychosis, affective) 296.2
        recurrent episode 296.3
        single episode 296.2
    nervous 300.4
    neurotic 300.4
    nose 738.0
    postpartum 648.4
    psychogenic 300.4
        reactive 298.0
    psychoneurotic 300.4
    psychotic (*see also* Psychosis, affective) 296.2
        reactive 298.0
        recurrent episode 296.3
        single episode 296.2
    reactive 300.4
        neurotic 300.4
        psychogenic 298.0
        psychoneurotic 300.4
        psychotic 298.0
    recurrent 296.3
    respiratory center 348.8
        newborn 770.89 ▲
    scapula 736.89
    senile 290.21
    situational (acute) (brief) 309.0
        prolonged 309.1
    skull 754.0
    sternum 738.3
    visual field 368.40

Depressive reaction — *see also* Reaction, depressive
    acute (transient) 309.0
        with anxiety 309.28
        prolonged 309.1
    situational (acute) 309.0
        prolonged 309.1

Deprivation
    cultural V62.4
    emotional V62.89
        affecting
            adult 995.82
            infant or child 995.51
    food 994.2
        specific substance NEC 269.8
    protein (familial) (kwashiorkor) 260
    social V62.4
        affecting
            adult 995.82
            infant or child 995.51

Deprivation — continued
symptoms, syndrome
alcohol 291.81
drug 292.0
vitamins (see also Deficiency, vitamin) 269.2
water 994.3
de Quervain's
disease (tendon sheath) 727.04
thyroiditis (subacute granulomatous thyroiditis) 245.1
Derangement
ankle (internal) 718.97
current injury (see also Dislocation, ankle) 837.0
recurrent 718.37
cartilage (articular) NEC (see also Disorder, cartilage, articular) 718.0 ✓5ᵗʰ
knee 717.9
recurrent 718.36
recurrent 718.3 ✓5ᵗʰ
collateral ligament (knee) (medial) (tibial) 717.82
current injury 844.1
lateral (fibular) 844.0
lateral (fibular) 717.81
current injury 844.0
cruciate ligament (knee) (posterior) 717.84
anterior 717.83
current injury 844.2
current injury 844.2
elbow (internal) 718.92
current injury (see also Dislocation, elbow) 832.00
recurrent 718.32
gastrointestinal 536.9
heart — see Disease, heart
hip (joint) (internal) (old) 718.95
current injury (see also Dislocation, hip) 835.00
recurrent 718.35
intervertebral disc — see Displacement, intervertebral disc
joint (internal) 718.90
ankle 718.97
current injury — see also Dislocation, by site
knee, meniscus or cartilage (see also Tear, meniscus) 836.2
elbow 718.92
foot 718.97
hand 718.94
hip 718.95
knee 717.9
multiple sites 718.99
pelvic region 718.95
recurrent 718.30
ankle 718.37
elbow 718.32
foot 718.37
hand 718.34
hip 718.35
knee 718.36
multiple sites 718.39
pelvic region 718.35
shoulder (region) 718.31
specified site NEC 718.38
temporomandibular (old) 524.69
wrist 718.33
shoulder (region) 718.91
specified site NEC 718.98
spine NEC 724.9

Derangement — continued
joint — continued
temporomandibular 524.69
wrist 718.93
knee (cartilage) (internal) 717.9
current injury (see also Tear, meniscus) 836.2
ligament 717.89
capsular 717.85
collateral — see Derangement, collateral ligament
cruciate — see Derangement, cruciate ligament
specified NEC 717.85
recurrent 718.36
low back NEC 724.9
meniscus NEC (knee) 717.5
current injury (see also Tear, meniscus) 836.2
lateral 717.40
anterior horn 717.42
posterior horn 717.43
specified NEC 717.49
medial 717.3
anterior horn 717.1
posterior horn 717.2
recurrent 718.3 ✓5ᵗʰ
site other than knee — see Disorder, cartilage, articular
mental (see also Psychosis) 298.9
rotator cuff (recurrent) (tear) 726.10
current 840.4
sacroiliac (old) 724.6
current — see Dislocation, sacroiliac
semilunar cartilage (knee) 717.5
current injury 836.2
lateral 836.1
medial 836.0
recurrent 718.3 ✓5ᵗʰ
shoulder (internal) 718.91
current injury (see also Dislocation, shoulder) 831.00
recurrent 718.31
spine (recurrent) NEC 724.9
current — see Dislocation, spine
temporomandibular (internal) (joint) (old) 524.69
current — see Dislocation, jaw
Dercum's disease or syndrome (adiposis dolorosa) 272.8
Derealization (neurotic) 300.6
Dermal — see condition
Dermaphytid — see Dermatophytosis
Dermatergosis — see Dermatitis
Dermatitis (allergic) (contact) (occupational) (venenata) 692.9
ab igne 692.82
acneiform 692.9
actinic (due to sun) 692.70
acute 692.72
chronic NEC 692.74
other than from sun NEC 692.82
ambustionis
due to
burn or scald — see Burn, by site
sunburn (see also Sunburn) 692.71
amebic 006.6
ammonia 691.0
anaphylactoid NEC 692.9
arsenical 692.4

Dermatitis — *continued*
  artefacta 698.4
    psychogenic 316 *[698.4]*
  asthmatic 691.8
  atopic (allergic) (intrinsic) 691.8
    psychogenic 316 *[691.8]*
  atrophicans 701.8
    diffusa 701.8
    maculosa 701.3
  berlock, berloque 692.72
  blastomycetic 116.0
  blister beetle 692.89
  Brucella NEC 023.9
  bullosa 694.9
    striata pratensis 692.6
  bullous 694.9
    mucosynechial, atrophic 694.60
      with ocular involvement 694.61
    seasonal 694.8
  calorica
    due to
      burn or scald — *see* Burn, by site
      cold 692.89
      sunburn (*see also* Sunburn) 692.71
  caterpillar 692.89
  cercarial 120.3
  combustionis
    due to
      burn or scald — *see* Burn, by site
      sunburn (*see also* Sunburn) 692.71
  congelationis 991.5
  contusiformis 695.2
  diabetic 250.8 ✓5ᵗʰ
  diaper 691.0
  diphtheritica 032.85
  due to
    acetone 692.2
    acids 692.4
    adhesive plaster 692.4
    alcohol (skin contact) (substances
        classifiable to 980.0-980.9) 692.4
      taken internally 693.8
    alkalis 692.4
    allergy NEC 692.9
    ammonia (household) (liquid) 692.4
    arnica 692.3
    arsenic 692.4
      taken internally 693.8
    blister beetle 692.89
    cantharides 692.3
    carbon disulphide 692.2
    caterpillar 692.89
    caustics 692.4
    cereal (ingested) 693.1
      contact with skin 692.5
    chemical(s) NEC 692.4
      internal 693.8
      irritant NEC 692.4
      taken internally 693.8
    chlorocompounds 692.2
    coffee (ingested) 693.1
      contact with skin 692.5
    cold weather 692.89
    cosmetics 692.81
    cyclohexanes 692.2
    deodorant 692.81
    detergents 692.0
    dichromate 692.4
    drugs and medicinals (correct substance
        properly administered) (internal use)
        693.0

Dermatitis — *continued*
  due to — *continued*
    drugs and medicinals — *continued*
      external (in contact with skin) 692.3
        wrong substance given or taken 976.9
          specified substance — *see* Table of
            Drugs and Chemicals
      wrong substance given or taken 977.9
        specified substance — *see* Table of
          Drugs and Chemicals
    dyes 692.89
      hair 692.89
    epidermophytosis — *see* Dermatophytosis
    esters 692.2
    external irritant NEC 692.9
      specified agent NEC 692.89
    eye shadow 692.81
    fish (ingested) 693.1
      contact with skin 692.5
    flour (ingested) 693.1
      contact with skin 692.5
    food (ingested) 693.1
      in contact with skin 692.5
    fruit (ingested) 693.1
      contact with skin 692.5
    fungicides 692.3
    furs 692.89
    glycols 692.2
    greases NEC 692.1
    hair dyes 692.89
    hot
      objects and materials — *see* Burn, by
        site
      weather or places 692.89
    hydrocarbons 692.2
    infrared rays, except from sun 692.82
      solar NEC (*see also* Dermatitis, due to,
        sun) 692.70
    ingested substance 693.9
      drugs and medicinals (*see also*
        Dermatitis, due to, drugs and
        medicinals) 693.0
      food 693.1
      specified substance NEC 693.8
    ingestion or injection of chemical 693.8
      drug (correct substance properly
        administered) 693.0
      wrong substance given or taken 977.9
        specified substance — *see* Table of
          Drugs and Chemicals
    insecticides 692.4
    internal agent 693.9
      drugs and medicinals (*see also*
        Dermatitis, due to, drugs and
        medicinals) 693.0
      food (ingested) 693.1
        in contact with skin 692.5
      specified agent NEC 693.8
    iodine 692.3
    iodoform 692.3
    irradiation 692.82
    jewelry 692.83
    keratolytics 692.3
    ketones 692.2
    lacquer tree (Rhus verniciflua) 692.6
    light NEC (*see also* Dermatitis, due to, sun)
      692.70
      other 692.82
    low temperature 692.89
    mascara 692.81

Index to Diseases — Dermatitis

Dermatitis — *continued*
  due to — *continued*
    meat (ingested) 693.1
      contact with skin 692.5
    mercury, mercurials 692.3
    metals 692.83
    milk (ingested) 693.1
      contact with skin 692.5
    Neomycin 692.3
    nylon 692.4
    oils NEC 692.1
    paint solvent 692.2
    pediculocides 692.3
    petroleum products (substances classifiable to 981) 692.4
    phenol 692.3
    photosensitiveness, photosensitivity (sun) 692.72
      other light 692.82
    plants NEC 692.6
    plasters, medicated (any) 692.3
    plastic 692.4
    poison
      ivy (Rhus toxicodendron) 692.6
      oak (Rhus diversiloba) 692.6
      plant or vine 692.6
      sumac (Rhus venenata) 692.6
      vine (Rhus radicans) 692.6
    preservatives 692.89
    primrose (primula) 692.6
    primula 692.6
    radiation 692.82
      sun NEC (*see also* Dermatitis, due to, sun) 692.70
      tanning bed 692.82
    radioactive substance 692.82
    radium 692.82
    ragweed (Senecio jacobae) 692.6
    Rhus (diversiloba) (radicans) (toxicodendron) (venenata) (verniciflua) 692.6
    rubber 692.4
    scabicides 692.3
    Senecio jacobae 692.6
    solar radiation — *see* Dermatitis, due to, sun
    solvents (any) (substances classifiable to 982.0-982.8) 692.2
      chlorocompound group 692.2
      cyclohexane group 692.2
      ester group 692.2
      glycol group 692.2
      hydrocarbon group 692.2
      ketone group 692.2
      paint 692.2
    specified agent NEC 692.89
    sun 692.70
      acute 692.72
      chronic NEC 692.74
      specified NEC 692.79
    sunburn (*see also* Sunburn) 692.71
    sunshine NEC (*see also* Dermatitis, due to, sun) 692.70
    tanning bed 692.82
    tetrachlorethylene 692.2
    toluene 692.2
    topical medications 692.3
    turpentine 692.2
    ultraviolet rays, except from sun 692.82
      sun NEC (*see also* Dermatitis, due to, sun) 692.82

Dermatitis — *continued*
  due to — *continued*
    vaccine or vaccination (correct substance properly administered) 693.0
    wrong substance given or taken
      bacterial vaccine 978.8
        specified — *see* Table of Drugs and Chemicals
      other vaccines NEC 979.9
        specified — *see* Table of Drugs and Chemicals
    varicose veins (*see also* Varicose, vein, inflamed or infected) 454.1
    x-rays 692.82
  dyshydrotic 705.81
  dysmenorrheica 625.8
  eczematoid NEC 692.9
    infectious 690.8
  eczematous NEC 692.9
  epidemica 695.89
  erysipelatosa 695.81
  escharotica — *see* Burn, by site
  exfoliativa, exfoliative 695.89
    generalized 695.89
    infantum 695.81
    neonatorum 695.81
  eyelid 373.31
    allergic 373.32
    contact 373.32
    eczematous 373.31
    herpes (zoster) 053.20
      simplex 054.41
    infective 373.5
      due to
        actinomycosis 039.3 [373.5]
        herpes
          simplex 054.41
          zoster 053.20
        impetigo 684 [373.5]
        leprosy (*see also* Leprosy) 030.0 [373.4]
        lupus vulgaris (tuberculous) (*see also* Tuberculosis) 017.0 ✓5ᵗʰ [373.4]
        mycotic dermatitis (*see also* Dermatomycosis) 111.9 [373.5]
        vaccinia 051.0 [373.5]
          postvaccination 999.0 [373.5]
        yaws (*see also* Yaws) 102.9 [373.4]
  facta, factitia 698.4
    psychogenic 316 [698.4]
  ficta 698.4
    psychogenic 316 [698.4]
  flexural 691.8
  follicularis 704.8
  friction 709.8
  fungus 111.9
    specified type NEC 111.8
  gangrenosa, gangrenous (infantum) (*see also* Gangrene) 785.4
  gestationis 646.8 ✓5ᵗʰ
  gonococcal 098.89
  gouty 274.89
  harvest mite 133.8
  heat 692.89
  herpetiformis (bullous) (erythematous) (pustular) (vesicular) 694.0
    juvenile 694.2
    senile 694.5
  hiemalis 692.89
  hypostatic, hypostatica 454.1
    with ulcer 454.2

✓4ᵗʰ Fourth-digit Required   ✓5ᵗʰ Fifth-digit Required

Dermatitis — continued
impetiginous 684
infantile (acute) (chronic) (intertriginous) (intrinsic) (seborrheic) 690.12
infectiosa eczematoides 690.8
infectious (staphylococcal) (streptococcal) 686.9
  eczematoid 690.8
infective eczematoid 690.8
Jacquet's (diaper dermatitis) 691.0
leptus 133.8
lichenified NEC 692.9
lichenoid, chronic 701.0
lichenoides purpurica pigmentosa 709.1
meadow 692.6
medicamentosa (correct substance properly administered) (internal use) (see also Dermatitis, due to, drugs, or medicinals) 693.0
  due to contact with skin 692.3
mite 133.8
multiformis 694.0
  juvenile 694.2
  senile 694.5
napkin 691.0
neuro 698.3
neurotica 694.0
nummular NEC 692.9
osteatosis, osteatotic 706.8
papillaris capillitii 706.1
pellagrous 265.2
perioral 695.3
perstans 696.1
photosensitivity (sun) 692.72
  other light 692.82
pigmented purpuric lichenoid 709.1
polymorpha dolorosa 694.0
primary irritant 692.9
pruriginosa 694.0
pruritic NEC 692.9
psoriasiform nodularis 696.2
psychogenic 316
purulent 686.00
pustular contagious 051.2
pyococcal 686.00
pyocyaneus 686.09
pyogenica 686.00
radiation 692.82
repens 696.1
Ritter's (exfoliativa) 695.81
Schamberg's (progressive pigmentary dermatosis) 709.09
schistosome 120.3
seasonal bullous 694.8
seborrheic 690.10
  infantile 690.12
sensitization NEC 692.9
septic (see also Septicemia) 686.00
  gonococcal 098.89
solar, solare NEC (see also Dermatitis, due to, sun) 692.70
stasis 459.81
  due to
    postphlebitic syndrome 459.12 ▲
      with ulcer 459.13 ●
    varicose veins — see Varicose
  ulcerated or with ulcer (varicose) 454.2
sunburn (see also Sunburn) 692.71
suppurative 686.00
traumatic NEC 709.8
trophoneurotica 694.0

Dermatitis — continued
ultraviolet, except from sun 692.82
  due to sun NEC (see also Dermatitis, due to, sun) 692.70
varicose 454.1
  with ulcer 454.2
vegetans 686.8
verrucosa 117.2
xerotic 706.8
Dermatoarthritis, lipoid 272.8 [713.0]
Dermatochalasia, dermatochalasis 374.87
Dermatofibroma (lenticulare) (M8832/0) — see also Neoplasm, skin, benign
  protuberans (M8832/1) — see Neoplasm, skin, uncertain behavior
Dermatofibrosarcoma (protuberans) (M8832/3) — see Neoplasm, skin, malignant
Dermatographia 708.3
Dermatolysis (congenital) (exfoliativa) 757.39
  acquired 701.8
  eyelids 374.34
  palpebrarum 374.34
  senile 701.8
Dermatomegaly NEC 701.8
Dermatomucomyositis 710.3
Dermatomycosis 111.9
  furfuracea 111.0
  specified type NEC 111.8
Dermatomyositis (acute) (chronic) 710.3
Dermatoneuritis of children 985.0
Dermatophiliasis 134.1
Dermatophytide — see Dermatophytosis
Dermatophytosis (Epidermophyton) (infection) (microsporum) (tinea) (Trichophyton) 110.9
  beard 110.0
  body 110.5
  deep seated 110.6
  fingernails 110.1
  foot 110.4
  groin 110.3
  hand 110.2
  nail 110.1
  perianal (area) 110.3
  scalp 110.0
  scrotal 110.8
  specified site NEC 110.8
  toenails 110.1
  vulva 110.8
Dermatopolyneuritis 985.0
Dermatorrhexis 756.83
  acquired 701.8
Dermatosclerosis (see also Scleroderma) 710.1
  localized 701.0
Dermatosis 709.9
  Andrews' 686.8
  atopic 691.8
  Bowen's (M8081/2) — see Neoplasm, skin, in situ
  bullous 694.9
    specified type NEC 694.8
  erythematosquamous 690.8
  exfoliativa 695.89
  factitial 698.4
  gonococcal 098.89
  herpetiformis 694.0
    juvenile 694.2
    senile 694.5
  hysterical 300.11

Dermatosis — *continued*
  Linear IgA 694.8
  menstrual NEC 709.8
  neutrophilic, acute febrile 695.89
  occupational (*see also* Dermatitis) 692.9
  papulosa nigra 709.8
  pigmentary NEC 709.00
    progressive 709.09
    Schamberg's 709.09
    Siemens-Bloch 757.33
  progressive pigmentary 709.09
  psychogenic 316
  pustular subcorneal 694.1
  Schamberg's (progressive pigmentary) 709.09
  senile NEC 709.3
  Unna's (seborrheic dermatitis) 690.10
Dermographia 708.3
Dermographism 708.3
Dermoid (cyst) (M9084/0) — *see also* Neoplasm, by site, benign
  with malignant transformation (M9084/3) 183.0
Dermopathy
  infiltrative, with throtoxicosis 242.0
  senile NEC 709.3
Dermophytosis — *see* Dermatophytosis
Descemet's membrane — *see* condition
Descemetocele 371.72
Descending — *see* condition
Descensus uteri (complete) (incomplete) (partial) (without vaginal wall prolapse) 618.1
  with mention of vaginal wall proplapse — *see* Prolapse, uterovaginal
Desensitization to allergens V07.1
Desert
  rheumatism 114.0
  sore (*see also* Ulcer, skin) 707.9
Desertion (child) (newborn) 995.52
  adult 995.84
Desmoid (extra-abdominal) (tumor) (M8821/1) — *see also* Neoplasm, connective tissue, uncertain behavior
  abdominal (M8822/1) — *see* Neoplasm, connective tissue, uncertain behavior
Despondency 300.4
Desquamative dermatitis NEC 695.89
Destruction
  articular facet (*see also* Derangement, joint) 718.9
    vertebra 724.9
  bone 733.90
    syphilitic 095.5
  joint (*see also* Derangement, joint) 718.9
    sacroiliac 724.6
  kidney 593.89
  live fetus to facilitate birth NEC 763.89
  ossicles (ear) 385.24
  rectal sphincter 569.49
  septum (nasal) 478.1
  tuberculous NEC (*see also* Tuberculosis) 011.9
  tympanic membrane 384.82
  tympanum 385.89
  vertebral disc — *see* Degeneration, intervertebral disc
Destructiveness (*see also* Disturbance, conduct) 312.9
  adjustment reaction 309.3

Detachment
  cartilage — *see also* Sprain, by site
    knee — *see* Tear, meniscus
  cervix, annular 622.8
    complicating delivery 665.3
  choroid (old) (postinfectional) (simple) (spontaneous) 363.70
    hemorrhagic 363.72
    serous 363.71
  knee, medial meniscus (old) 717.3
    current injury 836.0
  ligament — *see* Sprain, by site
  placenta (premature) — *see* Placenta, separation
  retina (recent) 361.9
    with retinal defect (rhegmatogenous) 361.00
      giant tear 361.03
      multiple 361.02
      partial
        with
          giant tear 361.03
          multiple defects 361.02
          retinal dialysis (juvenile) 361.04
          single defect 361.01
      retinal dialysis (juvenile) 361.04
      single 361.01
      subtotal 361.05
      total 361.05
    delimited (old) (partial) 361.06
    old
      delimited 361.06
      partial 361.06
      total or subtotal 361.07
    pigment epithelium (RPE) (serous) 362.42
      exudative 362.42
      hemorrhagic 362.43
    rhegmatogenous (*see also* Detachment, retina, with retinal defect) 361.00
    serous (without retinal defect) 361.2
    specified type NEC 361.89
    traction (with vitreoretinal organization) 361.81
  vitreous humor 379.21
Detergent asthma 507.8
Deterioration
  epileptic
    with behavioral disturbance 345.9 *[294.11]*
    without behavioral disturbance 345.9 *[294.10]*
  heart, cardiac (*see also* Degeneration, myocardial) 429.1
  mental (*see also* Psychosis) 298.9
  myocardium, myocardial (*see also* Degeneration, myocardial) 429.1
  senile (simple) 797
  transplanted organ — *see* Complications, transplant, organ, by site
de Toni-Fanconi syndrome (cystinosis) 270.0
Deuteranomaly 368.52
Deuteranopia (anomalous trichromat) (complete) (incomplete) 368.52
Deutschländer's disease — *see* Fracture, foot
Development
  abnormal, bone 756.9
  arrested 783.40
    bone 733.91
    child 783.40
    due to malnutrition (protein-calorie) 263.2
    fetus or newborn 764.9
  tracheal rings (congenital) 748.3

Development

Development — *continued*
  defective, congenital — *see also* Anomaly
    cauda equina 742.59
    left ventricle 746.9
      with atresia or hypoplasia of aortic orifice or valve with hypoplasia of ascending aorta 746.7
      in hypoplastic left heart syndrome 746.7
  delayed (*see also* Delay, development) 783.40
    arithmetical skills 315.1
    language (skills) 315.31
      expressive 315.31
      mixed receptive-expressive 315.32
    learning skill, specified NEC 315.2
    mixed skills 315.5
    motor coordination 315.4
    reading 315.00
    specified
      learning skill NEC 315.2
      type NEC, except learning 315.8
    speech 315.39
      associated with hyperkinesia 314.1
      phonological 315.39
    spelling 315.09
  imperfect, congenital — *see also* Anomaly
    heart 746.9
    lungs 748.60
  improper (fetus or newborn) 764.9 ✓5ᵗʰ
  incomplete (fetus or newborn) 764.9 ✓5ᵗʰ
    affecting management of pregnancy 656.5 ✓5ᵗʰ
    bronchial tree 748.3
    organ or site not listed — *see* Hypoplasia
    respiratory system 748.9
  sexual, precocious NEC 259.1
  tardy, mental (*see also* Retardation, mental) 319
  written expression 315.2

Developmental — *see* condition

Devergie's disease (pityriasis rubra pilaris) 696.4

Deviation
  conjugate (eye) 378.87
    palsy 378.81
    spasm, spastic 378.82
  esophagus 530.89
  eye, skew 378.87
  midline (jaw) (teeth) 524.2
    specified site NEC — *see* Malposition
  organ or site, congenital NEC — *see* Malposition, congenital
  septum (acquired) (nasal) 470
    congenital 754.0
  sexual 302.9
    bestiality 302.9
    coprophilia 302.89
    ego-dystonic
      homosexuality 302.0
      lesbianism 302.0
    erotomania 302.89
      Clérambault's 297.8
    exhibitionism (sexual) 302.4
    fetishism 302.81
      transvestic 302.3
    frotteurism 302.89
    homosexuality, ego-dystonic 302.0
      pedophilic 302.2
    lesbianism, ego-dystonic 302.0
    masochism 302.83
    narcissism 302.89
    necrophilia 302.89

Deviation — *continued*
  sexual — *continued*
    nymphomania 302.89
    pederosis 302.2
    pedophilia 302.2
    sadism 302.84
    sadomasochism 302.84
    satyriasis 302.89
    specified type NEC 302.89
    transvestic fetishism 302.3
    transvestism 302.3
    voyeurism 302.82
    zoophilia (erotica) 302.1
  teeth, midline 524.2
  trachea 519.1
  ureter (congenital) 753.4

Devic's disease 341.0

Device
  cerebral ventricle (communicating) in situ V45.2
  contraceptive — *see* Contraceptive, device
  drainage, cerebrospinal fluid V45.2

Devil's
  grip 074.1
  pinches (purpura simplex) 287.2

Devitalized tooth 522.9

Devonshire colic 984.9
  specified type of lead — *see* Table of Drugs and Chemicals

Dextraposition, aorta 747.21
  with ventricular septal defect, pulmonary stenosis or atresia, and hypertrophy of right ventricle 745.2
  in tetralogy of Fallot 745.2

Dextratransposition, aorta 745.11

Dextrinosis, limit (debrancher enzyme deficiency) 271.0

Dextrocardia (corrected) (false) (isolated) (secondary) (true) 746.87
  with
    complete transposition of viscera 759.3
    situs inversus 759.3

Dextroversion, kidney (left) 753.3

Dhobie itch 110.3

Diabetes, diabetic (brittle) (congenital) (familial) (mellitus) (severe) (slight) (without complication) 250.0 ✓5ᵗʰ

> Note — Use the following fifth-digit subclassification with category 250:
>
> 0   type II [non-insulin dependent type] [NIDDM type] [adult-onset type] or unspecified type, not stated as uncontrolled
>
> 1   type I [insulin dependent type] [IDDM type] [juvenile type], not stated as uncontrolled
>
> 2   type II [non-insulin dependent type] [NIDDM type] [adult-onset type] or unspecified type, uncontrolled
>
> 3   type I [insulin dependent type] [IDDM type] [juvenile type], uncontrolled

  with
    coma (with ketoacidosis) 250.3 ✓5ᵗʰ
      hyperosmolar (nonketotic) 250.2 ✓5ᵗʰ
    complication NEC 250.9 ✓5ᵗʰ
    specified NEC 250.8 ✓5ᵗʰ

Diabetes, diabetic — *continued*
with — *continued*
gangrene 250.7 ✓5ᵗʰ [785.4]
hyperosmolarity 250.2 ✓5ᵗʰ
ketosis, ketoacidosis 250.1 ✓5ᵗʰ
osteomyelitis 250.8 ✓5ᵗʰ [731.8]
specified manifestations NEC 250.8 ✓5ᵗʰ
acetonemia 250.1 ✓5ᵗʰ
acidosis 250.1 ✓5ᵗʰ
amyotrophy 250.6 ✓5ᵗʰ [358.1]
angiopathy, peripheral 250.7 ✓5ᵗʰ [443.81]
asymptomatic 790.2
autonomic neuropathy (peripheral) 250.6 ✓5ᵗʰ [337.1]
bone change 250.8 ✓5ᵗʰ [731.8]
bronze, bronzed 275.0
cataract 250.5 ✓5ᵗʰ [366.41]
chemical 790.2
complicating pregnancy, childbirth, or puerperium 648.8 ✓5ᵗʰ
coma (with ketoacidosis) 250.3 ✓5ᵗʰ
hyperglycemic 250.3 ✓5ᵗʰ
hyperosmolar (nonketotic) 250.2 ✓5ᵗʰ
hypoglycemic 250.3 ✓5ᵗʰ
insulin 250.3 ✓5ᵗʰ
complicating pregnancy, childbirth, or puerperium (maternal) 648.0 ✓5ᵗʰ
affecting fetus or newborn 775.0
complication NEC 250.9 ✓5ᵗʰ
specified NEC 250.8 ✓5ᵗʰ
dorsal sclerosis 250.6 ✓5ᵗʰ [340] ✓5ᵗʰ
dwarfism-obesity syndrome 258.1
gangrene 250.7 ✓5ᵗʰ [785.4]
gastroparesis 250.6 ✓5ᵗʰ [536.3]
gestational 648.8 ✓5ᵗʰ
complicating pregnancy, childbirth, or puerperium 648.8 ✓5ᵗʰ
glaucoma 250.5 ✓5ᵗʰ [365.44]
glomerulosclerosis (intercapillary) 250.4 ✓5ᵗʰ [581.81]
glycogenosis, secondary 250.8 ✓5ᵗʰ [259.8]
hemochromatosis 275.0
hyperosmolar coma 250.2 ✓5ᵗʰ
hyperosmolarity 250.2 ✓5ᵗʰ
hypertension-nephrosis syndrome 250.4 ✓5ᵗʰ [581.81]
hypoglycemia 250.8 ✓5ᵗʰ
hypoglycemic shock 250.8 ✓5ᵗʰ
insipidus 253.5
nephrogenic 588.1
pituitary 253.5
vasopressin-resistant 588.1
intercapillary glomerulosclerosis 250.4 ✓5ᵗʰ [581.81]
iritis 250.5 ✓5ᵗʰ [364.42]
ketosis, ketoacidosis 250.1 ✓5ᵗʰ
Kimmelstiel (-Wilson) disease or syndrome (intercapillary glomerulosclerosis) 250.4 ✓5ᵗʰ [581.81]
Lancereaux's (diabetes mellitus with marked emaciation) 250.8 ✓5ᵗʰ [261]
latent (chemical) 790.2
complicating pregnancy, childbirth, or puerperium 648.8 ✓5ᵗʰ
lipoidosis 250.8 ✓5ᵗʰ [272.7]
macular edema 250.5 ✓5ᵗʰ [362.01]
maternal
with manifest disease in the infant 775.1
affecting fetus or newborn 775.0
microaneurysms, retinal 250.5 ✓5ᵗʰ [362.01]
mononeuropathy 250.6 ✓5ᵗʰ [355.9]

Diabetes, diabetic — *continued*
neonatal, transient 775.1
nephropathy 250.4 ✓5ᵗʰ [583.81]
nephrosis (syndrome) 250.4 ✓5ᵗʰ [581.81]
neuralgia 250.6 ✓5ᵗʰ [357.2]
neuritis 250.6 ✓5ᵗʰ [357.2]
neurogenic arthropathy 250.6 ✓5ᵗʰ [713.5]
neuropathy 250.6 ✓5ᵗʰ [357.2]
nonclinical 790.2
osteomyelitis 250.8 ✓5ᵗʰ [731.8]
peripheral autonomic neuropathy 250.6 ✓5ᵗʰ [337.1]
phosphate 275.3
polyneuropathy 250.6 ✓5ᵗʰ [357.2]
renal (true) 271.4
retinal
edema 250.5 ✓5ᵗʰ [362.01]
hemorrhage 250.5 ✓5ᵗʰ [362.01]
microaneurysms 250.5 ✓5ᵗʰ [362.01]
retinitis 250.5 ✓5ᵗʰ [362.01]
retinopathy 250.5 ✓5ᵗʰ [362.01]
background 250.5 ✓5ᵗʰ [362.01]
proliferative 250.5 ✓5ᵗʰ [362.02]
steroid induced
correct substance properly administered 251.8
overdose or wrong substance given or taken 962.0
stress 790.2
subclinical 790.2
subliminal 790.2
sugar 250.0 ✓5ᵗʰ
ulcer (skin) 250.8 ✓5ᵗʰ [707.9]
lower extremity 250.8 ✓5ᵗʰ [707.10]
ankle 250.8 [707.13]
calf 250.8 [707.12]
foot 250.8 [707.15]
heel 250.8 [707.14]
knee 250.8 [707.19]
specified site NEC 250.8 [707.19]
thigh 250.8 [707.11]
toes 250.8 [707.15]
specified site NEC 250.8 ✓5ᵗʰ [707.8]
xanthoma 250.8 ✓5ᵗʰ [272.2]

Diacyclothrombopathia 287.1
Diagnosis deferred 799.9
Dialysis (intermittent) (treatment)
anterior retinal (juvenile) (with detachment) 361.04
extracorporeal V56.0
peritoneal V56.8
renal V56.0
status only V45.1
specified type NEC V56.8
Diamond-Blackfan anemia or syndrome (congenital hypoplastic anemia) 284.0
Diamond-Gardener syndrome (autoerythrocyte sensitization) 287.2
Diaper rash 691.0
Diaphoresis (excessive) NEC 780.8
Diaphragm — *see* condition
Diaphragmalgia 786.52
Diaphragmitis 519.4
Diaphyseal aclasis 756.4
Diaphysitis 733.99

Diarrhea, diarrheal (acute) (autumn) (bilious)
  (bloody) (catarrhal) (choleraic) (chronic)
  (gravis) (green) (infantile) (lienteric)
  (noninfectious) (presumed noninfectious)
  (putrefactive) (secondary) (sporadic)
  (summer) (symptomatic) (thermic) 787.91
  achlorhydric 536.0
  allergic 558.3
  amebic (see also Amebiasis) 006.9
    with abscess — see Abscess, amebic
    acute 006.0
    chronic 006.1
    nondysenteric 006.2
  bacillary — see Dysentery, bacillary
  bacterial NEC 008.5
  balantidial — 007.0
  bile salt-induced 579.8
  cachectic NEC 787.91
  chilomastix 007.8
  choleriformis 001.1
  coccidial 007.2
  Cochin-China 579.1
    anguilluliasis 127.2
    psilosis 579.1
  Dientamoeba 007.8
  dietetic 787.91
  due to
    achylia gastrica 536.8
    Aerobacter aerogenes 008.2 ✓5ᵗʰ
    Bacillus coli — see Enteritis, E. coli
    bacteria NEC 008.5
    bile salts 579.8
    Capillaria
      hepatica 128.8
      philippinensis 127.5
    Clostridium perfringens (C) (F) 008.46
    Enterobacter aerogenes 008.2 ✓5ᵗʰ
    enterococci 008.49
    Escherichia coli — see Enteritis, E. coli
    Giardia lamblia 007.1
    Heterophyes heterophyes 121.6
    irritating foods 787.91
    Metagonimus yokogawai 121.5
    Necator americanus 126.1
    Paracolobactrum arizonae 008.1
    Paracolon bacillus NEC 008.47
      Arizona 008.1
    Proteus (bacillus) (mirabilis) (Morganii) 008.3
    Pseudomonas aeruginosa 008.42
    S. japonicum 120.2
    specified organism NEC 008.8
      bacterial 008.49
      viral NEC 008.69
    Staphylococcus 008.41
    Streptococcus 008.49
      anaerobic 008.46
    Strongyloides stercoralis 127.2
    Trichuris trichiuria 127.3
    virus NEC (see also Enteritis, viral) 008.69
  dysenteric 009.2
    due to specified organism NEC 008.8
  dyspeptic 787.91
  endemic 009.3
    due to specified organism NEC 008.8
  epidemic 009.2
    due to specified organism NEC 008.8
  fermentative 787.91
  flagellate 007.9
  Flexner's (ulcerative) 004.1

Diarrhea, diarrheal — continued
  functional 564.5
    following gastrointestinal surgery 564.4
    psychogenic 306.4
  giardial 007.1
  Giardia lamblia 007.1
  hill 579.1
  hyperperistalsis (nervous) 306.4
  infectious 009.2
    due to specified organism NEC 008.8
    presumed 009.3
  inflammatory 787.91
    due to specified organism NEC 008.8
  malarial (see also Malaria) 084.6
  mite 133.8
  mycotic 117.9
  nervous 306.4
  neurogenic 564.5
  parenteral NEC 009.2
  postgastrectomy 564.4
  postvagotomy 564.4
  prostaglandin induced 579.8
  protozoal NEC 007.9
  psychogenic 306.4
  septic 009.2
    due to specified organism NEC 008.8
  specified organism NEC 008.8
    bacterial 008.49
    viral NEC 008.69
  Staphylococcus 008.41
  Streptococcus 008.49
    anaerobic 008.46
  toxic 558.2
  travelers' 009.2
    due to specified organism NEC 008.8
  trichomonal 007.3
  tropical 579.1
  tuberculous 014.8 ✓5ᵗʰ
  ulcerative (chronic) (see also Colitis, ulcerative) 556.9
  viral (see also Enteritis, viral) 008.8
  zymotic NEC 009.2

Diastasis
  cranial bones 733.99
    congenital 756.0
  joint (traumatic) — see Dislocation, by site
  muscle 728.84
    congenital 756.89
  recti (abdomen) 728.84
    complicating delivery 665.8 ✓5ᵗʰ
    congenital 756.79

Diastema, teeth, tooth 524.3
Diastematomyelia 742.51
Diataxia, cerebral, infantile 343.0
Diathesis
  allergic V15.09
  bleeding (familial) 287.9
  cystine (familial) 270.0
  gouty 274.9
  hemorrhagic (familial) 287.9
    newborn NEC 776.0
  oxalic 271.8
  scrofulous (see also Tuberculosis) 017.2 ✓5ᵗʰ
  spasmophilic (see also Tetany) 781.7
  ulcer 536.9
  uric acid 274.9

Diaz's disease or osteochondrosis 732.5
Dibothriocephaliasis 123.4
  larval 123.5

Index to Diseases

Dibothriocephalus (infection) (infestation) (latus) 123.4
   larval 123.5
Dicephalus 759.4
Dichotomy, teeth 520.2
Dichromat, dichromata (congenital) 368.59
Dichromatopsia (congenital) 368.59
Dichuchwa 104.0
Dicroceliasis 121.8
Didelphys, didelphic (see also Double uterus) 752.2
Didymitis (see also Epididymitis) 604.90
Died — see also Death
   without
      medical attention (cause unknown) 798.9
      sign of disease 798.2
Dientamoeba diarrhea 007.8
Dietary
   inadequacy or deficiency 269.9
   surveillance and counseling V65.3
Dietl's crisis 593.4
Dieulafoy ▶lesion (hemorrhagic)◀
   of
      duodenum 537.84
      intestine 569.86
      stomach 537.84
Difficult
   birth, affecting fetus or newborn 763.9
   delivery NEC 669.9 ✓5ᵗʰ
Difficulty
   feeding 783.3
      breast 676.8 ✓5ᵗʰ
      newborn 779.3
      nonorganic (infant) NEC 307.59
   mechanical, gastroduodenal stoma 537.89
   reading 315.00
   specific, spelling 315.09
   swallowing (see also Dysphagia) 787.2
   walking 719.7 ✓5ᵗʰ
Diffuse — see condition
Diffused ganglion 727.42
DiGeorge's syndrome (thymic hypoplasia) 279.11
Digestive — see condition
Di Guglielmo's disease or syndrome (M9841/3) 207.0 ✓5ᵗʰ
Diktyoma (M9051/3) — see Neoplasm, by site, malignant
Dilaceration, tooth 520.4
Dilatation
   anus 564.89
      venule — see Hemorrhoids
   aorta (focal) (general) (see also Aneurysm, aorta) 441.9
      congenital 747.29
      infectional 093.0
      ruptured 441.5
      syphilitic 093.0
   appendix (cystic) 543.9
   artery 447.8
   bile duct (common) (cystic) (congenital) 751.69
      acquired 576.8
   bladder (sphincter) 596.8
      congenital 753.8
      in pregnancy or childbirth 654.4 ✓5ᵗʰ
         causing obstructed labor 660.2 ✓5ᵗʰ
            affecting fetus or newborn 763.1

Dilatation — continued
   blood vessel 459.89
   bronchus, bronchi 494.0
      with acute exacerbation 494.1
   calyx (due to obstruction) 593.89
   capillaries 448.9
   cardiac (acute) (chronic) (see also Hypertrophy, cardiac) 429.3
      congenital 746.89
         valve NEC 746.89
            pulmonary 746.09
      hypertensive (see also Hypertension, heart) 402.90
   cavum septi pellucidi 742.4
   cecum 564.89
      psychogenic 306.4
   cervix (uteri) — see also Incompetency, cervix
      incomplete, poor, slow
         affecting fetus or newborn 763.7
         complicating delivery 661.0 ✓5ᵗʰ
            affecting fetus or newborn 763.7
   colon 564.7
      congenital 751.3
      due to mechanical obstruction 560.89
      psychogenic 306.4
   common bile duct (congenital) 751.69
      acquired 576.8
         with calculus, choledocholithiasis, or stones — see Choledocholithiasis
   cystic duct 751.69
      acquired (any bile duct) 575.8
   duct, mammary 610.4
   duodenum 564.89
   esophagus 530.89
      congenital 750.4
      due to
         achalasia 530.0
         cardiospasm 530.0
   Eustachian tube, congenital 744.24
   fontanel 756.0
   gallbladder 575.8
      congenital 751.69
   gastric 536.8
      acute 536.1
      psychogenic 306.4
   heart (acute) (chronic) (see also Hypertrophy, cardiac) 429.3
      congenital 746.89
      hypertensive (see also Hypertension, heart) 402.90
      valve — see also Endocarditis
         congenital 746.89
   ileum 564.89
      psychogenic 306.4
   inguinal rings — see Hernia, inguinal
   jejunum 564.89
      psychogenic 306.4
   kidney (calyx) (collecting structures) (cystic) (parenchyma) (pelvis) 593.89
   lacrimal passages 375.69
   lymphatic vessel 457.1
   mammary duct 610.4
   Meckel's diverticulum (congenital) 751.0
   meningeal vessels, congenital 742.8
   myocardium (acute) (chronic) (see also Hypertrophy, cardiac) 429.3
   organ or site, congenital NEC — see Distortion
   pancreatic duct 577.8
   pelvis, kidney 593.89
   pericardium — see Pericarditis
   pharynx 478.29

Dilatation — continued
  prostate 602.8
  pulmonary
    artery (idiopathic) 417.8
      congenital 747.3
    valve, congenital 746.09
  pupil 379.43
  rectum 564.89
  renal 593.89
  saccule vestibularis, congenital 744.05
  salivary gland (duct) 527.8
  sphincter ani 564.89
  stomach 536.8
    acute 536.1
    psychogenic 306.4
  submaxillary duct 527.8
  trachea, congenital 748.3
  ureter (idiopathic) 593.89
    congenital 753.20
    due to obstruction 593.5
  urethra (acquired) 599.84
  vasomotor 443.9
  vein 459.89
  ventricular, ventricle (acute) (chronic) (*see also* Hypertrophy, cardiac) 429.3
    cerebral, congenital 742.4
    hypertensive (*see also* Hypertension, heart) 402.90
  venule 459.89
    anus — *see* Hemorrhoids
  vesical orifice 596.8
Dilated, dilation — *see* Dilatation
Diminished
  hearing (acuity) (*see also* Deafness) 389.9
  pulse pressure 785.9
  vision NEC 369.9
  vital capacity 794.2
Diminuta taenia 123.6
Diminution, sense or sensation (cold) (heat) (tactile) (vibratory) (*see also* Disturbance, sensation) 782.0
Dimitri-Sturge-Weber disease (encephalocutaneous angiomatosis) 759.6
Dimple
  parasacral 685.1
    with abscess 685.0
  pilonidal 685.1
    with abscess 685.0
  postanal 685.1
    with abscess 685.0
Dioctophyma renale (infection) (infestation) 128.8
Dipetalonemiasis 125.4
Diphallus 752.69
Diphtheria, diphtheritic (gangrenous) (hemorrhagic) 032.9
  carrier (suspected) of V02.4
  cutaneous 032.85
  cystitis 032.84
  faucial 032.0
  infection of wound 032.85
  inoculation (anti) (not sick) V03.5
  laryngeal 032.3
  myocarditis 032.82
  nasal anterior 032.2
  nasopharyngeal 032.1
  neurological complication 032.89
  peritonitis 032.83
  specified site NEC 032.89

Diphyllobothriasis (intestine) 123.4
  larval 123.5
Diplacusis 388.41
Diplegia (upper limbs) 344.2
  brain or cerebral 437.8
  congenital 343.0
  facial 351.0
    congenital 352.6
  infantile or congenital (cerebral) (spastic) (spinal) 343.0
  lower limbs 344.1
  syphilitic, congenital 090.49
Diplococcus, diplococcal — *see* condition
Diplomyelia 742.59
Diplopia 368.2
  refractive 368.15
Dipsomania (*see also* Alcoholism) 303.9
  with psychosis (*see also* Psychosis, alcoholic) 291.9
Dipylidiasis 123.8
  intestine 123.8
Direction, teeth, abnormal 524.3
Dirt-eating child 307.52
Disability
  heart — *see* Disease, heart
  learning NEC 315.2
  special spelling 315.09
Disarticulation (*see also* Derangement, joint) 718.9
  meaning
    amputation
      status — *see* Absence, by site
      traumatic — *see* Amputation, traumatic
    dislocation, traumatic or congenital — *see* Dislocation
Disaster, cerebrovascular (*see also* Disease, cerebrovascular, acute) 436
Discharge
  anal NEC 787.99
  breast (female) (male) 611.79
  conjunctiva 372.89
  continued locomotor idiopathic (*see also* Epilepsy) 345.5
  diencephalic autonomic idiopathic (*see also* Epilepsy) 345.5
  ear 388.60
    blood 388.69
    cerebrospinal fluid 388.61
  excessive urine 788.42
  eye 379.93
  nasal 478.1
  nipple 611.79
  patterned motor idiopathic (*see also* Epilepsy) 345.5
  penile 788.7
  postnasal — *see* Sinusitis
  sinus, from mediastinum 510.0
  umbilicus 789.9
  urethral 788.7
    bloody 599.84
  vaginal 623.5
Discitis 722.90
  cervical, cervicothoracic 722.91
  lumbar, lumbosacral 722.93
  thoracic, thoracolumbar 722.92
Discogenic syndrome — *see* Displacement, intervertebral disc
Discoid
  kidney 753.3

Index to Diseases

Discoid — *continued*
  meniscus, congenital 717.5
  semilunar cartilage 717.5
Discoloration
  mouth 528.9
  nails 703.8
  teeth 521.7
    due to
      drugs 521.7
      metals (copper) (silver) 521.7
      pulpal bleeding 521.7
    during formation 520.8
    posteruptive 521.7
Discomfort
  chest 786.59
  visual 368.13
Discomycosis — *see* Actinomycosis
Discontinuity, ossicles, ossicular chain 385.23
Discrepancy
  leg length (acquired) 736.81
    congenital 755.30
  uterine size-date 646.8 ✓5ᵗʰ
Discrimination
  political V62.4
  racial V62.4
  religious V62.4
  sex V62.4
Disease, diseased — *see also* Syndrome
  Abrami's (acquired hemolytic jaundice) 283.9
  absorbent system 459.89
  accumulation — *see* Thesaurismosis
  acid-peptic 536.8
  Acosta's 993.2
  Adams-Stokes (-Morgagni) (syncope with heart block) 426.9
  Addison's (bronze) (primary adrenal insufficiency) 255.4
    anemia (pernicious) 281.0
    tuberculous (*see also* Tuberculosis) 017.6 ✓5ᵗʰ
  Addison-Gull — *see* Xanthoma
  adenoids (and tonsils) (chronic) 474.9
  adrenal (gland) (capsule) (cortex) 255.9
    hyperfunction 255.3
    hypofunction 255.4
    specified type NEC 255.8
  ainhum (dactylolysis spontanea) 136.0
  akamushi (scrub typhus) 081.2
  Akureyri (epidemic neuromyasthenia) 049.8
  Albarrán's (colibacilluria) 791.9
  Albers-Schönberg's (marble bones) 756.52
  Albert's 726.71
  Albright (-Martin) (-Bantam) 275.49
  Alibert's (mycosis fungoides) (M9700/3) 202.1 ✓5ᵗʰ
  Alibert-Bazin (M9700/3) 202.1 ✓5ᵗʰ
  alimentary canal 569.9
  alligator skin (ichthyosis congenita) 757.1
    acquired 701.1
  Almeida's (Brazilian blastomycosis) 116.1
  Alpers' 330.8
  alpine 993.2
  altitude 993.2
  alveoli, teeth 525.9
  Alzheimer's — *see* Alzheimer's
  amyloid (any site) 277.3
  anarthritic rheumatoid 446.5
  Anders' (adiposis tuberosa simplex) 272.8
  Andersen's (glycogenosis IV) 271.0

Disease, diseased — *continued*
  Anderson's (angiokeratoma corporis diffusum) 272.7
  Andes 993.2
  Andrews' (bacterid) 686.8
  angiospastic, angiospasmodic 443.9
    cerebral 435.9
      with transient neurologic deficit 435.9
    vein 459.89
  anterior
    chamber 364.9
    horn cell 335.9
      specified type NEC 335.8
  antral (chronic) 473.0
    acute 461.0
  anus NEC 569.49
  aorta (nonsyphilitic) 447.9
    syphilitic NEC 093.89
  aortic (heart) (valve) (*see also* Endocarditis, aortic) 424.1
  apollo 077.4
  aponeurosis 726.90
  appendix 543.9
  aqueous (chamber) 364.9
  arc-welders' lung 503
  Armenian 277.3
  Arnold-Chiari (*see also* Spina bifida) 741.0 ✓5ᵗʰ
  arterial 447.9
    occlusive (*see also* Occlusion, by site) 444.22
      with embolus or thrombus — *see* Occlusion, by site
    due to stricture or stenosis 447.1
    specified type NEC 447.8
  arteriocardiorenal (*see also* Hypertension, cardiorenal) 404.90
  arteriolar (generalized) (obliterative) 447.9
    specified type NEC 447.8
  arteriorenal — *see* Hypertension, kidney
  arteriosclerotic — *see also* Arteriosclerosis
    cardiovascular 429.2
    coronary — *see* Arteriosclerosis, coronary
    heart — *see* Arteriosclerosis, coronary
    vascular — *see* Arteriosclerosis
  artery 447.9
    cerebral 437.9
    coronary — *see* Arteriosclerosis, coronary
    specified type NEC 447.8
  arthropod-borne NEC 088.9
    specified type NEC 088.89
  Asboe-Hansen's (incontinentia pigmenti) 757.33
  atticoantral, chronic (with posterior or superior marginal perforation of ear drum) 382.2
  auditory canal, ear 380.9
  Aujeszky's 078.89
  auricle, ear NEC 380.30
  Australian X 062.4
  autoimmune NEC 279.4
    hemolytic (cold type) (warm type) 283.0
    parathyroid 252.1
    thyroid 245.2
  aviators' (*see also* Effect, adverse, high altitude) 993.2
  ax(e)-grinders' 502
  Ayala's 756.89
  Ayerza's (pulmonary artery sclerosis with pulmonary hypertension) 416.0
  Azorean (of the nervous system) 334.8

Disease, diseased — continued
- Babington's (familial hemorrhagic telangiectasia) 448.0
- back bone NEC 733.90
- bacterial NEC 040.89
  - zoonotic NEC 027.9
  - specified type NEC 027.8
- Baehr-Schiffrin (thrombotic thrombocytopenic purpura) 446.6
- Baelz's (cheilitis glandularis apostematosa) 528.5
- Baerensprung's (eczema marginatum) 110.3
- Balfour's (chloroma) 205.3
- balloon (see also Effect, adverse, high altitude 993.2
- Baló's 341.1
- Bamberger (-Marie) (hypertrophic pulmonary osteoarthropathy) 731.2
- Bang's (Brucella abortus) 023.1
- Bannister's 995.1
- Banti's (with cirrhosis) (with portal hypertension) — see Cirrhosis, liver
- Barcoo (see also Ulcer, skin) 707.9
- barium lung 503
- Barlow (-Möller) (infantile scurvy) 267
- barometer makers' 985.0
- Barraquer (-Simons) (progressive lipodystrophy) 272.6
- basal ganglia 333.90
  - degenerative NEC 333.0
  - specified NEC 333.89
- Basedow's (exophthalmic goiter) 242.0
- basement membrane NEC 583.89
  - with
    - pulmonary hemorrhage (Goodpasture's syndrome) 446.21 [583.81]
- Bateman's 078.0
  - purpura (senile) 287.2
- Batten's 330.1 [362.71]
- Batten-Mayou (retina) 330.1 [362.71]
- Batten-Steinert 359.2
- Battey 031.0
- Baumgarten-Cruveilhier (cirrhosis of liver) 571.5
- bauxite-workers' 503
- Bayle's (dementia paralytica) 094.1
- Bazin's (primary) (see also Tuberculosis) 017.1
- Beard's (neurasthenia) 300.5
- Beau's (see also Degeneration, myocardial) 429.1
- Bechterew's (ankylosing spondylitis) 720.0
- Becker's (idiopathic mural endomyocardial disease) 425.2
- Begbie's (exophthalmic goiter) 242.0
- Behr's 362.50
- Beigel's (white piedra) 111.2
- Bekhterev's (ankylosing spondylitis) 720.0
- Bell's (see also Psychosis, affective) 296.0
- Bennett's (leukemia) 208.9
- Benson's 379.22
- Bergeron's (hysteroepilepsy) 300.11
- Berlin's 921.3
- Bernard-Soulier (thrombopathy) 287.1
- Bernhardt (-Roth) 355.1
- beryllium 503
- Besnier-Boeck (-Schaumann) (sarcoidosis) 135
- Best's 362.76
- Beurmann's (sporotrichosis) 117.1
- Bielschowsky (-Jansky) 330.1
- Biermer's (pernicious anemia) 281.0

Disease, diseased — continued
- Biett's (discoid lupus erythematosus) 695.4
- bile duct (see also Disease, biliary) 576.9
- biliary (duct) (tract) 576.9
  - with calculus, choledocholithiasis, or stones — see Choledocholithiasis
- Billroth's (meningocele) (see also Spina bifida) 741.9
- Binswanger's 290.12
- Bird's (oxaluria) 271.8
- bird fanciers' 495.2
- black lung 500
- bladder 596.9
  - specified NEC 596.8
- bleeder's 286.0
- Bloch-Sulzberger (incontinentia pigmenti) 757.33
- Blocq's (astasia-abasia) 307.9
- blood (-forming organs) 289.9
  - specified NEC 289.8
  - vessel 459.9
- Bloodgood's 610.1
- Blount's (tibia vara) 732.4
- blue 746.9
- Bodechtel-Guttmann (subacute sclerosing panencephalitis) 046.2
- Boeck's (sarcoidosis) 135
- bone 733.90
  - fibrocystic NEC 733.29
  - jaw 526.2
  - marrow 289.9
  - Paget's (osteitis deformans) 731.0
  - specified type NEC 733.99
  - von Recklinghausen's (osteitis fibrosa cystica) 252.0
- Bonfils' — see Disease, Hodgkin's
- Borna 062.9
- Bornholm (epidemic pleurodynia) 074.1
- Bostock's (see also Fever, hay) 477.9
- Bouchard's (myopathic dilatation of the stomach) 536.1
- Bouillaud's (rheumatic heart disease) 391.9
- Bourneville (-Brissaud) (tuberous sclerosis) 759.5
- Bouveret (-Hoffmann) (paroxysmal tachycardia) 427.2
- bowel 569.9
  - functional 564.9
  - psychogenic 306.4
- Bowen's (M8081/2) — see Neoplasm, skin, in situ
- Bozzolo's (multiple myeloma) (M973/3) 203.0
- Bradley's (epidemic vomiting) 078.82
- Brailsford's 732.3
  - radius, head 732.3
  - tarsal, scaphoid 732.5
- Brailsford-Morquio (mucopolysaccharidosis IV) 277.5
- brain 348.9
  - Alzheimer's 331.0
    - with dementia — see Alzheimer's, dementia
  - arterial, artery 437.9
  - arteriosclerotic 437.0
  - congenital 742.9
  - degenerative — see Degeneration, brain
  - inflammatory — see also Encephalitis
  - late effect — see category 326
  - organic 348.9
    - arteriosclerotic 437.0

Index to Diseases

Disease, diseased — *continued*
  brain — *continued*
    parasitic NEC 123.9
    Pick's 331.1
      with dementia
        with behavioral disturbance 331.1
          [294.11]
        without behavioral disturbance 331.1
          [294.10]
    senile 331.2
  brazier's 985.8
  breast 611.9
    cystic (chronic) 610.1
    fibrocystic 610.1
    inflammatory 611.0
    Paget's (M8540/3) 174.0
    puerperal, postpartum NEC 676.3
    specified NEC 611.8
  Breda's (*see also* Yaws) 102.9
  Breisky's (kraurosis vulvae) 624.0
  Bretonneau's (diphtheritic malignant angina) 032.0
  Bright's (*see also* Nephritis) 583.9
    arteriosclerotic (*see also* Hypertension, kidney) 403.90
  Brill's (recrudescent typhus) 081.1
    flea-borne 081.0
    louse-borne 081.1
  Brill-Symmers (follicular lymphoma) (M9690/3) 202.0
  Brill-Zinsser (recrudescent typhus) 081.1
  Brinton's (leather bottle stomach) (M8142/3) 151.9
  Brion-Kayser (*see also* Fever, paratyphoid) 002.9
  broad
    beta 272.2
    ligament, noninflammatory 620.9
      specified NEC 620.8
  Brocq's 691.8
    meaning
      atopic (diffuse) neurodermatitis 691.8
      dermatitis herpetiformis 694.0
      lichen simplex chronicus 698.3
      parapsoriasis 696.2
      prurigo 698.2
  Brocq-Duhring (dermatitis herpetiformis) 694.0
  Brodie's (joint) (*see also* Osteomyelitis) 730.1
  bronchi 519.1
  bronchopulmonary 519.1
  bronze (Addison's) 255.4
    tuberculous (*see also* Tuberculosis) 017.6
  Brown-Séquard 344.89
  Bruck's 733.99
  Bruck-de Lange (Amsterdam dwarf, mental retardation and brachycephaly) 759.89
  Bruhl's (splenic anemia with fever) 285.8
  Bruton's (X-linked agammaglobulinemia) 279.04
  buccal cavity 528.9
  Buchanan's (juvenile osteochondrosis, iliac crest) 732.1
  Buchman's (osteochondrosis juvenile) 732.1
  Budgerigar-fanciers' 495.2
  Büdinger-Ludloff-Läwen 717.89
  Buerger's (thromboangiitis obliterans) 443.1
  Bürger-Grütz (essential familial hyperlipemia) 272.3

Disease, diseased — *continued*
  Burns' (lower ulna) 732.3
  bursa 727.9
  Bury's (erythema elevatum diutinum) 695.89
  Buschke's 710.1
  Busquet's (*see also* Osteomyelitis) 730.1
  Busse-Buschke (cryptococcosis) 117.5
  C_2 (*see also* Alcoholism) 303.9
  Caffey's (infantile cortical hyperostosis) 756.59
  caisson 993.3
  calculous 592.9
  California 114.0
  Calvé (-Perthes) (osteochondrosis, femoral capital) 732.1
  Camurati-Engelmann (diaphyseal sclerosis) 756.59
  Canavan's 330.0
  capillaries 448.9
  Carapata 087.1
  cardiac — *see* Disease, heart
  cardiopulmonary, chronic 416.9
  cardiorenal (arteriosclerotic) (hepatic) (hypertensive) (vascular) (*see also* Hypertension, cardiorenal) 404.90
  cardiovascular (arteriosclerotic) 429.2
    congenital 746.9
    hypertensive (*see also* Hypertension, heart) 402.90
      benign 402.10
      malignant 402.00
    renal (*see also* Hypertension, cardiorenal) 404.90
    syphilitic (asymptomatic) 093.9
  carotid gland 259.8
  Carrión's (Bartonellosis) 088.0
  cartilage NEC 733.90
    specified NEC 733.99
  Castellani's 104.8
  cat-scratch 078.3
  Cavare's (familial periodic paralysis) 359.3
  Cazenave's (pemphigus) 694.4
  cecum 569.9
  celiac (adult) 579.0
    infantile 579.0
  cellular tissue NEC 709.9
  central core 359.0
  cerebellar, cerebellum — *see* Disease, brain
  cerebral (*see also* Disease, brain) 348.9
    arterial, artery 437.9
    degenerative — *see* Degeneration, brain
  cerebrospinal 349.9
  cerebrovascular NEC 437.9
    acute 436
      embolic — *see* Embolism, brain
      late effect — *see* Late effect(s) (of) cerebrovascular disease
      puerperal, postpartum, childbirth 674.0
      thrombotic — *see* Thrombosis, brain
    arteriosclerotic 437.0
    embolic — *see* Embolism, brain
    ischemic, generalized NEC 437.1
    late effect — *see* Late effect(s) (of) cerebrovascular disease
    occlusive 437.1
    puerperal, postpartum, childbirth 674.0
    specified type NEC 437.8
    thrombotic — *see* Thrombosis, brain
  ceroid storage 272.7

Disease, diseased — continued
  cervix (uteri)
    inflammatory 616.9
      specified NEC 616.8
    noninflammatory 622.9
      specified NEC 622.8
  Chabert's 022.9
  Chagas' (see also Trypanosomiasis, American) 086.2
  Chandler's (osteochondritis dissecans, hip) 732.7
  Charcots' (joint) 094.0 [713.5]
    spinal cord 094.0
  Charcôt-Marie-Tooth 356.1
  Charlouis' (see also Yaws) 102.9
  Cheadle (-Möller) (-Barlow) (infantile scurvy) 267
  Chédiak-Steinbrinck (-Higashi) (congenital gigantism of peroxidase granules) 288.2
  cheek, inner 528.9
  chest 519.9
  Chiari's (hepatic vein thrombosis) 453.0
  Chicago (North American blastomycosis) 116.0
  chignon (white piedra) 111.2
  chigoe, chigo (jigger) 134.1
  childhood granulomatous 288.1
  Chinese liver fluke 121.1
  chlamydial NEC 078.88
  cholecystic (see also Disease, gallbladder) 575.9
  choroid 363.9
    degenerative (see also Degeneration, choroid) 363.40
    hereditary (see also Dystrophy, choroid) 363.50
    specified type NEC 363.8
  Christian's (chronic histiocytosis X) 277.8
  Christian-Weber (nodular nonsuppurative panniculitis) 729.30
  Christmas 286.1
  ciliary body 364.9
  circulatory (system) NEC 459.9
    chronic, maternal, affecting fetus or newborn 760.3
    specified NEC 459.89
    syphilitic 093.9
      congenital 090.5
  Civatte's (poikiloderma) 709.09
  climacteric 627.2
    male 608.89
  coagulation factor deficiency (congenital) (see also Defect, coagulation) 286.9
  Coats' 362.12
  coccidiodal pulmonary 114.5
    acute 114.0
    chronic 114.4
    primary 114.0
    residual 114.4
  Cockayne's (microcephaly and dwarfism) 759.89
  Cogan's 370.52
  cold
    agglutinin 283.0
      or hemoglobinuria 283.0
        paroxysmal (cold) (nocturnal) 283.2
    hemagglutinin (chronic) 283.0
  collagen NEC 710.9
    nonvascular 710.9
    specified NEC 710.8
    vascular (allergic) (see also Angiitis, hypersensitivity) 446.20

Disease, diseased — continued
  colon 569.9
    functional 564.9
      congenital 751.3
    ischemic 557.0
  combined system (of spinal cord) 266.2 [336.2]
    with anemia (pernicious) 281.0 [336.2]
  compressed air 993.3
  Concato's (pericardial polyserositis) 423.2
    peritoneal 568.82
    pleural — see Pleurisy
  congenital NEC 799.8
  conjunctiva 372.9
    chlamydial 077.98
      specified NEC 077.8
    specified type NEC 372.89
    viral 077.99
      specified NEC 077.8
  connective tissue, diffuse (see also Disease, collagen) 710.9
  Conor and Bruch's (boutonneuse fever) 082.1
  Conradi (-Hünermann) 756.59
  Cooley's (erythroblastic anemia) 282.4
  Cooper's 610.1
  Corbus' 607.1
  cork-handlers' 495.3
  cornea (see also Keratopathy) 371.9
  coronary (see also Ischemia, heart) 414.9
    congenital 746.85
    ostial, syphilitic 093.20
      aortic 093.22
      mitral 093.21
      pulmonary 093.24
      tricuspid 093.23
  Corrigan's — see Insufficiency, aortic
  Cotugno's 724.3
  Coxsackie (virus) NEC 074.8
  cranial nerve NEC 352.9
  Creutzfeldt-Jakob 046.1
    with dementia
      with behavioral disturbance 046.1 [294.11]
      without behavioral disturbance 046.1 [294.10]
  Crigler-Najjar (congenital hyperbilirubinemia) 277.4
  Crocq's (acrocyanosis) 443.89
  Crohn's (intestine) (see also Enteritis, regional) 555.9
  Crouzon's (craniofacial dysostosis) 756.0
  Cruchet's (encephalitis lethargica) 049.8
  Cruveilhier's 335.21
  Cruz-Chagas (see also Trypanosomiasis, American) 086.2
  crystal deposition (see also Arthritis, due to, crystals) 712.9
  Csillag's (lichen sclerosus et atrophicus) 701.0
  Curschmann's 359.2
  Cushing's (pituitary basophilism) 255.0
  cystic
    breast (chronic) 610.1
    kidney, congenital (see also Cystic, disease, kidney) 753.10
    liver, congenital 751.62
    lung 518.89
      congenital 748.4
    pancreas 577.2
      congenital 751.7
    renal, congenital (see also Cystic, disease, kidney) 753.10
    semilunar cartilage 717.5

Index to Diseases

Disease, diseased — *continued*
cysticercus 123.1
cystine storage (with renal sclerosis) 270.0
cytomegalic inclusion (generalized) 078.5
  with
    pneumonia 078.5 *[484.1]*
  congenital 771.1
Daae (-Finsen) (epidemic pleurodynia) 074.1
dancing 297.8
Danielssen's (anesthetic leprosy) 030.1
Darier's (congenital) (keratosis follicularis) 757.39
  erythema annulare centrifugum 695.0
  vitamin A deficiency 264.8
Darling's (histoplasmosis) (*see also* Histoplasmosis, American) 115.00
Davies' 425.0
de Beurmann-Gougerot (sporotrichosis) 117.1
Débove's (splenomegaly) 789.2
deer fly (*see also* Tularemia) 021.9
deficiency 269.9
degenerative — *see also* Degeneration
  disc — *see* Degeneration, intervertebral disc
Degos' 447.8
Déjérine (-Sottas) 356.0
Déleage's 359.89
demyelinating, demyelinizating (brain stem) (central nervous system) 341.9
  multiple sclerosis 340
  specified NEC 341.8
de Quervain's (tendon sheath) 727.04
  thyroid (subacute granulomatous thyroiditis) 245.1
Dercum's (adiposis dolorosa) 272.8
Deutschländer's — *see* Fracture, foot
Devergie's (pityriasis rubra pilaris) 696.4
Devic's 341.0
diaphorase deficiency 289.7
diaphragm 519.4
diarrheal, infectious 009.2
diatomaceous earth 502
Diaz's (osteochondrosis astragalus) 732.5
digestive system 569.9
Di Guglielmo's (erythemic myelosis) (M9841/3) 207.0
Dimitri-Sturge-Weber (encephalocutaneous angiomatosis) 759.6
disc, degenerative — *see* Degeneration, intervertebral disc
discogenic (*see also* Disease, intervertebral disc) 722.90
diverticular — *see* Diverticula
Down's (mongolism) 758.0
Dubini's (electric chorea) 049.8
Dubois' (thymus gland) 090.5
Duchenne's 094.0
  locomotor ataxia 094.0
  muscular dystrophy 359.1
  paralysis 335.22
  pseudohypertrophy, muscles 359.1
Duchenne-Griesinger 359.1
ductless glands 259.9
Duhring's (dermatitis herpetiformis) 694.0
Dukes (-Filatov) 057.8
duodenum NEC 537.9
  specified NEC 537.89
Duplay's 726.2
Dupré's (meningism) 781.6
Dupuytren's (muscle contracture) 728.6
Durand-Nicolas-Favre (climatic bubo) 099.1

Disease, diseased — *continued*
Duroziez's (congenital mitral stenosis) 746.5
Dutton's (trypanosomiasis) 086.9
Eales' 362.18
ear (chronic) (inner) NEC 388.9
  middle 385.9
    adhesive (*see also* Adhesions, middle ear) 385.10
  specified NEC 385.89
Eberth's (typhoid fever) 002.0
Ebstein's
  heart 746.2
  meaning diabetes 250.4 *[581.81]*
Echinococcus (*see also* Echinococcus) 122.9
ECHO virus NEC 078.89
Economo's (encephalitis lethargica) 049.8
Eddowes' (brittle bones and blue sclera) 756.51
Edsall's 992.2
Eichstedt's (pityriasis versicolor) 111.0
Ellis-van Creveld (chondroectodermal dysplasia) 756.55
endocardium — *see* Endocarditis
endocrine glands or system NEC 259.9
  specified NEC 259.8
endomyocardial, idiopathic mural 425.2
Engel-von Recklinghausen (osteitis fibrosa cystica) 252.0
Engelmann's (diaphyseal sclerosis) 756.59
English (rickets) 268.0
Engman's (infectious eczematoid dermatitis) 690.8
enteroviral, enterovirus NEC 078.89
  central nervous system NEC 048
epidemic NEC 136.9
epididymis 608.9
epigastric, functional 536.9
  psychogenic 306.4
Erb (-Landouzy) 359.1
Erb-Goldflam 358.0
Erichsen's (railway spine) 300.16
esophagus 530.9
  functional 530.5
  psychogenic 306.4
Eulenburg's (congenital paramyotonia) 359.2
Eustachian tube 381.9
Evans' (thrombocytopenic purpura) 287.3
external auditory canal 380.9
extrapyramidal NEC 333.90
eye 379.90
  anterior chamber 364.9
  inflammatory NEC 364.3
  muscle 378.9
eyeball 360.9
eyelid 374.9
eyeworm of Africa 125.2
Fabry's (angiokeratoma corporis diffusum) 272.7
facial nerve (seventh) 351.9
  newborn 767.5
Fahr-Volhard (malignant nephrosclerosis) 403.00
fallopian tube, noninflammatory 620.9
  specified NEC 620.8
familial periodic 277.3
  paralysis 359.3
Fanconi's (congenital pancytopenia) 284.0
Farber's (disseminated lipogranulomatosis) 272.8
fascia 728.9
  inflammatory 728.9

Disease, diseased — continued
   Fauchard's (periodontitis) 523.4
   Favre-Durand-Nicolas (climatic bubo) 099.1
   Favre-Racouchot (elastoidosis cutanea nodularis) 701.8
   Fede's 529.0
   Feer's 985.0
   Felix's (juvenile osteochondrosis, hip) 732.1
   Fenwick's (gastric atrophy) 537.89
   Fernels' (aortic aneurysm) 441.9
   fibrocaseous, of lung (*see also* Tuberculosis, pulmonary) 011.9 ✓5ᵗʰ
   fibrocystic — *see also* Fibrocystic, disease
      newborn 277.01
   Fiedler's (leptospiral jaundice) 100.0
   fifth 057.0
   Filatoff's (infectious mononucleosis) 075
   Filatov's (infectious mononucleosis) 075
   file-cutters' 984.9
      specified type of lead — *see* Table of Drugs and Chemicals
   filterable virus NEC 078.89
   fish skin 757.1
      acquired 701.1
   Flajani (-Basedow) (exophthalmic goiter) 242.0 ✓5ᵗʰ
   Flatau-Schilder 341.1
   flax-dressers' 504
   Fleischner's 732.3
   flint 502
   fluke — *see* Infestation, fluke
   Følling's (phenylketonuria) 270.1
   foot and mouth 078.4
   foot process 581.3
   Forbes' (glycogenosis III) 271.0
   Fordyce's (ectopic sebaceous glands) (mouth) 750.26
   Fordyce-Fox (apocrine miliaria) 705.82
   Fothergill's
      meaning scarlatina anginosa 034.1
      neuralgia (*see also* Neuralgia, trigeminal) 350.1
   Fournier's 608.83
   fourth 057.8
   Fox (-Fordyce) (apocrine miliaria) 705.82
   Francis' (*see also* Tularemia) 021.9
   Franklin's (heavy chain) 273.2
   Frei's (climatic bubo) 099.1
   Freiberg's (flattening metarsal) 732.5
   Friedländer's (endarteritis obliterans) — *see* Arteriosclerosis
   Friedreich's
      combined systemic or ataxia 334.0
      facial hemihypertrophy 756.0
      myoclonia 333.2
   Fröhlich's (adiposogenital dystrophy) 253.8
   Frommel's 676.6 ✓5ᵗʰ
   frontal sinus (chronic) 473.1
      acute 461.1
   Fuller's earth 502
   fungus, fungous NEC 117.9
   Gaisböck's (polycythemia hypertonica) 289.0
   gallbladder 575.9
      congenital 751.60
   Gamna's (siderotic splenomegaly) 289.51
   Gamstorp's (adynamia episodica hereditaria) 359.3
   Gandy-Nanta (siderotic splenomegaly) 289.51
   gannister (occupational) 502
   Garré's (*see also* Osteomyelitis) 730.1 ✓5ᵗʰ
   gastric (*see also* Disease, stomach) 537.9

Disease, diseased — continued
   gastrointestinal (tract) 569.9
      amyloid 277.3
      functional 536.9
      psychogenic 306.4
   Gaucher's (adult) (cerebroside lipidosis) (infantile) 272.7
   Gayet's (superior hemorrhagic polioencephalitis) 265.1
   Gee (-Herter) (-Heubner) (-Thaysen) (nontropical sprue) 579.0
   generalized neoplastic (M8000/6) 199.0
   genital organs NEC
      female 629.9
         specified NEC 629.8
      male 608.9
   Gerhardt's (erythromelalgia) 443.89
   Gerlier's (epidemic vertigo) 078.81
   Gibert's (pityriasis rosea) 696.3
   Gibney's (perispondylitis) 720.9
   Gierke's (glycogenosis I) 271.0
   Gilbert's (familial nonhemolytic jaundice) 277.4
   Gilchrist's (North American blastomycosis) 116.0
   Gilford (-Hutchinson) (progeria) 259.8
   Gilles de la Tourette's (motor-verbal tic) 307.23
   Giovannini's 117.9
   gland (lymph) 289.9
   Glanzmann's (hereditary hemorrhagic thrombasthenia) 287.1
   glassblowers' 527.1
   Glénard's (enteroptosis) 569.89
   Glisson's (*see also* Rickets) 268.0
   glomerular
      membranous, idiopathic 581.1
      minimal change 581.3
   glycogen storage (Andersen's) (Cori types 1-7) (Forbes') (McArdle-Schmid-Pearson) (Pompe's) (types I-VII) 271.0
      cardiac 271.0 *[425.7]*
      generalized 271.0
      glucose-6-phosphatase deficiency 271.0
      heart 271.0 *[425.7]*
      hepatorenal 271.0
      liver and kidneys 271.0
      myocardium 271.0 *[425.7]*
      von Gierke's (glycogenosis I) 271.0
   Goldflam-Erb 358.0
   Goldscheider's (epidermolysis bullosa) 757.39
   Goldstein's (familial hemorrhagic telangiectasia) 448.0
   gonococcal NEC 098.0
   Goodall's (epidemic vomiting) 078.82
   Gordon's (exudative enteropathy) 579.8
   Gougerot's (trisymptomatic) 709.1
   Gougerot-Carteaud (confluent reticulate papillomatosis) 701.8
   Gougerot-Hailey-Hailey (benign familial chronic pemphigus) 757.39
   graft-versus-host (bone marrow) 996.85
      due to organ transplant NEC — *see* Complications, transplant, organ
   grain-handlers' 495.8
   Grancher's (splenopneumonia) — *see* Pneumonia
   granulomatous (childhood) (chronic) 288.1
   graphite lung 503
   Graves' (exophthalmic goiter) 242.0 ✓5ᵗʰ
   Greenfield's 330.0

Index to Diseases

Disease, diseased — *continued*
  green monkey 078.89
  Griesinger's (*see also* Ancylostomiasis) 126.9
  grinders' 502
  Grisel's 723.5
  Gruby's (tinea tonsurans) 110.0
  Guertin's (electric chorea) 049.8
  Guillain-Barré 357.0
  Guinon's (motor-verbal tic) 307.23
  Gull's (thyroid atrophy with myxedema) 244.8
  Gull and Sutton's — *see* Hypertension, kidney
  gum NEC 523.9
  Günther's (congenital erythropoietic porphyria) 277.1
  gynecological 629.9
    specified NEC 629.8
  H 270.0
  Haas' 732.3
  Habermann's (acute parapsoriasis varioliformis) 696.2
  Haff 985.1
  Hageman (congenital factor XII deficiency) (*see also* Defect, congenital) 286.3
  Haglund's (osteochondrosis os tibiale externum) 732.5
  Hagner's (hypertrophic pulmonary osteoarthropathy) 731.2
  Hailey-Hailey (benign familial chronic pemphigus) 757.39
  hair (follicles) NEC 704.9
    specified type NEC 704.8
  Hallervorden-Spatz 333.0
  Hallopeau's (lichen sclerosus et atrophicus) 701.0
  Hamman's (spontaneous mediastinal emphysema) 518.1
  hand, foot, and mouth 074.3
  Hand-Schüller-Christian (chronic histiocytosis X) 277.8
  Hanot's — *see* Cirrhosis, biliary
  Hansen's (leprosy) 030.9
    benign form 030.1
    malignant form 030.0
  Harada's 363.22
  Harley's (intermittent hemoglobinuria) 283.2
  Hart's (pellagra-cerebellar ataxia renal aminoaciduria) 270.0
  Hartnup (pellagra-cerebellar ataxia renal aminoaciduria) 270.0
  Hashimoto's (struma lymphomatosa) 245.2
  Hb — *see* Disease, hemoglobin
  heart (organic) 429.9
    with
      acute pulmonary edema (*see also* Failure, ventricular, left) 428.1
      hypertensive 402.91
        with renal failure 404.91
        benign 402.11
          with renal failure 404.11
        malignant 402.01
          with renal failure 404.01
      kidney disease — *see* Hypertension, cardiorenal
      rheumatic fever (conditions classifiable to 390)
        active 391.9
          with chorea 392.0
        inactive or quiescent (with chorea) 398.90
      amyloid 277.3 [425.7]

Disease, diseased — *continued*
  heart — *continued*
    aortic (valve) (*see also* Endocarditis, aortic) 424.1
    arteriosclerotic or sclerotic (minimal) (senile) — *see* Arteriosclerosis, coronary
    artery — *see* Arteriosclerosis, coronary
    atherosclerotic — *see* Arteriosclerosis, coronary
    beer drinkers' 425.5
    beriberi 265.0 [425.7]
    black 416.0
    congenital NEC 746.9
      cyanotic 746.9
      maternal, affecting fetus or newborn 760.3
      specified type NEC 746.89
    congestive (*see also* Failure, heart) 428.0
    coronary 414.9
    cryptogenic 429.9
    due to
      amyloidosis 277.3 [425.7]
      beriberi 265.0 [425.7]
      cardiac glycogenosis 271.0 [425.7]
      Friedreich's ataxia 334.0 [425.8]
      gout 274.82
      mucopolysaccharidosis 277.5 [425.7]
      myotonia atrophica 359.2 [425.8]
      progressive muscular dystrophy 359.1 [425.8]
      sarcoidosis 135 [425.8]
    fetal 746.9
      inflammatory 746.89
    fibroid (*see also* Myocarditis) 429.0
    functional 427.9
      postoperative 997.1
      psychogenic 306.2
    glycogen storage 271.0 [425.7]
    gonococcal NEC 098.85
    gouty 274.82
    hypertensive (*see also* Hypertension, heart) 402.90
      benign 402.10
      malignant 402.00
    hyperthyroid (*see also* Hyperthyroidism) 242.9 ✓5ᵗʰ [425.7]
    incompletely diagnosed — *see* Disease, heart
    ischemic (chronic) (*see also* Ischemia, heart) 414.9
      acute (*see also* Infarct, myocardium)
        without myocardial infarction 411.89
          with coronary (artery) occlusion 411.81
      asymptomatic 412
      diagnosed on ECG or other special investigation but currently presenting no symptoms 412
    kyphoscoliotic 416.1
    mitral (*see also* Endocarditis, mitral) 394.9
    muscular (*see also* Degeneration, myocardial) 429.1
    postpartum 674.8 ✓5ᵗʰ
    psychogenic (functional) 306.2
    pulmonary (chronic) 416.9
      acute 415.0
      specified NEC 416.8
    rheumatic (chronic) (inactive) (old) (quiescent) (with chorea) 398.90

Disease, diseased — continued
- heart — continued
  - rheumatic — continued
    - active or acute 391.9
      - with chorea (active) (rheumatic) (Sydenham's) 392.0
    - specified type NEC 391.8
    - maternal, affecting fetus or newborn 760.3
  - rheumatoid — see Arthritis, rheumatoid
  - sclerotic — see Arteriosclerisis, coronary
  - senile (see also Myocarditis) 429.0
  - specified type NEC 429.89
  - syphilitic 093.89
    - aortic 093.1
      - aneurysm 093.0
    - asymptomatic 093.89
    - congenital 090.5
  - thyroid (gland) (see also Hyper-thyroidism) 242.9 [425.7]
  - thyrotoxic (see also Thyrotoxicosis) 242.9 [425.7]
  - tuberculous (see also Tuberculosis) 017.9 [425.8]
  - valve, valvular (obstructive) (regurgitant) — see also Endocarditis
    - congenital NEC (see also Anomaly, heart, valve) 746.9
      - pulmonary 746.00
      - specified type NEC 746.89
  - vascular — see Disease, cardiovascular
- heavy-chain (gamma G) 273.2
- Heberden's 715.04
- Hebra's
  - dermatitis exfoliativa 695.89
  - erythema multiforme exudativum 695.1
  - pityriasis
    - maculata et circinata 696.3
    - rubra 695.89
      - pilaris 696.4
  - prurigo 698.2
- Heerfordt's (uveoparotitis) 135
- Heidenhain's 290.10
  - with dementia 290.10
- Heilmeyer-Schöner (M9842/3) 207.1
- Heine-Medin (see also Poliomyelitis) 045.9
- Heller's (see also Psychosis, childhood) 299.1
- Heller-Döhle (syphilitic aortitis) 093.1
- hematopoietic organs 289.9
- hemoglobin (Hb) 282.7
  - with thalassemia 282.4
  - abnormal (mixed) NEC 282.7
    - with thalassemia 282.4
  - AS genotype 282.5
  - Bart's 282.7
  - C (Hb-C) 282.7
    - with other abnormal hemoglobin NEC 282.7
    - elliptocytosis 282.7
    - Hb-S 282.63
    - sickle-cell 282.63
    - thalassemia 282.4
  - constant spring 282.7
  - D (Hb-D) 282.7
    - with other abnormal hemoglobin NEC 282.7
    - Hb-S 282.69
    - sickle-cell 282.69
    - thalassemia 282.4

Disease, diseased — continued
- hemoglobin — continued
  - E (Hb-E) 282.7
    - with other abnormal hemoglobin NEC 282.7
    - Hb-S 282.69
    - sickle-cell 282.69
    - thalassemia 282.4
  - elliptocytosis 282.7
  - F (Hb-F) 282.7
  - G (Hb-G) 282.7
  - H (Hb-H) 282.4
  - hereditary persistence, fetal (HPFH) ("Swiss variety") 282.7
  - high fetal gene 282.7
  - I thalassemia 282.4
  - M 289.7
  - S — see Disease, sickle-cell, Hb-S
  - spherocytosis 282.7
  - unstable, hemolytic 282.7
  - Zurich (Hb-Zurich) 282.7
- hemolytic (fetus) (newborn) 773.2
  - autoimmune (cold type) (warm type) 283.0
  - due to or with
    - incompatibility
      - ABO (blood group) 773.1
      - blood (group) (Duffy) (Kell) (Kidd) (Lewis) (M) (S) NEC 773.2
      - Rh (blood group) (factor) 773.0
    - Rh negative mother 773.0
  - unstable hemoglobin 282.7
- hemorrhagic 287.9
  - newborn 776.0
- Henoch (-Schönlein) (purpura nervosa) 287.0
- hepatic — see Disease, liver
- hepatolenticular 275.1
- heredodegenerative NEC
  - brain 331.89
  - spinal cord 336.8
- Hers' (glycogenosis VI) 271.0
- Herter (-Gee) (-Heubner) (nontropical sprue) 579.0
- Herxheimer's (diffuse idiopathic cutaneous atrophy) 701.8
- Heubner's 094.89
- Heubner-Herter (nontropical sprue) 579.0
- high fetal gene or hemoglobin thalassemia 282.4
- Hildenbrand's (typhus) 081.9
- hip (joint) NEC 719.95
  - congenital 755.63
  - suppurative 711.05
  - tuberculous (see also Tuberculosis) 015.1 [730.85]
- Hippel's (retinocerebral angiomatosis) 759.6
- Hirschfield's (acute diabetes mellitus) (see also Diabetes) 250.0
- Hirschsprung's (congenital megacolon) 751.3
- His (-Werner) (trench fever) 083.1
- HIV 042

Index to Diseases

Disease, diseased — *continued*
  Hodgkin's (M9650/3) 201.9 ✓5ᵗʰ

> Note — Use the following fifth-digit subclassification with category 201:
>
> 0   unspecified site
> 1   lymph nodes of head, face, and neck
> 2   intrathoracic lymp nodes
> 3   intra-abdominal lymph nodes
> 4   lymph nodes of axilla and upper limb
> 5   lymph nodes of inguinal region and lower limb
> 6   intrapelvic lymph nodes
> 7   spleen
> 8   lymph nodes of multiple sites

  lymphocytic
    depletion (M9653/3) 201.7 ✓5ᵗʰ
     diffuse fibrosis (M9654/3) 201.7 ✓5ᵗʰ
     reticular type (M9655/3) 201.7 ✓5ᵗʰ
    predominance (M9651/3) 201.4 ✓5ᵗʰ
  lymphocytic-histiocytic predominance (M9651/3) 201.4 ✓5ᵗʰ
  mixed cellularity (M9652/3) 201.6 ✓5ᵗʰ
  nodular sclerosis (M9656/3) 201.5 ✓5ᵗʰ
    cellular phase (M9657/3) 201.5 ✓5ᵗʰ
Hodgson's 441.9
  ruptured 441.5
Hoffa (-Kastert) (liposynovitis prepatellaris) 272.8
Holla (see also Spherocytosis) 282.0
homozygous-Hb-S 282.61
hoof and mouth 078.4
hookworm (see also Ancylostomiasis) 126.9
Horton's (temporal arteritis) 446.5
host-versus-graft (immune or nonimmune cause) 996.80
  bone marrow 996.85
  heart 996.83
  intestines 996.87
  kidney 996.81
  liver 996.82
  lung 996.84
  pancreas 996.86
  specified NEC 996.89
HPFH (hereditary persistence of fetal hemoglobin) ("Swiss variety") 282.7
Huchard's (continued arterial hypertension) 401.9
Huguier's (uterine fibroma) 218.9
human immunodeficiency (virus) 042
hunger 251.1
Hunt's
  dyssynergia cerebellaris myoclonica 334.2
  herpetic geniculate ganglionitis 053.11
Huntington's 333.4
Huppert's (multiple myeloma) (M9730/3) 203.0 ✓5ᵗʰ
Hurler's (mucopolysaccharidosis I) 277.5
Hutchinson's, meaning
  angioma serpiginosum 709.1
  cheiropompholyx 705.81
  prurigo estivalis 692.72
Hutchinson-Boeck (sarcoidosis) 135
Hutchinson-Gilford (progeria) 259.8
hyaline (diffuse) (generalized) 728.9
  membrane (lung) (newborn) 769
hydatid (see also Echinococcus) 122.9

Disease, diseased — *continued*
Hyde's (prurigo nodularis) 698.3
hyperkinetic (see also Hyperkinesia) 314.9
  heart 429.82
hypertensive (see also Hypertension) 401.9
hypophysis 253.9
  hyperfunction 253.1
  hypofunction 253.2
Iceland (epidemic neuromyasthenia) 049.8
I cell 272.7
ill-defined 799.8
immunologic NEC 279.9
immunoproliferative 203.8 ✓5ᵗʰ
inclusion 078.5
  salivary gland 078.5
infancy, early NEC 779.9
infective NEC 136.9
inguinal gland 289.9
internal semilunar cartilage, cystic 717.5
intervertebral disc 722.90
  with myelopathy 722.70
  cervical, cervicothoracic 722.91
    with myelopathy 722.71
  lumbar, lumbosacral 722.93
    with myelopathy 722.73
  thoracic, thoracolumbar 722.92
    with myelopathy 722.72
intestine 569.9
  functional 564.9
    congenital 751.3
    psychogenic 306.4
  lardaceous 277.3
  organic 569.9
  protozoal NEC 007.9
iris 364.9
iron
  metabolism 275.0
  storage 275.0
Isambert's (see also Tuberculosis, larynx) 012.3 ✓5ᵗʰ
Iselin's (osteochondrosis, fifth metatarsal) 732.5
Island (scrub typhus) 081.2
itai-itai 985.5
Jadassohn's (maculopapular erythroderma) 696.2
Jadassohn-Pellizari's (anetoderma) 701.3
Jakob-Creutzfeldt 046.1
  with dementia
    with behavioral disturbance 046.1 *[294.11]*
    without behavioral disturbance 046.1 *[294.10]*
Jaksch (-Luzet) (pseudoleukemia infantum) 285.8
Janet's 300.89
Jansky-Bielschowsky 330.1
jaw NEC 526.9
  fibrocystic 526.2
Jensen's 363.05
Jeune's (asphyxiating thoracic dystrophy) 756.4
jigger 134.1
Johnson-Stevens (erythema multiforme exudativum) 695.1
joint NEC 719.9 ✓5ᵗʰ
  ankle 719.97
  Charcôt 094.0 *[713.5]*
  degenerative (see also Osteoarthrosis) 715.9 ✓5ᵗʰ

Disease, diseased — *continued*
  joint NEC — *continued*
   degenerative — *continued*
    multiple 715.09
    spine (*see also* Spondylosis) 721.90
   elbow 719.92
   foot 719.97
   hand 719.94
   hip 719.95
   hypertrophic (chronic) (degenerative) (*see also* Osteoarthrosis) 715.9 ✓5ᵗʰ
    spine (*see also* Spondylosis) 721.90
   knee 719.96
   Luschka 721.90
   multiple sites 719.99
   pelvic region 719.95
   sacroiliac 724.6
   shoulder (region) 719.91
   specified site NEC 719.98
   spine NEC 724.9
    pseudarthrosis following fusion 733.82
    sacroiliac 724.6
   wrist 719.93
  Jourdain's (acute gingivitis) 523.0
  Jüngling's (sarcoidosis) 135
  Kahler (-Bozzolo) (multiple myeloma) (M9730/3) 203.0 ✓5ᵗʰ
  Kalischer's 759.6
  Kaposi's 757.33
   lichen ruber 697.8
    acuminatus 696.4
    moniliformis 697.8
   xeroderma pigmentosum 757.33
  Kaschin-Beck (endemic polyarthritis) 716.00
   ankle 716.07
   arm 716.02
    lower (and wrist) 716.03
    upper (and elbow) 716.02
   foot (and ankle) 716.07
   forearm (and wrist) 716.03
   hand 716.04
   leg 716.06
    lower 716.06
    upper 716.05
   multiple sites 716.09
   pelvic region (hip) (thigh) 716.05
   shoulder region 716.01
   specified site NEC 716.08
  Katayama 120.2
  Kawasaki 446.1
  Kedani (scrub typhus) 081.2
  kidney (functional) (pelvis) (*see also* Disease, renal) 593.9
   cystic (congenital) 753.10
    multiple 753.19
    single 753.11
    specified NEC 753.19
   fibrocystic (congenital) 753.19
   in gout 274.10
   polycystic (congenital) 753.12
    adult type (APKD) 753.13
    autosomal dominant 753.13
    autosomal recessive 753.14
    childhood type (CPKD) 753.14
    infantile type 753.14
  Kienböck's (carpal lunate) (wrist) 732.3
  Kimmelstiel (-Wilson) (intercapillary glomerulosclerosis) 250.4 ✓5ᵗʰ [581.81]
  Kinnier Wilson's (hepatolenticular degeneration) 275.1
  kissing 075

Disease, diseased — *continued*
  Kleb's (*see also* Nephritis) 583.9
  Klinger's 446.4
  Klippel's 723.8
  Klippel-Feil (brevicollis) 756.16
  knight's 911.1
  Köbner's (epidermolysis bullosa) 757.39
  Koenig-Wichmann (pemphigus) 694.4
  Köhler's
   first (osteoarthrosis juvenilis) 732.5
   second (Freiberg's infraction, metatarsal head) 732.5
   patellar 732.4
   tarsal navicular (bone) (osteoarthrosis juvenilis) 732.5
  Köhler-Freiberg (infraction, metatarsal head) 732.5
  Köhler-Mouchet (osteoarthrosis juvenilis) 732.5
  Köhler-Pellegrini-Stieda (calcification, knee joint) 726.62
  König's (osteochondritis dissecans) 732.7
  Korsakoff's (nonalcoholic) 294.0
   alcoholic 291.1
  Kostmann's (infantile genetic agranulocytosis) 288.0
  Krabbe's 330.0
  Kraepelin-Morel (*see also* Schizophrenia) 295.9 ✓5ᵗʰ
  Kraft-Weber-Dimitri 759.6
  Kufs' 330.1
  Kugelberg-Welander 335.11
  Kuhnt-Junius 362.52
  Kümmell's (-Verneuil) (spondylitis) 721.7
  Kundrat's (lymphosarcoma) 200.1 ✓5ᵗʰ
  kuru 046.0
  Kussmaul (-Meier) (polyarteritis nodosa) 446.0
  Kyasanur Forest 065.2
  Kyrle's (hyperkeratosis follicularis in cutem penetrans) 701.1
  labia
   inflammatory 616.9
    specified NEC 616.8
   noninflammatory 624.9
    specified NEC 624.8
  labyrinth, ear 386.8
  lacrimal system (apparatus) (passages) 375.9
   gland 375.00
   specified NEC 375.89
  Lafora's 333.2
  Lagleyze-von Hippel (retinocerebral angiomatosis) 759.6
  Lancereaux-Mathieu (leptospiral jaundice) 100.0
  Landry's 357.0
  Lane's 569.89
  lardaceous (any site) 277.3
  Larrey-Weil (leptospiral jaundice) 100.0
  Larsen (-Johansson) (juvenile osteopathia patellae) 732.4
  larynx 478.70
  Lasègue's (persecution mania) 297.9
  Leber's 377.16
  Lederer's (acquired infectious hemolytic anemia) 283.19
  Legg's (capital femoral osteochondrosis) 732.1
  Legg-Calvé-Perthes (capital femoral osteochondrosis) 732.1
  Legg-Calvé-Waldenström (femoral capital osteochondrosis) 732.1

Disease, diseased — *continued*
  Legg-Perthes (femoral capital osteochrondosis) 732.1
  Legionnaires' 482.84
  Leigh's 330.8
  Leiner's (exfoliative dermatitis) 695.89
  Leloir's (lupus erythematosus) 695.4
  Lenegre's 426.0
  lens (eye) 379.39
  Leriche's (osteoporosis, post-traumatic) 733.7
  Letterer-Siwe (acute histiocytosis X) (M9722/3) 202.5 ✓5ᵗʰ
  Lev's (acquired complete heart block) 426.0
  Lewandowski's (*see also* Tuberculosis) 017.0 ✓5ᵗʰ
  Lewandowski-Lutz (epidermodysplasia verruciformis) 078.19
  Leyden's (periodic vomiting) 536.2
  Libman-Sacks (verrucous endocarditis) 710.0 *[424.91]*
  Lichtheim's (subacute combined sclerosis with pernicious anemia) 281.0 *[336.2]*
  ligament 728.9
  light chain 203.0 ✓5ᵗʰ
  Lightwood's (renal tubular acidosis) 588.8
  Lignac's (cystinosis) 270.0
  Lindau's (retinocerebral angiomatosis) 759.6
  Lindau-von Hippel (angiomatosis retinocerebellosa) 759.6
  lip NEC 528.5
  lipidosis 272.7
  lipoid storage NEC 272.7
  Lipschütz's 616.50
  Little's — *see* Palsy, cerebral
  liver 573.9
    alcoholic 571.3
      acute 571.1
      chronic 571.3
    chronic 571.9
      alcoholic 571.3
    cystic, congenital 751.62
    drug-induced 573.3
    due to
      chemicals 573.3
      fluorinated agents 573.3
      hypersensitivity drugs 573.3
      isoniazids 573.3
    fibrocystic (congenital) 751.62
    glycogen storage 271.0
    organic 573.9
    polycystic (congenital) 751.62
  Lobo's (keloid blastomycosis) 116.2
  Lobstein's (brittle bones and blue sclera) 756.51
  locomotor system 334.9
  Lorain's (pituitary dwarfism) 253.3
  Lou Gehrig's 335.20
  Lucas-Championnière (fibrinous bronchitis) 466.0
  Ludwig's (submaxillary cellulitis) 528.3
  luetic — *see* Syphilis
  lumbosacral region 724.6
  lung NEC 518.89
    black 500
    congenital 748.60
    cystic 518.89
      congenital 748.4
    fibroid (chronic) (*see also* Fibrosis, lung) 515
    fluke 121.2
      Oriental 121.2

Disease, diseased — *continued*
  lung NEC — *continued*
    in
      amyloidosis 277.3 *[517.8]*
      polymyositis 710.4 *[517.8]*
      sarcoidosis 135 *[517.8]*
      Sjögren's syndrome 710.2 *[517.8]*
      syphilis 095.1
      systemic lupus erythematosus 710.0 *[517.8]*
      systemic sclerosis 710.1 *[517.2]*
    interstitial (chronic) 515
      acute 136.3
    nonspecific, chronic 496
    obstructive (chronic) (COPD) 496
      with
        acute exacerbation NEC 491.21
        alveolitis, allergic (*see also* Alveolitis, allergic) 495.9
        asthma (chronic) (obstructive) 493.2 ✓5ᵗʰ
        bronchiectasis 494.0
          with acute exacerbation 494.1
        bronchitis (chronic) 491.20
          with acute exacerbation 491.21
        emphysema NEC 492.8
      diffuse (with fibrosis) 496
    polycystic 518.89
      asthma (chronic) (obstructive) 493.2 ✓5ᵗʰ
      congenital 748.4
      purulent (cavitary) 513.0
      restrictive 518.89
      rheumatoid 714.81
        diffuse interstitial 714.81
      specified NEC 518.89
  Lutembacher's (atrial septal defect with mitral stenosis) 745.5
  Lutz-Miescher (elastosis perforans serpiginosa) 701.1
  Lutz-Splendore-de Almeida (Brazilian blastomycosis) 116.1
  Lyell's (toxic epidermal necrolysis) 695.1
    due to drug
      correct substance properly administered 695.1
      overdose or wrong substance given or taken 977.9
      specific drug — *see* Table of Drugs and Chemicals
  Lyme 088.81
  lymphatic (gland) (system) 289.9
    channel (noninfective) 457.9
    vessel (noninfective) 457.9
    specified NEC 457.8
  lymphoproliferative (chronic) (M9970/1) 238.7
  Machado-Joseph 334.8
  Madelung's (lipomatosis) 272.8
  Madura (actinomycotic) 039.9
    mycotic 117.4
  Magitot's 526.4
  Majocchi's (purpura annularis telangiectodes) 709.1
  malarial (*see also* Malaria) 084.6
  Malassez's (cystic) 608.89
  Malibu 919.8
    infected 919.9
  malignant (M8000/3) — *see also* Neoplasm, by site, malignant
    previous, affecting management of pregnancy V23.8 ✓5ᵗʰ
  Manson's 120.1

Disease, diseased — *continued*
- maple bark 495.6
- maple syrup (urine) 270.3
- Marburg (virus) 078.89
- Marchiafava (-Bignami) 341.8
- Marfan's 090.49
  - congenital syphilis 090.49
  - meaning Marfan's syndrome 759.82
- Marie-Bamberger (hypertrophic pulmonary osteoarthropathy) (secondary) 731.2
  - primary or idiopathic (acropachyderma) 757.39
  - pulmonary (hypertrophic osteoarthropathy) 731.2
- Marie-Strümpell (ankylosing spondylitis) 720.0
- Marion's (bladder neck obstruction) 596.0
- Marsh's (exophthalmic goiter) 242.0
- Martin's 715.27
- mast cell 757.33
  - systemic (M9741/3) 202.6
- mastoid (*see also* Mastoiditis) 383.9
  - process 385.9
- maternal, unrelated to pregnancy NEC, affecting fetus or newborn 760.9
- Mathieu's (leptospiral jaundice) 100.0
- Mauclaire's 732.3
- Mauriac's (erythema nodosum syphiliticum) 091.3
- Maxcy's 081.0
- McArdle (-Schmid-Pearson) (glycogenosis V) 271.0
- mediastinum NEC 519.3
- Medin's (*see also* Poliomyelitis) 045.9
- Mediterranean (with hemoglobinopathy) 282.4
- medullary center (idiopathic) (respiratory) 348.8
- Meige's (chronic hereditary edema) 757.0
- Meleda 757.39
- Ménétrier's (hypertrophic gastritis) 535.2
- Ménière's (active) 386.00
  - cochlear 386.02
  - cochleovestibular 386.01
  - inactive 386.04
  - in remission 386.04
  - vestibular 386.03
- meningeal — *see* Meningitis
- mental (*see also* Psychosis) 298.9
- Merzbacher-Pelizaeus 330.0
- mesenchymal 710.9
- mesenteric embolic 557.0
- metabolic NEC 277.9
- metal polishers' 502
- metastatic — *see* Metastasis
- Mibelli's 757.39
- microdrepanocytic 282.4
- Miescher's 709.3
- Mikulicz's (dryness of mouth, absent or decreased lacrimation) 527.1
- Milkman (-Looser) (osteomalacia with pseudofractures) 268.2
- Miller's (osteomalacia) 268.2
- Mills' 335.29
- Milroy's (chronic hereditary edema) 757.0
- Minamata 985.0
- Minor's 336.1
- Minot's (hemorrhagic disease, newborn) 776.0
- Minot-von Willebrand-Jürgens (angiohemophilia) 286.4
- Mitchell's (erythromelalgia) 443.89
- mitral — *see* Endocarditis, mitral
- Mljet (mal de Meleda) 757.39

Disease, diseased — *continued*
- Möbius', Moebius' 346.8
- Moeller's 267
- Möller (-Barlow) (infantile scurvy) 267
- Mönckeberg's (*see also* Arteriosclerosis, extremities) 440.20
- Mondor's (thrombophlebitis of breast) 451.89
- Monge's 993.2
- Morel-Kraepelin (*see also* Schizophrenia) 295.9
- Morgagni's (syndrome) (hyperostosis frontalis interna) 733.3
- Morgagni-Adams-Stokes (syncope with heart block) 426.9
- Morquio (-Brailsford) (-Ullrich) (mucopolysaccharidosis IV) 277.5
- Morton's (with metatarsalgia) 355.6
- Morvan's 336.0
- motor neuron (bulbar) (mixed type) 335.20
- Mouchet's (juvenile osteochondrosis, foot) 732.5
- mouth 528.9
- Moyamoya 437.5
- Mucha's (acute parapsoriasis varioliformis) 696.2
- mu-chain 273.2
- mucolipidosis (I) (II) (III) 272.7
- Münchmeyer's (exostosis luxurians) 728.11
- Murri's (intermittent hemoglobinuria) 283.2
- muscle 359.9
  - inflammatory 728.9
  - ocular 378.9
- musculoskeletal system 729.9
- mushroom workers' 495.5
- Myà's (congenital dilation, colon) 751.3
- mycotic 117.9
- myeloproliferative (chronic) (M9960/1) 238.7
- myocardium, myocardial (*see also* Degeneration, myocardial) 429.1
  - hypertensive (*see also* Hypertension, heart 402.90
  - primary (idiopathic) 425.4
- myoneural 358.9
- Naegeli's 287.1
- nail 703.9
  - specified type NEC 703.8
- Nairobi sheep 066.1
- nasal 478.1
  - cavity NEC 478.1
  - sinus (chronic) — *see* Sinusitis
- navel (newborn) NEC 779.89 ▲
- nemaline body 359.0
- neoplastic, generalized (M8000/6) 199.0
- nerve — *see* Disorder, nerve
- nervous system (central) 349.9
  - autonomic, peripheral (*see also* Neuropathy, peripheral, autonomic) 337.9
  - congenital 742.9
  - inflammatory — *see* Encephalitis
  - parasympathetic (*see also* Neuropathy, peripheral, autonomic) 337.9
  - peripheral NEC 355.9
  - specified NEC 349.89
  - sympathetic (*see also* Neuropathy, peripheral, autonomic) 337.9
  - vegetative (*see also* Neuropathy, peripheral, autonomic) 337.9
- Nettleship's (urticaria pigmentosa) 757.33
- Neumann's (pemphigus vegetans) 694.4

Disease, diseased — *continued*
  neurologic (central) NEC (*see also* Disease, nervous system) 349.9
    peripheral NEC 355.9
  neuromuscular system NEC 358.9
  Newcastle 077.8
  Nicolas (-Durand) — Favre (climatic bubo) 099.1
  Niemann-Pick (lipid histiocytosis) 272.7
  nipple 611.9
    Paget's (M8540/3) 174.0
  Nishimoto (-Takeuchi) 437.5
  nonarthropod-borne NEC 078.89
    central nervous system NEC 049.9
    enterovirus NEC 078.89
  non-autoimmune hemolytic NEC 283.10
  Nonne-Milroy-Meige (chronic hereditary edema) 757.0
  Norrie's (congenital progressive oculoacousticocerebral degeneration) 743.8
  nose 478.1
  nucleus pulposus — *see* Disease, intervertebral disc
  nutritional 269.9
    maternal, affecting fetus or newborn 760.4
  oasthouse, urine 270.2
  obliterative vascular 447.1
  Odelberg's (juvenile osteochondrosis) 732.1
  Oguchi's (retina) 368.61
  Ohara's (*see also* Tularemia) 021.9
  Ollier's (chondrodysplasia) 756.4
  Opitz's (congestive splenomegaly) 289.51
  Oppenheim's 358.8
  Oppenheim-Urbach (necrobiosis lipoidica diabeticorum) 250.8 ✓5ᵗʰ [709.3]
  optic nerve NEC 377.49
  orbit 376.9
    specified NEC 376.89
  Oriental liver fluke 121.1
  Oriental lung fluke 121.2
  Ormond's 593.4
  Osgood's tibia (tubercle) 732.4
  Osgood-Schlatter 732.4
  Osler (-Vaquez) (polycythemia vera) (M9950/1) 238.4
  Osler-Rendu (familial hemorrhagic telangiectasia) 448.0
  osteofibrocystic 252.0
  Otto's 715.35
  outer ear 380.9
  ovary (noninflammatory) NEC 620.9
    cystic 620.2
    polycystic 256.4
    specified NEC 620.8
  Owren's (congenital) (*see also* Defect, coagulation) 286.3
  Paas' 756.59
  Paget's (osteitis deformans) 731.0
    with infiltrating duct carcinoma of the breast (M8541/3) — *see* Neoplasm, breast, malignant
    bone 731.0
      osteosarcoma in (M9184/3) — *see* Neoplasm, bone, malignant
    breast (M8540/3) 174.0
      extramammary (M8542/3) — *see also* Neoplasm, skin, malignant
        anus 154.3
        skin 173.5

Disease, diseased — *continued*
  Paget's — *continued*
    malignant (M8540/3)
      breast 174.0
      specified site NEC (M8542/3) — *see* Neoplasm, skin, malignant
      unspecified site 174.0
    mammary (M8540/3) 174.0
    nipple (M8540/3) 174.0
  palate (soft) 528.9
  Paltauf-Sternberg 201.9 ✓5ᵗʰ
  pancreas 577.9
    cystic 577.2
    congenital 751.7
    fibrocystic 277.00
  Panner's 732.3
    capitellum humeri 732.3
    head of humerus 732.3
    tarsal navicular (bone) (osteochondrosis) 732.5
  panvalvular — *see* Endocarditis, mitral
  parametrium 629.9
  parasitic NEC 136.9
    cerebral NEC 123.9
    intestinal NEC 129
    mouth 112.0
    skin NEC 134.9
    specified type — *see* Infestation
    tongue 112.0
  parathyroid (gland) 252.9
    specified NEC 252.8
  Parkinson's 332.0
  parodontal 523.9
  Parrot's (syphilitic osteochondritis) 090.0
  Parry's (exophthalmic goiter) 242.0 ✓5ᵗʰ
  Parson's (exophthalmic goiter) 242.0 ✓5ᵗʰ
  Pavy's 593.6
  Paxton's (white piedra) 111.2
  Payr's (splenic flexure syndrome) 569.89
  pearl-workers' (chronic osteomyelitis) (*see also* Osteomyelitis) 730.1 ✓5ᵗʰ
  Pel-Ebstein — *see* Disease, Hodgkin's
  Pelizaeus-Merzbacher 330.0
    with dementia
      with behavioral disturbance 330.0 [294.11]
      without behavioral disturbance 330.0 [294.10]
  Pellegrini-Stieda (calcification, knee joint) 726.62
  pelvis, pelvic
    female NEC 629.9
      specified NEC 629.8
    gonococcal (acute) 098.19
      chronic or duration of 2 months or over 098.39
    infection (*see also* Disease, pelvis, inflammatory) 614.9
    inflammatory (female) (PID) 614.9
      with
        abortion — *see* Abortion, by type, with sepsis
        ectopic pregnancy (*see also* categories 633.0-633.9) 639.0
        molar pregnancy (*see also* categories 630-632) 639.0
      acute 614.3
      chronic 614.4
      complicating pregnancy 646.6 ✓5ᵗʰ
        affecting fetus or newborn 760.8

Disease, diseased — *continued*
  pelvis, pelvic — *continued*
    inflammatory — *continued*
      following
        abortion 639.0
        ectopic or molar pregnancy 639.0
      peritonitis (acute) 614.5
        chronic NEC 614.7
      puerperal, postpartum, childbirth 670 ✓4ᵗʰ
      specified NEC 614.8
    organ, female NEC 629.9
      specified NEC 629.8
    peritoneum, female NEC 629.9
      specified NEC 629.8
  penis 607.9
    inflammatory 607.2
  peptic NEC 536.9
    acid 536.8
  periapical tissues NEC 522.9
  pericardium 423.9
    specified type NEC 423.8
  perineum
    female
      inflammatory 616.9
        specified NEC 616.8
      noninflammatory 624.9
        specified NEC 624.8
    male (inflammatory) 682.2
  periodic (familial) (Reimann's) NEC 277.3
    paralysis 359.3
  periodontal NEC 523.9
    specified NEC 523.8
  periosteum 733.90
  peripheral
    arterial 443.9
    autonomic nervous system (*see also* Neuropathy, autonomic) 337.9
    nerve NEC (*see also* Neuropathy) 356.9
      multiple — *see* Polyneuropathy
    vascular 443.9
      specified type NEC 443.89
  peritoneum 568.9
    pelvic, female 629.9
      specified NEC 629.8
  Perrin-Ferraton (snapping hip) 719.65
  persistent mucosal (middle ear) (with posterior or superior marginal perforation of ear drum) 382.2
  Perthes' (capital femoral osteochondrosis) 732.1
  Petit's (*see also* Hernia, lumbar) 553.8
  Peutz-Jeghers 759.6
  Peyronie's 607.89
  Pfeiffer's (infectious mononucleosis) 075
  pharynx 478.20
  Phocas' 610.1
  photochromogenic (acid-fast bacilli) (pulmonary) 031.0
    nonpulmonary 031.9
  Pick's
    brain 331.1
      with dementia
        with behavioral disturbance 331.1 [294.11]
        without behavioral disturbance 331.1 [294.10]
    cerebral atrophy 331.1
      with dementia
        with behavioral disturbance 331.1 [294.11]

Disease, diseased — *continued*
  Pick's — *continued*
    cerebral atrophy — *continued*
      with dementia — *continued*
        without behavioral disturbance 331.1 [294.10]
    lipid histiocytosis 272.7
    liver (pericardial pseudocirrhosis of liver) 423.2
    pericardium (pericardial pseudocirrhosis of liver) 423.2
    polyserositis (pericardial pseudocirrhosis of liver) 423.2
  Pierson's (osteochondrosis) 732.1
  pigeon fanciers' or breeders' 495.2
  pineal gland 259.8
  pink 985.0
  Pinkus' (lichen nitidus) 697.1
  pinworm 127.4
  pituitary (gland) 253.9
    hyperfunction 253.1
    hypofunction 253.2
  pituitary snuff-takers' 495.8
  placenta
    affecting fetus or newborn 762.2
    complicating pregnancy or childbirth 656.7 ✓5ᵗʰ
  pleura (cavity) (*see also* Pleurisy) 511.9
  Plummer's (toxic nodular goiter) 242.3 ✓5ᵗʰ
  pneumatic
    drill 994.9
    hammer 994.9
  policeman's 729.2
  Pollitzer's (hidradenitis suppurativa) 705.83
  polycystic (congenital) 759.89
    kidney or renal 753.12
      adult type (APKD) 753.13
      autosomal dominant 753.13
      autosomal recessive 753.14
      childhood type (CPKD) 753.14
      infantile type 753.14
    liver or hepatic 751.62
    lung or pulmonary 518.89
      congenital 748.4
    ovary, ovaries 256.4
    spleen 759.0
  Pompe's (glycogenosis II) 271.0
  Poncet's (tuberculous rheumatism) (*see also* Tuberculosis) 015.9 ✓5ᵗʰ
  Posada-Wernicke 114.9
  Potain's (pulmonary edema) 514
  Pott's (*see also* Tuberculosis) 015.0 ✓5ᵗʰ [730.88]
    osteomyelitis 015.0 ✓5ᵗʰ [730.88]
    paraplegia 015.0 ✓5ᵗʰ [730.88]
    spinal curvature 015.0 ✓5ᵗʰ [737.43]
    spondylitis 015.0 ✓5ᵗʰ [720.81]
  Potter's 753.0
  Poulet's 714.2
  pregnancy NEC (*see also* Pregnancy) 646.9 ✓5ᵗʰ
  Preiser's (osteoporosis) 733.09
  Pringle's (tuberous sclerosis) 759.5
  Profichet's 729.9
  prostate 602.9
    specified type NEC 602.8
  protozoal NEC 136.8
    intestine, intestinal NEC 007.9
  pseudo-Hurler's (mucolipidosis III) 272.7
  psychiatric (*see also* Psychosis) 298.9
  psychotic (*see also* Psychosis) 298.9
  Puente's (simple glandular cheilitis) 528.5

Index to Diseases

Disease, diseased — *continued*
  puerperal NEC (*see also* Puerperal) 674.9 ✓5ᵗʰ
  pulmonary — *see also* Disease, lung
    amyloid 277.3 *[517.8]*
    artery 417.9
    circulation, circulatory 417.9
      specified NEC 417.8
    diffuse obstructive (chronic) 496
      with
        acute exacerbation NEC 491.21
        asthma (chronic) (obstructive)
          493.2 ✓5ᵗʰ
    heart (chronic) 416.9
      specified NEC 416.8
    hypertensive (vascular) 416.0
      cardiovascular 416.0
    obstructive diffuse (chronic) 496
      with
        acute exacerbation NEC 491.21
        asthma (chronic) (obstructive)
          493.2 ✓5ᵗʰ
        bronchitis (chronic) 491.20
          with acute exacerbation 491.21
    valve (*see also* Endocarditis, pulmonary)
      424.3
  pulp (dental) NEC 522.9
  pulseless 446.7
  Putnam's (subacute combined sclerosis with pernicious anemia) 281.0 *[336.2]*
  Pyle (-Cohn) (craniometaphyseal dysplasia) 756.89
  pyramidal tract 333.90
  Quervain's
    tendon sheath 727.04
    thyroid (subacute granulomatous thyroiditis) 245.1
  Quincke's — *see* Edema, angioneurotic
  Quinquaud (acne decalvans) 704.09
  rag sorters' 022.1
  Raynaud's (paroxysmal digital cyanosis) 443.0
  reactive airway — *see* Asthma
  Recklinghausen's (M9540/1) 237.71
    bone (osteitis fibrosa cystica) 252.0
  Recklinghausen-Applebaum (hemochromatosis) 275.0
  Reclus' (cystic) 610.1
  rectum NEC 569.49
  Refsum's (heredopathia atactica polyneuritiformis) 356.3
  Reichmann's (gastrosuccorrhea) 536.8
  Reimann's (periodic) 277.3
  Reiter's 099.3
  renal (functional) (pelvis) 593.9
    with
      edema (*see also* Nephrosis) 581.9
      exudative nephritis 583.89
      lesion of interstitial nephritis 583.89
      stated generalized cause — *see* Nephritis
    acute — *see* Nephritis, acute
    basement membrane NEC 583.89
      with
        pulmonary hemorrhage (Goodpasture's syndrome) 446.21 *[583.81]*
    chronic — *see* Nephritis, chronic
    complicating pregnancy or puerperium NEC 646.2 ✓5ᵗʰ
      with hypertension — *see* Toxemia, of pregnancy
      affecting fetus or newborn 760.1

Disease, diseased — *continued*
  renal — *continued*
    cystic, congenital (*see also* Cystic, disease, kidney) 753.10
    diabetic 250.4 ✓5ᵗʰ *[583.81]*
    due to
      amyloidosis 277.3 *[583.81]*
      diabetes mellitus 250.4 ✓5ᵗʰ *[583.81]*
      systemic lupus erythematosis 710.0 *[583.81]*
    end-stage 585
    exudative 583.89
    fibrocystic (congenital) 753.19
    gonococcal 098.19 *[583.81]*
    gouty 274.10
    hypertensive (*see also* Hypertension, kidney) 403.90
    immune complex NEC 583.89
    interstitial (diffuse) (focal) 583.89
    lupus 710.0 *[583.81]*
    maternal, affecting fetus or newborn 760.1
      hypertensive 760.0
    phosphate-losing (tubular) 588.0
    polycystic (congenital) 753.12
      adult type (APKD) 753.13
      autosomal dominant 753.13
      autosomal recessive 753.14
      childhood type (CPKD) 753.14
      infantile type 753.14
    specified lesion or cause NEC (*see also* Glomerulonephritis) 583.89
    subacute 581.9
    syphilitic 095.4
    tuberculous (*see also* Tuberculosis) 016.0 ✓5ᵗʰ *[583.81]*
    tubular (*see also* Nephrosis, tubular) 584.5
  Rendu-Osler-Weber (familial hemorrhagic telangiectasia) 448.0
  renovascular (arteriosclerotic) (*see also* Hypertension, kidney) 403.90
  respiratory (tract) 519.9
    acute or subacute (upper) NEC 465.9
      due to fumes or vapors 506.3
      multiple sites NEC 465.8
      noninfectious 478.9
      streptococcal 034.0
    chronic 519.9
      arising in the perinatal period 770.7
      due to fumes or vapors 506.4
    due to
      aspiration of liquids or solids 508.9
      external agents NEC 508.9
        specified NEC 508.8
      fumes or vapors 506.9
        acute or subacute NEC 506.3
        chronic 506.4
    fetus or newborn NEC 770.9
    obstructive 496
    specified type NEC 519.8
    upper (acute) (infectious) NEC 465.9
      multiple sites NEC 465.8
      noninfectious NEC 478.9
      streptococcal 034.0
  retina, retinal NEC 362.9
    Batten's or Batten-Mayou 330.1 *[362.71]*
    degeneration 362.89
    vascular lesion 362.17
  rheumatic (*see also* Arthritis) 716.8 ✓5ᵗʰ
    heart — *see* Disease, heart, rheumatic
  rheumatoid (heart) — *see* Arthritis, rheumatoid

Disease, diseased — continued
rickettsial NEC 083.9
  specified type NEC 083.8
Riedel's (ligneous thyroiditis) 245.3
Riga (-Fede) (cachectic aphthae) 529.0
Riggs' (compound periodontitis) 523.4
Ritter's 695.81
Rivalta's (cervicofacial actinomycosis) 039.3
Robles' (onchocerciasis) 125.3 *[360.13]*
Roger's (congenital interventricular septal defect) 745.4
Rokitansky's (*see also* Necrosis, liver) 570
Romberg's 349.89
Rosenthal's (factor XI deficiency) 286.2
Rossbach's (hyperchlorhydria) 536.8
  psychogenic 306.4
Roth (-Bernhardt) 355.1
Runeberg's (progressive pernicious anemia) 281.0
Rust's (tuberculous spondylitis) (*see also* Tuberculosis) 015.0 ✓5ᵗʰ *[720.81]*
Rustitskii's (multiple myeloma) (M9730/3) 203.0 ✓5ᵗʰ
Ruysch's (Hirschsprung's disease) 751.3
Sachs (-Tay) 330.1
sacroiliac NEC 724.6
salivary gland or duct NEC 527.9
  inclusion 078.5
    streptococcal 034.0
  virus 078.5
Sander's (paranoia) 297.1
Sandhoff's 330.1
sandworm 126.9
Savill's (epidemic exfoliative dermatitis) 695.89
Schamberg's (progressive pigmentary dermatosis) 709.09
Schaumann's (sarcoidosis) 135
Schenck's (sporotrichosis) 117.1
Scheuermann's (osteochondrosis) 732.0
Schilder (-Flatau) 341.1
Schimmelbusch's 610.1
Schlatter's tibia (tubercle) 732.4
Schlatter-Osgood 732.4
Schmorl's 722.30
  cervical 722.39
  lumbar, lumbosacral 722.32
  specified region NEC 722.39
  thoracic, thoracolumbar 722.31
Scholz's 330.0
Schönlein (-Henoch) (purpura rheumatica) 287.0
Schottmüller's (*see also* Fever, paratyphoid) 002.9
Schüller-Christian (chronic histiocytosis X) 277.8
Schultz's (agranulocytosis) 288.0
Schwalbe-Ziehen-Oppenheimer 333.6
Schweninger-Buzzi (macular atrophy) 701.3
sclera 379.19
scrofulous (*see also* Tuberculosis) 017.2 ✓5ᵗʰ
scrotum 608.9
sebaceous glands NEC 706.9
Secretan's (posttraumatic edema) 782.3
semilunar cartilage, cystic 717.5
seminal vesicle 608.9
Senear-Usher (pemphigus erythematosus) 694.4
serum NEC 999.5
Sever's (osteochondrosis calcaneum) 732.5
Sézary's (reticulosis) (M9701/3) 202.2 ✓5ᵗʰ
Shaver's (bauxite pneumoconiosis) 503

Disease, diseased — continued
Sheehan's (postpartum pituitary necrosis) 253.2
shimamushi (scrub typus) 081.2
shipyard 077.1
sickle cell 282.60
  with
    crisis 282.62
    Hb-S disease 282.61
    other abnormal hemoglobin (Hb-D) (Hb-E) (Hb-G) (Hb-J) (Hb-K) (Hb-O) (Hb-P) (high fetal gene) 282.69
elliptocytosis 282.60
Hb-C 282.63
Hb-S 282.61
  with
    crisis 282.62
    Hb-C 282.63
    other abnormal hemoglobin (Hb-D) (Hb-E) (Hb-G) (Hb-J) (Hb-K) (Hb-O) (Hb-P) (high fetal gene) 282.69
spherocytosis 282.60
thalassemia 282.4
Siegal-Cattan-Mamou (periodic) 277.3
silo fillers' 506.9
Simian B 054.3
Simmonds' (pituitary cachexia) 253.2
Simons' (progressive lipodystrophy) 272.6
Sinding-Larsen (juvenile osteopathia patellae) 732.4
sinus — *see also* Sinusitis
  brain 437.9
  specified NEC 478.1
Sirkari's 085.0
sixth 057.8
Sjögren (-Gougerot) 710.2
  with lung involvement 710.2 *[517.8]*
Skevas-Zerfus 989.5
skin NEC 709.9
  due to metabolic disorder 277.9
  specified type NEC 709.8
sleeping 347
  meaning sleeping sickness (*see also* Trypanosomiasis) 086.5
small vessel 443.9
Smith-Strang (oasthouse urine) 270.2
Sneddon-Wilkinson (subcorneal pustular dermatosis) 694.1
South African creeping 133.8
Spencer's (epidemic vomiting) 078.82
Spielmeyer-Stock 330.1
Spielmeyer-Vogt 330.1
spine, spinal 733.90
  combined system (*see also* Degeneration, combined) 266.2 *[336.2]*
    with pernicious anemia 281.0 *[336.2]*
  cord NEC 336.9
    congenital 742.9
  demyelinating NEC 341.8
  joint (*see also* Disease, joint, spine) 724.9
  tuberculous 015.0 ✓5ᵗʰ *[730.8]* ✓5ᵗʰ
spinocerebellar 334.9
  specified NEC 334.8
spleen (organic) (postinfectional) 289.50
  amyloid 277.3
  lardaceous 277.3
  polycystic 759.0
  specified NEC 289.59
sponge divers' 989.5
Stanton's (melioidosis) 025

Disease, diseased — *continued*
- Stargardt's 362.75
- Steinert's 359.2
- Sternberg's — *see* Disease, Hodgkin's
- Stevens-Johnson (erythema multiforme exudativum) 695.1
- Sticker's (erythema infectiosum) 057.0
- Stieda's (calcification, knee joint) 726.62
- Still's (juvenile rheumatoid arthritis) 714.30
- Stiller's (asthenia) 780.79
- Stokes' (exophthalmic goiter) 242.0 ✓5th
- Stokes-Adams (syncope with heart block) 426.9
- Stokvis (-Talma) (enterogenous cyanosis) 289.7
- stomach NEC (organic) 537.9
  - functional 536.9
    - psychogenic 306.4
  - lardaceous 277.3
- stonemasons' 502
- storage
  - glycogen (*see also* Disease, glycogen storage) 271.0
  - lipid 272.7
  - mucopolysaccharide 277.5
- striatopallidal system 333.90
  - specified NEC 333.89
- Strümpell-Marie (ankylosing spondylitis) 720.0
- Stuart's (congenital factor X deficiency) (*see also* Defect, coagulation) 286.3
- Stuart-Prower (congenital factor X deficiency) (*see also* Defect, coagulation) 286.3
- Sturge (-Weber) (-Dimitri) (encephalocutaneous angiomatosis) 759.6
- Stuttgart 100.89
- Sudeck's 733.7
- supporting structures of teeth NEC 525.9
- suprarenal (gland) (capsule) 255.9
  - hyperfunction 255.3
  - hypofunction 255.4
- Sutton's 709.09
- Sutton and Gull's — *see* Hypertension, kidney
- sweat glands NEC 705.9
  - specified type NEC 705.89
- sweating 078.2
- Sweeley-Klionsky 272.4
- Swift (-Feer) 985.0
- swimming pool (bacillus) 031.1
- swineherd's 100.89
- Sylvest's (epidemic pleurodynia) 074.1
- Symmers (follicular lymphoma) (M9690/3) 202.0 ✓5th
- sympathetic nervous system (*see also* Neuropathy, peripheral, autonomic) 337.9
- synovium 727.9
- syphilitic — *see* Syphilis
- systemic tissue mast cell (M9741/3) 202.5 ✓5th
- Taenzer's 757.4
- Takayasu's (pulseless) 446.7
- Talma's 728.85
- Tangier (familial high-density lipoprotein deficiency) 272.5
- Tarral-Besnier (pityriasis rubra pilaris) 696.4
- Tay-Sachs 330.1
- Taylor's 701.8
- tear duct 375.69
- teeth, tooth 525.9
  - hard tissues NEC 521.9
  - pulp NEC 522.9

Disease, diseased — *continued*
- tendon 727.9
  - inflammatory NEC 727.9
- terminal vessel 443.9
- testis 608.9
- Thaysen-Gee (nontropical sprue) 579.0
- Thomsen's 359.2
- Thomson's (congenital poikiloderma) 757.33
- Thornwaldt's, Tornwaldt's (pharyngeal bursitis) 478.29
- throat 478.20
  - septic 034.0
- thromboembolic (*see also* Embolism) 444.9
- thymus (gland) 254.9
  - specified NEC 254.8
- thyroid (gland) NEC 246.9
  - heart (*see also* Hyperthyroidism) 242.9 ✓5th [425.7]
  - lardaceous 277.3
  - specified NEC 246.8
- Tietze's 733.6
- Tommaselli's
  - correct substance properly administered 599.7
  - overdose or wrong substance given or taken 961.4
- tongue 529.9
- tonsils, tonsillar (and adenoids) (chronic) 474.9
  - specified NEC 474.8
- tooth, teeth 525.9
  - hard tissues NEC 521.9
  - pulp NEC 522.9
- Tornwaldt's (pharyngeal bursitis) 478.29
- Tourette's 307.23
- trachea 519.1
- tricuspid — *see* Endocarditis, tricuspid
- triglyceride-storage, type I, II, III 272.7
- triple vessel (coronary arteries) — *see* Arteriosclerosis, coronary
- trisymptomatic, Gourgerot's 709.1
- trophoblastic (*see also* Hydatidiform mole) 630
  - previous, affecting management of pregnancy V23.1
- tsutsugamushi (scrub typhus) 081.2
- tube (fallopian), noninflammatory 620.9
  - specified NEC 620.8
- tuberculous NEC (*see also* Tuberculosis) 011.9 ✓5th
- tubo-ovarian
  - inflammatory (*see also* Salpingo-oophoritis) 614.2
  - noninflammatory 620.9
  - specified NEC 620.8
- tubotympanic, chronic (with anterior perforation of ear drum) 382.1
- tympanum 385.9
- Uhl's 746.84
- umbilicus (newborn) NEC 779.89 ▲
- Underwood's (sclerema neonatorum) 778.1
- undiagnosed 799.9
- Unna's (seborrheic dermatitis) 690.18
- unstable hemoglobin hemolytic 282.7
- Unverricht (-Lundborg) 333.2
- Urbach-Oppenheim (necrobiosis lipoidica diabeticorum) 250.8 ✓5th [709.3]
- Urbach-Wiethe (lipoid proteinosis) 272.8
- ureter 593.9
- urethra 599.9
  - specified type NEC 599.84

Disease, diseased

Disease, diseased — *continued*
  urinary (tract) 599.9
    bladder 596.9
      specified NEC 596.8
      maternal, affecting fetus or newborn 760.1
  Usher-Senear (pemphigus erythematosus) 694.4
  uterus (organic) 621.9
    infective (*see also* Endometritis) 615.9
    inflammatory (*see also* Endometritis) 615.9
    noninflammatory 621.9
    specified type NEC 621.8
  uveal tract
    anterior 364.9
    posterior 363.9
  vagabonds' 132.1
  vagina, vaginal
    inflammatory 616.9
      specified NEC 616.8
    noninflammatory 623.9
      specified NEC 623.8
  Valsuani's (progressive pernicious anemia, puerperal) 648.2
    complicating pregnancy or puerperium 648.2
  valve, valvular — *see* Endocarditis
  van Bogaert-Nijssen (-Peiffer) 330.0
  van Creveld-von Gierke (glycogenosis I) 271.0
  van den Bergh's (enterogenous cyanosis) 289.7
  van Neck's (juvenile osteochondrosis) 732.1
  Vaquez (-Osler) (polycythemia vera) (M9950/1) 238.4
  vascular 459.9
    arteriosclerotic — *see* Arteriosclerosis
    hypertensive — *see* Hypertension
    obliterative 447.1
      peripheral 443.9
    occlusive 459.9
    peripheral (occlusive) 443.9
      in diabetes mellitus 250.7 [443.81]
      specified type NEC 443.89
  vas deferens 608.9
  vasomotor 443.9
  vasopastic 443.9
  vein 459.9
  venereal 099.9
    chlamydial NEC 099.50
      anus 099.52
      bladder 099.53
      cervix 099.53
      epididymis 099.54
      genitourinary NEC 099.55
        lower 099.53
        specified NEC 099.54
      pelvic inflammatory disease 099.54
      perihepatic 099.56
      peritoneum 099.56
      pharynx 099.51
      rectum 099.52
      specified site NEC 099.54
      testis 099.54
      vagina 099.53
      vulva 099.53
    fifth 099.1
    sixth 099.1
    complicating pregnancy, childbirth, or puerperium 647.2
    specified nature or type NEC 099.8
      chlamydial — *see* Disease, venereal, chlamydial
  Verneuil's (syphilitic bursitis) 095.7

Disease, diseased — *continued*
  Verse's (calcinosis intervertebralis) 275.49 [722.90]
  vertebra, vertebral NEC 733.90
    disc — *see* Disease, Intervertebral disc
  vibration NEC 994.9
  Vidal's (lichen simplex chronicus) 698.3
  Vincent's (trench mouth) 101
  Virchow's 733.99
  virus (filterable) NEC 078.89
    arbovirus NEC 066.9
    arthropod-borne NEC 066.9
    central nervous system NEC 049.9
      specified type NEC 049.8
    complicating pregnancy, childbirth, or puerperium 647.6
    contact (with) V01.7
    exposure to V01.7
    Marburg 078.89
    maternal
      with fetal damage affecting management of pregnancy 655.3
    nonarthropod-borne NEC 078.89
      central nervous sytem NEC 049.9
      specified NEC 049.8
  vitreous 379.29
  vocal cords NEC 478.5
  Vogt's (Cecile) 333.7
  Vogt-Spielmeyer 330.1
  Volhard-Fahr (malignant nephrosclerosis) 403.00
  Volkmann's
    acquired 958.6
  von Bechterew's (ankylosing spondylitis) 720.0
  von Economo's (encephalitis lethargica) 049.8
  von Eulenburg's (congenital paramyotonia) 359.2
  von Gierke's (glycogenosis I) 271.0
  von Graefe's 378.72
  von Hippel's (retinocerebral angiomatosis) 759.6
  von Hippel-Lindau (angiomatosis retinocerebellosa) 759.6
  von Jaksch's (pseudoleukemia infantum) 285.8
  von Recklinghausen's (M9540/1) 237.71
    bone (osteitis fibrosa cystica) 252.0
  von Recklinghausen-Applebaum (hemochromatosis) 275.0
  von Willebrand (-Jürgens) (angiohemophilia) 286.4
  von Zambusch's (lichen sclerosus et atrophicus) 701.0
  Voorhoeve's (dyschondroplasia) 756.4
  Vrolik's (osteogenesis imperfecta) 756.51
  vulva
    noninflammatory 624.9
      specified NEC 624.8
  Wagner's (colloid milium) 709.3
  Waldenström's (osteochondrosis capital femoral) 732.1
  Wallgren's (obstruction of splenic vein with collateral circulation) 459.89
  Wardrop's (with lymphangitis) 681.9
    finger 681.02
    toe 681.11
  Wassilieff's (leptospiral jaundice) 100.0
  wasting NEC 799.4
    due to malnutrition 261
    paralysis 335.21
  Waterhouse-Friderichsen 036.3

Index to Diseases — Dislocation

Disease, diseased — *continued*
 waxy (any site) 277.3
 Weber-Christian (nodular nonsuppurative panniculitis) 729.30
 Wegner's (syphilitic osteochondritis) 090.0
 Weil's (leptospral jaundice) 100.0
  of lung 100.0
 Weir Mitchell's (erythromelalgia) 443.89
 Werdnig-Hoffmann 335.0
 Werlhof's (*see also* Purpura, thrombocytopenic) 287.3
 Wermer's 258.0
 Werner's (progeria adultorum) 259.8
 Werner-His (trench fever) 083.1
 Werner-Schultz (agranulocytosis) 288.0
 Wernicke's (superior hemorrhagic polioencephalitis) 265.1
 Wernicke-Posadas 114.9
 Whipple's (intestinal lipodystrophy) 040.2
 whipworm 127.3
 white
  blood cell 288.9
   specified NEC 288.8
  spot 701.0
 White's (congenital) (keratosis follicularis) 757.39
 Whitmore's (melioidosis) 025
 Widal-Abrami (acquired hemolytic jaundice) 283.9
 Wilkie's 557.1
 Wilkinson-Sneddon (subcorneal pustular dermatosis) 694.1
 Willis' (diabetes mellitus) (*see also* Diabetes) 250.0 ✓5ᵗʰ
 Wilson's (hepatolenticular degeneration) 275.1
 Wilson-Brocq (dermatitis exfoliativa) 695.89
 winter vomiting 078.82
 Wise's 696.2
 Wohlfart-Kugelberg-Welander 335.11
 Woillez's (acute idiopathic pulmonary congestion) 518.5
 Wolman's (primary familial xanthomatosis) 272.7
 wool-sorters' 022.1
 Zagari's (xerostomia) 527.7
 Zahorsky's (exanthem subitum) 057.8
 Ziehen-Oppenheim 333.6
 zoonotic, bacterial NEC 027.9
  specified type NEC 027.8
Disfigurement (due to scar) 709.2
 head V48.6
 limb V49.4
 neck V48.7
 trunk V48.7
Disgerminoma — *see* Dysgerminoma
Disinsertion, retina 361.04
Disintegration, complete, of the body 799.8
 traumatic 869.1
Disk kidney 753.3
Dislocatable hip, congenital (*see also* Dislocation, hip, congenital) 754.30
Dislocation (articulation) (closed) (displacement) (simple) (subluxation) 839.8

Dislocation — *continued*

> Note — "Closed" includes simple, complete, partial, uncomplicated, and unspecified dislocation.
>
> "Open" includes dislocation specified as infected or compound and dislocation with foreign body.
>
> "Chronic," "habitual," "old," or "recurrent" dislocations should be coded as indicated under the entry "Dislocation, recurrent," and "pathological" as indicated under the entry "Dislocation, pathological."
>
> For late effect of dislocation see Late, effect, dislocation.

 with fracture — *see* Fracture, by site
 acromioclavicular (joint) (closed) 831.04
  open 831.14
 anatomical site (closed)
  specified NEC 839.69
   open 839.79
  unspecified or ill-defined 839.8
   open 839.9
 ankle (scaphoid bone) (closed) 837.0
  open 837.1
 arm (closed) 839.8
  open 839.9
 astragalus (closed) 837.0
  open 837.1
 atlanto-axial (closed) 839.01
  open 839.11
 atlas (closed) 839.01
  open 839.11
 axis (closed) 839.02
  open 839.12
 back (closed) 839.8
  open 839.9
 Bell-Daly 723.8
 breast bone (closed) 839.61
  open 839.71
 capsule, joint — *see* Dislocation, by site
 carpal (bone) — *see* Dislocation, wrist
 carpometacarpal (joint) (closed) 833.04
  open 833.14
 cartilage (joint) — *see also* Dislocation, by site
  knee — *see* Tear, meniscus
 cervical, cervicodorsal, or cervicothoracic (spine) (vertebra) — *see* Dislocation, vertebra, cervical
 chiropractic (*see also* Lesion, nonallopathic) 739.9
 chondrocostal — *see* Dislocation, costochondral
 chronic — *see* Dislocation, recurrent
 clavicle (closed) 831.04
  open 831.14
 coccyx (closed) 839.41
  open 839.51
 collar bone (closed) 831.04
  open 831.14
 compound (open) NEC 839.9
 congenital NEC 755.8
  hip (*see also* Dislocation, hip, congenital) 754.30
  lens 743.37
  rib 756.3
  sacroiliac 755.69
  spine NEC 756.19
  vertebra 756.19

✓4ᵗʰ Fourth-digit Required   ✓5ᵗʰ Fifth-digit Required

Dislocation — continued
　coracoid (closed) 831.09
　　open 831.19
　costal cartilage (closed) 839.69
　　open 839.79
　costochondral (closed) 839.69
　　open 839.79
　cricoarytenoid articulation (closed) 839.69
　　open 839.79
　cricothyroid (cartilage) articulation (closed) 839.69
　　open 839.79
　dorsal vertebrae (closed) 839.21
　　open 839.31
　ear ossicle 385.23
　elbow (closed) 832.00
　　anterior (closed) 832.01
　　　open 832.11
　　congenital 754.89
　　divergent (closed) 832.09
　　　open 832.19
　　lateral (closed) 832.04
　　　open 832.14
　　medial (closed) 832.03
　　　open 832.13
　　open 832.10
　　posterior (closed) 832.02
　　　open 832.12
　　recurrent 718.32
　　specified type NEC 832.09
　　　open 832.19
　eye 360.81
　　lateral 376.36
　eyeball 360.81
　　lateral 376.36
　femur
　　distal end (closed) 836.50
　　　anterior 836.52
　　　　open 836.62
　　　lateral 836.53
　　　　open 836.63
　　　medial 836.54
　　　　open 836.64
　　　open 836.60
　　　posterior 836.51
　　　　open 836.61
　　proximal end (closed) 835.00
　　　anterior (pubic) 835.03
　　　　open 835.13
　　　obturator 835.02
　　　　open 835.12
　　　open 835.10
　　　posterior 835.01
　　　　open 835.11
　fibula
　　distal end (closed) 837.0
　　　open 837.1
　　proximal end (closed) 836.59
　　　open 836.69
　finger(s) (phalanx) (thumb) (closed) 834.00
　　interphalangeal (joint) 834.02
　　　open 834.12
　　metacarpal (bone), distal end 834.01
　　　open 834.11
　　metacarpophalangeal (joint) 834.01
　　　open 834.11
　　open 834.10
　　recurrent 718.34
　foot (closed) 838.00
　　open 838.10
　　recurrent 718.37

Dislocation — continued
　forearm (closed) 839.8
　　open 839.9
　fracture — see Fracture, by site
　glenoid (closed) 831.09
　　open 831.19
　habitual — see Dislocation, recurrent
　hand (closed) 839.8
　　open 839.9
　hip (closed) 835.00
　　anterior 835.03
　　　obturator 835.02
　　　　open 835.12
　　　open 835.13
　　congenital (unilateral) 754.30
　　　with subluxation of other hip 754.35
　　　bilateral 754.31
　　developmental 718.75
　　open 835.10
　　posterior 835.01
　　　open 835.11
　　recurrent 718.35
　humerus (closed) 831.00
　　distal end (see also Dislocation, elbow) 832.00
　　open 831.10
　　proximal end (closed) 831.00
　　　anterior (subclavicular) (subcoracoid) (subglenoid) (closed) 831.01
　　　　open 831.11
　　　inferior (closed) 831.03
　　　　open 831.13
　　　open 831.10
　　　posterior (closed) 831.02
　　　　open 831.12
　implant — see Complications, mechanical
　incus 385.23
　infracoracoid (closed) 831.01
　　open 831.11
　innominate (pubic juntion) (sacral junction) (closed) 839.69
　　acetabulum (see also Dislocation, hip) 835.00
　　open 839.79
　interphalangeal (joint)
　　finger or hand (closed) 834.02
　　　open 834.12
　　foot or toe (closed) 838.06
　　　open 838.16
　jaw (cartilage) (meniscus) (closed) 830.0
　　open 830.1
　　recurrent 524.69
　joint NEC (closed) 839.8
　　developmental 718.7 ✓5ᵗʰ
　　open 839.9
　　pathological — see Dislocation, pathological
　　recurrent — see Dislocation, recurrent
　knee (closed) 836.50
　　anterior 836.51
　　　open 836.61
　　congenital (with genu recurvatum) 754.41
　　habitual 718.36
　　lateral 836.54
　　　open 836.64
　　medial 836.53
　　　open 836.63
　　old 718.36
　　open 836.60
　　posterior 836.52
　　　open 836.62

Index to Diseases — Dislocation

Dislocation — *continued*
  knee — *continued*
    recurrent 718.36
    rotatory 836.59
      open 836.69
  lacrimal gland 375.16
  leg (closed) 839.8
    open 839.9
  lens (crystalline) (complete) (partial) 379.32
    anterior 379.33
    congenital 743.37
    ocular implant 996.53
    posterior 379.34
    traumatic 921.3
  ligament — *see* Dislocation, by site
  lumbar (vertebrae) (closed) 839.20
    open 839.30
  lumbosacral (vertebrae) (closed) 839.20
    congenital 756.19
    open 839.30
  mandible (closed) 830.0
    open 830.1
  maxilla (inferior) (closed) 830.0
    open 830.1
  meniscus (knee) — *see also* Tear, meniscus
    other sites — *see* Dislocation, by site
  metacarpal (bone)
    distal end (closed) 834.01
      open 834.11
    proximal end (closed) 833.05
      open 833.15
  metacarpophalangeal (joint) (closed) 834.01
    open 834.11
  metatarsal (bone) (closed) 838.04
    open 838.14
  metatarsophalangeal (joint) (closed) 838.05
    open 838.15
  midcarpal (joint) (closed) 833.03
    open 833.13
  midtarsal (joint) (closed) 838.02
    open 838.12
  Monteggia's — *see* Dislocation, hip
  multiple locations (except fingers only or toes only) (closed) 839.8
    open 839.9
  navicular (bone) foot (closed) 837.0
    open 837.1
  neck (*see also* Dislocation, vertebra, cervical) 839.00
  Nélaton's — *see* Dislocation, ankle
  nontraumatic (joint) — *see* Dislocation, pathological
  nose (closed) 839.69
    open 839.79
  not recurrent, not current injury — *see* Dislocation, pathological
  occiput from atlas (closed) 839.01
    open 839.11
  old — *see* Dislocation, recurrent
  open (compound) NEC 839.9
  ossicle, ear 385.23
  paralytic (flaccid) (spastic) — *see* Dislocation, pathological
  patella (closed) 836.3
    congenital 755.64
    open 836.4
  pathological NEC 718.20
    ankle 718.27
    elbow 718.22
    foot 718.27
    hand 718.24

Dislocation — *continued*
  pathological NEC — *continued*
    hip 718.25
    knee 718.26
    lumbosacral joint 724.6
    multiple sites 718.29
    pelvic region 718.25
    sacroiliac 724.6
    shoulder (region) 718.21
    specified site NEC 718.28
    spine 724.8
      sacroiliac 724.6
    wrist 718.23
  pelvis (closed) 839.69
    acetabulum (*see also* Dislocation, hip) 835.00
    open 839.79
  phalanx
    foot or toe (closed) 838.09
      open 838.19
    hand or finger (*see also* Dislocation, finger) 834.00
  postpoliomyelitic — *see* Dislocation, pathological
  prosthesis, internal — *see* Complications, mechanical
  radiocarpal (joint) (closed) 833.02
    open 833.12
  radioulnar (joint)
    distal end (closed) 833.01
      open 833.11
    proximal end (*see also* Dislocation, elbow) 832.00
  radius
    distal end (closed) 833.00
      open 833.10
    proximal end (closed) 832.01
      open 832.11
  recurrent (*see also* Derangement, joint, recurrent) 718.3 ✓5ᵗʰ
    elbow 718.32
    hip 718.35
    joint NEC 718.38
    knee 718.36
    lumbosacral (joint) 724.6
    patella 718.36
    sacroiliac 724.6
    shoulder 718.31
    temporomandibular 524.69
  rib (cartilage) (closed) 839.69
    congenital 756.3
    open 839.79
  sacrococcygeal (closed) 839.42
    open 839.52
  sacroiliac (joint) (ligament) (closed) 839.42
    congenital 755.69
    open 839.52
    recurrent 724.6
  sacrum (closed) 839.42
    open 839.52
  scaphoid (bone)
    ankle or foot (closed) 837.0
      open 837.1
    wrist (closed) (*see also* Dislocation, wrist) 833.00
      open 833.10
  scapula (closed) 831.09
    open 831.19
  semilunar cartilage, knee — *see* Tear, meniscus

Dislocation — *continued*
  septal cartilage (nose) (closed) 839.69
    open 839.79
  septum (nasal) (old) 470
  sesamoid bone — *see* Dislocation, by site
  shoulder (blade) (ligament) (closed) 831.00
    anterior (subclavicular) (subcoracoid)
      (subglenoid) (closed) 831.01
      open 831.11
    chronic 718.31
    inferior 831.03
      open 831.13
    open 831.10
    posterior (closed) 831.02
      open 831.12
    recurrent 718.31
  skull — *see* Injury, intracranial
  Smith's — *see* Dislocation, foot
  spine (articular process) (*see also* Dislocation,
    vertebra) (closed) 839.40
    atlanto-axial (closed) 839.01
      open 839.11
      recurrent 723.8
    cervical, cervicodorsal, cervicothoracic
      (closed) (*see also* Dislocation,
      vertebrae, cervical) 839.00
      open 839.10
      recurrent 723.8
    coccyx 839.41
      open 839.51
    congenital 756.19
    due to birth trauma 767.4
    open 839.50
    recurrent 724.9
    sacroiliac 839.42
      recurrent 724.6
    sacrum (sacrococcygeal) (sacroiliac) 839.42
      open 839.52
  spontaneous — *see* Dislocation, pathological
  sternoclavicular (joint) (closed) 839.61
    open 839.71
  sternum (closed) 839.61
    open 839.71
  subastragalar — *see* Dislocation, foot
  subglenoid (closed) 831.01
    open 831.11
  symphysis
    jaw (closed) 830.0
      open 830.1
    mandibular (closed) 830.0
      open 830.1
    pubis (closed) 839.69
      open 839.79
  tarsal (bone) (joint) 838.01
    open 838.11
  tarsometatarsal (joint) 838.03
    open 838.13
  temporomandibular (joint) (closed) 830.0
    open 830.1
    recurrent 524.69
  thigh
    distal end (*see also* Dislocation, femur,
      distal end) 836.50
    proximal end (*see also* Dislocation, hip)
      835.00
  thoracic (vertebrae) (closed) 839.21
    open 839.31
  thumb(s) (*see also* Dislocation, finger) 834.00
  thyroid cartilage (closed) 839.69
    open 839.79

Dislocation — *continued*
  tibia
    distal end (closed) 837.0
      open 837.1
    proximal end (closed) 836.50
      anterior 836.51
        open 836.61
      lateral 836.54
        open 836.64
      medial 836.53
        open 836.63
      open 836.60
      posterior 836.52
        open 836.62
      rotatory 836.59
        open 836.69
  tibiofibular
    distal (closed) 837.0
      open 837.1
    superior (closed) 836.59
      open 836.69
  toe(s) (closed) 838.09
    open 838.19
  trachea (closed) 839.69
    open 839.79
  ulna
    distal end (closed) 833.09
      open 833.19
    proximal end — *see* Dislocation, elbow
  vertebra (articular process) (body) (closed)
    839.40
    cervical, cervicodorsal or cervicothoracic
      (closed) 839.00
      first (atlas) 839.01
        open 839.11
      second (axis) 839.02
        open 839.12
      third 839.03
        open 839.13
      fourth 839.04
        open 839.14
      fifth 839.05
        open 839.15
      sixth 839.06
        open 839.16
      seventh 839.07
        open 839.17
      congenital 756.19
      multiple sites 839.08
        open 839.18
      open 839.10
    congenital 756.19
    dorsal 839.21
      open 839.31
      recurrent 724.9
    lumbar, lumbosacral 839.20
      open 839.30
    open NEC 839.50
    recurrent 724.9
    specified region NEC 839.49
      open 839.59
    thoracic 839.21
      open 839.31
  wrist (carpal bone) (scaphoid) (semilunar)
    (closed) 833.00
    carpometacarpal (joint) 833.04
      open 833.14
    metacarpal bone, proximal end 833.05
      open 833.15
    midcarpal (joint) 833.03
      open 833.13

Dislocation — *continued*
　wrist — *continued*
　　open 833.10
　　　radiocarpal (joint) 833.02
　　　　open 833.12
　　　radioulnar (joint) 833.01
　　　　open 833.11
　　　recurrent 718.33
　　　specified site NEC 833.09
　　　　open 833.19
　　xiphoid cartilage (closed) 839.61
　　　open 839.71

Dislodgement
　artificial skin graft 996.55
　decellularized allodermis graft 996.55

Disobedience, hostile (covert) (overt) (*see also* Disturbance, conduct) 312.0 ✓5ᵗʰ

Disorder — *see also* Disease
　academic underachievement, childhood and adolescence 313.83
　accommodation 367.51
　　drug-induced 367.89
　　toxic 367.89
　adjustment (*see also* Reaction, adjustment) 309.9
　adrenal (capsule) (cortex) (gland) 255.9
　　specified type NEC 255.8
　adrenogenital 255.2
　affective (*see also* Psychosis, affective) 296.90
　　atypical 296.81
　aggressive, unsocialized (*see also* Disturbance, conduct) 312.0 ✓5ᵗʰ
　alcohol, alcoholic (*see also* Alcohol) 291.9
　allergic — *see* Allergy
　amnestic (*see also* Amnestic syndrome) 294.0
　amino acid (metabolic) (*see also* Disturbance, metabolism, amino acid) 270.9
　　albinism 270.2
　　alkaptonuria 270.2
　　argininosuccinicaciduria 270.6
　　beta-amino-isobutyricaciduria 277.2
　　cystathioninuria 270.4
　　cystinosis 270.0
　　cystinuria 270.0
　　glycinuria 270.0
　　homocystinuria 270.4
　　imidazole 270.5
　　maple syrup (urine) disease 270.3
　　neonatal, transitory 775.8
　　oasthouse urine disease 270.2
　　ochronosis 270.2
　　phenylketonuria 270.1
　　phenylpyruvic oligophrenia 270.1
　　purine NEC 277.2
　　pyrimidine NEC 277.2
　　renal transport NEC 270.0
　　specified type NEC 270.8
　　transport NEC 270.0
　　　renal 270.0
　　xanthinuria 277.2
　anaerobic glycolysis with anemia 282.3
　anxiety (*see also* Anxiety) 300.00
　　due to or associated with physical condition 293.84
　arteriole 447.9
　　specified type NEC 447.8
　artery 447.9
　　specified type NEC 447.8
　articulation — *see* Disorder, joint
　Asperger's 299.8 ✓5ᵗʰ
　attachment of infancy 313.89

Disorder — *continued*
　attention deficit 314.00
　　with hyperactivity 314.01
　　predominantly
　　　combined hyperactive/inattentive 314.01
　　　hyperactive/impulsive 314.01
　　　inattentive 314.00
　　residual type 314.8
　autoimmune NEC 279.4
　　hemolytic (cold type) (warm type) 283.0
　　parathyroid 252.1
　　thyroid 245.2
　autistic 299.0 ✓5ᵗʰ
　avoidant, childhood or adolescence 313.21
　balance
　　acid-base 276.9
　　　mixed (with hypercapnia) 276.4
　　electrolyte 276.9
　　fluid 276.9
　behavior NEC (*see also* Disturbance, conduct) 312.9
　bilirubin excretion 277.4
　bipolar (affective) (alternating) (type I) (*see also* Psychosis, affective) 296.7
　　atypical 296.7
　　currently
　　　depressed 296.5 ✓5ᵗʰ
　　　hypomanic 296.4 ✓5ᵗʰ
　　　manic 296.4 ✓5ᵗʰ
　　mixed 296.6 ✓5ᵗʰ
　　type II (recurrent major depressive episodes with hypomania) 296.89
　bladder 596.9
　　functional NEC 596.59
　　specified NEC 596.8
　bone NEC 733.90
　　specified NEC 733.99
　brachial plexus 353.0
　branched-chain amino-acid degradation 270.3
　breast 611.9
　　puerperal, postpartum 676.3 ✓5ᵗʰ
　　specified NEC 611.8
　Briquet's 300.81
　bursa 727.9
　　shoulder region 726.10
　carbohydrate metabolism, congenital 271.9
　cardiac, functional 427.9
　　postoperative 997.1
　　psychogenic 306.2
　cardiovascular, psychogenic 306.2
　cartilage NEC 733.90
　　articular 718.00
　　　ankle 718.07
　　　elbow 718.02
　　　foot 718.07
　　　hand 718.04
　　　hip 718.05
　　　knee 717.9
　　　multiple sites 718.09
　　　pelvic region 718.05
　　　shoulder region 718.01
　　　specified
　　　　site NEC 718.08
　　　　type NEC 733.99
　　　wrist 718.03
　catatonic — *see* Catatonia
　cervical region NEC 723.9
　cervical root (nerve) NEC 353.2
　character NEC (*see also* Disorder, personality) 301.9

Disorder — continued
  coagulation (factor) (see also Defect,
      coagulation) 286.9
    factor VIII (congenital) (functional) 286.0
    factor IX (congenital) (functional) 286.1
    neonatal, transitory 776.3
  coccyx 724.70
    specified NEC 724.79
  colon 569.9
    functional 564.9
      congenital 751.3
  cognitive 294.9
  conduct (see also Disturbance, conduct) 312.9
    adjustment reaction 309.3
    adolescent onset type 312.82
    childhood onset type 312.81
    compulsive 312.30
      specified type NEC 312.39
    hyperkinetic 314.2
    socialized (type) 312.20
      aggressive 312.23
      unaggressive 312.21
    specified NEC 312.89
  conduction, heart 426.9
    specified NEC 426.89
  convulsive (secondary) (see also Convulsions)
      780.39
    due to injury at birth 767.0
    idiopathic 780.39
  coordination 781.3
  cornea NEC 371.89
    due to contact lens 371.82
  corticosteroid metabolism NEC 255.2
  cranial nerve — see Disorder, nerve, cranial
  cyclothymic 301.13
  degradation, branched-chain amino acid 270.3
  delusional 297.9
  dentition 520.6
  depressive NEC 311
    atypical 296.82
    major (see also Psychosis, affective)
        296.2 ✓5ᵗʰ
      recurrent episode 296.3 ✓5ᵗʰ
      single episode 296.2 ✓5ᵗʰ
  development, specific 315.9
    associated with hyperkinesia 314.1
    language 315.31
    learning 315.2
      arithmetical 315.1
      reading 315.00
    mixed 315.5
    motor coordination 315.4
    specified type NEC 315.8
    speech 315.39
  diaphragm 519.4
  digestive 536.9
    fetus or newborn 777.9
      specified NEC 777.8
    psychogenic 306.4
  disintegrative (childhood) 299.1 ✓5ᵗʰ
  dissociative 300.14
    identity 300.14
  dysmorphic body 300.7
  dysthymic 300.4
  ear 388.9
    degenerative NEC 388.00
    external 380.9
      specified 380.89
    pinna 380.30
    specified type NEC 388.8
    vascular NEC 388.00

Disorder — continued
  eating NEC 307.50
  electrolyte NEC 276.9
    with
      abortion — see Abortion, by type, with
          metabolic disorder
      ectopic pregnancy (see also categories
          633.0-633.9) 639.4
      molar pregnancy (see also categories
          630-632) 639.4
    acidosis 276.2
      metabolic 276.2
      respiratory 276.2
    alkalosis 276.3
      metabolic 276.3
      respiratory 276.3
    following
      abortion 639.4
      ectopic or molar pregnancy 639.4
    neonatal, transitory NEC 775.5
  emancipation as adjustment reaction 309.22
  emotional (see also Disorder, mental,
      nonpsychotic) V40.9
  endocrine 259.9
    specified type NEC 259.8
  esophagus 530.9
    functional 530.5
    psychogenic 306.4
  explosive
    intermittent 312.34
    isolated 312.35
  expressive language 315.31
  eye 379.90
    globe — see Disorder, globe
    ill-defined NEC 379.99
    limited duction NEC 378.63
    specified NEC 379.8
  eyelid 374.9
    degenerative 374.50
    sensory 374.44
    specified type NEC 374.89
    vascular 374.85
  factitious — see Illness, factitious
  factor, coagulation (see also Defect,
      coagulation) 286.9
    VIII (congenital) (functional) 286.0
    IX (congenital) (funcitonal) 286.1
  fascia 728.9
  feeding — see Feeding
  female sexual arousal 302.72
  fluid NEC 276.9
  gastric (functional) 536.9
    motility 536.8
    psychogenic 306.4
    secretion 536.8
  gastrointestinal (functional) NEC 536.9
    newborn (neonatal) 777.9
      specified NEC 777.8
    psychogenic 306.4
  gender (child) 302.6
    adult 302.85
  gender identity (childhood) 302.6
    adult-life 302.85
  genitourinary system, psychogenic 306.50
  globe 360.9
    degenerative 360.20
      specified NEC 360.29
    specified type NEC 360.89
  hearing — see also Deafness
    conductive type (air) (see also Deafness,
        conductive) 389.00

Disorder — continued
  hearing — continued
    mixed conductive and sensorineural 389.2
    nerve 389.12
    perceptive (see also Deafness, perceptive) 389.10
    sensorineural type NEC (see also Deafness, perceptive) 389.10
  heart action 427.9
    postoperative 997.1
  hematological, transient neonatal 776.9
    specified type NEC 776.8
  hematopoietic organs 289.9
  hemorrhagic NEC 287.9
    due to circulating anticoagulants 286.5
    specified type NEC 287.8
  hemostasis (see also Defect, coagulation) 286.9
  homosexual conflict 302.0
  hypomanic (chronic) 301.11
  identity
    childhood and adolescence 313.82
      gender 302.6
    gender 302.6
  immune mechanism (immunity) 279.9
    single complement (C-C) 279.8
    specified type NEC 279.8
  impulse control (see also Disturbance, conduct, compulsive) 312.30
  infant sialic acid storage 271.8
  integument, fetus or newborn 778.9
    specified type NEC 778.8
  interactional psychotic (childhood) (see also Psychosis, childhood) 299.1
  intermittent explosive 312.34
  intervertebral disc 722.90
    cervical, cervicothoracic 722.91
    lumbar, lumbosacral 722.93
    thoracic, thoracolumbar 722.92
  intestinal 569.9
    functional NEC 564.9
      congenital 751.3
      postoperative 564.4
    psychogenic 306.4
  introverted, of childhood and adolescence 313.22
  iron, metabolism 275.0
  isolated explosive 312.35
  joint NEC 719.90
    ankle 719.97
    elbow 719.92
    foot 719.97
    hand 719.94
    hip 719.95
    knee 719.96
    multiple sites 719.99
    pelvic region 719.95
    psychogenic 306.0
    shoulder (region) 719.91
    specified site NEC 719.98
    temporomandibular 524.60
      specified NEC 524.69
    wrist 719.93
  kidney 593.9
    functional 588.9
      specified NEC 588.8
  labyrinth, labyrinthine 386.9
    specified type NEC 386.8
  lactation 676.9

Disorder — continued
  language (developmental) (expressive) 315.31
    mixed (receptive) (receptive-expressive) 315.32
  ligament 728.9
  ligamentous attachments, peripheral — see also Enthesopathy
    spine 720.1
  limb NEC 729.9
    psychogenic 306.0
  lipid
    metabolism, congenital 272.9
    storage 272.7
  lipoprotein deficiency (familial) 272.5
  low back NEC 724.9
    psychogenic 306.0
  lumbosacral
    plexus 353.1
    root (nerve) NEC 353.4
  lymphoproliferative (chronic) NEC (M9970/1) 238.7
  male erectile 302.72
    organic origin 607.84
  major depressive (see also Psychosis, affective) 296.2
    recurrent episode 296.3
    single episode 296.2
  manic (see also Psychosis, affective) 296.0
    atypical 296.81
  meniscus NEC (see also Disorder, cartilage, articular) 718.0
  menopausal 627.9
    specified NEC 627.8
  menstrual 626.9
    psychogenic 306.52
    specified NEC 626.8
  mental (nonpsychotic) 300.9
    affecting management of pregnancy, childbirth, or puerperium 648.4
    drug-induced 292.9
      hallucinogen persisting perception 292.89
      specified type NEC 292.89
    due to or associated with
      alcoholism 291.9
      drug consumption NEC 292.9
        specified type NEC 292.89
      physical condition NEC 293.9
    induced by drug 292.9
      specified type NEC 292.89
    neurotic (see also Neurosis) 300.9
    presenile 310.1
      psychotic NEC 290.10
    previous, affecting management of pregnancy V23.8
    psychoneurotic (see also Neurosis) 300.9
    psychotic (see also Psychosis) 298.9
    senile 290.20
    specific, following organic brain damage 310.9
      cognitive or personality change of other type 310.1
      frontal lobe syndrome 310.0
      postconcussional syndrome 310.2
      specified type NEC 310.8
  metabolism NEC 277.9
    with
      abortion — see Abortion, by type with metabolic disorder
      ectopic pregnancy (see also categories 633.0-633.9) 639.4

Disorder — continued
- metabolism NEC — continued
  - with — continued
    - molar pregnancy (see also categories 630-632) 639.4
  - alkaptonuria 270.2
  - amino acid (see also Disorder, amino acid) 270.9
    - specified type NEC 270.8
  - ammonia 270.6
  - arginine 270.6
  - argininosuccinic acid 270.6
  - basal 794.7
  - bilirubin 277.4
  - calcium 275.40
  - carbohydrate 271.9
    - specified type NEC 271.8
  - cholesterol 272.9
  - citrulline 270.6
  - copper 275.1
  - corticosteroid 255.2
  - cystine storage 270.0
  - cystinuria 270.0
  - fat 272.9
  - following
    - abortion 639.4
    - ectopic or molar pregnancy 639.4
  - fructosemia 271.2
  - fructosuria 271.2
  - fucosidosis 271.8
  - galactose-1-phosphate uridyl transferase 271.1
  - glutamine 270.7
  - glycine 270.7
  - glycogen storage NEC 271.0
    - hepatorenal 271.0
  - hemochromatosis 275.0
  - in labor and delivery 669.0
  - iron 275.0
  - lactose 271.3
  - lipid 272.9
    - specified type NEC 272.8
    - storage 272.7
  - lipoprotein — see also Hyperlipemia
    - deficiency (familial) 272.5
  - lysine 270.7
  - magnesium 275.2
  - mannosidosis 271.8
  - mineral 275.9
    - specified type NEC 275.8
  - mucopolysaccharide 277.5
  - nitrogen 270.9
  - ornithine 270.6
  - oxalosis 271.8
  - pentosuria 271.8
  - phenylketonuria 270.1
  - phosphate 275.3
  - phosphorous 275.3
  - plasma protein 273.9
    - specified type NEC 273.8
  - porphyrin 277.1
  - purine 277.2
  - pyrimidine 277.2
  - serine 270.7
  - sodium 276.9
  - specified type NEC 277.8
  - steroid 255.2
  - threonine 270.7
  - urea cycle 270.6
  - xylose 271.8

Disorder — continued
- micturition NEC 788.69
  - psychogenic 306.53
- misery and unhappiness, of childhood and adolescence 313.1
- mitral valve 424.0
- mood — see Psychosis, affective
- motor tic 307.20
  - chronic 307.22
  - transient, childhood 307.21
- movement NEC 333.90
  - hysterical 300.11
  - specified type NEC 333.99
  - stereotypic 307.3
- mucopolysaccharide 277.5
- muscle 728.9
  - psychogenic 306.0
  - specified type NEC 728.3
- muscular attachments, peripheral — see also Enthesopathy
  - spine 720.1
- musculoskeletal system NEC 729.9
  - psychogenic 306.0
- myeloproliferative (chronic) NEC (M9960/1) 238.7
- myoneural 358.9
  - due to lead 358.2
  - specified type NEC 358.8
  - toxic 358.2
- myotonic 359.2
- neck region NEC 723.9
- nerve 349.9
  - abducens NEC 378.54
  - accessory 352.4
  - acoustic 388.5
  - auditory 388.5
  - auriculotemporal 350.8
  - axillary 353.0
  - cerebral — see Disorder, nerve, cranial
  - cranial 352.9
    - first 352.0
    - second 377.49
    - third
      - partial 378.51
      - total 378.52
    - fourth 378.53
    - fifth 350.9
    - sixth 378.54
    - seventh NEC 351.9
    - eighth 388.5
    - ninth 352.2
    - tenth 352.3
    - eleventh 352.4
    - twelfth 352.5
    - multiple 352.6
  - entrapment — see Neuropathy, entrapment
  - facial 351.9
    - specified NEC 351.8
  - femoral 355.2
  - glossopharyngeal NEC 352.2
  - hypoglossal 352.5
  - iliohypogastric 355.79
  - ilioinguinal 355.79
  - intercostal 353.8
  - lateral
    - cutaneous of thigh 355.1
    - popliteal 355.3
  - lower limb NEC 355.8
  - medial, popliteal 355.4
  - median NEC 354.1
  - obturator 355.79

Index to Diseases

Disorder — *continued*
nerve — *continued*
  oculomotor
    partial 378.51
    total 378.52
  olfactory 352.0
  optic 377.49
    ischemic 377.41
    nutritional 377.33
    toxic 377.34
  peroneal 355.3
  phrenic 354.8
  plantar 355.6
  pneumogastric 352.3
  posterior tibial 355.5
  radial 354.3
  recurrent laryngeal 352.3
  root 353.9
    specified NEC 353.8
  saphenous 355.79
  sciatic NEC 355.0
  specified NEC 355.9
    lower limb 355.79
    upper limb 354.8
  spinal 355.9
  sympathetic NEC 337.9
  trigeminal 350.9
    specified NEC 350.8
  trochlear 378.53
  ulnar 354.2
  upper limb NEC 354.9
  vagus 352.3
nervous system NEC 349.9
  autonomic (peripheral) (*see also*
      Neuropathy, peripheral, autonomic)
      337.9
  cranial 352.9
  parasympathetic (*see also* Neuropathy,
      peripheral, autonomic) 337.9
  specified type NEC 349.89
  sympathetic (*see also* Neuropathy,
      peripheral, autonomic) 337.9
  vegetative (*see also* Neuropathy, peripheral,
      autonomic) 337.9
neurohypophysis NEC 253.6
neurological NEC 781.99
  peripheral NEC 355.9
neuromuscular NEC 358.9
  hereditary NEC 359.1
  specified NEC 358.8
  toxic 358.2
neurotic 300.9
  specified type NEC 300.89
neutrophil, polymorphonuclear (functional)
    288.1
obsessive-compulsive 300.3
oppositional, childhood and adolescence
    313.81
optic
  chiasm 377.54
    associated with
      inflammatory disorders 377.54
      neoplasm NEC 377.52
        pituitary 377.51
      pituitary disorders 377.51
      vascular disorders 377.53
  nerve 377.49
  radiations 377.63
  tracts 377.63
orbit 376.9
  specified NEC 376.89

Disorder — *continued*
overanxious, of childhood and adolescence
    313.0
pancreas, internal secretion (other than
    diabetes mellitus) 251.9
  specified type NEC 251.8
panic 300.01
  with agoraphobia 300.21
papillary muscle NEC 429.81
paranoid 297.9
  induced 297.3
  shared 297.3
parathyroid 252.9
  specified type NEC 252.8
paroxysmal, mixed 780.39
pentose phosphate pathway with anemia
    282.2
personality 301.9
  affective 301.10
  aggressive 301.3
  amoral 301.7
  anancastic, anankastic 301.4
  antisocial 301.7
  asocial 301.7
  asthenic 301.6
  boderline 301.83
  compulsive 301.4
  cyclothymic 301.13
  dependent-passive 301.6
  dyssocial 301.7
  emotional instability 301.59
  epileptoid 301.3
  explosive 301.3
  following organic brain damage 310.1
  histrionic 301.50
  hyperthymic 301.11
  hypomanic (chronic) 301.11
  hypothymic 301.12
  hysterical 301.50
  immature 301.89
  inadequate 301.6
  introverted 301.21
  labile 301.59
  moral deficiency 301.7
  obsessional 301.4
  obsessive (-compulsive) 301.4
  overconscientious 301.4
  paranoid 301.0
  passive (-dependent) 301.6
  passive-aggressive 301.84
  pathological NEC 301.9
  pseudosocial 301.7
  psychopathic 301.9
  schizoid 301.20
    introverted 301.21
    schizotypal 301.22
  schizotypal 301.22
  seductive 301.59
  type A 301.4
  unstable 301.59
pervasive developmental, childhood-onset
    299.8 ✓5ᵗʰ
pigmentation, choroid (congenital) 743.53
pinna 380.30
  specified type NEC 380.39
pituitary, thalamic 253.9
  anterior NEC 253.4
  iatrogenic 253.7
  postablative 253.7
  specified NEC 253.8
pityriasis-like NEC 696.8

Disorder — continued
- platelets (blood) 287.1
- polymorphonuclear neutrophils (functional) 288.1
- porphyrin metabolism 277.1
- postmenopausal 627.9
  - specified type NEC 627.8
- posttraumatic stress 309.81
  - acute 308.3
  - brief 308.3
  - chronic 309.81
- premenstrual dysphoric 625.4
- psoriatic-like NEC 696.8
- psychic, with diseases classified elsewhere 316
- psychogenic NEC (see also condition) 300.9
  - allergic NEC
    - respiratory 306.1
  - anxiety 300.00
    - atypical 300.00
    - generalized 300.02
  - appetite 307.50
  - articulation, joint 306.0
  - asthenic 300.5
  - blood 306.8
  - cardiovascular (system) 306.2
  - compulsive 300.3
  - cutaneous 306.3
  - depressive 300.4
  - digestive (system) 306.4
  - dysmenorrheic 306.52
  - dyspneic 306.1
  - eczematous 306.3
  - endocrine (system) 306.6
  - eye 306.7
  - feeding 307.59
  - functional NEC 306.9
  - gastric 306.4
  - gastrointestinal (system) 306.4
  - genitourinary (system) 306.50
  - heart (function) (rhythm) 306.2
  - hemic 306.8
  - hyperventilatory 306.1
  - hypochondriacal 300.7
  - hysterical 300.10
  - intestinal 306.4
  - joint 306.0
  - learning 315.2
  - limb 306.0
  - lymphatic (system) 306.8
  - menstrual 306.52
  - micturition 306.53
  - monoplegic NEC 306.0
  - motor 307.9
  - muscle 306.0
  - musculoskeletal 306.0
  - neurocirculatory 306.2
  - obsessive 300.3
  - occupational 300.89
  - organ or part of body NEC 306.9
  - organs of special sense 306.7
  - paralytic NEC 306.0
  - phobic 300.20
  - physical NEC 306.9
  - pruritic 306.3
  - rectal 306.4
  - respiratory (system) 306.1
  - rheumatic 306.0
  - sexual (function) 302.70
    - specified type NEC 302.79
  - skin (allergic) (eczematous) (pruritic) 306.3

Disorder — continued
- psychogenic NEC — continued
  - sleep 307.40
    - initiation or maintenance 307.41
      - persistent 307.42
      - transient 307.41
    - specified type NEC 307.49
  - specified part of body NEC 306.8
  - stomach 306.4
- psychomotor NEC 307.9
  - hysterical 300.11
- psychoneurotic (see also Neurosis) 300.9
  - mixed NEC 300.89
- psychophysiologic (see also Disorder, psychosomatic) 306.9
- psychosexual identity (childhood) 302.6
  - adult-life 302.85
- psychosomatic NEC 306.9
  - allergic NEC
    - respiratory 306.1
  - articulation, joint 306.0
  - cardiovascular (system) 306.2
  - cutaneous 306.3
  - digestive (system) 306.4
  - dysmenorrheic 306.52
  - dyspneic 306.1
  - endocrine (system) 306.6
  - eye 306.7
  - gastric 306.4
  - gastrointestinal (system) 306.4
  - genitourinary (system) 306.50
  - heart (functional) (rhythm) 306.2
  - hyperventilatory 306.1
  - intestinal 306.4
  - joint 306.0
  - limb 306.0
  - lymphatic (system) 306.8
  - menstrual 306.52
  - micturition 306.53
  - monoplegic NEC 306.0
  - muscle 306.0
  - musculoskeletal 306.0
  - neurocirculatory 306.2
  - organs of special sense 306.7
  - paralytic NEC 306.0
  - pruritic 306.3
  - rectal 306.4
  - respiratory (system) 306.1
  - rheumatic 306.0
  - sexual (function) 302.70
  - specified type NEC 302.79
  - skin 306.3
  - specified part of body NEC 306.8
  - stomach 306.4
- psychotic — see Psychosis
- purine metabolism NEC 277.2
- pyrimidine metabolism NEC 277.2
- reactive attachment (of infancy or early childhood) 313.89
- reading, developmental 315.00
- reflex 796.1
- renal function, impaired 588.9
  - specified type NEC 588.8
- renal transport NEC 588.8
- respiration, respiratory NEC 519.9
  - due to
    - aspiration of liquids or solids 508.9
    - inhalation of fumes or vapors 506.9
  - psychogenic 306.1
- retina 362.9
  - specified type NEC 362.89

Disorder — continued
    sacroiliac joint NEC 724.6
    sacrum 724.6
    schizo-affective (see also Schizophrenia) 295.7 ✓5ᵗʰ
    schizoid, childhood or adolescence 313.22
    schizophreniform 295.4 ✓5ᵗʰ
    schizotypal personality 301.22
    secretion, thyrocalcitonin 246.0
    seizure 780.39
        recurrent 780.39
            epileptic — see Epilepsy
    sense of smell 781.1
        psychogenic 306.7
    separation anxiety 309.21
    sexual (see also Deviation, sexual) 302.9
        function, psychogenic 302.70
    shyness, of childhood and adolescence 313.21
    single complement (C-C) 279.8
    skin NEC 709.9
        fetus or newborn 778.9
            specified type 778.8
        psychogenic (allergic) (eczematous) (pruritic) 306.3
        specified type NEC 709.8
        vascular 709.1
    sleep 780.50
        with apnea — see Apnea, sleep
        circadian rhythm 307.45
        initiation or maintenance (see also Insomnia) 780.52
            nonorganic origin (transient) 307.41
            persistent 307.42
        nonorganic origin 307.40
            specified type NEC 307.49
        specified NEC 780.59
    social, of childhood and adolescence 313.22
        specified NEC 780.59
    soft tissue 729.9
    somatization 300.81
    somatoform (atypical) (undifferentiated) 300.82
        severe 300.81
    speech NEC 784.5
        nonorganic origin 307.9
    spine NEC 724.9
        ligamentous or muscular attachments, peripheral 720.1
    steroid metabolism NEC 255.2
    stomach (functional) (see also Disorder, gastric) 536.9
        psychogenic 306.4
    storage, iron 275.0
    stress (see also Reaction, stress, acute) 308.9
        posttraumatic
            acute 308.3
            brief 308.3
            chronic 309.81
    substitution 300.11
    suspected — see Observation
    synovium 727.9
    temperature regulation, fetus or newborn 778.4
    temporomandibular joint NEC 524.60
        specified NEC 524.69
    tendon 727.9
        shoulder region 726.10
    thoracic root (nerve) NEC 353.3
    thyrocalcitonin secretion 246.0
    thyroid (gland) NEC 246.9
        specified type NEC 246.8

Disorder — continued
    tic 307.20
        chronic (motor or vocal) 307.22
        motor-verbal 307.23
        organic origin 333.1
        transient of childhood 307.21
    tooth NEC 525.9
        development NEC 520.9
            specified type NEC 520.8
        eruption 520.6
            with abnormal position 524.3
        specified type NEC 525.8
    transport, carbohydrate 271.9
        specified type NEC 271.8
    tubular, phosphate-losing 588.0
    tympanic membrane 384.9
    unaggressive, unsocialized (see also Disturbance, conduct) 312.1 ✓5ᵗʰ
    undersocialized, unsocialized (see also Disturbance, conduct)
        aggressive (type) 312.0 ✓5ᵗʰ
        unaggressive (type) 312.1 ✓5ᵗʰ
    vision, visual NEC 368.9
        binocular NEC 368.30
        cortex 377.73
            associated with
                inflammatory disorders 377.73
                neoplasms 377.71
                vascular disorders 377.72
        pathway NEC 377.63
            associated with
                inflammatory disorders 377.63
                neoplasms 377.61
                vascular disorders 377.62
    wakefulness (see also Hypersomnia) 780.54
        nonorganic origin (transient) 307.43
        persistent 307.44
Disorganized globe 360.29
Displacement, displaced

> Note — For acquired displacement of bones, cartilage, joints, tendons, due to injury, see also Dislocation.
>
> Displacements at ages under one year should be considered congenital, provided there is no indication the condition was acquired after birth.

    acquired traumatic of bone, cartilage, joint, tendon NEC (without fracture) (see also Dislocation) 839.8
        with fracture — see Fracture, by site
    adrenal gland (congenital) 759.1
    appendix, retrocecal (congenital) 751.5
    auricle (congenital) 744.29
    bladder (acquired) 596.8
        congenital 753.8
    brachial plexus (congenital) 742.8
    brain stem, caudal 742.4
    canaliculus lacrimalis 743.65
    cardia, through esophageal hiatus 750.6
    cerebellum, caudal 742.4
    cervix (see also Malposition, uterus) 621.6
    colon (congenital) 751.4
    device, implant, or graft — see Complications, mechanical
    epithelium
        columnar of cervix 622.1
        cuboidal, beyond limits of external os (uterus) 752.49

Displacement, displaced — continued
　esophageal mucosa into cardia of stomach,
　　congenital 750.4
　esophagus (acquired) 530.89
　　congenital 750.4
　eyeball (acquired) (old) 376.36
　　congenital 743.8
　　current injury 871.3
　　lateral 376.36
　fallopian tube (acquired) 620.4
　　congenital 752.19
　　opening (congenital) 752.19
　gallbladder (congenital) 751.69
　gastric mucosa 750.7
　　into
　　　duodenum 750.7
　　　esophagus 750.7
　　　Meckel's diverticulum, congenital 750.7
　globe (acquired) (lateral) (old) 376.36
　　current injury 871.3
　graft
　　artificial skin graft 996.55
　　decellularized allodermis graft 996.55
　heart (congenital) 746.87
　　acquired 429.89
　hymen (congenital) (upward) 752.49
　internal prothesis NEC — see Complications,
　　mechanical
　intervertebral disc (with neuritis, radiculutis,
　　sciatica, or other pain) 722.2
　　with myelopathy 722.70
　　cervical, cervicodorsal, cervicothoracic
　　　722.0
　　　with myelopathy 722.71
　　　due to major trauma — see Dislocation,
　　　　vertebra, cervical
　　due to major trauma — see Dislocation,
　　　vertebra
　intervertebral disc
　　lumbar, lumbosacral 722.10
　　　with myelopathy 722.73
　　　due to major trauma — see Dislocation,
　　　　vertebra, lumbar
　　thoracic, thoracolumbar 722.11
　　　with myelopathy 722.72
　　　due to major trauma — see Dislocation,
　　　　vertebra, thoracic
　intrauterine device 996.32
　kidney (acquired) 593.0
　　congenital 753.3
　lacrimal apparatus or duct (congenital) 743.65
　macula (congenital) 743.55
　Meckel's diverticulum (congenital) 751.0
　nail (congenital) 757.5
　　acquired 703.8
　opening of Wharton's duct in mouth 750.26
　organ or site, congenital NEC — see
　　Malposition, congenital
　ovary (acquired) 620.4
　　congenital 752.0
　　free in peritoneal cavity (congenital) 752.0
　　into hernial sac 620.4
　oviduct (acquired) 620.4
　　congenital 752.19
　parathyroid (gland) 252.8
　parotid gland (congenital) 750.26
　punctum lacrimale (congenital) 743.65
　sacroiliac (congenital) (joint) 755.69
　　current injury — see Dislocation, sacroiliac
　　old 724.6
　spine (congenital) 756.19

Displacement, displaced — continued
　spleen, congenital 759.0
　stomach (congenital) 750.7
　　acquired 537.89
　subglenoid (closed) 831.01
　sublingual duct (congenital) 750.26
　teeth, tooth 524.3
　tongue (congenital) (downward) 750.19
　trachea (congenital) 748.3
　ureter or ureteric opening or orifice
　　(congenital) 753.4
　uterine opening of oviducts or fallopian tubes
　　752.19
　uterus, uterine (see also Malposition, uterus)
　　621.6
　　congenital 752.3
　ventricular septum 746.89
　　with rudimentary ventricle 746.89
　xyphoid bone (process) 738.3
Disproportion 653.9
　affecting fetus or newborn 763.1
　caused by
　　conjoined twins 653.7
　　contraction, pelvis (general) 653.1
　　　inlet 653.2
　　　midpelvic 653.8
　　　midplane 653.8
　　　outlet 653.3
　　fetal
　　　ascites 653.7
　　　hydrocephalus 653.6
　　　hydrops 653.7
　　　meningomyelocele 653.7
　　　sacral teratoma 653.7
　　　tumor 653.7
　　hydrocephalic fetus 653.6
　　pelvis, pelvic, abnormality (bony) NEC
　　　653.0
　　unusually large fetus 653.5
　　causing obstructed labor 660.1
　　cephalopelvic, normally formed fetus
　　　653.4
　　　causing obstructed labor 660.1
　　fetal NEC 653.5
　　　causing obstructed labor 660.1
　　fetopelvic, normally formed fetus 653.4
　　　causing obstructed labor 660.1
　　mixed maternal and fetal origin, normally
　　　formed fetus 653.4
　　pelvis, pelvic (bony) NEC 653.1
　　　causing obstructed labor 660.1
　　specified type NEC 653.8
Disruption
　cesarean wound 674.1
　family V61.0
　gastrointestinal anastomosis 997.4
　ligament(s) — see also Sprain
　　knee
　　　current injury — see Dislocation knee
　　　old 717.89
　　　　capsular 717.85
　　　　collateral (medial) 717.82
　　　　　lateral 717.81
　　　　cruciate (posterior) 717.84
　　　　　anterior 717.83
　　　　specified site NEC 717.85
　marital V61.10
　　involving divorce or estrangement V61.0
　operation wound ▶(external)◀ 998.32 ▲
　　internal 998.31 ●

Disruption — *continued*
  organ transplant, anastomosis site — *see* Complications, transplant, organ, by site
  ossicles, ossicular chain 385.23
    traumatic — *see* Fracture, skull, base
  parenchyma
    liver (hepatic) — *see* Laceration, liver, major
    spleen — *see* Laceration, spleen, parenchyma, massive
  phase-shift, of 24-hour sleep-wake cycle 780.55
    nonorganic origin 307.45
  sleep-wake cycle (24-hour) 780.55
    circadian rhythm 307.45
    nonorganic origin 307.45
  suture line (external) 998.32
    internal 998.31
  wound
    cesarean operation 674.1 ✔5ᵗʰ
    episiotomy 674.2 ✔5ᵗʰ
    operation 998.32
      cesarean 674.1 ✔5ᵗʰ
      internal 998.31
    perineal (obstetric) 674.2 ✔5ᵗʰ
    uterine 674.1 ✔5ᵗʰ
Disruptio uteri — *see also* Rupture, uterus
  complicating delivery — *see* Delivery, complicated, rupture, uterus
Dissatisfaction with
  employment V62.2
  school environment V62.3
Dissecting — *see* condition
Dissection
  aorta 441.00
    abdominal 441.02
    thoracic 441.01
    thoracoabdominal 441.03
  artery, arterial
    carotid 443.21
    coronary 414.12
    iliac 443.22
    renal 443.23
    specified NEC 443.29
    vertebral 443.24
  vascular 459.9
  wound — *see* Wound, open, by site
Disseminated — *see* condition
Dissociated personality NEC 300.15
Dissociation
  auriculoventricular or atrioventricular (any degree) (AV) 426.89
    with heart block 426.0
  interference 426.89
  isorhythmic 426.89
  rhythm
    atrioventricular (AV) 426.89
    interference 426.89
Dissociative
  identity disorder 300.14
  reaction NEC 300.15
Dissolution, vertebra (*see also* Osteoporosis) 733.00
Distention
  abdomen (gaseous) 787.3
  bladder 596.8
  cecum 569.89
  colon 569.89
  gallbladder 575.8
  gaseous (abdomen) 787.3
  intestine 569.89

Distention — *continued*
  kidney 593.89
  liver 573.9
  seminal vesicle 608.89
  stomach 536.8
    acute 536.1
    psychogenic 306.4
  ureter 593.5
  uterus 621.8
Distichia, distichiasis (eyelid) 743.63
Distoma hepaticum infestation 121.3
Distomiasis 121.9
  bile passages 121.3
    due to Clonorchis sinensis 121.1
  hemic 120.9
  hepatic (liver) 121.3
    due to Clonorchis sinensis (clonorchiasis) 121.1
  intestinal 121.4
  liver 121.3
    due to Clonorchis sinensis 121.1
  lung 121.2
  pulmonary 121.2
Distomolar (fourth molar) 520.1
  causing crowding 524.3
Disto-occlusion 524.2
Distortion (congenital)
  adrenal (gland) 759.1
  ankle (joint) 755.69
  anus 751.5
  aorta 747.29
  appendix 751.5
  arm 755.59
  artery (peripheral) NEC (*see also* Distortion, peripheral vascular system) 747.60
    cerebral 747.81
    coronary 746.85
    pulmonary 747.3
    retinal 743.58
    umbilical 747.5
  auditory canal 744.29
    causing impairment of hearing 744.02
  bile duct or passage 751.69
  bladder 753.8
  brain 742.4
  bronchus 748.3
  cecum 751.5
  cervix (uteri) 752.49
  chest (wall) 756.3
  clavicle 755.51
  clitoris 752.49
  coccyx 756.19
  colon 751.5
  common duct 751.69
  cornea 743.41
  cricoid cartilage 748.3
  cystic duct 751.69
  duodenum 751.5
  ear 744.29
    auricle 744.29
      causing impairment of hearing 744.02
    causing impairment of hearing 744.09
    external 744.29
      causing impairment of hearing 744.02
    inner 744.05
    middle, except ossicles 744.03
      ossicles 744.04
    ossicles 744.04
  endocrine (gland) NEC 759.2
  epiglottis 748.3

Distortion — *continued*
Eustachian tube 744.24
eye 743.8
    adnexa 743.69
face bone(s) 756.0
fallopian tube 752.19
femur 755.69
fibula 755.69
finger(s) 755.59
foot 755.67
gallbladder 751.69
genitalia, genital organ(s)
    female 752.8
        external 752.49
        internal NEC 752.8
    male 752.8
        penis 752.69
glottis 748.3
gyri 742.4
hand bone(s) 755.59
heart (auricle) (ventricle) 746.89
    valve (cusp) 746.89
hepatic duct 751.69
humerus 755.59
hymen 752.49
ileum 751.5
intestine (large) (small) 751.5
    with anomalous adhesions, fixation or malrotation 751.4
jaw NEC 524.8
jejunum 751.5
kidney 753.3
knee (joint) 755.64
labium (majus) (minus) 752.49
larynx 748.3
leg 755.69
lens 743.36
liver 751.69
lumbar spine 756.19
    with disproportion (fetopelvic) 653.0 ✓5ᵗʰ
        affecting fetus or newborn 763.1
        causing obstructed labor 660.1 ✓5ᵗʰ
lumbosacral (joint) (region) 756.19
lung (fissures) (lobe) 748.69
nerve 742.8
nose 748.1
organ
    of Corti 744.05
    or site not listed — *see* Anomaly, specified type NEC
ossicles, ear 744.04
ovary 752.0
oviduct 752.19
pancreas 751.7
parathyroid (gland) 759.2
patella 755.64
peripheral vascular system NEC 747.60
    gastrointestinal 747.61
    lower limb 747.64
    renal 747.62
    spinal 747.82
    upper limb 747.63
pituitary (gland) 759.2
radius 755.59
rectum 751.5
rib 756.3
sacroiliac joint 755.69
sacrum 756.19
scapula 755.59
shoulder girdle 755.59

Distortion — *continued*
site not listed — *see* Anomaly, specified type NEC
skull bone(s) 756.0
    with
        anencephalus 740.0
        encephalocele 742.0
        hydrocephalus 742.3
            with spina bifida (*see also* Spina bifida) 741.0 ✓5ᵗʰ
        microcephalus 742.1
spinal cord 742.59
spine 756.19
spleen 759.0
sternum 756.3
thorax (wall) 756.3
thymus (gland) 759.2
thyroid (gland) 759.2
    cartilage 748.3
tibia 755.69
toe(s) 755.66
tongue 750.19
trachea (cartilage) 748.3
ulna 755.59
ureter 753.4
    causing obstruction 753.20
urethra 753.8
    causing obstruction 753.6
uterus 752.3
vagina 752.49
vein (peripheral) NEC (*see also* Distortion, peripheral vascular system) 747.60
    great 747.49
    portal 747.49
    pulmonary 747.49
vena cava (inferior) (superior) 747.49
vertebra 756.19
visual NEC 368.15
    shape or size 368.14
vulva 752.49
wrist (bones) (joint) 755.59

Distress
abdomen 789.0 ✓5ᵗʰ
colon 789.0 ✓5ᵗʰ
emotional V40.9
epigastric 789.0 ✓5ᵗʰ
fetal (syndrome) 768.4
    affecting management of pregnancy or childbirth 656.8 ✓5ᵗʰ ▲
    liveborn infant 768.4
        first noted
            before onset of labor 768.2
            during labor or delivery 768.3
    stillborn infant (death before onset of labor) 768.0
        death during labor 768.1
gastrointestinal (functional) 536.9
    psychogenic 306.4
intestinal (functional) NEC 564.9
    psychogenic 306.4
intrauterine — *see* Distress, fetal
leg 729.5
maternal 669.0 ✓5ᵗʰ
mental V40.9
respiratory 786.09
    acute (adult) 518.82
    adult syndrome (following shock, surgery, or trauma) 518.5
        specified NEC 518.82
    fetus or newborn 770.89 ▲
    syndrome (idiopathic) (newborn) 769

Index to Diseases

Distress — *continued*
  stomach 536.9
    psychogenic 306.4
Distribution vessel, atypical NEC 747.60
  coronary artery 746.85
  spinal 747.82
Districhiasis 704.2
Disturbance — *see also* Disease
  absorption NEC 579.9
    calcium 269.3
    carbohydrate 579.8
    fat 579.8
    protein 579.8
    specified type NEC 579.8
    vitamin (*see also* Deficiency, vitamin) 269.2
  acid-base equilibrium 276.9
  activity and attention, simple, with hyperkinesis 314.01
  amino acid (metabolic) (*see also* Disorder, amino acid) 270.9
    imidazole 270.5
    maple syrup (urine) disease 270.3
    transport 270.0
  assimilation, food 579.9
  attention, simple 314.00
    with hyperactivity 314.01
  auditory, nerve, except deafness 388.5
  behavior (*see also* Disturbance, conduct) 312.9
  blood clotting (hypoproteinemia) (mechanism) (*see also* Defect, coagulation) 286.9
  central nervous system NEC 349.9
  cerebral nerve NEC 352.9
  circulatory 459.9
  conduct 312.9
    adjustment reaction 309.3
    adolescent onset type 312.82
    childhood onset type 312.81

Note — Use the following fifth-digit subclassification with categories 312.0–312.2:

0	unspecified
1	mild
2	moderate
3	severe

    compulsive 312.30
      intermittent explosive disorder 312.34
      isolated explosive disorder 312.35
      kleptomania 312.32
      pathological gambling 312.31
      pyromania 312.33
    hyperkinetic 314.2
    intermittent explosive 312.34
    isolated explosive 312.35
    mixed with emotions 312.4
    socialized (type) 312.20
      aggressive 312.23
      unaggressive 312.21
    specified type NEC 312.89
    undersocialized, unsocialized
      aggressive (type) 312.0 ▪5▪
      unaggressive (type) 312.1 ▪5▪
  coordination 781.3
  cranial nerve NEC 352.9
  deep sensibility — *see* Disturbance, sensation
  digestive 536.9
    psychogenic 306.4
  electrolyte — *see* Imbalance, electrolyte

Disturbance — *continued*
  emotions specific to childhood and adolescence 313.9
    with
      academic underachievement 313.83
      anxiety and fearfulness 313.0
      elective mutism 313.23
      identity disorder 313.82
      jealousy 313.3
      misery and unhappiness 313.1
      oppositional disorder 313.81
      overanxiousness 313.0
      sensitivity 313.21
      shyness 313.21
      social withdrawal 313.22
      withdrawal reaction 313.22
    involving relationship problems 313.3
    mixed 313.89
    specified type NEC 313.89
  endocrine (gland) 259.9
    neonatal, transitory 775.9
      specified NEC 775.8
  equilibrium 780.4
  feeding (elderly) (infant) 783.3
    newborn 779.3
    nonorganic origin NEC 307.59
    psychogenic NEC 307.59
  fructose metabolism 271.2
  gait 781.2
    hysterical 300.11
  gastric (functional) 536.9
    motility 536.8
    psychogenic 306.4
    secretion 536.8
  gastrointestinal (functional) 536.9
    psychogenic 306.4
  habit, child 307.9
  hearing, except deafness 388.40
  heart, functional (conditions classifiable to 426, 427, 428)
    due to presence of (cardiac) prosthesis 429.4
    postoperative (immediate) 997.1
      long-term effect of cardiac surgery 429.4
    psychogenic 306.2
  hormone 259.9
  innervation uterus, sympathetic, parasympathetic 621.8
  keratinization NEC
    gingiva 523.1
    lip 528.5
    oral (mucosa) (soft tissue) 528.7
    tongue 528.7
  labyrinth, labyrinthine (vestibule) 386.9
  learning, specific NEC 315.2
  memory (*see also* Amnesia) 780.99 ▲
    mild, following organic brain damage 310.1
  mental (*see also* Disorder, mental) 300.9
    associated with diseases classified elsewhere 316
  metabolism (acquired) (congenital) (*see also* Disorder, metabolism) 277.9
    with
      abortion — *see* Abortion, by type, with metabolic disorder
      ectopic pregnancy (*see also* categories 633.0-633.9) 639.4
      molar pregnancy (*see also* categories 630-632) 639.4

Disturbance — continued
  metabolism — continued
    amino acid (see also Disorder, amino acid) 270.9
      aromatic NEC 270.2
      branched-chain 270.3
      specified type NEC 270.8
      straight-chain NEC 270.7
      sulfur-bearing 270.4
      transport 270.0
    ammonia 270.6
    arginine 270.6
    argininosuccinic acid 270.6
    carbohydrate NEC 271.9
    cholesterol 272.9
    citrulline 270.6
    cystathionine 270.4
    fat 272.9
    following
      abortion 639.4
      ectopic or molar pregnancy 639.4
    general 277.9
      carbohydrate 271.9
      iron 275.0
      phosphate 275.3
      sodium 276.9
    glutamine 270.7
    glycine 270.7
    histidine 270.5
    homocystine 270.4
    in labor or delivery 669.0 ◢5ᵗʰ
    iron 275.0
    isoleucine 270.3
    leucine 270.3
    lipoid 272.9
      specified type NEC 272.8
    lysine 270.7
    methionine 270.4
    neonatal, transitory 775.9
      specified type NEC 775.8
    nitrogen 788.9
    ornithine 270.6
    phosphate 275.3
    phosphatides 272.7
    serine 270.7
    sodium NEC 276.9
    threonine 270.7
    tryptophan 270.2
    tyrosine 270.2
    urea cycle 270.6
    valine 270.3
  motor 796.1
  nervous functional 799.2
  neuromuscular mechanism (eye) due to syphilis 094.84
  nutritional 269.9
    nail 703.8
  ocular motion 378.87
    psychogenic 306.7
  oculogyric 378.87
    psychogenic 306.7
  oculomotor NEC 378.87
    psychogenic 306.7
  olfactory nerve 781.1
  optic nerve NEC 377.49
  oral epithelium, including tongue 528.7
  personality (pattern) (trait) (see also Disorder, personality) 301.9
    following organic brain damage 310.1
  polyglandular 258.9
  psychomotor 307.9

Disturbance — continued
  pupillary 379.49
  reflex 796.1
  rhythm, heart 427.9
    postoperative (immediate) 997.1
      long-term effect of cardiac surgery 429.4
    psychogenic 306.2
  salivary secretion 527.7
  sensation (cold) (heat) (localization) (tactile discrimination localization) (texture) (vibratory) NEC 782.0
    hysterical 300.11
    skin 782.0
    smell 781.1
    taste 781.1
  sensory (see also Disturbance, sensation) 782.0
    innervation 782.0
  situational (transient) (see also Reaction, adjustment) 309.9
    acute 308.3
  sleep 780.50
    with apnea — see Apnea, sleep
    initiation or maintenance (see also Insomnia) 780.52
      nonorganic origin 307.41
    nonorganic origin 307.40
      specified type NEC 307.49
    specified NEC 780.59
      nonorganic origin 307.49
    wakefulness (see also Hypersomnia) 780.54
      nonorganic origin 307.43
  sociopathic 301.7
  speech NEC 784.5
    developmental 315.39
      associated with hyperkinesis 314.1
    secondary to organic lesion 784.5
  stomach (functional) (see also Disturbance, gastric) 536.9
  sympathetic (nerve) (see also Neuropathy, peripheral, autonomic) 337.9
  temperature sense 782.0
    hysterical 300.11
  tooth
    eruption 520.6
    formation 520.4
    structure, hereditary NEC 520.5
  touch (see also Disturbance, sensation) 782.0
  vascular 459.9
    arteriosclerotic — see Arteriosclerosis
  vasomotor 443.9
  vasospastic 443.9
  vestibular labyrinth 386.9
  vision, visual NEC 368.9
    psychophysical 368.16
    specified NEC 368.8
    subjective 368.10
  voice 784.40
  wakefulness (initiation or maintenance) (see also Hypersomnia) 780.54
    nonorganic origin 307.43

Disulfiduria, beta-mercaptolactate-cysteine 270.0

Disuse atrophy, bone 733.7

Ditthomska syndrome 307.81

Diuresis 788.42

Divers'
  palsy or paralysis 993.3
  squeeze 993.3

Index to Diseases

Diverticulitis

Diverticula, diverticulosis, diverticulum
(acute) (multiple) (perforated) (ruptured) 562.10
with diverticulitis 562.11
aorta (Kommerell's) 747.21
appendix (noninflammatory) 543.9
bladder (acquired) (sphincter) 596.3
  congenital 753.8
broad ligament 620.8
bronchus (congenital) 748.3
  acquired 494.0
    with acute exacerbation 494.1
calyx, calyceal (kidney) 593.89
cardia (stomach) 537.1
cecum 562.10
  with
    diverticulitis 562.11
      with hemorrhage 562.13
    hemorrhage 562.12
  congenital 751.5
colon (acquired) 562.10
  with
    diverticulitis 562.11
      with hemorrhage 562.13
    hemorrhage 562.12
  congenital 751.5
duodenum 562.00
  with
    diverticulitis 562.01
      with hemorrhage 562.03
    hemorrhage 562.02
  congenital 751.5
epiphrenic (esophagus) 530.6
esophagus (congenital) 750.4
  acquired 530.6
  epiphrenic 530.6
  pulsion 530.6
  traction 530.6
  Zenker's 530.6
Eustachian tube 381.89
fallopian tube 620.8
gallbladder (congenital) 751.69
gastric 537.1
heart (congenital) 746.89
ileum 562.00
  with
    diverticulitis 562.01
      with hemorrhage 562.03
    hemorrhage 562.02
intestine (large) 562.10
  with
    diverticulitis 562.11
      with hemorrhage 562.13
    hemorrhage 562.12
  congenital 751.5
  small 562.00
    with
      diverticulitis 562.01
        with hemorrhage 562.03
      hemorrhage 562.02
    congenital 751.5
jejunum 562.00
  with
    diverticulitis 562.01
      with hemorrhage 562.03
    hemorrhage 562.02
kidney (calyx) (pelvis) 593.89
  with calculus 592.0
Kommerell's 747.21
laryngeal ventricle (congenital) 748.3
Meckel's (displaced) (hypertrophic) 751.0

Diverticula, diverticulosis, diverticulum — *continued*
midthoracic 530.6
organ or site, congenital NEC — *see* Distortion
pericardium (congenital) (cyst) 746.89
  acquired (true) 423.8
pharyngoesophageal (pulsion) 530.6
pharynx (congenital) 750.27
pulsion (esophagus) 530.6
rectosigmoid 562.10
  with
    diverticulitis 562.11
      with hemorrhage 562.13
    hemorrhage 562.12
  congenital 751.5
rectum 562.10
  with
    diverticulitis 562.11
      with hemorrhage 562.13
    hemorrhage 562.12
renal (calyces) (pelvis) 593.89
  with calculus 592.0
Rokitansky's 530.6
seminal vesicle 608.0
sigmoid 562.10
  with
    diverticulitis 562.11
      with hemorrhage 562.13
    hemorrhage 562.12
  congenital 751.5
small intestine 562.00
  with
    diverticulitis 562.01
      with hemorrhage 562.03
    hemorrhage 562.02
stomach (cardia) (juxtacardia) (juxtapyloric) (acquired) 537.1
  congenital 750.7
subdiaphragmatic 530.6
trachea (congenital) 748.3
  acquired 519.1
traction (esophagus) 530.6
ureter (acquired) 593.89
  congenital 753.4
ureterovesical orifice 593.89
urethra (acquired) 599.2
  congenital 753.8
ventricle, left (congenital) 746.89
vesical (urinary) 596.3
  congenital 753.8
Zenker's (esophagus) 530.6
Diverticulitis (acute) (*see also* Diverticula) 562.11
with hemorrhage 562.13
bladder (urinary) 596.3
cecum (perforated) 562.11
  with hemorrhage 562.13
colon (perforated) 562.11
  with hemorrhage 562.13
duodenum 562.01
  with hemorrhage 562.03
esophagus 530.6
ileum (perforated) 562.01
  with hemorrhage 562.03
intestine (large) (perforated) 562.11
  with hemorrhage 562.13
  small 562.01
    with hemorrhage 562.03
jejunum (perforated) 562.01
  with hemorrhage 562.03
Meckel's (perforated) 751.0

Diverticulitis — continued
  pharyngoesophageal 530.6
  rectosigmoid (perforated) 562.11
    with hemorrhage 562.13
  rectum 562.11
    with hemorrhage 562.13
  sigmoid (old) (perforated) 562.11
    with hemorrhage 562.13
  small intestine (perforated) 562.01
    with hemorrhage 562.03
  vesical (urinary) 596.3
Diverticulosis — see Diverticula
Division
  cervix uteri 622.8
    external os into two openings by frenum 752.49
  external (cervical) into two openings by frenum 752.49
  glans penis 752.69
  hymen 752.49
  labia minora (congenital) 752.49
  ligament (partial or complete) (current) — see also Sprain, by site
    with open wound — see Wound, open, by site
  muscle (partial or complete) (current) — see also Sprain, by site
    with open wound — see Wound, open, by site
  nerve — see Injury, nerve, by site
  penis glans 752.69
  spinal cord — see Injury, spinal, by site
  vein 459.9
    traumatic — see Injury, vascular, by site
Divorce V61.0
Dix-Hallpike neurolabyrinthitis 386.12
Dizziness 780.4
  hysterical 300.11
  psychogenic 306.9
Doan-Wiseman syndrome (primary splenic neutropenia) 288.0
Dog bite — see Wound, open, by site
Döhle-Heller aortitis 093.1
Döhle body-panmyelopathic syndrome 288.2
Dolichocephaly, dolichocephalus 754.0
Dolichocolon 751.5
Dolichostenomelia 759.82
Donohue's syndrome (leprechaunism) 259.8
Donor
  blood V59.01
    other blood components V59.09
    stem cells V59.02
    whole blood V59.01
  bone V59.2
    marrow V59.3
  cornea V59.5
  heart V59.8
  kidney V59.4
  liver V59.6
  lung V59.8
  lymphocyte V59.8
  organ V59.9
    specified NEC V59.8
  potential, examination of V70.8
  skin V59.1
  specified organ or tissue NEC V59.8
  stem cells V59.02

Donor — continued
  tissue V59.9
    specified type NEC V59.8
Donovanosis (granuloma venereum) 099.2
DOPS (diffuse obstructive pulmonary syndrome) 496
Double
  albumin 273.8
  aortic arch 747.21
  auditory canal 744.29
  auricle (heart) 746.82
  bladder 753.8
  external (cervical) os 752.49
  kidney with double pelvis (renal) 753.3
  larynx 748.3
  meatus urinarius 753.8
  organ or site NEC — see Accessory
  orifice
    heart valve NEC 746.89
      pulmonary 746.09
  outlet, right ventricle 745.11
  pelvis (renal) with double ureter 753.4
  penis 752.69
  tongue 750.13
  ureter (one or both sides) 753.4
    with double pelvis (renal) 753.4
  urethra 753.8
  urinary meatus 753.8
  uterus (any degree) 752.2
    with doubling of cervix and vagina 752.2
    in pregnancy or childbirth 654.0
      affecting fetus or newborn 763.89
  vagina 752.49
    with doubling of cervix and uterus 752.2
  vision 368.2
  vocal cords 748.3
  vulva 752.49
  whammy (syndrome) 360.81
Douglas' pouch, cul-de-sac — see condition
Down's disease or syndrome (mongolism) 758.0
Down-growth, epithelial (anterior chamber) 364.61
Dracontiasis 125.7
Dracunculiasis 125.7
Drancunculosis 125.7
Drainage
  abscess (spontaneous) — see Abscess
  anomalous pulmonary veins to hepatic veins or right atrium 747.41
  stump (amputation) (surgical) 997.62
  suprapubic, bladder 596.8
Dream state, hysterical 300.13
Drepanocytic anemia (see also Disease, sickle cell) 282.60
Dresbach's syndrome (elliptocytosis) 282.1
Dreschlera (infection) 118
  hawaiiensis 117.8
Dressler's syndrome (postmyocardial infarction) 411.0
Dribbling (post-void) 788.35
Drift, ulnar 736.09
Drinking (alcohol) — see also Alcoholism
  excessive, to excess NEC (see also Abuse, drugs, nondependent) 305.0
    bouts, periodic 305.0
    continual 303.9
    episodic 305.0
    habitual 303.9

Drinking — continued
excessive, to excess NEC — continued
periodic 305.0
Drip, postnasal (chronic) — see Sinusitis
Drivers' license examination V70.3
Droop
Cooper's 611.8
facial 781.99
Drop
finger 736.29
foot 736.79
hematocrit (precipitous) 790.01
toe 735.8
wrist 736.05
Dropped
dead 798.1
heart beats 426.6
Dropsy, dropsical (see also Edema) 782.3
abdomen 789.5
amnion (see also Hydramnios) 657
brain — see Hydrocephalus
cardiac (see also Failure, heart) 428.0
cardiorenal (see also Hypertension,
cardiorenal) 404.90
chest 511.9
fetus or newborn 778.0
due to isoimmunization 773.3
gangrenous (see also Gangrene) 785.4
heart (see also Failure, heart) 428.0
hepatic — see Cirrhosis, liver
infantile — see Hydrops, fetalis
kidney (see also Nephrosis) 581.9
liver — see Cirrhosis, liver
lung 514
malarial (see also Malaria) 084.9
neonatorum — see Hydrops, fetalis
nephritic 581.9
newborn — see Hydrops, fetalis
nutritional 269.9
ovary 620.8
pericardium (see also Pericarditis) 423.9
renal (see also Nephrosis) 581.9
uremic — see Uremia
Drowned, drowning 994.1
lung 518.5
Drowsiness 780.09
Drug — see also condition
addiction (see also listing under Dependence) 304.9
adverse effect NEC, correct substance properly administered 995.2
dependence (see also listing under Dependence) 304.9
habit (see also listing under Dependence) 304.9
overdose — see Table of Drugs and Chemicals
poisoning — see Table of Drugs and Chemicals
therapy (maintenance) status NEC V58.1
anticoagulant V58.61
long-term (current) use V58.69
antibiotics V58.62
wrong substance given or taken in error — see Table of Drugs and Chemicals
Drunkenness (see also Abuse, drugs, nondependent) 305.0
acute in alcoholism (see also Alcoholism) 303.0
chronic (see also Alcoholism) 303.9
pathologic 291.4

Drunkenness — continued
simple (acute) 305.0
in alcoholism 303.0
sleep 307.47
Drusen
optic disc or papilla 377.21
retina (colloid) (hyaloid degeneration) 362.57
hereditary 362.77
Drusenfieber 075
Dry, dryness — see also condition
eye 375.15
syndrome 375.15
larynx 478.79
mouth 527.7
nose 478.1
skin syndrome 701.1
socket (teeth) 526.5
throat 478.29
DSAP (disseminated superficial actinic porokeratosis) 692.75
Duane's retraction syndrome 378.71
Duane-Stilling-Türk syndrome (ocular retraction syndrome) 378.71
Dubin-Johnson disease or syndrome 277.4
Dubini's disease (electric chorea) 049.8
Dubois' abscess or disease 090.5
Duchenne's
disease 094.0
locomotor ataxia 094.0
muscular dystrophy 359.1
pseudohypertrophy, muscles 359.1
paralysis 335.22
syndrome 335.22
Duchenne-Aran myelopathic, muscular atrophy (nonprogressive) (progressive) 335.21
Duchenne-Griesinger disease 359.1
Ducrey's
bacillus 099.0
chancre 099.0
disease (chancroid) 099.0
Duct, ductus — see condition
Duengero 061
Duhring's disease (dermatitis herpetiformis) 694.0
Dukes (-Filatov) disease 057.8
Dullness
cardiac (decreased) (increased) 785.3
Dumb ague (see also Malaria) 084.6
Dumbness (see also Aphasia) 784.3
Dumdum fever 085.0
Dumping syndrome (postgastrectomy) 564.2
nonsurgical 536.8
Duodenitis (nonspecific) (peptic) 535.60
with hemorrhage 535.61
due to
Strongyloides stercoralis 127.2
Duodenocholangitis 575.8
Duodenum, duodenal — see condition
Duplay's disease, periarthritis, or syndrome 726.0
Duplex — see also Accessory
kidney 753.3
placenta — see Placenta, abnormal
uterus 752.2

Duplication — *see also* Accessory
- anus 751.5
- aortic arch 747.21
- appendix 751.5
- biliary duct (any) 751.69
- bladder 753.8
- cecum 751.5
  - and appendix 751.5
- clitoris 752.49
- cystic duct 751.69
- digestive organs 751.8
- duodenum 751.5
- esophagus 750.4
- fallopian tube 752.19
- frontonasal process 756.0
- gallbladder 751.69
- ileum 751.5
- intestine (large) (small) 751.5
- jejunum 751.5
- kidney 753.3
- liver 751.69
- nose 748.1
- pancreas 751.7
- penis 752.69
- respiratory organs NEC 748.9
- salivary duct 750.22
- spinal cord (incomplete) 742.51
- stomach 750.7
- ureter 753.4
- vagina 752.49
- vas deferens 752.8
- vocal cords 748.3

Dupré's disease or syndrome (meningism) 781.6

Dupuytren's
- contraction 728.6
- disease (muscle contracture) 728.6
- fracture (closed) 824.4
  - ankle (closed) 824.4
    - open 824.5
  - fibula (closed) 824.4
    - open 824.5
  - radius (closed) 813.42
    - open 813.52
- muscle contracture 728.6

Durand-Nicolas-Favre disease (climatic bubo) 099.1

Duroziez's disease (congenital mitral stenosis) 746.5

Dust
- conjunctivitis 372.05
- reticulation (occupational) 504

Dutton's
- disease (trypanosomiasis) 086.9
- relapsing fever (West African) 087.1

Dwarf, dwarfism 259.4
- with infantilism (hypophyseal) 253.3
- achondroplastic 756.4
- Amsterdam 759.89
- bird-headed 759.89
- congenital 259.4
- constitutional 259.4
- hypophyseal 253.3
- infantile 259.4
- Levi type 253.3
- Lorain-Levi (pituitary) 253.3
- Lorain type (pituitary) 253.3
- metatropic 756.4
- nephrotic-glycosuric, with hypophosphatemic rickets 270.0

Dwarf, dwarfism — *continued*
- nutritional 263.2
- ovarian 758.6
- pancreatic 577.8
- pituitary 253.3
- polydystrophic 277.5
- primordial 253.3
- psychosocial 259.4
- renal 588.0
  - with hypertension — *see* Hypertension, kidney
- Russell's (uterine dwarfism and craniofacial dysostosis) 759.89

Dyke-Young anemia or syndrome (acquired macrocytic hemolytic anemia) (secondary) (symptomatic) 283.9

Dynia abnormality (*see also* Defect, coagulation) 286.9

Dysacousis 388.40

Dysadrenocortism 255.9
- hyperfunction 255.3
- hypofunction 255.4

Dysarthria 784.5

Dysautonomia (*see also* Neuropathy, peripheral, autonomic) 337.9
- familial 742.8

Dysbarism 993.3

Dysbasia 719.7
- angiosclerotica intermittens 443.9
  - due to atherosclerosis 440.21
- hysterical 300.11
- lordotica (progressiva) 333.6
- nonorganic origin 307.9
- psychogenic 307.9

Dysbetalipoproteinemia (familial) 272.2

Dyscalculia 315.1

Dyschezia (*see also* Constipation) 564.00

Dyschondroplasia (with hemangiomata) 756.4
- Voorhoeve's 756.4

Dyschondrosteosis 756.59

Dyschromia 709.00

Dyscollagenosis 710.9

Dyscoria 743.41

Dyscraniopyophalangy 759.89

Dyscrasia
- blood 289.9
  - with antepartum hemorrhage 641.3
  - fetus or newborn NEC 776.9
  - hemorrhage, subungual 287.8
  - puerperal, postpartum 666.3
- ovary 256.8
- plasma cell 273.9
- pluriglandular 258.9
- polyglandular 258.9

Dysdiadochokinesia 781.3

Dysectasia, vesical neck 596.8

Dysendocrinism 259.9

Dysentery, dysenteric (bilious) (catarrhal) (diarrhea) (epidemic) (gangrenous) (hemorrhagic) (infectious) (sporadic) (tropical) (ulcerative) 009.0
- abscess, liver (*see also* Abscess, amebic) 006.3
- amebic (*see also* Amebiasis) 006.9
  - with abscess — *see* Abscess, amebic
  - acute 006.0
  - carrier (suspected) of V02.2
  - chronic 006.1

Dysentery, dysenteric — *continued*
  arthritis (*see also* Arthritis, due to, dysentery) 009.0 *[711.3]*
    bacillary 004.9 *[711.3]*
  asylum 004.9
  bacillary 004.9
    arthritis 004.9 *[711.3]*
    Boyd 004.2
    Flexner 004.1
    Schmitz (-Stutzer) 004.0
    Shiga 004.0
    Shigella 004.9
      group A 004.0
      group B 004.1
      group C 004.2
      group D 004.3
      specified type NEC 004.8
    Sonne 004.3
    specified type NEC 004.8
  bacterium 004.9
  balantidial 007.0
  Balantidium coli 007.0
  Boyd's 004.2
  Chilomastix 007.8
  Chinese 004.9
  choleriform 001.1
  coccidial 007.2
  Dientamoeba fragilis 007.8
  due to specified organism NEC — *see* Enteritis, due to, by organism
  Embadomonas 007.8
  Endolimax nana — *see* Dysentery, amebic
  Entamoba, entamebic — *see* Dysentery, amebic
  Flexner's 004.1
  Flexner-Boyd 004.2
  giardial 007.1
  Giardia lamblia 007.1
  Hiss-Russell 004.1
  lamblia 007.1
  leishmanial 085.0
  malarial (*see also* Malaria) 084.6
  metazoal 127.9
  Monilia 112.89
  protozoal NEC 007.9
  Russell's 004.8
  salmonella 003.0
  schistosomal 120.1
  Schmitz (-Stutzer) 004.0
  Shiga 004.0
  Shigella NEC (*see also* Dysentery, bacillary) 004.9
    boydii 004.2
    dysenteriae 004.0
      Schmitz 004.0
      Shiga 004.0
    flexneri 004.1
    Group A 004.0
    Group B 004.1
    Group C 004.2
    Group D 004.3
    Schmitz 004.0
    Shiga 004.0
    Sonnei 004.3
  Sonne 004.3
  strongyloidiasis 127.2
  trichomonal 007.3
  tuberculous (*see also* Tuberculosis) 014.8
  viral (*see also* Enteritis, viral) 008.8
Dysequilibrium 780.4

Dysesthesia 782.0
  hysterical 300.11
Dysfibrinogenemia (congenital) (*see also* Defect, coagulation) 286.3
Dysfunction
  adrenal (cortical) 255.9
    hyperfunction 255.3
    hypofunction 255.4
  associated with sleep stages or arousal from sleep 780.56
    nonorganic origin 307.47
  bladder NEC 596.59
  bleeding, uterus 626.8
  brain, minimal (*see also* Hyperkinesia) 314.9
  cerebral 348.3
  colon 564.9
    psychogenic 306.4
  colostomy or enterostomy 569.62
  cystic duct 575.8
  diastolic 429.9
    with heart failure — *see* Failure, heart
    due to
      cardiomyopathy — *see* Cardiomyopathy
      hypertension — *see* Hypertension, heart
  endocrine NEC 259.9
  endometrium 621.8
  enteric stoma 569.62
  enterostomy 569.62
  Eustachian tube 381.81
  gallbladder 575.8
  gastrointestinal 536.9
  gland, glandular NEC 259.9
  heart 427.9
    postoperative (immediate) 997.1
      long-term effect of cardiac surgery 429.4
  hemoglobin 288.8
  hepatic 573.9
  hepatocellular NEC 573.9
  hypophysis 253.9
    hyperfunction 253.1
    hypofunction 253.2
    posterior lobe 253.6
      hypofunction 253.5
  kidney (*see also* Disease, renal) 593.9
  labyrinthine 386.50
    specified NEC 386.58
  liver 573.9
    constitutional 277.4
  minimal brain (child) (*see also* Hyperkinesia) 314.9
  ovary, ovarian 256.9
    hyperfunction 256.1
      estrogen 256.0
    hypofunction 256.39
      postablative 256.2
    postablative 256.2
    specified NEC 256.8
  papillary muscle 429.81
    with myocardial infarction 410.8
  parathyroid 252.8
    hyperfunction 252.0
    hypofunction 252.1
  pineal gland 259.8
  pituitary (gland) 253.9
    hyperfunction 253.1
    hypofunction 253.2
    posterior 253.6
      hypofunction 253.5
  placental — *see* Placenta, insufficiency
  platelets (blood) 287.1

Dysfunction — continued
  polyglandular 258.9
    specified NEC 258.8
  psychosexual 302.70
    with
      dyspareunia (functional) (psychogenic) 302.76
      frigidity 302.72
      impotence 302.72
      inhibition
        orgasm
          female 302.73
          male 302.74
        sexual
          desire 302.71
          excitement 302.72
      premature ejaculation 302.75
      sexual aversion 302.79
      specified disorder NEC 302.79
      vaginismus 306.51
  pylorus 537.9
  rectum 564.9
    psychogenic 306.4
  segmental (see also Dysfunction, somatic) 739.9
  senile 797
  sinoatrial node 427.81
  somatic 739.9
    abdomen 739.9
    acromioclavicular 739.7
    cervical 739.1
    cervicothoracic 739.1
    costochondral 739.8
    costovertebral 739.8
    extremities
      lower 739.6
      upper 739.7
    head 739.0
    hip 739.5
    lumbar, lumbosacral 739.3
    occipitocervical 739.0
    pelvic 739.5
    pubic 739.5
    rib cage 739.8
    sacral 739.4
    sacrococcygeal 739.4
    sacroiliac 739.4
    specified site NEC 739.9
    sternochondral 739.8
    sternoclavicular 739.7
    temporomandibular 739.0
    thoracic, thoracolumbar 739.2
  stomach 536.9
    psychogenic 306.4
  suprarenal 255.9
    hyperfunction 255.3
    hypofunction 255.4
  symbolic NEC 784.60
    specified type NEC 784.69
  temporomandibular (joint) (joint-pain-syndrome) NEC 524.60
    specified NEC 524.69
  testicular 257.9
    hyperfunction 257.0
    hypofunction 257.2
    specified type NEC 257.8
  thymus 254.9
  thyroid 246.9
    complicating pregnancy, childbirth or puerperium 648.1
    hyperfunction — see Hyperthyroidism

Dysfunction — continued
  thyroid — continued
    hypofunction — see Hypothyroidism
  uterus, complicating delivery 661.9
    affecting fetus or newborn 763.7
    hypertonic 661.4
    hypotonic 661.2
      primary 661.0
      secondary 661.1
  velopharyngeal (acquired) 528.9
    congenital 750.29
  ventricular 429.9
    with congestive heart failure (see also Failure, heart) 428.0
    due to
      cardiomyopathy — see Cardiomyopathy
      hypertension — see Hypertension, heart
  vesicourethral NEC 596.59
  vestibular 386.50
    specified type NEC 386.58
Dysgammaglobulinemia 279.06
Dysgenesis
  gonadal (due to chromosomal anomaly) 758.6
    pure 752.7
  kidney(s) 753.0
  ovarian 758.6
  renal 753.0
  reticular 279.2
  seminiferous tubules 758.6
  tidal platelet 287.3
Dysgerminoma (M9060/3)
  specified site — see Neoplasm, by site, malignant
  unspecified site
    female 183.0
    male 186.9
Dysgeusia 781.1
Dysgraphia 781.3
Dyshidrosis 705.81
Dysidrosis 705.81
Dysinsulinism 251.8
Dyskaryotic cervical smear 795.09 ▲
Dyskeratosis (see also Keratosis) 701.1
  bullosa hereditaria 757.39
  cervix 622.1
  congenital 757.39
  follicularis 757.39
    vitamin A deficiency 264.8
  gingiva 523.8
  oral soft tissue NEC 528.7
  tongue 528.7
  uterus NEC 621.8
Dyskinesia 781.3
  biliary 575.8
  esophagus 530.5
  hysterical 300.11
  intestinal 564.89
  nonorganic origin 307.9
  orofacial 333.82
  psychogenic 307.9
  tardive (oral) 333.82
Dyslalia 784.5
  developmental 315.39
Dyslexia 784.61
  developmental 315.02
  secondary to organic lesion 784.61
Dysmaturity (see also Immaturity) 765.1
  lung 770.4
  pulmonary 770.4

Index to Diseases

Dysmenorrhea (essential) (exfoliative) (functional) (intrinsic) (membranous) (primary) (secondary) 625.3
   psychogenic 306.52
Dysmetabolic syndrome X 277.7
Dysmetria 781.3
Dysmorodystrophia mesodermalis congenita 759.82
Dysnomia 784.3
Dysorexia 783.0
   hysterical 300.11
Dysostosis
   cleidocranial, cleidocranialis 755.59
   craniofacial 756.0
   Fairbank's (idiopathic familial generalized osteophytosis) 756.50
   mandibularis 756.0
   mandibulofacial, incomplete 756.0
   multiplex 277.5
   orodigitofacial 759.89
Dyspareunia (female) 625.0
   male 608.89
   psychogenic 302.76
Dyspepsia (allergic) (congenital) (fermentative) (flatulent) (functional) (gastric) (gastrointestinal) (neurogenic) (occupational) (reflex) 536.8
   acid 536.8
   atonic 536.3
      psychogenic 306.4
   diarrhea 787.91
      psychogenic 306.4
   intestinal 564.89
      psychogenic 306.4
   nervous 306.4
   neurotic 306.4
   psychogenic 306.4
Dysphagia 787.2
   functional 300.11
   hysterical 300.11
   nervous 300.11
   psychogenic 306.4
   sideropenic 280.8
   spastica 530.5
Dysphagocytosis, congenital 288.1
Dysphasia 784.5
Dysphonia 784.49
   clericorum 784.49
   functional 300.11
   hysterical 300.11
   psychogenic 306.1
   spastica 478.79
Dyspigmentation — see also Pigmentation
   eyelid (acquired) 374.52
Dyspituitarism 253.9
   hyperfunction 253.1
   hypofunction 253.2
   posterior lobe 253.6
Dysplasia — see also Anomaly
   artery
      fibromuscular NEC 447.8
         carotid 447.8
         renal 447.3
   bladder 596.8
   bone (fibrous) NEC 733.29
      diaphyseal, progressive 756.59
      jaw 526.89
      monostotic 733.29
      polyostotic 756.54

Dysplasia — continued
   bone NEC — continued
      solitary 733.29
   brain 742.9
   bronchopulmonary, fetus or newborn 770.7
   cervix (uteri) 622.1
      cervical intraepithelial neoplasia I [CIN I] 622.1
      cervical intraepithelial neoplasia II [CIN II] 622.1
      cervical intraepithelial neoplasia III [CIN III] 233.1
      CIN I 622.1
      CIN II 622.1
      CIN III 233.1
   chondroectodermal 756.55
   chondromatose 756.4
   craniocarpotarsal 759.89
   craniometaphyseal 756.89
   dentinal 520.5
   diaphyseal, progressive 756.59
   ectodermal (anhidrotic) (Bason) (Clouston's) (congenital) (Feinmesser) (hereditary) (hidrotic) (Marshall) (Robinson's) 757.31
   epiphysealis 756.9
      multiplex 756.56
      punctata 756.59
   epiphysis 756.9
      multiple 756.56
   epithelial
      epiglottis 478.79
      uterine cervix 622.1
   erythroid NEC 289.8
   eye (see also Microphthalmos) 743.10
   familial metaphyseal 756.89
   fibromuscular, artery NEC 447.8
      carotid 447.8
      renal 447.3
   fibrous
      bone NEC 733.29
      diaphyseal, progressive 756.59
      jaw 526.89
      monostotic 733.29
      polyostotic 756.54
      solitary 733.29
   high grade squamous intraepithelial (HGSIL) 622.1
   hip (congenital) 755.63
      with dislocation (see also Dislocation, hip, congenital) 754.30
   hypohidrotic ectodermal 757.31
   joint 755.8
   kidney 753.15
   leg 755.69
   linguofacialis 759.89
   low grade squamous intraepithelial (LGSIL) 622.1
   lung 748.5
   macular 743.55
   mammary (benign) (gland) 610.9
      cystic 610.1
      specified type NEC 610.8
   metaphyseal 756.9
      familial 756.89
   monostotic fibrous 733.29
   muscle 756.89
   myeloid NEC 289.8
   nervous system (general) 742.9
   neuroectodermal 759.6
   oculoauriculovertebral 756.0
   oculodentodigital 759.89

Dysplasia — continued
  olfactogenital 253.4
  osteo-onycho-arthro (hereditary) 756.89
  periosteum 733.99
  polyostotic fibrous 756.54
  progressive diaphyseal 756.59
  prostate 602.3
    intraepithelial neoplasia I [PIN I] 602.3
    intraepithelial neoplasia II [PIN II] 602.3
    intraepithelial neoplasia III [PIN III] 233.4
  renal 753.15
  renofacialis 753.0
  retinal NEC 743.56
  retrolental 362.21
  spinal cord 742.9
  thymic, with immunodeficiency 279.2
  vagina 623.0
  vocal cord 478.5
  vulva 624.8
    intraepithelial neoplasia I [VIN I] 624.8
    intraepithelial neoplasia II [VIN II] 624.8
    intraepithelial neoplasia III [VIN III] 233.3
    VIN I 624.8
    VIN II 624.8
    VIN III 233.3
Dyspnea (nocturnal) (paroxysmal) 786.09
  asthmatic (bronchial) (*see also* Asthma) 493.9
    with bronchitis (*see also* Asthma) 493.9
      chronic 493.2
  cardiac (*see also* Failure, ventricular, left) 428.1
  cardiac (*see also* Failure, ventricular, left) 428.1
  functional 300.11
  hyperventilation 786.01
  hysterical 300.11
  Monday morning 504
  newborn 770.89
  psychogenic 306.1
  uremic — *see* Uremia
Dyspraxia 781.3
  syndrome 315.4
Dysproteinemia 273.8
  transient with copper deficiency 281.4
Dysprothrombinemia (constitutional) (*see also* Defect, coagulation) 286.3
Dysreflexia, autonomic 337.3
Dysrhythmia
  cardiac 427.9
    postoperative (immediate) 997.1
      long-term effect of cardiac surgery 429.4
    specified type NEC 427.89
  cerebral or cortical 348.3
Dyssecretosis, mucoserous 710.2
Dyssocial reaction, without manifest psychiatric disorder
  adolescent V71.02
  adult V71.01
  child V71.02
Dyssomnia NEC 780.56
  nonorganic origin 307.47
Dyssplenism 289.4
Dyssynergia
  biliary (*see also* Disease, biliary) 576.8
  cerebellaris myoclonica 334.2
  detrusor sphincter (bladder) 596.55
  ventricular 429.89
Dystasia, hereditary areflexic 334.3

Dysthymia 300.4
Dysthymic disorder 300.4
Dysthyroidism 246.9
Dystocia 660.9
  affecting fetus or newborn 763.1
  cervical 661.0
    affecting fetus or newborn 763.7
  contraction ring 661.4
    affecting fetus or newborn 763.7
  fetal 660.9
    abnormal size 653.5
      affecting fetus or newborn 763.1
    deformity 653.7
  maternal 660.9
    affecting fetus or newborn 763.1
  positional 660.0
    affecting fetus or newborn 763.1
  shoulder (girdle) 660.4
    affecting fetus or newborn 763.1
  uterine NEC 661.4
    affecting fetus or newborn 763.7
Dystonia
  deformans progressiva 333.6
  due to drugs 333.7
  lenticularis 333.6
  musculorum deformans 333.6
  torsion (idiopathic) 333.6
    fragments (of) 333.89
    symptomatic 333.7
Dystonic
  movements 781.0
Dystopia kidney 753.3
Dystrophy, dystrophia 783.9
  adiposogenital 253.8
  asphyxiating thoracic 756.4
  Becker's type 359.1
  brevicollis 756.16
  Bruch's membrane 362.77
  cervical (sympathetic) NEC 337.0
  chondro-osseus with punctate epiphyseal dysplasia 756.59
  choroid (hereditary) 363.50
    central (areolar) (partial) 363.53
      total (gyrate) 363.54
    circinate 363.53
    circumpapillary (partial) 363.51
      total 363.52
    diffuse
      partial 363.56
      total 363.57
    generalized
      partial 363.56
      total 363.57
    gyrate
      central 363.54
      generalized 363.57
    helicoid 363.52
    peripapillary — *see* Dystrophy, choroid, circumpapillary
    serpiginous 363.54
  cornea (hereditary) 371.50
    anterior NEC 371.52
    Cogan's 371.52
    combined 371.57
    crystalline 371.56
    endothelial (Fuchs') 371.57
    epithelial 371.50
      juvenile 371.51
      microscopic cystic 371.52
    granular 371.53

Dystrophy, dystrophia — continued
  cornea — continued
    lattice 371.54
    macular 371.55
    marginal (Terrien's) 371.48
    Meesman's 371.51
    microscopic cystic (epithelial) 371.52
    nodular, Salzmann's 371.46
    polymorphous 371.58
    posterior NEC 371.58
    ring-like 371.52
    Salzmann's nodular 371.46
    stromal NEC 371.56
  dermatochondrocorneal 371.50
  Duchenne's 359.1
  due to malnutrition 263.9
  Erb's 359.1
  familial
    hyperplastic periosteal 756.59
    osseous 277.5
  foveal 362.77
  Fuchs', cornea 371.57
  Gowers' muscular 359.1
  hair 704.2
  hereditary, progressive muscular 359.1
  hypogenital, with diabetic tendency 759.81
  Landouzy-Déjérine 359.1
  Leyden-Möbius 359.1
  mesodermalis congenita 759.82
  muscular 359.1
    congenital (hereditary) 359.0
      myotonic 359.2
    distal 359.1
    Duchenne's 359.1
    Erb's 359.1
    fascioscapulohumeral 359.1
    Gowers' 359.1
    hereditary (progressive) 359.1
    Landouzy-Déjérine 359.1
    limb-girdle 359.1
    myotonic 359.2
    progressive (hereditary) 359.1
      Charcôt-Marie-Tooth 356.1
    pseudohypertrophic (infantile) 359.1
  myocardium, myocardial (see also
      Degeneration, myocardial) 429.1
  myotonic 359.2
  myotonica 359.2
  nail 703.8
    congenital 757.5
  neurovascular (traumatic) (see also
      Neuropathy, peripheral, autonomic)
      337.9
  nutritional 263.9
  ocular 359.1
  oculocerebrorenal 270.8
  oculopharyngeal 359.1
  ovarian 620.8
  papillary (and pigmentary) 701.1
  pelvicrural atrophic 359.1
  pigmentary (see also Acanthosis) 701.2
  pituitary (gland) 253.8
  polyglandular 258.8
  posttraumatic sympathetic — see Dystrophy,
      sympathetic
  progressive ophthalmoplegic 359.1
  retina, retinal (hereditary) 362.70
    albipunctate 362.74
    Bruch's membrane 362.77
    cone, progressive 362.75
    hyaline 362.77

Dystrophy, dystrophia — continued
  retina, retinal — continued
    in
      Bassen-Kornzweig syndrome 272.5
        [362.72]
      cerebroretinal lipidosis 330.1 [362.71]
      Refsum's disease 356.3 [362.72]
      systemic lipidosis 272.7 [362.71]
    juvenile (Stargardt's) 362.75
    pigmentary 362.74
    pigment epithelium 362.76
    progressive cone (-rod) 362.75
    pseudoinflammatory foveal 362.77
    rod, progressive 362.75
    sensory 362.75
    vitelliform 362.76
  Salzmann's nodular 371.46
  scapuloperoneal 359.1
  skin NEC 709.9
  sympathetic (posttraumatic) (reflex) 337.20
    lower limb 337.22
    specified NEC 337.29
    upper limb 337.21
  tapetoretinal NEC 362.74
  thoracic asphyxiating 756.4
  unguium 703.8
    congenital 757.5
  vitreoretinal (primary) 362.73
    secondary 362.66
  vulva 624.0

Dysuria 788.1
  psychogenic 306.53

E

Eagle-Barrett syndrome 756.71
Eales' disease (syndrome) 362.18
Ear — see also condition
  ache 388.70
    otogenic 388.71
    referred 388.72
  lop 744.29
  piercing V50.3
  swimmers' acute 380.12
  tank 380.12
  tropical 111.8 [380.15]
  wax 380.4
Earache 388.70
  otogenic 388.71
  referred 388.72
Eaton-Lambert syndrome (see also Neoplasm,
    by site, malignant) 199.1 [358.1]
Eberth's disease (typhoid fever) 002.0
Ebstein's
  anomaly or syndrome (downward
      displacement, tricuspid valve into right
      ventricle) 746.2
  disease (diabetes) 250.4 [581.81]
Eccentro-osteochondrodysplasia 277.5
Ecchondroma (M9210/0) — see Neoplasm, bone,
    benign
Ecchondrosis (M9210/1) 238.0
Ecchordosis physaliphora 756.0
Ecchymosis (multiple) 459.89
  conjunctiva 372.72
  eye (traumatic) 921.0
  eyelids (traumatic) 921.1
  newborn 772.6
  spontaneous 782.7

Ecchymosis — continued
  traumatic — see Contusion
Echinococciasis — see Echinococcus
Echinococcosis — see Echinococcus
Echinococcus (infection) 122.9
  granulosus 122.4
    liver 122.0
    lung 122.1
    orbit 122.3 [376.13]
    specified site NEC 122.3
    thyroid 122.2
  liver NEC 122.8
    granulosus 122.0
    multilocularis 122.5
  lung NEC 122.9
    granulosus 122.1
    multilocularis 122.6
  multilocularis 122.7
    liver 122.5
    specified site NEC 122.6
  orbit 122.9 [376.13]
    granulosus 122.3 [376.13]
    multilocularis 122.6 [376.13]
  specified site NEC 122.9
    granulosus 122.3
    multilocularis 122.6 [376.13]
  thyroid NEC 122.9
    granulosus 122.2
    multilocularis 122.6
Echinorhynchiasis 127.7
Echinostomiasis 121.8
Echolalia 784.69
ECHO virus infection NEC 079.1
Eclampsia, eclamptic (coma) (convulsions) (delirium) 780.39
  female, child-bearing age NEC — see Eclampsia, pregnancy
  gravidarum — see Eclampsia, pregnancy
  male 780.39
  not associated with pregnancy or childbirth 780.39
  pregnancy, childbirth, or puerperium 642.6
    with pre-existing hypertension 642.7
    affecting fetus or newborn 760.0
  uremic 586
Eclipse blindness (total) 363.31
Economic circumstance affecting care V60.9
  specified type NEC V60.8
Economo's disease (encephalitis lethargica) 049.8
Ectasia, ectasis
  aorta (see also Aneurysm, aorta) 441.9
    ruptured 441.5
  breast 610.4
  capillary 448.9
  cornea (marginal) (postinfectional) 371.71
  duct (mammary) 610.4
  kidney 593.89
  mammary duct (gland) 610.4
  papillary 448.9
  renal 593.89
  salivary gland (duct) 527.8
  scar, cornea 371.71
  sclera 379.11
Ecthyma 686.8
  contagiosum 051.2
  gangrenosum 686.09
  infectiosum 051.2

Ectocardia 746.87
Ectodermal dysplasia, congenital 757.31
Ectodermosis erosiva pluriorificialis 695.1
Ectopic, ectopia (congenital) 759.89
  abdominal viscera 751.8
    due to defect in anterior abdominal wall 756.79
  ACTH syndrome 255.0
  adrenal gland 759.1
  anus 751.5
  auricular beats 427.61
  beats 427.60
  bladder 753.5
  bone and cartilage in lung 748.69
  brain 742.4
  breast tissue 757.6
  cardiac 746.87
  cerebral 742.4
  cordis 746.87
  endometrium 617.9
  gallbladder 751.69
  gastric mucosa 750.7
  gestation — see Pregnancy, ectopic
  heart 746.87
  hormone secretion NEC 259.3
  hyperparathyroidism 259.3
  kidney (crossed) (intrathoracic) (pelvis) 753.3
    in pregnancy or childbirth 654.4
      causing obstructed labor 660.2
  lens 743.37
  lentis 743.37
  mole — see Pregnancy, ectopic
  organ or site NEC — see Malposition, congenital
  ovary 752.0
  pancreas, pancreatic tissue 751.7
  pregnancy — see Pregnancy, ectopic
  pupil 364.75
  renal 753.3
  sebaceous glands of mouth 750.26
  secretion
    ACTH 255.0
    adrenal hormone 259.3
    adrenalin 259.3
    adrenocorticotropin 255.0
    antidiuretic hormone (ADH) 259.3
    epinephrine 259.3
    hormone NEC 259.3
    norepinephrine 259.3
    pituitary (posterior) 259.3
  spleen 759.0
  testis 752.51
  thyroid 759.2
  ureter 753.4
  ventricular beats 427.69
  vesicae 753.5
Ectrodactyly 755.4
  finger (see also Absence, finger, congenital) 755.29
  toe (see also Absence, toe, congenital) 755.39
Ectromelia 755.4
  lower limb 755.30
  upper limb 755.20
Ectropion 374.10
  anus 569.49
  cervix 622.0
    with mention of cervicitis 616.0
  cicatricial 374.14
  congenital 743.62

Ectropion — *continued*
  eyelid 374.10
    cicatricial 374.14
    congenital 743.62
    mechanical 374.12
    paralytic 374.12
    senile 374.11
    spastic 374.13
  iris (pigment epithelium) 364.54
  lip (congenital) 750.26
    acquired 528.5
  mechanical 374.12
  paralytic 374.12
  rectum 569.49
  senile 374.11
  spastic 374.13
  urethra 599.84
  uvea 364.54
Eczema (acute) (allergic) (chronic) (erythematous) (fissum) (occupational) (rubrum) (squamous) 692.9
  asteatotic 706.8
  atopic 691.8
  contact NEC 692.9
  dermatitis NEC 692.9
  due to specified cause — *see* Dermatitis, due to
  dyshidrotic 705.81
  external ear 380.22
  flexural 691.8
  gouty 274.89
  herpeticum 054.0
  hypertrophicum 701.8
  hypostatic — *see* Varicose, vein
  impetiginous 684
  infantile (acute) (chronic) (due to any substance) (intertriginous) (seborrheic) 690.12
  intertriginous NEC 692.9
    infantile 690.12
  intrinsic 691.8
  lichenified NEC 692.9
  marginatum 110.3
  nummular 692.9
  pustular 686.8
  seborrheic 690.18
    infantile 690.12
  solare 692.72
  stasis (lower extremity) 454.1
    ulcerated 454.2
  vaccination, vaccinatum 999.0
  varicose (lower extremity) — *see* Varicose, vein
  verrucosum callosum 698.3
Eczematoid, exudative 691.8
Eddowes' syndrome (brittle bone and blue sclera) 756.51
Edema, edematous 782.3
  with nephritis (*see also* Nephrosis) 581.9
  allergic 995.1
  angioneurotic (allergic) (any site) (with urticaria) 995.1
    hereditary 277.6
  angiospastic 443.9
  Berlin's (traumatic) 921.3
  brain 348.5
    due to birth injury 767.8
    fetus or newborn 767.8
  cardiac (*see also* Failure, heart) 428.0
  cardiovascular (*see also* Failure, heart) 428.0
  cerebral — *see* Edema, brain
  cerebrospinal vessel — *see* Edema, brain

Edema, edematous — *continued*
  cervix (acute) (uteri) 622.8
    puerperal, postpartum 674.8
  chronic hereditary 757.0
  circumscribed, acute 995.1
    hereditary 277.6
  complicating pregnancy (gestational) 646.1
    with hypertension — *see* Toxemia, of pregnancy
  conjunctiva 372.73
  connective tissue 782.3
  cornea 371.20
    due to contact lenses 371.24
    idiopathic 371.21
    secondary 371.22
  due to
    lymphatic obstruction — *see* Edema, lymphatic
    salt retention 276.0
  epiglottis — *see* Edema, glottis
  essential, acute 995.1
    hereditary 277.6
  extremities, lower — *see* Edema, legs
  eyelid NEC 374.82
  familial, hereditary (legs) 757.0
  famine 262
  fetus or newborn 778.5
  genital organs
    female 629.8
    male 608.86
  gestational 646.1
    with hypertension — *see* Toxemia, of pregnancy
  glottis, glottic, glottides (obstructive) (passive) 478.6
    allergic 995.1
      hereditary 277.6
    due to external agent — *see* Condition, respiratory, acute, due to specified agent
  heart (*see also* Failure, heart) 428.0
    newborn 779.89
  heat 992.7
  hereditary (legs) 757.0
  inanition 262
  infectious 782.3
  intracranial 348.5
    due to injury at birth 767.8
  iris 364.8
  joint (*see also* Effusion, joint) 719.0
  larynx (*see also* Edema, glottis) 478.6
  legs 782.3
    due to venous obstruction 459.2
    hereditary 757.0
  localized 782.3
    due to venous obstruction 459.2
      lower extremity 459.2
  lower extremities — *see* Edema, legs
  lung 514
    acute 518.4
      with heart disease or failure (*see also* Failure, ventricular, left) 428.1
      congestive 428.0
    chemical (due to fumes or vapors) 506.1
    due to
      external agent(s) NEC 508.9
        specified NEC 508.8
      fumes and vapors (chemical) (inhalation) 506.1
      radiation 508.0

Edema, edematous — *continued*
　lung — *continued*
　　chemical (acute) 506.1
　　　chronic 506.4
　　chronic 514
　　　chemical (due to fumes or vapors) 506.4
　　　due to
　　　　external agent(s) NEC 508.9
　　　　　specified NEC 508.8
　　　　fumes or vapors (chemical)
　　　　　(inhalation) 506.4
　　　　radiation 508.1
　　due to
　　　external agent 508.9
　　　　specified NEC 508.8
　　high altitude 993.2
　　near drowning 994.1
　　postoperative 518.4
　　terminal 514
　lymphatic 457.1
　　due to mastectomy operation 457.0
　macula 362.83
　　cystoid 362.53
　　diabetic 250.5 [362.01]
　malignant (*see also* Gangrene, gas) 040.0
　Milroy's 757.0
　nasopharynx 478.25
　neonatorum 778.5
　nutritional (newborn) 262
　　with dyspigmentation, skin and hair 260
　optic disc or nerve — *see* Papilledema
　orbit 376.33
　　circulatory 459.89
　palate (soft) (hard) 528.9
　pancreas 577.8
　penis 607.83
　periodic 995.1
　　hereditary 277.6
　pharynx 478.25
　pitting 782.3
　pulmonary — *see* Edema, lung
　Quincke's 995.1
　　hereditary 277.6
　renal (*see also* Nephrosis) 581.9
　retina (localized) (macular) (perepheral) 362.83
　　cystoid 362.53
　　diabetic 250.5 [362.01]
　salt 276.0
　scrotum 608.86
　seminal vesicle 608.86
　spermatic cord 608.86
　spinal cord 336.1
　starvation 262
　stasis (*see also* Hypertension, venous)
　　459.30
　subconjunctival 372.73
　subglottic (*see also* Edema, glottis) 478.6
　supraglottic (*see also* Edema, glottis) 478.6
　testis 608.86
　toxic NEC 782.3
　traumatic NEC 782.3
　tunica vaginalis 608.86
　vas deferens 608.86
　vocal cord — *see* Edema, glottis
　vulva (acute) 624.8
Edentia (complete) (partial) (*see also* Absence, tooth) 520.0
　acquired 525.10
　　due to
　　　caries 525.13
　　　extraction 525.10

Edentia — *continued*
　acquired — *continued*
　　due to — *continued*
　　　periodontal disease 525.12
　　　specified NEC 525.19
　　　trauma 525.11
　　causing malocclusion 524.3
　　congenital (deficiency of tooth buds) 520.0
Edentulism 525.10
Edsall's disease 992.2
Educational handicap V62.3
Edwards' syndrome 758.2
Effect, adverse NEC
　abnormal gravitation (G) forces or states 994.9
　air pressure — *see* Effect, adverse, atmospheric pressure
　altitude (high) — *see* Effect, adverse, high altitude
　anesthetic
　　in labor and delivery NEC 668.9
　　affecting fetus or newborn 763.5
　antitoxin — *see* Complications, vaccination
　atmospheric pressure 993.9
　　due to explosion 993.4
　　high 993.3
　　low — *see* Effect, adverse, high altitude
　　specified effect NEC 993.8
　biological, correct substance properly administered (*see also* Effect, adverse, drug) 995.2
　blood (derivatives) (serum) (transfusion) — *see* Complications, transfusion
　chemical substance NEC 989.9
　　specified — *see* Table of Drugs and Chemicals
　cobalt, radioactive (*see also* Effect, adverse, radioactive substance) 990
　cold (temperature) (weather) 991.9
　　chilblains 991.5
　　frostbite — *see* Frostbite
　　specified effect NEC 991.8
　drugs and medicinals NEC 995.2
　　correct substance properly administered 995.2
　　overdose or wrong substance given or taken 977.9
　　specified drug — *see* Table of Drugs and Chemicals
　electric current (shock) 994.8
　　burn — *see* Burn, by site
　electricity (electrocution) (shock) 994.8
　　burn — *see* Burn, by site
　exertion (excessive) 994.5
　exposure 994.9
　　exhaustion 994.4
　external cause NEC 994.9
　fallout (radioactive) NEC 990
　fluoroscopy NEC 990
　foodstuffs
　　allergic reaction (*see also* Allergy, food) 693.1
　　anaphylactic shock due to food NEC 995.60
　　noxious 988.9
　　specified type NEC (*see also* Poisoning, by name of noxious foodstuff) 988.8
　gases, fumes, or vapors — *see* Table of Drugs and Chemicals
　glue (airplane) sniffing 304.6
　heat — *see* Heat

Effect, adverse NEC — *continued*
  high altitude NEC 993.2
    anoxia 993.2
    on
      ears 993.0
      sinuses 993.1
    polycythemia 289.0
  hot weather — *see* Heat
  hunger 994.2
  immersion, foot 991.4
  immunization — *see* Complications, vaccination
  immunological agents — *see* Complications, vaccination
  implantation (removable) of isotope or radium NEC 990
  infrared (radiation) (rays) NEC 990
    burn — *see* Burn, by site
    dermatitis or eczema 692.82
  infusion — *see* Complications, infusion
  ingestion or injection of isotope (therapeutic) NEC 990
  irradiation NEC (*see also* Effect, adverse, radiation) 990
  isotope (radioactive) NEC 990
  lack of care (child) (infant) (newborn) 995.52
    adult 995.84
  lightning 994.0
    burn — *see* Burn, by site
  Lirugin — *see* Complications, vaccination
  medicinal substance, correct, properly administered (*see also* Effect, adverse, drugs) 995.2
  mesothorium NEC 990
  motion 994.6
  noise, inner ear 388.10
  overheated places — *see* Heat
  polonium NEC 990
  psychosocial, of work environment V62.1
  radiation (diagnostic) (fallout) (infrared) (natural source) (therapeutic) (tracer) (ultraviolet) (x-ray) NEC 990
    with pulmonary manifestations
      acute 508.0
      chronic 508.1
    dermatitis or eczema 692.82
      due to sun NEC (*see also* Dermatitis, due to, sun) 692.70
    fibrosis of lungs 508.1
    maternal with suspected damage to fetus affecting management of pregnancy 655.6 [5]
    pneumonitis 508.0
  radioactive substance NEC 990
    dermatitis or eczema 692.82
  radioactivity NEC 990
  radiotherapy NEC 990
    dermatitis or eczema 692.82
  radium NEC 990
  reduced temperature 991.9
    frostbite — *see* Frostbite
    immersion, foot (hand) 991.4
    specified effect NEC 991.8
  roentgenography NEC 990
  roentgenoscopy NEC 990
  roentgen rays NEC 990
  serum (prophylactic) (therapeutic) NEC 999.5
  specified NEC 995.89
    external cause NEC 994.9
  strangulation 994.7
  submersion 994.1

Effect, adverse NEC — *continued*
  teletherapy NEC 990
  thirst 994.3
  transfusion — *see* Complications, transfusion
  ultraviolet (radiation) (rays) NEC 990
    burn — *see also* Burn, by site
      from sun (*see also* Sunburn) 692.71
    dermatitis or eczema 692.82
      due to sun NEC (*see also* Dermatitis, due to, sun) 692.70
  uranium NEC 990
  vaccine (any) — *see* Complications, vaccination
  weightlessness 994.9
  whole blood — *see also* Complications, transfusion
    overdose or wrong substance given (*see also* Table of Drugs and Chemicals) 964.7
  working environment V62.1
  x-rays NEC 990
    dermatitis or eczema 692.82
Effects, late — *see* Late, effect (of)
Effect, remote
  of cancer — *see* condition
Effluvium, telogen 704.02
Effort
  intolerance 306.2
  syndrome (aviators) (psychogenic) 306.2
Effusion
  amniotic fluid (*see also* Rupture, membranes, premature) 658.1 [5]
  brain (serous) 348.5
  bronchial (*see also* Bronchitis) 490
  cerebral 348.5
  cerebrospinal (*see also* Meningitis) 322.9
    vessel 348.5
  chest — *see* Effusion, pleura
  intracranial 348.5
  joint 719.00
    ankle 719.07
    elbow 719.02
    foot 719.07
    hand 719.04
    hip 719.05
    knee 719.06
    multiple sites 719.09
    pelvic region 719.05
    shoulder (region) 719.01
    specified site NEC 719.08
    wrist 719.03
  meninges (*see also* Meningitis) 322.9
  pericardium, pericardial (*see also* Pericarditis) 423.9
    acute 420.90
  peritoneal (chronic) 568.82
  pleura, pleurisy, pleuritic, pleuropericardial 511.9
    bacterial, nontuberculous 511.1
    fetus or newborn 511.9
    malignant 197.2
    nontuberculous 511.9
      bacterial 511.1
    pneumococcal 511.1
    staphylococcal 511.1
    streptococcal 511.1
    traumatic 862.29
      with open wound 862.39
    tuberculous (*see also* Tuberculosis, pleura) 012.0 [5]
      primary progressive 010.1 [5]

Effusion — *continued*
  pulmonary — *see* Effusion, pleura
  spinal (*see also* Meningitis) 322.9
  thorax, thoracic — *see* Effusion, pleura
Eggshell nails 703.8
  congenital 757.5
Ego-dystonic
  homosexuality 302.0
  lesbianism 302.0
Egyptian splenomegaly 120.1
Ehlers-Danlos syndrome 756.83
Ehrlichiosis 082.40
  chaffeensis 082.41
  specified type NEC 082.49
Eichstedt's disease (pityriasis versicolor) 111.0
Eisenmenger's complex or syndrome
  (ventricular septal defect) 745.4
Ejaculation, semen
  painful 608.89
    psychogenic 306.59
  premature 302.75
  retrograde 608.87
Ekbom syndrome (restless legs) 333.99
Ekman's syndrome (brittle bones and blue sclera) 756.51
Elastic skin 756.83
  acquired 701.8
Elastofibroma (M8820/0) — *see* Neoplasm, connective tissue, benign
Elastoidosis
  cutanea nodularis 701.8
  cutis cystica et comedonica 701.8
Elastoma 757.39
  juvenile 757.39
  Miescher's (elastosis perforans serpiginosa) 701.1
Elastomyofibrosis 425.3
Elastosis 701.8
  atrophicans 701.8
  perforans serpiginosa 701.1
  reactive perforating 701.1
  senilis 701.8
  solar (actinic) 692.74
Elbow — *see* condition
Electric
  current, electricity, effects (concussion) (fatal) (nonfatal) (shock) 994.8
    burn — *see* Burn, by site
  feet (foot) syndrome 266.2
Electrocution 994.8
Electrolyte imbalance 276.9
  with
    abortion — *see* Abortion, by type with metabolic disorder
    ectopic pregnancy (*see also* categories 633.0-633.9) 639.4
    hyperemesis gravidarum (before 22 completed weeks gestation) 643.1
    molar pregnancy (*see also* categories 630-632) 639.4
  following
    abortion 639.4
    ectopic or molar pregnancy 639.4
Elephant man syndrome 237.71
Elephantiasis (nonfilarial) 457.1
  arabicum (*see also* Infestation, filarial) 125.9
  congenita hereditaria 757.0

Elephantiasis — *continued*
  congenital (any site) 757.0
  due to
    Brugia (malayi) 125.1
    mastectomy operation 457.0
    Wuchereria (bancrofti) 125.0
      malayi 125.1
  eyelid 374.83
  filarial (*see also* Infestation, filarial) 125.9
  filariensis (*see also* Infestation, filarial) 125.9
  gingival 523.8
  glandular 457.1
  graecorum 030.9
  lymphangiectatic 457.1
  lymphatic vessel 457.1
    due to mastectomy operation 457.0
  neuromatosa 237.71
  postmastectomy 457.0
  scrotum 457.1
  streptococcal 457.1
  surgical 997.99
    postmastectomy 457.0
  telangiectodes 457.1
  vulva (nonfilarial) 624.8
Elevated — *see* Elevation
Elevation
  17-ketosteroids 791.9
  acid phosphatase 790.5
  alkaline phosphatase 790.5
  amylase 790.5
  antibody titers 795.79
  basal metabolic rate (BMR) 794.7
  blood pressure (*see also* Hypertension) 401.9
    reading (incidental) (isolated) (nonspecific), no diagnosis or hypertension 796.2
  body temperature (of unknown origin) (*see also* Pyrexia) 780.6
  conjugate, eye 378.81
  diaphragm, congenital 756.6
  immunoglobulin level 795.79
  indolacetic acid 791.9
  lactic acid dehydrogenase (LDH) level 790.4
  lipase 790.5
  prostate specific antigen (PSA) 790.93
  renin 790.99
    in hypertension (*see also* Hypertension, renovascular) 405.91
  Rh titer 999.7
  scapula, congenital 755.52
  sedimentation rate 790.1
  SGOT 790.4
  SGPT 790.4
  transaminase 790.4
  vanillylmandelic acid 791.9
  venous pressure 459.89
  VMA 791.9
Elliptocytosis (congenital) (hereditary) 282.1
  Hb-C (disease) 282.7
  hemoglobin disease 282.7
  sickle-cell (disease) 282.60
    trait 282.5
Ellis-van Creveld disease or syndrome (chondroectodermal dysplasia) 756.55
Ellison-Zollinger syndrome (gastric hypersecretion with pancreatic islet cell tumor) 251.5
Elongation, elongated (congenital) — *see also* Distortion
  bone 756.9
  cervix (uteri) 752.49

Elongation, elongated — *continued*
  cervix — *continued*
    acquired 622.6
    hypertrophic 622.6
  colon 751.5
  common bile duct 751.69
  cystic duct 751.69
  frenulum, penis 752.69
  labia minora, acquired 624.8
  ligamentum patellae 756.89
  petiolus (epiglottidis) 748.3
  styloid bone (process) 733.99
  tooth, teeth 520.2
  uvula 750.26
    acquired 528.9

Elschnig bodies or pearls 366.51
El Tor cholera 001.1
Emaciation (due to malnutrition) 261
Emancipation disorder 309.22
Embadomoniasis 007.8
Embarrassment heart, cardiac — *see* Disease, heart
Embedded tooth, teeth 520.6
  with abnormal position (same or adjacent tooth) 524.3
  root only 525.3
Embolic — *see* conditon
Embolism 444.9
  with
    abortion — *see* Abortion, by type, with embolism
    ectopic pregnancy (*see also* categories 633.0-633.9) 639.6
    molar pregnancy (*see also* categories 630-632) 639.6
  air (any site) 958.0
    with
      abortion — *see* Abortion, by type, with embolism
      ectopic pregnancy (*see also* categories 633.0-633.9) 639.6
      molar pregnancy (*see also* categories 630-632) 639.6
    due to implanted device — *see* Complications, due to (presence of) any device, implant, or graft classified to 996.0-996.5 NEC
    following
      abortion 639.6
      ectopic or molar pregnancy 639.6
      infusion, perfusion, or transfusion 999.1
    in pregnancy, childbirth, or puerperium 673.0
    traumatic 958.0
  amniotic fluid (pulmonary) 673.1
    with
      abortion — *see* Abortion, by type, with embolism
      ectopic pregnancy (*see also* categories 633.0-633.9) 639.6
      molar pregnancy (*see also* categories 630-632) 639.6
    following
      abortion 639.6
      ectopic or molar pregnancy 639.6
  aorta, aortic 444.1
    abdominal 444.0
    bifurcation 444.0
    saddle 444.0
    thoracic 444.1

Embolism — *continued*
  artery 444.9
    auditory, internal 433.8
    basilar (*see also* Occlusion, artery, basilar) 433.0
    bladder 444.89
    carotid (common) (internal) (*see also* Occlusion, artery, carotid) 433.1
    cerebellar (anterior inferior) (posterior inferior) (superior) 433.8
    cerebral (*see also* Embolism, brain) 434.1
    choroidal (anterior) 433.8
    communicating posterior 433.8
    coronary (*see also* Infarct, myocardium) 410.9
      without myocardial infarction 411.81
    extremity 444.22
      lower 444.22
      upper 444.21
    hypophyseal 433.8
    mesenteric (with gangrene) 557.0
    ophthalmic (*see also* Occlusion, retina) 362.30
    peripheral 444.22
    pontine 433.8
    precerebral NEC — *see* Occlusion, artery, precerebral
    pulmonary — *see* Embolism, pulmonary
    renal 593.81
    retinal (*see also* Occlusion, retina) 362.30
    specified site NEC 444.89
    vertebral (*see also* Occlusion, artery, vertebral) 433.2
  auditory, internal 433.8
  basilar (artery) (*see also* Occlusion, artery, basilar) 433.0
  birth, mother — *see* Embolism, obstetrical
  blood-clot
    with
      abortion — *see* Abortion, by type, with embolism
      ectopic pregnancy (*see also* categories 633.0-633.9) 639.6
      molar pregnancy (*see also* categories 630-632) 639.6
    following
      abortion 639.6
      ectopic or molar pregnancy 639.6
    in pregnancy, childbirth, or puerperium 673.2
  brain 434.1
    with
      abortion — *see* Abortion, by type, with embolism
      ectopic pregnancy (*see also* categories 633.0-633.9) 639.6
      molar pregnancy (*see also* categories 630-632) 639.6
    following
      abortion 639.6
      ectopic or molar pregnancy 639.6
    late effect — *see* Late effect(s) (of) cerebrovascular disease
    puerperal, postpartum, childbirth 674.0
  capillary 448.9
  cardiac (*see also* Infarct, myocardium) 410.9
  carotid (artery) (common) (internal) (*see also* Occlusion, artery, carotid) 433.1

Embolism

Embolism — *continued*
- cavernous sinus (venous) — *see* Embolism, intracranial venous sinus
- cerebral (*see also* Embolism, brain) 434.1
- cholesterol — *see* Atheroembolism
- choroidal (anterior) (artery) 433.8
- coronary (artery or vein) (systemic) (*see also* Infarct, myocardium) 410.9
  - without myocardial infarction 411.81
- due to (presence of) any device, implant, or graft classifiable to 996.0-996.5 — *see* Complications, due to (presence of) any device, implant, or graft classified to 996.0-996.5 NEC
- encephalomalacia (*see also* Embolism, brain) 434.1
- extremities 444.22
  - lower 444.22
  - upper 444.21
- eye 362.30
- fat (cerebral) (pulmonary) (systemic) 958.1
  - with
    - abortion — *see* Abortion, by type, with embolism
    - ectopic pregnancy (*see also* categories 633.0-633.9) 639.6
    - molar pregnancy (*see also* categories 630-632) 639.6
  - complicating delivery or puerperium 673.8
  - following
    - abortion 639.6
    - ectopic or molar pregnancy 639.6
  - in pregnancy, childbirth, or the puerperium 673.8
- femoral (artery) 444.22
  - vein 453.8
- following
  - abortion 639.6
  - ectopic or molar pregnancy 639.6
  - infusion, perfusion, or transfusion
    - air 999.1
    - thrombus 999.2
- heart (fatty) (*see also* Infarct, myocardium) 410.9
- hepatic (vein) 453.0
- iliac (artery) 444.81
- iliofemoral 444.81
- in pregnancy, childbirth, or puerperium (pulmonary) — *see* Embolism, obstetrical
- intestine (artery) (vein) (with gangrene) 557.0
- intracranial (*see also* Embolism, brain) 434.1
  - venous sinus (any) 325
    - late effect — *see* category 326
    - nonpyogenic 437.6
      - in pregnancy or puerperium 671.5
- kidney (artery) 593.81
- lateral sinus (venous) — *see* Embolism, intracranial venous sinus
- longitudinal sinus (venous) — *see* Embolism, intracranial venous sinus
- lower extremity 444.22
- lung (massive) — *see* Embolism, pulmonary
- meninges (*see also* Embolism, brain) 434.1
- mesenteric (artery) (with gangrene) 557.0
- multiple NEC 444.9

Embolism — *continued*
- obstetrical (pulmonary) 673.2
  - air 673.0
  - amniotic fluid (pulmonary) 673.1
  - blood-clot 673.2
  - cardiac 674.8
  - fat 673.8
  - heart 674.8
  - pyemic 673.3
  - septic 673.3
  - specified NEC 674.8
- ophthalmic (*see also* Occlusion, retina) 362.30
- paradoxical NEC 444.9
- penis 607.82
- peripheral arteries NEC 444.22
  - lower 444.22
  - upper 444.21
- pituitary 253.8
- popliteal (artery) 444.22
- portal (vein) 452
- postoperative NEC 997.2
  - cerebral 997.02
  - mesenteric artery 997.71
  - other vessels 997.79
  - peripheral vascular 997.2
  - pulmonary 415.11
  - renal artery 997.72
- precerebral artery (*see also* Occlusion, artery, precerebral) 433.9
- puerperal — *see* Embolism, obstetrical
- pulmonary (artery) (vein) 415.1
  - with
    - abortion — *see* Abortion, by type, with embolism
    - ectopic pregnancy (*see also* categories 633.0-633.9) 639.6
    - molar pregnancy (*see also* categories 630-632) 639.6
  - following
    - abortion 639.6
    - ectopic or molar pregnancy 639.6
  - iatrogenic 415.11
  - in pregnancy, childbirth, or puerperium — *see* Embolism, obstetrical
  - postoperative 415.11
- pyemic (multiple) 038.9
  - with
    - abortion — *see* Abortion, by type, with embolism
    - ectopic pregnancy (*see also* categories 633.0-633.9) 639.6
    - molar pregnancy (*see also* categories 630-632) 639.6
  - Aerobacter aerogenes 038.49
  - enteric gram-negative bacilli 038.40
  - Enterobacter aerogenes 038.49
  - Escherichia coli 038.42
  - following
    - abortion 639.6
    - ectopic or molar pregnancy 639.6
  - Hemophilus influenzae 038.41
  - pneumococcal 038.2
  - Proteus vulgaris 038.49
  - Pseudomonas (aeruginosa) 038.43
  - puerperal, postparztum, childbirth (any organism) 673.3
  - Serratia 038.44
  - specified organism NEC 038.8
  - staphylococcal 038.10
    - aureus 038.11
    - specified organism NEC 038.19

Index to Diseases

Embolism — *continued*
  pyemic — *continued*
    streptococcal 038.0
    renal (artery) 593.81
      vein 453.3
    retina, retinal (*see also* Occlusion, retina) 362.30
    saddle (aorta) 444.0
    septicemic — *see* Embolism, pyemic
    sinus — *see* Embolism, intracranial venous sinus
  soap
    with
      abortion — *see* Abortion, by type, with embolism
      ectopic pregnancy (*see also* categories 633.0-633.9) 639.6
      molar pregnancy (*see also* categories 630-632) 639.6
    following
      abortion 639.6
      ectopic or molar pregnancy 639.6
  spinal cord (nonpyogenic) 336.1
    in pregnancy or puerperium 671.5 ✓5ᵗʰ
    pyogenic origin 324.1
    late effect — *see* category 326
  spleen, splenic (artery) 444.89
  thrombus (thromboembolism) following infusion, perfusion, or transfusion 999.2
  upper extremity 444.21
  vein 453.9
    with inflammation or phlebitis — *see* Thrombophlebitis
    cerebral (*see also* Embolism, brain) 434.1 ✓5ᵗʰ
    coronary (*see also* Infarct, myocardium) 410.9 ✓5ᵗʰ
      without myocardial infarction 411.81
    hepatic 453.0
    mesenteric (with gangrene) 557.0
    portal 452
    pulmonary — *see* Embolism, pulmonary
    renal 453.3
    specified NEC 453.8
      with inflammation or phlebitis — *see* Thrombophlebitis
    vena cava (inferior) (superior) 453.2
    vessels of brain (*see also* Embolism, brain) 434.1 ✓5ᵗʰ

Embolization — *see* Embolism

Embolus — *see* Embolism

Embryoma (M9080/1) — *see also* Neoplasm, by site, uncertain behavior
  benign (M9080/0 — *see* Neoplasm, by site, benign
  kidney (M8960/3) 189.0
  liver (M8970/3) 155.0
  malignant (M9080/3) — *see also* Neoplasm, by site, malignant
    kidney (M8960/3) 189.0
    liver (M8970/3) 155.0
    testis (M9070/3) 186.9
      undescended 186.0
  testis (M9070/3) 186.9
    undescended 186.0

Embryonic
  circulation 747.9
  heart 747.9
  vas deferens 752.8

Embryopathia NEC 759.9

Embryotomy, fetal 763.89

Embryotoxon 743.43
  interfering with vision 743.42

Emesis — *see also* Vomiting
  gravidarum — *see* Hyperemesis, gravidarum

Emissions, nocturnal (semen) 608.89

Emotional
  crisis — *see* Crisis, emotional
  disorder (*see also* Disorder, mental) 300.9
  instability (excessive) 301.3
  overlay — *see* Reaction, adjustment
  upset 300.9

Emotionality, pathological 301.3

Emotogenic disease (*see also* Disorder, psychogenic) 306.9

Emphysema (atrophic) (centriacinar) (centrilobular) (chronic) (diffuse) (essential) (hypertrophic) (interlobular) (lung) (obstructive) (panlobular) (paracicatricial) (paracinar) (postural) (pulmonary) (senile) (subpleural) (traction) (unilateral) (unilobular) (vesicular) 492.8
  with
    bronchitis
      acute and chronic 491.21
      chronic 491.20
        with acute bronchitis or acute exacerbation 491.21
  bullous (giant) 492.0
  cellular tissue 958.7
    surgical 998.81
  compensatory 518.2
  congenital 770.2
  conjunctiva 372.89
  connective tissue 958.7
    surgical 998.81
  due to fumes or vapors 506.4
  eye 376.89
  eyelid 374.85
    surgical 998.81
    traumatic 958.7
  fetus or newborn (interstitial) (mediastinal) (unilobular) 770.2
  heart 416.9
  interstitial 518.1
    congenital 770.2
    fetus or newborn 770.2
  laminated tissue 958.7
    surgical 998.81
  mediastinal 518.1
    fetus or newborn 770.2
  newborn (interstitial) (mediastinal) (unilobular) 770.2
  obstructive diffuse with fibrosis 492.8
  orbit 376.89
  subcutaneous 958.7
    due to trauma 958.7
    nontraumatic 518.1
    surgical 998.81
  surgical 998.81
  thymus (gland) (congenital) 254.8
  traumatic 958.7
  tuberculous (*see also* Tuberculosis, pulmonary) 011.9 ✓5ᵗʰ

Employment examination (certification) V70.5

Empty sella (turcica) syndrome 253.8

Empyema

Empyema (chest) (diaphragmatic) (double) (encapsulated) (general) (interlobar) (lung) (medial) (necessitatis) (perforating chest wall) (pleura) (pneumococcal) (residual) (sacculated) (streptococcal) (supradiaphragmatic) 510.9
  with fistula 510.0
  accessory sinus (chronic) (see also Sinusitis) 473.9
  acute 510.9
    with fistula 510.0
  antrum (chronic) (see also Sinusitis, maxillary) 473.0
  brain (any part) (see also Abcess, brain) 324.0
  ethmoidal (sinus) (chronic) (see also Sinusitis, ethmoidal) 473.2
  extradural (see also Abscess, extradural) 324.9
  frontal (sinus) (chronic) (see also Sinusitis, frontal) 473.1
  gallbladder (see also Cholecystitis, acute) 575.0
  mastoid (process) (acute) (see also Mastoiditis, acute) 383.00
  maxilla, maxillary 526.4
    sinus (chronic) (see also Sinusitis, maxillary) 473.0
  nasal sinus (chronic) (see also Sinusitis) 473.9
  sinus (accessory) (nasal) (see also Sinusitis) 473.9
  sphenoidal (chronic) (sinus) (see also Sinusitis, sphenoidal) 473.3
  subarachnoid (see also Abscess, extradural) 324.9
  subdural (see also Abscess, extradural) 324.9
  tuberculous (see also Tuberculosis, pleura) 012.0 ✓5ᵗʰ
  ureter (see also Ureteritis) 593.89
  ventricular (see also Abscess, brain) 324.0
Enameloma 520.2
Encephalitis (bacterial) (chronic) (hemorrhagic) (idiopathic) (nonepidemic) (spurious) (subacute) 323.9
  acute — see also Encephalitis, viral
    disseminated (postinfectious) NEC 136.9 [323.6]
      postimmunization or postvaccination 323.5
    inclusional 049.8
    inclusion body 049.8
    necrotizing 049.8
  arboviral, arbovirus NEC 064
  arthropod-borne (see also Encephalitis, viral, arthropod-borne) 064
  Australian X 062.4
  Bwamba fever 066.3
  California (virus) 062.5
  Central European 063.2
  Czechoslovakian 063.2
  Dawson's (inclusion body) 046.2
  diffuse sclerosing 046.2
  due to
    actinomycosis 039.8 [323.4]
    cat-scratch disease 078.3 [323.0]
    infectious mononucleosis 075 [323.0]
    malaria (see also Malaria) 084.6 [323.2]
    Negishi virus 064
    ornithosis 073.7 [323.0]
    prophylactic inoculation against smallpox 323.5

Encephalitis — continued
  due to — continued
    rickettsiosis (see also Rickettsiosis) 083.9 [323.1]
    rubella 056.01
    toxoplasmosis (acquired) 130.0
      congenital (active) 771.2 [323.4]
    typhus (fever) (see also Typhus) 081.9 [323.1]
    vaccination (smallpox) 323.5
  Eastern equine 062.2
  endemic 049.8
  epidemic 049.8
  equine (acute) (infectious) (viral) 062.9
    Eastern 062.2
    Venezuelan 066.2
    Western 062.1
  Far Eastern 063.0
  following vaccination or other immunization procedure 323.5
  herpes 054.3
  Ilheus (virus) 062.8
  inclusion body 046.2
  infectious (acute) (virus) NEC 049.8
  influenzal 487.8 [323.4]
    lethargic 049.8
  Japanese (B type) 062.0
  La Crosse 062.5
  Langat 063.8
  late effect — see Late, effect, encephalitis
  lead 984.9 [323.7]
  lethargic (acute) (infectious) (influenzal) 049.8
  lethargica 049.8
  louping ill 063.1
  lupus 710.0 [323.8]
  lymphatica 049.0
  Mengo 049.8
  meningococcal 036.1
  mumps 072.2
  Murray Valley 062.4
  myoclonic 049.8
  Negishi virus 064
  otitic NEC 382.4 [323.4]
  parasitic NEC 123.9 [323.4]
  periaxialis (concentrica) (diffusa) 341.1
  postchickenpox 052.0
  postexanthematous NEC 057.9 [323.6]
  postimmunization 323.5
  postinfectious NEC 136.9 [323.6]
  postmeasles 055.0
  posttraumatic 323.8
  postvaccinal (smallpox) 323.5
  postvaricella 052.0
  postviral NEC 079.99 [323.6]
    postexanthematous 057.9 [323.6]
    specified NEC 057.8 [323.6]
  Powassan 063.8
  progressive subcortical (Binswanger's) 290.12
  Rio Bravo 049.8
  rubella 056.01
  Russian
    autumnal 062.0
    spring-summer type (taiga) 063.0
  saturnine 984.9 [323.7]
  Semliki Forest 062.8
  serous 048
  slow-acting virus NEC 046.8
  specified cause NEC 323.8
  St. Louis type 062.3
  subacute sclerosing 046.2
  subcorticalis chronica 290.12

Encephalitis — continued
  summer 062.0
  suppurative 324.0
  syphilitic 094.81
    congenital 090.41
  tick-borne 063.9
  torula, torular 117.5 *[323.4]*
  toxic NEC 989.9 *[323.7]*
  toxoplasmic (acquired) 130.0
    congenital (active) 771.2 *[323.4]*
  trichinosis 124 *[323.4]*
  Trypanosomiasis (*see also* Trypanosomiasis) 086.9 *[323.2]*
  tuberculous (*see also* Tuberculosis) 013.6 ✓5ᵗʰ
  type B (Japanese) 062.0
  type C 062.3
  van Bogaert's 046.2
  Venezuelan 066.2
  Vienna type 049.8
  viral, virus 049.9
    arthropod-borne NEC 064
      mosquito-borne 062.9
        Australian X disease 062.4
        California virus 062.5
        Eastern equine 062.2
        Ilheus virus 062.8
        Japanese (B type) 062.0
        Murray Valley 062.4
        specified type NEC 062.8
        St. Louis 062.3
        type B 062.0
        type C 062.3
        Western equine 062.1
      tick-borne 063.9
        biundulant 063.2
        Central European 063.2
        Czechoslovakian 063.2
        diphasic meningoencephalitis 063.2
        Far Eastern 063.0
        Langat 063.8
        louping ill 063.1
        Powassan 063.8
        Russian spring-summer (taiga) 063.0
        specified type NEC 063.8
      vector unknown 064
    slow acting NEC 046.8
    specified type NEC 049.8
    vaccination, prophylactic (against) V05.0
  von Economo's 049.8
  Western equine 062.1
  West Nile type 066.4 ▲
Encephalocele 742.0
  orbit 376.81
Encephalocystocele 742.0
Encephalomalacia (brain) (cerebellar) (cerebral) (cerebrospinal) (*see also* Softening, brain) 434.9 ✓5ᵗʰ
  due to
    hemorrhage (*see also* Hemorrhage, brain) 431
    recurrent spasm of artery 435.9
  embolic (cerebral) (*see also* Embolism, brain) 434.1 ✓5ᵗʰ
  subcorticalis chronicus arteriosclerotica 290.12
  thrombotic (*see also* thrombosis, brain) 434.0 ✓5ᵗʰ
Encephalomeningitis — *see* Meningoencephalitis
Encephalomeningocele 742.0

Encephalomeningomyelitis — *see* Meningoencephalitis
Encephalomeningopathy (*see also* Meningoencephalitis) 349.9
Encephalomyelitis (chronic) (granulomatous) (hemorrhagic necrotizing, acute) (myalgic, benign) (*see also* Encephalitis) 323.9
  abortive disseminated 049.8
  acute disseminated (postinfectious) 136.9 *[323.6]*
    postimmunization 323.5
  due to or resulting from vaccination (any) 323.5
  equine (acute) (infectious) 062.9
    Eastern 062.2
    Venezuelan 066.2
    Western 062.1
  funicularis infectiosa 049.8
  late effect — *see* Late, effect, encephalitis
  Munch-Peterson's 049.8
  postchickenpox 052.0
  postimmunization 323.5
  postmeasles 055.0
  postvaccinal (smallpox) 323.5
  rubella 056.01
  specified cause NEC 323.8
  syphilitic 094.81
Encephalomyelocele 742.0
Encephalomyelomeningitis — *see* Meningoencephalitis
Encephalomyeloneuropathy 349.9
Encephalomyelopathy 349.9
  subacute necrotizing (infantile) 330.8
Encephalomyeloradiculitis (acute) 357.0
Encephalomyeloradiculoneuritis (acute) 357.0
Encephalomyeloradiculopathy 349.9
Encephalomyocarditis 074.23
Encephalopathia hyperbilirubinemica, newborn 774.7
  due to isoimmunization (conditions classifiable to 773.0-773.2) 773.4
Encephalopathy (acute) 348.3
  alcoholic 291.2
  anoxic — *see* Damage, brain, anoxic
  arteriosclerotic 437.0
    late effect — *see* Late effect(s) (of) cerebrovascular disease
  bilirubin, newborn 774.7
    due to isoimmunization 773.4
  congenital 742.9
  demyelinating (callosal) 341.8
  due to
    birth injury (intracranial) 767.8
    dialysis 294.8
      transient 293.9
    hyperinsulinism — *see* Hyperinsulinism
    influenza (virus) 487.8
    lack of vitamin (*see also* Deficiency, vitamin) 269.2
    nicotinic acid deficiency 291.2
    serum (nontherapeutic) (therapeutic) 999.5
    syphilis 094.81
    trauma (postconcussional) 310.2
      current (*see also* Concussion, brain) 850.9
        with skull fracture — *see* Fracture, skull, by site, with intracranial injury
    vaccination 323.5

Encephalopathy — continued
  hepatic 572.2
  hyperbilirubinemic, newborn 774.7
    due to isoimmunization (conditions
      classifiable to 773.0-773.2) 773.4
  hypertensive 437.2
  hypoglycemic 251.2
  hypoxic — see Damage, brain, anoxic
  infantile cystic necrotizing (congenital) 341.8
  lead 984.9 [323.7]
  leukopolio 330.0
  metabolic (toxic) — see Delirium
  necrotizing, subacute 330.8
  pellagrous 265.2
  portal-systemic 572.2
  postcontusional 310.2
  posttraumatic 310.2
  saturnine 984.9 [323.7]
  spongioform, subacute (viral) 046.1
  subacute
    necrotizing 330.8
    spongioform 046.1
    viral, spongioform 046.1
  subcortical progressive (Schilder) 341.1
    chronic (Binswanger's) 290.12
  toxic 349.82
    metabolic — see Delirium
  traumatic (postconcussional) 310.2
    current (see also Concussion, brain) 850.9
      with skull fracture — see Fracture,
        skull, by site, with intracranial
        injury
  vitamin B deficiency NEC 266.9
  Wernicke's (superior hemorrhagic
    polioencephalitis) 265.1
Encephalorrhagia (see also Hemorrhage, brain)
  432.9
  healed or old V12.59
  late effect — see Late effect(s) (of)
    cerebrovascular disease
Encephalosis, posttraumatic 310.2
Enchondroma (M9220/0) — see also Neoplasm,
  bone, benign
  multiple, congenital 756.4
Enchondromatosis (cartilaginous) (congenital)
  (multiple) 756.4
Enchondroses, multiple (cartilaginous)
  (congenital) 756.4
Encopresis (see also Incontinence, feces) 787.6
  nonorganic origin 307.7
Encounter for — see also Admission for
  administrative purpose only V68.9
    referral of patient without examination or
      treatment V68.81
    specified purpose NEC V68.89
  chemotherapy V58.1
  end-of-life care V66.7
  hospice care V66.7
  palliative care V66.7
  paternity testing V70.4
  radiotherapy V58.0
  screening mammogram NEC V76.12
    for high-risk patient V76.11
  terminal care V66.7
Encystment — see Cyst
End-of-life care V66.7
Endamebiasis — see Amebiasis
Endamoeba — see Amebiasis

Endarteritis (bacterial, subacute) (infective)
  (septic) 447.6
  brain, cerebral or cerebrospinal 437.4
    late effect — see Late effect(s) (of)
      cerebrovascular disease
  coronary (artery) — see Arteriosclerosis,
    coronary
  deformans — see Arteriosclerosis
  embolic (see also Embolism) 444.9
  obliterans — see also Arteriosclerosis
    pulmonary 417.8
  pulmonary 417.8
  retina 362.18
  senile — see Arteriosclerosis
  syphilitic 093.89
    brain or cerebral 094.89
    congenital 090.5
    spinal 094.89
  tuberculous (see also Tuberculosis) 017.9 ✓5ᵗʰ
Endemic — see condition
Endocarditis (chronic) (indeterminate)
  (interstitial) (marantis) (nonbacterial
  thrombotic) (residual) (sclerotic) (sclerous)
  (senile) (valvular) 424.90
  with
    rheumatic fever (conditions classifiable to
      390)
      active — see Endocarditis, acute,
        rheumatic
      inactive or quiescent (with chorea) 397.9
  acute or subacute 421.9
    rheumatic (aortic) (mitral) (pulmonary)
      (tricuspid) 391.1
      with chorea (acute) (rheumatic)
        (Sydenham's) 392.0
  aortic (heart) (nonrheumatic) (valve) 424.1
  with
    mitral (valve) disease 396.9
      active or acute 391.1
        with chorea (acute) (rheumatic)
          (Sydenham's) 392.0
    rheumatic fever (conditions classifiable
      to 390)
      active — see Endocarditis, acute,
        rheumatic
      inactive or quiescent (with chorea)
        395.9
        with mitral disease 396.9
  acute or subacute 421.9
  arteriosclerotic 424.1
  congenital 746.89
  hypertensive 424.1
  rheumatic (chronic) (inactive) 395.9
    with mitral (valve) disease 396.9
      active or acute 391.1
        with chorea (acute) (rheumatic)
          (Sydenham's) 392.0
    active or acute 391.1
      with chorea (acute) (rheumatic)
        (Sydenham's) 392.0
  specified cause, except rheumatic 424.1
  syphilitic 093.22
  arteriosclerotic or due to arteriosclerosis
    424.99
  atypical verrucous (Libman-Sacks) 710.0
    [424.91]
  bacterial (acute) (any valve) (chronic)
    (subacute) 421.0
  blastomycotic 116.0 [421.1]
  candidal 112.81
  congenital 425.3

Endocarditis — continued
  constrictive 421.0
  Coxsackie 074.22
  due to
    blastomycosis 116.0 *[421.1]*
    candidiasis 112.81
    Coxsackie (virus) 074.22
    disseminated lupus erythematosus 710.0 *[424.91]*
    histoplasmosis (*see also* Histoplasmosis) 115.94
    hypertension (benign) 424.99
    moniliasis 112.81
    prosthetic cardiac valve 996.61
    Q fever 083.0 *[421.1]*
    serratia marcescens 421.0
    typhoid (fever) 002.0 *[421.1]*
  fetal 425.3
  gonococcal 098.84
  hypertensive 424.99
  infectious or infective (acute) (any valve) (chronic) (subacute) 421.0
  lenta (acute) (any valve) (chronic) (subacute) 421.0
  Libman-Sacks 710.0 *[424.91]*
  Loeffler's (parietal fibroplastic) 421.0
  malignant (acute) (any valve) (chronic) (subacute) 421.0
  meningococcal 036.42
  mitral (chronic) (double) (fibroid) (heart) (inactive) (valve) (with chorea) 394.9
    with
      aortic (valve) disease 396.9
        active or acute 391.1
          with chorea (acute) (rheumatic) (Sydenham's) 392.0
        rheumatic fever (conditions classifiable to 390)
          active — *see* Endocarditis, acute, rheumatic
          inactive or quiescent (with chorea) 394.9
      with aortic valve disease 396.9
    active or acute 391.1
      with chorea (acute) (rheumatic) (Sydenham's) 392.0
    bacterial 421.0
    arteriosclerotic 424.0
    congenital 746.89
    hypertensive 424.0
    nonrheumatic 424.0
      acute or subacute 421.9
    syphilitic 093.21
  monilial 112.81
  mycotic (acute) (any valve) (chronic) (subacute) 421.0
  pneumococcic (acute) (any valve) (chronic) (subacute) 421.0
  pulmonary (chronic) (heart) (valve) 424.3
    with
      rheumatic fever (conditions classifiable to 390)
        active — *see* Endocarditis, acute, rheumatic
        inactive or quiescent (with chorea) 397.1
    acute or subacute 421.9
      rheumatic 391.1
        with chorea (acute) (rheumatic) (Sydenham's) 392.0

Endocarditis — continued
  pulmonary — *continued*
    arteriosclerotic or due to arteriosclerosis 424.3
    congenital 746.09
    hypertensive or due to hypertension (benign) 424.3
    rheumatic (chronic) (inactive) (with chorea) 397.1
      active or acute 391.1
        with chorea (acute) (rheumatic) (Sydenham's) 392.0
    syphilitic 093.24
  purulent (acute) (any valve) (chronic) (subacute) 421.0
  rheumatic (chronic) (inactive) (with chorea) 397.9
    active or acute (aortic) (mitral) (pulmonary) (tricuspid) 391.1
      with chorea (acute) (rheumatic) (Sydenham's) 392.0
  septic (acute) (any valve) (chronic) (subacute) 421.0
  specified cause, except rheumatic 424.99
  streptococcal (acute) (any valve) (chronic) (subacute) 421.0
  subacute — *see* Endocarditis, acute
  suppurative (any valve) (acute) (chronic) (subacute) 421.0
  syphilitic NEC 093.20
  toxic (*see also* Endocarditis, acute) 421.9
  tricuspid (chronic) (heart) (inactive) (rheumatic) (valve) (with chorea) 397.0
    with
      rheumatic fever (conditions classifiable to 390)
        active — *see* Endocarditis, acute, rheumatic
        inactive or quiescent (with chorea) 397.0
    active or acute 391.1
      with chorea (acute) (rheumatic) (Sydenham's) 392.0
    arteriosclerotic 424.2
    congenital 746.89
    hypertensive 424.2
    nonrheumatic 424.2
      acute or subacute 421.9
    specified cause, except rheumatic 424.2
    syphilitic 093.23
  tuberculous (*see also* Tuberculosis) 017.9 *[424.91]*
  typhoid 002.0 *[421.1]*
  ulcerative (acute) (any valve) (chronic) (subacute) 421.0
  vegetative (acute) (any valve) (chronic) (subacute) 421.0
  verrucous (acute) (any valve) (chronic) (subacute) NEC 710.0 *[424.91]*
    nonbacterial 710.0 *[424.91]*
    nonrheumatic 710.0 *[424.91]*

Endocardium, endocardial — *see also* condition
  cushion defect 745.60
  specified type NEC 745.69

Endocervicitis (*see also* Cervicitis) 616.0
  due to
    intrauterine (contraceptive) device 996.65
  gonorrheal (acute) 098.15
    chronic or duration of 2 months or over 098.35
  hyperplastic 616.0

Endocervicitis — continued
    syphilitic 095.8
    trichomonal 131.09
    tuberculous (see also Tuberculosis) 016.7
Endocrine — see condition
Endocrinopathy, pluriglandular 258.9
Endodontitis 522.0
Endomastoiditis (see also Mastoiditis) 383.9
Endometrioma 617.9
Endometriosis 617.9
    appendix 617.5
    bladder 617.8
    bowel 617.5
    broad ligament 617.3
    cervix 617.0
    colon 617.5
    cul-de-sac (Douglas') 617.3
    exocervix 617.0
    fallopian tube 617.2
    female genital organ NEC 617.8
    gallbladder 617.8
    in scar of skin 617.6
    internal 617.0
    intestine 617.5
    lung 617.8
    myometrium 617.0
    ovary 617.1
    parametrium 617.3
    pelvic peritoneum 617.3
    peritoneal (pelvic) 617.3
    rectovaginal septum 617.4
    rectum 617.5
    round ligament 617.3
    skin 617.6
    specified site NEC 617.8
    stromal (M8931/1) 236.0
    umbilicus 617.8
    uterus 617.0
        internal 617.0
    vagina 617.4
    vulva 617.8
Endometritis (nonspecific) (purulent) (septic) (suppurative) 615.9
    with
        abortion — see Abortion, by type, with sepsis
        ectopic pregnancy (see also categories 633.0-633.9) 639.0
        molar pregancy (see also categories 630-632) 639.0
    acute 615.0
    blennorrhagic 098.16
        acute 098.16
        chronic or duration of 2 months or over 098.36
    cervix, cervical (see also Cervicitis) 616.0
        hyperplastic 616.0
    chronic 615.1
    complicating pregnancy 646.6
        affecting fetus or newborn 760.8
    decidual 615.9
    following
        abortion 639.0
        ectopic or molar pregnancy 639.0
    gonorrheal (acute) 098.16
        chronic or duration of 2 months or over 098.36
    hyperplastic 621.3
        cervix 616.0
    polypoid — see Endometritis, hyperplastic

Endometritis — continued
    puerperal, postpartum, childbirth 670
    senile (atrophic) 615.9
    subacute 615.0
    tuberculous (see also Tuberculosis) 016.7
Endometrium — see condition
Endomyocardiopathy, South African 425.2
Endomyocarditis — see Endocarditis
Endomyofibrosis 425.0
Endomyometritis (see also Endometritis) 615.9
Endopericarditis — see Endocarditis
Endoperineuritis — see Disorder, nerve
Endophlebitis (see also Phlebitis) 451.9
    leg 451.2
        deep (vessels) 451.19
        superficial (vessels) 451.0
    portal (vein) 572.1
    retina 362.18
    specified site NEC 451.89
    syphilitic 093.89
Endophthalmia (see also Endophthalmitis) 360.00
    gonorrheal 098.42
Endophthalmitis (globe) (infective) (metastatic) (purulent) (subacute) 360.00
    acute 360.01
    chronic 360.03
    parasitis 360.13
    phacoanaphylactic 360.19
    specified type NEC 360.19
    sympathetic 360.11
Endosalpingioma (M9111/1) 236.2
Endosteitis — see Osteomyelitis
Endothelioma, bone (M9260/3) — see Neoplasm, bone, malignant
Endotheliosis 287.8
    hemorrhagic infectional 287.8
Endotoxic shock 785.59
Endotrachelitis (see also Cervicitis) 616.0
Enema rash 692.89
Engel-von Recklinghausen disease or syndrome (osteitis fibrosa cystica) 252.0
Engelmann's disease (diaphyseal sclerosis) 756.9
English disease (see also Rickets) 268.0
Engman's disease (infectious eczematoid dermatitis) 690.8
Engorgement
    breast 611.79
        newborn 778.7
        puerperal, postpartum 676.2
    liver 573.9
    lung 514
    pulmonary 514
    retina, venous 362.37
    stomach 536.8
    venous, retina 362.37
Enlargement, enlarged — see also Hypertrophy
    abdomen 789.3
    adenoids 474.12
        and tonsils 474.10
    alveolar process or ridge 525.8
    apertures of diaphragm (congenital) 756.6
    blind spot, visual field 368.42
    gingival 523.8
    heart, cardiac (see also Hypertrophy, cardiac) 429.3

Enlargement, enlarged — *continued*
  lacrimal gland, chronic 375.03
  liver (*see also* Hypertrophy, liver) 789.1
  lymph gland or node 785.6
  orbit 376.46
  organ or site, congenital NEC — *see* Anomaly, specified type NEC
  parathyroid (gland) 252.0
  pituitary fossa 793.0
  prostate ▶(simple) (soft)◀ 600.0
  sella turcica 793.0
  spleen (*see also* Splenomegaly) 789.2
    congenital 759.0
  thymus (congenital) (gland) 254.0
  thyroid (gland) (*see also* Goiter) 240.9
  tongue 529.8
  tonsils 474.11
    and adenoids 474.10
  uterus 621.2
Enophthalmos 376.50
  due to
    atrophy of orbital tissue 376.51
    surgery 376.52
    trauma 376.52
Enostosis 526.89
Entamebiasis — *see* Amebiasis
Entamebic — *see* Amebiasis
Entanglement, umbilical cord(s) 663.3
  with compression 663.2
    affecting fetus or newborn 762.5
  around neck with compression 663.1
  twins in monoamniotic sac 663.2
Enteralgia 789.0
Enteric — *see* condition
Enteritis (acute) (catarrhal) (choleraic) (chronic) (congestive) (diarrheal) (exudative) (follicular) (hemorrhagic) (infantile) (lienteric) (noninfectious) (perforative) (phlegmonous) (presumed noninfectious) (pseudomembranous) 558.9
  adaptive 564.9
  aertrycke infection 003.0
  allergic 558.3
  amebic (*see also* Amebiasis) 006.9
    with abscess — *see* Abscess, amebic
    acute 006.0
      with abscess — *see* Abscess, amebic
      nondysenteric 006.2
    chronic 006.1
      with abscess — *see* Abscess, amebic
      nondysenteric 006.2
    nondysenteric 006.2
  anaerobic (cocci) (gram-negative) (gram-positive) (mixed) NEC 008.46
  bacillary NEC 004.9
  bacterial NEC 008.5
    specified NEC 008.49
  Bacteroides (fragilis) (melaninogeniscus) (oralis) 008.46
  Butyrivibrio (fibriosolvens) 008.46
  Campylobacter 008.43
  Candida 112.85
  Chilomastix 007.8
  choleriformis 001.1
  chronic 558.9
    ulcerative (*see also* Colitis, ulcerative) 556.9
  cicatrizing (chronic) 555.0
  Clostridium
    botulinum 005.1
    difficile 008.45

Enteritis — *continued*
  Clostridium — *continued*
    haemolyticum 008.46
    novyi 008.46
    perfringens (C) (F) 008.46
    specified type NEC 008.46
  coccidial 007.2
  dietetic 558.9
  due to
    achylia gastrica 536.8
    adenovirus 008.62
    Aerobacter aerogenes 008.2
    anaerobes — *see* Enteritis, anaerobic
    Arizona (bacillus) 008.1
    astrovirus 008.66
    Bacillus coli — *see* Enteritis, E. coli 008.0
    bacteria NEC 008.5
      specified NEC 008.49
    Bacteroides 008.46
    Butyrivibrio (fibriosolvens)
    Calcivirus 008.65
    Camplyobacter 008.43
    Clostridium — *see* Enteritis, Clostridium
    Cockle agent 008.64
    Coxsackie (virus) 008.67
    Ditchling agent 008.64
    ECHO virus 008.67
    Enterobacter aerogenes 008.2
    enterococci 008.49
    enterovirus NEC 008.67
    Escherichia coli — *see* Enteritis, E. coli 008.0
    Eubacterium 008.46
    Fusobacterium (nucleatum) 008.46
    gram-negative bacteria NEC 008.47
      anaerobic NEC 008.46
    Hawaii agent 008.63
    irritating foods 558.9
    Klebsiella aerogenes 008.47
    Marin County agent 008.66
    Montgomery County agent 008.63
    Norwalk-like agent 008.63
    Norwalk virus 008.63
    Otofuke agent 008.63
    Paracolobactrum arizonae 008.1
    paracolon bacillus NEC 008.47
      Arizona 008.1
    Paramatta agent 008.64
    Peptococcus 008.46
    Peptostreptococcus 008.46
    Proprionibacterium 008.46
    Proteus (bacillus) (mirabilis) (morganii) 008.3
    Pseudomonas aeruginosa 008.42
    Rotavirus 008.61
    Sapporo agent 008.63
    small round virus (SRV) NEC 008.64
      featureless NEC 008.63
      structured NEC 008.63
    Snow Mountain (SM) agent 008.63
    specified
      bacteria NEC 008.49
      organism, nonbacterial NEC 008.8
      virus (NEC) 008.69
    Staphylococcus 008.41
    Streptococcus 008.49
      anaerobic 008.46
    Taunton agent 008.63
    Torovirus 008.69
    Treponema 008.46

Enteritis — continued
  due to — continued
    Veillonella 008.46
    virus 008.8
      specified type NEC 008.69
    Wollan (W) agent 008.64
    Yersinia enterocolitica 008.44
  dysentery — see Dysentery
  E. coli 008.00
    enterohemorrhagic 008.04
    enteroinvasive 008.03
    enteropathogenic 008.01
    enterotoxigenic 008.02
    specified type NEC 008.09
  el tor 001.1
  embadomonial 007.8
  epidemic 009.0
  Eubacterium 008.46
  fermentative 558.9
  fulminant 557.0
  Fusobacterium (nucleatum) 008.46
  gangrenous (see also Enteritis, due to, by organism) 009.0
  giardial 007.1
  gram-negative bacteria NEC 008.47
    anaerobic NEC 008.46
  infectious NEC (see also Enteritis, due to, by organism) 009.0
    presumed 009.1
  influenzal 487.8
  ischemic 557.9
    acute 557.0
    chronic 557.1
    due to mesenteric artery insufficiency 557.1
  membranous 564.9
  mucous 564.9
  myxomembranous 564.9
  necrotic (see also Enteritis, due to, by organism) 009.0
  necroticans 005.2
  necrotizing of fetus or newborn 777.5
  neurogenic 564.9
  newborn 777.8
    necrotizing 777.5
  parasitic NEC 129
  paratyphoid (fever) (see also Fever, paratyphoid) 002.9
  Peptococcus 008.46
  Peptostreptococcus 008.46
  Proprionibacterium 008.46
  protozoal NEC 007.9
  radiation 558.1
  regional (of) 555.9
    intestine
      large (bowel, colon, or rectum) 555.1
        with small intestine 555.2
      small (duodenum, ileum, or jejunum) 555.0
        with large intestine 555.2
  Salmonella infection 003.0
  salmonellosis 003.0
  segmental (see also Enteritis, regional) 555.9
  septic (see also Enteritis, due to, by organism) 009.0
  Shigella 004.9
  simple 558.9
  spasmodic 564.9
  spastic 564.9
  staphylococcal 008.41
    due to food 005.0

Enteritis — continued
  streptococcal 008.49
    anaerobic 008.46
  toxic 558.2
  Treponema (denticola) (macrodentium) 008.46
  trichomonal 007.3
  tuberculous (see also Tuberculosis) 014.8
  typhosa 002.0
  ulcerative (chronic) (see also Colitis, ulcerative) 556.9
  Veillonella 008.46
  viral 008.8
    adenovirus 008.62
    enterovirus 008.67
    specified virus NEC 008.69
  Yersinia enterocolitica 008.44
  zymotic 009.0
Enteroarticular syndrome 099.3
Enterobiasis 127.4
Enterobius vermicularis 127.4
Enterocele (see also Hernia) 553.9
  pelvis, pelvic (acquired) (congenital) 618.6
  vagina, vaginal (acquired) (congenital) 618.6
Enterocolitis — see also Enteritis
  fetus or newborn 777.8
    necrotizing 777.5
  fulminant 557.0
  granulomatous 555.2
  hemorrhagic (acute) 557.0
    chronic 557.1
  necrotizing (acute) membranous) 557.0
  primary necrotizing 777.5
  pseudomembranous 008.45
  radiation 558.1
    newborn 777.5
  ulcerative 556.0
Enterocystoma 751.5
Enterogastritis — see Enteritis
Enterogenous cyanosis 289.7
Enterolith, enterolithiasis (impaction) 560.39
  with hernia — see also Hernia, by site, with obstruction
    gangrenous — see Hernia, by site, with gangrene
Enteropathy 569.9
  exudative (of Gordon) 579.8
  gluten 579.0
  hemorrhagic, terminal 557.0
  protein-losing 579.8
Enteroperitonitis (see also Peritonitis) 567.9
Enteroptosis 569.89
Enterorrhagia 578.9
Enterospasm 564.9
  psychogenic 306.4
Enterostenosis (see also Obstruction, intestine) 560.9
Enterostomy status V44.4
  with complication 569.60
Enthesopathy 726.39
  ankle and tarsus 726.70
  elbow region 726.30
    specified NEC 726.39
  hip 726.5
  knee 726.60
  peripheral NEC 726.8
  shoulder region 726.10
    adhesive 726.0
  spinal 720.1

Enthesopathy — *continued*
  wrist and carpus 726.4
Entrance, air into vein — *see* Embolism, air
Entrapment, nerve — *see* Neuropathy, entrapment
Entropion (eyelid) 374.00
  cicatricial 374.04
  congenital 743.62
  late effect of trachoma (healed) 139.1
  mechanical 374.02
  paralytic 374.02
  senile 374.01
  spastic 374.03
Enucleation of eye (current) (traumatic) 871.3
Enuresis 788.30
  habit disturbance 307.6
  nocturnal 788.36
    psychogenic 307.6
  nonorganic origin 307.6
  psychogenic 307.6
Enzymopathy 277.9
Eosinopenia 288.0
Eosinophilia 288.3
  allergic 288.3
  hereditary 288.3
  idiopathic 288.3
  infiltrative 518.3
  Loeffler's 518.3
  myalgia syndrome 710.5
  pulmonary (tropical) 518.3
  secondary 288.3
  tropical 518.3
Eosinophilic — *see also* condition
  fasciitis 728.89
  granuloma (bone) 277.8
  infiltration lung 518.3
Ependymitis (acute) (cerebral) (chronic) (granular) (*see also* Meningitis) 322.9
Ependymoblastoma (M9392/3)
  specified site — *see* Neoplasm, by site, malignant
  unspecified site 191.9
Ependymoma (epithelial) (malignant) (M9391/3)
  anaplastic type (M9392/3)
    specified site — *see* Neoplasm, by site, malignant
    unspecified site 191.9
  benign (M9391/0)
    specified site — *see* Neoplasm, by site, benign
    unspecified site 225.0
  myxopapillary (M9394/1) 237.5
  papillary (M9393/1) 237.5
  specified site — *see* Neoplasm, by site, malignant
  unspecified site 191.9
Ependymopathy 349.2
  spinal cord 349.2
Ephelides, ephelis 709.09
Ephemeral fever (*see also* Pyrexia) 780.6
Epiblepharon (congenital) 743.62
Epicanthus, epicanthic fold (congenital) (eyelid) 743.63
Epicondylitis (elbow) (lateral) 726.32
  medial 726.31
Epicystitis (*see also* Cystitis) 595.9
Epidemic — *see* condition
Epidermidalization, cervix — *see* condition

Epidermidization, cervix — *see* condition
Epidermis, epidermal — *see* condition
Epidermization, cervix — *see* condition
Epidermodysplasia verruciformis 078.19
Epidermoid
  cholesteatoma — *see* Cholesteatoma
  inclusion (*see also* Cyst, skin) 706.2
Epidermolysis
  acuta (combustiformis) (toxica) 695.1
  bullosa 757.39
  necroticans combustiformis 695.1
    due to drug
      correct substance properly administered 695.1
      overdose or wrong substance given or taken 977.9
        specified drug — *see* Table of Drugs and Chemicals
Epidermophytid — *see* Dermatophytosis
Epidermophytosis (infected) — *see* Dermatophytosis
Epidermosis, ear (middle) (*see also* Cholesteatoma) 385.30
Epididymis — *see* condition
Epididymitis (nonvenereal) 604.90
  with abscess 604.0
  acute 604.99
  blennorrhagic (acute) 098.0
    chronic or duration of 2 months or over 098.2
  caseous (*see also* Tuberculosis) 016.4 ✓5ᵗʰ
  chlamydial 099.54
  diphtheritic 032.89 [604.91]
  filarial 125.9 [604.91]
  gonococcal (acute) 098.0
    chronic or duration of 2 months or over 098.2
  recurrent 604.99
  residual 604.99
  syphilitic 095.8 [604.91]
  tuberculous (*see also* Tuberculosis) 016.4 ✓5ᵗʰ
Epididymo-orchitis (*see also* Epididymitis) 604.90
  with abscess 604.0
  chlamydial 099.54
  gonococcal (acute) 098.13
    chronic or duration of 2 months or over 098.33
Epidural — *see* condition
Epigastritis (*see also* Gastritis) 535.5 ✓5ᵗʰ
Epigastrium, epigastric — *see* condition
Epigastrocele (*see also* Hernia, epigastric) 553.29
Epiglottiditis (acute) 464.30
  with obstruction 464.31
  chronic 476.1
  viral 464.30
    with obstruction 464.31
Epiglottis — *see* condition
Epiglottitis (acute) 464.30
  with obstruction 464.31
  chronic 476.1
  viral 464.30
    with obstruction 464.31
Epignathus 759.4
Epilepsia
  partialis continua (*see also* Epilepsy) 345.7 ✓5ᵗʰ

Epilepsia — continued
  procursiva (see also Epilepsy) 345.8 ✓5ᵗʰ
Epilepsy, epileptic (idiopathic) 345.9 ✓5ᵗʰ

> Note — use the following fifth-digit subclassification with categories 345.0, 345.1, 345.4–345.9:
> 0 without mention of intractable epilepsy
> 1 with intractable epilepsy

  abdominal 345.5 ✓5ᵗʰ
  absence (attack) 345.0 ✓5ᵗʰ
  akinetic 345.0 ✓5ᵗʰ
    psychomotor 345.4 ✓5ᵗʰ
  automatism 345.4 ✓5ᵗʰ
  autonomic diencephalic 345.5 ✓5ᵗʰ
  brain 345.9 ✓5ᵗʰ
  Bravais-Jacksonian 345.5 ✓5ᵗʰ
  cerebral 345.9 ✓5ᵗʰ
  climacteric 345.9 ✓5ᵗʰ
  clonic 345.1 ✓5ᵗʰ
  clouded state 345.9 ✓5ᵗʰ
  coma 345.3
  communicating 345.4 ✓5ᵗʰ
  congenital 345.9 ✓5ᵗʰ
  convulsions 345.9 ✓5ᵗʰ
  cortical (focal) (motor) 345.5 ✓5ᵗʰ
  cursive (running) 345.8 ✓5ᵗʰ
  cysticercosis 123.1
  deterioration
    with behavioral disturbance 345.9 ✓5ᵗʰ [294.11]
    without behavioral disturbance 345.9 ✓5ᵗʰ [294.10]
  due to syphilis 094.89
  equivalent 345.5 ✓5ᵗʰ
  fit 345.9 ✓5ᵗʰ
  focal (motor) 345.5 ✓5ᵗʰ
  gelastic 345.8 ✓5ᵗʰ
  generalized 345.9 ✓5ᵗʰ
    convulsive 345.1 ✓5ᵗʰ
    flexion 345.1 ✓5ᵗʰ
    nonconvulsive 345.0 ✓5ᵗʰ
  grand mal (idiopathic) 345.1 ✓5ᵗʰ
  Jacksonian (motor) (sensory) 345.5 ✓5ᵗʰ
  Kojevnikoff's, Kojevnikov's, Kojewnikoff's 345.7 ✓5ᵗʰ
  laryngeal 786.2
  limbic system 345.4 ✓5ᵗʰ
  major (motor) 345.1 ✓5ᵗʰ
  minor 345.0 ✓5ᵗʰ
  mixed (type) 345.9 ✓5ᵗʰ
  motor partial 345.5 ✓5ᵗʰ
  musicogenic 345.1 ✓5ᵗʰ
  myoclonus, myoclonic 345.1 ✓5ᵗʰ
    progressive (familial) 333.2
  nonconvulsive, generalized 345.0 ✓5ᵗʰ
  parasitic NEC 123.9
  partial (focalized) 345.5 ✓5ᵗʰ
    with
      impairment of consciousness 345.4 ✓5ᵗʰ
      memory and ideational disturbances 345.4 ✓5ᵗʰ
      abdominal type 345.5 ✓5ᵗʰ
      motor type 345.5 ✓5ᵗʰ
      psychomotor type 345.4 ✓5ᵗʰ
      psychosensory type 345.4 ✓5ᵗʰ
      secondarily generalized 345.4 ✓5ᵗʰ
      sensory type 345.5 ✓5ᵗʰ
      somatomotor type 345.5 ✓5ᵗʰ

Epilepsy, epileptic — continued
  partial — continued
    somatosensory type 345.5 ✓5ᵗʰ
    temporal lobe type 345.4 ✓5ᵗʰ
    visceral type 345.5 ✓5ᵗʰ
    visual type 345.5 ✓5ᵗʰ
  peripheral 345.9 ✓5ᵗʰ
  petit mal 345.0 ✓5ᵗʰ
  photokinetic 345.8 ✓5ᵗʰ
  progressive myoclonic (familial) 333.2
  psychic equivalent 345.5 ✓5ᵗʰ
  psychomotor 345.4 ✓5ᵗʰ
  psychosensory 345.4 ✓5ᵗʰ
  reflex 345.1 ✓5ᵗʰ
  seizure 345.9 ✓5ᵗʰ
  senile 345.9 ✓5ᵗʰ
  sensory-induced 345.5 ✓5ᵗʰ
  sleep 347
  somatomotor type 345.5 ✓5ᵗʰ
  somatosensory 345.5 ✓5ᵗʰ
  specified type NEC 345.8 ✓5ᵗʰ
  status (grand mal) 345.3
    focal motor 345.7 ✓5ᵗʰ
    petit mal 345.2
    psychomotor 345.7 ✓5ᵗʰ
    temporal lobe 345.7 ✓5ᵗʰ
  symptomatic 345.9 ✓5ᵗʰ
  temporal lobe 345.4 ✓5ᵗʰ
  tonic (-clonic) 345.1 ✓5ᵗʰ
  traumatic (injury unspecified) 907.0
    injury specified — see Late, effect (of) specified injury
  twilight 293.0
  uncinate (gyrus) 345.4 ✓5ᵗʰ
  Unverricht (-Lundborg) (familial myoclonic) 333.2
  visceral 345.5 ✓5ᵗʰ
  visual 345.5 ✓5ᵗʰ
Epileptiform
  convulsions 780.39
  seizure 780.39
Epiloia 759.5
Epimenorrhea 626.2
Epipharyngitis (see also Nasopharyngitis) 460
Epiphora 375.20
  due to
    excess lacrimation 375.21
    insufficient drainage 375.22
Epiphyseal arrest 733.91
  femoral head 732.2
Epiphyseolysis, epiphysiolysis (see also Osteochondrosis) 732.9
Epiphysitis (see also Osteochondrosis) 732.9
  juvenile 732.6
  marginal (Scheuermann's) 732.0
  os calcis 732.5
  syphilitic (congenital) 090.0
  vertebral (Scheuermann's) 732.0
Epiplocele (see also Hernia) 553.9
Epiploitis (see also Peritonitis) 567.9
Epiplosarcomphalocele (see also Hernia, umbilicus) 553.1
Episcleritis 379.00
  gouty 274.89 [379.09]
  nodular 379.02
  periodica fugax 379.01
    angioneurotic — see Edema, angioneurotic
  specified NEC 379.09
  staphylococcal 379.00

Episcleritis — *continued*
  suppurative 379.00
  syphilitic 095.0
  tuberculous (*see also* Tuberculosis) 017.3 ✓5ᵗʰ
    [379.09]

Episode
  brain (*see also* Disease, cerebrovascular, acute) 436
  cerebral (*see also* Disease, cerebrovascular, acute) 436
  depersonalization (in neurotic state) 300.6
  hyporesponsive 780.09
  psychotic (*see also* Psychosis) 298.9
    organic, transient 293.9
  schizophrenic (acute) NEC (*see also* Schizophrenia) 295.4 ✓5ᵗʰ

Epispadias
  female 753.8
  male 752.62

Episplenitis 289.59

Epistaxis (multiple) 784.7
  hereditary 448.0
  vicarious menstruation 625.8

Epithelioma (malignant) (M8011/3) — *see also* Neoplasm, by site, malignant
  adenoides cysticum (M8100/0) — *see* Neoplasm, skin, benign
  basal cell (M8090/3) — *see* Neoplasm, skin, malignant
  benign (M8011/0) — *see* Neoplasm, by site, benign
  Bowen's (M8081/2) — *see* Neoplasm, skin, in situ
  calcifying (benign) (Malherbe's) (M8110/0) — *see* Neoplasm, skin, benign
  external site — *see* Neoplasm, skin, malignant
  intraepidermal, Jadassohn (M8096/0) — *see* Neoplasm, skin, benign
  squamous cell (M8070/3) — *see* Neoplasm, by site, malignant

Epitheliopathy
  pigment, retina 363.15
  posterior multifocal placoid (acute) 363.15

Epithelium, epithelial — *see* condition

Epituberculosis (allergic) (with atelectasis) (*see also* Tuberculosis) 010.8 ✓5ᵗʰ

Eponychia 757.5

Epstein's
  nephrosis or syndrome (*see also* Nephrosis) 581.9
  pearl (mouth) 528.4

Epstein-Barr infection (viral) 075
  chronic 780.79 *[139.8]*

Epulis (giant cell) (gingiva) 523.8

Equinia 024

Equinovarus (congenital) 754.51
  acquired 736.71

Equivalent
  convulsive (abdominal) (*see also* Epilepsy) 345.5 ✓5ᵗʰ
  epileptic (psychic) (*see also* Epilepsy) 345.5 ✓5ᵗʰ

Erb's
  disease 359.1
  palsy, paralysis (birth) (brachial) (newborn) 767.6
    spinal (spastic) syphilitic 094.89
  pseudohypertrophic muscular dystrophy 359.1

Erb (-Duchenne) paralysis (birth injury) (newborn) 767.6

Erb-Goldflam disease or syndrome 358.0

Erdheim's syndrome (acromegalic macrospondylitis) 253.0

Erection, painful (persistent) 607.3

Ergosterol deficiency (vitamin D) 268.9
  with
    osteomalacia 268.2
    rickets (*see also* Rickets) 268.0

Ergotism (ergotized grain) 988.2
  from ergot used as drug (migraine therapy)
    correct substance properly administered 349.82
    overdose or wrong substance given or taken 975.0

Erichsen's disease (railway spine) 300.16

Erlacher-Blount syndrome (tibia vara) 732.4

Erosio interdigitalis blastomycetica 112.3

Erosion
  artery NEC 447.2
    without rupture 447.8
  arteriosclerotic plaque — *see* Arteriosclerosis, by site
  bone 733.99
  bronchus 519.1
  cartilage (joint) 733.99
  cervix (uteri) (acquired) (chronic) (congenital) 622.0
    with mention of cervicitis 616.0
  cornea (recurrent) (*see also* Keratitis) 371.42
    traumatic 918.1
  dental (idiopathic) (occupational) 521.3
  duodenum, postpyloric — *see* Ulcer, duodenum
  esophagus 530.89
  gastric 535.4 ✓5ᵗʰ
  intestine 569.89
  lymphatic vessel 457.8
  pylorus, pyloric (ulcer) 535.4 ✓5ᵗʰ
  sclera 379.16
  spine, aneurysmal 094.89
  spleen 289.59
  stomach 535.4 ✓5ᵗʰ
  teeth (idiopathic) (occupational) 521.3
    due to
      medicine 521.3
      persistent vomiting 521.3
  urethra 599.84
  uterus 621.8
  vertebra 733.99

Erotomania 302.89
  Clérambault's 297.8

Error
  in diet 269.9
  refractive 367.9
    astigmatism (*see also* Astigmatism) 367.20
    drug-induced 367.89
    hypermetropia 367.0
    hyperopia 367.0
    myopia 367.1
    presbyopia 367.4
    toxic 367.89

Eructation 787.3
  nervous 306.4
  psychogenic 306.4

Eruption
  creeping 126.9
  drug — *see* Dermatitis, due to, drug

Eruption — continued
  Hutchinson, summer 692.72
  Kaposi's varicelliform 054.0
  napkin (psoriasiform) 691.0
  polymorphous
    light (sun) 692.72
      other source 692.82
  psoriasiform, napkin 691.0
  recalcitrant pustular 694.8
  ringed 695.89
  skin (see also Dermatitis) 782.1
    creeping (meaning hookworm) 126.9
    due to
      chemical(s) NEC 692.4
        internal use 693.8
      drug — see Dermatitis, due to, drug
      prophylactic inoculation or vaccination
        against disease — see Dermatitis,
        due to, vaccine
      smallpox vaccination NEC — see
        Dermatitis, due to, vaccine
    erysipeloid 027.1
    feigned 698.4
    Hutchinson, summer 692.72
    Kaposi's, varicelliform 054.0
      vaccinia 999.0
    lichenoid, axilla 698.3
    polymorphous, due to light 692.72
    toxic NEC 695.0
    vesicular 709.8
  teeth, tooth
    accelerated 520.6
    delayed 520.6
    difficult 520.6
    disturbance of 520.6
    in abnormal sequence 520.6
    incomplete 520.6
    late 520.6
    natal 520.6
    neonatal 520.6
    obstructed 520.6
    partial 520.6
    persistent primary 520.6
    premature 520.6
  vesicular 709.8
Erysipelas (gangrenous) (infantile) (newborn)
    (phlegmonous) (suppurative) 035
  external ear 035 [380.13]
  puerperal, postpartum, childbirth 670 ✓5ᵗʰ
Erysipelatoid (Rosenbach's) 027.1
Erysipeloid (Rosenbach's) 027.1
Erythema, erythematous (generalized) 695.9
  ab igne — see Burn, by site, first degree
  annulare (centrifugum) (rheumaticum) 695.0
  arthriticum epidemicum 026.1
  brucellum (see also Brucellosis) 023.9
  bullosum 695.1
  caloricum — see Burn, by site, first degree
  chronicum migrans 088.81
    chronicum 088.81
  circinatum 695.1
  diaper 691.0
  due to
    chemical (contact) NEC 692.4
      internal 693.8
    drug (internal use) 693.0
      contact 692.3
  elevatum diutinum 695.89
  endemic 265.2
  epidemic, arthritic 026.1
  figuratum perstans 695.0

Erythema, erythematous — continued
  gluteal 691.0
  gyratum (perstans) (repens) 695.1
  heat — see Burn, by site, first degree
  ichthyosiforme congenitum 757.1
  induratum (primary) (scrofulosorum) (see also
      Tuberculosis) 017.1 ✓5ᵗʰ
    nontuberculous 695.2
  infantum febrile 057.8
  infectional NEC 695.9
  infectiosum 057.0
  inflammation NEC 695.9
  intertrigo 695.89
  iris 695.1
  lupus (discoid) (localized) (see also Lupus
      erythematosus) 695.4
  marginatum 695.0
    rheumaticum — see Fever, rheumatic
  medicamentosum — see Dermatitis, due to,
      drug
  migrans 529.1
    chronicum 088.81
  multiforme 695.1
    bullosum 695.1
    conjunctiva 695.1
    exudativum (Hebra) 695.1
    pemphigoides 694.5
  napkin 691.0
  neonatorum 778.8
  nodosum 695.2
    tuberculous (see also Tuberculosis)
        017.1 ✓5ᵗʰ
  nummular, nummulare 695.1
  palmar 695.0
  palmaris hereditarium 695.0
  pernio 991.5
  perstans solare 692.72
  rash, newborn 778.8
  scarlatiniform (exfoliative) (recurrent) 695.0
  simplex marginatum 057.8
  solare (see also Sunburn) 692.71
  streptogenes 696.5
  toxic, toxicum NEC 695.0
    newborn 778.8
  tuberculous (primary) (see also Tuberculosis)
      017.0 ✓5ᵗʰ
  venenatum 695.0
Erythematosus — see condition
Erythematous — see condition
Erythermalgia (primary) 443.89
Erythralgia 443.89
Erythrasma 039.0
Erythredema 985.0
  polyneuritica 985.0
  polyneuropathy 985.0
Erythremia (acute) (M9841/3) 207.0 ✓5ᵗʰ
  chronic (M9842/3) 207.1 ✓5ᵗʰ
  secondary 289.0
Erythroblastopenia (acquired) 284.8
  congenital 284.0
Erythroblastophthisis 284.0
Erythroblastosis (fetalis) (newborn) 773.2
  due to
    ABO
      antibodies 773.1
      incompatibility, maternal/fetal 773.1
      isoimmunization 773.1
    Rh
      antibodies 773.0
      incompatibility, maternal/fetal 773.0
      isoimmunization 773.0

Erythrocyanosis (crurum) 443.89
Erythrocythemia — see Erythremia
Erythrocytopenia 285.9
Erythrocytosis (megalosplenic)
 familial 289.6
 oval, hereditary (see also Elliptocytosis) 282.1
 secondary 289.0
 stress 289.0
Erythroderma (see also Erythema) 695.9
 desquamativa (in infants) 695.89
 exfoliative 695.89
 ichthyosiform, congenital 757.1
 infantum 695.89
 maculopapular 696.2
 neonatorum 778.8
 psoriaticum 696.1
 secondary 695.9
Erythrogenesis imperfecta 284.0
Erythroleukemia (M9840/3) 207.0 ✓5ᵗʰ
Erythromelalgia 443.89
Erythromelia 701.8
Erythropenia 285.9
Erythrophagocytosis 289.9
Erythrophobia 300.23
Erythroplakia
 oral mucosa 528.7
 tongue 528.7
Erythroplasia (Queyrat) (M8080/2)
 specified site — see Neoplasm, skin, in situ
 unspecified site 233.5
Erythropoiesis, idiopathic ineffective 285.0
Escaped beats, heart 427.60
 postoperative 997.1
Esoenteritis — see Enteritis
Esophagalgia 530.89
Esophagectasis 530.89
 due to cardiospasm 530.0
Esophagismus 530.5
Esophagitis (alkaline) (chemical) (chronic) (infectional) (necrotic) (peptic) (postoperative) (regurgitant) 530.10
 acute 530.12
 candidal 112.84
 reflux 530.11
 specified NEC 530.19
 tuberculous (see also Tuberculosis) 017.8 ✓5ᵗʰ
 ulcerative 530.19
Esophagocele 530.6
Esophagodynia 530.89
Esophagomalacia 530.89
Esophagoptosis 530.89
Esophagospasm 530.5
Esophagostenosis 530.3
Esophagostomiasis 127.7
Esophagotracheal — see condition
Esophagus — see condition
Esophoria 378.41
 convergence, excess 378.84
 divergence, insufficiency 378.85
Esotropia (nonaccommodative) 378.00
 accommodative 378.35
 alternating 378.05
  with
   A pattern 378.06
   specified noncomitancy NEC 378.08
   V pattern 378.07

Esotropia — continued
 alternating — continued
  with — continued
   X pattern 378.08
   Y pattern 378.08
  intermittent 378.22
 intermittent 378.20
  alternating 378.22
  monocular 378.21
 monocular 378.01
  with
   A pattern 378.02
   specified noncomitancy NEC 378.04
   V pattern 378.03
   X pattern 378.04
   Y pattern 378.04
  intermittent 378.21
Espundia 085.5
Essential — see condition
Esterapenia 289.8
Esthesioneuroblastoma (M9522/3) 160.0
Esthesioneurocytoma (M9521/3) 160.0
Esthesioneuroepithelioma (M9523/3) 160.0
Esthiomene 099.1
Estivo-autumnal
 fever 084.0
 malaria 084.0
Estrangement V61.0
Estriasis 134.0
Ethanolaminuria 270.8
Ethanolism (see also Alcoholism) 303.9 ✓5ᵗʰ
Ether dependence, dependency (see also Dependence) 304.6 ✓5ᵗʰ
Etherism (see also Dependence) 304.6 ✓5ᵗʰ
Ethmoid, ethmoidal — see condition
Ethmoiditis (chronic) (nonpurulent) (purulent) (see also Sinusitis, ethmoidal) 473.2
 influenzal 487.1
 Woakes' 471.1
Ethylism (see also Alcoholism) 303.9 ✓5ᵗʰ
Eulenburg's disease (congenital paramyotonia) 359.2
Eunuchism 257.2
Eunuchoidism 257.2
 hypogonadotropic 257.2
European blastomycosis 117.5
Eustachian — see condition
Euthyroid sick syndrome 790.94
Euthyroidism 244.9
Evaluation
 fetal lung maturity 659.8
 for suspected condition (see also Observation) V71.9
  abuse V71.81
  exposure
   anthrax V71.82
   biologic agent NEC V71.83
  neglect V71.81
  newborn — see Observation, suspected, condition, newborn
  specified condition NEC V71.89
 mental health V70.2
 requested by authority V70.1
 nursing care V63.8
 social service V63.8
Evan's syndrome (thrombocytopenic purpura) 287.3

Eventration
  colon into chest — *see* Hernia, diaphragm
  diaphragm (congenital) 756.6
Eversion
  bladder 596.8
  cervix (uteri) 622.0
    with mention of cervicitis 616.0
  foot NEC 736.79
    congenital 755.67
  lacrimal punctum 375.51
  punctum lacrimale (postinfectional) (senile) 375.51
  ureter (meatus) 593.89
  urethra (meatus) 599.84
  uterus 618.1
    complicating delivery 665.2
      affecting fetus or newborn 763.89
    puerperal, postpartum 674.8
Evisceration
  birth injury 767.8
  bowel (congenital) — *see* Hernia, ventral
  congenital (*see also* Hernia, ventral) 553.29
  operative wound 998.32 ▲
  traumatic NEC 869.1
    eye 871.3
Evulsion — *see* Avulsion
Ewing's
  angioendothelioma (M9260/3) — *see* Neoplasm, bone, malignant
  sarcoma (M9260/3) — *see* Neoplasm, bone, malignant
  tumor (M9260/3) — *see* Neoplasm, bone, malignant
Exaggerated lumbosacral angle (with impinging spine) 756.12
Examination (general) (routine) (of) (for) V70.9
  allergy V72.7
  annual V70.0
  cardiovascular preoperative V72.81
  cervical Papanicolaou smear V76.2
    as a part of routine gynecological examination V72.3
  child care (routine) V20.2
  clinical research investigation (normal control patient) (participant) V70.7
  dental V72.2
  developmental testing (child) (infant) V20.2
  donor (potential) V70.8
  ear V72.1
  eye V72.0
  following
    accident (motor vehicle) V71.4
    alleged rape or seduction (victim or culprit) V71.5
    inflicted injury (victim or culprit) NEC V71.6
    rape or seduction, alleged (victim or culprit) V71.5
    treatment (for) V67.9
      combined V67.6
      fracture V67.4
      involving high-risk medication NEC V67.51
      mental disorder V67.3
      specified condition NEC V67.59
  follow-up (routine) (following) V67.9
    cancer chemotherapy V67.2
    chemotherapy V67.2
    disease NEC V67.59
    high-risk medication NEC V67.51

Examination — *continued*
  follow-up — *continued*
    injury NEC V67.59
    population survey V70.6
    postpartum V24.2
    psychiatric V67.3
    psychotherapy V67.3
    radiotherapy V67.1
    specified surgery NEC V67.09
    surgery V67.00
      vaginal pap smear V67.01
  gynecological V72.3
    for contraceptive maintenance V25.40
      intrauterine device V25.42
      pill V25.41
      specified method NEC V25.49
  health (of)
    armed forces personnel V70.5
    checkup V70.0
    child, routine V20.2
    defined subpopulation NEC V70.5
    inhabitants of institutions V70.5
    occupational V70.5
    pre-employment screening V70.5
    preschool children V70.5
      for admission to school V70.3
    prisoners V70.5
      for entrance into prison V70.3
    prostitutes V70.5
    refugees V70.5
    school children V70.5
    students V70.5
  hearing V72.1
  infant V20.2
  laboratory V72.6
  lactating mother V24.1
  medical (for) (of) V70.9
    administrative purpose NEC V70.3
    admission to
      old age home V70.3
      prison V70.3
      school V70.3
    adoption V70.3
    armed forces personnel V70.5
    at health care facility V70.0
    camp V70.3
    child, routine V20.2
    clinical research investigation (control) (normal comparison) (participant) V70.7
    defined subpopulation NEC V70.5
    donor (potential) V70.8
    driving license V70.3
    general V70.9
      routine V70.0
      specified reason NEC V70.8
    immigration V70.3
    inhabitants of institutions V70.5
    insurance certification V70.3
    marriage V70.3
    medicolegal reasons V70.4
    naturalization V70.3
    occupational V70.5
    population survey V70.6
    pre-employment V70.5
    preschool children V70.5
      for admission to school V70.3
    prison V70.3
    prisoners V70.5
      for entrance into prison V70.3
    prostitutes V70.5

Examination — *continued*
  medical — *continued*
    refugees V70.5
    school children V70.5
    specified reason NEC V70.8
    sport competition V70.3
    students V70.5
  medicolegal reason V70.4
  pelvic (annual) (periodic) V72.3
  periodic (annual) (routine) V70.0
  postpartum
    immediately after delivery V24.0
    routine follow-up V24.2
  pregnancy (unconfirmed) (possible) V72.4
  prenatal V22.1
    first pregnancy V22.0
    high-risk pregnancy V23.9
      specified problem NEC V23.8 ✓5ᵗʰ
  preoperative V72.84
    cardiovascular V72.81
    respiratory V72.82
    specified NEC V72.83
  psychiatric V70.2
    follow-up not needing further care V67.3
    requested by authority V70.1
  radiological NEC V72.5
  respiratory preoperative V72.82
  screening — *see* Screening
  sensitization V72.7
  skin V72.7
    hypersensitivity V72.7
  special V72.9
  specified type or reason NEC V72.85
    preoperative V72.83
      specified NEC V72.83
  teeth V72.2
  victim or culprit following
    alleged rape or seduction V71.5
    inflicted injury NEC V71.6
  vaginal Papanicolaou smear V76.47
    following hysterectomy for malignant
      condition V67.01
  vision V72.0
  well baby V20.2
Exanthem, exanthema (*see also* Rash) 782.1
  Boston 048
  epidemic, with meningitis 048
  lichenoid psoriasiform 696.2
  subitum 057.8
  viral, virus NEC 057.9
    specified type NEC 057.8
Excess, excessive, excessively
  alcohol level in blood 790.3
  carbohydrate tissue, localized 278.1
  carotene (dietary) 278.3
  cold 991.9
    specified effect NEC 991.8
  convergence 378.84
  crying of infant (baby) 780.92
  development, breast 611.1
  diaphoresis 780.8
  divergence 378.85
  drinking (alcohol) NEC (*see also* Abuse, drugs,
    nondependent) 305.0 ✓5ᵗʰ
    continual (*see also* Alcoholism) 303.9 ✓5ᵗʰ
    habitual (*see also* Alcoholism) 303.9 ✓5ᵗʰ
  eating 783.6
  eyelid fold (congenital) 743.62
  fat 278.00
    in heart (*see also* Degeneration, myocardial)
      429.1

Excess, excessive, excessively — *continued*
  fat — *continued*
    tissue, localized 278.1
  foreskin 605
  gas 787.3
  gastrin 251.5
  glucagon 251.4
  heat (*see also* Heat) 992.9
  large
    colon 564.7
      congenital 751.3
    fetus or infant 766.0
      with obstructed labor 660.1 ✓5ᵗʰ
      affecting management of pregnancy
        656.6 ✓5ᵗʰ
      causing disproportion 653.5 ✓5ᵗʰ
      newborn (weight of 4500 grams or more)
        766.0
    organ or site, congenital NEC — *see*
      Anomaly, specified type NEC
  lid fold (congenital) 743.62
  long
    colon 751.5
    organ or site, congenital NEC — *see*
      Anomaly, specified type NEC
    umbilical cord (entangled)
      affecting fetus or newborn 762.5
      in pregnancy or childbirth 663.3 ✓5ᵗʰ
        with compression 663.2 ✓5ᵗʰ
  menstruation 626.2
  number of teeth 520.1
    causing crowding 524.3
  nutrients (dietary) NEC 783.6
  potassium (K) 276.7
  salivation (*see also* Ptyalism) 527.7
  secretion — *see also* Hypersecretion
    milk 676.6 ✓5ᵗʰ
    sputum 786.4
    sweat 780.8
  short
    organ or site, congenital NEC — *see*
      Anomaly, specified type NEC
    umbilical cord
      affecting fetus or newborn 762.6
      in pregnancy or childbirth 663.4 ✓5ᵗʰ
  skin NEC 701.9
    eyelid 743.62
      acquired 374.30
  sodium (Na) 276.0
  sputum 786.4
  sweating 780.8
  tearing (ducts) (eye) (*see also* Epiphora) 375.20
  thirst 783.5
    due to deprivation of water 994.3
  vitamin
    A (dietary) 278.2
      administered as drug (chronic)
        (prolonged excessive intake) 278.2
        reaction to sudden overdose 963.5
    D (dietary) 278.4
      administered as drug (chronic)
        (prolonged excessive intake) 278.4
        reaction to sudden overdose 963.5
  weight 278.00
    gain 783.1
      of pregnancy 646.1 ✓5ᵗʰ
    loss 783.21
Excitability, abnormal, under minor stress
  309.29
Excitation
  catatonic (*see also* Schizophrenia) 295.2 ✓5ᵗʰ

Excitation — *continued*
  psychogenic 298.1
  reactive (from emotional stress, psychological trauma) 298.1
Excitement
  manic (*see also* Psychosis, affective) 296.0 ⚠5ᵗʰ
    recurrent episode 296.1 ⚠5ᵗʰ
    single episode 296.0 ⚠5ᵗʰ
  mental, reactive (from emotional stress, psychological trauma) 298.1
  state, reactive (from emotional stress, psychological trauma) 298.1
Excluded pupils 364.76
Excoriation (traumatic) (*see also* Injury, superficial, by site) 919.8
  neurotic 698.4
Excyclophoria 378.44
Excyclotropia 378.33
Exencephalus, exencephaly 742.0
Exercise
  breathing V57.0
  remedial NEC V57.1
  therapeutic NEC V57.1
Exfoliation, teeth due to systemic causes 525.0
Exfoliative — *see also* condition dermatitis 695.89
Exhaustion, exhaustive (physical NEC) 780.79
  battle (*see also* Reaction, stress, acute) 308.9
  cardiac (*see also* Failure, heart) 428.9
  delirium (*see also* Reaction, stress, acute) 308.9
  due to
    cold 991.8
    excessive exertion 994.5
    exposure 994.4
  fetus or newborn 779.89 ▲
  heart (*see also* Failure, heart) 428.9
  heat 992.5
    due to
      salt depletion 992.4
      water depletion 992.3
  manic (*see also* Psychosis, affective) 296.0 ⚠5ᵗʰ
    recurrent episode 296.1 ⚠5ᵗʰ
    single episode 296.0 ⚠5ᵗʰ
  maternal, complicating delivery 669.8 ⚠5ᵗʰ
    affecting fetus or newborn 763.89
  mental 300.5
  myocardium, myocardial (*see also* Failure, heart) 428.9
  nervous 300.5
  old age 797
  postinfectional NEC 780.79
  psychogenic 300.5
  psychosis (*see also* Reaction, stress, acute) 308.9
  senile 797
    dementia 290.0
Exhibitionism (sexual) 302.4
Exomphalos 756.79
Exophoria 378.42
  convergence, insufficiency 378.83
  divergence, excess 378.85
Exophthalmic
  cachexia 242.0 ⚠5ᵗʰ
  goiter 242.0 ⚠5ᵗʰ
  ophthalmoplegia 242.0 ⚠5ᵗʰ *[376.22]*
Exophthalmos 376.30
  congenital 743.66

Exophthalmos — *continued*
  constant 376.31
  endocrine NEC 259.9 *[376.22]*
  hyperthyroidism 242.0 ⚠5ᵗʰ *[376.21]*
  intermittent NEC 376.34
  malignant 242.0 ⚠5ᵗʰ *[376.21]*
  pulsating 376.35
    endocrine NEC 259.9 *[376.22]*
  thyrotoxic 242.0 ⚠5ᵗʰ *[376.21]*
Exostosis 726.91
  cartilaginous (M9210/0) — *see* Neoplasm, bone, benign
  congenital 756.4
  ear canal, external 380.81
  gonococcal 098.89
  hip 726.5
  intracranial 733.3
  jaw (bone) 526.81
  luxurians 728.11
  multiple (cancellous) (congenital) (hereditary) 756.4
  nasal bones 726.91
  orbit, orbital 376.42
  osteocartilaginous (M9210/0) — *see* Neoplasm, bone, benign
  spine 721.8
    with spondylosis — *see* Spondylosis
  syphilitic 095.5
  wrist 726.4
Exotropia 378.10
  alternating 378.15
    with
      A pattern 378.16
      specified noncomitancy NEC 378.18
      V pattern 378.17
      X pattern 378.18
      Y pattern 378.18
    intermittent 378.24
  intermittent 378.20
    alternating 378.24
    monocular 378.23
  monocular 378.11
    with
      A pattern 378.12
      specified noncomitancy NEC 378.14
      V pattern 378.13
      X pattern 378.14
      Y pattern 378.14
    intermittent 378.23
Explanation of
  investigation finding V65.4
  medication V65.4
Exposure 994.9
  cold 991.9
    specified effect NEC 991.8
  effects of 994.9
  exhaustion due to 994.4
  to
    AIDS virus V01.7
    anthrax V01.81 ●
    asbestos V15.84
    body fluids (hazardous) V15.85
    cholera V01.0
    communicable disease V01.9
      specified type NEC V01.89 ▲
    German measles V01.4
    gonorrhea V01.6
    hazardous body fluids V15.85
    HIV V01.7
    human immunodeficiency virus V01.7
    lead V15.86

Exposure — *continued*
  to — *continued*
    parasitic disease V01.89
    poliomyelitis V01.2
    potentially hazardous body fluids V15.85
    rabies V01.5
    rubella V01.4
    smallpox V01.3
    syphilis V01.6
    tuberculosis V01.1
    venereal disease V01.6
    viral disease NEC V01.7
Exsanguination, fetal 772.0
Exstrophy
  abdominal content 751.8
  bladder (urinary) 753.5
Extensive — *see* condition
Extra — *see also* Accessory
  rib 756.3
    cervical 756.2
Extraction
  with hook 763.89
  breech NEC 669.6
    affecting fetus or newborn 763.0
  cataract postsurgical V45.61
  manual NEC 669.8
    affecting fetus or newborn 763.89
Extrasystole 427.60
  atrial 427.61
  postoperative 997.1
  ventricular 427.69
Extrauterine gestation or pregnancy — *see* Pregnancy, ectopic
Extravasation
  blood 459.0
    lower extremity 459.0
  chyle into mesentery 457.8
  pelvicalyceal 593.4
  pyelosinus 593.4
  urine 788.8
    from ureter 788.8
Extremity — *see* condition
Extrophy — *see* Exstrophy
Extroversion
  bladder 753.5
  uterus 618.1
    complicating delivery 665.2
      affecting fetus or newborn 763.89
    postpartal (old) 618.1
Extrusion
  breast implant (prosthetic) 996.54
  device, implant, or graft — *see* Complications, mechanical
  eye implant (ball) (globe) 996.59
  intervertebral disc — *see* Displacement, intervertebral disc
  lacrimal gland 375.43
  mesh (reinforcing) 996.59
  ocular lens implant 996.53
  prosthetic device NEC — *see* Complications, mechanical
  vitreous 379.26
Exudate, pleura — *see* Effusion, pleura
Exudates, retina 362.82
Exudative — *see* condition
Eye, eyeball, eyelid — *see* condition
Eyestrain 368.13
Eyeworm disease of Africa 125.2

F

Faber's anemia or syndrome (achlorhydric anemia) 280.9
Fabry's disease (angiokeratoma corporis diffusum) 272.7
Face, facial — *see* condition
Facet of cornea 371.44
Faciocephalalgia, autonomic (*see also* Neuropathy, peripheral, autonomic) 337.9
Facioscapulohumeral myopathy 359.1
Factitious disorder, illness — *see* Illness, factitious
Factor
  deficiency — *see* Deficiency, factor
  psychic, associated with diseases classified elsewhere 316
  risk — *see* Problem
Fahr-Volhard disease (malignant nephrosclerosis) 403.00
Failure, failed
  adenohypophyseal 253.2
  attempted abortion (legal) (*see also* Abortion, failed) 638.9
  bone marrow (anemia) 284.9
    acquired (secondary) 284.8
    congenital 284.0
    idiopathic 284.9
  cardiac (*see also* Failure, heart) 428.9
    newborn 779.89
  cardiorenal (chronic) 428.9
    hypertensive (*see also* Hypertension, cardiorenal) 404.93
  cardiorespiratory 799.1
    specified during or due to a procedure 997.1
      long-term effect of cardiac surgery 429.4
  cardiovascular (chronic) 428.9
  cerebrovascular 437.8
  cervical dilatation in labor 661.0
    affecting fetus or newborn 763.7
  circulation, circulatory 799.8
    fetus or newborn 779.89
    peripheral 785.50
  compensation — *see* Disease, heart
  congestive (*see also* Failure, heart) 428.0
  coronary (*see also* Insufficiency, coronary) 411.89
  descent of head (at term) 652.5
    affecting fetus or newborn 763.1
    in labor 660.0
      affecting fetus or newborn 763.1
  device, implant, or graft — *see* Complications, mechanical
  engagement of head NEC 652.5
    in labor 660.0
  extrarenal 788.9
  fetal head to enter pelvic brim 652.5
    affecting fetus or newborn 763.1
    in labor 660.0
      affecting fetus or newborn 763.1
  forceps NEC 660.7
    affecting fetus or newborn 763.1
  fusion (joint) (spinal) 996.4
  growth in childhood 783.43
  heart (acute) (sudden) 428.9
    with
      abortion — *see* Abortion, by type, with specified complication NEC

Failure, failed — continued
  heart — continued
    with — continued
      acute pulmonary edema (see also
        Failure, ventricular, left) 428.1
        with congestion ▶(see also Failure,
          heart)◀ 428.0
      decompensation (see also Failure, heart)
        428.0
      dilation — see Disease, heart
      ectopic pregnancy (see also categories
        633.0-633.9) 639.8
      molar pregnancy (see also categories
        630-632) 639.8
    arteriosclerotic 440.9
    combined left-right sided 428.0
    combined systolic and diastolic 428.40 ●
      acute 428.41 ●
      acute on chronic 428.43 ●
      chronic 428.42 ●
    compensated (see also Failure, heart) 428.0
    complicating
      abortion — see Abortion, by type, with
        specified complication NEC
      delivery (cesarean) (instrumental)
        669.4 ✓5ᵗʰ
      ectopic pregnancy (see also categories
        633.0-633.9) 639.8
      molar pregnancy (see also categories
        630-632) 639.8
      obstetric anesthesia or sedation
        668.1 ✓5ᵗʰ
      surgery 997.1
    congestive (compensated) (decompensated)
      ▶(see also Failure, heart)◀ 428.0
      with rheumatic fever (conditions
        classifiable to 390)
        active 391.8
        inactive or quiescent (with chorea)
          398.91
      fetus or newborn 779.89 ▲
      hypertensive (see also Hypertension,
        heart) 402.90
        with renal disease (see also
          Hypertension, cardiorenal)
          404.91
          with renal failure 404.93
          benign 402.11
          malignant 402.01
        rheumatic (chronic) (inactive) (with
          chorea) 398.91
          active or acute 391.8
          with chorea (Sydenham's) 392.0
    decompensated (see also Failure, heart)
      428.0
    degenerative (see also Degeneration,
      myocardial) 429.1
    diastolic 428.30 ●
      acute 428.31 ●
      acute on chronic 428.33 ●
      chronic 428.32 ●
    due to presence of (cardiac) prosthesis
      429.4
    fetus or newborn 779.89 ▲
    following
      abortion 639.8
      cardiac surgery 429.4
      ectopic or molar pregnancy 639.8
    high output NEC 428.9
    hypertensive (see also Hypertension, heart)
      402.91

Failure, failed — continued
  heart — continued
    hypertensive — continued
      with renal disease (see also
        Hypertension, cardiorenal) 404.91
        with renal failure 404.93
        benign 402.11
        malignant 402.01
      left (ventricular) (see also Failure,
        ventricular, left) 428.1
        with right-sided failure ▶(see also
          Failure, heart)◀ 428.0
    low output (syndrome) NEC 428.9
    organic — see Disease, heart
    postoperative (immediate) 997.1
      long term effect of cardiac surgery 429.4
    rheumatic (chronic) (congestive) (inactive)
      398.91
    right (secondary to left heart failure,
      conditions classifiable to 428.1)
      (ventricular) (see also Failure, heart)
      428.0
    senile 797
    specified during or due to a procedure
      997.1
      long-term effect of cardiac surgery 429.4
    systolic 428.20 ●
      acute 428.21 ●
      acute on chronic 428.23 ●
      chronic 428.22 ●
    thyrotoxic (see also Thyrotoxicosis)
      242.9 ✓5ᵗʰ [425.7]
    valvular — see Endocarditis
  hepatic 572.8
    acute 570
    due to a procedure 997.4
  hepatorenal 572.4
  hypertensive heart (see also Hypertension,
    heart) 402.91
    benign 402.11
    malignant 402.01
  induction (of labor) 659.1 ✓5ᵗʰ
    abortion (legal) (see also Abortion, failed)
      638.9
    affecting fetus or newborn 763.89
    by oxytocic drugs 659.1 ✓5ᵗʰ
    instrumental 659.0 ✓5ᵗʰ
    mechanical 659.0 ✓5ᵗʰ
    medical 659.1 ✓5ᵗʰ
    surgical 659.0 ✓5ᵗʰ
  initial alveolar expansion, newborn 770.4
  involution, thymus (gland) 254.8
  kidney — see Failure, renal
  lactation 676.4 ✓5ᵗʰ
  Leydig's cell, adult 257.2
  liver 572.8
    acute 570
  medullary 799.8
  mitral — see Endocarditis, mitral
  myocardium, myocardial (see also Failure,
    heart) 428.9
    chronic (see also Failure, heart) 428.0
    congestive (see also Failure, heart) 428.0
  ovarian (primary) 256.39
    iatrogenic 256.2
    postablative 256.2
    postirradiation 256.2
    postsurgical 256.2
  ovulation 628.0
  prerenal 788.9

Index to Diseases

Failure, failed — *continued*
  renal 586
    with
      abortion — *see* Abortion, by type, with renal failure
      ectopic pregnancy (*see also* categories 633.0-633.9) 639.3
      edema (*see also* Nephrosis) 581.9
      hypertension (*see also* Hypertension, kidney) 403.91
      hypertensive heart disease (conditions classifiable to 402) 404.92
        with heart failure 404.93
        benign 404.12
          with heart failure 404.13
        malignant 404.02
          with heart failure 404.03
      molar pregnancy (*see also* categories 630-632) 639.3
      tubular necrosis (acute) 584.5
    acute 584.9
      with lesion of
        necrosis
          cortical (renal) 584.6
          medullary (renal) (papillary) 584.7
          tubular 584.5
      specified pathology NEC 584.8
    chronic 585
      hypertensive or with hypertension (*see also* Hypertension, kidney) 403.91
    due to a procedure 997.5
    following
      abortion 639.3
      crushing 958.5
      ectopic or molar pregnancy 639.3
      labor and delivery (acute) 669.3 ✓5ᵗʰ
    hypertensive (*see also* Hypertension, kidney) 403.91
    puerperal, postpartum 669.3 ✓5ᵗʰ
  respiration, respiratory 518.81
    acute 518.81
    acute and chronic 518.84
    center 348.8
      newborn 770.84 ▲
    chronic 518.83
    due to trauma, surgery or shock 518.5
    newborn 770.84 ▲
  rotation
    cecum 751.4
    colon 751.4
    intestine 751.4
    kidney 753.3
  segmentation — *see also* Fusion
    fingers (*see also* Syndactylism, fingers) 755.11
    toes (*see also* Syndactylism, toes) 755.13
  seminiferous tubule, adult 257.2
  senile (general) 797
    with psychosis 290.20
  testis, primary (seminal) 257.2
  to progress 661.2 ✓5ᵗʰ
  to thrive
    adult 783.7
    child 783.41
  transplant 996.80
    bone marrow 996.85
    organ (immune or nonimmune cause) 996.80
      bone marrow 996.85
      heart 996.83
      intestines 996.87

Failure, failed — *continued*
  transplant — *continued*
    organ — *continued*
      kidney 996.81
      liver 996.82
      lung 996.84
      pancreas 996.86
      specified NEC 996.89
    skin 996.52
      artificial 996.55
      decellularized allodermis 996.55
      temporary allograft or pigskin graft — *omit code*
  trial of labor NEC 660.6 ✓5ᵗʰ
    affecting fetus or newborn 763.1
  urinary 586
  vacuum extraction
    abortion — *see* Abortion, failed
    delivery NEC 660.7 ✓5ᵗʰ
      affecting fetus or newborn 763.1
  ventouse NEC 660.7 ✓5ᵗʰ
    affecting fetus or newborn 763.1
  ventricular (*see also* Failure, heart) 428.9
    left 428.1
      with rheumatic fever (conditions classifiable to 390)
        active 391.8
          with chorea 392.0
        inactive or quiescent (with chorea) 398.91
      hypertensive (*see also* Hypertension, heart) 402.91
        benign 402.11
        malignant 402.01
      rheumatic (chronic) (inactive) (with chorea) 398.91
        active or acute 391.8
          with chorea 392.0
    right (*see also* Failure, heart) 428.0
  vital centers, fetus or newborn 779.8
  weight gain in childhood 783.41

Fainting (fit) (spell) 780.2
Falciform hymen 752.49
Fall, maternal, affecting fetus or newborn 760.5
Fallen arches 734
Falling, any organ or part — *see* Prolapse
Fallopian
  insufflation
    fertility testing V26.21
    following sterilization reversal V26.22
  tube — *see* condition
Fallot's
  pentalogy 745.2
  tetrad or tetralogy 745.2
  triad or trilogy 746.09
Fallout, radioactive (adverse effect) NEC 990
False — *see also* condition
  bundle branch block 426.50
  bursa 727.89
  croup 478.75
  joint 733.82
  labor (pains) 644.1 ✓5ᵗʰ
  opening, urinary, male 752.69
  passage, urethra (prostatic) 599.4
  positive
    serological test for syphilis 795.6
    Wassermann reaction 795.6
  pregnancy 300.11

Family, familial — *see also* condition
  disruption V61.0
  planning advice V25.09
  problem V61.9
    specified circumstance NEC V61.8
Famine 994.2
  edema 262
Fanconi's anemia (congenital pancytopenia) 284.0
Fanconi (-de Toni) (-Debré) syndrome (cystinosis) 270.0
Farber (-Uzman) syndrome or disease (disseminated lipogranulomatosis) 272.8
Farcin 024
Farcy 024
Farmers'
  lung 495.0
  skin 692.74
Farsightedness 367.0
Fascia — *see* condition
Fasciculation 781.0
Fasciculitis optica 377.32
Fasciitis 729.4
  eosinophilic 728.89
  necrotizing 728.86
  nodular 728.79
  perirenal 593.4
  plantar 728.71
  pseudosarcomatous 728.79
  traumatic (old) NEC 728.79
    current — *see* Sprain, by site
Fasciola hepatica infestation 121.3
Fascioliasis 121.3
Fasciolopsiasis (small intestine) 121.4
Fasciolopsis (small intestine) 121.4
Fast pulse 785.0
Fat
  embolism (cerebral) (pulmonary) (systemic) 958.1
    with
      abortion — *see* Abortion, by type, with embolism
      ectopic pregnancy (*see also* categories 633.0-633.9) 639.6
      molar pregnancy (*see also* categories 630-632) 639.6
    complicating delivery or puerperium 673.8
    following
      abortion 639.6
      ectopic or molar pregnancy 639.6
    in pregnancy, childbirth, or the puerperium 673.8
  excessive 278.00
    in heart (*see also* Degeneration, myocardial) 429.1
  general 278.00
  hernia, herniation 729.30
    eyelid 374.34
    knee 729.31
    orbit 374.34
    retro-orbital 374.34
    retropatellar 729.31
    specified site NEC 729.39
  indigestion 579.8
  in stool 792.1
  localized (pad) 278.1

Fat — *continued*
  localized — *continued*
    heart (*see also* Degeneration, myocardial) 429.1
    knee 729.31
    retropatellar 729.31
    necrosis — *see also* Fatty, degeneration breast (aseptic) (segmental) 611.3
    mesentery 567.8
    omentum 567.8
  pad 278.1
Fatal syncope 798.1
Fatigue 780.79
  auditory deafness (*see also* Deafness) 389.9
  chronic 780.7
  chronic, syndrome 780.71
  combat (*see also* Reaction, stress, acute) 308.9
  during pregnancy 646.8
  general 780.79
    psychogenic 300.5
  heat (transient) 992.6
  muscle 729.89
  myocardium (*see also* Failure, heart) 428.9
  nervous 300.5
  neurosis 300.5
  operational 300.89
  postural 729.89
  posture 729.89
  psychogenic (general) 300.5
  senile 797
  syndrome NEC 300.5
    chronic 780.71
  undue 780.79
  voice 784.49
Fatness 278.00
Fatty — *see also* condition
  apron 278.1
  degeneration (diffuse) (general) NEC 272.8
    localized — *see* Degeneration, by site, fatty
    placenta — *see* Placenta, abnormal
  heart (enlarged) (*see also* Degeneration, myocardial) 429.1
  infiltration (diffuse) (general) (*see also* Degeneration, by site, fatty) 272.8
    heart (enlarged) (*see also* Degeneration, myocardial) 429.1
  liver 571.8
    alcoholic 571.0
  necrosis — *see* Degeneration, fatty
  phanerosis 272.8
Fauces — *see* condition
Fauchard's disease (periodontitis) 523.4
Faucitis 478.29
Faulty — *see also* condition
  position of teeth 524.3
Favism (anemia) 282.2
Favre-Racouchot disease (elastoidosis cutanea nodularis) 701.8
Favus 110.9
  beard 110.0
  capitis 110.0
  corporis 110.5
  eyelid 110.8
  foot 110.4
  hand 110.2
  scalp 110.0
  specified site NEC 110.8

Fear, fearfullness (complex) (reaction) 300.20
  child 313.0
  of
    animals 300.29
    closed spaces 300.29
    crowds 300.29
    eating in public 300.23
    heights 300.29
    open spaces 300.22
      with panic attacks 300.21
    public speaking 300.23
    streets 300.22
      with panic attacks 300.21
    travel 300.22
      with panic attacks 300.21
    washing in public 300.23
  transient 308.0
Feared complaint unfounded V65.5
Febricula (continued) (simple) (see also Pyrexia) 780.6
Febrile (see also Pyrexia) 780.6
  convulsion 780.31
  seizure 780.31
Febris (see also Fever) 780.6
  aestiva (see also Fever, hay) 477.9
  flava (see also Fever, yellow) 060.9
  melitensis 023.0
  pestis (see also Plague) 020.9
  puerperalis 672 ▨4▥
  recurrens (see also Fever, relapsing) 087.9
    pediculo vestimenti 087.0
  rubra 034.1
  typhoidea 002.0
  typhosa 002.0
Fecal — see condition
Fecalith (impaction) 560.39
  with hernia — see also Hernia, by site, with obstruction
    gangrenous — see Hernia, by site, with gangrene
  appendix 543.9
  congenital 777.1
Fede's disease 529.0
Feeble-minded 317
Feeble rapid pulse due to shock following injury 958.4
Feeding
  faulty (elderly) (infant) 783.3
    newborn 779.3
  formula check V20.2
  improper (elderly) (infant) 783.3
    newborn 779.3
  problem (elderly) (infant) 783.3
    newborn 779.3
    nonorganic origin 307.59
Feer's disease 985.0
Feet — see condition
Feigned illness V65.2
Feil-Klippel syndrome (brevicollis) 756.16
Feinmesser's (hidrotic) ectodermal dysplasia 757.31
Felix's disease (juvenile osteochondrosis, hip) 732.1
Felon (any digit) (with lymphangitis) 681.01
  herpetic 054.6
Felty's syndrome (rheumatoid arthritis with splenomegaly and leukopenia) 714.1
Feminism in boys 302.6

Feminization, testicular 257.8
  with pseudohermaphroditism, male 257.8
Femoral hernia — see Hernia, femoral
Femora vara 736.32
Femur, femoral — see condition
Fenestrata placenta — see Placenta, abnormal
Fenestration, fenestrated — see also Imperfect, closure
  aorta-pulmonary 745.0
  aorticopulmonary 745.0
  aortopulmonary 745.0
  cusps, heart valve NEC 746.89
    pulmonary 746.09
  hymen 752.49
  pulmonic cusps 746.09
Fenwick's disease 537.89
Fermentation (gastric) (gastrointestinal) (stomach) 536.8
  intestine 564.89
    psychogenic 306.4
  psychogenic 306.4
Fernell's disease (aortic aneurysm) 441.9
Fertile eunuch syndrome 257.2
Fertility, meaning multiparity — see Multiparity
Fetal alcohol syndrome 760.71
Fetalis uterus 752.3
Fetid
  breath 784.9
  sweat 705.89
Fetishism 302.81
  transvestic 302.3
Fetomaternal hemorrhage
  affecting management of pregnancy 656.0 ▨5▥
  fetus or newborn 772.0
Fetus, fetal — see also condition
  papyraceous 779.89
  type lung tissue 770.4
Fever 780.6
  with chills 780.6
    in malarial regions (see also Malaria) 084.6
  abortus NEC 023.9
  Aden 061
  African tick-borne 087.1
  American
    mountain tick 066.1
    spotted 082.0
  and ague (see also Malaria) 084.6
  aphthous 078.4
  arbovirus hemorrhagic 065.9
  Assam 085.0
  Australian A or Q 083.0
  Bangkok hemorrhagic 065.4
  biliary, Charcôt's intermittent — see Choledocholithiasis
  bilious, hemoglobinuric 084.8
  blackwater 084.8
  blister 054.9
  Bonvale Dam 780.79
  boutonneuse 082.1
  brain 323.9
    late effect — see category 326
  breakbone 061
  Bullis 082.8
  Bunyamwera 066.3
  Burdwan 085.0
  Bwamba (encephalitis) 066.3
  Cameroon (see also Malaria) 084.6

Fever — *continued*
- Canton 081.9
- catarrhal (acute) 460
    - chronic 472.0
- cat-scratch 078.3
- cerebral 323.9
    - late effect — *see* category 326
- cerebrospinal (meningococcal) (*see also* Meningitis, cerebrospinal) 036.0
- Chagres 084.0
- Chandipura 066.8
- changuinola 066.0
- Charcôt's (biliary) (hepatic) (intermittent) *see* Choledocholithiasis
- Chikungunya (viral) 066.3
    - hemorrhagic 065.4
- childbed 670 ✓4ᵗʰ
- Chitral 066.0
- Colombo (*see also* Fever, paratyphoid) 002.9
- Colorado tick (virus) 066.1
- congestive
    - malarial (*see also* Malaria) 084.6
    - remittent (*see also* Malaria) 084.6
- Congo virus 065.0
- continued 780.6
    - malarial 084.0
- Corsican (*see also* Malaria) 084.6
- Crimean hemorrhagic 065.0
- Cyprus (*see also* Brucellosis) 023.9
- dandy 061
- deer fly (*see also* Tularemia) 021.9
- dehydration, newborn 778.4
- dengue (virus) 061
    - hemorrhagic 065.4
- desert 114.0
- due to heat 992.0
- Dumdum 085.0
- enteric 002.0
- ephemeral (of unknown origin) (*see also* Pyrexia) 780.6
- epidemic, hemorrhagic of the Far East 065.0
- erysipelatous (*see also* Erysipelas) 035
- estivo-autumnal (malarial) 084.0
- etiocholanolone 277.3
- famine — *see also* Fever, relapsing
    - meaning typhus — *see* Typhus
- Far Eastern hemorrhagic 065.0
- five day 083.1
- Fort Bragg 100.89
- gastroenteric 002.0
- gastromalarial (*see also* Malaria) 084.6
- Gibraltar (*see also* Brucellosis) 023.9
- glandular 075
- Guama (viral) 066.3
- Haverhill 026.1
- hay (allergic) (with rhinitis) 477.9
    - with
        - asthma (bronchial) (*see also* Asthma) 493.0 ✓5ᵗʰ
        - due to
            - dander 477.8
            - dust 477.8
            - fowl 477.8
            - pollen, any plant or tree 477.0
            - specified allergen other than pollen 477.8
- heat (effects) 992.0
- hematuric, bilious 084.8
- hemoglobinuric (malarial) 084.8
    - bilious 084.8

Fever — *continued*
- hemorrhagic (arthropod-borne) NEC 065.9
    - with renal syndrome 078.6
    - arenaviral 078.7
    - Argentine 078.7
    - Bangkok 065.4
    - Bolivian 078.7
    - Central Asian 065.0
    - chikungunya 065.4
    - Crimean 065.0
    - dengue (virus) 065.4
    - Ebola 065.8
    - epidemic 078.6
        - of Far East 065.0
    - Far Eastern 065.0
    - Junin virus 078.7
    - Korean 078.6
    - Kyasanur forest 065.2
    - Machupo virus 078.7
    - mite-borne NEC 065.8
    - mosquito-borne 065.4
    - Omsk 065.1
    - Philippine 065.4
    - Russian (Yaroslav) 078.6
    - Singapore 065.4
    - Southeast Asia 065.4
    - Thailand 065.4
    - tick-borne NEC 065.3
- hepatic (*see also* Cholecystitis) 575.8
    - intermittent (Charcôt's) — *see* Choledocholithiasis
- herpetic (*see also* Herpes) 054.9
- Hyalomma tick 065.0
- icterohemorrhagic 100.0
- inanition 780.6
    - newborn 778.4
- infective NEC 136.9
- intermittent (bilious) (*see also* Malaria) 084.6
    - hepatic (Charcôt) — *see* Choledocholithiasis
    - of unknown origin (*see also* Pyrexia) 780.6
    - pernicious 084.0
- iodide
    - correct substance properly administered 780.6
    - overdose or wrong substance given or taken 975.5
- Japanese river 081.2
- jungle yellow 060.0
- Junin virus, hemorrhagic 078.7
- Katayama 120.2
- Kedani 081.2
- Kenya 082.1
- Korean hemorrhagic 078.6
- Lassa 078.89
- Lone Star 082.8
- lung — *see* Pneumonia
- Machupo virus, hemorrhagic 078.7
- malaria, malarial (*see also* Malaria) 084.6
- Malta (*see also* Brucellosis) 023.9
- Marseilles 082.1
- marsh (*see also* Malaria) 084.6
- Mayaro (viral) 066.3
- Mediterranean (*see also* Brucellosis) 023.9
    - familial 277.3
    - tick 082.1
- meningeal — *see* Meningitis
- metal fumes NEC 985.8
- Meuse 083.1
- Mexican — *see* Typhus, Mexican
- Mianeh 087.1
- miasmatic (*see also* Malaria) 084.6

Index to Diseases — Fever

Fever — continued
- miliary 078.2
- milk, female 672 ◢4ᵗʰ
- mill 504
- mite-borne hemorrhagic 065.8
- Monday 504
- mosquito-borne NEC 066.3
  - hemorrhagic NEC 065.4
- mountain 066.1
  - meaning
    - Rocky Mountain spotted 082.0
    - undulant fever (see also Brucellosis) 023.9
    - tick (American) 066.1
- Mucambo (viral) 066.3
- mud 100.89
- Neapolitan (see also Brucellosis) 023.9
- neutropenic 288.0
- nine-mile 083.0
- nonexanthematous tick 066.1
- North Asian tick-borne typhus 082.2
- Omsk hemorrhagic 065.1
- O'nyong-nyong (viral) 066.3
- Oropouche (viral) 066.3
- Oroya 088.0
- paludal (see also Malaria) 084.6
- Panama 084.0
- pappataci 066.0
- paratyphoid 002.9
  - A 002.1
  - B (Schottmüller's) 002.2
  - C (Hirschfeld) 002.3
- parrot 073.9
- periodic 277.3
- pernicious, acute 084.0
- persistent (of unknown origin) (see also Pyrexia) 780.6
- petechial 036.0
- pharyngoconjunctival 077.2
  - adenoviral type 3 077.2
- Philippine hemorrhagic 065.4
- phlebotomus 066.0
- Piry 066.8
- Pixuna (viral) 066.3
- Plasmodium ovale 084.3
- pleural (see also Pleurisy) 511.0
- pneumonic — see Pneumonia
- polymer fume 987.8
- postoperative 998.89
  - due to infection 998.59
- pretibial 100.89
- puerperal, postpartum 672 ◢4ᵗʰ
- putrid — see Septicemia
- pyemic — see Septicemia
- Q 083.0
  - with pneumonia 083.0 [484.8]
- quadrilateral 083.0
- quartan (malaria) 084.2
- Queensland (coastal) 083.0
  - seven-day 100.89
- Quintan (A) 083.1
- quotidian 084.0
- rabbit (see also Tularemia) 021.9
- rat-bite 026.9
  - due to
    - Spirillum minor or minus 026.0
    - Spirochaeta morsus muris 026.0
    - Streptobacillus moniliformis 026.1
- recurrent — see Fever, relapsing
- relapsing 087.9
  - Carter's (Asiatic) 087.0

Fever — continued
- relapsing — continued
  - Dutton's (West African) 087.1
  - Koch's 087.9
  - louse-borne (epidemic) 087.0
  - Novy's (American) 087.1
  - Obermeyer's (European) 087.0
  - spirillum NEC 087.9
  - tick-borne (endemic) 087.1
- remittent (bilious) (congestive) (gastric) (see also Malaria) 084.6
- rheumatic (active) (acute) (chronic) (subacute) 390
  - with heart involvement 391.9
    - carditis 391.9
    - endocarditis (aortic) (mitral) (pulmonary) (tricuspid) 391.1
    - multiple sites 391.8
    - myocarditis 391.2
    - pancarditis, acute 391.8
    - pericarditis 391.0
    - specified type NEC 391.8
    - valvulitis 391.1
  - inactive or quiescent with cardiac hypertrophy 398.99
    - carditis 398.90
    - endocarditis 397.9
      - aortic (valve) 395.9
        - with mitral (valve) disease 396.9
      - mitral (valve) 394.9
        - with aortic (valve) disease 396.9
      - pulmonary (valve) 397.1
      - tricuspid (valve) 397.0
    - heart conditions (classifiable to 429.3, 429.6, 429.9) 398.99
      - failure (congestive) (conditions classifiable to 428.0, 428.9) 398.91
    - left ventricular failure (conditions classifiable to 428.1) 398.91
    - myocardial degeneration (conditions classifiable to 429.1) 398.0
    - myocarditis (conditions classifiable to 429.0) 398.0
    - pancarditis 398.99
    - pericarditis 393
- Rift Valley (viral) 066.3
- Rocky Mountain spotted 082.0
- rose 477.0
- Ross river (viral) 066.3
- Russian hemorrhagic 078.6
- sandfly 066.0
- San Joaquin (valley) 114.0
- São Paulo 082.0
- scarlet 034.1
- septic — see Septicemia
- seven-day 061
  - Japan 100.89
  - Queensland 100.89
- shin bone 083.1
- Singapore hemorrhagic 065.4
- solar 061
- sore 054.9
- South African tick-bite 087.1
- Southeast Asia hemorrhagic 065.4
- spinal — see Meningitis
- spirillary 026.0
- splenic (see also Anthrax) 022.9
- spotted (Rocky Mountain) 082.0
  - American 082.0
  - Brazilian 082.0

Fever — *continued*
  spotted — *continued*
    Colombian 082.0
    meaning
      cerebrospinal meningitis 036.0
      typhus 082.9
  spring 309.23
  steroid
    correct substance properly administered 780.6
    overdose or wrong substance given or taken 962.0
  streptobacillary 026.1
  subtertian 084.0
  Sumatran mite 081.2
  sun 061
  swamp 100.89
  sweating 078.2
  swine 003.8
  sylvatic yellow 060.0
  Tahyna 062.5
  tertian — *see* Malaria, tertian
  Thailand hemorrhagic 065.4
  thermic 992.0
  three day 066.0
    with Coxsackie exanthem 074.8
  tick
    American mountain 066.1
    Colorado 066.1
    Kemerovo 066.1
    Mediterranean 082.1
    mountain 066.1
    nonexanthematous 066.1
    Quaranfil 066.1
  tick-bite NEC 066.1
  tick-borne NEC 066.1
    hemorrhagic NEC 065.3
  transitory of newborn 778.4
  trench 083.1
  tsutsugamushi 081.2
  typhogastric 002.0
  typhoid (abortive) (ambulant) (any site) (hemorrhagic) (infection) (intermittent) (malignant) (rheumatic) 002.0
  typhomalarial (*see also* Malaria) 084.6
  typhus — *see* Typhus
  undulant (*see also* Brucellosis) 023.9
  unknown origin (*see also* Pyrexia) 780.6
  uremic — *see* Uremia
  uveoparotid 135
  valley (Coccidioidomycosis) 114.0
  Venezuelan equine 066.2
  Volhynian 083.1
  Wesselsbron (viral) 066.3
  West
    African 084.8
    Nile (viral) 066.4 ▲
  Whitmore's 025
  Wolhynian 083.1
  worm 128.9
  Yaroslav hemorrhagic 078.6
  yellow 060.9
    jungle 060.0
    sylvatic 060.0
    urban 060.1
    vaccination, prophylactic (against) V04.4
  Zika (viral) 066.3
Fibrillation
  atrial (established) (paroxysmal) 427.31
  auricular (atrial) (established) 427.31
  cardiac (ventricular) 427.41

Fibrillation — *continued*
  coronary (*see also* Infarct, myocardium) 410.9 ✓5ᵗʰ
  heart (ventricular) 427.41
  muscular 728.9
  postoperative 997.1
  ventricular 427.41
Fibrin
  ball or bodies, pleural (sac) 511.0
  chamber, anterior (eye) (gelatinous exudate) 364.04
Fibrinogenolysis (hemorrhagic) — *see* Fibrinolysis
Fibrinogenopenia (congenital) (hereditary) (*see also* Defect, coagulation) 286.3
  acquired 286.6
Fibrinolysis (acquired) (hemorrhagic) (pathologic) 286.6
  with
    abortion — *see* Abortion, by type, with hemorrhage, delayed or excessive
    ectopic pregnancy (*see also* categories 633.0-633.9) 639.1
    molar pregnancy (*see also* categories 630-632) 639.1
  antepartum or intrapartum 641.3 ✓5ᵗʰ
    affecting fetus or newborn 762.1
  following
    abortion 639.1
    ectopic or molar pregnancy 639.1
  newborn, transient 776.2
  postpartum 666.3 ✓5ᵗʰ
Fibrinopenia (hereditary) (*see also* Defect, coagulation) 286.3
  acquired 286.6
Fibrinopurulent — *see* condition
Fibrinous — *see* condition
Fibroadenoma (M9010/0)
  cellular intracanalicular (M9020/0) 217
  giant (intracanalicular) (M9020/0) 217
  intracanalicular (M9011/0)
    cellular (M9020/0) 217
    giant (M9020/0) 217
    specified site — *see* Neoplasm, by site, benign
    unspecified site 217
  juvenile (M9030/0) 217
  pericanicular (M9012/0)
    specified site — *see* Neoplasm, by site, benign
    unspecified site 217
  phyllodes (M9020/0) 217
  prostate 600.2
  specified site — *see* Neoplasm, by site, benign
  unspecified site 217
Fibroadenosis, breast (chronic) (cystic) (diffuse) (periodic) (segmental) 610.2
Fibroangioma (M9160/0) — *see also* Neoplasm, by site, benign
  juvenile (M9160/0)
    specified site — *see* Neoplasm, by site, benign
    unspecified site 210.7
Fibrocellulitis progressiva ossificans 728.11
Fibrochondrosarcoma (M9220/3) — *see* Neoplasm, cartilage, malignant
Fibrocystic
  disease 277.00
    bone NEC 733.29
    breast 610.1

Fibrocystic — *continued*
  disease — *continued*
    jaw 526.2
    kidney (congenital) 753.19
    liver 751.62
    lung 518.89
      congenital 748.4
    pancreas 277.00
  kidney (congenital) 753.19
Fibrodysplasia ossificans multiplex
    (progressiva) 728.11
Fibroelastosis (cordis) (endocardial)
    (endomyocardial) 425.3
Fibroid (tumor) (M8890/0) — *see also* Neoplasm,
    connective tissue, benign
  disease, lung (chronic) (*see also* Fibrosis, lung)
    515
  heart (disease) (*see also* Myocarditis) 429.0
  induration, lung (chronic) (*see also* Fibrosis,
    lung) 515
  in pregnancy or childbirth 654.1 ✓5ᵗʰ
    affecting fetus or newborn 763.89
    causing obstructed labor 660.2 ✓5ᵗʰ
      affecting fetus or newborn 763.1
  liver — *see* Cirrhosis, liver
  lung (*see also* Fibrosis, lung) 515
  pneumonia (chronic) (*see also* Fibrosis, lung)
    515
  uterus (M8890/0) (*see also* Leiomyoma,
    uterus) 218.9
Fibrolipoma (M8851/0) (*see also* Lipoma, by site)
    214.9
Fibroliposarcoma (M8850/3) — *see* Neoplasm,
    connective tissue, malignant
Fibroma (M8810/0) — *see also* Neoplasm,
    connective tissue, benign
  ameloblastic (M9330/0) 213.1
    upper jaw (bone) 213.0
  bone (nonossifying) 733.99
    ossifying (M9262/0) — *see* Neoplasm, bone,
      benign
  cementifying (M9274/0) — *see* Neoplasm,
    bone, benign
  chondromyxoid (M9241/0) — *see* Neoplasm,
    bone, benign
  desmoplastic (M8823/1) — *see* Neoplasm,
    connective tissue, uncertain behavior
  facial (M8813/0) — *see* Neoplasm, connective
    tissue, benign
  invasive (M8821/1) — *see* Neoplasm,
    connective tissue, uncertain behavior
  molle (M8851/0) (*see also* Lipoma, by site)
    214.9
  myxoid (M8811/0) — *see* Neoplasm,
    connective tissue, benign
  nasopharynx, nasopharyngeal (juvenile)
    (M9160/0) 210.7
  nonosteogenic (nonossifying) — *see* Dysplasia,
    fibrous
  odontogenic (M9321/0) 213.1
    upper jaw (bone) 213.0
  ossifying (M9262/0) — *see* Neoplasm, bone,
    benign
  periosteal (M8812/0) — *see* Neoplasm, bone,
    benign
  prostate 600.2
  soft (M8851/0) (*see also* Lipoma, by site)
    214.9

Fibromatosis
  abdominal (M8822/1) — *see* Neoplasm,
    connective tissue, uncertain behavior
  aggressive (M8821/1) — *see* Neoplasm,
    connective tissue, uncertain behavior
  Dupuytren's 728.6
  gingival 523.8
  plantar fascia 728.71
  proliferative 728.79
  pseudosarcomatous (proliferative)
    (subcutaneous) 728.79
  subcutaneous pseudosarcomatous
    (proliferative) 728.79
Fibromyalgia 729.1
Fibromyoma (M8890/0) — *see also* Neoplasm,
    connective tissue, benign
  uterus (corpus) (*see also* Leiomyoma, uterus)
    218.9
    in pregnancy or childbirth 654.1 ✓5ᵗʰ
      affecting fetus or newborn 763.89
      causing obstructed labor 660.2 ✓5ᵗʰ
        affecting fetus or newborn 763.1
Fibromyositis (*see also* Myositis) 729.1
  scapulohumeral 726.2
Fibromyxolipoma (M8852/0) (*see also* Lipoma,
    by site) 214.9
Fibromyxoma (M8811/0) — *see* Neoplasm,
    connective tissue, benign
Fibromyxosarcoma (M8811/3) — *see* Neoplasm,
    connective tissue, malignant
Fibro-odontoma, ameloblastic (M9290/0) 213.1
  upper jaw (bone) 213.0
Fibro-osteoma (M9262/0) — *see* Neoplasm,
    bone, benign
Fibroplasia, retrolental 362.21
Fibropurulent — *see* condition
Fibrosarcoma (M8810/3) — *see also* Neoplasm,
    connective tissue, malignant
  ameloblastic (M9330/3) 170.1
    upper jaw (bone) 170.0
  congenital (M8814/3) — *see* Neoplasm,
    connective tissue, malignant
  fascial (M8813/3) — *see* Neoplasm, connective
    tissue, malignant
  infantile (M8814/3) — *see* Neoplasm,
    connective tissue, malignant
  odontogenic (M9330/3) 170.1
    upper jaw (bone) 170.0
  periosteal (M8812/3) — *see* Neoplasm, bone,
    malignant
Fibrosclerosis
  breast 610.3
  corpora cavernosa (penis) 607.89
  familial multifocal NEC 710.8
  multifocal (idiopathic) NEC 710.8
  penis (corpora cavernosa) 607.89
Fibrosis, fibrotic
  adrenal (gland) 255.8
  alveolar (diffuse) 516.3
  amnion 658.8 ✓5ᵗʰ
  anal papillae 569.49
  anus 569.49
  appendix, appendiceal, noninflammatory
    543.9
  arteriocapillary — *see* Arteriosclerosis
  bauxite (of lung) 503
  biliary 576.8
    due to Clonorchis sinensis 121.1

Fibrosis, fibrotic — *continued*
- bladder 596.8
  - interstitial 595.1
  - localized submucosal 595.1
  - panmural 595.1
- bone, diffuse 756.59
- breast 610.3
- capillary — *see also* Arteriosclerosis
  - lung (chronic) (*see also* Fibrosis, lung) 515
- cardiac (*see also* Myocarditis) 429.0
- cervix 622.8
- chorion 658.8 ✓5ᵗʰ
- corpus cavernosum 607.89
- cystic (of pancreas) 277.00
  - with •
    - manifestations •
      - gastrointestinal 277.03 •
      - pulmonary 277.02 •
      - specified NEC 277.09 •
    - meconium ileus 277.01 •
    - pulmonary exacerbation 277.02 •
- due to (presence of) any device, implant, or graft — *see* Complications, due to (presence of) any device, implant, or graft classified to 996.0-996.5 NEC
- ejaculatory duct 608.89
- endocardium (*see also* Endocarditis) 424.90
- endomyocardial (African) 425.0
- epididymis 608.89
- eye muscle 378.62
- graphite (of lung) 503
- heart (*see also* Myocarditis) 429.0
- hepatic — *see also* Cirrhosis, liver due to Clonorchis sinensis 121.1
- hepatolienal — *see* Cirrhosis, liver
- hepatosplenic — *see* Cirrhosis, liver
- infrapatellar fat pad 729.31
- interstitial pulmonary, newborn 770.7
- intrascrotal 608.89
- kidney (*see also* Sclerosis, renal) 587
- liver — *see* Cirrhosis, liver
- lung (atrophic) (capillary) (chronic) (confluent) (massive) (perialveolar) (peribronchial) 515
  - with
    - anthracosilicosis (occupational) 500
    - anthracosis (occupational) 500
    - asbestosis (occupational) 501
    - bagassosis (occupational) 495.1
    - bauxite 503
    - berylliosis (occupational) 503
    - byssinosis (occupational) 504
    - calcicosis (occupational) 502
    - chalicosis (occupational) 502
    - dust reticulation (occupational) 504
    - farmers' lung 495.0
    - gannister disease (occupational) 502
    - graphite 503
    - pneumonoconiosis (occupational) 505
    - pneumosiderosis (occupational) 503
    - siderosis (occupational) 503
    - silicosis (occupational) 502
    - tuberculosis (*see also* Tuberculosis) 011.4 ✓5ᵗʰ
  - diffuse (idiopathic) (interstitial) 516.3
  - due to
    - bauxite 503
    - fumes or vapors (chemical) inhalation 506.4
    - graphite 503
  - following radiation 508.1

Fibrosis, fibrotic — *continued*
- lung — *continued*
  - postinflammatory 515
  - silicotic (massive) (occupational) 502
  - tuberculous (*see also* Tuberculosis) 011.4 ✓5ᵗʰ
- lymphatic gland 289.3
- median bar 600.9
- mediastinum (idiopathic) 519.3
- meninges 349.2
- muscle NEC 728.2
  - iatrogenic (from injection) 999.9
- myocardium, myocardial (*see also* Myocarditis) 429.0
- oral submucous 528.8
- ovary 620.8
- oviduct 620.8
- pancreas 577.8
  - cystic 277.00
    - with •
      - manifestations •
        - gastrointestinal 277.03 •
        - pulmonary 277.02 •
        - specified NEC 277.09 •
      - meconium ileus 277.01 •
      - pulmonary exacerbation 277.02 •
- penis 607.89
- periappendiceal 543.9
- periarticular (*see also* Ankylosis) 718.5 ✓5ᵗʰ
- pericardium 423.1
- perineum, in pregnancy or childbirth 654.8 ✓5ᵗʰ
  - affecting fetus or newborn 763.89
  - causing obstructed labor 660.2 ✓5ᵗʰ
    - affecting fetus or newborn 763.1
- perineural NEC 355.9
  - foot 355.6
- periureteral 593.89
- placenta — *see* Placenta, abnormal
- pleura 511.0
- popliteal fat pad 729.31
- preretinal 362.56
- prostate (chronic) 600.9
- pulmonary (chronic) (*see also* Fibrosis, lung) 515
  - alveolar capillary block 516.3
  - interstitial
    - diffuse (idiopathic) 516.3
    - newborn 770.7
- radiation — *see* Effect, adverse, radiation
- rectal sphincter 569.49
- retroperitoneal, idiopathic 593.4
- scrotum 608.89
- seminal vesicle 608.89
- senile 797
- skin NEC 709.2
- spermatic cord 608.89
- spleen 289.59
  - bilharzial (*see also* Schistosomiasis) 120.9
- subepidermal nodular (M8832/0) — *see* Neoplasm, skin, benign
- submucous NEC 709.2
  - oral 528.9
  - tongue 528.8
- syncytium — *see* Placenta, abnormal
- testis 608.89
  - chronic, due to syphilis 095.8
- thymus (gland) 254.8
- tunica vaginalis 608.89
- ureter 593.89
- urethra 599.84

Fibrosis, fibrotic — *continued*
   uterus (nonneoplastic) 621.8
      bilharzial (*see also* Schistosomiasis) 120.9
      neoplastic (*see also* Leiomyoma, uterus) 218.9
   vagina 623.8
   valve, heart (*see also* Endocarditis) 424.90
   vas deferens 608.89
   vein 459.89
      lower extremities 459.89
   vesical 595.1
Fibrositis (periarticular) (rheumatoid) 729.0
   humeroscapular region 726.2
   nodular, chronic
      Jaccoud's 714.4
      rheumatoid 714.4
   ossificans 728.11
   scapulohumeral 726.2
Fibrothorax 511.0
Fibrotic — *see* Fibrosis
Fibrous — *see* condition
Fibroxanthoma (M8831/0) — *see also* Neoplasm, connective tissue, benign
   atypical (M8831/1) — *see* Neoplasm, connective tissue, uncertain behavior
   malignant (M8831/3) — *see* Neoplasm, connective tissue, malignant
Fibroxanthosarcoma (M8831/3) — *see* Neoplasm, connective tissue, malignant
Fiedler's
   disease (leptospiral jaundice) 100.0
   myocarditis or syndrome (acute isolated myocarditis) 422.91
Fiessinger-Leroy (-Reiter) syndrome 099.3
Fiessinger-Rendu syndrome (erythema muliforme exudativum) 695.1
Fifth disease (eruptive) 057.0
   venereal 099.1
Filaria, filarial — *see* Infestation, filarial
Filariasis (*see also* Infestation, filarial) 125.9
   bancroftian 125.0
   Brug's 125.1
   due to
      bancrofti 125.0
      Brugia (Wuchereria) (malayi) 125.1
      Loa loa 125.2
      malayi 125.1
      organism NEC 125.6
      Wuchereria (bancrofti) 125.0
         malayi 125.1
   Malayan 125.1
   ozzardi 125.1
   specified type NEC 125.6
Filatoff's, Filatov's, Filatow's disease (infectious mononucleosis) 075
File-cutters' disease 984.9
   specified type of lead — *see* Table of Drugs and Chemicals
Filling defect
   biliary tract 793.3
   bladder 793.5
   duodenum 793.4
   gallbladder 793.3
   gastrointestinal tract 793.4
   intestine 793.4
   kidney 793.5
   stomach 793.4
   ureter 793.5

Filtering bleb, eye (postglaucoma) (status) V45.69
   with complication or rupture 997.99
   postcataract extraction (complication) 997.99
Fimbrial cyst (congenital) 752.11
Fimbriated hymen 752.49
Financial problem affecting care V60.2
Findings, abnormal, without diagnosis (examination) (laboratory test) 796.4
   17-ketosteroids, elevated 791.9
   acetonuria 791.6
   acid phosphatase 790.5
   albumin-globulin ratio 790.99
   albuminuria 791.0
   alcohol in blood 790.3
   alkaline phosphatase 790.5
   amniotic fluid 792.3
   amylase 790.5
   anisocytosis 790.09
   antenatal screening 796.5
   anthrax, positive 795.31 ●
   antibody titers, elevated 795.79
   anticardiolipin antibody 795.79
   antigen-antibody reaction 795.79
   antiphospholipid antibody 795.79
   bacteriuria 791.9
   ballistocardiogram 794.39
   bicarbonate 276.9
   bile in urine 791.4
   bilirubin 277.4
   bleeding time (prolonged) 790.92
   blood culture, positive 790.7
   blood gas level 790.91
   blood sugar level 790.2
      high 790.2
      low 251.2
   calcium 275.40
   carbonate 276.9
   casts, urine 791.7
   catecholamines 791.9
   cells, urine 791.7
   cerebrospinal fluid (color) (content) (pressure) 792.0
   chloride 276.9
   cholesterol 272.9
   chromosome analysis 795.2
   chyluria 791.1
   circulation time 794.39
   cloudy dialysis effluent 792.5
   cloudy urine 791.9
   coagulation study 790.92
   cobalt, blood 790.6
   color of urine (unusual) NEC 791.9
   copper, blood 790.6
   crystals, urine 791.9
   culture, positive NEC 795.39 ▲
      blood 790.7
      HIV V08
      human immunodeficiency virus V08
      nose 795.39 ▲
      skin lesion NEC 795.39 ▲
      spinal fluid 792.0
      sputum 795.39 ▲
      stool 792.1
      throat 795.39 ▲
      urine 791.9
      viral
         human immunodeficiency V08
      wound 795.39 ▲
   echocardiogram 793.2
   echoencephalogram 794.01

Findings, abnormal, without diagnosis —
continued
- echogram NEC — *see* Findings, abnormal, structure
- electrocardiogram (ECG) (EKG) 794.31
- electroencephalogram (EEG) 794.02
- electrolyte level, urinary 791.9
- electromyogram (EMG) 794.17
  - ocular 794.14
- electro-oculogram (EOG) 794.12
- electroretinogram (ERG) 794.11
- enzymes, serum NEC 790.5
- fibrinogen titer coagulation study 790.92
- filling defect — *see* Filling defect
- function study NEC 794.9
  - auditory 794.15
  - bladder 794.9
  - brain 794.00
  - cardiac 794.30
  - endocrine NEC 794.6
    - thyroid 794.5
  - kidney 794.4
  - liver 794.8
  - nervous system
    - central 794.00
    - peripheral 794.19
  - oculomotor 794.14
  - pancreas 794.9
  - placenta 794.9
  - pulmonary 794.2
  - retina 794.11
  - special senses 794.19
  - spleen 794.9
  - vestibular 794.16
- gallbladder, nonvisualization 793.3
- glucose 790.2
  - tolerance test 790.2
- glycosuria 791.5
- heart
  - shadow 793.2
  - sounds 785.3
- hematinuria 791.2
- hematocrit
  - drop (precipitous) 790.01
  - elevated 282.7
  - low 285.9
- hematologic NEC 790.99
- hematuria 599.7
- hemoglobin
  - elevated 282.7
  - low 285.9
- hemoglobinuria 791.2
- histological NEC 795.4
- hormones 259.9
- immunoglobulins, elevated 795.79
- indolacetic acid, elevated 791.9
- iron 790.6
- karyotype 795.2
- ketonuria 791.6
- lactic acid dehydrogenase (LDH) 790.4
- lipase 790.5
- lipids NEC 272.9
- lithium, blood 790.6
- lung field (coin lesion) (shadow) 793.1
- magnesium, blood 790.6
- mammogram 793.80
  - microcalcification 793.81
- mediastinal shift 793.2
- melanin, urine 791.9
- microbiologic NEC 795.39 ▲
- mineral, blood NEC 790.6

Findings, abnormal, without diagnosis —
continued
- myoglobinuria 791.3
- nasal swab, anthrax 795.31 ●
- nitrogen derivatives, blood 790.6
- nonvisualization of gallbladder 793.3
- nose culture, positive 795.39 ▲
- odor of urine (unusual) NEC 791.9
- oxygen saturation 790.91
- Papanicolaou (smear) 795.1
  - cervix 795.00 ●
    - atypical squamous cell changes of undetermined significance ●
      - favor benign (ASCUS favor benign) ●
        795.01
      - favor dysplasia (ASCUS favor dysplasia) 795.02 ●
    - dyskaryotic 795.09 ●
    - nonspecific finding NEC 795.09 ●
  - other site 795.1
- peritoneal fluid 792.9
- phonocardiogram 794.39
- phosphorus 275.3
- pleural fluid 792.9
- pneumoencephalogram 793.0
- PO$_2$-oxygen ratio 790.91
- poikilocytosis 790.09
- potassium
  - deficiency 276.8
  - excess 276.7
- PPD 795.5
- prostate specific antigen (PSA) 790.93
- protein, serum NEC 790.99
- proteinuria 791.0
- prothrombin time (partial) (prolonged) (PT) (PTT) 790.92
- pyuria 791.9
- radiologic (x-ray) 793.9
  - abdomen 793.6
  - biliary tract 793.3
  - breast 793.89
    - abnormal mammogram NOS 793.80
    - mammographic microcalcification 793.81
  - gastrointestinal tract 793.4
  - genitourinary organs 793.5
  - head 793.0
  - intrathoracic organs NEC 793.2
  - lung 793.1
  - musculoskeletal 793.7
  - placenta 793.9
  - retroperitoneum 793.6
  - skin 793.9
  - skull 793.0
  - subcutaneous tissue 793.9
- red blood cell 790.09
  - count 790.09
  - morphology 790.09
  - sickling 790.09
  - volume 790.09
- saliva 792.4
- scan NEC 794.9
  - bladder 794.9
  - bone 794.9
  - brain 794.09
  - kidney 794.4
  - liver 794.8
  - lung 794.2
  - pancreas 794.9
  - placental 794.9
  - spleen 794.9

Index to Diseases

Findings, abnormal, without diagnosis — *continued*
  scan NEC — *continued*
    thyroid 794.5
  sedimentation rate, elevated 790.1
  semen 792.2
  serological (for)
    human immunodeficiency virus (HIV)
      inconclusive 795.71
      positive V08
    syphilis — *see* Findings, serology for syphilis
  serology for syphilis
    false positive 795.6
    positive 097.1
      false 795.6
      follow-up of latent syphilis — *see* Syphilis, latent
      only finding — *see* Syphilis, latent
  serum 790.99
    blood NEC 790.99
    enzymes NEC 790.5
    proteins 790.99
  SGOT 790.4
  SGPT 790.4
  sickling of red blood cells 790.09
  skin test, positive 795.79
    tuberculin (without active tuberculosis) 795.5
  sodium 790.6
    deficiency 276.1
    excess 276.0
  spermatozoa 792.2
  spinal fluid 792.0
    culture, positive 792.0
  sputum culture, positive 795.39 ▲
    for acid-fast bacilli 795.39 ▲
  stool NEC 792.1
    bloody 578.1
      occult 792.1
    color 792.1
    culture, positive 792.1
    occult blood 792.1
  structure, body (echogram) (thermogram) (ultrasound) (x-ray) NEC 793.9
    abdomen 793.6
    breast 793.89
      abnormal mammogram 793.80
      mammographic microcalcification 793.81
    gastrointestinal tract 793.4
    genitourinary organs 793.5
    head 793.0
      echogram (ultrasound) 794.01
    intrathoracic organs NEC 793.2
    lung 793.1
    musculoskeletal 793.7
    placenta 793.9
    retroperitoneum 793.6
    skin 793.9
    subcutaneous tissue NEC 793.9
  synovial fluid 792.9
  thermogram — *see* Finding, abnormal, structure
  throat culture, positive 795.39 ▲
  thyroid (function) 794.5
    metabolism (rate) 794.5
    scan 794.5
    uptake 794.5
  total proteins 790.99
  toxicology (drugs) (heavy metals) 796.0

Findings, abnormal, without diagnosis — *continued*
  transaminase (level) 790.4
  triglycerides 272.9
  tuberculin skin test (without active tuberculosis) 795.5
  ultrasound — *see also* Finding, abnormal, structure
    cardiogram 793.2
  uric acid, blood 790.6
  urine, urinary constituents 791.9
    acetone 791.6
    albumin 791.0
    bacteria 791.9
    bile 791.4
    blood 599.7
    casts or cells 791.7
    chyle 791.1
    culture, positive 791.9
    glucose 791.5
    hemoglobin 791.2
    ketone 791.6
    protein 791.0
    pus 791.9
    sugar 791.5
  vaginal fluid 792.9
  vanillylmandelic acid, elevated 791.9
  vectorcardiogram (VCG) 794.39
  ventriculogram (cerebral) 793.0
  VMA, elevated 791.9
  Wassermann reaction
    false positive 795.6
    positive 097.1
      follow-up of latent syphilis — *see* Syphilis, latent
      only finding — *see* Syphilis, latent
  white blood cell 288.9
    count 288.9
      elevated 288.8
      low 288.0
    differential 288.9
    morphology 288.9
  wound culture 795.39 ▲
  xerography 793.89
  zinc, blood 790.6

Finger — *see* condition
Fire, St. Anthony's (*see also* Erysipelas) 035
Fish
  hook stomach 537.89
  meal workers' lung 495.8
Fisher's syndrome 357.0
Fissure, fissured
  abdominal wall (congenital) 756.79
  anus, anal 565.0
    congenital 751.5
  buccal cavity 528.9
  clitoris (congenital) 752.49
  ear, lobule (congenital) 744.29
  epiglottis (congenital) 748.3
  larynx 478.79
    congenital 748.3
  lip 528.5
    congenital (*see also* Cleft, lip) 749.10
  nipple 611.2
    puerperal, postpartum 676.1 ✓5ᵗʰ
  palate (congenital) (*see also* Cleft, palate) 749.00
  postanal 565.0
  rectum 565.0
  skin 709.8
    streptococcal 686.9

✓4ᵗʰ Fourth-digit Required
✓5ᵗʰ Fifth-digit Required

Fissure, fissured — *continued*
   spine (congenital) (*see also* Spina bifida) 741.9
   sternum (congenital) 756.3
   tongue (acquired) 529.5
      congenital 750.13

Fistula (sinus) 686.9
   abdomen (wall) 569.81
      bladder 596.2
      intestine 569.81
      ureter 593.82
      uterus 619.2
   abdominorectal 569.81
   abdominosigmoidal 569.81
   abdominothoracic 510.0
   abdominouterine 619.2
      congenital 752.3
   abdominovesical 596.2
   accessory sinuses (*see also* Sinusitis) 473.9
   actinomycotic — *see* Actinomycosis
   alveolar
      antrum (*see also* Sinusitis, maxillary) 473.0
      process 522.7
   anorectal 565.1
   antrobuccal (*see also* Sinusitis, maxillary) 473.0
   antrum (*see also* Sinusitis, maxillary) 473.0
   anus, anal (infectional) (recurrent) 565.1
      congenital 751.5
      tuberculous (*see also* Tuberculosis) 014.8
   aortic sinus 747.29
   aortoduodenal 447.2
   appendix, appendicular 543.9
   arteriovenous (acquired) 447.0
      brain 437.3
         congenital 747.81
            ruptured (*see also* Hemorrhage, subarachnoid) 430
         ruptured (*see also* Hemorrhage, subarachnoid) 430
      cerebral 437.3
         congenital 747.81
      congenital (peripheral) 747.60
         brain — *see* Fistula, arteriovenous, brain, congenital
         coronary 746.85
         gastrointestinal 747.61
         lower limb 747.64
         pulmonary 747.3
         renal 747.62
         specified NEC 747.69
         upper limb 747.63
      coronary 414.19
         congenital 746.85
      heart 414.19
      pulmonary (vessels) 417.0
         congenital 747.3
      surgically created (for dialysis) V45.1
         complication NEC 996.73
            atherosclerosis — *see* Arteriosclerosis, extremities
            embolism 996.74
            infection or inflammation 996.62
            mechanical 996.1
            occlusion NEC 996.74
            thrombus 996.74
      traumatic — *see* Injury, blood vessel, by site
   artery 447.2

Fistula — *continued*
   aural 383.81
      congenital 744.49
   auricle 383.81
      congenital 744.49
   Bartholin's gland 619.8
   bile duct (*see also* Fistula, biliary) 576.4
   biliary (duct) (tract) 576.4
      congenital 751.69
   bladder (neck) (sphincter) 596.2
      into seminal vesicle 596.2
   bone 733.99
   brain 348.8
      arteriovenous — *see* Fistula, arteriovenous, brain
   branchial (cleft) 744.41
   branchiogenous 744.41
   breast 611.0
      puerperal, postpartum 675.1
   bronchial 510.0
   bronchocutaneous, bronchomediastinal, bronchopleural, bronchopleuromediastinal (infective) 510.0
      tuberculous (*see also* Tuberculosis) 011.3
   bronchoesophageal 530.89
      congenital 750.3
   buccal cavity (infective) 528.3
   canal, ear 380.89
   carotid-cavernous
      congenital 747.81
         with hemorrhage 430
      traumatic 900.82
         with hemorrhage (*see also* Hemorrhage, brain, traumatic) 853.0
         late effect 908.3
   cecosigmoidal 569.81
   cecum 569.81
   cerebrospinal (fluid) 349.81
   cervical, lateral (congenital) 744.41
   cervicoaural (congenital) 744.49
   cervicosigmoidal 619.1
   cervicovesical 619.0
   cervix 619.8
   chest (wall) 510.0
   cholecystocolic (*see also* Fistula, gallbladder) 575.5
   cholecystocolonic (*see also* Fistula, gallbladder) 575.5
   cholecystoduodenal (*see also* Fistula, gallbladder) 575.5
   cholecystoenteric (*see also* Fistula, gallbladder) 575.5
   cholecystogastric (*see also* Fistula, gallbladder) 575.5
   cholecystointestinal (*see also* Fistula, gallbladder) 575.5
   choledochoduodenal 576.4
   cholocolic (*see also* Fistula, gallbladder) 575.5
   coccyx 685.1
      with abscess 685.0
   colon 569.81
   colostomy 569.69
   colovaginal (acquired) 619.1
   common duct (bile duct) 576.4
   congenital, NEC — *see* Anomaly, specified type NEC
   cornea, causing hypotony 360.32
   coronary, arteriovenous 414.19
      congenital 746.85

Fistula — *continued*
- costal region 510.0
- cul-de-sac, Douglas' 619.8
- cutaneous 686.9
- cystic duct (*see also* Fistula, gallbladder) 575.5
  - congenital 751.69
- dental 522.7
- diaphragm 510.0
  - bronchovisceral 510.0
  - pleuroperitoneal 510.0
  - pulmonoperitoneal 510.0
- duodenum 537.4
- ear (canal) (external) 380.89
- enterocolic 569.81
- enterocutaneous 569.81
- enteroenteric 569.81
- entero-uterine 619.1
  - congenital 752.3
- enterovaginal 619.1
  - congenital 752.49
- enterovesical 596.1
- epididymis 608.89
  - tuberculous (*see also* Tuberculosis) 016.4 ✓5ᵗʰ
- esophagobronchial 530.89
  - congenital 750.3
- esophagocutaneous 530.89
- esophagopleurocutaneous 530.89
- esophagotracheal 530.84
  - congenital 750.3
- esophagus 530.89
  - congenital 750.4
- ethmoid (*see also* Sinusitis, ethmoidal) 473.2
- eyeball (cornea) (sclera) 360.32
- eyelid 373.11
- fallopian tube (external) 619.2
- fecal 569.81
  - congenital 751.5
- from periapical lesion 522.7
- frontal sinus (*see also* Sinusitis, frontal) 473.1
- gallbladder 575.5
  - with calculus, cholelithiasis, stones (*see also* Cholelithiasis) 574.2 ✓5ᵗʰ
  - congenital 751.69
- gastric 537.4
- gastrocolic 537.4
  - congenital 750.7
  - tuberculous (*see also* Tuberculosis) 014.8 ✓5ᵗʰ
- gastroenterocolic 537.4
- gastroesophageal 537.4
- gastrojejunal 537.4
- gastrojejunocolic 537.4
- genital
  - organs
    - female 619.9
      - specified site NEC 619.8
    - male 608.89
  - tract-skin (female) 619.2
- hepatopleural 510.0
- hepatopulmonary 510.0
- horseshoe 565.1
- ileorectal 569.81
- ileosigmoidal 569.81
- ileostomy 569.69
- ileovesical 596.1
- ileum 569.81
- in ano 565.1
  - tuberculous (*see also* Tuberculosis) 014.8 ✓5ᵗʰ

Fistula — *continued*
- inner ear (*see also* Fistula, labyrinth) 386.40
- intestine 569.81
- intestinocolonic (abdominal) 569.81
- intestinoureteral 593.82
- intestinouterine 619.1
- intestinovaginal 619.1
  - congenital 752.49
- intestinovesical 596.1
- involving female genital tract 619.9
  - digestive-genital 619.1
  - genital tract-skin 619.2
  - specified site NEC 619.8
  - urinary-genital 619.0
- ischiorectal (fossa) 566
- jejunostomy 569.69
- jejunum 569.81
- joint 719.89
  - ankle 719.87
  - elbow 719.82
  - foot 719.87
  - hand 719.84
  - hip 719.85
  - knee 719.86
  - multiple sites 719.89
  - pelvic region 719.85
  - shoulder (region) 719.81
  - specified site NEC 719.88
  - tuberculous — *see* Tuberculosis, joint
  - wrist 719.83
- kidney 593.89
- labium (majus) (minus) 619.8
- labyrinth, labyrinthine NEC 386.40
  - combined sites 386.48
  - multiple sites 386.48
  - oval window 386.42
  - round window 386.41
  - semicircular canal 386.43
- lacrimal, lachrymal (duct) (gland) (sac) 375.61
- lacrimonasal duct 375.61
- laryngotracheal 748.3
- larynx 478.79
- lip 528.5
  - congenital 750.25
- lumbar, tuberculous (*see also* Tuberculosis) 015.0 ✓5ᵗʰ [730.8] ✓5ᵗʰ
- lung 510.0
- lymphatic (node) (vessel) 457.8
- mamillary 611.0
- mammary (gland) 611.0
  - puerperal, postpartum 675.1 ✓5ᵗʰ
- mastoid (process) (region) 383.1
- maxillary (*see also* Sinusitis, maxillary) 473.0
- mediastinal 510.0
- mediastinobronchial 510.0
- mediastinocutaneous 510.0
- middle ear 385.89
- mouth 528.3
- nasal 478.1
  - sinus (*see also* Sinusitis) 473.9
- nasopharynx 478.29
- nipple — *see* Fistula, breast
- nose 478.1
- oral (cutaneous) 528.3
  - maxillary (*see also* Sinusitis, maxillary) 473.0
  - nasal (with cleft palate) (*see also* Cleft, palate) 749.00
- orbit, orbital 376.10
- oro-antral (*see also* Sinusitis, maxillary) 473.0
- oval window (internal ear) 386.42

Fistula — *continued*
- oviduct (external) 619.2
- palate (hard) 526.89
  - soft 528.9
- pancreatic 577.8
- pancreaticoduodenal 577.8
- parotid (gland) 527.4
  - region 528.3
- pelvoabdominointestinal 569.81
- penis 607.89
- perianal 565.1
- pericardium (pleura) (sac) (*see also* Pericarditis) 423.8
- pericecal 569.81
- perineal — *see* Fistula, perineum
- perineorectal 569.81
- perineosigmoidal 569.81
- perineo-urethroscrotal 608.89
- perineum, perineal (with urethral involvement) NEC 599.1
  - tuberculous (*see also* Tuberculosis) 017.9
  - ureter 593.82
- perirectal 565.1
  - tuberculous (*see also* Tuberculosis) 014.8
- peritoneum (*see also* Peritonitis) 567.2
- periurethral 599.1
- pharyngo-esophageal 478.29
- pharynx 478.29
  - branchial cleft (congenital) 744.41
- pilonidal (infected) (rectum) 685.1
  - with abscess 685.0
- pleura, pleural, pleurocutaneous, pleuroperitoneal 510.0
  - stomach 510.0
  - tuberculous (*see also* Tuberculosis) 012.0
- pleuropericardial 423.8
- postauricular 383.81
- postoperative, persistent 998.6
- preauricular (congenital) 744.46
- prostate 602.8
- pulmonary 510.0
  - arteriovenous 417.0
    - congenital 747.3
  - tuberculous (*see also* Tuberculosis, pulmonary) 011.9
- pulmonoperitoneal 510.0
- rectolabial 619.1
- rectosigmoid (intercommunicating) 569.81
- rectoureteral 593.82
- rectourethral 599.1
  - congenital 753.8
- rectouterine 619.1
  - congenital 752.3
- rectovaginal 619.1
  - congenital 752.49
  - old, postpartal 619.1
  - tuberculous (*see also* Tuberculosis) 014.8
- rectovesical 596.1
  - congenital 753.8
- rectovesicovaginal 619.1
- rectovulvar 619.1
  - congenital 752.49
- rectum (to skin) 565.1
  - tuberculous (*see also* Tuberculosis) 014.8
- renal 593.89
- retroauricular 383.81

Fistula — *continued*
- round window (internal ear) 386.41
- salivary duct or gland 527.4
  - congenital 750.24
- sclera 360.32
- scrotum (urinary) 608.89
  - tuberculous (*see also* Tuberculosis) 016.5
- semicircular canals (internal ear) 386.43
- sigmoid 569.81
  - vesicoabdominal 596.1
- sigmoidovaginal 619.1
  - congenital 752.49
- skin 686.9
  - ureter 593.82
  - vagina 619.2
- sphenoidal sinus (*see also* Sinusitis, sphenoidal) 473.3
- splenocolic 289.59
- stercoral 569.81
- stomach 537.4
- sublingual gland 527.4
  - congenital 750.24
- submaxillary
  - gland 527.4
    - congenital 750.24
  - region 528.3
- thoracic 510.0
  - duct 457.8
- thoracoabdominal 510.0
- thoracicogastric 510.0
- thoracicointestinal 510.0
- thoracoabdominal 510.0
- thoracogastric 510.0
- thorax 510.0
- thyroglossal duct 759.2
- thyroid 246.8
- trachea (congenital) (external) (internal) 748.3
- tracheoesophageal 530.84
  - congenital 750.3
  - following tracheostomy 519.09
- traumatic
  - arteriovenous (*see also* Injury, blood vessel, by site) 904.9
  - brain — *see* Injury, intracranial
- tuberculous — *see* Tuberculosis, by site
- typhoid 002.0
- umbilical 759.89
- umbilico-urinary 753.8
- urachal, urachus 753.7
- ureter (persistent) 593.82
- ureteroabdominal 593.82
- ureterocervical 593.82
- ureterorectal 593.82
- ureterosigmoido-abdominal 593.82
- ureterovaginal 619.0
- ureterovesical 596.2
- urethra 599.1
  - congenital 753.8
  - tuberculous (*see also* Tuberculosis) 016.3
- urethroperineal 599.1
- urethroperineovesical 596.2
- urethrorectal 599.1
  - congenital 753.8
- urethroscrotal 608.89
- urethrovaginal 619.0
- urethrovesical 596.2
- urethrovesicovaginal 619.0
- urinary (persistent) (recurrent) 599.1

Fistula — continued
  uteroabdominal (anterior wall) 619.2
    congenital 752.3
  uteroenteric 619.1
  uterofecal 619.1
  uterointestinal 619.1
    congenital 752.3
  uterorectal 619.1
    congenital 752.3
  uteroureteric 619.0
  uterovaginal 619.8
  uterovesical 619.0
    congenital 752.3
  uterus 619.8
  vagina (wall) 619.8
    postpartal, old 619.8
  vaginocutaneous (postpartal) 619.2
  vaginoileal (acquired) 619.1
  vaginoperineal 619.2
  vesical NEC 596.2
  vesicoabdominal 596.2
  vesicocervicovaginal 619.0
  vesicocolic 596.1
  vesicocutaneous 596.2
  vesicoenteric 596.1
  vesicointestinal 596.1
  vesicometrorectal 619.1
  vesicoperineal 596.2
  vesicorectal 596.1
    congenital 753.8
  vesicosigmoidal 596.1
  vesicosigmoidovaginal 619.1
  vesicoureteral 596.2
  vesicoureterovaginal 619.0
  vesicourethral 596.2
  vesicourethrorectal 596.1
  vesicouterine 619.0
    congenital 752.3
  vesicovaginal 619.0
  vulvorectal 619.1
    congenital 752.49
Fit 780.39
  apoplectic (see also Disease, cerebrovascular, acute) 436
    late effect — see Late effect(s) (of) cerebrovascular disease
  epileptic (see also Epilepsy) 345.9
  fainting 780.2
  hysterical 300.11
  newborn 779.0
Fitting (of)
  artificial
    arm (complete) (partial) V52.0
    breast V52.4
    eye(s) V52.2
    leg(s) (complete) (partial) V52.1
  brain neuropacemaker V53.02
  cardiac pacemaker V53.31
  carotid sinus pacemaker V53.39
  cerebral ventricle (communicating) shunt V53.01
  colostomy belt V53.5
  contact lenses V53.1
  cystostomy device V53.6
  defibrillator, automatic implantable cardiac V53.32
  dentures V52.3
  device NEC V53.9
    abdominal V53.5

Fitting (of) — continued
  device NEC — continued
    cardiac
      defibrillator, automatic implantable V53.32
      pacemaker V53.31
      specified NEC V53.39
    cerebral ventricle (communicating) shunt V53.01
    intrauterine contraceptive V25.1
    nervous system V53.09
    orthodontic V53.4
    orthoptic V53.1
    prosthetic V52.9
      breast V52.4
      dental V52.3
      eye V52.2
      specified type NEC V52.8
    special senses V53.09
    substitution
      auditory V53.09
      nervous system V53.09
      visual V53.09
    urinary V53.6
  diaphragm (contraceptive) V25.02
  glasses (reading) V53.1
  hearing aid V53.2
  ileostomy device V53.5
  intestinal appliance or device NEC V53.5
  intrauterine contraceptive device V25.1
  neuropacemaker (brain) (peripheral nerve) (spinal cord) V53.02
  orthodontic device V53.4
  orthopedic (device) V53.7
    brace V53.7
    cast V53.7
    corset V53.7
    shoes V53.7
  pacemaker (cardiac) V53.31
    brain V53.02
    carotid sinus V53.39
    peripheral nerve V53.02
    spinal cord V53.02
  prosthesis V52.9
    arm (complete) (partial) V52.0
    breast V52.4
    dental V52.3
    eye V52.2
    leg (complete) (partial) V52.1
    specified type NEC V52.8
  spectacles V53.1
  wheelchair V53.8
Fitz's syndrome (acute hemorrhagic pancreatitis) 577.0
Fitz-Hugh and Curtis syndrome (gonococcal peritonitis) 098.86
Fixation
  joint — see Ankylosis
  larynx 478.79
  pupil 364.76
  stapes 385.22
    deafness (see also Deafness, conductive) 389.04
  uterus (acquired) — see Malposition, uterus
  vocal cord 478.5
Flaccid — see also condition
  foot 736.79
  forearm 736.09
  palate, congenital 750.26

Flail
chest 807.4
  newborn 767.3
joint (paralytic) 718.80
  ankle 718.87
  elbow 718.82
  foot 718.87
  hand 718.84
  hip 718.85
  knee 718.86
  multiple sites 718.89
  pelvic region 718.85
  shoulder (region) 718.81
  specified site NEC 718.88
  wrist 718.83

Flajani (-Basedow) syndrome or disease (exophthalmic goiter) 242.0

Flap, liver 572.8

Flare, anterior chamber (aqueous) (eye) 364.04

Flashback phenomena (drug) (hallucinogenic) 292.89

Flat
chamber (anterior) (eye) 360.34
chest, congenital 754.89
electroencephalogram (EEG) 348.8
foot (acquired) (fixed type) (painful) (postural) (spastic) 734
  congenital 754.61
    rocker bottom 754.61
    vertical talus 754.61
  rachitic 268.1
  rocker bottom (congenital) 754.61
  vertical talus, congenital 754.61
organ or site, congenital NEC — see Anomaly, specified type NEC
pelvis 738.6
  with disproportion (fetopelvic) 653.2
    affecting fetus or newborn 763.1
    causing obstructed labor 660.1
      affecting fetus or newborn 763.1
  congenital 755.69

Flatau-Schilder disease 341.1

Flattening
head, femur 736.39
hip 736.39
lip (congenital) 744.89
nose (congenital) 754.0
  acquired 738.0

Flatulence 787.3

Flatus 787.3
vaginalis 629.8

Flax dressers' disease 504

Flea bite — see Injury, superficial, by site

Fleischer (-Kayser) ring (corneal pigmentation) 275.1 [371.14]

Fleischner's disease 732.3

Fleshy mole 631

Flexibilitas cerea (see also Catalepsy) 300.11

Flexion
cervix (see also Malposition, uterus) 621.6
contracture, joint (see also Contraction, joint) 718.4
deformity, joint (see also Contraction, joint) 718.4
hip, congenital (see also Subluxation, congenital, hip) 754.32
uterus (see also Malposition, uterus) 621.6

Flexner's
bacillus 004.1
diarrhea (ulcerative) 004.1
dysentery 004.1

Flexner-Boyd dysentery 004.2

Flexure — see condition

Floater, vitreous 379.24

Floating
cartilage (joint) (see also Disorder, cartilage, articular) 718.0
  knee 717.6
gallbladder (congenital) 751.69
kidney 593.0
  congenital 753.3
liver (congenital) 751.69
rib 756.3
spleen 289.59

Flooding 626.2

Floor — see condition

Floppy
infant NEC 781.99
valve syndrome (mitral) 424.0

Flu — see also Influenza
gastric NEC 008.8

Fluctuating blood pressure 796.4

Fluid
abdomen 789.5
chest (see also Pleurisy, with effusion) 511.9
heart (see also Failure, heart) 428.0
joint (see also Effusion, joint) 719.0
loss (acute) 276.5
  with
    hypernatremia 276.0
    hyponatremia 276.1
lung — see also Edema, lung encysted 511.8
peritoneal cavity 789.5
pleural cavity (see also Pleurisy, with effusion) 511.9
retention 276.6

Flukes NEC (see also Infestation, fluke) 121.9
blood NEC (see also Infestation, Schistosoma) 120.9
liver 121.3

Fluor (albus) (vaginalis) 623.5
trichomonal (Trichomonas vaginalis) 131.00

Fluorosis (dental) (chronic) 520.3

Flushing 782.62
menopausal 627.2

Flush syndrome 259.2

Flutter
atrial or auricular 427.32
heart (ventricular) 427.42
  atrial 427.32
impure 427.32
postoperative 997.1
ventricular 427.42

Flux (bloody) (serosanguineous) 009.0

Focal — see condition

Fochier's abscess — see Abscess, by site

Focus, Assmann's (see also Tuberculosis) 011.0

Fogo selvagem 694.4

Foix-Alajouanine syndrome 336.1

Folds, anomalous — see also Anomaly, specified type NEC
Bowman's membrane 371.31
Descemet's membrane 371.32

Folds, anomalous — *continued*
  epicanthic 743.63
  heart 746.89
  posterior segment of eye, congenital 743.54
Folie à deux 297.3
Follicle
  cervix (nabothian) (ruptured) 616.0
  graafian, ruptured, with hemorrhage 620.0
  nabothian 616.0
Folliclis (primary) (*see also* Tuberculosis) 017.0 ✓5
Follicular — *see also* condition
  cyst (atretic) 620.0
Folliculitis 704.8
  abscedens et suffodiens 704.8
  decalvans 704.09
  gonorrheal (acute) 098.0
    chronic or duration of 2 months or more 098.2
  keloid, keloidalis 706.1
  pustular 704.8
  ulerythematosa reticulata 701.8
Folliculosis, conjunctival 372.02
Følling's disease (phenylketonuria) 270.1
Follow-up (examination) (routine) (following) V67.9
  cancer chemotherapy V67.2
  chemotherapy V67.2
  fracture V67.4
  high-risk medication V67.51
  injury NEC V67.59
  postpartum
    immediately after delivery V24.0
    routine V24.2
  psychiatric V67.3
  psychotherapy V67.3
  radiotherapy V67.1
  specified condition NEC V67.59
  specified surgery NEC V67.09
  surgery V67.00
    vaginal pap smear V67.01
  treatment V67.9
    combined NEC V67.6
    fracture V67.4
    involving high-risk medication NEC V67.51
    mental disorder V67.3
    specified NEC V67.59
Fong's syndrome (hereditary osteoonychodysplasia) 756.89
Food
  allergy 693.1
  anaphylactic shock — *see* Anaphylactic shock, due to, food
  asphyxia (from aspiration or inhalation) (*see also* Asphyxia, food) 933.1
  choked on (*see also* Asphyxia, food) 933.1
  deprivation 994.2
    specified kind of food NEC 269.8
  intoxication (*see also* Poisoning, food) 005.9
  lack of 994.2
  poisoning (*see also* Poisoning, food) 005.9
  refusal or rejection NEC 307.59
  strangulation or suffocation (*see also* Asphyxia, food) 933.1
  toxemia (*see also* Poisoning, food) 005.9
Foot — *see also* condition
  and mouth disease 078.4
  process disease 581.3

Foramen ovale (nonclosure) (patent) (persistent) 745.5
Forbes' (glycogen storage) disease 271.0
Forbes-Albright syndrome (nonpuerperal amenorrhea and lactation associated with pituitary tumor) 253.1
Forced birth or delivery NEC 669.8 ✓5
  affecting fetus or newborn NEC 763.89
Forceps
  delivery NEC 669.6 ✓5
  affecting fetus or newborn 763.2
Fordyce's disease (ectopic sebaceous glands) (mouth) 750.26
Fordyce-Fox disease (apocrine miliaria) 705.82
Forearm — *see* condition
Foreign body

> Note — For foreign body with open wound or other injury, see Wound, open, or the type of injury specified.

  accidentally left during a procedure 998.4
  anterior chamber (eye) 871.6
    magnetic 871.5
      retained or old 360.51
    retained or old 360.61
  ciliary body (eye) 871.6
    magnetic 871.5
      retained or old 360.52
    retained or old 360.62
  entering through orifice (current) (old)
    accessory sinus 932
    air passage (upper) 933.0
      lower 934.8
    alimentary canal 938
    alveolar process 935.0
    antrum (Highmore) 932
    anus 937
    appendix 936
    asphyxia due to (*see also* Asphyxia, food) 933.1
    auditory canal 931
    auricle 931
    bladder 939.0
    bronchioles 934.8
    bronchus (main) 934.1
    buccal cavity 935.0
    canthus (inner) 930.1
    cecum 936
    cervix (canal) uterine 939.1
    coil, ileocecal 936
    colon 936
    conjunctiva 930.1
    conjunctival sac 930.1
    cornea 930.0
    digestive organ or tract NEC 938
    duodenum 936
    ear (external) 931
    esophagus 935.1
    eye (external) 930.9
      combined sites 930.8
      intraocular — *see* Foreign body, by site
      specified site NEC 930.8
    eyeball 930.8
      intraocular — *see* Foreign body, intraocular
    eyelid 930.1
      retained or old 374.86
    frontal sinus 932
    gastrointestinal tract 938

Foreign body — *continued*
  entering through orifice — *continued*
    genitourinary tract 939.9
    globe 930.8
      penetrating 871.6
        magnetic 871.5
          retained or old 360.50
        retained or old 360.60
    gum 935.0
    Highmore's antrum 932
    hypopharynx 933.0
    ileocecal coil 936
    ileum 936
    inspiration (of) 933.1
    intestine (large) (small) 936
    lacrimal apparatus, duct, gland, or sac 930.2
    larynx 933.1
    lung 934.8
    maxillary sinus 932
    mouth 935.0
    nasal sinus 932
    nasopharynx 933.0
    nose (passage) 932
    nostril 932
    oral cavity 935.0
    palate 935.0
    penis 939.3
    pharynx 933.0
    pyriform sinus 933.0
    rectosigmoid 937
      junction 937
    rectum 937
    respiratory tract 934.9
      specified part NEC 934.8
    sclera 930.1
    sinus 932
      accessory 932
      frontal 932
      maxillary 932
      nasal 932
      pyriform 933.0
    small intestine 936
    stomach (hairball) 935.2
    suffocation by (*see also* Asphyxia, food) 933.1
    swallowed 938
      tongue 933.0
    tear ducts or glands 930.2
    throat 933.0
    tongue 935.0
      swallowed 933.0
    tonsil, tonsillar 933.0
      fossa 933.0
    trachea 934.0
    ureter 939.0
    urethra 939.0
    uterus (any part) 939.1
    vagina 939.2
    vulva 939.2
    wind pipe 934.0
  granuloma (old) 728.82
    bone 733.99
    in operative wound (inadvertently left) 998.4
      due to surgical material intentionally left — *see* Complications, due to (presence of) any device, implant, or graft classified to 996.0-996.5 NEC
    muscle 728.82

Foreign body — *continued*
  granuloma — *continued*
    skin 709.4
    soft tissue 709.4
    subcutaneous tissue 709.4
  in
    bone (residual) 733.99
    open wound — *see* Wound, open, by site complicated
    soft tissue (residual) 729.6
  inadvertently left in operation wound (causing adhesions, obstruction, or perforation) 998.4
  ingestion, ingested NEC 938
  inhalation or inspiration (*see also* Asphyxia, food) 933.1
  internal organ, not entering through an orifice — *see* Injury, internal, by site, with open wound
  intraocular (nonmagnetic) 871.6
    combined sites 871.6
      magnetic 871.5
        retained or old 360.59
      retained or old 360.69
    magnetic 871.5
      retained or old 360.50
    retained or old 360.60
    specified site NEC 871.6
      magnetic 871.5
        retained or old 360.59
      retained or old 360.69
  iris (nonmagnetic) 871.6
    magnetic 871.5
      retained or old 360.52
    retained or old 360.62
  lens (nonmagnetic) 871.6
    magnetic 871.5
      retained or old 360.53
    retained or old 360.63
  lid, eye 930.1
  ocular muscle 870.4
    retained or old 376.6
  old or residual
    bone 733.99
    eyelid 374.86
    middle ear 385.83
    muscle 729.6
      ocular 376.6
    retrobulbar 376.6
    skin 729.6
      with granuloma 709.4
    soft tissue 729.6
      with granuloma 709.4
    subcutaneous tissue 729.6
      with granuloma 709.4
  operation wound, left accidentally 998.4
  orbit 870.4
    retained or old 376.6
  posterior wall, eye 871.6
    magnetic 871.5
      retained or old 360.55
    retained or old 360.65
  respiratory tree 934.9
    specified site NEC 934.8
  retained (old) (nonmagnetic) (in)
    anterior chamber (eye) 360.61
      magnetic 360.51
    ciliary body 360.62
      magnetic 360.52
    eyelid 374.86

Index to Diseases — Fracture

Foreign body — *continued*
  retained — *continued*
    globe 360.60
      magnetic 360.50
    intraocular 360.60
      magnetic 360.50
      specified site NEC 360.69
        magnetic 360.59
    iris 360.62
      magnetic 360.52
    lens 360.63
      magnetic 360.53
    muscle 729.6
    orbit 376.6
    posterior wall of globe 360.65
      magnetic 360.55
    retina 360.65
      magnetic 360.55
    retrobulbar 376.6
    soft tissue 729.6
    vitreous 360.64
      magnetic 360.54
    skin 729.6
      with granuloma 709.4
    soft tissue 729.6
      with granuloma 709.4
    subcutaneous tissue 729.6
      with granuloma 709.4
  retina 871.6
    magnetic 871.5
    retained or old 360.55
    retained or old 360.65
  superficial, without major open wound (*see also* Injury, superficial, by site) 919.6
  swallowed NEC 938
  vitreous (humor) 871.6
    magnetic 871.5
    retained or old 360.54
    retained or old 360.64
Forking, aqueduct of Sylvius 742.3
  with spina bifida (*see also* Spina bifida) 741.0
Formation
  bone in scar tissue (skin) 709.3
  connective tissue in vitreous 379.25
  Elschnig pearls (postcataract extraction) 366.51
  hyaline in cornea 371.49
  sequestrum in bone (due to infection) (*see also* Osteomyelitis) 730.1
  valve
    colon, congenital 751.5
    ureter (congenital) 753.29
Formication 782.0
Fort Bragg fever 100.89
Fossa — *see also* condition
  pyriform — *see* condition
Foster-Kennedy syndrome 377.04
Fothergill's
  disease, meaning scarlatina anginosa 034.1
  neuralgia (*see also* Neuralgia, trigeminal) 350.2
Foul breath 784.9
Found dead (cause unknown) 798.9
Foundling V20.0
Fournier's disease (idiopathic gangrene) 608.83
Fourth
  cranial nerve — *see* condition
  disease 057.8

Fourth — *continued*
  molar 520.1
Foville's syndrome 344.89
Fox's
  disease (apocrine miliaria) 705.82
  impetigo (contagiosa) 684
Fox-Fordyce disease (apocrine miliaria) 705.82
Fracture (abduction) (adduction) (avulsion) (compression) (crush) (dislocation) (oblique) (separation) (closed) 829.0

> Note — For fracture of any of the following sites with fracture of other bones — *see* Fracture, multiple.
> "Closed" includes the following descriptions of fractures, with or without delayed healing, unless they are specified as open or compound:
>
> | comminuted | linear |
> |---|---|
> | depressed | simple |
> | elevated | slipped epiphysis |
> | fissured | spiral |
> | greenstick | unspecified |
> | impacted | |
>
> "Open" includes the following descriptions of fractures, with or without delayed healing:
>
> | compound | puncture |
> |---|---|
> | infected | with foreign body |
> | missile | |
>
> For late effect of fracture, *see* Late, effect, fracture, by site.

  with
    internal injuries in same region (conditions classifiable to 860-869) — *see also* Injury, internal, by site pelvic region — *see* Fracture, pelvis
  acetabulum (with visceral injury) (closed) 808.0
    open 808.1
  acromion (process) (closed) 811.01
    open 811.11
  alveolus (closed) 802.8
    open 802.9
  ankle (malleolus) (closed) 824.8
    bimalleolar (Dupuytren's) (Pott's) 824.4
      open 824.5
    bone 825.21
      open 825.31
    lateral malleolus only (fibular) 824.2
      open 824.3
    medial malleolus only (tibial) 824.0
      open 824.1
    open 824.9
    pathologic 733.16
    talus 825.21
      open 825.31
    trimalleolar 824.6
      open 824.7
  antrum — *see* Fracture, skull, base
  arm (closed) 818.0
    and leg(s) (any bones) 828.0
      open 828.1
    both (any bones) (with rib(s)) (with sternum) 819.0
      open 819.1
    lower 813.80
      open 813.90
    open 818.1
    upper — *see* Fracture, humerus

Fourth-digit Required   Fifth-digit Required

Fracture — *continued*
  astragalus (closed) 825.21
    open 825.31
  atlas — *see* Fracture, vertebra, cervical, first
  axis — *see* Fracture, vertebra, cervical, second
  back — *see* Fracture, vertebra, by site
  Barton's — *see* Fracture, radius, lower end
  basal (skull) — *see* Fracture, skull, base
  Bennett's (closed) 815.01
    open 815.11
  bimalleolar (closed) 824.4
    open 824.5
  bone (closed) NEC 829.0
    birth injury NEC 767.3
    open 829.1
    pathologic NEC (*see also* Fracture, pathologic) 733.10
    stress NEC (*see also* Fracture, stress) 733.95
  boot top — *see* Fracture, fibula
  boxers' — *see* Fracture, metacarpal bone(s)
  breast bone — *see* Fracture, sternum
  bucket handle (semilunar cartilage) — *see* Tear, meniscus
  bursting — *see* Fracture, phalanx, hand, distal
  calcaneus (closed) 825.0
    open 825.1
  capitate (bone) (closed) 814.07
    open 814.17
  capitellum (humerus) (closed) 812.49
    open 812.59
  carpal bone(s) (wrist NEC) (closed) 814.00
    open 814.10
    specified site NEC 814.09
      open 814.19
  cartilage, knee (semilunar) — *see* Tear, meniscus
  cervical — *see* Fracture, vertebra, cervical
  chauffeur's — *see* Fracture, ulna, lower end
  chisel — *see* Fracture, radius, upper end
  clavicle (interligamentous part) (closed) 810.00
    acromial end 810.03
      open 810.13
    due to birth trauma 767.2
    open 810.10
    shaft (middle third) 810.02
      open 810.12
    sternal end 810.01
      open 810.11
  clayshovelers' — *see* Fracture, vertebra, cervical
  coccyx — *see also* Fracture, vertebra, coccyx
    complicating delivery 665.6
  collar bone — *see* Fracture, clavicle
  Colles' (reversed) (closed) 813.41
    open 813.51
  comminuted — *see* Fracture, by site
  compression — *see also* Fracture, by site
    nontraumatic — *see* Fracture, pathologic
  congenital 756.9
  coracoid process (closed) 811.02
    open 811.12
  coronoid process (ulna) (closed) 813.02
    mandible (closed) 802.23
      open 802.33
    open 813.12
  costochondral junction — *see* Fracture, rib
  costosternal junction — *see* Fracture, rib
  cranium — *see* Fracture, skull, by site

Fracture — *continued*
  cricoid cartilage (closed) 807.5
    open 807.6
  cuboid (ankle) (closed) 825.23
    open 825.33
  cuneiform
    foot (closed) 825.24
      open 825.34
    wrist (closed) 814.03
      open 814.13
  due to
    birth injury — *see* Birth injury, fracture
    gunshot — *see* Fracture, by site, open
    neoplasm — *see* Fracture, pathologic
    osteoporosis — *see* Fracture, pathologic
  Dupuytren's (ankle) (fibula) (closed) 824.4
    open 824.5
  radius 813.42
    open 813.52
  Duverney's — *see* Fracture, ilium
  elbow — *see also* Fracture, humerus, lower end
    olecranon (process) (closed) 813.01
      open 813.11
    supracondylar (closed) 812.41
      open 812.51
  ethmoid (bone) (sinus) — *see* Fracture, skull, base
  face bone(s) (closed) NEC 802.8
    with
      other bone(s) — *see* Fracture, multiple, skull
      skull — *see also* Fracture, skull
        involving other bones — *see* Fracture, multiple, skull
    open 802.9
  fatigue — *see* Fracture, march
  femur, femoral (closed) 821.00
    cervicotrochanteric 820.03
      open 820.13
    condyles, epicondyles 821.21
      open 821.31
    distal end — *see* Fracture, femur, lower end
    epiphysis (separation)
      capital 820.01
        open 820.11
      head 820.01
        open 820.11
      lower 821.22
        open 821.32
      trochanteric 820.01
        open 820.11
      upper 820.01
        open 820.11
    head 820.09
      open 820.19
    lower end or extremity (distal end) (closed) 821.20
      condyles, epicondyles 821.21
        open 821.31
      epiphysis (separation) 821.22
        open 821.32
      multiple sites 821.29
        open 821.39
      open 821.30
      specified site NEC 821.29
        open 821.39
      supracondylar 821.23
        open 821.33
      T-shaped 821.21
        open 821.31

Fracture — *continued*
  femur, femoral — *continued*
    neck (closed) 820.8
      base (cervicotrochanteric) 820.03
        open 820.13
      extracapsular 820.20
        open 820.30
      intertrochanteric (section) 820.21
        open 820.31
      intracapsular 820.00
        open 820.10
      intratrochanteric 820.21
        open 820.31
      midcervical 820.02
        open 820.12
      open 820.9
      pathologic 733.14
        specified part NEC 733.15
      specified site NEC 820.09
        open 820.19
      transcervical 820.02
        open 820.12
      transtrochanteric 820.20
        open 820.30
    open 821.10
    pathologic 733.14
      specified part NEC 733.15
    peritrochanteric (section) 820.20
      open 820.30
    shaft (lower third) (middle third) (upper third) 821.01
      open 821.11
    subcapital 820.09
      open 820.19
    subtrochanteric (region) (section) 820.22
      open 820.32
    supracondylar 821.23
      open 821.33
    transepiphyseal 820.01
      open 820.11
    trochanter (greater) (lesser) (*see also* Fracture, femur, neck, by site) 820.20
      open 820.30
    T-shaped, into knee joint 821.21
      open 821.31
    upper end 820.8
      open 820.9
  fibula (closed) 823.81
    with tibia 823.82
      open 823.92
    distal end 824.8
      open 824.9
    epiphysis
      lower 824.8
        open 824.9
      upper — *see* Fracture, fibula, upper end
    head — *see* Fracture, fibula, upper end
    involving ankle 824.2
      open 824.3
    lower end or extremity 824.8
      open 824.9
    malleolus (external) (lateral) 824.2
      open 824.3
    open NEC 823.91
    pathologic 733.16
    proximal end — *see* Fracture, fibula, upper end
    shaft 823.21
      with tibia 823.22
        open 823.32
      open 823.31

Fracture — *continued*
  fibula — *continued*
    stress 733.93
    torus 823.41 ●
      with tibia 823.42 ●
    upper end or extremity (epiphysis) (head) (proximal end) (styloid) 823.01
      with tibia 823.02
        open 823.12
      open 823.11
  finger(s), of one hand (closed) (*see also* Fracture, phalanx, hand) 816.00
    with
      metacarpal bone(s), of same hand 817.0
        open 817.1
      thumb of same hand 816.03
        open 816.13
    open 816.10
  foot, except toe(s) alone (closed) 825.20
    open 825.30
  forearm (closed) NEC 813.80
    lower end (distal end) (lower epiphysis) 813.40
      open 813.50
    open 813.90
    shaft 813.20
      open 813.30
    upper end (proximal end) (upper epiphysis) 813.00
      open 813.10
  fossa, anterior, middle, or posterior — *see* Fracture, skull, base
  frontal (bone) — *see also* Fracture, skull, vault
    sinus — *see* Fracture, skull, base
  Galeazzi's — *see* Fracture, radius, lower end
  glenoid (cavity) (fossa) (scapula) (closed) 811.03
    open 811.13
  Gosselin's — *see* Fracture, ankle
  greenstick — *see* Fracture, by site
  grenade-throwers' — *see* Fracture, humerus, shaft
  gutter — *see* Fracture, skull, vault
  hamate (closed) 814.08
    open 814.18
  hand, one (closed) 815.00
    carpals 814.00
      open 814.10
      specified site NEC 814.09
        open 814.19
    metacarpals 815.00
      open 815.10
    multiple, bones of one hand 817.0
      open 817.1
    open 815.10
    phalanges (*see also* Fracture, phalanx, hand) 816.00
      open 816.10
  healing
    aftercare ▶(*see also* Aftercare, fracture)◀ V54.89 ▲
    change of cast V54.89 ▲
    complications — *see* condition
    convalescence V66.4 ●
    removal of
      cast V54.89 ▲
      fixation device
        external V54.89 ▲
        internal V54.0
  heel bone (closed) 825.0
    open 825.1

Fracture — *continued*
  hip (closed) (*see also* Fracture, femur, neck) 820.8
    open 820.9
    pathologic 733.14
  humerus (closed) 812.20
    anatomical neck 812.02
      open 812.12
    articular process (*see also* Fracture humerus, condyle(s)) 812.44
      open 812.54
    capitellum 812.49
      open 812.59
    condyle(s) 812.44
      lateral (external) 812.42
        open 812.52
      medial (internal epicondyle) 812.43
        open 812.53
      open 812.54
    distal end — *see* Fracture, humerus, lower end
    epiphysis
      lower (*see also* Fracture, humerus, condyle(s)) 812.44
        open 812.54
      upper 812.09
        open 812.19
    external condyle 812.42
      open 812.52
    great tuberosity 812.03
      open 812.13
    head 812.09
      open 812.19
    internal epicondyle 812.43
      open 812.53
    lesser tuberosity 812.09
      open 812.19
    lower end or extremity (distal end) (*see also* Fracture, humerus, by site) 812.40
      multiple sites NEC 812.49
        open 812.59
      open 812.50
      specified site NEC 812.49
        open 812.59
    neck 812.01
      open 812.11
    open 812.30
    pathologic 733.11
    proximal end — *see* Fracture, humerus, upper end
    shaft 812.21
      open 812.31
    supracondylar 812.41
      open 812.51
    surgical neck 812.01
      open 812.11
    trochlea 812.49
      open 812.59
    T-shaped 812.44
      open 812.54
    tuberosity — *see* Fracture, humerus, upper end
    upper end or extremity (proximal end) (*see also* Fracture, humerus, by site) 812.00
      open 812.10
      specified site NEC 812.09
        open 812.19
  hyoid bone (closed) 807.5
    open 807.6

Fracture — *continued*
  hyperextension — *see* Fracture, radius, lower end
  ilium (with visceral injury) (closed) 808.41
    open 808.51
  impaction, impacted — *see* Fracture, by site
  incus — *see* Fracture, skull, base
  innominate bone (with visceral injury) (closed) 808.49
    open 808.59
  instep, of one foot (closed) 825.20
    with toe(s) of same foot 827.0
      open 827.1
    open 825.30
  internal
    ear — *see* Fracture, skull, base
    semilunar cartilage, knee — *see* Tear, meniscus, medial
  intertrochanteric — *see* Fracture, femur, neck, intertrochanteric
  ischium (with visceral injury) (closed) 808.42
    open 808.52
  jaw (bone) (lower) (closed) (*see also* Fracture, mandible) 802.20
    angle 802.25
      open 802.35
    open 802.30
    upper — *see* Fracture, maxilla
  knee
    cap (closed) 822.0
      open 822.1
    cartilage (semilunar) — *see* Tear, meniscus
  labyrinth (osseous) — *see* Fracture, skull, base
  larynx (closed) 807.5
    open 807.6
  late effect — *see* Late, effects (of), fracture
  Le Fort's — *see* Fracture, maxilla
  leg (closed) 827.0
    with rib(s) or sternum 828.0
      open 828.1
    both (any bones) 828.0
      open 828.1
    lower — *see* Fracture, tibia
    open 827.1
    upper — *see* Fracture, femur
  limb
    lower (multiple) (closed) NEC 827.0
      open 827.1
    upper (multiple) (closed) NEC 818.0
      open 818.1
  long bones, due to birth trauma — *see* Birth injury, fracture
  lumbar — *see* Fracture, vertebra, lumbar
  lunate bone (closed) 814.02
    open 814.12
  malar bone (closed) 802.4
    open 802.5
  Malgaigne's (closed) 808.43
    open 808.53
  malleolus (closed) 824.8
    bimalleolar 824.4
      open 824.5
    lateral 824.2
      and medial — *see also* Fracture, malleolus, bimalleolar
        with lip of tibia — *see* Fracture, malleolus, trimalleolar
    open 824.3

Fracture — *continued*
  malleolus — *continued*
    medial (closed) 824.0
      and lateral — *see also* Fracture,
        malleolus, bimalleolar
      with lip of tibia — *see* Fracture,
        malleolus, trimalleolar
      open 824.1
    open 824.9
    trimalleolar (closed) 824.6
      open 824.7
  malleus — *see* Fracture, skull, base
  malunion 733.81
  mandible (closed) 802.20
    angle 802.25
      open 802.35
    body 802.28
      alveolar border 802.27
        open 802.37
      open 802.38
      symphysis 802.26
        open 802.36
    condylar process 802.21
      open 802.31
    coronoid process 802.23
      open 802.33
    multiple sites 802.29
      open 802.39
    open 802.30
    ramus NEC 802.24
      open 802.34
    subcondylar 802.22
      open 802.32
  manubrium — *see* Fracture, sternum
  march 733.95
    fibula 733.94
    metatarsals 733.94
    tibia 733.94
  maxilla, maxillary (superior) (upper jaw)
    (closed) 802.4
    inferior — *see* Fracture, mandible
    open 802.5
  meniscus, knee — *see* Tear, meniscus
  metacarpus, metacarpal (bone(s)), of one hand
    (closed) 815.00
    with phalanx, phalanges, hand (finger(s))
      (thumb) of same hand 817.0
      open 817.1
    base 815.02
      first metacarpal 815.01
        open 815.11
      open 815.12
      thumb 815.01
        open 815.11
    multiple sites 815.09
      open 815.19
    neck 815.04
      open 815.14
    open 815.10
    shaft 815.03
      open 815.13
  metatarsus, metatarsal (bone(s)), of one foot
    (closed) 825.25
    with tarsal bone(s) 825.29
      open 825.39
    open 825.35
  Monteggia's (closed) 813.03
    open 813.13
  Moore's — *see* Fracture, radius, lower end
    multangular bone (closed)
      larger 814.05

Fracture — *continued*
  Moore's — *continued*
    larger — *continued*
      open 814.15
    smaller 814.06
      open 814.16
  multiple (closed) 829.0

> **Note** — *Multiple fractures of sites classifiable to the same three- or four-digit category are coded to that category, except for sites classifiable to 810-818 or 820-827 in different limbs.*
>
> *Multiple fractures of sites classifiable to different fourth-digit subdivisions within the same three-digit category should be dealt with according to coding rules.*
>
> *Multiple fractures of sites classifiable to different three-digit categories (identifiable from the listing under "Fracture"), and of sites classifiable to 810-818 or 820-827 in different limbs should be coded according to the following list, which should be referred to in the following priority order: skull or face bones, pelvis or vertebral column, legs, arms.*

    arm (multiple bones in same arm except in
      hand alone) (sites classifiable to 810-
      817 with sites classifiable to a
      different three-digit category in 810-
      817 in same arm) (closed) 818.0
      open 818.1
    arms, both or arm(s) with rib(s) or sternum
      (sites classifiable to 810-818 with
      sites classifiable to same range of
      categories in other limb or to 807)
      (closed) 819.0
      open 819.1
    bones of trunk NEC (closed) 809.0
      open 809.1
    hand, metacarpal bone(s) with phalanx or
      phalanges of same hand (sites
      classifiable to 815 with sites
      classifiable to 816 in same hand)
      (closed) 817.0
      open 817.1
    leg (multiple bones in same leg) (sites
      classifiable to 820-826 with sites
      classifiable to a different three-digit
      category in that range in same leg)
      (closed) 827.0
      open 827.1
    legs, both or leg(s) with arm(s), rib(s), or
      sternum (sites classifiable to 820-827
      with sites classifiable to same range
      of categories in other leg or to 807 or
      810-819) (closed) 828.0
      open 828.1
    open 829.1
    pelvis with other bones except skull or face
      bones (sites classifiable to 808 with
      sites classifiable to 805-807 or 810-
      829) (closed) 809.0
      open 809.1
    skull, specified or unspecified bones, or
      face bone(s) with any other bone(s)
      (sites classifiable to 800-803 with
      sites classifiable to 805-829) (closed)
      804.0

Fracture

Fracture — *continued*
　multiple — *continued*
　　skull, specified or unspecified bones, or face bone(s) with any other bone(s) — *continued*

> Note — Use the following fifth-digit subclassification with categories 800, 801, 803, and 804:
>
> 0　unspecified state of consciousness
> 1　with no loss of consciousness
> 2　with brief [less than one hour] loss of consciousness
> 3　with moderate [1-24 hours] loss of consciousness
> 4　with prolonged [more than 24 hours] loss of consciousness and return to pre-existing conscious level
> 5　with prolonged [more than 24 hours] loss of consciousness, without return to pre-existing conscious level
>
> Use fifth-digit 5 to designate when a patient is unconscious and dies before regaining consciousness, regardless of the duration of the loss of consciousness
>
> 6　with loss of consciousness of unspecified duration
> 9　with concussion, unspecified

　　　with
　　　　contusion, cerebral 804.1 ✓5ᵗʰ
　　　　epidural hemorrhage 804.2 ✓5ᵗʰ
　　　　extradural hemorrhage 804.2 ✓5ᵗʰ
　　　　hemorrhage (intracranial) NEC 804.3 ✓5ᵗʰ
　　　　intracranial injury NEC 804.4 ✓5ᵗʰ
　　　　laceration, cerebral 804.1 ✓5ᵗʰ
　　　　subarachnoid hemorrhage 804.2 ✓5ᵗʰ
　　　　subdural hemorrhage 804.2 ✓5ᵗʰ
　　　open 804.5 ✓5ᵗʰ
　　　　with
　　　　　contusion, cerebral 804.6 ✓5ᵗʰ
　　　　　epidural hemorrhage 804.7 ✓5ᵗʰ
　　　　　extradural hemorrhage 804.7 ✓5ᵗʰ
　　　　　hemorrhage (intracranial) NEC 804.8 ✓5ᵗʰ
　　　　　intracranial injury NEC 804.9 ✓5ᵗʰ
　　　　　laceration, cerebral 804.6 ✓5ᵗʰ
　　　　　subarachnoid hemorrhage 804.7 ✓5ᵗʰ
　　　　　subdural hemorrhage 804.7 ✓5ᵗʰ
　　vertebral column with other bones, except skull or face bones (sites classifiable to 805 or 806 with sites classifiable to 807-808 or 810-829) (closed) 809.0
　　　open 809.1
　nasal (bone(s)) (closed) 802.0
　　open 802.1
　　sinus — *see* Fracture, skull, base
　navicular
　　carpal (wrist) (closed) 814.01
　　　open 814.11
　　tarsal (ankle) (closed) 825.22
　　　open 825.32
　neck — *see* Fracture, vertebra, cervical
　neural arch — *see* Fracture, vertebra, by site
　nonunion 733.82

Fracture — *continued*
　nose, nasal, (bone) (septum) (closed) 802.0
　　open 802.1
　occiput — *see* Fracture, skull, base
　odontoid process — *see* Fracture, vertebra, cervical
　olecranon (process) (ulna) (closed) 813.01
　　open 813.11
　open 829.1
　orbit, orbital (bone) (region) (closed) 802.8
　　floor (blow-out) 802.6
　　　open 802.7
　　　open 802.9
　　roof — *see* Fracture, skull, base
　　specified part NEC 802.8
　　　open 802.9
　os
　　calcis (closed) 825.0
　　　open 825.1
　　magnum (closed) 814.07
　　　open 814.17
　　pubis (with visceral injury) (closed) 808.2
　　　open 808.3
　　triquetrum (closed) 814.03
　　　open 814.13
　osseous
　　auditory meatus — *see* Fracture, skull, base
　　labyrinth — *see* Fracture, skull, base
　　ossicles, auditory (incus) (malleus) (stapes) — *see* Fracture, skull, base
　osteoporotic — *see* Fracture, pathologic
　palate (closed) 802.8
　　open 802.9
　paratrooper — *see* Fracture, tibia, lower end
　parietal bone — *see* Fracture, skull, vault
　parry — *see* Fracture, Monteggia's
　patella (closed) 822.0
　　open 822.1
　pathologic (cause unknown) 733.10
　　ankle 733.16
　　femur (neck) 733.14
　　　specified NEC 733.15
　　fibula 733.16
　　hip 733.14
　　humerus 733.11
　　radius 733.12
　　specified site NEC 733.19
　　tibia 733.16
　　ulna 733.12
　　vertebrae (collapse) 733.13
　　wrist 733.12
　pedicle (of vertebral arch) — *see* Fracture, vertebra, by site
　pelvis, pelvic (bone(s)) (with visceral injury) (closed) 808.8
　　multiple (with disruption of pelvic circle) 808.43
　　　open 808.53
　　open 808.9
　　rim (closed) 808.49
　　　open 808.59
　peritrochanteric (closed) 820.20
　　open 820.30
　phalanx, phalanges, of one
　　foot (closed) 826.0
　　　with bone(s) of same lower limb 827.0
　　　　open 827.1
　　　open 826.1

Index to Diseases

Fracture

Fracture — *continued*
  phalanx, phalanges, of one — *continued*
    hand (closed) 816.00
      with metacarpal bone(s) of same hand 817.0
        open 817.1
      distal 816.02
        open 816.12
      middle 816.01
        open 816.11
      multiple sites NEC 816.03
        open 816.13
      open 816.10
      proximal 816.01
        open 816.11
  pisiform (closed) 814.04
    open 814.14
  pond — *see* Fracture, skull, vault
  Pott's (closed) 824.4
    open 824.5
  prosthetic device, internal — *see* Complications, mechanical
  pubis (with visceral injury) (closed) 808.2
    open 808.3
  Quervain's (closed) 814.01
    open 814.11
  radius (alone) (closed) 813.81
    with ulna NEC 813.83
      open 813.93
    distal end — *see* Fracture, radius, lower end
    epiphysis
      lower — *see* Fracture, radius, lower end
      upper — *see* Fracture, radius, upper end
    head — *see* Fracture, radius, upper end
    lower end or extremity (distal end) (lower epiphysis) 813.42
      with ulna (lower end) 813.44
        open 813.54
      open 813.52
      torus 813.45
    neck — *see* Fracture, radius, upper end
    open NEC 813.91
    pathologic 733.12
    proximal end — *see* Fracture, radius, upper end
    shaft (closed) 813.21
      with ulna (shaft) 813.23
        open 813.33
      open 813.31
    upper end 813.07
      with ulna (upper end) 813.08
        open 813.18
      epiphysis 813.05
        open 813.15
      head 813.05
        open 813.15
      multiple sites 813.07
        open 813.17
      neck 813.06
        open 813.16
      open 813.17
      specified site NEC 813.07
        open 813.17
  ramus
    inferior or superior (with visceral injury) (closed) 808.2
      open 808.3
    ischium — *see* Fracture, ischium
    mandible 802.24
      open 802.34

Fracture — *continued*
  rib(s) (closed) 807.0

> **Note** — *Use the following fifth-digit subclassification with categories 807.0-807.1:*
>
> 0   rib(s), unspecified
> 1   one rib
> 2   two ribs
> 3   three ribs
> 4   four ribs
> 5   five ribs
> 6   six ribs
> 7   seven ribs
> 8   eight or more ribs
> 9   multiple ribs, unspecified

    with flail chest (open) 807.4
    open 807.1 ✓5ᵗʰ
  root, tooth 873.63
    complicated 873.73
  sacrum — *see* Fracture, vertebra, sacrum
  scaphoid
    ankle (closed) 825.22
      open 825.32
    wrist (closed) 814.01
      open 814.11
  scapula (closed) 811.00
    acromial, acromion (process) 811.01
      open 811.11
    body 811.09
      open 811.19
    coracoid process 811.02
      open 811.12
    glenoid (cavity) (fossa) 811.03
      open 811.13
    neck 811.03
      open 811.13
    open 811.10
  semilunar
    bone, wrist (closed) 814.02
      open 814.12
    cartilage (interior) (knee) — *see* Tear, meniscus
  sesamoid bone — *see* Fracture, by site
  Shepherd's (closed) 825.21
    open 825.31
  shoulder — *see also* Fracture, humerus, upper end
    blade — *see* Fracture, scapula
  silverfork — *see* Fracture, radius, lower end
  sinus (ethmoid) (frontal) (maxillary) (nasal) (sphenoidal) — *see* Fracture, skull, base
  Skillern's — *see* Fracture, radius, shaft
  skull (multiple NEC) (with face bones) (closed) 803.0 ✓5ᵗʰ

✓4ᵗʰ Fourth-digit Required   ✓5ᵗʰ Fifth-digit Required

Fracture — continued
  skull — continued

> Note — Use the following fifth digit subclassification with categories 800, 801, 803, and 804:
>
> 0 unspecified state of consciousness
> 1 with no loss of consciousness
> 2 with brief [less than one hour] loss of consciousness
> 3 with moderate [1-24 hours] loss of consciousness
> 4 with prolonged [more than 24 hours] loss of consciousness and return to pre-existing conscious level
> 5 with prolonged [more than 24 hours] loss of consciousness, without return to pre-existing conscious level
>
> Use fifth-digit 5 to designate when a patient is unconscious and dies before regaining consciousness, regardless of the duration of loss of consciousness
>
> 6 with loss of consciousness of unspecified duration
> 9 with concussion, unspecified

    with
        contusion, cerebral 803.1 ✓5ᵗʰ
        epidural hemorrhage 803.2 ✓5ᵗʰ
        extradural hemorrhage 803.2 ✓5ᵗʰ
        hemorrhage (intracranial) NEC 803.3 ✓5ᵗʰ
        intracranial injury NEC 803.4 ✓5ᵗʰ
        laceration, cerebral 803.1 ✓5ᵗʰ
        other bones — see Fracture, multiple, skull
        subarachnoid hemorrhage 803.2 ✓5ᵗʰ
        subdural hemorrhage 803.2 ✓5ᵗʰ
    base (antrum) (ethmoid bone) (fossa) (internal ear) (nasal sinus) (occiput) (sphenoid) (temporal bone) (closed) 801.0 ✓5ᵗʰ
        with
            contusion, cerebral 801.1 ✓5ᵗʰ
            epidural hemorrhage 801.2 ✓5ᵗʰ
            extradural hemorrhage 801.2 ✓5ᵗʰ
            hemorrhage (intracranial) NEC 801.3 ✓5ᵗʰ
            intracranial injury NEC 801.4 ✓5ᵗʰ
            laceration, cerebral 801.1 ✓5ᵗʰ
            subarachnoid hemorrhage 801.2 ✓5ᵗʰ
            subdural hemorrhage 801.2 ✓5ᵗʰ
        open 801.5 ✓5ᵗʰ
            with
                contusion, cerebral 801.6 ✓5ᵗʰ
                epidural hemorrhage 801.7 ✓5ᵗʰ
                extradural hemorrhage 801.7 ✓5ᵗʰ
                hemorrhage (intracranial) NEC 801.8 ✓5ᵗʰ
                intracranial injury NEC 801.9 ✓5ᵗʰ
                laceration, cerebral 801.6 ✓5ᵗʰ
                subarachnoid hemorrhage 801.7 ✓5ᵗʰ
                subdural hemorrhage 801.7 ✓5ᵗʰ
    birth injury 767.3
    face bones — see Fracture, face bones
    open 803.5 ✓5ᵗʰ
        with
            contusion, cerebral 803.6 ✓5ᵗʰ

Fracture — continued
  skull — continued
    open — continued
        with — continued
            epidural hemorrhage 803.7 ✓5ᵗʰ
            extradural hemorrhage 803.7 ✓5ᵗʰ
            hemorrhage (intracranial) NEC 803.8 ✓5ᵗʰ
            intracranial injury NEC 803.9 ✓5ᵗʰ
            laceration, cerebral 803.6 ✓5ᵗʰ
            subarachnoid hemorrhage 803.7 ✓5ᵗʰ
            subdural hemorrhage 803.7 ✓5ᵗʰ
    vault (frontal bone) (parietal bone) (vertex) (closed) 800.0 ✓5ᵗʰ
        with
            contusion, cerebral 800.1 ✓5ᵗʰ
            epidural hemorrhage 800.2 ✓5ᵗʰ
            extradural hemorrhage 800.2 ✓5ᵗʰ
            hemorrhage (intracranial) NEC 800.3 ✓5ᵗʰ
            intracranial injury NEC 800.4 ✓5ᵗʰ
            laceration, cerebral 800.1 ✓5ᵗʰ
            subarachnoid hemorrhage 800.2 ✓5ᵗʰ
            subdural hemorrhage 800.2 ✓5ᵗʰ
        open 800.5 ✓5ᵗʰ
            with
                contusion, cerebral 800.6 ✓5ᵗʰ
                epidural hemorrhage 800.7 ✓5ᵗʰ
                extradural hemorrhage 800.7 ✓5ᵗʰ
                hemorrhage (intracranial) NEC 800.8 ✓5ᵗʰ
                intracranial injury NEC 800.9 ✓5ᵗʰ
                laceration, cerebral 800.6 ✓5ᵗʰ
                subarachnoid hemorrhage 800.7 ✓5ᵗʰ
                subdural hemorrhage 800.7 ✓5ᵗʰ
  Smith's 813.41
    open 813.51
  sphenoid (bone) (sinus) — see Fracture, skull, base
  spine — see also Fracture, vertebra, by site
    due to birth trauma 767.4
  spinous process — see Fracture, vertebra, by site
  spontaneous — see Fracture, pathologic
  sprinters' — see Fracture, ilium
  stapes — see Fracture, skull, base
  stave — see also Fracture, metacarpus, metacarpal bone(s)
    spine — see Fracture, tibia, upper end
  sternum (closed) 807.2
    with flail chest (open) 807.4
    open 807.3
  Stieda's — see Fracture, femur, lower end
  stress 733.95
    fibula 733.93
    metatarsals 733.94
    specified site NEC 733.95
    tibia 733.93
  styloid process
    metacarpal (closed) 815.02
        open 815.12
    radius — see Fracture, radius, lower end
    temporal bone — see Fracture, skull, base
    ulna — see Fracture, ulna, lower end
  supracondylar, elbow 812.41
    open 812.51
  symphysis pubis (with visceral injury) (closed) 808.2
    open 808.3

Fracture — *continued*
  talus (ankle bone) (closed) 825.21
    open 825.31
  tarsus, tarsal bone(s) (with metatarsus) of one foot (closed) NEC 825.29
    open 825.39
  temporal bone (styloid) — *see* Fracture, skull, base
  tendon — *see* Sprain, by site
  thigh — *see* Fracture, femur, shaft
  thumb (and finger(s)) of one hand (closed) (*see also* Fracture, phalanx, hand) 816.00
    with metacarpal bone(s) of same hand 817.0
      open 817.1
    metacarpal(s) — *see* Fracture, metacarpus
    open 816.10
  thyroid cartilage (closed) 807.5
    open 807.6
  tibia (closed) 823.80
    with fibula 823.82
      open 823.92
    condyles — *see* Fracture, tibia, upper end
    distal end 824.8
      open 824.9
    epiphysis
      lower 824.8
        open 824.9
      upper — *see* Fracture, tibia, upper end
    head (involving knee joint) — *see* Fracture, tibia, upper end
    intercondyloid eminence — *see* Fracture, tibia, upper end
    involving ankle 824.0
      open 824.9
    malleolus (internal) (medial) 824.0
      open 824.1
    open NEC 823.90
    pathologic 733.16
    proximal end — *see* Fracture, tibia, upper end
    shaft 823.20
      with fibula 823.22
        open 823.32
      open 823.30
    spine — *see* Fracture, tibia, upper end
    stress 733.93
    torus 823.40 •
      with tibia 823.42 •
    tuberosity — *see* Fracture, tibia, upper end
    upper end or extremity (condyle) (epiphysis) (head) (spine) (proximal end) (tuberosity) 823.00
      with fibula 823.02
        open 823.12
      open 823.10
  toe(s), of one foot (closed) 826.0
    with bone(s) of same lower limb 827.0
      open 827.1
    open 826.1
  tooth (root) 873.63
    complicated 873.73
  torus •
    fibula 823.41 •
      with tibia 823.42 •
    radius 813.45 •
    tibia 823.40 •
      with fibula 823.42 •
  trachea (closed) 807.5
    open 807.6

Fracture — *continued*
  transverse process — *see* Fracture, vertebra, by site
  trapezium (closed) 814.05
    open 814.15
  trapezoid bone (closed) 814.06
    open 814.16
  trimalleolar (closed) 824.6
    open 824.7
  triquetral (bone) (closed) 814.03
    open 814.13
  trochanter (greater) (lesser) (closed) (*see also* Fracture, femur, neck, by site) 820.20
    open 820.30
  trunk (bones) (closed) 809.0
    open 809.1
  tuberosity (external) — *see* Fracture, by site
  ulna (alone) (closed) 813.82
    with radius NEC 813.83
      open 813.93
    coronoid process (closed) 813.02
      open 813.12
    distal end — *see* Fracture, ulna, lower end
    epiphysis
      lower — *see* Fracture, ulna, lower end
      upper — *see* Fracture, ulna, upper end
    head — *see* Fracture, ulna, lower end
    lower end (distal end) (head) (lower epiphysis) (styloid process) 813.43
      with radius (lower end) 813.44
        open 813.54
      open 813.53
    olecranon process (closed) 813.01
      open 813.11
    open NEC 813.92
    pathologic 733.12
    proximal end — *see* Fracture, ulna, upper end
    shaft 813.22
      with radius (shaft) 813.23
        open 813.33
      open 813.32
    styloid process — *see* Fracture, ulna, lower end
    transverse — *see* Fracture, ulna, by site
    upper end (epiphysis) 813.04
      with radius (upper end) 813.08
        open 813.18
      multiple sites 813.04
        open 813.14
      open 813.14
      specified site NEC 813.04
        open 813.14
  unciform (closed) 814.08
    open 814.18
  vertebra, vertebral (back) (body) (column) (neural arch) (pedicle) (spine) (spinous process) (transverse process) (closed) 805.8
    with
      hematomyelia — *see* Fracture, vertebra, by site, with spinal cord injury
      injury to
        cauda equina — *see* Fracture, vertebra, sacrum, with spinal cord injury
        nerve — *see* Fracture, vertebra, by site, with spinal cord injury
        paralysis — *see* Fracture, vertebra, by site, with spinal cord injury

Fracture — continued
  vertebra, vertebral — continued
    with — continued
      paraplegia — see Fracture, vertebra, by site, with spinal cord injury
      quadriplegia — see Fracture, vertebra, by site, with spinal cord injury
      spinal concussion — see Fracture, vertebra, by site, with spinal cord injury
      spinal cord injury (closed) NEC 806.8

Note — Use the following fifth-digit subclassification with categories 806.0-806.3:

C_1-C_4 or unspecified level and D_1-D_6 (T_1-T_6) or unspecified level with
  0 unspecified spinal cord injury
  1 complete lesion of cord
  2 anterior cord syndrome
  3 central cord syndrome
  4 specified injury NEC

C_5-C_7 level and D_7-D_{12} level with:
  5 unspecified spinal cord injury
  6 complete lesion of cord
  7 anterior cord syndrome
  8 central cord syndrome
  9 specified injury NEC

---

        cervical 806.0 ✓5ᵗʰ
          open 806.1 ✓5ᵗʰ
        dorsal, dorsolumbar 806.2 ✓5ᵗʰ
          open 806.3 ✓5ᵗʰ
        open 806.9
        thoracic, thoracolumbar 806.2 ✓5ᵗʰ
          open 806.3 ✓5ᵗʰ
    atlanto-axial — see Fracture, vertebra, cervical
    cervical (hangman) (teardrop) (closed) 805.00
      with spinal cord injury — see Fracture, vertebra, with spinal cord injury, cervical
      first (atlas) 805.01
        open 805.11
      second (axis) 805.02
        open 805.12
      third 805.03
        open 805.13
      fourth 805.04
        open 805.14
      fifth 805.05
        open 805.15
      sixth 805.06
        open 805.16
      seventh 805.07
        open 805.17
      multiple sites 805.08
        open 805.18
      open 805.10
    coccyx (closed) 805.6
      with spinal cord injury (closed) 806.60
        cauda equina injury 806.62
          complete lesion 806.61
            open 806.71
          open 806.72
        open 806.70

Fracture — continued
  vertebra, vertebral — continued
    coccyx — continued
      with spinal cord injury — continued
        specified type NEC 806.69
          open 806.79
      open 805.7
    collapsed 733.13
    compression, not due to trauma 733.13
    dorsal (closed) 805.2
      with spinal cord injury — see Fracture, vertebra, with spinal cord injury, dorsal
      open 805.3
    dorsolumbar (closed) 805.2
      with spinal cord injury — see Fracture, vertebra, with spinal cord injury, dorsal
      open 805.3
    due to osteoporosis 733.13
    fetus or newborn 767.4
    lumbar (closed) 805.4
      with spinal cord injury (closed) 806.4
        open 806.5
      open 805.5
    nontraumatic 733.13
    open NEC 805.9
    pathologic (any site) 733.13
    sacrum (closed) 805.6
      with spinal cord injury 806.60
        cauda equina injury 806.62
          complete lesion 806.61
            open 806.71
          open 806.72
        open 806.70
        specified type NEC 806.69
          open 806.79
      open 805.7
    site unspecified (closed) 805.8
      with spinal cord injury (closed) 806.8
        open 806.9
      open 805.9
    stress (any site) 733.95
    thoracic (closed) 805.2
      with spinal cord injury — see Fracture, vertebra, with spinal cord injury, thoracic
      open 805.3
  vertex — see Fracture, skull, vault
  vomer (bone) 802.0
    open 802.1
  Wagstaffe's — see Fracture, ankle
  wrist (closed) 814.00
    open 814.10
    pathologic 733.12
  xiphoid (process) — see Fracture, sternum
  zygoma (zygomatic arch) (closed) 802.4
    open 802.5

Fragile X syndrome 759.83
Fragilitas
  crinium 704.2
  hair 704.2
  ossium 756.51
    with blue sclera 756.51
  unguium 703.8
    congenital 757.5
Fragility
  bone 756.51
    with deafness and blue sclera 756.51
  capillary (hereditary) 287.8
  hair 704.2

Fragility — continued
  nails 703.8
Fragmentation — see Fracture, by site
Frambesia, frambesial (tropica) (see also Yaws) 102.9
  initial lesion or ulcer 102.0
  primary 102.0
Frambeside
  gummatous 102.4
  of early yaws 102.2
Frambesioma 102.1
Franceschetti's syndrome (mandibulofacial dysotosis) 756.0
Francis' disease (see also Tularemia) 021.9
Frank's essential thrombocytopenia (see also Purpura, thrombocytopenic) 287.3
Franklin's disease (heavy chain) 273.2
Fraser's syndrome 759.89
Freckle 709.09
  malignant melanoma in (M8742/3) — see Melanoma
  melanotic (of Hutchinson) (M8742/2) — see Neoplasm, skin, in situ
Freeman-Sheldon syndrome 759.89
Freezing 991.9
  specified effect NEC 991.8
Frei's disease (climatic bubo) 099.1
Freiberg's
  disease (osteochondrosis, second metatarsal) 732.5
  infraction of metatarsal head 732.5
  osteochondrosis 732.5
Fremitus, friction, cardiac 785.3
Frenulum linguae 750.0
Frenum
  external os 752.49
  tongue 750.0
Frequency (urinary) NEC 788.41
  micturition 788.41
  nocturnal 788.43
  psychogenic 306.53
Frey's syndrome (auriculotemporal syndrome) 350.8
Friction
  burn (see also Injury, superficial, by site) 919.0
  fremitus, cardiac 785.3
  precordial 785.3
  sounds, chest 786.7
Friderichsen-Waterhouse syndrome or disease 036.3
Friedländer's
  B (bacillus) NEC (see also condition) 041.3
  sepsis or septicemia 038.49
  disease (endarteritis obliterans) — see Arteriosclerosis
Friedreich's
  ataxia 334.0
  combined systemic disease 334.0
  disease 333.2
    combined systemic 334.0
  myoclonia 333.2
  sclerosis (spinal cord) 334.0
Friedrich-Erb-Arnold syndrome (acropachyderma) 757.39
Frigidity 302.72
  psychic or psychogenic 302.72

Fröhlich's disease or syndrome (adiposogenital dystrophy) 253.8
Froin's syndrome 336.8
Frommel's disease 676.6
Frommel-Chiari syndrome 676.6
Frontal — see also condition
  lobe syndrome 310.0
Frostbite 991.3
  face 991.0
  foot 991.2
  hand 991.1
  specified site NEC 991.3
Frotteurism 302.89
Frozen 991.9
  pelvis 620.8
  shoulder 726.0
Fructosemia 271.2
Fructosuria (benign) (essential) 271.2
Fuchs'
  black spot (myopic) 360.21
  corneal dystrophy (endothelial) 371.57
  heterochromic cyclitis 364.21
Fucosidosis 271.8
Fugue 780.99
  hysterical (dissociative) 300.13
  reaction to exceptional stress (transient) 308.1
Fuller Albright's syndrome (osteitis fibrosa disseminata) 756.59
Fuller's earth disease 502
Fulminant, fulminating — see condition
Functional — see condition
Fundus — see also condition
  flavimaculatus 362.76
Fungemia 117.9
Fungus, fungous
  cerebral 348.8
  disease NEC 117.9
  infection — see Infection, fungus
  testis (see also Tuberculosis) 016.5 [608.81]
Funiculitis (acute) 608.4
  chronic 608.4
  endemic 608.4
  gonococcal (acute) 098.14
    chronic or duration of 2 months or over 098.34
  tuberculous (see also Tuberculosis) 016.5
Funnel
  breast (acquired) 738.3
    congenital 754.81
    late effect of rickets 268.1
  chest (acquired) 738.3
    congenital 754.81
    late effect of rickets 268.1
  pelvis (acquired) 738.6
    with disproportion (fetopelvic) 653.3
      affecting fetus or newborn 763.1
      causing obstructed labor 660.1
        affecting fetus or newborn 763.1
    congenital 755.69
    tuberculous (see also Tuberculosis) 016.9
F.U.O. (see also Pyrexia) 780.6
Furfur 690.18
  microsporon 111.0
Furor, paroxysmal (idiopathic) (see also Epilepsy) 345.8

Furriers' lung 495.8
Furrowed tongue 529.5
   congenital 750.13
Furrowing nail(s) (transverse) 703.8
   congenital 757.5
Furuncle 680.9
   abdominal wall 680.2
   ankle 680.6
   anus 680.5
   arm (any part, above wrist) 680.3
   auditory canal, external 680.0
   axilla 680.3
   back (any part) 680.2
   breast 680.2
   buttock 680.5
   chest wall 680.2
   corpus cavernosum 607.2
   ear (any part) 680.0
   eyelid 373.13
   face (any part, except eye) 680.0
   finger (any) 680.4
   flank 680.2
   foot (any part) 680.7
   forearm 680.3
   gluteal (region) 680.5
   groin 680.2
   hand (any part) 680.4
   head (any part, except face) 680.8
   heel 680.7
   hip 680.6
   kidney (*see also* Abscess, kidney) 590.2
   knee 680.6
   labium (majus) (minus) 616.4
   lacrimal
      gland (*see also* Dacryoadenitis) 375.00
      passages (duct) (sac) (*see also* Dacryocystitis) 375.30
   leg, any part except foot 680.6
   malignant 022.0
   multiple sites 680.9
   neck 680.1
   nose (external) (septum) 680.0
   orbit 376.01
   partes posteriores 680.5
   pectoral region 680.2
   penis 607.2
   perineum 680.2
   pinna 680.0
   scalp (any part) 680.8
   scrotum 608.4
   seminal vesicle 608.0
   shoulder 680.3
   skin NEC 680.9
   specified site NEC 680.8
   spermatic cord 608.4
   temple (region) 680.0
   testis 604.90
   thigh 680.6
   thumb 680.4
   toe (any) 680.7
   trunk 680.2
   tunica vaginalis 608.4
   umbilicus 680.2
   upper arm 680.3
   vas deferens 608.4
   vulva 616.4
   wrist 680.4
Furunculosis (*see also* Furuncle) 680.9
   external auditory meatus 680.0 *[380.13]*
Fusarium (infection) 118

Fusion, fused (congenital)
   anal (with urogenital canal) 751.5
   aorta and pulmonary artery 745.0
   astragaloscaphoid 755.67
   atria 745.5
   atrium and ventricle 745.69
   auditory canal 744.02
   auricles, heart 745.5
   binocular, with defective stereopsis 368.33
   bone 756.9
   cervical spine — *see* Fusion, spine
   choanal 748.0
   commissure, mitral valve 746.5
   cranial sutures, premature 756.0
   cusps, heart valve NEC 746.89
      mitral 746.5
      tricuspid 746.89
   ear ossicles 744.04
   fingers (*see also* Syndactylism, fingers) 755.11
   hymen 752.42
   hymeno-urethral 599.89
      causing obstructed labor 660.1 ✓5ᵗʰ
      affecting fetus or newborn 763.1
   joint (acquired) — *see also* Ankylosis
      congenital 755.8
   kidneys (incomplete) 753.3
   labium (majus) (minus) 752.49
   larynx and trachea 748.3
   limb 755.8
      lower 755.69
      upper 755.59
   lobe, lung 748.5
   lumbosacral (acquired) 724.6
      congenital 756.15
      surgical V45.4
   nares (anterior) (posterior) 748.0
   nose, nasal 748.0
   nostril(s) 748.0
   organ or site NEC — *see* Anomaly, specified type NEC
   ossicles 756.9
      auditory 744.04
   pulmonary valve segment 746.02
   pulmonic cusps 746.02
   ribs 756.3
   sacroiliac (acquired) (joint) 724.6
      congenital 755.69
      surgical V45.4
   skull, imperfect 756.0
   spine (acquired) 724.9
      arthrodesis status V45.4
      congenital (vertebra) 756.15
   postoperative status V45.4
   sublingual duct with submaxillary duct at opening in mouth 750.26
   talonavicular (bar) 755.67
   teeth, tooth 520.2
   testes 752.8
   toes (*see also* Syndactylism, toes) 755.13
   trachea and esophagus 750.3
   twins 759.4
   urethral-hymenal 599.89
   vagina 752.49
   valve cusps — *see* Fusion, cusps, heart valve
   ventricles, heart 745.4
   vertebra (arch) — *see* Fusion, spine
   vulva 752.49
Fusospirillosis (mouth) (tongue) (tonsil) 101
Fussy infant (baby) 780.91

G

Gafsa boil 085.1
Gain, weight (abnormal) (excessive) (see also Weight, gain) 783.1
Gaisböck's disease or syndrome (polycythemia hypertonica) 289.0
Gait
   abnormality 781.2
     hysterical 300.11
   ataxic 781.2
     hysterical 300.11
   disturbance 781.2
     hysterical 300.11
   paralytic 781.2
   scissor 781.2
   spastic 781.2
   staggering 781.2
     hysterical 300.11
Galactocele (breast) (infected) 611.5
   puerperal, postpartum 676.8
Galactophoritis 611.0
   puerperal, postpartum 675.2
Galactorrhea 676.6
   not associated with childbirth 611.6
Galactosemia (classic) (congenital) 271.1
Galactosuria 271.1
Galacturia 791.1
   bilharziasis 120.0
Galen's vein — see condition
Gallbladder — see also condition
   acute (see also Disease, gallbladder) 575.0
Gall duct — see condition
Gallop rhythm 427.89
Gallstone (cholemic) (colic) (impacted) — see also Cholelithiasis
   causing intestinal obstruction 560.31
Gambling, pathological 312.31
Gammaloidosis 277.3
Gammopathy 273.9
   macroglobulinemia 273.3
   monoclonal (benign) (essential) (idiopathic) (with lymphoplasmacytic dyscrasia) 273.1
Gamna's disease (siderotic splenomegaly) 289.51
Gampsodactylia (congenital) 754.71
Gamstorp's disease (adynamia episodica hereditaria) 359.3
Gandy-Nanta disease (siderotic splenomegaly) 289.51
Gang activity, without manifest psychiatric disorder V71.09
   adolescent V71.02
   adult V71.01
   child V71.02
Gangliocytoma (M9490/0) — see Neoplasm, connective tissue, benign
Ganglioglioma (M9505/1) — see Neoplasm, by site, uncertain behavior
Ganglion 727.43
   joint 727.41
   of yaws (early) (late) 102.6
   periosteal (see also Periostitis) 730.3
   tendon sheath (compound) (diffuse) 727.42
   tuberculous (see also Tuberculosis) 015.9
Ganglioneuroblastoma (M9490/3) — see Neoplasm, connective tissue, malignant
Ganglioneuroma (M9490/0) — see also Neoplasm, connective tissue, benign
   malignant (M9490/3) — see Neoplasm, connective tissue, malignant
Ganglioneuromatosis (M9491/0) — see Neoplasm, connective tissue, benign
Ganglionitis
   fifth nerve (see also Neuralgia, trigeminal) 350.1
   gasserian 350.1
   geniculate 351.1
     herpetic 053.11
     newborn 767.5
   herpes zoster 053.11
   herpetic geniculate (Hunt's syndrome) 053.11
Gangliosidosis 330.1
Gangosa 102.5
Gangrene, gangrenous (anemia) (artery) (cellulitis) (dermatitis) (dry) (infective) (moist) (pemphigus) (septic) (skin) (stasis) (ulcer) 785.4
   with
     arteriosclerosis (native artery) 440.24
       bypass graft 440.30
         autologous vein 440.31
         nonautologous biolog-ical 440.32
     diabetes (mellitus) 250.7 [785.4]
   abdomen (wall) 785.4
     arteriosclerosis 440.29 [785.4]
   adenitis 683
   alveolar 526.5
   angina 462
     diphtheritic 032.0
   anus 569.49
   appendices epiploicae — see Gangrene, mesentery
   appendix — see Appendicitis, acute
   arteriosclerotic — see Arteriosclerosis, with, gangrene
   auricle 785.4
   Bacillus welchii (see also Gangrene, gas) 040.0
   bile duct (see also Cholangitis) 576.8
   bladder 595.89
   bowel — see Gangrene, intestine
   cecum — see Gangrene, intestine
   Clostridium perfringens or welchii (see also Gangrene, gas) 040.0
   colon — see Gangrene, intestine
   connective tissue 785.4
   cornea 371.40
   corpora cavernosa (infective) 607.2
     noninfective 607.89
   cutaneous, spreading 785.4
   decubital 707.0 [785.4]
   diabetic (any site) 250.7 [785.4]
   dropsical 785.4
   emphysematous (see also Gangrene, gas) 040.0
   epidemic (ergotized grain) 988.2
   epididymis (infectional) (see also Epididymitis) 604.99
   erysipelas (see also Erysipelas) 035
   extremity (lower) (upper) 785.4
   gallbladder or duct (see also Cholecystitis, acute) 575.0
   gas (bacillus) 040.0
     with
       abortion — see Abortion, by type, with sepsis
       ectopic pregnancy (see also categories 633.0-633.9) 639.0

Gangrene, gangrenous — continued
  gas — continued
    with — continued
      molar pregnancy (see also categories 630-632) 639.0
    following
      abortion 639.0
      ectopic or molar pregnancy 639.0
    puerperal, postpartum, childbirth 670 ✓4ᵗʰ
  glossitis 529.0
  gum 523.8
  hernia — see Hernia, by site, with gangrene
  hospital noma 528.1
  intestine, intestinal (acute) (hemorrhagic) (massive) 557.0
    with
      hernia — see Hernia, by site, with gangrene
      mesenteric embolism or infarction 557.0
      obstruction (see also Obstruction, intestine) 560.9
  laryngitis 464.00
    with obstruction 464.01
  liver 573.8
  lung 513.0
    spirochetal 104.8
  lymphangitis 457.2
  Meleney's (cutaneous) 686.09
  mesentery 557.0
    with
      embolism or infarction 557.0
      intestinal obstruction (see also Obstruction, intestine) 560.9
  mouth 528.1
  noma 528.1
  orchitis 604.90
  ovary (see also Salpingo-oophoritis) 614.2
  pancreas 577.0
  penis (infectional) 607.2
    noninfective 607.89
  perineum 785.4
  pharynx 462
  septic 034.0
  pneumonia 513.0
  Pott's 440.24
  presenile 443.1
  pulmonary 513.0
  pulp, tooth 522.1
  quinsy 475
  Raynaud's (symmetric gangrene) 443.0 [785.4]
  rectum 569.49
  retropharyngeal 478.24
  rupture — see Hernia, by site, with gangrene
  scrotum 608.4
    noninfective 608.83
  senile 440.24
  sore throat 462
  spermatic cord 608.4
    noninfective 608.89
  spine 785.4
  spirochetal NEC 104.8
  spreading cutaneous 785.4
  stomach 537.89
  stomatitis 528.1
  symmetrical 443.0 [785.4]
  testis (infectional) (see also Orchitis) 604.99
    noninfective 608.89
  throat 462
    diphtheritic 032.0
  thyroid (gland) 246.8
  tonsillitis (acute) 463

Gangrene, gangrenous — continued
  tooth (pulp) 522.1
  tuberculous NEC (see also Tuberculosis) 011.9 ✓5ᵗʰ
  tunica vaginalis 608.4
    noninfective 608.89
  umbilicus 785.4
  uterus (see also Endometritis) 615.9
  uvulitis 528.3
  vas deferens 608.4
    noninfective 608.89
  vulva (see also Vulvitis) 616.10
Gannister disease (occupational) 502
  with tuberculosis — see Tuberculosis, pulmonary
Ganser's syndrome, hysterical 300.16
Gardner-Diamond syndrome (autoerythrocyte sensitization) 287.2
Gargoylism 277.5
Garré's
  disease (see also Osteomyelitis) 730.1 ✓5ᵗʰ
  osteitis (sclerosing) (see also Osteomyelitis) 730.1 ✓5ᵗʰ
  osteomyelitis (see also Osteomyelitis) 730.1 ✓5ᵗʰ
Garrod's pads, knuckle 728.79
Gartner's duct
  cyst 752.11
  persistent 752.11
Gas
  asphyxia, asphyxiation, inhalation, poisoning, suffocation NEC 987.9
    specified gas — see Table of Drugs and Chemicals
  bacillus gangrene or infection — see Gas, gangrene
  cyst, mesentery 568.89
  excessive 787.3
  gangrene 040.0
    with
      abortion — see Abortion, by type, with sepsis
      ectopic pregnancy (see also categories 633.0-633.9) 639.0
      molar pregnancy (see also categories 630-632) 639.0
    following
      abortion 639.0
      ectopic or molar pregnancy 639.0
    puerperal, postpartum, childbirth 670 ✓4ᵗʰ
  on stomach 787.3
  pains 787.3
Gastradenitis 535.0 E
Gastralgia 536.8
  psychogenic 307.89
Gastrectasis, gastrectasia 536.1
  psychogenic 306.4
Gastric — see condition
Gastrinoma (M8153/1)
  malignant (M8153/3)
    pancreas 157.4
    specified site NEC — see Neoplasm, by site, malignant
    unspecified site 157.4
  specified site — see Neoplasm, by site, uncertain behavior
  unspecified site 235.5

Index to Diseases

Gastritis 535.5 ✓5ᵗʰ

> Note — Use the following fifth-digit subclassification for category 535:
>
> 0   without mention of hemorrhage
> 1   with hemorrhage

    acute 535.0 ✓5ᵗʰ
    alcoholic 535.3 ✓5ᵗʰ
    allergic 535.4 ✓5ᵗʰ
    antral 535.4 ✓5ᵗʰ
    atrophic 535.1 ✓5ᵗʰ
    atrophic-hyperplastic 535.1 ✓5ᵗʰ
    bile-induced 535.4 ✓5ᵗʰ
    catarrhal 535.0 ✓5ᵗʰ
    chronic (atrophic) 535.1 ✓5ᵗʰ
    cirrhotic 535.4 ✓5ᵗʰ
    corrosive (acute) 535.4 ✓5ᵗʰ
    dietetic 535.4 ✓5ᵗʰ
    due to diet deficiency 269.9 [535.4]
    eosinophilic 535.4 ✓5ᵗʰ
    erosive 535.4 ✓5ᵗʰ
    follicular 535.4 ✓5ᵗʰ
        chronic 535.1 ✓5ᵗʰ
    giant hypertrophic 535.2 ✓5ᵗʰ
    glandular 535.4 ✓5ᵗʰ
        chronic 535.1 ✓5ᵗʰ
    hypertrophic (mucosa) 535.2 ✓5ᵗʰ
        chronic giant 211.1
    irritant 535.4 ✓5ᵗʰ
    nervous 306.4
    phlegmonous 535.0 ✓5ᵗʰ
    psychogenic 306.4
    sclerotic 535.4 ✓5ᵗʰ
    spastic 536.8
    subacute 535.0 ✓5ᵗʰ
    superficial 535.4 ✓5ᵗʰ
    suppurative 535.0 ✓5ᵗʰ
    toxic 535.4 ✓5ᵗʰ
    tuberculous (*see also* Tuberculosis) 017.9 ✓5ᵗʰ

Gastrocarcinoma (M8010/3) 151.9
Gastrocolic — *see* condition
Gastrocolitis — *see* Enteritis
Gastrodisciasis 121.8
Gastroduodenitis (*see also* Gastritis) 535.5 ✓5ᵗʰ
    catarrhal 535.0 ✓5ᵗʰ
    infectional 535.0 ✓5ᵗʰ
    virus, viral 008.8
        specified type NEC 008.69

Gastrodynia 536.8
Gastroenteritis (acute) (catarrhal) (congestive) (hemorrhagic) (noninfectious) (*see also* Enteritis) 558.9
    aertrycke infection 003.0
    allergic 558.3
    chronic 558.9
        ulcerative (*see also* Colitis, ulcerative) 556.9
    dietetic 558.9
    due to
        food poisoning (*see also* Poisoning, food) 005.9
        radiation 558.1
    epidemic 009.0
    functional 558.9
    infectious (*see also* Enteritis, due to, by organism) 009.0
        presumed 009.1
    salmonella 003.0

Gastroenteritis — *continued*
    septic (*see also* Enteritis, due to, by organism) 009.0
    toxic 558.2
    tuberculous (*see also* Tuberculosis) 014.8 ✓5ᵗʰ
    ulcerative (*see also* Colitis, ulcerative) 556.9
    viral NEC 008.8
        specified type NEC 008.69
    zymotic 009.0

Gastroenterocolitis — *see* Enteritis
Gastroenteropathy, protein-losing 579.8
Gastroenteroptosis 569.89
Gastroesophageal laceration-hemorrhage syndrome 530.7
Gastroesophagitis 530.19
Gastrohepatitis (*see also* Gastritis) 535.5 ✓5ᵗʰ
Gastrointestinal — *see* condition
Gastrojejunal — *see* condition
Gastrojejunitis (*see also* Gastritis) 535.5 ✓5ᵗʰ
Gastrojejunocolic — *see* condition
Gastroliths 537.89
Gastromalacia 537.89
Gastroparalysis 536.8
    diabetic 250.6 ✓5ᵗʰ [536.3]
Gastroparesis 536.3
    diabetic 250.6 ✓5ᵗʰ [536.3]
Gastropathy, exudative 579.8
Gastroptosis 537.5
Gastrorrhagia 578.0
Gastorrhea 536.8
    psychogenic 306.4
Gastroschisis (congenital) 756.79
    acquired 569.89
Gastrospasm (neurogenic) (reflex) 536.8
    neurotic 306.4
    psychogenic 306.4
Gastrostaxis 578.0
Gastrostenosis 537.89
Gastrostomy
    attention to V55.1
    complication 536.40
        specified type 536.49
    infection 536.41
    malfunctioning 536.42
    status V44.1
Gastrosuccorrhea (continous) (intermittent) 536.8
    neurotic 306.4
    psychogenic 306.4
Gaucher's
    disease (adult) (cerebroside lipidosis) (infantile) 272.7
    hepatomegaly 272.7
    splenomegaly (cerebroside lipidosis) 272.7
Gayet's disease (superior hemorrhagic polioencephalitis) 265.1
Gayet-Wernicke's syndrome (superior hemorrhagic polioencephalitis) 265.1
Gee (-Herter) (-Heubner) (-Thaysen) disease or syndrome (nontropical sprue) 579.0
Gélineau's syndrome 347
Gemination, teeth 520.2
Gemistocytoma (M9411/3)
    specified site — *see* Neoplasm, by site, malignant
    unspecified site 191.9

General, generalized — see condtion
Genital — see condition
Genito-anorectal syndrome 099.1
Genitourinary system — see condition
Genu
  congenital 755.64
  extrorsum (acquired) 736.42
    congential 755.64
    late effects of rickets 268.1
  introrsum (acquired) 736.41
    congenital 755.64
    late effects of rickets 268.1
  rachitic (old) 268.1
  recurvatum (acquired) 736.5
    congenital 754.40
      with dislocation of knee 754.41
    late effects or rickets 268.1
  valgum (acquired) (knock-knee) 736.41
    congenital 755.64
    late effects of rickets 268.1
  varum (acquired) (bowleg) 736.42
    congenital 755.64
    late effect of rickets 268.1
Geographic tongue 529.1
Geophagia 307.52
Geotrichosis 117.9
  intestine 117.9
  lung 117.9
  mouth 117.9
Gephyrophobia 300.29
Gerbode defect 745.4
Gerhardt's
  disease (erythromelalgia) 443.89
  syndrome (vocal cord paralysis) 478.30
Gerlier's disease (epidemic vertigo) 078.81
German measles 056.9
  exposure to V01.4
Germinoblastoma (diffuse) (M9614/3) 202.8
  follicular (M9692/3) 202.0
Germinoma (M9064/3) — see Neoplasm, by site, malignant
Gerontoxon 371.41
Gerstmann's syndrome (finger agnosia) 784.69
Gestation (period) — see also Pregnancy
  ectopic NEC (see also Pregnancy, ectopic) 633.90
    with intrauterine pregnancy 633.91
Gestational proteinuria 646.2
  with hypertension — see Toxemia, of pregnancy
Ghon tubercle primary infection (see also Tuberculosis) 010.0
Ghost
  teeth 520.4
  vessels, cornea 370.64
Ghoul hand 102.3
Giant
  cell
    epulis 523.8
    peripheral (gingiva) 523.8
    tumor, tendon sheath 727.02
  colon (congenital) 751.3
  esophagus (congenital) 750.4
  kidney 753.3
  urticaria 995.1
    hereditary 277.6
Giardia lamblia infestation 007.1

Giardiasis 007.1
Gibert's disease (pityriasis rosea) 696.3
Gibraltar fever — see Brucellosis
Giddiness 780.4
  hysterical 300.11
  psychogenic 306.9
Gierke's disease (glycogenosis I) 271.0
Gigantism (cerebral) (hypophyseal) (pituitary) 253.0
Gilbert's disease or cholemia (familial nonhemolytic jaundice) 277.4
Gilchrist's disease (North American blastomycosis) 116.0
Gilford (-Hutchinson) disease or syndrome (progeria) 259.8
Gilles de la Tourette's disease (motor-verbal tic) 307.23
Gillespie's syndrome (dysplasia oculodentodigitalis) 759.89
Gingivitis 523.1
  acute 523.0
    necrotizing 101
  catarrhal 523.0
  chronic 523.1
  desquamative 523.1
  expulsiva 523.4
  hyperplastic 523.1
  marginal, simple 523.1
  necrotizing, acute 101
  pellagrous 265.2
  ulcerative 523.1
    acute necrotizing 101
  Vincent's 101
Gingivoglossitis 529.0
Gingivopericementitis 523.4
Gingivosis 523.1
Gingivostomatitis 523.1
  herpetic 054.2
Giovannini's disease 117.9
Gland, glandular — see condition
Glanders 024
Glanzmann (-Naegeli) disease or thrombasthenia 287.1
Glassblowers' disease 527.1
Glaucoma (capsular) (inflammatory) (noninflammatory) (primary) 365.9
  with increased episcleral venous pressure 365.82
  absolute 360.42
  acute 365.22
    narrow angle 365.22
    secondary 365.60
  angle closure 365.20
    acute 365.22
    chronic 365.23
    intermittent 365.21
    interval 365.21
    residual stage 365.24
    subacute 365.21
  borderline 365.00
  chronic 365.11
    noncongestive 365.11
    open angle 365.11
    simple 365.11
  closed angle — see Glaucoma, angle closure
  congenital 743.20
    associated with other eye anomalies 743.22
    simple 743.21

Glaucoma — *continued*
  congestive — *see* Glaucoma, narrow angle
  corticosteroid-induced (glaucomatous stage) 365.31
    residual stage 365.32
  hemorrhagic 365.60
  hypersecretion 365.81
  in or with
    aniridia 743.45 *[365.42]*
    Axenfeld's anomaly 743.44 *[365.41]*
    concussion of globe 921.3 *[365.65]*
    congenital syndromes NEC 759.89 *[365.44]*
    dislocation of lens
      anterior 379.33 *[365.59]*
      posterior 379.34 *[365.59]*
    disorder of lens NEC 365.59
    epithelial down-growth 364.61 *[365.64]*
    glaucomatocyclitic crisis 364.22 *[365.62]*
    hypermature cataract 366.18 *[365.51]*
    hyphema 364.41 *[365.63]*
    inflammation, ocular 365.62
    iridocyclitis 364.3 *[365.62]*
    iris
      anomalies NEC 743.46 *[365.42]*
      atrophy, essential 364.51 *[365.42]*
      bombé 364.74 *[365.61]*
      rubeosis 364.42 *[365.63]*
    microcornea 743.41 *[365.43]*
    neurofibromatosis 237.71 *[365.44]*
    ocular
      cysts NEC 365.64
      disorders NEC 365.60
      trauma 365.65
      tumors NEC 365.64
    postdislocation of lens
      anterior 379.33 *[365.59]*
      posterior 379.34 *[365.59]*
    pseudoexfoliation of capsule 366.11 *[365.52]*
    pupillary block or seclusion 364.74 *[365.61]*
    recession of chamber angle 364.77 *[365.65]*
    retinal vein occlusion 362.35 *[365.63]*
    Rieger's anomaly or syndrome 743.44 *[365.41]*
    rubeosis of iris 364.42 *[365.63]*
    seclusion of pupil 364.74 *[365.61]*
    spherophakia 743.36 *[365.59]*
    Sturge-Weber (-Dimitri) syndrome 759.6 *[365.44]*
    systemic syndrome NEC 365.44
    tumor of globe 365.64
    vascular disorders NEC 365.63
  infantile 365.14
    congenital 743.20
      associated with other eye anomalies 743.22
      simple 743.21
  juvenile 365.14
  low tension 365.12
  malignant 365.83 ▲
  narrow angle (primary) 365.20
    acute 365.22
    chronic 365.23
    intermittent 365.21
    interval 365.21
    residual stage 365.24
    subacute 365.21
  newborn 743.20
    associated with other eye anomalies 743.22
    simple 743.21
  noncongestive (chronic) 365.11

Glaucoma — *continued*
  nonobstructive (chronic) 365.11
  obstructive 365.60
    due to lens changes 365.59
  open angle 365.10
    with
      borderline intraocular pressure 365.01
      cupping of optic discs 365.01
    primary 365.11
    residual stage 365.15
  phacolytic 365.51
    with hypermature cataract 366.18 *[365.51]*
  pigmentary 365.13
  postinfectious 365.60
  pseudoexfoliation 365.52
    with pseudoexfoliation of capsule 366.11 *[365.52]*
  secondary NEC 365.60
  simple (chronic) 365.11
  simplex 365.11
  steroid responders 365.03
  suspect 365.00
  syphilitic 095.8
  traumatic NEC 365.65
    newborn 767.8
  tuberculous (*see also* Tuberculosis) 017.3 ✓5ᵗʰ *[365.62]*
  wide angle (*see also* Glaucoma, open angle) 365.10

Glaucomatous flecks (subcapsular) 366.31

Glazed tongue 529.4

Gleet 098.2

Glénard's disease or syndrome (enteroptosis) 569.89

Glinski-Simmonds syndrome (pituitary cachexia) 253.2

Glioblastoma (multiforme) (M9440/3)
  with sarcomatous component (M9442/3)
    specified site — *see* Neoplasm, by site, malignant
    unspecified site 191.9
  giant cell (M9441/3)
    specified site — *see* Neoplasm, by site, malignant
    unspecified site 191.9
  specified site — *see* Neoplasm, by site, malignant
  unspecified site 191.9

Glioma (malignant) (M9380/3)
  astrocytic (M9400/3)
    specified site — *see* Neoplasm, by site, malignant
    unspecified site 191.9
  mixed (M9382/3)
    specified site — *see* Neoplasm, by site, malignant
    unspecified site 191.9
  nose 748.1
  specified site NEC — *see* Neoplasm, by site, malignant
  subependymal (M9383/1) 237.5
  unspecified site 191.9

Gliomatosis cerebri (M9381/3) 191.0

Glioneuroma (M9505/1) — *see* Neoplasm, by site, uncertain behavior

Gliosarcoma (M9380/3)
  specified site — *see* Neoplasm, by site, malignant
  unspecified site 191.9

Gliosis (cerebral) 349.89
    spinal 336.0
Glisson's
    cirrhosis — *see* Cirrhosis, portal
    disease (*see also* Rickets) 268.0
Glissonitis 573.3
Globinuria 791.2
Globus 306.4
    hystericus 300.11
Glomangioma (M8712/0) (*see also* Hemangioma)
    228.00
Glomangiosarcoma (M8710/3) — *see* Neoplasm,
    connective tissue, malignant
Glomerular nephritis (*see also* Nephritis) 583.9
Glomerulitis (*see also* Nephritis) 583.9
Glomerulonephritis (*see also* Nephritis) 583.9
    with
        edema (*see also* Nephrosis) 581.9
        lesion of
            exudative nephritis 583.89
            interstitial nephritis (diffuse) (focal)
                583.89
            necrotizing glomerulitis 583.4
                acute 580.4
                chronic 582.4
            renal necrosis 583.9
                cortical 583.6
                medullary 583.7
            specified pathology NEC 583.89
                acute 580.89
                chronic 582.89
        necrosis, renal 583.9
            cortical 583.6
            medullary (papillary) 583.7
        specified pathology or lesion NEC 583.89
    acute 580.9
        with
            exudative nephritis 580.89
            interstitial nephritis (diffuse) (focal)
                580.89
            necrotizing glomerulitis 580.4
            extracapillary with epithelial crescents
                580.4
            poststreptococcal 580.0
            proliferative (diffuse) 580.0
            rapidly progressive 580.4
            specified pathology NEC 580.89
    arteriolar (*see also* Hypertension, kidney)
        403.90
    arteriosclerotic (*see also* Hypertension, kidney)
        403.90
    ascending (*see also* Pyelitis) 590.80
    basement membrane NEC 583.89
        with
            pulmonary hemorrhage (Goodpasture's
                syndrome) 446.21 *[583.81]*
    chronic 582.9
        with
            exudative nephritis 582.89
            interstitial nephritis (diffuse) (focal)
                582.89
            necrotizing glomerulitis 582.4
            specified pathology or lesion NEC 582.89
        endothelial 582.2
        extracapillary with epithelial crescents
            582.4
        hypocomplementemic persistent 582.2
        lobular 582.2
        membranoproliferative 582.2

Glomerulonephritis — *continued*
    chronic — *continued*
        membranous 582.1
            and proliferative (mixed) 582.2
            sclerosing 582.1
        mesangiocapillary 582.2
        mixed membranous and proliferative 582.2
        proliferative (diffuse) 582.0
        rapidly progressive 582.4
        sclerosing 582.1
    cirrhotic — *see* Sclerosis, renal
    desquamative — *see* Nephrosis
    due to or associated with
        amyloidosis 277.3 *[583.81]*
            with nephrotic syndrome 277.3 *[581.81]*
            chronic 277.3 *[582.81]*
        diabetes mellitus 250.4 ■5■ *[583.81]*
            with nephrotic syndrome 250.4 ■5■
                [581.81]
        diphtheria 032.89 *[580.81]*
        gonococcal infection (acute) 098.19 *[583.81]*
            chronic or duration of 2 months or over
                098.39 *[583.81]*
        infectious hepatitis 070.9 *[580.81]*
        malaria (with nephrotic syndrome) 084.9
            [581.81]
        mumps 072.79 *[580.81]*
        polyarteritis (nodosa) (with nephrotic
            syndrome) 446.0 *[581.81]*
        specified pathology NEC 583.89
            acute 580.89
            chronic 582.89
        streptotrichosis 039.8 *[583.81]*
        subacute bacterial endocarditis 421.0
            [580.81]
        syphilis (late) 095.4
            congenital 090.5 *[583.81]*
            early 091.69 *[583.81]*
        systemic lupus erythematosus 710.0
            [583.81]
            with nephrotic syndrome 710.0 *[581.81]*
            chronic 710.0 *[582.81]*
        tuberculosis (*see also* Tuberculosis)
            016.0 ■5■ *[583.81]*
        typhoid fever 002.0 *[580.81]*
    extracapillary with epithelial crescents 583.4
        acute 580.4
        chronic 582.4
    exudative 583.89
        acute 580.89
        chronic 582.89
    focal (*see also* Nephritis) 583.9
        embolic 580.4
    granular 582.89
    granulomatous 582.89
    hydremic (*see also* Nephrosis) 581.9
    hypocomplementemic persistent 583.2
        with nephrotic syndrome 581.2
        chronic 582.2
    immune complex NEC 583.89
    infective (*see also* Pyelitis) 590.80
    interstitial (diffuse) (focal) 583.89
        with nephrotic syndrome 581.89
        acute 580.89
        chronic 582.89
    latent or quiescent 582.9
    lobular 583.2
        with nephrotic syndrome 581.2
        chronic 582.2
    membranoproliferative 583.2
        with nephrotic syndrome 581.2

Glomerulonephritis — continued
  membranoproliferative — continued
    chronic 582.2
  membranous 583.1
    with nephrotic syndrome 581.1
    and proliferative (mixed) 583.2
      with nephrotic syndrome 581.2
        chronic 582.2
    chronic 582.1
    sclerosing 582.1
      with nephrotic syndrome 581.1
  mesangiocapillary 583.2
    with nephrotic syndrome 581.2
    chronic 582.2
  minimal change 581.3
  mixed membranous and proliferative 583.2
    with nephrotic syndrome 581.2
    chronic 582.2
  necrotizing 583.4
    acute 580.4
    chronic 582.4
  nephrotic (see also Nephrosis) 581.9
  old — see Glomerulonephritis, chronic
  parenchymatous 581.89
  poststreptococcal 580.0
  proliferative (diffuse) 583.0
    with nephrotic syndrome 581.0
    acute 580.0
    chronic 582.0
  purulent (see also Pyelitis) 590.80
  quiescent — see Nephritis, chronic
  rapidly progressive 583.4
    acute 580.4
    chronic 582.4
  sclerosing membranous (chronic) 582.1
    with nephrotic syndrome 581.1
  septic (see also Pyelitis) 590.80
  specified pathology or lesion NEC 583.89
    with nephrotic syndrome 581.89
    acute 580.89
    chronic 582.89
  suppurative (acute) (disseminated) (see also Pyelitis) 590.80
  toxic — see Nephritis, acute
  tubal, tubular — see Nephrosis, tubular
  type II (Ellis) — see Nephrosis
  vascular — see Hypertension, kidney
Glomerulosclerosis (see also Sclerosis, renal) 587
  focal 582.1
    with nephrotic syndrome 581.1
  intercapillary (nodular) (with diabetes) 250.4 ☒ [581.81]
Glossagra 529.6
Glossalgia 529.6
Glossitis 529.0
  areata exfoliativa 529.1
  atrophic 529.4
  benign migratory 529.1
  gangrenous 529.0
  Hunter's 529.4
  median rhomboid 529.2
  Moeller's 529.4
  pellagrous 265.2
Glossocele 529.8
Glossodynia 529.6
  exfoliativa 529.4
Glossoncus 529.8
Glossophytia 529.3
Glossoplegia 529.8

Glossoptosis 529.8
Glossopyrosis 529.6
Glossotrichia 529.3
Glossy skin 710.9
Glottis — see condition
Glottitis — see Glossitis
Glucagonoma (M8152/0)
  malignant (M8152/3)
    pancreas 157.4
    specified site NEC — see Neoplasm, by site, malignant
    unspecified site 157.4
  pancreas 211.7
    specified site NEC — see Neoplasm, by site, benign
    unspecified site 211.7
Glucoglycinuria 270.7
Glue ear syndrome 381.20
Glue sniffing (airplane glue) (see also Dependence) 304.6 ☒
Glycinemia (with methylmalonic acidemia) 270.7
Glycinuria (renal) (with ketosis) 270.0
Glycogen
  infiltration (see also Disease, glycogen storage) 271.0
  storage disease (see also Disease, glycogen storage) 271.0
Glycogenosis (see also Disease, glycogen storage) 271.0
  cardiac 271.0 [425.7]
  Cori, types I-VII 271.0
  diabetic, secondary 250.8 ☒ [259.8]
  diffuse (with hepatic cirrhosis) 271.0
  generalized 271.0
  glucose-6-phosphatase deficiency 271.0
  hepatophosphorylase deficiency 271.0
  hepatorenal 271.0
  myophosphorylase deficiency 271.0
Glycopenia 251.2
Glycoprolinuria 270.8
Glycosuria 791.5
  renal 271.4
Gnathostoma (spinigerum) (infection) (infestation) 128.1
  wandering swellings from 128.1
Gnathostomiasis 128.1
Goiter (adolescent) (colloid) (diffuse) (dipping) (due to iodine deficiency) (endemic) (euthyroid) (heart) (hyperplastic) (internal) (intrathoracic) (juvenile) (mixed type) (nonendemic) (parenchymatous) (plunging) (sporadic) (subclavicular) (substernal) 240.9
  with
    hyperthyroidism (recurrent) (see also Goiter, toxic) 242.0 ☒
    thyrotoxicosis (see also Goiter, toxic) 242.0 ☒
  adenomatous (see also Goiter, nodular) 241.9
  cancerous (M8000/3) 193
  complicating pregnancy, childbirth, or puerperium 648.1 ☒
  congenital 246.1
  cystic (see also Goiter, nodular) 241.9
  due to enzyme defect in synthesis of thyroid hormone (butane-insoluble iodine) (coupling) (deiodinase) (iodide trapping or organificaiton) (iodotyrosine dehalogenase) (peroxidase) 246.1

Goiter — continued
 dyshormonogenic 246.1
 exophthalmic (see also Goiter, toxic) 242.0 ✓5th
 familial (with deaf-mutism) 243
 fibrous 245.3
 lingual 759.2
 lymphadenoid 245.2
 malignant (M8000/3) 193
 multinodular (nontoxic) 241.1
  toxic or with hyperthyroidism (see also Goiter, toxic) 242.2 ✓5th
 nodular (nontoxic) 241.9
  with
   hyperthyroidism (see also Goiter, toxic) 242.3 ✓5th
   thyrotoxicosis (see also Goiter, toxic) 242.3 ✓5th
  endemic 241.9
  exophthalmic (diffuse) (see also Goiter, toxic) 242.0 ✓5th
  multinodular (nontoxic) 241.1
  sporadic 241.9
  toxic (see also Goiter, toxic) 242.3 ✓5th
  uninodular (nontoxic) 241.0
 nontoxic (nodular) 241.9
  multinodular 241.1
  uninodular 241.0
 pulsating (see also Goiter, toxic) 242.0 ✓5th
 simple 240.0
 toxic 242.0 ✓5th

> Note — Use the following fifth-digit subclassification with category 242:
>
> 0 without mention of thyrotoxic crisis or storm
> 1 with mention of thyrotoxic crisis or storm

  adenomatous 242.3 ✓5th
   multinodular 242.2 ✓5th
   uninodular 242.1 ✓5th
  multinodular 242.2 ✓5th
  nodular 242.3 ✓5th
   multinodular 242.2 ✓5th
   uninodular 242.1 ✓5th
  uninodular 242.1 ✓5th
 uninodular (nontoxic) 241.0
  toxic or with hyperthyroidism (see also Goiter, toxic) 242.1 ✓5th
Goldberg (-Maxwell) (-Morris) syndrome (testicular feminization) 257.8
Goldblatt's
 hypertension 440.1
 kidney 440.1
Goldenhar's syndrome (oculoauriculovertebral dysplasia) 756.0
Goldflam-Erb disease or syndrome 358.0
Goldscheider's disease (epidermolysis bullosa) 757.39
Goldstein's disease (familial hemorrhagic telangiectasia) 448.0
Golfer's elbow 726.32
Goltz-Gorlin syndrome (dermal hypoplasia) 757.39
Gonadoblastoma (M9073/1)
 specified site — see Neoplasm, by site, uncertain behavior
 unspecified site
  female 236.2

Gonadoblastoma — continued
 unspecified site — continued
  male 236.4
Gonecystitis (see also Vesiculitis) 608.0
Gongylonemiasis 125.6
 mouth 125.6
Goniosynechiae 364.73
Gonococcemia 098.89
Gonococcus, gonococcal (disease) (infection) (see also condition) 098.0
 anus 098.7
 bursa 098.52
 chronic NEC 098.2
 complicating pregnancy, childbirth, or puerperium 647.1 ✓5th
  affecting fetus or newborn 760.2
 conjunctiva, conjunctivitis (neonatorum) 098.40
 dermatosis 098.89
 endocardium 098.84
 epididymo-orchitis 098.13
  chronic or duration of 2 months or over 098.33
 eye (newborn) 098.40
 fallopian tube (chronic) 098.37
  acute 098.17
 genitourinary (acute) (organ) (system) (tract) (see also Gonnorrhea) 098.0
  lower 098.0
   chronic 098.2
  upper 098.10
   chronic 098.30
 heart NEC 098.85
 joint 098.50
 keratoderma 098.81
 keratosis (blennorrhagica) 098.81
 lymphatic (gland) (node) 098.89
 meninges 098.82
 orchitis (acute) 098.13
  chronic or duration of 2 months or over 098.33
 pelvis (acute) 098.19
  chronic or duration of 2 months or over 098.39
 pericarditis 098.83
 peritonitis 098.86
 pharyngitis 098.6
 pharynx 098.6
 proctitis 098.7
 pyosalpinx (chronic) 098.37
  acute 098.17
 rectum 098.7
 septicemia 098.89
 skin 098.89
 specified site NEC 098.89
 synovitis 098.51
 tendon sheath 098.51
 throat 098.6
 urethra (acute) 098.0
  chronic or duration of 2 months or over 098.2
 vulva (acute) 098.0
  chronic or duration of 2 months or over 098.2
Gonocytoma (M9073/1)
 specified site — see Neoplasm, by site, uncertain behavior
 unspecified site
  female 236.2
  male 236.4

Index to Diseases

Gonorrhea 098.0
  acute 098.0
  Bartholin's gland (acute) 098.0
    chronic or duration of 2 months or over 098.2
  bladder (acute) 098.11
    chronic or duration of 2 months or over 098.31
  carrier (suspected of) V02.7
  cervix (acute) 098.15
    chronic or duration of 2 months or over 098.35
  chronic 098.2
  complicating pregnancy, childbirth, or puerperium 647.1 ☑5ᵗʰ
    affecting fetus or newborn 760.2
  conjunctiva, conjunctivitis (neonatorum) 098.40
  contact V01.6
  Cowper's gland (acute) 098.0
    chronic or duration of 2 months or over 098.2
  duration of two months or over 098.2
  exposure to V01.6
  fallopian tube (chronic) 098.37
    acute 098.17
  genitourinary (acute) (organ) (system) (tract) 098.0
    chronic 098.2
    duration of two months or over 098.2
  kidney (acute) 098.19
    chronic or duration of 2 months or over 098.39
  ovary (acute) 098.19
    chronic or duration of 2 months or over 098.39
  pelvis (acute) 098.19
    chronic or duration of 2 months or over 098.39
  penis (acute) 098.0
    chronic or duration of 2 months or over 098.2
  prostate (acute) 098.12
    chronic or duration of 2 months or over 098.32
  seminal vesicle (acute) 098.14
    chronic or duration of 2 months or over 098.34
  specified site NEC — *see* Gonococcus
  spermatic cord (acute) 098.14
    chronic or duration of 2 months or over 098.34
  urethra (acute) 098.0
    chronic or duration of 2 months or over 098.2
  vagina (acute) 098.0
    chronic or duration of 2 months or over 098.2
  vas deferens (acute) 098.14
    chronic or duration of 2 months or over 098.34
  vulva (acute) 098.0
    chronic or duration of 2 months or over 098.2
Goodpasture's syndrome (pneumorenal) 446.21
Gopalan's syndrome (burning feet) 266.2
Gordon's disease (exudative enteropathy) 579.8
Gorlin-Chaudhry-Moss syndrome 759.89
Gougerot's syndrome (trisymptomatic) 709.1

Gougerot-Blum syndrome (pigmented purpuric lichenoid dermatitis) 709.1
Gougerot-Carteaud disease or syndrome (confluent reticulate papillomatosis) 701.8
Gougerot-Hailey-Hailey disease (benign familial chronic pemphigus) 757.39
Gougerot (-Houwer) - Sjögren syndrome (keratoconjunctivitis sicca) 710.2
Gouley's syndrome (constrictive pericarditis) 423.2
Goundou 102.6
Gout, gouty 274.9
  with specified manifestations NEC 274.89
  arthritis (acute) 274.0
  arthropathy 274.0
  degeneration, heart 274.82
  diathesis 274.9
  eczema 274.89
  episcleritis 274.89 *[379.09]*
  external ear (tophus) 274.81
  glomerulonephritis 274.10
  iritis 274.89 *[364.11]*
  joint 274.0
  kidney 274.10
  lead 984.9
    specified type of lead — *see* Table of Drugs and Chemicals
  nephritis 274.10
  neuritis 274.89 *[357.4]*
  phlebitis 274.89 *[451.9]*
  rheumatic 714.0
  saturnine 984.9
    specified type of lead — *see* Table of Drugs and Chemicals
  spondylitis 274.0
  synovitis 274.0
  syphilitic 095.8
  tophi 274.0
    ear 274.81
    heart 274.82
    specified site NEC 274.82
Gowers'
  muscular dystrophy 359.1
  syndrome (vasovagal attack) 780.2
Gowers-Paton-Kennedy syndrome 377.04
Gradenigo's syndrome 383.02
Graft-versus-host disease (bone marrow) 996.85
  due to organ transplant NEC — *see* Complications, transplant, organ
Graham Steell's murmur (pulmonic regurgitation) (*see also* Endocarditis, pulmonary) 424.3
Grain-handlers' disease or lung 495.8
Grain mite (itch) 133.8
Grand
  mal (idiopathic) (*see also* Epilepsy) 345.1 ☑5ᵗʰ
    hysteria of Charcôt 300.11
    nonrecurrent or isolated 780.39
  multipara
    affecting management of labor and delivery 659.4 ☑5ᵗʰ
    status only (not pregnant) V61.5
Granite workers' lung 502
Granular — *see also* condition
  inflammation, pharynx 472.1
  kidney (contracting) (*see also* Sclerosis, renal) 587
  liver — *see* Cirrhosis, liver
  nephritis — *see* Nephritis

Granulation tissue, abnormal — see also
  Granuloma
  abnormal or excessive 701.5
  postmastoidectomy cavity 383.33
  postoperative 701.5
  skin 701.5
Granulocytopenia, granulocytopenic (primary) 288.0
  malignant 288.0
Granuloma NEC 686.1
  abdomen (wall) 568.89
    skin (pyogenicum) 686.1
      from residual foreign body 709.4
  annulare 695.89
  anus 569.49
  apical 522.6
  appendix 543.9
  aural 380.23
  beryllium (skin) 709.4
    lung 503
  bone (see also Osteomyelitis) 730.1
    eosinophilic 277.8
    from residual foreign body 733.99
  canaliculus lacrimalis 375.81
  cerebral 348.8
  cholesterin, middle ear 385.82
  coccidioidal (progressive) 114.3
    lung 114.4
    meninges 114.2
    primary (lung) 114.0
  colon 569.89
  conjunctiva 372.61
  dental 522.6
  ear, middle (cholesterin) 385.82
    with otitis media — see Otitis media
  eosinophilic 277.8
    bone 277.8
    lung 277.8
    oral mucosa 528.9
  exuberant 701.5
  eyelid 374.89
  facial
    lethal midline 446.3
    malignant 446.3
  faciale 701.8
  fissuratum (gum) 523.8
  foot NEC 686.1
  foreign body (in soft tissue) NEC 728.82
    bone 733.99
    in operative wound 998.4
    muscle 728.82
    skin 709.4
    subcutaneous tissue 709.4
  fungoides 202.1
  gangraenescens 446.3
  giant cell (central) (jaw) (reparative) 526.3
    gingiva 523.8
    peripheral (gingiva) 523.8
  gland (lymph) 289.3
  Hodgkin's (M9661/3) 201.1
  ileum 569.89
  infectious NEC 136.9
  inguinale (Donovan) 099.2
    venereal 099.2
  intestine 569.89
  iridocyclitis 364.10
  jaw (bone) 526.3
    reparative giant cell 526.3
  kidney (see also Infection, kidney) 590.9
  lacrimal sac 375.81
  larynx 478.79

Granuloma NEC — continued
  lethal midline 446.3
  lipid 277.8
  lipoid 277.8
  liver 572.8
  lung (infectious) (see also Fibrosis, lung) 515
    coccidioidal 114.4
    eosinophilic 277.8
  lymph gland 289.3
  Majocchi's 110.6
  malignant, face 446.3
  mandible 526.3
  mediastinum 519.3
  midline 446.3
  monilial 112.3
  muscle 728.82
    from residual foreign body 728.82
  nasal sinus (see also Sinusitis) 473.9
  operation wound 998.59
    foreign body 998.4
    stitch (external) 998.89
      internal organ 996.7
      internal wound 998.89
    talc 998.7
  oral mucosa, eosinophilic or pyogenic 528.9
  orbit, orbital 376.11
  paracoccidiodal 116.1
  penis, venereal 099.2
  periapical 522.6
  peritoneum 568.89
    due to ova of helminths NEC (see also Helminthiasis) 128.9
  postmastoidectomy cavity 383.33
  postoperative — see Granuloma, operation wound
  prostate 601.8
  pudendi (ulcerating) 099.2
  pudendorum (ulcerative) 099.2
  pulp, internal (tooth) 521.4
  pyogenic, pyogenicum (skin) 686.1
    maxillary alveolar ridge 522.6
    oral mucosa 528.9
  rectum 569.49
  reticulohistiocytic 277.8
  rubrum nasi 705.89
  sarcoid 135
  Schistosoma 120.9
  septic (skin) 686.1
  silica (skin) 709.4
  sinus (accessory) (infectional) (nasal) (see also Sinusitis) 473.9
  skin (pyogenicum) 686.1
    from foreign body or material 709.4
  sperm 608.89
  spine
    syphilitic (epidural) 094.89
    tuberculous (see also Tuberculosis) 015.0 [730.88]
  stitch (postoperative) 998.89
    internal wound 998.89
  suppurative (skin) 686.1
  suture (postoperative) 998.89
    internal wound 998.89
  swimming pool 031.1
  talc 728.82
    in operation wound 998.7
  telangiectaticum (skin) 686.1
  trichophyticum 110.6
  tropicum 102.4
  umbilicus 686.1
    newborn 771.4

Granuloma NEC — *continued*
  urethra 599.84
  uveitis 364.10
  vagina 099.2
  venereum 099.2
  vocal cords 478.5
  Wegener's (necrotizing respiratory granulomatosis) 446.4
Granulomatosis NEC 686.1
  disciformis chronica et progressiva 709.3
  infantiseptica 771.2
  lipoid 277.8
  lipohagic, intestinal 040.2
  miliary 027.0
  necrotizing, respiratory 446.4
  progressive, septic 288.1
  Wegener's (necrotizing respiratory) 446.4
Granulomatous tissue — *see* Granuloma
Granulosis rubra nasi 705.89
Graphite fibrosis (of lung) 503
Graphospasm 300.89
  organic 333.84
Grating scapula 733.99
Gravel (urinary) (*see also* Calculus) 592.9
Graves' disease (exophthalmic goiter) (*see also* Goiter, toxic) 242.0
Gravis — *see* condition
Grawitz's tumor (hypernephroma) (M8312/3) 189.0
Grayness, hair (premature) 704.3
  congenital 757.4
Gray or grey syndrome (chloramphenicol) (newborn) 779.4
Greenfield's disease 330.0
Green sickness 280.9
Greenstick fracture — *see* Fracture, by site
Greig's syndrome (hypertelorism) 756.0
Griesinger's disease (*see also* Ancylostomiasis) 126.9
Grinders'
  asthma 502
  lung 502
  phthisis (*see also* Tuberculosis) 011.4
Grinding, teeth 306.8
Grip
  Dabney's 074.1
  devil's 074.1
Grippe, grippal — *see also* Influenza
  Balkan 083.0
  intestinal 487.8
  summer 074.8
Grippy cold 487.1
Grisel's disease 723.5
Groin — *see* condition
Grooved
  nails (transverse) 703.8
  tongue 529.5
    congenital 750.13
Ground itch 126.9
Growing pains, children 781.99
Growth (fungoid) (neoplastic) (new) (M8000/1) — *see also* Neoplasm, by site, unspecified nature
  adenoid (vegetative) 474.12
  benign (M8000/0) — *see* Neoplasm, by site, benign

Growth — *continued*
  fetal, poor 764.9
    affecting management of pregnancy 656.5
  malignant (M8000/3) — *see* Neoplasm, by site, malignant
  rapid, childhood V21.0
  secondary (M8000/6) — *see* Neoplasm, by site, malignant, secondary
Gruber's hernia — *see* Hernia, Gruber's
Gruby's disease (tinea tonsurans) 110.0
G-trisomy 758.0
Guama fever 066.3
Gubler (-Millard) paralysis or syndrome 344.89
Guérin-Stern syndrome (arthorgryposis multiplex congenita) 754.89
Guertin's disease (electric chorea) 049.8
Guillain-Barré disease or syndrome 357.0
Guinea worms (infection) (infestation) 125.7
Guinon's disease (motor-verbal tic) 307.23
Gull's disease (thyroid atrophy with myxedema) 244.8
Gull and Sutton's disease — *see* Hypertension, kidney
Gum — *see* condition
Gumboil 522.7
Gumma (syphilitic) 095.9
  artery 093.89
    cerebral or spinal 094.89
  bone 095.5
    of yaws (late) 102.6
  brain 094.89
  cauda equina 094.89
  central nervous system NEC 094.9
  ciliary body 095.8 [364.11]
  congenital 090.5
    testis 090.5
  eyelid 095.8 [373.5]
  heart 093.89
  intracranial 094.89
  iris 095.8 [364.11]
  kidney 095.4
  larynx 095.8
  leptomeninges 094.2
  liver 095.3
  meninges 094.2
  myocardium 093.82
  nasopharynx 095.8
  neurosyphilitic 094.9
  nose 095.8
  orbit 095.8
  palate (soft) 095.8
  penis 095.8
  pericardium 093.81
  pharynx 095.8
  pituitary 095.8
  scrofulous (*see also* Tuberculosis) 017.0
  skin 095.8
  specified site NEC 095.8
  spinal cord 094.89
  tongue 095.8
  tonsil 095.8
  trachea 095.8
  tuberculous (*see also* Tuberculosis) 017.0
  ulcerative due to yaws 102.4
  ureter 095.8
  yaws 102.4
    bone 102.6
Gunn's syndrome (jaw-winking syndrome) 742.8

Gunshot wound — *see also* Wound, open, by site
  fracture — *see* Fracture, by site, open
  internal organs (abdomen, chest, or pelvis) — *see* Injury, internal, by site, with open wound
  intracranial — *see* Laceration, brain, with open intracranial wound
Günther's disease or syndrome (congenital erythropoietic porphyria) 277.1
Gustatory hallucination 780.1
Gynandrism 752.7
Gynanadroblastoma (M8632/1)
  specified site — *see* Neoplasm, by site, uncertain behavior
  unspecified site
    female 236.2
    male 236.4
Gynandromorphism 752.7
Gynatresia (congenital) 752.49
Gynecoid pelvis, male 738.6
Gynecological examination V72.3
  for contraceptive maintenance V25.40
Gynecomastia 611.1
Gynephobia 300.29
Gyrate scalp 757.39

H

Haas' disease (osteochondrosis head of humerus) 732.3
Habermann's disease (acute parapsoriasis varioliformis) 696.2
Habit, habituation
  chorea 307.22
  disturbance, child 307.9
  drug (*see also* Dependence) 304.9
  laxative (*see also* Abuse, drugs, nondependent) 305.9
  spasm 307.20
    chronic 307.22
    transient of childhood 307.21
  tic 307.20
    chronic 307.22
    transient of childhood 307.21
  use of
    nonprescribed drugs (*see also* Abuse, drugs, nondependent) 305.9
    patent medicines (*see also* Abuse, drugs, nondependent) 305.9
  vomiting 536.2
Hadfield-Clarke syndrome (pancreatic infantilism) 577.8
Haff disease 985.1
Hageman factor defect, deficiency, or disease (*see also* Defect, coagulation) 286.3
Haglund's disease (osteochondrosis os tibiale externum) 732.5
Haglund-Läwen-Fründ syndrome 717.89
Hagner's disease (hypertrophic pulmonary osteoarthropathy) 731.2
Hag teeth, tooth 524.3
Hailey-Hailey disease (benign familial chronic pemphigus) 757.39
Hair — *see also* condition
  plucking 307.9
Hairball in stomach 935.2
Hairy black tongue 529.3

Half vertebra 756.14
Halitosis 784.9
Hallermann-Streiff syndrome 756.0
Hallervorden-Spatz disease or syndrome 333.0
Hallopeau's
  acrodermatitis (continua) 696.1
  disease (lichen sclerosis et atrophicus) 701.0
Hallucination (auditory) (gustatory) (olfactory) (tactile) 780.1
  alcoholic 291.3
  drug-induced 292.12
  visual 368.16
Hallucinosis 298.9
  alcoholic (acute) 291.3
  drug-induced 292.12
Hallus — *see* Hallux
Hallux 735.9
  malleus (acquired) 735.3
  rigidus (acquired) 735.2
    congenital 755.66
    late effects of rickets 268.1
  valgus (acquired) 735.0
    congenital 755.66
  varus (acquired) 735.1
    congenital 755.66
Halo, visual 368.15
Hamartoblastoma 759.6
Hamartoma 759.6
  epithelial (gingival), odontogenic, central, or peripheral (M9321/0) 213.1
  upper jaw (bone) 213.0
  vascular 757.32
Hamartosis, hamartoses NEC 759.6
Hamman's disease or syndrome (spontaneous mediastinal emphysema) 518.1
Hamman-Rich syndrome (diffuse interstitial pulmonary fibrosis) 516.3
Hammer toe (acquired) 735.4
  congenital 755.66
  late effects of rickets 268.1
Hand — *see* condition
Hand-Schüller-Christian disease or syndrome (chronic histiocytosis x) 277.8
Hand-foot syndrome 282.61
Hanging (asphyxia) (strangulation) (suffocation) 994.7
Hangnail (finger) (with lymphangitis) 681.02
Hangover (alcohol) (*see also* Abuse, drugs, nondependent) 305.0
Hanot's cirrhosis or disease — *see* Cirrhosis, biliary
Hanot-Chauffard (-Troisier) syndrome (bronze diabetes) 275.0
Hansen's disease (leprosy) 030.9
  benign form 030.1
  malignant form 030.0
Harada's disease or syndrome 363.22
Hard chancre 091.0
Hard firm prostate 600.1
Hardening
  artery — *see* Arteriosclerosis
  brain 348.8
  liver 571.8
Hare's syndrome (M8010/3) (carcinoma, pulmonary apex) 162.3
Harelip (*see also* Cleft, lip) 749.10

Harkavy's syndrome 446.0
Harlequin (fetus) 757.1
  color change syndrome 779.89
Harley's disease (intermittent hemoglobinuria) 283.2
Harris'
  lines 733.91
  syndrome (organic hyperinsulinism) 251.1
Hart's disease or syndrome (pellagra-cerebellar ataxia-renal aminoaciduria) 270.0
Hartmann's pouch (abnormal sacculation of gallbladder neck) 575.8
  of intestine V44.3
    attention to V55.3
Hartnup disease (pellagra-cerebellar ataxia-renal aminoaciduria) 270.0
Harvester lung 495.0
Hashimoto's disease or struma (struma lymphomatosa) 245.2
Hassell-Henle bodies (corneal warts) 371.41
Haut mal (see also Epilepsy) 345.1 ✓5ᵗʰ
Haverhill fever 026.1
Hawaiian wood rose dependence 304.5 ✓5ᵗʰ
Hawkins' keloid 701.4
Hay
  asthma (see also Asthma) 493.0 ✓5ᵗʰ
  fever (allergic) (with rhinitis) 477.9
    with asthma (bronchial) (see also Asthma) 493.0 ✓5ᵗʰ
    allergic, due to grass, pollen, ragweed, or tree 477.0
    conjunctivitis 372.05
    due to
      dander 477.8
      dust 477.8
      fowl 477.8
      pollen 477.0
      specified allergen other than pollen 477.8
Hayem-Faber syndrome (achlorhydric anemia) 280.9
Hayem-Widal syndrome (acquired hemolytic jaundice) 283.9
Haygarth's nodosities 715.04
Hazard-Crile tumor (M8350/3) 193
Hb (abnormal)
  disease — see Disease, hemoglobin
  trait — see Trait
H disease 270.0
Head — see also condition
  banging 307.3
Headache 784.0
  allergic 346.2 ✓5ᵗʰ
  cluster 346.2 ✓5ᵗʰ
  due to
    loss, spinal fluid 349.0
    lumbar puncture 349.0
    saddle block 349.0
  emotional 307.81
  histamine 346.2 ✓5ᵗʰ
  lumbar puncture 349.0
  menopausal 627.2
  migraine 346.9 ✓5ᵗʰ
  nonorganic origin 307.81
  postspinal 349.0
  psychogenic 307.81
  psychophysiologic 307.81

Headache — continued
  sick 346.1 ✓5ᵗʰ
  spinal 349.0
    complicating labor and delivery 668.8 ✓5ᵗʰ
    postpartum 668.8 ✓5ᵗʰ
  spinal fluid loss 349.0
  tension 307.81
  vascular 784.0
    migraine type 346.9 ✓5ᵗʰ
  vasomotor 346.9 ✓5ᵗʰ
Health
  advice V65.4
  audit V70.0
  checkup V70.0
  education V65.4
  hazard (see also History of) V15.9
    specified cause NEC V15.89
  instruction V65.4
  services provided because (of)
    boarding school residence V60.6
    holiday relief for person providing home care V60.5
    inadequate
      housing V60.1
      resources V60.2
    lack of housing V60.0
    no care available in home V60.4
    person living alone V60.3
    poverty V60.3
    residence in institution V60.6
    specified cause NEC V60.8
    vacation relief for person providing home care V60.5
Healthy
  donor (see also Donor) V59.9
  infant or child
    accompanying sick mother V65.0
    receiving care V20.1
  person
    accompanying sick relative V65.0
    admitted for sterilization V25.2
    receiving prophylactic inoculation or vaccination (see also Vaccination, prophylactic) V05.9
Hearing examination V72.1
Heart — see condition
Heartburn 787.1
  psychogenic 306.4
Heat (effects) 992.9
  apoplexy 992.0
  burn — see also Burn, by site
    from sun (see also Sunburn) 692.71
  collapse 992.1
  cramps 992.2
  dermatitis or eczema 692.89
  edema 992.7
  erythema — see Burn, by site
  excessive 992.9
    specified effect NEC 992.8
  exhaustion 992.5
    anhydrotic 992.3
    due to
      salt (and water) depletion 992.4
      water depletion 992.3
  fatigue (transient) 992.6
  fever 992.0
  hyperpyrexia 992.0
  prickly 705.1
  prostration — see Heat, exhaustion
  pyrexia 992.0

Heat — *continued*
   rash 705.1
   specified effect NEC 992.8
   stroke 992.0
   sunburn (*see also* Sunburn) 692.71
   syncope 992.1
Heavy-chain disease 273.2
Heavy-for-dates (fetus or infant) 766.1
   4500 grams or more 766.0
   exceptionally 766.0
Hebephrenia, hebephrenic (acute) (*see also* Schizophrenia) 295.1
   dementia (praecox) (*see also* Schizophrenia) 295.1
   schizophrenia (*see also* Schizophrenia) 295.1
Heberden's
   disease or nodes 715.04
   syndrome (angina pectoris) 413.9
Hebra's disease
   dermatitis exfoliativa 695.89
   erythema multiforme exudativum 695.1
   pityriasis 695.89
     maculata et circinata 696.3
     rubra 695.89
       pilaris 696.4
   prurigo 698.2
Hebra, nose 040.1
Hedinger's syndrome (malignant carcinoid) 259.2
Heel — *see* condition
Heerfordt's disease or syndrome (uveoparotitis) 135
Hegglin's anomaly or syndrome 288.2
Heidenhain's disease 290.10
   with dementia 290.10
Heilmeyer-Schöner disease (M9842/3) 207.1
Heine-Medin disease (*see also* Poliomyelitis) 045.9
Heinz-body anemia, congenital 282.7
Heller's disease or syndrome (infantile psychosis) (*see also* Psychosis, childhood) 299.1
H.E.L.L.P 642.5
Helminthiasis (*see also* Infestation, by specific parasite) 128.9
   Ancylostoma (*see also* Ancylostoma) 126.9
   intestinal 127.9
     mixed types (types classifiable to more than one of the titles 120.0-127.7) 127.8
     specified type 127.7
   mixed types (intestinal) (types classifiable to more than one of the titles 120.0-127.7) 127.8
   Necator americanus 126.1
   specified type NEC 128.8
   Trichinella 124
Heloma 700
Hemangioblastoma (M9161/1) — *see also* Neoplasm, connective tissue, uncertain behavior
   malignant (M9161/3) — *see* Neoplasm, connective tissue, malignant
Hemangioblastomatosis, cerebelloretinal 759.6
Hemangioendothelioma (M9130/1) — *see also* Neoplasm, by site, uncertain behavior
   benign (M9130/0) 228.00

Hemangioendothelioma — *continued*
   bone (diffuse) (M9130/3) — *see* Neoplasm, bone, malignant
   malignant (M9130/3) — *see* Neoplasm, connective tissue, malignant
   nervous system (M9130/0) 228.09
Hemangioendotheliosarcoma (M9130/3) — *see* Neoplasm, connective tissue, malignant
Hemangiofibroma (M9160/0) — *see* Neoplasm, by site, benign
Hemangiolipoma (M8861/0) — *see* Lipoma
Hemangioma (M9120/0) 228.00
   arteriovenous (M9123/0) — *see* Hemangioma, by site
   brain 228.02
   capillary (M9131/0) — *see* Hemangioma, by site
   cavernous (M9121/0) — *see* Hemangioma, by site
   central nervous system NEC 228.09
   choroid 228.09
   heart 228.09
   infantile (M9131/0) — *see* Hemangioma, by site
   intra-abdominal structures 228.04
   intracranial structures 228.02
   intramuscular (M9132/0) — *see* Hemangioma, by site
   iris 228.09
   juvenile (M9131/0) — *see* Hemangioma, by site
   malignant (M9120/3) — *see* Neoplasm, connective tissue, malignant
   meninges 228.09
     brain 228.02
     spinal cord 228.09
   peritoneum 228.04
   placenta — *see* Placenta, abnormal
   plexiform (M9131/0) — *see* Hemangioma, by site
   racemose (M9123/0) — *see* Hemangioma, by site
   retina 228.03
   retroperitoneal tissue 228.04
   sclerosing (M8832/0) — *see* Neoplasm, skin, benign
   simplex (M9131/0) — *see* Hemangioma, by site
   skin and subcutaneous tissue 228.01
   specified site NEC 228.09
   spinal cord 228.09
   venous (M9122/0) — *see* Hemangioma, by site
   verrucous keratotic (M9142/0) — *see* Hemangioma, by site
Hemangiomatosis (systemic) 757.32
   involving single site — *see* Hemangioma
Hemangiopericytoma (M9150/1) — *see also* Neoplasm, connective tissue, uncertain behavior
   benign (M9150/0) — *see* Neoplasm, connective tissue, benign
   malignant (M9150/3) — *see* Neoplasm, connective tissue, malignant
Hemangiosarcoma (M9120/3) — *see* Neoplasm, connective tissue, malignant
Hemarthrosis (nontraumatic) 719.10
   ankle 719.17
   elbow 719.12
   foot 719.17
   hand 719.14

Index to Diseases — Hematoma

Hemarthrosis — *continued*
  hip 719.15
  knee 719.16
  multiple sites 719.19
  pelvic region 719.15
  shoulder (region) 719.11
  specified site NEC 719.18
  traumatic — *see* Sprain, by site
  wrist 719.13
Hematemesis 578.0
  with ulcer — *see* Ulcer, by site, with hemorrhage
  due to S. japonicum 120.2
  Goldstein's (familial hemorrhagic telangiectasia) 448.0
  newborn 772.4
    due to swallowed maternal blood 777.3
Hematidrosis 705.89
Hematinuria (*see also* Hemoglobinuria) 791.2
  malarial 084.8
  paroxysmal 283.2
Hematite miners' lung 503
Hematobilia 576.8
Hematocele (congenital) (diffuse) (idiopathic) 608.83
  broad ligament 620.7
  canal of Nuck 629.0
  cord male 608.83
  fallopian tube 620.8
  female NEC 629.0
  ischiorectal 569.89
  male NEC 608.83
  ovary 629.0
  pelvis, pelvic
    female 629.0
      with ectopic pregnancy (*see also* Pregnancy, ectopic) 633.90 ▲
        with intrauterine pregnancy 633.91 ●
    male 608.83
  periuterine 629.0
  retrouterine 629.0
  scrotum 608.83
  spermatic cord (diffuse) 608.83
  testis 608.84
  traumatic — *see* Injury, internal, pelvis
  tunica vaginalis 608.83
  uterine ligament 629.0
  uterus 621.4
  vagina 623.6
  vulva 624.5
Hematocephalus 742.4
Hematochezia (*see also* Melena) 578.1
Hematochyluria (*see also* Infestation, filarial) 125.9
Hematocolpos 626.8
Hematocornea 371.12
Hematogenous — *see* condition
Hematoma (skin surface intact) (traumatic) — *see also* Contusion

Hematoma — *continued*

> Note — Hematomas are coded according to origin and the nature and site of the hematoma or the accompanying injury. Hematomas of unspecified origin are coded as injuries of the sites involved, except:
>
> (a) hematomas of genital organs which are coded as diseases of the organ involved unless they complicate pregnancy or delivery
>
> (b) hematomas of the eye which are coded as diseases of the eye.
>
> For late effect of hematoma classifiable to 920-924 see Late, effect, contusion

  with
    crush injury — *see* Crush
    fracture — *see* Fracture, by site
    injury of internal organs — *see also* Injury, internal, by site
      kidney — *see* Hematoma, kidney traumatic
      liver — *see* Hematoma, liver, traumatic
      spleen — *see* Hematoma, spleen
    nerve injury — *see* Injury, nerve
    open wound — *see* Wound, open, by site
    skin surface intact — *see* Contusion
  abdomen (wall) — *see* Contusion, abdomen
  amnion 658.8
  aorta, dissecting 441.00
    abdominal 441.02
    thoracic 441.01
    thoracoabdominal 441.03
  arterial (complicating trauma) 904.9
    specified site — *see* Injury, blood vessel, by site
  auricle (ear) 380.31
  birth injury 767.8
    skull 767.1
  brain (traumatic) 853.0

> Note — Use the following fifth-digit subclassification with categories 851-854:
>
> 0 unspecified state of consciousness
> 1 with no loss of consciousness
> 2 with brief [less than one hour] loss of consciousness
> 3 with moderate [1-24 hours] loss of consciousness
> 4 with prolonged [more than 24 hours] loss of consciousness and return to pre-existing conscious level
> 5 with prolonged [more than 24 hours] loss of consciousness, without return to pre-existing conscious level
>
> Use fifth-digit 5 to designate when a patient is unconscious and dies before regaining consciousness, regardless of the duration of the loss of consciousness
>
> 6 with loss of consciousness of unspecified duration
> 9 with concussion, unspecified

Hematoma — continued
　brain — continued
　　with
　　　cerebral
　　　　contusion — see Contusion, brain
　　　　laceration — see Laceration, brain
　　　open intracranial wound 853.1 ✓5ᵗʰ
　　　skull fracture — see Fracture, skull, by site
　　extradural or epidural 852.4 ✓5ᵗʰ
　　　with open intracranial wound 852.5 ✓5ᵗʰ
　　　fetus or newborn 767.0
　　　nontraumatic 432.0
　　fetus or newborn NEC 767.0
　　nontraumatic (see also Hemorrhage, brain) 431
　　　epidural or extradural 432.0
　　　newborn NEC 772.8
　　　subarachnoid, arachnoid, or meningeal (see also Hemorrhage, subarachnoid) 430
　　　subdural (see also Hemorrhage, subdural) 432.1
　　subarachnoid, arachnoid, or meningeal 852.0 ✓5ᵗʰ
　　　with open intracranial wound 852.1 ✓5ᵗʰ
　　　fetus or newborn 772.2
　　　nontraumatic (see also Hemorrhage, subarachnoid) 430
　　subdural 852.2 ✓5ᵗʰ
　　　with open intracranial wound 852.3 ✓5ᵗʰ
　　　fetus or newborn (localized) 767.0
　　　nontraumatic (see also Hemorrhage, subdural) 432.1
　breast (nontraumatic) 611.8
　broad ligament (nontraumatic) 620.7
　　complicating delivery 665.7 ✓5ᵗʰ
　　traumatic — see Injury, internal, broad ligament
　calcified NEC 959.9
　capitis 920
　　due to birth injury 767.1
　　newborn 767.1
　cerebral — see Hematoma, brain
　cesarean section wound 674.3 ✓5ᵗʰ
　chorion — see Placenta, abnormal
　complicating delivery (perineum) (vulva) 664.5 ✓5ᵗʰ
　　pelvic 665.7 ✓5ᵗʰ
　　vagina 665.7 ✓5ᵗʰ
　corpus
　　cavernosum (nontraumatic) 607.82
　　luteum (nontraumatic) (ruptured) 620.1
　dura (mater) — see Hematoma, brain, subdural
　epididymis (nontraumatic) 608.83
　epidural (traumatic) — see also Hematoma, brain, extradural
　　spinal — see Injury, spinal, by site
　episiotomy 674.3 ✓5ᵗʰ
　external ear 380.31
　extradural — see also Hematoma, brain, extradural
　　fetus or newborn 767.0
　　nontraumatic 432.0
　　　fetus or newborn 767.0
　fallopian tube 620.8
　genital organ (nontraumatic)
　　female NEC 629.8
　　male NEC 608.83

Hematoma — continued
　genital organ — continued
　　traumatic (external site) 922.4
　　　internal — see Injury, internal, genital organ
　graafian follicle (ruptured) 620.0
　internal organs (abdomen, chest, or pelvis) — see also Injury, internal, by site
　　kidney — see Hematoma, kidney, traumatic
　　liver — see Hematoma, liver, traumatic
　　spleen — see Hematoma, brain
　intracrainal — see Hematoma, brain
　kidney, cystic 593.81
　　traumatic 866.01
　　　with open wound into cavity 866.11
　labia (nontraumatic) 624.5
　lingual (and other parts of neck, scalp, or face, except eye) 920
　liver (subcapsular) 573.8
　　birth injury 767.8
　　fetus or newborn 767.8
　　traumatic NEC 864.01
　　　with
　　　　laceration — see Laceration, liver
　　　　open wound into cavity 864.11
　mediastinum — see Injury, internal, mediastinum
　meninges, meningeal (brain) — see also Hematoma, brain, subarachnoid
　　spinal — see Injury, spinal, by site
　mesosalpinx (nontraumatic) 620.8
　　traumatic — see Injury, internal, pelvis
　muscle (traumatic — see Contusion, by site
　nasal (septum) (and other part(s) of neck, scalp, or face, except eye) 920
　obstetrical surgical wound 674.3 ✓5ᵗʰ
　orbit, orbital (nontraumatic) 376.32
　　traumatic 921.2
　ovary (corpus luteum) (nontraumatic) 620.1
　　traumatic — see Injury, internal, ovary
　pelvis (female) (nontraumatic) 629.8
　　complicating delivery 665.7 ✓5ᵗʰ
　　male 608.83
　　traumatic — see also Injury, internal, pelvis
　　　specified organ NEC (see also Injury, internal, pelvis) 867.6
　penis (nontraumatic) 607.82
　pericranial (and neck, or face any part, except eye) 920
　　due to injury at birth 767.1
　perineal wound (obstetrical) 674.3 ✓5ᵗʰ
　　complicating delivery 664.5 ✓5ᵗʰ
　perirenal, cystic 593.81
　pinna 380.31
　placenta — see Placenta, abnormal
　postoperative 998.12
　retroperitoneal (nontraumatic) 568.81
　　traumatic — see Injury, internal, retroperitoneum
　retropubic, male 568.81
　scalp (and neck, or face any part, except eye) 920
　　fetus or newborn 767.1
　scrotum (nontraumatic) 608.83
　　traumatic 922.4
　seminal vesicle (nontraumatic) 608.83
　　traumatic — see Injury, internal, seminal, vesicle

Hematoma — *continued*
  spermatic cord — *see also* Injury, internal, spermatic cord
    nontraumatic 608.83
  spinal (cord) (meninges) — *see also* Injury, spinal, by site
    fetus or newborn 767.4
    nontraumatic 336.1
  spleen 865.01
    with
      laceration — *see* Laceration, spleen
      open wound into cavity 865.11
  sternocleidomastoid, birth injury 767.8
  sternomastoid, birth injury 767.8
  subarachnoid — *see also* Hematoma, brain, subarachnoid
    fetus or newborn 772.2
    nontraumatic (*see also* Hemorrhage, subarachnoid) 430
      newborn 772.2
  subdural — *see also* Hematoma, brain, subdural
    fetus or newborn (localized) 767.0
    nontraumatic (*see also* Hemorrhage, subdural) 432.1
  subperiosteal (syndrome) 267
    traumatic — *see* Hematoma, by site
  superficial, fetus or newborn 772.6
  syncytium — *see* Placenta, abnormal
  testis (nontraumatic) 608.83
    birth injury 767.8
    traumatic 922.4
  tunica vaginalis (nontraumatic) 608.83
  umbilical cord 663.6 ✓5ᵗʰ
    affecting fetus or newborn 762.6
  uterine ligament (nontraumatic) 620.7
    traumatic — *see* Injury, internal, pelvis
  uterus 621.4
    traumatic — *see* Injury, internal, pelvis
  vagina (nontraumatic) (ruptured) 623.6
    complicating delivery 665.7 ✓5ᵗʰ
    traumatic 922.4
  vas deferens (nontraumatic) 608.83
    traumatic — *see* Injury, internal, vas deferens
  vitreous 379.23
  vocal cord 920
  vulva (nontraumatic) 624.5
    complicating delivery 664.5 ✓5ᵗʰ
    fetus or newborn 767.8
    traumatic 922.4
Hematometra 621.4
Hematomyelia 336.1
  with fracture of vertebra (*see also* Fracture, vertebra, by site, with spinal cord injury) 806.8
  fetus or newborn 767.4
Hematomyelitis 323.9
  late effect — *see* category 326
Hematoperitoneum (*see also* Hemoperitoneum) 568.81
Hematopneumothorax (*see also* Hemothorax) 511.8
Hematoporphyria (acquired) (congenital) 277.1
Hematoporphyrinuria (acquired) (congenital) 277.1
Hematorachis, hematorrhachis 336.1
  fetus or newborn 767.4

Hematosalpinx 620.8
  with
    ectopic pregnancy (*see also* categories 633.0-633.9) 639.2
    molar pregnancy (*see also* categories 630-632) 639.2
    infectional (*see also* Salpingo-oophoritis) 614.2
Hematospermia 608.82
Hematothorax (*see also* Hemothorax) 511.8
Hematotympanum 381.03
Hematuria (benign) (essential) (idiopathic) 599.7
  due to S. hematobium 120.0
  endemic 120.0
  intermittent 599.7
  malarial 084.8
  paroxysmal 599.7
  sulfonamide
    correct substance properly administered 599.7
    overdose or wrong substance given or taken 961.0
  tropical (bilharziasis) 120.0
  tuberculous (*see also* Tuberculosis) 016.9 ✓5ᵗʰ
Hematuric bilious fever 084.8
Hemeralopia 368.10
Hemiabiotrophy 799.8
Hemi-akinesia 781.8
Hemianalgesia (*see also* Disturbance, sensation) 782.0
Hemianencephaly 740.0
Hemianesthesia (*see also* Disturbance, sensation) 782.0
Hemianopia, hemianopsia (altitudinal) (homonymous) 368.46
  binasal 368.47
  bitemporal 368.47
  heteronymous 368.47
  syphilitic 095.8
Hemiasomatognosia 307.9
Hemiathetosis 781.0
Hemiatrophy 799.8
  cerebellar 334.8
  face 349.89
    progressive 349.89
  fascia 728.9
  leg 728.2
  tongue 529.8
Hemiballism(us) 333.5
Hemiblock (cardiac) (heart) (left) 426.2
Hemicardia 746.89
Hemicephalus, hemicephaly 740.0
Hemichorea 333.5
Hemicrania 346.9 ✓5ᵗʰ
  congenital malformation 740.0
Hemidystrophy — *see* Hemiatrophy
Hemiectromelia 755.4
Hemihypalgesia (*see also* Disturbance, sensation) 782.0
Hemihypertrophy (congenital) 759.89
  cranial 756.0
Hemihypesthesia (*see also* Disturbance, sensation) 782.0
Hemi-inattention 781.8

Hemimelia 755.4
  lower limb 755.30
    paraxial (complete) (incomplete)
      (intercalary) (terminal) 755.32
      fibula 755.37
      tibia 755.36
    transverse (complete) (partial) 755.31
  upper limb 755.20
    paraxial (complete) (incomplete)
      (intercalary) (terminal) 755.22
      radial 755.26
      ulnar 755.27
    transverse (complete) (partial) 755.21
Hemiparalysis (see also Hemiplegia) 342.9 ✓5ᵗʰ
Hemiparesis (see also Hemiplegia) 342.9 ✓5ᵗʰ
Hemiparesthesia (see also Disturbance, sensation) 782.0
Hemiplegia 342.9 ✓5ᵗʰ
  acute (see also Disease, cerebrovascular, acute) 436
  alternans facialis 344.89
  apoplectic (see also Disease, cerebrovascular, acute) 436
    late effect or residual
      affecting
        dominant side 438.21
        nondominant side 438.22
        unspecified side 438.20
  arteriosclerotic 437.0
    late effect or residual
      affecting
        dominant side 438.21
        nondominant side 438.22
        unspecified side 438.20
  ascending (spinal) NEC 344.89
  attack (see also Disease, cerebrovascular, acute) 436
  brain, cerebral (current episode) 437.8
    congenital 343.1
  cerebral — see Hemiplegia, brain
  congenital (cerebral) (spastic) (spinal) 343.1
  conversion neurosis (hysterical) 300.11
  cortical — see Hemiplegia, brain
  due to
    arteriosclerosis 437.0
      late effect or residual
        affecting
          dominant side 438.21
          nondominant side 438.22
          unspecified side 438.20
    cerebrovascular lesion (see also Disease, cerebrovascular, acute) 436
      late effect
        affecting
          dominant side 438.21
          nondominant side 438.22
          unspecified side 438.20
  embolic (current) (see also Embolism, brain) 434.1 ✓5ᵗʰ
    late effect
      affecting
        dominant side 438.21
        nondominant side 438.22
        unspecified side 438.20
  flaccid 342.0
  hypertensive (current episode) 437.8
  infantile (postnatal) 343.4
  late effect
    birth injury, intracranial or spinal 343.4
    cerebrovascular lesion — see Late effect(s) (of) cerebrovascular disease

Hemiplegia — continued
  late effect — continued
    viral encephalitis 139.0
  middle alternating NEC 344.89
  newborn NEC 767.0
  seizure (current episode) (see also Disease, cerebrovascular, acute) 436
  spastic 342.1
    congenital or infantile 343.1
  specified NEC 342.8
  thrombotic (current) (see also Thrombosis, brain) 434.0 ✓5ᵗʰ
    late effect — see Late effect(s) (of) cerebrovascular disease
Hemisection, spinal cord — see Fracture, vertebra, by site, with spinal cord injury
Hemispasm 781.0
  facial 781.0
Hemispatial neglect 781.8
Hemisporosis 117.9
Hemitremor 781.0
Hemivertebra 756.14
Hemobilia 576.8
Hemocholecyst 575.8
Hemochromatosis (acquired) (diabetic) (hereditary) (liver) (myocardium) (primary idiopathic) (secondary) 275.0
  with refractory anemia 285.0
Hemodialysis V56.0
Hemoglobin — see also condition
  abnormal (disease) — see Disease, hemoglobin
  AS genotype 282.5
  fetal, hereditary persistence 282.7
  high-oxygen-affinity 289.0
  low NEC 285.9
  S (Hb-S), heterozygous 282.5
Hemoglobinemia 283.2
  due to blood transfusion NEC 999.8
    bone marrow 996.85
  paroxysmal 283.2
Hemoglobinopathy (mixed) (see also Disease, hemoblobin) 282.7
  with thalassemia 282.4
  sickle-cell 282.60
    with thalassemia 282.4
Hemoglobinuria, hemoglobinuric 791.2
  with anemia, hemolytic, acquired (chronic) NEC 283.2
  cold (agglutinin) (paroxysmal) (with Raynaud's syndrome) 283.2
  due to
    exertion 283.2
    hemolysis (from external causes) NEC 283.2
  exercise 283.2
  fever (malaria) 084.8
  infantile 791.2
  intermittent 283.2
  malarial 084.8
  march 283.2
  nocturnal (paroxysmal) 283.2
  paroxysmal (cold) (nocturnal) 283.2
Hemolymphangioma (M9175/0) 228.1
Hemolysis
  fetal — see Jaundice, fetus or newborn
  intravascular (disseminated) NEC 286.6
    with
      abortion — see Abortion, by type, with hemorrhage, delayed or excessive

Hemolysis — continued
  intravascular — continued
    with — continued
      ectopic pregnancy (see also categories 633.0-633.9) 639.1
      hemorrhage of pregnancy 641.3 ✓5ᵗʰ
        affecting fetus or newborn 762.1
      molar pregnancy (see also categories 630-632) 639.1
    acute 283.2
    following
      abortion 639.1
      ectopic or molar pregnancy 639.1
    neonatal — see Jaundice, fetus or newborn
    transfusion NEC 999.8
      bone marrow 996.85
Hemolytic — see also condition
  anemia — see Anemia, hemolytic
  uremic syndrome 283.11
Hemometra 621.4
Hemopericardium (with effusion) 423.0
  newborn 772.8
  traumatic (see also Hemothorax, traumatic) 860.2
    with open wound into thorax 860.3
Hemoperitoneum 568.81
  infectional (see also Peritonitis) 567.2
  traumatic — see Injury, internal, peritoneum
Hemophilia (familial) (hereditary) 286.0
  A 286.0
    carrier (asymptomatic) V83.01
      symptomatic V83.02
  acquired 286.5
  B (Leyden) 286.1
  C 286.2
  calcipriva (see also Fibrinolysis) 286.7
  classical 286.0
  nonfamilial 286.7
  vascular 286.4
Hemophilus influenzae NEC 041.5
  arachnoiditis (basic) (brain) (spinal) 320.0
    late effect — see category 326
  bronchopneumonia 482.2
  cerebral ventriculitis 320.0
    late effect — see category 326
  cerebrospinal inflammation 320.0
    late effect — see category 326
  infection NEC 041.5
  leptomeningitis 320.0
    late effect — see category 326
  meningitis (cerebral) (cerebrospinal) (spinal) 320.0
    late effect — see category 326
  meningomyelitis 320.0
    late effect — see category 326
  pachymeningitis (adhesive) (fibrous) (hemorrhagic) (hypertrophic) (spinal) 320.0
    late effect — see category 326
  pneumonia (broncho-) 482.2
Hemophthalmos 360.43
Hemopneumothorax (see also Hemothorax) 511.8
  traumatic 860.4
    with open wound into thorax 860.5
Hemoptysis 786.3
  due to Paragonimus (westermani) 121.2
  newborn 770.3
  tuberculous (see also Tuberculosis, pulmonary) 011.9 ✓5ᵗʰ

Hemorrhage, hemorrhagic (nontraumatic) 459.0
  abdomen 459.0
  accidental (antepartum) 641.2 ✓5ᵗʰ
    affecting fetus or newborn 762.1
  adenoid 474.8
  adrenal (capsule) (gland) (medulla) 255.4
    newborn 772.5
  after labor — see Hemorrhage, postpartum
  alveolar
    lung, newborn 770.3
    process 525.8
  alveolus 525.8
  amputation stump (surgical) 998.11
    secondary, delayed 997.69
  anemia (chronic) 280.0
    acute 285.1
  antepartum — see Hemorrhage, pregnancy
  anus (sphincter) 569.3
  apoplexy (stroke) 432.9
  arachnoid — see Hemorrhage, subarachnoid
  artery NEC 459.0
    brain (see also Hemorrhage, brain) 431
    middle meningeal — see Hemorrhage, subarachnoid
  basilar (ganglion) (see also Hemorrhage, brain) 431
  bladder 596.8
  blood dyscrasia 289.9
  bowel 578.9
    newborn 772.4
  brain (miliary) (nontraumatic) 431
    with
      birth injury 767.0
      arachnoid — see Hemorrhage, subarachnoid
      due to
        birth injury 767.0
        rupture of aneurysm (congenital) (see also Hemorrhage, subarachnoid) 430
      mycotic 431
      syphilis 094.89
    epidural or extradural — see Hemorrhage, extradural
    fetus or newborn (anoxic) (hypoxic) (due to birth trauma) (nontraumatic) 767.0
      intraventricular 772.10
        grade I 772.11
        grade II 772.12
        grade III 772.13
        grade IV 772.14
    iatrogenic 997.02
    postoperative 997.02
    puerperal, postpartum, childbirth 674.0 ✓5ᵗʰ
    stem 431
    subarachnoid, arachnoid, or meningeal — see Hemorrhage, subarachnoid
    subdural — see Hemorrhage, subdural
  traumatic NEC 853.0 ✓5ᵗʰ

Hemorrhage, hemorrhagic — continued
  brain — continued

> Note — Use the following fifth-digit subclassification with categories 851-854:
>
> 0   unspecified state of consciousness
> 1   with no loss of consciousness
> 2   with brief [less than one hour] loss of consciousness
> 3   with moderate [1-24 hours] loss of consciousness
> 4   with prolonged [more than 24 hours] loss of consciousness and return to pre-existing conscious level
> 5   with prolonged [more than 24 hours] loss of consciousness, without return to pre-existing conscious level
>
> Use fifth-digit 5 to designate when a patient is unconscious and dies before regaining consciousness, regardless of the duration of the loss of consciousness
>
> 6   with loss of consciousness of unspecified duration
> 9   with concussion, unspecified

    with
      cerebral
        contusion — see Contusion, brain
        laceration — see Laceration, brain
      open intracranial wound 853.1
      skull fracture — see Fracture, skull, by site
    extradural or epidural 852.4
      with open intracranial wound 852.5
    subarachnoid 852.0
      with open intracranial wound 852.1
    subdural 852.2
      with open intracranial wound 852.3
  breast 611.79
  bronchial tube — see Hemorrhage, lung
  bronchopulmonary — see Hemorrhage, lung
  bronchus (cause unknown) (see also Hemorrhage, lung) 786.3
  bulbar (see also Hemorrhage, brain) 431
  bursa 727.89
  capillary 448.9
    primary 287.8
  capsular — see Hemorrhage, brain
  cardiovascular 429.89
  cecum 578.9
  cephalic (see also Hemorrhage, brain) 431
  cerebellar (see also Hemorrhage, brain) 431
  cerebellum (see also Hemorrhage, brain) 431
  cerebral (see also Hemorrhage, brain) 431
    fetus or newborn (anoxic) (traumatic) 767.0
  cerebromeningeal (see also Hemorrhage, brain) 431
  cerebrospinal (see also Hemorrhage, brain) 431
  cerebrum (see also Hemorrhage, brain) 431
  cervix (stump) (uteri) 622.8
  cesarean section wound 674.3
  chamber, anterior (eye) 364.41
  childbirth — see Hemorrhage, complicating, delivery

Hemorrhage, hemorrhagic — continued
  choroid 363.61
    expulsive 363.62
  ciliary body 364.41
  cochlea 386.8
  colon — see Hemorrhage, intestine
  complicating
    delivery 641.9
      affecting fetus or newborn 762.1
      associated with
        afibrinogenemia 641.3
          affecting fetus or newborn 763.89
        coagulation defect 641.3
          affecting fetus or newborn 763.89
        hyperfibrinolysis 641.3
          affecting fetus or newborn 763.89
        hypofibrinogenemia 641.3
          affecting fetus or newborn 763.89
      due to
        low-lying placenta 641.1
          affecting fetus or newborn 762.0
        placenta previa 641.1
          affecting fetus or newborn 762.0
        premature separation of placenta 641.2
          affecting fetus or newborn 762.1
      retained
        placenta 666.0
        secundines 666.2
      trauma 641.8
        affecting fetus or newborn 763.89
      uterine leiomyoma 641.8
        affecting fetus or newborn 763.89
    surgical procedure 998.11
  concealed NEC 459.0
  congenital 772.9
  conjunctiva 372.72
    newborn 772.8
  cord, newborn 772.0
    slipped ligature 772.3
    stump 772.3
  corpus luteum (ruptured) 620.1
  cortical (see also Hemorrhage, brain) 431
  cranial 432.9
  cutaneous 782.7
    newborn 772.6
  cyst, pancreas 577.2
  cystitis — see Cystitis
  delayed
    with
      abortion — see Abortion, by type, with hemorrhage, delayed or excessive
      ectopic pregnancy (see also categories 633.0-633.9) 639.1
      molar pregnancy (see also categories 630-632) 639.1
    following
      abortion 639.1
      ectopic or molar pregnancy 639.1
    postpartum 666.2
  diathesis (familial) 287.9
    newborn 776.0
  disease 287.9
    newborn 776.0
    specified type NEC 287.8
  disorder 287.9
    due to circulating anticoagulants 286.5
    specified type NEC 287.8

Hemorrhage, hemorrhagic — *continued*
  due to
    any device, implant or graft (presence of)
      classifiable to 996.0-996.5 — *see*
      Complications, due to (presence of)
      any device, implant, or graft classified
      to 996.0-996.5 NEC
    circulating anticoagulant 286.5
  duodenum, duodenal 537.89
    ulcer — *see* Ulcer, duodenum, with
      hemorrhage
  dura mater — *see* Hemorrhage, subdural
  endotracheal — *see* Hemorrhage, lung
  epidural — *see* Hemorrhage, extradural
  episiotomy 674.3 ✓5ᵗʰ
  esophagus 530.82
    varix (*see also* Varix, esophagus, bleeding)
      456.0
  excessive
    with
      abortion — *see* Abortion, by type, with
        hemorrhage, delayed or excessive
      ectopic pregnancy (*see also* categories
        633.0-633.9) 639.1
      molar pregnancy (*see also* categories
        630-632) 639.1
    following
      abortion 639.1
      ectopic or molar pregnancy 639.1
  external 459.0
  extradural (traumatic) — *see also* Hemorrhage,
    brain, traumatic, extradural
    birth injury 767.0
    fetus or newborn (anoxic) (traumatic) 767.0
    nontraumatic 432.0
  eye 360.43
    chamber (anterior) (aqueous) 364.41
    fundus 362.81
  eyelid 374.81
  fallopian tube 620.8
  fetomaternal 772.0
    affecting management of pregnancy or
      puerperium 656.0 ✓5ᵗʰ
  fetus, fetal 772.0
    from
      cut end of co-twin's cord 772.0
      placenta 772.0
      ruptured cord 772.0
      vasa previa 772.0
    into
      co-twin 772.0
      mother's circulation 772.0
        affecting management of pregnancy
          or puerperium 656.0 ✓5ᵗʰ
  fever (*see also* Fever, hemorrhagic) 065.9
    with renal syndrome 078.6
    arthropod-borne NEC 065.9
    Bangkok 065.4
    Crimean 065.0
    dengue virus 065.4
    epidemic 078.6
    Junin virus 078.7
    Korean 078.6
    Machupo virus 078.7
    mite-borne 065.8
    mosquito-borne 065.4
    Philippine 065.4
    Russian (Yaroslav) 078.6
    Singapore 065.4
    southeast Asia 065.4
    Thailand 065.4

Hemorrhage, hemorrhagic — *continued*
  fever — *continued*
    tick-borne NEC 065.3
  fibrinogenolysis (*see also* Fibrinolysis) 286.6
  fibrinolytic (acquired) (*see also* Fibrinolysis)
    286.6
  fontanel 767.1
  from tracheostomy stoma 519.09
  fundus, eye 362.81
  funis
    affecting fetus or newborn 772.0
    complicating delivery 663.8 ✓5ᵗʰ
  gastric (*see also* Hemorrhage, stomach) 578.9
  gastroenteric 578.9
    newborn 772.4
  gastrointestinal (tract) 578.9
    newborn 772.4
  genitourinary (tract) NEC 599.89
  gingiva 523.8
  globe 360.43
  gravidarum — *see* Hemorrhage, pregnancy
  gum 523.8
  heart 429.89
  hypopharyngeal (throat) 784.8
  intermenstrual 626.6
    irregular 626.6
    regular 626.5
  internal (organs) 459.0
    capsule (*see also* Hemorrhage, brain) 431
    ear 386.8
    newborn 772.8
  intestine 578.9
    congenital 772.4
    newborn 772.4
  into
    bladder wall 596.7
    bursa 727.89
    corpus luysii (*see also* Hemorrhage, brain)
      431
  intra-abdominal 459.0
    during or following surgery 998.11
  intra-alveolar, newborn (lung) 770.3
  intracerebral (*see also* Hemorrhage, brain) 431
  intracranial NEC 432.9
    puerperal, postpartum, childbirth 674.0
      ✓5ᵗʰ
    traumatic — *see* Hemorrhage, brain,
      traumatic
  intramedullary NEC 336.1
  intraocular 360.43
  intraoperative 998.11
  intrapartum — *see* Hemorrhage, complicating,
    delivery
  intrapelvic
    female 629.8
    male 459.0
  intraperitoneal 459.0
  intrapontine (*see also* Hemorrhage, brain) 431
  intrauterine 621.4
    complicating delivery — *see* Hemorrhage,
      complicating, delivery
    in pregnancy or childbirth — *see*
      Hemorrhage, pregnancy
    postpartum (*see also* Hemorrhage,
      postpartum) 666.1 ✓5ᵗʰ
  intraventricular (*see also* Hemorrhage, brain)
    431
    fetus or newborn (anoxic) (traumatic)
      772.10
      grade I 772.11
      grade II 772.12

Hemorrhage, hemorrhagic — continued
  intraventricular — continued
    fetus or newborn — continued
      grade III 772.13
      grade IV 772.14
  intravesical 596.7
  iris (postinfectional) (postinflammatory) (toxic) 364.41
  joint (nontraumatic) 719.10
    ankle 719.17
    elbow 719.12
    foot 719.17
    forearm 719.13
    hand 719.14
    hip 719.15
    knee 719.16
    lower leg 719.16
    multiple sites 719.19
    pelvic region 719.15
    shoulder (region) 719.11
    specified site NEC 719.18
    thigh 719.15
    upper arm 719.12
    wrist 719.13
  kidney 593.81
  knee (joint) 719.16
  labyrinth 386.8
  leg NEC 459.0
  lenticular striate artery (see also Hemorrhage, brain) 431
  ligature, vessel 998.11
  liver 573.8
  lower extremity NEC 459.0
  lung 786.3
    newborn 770.3
    tuberculous (see also Tuberculosis, pulmonary) 011.9
  malaria 084.8
  marginal sinus 641.2
  massive subaponeurotic, birth injury 767.1
  maternal, affecting fetus or newborn 762.1
  mediastinum 786.3
  medulla (see also Hemorrhage, brain) 431
  membrane (brain) (see also Hemorrhage, subarachnoid) 430
    spinal cord — see Hemorrhage, spinal cord
  meninges, meningeal (brain) (middle) (see also Hemorrhage, subarachnoid) 430
    spinal cord — see Hemorrhage, spinal cord
  mesentery 568.81
  metritis 626.8
  midbrain (see also Hemorrhage, brain) 431
  mole 631
  mouth 528.9
  mucous membrane NEC 459.0
    newborn 728.8
  muscle 728.89
  nail (subungual) 703.8
  nasal turbinate 784.7
    newborn 772.8
  nasopharynx 478.29
  navel, newborn 772.3
  newborn 772.9
    adrenal 772.5
    alveolar (lung) 770.3
    brain (anoxic) (hypoxic) (due to birth trauma) 767.0
    cerebral (anoxic) (hypoxic) (due to birth trauma) 767.0
    conjunctiva 772.8
    cutaneous 772.6

Hemorrhage, hemorrhagic — continued
  newborn — continued
    diathesis 776.0
    due to vitamin K deficiency 776.0
    gastrointestinal 772.4
    internal (organs) 772.8
    intestines 772.4
    intra-alveolar (lung) 770.3
    intracranial (from any perinatal cause) 767.0
    intraventricular (from any perinatal cause) 772.10
      grade I 772.11
      grade II 772.12
      grade III 772.13
      grade IV 772.14
    lung 770.3
    pulmonary (massive) 770.3
    spinal cord, traumatic 767.4
    stomach 772.4
    subaponeurotic (massive) 767.1
    subarachnoid (from any perinatal cause) 772.2
    subconjunctival 772.8
    umbilicus 772.0
      slipped ligature 772.3
      vasa previa 772.0
  nipple 611.79
  nose 784.7
    newborn 772.8
  obstetrical surgical wound 674.3
  omentum 568.89
    newborn 772.4
  optic nerve (sheath) 377.42
  orbit 376.32
  ovary 620.1
  oviduct 620.8
  pancreas 577.8
  parathyroid (gland) (spontaneous) 252.8
  parturition — see Hemorrhage, complicating, delivery
  penis 607.82
  pericardium, paricarditis 423.0
  perineal wound (obstetrical) 674.3
  peritoneum, peritoneal 459.0
  peritonsillar tissue 474.8
    after operation on tonsils 998.11
    due to infection 475
  petechial 782.7
  pituitary (gland) 253.8
  placenta NEC 641.9
    affecting fetus or newborn 762.1
    from surgical or instrumental damage 641.8
      affecting fetus or newborn 762.1
    previa 641.8
      affecting fetus or newborn 762.0
  pleura — see Hemorrhage, lung
  polioencephalitis, superior 265.1
  polymyositis — see Polymyositis
  pons (see also Hemorrhage, brain) 431
  pontine (see also Hemorrhage, brain) 431
  popliteal 459.0
  postcoital 626.7
  postextraction (dental) 998.11
  postmenopausal 627.1
  postnasal 784.7
  postoperative 998.11
  postpartum (atonic) (following delivery of placenta) 666.1

Hemorrhage, hemorrhagic — *continued*
   postpartum — *continued*
      delayed or secondary (after 24 hours) 666.2 ⬛5ᴵᴵᴵ
      retained placenta 666.0 ⬛5ᴵᴵᴵ
      third stage 666.0 ⬛5ᴵᴵᴵ
   pregnancy (concealed) 641.9 ⬛5ᴵᴵᴵ
      accidental 641.2 ⬛5ᴵᴵᴵ
         affecting fetus or newborn 762.1
      affecting fetus or newborn 762.1
      before 22 completed weeks gestation 640.9 ⬛5ᴵᴵᴵ
         affecting fetus or newborn 762.1
      due to
         abruptio placenta 641.2 ⬛5ᴵᴵᴵ
            affecting fetus or newborn 762.1
         afibrinogenemia or other coagulation defect (conditions classifiable to 286.0-286.9) 641.3 ⬛5ᴵᴵᴵ
            affecting fetus or newborn 762.1
         coagulation defect 641.3 ⬛5ᴵᴵᴵ
            affecting fetus or newborn 762.1
         hyperfibrinolysis 641.3 ⬛5ᴵᴵᴵ
            affecting fetus or newborn 762.1
         hypofibrinogenemia 641.3 ⬛5ᴵᴵᴵ
            affecting fetus or newborn 762.1
         leiomyoma, uterus 641.8 ⬛5ᴵᴵᴵ
            affecting fetus or newborn 762.1
         low-lying placenta 641.1 ⬛5ᴵᴵᴵ
            affecting fetus or newborn 762.1
         marginal sinus (rupture) 641.2 ⬛5ᴵᴵᴵ
            affecting fetus or newborn 762.1
         placenta previa 641.1 ⬛5ᴵᴵᴵ
            affecting fetus or newborn 762.0
         premature separation of placenta (normally implanted) 641.2 ⬛5ᴵᴵᴵ
            affecting fetus or newborn 762.1
         threatend abortion 640.0 ⬛5ᴵᴵᴵ
            affecting fetus or newborn 762.1
         trauma 641.8 ⬛5ᴵᴵᴵ
            affecting fetus or newborn 762.1
      early (before 22 completed weeks gestation) 640.9 ⬛5ᴵᴵᴵ
         affecting fetus or newborn 762.1
      previous, affecting management of pregnancy or childbirth V23.49 ▲
      unavoidable — *see* Hemorrhage, pregnancy, due to placenta previa
   prepartum (mother) — *see* Hemorrhage, pregnancy
   preretinal, cause unspecified 362.81
   prostate 602.1
   puerperal (*see also* Hemorrhage, postpartum) 666.1 ⬛5ᴵᴵᴵ
   pulmonary — *see also* Hemorrhage, lung
      newborn (massive) 770.3
      renal syndrome 446.21
   purpura (primary) (*see also* Purpura, thrombocytopenic) 287.3
   rectum (sphincter) 569.3
   recurring, following initial hemorrhage at time of injury 958.2
   renal 593.81
      pulmonary syndrome 446.21
   respiratory tract (*see also* Hemorrhage, lung) 786.3
   retina, retinal (deep) (superficial) (vessels) 362.81
      diabetic 250.5 ⬛5ᴵᴵᴵ *[362.01]*
      due to birth injury 772.8
   retrobulbar 376.89

Hemorrhage, hemorrhagic — *continued*
   retroperitoneal 459.0
   retroplacental (*see also* Placenta, separation) 641.2 ⬛5ᴵᴵᴵ
   scalp 459.0
      due to injury at birth 767.1
   scrotum 608.83
   secondary (nontraumatic) 459.0
      following initial hemorrhage at time of injury 958.2
   seminal vesicle 608.83
   skin 782.7
      newborn 772.6
   spermatic cord 608.83
   spinal (cord) 336.1
      aneurysm (ruptured) 336.1
         syphilitic 094.89
      due to birth injury 767.4
      fetus or newborn 767.4
   spleen 289.59
   spontaneous NEC 459.0
      petechiae 782.7
   stomach 578.9
      newborn 772.4
      ulcer — *see* Ulcer, stomach, with hemorrhage
   subaponeurotic, newborn 767.1
      massive (birth injury) 767.1
   subarachnoid (nontraumatic) 430
      fetus or newborn (anoxic) (traumatic) 772.2
      puerperal, postpartum, childbirth 674.0 ⬛5ᴵᴵᴵ
      traumatic — *see* Hemorrhage, brain, traumatic, subarachnoid
   subconjunctival 372.72
      due to birth injury 772.8
      newborn 772.8
   subcortical (*see also* Hemorrhage, brain) 431
   subcutaneous 782.7
   subdiaphragmatic 459.0
   subdural (nontraumatic) 432.1
      due to birth injury 767.0
      fetus or newborn (anoxic) (hypoxic) (due to birth trauma) 767.0
      puerperal, postpartum, childbirth 674.0 ⬛5ᴵᴵᴵ
      spinal 336.1
      traumatic — *see* Hemorrhage, brain, traumatic, subdural
   subhyaloid 362.81
   subperiosteal 733.99
   subretinal 362.81
   subtentorial (*see also* Hemorrhage, subdural) 432.1
   subungual 703.8
      due to blood dyscrasia 287.8
   suprarenal (capsule) (gland) 255.4
      fetus or newborn 772.5
   tentorium (traumatic) — *see also* Hemorrhage, brain, traumatic
      fetus or newborn 767.0
      nontraumatic — *see* Hemorrhage, subdural
   testis 608.83
   thigh 459.0
   third stage 666.0 ⬛5ᴵᴵᴵ
   thorax — *see* Hemorrhage, lung
   throat 784.8
   thrombocythemia 238.7
   thymus (gland) 254.8
   thyroid (gland) 246.3
      cyst 246.3

Hemorrhage, hemorrhagic — *continued*
   tongue 529.8
   tonsil 474.8
      postoperative 998.11
   tooth socket (postextraction) 998.11
   trachea — *see* Hemorrhage, lung
   traumatic — *see also* nature of injury
      brain — *see* Hemorrhage, brain, traumatic
      recurring or secondary (following initial hemorrhage at time of injury) 958.2
   tuberculous NEC (*see also* Tuberculosis, pulmonary) 011.9 ✓5ᵗʰ
   tunica vaginalis 608.83
   ulcer — *see* Ulcer, by site, with hemorrhage
   umbilicus, umbilical cord 772.0
      after birth, newborn 772.3
      complicating delivery 663.8 ✓5ᵗʰ
         affecting fetus or newborn 772.0
      slipped ligature 772.3
      stump 772.3
   unavoidable (due to placenta previa) 641.1 ✓5ᵗʰ
      affecting fetus or newborn 762.0
   upper extremity 459.0
   urethra (idiopathic) 599.84
   uterus, uterine (abnormal) 626.9
      climacteric 627.0
      complicating delivery — *see* Hemorrhage, complicating delivery
      due to
         intrauterine contraceptive device 996.76
            perforating uterus 996.32
      functional or dysfunctional 626.8
      in pregnancy — *see* Hemorrhage, pregnancy
      intermenstrual 626.6
         irregular 626.6
         regular 626.5
      postmenopausal 627.1
      postpartum (*see also* Hemorrhage, postpartum) 666.1 ✓5ᵗʰ
      prepubertal 626.8
      pubertal 626.3
      puerperal (immediate) 666.1 ✓5ᵗʰ
   vagina 623.8
   vasa previa 663.5 ✓5ᵗʰ
      affecting fetus or newborn 772.0
   vas deferens 608.83
   ventricular (*see also* Hemorrhage, brain) 431
   vesical 596.8
   viscera 459.0
      newborn 772.8
   vitreous (humor) (intraocular) 379.23
   vocal cord 478.5
   vulva 624.8
Hemorrhoids (anus) (rectum) (without complication) 455.6
   bleeding, prolapsed, strangulated, or ulcerated NEC 455.8
      external 455.5
      internal 455.2
   complicated NEC 455.8
   complicating pregnancy and puerperium 671.8 ✓5ᵗʰ
   external 455.3
      with complication NEC 455.5
      bleeding, prolapsed, strangulated, or ulcerated 455.5
         thrombosed 455.4
   internal 455.0
      with complication NEC 455.2

Hemorrhoids — *continued*
   internal — *continued*
      bleeding, prolapsed, strangulated, or ulcerated 455.2
         thrombosed 455.1
   residual skin tag 455.9
   sentinel pile 455.9
   thrombosed NEC 455.7
      external 455.4
      internal 455.1
Hemosalpinx 620.8
Hemosiderosis 275.0
   dietary 275.0
   pulmonary (idiopathic) 275.0 *[516.1]*
   transfusion NEC 999.8
      bone marrow 996.85
Hemospermia 608.82
Hemothorax 511.8
   bacterial, nontuberculous 511.1
   newborn 772.8
   nontuberculous 511.8
      bacterial 511.1
   pneumococcal 511.1
   postoperative 998.11
   staphylococcal 511.1
   streptococcal 511.1
   traumatic 860.2
      with
         open wound into thorax 860.3
         pneumothorax 860.4
            with open wound into thorax 860.5
   tuberculous (*see also* Tuberculosis, pleura) 012.0 ✓5ᵗʰ
Hemotympanum 385.89
Hench-Rosenberg syndrome (palindromic arthritis) (*see also* Rheumatism, palindromic) 719.3 ✓5ᵗʰ
Henle's warts 371.41
Henoch (-Schönlein)
   disease or syndrome (allergic purpura) 287.0
   purpura (allergic) 287.0
Henpue, henpuye 102.6
Heparitinuria 277.5
Hepar lobatum 095.3
Hepatalgia 573.8
Hepatic — *see also* conditon
   flexure syndrome 569.89
Hepatitis 573.3
   acute (*see also* Necrosis, liver) 570
      alcoholic 571.1
      infective 070.1
         with hepatic coma 070.0
   alcoholic 571.1
   amebic — *see* Abscess, liver, amebic
   anicteric (acute) — *see* Hepatitis, viral
   antigen-associated (HAA) — *see* Hepatitis, viral, type B
   Australian antigen (positive) — *see* Hepatitis, viral, type B
   catarrhal (acute) 070.1
      with hepatic coma 070.0
      chronic 571.40
      newborn 070.1
         with hepatic coma 070.0
   chemical 573.3
   cholangiolitic 573.8
   cholestatic 573.8
   chronic 571.40
      active 571.49

Hepatitis — continued
  chronic — continued
    active — continued
      viral — see Hepatitis, viral
    aggressive 571.49
    persistent 571.41
    viral — see Hepatitis, viral
  cytomegalic inclusion virus 078.5 [573.1]
  diffuse 573.3
  "dirty needle" — see Hepatitis, viral
    with hepatic coma 070.2 ✓5ᵗʰ
  drug-induced 573.3
  due to
    Coxsackie 074.8 [573.1]
    cytomegalic inclusion virus 078.5 [573.1]
    infectious mononucleosis 075 [573.1]
    malaria 084.9 [573.2]
    mumps 072.71
    secondary syphilis 091.62
    toxoplasmosis (acquired) 130.5
      congenital (active) 771.2
  epidemic — see Hepatitis, viral, type A
  fetus or newborn 774.4
  fibrous (chronic) 571.49
    acute 570
  from injection, inoculation, or transfusion (blood) (other substance) (plasma) (serum) (onset within 8 months after administration) — see Hepatitis, viral
  fulminant (viral) (see also Hepatitis, viral) 070.9
    with hepatic coma 070.6
    type A 070.1
      with hepatic coma 070.0
    type B — see Hepatitis, viral, type B
  giant cell (neonatal) 774.4
  hemorrhagic 573.8
  homologous serum — see Hepatitis, viral
  hypertrophic (chronic) 571.49
    acute 570
  infectious, infective (acute) (chronic) (subacute) 070.1
    with hepatic coma 070.0
  inoculation — see Hepatitis, viral
  interstitial (chronic) 571.49
    acute 570
  lupoid 571.49
  malarial 084.9 [573.2]
  malignant (see also Necrosis, liver) 570
  neonatal (toxic) 774.4
  newborn 774.4
  parenchymatous (acute) (see also Necrosis, liver) 570
  peliosis 573.3
  persistent, chronic 571.41
  plasma cell 571.49
  postimmunization — see Hepatitis, viral
  postnecrotic 571.49
  posttransfusion — see Hepatitis, viral
  recurrent 571.49
  septic 573.3
  serum — see Hepatitis, viral
    carrier (suspected of) V02.61
  subacute (see also Necrosis, liver) 570
  suppurative (diffuse) 572.0
  syphilitic (late) 095.3
    congenital (early) 090.0 [573.2]
      late 090.5 [573.2]
    secondary 091.62
  toxic (noninfectious) 573.3
    fetus or newborn 774.4

Hepatitis — continued
  tuberculous (see also Tuberculosis) 017.9 ✓5ᵗʰ
  viral (acute) (anicteric) (cholangiolitic) (cholestatic) (chronic) (subacute) 070.9
    with hepatic coma 070.6
    AU-SH type virus — see Hepatitis, viral, type B
    Australian antigen — see Hepatitis, viral, type B
    B-antigen — see Hepatitis, viral, type B
    Coxsackie 074.8 [573.1]
    cytomegalic inclusion 078.5 [573.1]
    IH (virus) — see Hepatitis, viral, type A
    infectious hepatitis, viral, type A
    serum hepatitis virus — see Hepatitis, viral, type B
    SH — see Hepatitis, viral, type B
    specified type NEC 070.59
      with hepatic coma 070.49
    type A 070.1
      with hepatic coma 070.0
    type B (acute) 070.30
      with
        hepatic coma 070.20
          with hepatitis delta 070.21
        hepatitis delta 070.31
          with hepatic coma 070.21
      carrier status V02.61
      chronic 070.32
        with
          hepatic coma 070.22
            with hepatitis delta 070.23
          hepatitis delta 070.33
            with hepatic coma 070.23
    type C (acute) 070.51
      with hepatic coma 070.41
      carrier status V02.62
      chronic 070.54
        with hepatic coma 070.44
    type delta (with hepatitis B carrier state) 070.52
      with
        active hepatitis B disease — see Hepatitis, viral, type B
        hepatic coma 070.42
    type E 070.53
      with hepatic coma 070.43
    vaccination and inoculation (prophylactic) V05.3
  Waldenstrom's (lupoid hepatitis) 571.49
Hepatization, lung (acute) — see also Pneumonia, lobar
  chronic (see also Fibrosis, lung) 515
Hepatoblastoma (M8970/3) 155.0
Hepatocarcinoma (M8170/3) 155.0
Hepatocholangiocarcinoma (M8180/3) 155.0
Hepatocholangioma, benign (M8180/0) 211.5
Hepatocholangitis 573.8
Hepatocystitis (see also Cholecystitis) 575.10
Hepatodystrophy 570
Hepatolenticular degeneration 275.1
Hepatolithiasis — see Choledocholithiasis
Hepatoma (malignant) (M8170/3) 155.0
  benign (M8170/0) 211.5
  congenital (M8970/3) 155.0
  embryonal (M8970/3) 155.0
Hepatomegalia glycogenica diffusa 271.0
Hepatomegaly (see also Hypertrophy, liver) 789.1

Hepatomegaly — *continued*
  congenital 751.69
    syphilitic 090.0
  due to Clonorchis sinensis 121.1
  Gaucher's 272.7
  syphilitic (congenital) 090.0
Hepatoptosis 573.8
Hepatorrhexis 573.8
Hepatosis, toxic 573.8
Hepatosplenomegaly 571.8
  due to S. japonicum 120.2
  hyperlipemic (Burger-Grutz type) 272.3
Herald patch 696.3
Hereditary — *see* condition
Heredodegeneration 330.9
  macular 362.70
Heredopathia atactica polyneuritiformis 356.3
Heredosyphilis (*see also* Syphilis, congenital) 090.9
Hermaphroditism (true) 752.7
  with specified chromosomal anomaly — *see* Anomaly, chromosomes, sex
Hernia, hernial (acquired) (recurrent) 553.9
  with
    gangrene (obstructed) NEC 551.9
    obstruction NEC 552.9
      and gangrene 551.9
  abdomen (wall) — *see* Hernia, ventral
  abdominal, specified site NEC 553.8
    with
      gangrene (obstructed) 551.8
      obstruction 552.8
        and gangrene 551.8
  appendix 553.8
    with
      gangrene (obstructed) 551.8
      obstruction 552.8
        and gangrene 551.8
  bilateral (inguinal) — *see* Hernia, inguinal
  bladder (sphincter)
    congenital (female) (male) 756.71
    female 618.0
    male 596.8
  brain 348.4
    congenital 742.0
  broad ligament 553.8
  cartilage, vertebral — *see* Displacement, intervertebral disc
  cerebral 348.4
    congenital 742.0
    endaural 742.0
  ciliary body 364.8
    traumatic 871.1
  colic 553.9
    with
      gangrene (obstructed) 551.9
      obstruction 552.9
        and gangrene 551.9
  colon 553.9
    with
      gangrene (obstructed) 551.9
      obstruction 552.9
        and gangrene 551.9
  colostomy (stoma) 569.69
  Cooper's (retroperitoneal) 553.8
    with
      gangrene (obstructed) 551.8
      obstruction 552.8
        and gangrene 551.8

Hernia, hernial — *continued*
  crural — *see* Hernia, femoral
  diaphragm, diaphragmatic 553.3
    with
      gangrene (obstructed) 551.3
      obstruction 552.3
        and gangrene 551.3
    congenital 756.6
    due to gross defect of diaphragm 756.6
    traumatic 862.0
      with open wound into cavity 862.1
  direct (inguinal) — *see* Hernia, inguinal
  disc, intervertebral — *see* Displacement, intervertebral disc
  diverticulum, intestine 553.9
    with
      gangrene (obstructed) 551.9
      obstruction 552.9
        and gangrene 551.9
  double (inguinal) — *see* Hernia, inguinal
  duodenojejunal 553.8
    with
      gangrene (obstructed) 551.8
      obstruction 552.8
        and gangrene 551.8
  en glissade — *see* Hernia, inguinal
  enterostomy (stoma) 569.69
  epigastric 553.29
    with
      gangrene (obstruction) 551.29
      obstruction 552.29
        and gangrene 551.29
    recurrent 553.21
      with
        gangrene (obstructed) 551.21
        obstruction 552.21
          and gangrene 551.21
  esophageal hiatus (sliding) 553.3
    with
      gangrene (obstructed) 551.3
      obstruction 552.3
        and gangrene 551.3
    congenital 750.6
  external (inguinal) — *see* Hernia, inguinal
  fallopian tube 620.4
  fascia 728.89
  fat 729.30
    eyelid 374.34
    orbital 374.34
    pad 729.30
      eye, eyelid 374.34
      knee 729.31
      orbit 374.34
      popliteal (space) 729.31
      specified site NEC 729.39
  femoral (unilateral) 553.00
    with
      gangrene (obstructed) 551.00
      obstruction 552.00
        with gangrene 551.0
    bilateral 553.02
      gangrenous (obstructed) 551.02
      obstructed 552.02
        with gangrene 551.02
      recurrent 553.03
        gangrenous (obstructed) 551.03
        obstructed 552.03
          with gangrene 551.03
    recurrent (unilateral) 553.01
      bilateral 553.03
        gangrenous (obstructed) 551.03

Index to Diseases — Hernia, hernial

Hernia, hernial — *continued*
  femoral — *continued*
    recurrent — *continued*
      bilateral — *continued*
        obstructed 552.03
          with gangrene 551.03
      gangrenous (obstructed) 551.01
      obstructed 552.01
        with gangrene
  foramen
    Bochdalek 553.3
      with
        gangrene (obstructed) 551.3
        obstruction 552.3
          and gangrene 551.3
      congenital 756.6
    magnum 348.4
    Morgagni, Morgagnian 553.3
      with
        gangrene 551.3
        obstruction 552.3
          and gangrene 551.3
      congenital 756.6
  funicular (umbilical) 553.1
    with
      gangrene (obstructed) 551.1
      obstruction 552.1
        and gangrene 551.1
    spermatic cord — *see* Hernia, inguinal
  gangrenous — *see* Hernia, by site, with gangrene
  gastrointestinal tract 553.9
    with
      gangrene (obstructed) 551.9
      obstruction 552.9
        and gangrene 551.9
  gluteal — *see* Hernia, femoral
  Gruber's (internal mesogastric) 553.8
    with
      gangrene (obstructed) 551.8
      obstruction 552.8
        and gangrene 551.8
  Hesselbach's 553.8
    with
      gangrene (obstructed) 551.8
      obstruction 552.8
        and gangrene 551.8
  hiatal (esophageal) (sliding) 553.3
    with
      gangrene (obstructed) 551.3
      obstruction 552.3
        and gangrene 551.3
    congenital 750.6
  incarcerated (*see also* Hernia, by site, with obstruction) 552.9
    gangrenous (*see also* Hernia, by site, with gangrene) 551.9
  incisional 553.21
    with
      gangrene (obstructed) 551.21
      obstruction 552.21
        and gangrene 551.21
    lumbar — *see* Hernia, lumbar
    recurrent 553.21
      with
        gangrene (obstructed) 551.21
        obstruction 552.21
          and gangrene 551.21
  indirect (inguinal) — *see* Hernia, inguinal
  infantile — *see* Hernia, inguinal
  infrapatellar fat pad 729.31

Hernia, hernial — *continued*
  inguinal (direct) (double) (encysted) (external) (funicular) (indirect) (infantile) (internal) (interstitial) (oblique) (scrotal) (sliding) 550.9

> *Note* — Use the following fifth-digit subclassification with category 550:
>
> 0   unilateral or unspecified (not specified as recurrent)
> 1   unilateral or unspecified, recurrent
> 2   bilateral (not specified as recurrent)
> 3   bilateral, recurrent

    with
      gangrene (obstructed) 550.0
      obstruction 550.1
        and gangrene 550.0
    internal 553.8
      with
        gangrene (obstructed) 551.8
        obstruction 552.8
          and gangrene 551.8
    inguinal — *see* Hernia, inguinal
  interstitial 553.9
    with
      gangrene (obstructed) 551.9
      obstruction 552.9
        and gangrene 551.9
    inguinal — *see* Hernia, inguinal
  intervertebral cartilage or disc — *see* Displacement, intervertebral disc
  intestine, intestinal 553.9
    with
      gangrene (obstructed) 551.9
      obstruction 552.9
        and gangrene 551.9
  intra-abdominal 553.9
    with
      gangrene (obstructed) 551.9
      obstruction 552.9
        and gangrene 551.9
  intraparietal 553.9
    with
      gangrene (obstructed) 551.9
      obstruction 552.9
        and gangrene 551.9
  iris 364.8
    traumatic 871.1
  irreducible (*see also* Hernia, by site, with obstruction) 552.9
    gangrenous (with obstruction) (*see also* Hernia, by site, with gangrene) 551.9
  ischiatic 553.8
    with
      gangrene (obstructed) 551.8
      obstruction 552.8
        and gangrene 551.8
  ischiorectal 553.8
    with
      gangrene (obstructed) 551.8
      obstruction 552.8
        and gangrene 551.8
  lens 379.32
    traumatic 871.1
  linea
    alba — *see* Hernia, epigastric
    semilunaris — *see* Hernia, spigelian
  Littre's (diverticular) 553.9
    with
      gangrene (obstructed) 551.9

Hernia, hernial — continued
  Littre's — continued
    with — continued
      obstruction 552.9
        and gangrene 551.9
  lumbar 553.8
    with
      gangrene (obstructed) 551.8
      obstruction 552.8
        and gangrene 551.8
    intervertebral disc 722.10
  lung (subcutaneous) 518.89
    congenital 748.69
  mediastinum 519.3
  mesenteric (internal) 553.8
    with
      gangrene (obstructed) 551.8
      obstruction 552.8
        and gangrene 551.8
  mesocolon 553.8
    with
      gangrene (obstructed) 551.8
      obstruction 552.8
        and gangrene 551.8
  muscle (sheath) 728.89
  nucleus pulposus — *see* Displacement, intervertebral disc
  oblique (inguinal) — *see* Hernia, inguinal
  obstructive (*see also* Hernia, by site, with obstruction) 552.9
    gangrenous (with obstruction) (*see also* Hernia, by site, with gangrene) 551.9
  obturator 553.8
    with
      gangrene (obstructed) 551.8
      obstruction 552.8
        and gangrene 551.8
  omental 553.8
    with
      gangrene (obstructed) 551.8
      obstruction 552.8
        and gangrene 551.8
  orbital fat (pad) 374.34
  ovary 620.4
  oviduct 620.4
  paracolostomy (stoma) 569.69
  paraduodenal 553.8
    with
      gangrene (obstructed) 551.8
      obstruction 552.8
        and gangrene 551.8
  paraesophageal 553.3
    with
      gangrene (obstructed) 551.3
      obstruction 552.3
        and gangrene 551.3
    congenital 750.6
  parahiatal 553.3
    with
      gangrene (obstructed) 551.3
      obstruction 552.3
        and gangrene 551.3
  paraumbilical 553.1
    with
      gangrene (obstructed) 551.1
      obstruction 552.1
        and gangrene 551.1
  parietal 553.9
    with
      gangrene (obstructed) 551.9
      obstruction 552.9
        and gangrene 551.9

Hernia, hernial — continued
  perineal 553.8
    with
      gangrene (obstructed) 551.8
      obstruction 552.8
        and gangrene 551.8
  peritoneal sac, lesser 553.8
    with
      gangrene (obstructed) 551.8
      obstruction 552.8
        and gangrene 551.8
  popliteal fat pad 729.31
  postoperative 553.21
    with
      gangrene (obstructed) 551.21
      obstruction 552.21
        and gangrene 551.21
  pregnant uterus 654.4
  prevesical 596.8
  properitoneal 553.8
    with
      gangrene (obstructed) 551.8
      obstruction 552.8
        and gangrene 551.8
  pudendal 553.8
    with
      gangrene (obstructed) 551.8
      obstruction 552.8
        and gangrene 551.8
  rectovaginal 618.6
  retroperitoneal 553.8
    with
      gangrene (obstructed) 551.8
      obstruction 552.8
        and gangrene 551.8
  Richter's (parietal) 553.9
    with
      gangrene (obstructed) 551.9
      obstruction 552.9
        and gangrene 551.9
  Rieux's, Riex's (retrocecal) 553.8
    with
      gangrene (obstructed) 551.8
      obstruction 552.8
        and gangrene 551.8
  sciatic 553.8
    with
      gangrene (obstructed) 551.8
      obstruction 552.8
        and gangrene 551.8
  scrotum, scrotal — *see* Hernia, inguinal
  sliding (inguinal) — *see also* Hernia, inguinal
  hiatus — *see* Hernia, hiatal
  spigelian 553.29
    with
      gangrene (obstructed) 551.29
      obstruction 552.29
        and gangrene 551.29
  spinal (*see also* Spina bifida) 741.9
    with hydrocephalus 741.0
  strangulated (*see also* Hernia, by site, with obstruction) 552.9
    gangrenous (with obstruction) (*see also* Hernia, by site, with gangrene) 551.9
  supraumbilicus (linea alba) — *see* Hernia, epigastric
  tendon 727.9
  testis (nontraumatic) 550.9
    meaning
      scrotal hernia 550.9
      symptomatic late syphilis 095.8

Hernia, hernial — *continued*
  Treitz's (fossa) 553.8
    with
      gangrene (obstructed) 551.8
      obstruction 552.8
        and gangrene 551.8
  tunica
    albuginea 608.89
    vaginalis 752.8
  umbilicus, umbilical 553.1
    with
      gangrene (obstructed) 551.1
      obstruction 552.1
        and gangrene 551.1
  ureter 593.89
    with obstruction 593.4
  uterus 621.8
    pregnant 654.4 ✓5th
  vaginal (posterior) 618.6
  Velpeau's (femoral) (*see also* Hernia, femoral) 553.00
  ventral 553.20
    with
      gangrene (obstructed) 551.20
      obstruction 552.20
        and gangrene 551.20
    recurrent 553.21
      with
        gangrene (obstructed) 551.21
        obstruction 552.21
          and gangrene 551.21
  vesical
    congenital (female) (male) 756.71
    female 618.0
    male 596.8
  vitreous (into anterior chamber) 379.21
    traumatic 871.1
Herniation — *see also* Hernia
  brain (stem) 348.4
  cerebral 348.4
  gastric mucosa (into duodenal bulb) 537.89
  mediastinum 519.3
  nucleus pulposus — *see* Displacement, intervertebral disc
Herpangina 074.0
Herpes, herpetic 054.9
  auricularis (zoster) 053.71
    simplex 054.73
  blepharitis (zoster) 053.20
    simplex 054.41
  circinate 110.5
  circinatus 110.5
    bullous 694.5
  conjunctiva (simplex) 054.43
    zoster 053.21
  cornea (simplex) 054.43
    disciform (simplex) 054.43
    zoster 053.21
  encephalitis 054.3
  eye (zoster) 053.29
    simplex 054.40
  eyelid (zoster) 053.20
    simplex 054.41
  febrilis 054.9
  fever 054.9
  geniculate ganglionitis 053.11
  genital, genitalis 054.10
    specified site NEC 054.19
  gestationis 646.8 ✓5th
  gingivostomatitis 054.2

Herpes, herpetic — *continued*
  iridocyclitis (simplex) 054.44
    zoster 053.22
  iris (any site) 695.1
  iritis (simplex) 054.44
  keratitis (simplex) 054.43
    dendritic 054.42
    disciform 054.43
    interstitial 054.43
    zoster 053.21
  keratoconjunctivitis (simplex) 054.43
    zoster 053.21
  labialis 054.9
    meningococcal 036.89
  lip 054.9
  meningitis (simplex) 054.72
    zoster 053.0
  ophthalmicus (zoster) 053.20
    simplex 054.40
  otitis externa (zoster) 053.71
    simplex 054.73
  penis 054.13
  perianal 054.10
  pharyngitis 054.79
  progenitalis 054.10
  scrotum 054.19
  septicemia 054.4 ✓5th
  simplex 054.9
    complicated 054.8
      ophthalmic 054.40
        specified NEC 054.49
      specified NEC 054.79
    congenital 771.2
    external ear 054.73
    keratitis 054.43
      dendritic 054.42
    meningitis 054.72
    neuritis 054.79
    specified complication NEC 054.79
      ophthalmic 054.49
    visceral 054.71
  stomatitis 054.2
  tonsurans 110.0
    maculosus (of Hebra) 696.3
  visceral 054.71
  vulva 054.12
  vulvovaginitis 054.11
  whitlow 054.6
  zoster 053.9
    auricularis 053.71
    complicated 053.8
      specified NEC 053.79
    conjunctiva 053.21
    cornea 053.21
    ear 053.71
    eye 053.29
    geniculate 053.11
    keratitis 053.21
      interstitial 053.21
    neuritis 053.10
    ophthalmicus(a) 053.20
    oticus 053.71
    otitis externa 053.71
    specified complication NEC 053.79
    specified site NEC 053.9
  zosteriform, intermediate type 053.9
Herrick's
  anemia (hemoglobin S disease) 282.61
  syndrome (hemoglobin S disease) 282.61
Hers' disease (glycogenosis VI) 271.0
Herter's infantilism (nontropical sprue) 579.0

Herter (-Gee) disease or syndrome (nontropical sprue) 579.0
Herxheimer's disease (diffuse idiopathic cutaneous atrophy) 701.8
Herxheimer's reaction 995.0
Hesselbach's hernia — see Hernia, Hesselbach's
Heterochromia (congenital) 743.46
   acquired 364.53
   cataract 366.33
   cyclitis 364.21
   hair 704.3
   iritis 364.21
   retained metallic foreign body 360.62
      magnetic 360.52
   uveitis 364.21
Heterophoria 378.40
   alternating 378.45
   vertical 378.43
Heterophyes, small intestine 121.6
Heterophyiasis 121.6
Heteropsia 368.8
Heterotopia, heterotopic — see also Malposition, congenital
   cerebralis 742.4
   pancreas, pancreatic 751.7
   spinalis 742.59
Heterotropia 378.30
   intermittent 378.20
      vertical 378.31
   vertical (constant) (intermittent) 378.31
Heubner's disease 094.89
Heubner-Herter disease or syndrome (nontropical sprue) 579.0
Hexadactylism 755.0
Heyd's syndrome (hepatorenal) 572.4
HGSIL (high grade squamous intraepithelial dysplasia) 622.1
Hibernoma (M8880/0) — see Lipoma
Hiccough 786.8
   epidemic 078.89
   psychogenic 306.1
Hiccup (see also Hiccough) 786.8
Hicks (-Braxton) contractures 644.1
Hidden penis 752.65
Hidradenitis (axillaris) (suppurative) 705.83
Hidradenoma (nodular) (M8400/0) — see also Neoplasm, skin, benign
   clear cell (M8402/0) — see Neoplasm, skin, benign
   papillary (M8405/0) — see Neoplasm, skin, benign
Hidrocystoma (M8404/0) — see Neoplasm, skin, benign
High
   A_2 anemia 282.4
   altitude effects 993.2
      anoxia 993.2
      on
         ears 993.0
         sinuses 993.1
      polycythemia 289.0
   arch
      foot 755.67
      palate 750.26
   artery (arterial) tension (see also Hypertension) 401.9
      without diagnosis of hypertension 796.2

High — continued
   basal metabolic rate (BMR) 794.7
   blood pressure (see also Hypertension) 401.9
      incidental reading (isolated) (nonspecific), no diagnosis of hypertension 796.2
   compliance bladder 596.4
   diaphragm (congenital) 756.6
   frequency deafness (congenital) (regional) 389.8
   head at term 652.5
      affecting fetus or newborn 763.1
   output failure (cardiac) (see also Failure, heart) 428.9
   oxygen-affinity hemoglobin 289.0
   palate 750.26
   risk
      behavior — see Problem
      family situation V61.9
         specified circumstance NEC V61.8
      individual NEC V62.89
      infant NEC V20.1
      patient taking drugs (prescribed) V67.51
         nonprescribed (see also Abuse, drugs, nondependent) 305.9
      pregnancy V23.9
         inadequate prenatal care V23.7
         specified problem NEC V23.8
   temperature (of unknown origin) (see also Pyrexia) 780.6
   thoracic rib 756.3
Hildenbrand's disease (typhus) 081.9
Hilger's syndrome 337.0
Hill diarrhea 579.1
Hilliard's lupus (see also Tuberculosis) 017.0
Hilum — see condition
Hip — see condition
Hippel's disease (retinocerebral angiomatosis) 759.6
Hippus 379.49
Hirschfeld's disease (acute diabetes mellitus) (see also Diabetes) 250.0
Hirschsprung's disease or megacolon (congenital) 751.3
Hirsuties (see also Hypertrichosis) 704.1
Hirsutism (see also Hypertrichosis) 704.1
Hirudiniasis (external) (internal) 134.2
His-Werner disease (trench fever) 083.1
Hiss-Russell dysentery 004.1
Histamine cephalgia 346.2
Histidinemia 270.5
Histidinuria 270.5
Histiocytoma (M8832/0) — see also Neoplasm, skin, benign
   fibrous (M8830/0) — see also Neoplasm, skin, benign
      atypical (M8830/1) — see Neoplasm, connective tissue, uncertain behavior
      malignant (M8830/3) — see Neoplasm, connective tissue, malignant
Histiocytosis (acute) (chronic) (subacute) 277.8
   acute differentiated progressive (M9722/3) 202.5
   cholesterol 277.8
   essential 277.8
   lipid, lipoid (essential) 272.7
   lipochrome (familial) 288.1
   malignant (M9720/3) 202.3

Histiocytosis — *continued*
   X (chronic) 277.8
      acute (progressive) (M9722/3) 202.5
Histoplasmosis 115.90
   with
      endocarditis 115.94
      meningitis 115.91
      pericarditis 115.93
      pneumonia 115.95
      retinitis 115.92
      specified manifestation NEC 115.99
   African (due to Histoplasma duboisii) 115.10
      with
         endocarditis 115.14
         meningitis 115.11
         pericarditis 115.13
         pneumonia 115.15
         retinitis 115.12
         specified manifestation NEC 115.19
   American (due to Histoplasma capsulatum) 115.00
      with
         endocarditis 115.04
         meningitis 115.01
         pericarditis 115.03
         pneumonia 115.05
         retinitis 115.02
         specified manifestation NEC 115.09
   Darling's — *see* Histoplasmosis, American
   large form (*see also* Histoplasmosis, African) 115.10
   lung 115.05
   small form (*see also* Histoplasmosis, American) 115.00
History (personal) of
   abuse
      emotional V15.42
      neglect V15.42
      physical V15.41
      sexual V15.41
   affective psychosis V11.1
   alcoholism V11.3
      specified as drinking problem (*see also* Abuse, drugs, nondependent) 305.0
   allergy to
      analgesic agent NEC V14.6
      anesthetic NEC V14.4
      antibiotic agent NEC V14.1
         penicillin V14.0
      anti-infective agent NEC V14.3
      diathesis V15.09
      drug V14.9
         specified type NEC V14.8
      eggs V15.03
      food additives V15.05
      insect bite V15.06
      latex V15.07
      medicinal agents V14.9
         specified type NEC V14.8
      milk products V15.02
      narcotic agent NEC V14.5
      nuts V15.05
         peanuts V15.01
      penicillin V14.0
      radiographic dye V15.08
      seafood V15.04
      serum V14.7
      specified food NEC V15.05
      specified nonmedicinal agents NEC V15.09
      spider bite V15.06

History (personal) of — *continued*
   allergy to — *continued*
      sulfa V14.2
      sulfonamides V14.2
      therapeutic agent NEC V15.09
      vaccine V14.7
   anemia V12.3
   arthritis V13.4
   benign neoplasm of brain V12.41
   blood disease V12.3
   calculi, urinary V13.01
   cardiovascular disease V12.50
      myocardial infarction 412
   child abuse V15.41
   cigarette smoking V15.82
   circulatory system disease V12.50
      myocardial infarction 412
   congenital malformation V13.69
   contraception V15.7
   diathesis, allergic V15.09
   digestive system disease V12.70
      peptic ulcer V12.71
      polyps, colonic V12.72
      specified NEC V12.79
   disease (of) V13.9
      blood V12.3
      blood-forming organs V12.3
      cardiovascular system V12.50
      circulatory system V12.50
      digestive system V12.70
         peptic ulcer V12.71
         polyps, colonic V12.72
         specified NEC V12.79
      infectious V12.00
         malaria V12.03
         poliomyelitis V12.02
         specified NEC V12.09
         tuberculosis V12.01
      parasitic V12.00
         specified NEC V12.09
      respiratory system V12.6
      skin V13.3
      specified site NEC V13.8
      subcutaneous tissue V13.3
      trophoblastic V13.1
         affecting management of pregnant V23.1
   disorder (of) V13.9
      endocrine V12.2
      genital system V13.29
      hematological V12.3
      immunity V12.2
      mental V11.9
         affective type V11.1
         manic-depressive V11.1
         neurosis V11.2
         schizophrenia V11.0
         specified type NEC V11.8
      metabolic V12.2
      musculoskeletal NEC V13.5
      nervous system V12.40
         specified type NEC V12.49
      obstetric V13.29
         affecting management of current pregnancy V23.49
            pre-term labor V23.41
         pre-term labor V13.21
      sense organs V12.40
         specified type NEC V12.49
      specified site NEC V13.8
      urinary system V13.00
         calculi V13.01

History (personal) of — *continued*
   disorder — *continued*
     urinary system — *continued*
      specified NEC V13.09
   drug use
     nonprescribed (*see also* Abuse, drugs,
       nondependent) 305.9
     patent (*see also* Abuse, drugs,
       nondependent) 305.9
   effect NEC of external cause V15.89
   embolism (pulmonary) V12.51
   emotional abuse V15.42
   endocrine disorder V12.2
   family
     allergy V19.6
     anemia V18.2
     arteriosclerosis V17.4
     arthritis V17.7
     asthma V17.5
     blindness V19.0
     blood disorder NEC V18.3
     cardiovascular disease V17.4
     cerebrovascular disease V17.1
     chronic respiratory condition NEC V17.6
     congenital anomalies V19.5
     consanguinity V19.7
     coronary artery disease V17.3
     cystic fibrosis V18.1
     deafness V19.2
     diabetes mellitus V18.0
     digestive disorders V18.5
     disease or disorder (of)
       allergic V19.6
       blood NEC V18.3
       cardiovascular NEC V17.4
       cerebrovascular V17.1
       coronary artery V17.3
       digestive V18.5
       ear NEC V19.3
       endocrine V18.1
       eye NEC V19.1
       genitourinary NEC V18.7
       hypertensive V17.4
       infectious V18.8
       ischemic heart V17.3
       kidney V18.69
         polycystic V18.61
       mental V17.0
       metabolic V18.1
       musculoskeletal NEC V17.8
       neurological NEC V17.2
       parasitic V18.8
       psychiatric condition V17.0
       skin condition V19.4
     ear disorder NEC V19.3
     endocrine disease V18.1
     epilepsy V17.2
     eye disorder NEC V19.1
     genitourinary disease NEC V18.7
     glomerulonephritis V18.69
     gout V18.1
     hay fever V17.6
     hearing loss V19.2
     hematopoietic neoplasia V16.7
     Hodgkin's disease V16.7
     Huntington's chorea V17.2
     hydrocephalus V19.5
     hypertension V17.4
     hypospadias V13.61
     infectious disease V18.8
     ischemia heart disease V17.3

History (personal) of — *continued*
   family — *continued*
     kidney disease V18.69
       polycystic V18.61
     leukemia V16.6
     lymphatic malignant neoplasia NEC V16.7
     malignant neoplasm (of) NEC V16.9
       anorectal V16.0
       anus V16.0
       appendix V16.0
       bladder V16.59
       bone V16.8
       brain V16.8
       breast V16.3
         male V16.8
       bronchus V16.1
       cecum V16.0
       cervix V16.49
       colon V16.0
       duodenum V16.0
       esophagus V16.0
       eye V16.8
       gallbladder V16.0
       gastrointestinal tract V16.0
       genital organs V16.40
       hemopoietic NEC V16.7
       ileum V16.0
       ilium V16.8
       intestine V16.0
       intrathoracic organs NEC V16.2
       kidney V16.51
       larynx V16.2
       liver V16.0
       lung V16.1
       lymphatic NEC V16.7
       ovary V16.41
       oviduct V16.41
       pancreas V16.0
       penis V16.49
       prostate V16.42
       rectum V16.0
       respiratory organs NEC V16.2
       skin V16.8
       specified site NEC V16.8
       stomach V16.0
       testis V16.43
       trachea V16.1
       ureter V16.59
       urethra V16.59
       urinary organs V16.59
       uterus V16.49
       vagina V16.49
       vulva V16.49
     mental retardation V18.4
     metabolic disease NEC V18.1
     mongolism V19.5
     multiple myeloma V16.7
     musculoskeletal disease NEC V17.8
     nephritis V18.69
     nephrosis V18.69
     parasitic disease V18.8
     polycystic kidney disease V18.61
     psychiatric disorder V17.0
     psychosis V17.0
     retardation, mental V18.4
     retinitis pigmentosa V19.1
     schizophrenia V17.0
     skin conditions V19.4
     specified condition NEC V19.8
     stroke (cerebrovascular) V17.1
     visual loss V19.0

History (personal) of — *continued*
  genital system disorder V13.29 ▲
    pre-term labor V13.21 ●
  health hazard V15.9
    specified cause NEC V15.89
  Hodgkin's disease V10.72
  immunity disorder V12.2
  infectious disease V12.00
    malaria V12.03
    poliomyelitis V12.02
    specified NEC V12.09
    tuberculosis V12.01
  injury NEC V15.5
  insufficient prenatal care V23.7
  irradiation V15.3
  leukemia V10.60
    lymphoid V10.61
    monocytic V10.63
    myeloid V10.62
    specified type NEC V10.69
  little or no prenatal care V23.7
  low birth weight (*see also* Status, low birth weight) V21.30
  lymphosarcoma V10.71
  malaria V12.03
  malignant neoplasm (of) V10.9
    accessory sinus V10.22
    adrenal V10.88
    anus V10.06
    bile duct V10.09
    bladder V10.51
    bone V10.81
    brain V10.85
    breast V10.3
    bronchus V10.11
    cervix uteri V10.41
    colon V10.05
    connective tissue NEC V10.89
    corpus uteri V10.42
    digestive system V10.00
      specified part NEC V10.09
    duodenum V10.09
    endocrine gland NEC V10.88
    epididymis V10.48
    esophagus V10.03
    eye V10.84
    fallopian tube V10.44
    female genital organ V10.40
      specified site NEC V10.44
    gallbladder V10.09
    gastrointestinal tract V10.00
    gum V10.02
    hematopoietic NEC V10.79
    hypopharynx V10.02
    ileum V10.09
    intrathoracic organs NEC V10.20
    jejunum V10.09
    kidney V10.52
    large intestine V10.05
    larynx V10.21
    lip V10.02
    liver V10.07
    lung V10.11
    lymphatic NEC V10.79
    lymph glands or nodes NEC V10.79
    male genital organ V10.45
      specified site NEC V10.49
    mediastinum V10.29
    melanoma (of skin) V10.82
    middle ear V10.22

History (personal) of — *continued*
  malignant neoplasm — *continued*
    mouth V10.02
      specified part NEC V10.02
    nasal cavities V10.22
    nasopharynx V10.02
    nervous system NEC V10.86
    nose V10.22
    oropharynx V10.02
    ovary V10.43
    pancreas V10.09
    parathyroid V10.88
    penis V10.49
    pharynx V10.02
    pineal V10.88
    pituitary V10.88
    placenta V10.44
    pleura V10.29
    prostate V10.46
    rectosigmoid junction V10.06
    rectum V10.06
    renal pelvis V10.53
    respiratory organs NEC V10.20
    salivary gland V10.02
    skin V10.83
      melanoma V10.82
    small intestine NEC V10.09
    soft tissue NEC V10.89
    specified site NEC V10.89
    stomach V10.04
    testis V10.47
    thymus V10.29
    thyroid V10.87
    tongue V10.01
    trachea V10.12
    ureter V10.59
    urethra V10.59
    urinary organ V10.50
    uterine adnexa V10.44
    uterus V10.42
    vagina V10.44
    vulva V10.44
  manic-depressive psychosis V11.1
  mental disorder V11.9
    affective type V11.1
    manic-depressive V11.1
    neurosis V11.2
    schizophrenia V11.0
    specified type NEC V11.8
  metabolic disorder V12.2
  musculoskeletal disorder NEC V13.5
  myocardial infarction 412
  neglect (emotional) V15.42
  nervous system disorder V12.40
    specified type NEC V12.49
  neurosis V11.2
  noncompliance with medical treatment V15.81
  nutritional deficiency V12.1
  obstetric disorder V13.29 ▲
    affecting management of current pregnancy V23.49 ▲
      pre-term labor V23.41 ●
    pre-term labor V13.41 ●
  parasitic disease V12.00
    specified NEC V12.09
  perinatal problems V13.7
    low birth weight (*see also* Status, low birth weight) V21.30
  physical abuse V15.41
  poisoning V15.6
  poliomyelitis V12.02

History (personal) of — continued
  polyps, colonic V12.72
  poor obstetric V23.49
    affecting management of current pregnancy V23.49
      pre-term labor V23.41
      pre-term labor V13.41
  psychiatric disorder V11.9
    affective type V11.1
    manic-depressive V11.1
    neurosis V11.2
    schizophrenia V11.0
    specified type NEC V11.8
  psychological trauma V15.49
    emotional abuse V15.42
    neglect V15.42
    physical abuse V15.41
    rape V15.41
  psychoneurosis V11.2
  radiation therapy V15.3
  rape V15.41
  respiratory system disease V12.6
  reticulosarcoma V10.71
  schizophrenia V11.0
  skin disease V13.3
  smoking (tobacco) V15.82
  subcutaneous tissue disease V13.3
  surgery (major) to
    great vessels V15.1
    heart V15.1
    major organs NEC V15.2
  thrombophlebitis V12.52
  thrombosis V12.51
  tobacco use V15.82
  trophoblastic disease V13.1
    affecting management of pregnancy V23.1
  tuberculosis V12.01
  ulcer, peptic V12.71
  urinary system disorder V13.00
    calculi V13.01
    specified NEC V13.09
HIV infection (disease) (illness) — see Human immunodeficiency virus (disease) (illness) (infection)
Hives (bold) (see also Urticaria) 708.9
Hoarseness 784.49
Hobnail liver — see Cirrhosis, portal
Hobo, hoboism V60.0
Hodgkins
  disease (M9650/3) 201.9
    lymphocytic
      depletion (M9653/3) 201.7
        diffuse fibrosis (M9654/3) 201.7
        reticular type (M9655/3) 201.7
      predominance (M9651/3) 201.4
    lymphocytic-histiocytic predominance (M9651/3) 201.4
    mixed cellularity (M9652/3) 201.6
    nodular sclerosis (M9656/3) 201.5
      cellular phase (M9657/3) 201.5
  granuloma (M9661/3) 201.1
  lymphogranulomatosis (M9650/3) 201.9
  lymphoma (M9650/3) 201.9
  lymphosarcoma (M9650/3) 201.9
  paragranuloma (M9660/3) 201.0
  sarcoma (M9662/3) 201.2
Hodgson's disease (aneurysmal dilatation of aorta) 441.9
  ruptured 441.5
Hodi-potsy 111.0

Hoffa (-Kastert) disease or syndrome (liposynovitis prepatellaris) 272.8
Hoffman's syndrome 244.9 [359.5]
Hoffmann-Bouveret syndrome (paroxysmal tachycardia) 427.2
Hole
  macula 362.54
  optic disc, crater-like 377.22
  retina (macula) 362.54
    round 361.31
      with detachment 361.01
Holla disease (see also Spherocytosis) 282.0
Holländer-Simons syndrome (progressive lipodystrophy) 272.6
Hollow foot (congenital) 754.71
  acquired 736.73
Holmes' syndrome (visual disorientation) 368.16
Holoprosencephaly 742.2
  due to
    trisomy 13 758.1
    trisomy 18 758.2
Holthouse's hernia — see Hernia, inguinal
Homesickness 309.89
Homocystinemia 270.4
Homocystinuria 270.4
Homologous serum jaundice (prophylactic) (therapeutic) — see Hepatitis, viral
Homosexuality — omit code
  ego-dystonic 302.0
  pedophilic 302.2
  problems with 302.0
Homozygous Hb-S disease 282.61
Honeycomb lung 518.89
  congenital 748.4
Hong Kong ear 117.3
HOOD (hereditary osteo-onychodyplasia) 756.89
Hooded
  clitoris 752.49
  penis 752.69
Hookworm (anemia) (disease) (infestation) — see Ancylostomiasis
Hoppe-Goldflam syndrome 358.0
Hordeolum (external) (eyelid) 373.11
  internal 373.12
Horn
  cutaneous 702.8
    cheek 702.8
    eyelid 702.8
    penis 702.8
  iliac 756.89
  nail 703.8
    congenital 757.5
  papillary 700
Horner's
  syndrome (see also Neuropathy, peripheral, autonomic) 337.9
    traumatic 954.0
  teeth 520.4
Horseshoe kidney (congenital) 753.3
Horton's
  disease (temporal arteritis) 446.5
  headache or neuralgia 346.2
Hospice care V66.7
Hospitalism (in children) NEC 309.83
Hourglass contraction, contracture
  bladder 596.8

Hourglass contraction, contracture —
continued
  gallbladder 575.2
    congenital 751.69
  stomach 536.8
    congenital 750.7
    psychogenic 306.4
  uterus 661.4
    affecting fetus or newborn 763.7
Household circumstance affecting care V60.9
  specified type NEC V60.8
Housemaid's knee 727.2
Housing circumstance affecting care V60.9
  specified type NEC V60.8
Huchard's disease (continued arterial hypertension) 401.9
Hudson-Stähli lines 371.11
Huguier's disease (uterine fibroma) 218.9
Hum, venous — *omit code*
Human bite (open wound) — *see also* Wound, open, by site
  intact skin surface — *see* Contusion
Human immunodeficiency virus (disease) (illness) 042
  infection V08
    with symptoms, symptomatic 042
Human immunodeficiency virus-2 infection 079.53
Human immunovirus (disease) (illness) (infection) — *see* Human immunodeficiency virus (disease) (illness) (infection)
Human papillomavirus 079.4
Human T-cell lymphotrophic virus-I infection 079.51
Human T-cell lymphotrophic virus-II infection 079.52
Human T-cell lymphotrophic virus-III (disease) (illness) (infection) — *see* Human immunodeficiency virus (disease) (illness) (infection)
HTLV-I infection 079.51
HTLV-II infection 079.52
HTLV-III (disease) (illness) (infection) — *see* Human immunodeficiency virus (disease) (illness) (infection)
HTLV-III/LAV (disease) (illness) (infection) — *see* Human immunodeficiency virus (disease) (illness) (infection)
Humpback (acquired) 737.9
  congenital 756.19
Hunchback (acquired) 737.9
  congenital 756.19
Hunger 994.2
  air, psychogenic 306.1
  disease 251.1
Hunner's ulcer (*see also* Cystitis) 595.1
Hunt's
  neuralgia 053.11
  syndrome (herpetic geniculate ganglionitis) 053.11
    dyssynergia cerebellaris myoclonica 334.2
Hunter's glossitis 529.4
Hunter (-Hurler) syndrome (mucopolysaccharidosis II) 277.5
Hunterian chancre 091.0

Huntington's
  chorea 333.4
  disease 333.4
Huppert's disease (multiple myeloma) (M9730/3) 203.0
Hurler (-Hunter) disease or syndrome (mucopolysaccharidosis II) 277.5
Hürthle cell
  adenocarcinoma (M8290/3) 193
  adenoma (M8290/0) 226
  carcinoma (M8290/3) 193
  tumor (M8290/0) 226
Hutchinson's
  disease meaning
    angioma serpiginosum 709.1
    cheiropompholyx 705.81
    prurigo estivalis 692.72
    summer eruption, or summer prurigo 692.72
  incisors 090.5
  melanotic freckle (M8742/2) — *see also* Neoplasm, skin, in situ
    malignant melanoma in (M8742/3) — *see* Melanoma
  teeth or incisors (congenital syphilis) 090.5
Hutchinson-Boeck disease or syndrome (sarcoidosis) 135
Hutchinson-Gilford disease or syndrome (progeria) 259.8
Hyaline
  degeneration (diffuse) (generalized) 728.9
    localized — *see* Degeneration, by site
  membrane (disease) (lung) (newborn) 769
Hyalinosis cutis et mucosae 272.8
Hyalin plaque, sclera, senile 379.16
Hyalitis (asteroid) 379.22
  syphilitic 095.8
Hydatid
  cyst or tumor — *see also* Echinococcus
    fallopian tube 752.11
  mole — *see* Hydatidiform mole
  Morgagni (congenital) 752.8
    fallopian tube 752.11
Hydatidiform mole (benign) (complicating pregnancy) (delivered) (undelivered) 630
  invasive (M9100/1) 236.1
  malignant (M9100/1) 236.1
  previous, affecting management of pregnancy V23.1
Hydatidosis — *see* Echinococcus
Hyde's disease (prurigo nodularis) 698.3
Hydradenitis 705.83
Hydradenoma (M8400/0) — *see* Hidradenoma
Hydralazine lupus or syndrome
  correct substance properly administered 695.4
  overdose or wrong substance given or taken 972.6
Hydramnios 657
  affecting fetus or newborn 761.3
Hydrancephaly 742.3
  with spina bifida (*see also* Spina bifida) 741.0
Hydranencephaly 742.3
  with spina bifida (*see also* Spina bifida) 741.0
Hydrargyrism NEC 985.0

Hydrarthrosis

Hydrarthrosis (*see also* Effusion, joint) 719.0 ✓5ᵗʰ
  gonococcal 098.50
  intermittent (*see also* Rheumatism, palindromic) 719.3 ✓5ᵗʰ
  of yaws (early) (late) 102.6
  syphilitic 095.8
    congenital 090.5
Hydremia 285.9
Hydrencephalocele (congenital) 742.0
Hydrencephalomeningocele (congenital) 742.0
Hydroa 694.0
  aestivale 692.72
  gestationis 646.8 ✓5ᵗʰ
  herpetiformis 694.0
  pruriginosa 694.0
  vacciniforme 692.72
Hydroadenitis 705.83
Hydrocalycosis (*see also* Hydronephrosis) 591
  congenital 753.29
Hydrocalyx (*see also* Hydronephrosis) 591
Hydrocele (calcified) (chylous) (idiopathic) (infantile) (inguinal canal) (recurrent) (senile) (spermatic cord) (testis) (tunica vaginalis) 603.9
  canal of Nuck (female) 629.1
    male 603.9
  congenital 778.6
  encysted 603.0
    congenital 778.6
  female NEC 629.8
  infected 603.1
  round ligament 629.8
  specified type NEC 603.8
    congenital 778.6
  spinalis (*see also* Spina bifida) 741.9 ✓5ᵗʰ
  vulva 624.8
Hydrocephalic fetus
  affecting management or pregnancy 655.0 ✓5ᵗʰ
  causing disproportion 653.6 ✓5ᵗʰ
    with obstructed labor 660.1 ✓5ᵗʰ
      affecting fetus or newborn 763.1
Hydrocephalus (acquired) (external) (internal) (malignant) (noncommunicating) (obstructive) (recurrent) 331.4
  aqueduct of Sylvius structure 742.3
    with spina bifida (*see also* Spina bifida) 741.0 ✓5ᵗʰ
  chronic 742.3
    with spina bifida (*see also* Spina bifida) 741.0 ✓5ᵗʰ
  communicating 331.3
  congenital (external) (internal) 742.3
    with spina bifida (*see also* Spina bifida) 741.0 ✓5ᵗʰ
  due to
    structure of aqueduct of Sylvius 742.3
      with spina bifida (*see also* Spina bifida) 741.0 ✓5ᵗʰ
    toxoplasmosis (congenital) 771.2
  fetal affecting management of pregnancy 655.0 ✓5ᵗʰ
  foramen Magendie block (acquired) 331.3
    congenital 742.3
      with spina bifida (*see also* Spina bifida) 741.0 ✓5ᵗʰ
  newborn 742.3
    with spina bifida (*see also* Spina bifida) 741.0 ✓5ᵗʰ
  otitic 331.4

Hydrocephalus — *continued*
  syphilitic, congenital 090.49
  tuberculous (*see also* Tuberculosis) 013.8 ✓5ᵗʰ
Hydrocolpos (congenital) 623.8
Hydrocystoma (M8404/0) — *see* Neoplasm, skin, benign
Hydroencephalocele (congenital) 742.0
Hydroencephalomeningocele (congenital) 742.0
Hydrohematopneumothorax (*see also* Hemothorax) 511.8
Hydromeningitis — *see* Meningitis
Hydromeningocele (spinal) (*see also* Spina bifida) 741.9 ✓5ᵗʰ
  cranial 742.0
Hydrometra 621.8
Hydrometrocolpos 623.8
Hydromicrocephaly 742.1
Hydromphalus (congenital) (since birth) 757.39
Hydromyelia 742.53
Hydromyelocele (*see also* Spina bifida) 741.9 ✓5ᵗʰ
Hydronephrosis 591
  atrophic 591
  congenital 753.29
  due to S. hematobium 120.0
  early 591
  functionless (infected) 591
  infected 591
  intermittent 591
  primary 591
  secondary 591
  tuberculous (*see also* Tuberculosis) 016.0 ✓5ᵗʰ
Hydropericarditis (*see also* Pericarditis) 423.9
Hydropericardium (*see also* Pericarditis) 423.9
Hydroperitoneum 789.5
Hydrophobia 071
Hydrophthalmos (*see also* Buphthalmia) 743.20
Hydropneumohemothorax (*see also* Hemothorax) 511.8
Hydropneumopericarditis (*see also* Pericarditis) 423.9
Hydropneumopericardium (*see also* Pericarditis) 423.9
Hydropneumothorax 511.8
  nontuberculous 511.8
    bacterial 511.1
  pneumococcal 511.1
  staphylococcal 511.1
  streptococcal 511.1
  traumatic 860.0
    with open wound into thorax 860.1
  tuberculous (*see also* Tuberculosis, pleura) 012.0 ✓5ᵗʰ
Hydrops 782.3
  abdominis 789.5
  amnii (complicating pregnancy) (*see also* Hydramnios) 657 ✓4ᵗʰ
  articulorum intermittens (*see also* Rheumatism, palindromic) 719.3 ✓5ᵗʰ
  cardiac (*see also* Failure, heart) 428.0
  congenital — *see* Hydrops, fetalis
  endolymphatic (*see also* Disease, Ménière's) 386.00
  fetal(is) or newborn 778.0
    due to isoimmunization 773.3
    not due to isoimmunization 778.0
  gallbladder 575.3

Hydrops — *continued*
  idiopathic (fetus or newborn) 778.0
  joint (see also Effusion, joint) 719.0 [5]
  labyrinth (see also Disease, Ménière's) 386.00
  meningeal NEC 331.4
  nutritional 262
  pericardium — see Pericarditis
  pleura (see also Hydrothorax) 511.8
  renal (see also Nephrosis) 581.9
  spermatic cord (see also Hydrocele) 603.9
Hydropyonephrosis (see also Pyelitis) 590.80
  chronic 590.00
Hydrorachis 742.53
Hydrorrhea (nasal) 478.1
  gravidarum 658.1 [5]
  pregnancy 658.1 [5]
Hydrosadenitis 705.83
Hydrosalpinx (fallopian tube) (follicularis) 614.1
Hydrothorax (double) (pleural) 511.8
  chylous (nonfilarial) 457.8
    filaria (see also Infestation, filarial) 125.9
  nontuberculous 511.8
    bacterial 511.1
    pneumococcal 511.1
    staphylococcal 511.1
    streptococcal 511.1
  traumatic 862.29
    with open wound into thorax 862.39
  tuberculous (see also Tuberculosis, pleura) 012.0 [5]
Hydroureter 593.5
  congenital 753.22
Hydroureteronephrosis (see also Hydronephrosis) 591
Hydrourethra 599.84
Hydroxykynureninuria 270.2
Hydroxyprolinemia 270.8
Hydroxyprolinuria 270.8
Hygroma (congenital) (cystic) (M9173/0) 228.1
  prepatellar 727.3
  subdural — see Hematoma, subdural
Hymen — see condition
Hymenolepiasis (diminuta) (infection) (infestation) (nana) 123.6
Hymenolepis (diminuta) (infection) (infestation) (nana) 123.6
Hypalgesia (see also Disturbance, sensation) 782.0
Hyperabduction syndrome 447.8
Hyperacidity, gastric 536.8
  psychogenic 306.4
Hyperactive, hyperactivity
  basal cell, uterine cervix 622.1
  bladder 596.51
  bowel (syndrome) 564.9
    sounds 787.5
  cervix epithelial (basal) 622.1
    child 314.01
  colon 564.9
  gastrointestinal 536.8
    psychogenic 306.4
  intestine 564.9
  labyrinth (unilateral) 386.51
    with loss of labyrinthine reactivity 386.58
    bilateral 386.52
  nasal mucous membrane 478.1
  stomach 536.8

Hyperactive, hyperactivity — *continued*
  thyroid (gland) (see also Thyrotoxicosis) 242.9 [5]
Hyperacusis 388.42
Hyperadrenalism (cortical) 255.3
  medullary 255.6
Hyperadrenocorticism 255.3
  congenital 255.2
  iatrogenic
    correct substance properly administered 255.3
    overdose or wrong substance given or taken 962.0
Hyperaffectivity 301.11
Hyperaldosteronism (atypical) (hyperplastic) (normoaldosteronal) (normotensive) (primary) (secondary) 255.1
Hyperalgesia (see also Disturbance, sensation) 782.0
Hyperalimentation 783.6
  carotene 278.3
  specified NEC 278.8
  vitamin A 278.2
  vitamin D 278.4
Hyperaminoaciduria 270.9
  arginine 270.6
  citrulline 270.6
  cystine 270.0
  glycine 270.0
  lysine 270.7
  ornithine 270.6
  renal (types I, II, III) 270.0
Hyperammonemia (congenital) 270.6
Hyperamnesia 780.99 ▲
Hyperamylasemia 790.5
Hyperaphia 782.0
Hyperazotemia 791.9
Hyperbetalipoproteinemia (acquired) (essential) (familial) (hereditary) (primary) (secondary) 272.0
  with prebetalipoproteinemia 272.2
Hyperbilirubinemia 782.4
  congenital 277.4
  constitutional 277.4
  neonatal (transient) (see also Jaundice, fetus or newborn) 774.6
  of prematurity 774.2
Hyperbilirubinemica encephalopathia, newborn 774.7
  due to isoimmunization 773.4
Hypercalcemia, hypercalcemic (idiopathic) 275.42
  nephropathy 588.8
Hypercalcinuria 275.40
Hypercapnia 786.09
  with mixed acid-base disorder 276.4
  fetal, affecting newborn 770.89 ▲
Hypercarotinemia 278.3
Hypercementosis 521.5
Hyperchloremia 276.9
Hyperchlorhydria 536.8
  neurotic 306.4
  psychogenic 306.4
Hypercholesterinemia — see Hypercholesterolemia
Hypercholesterolemia 272.0
  with hyperglyceridemia, endogenous 272.2

Hypercholesterolemia — *continued*
  essential 272.0
  familial 272.0
  hereditary 272.0
  primary 272.0
  pure 272.0
Hypercholesterolosis 272.0
Hyperchylia gastrica 536.8
  psychogenic 306.4
Hyperchylomicronemia (familial) (with hyperbetalipoproteinemia) 272.3
Hypercoagulation syndrome 289.8
Hypercorticosteronism
  correct substance properly administered 255.3
  overdose or wrong substance given or taken 962.0
Hypercortisonism
  correct substance properly administered 255.3
  overdose or wrong substance given or taken 962.0
Hyperdynamic beta-adrenergic state or syndrome (circulatory) 429.82
Hyperelectrolytemia 276.9
Hyperemesis 536.2
  arising during pregnancy — *see* Hyperemesis, gravidarum
  gravidarum (mild) (before 22 completed weeks gestation) 643.0
    with
      carbohydrate depletion 643.1
      dehydration 643.1
      electrolyte imbalance 643.1
      metabolic disturbance 643.1
      affecting fetus or newborn 761.8
      severe (with metabolic disturbance) 643.1
  psychogenic 306.4
Hyperemia (acute) 780.99 ▲
  anal mucosa 569.49
  bladder 596.7
  cerebral 437.8
  conjunctiva 372.71
  ear, internal, acute 386.30
  enteric 564.89
  eye 372.71
  eyelid (active) (passive) 374.82
  intestine 564.89
  iris 364.41
  kidney 593.81
  labyrinth 386.30
  liver (active) (passive) 573.8
  lung 514
  ovary 620.8
  passive 780.99 ▲
  pulmonary 514
  renal 593.81
  retina 362.89
  spleen 289.59
  stomach 537.89
Hyperesthesia (body surface) (*see also* Disturbance, sensation) 782.0
  larynx (reflex) 478.79
    hysterical 300.11
  pharynx (reflex) 478.29
Hyperestrinism 256.0
Hyperestrogenism 256.0
Hyperestrogenosis 256.0

Hyperextension, joint 718.80
  ankle 718.87
  elbow 718.82
  foot 718.87
  hand 718.84
  hip 718.85
  knee 718.86
  multiple sites 718.89
  pelvic region 718.85
  shoulder (region) 718.81
  specified site NEC 718.88
  wrist 718.83
Hyperfibrinolysis — *see* Fibrinolysis
Hyperfolliculinism 256.0
Hyperfructosemia 271.2
Hyperfunction
  adrenal (cortex) 255.3
    androgenic, acquired benign 255.3
    medulla 255.6
    virilism 255.2
  corticoadrenal NEC 255.3
  labyrinth — *see* Hyperactive, labyrinth
  medulloadrenal 255.6
  ovary 256.1
    estrogen 256.0
  pancreas 577.8
  parathyroid (gland) 252.0
  pituitary (anterior) (gland) (lobe) 253.1
  testicular 257.0
Hypergammaglobulinemia 289.8
  monoclonal, benign (BMH) 273.1
  polyclonal 273.0
  Waldenström's 273.0
Hyperglobulinemia 273.8
Hyperglycemia 790.6
  maternal
    affecting fetus or newborn 775.0
    manifest diabetes in infant 775.1
  postpancreatectomy (complete) (partial) 251.3
Hyperglyceridemia 272.1
  endogenous 272.1
  essential 272.1
  familial 272.1
  hereditary 272.1
  mixed 272.3
  pure 272.1
Hyperglycinemia 270.7
Hypergonadism
  ovarian 256.1
  testicular (infantile) (primary) 257.0
Hyperheparinemia (*see also* Circulating anticoagulants) 286.5
Hyperhidrosis, hyperidrosis 780.8
  psychogenic 306.3
Hyperhistidinemia 270.5
Hyperinsulinism (ectopic) (functional) (organic) NEC 251.1
  iatrogenic 251.0
  reactive 251.2
  spontaneous 251.2
  therapeutic misadventure (from administration of insulin) 962.3
Hyperiodemia 276.9
Hyperirritability (cerebral), in newborn 779.1
Hyperkalemia 276.7
Hyperkeratosis (*see also* Keratosis) 701.1
  cervix 622.1
  congenital 757.39
  cornea 371.89

Hyperkeratosis — *continued*
  due to yaws (early) (late) (palmar or plantar) 102.3
  eccentrica 757.39
  figurata centrifuga atrophica 757.39
  follicularis 757.39
    in cutem penetrans 701.1
  limbic (cornea) 371.89
  palmoplantaris climacterica 701.1
  pinta (carate) 103.1
  senile (with pruritus) 702.0
  tongue 528.7
  universalis congenita 757.1
  vagina 623.1
  vocal cord 478.5
  vulva 624.0
Hyperkinesia, hyperkinetic (disease) (reaction) (syndrome) 314.9
  with
    attention deficit — *see* Disorder, attention deficit
    conduct disorder 314.2
    developmental delay 314.1
    simple disturbance of activity and attention 314.01
    specified manifestation NEC 314.8
  heart (disease) 429.82
  of childhood or adolescence NEC 314.9
Hyperlacrimation (*see also* Epiphora) 375.20
Hyperlipemia (*see also* Hyperlipidemia) 272.4
Hyperlipidemia 272.4
  carbohydrate-induced 272.1
  combined 272.4
  endogenous 272.1
  exogenous 272.3
  fat-induced 272.3
  group
    A 272.0
    B 272.1
    C 272.2
    D 272.3
  mixed 272.2
  specified type NEC 272.4
Hyperlipidosis 272.7
  hereditary 272.7
Hyperlipoproteinemia (acquired) (essential) (familial) (hereditary) (primary) (secondary) 272.4
  Fredrickson type
    I 272.3
    IIa 272.0
    IIb 272.2
    III 272.2
    IV 272.1
    V 272.3
  low-density-lipoid-type (LDL) 272.0
  very-low-density-lipoid-type (VLDL) 272.1
Hyperlucent lung, unilateral 492.8
Hyperluteinization 256.1
Hyperlysinemia 270.7
Hypermagnesemia 275.2
  neonatal 775.5
Hypermaturity (fetus or newborn) 766.2
Hypermenorrhea 626.2
Hypermetabolism 794.7
Hypermethioninemia 270.4
Hypermetropia (congenital) 367.0

Hypermobility
  cecum 564.9
  coccyx 724.71
  colon 564.9
    psychogenic 306.4
  ileum 564.89
  joint (acquired) 718.80
    ankle 718.87
    elbow 718.82
    foot 718.87
    hand 718.84
    hip 718.85
    knee 718.86
    multiple sites 718.89
    pelvic region 718.85
    shoulder (region) 718.81
    specified site NEC 718.88
    wrist 718.83
  kidney, congenital 753.3
  meniscus (knee) 717.5
  scapula 718.81
  stomach 536.8
    psychogenic 306.4
  syndrome 728.5
  testis, congenital 752.52
  urethral 599.81
Hypermotility
  gastrointestinal 536.8
  intestine 564.9
    psychogenic 306.4
  stomach 536.8
Hypernasality 784.49
Hypernatremia 276.0
  with water depletion 276.0
Hypernephroma (M8312/3) 189.0
Hyperopia 367.0
Hyperorexia 783.6
Hyperornithinemia 270.6
Hyperosmia (*see also* Disturbance, sensation) 781.1
Hyperosmolality 276.0
Hyperosteogenesis 733.99
Hyperostosis 733.99
  calvarial 733.3
  cortical 733.3
    infantile 756.59
  frontal, internal of skull 733.3
  interna frontalis 733.3
  monomelic 733.99
  skull 733.3
    congenital 756.0
  vertebral 721.8
    with spondylosis — *see* Spondylosis
    ankylosing 721.6
Hyperovarianism 256.1
Hyperovarism, hyperovaria 256.1
Hyperoxaluria (primary) 271.8
Hyperoxia 987.8
Hyperparathyroidism 252.0
  ectopic 259.3
  secondary, of renal origin 588.8
Hyperpathia (*see also* Disturbance, sensation) 782.0
  psychogenic 307.80
Hyperperistalsis 787.4
  psychogenic 306.4
Hyperpermeability, capillary 448.9
Hyperphagia 783.6

Hyperphenylalaninemia 270.1
Hyperphoria 378.40
   alternating 378.45
Hyperphosphatemia 275.3
Hyperpiesia (see also Hypertension) 401.9
Hyperpiesis (see also Hypertension) 401.9
Hyperpigmentation — see Pigmentation
Hyperpinealism 259.8
Hyperpipecolatemia 270.7
Hyperpituitarism 253.1
Hyperplasia, hyperplastic
   adenoids (lymphoid tissue) 474.12
      and tonsils 474.10
   adrenal (capsule) (cortex) (gland) 255.8
      with
         sexual precocity (male) 255.2
         virilism, adrenal 255.2
         virilization (female) 255.2
      congenital 255.2
      due to excess ACTH (ectopic) (pituitary) 255.0
      medulla 255.8
   alpha cells (pancreatic)
      with
         gastrin excess 251.5
         glucagon excess 251.4
   appendix (lymphoid) 543.0
   artery, fibromuscular NEC 447.8
      carotid 447.8
      renal 447.3
   bone 733.99
      marrow 289.9
   breast (see also Hypertrophy, breast) 611.1
   carotid artery 447.8
   cementation, cementum (teeth) (tooth) 521.5
   cervical gland 785.6
   cervix (uteri) 622.1
      basal cell 622.1
      congenital 752.49
      endometrium 622.1
      polypoid 622.1
   chin 524.05
   clitoris, congenital 752.49
   dentin 521.5
   endocervicitis 616.0
   endometrium, endometrial (adenomatous) (atypical) (cystic) (glandular) (polypoid) (uterus) 621.3
      cervix 622.1
   epithelial 709.8
      focal, oral, including tongue 528.7
      mouth (focal) 528.7
      nipple 611.8
      skin 709.8
      tongue (focal) 528.7
      vaginal wall 623.0
   erythroid 289.9
   fascialis ossificans (progressiva) 728.11
   fibromuscular, artery NEC 447.8
      carotid 447.8
      renal 447.3
   genital
      female 629.8
      male 608.89
   gingiva 523.8
   glandularis
      cystica uteri 621.3
      endometrium (uterus) 621.3
      interstitialis uteri 621.3
   granulocytic 288.8

Hyperplasia, hyperplastic — continued
   gum 523.8
   hymen, congenital 752.49
   islands of Langerhans 251.1
   islet cell (pancreatic) 251.9
      alpha cells
         with excess
            gastrin 251.5
            glucagon 251.4
      beta cells 251.1
   juxtaglomerular (complex) (kidney) 593.89
   kidney (congenital) 753.3
   liver (congenital) 751.69
   lymph node (gland) 785.6
   lymphoid (diffuse) (nodular) 785.6
      appendix 543.0
      intestine 569.89
   mandibular 524.02
      alveolar 524.72
      unilateral condylar 526.89
   Marchand multiple nodular (liver) — see Cirrhosis, postnecrotic
   maxillary 524.01
      alveolar 524.71
   medulla, adrenal 255.8
   myometrium, myometrial 621.2
   nose (lymphoid) (polypoid) 478.1
   oral soft tissue (inflammatory) (irritative) (mucosa) NEC 528.9
      gingiva 523.8
      tongue 529.8
   organ or site, congenital NEC — see Anomaly, specified type NEC
   ovary 620.8
   palate, papillary 528.9
   pancreatic islet cells 251.9
      alpha
         with excess
            gastrin 251.5
            glucagon 251.4
      beta 251.1
   parathyroid (gland) 252.0
   persistent, vitreous (primary) 743.51
   pharynx (lymphoid) 478.29
   prostate 600.9 ▲
      adenofibromatous 600.2
      nodular 600.1
   renal artery (fibromuscular) 447.3
   reticuloendothelial (cell) 289.9
   salivary gland (any) 527.1
   Schimmelbusch's 610.1
   suprarenal (capsule) (gland) 255.8
   thymus (gland) (persistent) 254.0
   thyroid (see also Goiter) 240.9
      primary 242.0 ✓5
      secondary 242.2 ✓5
   tonsil (lymphoid tissue) 474.11
      and adenoids 474.10
   urethrovaginal 599.89
   uterus, uterine (myometrium) 621.2
      endometrium 621.3
   vitreous (humor), primary persistent 743.51
   vulva 624.3
   zygoma 738.11
Hyperpnea (see also Hyperventilation) 786.01
Hyperpotassemia 276.7
Hyperprebetalipoproteinemia 272.1
   with chylomicronemia 272.3
   familial 272.1
Hyperprolactinemia 253.1
Hyperprolinemia 270.8

Hyperproteinemia 273.8
Hyperprothrombinemia 289.8
Hyperpselaphesia 782.0
Hyperpyrexia 780.6
  heat (effects of) 992.0
  malarial (*see also* Malaria) 084.6
  malignant, due to anesthetic 995.86
  rheumatic — *see* Fever, rheumatic
  unknown origin (*see also* Pyrexia) 780.6
Hyperreactor, vascular 780.2
Hyperreflexia 796.1
  bladder, autonomic 596.54
    with cauda equina 344.61
  detrusor 344.61
Hypersalivation (*see also* Ptyalism) 527.7
Hypersarcosinemia 270.8
Hypersecretion
  ACTH 255.3
  androgens (ovarian) 256.1
  calcitonin 246.0
  corticoadrenal 255.3
  cortisol 255.0
  estrogen 256.0
  gastric 536.8
    psychogenic 306.4
  gastrin 251.5
  glucagon 251.4
  hormone
    ACTH 255.3
    anterior pituitary 253.1
    growth NEC 253.0
    ovarian androgen 256.1
    testicular 257.0
    thyroid stimulating 242.8 ✓5ᵗʰ
  insulin — *see* Hyperinsulinism
  lacrimal glands (*see also* Epiphora) 375.20
  medulloadrenal 255.6
  milk 676.6 ✓5ᵗʰ
  ovarian androgens 256.1
  pituitary (anterior) 253.1
  salivary gland (any) 527.7
  testicular hormones 257.0
  thyrocalcitonin 246.0
  upper respiratory 478.9
Hypersegmentation, hereditary 288.2
  eosinophils 288.2
  neutrophil nuclei 288.2
Hypersensitive, hypersensitiveness, hypersensitivity — *see also* Allergy
  angiitis 446.20
    specified NEC 446.29
  carotid sinus 337.0
  colon 564.9
    psychogenic 306.4
  DNA (deoxyribonucleic acid) NEC 287.2
  drug (*see also* Allergy, drug) 995.2
  esophagus 530.89
  insect bites — *see* Injury, superficial, by site
  labyrinth 386.58
  pain (*see also* Disturbance, sensation) 782.0
  pneumonitis NEC 495.9
  reaction (*see also* Allergy) 995.3
    upper respiratory tract NEC 478.8
  stomach (allergic) (nonallergic) 536.8
    psychogenic 306.4
Hypersomatotropism (classic) 253.0
Hypersomnia 780.54
  with sleep apnea 780.53

Hypersomnia — *continued*
  nonorganic origin 307.43
    persistent (primary) 307.44
    transient 307.43
Hypersplenia 289.4
Hypersplenism 289.4
Hypersteatosis 706.3
Hyperstimulation, ovarian 256.1
Hypersuprarenalism 255.3
Hypersusceptibility — *see* Allergy
Hyper-TBG-nemia 246.8
Hypertelorism 756.0
  orbit, orbital 376.41

Hypertension

	Malignant	Benign	Unspecified
Hypertension, hypertensive (arterial) (arteriolar) (crisis) (degeneration) (disease) (essential) (fluctuating) (idiopathic) (intermittent) (labile) (low renin) (orthostatic) (paroxysmal) (primary) (systemic) (uncontrolled) (vascular)	401.0	401.1	401.9
with			
heart involvement (conditions classifiable to 425.8, 428, 429.0-429.3, 429.8, 429.9 due to hypertension) (see also Hypertension, heart)	402.00	402.10	402.90
with kidney involvement — see Hypertension, cardiorenal			
renal involvement (only conditions classifiable to 585, 586, 587) (excludes conditions classifiable to 584) (see also Hypertension, kidney)	403.00	403.10	403.90
renal sclerosis or failure	403.00	403.10	403.90
with heart involvement — see Hypertension, cardiorenal			
failure (and sclerosis) (see also Hypertension, kidney)	403.01	403.11	403.91
sclerosis without failure (see also Hypertension, kidney)	403.00	403.10	403.90
accelerated — (see also Hypertension, by type, malignant)	401.0	—	—
antepartum — see Hypertension, complicating pregnancy, childbirth, or the puerperium			
cardiorenal (disease)	404.00	404.10	404.90
with			
heart failure	404.01	404.11	404.91
and renal failure	404.03	404.13	404.93
renal failure	404.02	404.12	404.92
and heart failure	404.03	404.13	404.93
cardiovascular disease (arteriosclerotic) (sclerotic)	402.00	402.10	402.90
with			
heart failure	402.01	402.11	402.91
renal involvement (conditions classifiable to 403) (see also Hypertension, cardiorenal)	404.00	404.10	404.90
cardiovascular renal (disease) (sclerosis) (see also Hypertension, cardiorenal)	404.00	404.10	404.90
cerebrovascular disease NEC	437.2	437.2	437.2
complicating pregnancy, childbirth, or the puerperium	642.2 ✓5ᵗʰ	642.0	642.9 ✓5ᵗʰ
with			
albuminuria (and edema) (mild)	—	—	642.4 ✓5ᵗʰ
severe	—	—	642.5 ✓5ᵗʰ
edema (mild)	—	—	642.4 ✓5ᵗʰ
severe	—	—	642.5 ✓5ᵗʰ
heart disease	642.2 ✓5ᵗʰ	642.2 ✓5ᵗʰ	642.2 ✓5ᵗʰ
and renal disease	642.2 ✓5ᵗʰ	642.2 ✓5ᵗʰ	642.2 ✓5ᵗʰ
renal disease	642.2 ✓5ᵗʰ	642.2 ✓5ᵗʰ	642.2 ✓5ᵗʰ
and heart disease	642.2 ✓5ᵗʰ	642.2 ✓5ᵗʰ	642.2 ✓5ᵗʰ
chronic	642.2 ✓5ᵗʰ	642.0 ✓5ᵗʰ	642.0 ✓5ᵗʰ
with pre-eclampsia or eclampsia	642.7 ✓5ᵗʰ	642.7 ✓5ᵗʰ	642.7 ✓5ᵗʰ
fetus or newborn	760.0	760.0	760.0
essential	—	642.0	642.0 ✓5ᵗʰ
with pre-eclampsia or eclampsia	—	642.7 ✓5ᵗʰ	642.7 ✓5ᵗʰ
fetus or newborn	760.0	760.0	760.0
fetus or newborn	760.0	760.0	760.0
gestational	—	—	642.3 ✓5ᵗʰ
pre-existing	642.2 ✓5ᵗʰ	642.0	642.0 ✓5ᵗʰ
with pre-eclampsia or eclampsia	642.7 ✓5ᵗʰ	642.7 ✓5ᵗʰ	642.7 ✓5ᵗʰ
fetus or newborn	760.0	760.0	760.0
secondary to renal disease	642.1 ✓5ᵗʰ	642.1 ✓5ᵗʰ	642.1 ✓5ᵗʰ
with pre-eclampsia or eclampsia	642.7 ✓5ᵗʰ	642.7 ✓5ᵗʰ	642.7 ✓5ᵗʰ
fetus or newborn	760.0	760.0	760.0
transient	—	—	642.3 ✓5ᵗʰ

Index to Diseases — Hypertension

	Malignant	Benign	Unspecified
Hypertension, hypertensive — *continued*			
due to			
aldosteronism, primary	405.09	405.19	405.99
brain tumor	405.09	405.19	405.99
bulbar poliomyelitis	405.09	405.19	405.99
calculus			
kidney	405.09	405.19	405.99
ureter	405.09	405.19	405.99
coarctation, aorta	405.09	405.19	405.99
Cushing's disease	405.09	405.19	405.99
glomerulosclerosis (*see also* Hypertension, kidney)	403.00	403.10	403.90
periarteritis nodosa	405.09	405.19	405.99
pheochromocytoma	405.09	405.19	405.99
polycystic kidney(s)	405.09	405.19	405.99
polycythemia	405.09	405.19	405.99
porphyria	405.09	405.19	405.99
pyelonephritis	405.09	405.19	405.99
renal (artery)			
aneurysm	405.01	405.11	405.91
anomaly	405.01	405.11	405.91
embolism	405.01	405.11	405.91
fibromuscular hyperplasia	405.01	405.11	405.91
occlusion	405.01	405.11	405.91
stenosis	405.01	405.11	405.91
thrombosis	405.01	405.11	405.91
encephalopathy	437.2	437.2	437.2
gestational (transient) NEC	—	—	642.3 ▓5▓
Goldblatt's	440.1	440.1	440.1
heart (disease) (conditions classifiable to 425.8, 428, 429.0-429.3, 429.8, 429.9 due to hypertension)	402.00	402.10	402.90
with heart failure	402.01	402.11	402.91
hypertensive kidney disease (conditions classifiable to 403) (*see also* Hypertension, cardiorenal)	404.00	404.10	404.90
renal sclerosis (*see also* Hypertension, cardiorenal)	404.00	404.10	404.90
intracranial, benign	—	348.2	—
intraocular	—	—	365.04
kidney	403.00	403.10	403.90
with			
heart involvement (conditions classifiable to 425.8, 428, 429.0-429.3, 429.8, 429.9 due to hypertension) (*see also* Hypertension, cardiorenal)	404.00	404.10	404.90
hypertensive heart (disease) (conditions classifiable to 402) (*see also* Hypertension, cardiorenal)	404.00	404.10	404.90
lesser circulation	—	—	416.0
necrotizing	401.0	—	—
ocular	—	—	365.04
portal (due to chronic liver disease)	—	—	572.3
postoperative	—	—	997.91
psychogenic	—	—	306.2
puerperal, postpartum — *see* Hypertension, complicating pregnancy, childbirth, or the puerperium			
pulmonary (artery)	—	—	416.8
with cor pulmonale (chronic)	—	—	416.8
acute	—	—	415.0
idiopathic	—	—	416.0
primary	—	—	416.0
of newborn	—	—	747.83 ●
secondary	—	—	416.8
renal (disease) (*see also* Hypertension, kidney)	403.00	403.10	403.90

▓4▓ Fourth-digit Required   ▓5▓ Fifth-digit Required

Hypertension

Hypertension, hypertensive — *continued*

	Malignant	Benign	Unspecified
renovascular NEC	405.01	405.11	405.91
secondary NEC	405.09	405.19	405.99
due to			
aldosteronism, primary	405.09	405.19	405.99
brain tumor	405.09	405.19	405.99
bulbar poliomyelitis	405.09	405.19	405.99
calculus			
kidney	405.09	405.19	405.99
ureter	405.09	405.19	405.99
coarctation, aorta	405.09	405.19	405.99
Cushing's disease	405.09	405.19	405.99
glomerulosclerosis (*see also* Hypertension,			
kidney)	403.00	403.10	403.90
periarteritis nodosa	405.09	405.19	405.99
pheochromocytoma	405.09	405.19	405.99
polycystic kidney(s)	405.09	405.19	405.99
polycythemia	405.09	405.19	405.99
porphyria	405.09	405.19	405.99
pyelonephritis	405.09	405.19	405.99
renal (artery)			
aneurysm	405.01	405.11	405.91
anomaly	405.01	405.11	405.91
embolism	405.01	405.11	405.91
fibromuscular hyperplasia	405.01	405.11	405.91
occlusion	405.01	405.11	405.91
stenosis	405.01	405.11	405.91
thrombosis	405.01	405.11	405.91
transient	—	—	796.2
of pregnancy	—	—	642.3
venous, chronic (asymptomatic) (idiopathic)	—	—	459.30 ●
due to			
deep vein thrombosis (*see also* Syndrome,			
postphlebetic)	—	—	459.10 ●
with			
complication, NEC	—	—	459.39 ●
inflammation	—	—	459.32 ●
with ulcer	—	—	459.33 ●
ulcer	—	—	459.31 ●
with inflammation	—	—	459.33 ●

Hyperthecosis, ovary 256.8
Hyperthermia (of unknown origin) (*see also* Pyrexia) 780.6
    malignant (due to anesthesia) 995.86
    newborn 778.4
Hyperthymergasia (*see also* Psychosis, affective) 296.0 ✓5ᵗʰ
    reactive (from emotional stress, psychological trauma) 298.1
    recurrent episode 296.1 ✓5ᵗʰ
    single episode 296.0 ✓5ᵗʰ
Hyperthymism 254.8
Hyperthyroid (recurrent) — *see* Hyperthyroidism
Hyperthyroidism (latent) (preadult) (recurrent) (without goiter) 242.9 ✓5ᵗʰ

> Note — *Use the following fifth-digit subclassification with category 242:*
>
> 0   *without mention of thyrotoxic crisis or storm*
>
> 1   *with mention of thyrotoxic crisis or storm*

    with
        goiter (diffuse) 242.0 ✓5ᵗʰ
            adenomatous 242.3 ✓5ᵗʰ
                multinodular 242.2 ✓5ᵗʰ
                uninodular 242.1 ✓5ᵗʰ
            nodular 242.3 ✓5ᵗʰ
                multinodular 242.2 ✓5ᵗʰ
                uninodular 242.1 ✓5ᵗʰ
        thyroid nodule 242.1 ✓5ᵗʰ
    complicating pregnancy, childbirth, or puerperium 648.1 ✓5ᵗʰ
    neonatal (transient) 775.3
Hypertonia — *see* Hypertonicity
Hypertonicity
    bladder 596.51
    fetus or newborn 779.89 ▲
    gastrointestinal (tract) 536.8
    infancy 779.89 ▲
        due to electrolyte imbalance 779.89 ▲
    muscle 728.85
    stomach 536.8
        psychogenic 306.4
    uterus, uterine (contractions) 661.4 ✓5ᵗʰ
        affecting fetus or newborn 763.7
Hypertony — *see* Hypertonicity
Hypertransaminemia 790.4
Hypertrichosis 704.1
    congenital 757.4
    eyelid 374.54
    lanuginosa 757.4
        acquired 704.1
Hypertriglyceridemia, essential 272.1
Hypertrophy, hypertrophic
    adenoids (infectional) 474.12
        and tonsils (faucial) (infective) (lingual) (lymphoid) 474.10
    adrenal 255.8
    alveolar process or ridge 525.8
    anal papillae 569.49
    apocrine gland 705.82
    artery NEC 447.8
        carotid 447.8
        congenital (peripheral) NEC 747.60
            gastrointestinal 747.61
            lower limb 747.64

Hypertrophy, hypertrophic — *continued*
    artery NEC — *continued*
        congenital — *continued*
            renal 747.62
            specified NEC 747.69
            spinal 747.82
            upper limb 747.63
    arthritis (chronic) (*see also* Osteoarthrosis) 715.9 ✓5ᵗʰ
        spine (*see also* Spondylosis) 721.90
    arytenoid 478.79
    asymmetrical (heart) 429.9
    auricular — *see* Hypertrophy, cardiac
    Bartholin's gland 624.8
    bile duct 576.8
    bladder (sphincter) (trigone) 596.8
    blind spot, visual field 368.42
    bone 733.99
    brain 348.8
    breast 611.1
        cystic 610.1
        fetus or newborn 778.7
        fibrocystic 610.1
        massive pubertal 611.1
        puerperal, postpartum 676.3 ✓5ᵗʰ
        senile (parenchymatous) 611.1
    cardiac (chronic) (idiopathic) 429.3
        with
            rheumatic fever (conditions classifiable to 390)
                active 391.8
                    with chorea 392.0
                inactive or quiescent (with chorea) 398.99
        congenital NEC 746.89
        fatty (*see also* Degeneration, myocardial) 429.1
        hypertensive (*see also* Hypertension, heart) 402.90
        rheumatic (with chorea) 398.99
            active or acute 391.8
                with chorea 392.0
        valve (*see also* Endocarditis) 424.90
            congenital NEC 746.89
    cartilage 733.99
    cecum 569.89
    cervix (uteri) 622.6
        congenital 752.49
        elongation 622.6
    clitoris (cirrhotic) 624.2
        congenital 752.49
    colon 569.89
        congenital 751.3
    conjunctiva, lymphoid 372.73
    cornea 371.89
    corpora cavernosa 607.89
    duodenum 537.89
    endometrium (uterus) 621.3
        cervix 622.6
    epididymis 608.89
    esophageal hiatus (congenital) 756.6
        with hernia — *see* Hernia, diaphragm
    eyelid 374.30
    falx, skull 733.99
    fat pad 729.30
        infrapatellar 729.31
        knee 729.31
        orbital 374.34
        popliteal 729.31
        prepatellar 729.31
        retropatellar 729.31

Hypertrophy, hypertrophic — continued
  fat pad — continued
    specified site NEC 729.39
  foot (congenital) 755.67
  frenum, frenulum (tongue) 529.8
    linguae 529.8
    lip 528.5
  gallbladder or cystic duct 575.8
  gastric mucosa 535.2
  gingiva 523.8
  gland, glandular (general) NEC 785.6
  gum (mucous membrane) 523.8
  heart (idiopathic) — see also Hypertrophy, cardiac
    valve — see also Endocarditis
      congenital NEC 746.89
  hemifacial 754.0
  hepatic — see Hypertrophy, liver
  hiatus (esophageal) 756.6
  hilus gland 785.6
  hymen, congenital 752.49
  ileum 569.89
  infrapatellar fat pad 729.31
  intestine 569.89
  jejunum 569.89
  kidney (compensatory) 593.1
    congenital 753.3
  labial frenulum 528.5
  labium (majus) (minus) 624.3
  lacrimal gland, chronic 375.03
  ligament 728.9
    spinal 724.8
  linguae frenulum 529.8
  lingual tonsil (infectional) 474.11
  lip (frenum) 528.5
    congenital 744.81
  liver 789.1
    acute 573.8
    cirrhotic — see Cirrhosis, liver
    congenital 751.69
    fatty — see Fatty, liver
  lymph gland 785.6
    tuberculous — see Tuberculosis, lymph gland
  mammary gland — see Hypertrophy, breast
  maxillary frenulum 528.5
  Meckel's diverticulum (congenital) 751.0
  medial meniscus, acquired 717.3
  median bar 600.9
  mediastinum 519.3
  meibomian gland 373.2
  meniscus, knee, congenital 755.64
  metatarsal head 733.99
  metatarsus 733.99
  mouth 528.9
  mucous membrane
    alveolar process 523.8
    nose 478.1
    turbinate (nasal) 478.0
  muscle 728.9
  muscular coat, artery NEC 447.8
    carotid 447.8
    renal 447.3
  myocardium (see also Hypertrophy, cardiac) 429.3
    idiopathic 425.4
  myometrium 621.2
  nail 703.8
    congenital 757.5
  nasal 478.1
    alae 478.1

Hypertrophy, hypertrophic — continued
  nasal — continued
    bone 738.0
    cartilage 478.1
    mucous membrane (septum) 478.1
    sinus (see also Sinusitis) 473.9
    turbinate 478.0
  nasopharynx, lymphoid (infectional) (tissue) (wall) 478.29
  neck, uterus 622.6
  nipple 611.1
  normal aperture diaphragm (congenital) 756.6
  nose (see also Hypertrophy, nasal) 478.1
  orbit 376.46
  organ or site, congenital NEC — see Anomaly, specified type NEC
  osteoarthropathy (pulmonary) 731.2
  ovary 620.8
  palate (hard) 526.89
    soft 528.9
  pancreas (congenital) 751.7
  papillae
    anal 569.49
    tongue 529.3
  parathyroid (gland) 252.0
  parotid gland 527.1
  penis 607.89
  phallus 607.89
    female (clitoris) 624.2
  pharyngeal tonsil 474.12
  pharyngitis 472.1
  pharynx 478.29
    lymphoid (infectional) (tissue) (wall) 478.29
  pituitary (fossa) (gland) 253.8
  popliteal fat pad 729.31
  preauricular (lymph) gland (Hampstead) 785.6
  prepuce (congenital) 605
    female 624.2
  prostate (asymptomatic) (early) (recurrent) 600.9
    adenofibromatous 600.2
    benign 600.0
    congenital 752.8
  pseudoedematous hypodermal 757.0
  pseudomuscular 359.1
  pylorus (muscle) (sphincter) 537.0
    congenital 750.5
    infantile 750.5
  rectal sphincter 569.49
  rectum 569.49
  renal 593.1
  rhinitis (turbinate) 472.0
  salivary duct or gland 527.1
    congenital 750.26
  scaphoid (tarsal) 733.99
  scar 701.4
  scrotum 608.89
  sella turcica 253.8
  seminal vesicle 608.89
  sigmoid 569.89
  skin condition NEC 701.9
  spermatic cord 608.89
  spinal ligament 728.9
  spleen — see Splenomegaly
  spondylitis (spine) (see also Spondylosis) 721.90
  stomach 537.89
  subaortic stenosis (idiopathic) 425.1
  sublingual gland 527.1
    congenital 750.26
  submaxillary gland 527.1

Hypertrophy, hypertrophic — *continued*
  suprarenal (gland) 255.8
  tendon 727.9
  testis 608.89
    congenital 752.8
  thymic, thymus (congenital) (gland) 254.0
  thyroid (gland) (*see also* Goiter) 240.9
    primary 242.0
    secondary 242.2
  toe (congenital) 755.65
    acquired 735.8
  tongue 529.8
    congenital 750.15
    frenum 529.8
    papillae (foliate) 529.3
  tonsil (faucial) (infective) (lingual) (lymphoid) 474.11
    with
      adenoiditis 474.01
      tonsillitis 474.00
        and adenoiditis 474.02
    and adenoids 474.10
  tunica vaginalis 608.89
  turbinate (mucous membrane) 478.0
  ureter 593.89
  urethra 599.84
  uterus 621.2
    puerperal, postpartum 674.8
  uvula 528.9
  vagina 623.8
  vas deferens 608.89
  vein 459.89
  ventricle, ventricular (heart) (left) (right) — *see also* Hypertrophy, cardiac
    congenital 746.89
    due to hypertension (left) (right) (*see also* Hypertension, heart) 402.90
      benign 402.10
      malignant 402.00
    right with ventricular septal defect, pulmonary stenosis or atresia, and dextraposition of aorta 745.2
  verumontanum 599.89
  vesical 596.8
  vocal cord 478.5
  vulva 624.3
    stasis (nonfilarial) 624.3
Hypertropia (intermittent) (periodic) 378.31
Hypertyrosinemia 270.2
Hyperuricemia 790.6
Hypervalinemia 270.3
Hyperventilation (tetany) 786.01
  hysterical 300.11
  psychogenic 306.1
  syndrome 306.1
Hyperviscidosis 277.00
Hyperviscosity (of serum) (syndrome) NEC 273.3
  polycythemic 289.0
  sclerocythemic 282.8
Hypervitaminosis (dietary) NEC 278.8
  A (dietary) 278.2
  D (dietary) 278.4
  from excessive administration or use of vitamin preparations (chronic) 278.8
    reaction to sudden overdose 963.5
    vitamin A 278.2
      reaction to sudden overdose 963.5
    vitamin D 278.4
      reaction to sudden overdose 963.5

Hypervitaminosis — *continued*
  from excessive administration or use of vitamin preparations — *continued*
    vitamin K
      correct substance properly administered 278.8
      overdose or wrong substance given or taken 964.3
Hypervolemia 276.6
Hypesthesia (*see also* Disturbance, sensation) 782.0
  cornea 371.81
Hyphema (anterior chamber) (ciliary body) (iris) 364.41
  traumatic 921.3
Hyphemia — *see* Hyphema
Hypoacidity, gastric 536.8
  psychogenic 306.4
Hypoactive labyrinth (function) — *see* Hypofunction, labyrinth
Hypoadrenalism 255.4
  tuberculous (*see also* Tuberculosis) 017.6
Hypoadrenocorticism 255.4
  pituitary 253.4
Hypoalbuminemia 273.8
Hypoalphalipoproteinemia 272.5
Hypobarism 993.2
Hypobaropathy 993.2
Hypobetalipoproteinemia (familial) 272.5
Hypocalcemia 275.41
  cow's milk 775.4
  dietary 269.3
  neonatal 775.4
  phosphate-loading 775.4
Hypocalcification, teeth 520.4
Hypochloremia 276.9
Hypochlorhydria 536.8
  neurotic 306.4
  psychogenic 306.4
Hypocholesteremia 272.5
Hypochondria (reaction) 300.7
Hypochondriac 300.7
Hyponchondriasis 300.7
Hypochromasia blood cells 280.9
Hypochromic anemia 280.9
  due to blood loss (chronic) 280.0
    acute 285.1
  microcytic 280.9
Hypocoagulability (*see also* Defect, coagulation) 286.9
Hypocomplementemia 279.8
Hypocythemia (progressive) 284.9
Hypodontia (*see also* Anodontia) 520.0
Hypoeosinophilia 288.8
Hypoesthesia (*see also* Disturbance, sensation) 782.0
  cornea 371.81
  tactile 782.0
Hypoestrinism 256.39
Hypoestrogenism 256.39
Hypoferremia 280.9
  due to blood loss (chronic) 280.0
Hypofertility
  female 628.9
  male 606.1

Hypofibrinogenemia

Hypofibrinogenemia 286.3
- acquired 286.6
- congenital 286.3

Hypofunction
- adrenal (gland) 255.4
  - cortex 255.4
  - medulla 255.5
  - specified NEC 255.5
- cerebral 331.9
- corticoadrenal NEC 255.4
- intestinal 564.89
- labyrinth (unilateral) 386.53
  - with loss of labyrinthine reactivity 386.55
  - bilateral 386.54
    - with loss of labyrinthine reactivity 386.56
- Leydig cell 257.2
- ovary 256.39
  - postablative 256.2
- pituitary (anterior) (gland) (lobe) 253.2
  - posterior 253.5
- testicular 257.2
  - iatrogenic 257.1
  - postablative 257.1
  - postirradiation 257.1
  - postsurgical 257.1

Hypogammaglobulinemia 279.00
- acquired primary 279.06
- non-sex-linked, congenital 279.06
- sporadic 279.06
- transient of infancy 279.09

Hypogenitalism (congenital) (female) (male) 752.8
- penis 752.69

Hypoglycemia (spontaneous) 251.2
- coma 251.0
  - diabetic 250.3
- diabetic 250.8
- due to insulin 251.0
  - therapeutic misadventure 962.3
- familial (idiopathic) 251.2
- following gastrointestinal surgery 579.3
- infantile (idiopathic) 251.2
- in infant of diabetic mother 775.0
- leucine-induced 270.3
- neonatal 775.6
- reactive 251.2
- specified NEC 251.1

Hypoglycemic shock 251.0
- diabetic 250.8
- due to insulin 251.0
- functional (syndrome) 251.1

Hypogonadism
- female 256.39
- gonadotrophic (isolated) 253.4
- hypogonadotropic (isolated) (with anosmia) 253.4
- isolated 253.4
- male 257.2
- ovarian (primary) 256.39
- pituitary (secondary) 253.4
- testicular (primary) (secondary) 257.2

Hypohidrosis 705.0
Hypohidrotic ectodermal dysplasia 757.31
Hypoidrosis 705.0
Hypoinsulinemia, postsurgical 251.3
- postpancreatectomy (complete) (partial) 251.3

Hypokalemia 276.8
Hypokinesia 780.99

Hypoleukia splenica 289.4
Hypoleukocytosis 288.8
Hypolipidemia 272.5
Hypolipoproteinemia 272.5
Hypomagnesemia 275.2
- neonatal 775.4

Hypomania, hypomanic reaction (see also Psychosis, affective) 296.0
- recurrent episode 296.1
- single episode 296.0

Hypomastia (congenital) 757.6
Hypomenorrhea 626.1
Hypometabolism 783.9
Hypomotility
- gastrointestinal tract 536.8
  - psychogenic 306.4
- intestine 564.89
  - psychogenic 306.4
- stomach 536.8
  - psychogenic 306.4

Hyponasality 784.49
Hyponatremia 276.1
Hypo-ovarianism 256.39
Hypo-ovarism 256.39
Hypoparathyroidism (idiopathic) (surgically induced) 252.1
- neonatal 775.4

Hypopharyngitis 462
Hypophoria 378.40
Hypophosphatasia 275.3
Hypophosphatemia (acquired) (congenital) (familial) 275.3
- renal 275.3

Hypophyseal, hypophysis — see also condition
- dwarfism 253.3
- gigantism 253.0
- syndrome 253.8

Hypophyseothalamic syndrome 253.8
Hypopiesis — see Hypotension
Hypopigmentation 709.00
- eyelid 374.53

Hypopinealism 259.8
Hypopituitarism (juvenile) (syndrome) 253.2
- due to
  - hormone therapy 253.7
  - hypophysectomy 253.7
  - radiotherapy 253.7
- postablative 253.7
- postpartum hemorrhage 253.2

Hypoplasia, hypoplasis 759.89
- adrenal (gland) 759.1
- alimentary tract 751.8
  - lower 751.2
  - upper 750.8
- anus, anal (canal) 751.2
- aorta 747.22
- aortic
  - arch (tubular) 747.10
  - orifice or valve with hypoplasia of ascending aorta and defective development of left ventricle (with mitral valve atresia) 746.7
- appendix 751.2
- areola 757.6
- arm (see also Absence, arm, congenital) 755.20

Hypoplasia, hypoplasis — *continued*
  artery (congenital) (peripheral) NEC 747.60
    brain 747.81
    cerebral 747.81
    coronary 746.85
    gastrointestinal 747.61
    lower limb 747.64
    pulmonary 747.3
    renal 747.62
    retinal 743.58
    specified NEC 747.69
    spinal 747.82
    umbilical 747.5
    upper limb 747.63
  auditory canal 744.29
    causing impairment of hearing 744.02
  biliary duct (common) or passage 751.61
  bladder 753.8
  bone NEC 756.9
    face 756.0
    malar 756.0
    mandible 524.04
      alveolar 524.74
    marrow 284.9
      acquired (secondary) 284.8
      congenital 284.0
      idiopathic 284.9
    maxilla 524.03
      alveolar 524.73
    skull (*see also* Hypoplasia, skull) 756.0
  brain 742.1
    gyri 742.2
    specified part 742.2
  breast (areola) 757.6
  bronchus (tree) 748.3
  cardiac 746.89
    valve — *see* Hypoplasia, heart, valve
    vein 746.89
  carpus (*see also* Absence, carpal, congenital) 755.28
  cartilaginous 756.9
  cecum 751.2
  cementum 520.4
    hereditary 520.5
  cephalic 742.1
  cerebellum 742.2
  cervix (uteri) 752.49
  chin 524.06
  clavicle 755.51
  coccyx 756.19
  colon 751.2
  corpus callosum 742.2
  cricoid cartilage 748.3
  dermal, focal (Goltz) 757.39
  digestive organ(s) or tract NEC 751.8
    lower 751.2
    upper 750.8
  ear 744.29
    auricle 744.23
    lobe 744.29
    middle, except ossicles 744.03
      ossicles 744.04
    ossicles 744.04
  enamel of teeth (neonatal) (postnatal) (prenatal) 520.4
    hereditary 520.5
  endocrine (gland) NEC 759.2
  endometrium 621.8
  epididymis 752.8
  epiglottis 748.3
  erythroid, congenital 284.0

Hypoplasia, hypoplasis — *continued*
  erythropoietic, chronic acquired 284.8
  esophagus 750.3
  Eustachian tube 744.24
  eye (*see also* Microphthalmos) 743.10
    lid 743.62
  face 744.89
    bone(s) 756.0
  fallopian tube 752.19
  femur (*see also* Absence, femur, congenital) 755.34
  fibula (*see also* Absence, fibula, congenital) 755.37
  finger (*see also* Absence, finger, congenital) 755.29
  focal dermal 757.39
  foot 755.31
  gallbladder 751.69
  genitalia, genital organ(s)
    female 752.8
      external 752.49
      internal NEC 752.8
    in adiposogenital dystrophy 253.8
    male 752.8
      penis 752.69
  glottis 748.3
  hair 757.4
  hand 755.21
  heart 746.89
    left (complex) (syndrome) 746.7
    valve NEC 746.89
      pulmonary 746.01
  humerus (*see also* Absence, humerus, congenital) 755.24
  hymen 752.49
  intestine (small) 751.1
    large 751.2
  iris 743.46
  jaw 524.09
  kidney(s) 753.0
  labium (majus) (minus) 752.49
  labyrinth, membranous 744.05
  lacrimal duct (apparatus) 743.65
  larynx 748.3
  leg (*see also* Absence, limb, congenital, lower) 755.30
  limb 755.4
    lower (*see also* Absence, limb, congenital, lower) 755.30
    upper (*see also* Absence, limb, congenital, upper) 755.20
  liver 751.69
  lung (lobe) 748.5
  mammary (areolar) 757.6
  mandibular 524.04
    alveolar 524.74
    unilateral condylar 526.89
  maxillary 524.03
    alveolar 524.73
  medullary 284.9
  megakaryocytic 287.3
  metacarpus (*see also* Absence, metacarpal, congenital) 755.28
  metatarsus (*see also* Absence, metatarsal, congenital) 755.38
  muscle 756.89
    eye 743.69
  myocardium (congenital) (Uhl's anomaly) 746.84
  nail(s) 757.5
  nasolacrimal duct 743.65

Hypoplasia, hypoplasis — continued
- nervous system NEC 742.8
- neural 742.8
- nose, nasal 748.1
- ophthalmic (see also Microphthalmos) 743.10
- organ
  - of Corti 744.05
  - or site NEC — see Anomaly, by site
- osseous meatus (ear) 744.03
- ovary 752.0
- oviduct 752.19
- pancreas 751.7
- parathyroid (gland) 759.2
- parotid gland 750.26
- patella 755.64
- pelvis, pelvic girdle 755.69
- penis 752.69
- peripheral vascular system (congenital) NEC 747.60
  - gastrointestinal 747.61
  - lower limb 747.64
  - renal 747.62
  - specified NEC 747.69
  - spinal 747.82
  - upper limb 747.63
- pituitary (gland) 759.2
- pulmonary 748.5
  - arteriovenous 747.3
  - artery 747.3
  - valve 746.01
- punctum lacrimale 743.65
- radioulnar (see also Absence, radius, congenital, with ulna) 755.25
- radius (see also Absence, radius, congenital) 755.26
- rectum 751.2
- respiratory system NEC 748.9
- rib 756.3
- sacrum 756.19
- scapula 755.59
- shoulder girdle 755.59
- skin 757.39
- skull (bone) 756.0
  - with
    - anencephalus 740.0
    - encephalocele 742.0
    - hydrocephalus 742.3
      - with spina bifida (see also Spina bifida) 741.0 ✓5ᵗʰ
    - microcephalus 742.1
- spinal (cord) (ventral horn cell) 742.59
  - vessel 747.82
- spine 756.19
- spleen 759.0
- sternum 756.3
- tarsus (see also Absence, tarsal, congenital) 755.38
- testis, testicle 752.8
- thymus (gland) 279.11
- thyroid (gland) 243
  - cartilage 748.3
- tibiofibular (see also Absence, tibia, congenital, with fibula) 755.35
- toe (see also Absence, toe, congenital) 755.39
- tongue 750.16
- trachea (cartilage) (rings) 748.3
- Turner's (tooth) 520.4
- ulna (see also Absence, ulna, congenital) 755.27
- umbilical artery 747.5
- ureter 753.29

Hypoplasia, hypoplasis — continued
- uterus 752.3
- vagina 752.49
- vascular (peripheral) NEC (see also Hypoplasia, peripheral vascular system) 747.60
  - brain 747.81
- vein(s) (peripheral) NEC (see also Hypoplasia, peripheral vascular system) 747.60
  - brain 747.81
  - cardiac 746.89
  - great 747.49
  - portal 747.49
  - pulmonary 747.49
  - vena cava (inferior) (superior) 747.49
- vertebra 756.19
- vulva 752.49
- zonule (ciliary) 743.39
- zygoma 738.12

Hypopotassemia 276.8

Hypoproaccelerinemia (see also Defect, coagulation) 286.3

Hypoproconvertinemia (congenital) (see also Defect, coagulation) 286.3

Hypoproteinemia (essential) (hypermetabolic) (idiopathic) 273.8

Hypoproteinosis 260

Hypoprothrombinemia (congenital) (hereditary) (idiopathic) (see also Defect, coagulation) 286.3
- acquired 286.7
- newborn 776.3

Hypopselaphesia 782.0

Hypopyon (anterior chamber) (eye) 364.05
- iritis 364.05
- ulcer (cornea) 370.04

Hypopyrexia 780.99 ▲

Hyporeflex 796.1

Hyporeninemia, extreme 790.99
- in primary aldosteronism 255.1

Hyporesponsive episode 780.09

Hyposecretion
- ACTH 253.4
- ovary 256.39
  - postblative 256.2
- salivary gland (any) 527.7

Hyposegmentation of neutrophils, hereditary 288.2

Hyposiderinemia 280.9

Hyposmolality 276.1
- syndrome 276.1

Hyposomatotropism 253.3

Hyposomnia (see also Insomnia) 780.52

Hypospadias (male) 752.61
- female 753.8

Hypospermatogenesis 606.1

Hyposphagma 372.72

Hyposplenism 289.59

Hypostasis, pulmonary 514

Hypostatic — see condition

Hyposthenuria 593.89

Hyposuprarenalism 255.4

Hypo-TBG-nemia 246.8

Hypotension (arterial) (constitutional) 458.9
- chronic 458.1
- iatrogenic 458.2

Hypotension — continued
  maternal, syndrome (following labor and delivery) 669.2 ✓5ᵗʰ
  orthostatic (chronic) 458.0
    dysautonomic-dyskinetic syndrome 333.0
  permanent idiopathic 458.1
  postoperative 458.2
  postural 458.0
  specified type NEC 458.8
  transient 796.3
Hypothermia (accidental) 991.6
  anesthetic 995.89
  newborn NEC 778.3
  not associated with low environmental temperature 780.99 ▲
Hypothymergasia (see also Psychosis, affective) 296.2 ✓5ᵗʰ
  recurrent episode 296.3 ✓5ᵗʰ
  single episode 296.2 ✓5ᵗʰ
Hypothyroidism (acquired) 244.9
  complicating pregnancy, childbirth, or puerperium 648.1 ✓5ᵗʰ
  congenital 243
  due to
    ablation 244.1
      radioactive iodine 244.1
      surgical 244.0
    iodine (administration) (ingestion) 244.2
      radioactive 244.1
    irradiation therapy 244.1
    p-aminosalicylic acid (PAS) 244.3
    phenylbutazone 244.3
    resorcinol 244.3
    specified cause NEC 244.8
    surgery 244.0
  goitrous (sporadic) 246.1
  iatrogenic NEC 244.3
  iodine 244.2
  pituitary 244.8
  postablative NEC 244.1
  postsurgical 244.0
  primary 244.9
  secondary NEC 244.8
  specified cause NEC 244.8
  sporadic goitrous 246.1
Hypotonia, hypotonicity, hypotony 781.3
  benign congenital 358.8
  bladder 596.4
  congenital 779.89 ▲
    benign 358.8
  eye 360.30
    due to
      fistula 360.32
      ocular disorder NEC 360.33
      following loss of aqueous or vitreous 360.33
    primary 360.31
  infantile muscular (benign) 359.0
  muscle 728.9
  uterus, uterine (contractions) — see Inertia, uterus
Hypotrichosis 704.09
  congenital 757.4
  lid (congenital) 757.4
    acquired 374.55
  postinfectional NEC 704.09
Hypotropia 378.32
Hypoventilation 786.09
Hypovitaminosis (see also Deficiency, vitamin) 269.2

Hypovolemia 276.5
  surgical shock 998.0
  traumatic (shock) 958.4
Hypoxemia (see also Anoxia) 799.0
Hypoxia (see also Anoxia) 799.0
  cerebral 348.1
    during or resulting from a procedure 997.01
    newborn 768.9
      mild or moderate 768.6
      severe 768.5
  fetal, affecting newborn 768.9 ▲
  intrauterine — see Distress, fetal
  myocardial (see also Insufficiency, coronary) 411.89
    arteriosclerotic — see Arteriosclerosis, coronary
  newborn 768.9 ▲
Hypsarrhythmia (see also Epilepsy) 345.6 ✓5ᵗʰ
Hysteralgia, pregnant uterus 646.8 ✓5ᵗʰ
Hysteria, hysterical 300.10
  anxiety 300.20
  Charcôt's gland 300.11
  conversion (any manifestation) 300.11
  dissociative type NEC 300.15
  psychosis, acute 298.1
Hysteroepilepsy 300.11
Hysterotomy, affecting fetus or newborn 763.89

I

Iatrogenic syndrome of excess cortisol 255.0
Iceland disease (epidemic neuromyasthenia) 049.8
Ichthyosis (congenita) 757.1
  acquired 701.1
  fetalis gravior 757.1
  follicularis 757.1
  hystrix 757.39
  lamellar 757.1
  lingual 528.6
  palmaris and plantaris 757.39
  simplex 757.1
  vera 757.1
  vulgaris 757.1
Ichthyotoxism 988.0
  bacterial (see also Poisoning, food) 005.9
Icteroanemia, hemolytic (acquired) 283.9
  congenital (see also Spherocytosis) 282.0
Icterus (see also Jaundice) 782.4
  catarrhal — see Icterus, infectious
  conjunctiva 782.4
    newborn 774.6
  epidemic — see Icterus, infectious
  febrilis — see Icterus, infectious
  fetus or newborn — see Jaundice, fetus or newborn
  gravis (see also Necrosis, liver) 570
    complicating pregnancy 646.7 ✓5ᵗʰ
      affecting fetus or newborn 760.8
    fetus or newborn NEC 773.0
    obstetrical 646.7 ✓5ᵗʰ
      affecting fetus or newborn 760.8
  hematogenous (acquired) 283.9
  hemolytic (acquired) 283.9
    congenital (see also Spherocytosis) 282.0
  hemorrhagic (acute) 100.0
    leptospiral 100.0

Icterus — *continued*
  hemorrhagic — *continued*
    newborn 776.0
      spirochetal 100.0
    infectious 070.1
      with hepatic coma 070.0
    leptospiral 100.0
      spirochetal 100.0
  intermittens juvenilis 277.4
  malignant (*see also* Necrosis, liver) 570
  neonatorum (*see also* Jaundice, fetus or newborn) 774.6
  pernicious (*see also* Necrosis, liver) 570
  spirochetal 100.0
Ictus solaris, solis 992.0
Identity disorder 313.82
  dissociative 300.14
  gender role (child) 302.6
    adult 302.85
  psychosexual (child) 302.6
    adult 302.85
Idioglossia 307.9
Idiopathic — *see* condition
Idiosyncrasy (*see also* Allergy) 995.3
  drug, medicinal substance, and biological — *see* Allergy, drug
Idiot, idiocy (congenital) 318.2
  amaurotic (Bielschowsky) (-Jansky) (family) (infantile (late)) (juvenile (late)) (Vogt-Spielmeyer) 330.1
  microcephalic 742.1
  Mongolian 758.0
  oxycephalic 756.0
Id reaction (due to bacteria) 692.89
IgE asthma 493.0
Ileitis (chronic) (*see also* Enteritis) 558.9
  infectious 009.0
  noninfectious 558.9
  regional (ulcerative) 555.0
    with large intestine 555.2
  segmental 555.0
    with large intestine 555.2
  terminal (ulcerative) 555.0
    with large intestine 555.2
Ileocolitis (*see also* Enteritis) 558.9
  infectious 009.0
  regional 555.2
  ulcerative 556.1
Ileostomy status V44.2
  with complication 569.60
Ileotyphus 002.0
Ileum — *see* condition
Ileus (adynamic) (bowel) (colon) (inhibitory) (intestine) (neurogenic) (paralytic) 560.1
  arteriomesenteric duodenal 537.2
  due to gallstone (in intestine) 560.31
  duodenal, chronic 537.2
  following gastrointestinal surgery 997.4
  gallstone 560.31
  mechanical (*see also* Obstruction, intestine) 560.9
  meconium 777.1
    due to cystic fibrosis 277.01
  myxedema 564.89
  postoperative 997.4
  transitory, newborn 777.4
Iliac — *see* condition
Iliotibial band friction syndrome 728.89

Ill, louping 063.1
Illegitimacy V61.6
Illness — *see also* Disease
  factitious 300.19
    with
      combined physical and psychological symptoms 300.19
      physical symptoms 300.19
      psychological symptoms 300.16
    chronic (with physical symptoms) 301.51
  heart — *see* Disease, heart
  manic-depressive (*see also* Psychosis, affective) 296.80
  mental (*see also* Disorder, mental) 300.9
Imbalance 781.2
  autonomic (*see also* Neuropathy, peripheral, autonomic) 337.9
  electrolyte 276.9
    with
      abortion — *see* Abortion, by type, with metabolic disorder
      ectopic pregnancy (*see also* categories 633.0-633.9) 639.4
      hyperemesis gravidarum (before 22 completed weeks gestation) 643.1
      molar pregnancy (*see also* categories 630-632) 639.4
    following
      abortion 639.4
      ectopic or molar pregnancy 639.4
    neonatal, transitory NEC 775.5
  endocrine 259.9
  eye muscle NEC 378.9
    heterophoria — *see* Heterophoria
  glomerulotubular NEC 593.89
  hormone 259.9
  hysterical (*see also* Hysteria) 300.10
  labyrinth NEC 386.50
  posture 729.9
  sympathetic (*see also* Neuropathy, peripheral, autonomic) 337.9
Imbecile, imbecility 318.0
  moral 301.7
  old age 290.9
  senile 290.9
  specified IQ — *see* IQ
  unspecified IQ 318.0
Imbedding, intrauterine device 996.32
Imbibition, cholesterol (gallbladder) 575.6
Imerslund (-Gräsbeck) syndrome (anemia due to familial selective vitamin B_{12} malabsorption) 281.1
Iminoacidopathy 270.8
Iminoglycinuria, familial 270.8
Immature — *see also* Immaturity
  personality 301.89
Immaturity 765.1
  extreme 765.0
  fetus or infant light-for-dates — *see* Light-for-dates
  lung, fetus or newborn 770.4
  organ or site NEC — *see* Hypoplasia
  pulmonary, fetus or newborn 770.4
  reaction 301.89
  sexual (female) (male) 259.0
Immersion 994.1
  foot 991.4
  hand 991.4

Index to Diseases

Immobile, immobility
- intestine 564.89
- joint — *see* Ankylosis
- syndrome (paraplegic) 728.3

Immunization
- ABO
  - affecting management of pregnancy 656.2
    - fetus or newborn 773.1
- complication — *see* Complications, vaccination
- Rh factor
  - affecting management of pregnancy 656.1
    - fetus or newborn 773.0
  - from transfusion 999.7

Immunodeficiency 279.3
- with
  - adenosine-deaminase deficiency 279.2
  - defect, predominant
    - B-cell 279.00
    - T-cell 279.10
  - hyperimmunoglobulinemia 279.2
  - lymphopenia, hereditary 279.2
  - thrombocytopenia and eczema 279.12
  - thymic
    - aplasia 279.2
    - dysplasia 279.2
- autosomal recessive, Swiss-type 279.2
- common variable 279.06
- severe combined (SCID) 279.2
- to Rh factor
  - affecting management of pregnancy 656.1
    - fetus or newborn 773.0
- X-linked, with increased IgM 279.05

Immunotherapy, prophylactic V07.2

Impaction, impacted
- bowel, colon, rectum 560.30
  - with hernia — *see also* Hernia, by site, with obstruction
    - gangrenous — *see* Hernia, by site, with gangrene
  - by
    - calculus 560.39
    - gallstone 560.31
  - fecal 560.39
  - specified type NEC 560.39
- calculus — *see* Calculus
- cerumen (ear) (external) 380.4
- cuspid 520.6
  - with abnormal position (same or adjacent tooth) 524.3
- dental 520.6
  - with abnormal position (same or adjacent tooth) 524.3
- fecal, feces 560.39
  - with hernia — *see also* Hernia, by site, with obstruction
    - gangrenous — *see* Hernia, by site, with gangrene
- fracture — *see* Fracture, by site
- gallbladder — *see* Cholelithiasis
- gallstone(s) — *see* Cholelithiasis
  - in intestine (any part) 560.31
- intestine(s) 560.30
  - with hernia — *see also* Hernia, by site, with obstruction
    - grangrenous — *see* Hernia, by site, with gangrene

Impaired, impairment

Impaction, impacted — *continued*
- intestine(s) — *continued*
  - by
    - calculus 560.39
    - gallstone 560.31
  - fecal 560.39
  - specified type NEC 560.39
- intrauterine device (IUD) 996.32
- molar 520.6
  - with abnormal position (same or adjacent tooth) 524.3
- shoulder 660.4
  - affecting fetus or newborn 763.1
- tooth, teeth 520.6
  - with abnormal position (same or adjacent tooth) 524.3
- turbinate 733.99

Impaired, impairment (function)
- arm V49.1
  - movement, involving
    - musculoskeletal system V49.1
    - nervous system V49.2
- auditory discrimination 388.43
- back V48.3
- body (entire) V49.89
- hearing (*see also* Deafness) 389.9
- heart — *see* Disease, heart
- kidney (*see also* Disease, renal) 593.9
  - disorder resulting from 588.9
    - specified NEC 588.8
- leg V49.1
  - movement, involving
    - musculoskeletal system V49.1
    - nervous system V49.2
- limb V49.1
  - movement, involving
    - musculoskeletal system V49.1
    - nervous system V49.2
- liver 573.8
- mastication 524.9
- mobility
  - ear ossicles NEC 385.22
  - incostapedial joint 385.22
  - malleus 385.21
- myocardium, myocardial (*see also* Insufficiency, myocardial) 428.0
- neuromusculoskeletal NEC V49.89
  - back V48.3
  - head V48.2
  - limb V49.2
  - neck V48.3
  - spine V48.3
  - trunk V48.3
- rectal sphincter 787.99
- renal (*see also* Disease, renal) 593.9
  - disorder resulting from 588.9
    - specified NEC 588.8
- spine V48.3
- vision NEC 369.9
  - both eyes NEC 369.3
  - moderate 369.74
    - both eyes 369.25
      - with impairment of lesser eye (specified as)
        - blind, not further specified 369.15
        - low vision, not further specified 369.23
        - near-total 369.17
        - profound 369.18
        - severe 369.24
        - total 369.16

Impaired, impairment — *continued*
  vision NEC — *continued*
    moderate — *continued*
      one eye 369.74
        with vision of other eye (specified as)
          near-normal 369.75
          normal 369.76
    near-total 369.64
      both eyes 369.04
        with impairment of lesser eye (specified as)
          blind, not further specified 369.02
          total 369.03
      one eye 369.64
        with vision of other eye (specified as)
          near normal 369.65
          normal 369.66
    one eye 369.60
      with low vision of other eye 369.10
    profound 369.67
      both eyes 369.08
        with impairment of lesser eye (specified as)
          blind, not further specified 369.05
          near-total 369.07
          total 369.06
      one eye 369.67
        with vision of other eye (specified as)
          near-normal 369.68
          normal 369.69
    severe 369.71
      both eyes 369.22
        with impairment of lesser eye (specified as)
          blind, not further specified 369.11
          low vision, not further specified 369.21
          near-total 369.13
          profound 369.14
          total 369.12
      one eye 369.71
        with vision of other eye (specified as)
          near-normal 369.72
          normal 369.73
    total
      both eyes 369.01
      one eye 369.61
        with vision of other eye (specified as)
          near-normal 369.62
          normal 369.63

Impaludism — *see* Malaria

Impediment, speech NEC 784.5
  psychogenic 307.9
  secondary to organic lesion 784.5

Impending
  cerebrovascular accident or attack 435.9
  coronary syndrome 411.1
  delirium tremens 291.0
  myocardial infarction 411.1

Imperception, auditory (acquired) (congenital) 389.9

Imperfect
  aeration, lung (newborn) 770.5
  closure (congenital)
    alimentary tract NEC 751.8
      lower 751.5
      upper 750.8
    atrioventricular ostium 745.69
    atrium (secundum) 745.5
      primum 745.61
    branchial cleft or sinus 744.41

Imperfect — *continued*
  closure — *continued*
    choroid 743.59
    cricoid cartilage 748.3
    cusps, heart valve NEC 746.89
      pulmonary 746.09
    ductus
      arteriosus 747.0
      Botalli 747.0
    ear drum 744.29
      causing impairment of hearing 744.03
    endocardial cushion 745.60
    epiglottis 748.3
    esophagus with communication to bronchus or trachea 750.3
    Eustachian valve 746.89
    eyelid 743.62
    face, facial (*see also* Cleft, lip) 749.10
    foramen
      Botalli 745.5
      ovale 745.5
    genitalia, genital organ(s) or system
      female 752.8
        external 752.49
        internal NEC 752.8
        uterus 752.3
      male 752.8
        penis 752.69
    glottis 748.3
    heart valve (cusps) NEC 746.89
    interatrial ostium or septum 745.5
    interauricular ostium or septum 745.5
    interventricular ostium or septum 745.4
    iris 743.46
    kidney 753.3
    larynx 748.3
    lens 743.36
    lip (*see also* Cleft, lip) 749.10
    nasal septum or sinus 748.1
    nose 748.1
    omphalomesenteric duct 751.0
    optic nerve entry 743.57
    organ or site NEC — *see* Anomaly, specified type, by site
    ostium
      interatrial 745.5
      interauricular 745.5
      interventricular 745.4
    palate (*see also* Cleft, palate) 749.00
    preauricular sinus 744.46
    retina 743.56
    roof of orbit 742.0
    sclera 743.47
    septum
      aortic 745.0
      aorticopulmonary 745.0
      atrial (secundum) 745.5
        primum 745.61
      between aorta and pulmonary artery 745.0
      heart 745.9
      interatrial (secundum) 745.5
        primum 745.61
      interauricular (secundum) 745.5
        primum 745.61
      interventricular 745.4
        with pulmonary stenosis or atresia, dextraposition of aorta, and hypertrophy of right ventricle 745.2
        in tetralogy of Fallot 745.2

Imperfect — *continued*
　closure — *continued*
　　septum — *continued*
　　　nasal 748.1
　　　ventricular 745.4
　　　　with pulmonary stenosis or atresia, dextraposition of aorta, and hypertrophy of right ventricle 745.2
　　　　in tetralogy of Fallot 745.2
　　skull 756.0
　　　with
　　　　anencephalus 740.0
　　　　encephalocele 742.0
　　　　hydrocephalus 742.3
　　　　　with spina bifida (*see also* Spina bifida) 741.0
　　　　microcephalus 742.1
　　spine (with meningocele) (*see also* Spina bifida) 741.90
　　thyroid cartilage 748.3
　　trachea 748.3
　　tympanic membrane 744.29
　　　causing impairment of hearing 744.03
　　uterus (with communication to bladder, intestine, or rectum) 752.3
　　uvula 749.02
　　　with cleft lip (*see also* Cleft, palate, with cleft lip) 749.20
　　vitelline duct 751.0
　development — *see* Anomaly, by site
　erection 607.84
　fusion — *see* Imperfect, closure
　inflation lung (newborn) 770.5
　intestinal canal 751.5
　poise 729.9
　rotation — *see* Malrotation
　septum, ventricular 745.4
Imperfectly descended testis 752.51
Imperforate (congenital) — *see also* Atresia
　anus 751.2
　bile duct 751.61
　cervix (uteri) 752.49
　esophagus 750.3
　hymen 752.42
　intestine (small) 751.1
　　large 751.2
　jejunum 751.1
　pharynx 750.29
　rectum 751.2
　salivary duct 750.23
　urethra 753.6
　urinary meatus 753.6
　vagina 752.49
Impervious (congenital) — *see also* Atresia
　anus 751.2
　bile duct 751.61
　esophagus 750.3
　intestine (small) 751.1
　　large 751.5
　rectum 751.2
　urethra 753.6
Impetiginization of other dermatoses 684
Impetigo (any organism) (any site) (bullous) (circinate) (contagiosa) (neonatorum) (simplex) 684
　Bockhart's (superficial folliculitis) 704.8
　external ear 684 *[380.13]*
　eyelid 684 *[373.5]*
　Fox's (contagiosa) 684
　furfuracea 696.5

Impetigo — *continued*
　herpetiformis 694.3
　　nonobstetrical 694.3
　staphylococcal infection 684
　ulcerative 686.8
　vulgaris 684
Impingement, soft tissue between teeth 524.2
Implant, endometrial 617.9
Implantation
　anomalous — *see also* Anomaly, specified type, by site
　　ureter 753.4
　cyst
　　external area or site (skin) NEC 709.8
　　iris 364.61
　　vagina 623.8
　　vulva 624.8
　dermoid (cyst)
　　external area or site (skin) NEC 709.8
　　iris 364.61
　　vagina 623.8
　　vulva 624.8
　placenta, low or marginal — *see* Placenta previa
Impotence (sexual) (psychogenic) 302.72
　organic origin NEC 607.84
Impoverished blood 285.9
Impression, basilar 756.0
Imprisonment V62.5
Improper
　development, infant 764.9
Improperly tied umbilical cord (causing hemorrhage) 772.3
Impulses, obsessional 300.3
Impulsive neurosis 300.3
Inaction, kidney (*see also* Disease, renal) 593.9
Inactive — *see* condition
Inadequate, inadequacy
　biologic 301.6
　cardiac and renal — *see* Hypertension, cardiorenal
　constitutional 301.6
　development
　　child 783.40
　　fetus 764.9
　　　affecting management of pregnancy 656.5
　　genitalia
　　　after puberty NEC 259.0
　　　congenital — *see* Hypoplasia, genitalia
　　lungs 748.5
　　organ or site NEC — *see* Hypoplasia, by site
　dietary 269.9
　education V62.3
　environment
　　economic problem V60.2
　　household condition NEC V60.1
　　poverty V60.2
　　unemployment V62.0
　functional 301.6
　household care, due to
　　family member
　　　handicapped or ill V60.4
　　　temporarily away from home V60.4
　　　　on vacation V60.5
　　technical defects in home V60.1
　　temporary absence from home of person rendering care V60.4

Inadequate, inadequacy — continued
　housing (heating) (space) V60.1
　material resources V60.2
　mental (see also Retardation, mental) 319
　nervous system 799.2
　personality 301.6
　prenatal care in current pregnancy V23.7
　pulmonary
　　function 786.09
　　　newborn 770.89　▲
　　ventilation, newborn 770.89　▲
　respiration 786.09
　　newborn 770.89　▲
　social 301.6

Inanition 263.9
　with edema 262
　due to
　　deprivation of food 994.2
　　malnutrition 263.9
　fever 780.6

Inappropriate secretion
　ACTH 255.0
　antidiuretic hormone (ADH) (excessive) 253.6
　　deficiency 253.5
　ectopic hormone NEC 259.3
　pituitary (posterior) 253.6

Inattention after or at birth 995.52

Inborn errors of metabolism — see Disorder, metabolism

Incarceration, incarcerated
　bubonocele — see also Hernia, inguinal, with obstruction
　　gangrenous — see Hernia, inguinal, with gangrene
　colon (by hernia) — see also Hernia, by site with obstruction
　　gangrenous — see Hernia, by site, with gangrene
　enterocele 552.9
　　gangrenous 551.9
　epigastrocele 552.29
　　gangrenous 551.29
　epiplocele 552.9
　　gangrenous 551.9
　exomphalos 552.1
　　gangrenous 551.1
　fallopian tube 620.8
　hernia — see also Hernia, by site, with obstruction
　　gangrenous — see Hernia, by site, with gangrene
　iris, in wound 871.1
　lens, in wound 871.1
　merocele (see also Hernia, femoral, with obstruction) 552.00
　omentum (by hernia) — see also Hernia, by site, with obstruction
　　gangrenous — see Hernia, by site, with gangrene
　omphalocele 756.79
　rupture (meaning hernia) (see also Hernia, by site, with obstruction) 552.9
　　gangrenous (see also Hernia, by site, with gangrene) 551.9
　sarcoepiplocele 552.9
　　gangrenous 551.9
　sarcoepiplomphalocele 552.1
　　with gangrene 551.1

Incarceration, incarcerated — continued
　uterus 621.8
　　gravid 654.3
　　　causing obstructed labor 660.2
　　　affecting fetus or newborn 763.1

Incident, cerebrovascular (see also Disease, cerebrovascular, acute) 436

Incineration (entire body) (from fire, conflagration, electricity, or lightning) — see Burn, multiple, specified sites

Incised wound
　external — see Wound, open, by site
　internal organs (abdomen, chest, or pelvis) — see Injury, internal, by site, with open wound

Incision, incisional
　hernia — see Hernia, incisional
　surgical, complication — see Complications, surgical procedures
　traumatic
　　external — see Wound, open, by site
　　internal organs (abdomen, chest, or pelvis) — see Injury, internal, by site, with open wound

Inclusion
　azurophilic leukocytic 288.2
　blennorrhea (neonatal) (newborn) 771.6
　cyst — see Cyst, skin
　gallbladder in liver (congenital) 751.69

Incompatibility
　ABO
　　affecting management of pregnancy 656.2
　　fetus or newborn 773.1
　　infusion or transfusion reaction 999.6
　blood (group) (Duffy) (E) (K(ell)) (Kidd) (Lewis) (M) (N) (P) (S) NEC
　　affecting management of pregnancy 656.2
　　fetus or newborn 773.2
　　infusion or transfusion reaction 999.6
　marital V61.10
　　involving divorce or estrangement V61.0
　Rh (blood group) (factor)
　　affecting management of pregnancy 656.1
　　fetus or newborn 773.0
　　infusion or transfusion reaction 999.7
　Rhesus — see Incompatibility, Rh

Incompetency, incompetence, incompetent
　annular
　　aortic (valve) (see also Insufficiency, aortic) 424.1
　　mitral (valve) — (see also Insufficiency, mitral) 424.0
　　pulmonary valve (heart) (see also Endocarditis, pulmonary) 424.3
　aortic (valve) (see also Insufficiency, aortic) 424.1
　　syphilitic 093.22
　cardiac (orifice) 530.0
　　valve — see Endocarditis
　cervix, cervical (os) 622.5
　　in pregnancy 654.5
　　　affecting fetus or newborn 761.0
　esophagogastric (junction) (sphincter) 530.0
　heart valve, congenital 746.89
　mitral (valve) — see Insufficiency, mitral
　papillary muscle (heart) 429.81
　pelvic fundus 618.8

Index to Diseases

Incompetency, incompetence, incompetent — *continued*
  pulmonary valve (heart) (*see also* Endocarditis, pulmonary) 424.3
    congenital 746.09
  tricuspid (annular) (rheumatic) (valve) (*see also* Endocarditis, tricuspid) 397.0
  valvular — *see* Endocarditis
  vein, venous (saphenous) (varicose) (*see also* Varicose, vein) 454.9
  velopharyngeal (closure)
    acquired 528.9
    congenital 750.29

Incomplete — *see also* condition
  bladder emptying 788.21
  expansion lungs (newborn) 770.5
  gestation (liveborn) — *see* Immaturity
  rotation — *see* Malrotation

Incontinence 788.30
  without sensory awareness 788.34
  anal sphincter 787.6
  continuous leakage 788.37
  feces 787.6
    due to hysteria 300.11
    nonorganic origin 307.7
  hysterical 300.11
  mixed (male) (female) (urge and stress) 788.33
  overflow 788.39
  paradoxical 788.39
  rectal 787.6
  specified NEC 788.39
  stress (female) 625.6
    male NEC 788.32
  urethral sphincter 599.84
  urge 788.31
    and stress (male) (female) 788.33
  urine 788.30
    active 788.30
    male 788.30
      stress 788.32
        and urge 788.33
    neurogenic 788.39
    nonorganic origin 307.6
    stress (female) 625.6
      male NEC 788.32
    urge 788.31
      and stress 788.33

Incontinentia pigmenti 757.33

Incoordinate
  uterus (action) (contractions) 661.4 ✓5ᵗʰ
    affecting fetus or newborn 763.7

Incoordination
  esophageal-pharyngeal (newborn) 787.2
  muscular 781.3
  papillary muscle 429.81

Increase, increased
  abnormal, in development 783.9
  androgens (ovarian) 256.1
  anticoagulants (antithrombin) (anti-VIIIa) (anti-IXa) (anti-Xa) (anti-XIa) 286.5
    postpartum 666.3 ✓5ᵗʰ
  cold sense (*see also* Disturbance, sensation) 782.0
  estrogen 256.0
  function
    adrenal (cortex) 255.3
      medulla 255.6
    pituitary (anterior) (gland) (lobe) 253.1
      posterior 253.6

Increase, increased — *continued*
  heat sense (*see also* Disturbance, sensation) 782.0
  intracranial pressure 781.99
    injury at birth 767.8
  light reflex of retina 362.13
  permeability, capillary 448.9
  pressure
    intracranial 781.99
      injury at birth 767.8
    intraocular 365.00
  pulsations 785.9
  pulse pressure 785.9
  sphericity, lens 743.36
  splenic activity 289.4
  venous pressure 459.89
    portal 572.3

Incrustation, cornea, lead or zinc 930.0

Incyclophoria 378.44

Incyclotropia 378.33

Indeterminate sex 752.7

India rubber skin 756.83

Indicanuria 270.2

Indigestion (bilious) (functional) 536.8
  acid 536.8
  catarrhal 536.8
  due to decomposed food NEC 005.9
  fat 579.8
  nervous 306.4
  psychogenic 306.4

Indirect — *see* condition

Indolent bubo NEC 099.8

Induced
  abortion — *see* Abortion, induced
  birth, affecting fetus or newborn 763.89
  delivery — *see* Delivery
  labor — *see* Delivery

Induration, indurated
  brain 348.8
  breast (fibrous) 611.79
    puerperal, postpartum 676.3 ✓5ᵗʰ
  broad ligament 620.8
  chancre 091.0
    anus 091.1
    congenital 090.0
    extragenital NEC 091.2
  corpora cavernosa (penis) (plastic) 607.89
  liver (chronic) 573.8
    acute 573.8
  lung (black) (brown) (chronic) (fibroid) (*see also* Fibrosis, lung) 515
    essential brown 275.0 [516.1]
  penile 607.89
  phlebitic — *see* Phlebitis
  skin 782.8
  stomach 537.89

Induratio penis plastica 607.89

Industrial — *see* condition

Inebriety (*see also* Abuse, drugs, nondependent) 305.0 ✓5ᵗʰ

Inefficiency
  kidney (*see also* Disease, renal) 593.9
  thyroid (acquired) (gland) 244.9

Inelasticity, skin 782.8

Inequality, leg (acquired) (length) 736.81
  congenital 755.30

Inertia
bladder 596.4
  neurogenic 596.54
    with cauda equina syndrome 344.61
  stomach 536.8
    psychogenic 306.4
  uterus, uterine 661.2 ✓5ᵗʰ
    affecting fetus or newborn 763.7
    primary 661.0 ✓5ᵗʰ
    secondary 661.1 ✓5ᵗʰ
  vesical 596.4
    neurogenic 596.54
      with cauda equina 344.61
Infant — see also condition
  excessive crying of 780.92
  fussy (baby) 780.91
  held for adoption V68.89
  newborn — see Newborn
  syndrome of diabetic mother 775.0
"Infant Hercules" syndrome 255.2
Infantile — see also condition
  genitalia, genitals 259.0
    in pregnancy or childbirth NEC 654.4 ✓5ᵗʰ
      affecting fetus or newborn 763.89
      causing obstructed labor 660.2 ✓5ᵗʰ
        affecting fetus or newborn 763.1
  heart 746.9
  kidney 753.3
  lack of care 995.52
  macula degeneration 362.75
  melanodontia 521.05
  os, uterus (see also Infantile, genitalia) 259.0
  pelvis 738.6
    with disproportion (fetopelvic) 653.1 ✓5ᵗʰ
      affecting fetus or newborn 763.1
      causing obstructed labor 660.1 ✓5ᵗʰ
        affecting fetus or newborn 763.1
  penis 259.0
  testis 257.2
  uterus (see also Infantile, genitalia) 259.0
  vulva 752.49
Infantilism 259.9
  with dwarfism (hypophyseal) 253.3
  Brissaud's (infantile myxedema) 244.9
  celiac 579.0
  Herter's (nontropical sprue) 579.0
  hypophyseal 253.3
  hypothalamic (with obesity) 253.8
  idiopathic 259.9
  intestinal 579.0
  pancreatic 577.8
  pituitary 253.3
  renal 588.0
  sexual (with obesity) 259.0
Infants, healthy liveborn — see Newborn
Infarct, infarction
  adrenal (capsule) (gland) 255.4
  amnion 658.8 ✓5ᵗʰ
  anterior (with contiguous portion of
      intraventricular septum) NEC (see also
      Infarct, myocardium) 410.1 ✓5ᵗʰ
  appendices epiploicae 557.0
  bowel 557.0
  brain (stem) 434.91
    embolic (see also Embolism, brain) 434.11
    healed or old without residuals V12.59
    iatrogenic 997.02
    postoperative 997.02
    puerperal, postpartum, childbirth 674.0
      ✓5ᵗʰ

Infarct, infarction — continued
  brain — continued
    thrombotic (see also Thrombosis, brain)
      434.01
  breast 611.8
  Brewer's (kidney) 593.81
  cardiac (see also Infarct, myocardium)
    410.9 ✓5ᵗʰ
  cerebellar (see also Infarct, brain) 434.91
    embolic (see also Embolism, brain) 434.11
  cerebral (see also Infarct, brain) 434.91
    embolic (see also Embolism, brain) 434.11
  chorion 658.8 ✓5ᵗʰ
  colon (acute) (agnogenic) (embolic)
      (hemorrhagic) (nonocclusive)
      (nonthrombotic) (occlusive) (segmental)
      (thrombotic) (with gangrene) 557.0
  coronary artery (see also Infarct, myocardium)
    410.9 ✓5ᵗʰ
  embolic (see also Embolism) 444.9
  fallopian tube 620.8
  gallbladder 575.8
  heart (see also Infarct, myocardium) 410.9 ✓5ᵗʰ
  hepatic 573.4
  hypophysis (anterior lobe) 253.8
  impending (myocardium) 411.1
  intestine (acute) (agnogenic) (embolic)
      (hemorrhagic) (nonocclusive)
      (nonthrombotic) (occlusive) (thrombotic)
      (with gangrene) 557.0
  kidney 593.81
  liver 573.4
  lung (embolic) (thrombotic) 415.1 ✓5ᵗʰ
    with
      abortion — see Abortion, by type, with
        embolism
      ectopic pregnancy (see also categories
        633.0-633.9) 639.6
      molar pregnancy (see also categories
        630-632) 639.6
    following
      abortion 639.6
      ectopic or molar pregnancy 639.6
    iatrogenic 415.11
    in pregnancy, childbirth, or puerperium —
      see Embolism, obstetrical
    postoperative 415.11
  lymph node or vessel 457.8
  medullary (brain) — see Infarct, brain
  meibomian gland (eyelid) 374.85
  mesentary, mesenteric (embolic) (thrombotic)
      (with gangrene) 557.0
  midbrain — see Infarct, brain
  myocardium, myocardial (acute or with a
      stated duration of 8 weeks or less) (with
      hypertension) 410.9 ✓5ᵗʰ

> Note — Use the following fifth-digit
> subclassification with category 410:
>
> 0 episode unspecified
> 1 initial episode
> 2 subsequent episode without
>   recurrence

  with symptoms after 8 weeks from date of
    infarction 414.8
  anterior (wall) (with contiguous portion of
      intraventricular septum) NEC
      410.1 ✓5ᵗʰ
  anteroapical (with contiguous portion of
      intraventricular septum) 410.1 ✓5ᵗʰ

Index to Diseases

Infarct, infarction — *continued*
- myocardium, myocardial — *continued*
  - anterolateral (wall) 410.0 ✓5ᵗʰ
  - anteroseptal (with contiguous portion of intraventricular septum) 410.1 ✓5ᵗʰ
  - apical-lateral 410.5 ✓5ᵗʰ
  - atrial 410.8 ✓5ᵗʰ
  - basal-lateral 410.5 ✓5ᵗʰ
  - chronic (with symptoms after 8 weeks from date of infarction) 414.8
  - diagnosed on ECG, but presenting no symptoms 412
  - diaphragmatic wall (with contiguous portion of intraventricular septum) 410.4 ✓5ᵗʰ
  - healed or old, currently presenting no symptoms 412
  - high lateral 410.5 ✓5ᵗʰ
  - impending 411.1
  - inferior (wall) (with contiguous portion of intraventricular septum) 410.4 ✓5ᵗʰ
  - inferolateral (wall) 410.2 ✓5ᵗʰ
  - inferoposterior wall 410.3 ✓5ᵗʰ
  - lateral wall 410.5 ✓5ᵗʰ
  - nontransmural 410.7 ✓5ᵗʰ
  - papillary muscle 410.8 ✓5ᵗʰ
  - past (diagnosed on ECG or other special investigation, but currently presenting no symptoms) 412
    - with symptoms NEC 414.8
  - posterior (strictly) (true) (wall) 410.6 ✓5ᵗʰ
  - posterobasal 410.6 ✓5ᵗʰ
  - posteroinferior 410.3 ✓5ᵗʰ
  - posterolateral 410.5 ✓5ᵗʰ
  - previous, currently presenting no symptoms 412
  - septal 410.8 ✓5ᵗʰ
  - specified site NEC 410.8 ✓5ᵗʰ
  - subendocardial 410.7 ✓5ᵗʰ
  - syphilitic 093.82
- nontransmural 410.7 ✓5ᵗʰ
- omentum 557.0
- ovary 620.8
- pancreas 577.8
- papillary muscle (*see also* Infarct, myocardium) 410.8 ✓5ᵗʰ
- parathyroid gland 252.8
- pituitary (gland) 253.8
- placenta (complicating pregnancy) 656.7 ✓5ᵗʰ
  - affecting fetus or newborn 762.2
- pontine — *see* Infarct, brain
- posterior NEC (*see also* Infarct, myocardium) 410.6 ✓5ᵗʰ
- prostate 602.8
- pulmonary (artery) (hemorrhagic) (vein) 415.1 ✓5ᵗʰ
  - with
    - abortion — *see* Abortion, by type, with embolism
    - ectopic pregnancy (*see also* categories 633.0-633.9) 639.6
    - molar pregnancy (*see also* categories 630-632) 639.6
  - following
    - abortion 639.6
    - ectopic or molar pregnancy 639.6
  - iatrogenic 415.11
  - in pregnancy, childbirth, or puerperium — *see* Embolism, obstetrical
  - postoperative 415.11

Infarct, infarction — *continued*
- renal 593.81
  - embolic or thrombotic 593.81
- retina, retinal 362.84
  - with occlusion — *see* Occlusion, retina
- spinal (acute) (cord) (embolic) (nonembolic) 336.1
- spleen 289.59
  - embolic or thrombotic 444.89
- subchorionic — *see* Infarct, placenta
- subendocardial (*see also* Infarct, myocardium) 410.7 ✓5ᵗʰ
- suprarenal (capsule) (gland) 255.4
- syncytium — *see* Infarct, placenta
- testis 608.83
- thrombotic (*see also* Thrombosis) 453.9
  - artery, arterial — *see* Embolism
- thyroid (gland) 246.3
- ventricle (heart) (*see also* Infarct, myocardium) 410.9 ✓5ᵗʰ

Infecting — *see* condition

Infection, infected, infective (opportunistic) 136.9
- with lymphangitis — *see* Lymphangitis
- abortion — *see* Abortion, by type, with sepsis
- abscess (skin) — *see* Abscess, by site
- Absidia 117.7
- Acanthocheilonema (perstans) 125.4
  - streptocerca 125.6
- accessory sinus (chronic) (*see also* Sinusitis) 473.9
- Achorion — *see* Dermatophytosis
- Acremonium falciforme 117.4
- acromioclavicular (joint) 711.91
- actinobacillus
  - lignieresii 027.8
  - mallei 024
  - muris 026.1
- actinomadura — *see* Actinomycosis
- Actinomyces (israelii) — *see also* Actinomycosis
- muris-ratti 026.1
- Actinomycetales (actinomadura) (Actinomyces) (Nocardia) (Streptomyces) — *see* Actinomycosis
- actinomycotic NEC (*see also* Actinomycosis) 039.9
- adenoid (chronic) 474.01
  - acute 463
  - and tonsil (chronic) 474.02
  - acute or subacute 463
- adenovirus NEC 079.0
  - in diseases classified elsewhere — *see* category 079 ✓4ᵗʰ
  - unspecified nature or site 079.0
- Aerobacter aerogenes NEC 041.85
  - enteritis 008.2
- aerogenes capsulatus (*see also* Gangrene, gas) 040.0
- aertrycke (*see also* Infection, Salmonella) 003.9
- ajellomyces dermatitidis 116.0
- alimentary canal NEC (*see also* Enteritis, due to, by organism) 009.0
- Allescheria boydii 117.6
- Alternaria 118
- alveolus, alveolar (process) (pulpal origin) 522.4
- ameba, amebic (histolytica) (*see also* Amebiasis) 006.9
  - acute 006.0

Infection, infected, infective — *continued*
  ameba, amebic — *continued*
    chronic 006.1
    free-living 136.2
    hartmanni 007.8
    specified
      site NEC 006.8
      type NEC 007.8
  amniotic fluid or cavity 658.4 ✓5ᵗʰ
    affecting fetus or newborn 762.7
  anaerobes (cocci) (gram-negative) (gram-positive) (mixed) NEC 041.84
  anal canal 569.49
  Ancylostoma braziliense 126.2
  Angiostrongylus cantonensis 128.8
  anisakiasis 127.1
  Anisakis larva 127.1
  anthrax (*see also* Anthrax) 022.9
  antrum (chronic) (*see also* Sinusitis, maxillary) 473.0
  anus (papillae) (sphincter) 569.49
  arbor virus NEC 066.9
  arbovirus NEC 066.9
  argentophil-rod 027.0
  Ascaris lumbricoides 127.0
  ascomycetes 117.4
  Aspergillus (flavus) (fumigatus) (terreus) 117.3
  atypical
    acid-fast (bacilli) (*see also* Mycobacterium, atypical) 031.9
    mycobacteria (*see also* Mycobacterium, atypical) 031.9
  auditory meatus (circumscribed) (diffuse) (external) (*see also* Otitis, externa) 380.10
  auricle (ear) (*see also* Otitis, externa) 380.10
  axillary gland 683
  Babesiasis 088.82
  Babesiosis 088.82
  Bacillus NEC 041.89
    abortus 023.1
    anthracis (*see also* Anthrax) 022.9
    cereus (food poisoning) 005.89
    coli — *see* Infection, Escherichia coli
    coliform NEC 041.85
    Ducrey's (any location) 099.0
    Flexner's 004.1
    fragilis NEC 041.82
    Friedländer's NEC 041.3
    fusiformis 101
    gas (gangrene) (*see also* Gangrene, gas) 040.0
    mallei 024
    melitensis 023.0
    paratyphoid, paratyphosus 002.9
      A 002.1
      B 002.2
      C 002.3
    Schmorl's 040.3
    Shiga 004.0
    suipestifer (*see also* Infection, Salmonella) 003.9
    swimming pool 031.1
    typhosa 002.0
    welchii (*see also* Gangrene, gas) 040.0
    Whitmore's 025
  bacterial NEC 041.9
    specified NEC 041.89
      anaerobic NEC 041.84
      gram-negative NEC 041.85
        anaerobic NEC 041.84

Infection, infected, infective — *continued*
  Bacterium
    paratyphosum 002.9
      A 002.1
      B 002.2
      C 002.3
    typhosum 002.0
  Bacteroides (fragilis) (melaninogenicus) (oralis) NEC 041.84
  balantidium coli 007.0
  Bartholin's gland 616.8
  Basidiobolus 117.7
  Bedsonia 079.98
    specified NEC 079.88
  bile duct 576.1
  bladder (*see also* Cystitis) 595.9
  Blastomyces, blastomycotic 116.0
    brasiliensis 116.1
    dermatitidis 116.0
    European 117.5
    Loboi 116.2
    North American 116.0
    South American 116.1
  blood stream — *see* Septicemia
  bone 730.9 ✓5ᵗʰ
    specified — *see* Osteomyelitis
  Bordetella 033.9
    bronchiseptica 033.8
    parapertussis 033.1
    pertussis 033.0
  Borrelia
    bergdorfi 088.81
    vincentii (mouth) (pharynx) (tonsil) 101
  brain (*see also* Encephalitis) 323.9
    late effect — *see* category 326
    membranes — (*see also* Meningitis) 322.9
    septic 324.0
      late effect — *see* category 326
    meninges (*see also* Meningitis) 320.9
  branchial cyst 744.42
  breast 611.0
    puerperal, postpartum 675.2 ✓5ᵗʰ
      with nipple 675.9 ✓5ᵗʰ
        specified type NEC 675.8 ✓5ᵗʰ
      nonpurulent 675.2 ✓5ᵗʰ
      purulent 675.1 ✓5ᵗʰ
  bronchus (*see also* Bronchitis) 490
    fungus NEC 117.9
  Brucella 023.9
    abortus 023.1
    canis 023.3
    melitensis 023.0
    mixed 023.8
    suis 023.2
  Brugia (Wuchereria) malayi 125.1
  bursa — *see* Bursitis
  buttocks (skin) 686.9
  Candida (albicans) (tropicalis) (*see also* Candidiasis) 112.9
    congenital 771.7
  Candiru 136.8
  Capillaria
    hepatica 128.8
    philippinensis 127.5
  cartilage 733.99
  cat liver fluke 121.0
  cellulitis — *see* Cellulitis, by site
  Cephalosporum falciforme 117.4
  Cercomonas hominis (intestinal) 007.3
  cerebrospinal (*see also* Meningitis) 322.9
    late effect — *see* category 326

Infection, infected, infective — continued
- cervical gland 683
- cervix (see also Cervicitis) 616.0
- cesarean section wound 674.3 ✓5ᵗʰ
- Chilomastix (intestinal) 007.8
- Chlamydia 079.98
  - specified NEC 079.88
- cholera (see also Cholera) 001.9
- chorionic plate 658.8 ✓5ᵗʰ
- Cladosporium
  - bantianum 117.8
  - carrionii 117.2
  - mansoni 111.1
  - trichoides 117.8
  - wernecki 111.1
- Clonorchis (sinensis) (liver) 121.1
- Clostridium (haemolyticum) (novyi) NEC 041.84
  - botulinum 005.1
  - congenital 771.89 ▲
  - histolyticum (see also Gangrene, gas) 040.0
  - oedematiens (see also Gangrene, gas) 040.0
  - perfringens 041.83
    - due to food 005.2
  - septicum (see also Gangrene, gas) 040.0
  - sordellii (see also Gangrene, gas) 040.0
  - welchii (see also Gangrene, gas) 040.0
    - due to food 005.2
- Coccidioides (immitis) (see also Coccidioidomycosis) 114.9
- coccus NEC 041.89
- colon (see also Enteritis, due to, by organism) 009.0
  - bacillus — see Infection, Escherichia coli
- colostomy or enterostomy 569.61
- common duct 576.1
- complicating pregnancy, childbirth, or puerperium NEC 647.9 ✓5ᵗʰ
  - affecting fetus or newborn 760.2
- Condiobolus 117.7
- congenital NEC 771.89 ▲
  - Candida albicans 771.7
  - chronic 771.2
  - clostridial 771.89 ▲
  - cytomegalovirus 771.1
  - Escherichia coli 771.89 ▲
  - hepatitis, viral 771.2
  - herpes simplex 771.2
  - listeriosis 771.2
  - malaria 771.2
  - poliomyelitis 771.2
  - rubella 771.0
  - Salmonella 771.89 ▲
  - streptococcal 771.89 ▲
  - toxoplasmosis 771.2
  - tuberculosis 771.2
  - urinary (tract) 771.82 ▲
  - vaccinia 771.2
- corpus luteum (see also Salpingo-oophoritis) 614.2
- Corynebacterium diphtheriae — see Diphtheria
- Coxsackie (see also Coxsackie) 079.2
  - endocardium 074.22
  - heart NEC 074.20
  - in diseases classified elsewhere — see category 079 ✓5ᵗʰ
  - meninges 047.0
  - myocardium 074.23
  - pericardium 074.21
  - pharynx 074.0

Infection, infected, infective — continued
- Coxsackie — continued
  - specified disease NEC 074.8
  - unspecified nature or site 079.2
- Cryptococcus neoformans 117.5
- Cryptosporidia 007.4
- Cunninghamella 117.7
- cyst — see Cyst
- Cysticercus cellulosae 123.1
- cytomegalovirus 078.5
  - congenital 771.1
- dental (pulpal origin) 522.4
- deuteromycetes 117.4
- Dicrocoelium dendriticum 121.8
- Dipetalonema (perstans) 125.4
  - streptocerca 125.6
- diphtherial — see Diphtheria
- Diphyllobothrium (adult) (latum) (pacificum) 123.4
  - larval 123.5
- Diplogonoporus (grandis) 123.8
- Dipylidium (caninum) 123.8
- Dirofilaria 125.6
- dog tapeworm 123.8
- Dracunculus medinensis 125.7
- Dreschlera 118
  - hawaiiensis 117.8
- Ducrey's bacillus (any site) 099.0
- due to or resulting from
  - device, implant, or graft (any) (presence of) — see Complications, infection and inflammation, due to (presence of) any device, implant, or graft classified to 996.0-996.5 NEC
  - injection, inoculation, infusion, transfusion, or vaccination (prophylactic) (therapeutic) 999.3
  - injury NEC — see Wound, open, by site, complicated
  - surgery 998.59
- duodenum 535.6 ✓5ᵗʰ
- ear — see also Otitis
  - external (see also Otitis, externa) 380.10
  - inner (see also Labyrinthitis) 386.30
  - middle — see Otitis, media
- Eaton's agent NEC 041.81
- Eberthella typhosa 002.0
- Ebola 065.8
- echinococcosis 122.9
- Echinococcus (see also Echinococcus) 122.9
- Echinostoma 121.8
- ECHO virus 079.1
  - in diseases classified elsewhere — see category 079 ✓4ᵗʰ
  - unspecified nature or site 079.1
- Ehrlichiosis 082.40
  - chaffeensis 082.41
  - specified type NEC 082.49
- Endamoeba — see Infection, ameba
- endocardium (see also Endocarditis) 421.0
- endocervix (see also Cervicitis) 616.0
- Entamoeba — see Infection, ameba
- enteric (see also Enteritis, due to, by organism) 009.0
- Enterobacter aerogenes NEC 041.85
- Enterobius vermicularis 127.4
- enterococcus NEC 041.04
- enterovirus NEC 079.89
  - central nervous system NEC 048
  - enteritis 008.67
  - meningitis 047.9

Infection, infected, infective — *continued*
  Entomophthora 117.7
  Epidermophyton — *see* Dermatophytosis
  epidermophytosis — *see* Dermatophytosis
  episiotomy 674.3 ✓5ᵗʰ
  Epstein-Barr virus 075
    chronic 780.79 *[139.8]*
  erysipeloid 027.1
  Erysipelothrix (insidiosa) (rhusiopathiae) 027.1
  erythema infectiosum 057.0
  Escherichia coli NEC 041.4
    congenital 771.89 ▲
    enteritis — *see* Enteritis, E. coli
    generalized 038.42
    intestinal — *see* Enteritis, E. coli
  ethmoidal (chronic) (sinus) (*see also* Sinusitis, ethmoidal) 473.2
  Eubacterium 041.84
  Eustachian tube (ear) 381.50
    acute 381.51
    chronic 381.52
  exanthema subitum 057.8
  external auditory canal (meatus) (*see also* Otitis, externa) 380.10
  eye NEC 360.00
  eyelid 373.9
    specified NEC 373.8
  fallopian tube (*see also* Salpingo-oophoritis) 614.2
  fascia 728.89
  Fasciola
    gigantica 121.3
    hepatica 121.3
  Fasciolopsis (buski) 121.4
  fetus (intra-amniotic) — *see* Infection, congenital
  filarial — *see* Infestation, filarial
  finger (skin) 686.9
    abscess (with lymphangitis) 681.00
      pulp 681.01
    cellulitis (with lymphangitis) 681.00
    distal closed space (with lymphangitis) 681.00
    nail 681.02
      fungus 110.1
  fish tapeworm 123.4
    larval 123.5
  flagellate, intestinal 007.9
  fluke — *see* Infestation, fluke
  focal
    teeth (pulpal origin) 522.4
    tonsils 474.00
      and adenoids 474.02
  Fonsecaea
    compactum 117.2
    pedrosoi 117.2
  food (*see also* Poisoning, food) 005.9
  foot (skin) 686.9
    fungus 110.4
  Francisella tularensis (*see also* Tularemia) 021.9
  frontal sinus (chronic) (*see also* Sinusitis, frontal) 473.1
  fungus NEC 117.9
    beard 110.0
    body 110.2
    dermatiacious NEC 117.8
    foot 110.4
    groin 110.3
    hand 110.2
    nail 110.1

Infection, infected, infective — *continued*
  fungus NEC — *continued*
    pathogenic to compromised host only 118
    perianal (area) 110.3
    scalp 110.0
    scrotum 110.8
    skin 111.9
      foot 110.4
      hand 110.2
    toenails 110.1
    trachea 117.9
  Fusarium 118
  Fusobacterium 041.84
  gallbladder (*see also* Cholecystitis, acute) 575.0
  Gardnerella vaginalis 041.89 ●
  gas bacillus (*see also* Gas, gangrene) 040.0
  gastric (*see also* Gastritis) 535.5 ✓5ᵗʰ
  Gastrodiscoides hominis 121.8
  gastroenteric (*see also* Enteritis, due to, by organism) 009.0
  gastrointestinal (*see also* Enteritis, due to, by organism) 009.0
  gastrostomy 536.41
  generalized NEC (*see also* Septicemia) 038.9
  genital organ or tract NEC
    female 614.9
      with
        abortion — *see* Abortion, by type, with sepsis
        ectopic pregnancy (*see also* categories 633.0-633.9) 639.0
        molar pregnancy (*see also* categories 630-632) 639.0
      complicating pregnancy 646.6 ✓5ᵗʰ
        affecting fetus or newborn 760.8
      following
        abortion 639.0
        ectopic or molar pregnancy 639.0
      puerperal, postpartum, childbirth 670 ✓4ᵗʰ
      minor or localized 646.6 ✓5ᵗʰ
        affecting fetus or newborn 760.8
    male 608.4
  genitourinary tract NEC 599.0
  Ghon tubercle, primary (*see also* Tuberculosis) 010.0 ✓5ᵗʰ
  Giardia lamblia 007.1
  gingival (chronic) 523.1
    acute 523.0
    Vincent's 101
  glanders 024
  Glenosporopsis amazonica 116.2
  Gnathostoma spinigerum 128.1
  Gongylonema 125.6
  gonococcal NEC (*see also* Gonococcus) 098.0
  gram-negative bacilli NEC 041.85
    anaerobic 041.84
  guinea worm 125.7
  gum (*see also* Infection, gingival) 523.1
  Hantavirus 079.81
  heart 429.89
  Helicobacter pylori (H. pylori) 041.86
  helminths NEC 128.9
    intestinal 127.9
      mixed (types classifiable to more than one category in 120.0-127.7) 127.8
      specified type NEC 127.7
    specified type NEC 128.8
  Hemophilus influenzae NEC 041.5
    generalized 038.41

Infection, infected, infective — *continued*
- herpes (simplex) (*see also* Herpes, simplex) 054.9
  - congenital 771.2
  - zoster (*see also* Herpes, zoster) 053.9
  - eye NEC 053.29
- Heterophyes heterophyes 121.6
- Histoplasma (*see also* Histoplasmosis) 115.90
  - capsulatum (*see also* Histoplasmosis, American) 115.00
  - duboisii (*see also* Histoplasmosis, African) 115.10
- HIV V08
  - with symptoms, symptomatic 042
- hookworm (*see also* Ancylostomiasis) 126.9
- human immunodeficiency virus V08
  - with symptoms, symptomatic 042
- human papillomavirus 079.4
- hydrocele 603.1
- hydronephrosis 591
- Hymenolepis 123.6
- hypopharynx 478.29
- inguinal glands 683
  - due to soft chancre 099.0
- intestine, intestinal (*see also* Enteritis, due to, by organism) 009.0
- intrauterine (*see also* Endometritis) 615.9
  - complicating delivery 646.6 ▲5ᵗʰ
- isospora belli or hominis 007.2
- Japanese B encephalitis 062.0
- jaw (bone) (acute) (chronic) (lower) (subacute) (upper) 526.4
- joint — *see* Arthritis, infectious or infective
- kidney (cortex) (hematogenous) 590.9
  - with
    - abortion — *see* Abortion, by type, with urinary tract infection
    - calculus 592.0
    - ectopic pregnancy (*see also* categories 633.0-633.9) 639.8
    - molar pregnancy (*see also* categories 630-632) 639.8
  - complicating pregnancy or puerperium 646.6 ▲5ᵗʰ
    - affecting fetus or newborn 760.1
  - following
    - abortion 639.8
    - ectopic or molar pregnancy 639.8
  - pelvis and ureter 590.3
- Klebsiella pneumoniae NEC 041.3
- knee (skin) NEC 686.9
  - joint — *see* Arthritis, infectious
- Koch's (*see also* Tuberculosis, pulmonary) 011.9 ▲5ᵗʰ
- labia (majora) (minora) (*see also* Vulvitis) 616.10
- lacrimal
  - gland (*see also* Dacryoadenitis) 375.00
  - passages (duct) (sac) (*see also* Dacryocystitis) 375.30
- larynx NEC 478.79
- leg (skin) NEC 686.9
- Leishmania (*see also* Leishmaniasis) 085.9
  - braziliensis 085.5
  - donovani 085.0
  - Ethiopica 085.3
  - furunculosa 085.1
  - infantum 085.0
  - mexicana 085.4
  - tropica (minor) 085.1
    - major 085.2

Infection, infected, infective — *continued*
- Leptosphaeria senegalensis 117.4
- leptospira (*see also* Leptospirosis) 100.9
  - Australis 100.89
  - Bataviae 100.89
  - pyrogenes 100.89
  - specified type NEC 100.89
- leptospirochetal NEC (*see also* Leptospirosis) 100.9
- Leptothrix — *see* Actinomycosis
- Listeria monocytogenes (listeriosis) 027.0
  - congenital 771.2
- liver fluke — *see* Infestation, fluke, liver
- Loa loa 125.2
  - eyelid 125.2 [373.6]
- Loboa loboi 116.2
- local, skin (staphylococcal) (streptococcal) NEC 686.9
  - abscess — *see* Abscess, by site
  - cellulitis — *see* Cellulitis, by site
  - ulcer (*see also* Ulcer, skin) 707.9
- Loefflerella
  - mallei 024
  - whitmori 025
- lung 518.89
  - atypical Mycobacterium 031.0
    - tuberculous (*see also* Tuberculosis, pulmonary) 011.9 ▲5ᵗʰ
  - basilar 518.89
  - chronic 518.89
  - fungus NEC 117.9
  - spirochetal 104.8
  - virus — *see* Pneumonia, virus
- lymph gland (axillary) (cervical) (inguinal) 683
  - mesenteric 289.2
- lymphoid tissue, base of tongue or posterior pharynx, NEC 474.00
- madurella
  - grisea 117.4
  - mycetomii 117.4
- major
  - with
    - abortion — *see* Abortion, by type, with sepsis
    - ectopic pregnancy (*see also* categories 633.0-633.9) 639.0
    - molar pregnancy (*see also* categories 630-632) 639.0
  - following
    - abortion 639.0
    - ectopic or molar pregnancy 639.0
  - puerperal, postpartum, childbirth 670 ▲4ᵗʰ
- Malassezia furfur 111.0
- Malleomyces
  - mallei 024
  - pseudomallei 025
- mammary gland 611.0
  - puerperal, postpartum 675.2 ▲5ᵗʰ
- Mansonella (ozzardi) 125.5
- mastoid (suppurative) — *see* Mastoiditis
- maxilla, maxillary 526.4
  - sinus (chronic) (*see also* Sinusitis, maxillary) 473.0
- mediastinum 519.2
- medina 125.7
- meibomian
  - cyst 373.12
  - gland 373.12
- melioidosis 025
- meninges (*see also* Meningitis) 320.9

Infection, infected, infective — continued
  meningococcal (see also condition) 036.9
    brain 036.1
    cerebrospinal 036.0
    endocardium 036.42
    generalized 036.2
    meninges 036.0
    meningococcemia 036.2
    specified site NEC 036.89
  mesenteric lymph nodes or glands NEC 289.2
  Metagonimus 121.5
  metatarsophalangeal 711.97
  microorganism resistant to drugs — see Resistance (to), drugs by microorganisms
  Microsporidia 136.8
  microsporum, microsporic — see Dermatophytosis
  Mima polymorpha NEC 041.85
  mixed flora NEC 041.89
  Monilia (see also Candidiasis) 112.9
    neonatal 771.7
  Monosporium apiospermum 117.6
  mouth (focus) NEC 528.9
    parasitic 112.0
  Mucor 117.7
  muscle NEC 728.89
  mycelium NEC 117.9
  mycetoma
    actinomycotic NEC (see also Actinomycosis) 039.9
    mycotic NEC 117.4
  Mycobacterium, mycobacterial (see also Mycobacterium) 031.9
  mycoplasma NEC 041.81
  mycotic NEC 117.9
    pathogenic to compromised host only 118
    skin NEC 111.9
    systemic 117.9
  myocardium NEC 422.90
  nail (chronic) (with lymphangitis) 681.9
    finger 681.02
      fungus 110.1
      ingrowing 703.0
    toe 681.11
      fungus 110.1
  nasal sinus (chronic) (see also Sinusitis) 473.9
  nasopharynx (chronic) 478.29
    acute 460
  navel 686.9
    newborn 771.4
  Neisserian — see Gonococcus
  Neotestudina rosatii 117.4
  newborn, generalized 771.89 ▲
  nipple 611.0
    puerperal, postpartum 675.0
      with breast 675.9
        specified type NEC 675.8
  Nocardia — see Actinomycosis
  nose 478.1
  nostril 478.1
  obstetrical surgical wound 674.3
  Oesophagostomum (apiostomum) 127.7
  Oestrus ovis 134.0
  Oidium albicans (see also Candidiasis) 112.9
  Onchocerca (volvulus) 125.3
    eye 125.3 [360.13]
    eyelid 125.3 [373.6]
  operation wound 998.59
  Opisthorchis (felineus) (tenuicollis) (viverrini) 121.0

Infection, infected, infective — continued
  orbit 376.00
    chronic 376.10
  ovary (see also Salpingo-oophoritis) 614.2
  Oxyuris vermicularis 127.4
  pancreas 577.0
  Paracoccidioides brasiliensis 116.1
  Paragonimus (westermani) 121.2
  parainfluenza virus 079.89
  parameningococcus NEC 036.9
    with meningitis 036.0
  parasitic NEC 136.9
  paratyphoid 002.9
    Type A 002.1
    Type B 002.2
    Type C 002.3
  paraurethral ducts 597.89
  parotid gland 527.2
  Pasteurella NEC 027.2
    multocida (cat-bite) (dog-bite) 027.2
    pestis (see also Plague) 020.9
    pseudotuberculosis 027.2
    septica (cat-bite) (dog-bite) 027.2
    tularensis (see also Tularemia) 021.9
  pelvic, female (see also Disease, pelvis, inflammatory) 614.9
  penis (glans) (retention) NEC 607.2
    herpetic 054.13
  Peptococcus 041.84
  Peptostreptococcus 041.84
  periapical (pulpal origin) 522.4
  peridental 523.3
  perineal wound (obstetrical) 674.3
  periodontal 523.3
  periorbital 376.00
    chronic 376.10
  perirectal 569.49
  perirenal (see also Infection, kidney) 590.9
  peritoneal (see also Peritonitis) 567.9
  periureteral 593.89
  periurethral 597.89
  Petriellidium boydii 117.6
  pharynx 478.29
    Coxsackievirus 074.0
    phlegmonous 462
    posterior, lymphoid 474.00
  Phialophora
    gougerotii 117.8
    jeanselmei 117.8
    verrucosa 117.2
  Piedraia hortai 111.3
  pinna, acute 380.11
  pinta 103.9
    intermediate 103.1
    late 103.2
    mixed 103.3
    primary 103.0
  pinworm 127.4
  pityrosporum furfur 111.0
  pleuropneumonia-like organisms NEC (PPLO) 041.81
  pneumococcal NEC 041.2
    generalized (purulent) 038.2
  Pneumococcus NEC 041.2
  postoperative wound 998.59
  posttraumatic NEC 958.3
  postvaccinal 999.3
  prepuce NEC 607.1
  Proprionibacterium 041.84
  prostate (capsule) (see also Prostatitis) 601.9

Infection, infected, infective — continued
   Proteus (mirabilis) (morganii) (vulgaris) NEC 041.6
      enteritis 008.3
   protozoal NEC 136.8
      intestinal NEC 007.9
   Pseudomonas NEC 041.7
      mallei 024
      pneumonia 482.1
      pseudomallei 025
   psittacosis 073.9
   puerperal, postpartum (major) 670 ✓4ᵗʰ
      minor 646.6 ✓5ᵗʰ
   pulmonary — see Infection, lung
   purulent — see Abscess
   putrid, generalized — see Septicemia
   pyemic — see Septicemia
   Pyrenochaeta romeroi 117.4
   Q fever 083.0
   rabies 071
   rectum (sphincter) 569.49
   renal (see also Infection, kidney) 590.9
      pelvis and ureter 590.3
   resistant to drugs — see Resistance (to), drugs by microorganisms
   respiratory 519.8
      chronic 519.8
      influenzal (acute) (upper) 487.1
      lung 518.89
      rhinovirus 460
      syncytial virus 079.6
      upper (acute) (infectious) NEC 465.9
         with flu, grippe, or influenza 487.1
            influenzal 487.1
         multiple sites NEC 465.8
         streptococcal 034.0
         viral NEC 465.9
   respiratory syncytial virus (RSV) 079.6
   resulting from presence of shunt or other internal prosthetic device — see Complications, infection and inflammation, due to (presence of) any device, implant, or graft classified to 996.0-996.5 NEC
   retrovirus 079.50
      human immunodeficiency virus type 2 [HIV 2] 079.53
      human T-cell lymphotrophic virus type I [HTLV-I] 079.51
      human T-cell lymphotrophic virus type II [HTLV-II] 079.52
      specified NEC 079.59
   Rhinocladium 117.1
   Rhinosporidium (seeberi) 117.0
   rhinovirus
      in diseases classified elsewhere — see category 079 ✓4ᵗʰ
      unspecified nature or site 079.3
   Rhizopus 117.7
   rickettsial 083.9
   rickettsialpox 083.2
   rubella (see also Rubella) 056.9
      congenital 771.0
   Saccharomyces (see also Candidiasis) 112.9
   Saksenaea 117.7
   salivary duct or gland (any) 527.2
   Salmonella (aertrycke) (callinarum) (choleraesuis) (enteritidis) (suipestifer) (typhimurium) 003.9
      with
         arthritis 003.23
         gastroenteritis 003.0

Infection, infected, infective — continued
   Salmonella — continued
      with — continued
         localized infection 003.20
            specified type NEC 003.29
         meningitis 003.21
         osteomyelitis 003.24
         pneumonia 003.22
         septicemia 003.1
         specified manifestation NEC 003.8
      congenital 771.89 ▲
      due to food (poisoning) (any serotype) (see also Poisoning, food, due to, Salmonella)
      hirschfeldii 002.3
      localized 003.20
         specified type NEC 003.29
      paratyphi 002.9
         A 002.1
         B 002.2
         C 002.3
      schottmuelleri 002.2
      specified type NEC 003.8
      typhi 002.0
      typhosa 002.0
   saprophytic 136.8
   Sarcocystis, lindemanni 136.5
   scabies 133.0
   Schistosoma — see Infestation, Schistosoma
   Schmorl's bacillus 040.3
   scratch or other superficial injury — see Injury, superficial, by site
   scrotum (acute) NEC 608.4
   secondary, burn or open wound (dislocation) (fracture) 958.3
   seminal vesicle (see also Vesiculitis) 608.0
   septic
      generalized — see Septicemia
      localized, skin (see also Abscess) 682.9
   septicemic — see Septicemia
   seroma 998.51
   Serratia (marcescens) 041.85
      generalized 038.44
   sheep liver fluke 121.3
   Shigella 004.9
      boydii 004.2
      dysenteriae 004.0
      flexneri 004.1
      group
         A 004.0
         B 004.1
         C 004.2
         D 004.3
      Schmitz (-Stutzer) 004.0
      schmitzii 004.0
      shiga 004.0
      sonnei 004.3
      specified type NEC 004.8
   Sin Nombre virus 079.81
   sinus (see also Sinusitis) 473.9
      pilonidal 685.1
         with abscess 685.0
      skin NEC 686.9
   Skene's duct or gland (see also Urethritis) 597.89
   skin (local) (staphylococcal) (streptococcal) NEC 686.9
      abscess — see Abscess, by site
      cellulitis — see Cellulitis, by site
      due to fungus 111.9
         specified type NEC 111.8

Infection, infected, infective — continued
  skin — continued
    mycotic 111.9
      specified type NEC 111.8
    ulcer (see also Ulcer, skin) 707.9
  slow virus 046.9
    specified condition NEC 046.8
  Sparganum (mansoni) (proliferum) 123.5
  spermatic cord NEC 608.4
  sphenoidal (chronic) (sinus) (see also
      Sinusitis, sphenoidal 473.3)
  Spherophorus necrophorus 040.3
  spinal cord NEC (see also Encephalitis) 323.9
    abscess 324.1
      late effect — see category 326
    late effect — see category 326
    meninges — see Meningitis
    streptococcal 320.2
  Spirillum
    minus or minor 026.0
    morsus muris 026.0
    obermeieri 087.0
  spirochetal NEC 104.9
    lung 104.8
    specified nature or site NEC 104.8
  spleen 289.59
  Sporothrix schenckii 117.1
  Sporotrichum (schenckii) 117.1
  Sporozoa 136.8
  staphylococcal NEC 041.10
    aureus 041.11
    food poisoning 005.0
    generalized (purulent) 038.10
      aureus 038.11
      specified organism NEC 038.19
    pneumonia 482.40
      aureus 482.41
      specified type NEC 482.49
    septicemia 038.10
      aureus 038.11
      specified organism NEC 038.19
    specified NEC 041.19
  steatoma 706.2
  Stellantchasmus falcatus 121.6
  Streptobacillus moniliformis 026.1
  streptococcal NEC 041.00
    congenital 771.89 ▲
    generalized (purulent) 038.0
    Group
      A 041.01
      B 041.02
      C 041.03
      D [enterococcus] 041.04
      G 041.05
    pneumonia — see Pneumonia,
        streptococcal 482.3 ✓5ᵗʰ
    septicemia 038.0
    sore throat 034.0
    specified NEC 041.09
  Streptomyces — see Actinomycosis
  streptotrichosis — see Actinomycosis
  Strongyloides (stercoralis) 127.2
  stump (amputation) (posttraumatic) (surgical)
      997.62
    traumatic — see Amputation, traumatic, by
        site, complicated
  subcutaneous tissue, local NEC 686.9
  submaxillary region 528.9
  suipestifer (see also Infection, Salmonella)
      003.9
  swimming pool bacillus 031.1

Infection, infected, infective — continued
  syphilitic — see Syphilis
  systemic — see Septicemia
  Taenia — see Infestation, Taenia
  Taeniarhynchus saginatus 123.2
  tapeworm — see Infestation, tapeworm
  tendon (sheath) 727.89
  Ternidens diminutus 127.7
  testis (see also Orchitis) 604.90
  thigh (skin) 686.9
  threadworm 127.4
  throat 478.29
    pneumococcal 462
    staphylococcal 462
    streptococcal 034.0
    viral NEC (see also Pharyngitis) 462
  thumb (skin) 686.9
    abscess (with lymphangitis) 681.00
      pulp 681.01
    cellulitis (with lymphangitis) 681.00
    nail 681.02
  thyroglossal duct 529.8
  toe (skin) 686.9
    abscess (with lymphangitis) 681.10
    cellulitis (with lymphangitis) 681.10
    nail 681.11
      fungus 110.1
  tongue NEC 529.0
    parasitic 112.0
  tonsil (faucial) (lingual) (pharyngeal) 474.00
    acute or subacute 463
    and adenoid 474.02
    tag 474.00
  tooth, teeth 522.4
    periapical (pulpal origin) 522.4
    peridental 523.3
    periodontal 523.3
    pulp 522.0
    socket 526.5
  Torula histolytica 117.5
  Toxocara (cani) (cati) (felis) 128.0
  Toxoplasma gondii (see also Toxoplasmosis)
      130.9
  trachea, chronic 491.8
    fungus 117.9
  traumatic NEC 958.3
  trematode NEC 121.9
  trench fever 083.1
  Treponema
    denticola 041.84
    macrodenticum 041.84
    pallidum (see also Syphillis) 097.9
  Trichinella (spiralis) 124
  Trichomonas 131.9
    bladder 131.09
    cervix 131.09
    hominis 007.3
    intestine 007.3
    prostate 131.03
    specified site NEC 131.8
    urethra 131.02
    urogenitalis 131.00
    vagina 131.01
    vulva 131.01
  Trichophyton, trichophytid — see
      Dermatophytosis
  Trichosporon (beigelii) cutaneum 111.2
  Trichostrongylus 127.6
  Trichuris (trichiuria) 127.3
  Trombicula (irritans) 133.8

Infection, infected, infective — *continued*
　Trypanosoma (*see also* Trypanosomiasis) 086.9
　　cruzi 086.2
　tubal (*see also* Salpingo-oophoritis) 614.2
　tuberculous NEC (*see also* Tuberculosis) 011.9 ✓5ᵗʰ
　tubo-ovarian (*see also* Salpingo-oophoritis) 614.2
　tunica vaginalis 608.4
　tympanic membrane — *see* Myringitis
　typhoid (abortive) (ambulant) (bacillus) 002.0
　typhus 081.9
　　flea-borne (endemic) 081.0
　　louse-borne (epidemic) 080
　　mite-borne 081.2
　　recrudescent 081.1
　　tick-borne 082.9
　　　African 082.1
　　　North Asian 082.2
　umbilicus (septic) 686.9
　　newborn NEC 771.4
　ureter 593.89
　urethra (*see also* Urethritis) 597.80
　urinary (tract) NEC 599.0
　　with
　　　abortion — *see* Abortion, by type, with urinary tract infection
　　　ectopic pregnancy (*see also* categories 633.0-633.9) 639.8
　　　molar pregnancy (*see also* categories 630-632) 639.8
　　candidal 112.2
　　complicating pregnancy, childbirth, or puerperium 646.6 ✓5ᵗʰ
　　　affecting fetus or newborn 760.1
　　　asymptomatic 646.5 ✓5ᵗʰ
　　　　affecting fetus or newborn 760.1
　　diplococcal (acute) 098.0
　　　chronic 098.2
　　due to Trichomonas (vaginalis) 131.00
　　following
　　　abortion 639.8
　　　ectopic or molar pregnancy 639.8
　　gonococcal (acute) 098.0
　　　chronic or duration of 2 months or over 098.2
　　newborn 771.82　▲
　　trichomonal 131.00
　　tuberculous (*see also* Tuberculosis) 016.3 ✓5ᵗʰ
　　uterus, uterine (*see also* Endometritis) 615.9
　　utriculus masculinus NEC 597.89
　vaccination 999.3
　vagina (granulation tissue) (wall) (*see also* Vaginitis) 616.10
　varicella 052.9
　varicose veins — *see* Varicose, veins
　variola 050.9
　　major 050.0
　　minor 050.1
　vas deferens NEC 608.4
　Veillonella 041.84
　verumontanum 597.89
　vesical (*see also* Cystitis) 595.9
　Vibrio
　　cholerae 001.0
　　　El Tor 001.1
　　parahaemolyticus (food poisoning) 005.4
　　vulnificus 041.85

Infection, infected, infective — *continued*
　urinary NEC — *continued*
　　Vincent's (gums) (mouth) (tonsil) 101
　virus, viral 079.99
　　adenovirus
　　　in diseases classified elsewhere — *see* category 079 ✓4ᵗʰ
　　　unspecified nature or site 079.0
　　central nervous system NEC 049.9
　　　enterovirus 048
　　　　meningitis 047.9
　　　　　specified type NEC 047.8
　　　slow virus 046.9
　　　　specified condition NEC 046.8
　　chest 519.8
　　conjunctivitis 077.99
　　　specified type NEC 077.8
　　Coxsackie (*see also* Infection, Coxsackie) 079.2
　　Ebola 065.8
　　ECHO
　　　in diseases classified elsewhere — *see* category 079 ✓4ᵗʰ
　　　unspecified nature or site 079.1
　　encephalitis 049.9
　　　arthropod-borne NEC 064
　　　tick-borne 063.9
　　　　specified type NEC 063.8
　　enteritis NEC (*see also* Enteritis, viral) 008.8
　　exanthem NEC 057.9
　　Hantavirus 079.81
　　human papilloma 079.4
　　　in diseases classified elsewhere — *see* category 079 ✓4ᵗʰ
　　intestine (*see also* Enteritis, viral) 008.8
　　lung — *see* Pneumonia, viral
　　respiratory syncytial (RSV) 079.6
　　retrovirus 079.50
　　rhinovirus
　　　in diseases classified elsewhere — *see* category 079 ✓4ᵗʰ
　　　unspecified nature or site 079.3
　　salivary gland disease 078.5
　　slow 046.9
　　　specified condition NEC 046.8
　　specified type NEC 079.89
　　　in diseases classified elsewhere — *see* category 079 ✓4ᵗʰ
　　unspecified nature or site 079.99
　warts NEC 078.10
　vulva (*see also* Vulvitis) 616.10
　whipworm 127.3
　Whitmore's bacillus 025
　wound (local) (posttraumatic) NEC 958.3
　　with
　　　dislocation — *see* Dislocation, by site, open
　　　fracture — *see* Fracture, by site, open
　　　open wound — *see* Wound, open, by site, complicated
　　postoperative 998.59
　　surgical 998.59
　Wuchereria 125.0
　　bancrofti 125.0
　　malayi 125.1
　yaws — *see* Yaws
　yeast (*see also* Candidiasis) 112.9
　yellow fever (*see also* Fever, yellow) 060.9
　Yersinia pestis (*see also* Plague) 020.9
　Zeis' gland 373.12

Infection, infected, infective — *continued*
  zoonotic bacterial NEC 027.9
  Zopfia senegalensis 117.4
Infective, infectious — *see* condition
Inferiority complex 301.9
  constitutional psychopathic 301.9
Infertility
  female 628.9
    associated with
      adhesions, peritubal 614.6 *[628.2]*
      anomaly
        cervical mucus 628.4
        congenital
          cervix 628.4
          fallopian tube 628.2
          uterus 628.3
          vagina 628.4
      anovulation 628.0
      dysmucorrhea 628.4
      endometritis, tuberculous (*see also*
          Tuberculosis) 016.7 ✓5ᵗʰ *[628.3]*
      Stein-Leventhal syndrome 256.4 *[628.0]*
    due to
      adiposogenital dystrophy 253.8 *[628.1]*
      anterior pituitary disorder NEC 253.4
          [628.1]
        hyperfunction 253.1 *[628.1]*
      cervical anomaly 628.4
      fallopian tube anomaly 628.2
      ovarian failure 256.39 *[628.0]*
      Stein-Leventhal syndrome 256.4 *[628.0]*
      uterine anomaly 628.3
      vaginal anomaly 628.4
    nonimplantation 628.3
    origin
      cervical 628.4
      pituitary-hypothalamus NEC 253.8
          [628.1]
        anterior pituitary NEC 253.4 *[628.1]*
          hyperfunction NEC 253.1 *[628.1]*
        dwarfism 253.3 *[628.1]*
        panhypopituitarism 253.2 *[628.1]*
      specified NEC 628.8
      tubal (block) (occlusion) (stenosis) 628.2
        adhesions 614.6 *[628.2]*
        uterine 628.3
        vaginal 628.4
    previous, requiring supervision of
        pregnancy V23.0
  male 606.9
    absolute 606.0
    due to
      azoospermia 606.0
      drug therapy 606.8
      extratesticular cause NEC 606.8
      germinal cell
        aplasia 606.0
        desquamation 606.1
      hypospermatogenesis 606.1
      infection 606.8
      obstruction, afferent ducts 606.8
      oligospermia 606.1
      radiation 606.8
      spermatogenic arrest (complete) 606.0
        incomplete 606.1
      systemic disease 606.8
Infestation 134.9
  Acanthocheilonema (perstans) 125.4
    streptocerca 125.6
  Acariasis 133.9
    demodex folliculorum 133.8

Infestation — *continued*
  Acariasis — *continued*
    Sarcoptes scabiei 133.0
    trombiculae 133.8
  Agamofilaria streptocerca 125.6
  Ancylostoma, Ankylostoma 126.9
    americanum 126.1
    braziliense 126.2
    canium 126.8
    ceylanicum 126.3
    duodenale 126.0
    new world 126.1
    old world 126.0
  Angiostrongylus cantonensis 128.8
  anisakiasis 127.1
  Anisakis larva 127.1
  arthropod NEC 134.1
  Ascaris lumbricoides 127.0
  Bacillus fusiformis 101
  Balantidium coli 007.0
  beef tapeworm 123.2
  Bothriocephalus (latus) 123.4
    larval 123.5
  broad tapeworm 123.4
    larval 123.5
  Brugia malayi 125.1
  Candiru 136.8
  Capillaria
    hepatica 128.8
    philippinensis 127.5
  cat liver fluke 121.0
  Cercomonas hominis (intestinal) 007.3
  cestodes 123.9
    specified type NEC 123.8
  chigger 133.8
  chigoe 134.1
  Chilomastix 007.8
  Clonorchis (sinensis) (liver) 121.1
  coccidia 007.2
  complicating pregnancy, childbirth, or
      puerperium 647.9 ✓5ᵗʰ
    affecting fetus or newborn 760.8
  Cysticercus cellulosae 123.1
  Demodex folliculorum 133.8
  Dermatobia (hominis) 134.0
  Dibothriocephalus (latus) 123.4
    larval 123.5
  Dicrocoelium dendriticum 121.8
  Diphyllobothrium (adult) (intestinal) (latum)
      (pacificum) 123.4
    larval 123.5
  Diplogonoporus (grandis) 123.8
  Dipylidium (caninum) 123.8
  Distoma hepaticum 121.3
  dog tapeworm 123.8
  Dracunculus medinensis 125.7
  dragon worm 125.7
  dwarf tapeworm 123.6
  Echinococcus (*see also* Echinococcus) 122.9
  Echinostoma ilocanum 121.8
  Embadomonas 007.8
  Endamoeba (histolytica) — *see* Infection,
      ameba
  Entamoeba (histolytica) — *see* Infection,
      ameba
  Enterobius vermicularis 127.4
  Epidermophyton — *see* Dermatophytosis
  eyeworm 125.2
  Fasciola
    gigantica 121.3
    hepatica 121.3

Index to Diseases

Infestation — *continued*
Fasciolopsis (buski) (small intestine) 121.4
  filarial 125.9
    due to
      Acanthocheilonema (perstans) 125.4
        streptocerca 125.6
      Brugia (Wuchereria) malayi 125.1
      Dracunculus medinensis 125.7
      guinea worms 125.7
      Mansonella (ozzardi) 125.5
      Onchocerca volvulus 125.3
        eye 125.3 *[360.13]*
        eyelid 125.3 *[373.6]*
      Wuchereria (bancrofti) 125.0
        malayi 125.1
  specified type NEC 125.6
fish tapeworm 123.4
  larval 123.5
fluke 121.9
  blood NEC (*see also* Schistosomiasis) 120.9
  cat liver 121.0
  intestinal (giant) 121.4
  liver (sheep) 121.3
    cat 121.0
    Chinese 121.1
    clonorchiasis 121.1
    fascioliasis 121.3
    Oriental 121.1
  lung (oriental) 121.2
  sheep liver 121.3
fly larva 134.0
Gasterophilus (intestinalis) 134.0
Gastrodiscoides hominis 121.8
Giardia lamblia 007.1
Gnathostoma (spinigerum) 128.1
Gongylonema 125.6
guinea worm 125.7
helminth NEC 128.9
  intestinal 127.9
    mixed (types classifiable to more than
      one category in 120.0-127.7) 127.8
    specified type NEC 127.7
  specified type NEC 128.8
Heterophyes heterophyes (small intestine)
    121.6
hookworm (*see also* Infestation, ancylostoma)
    126.9
Hymenolepis (diminuta) (nana) 123.6
intestinal NEC 129
leeches (aquatic) (land) 134.2
Leishmania — *see* Leishmaniasis
lice (*see also* Infestation, pediculus) 132.9
Linguatulidae, linguatula (pentastoma)
    (serrata) 134.1
Loa loa 125.2
  eyelid 125.2 *[373.6]*
louse (*see also* Infestation, pediculus) 132.9
  body 132.1
  head 132.0
  pubic 132.2
maggots 134.0
Mansonella (ozzardi) 125.5
medina 125.7
Metagonimus yokogawai (small intestine)
    121.5
Microfilaria streptocerca 125.3
  eye 125.3 *[360.13]*
  eyelid 125.3 *[373.6]*
Microsporon furfur 111.0
microsporum — *see* Dermatophytosis

Infestation — *continued*
mites 133.9
  scabic 133.0
  specified type NEC 133.8
Monilia (albicans) (*see also* Candidiasis) 112.9
  vagina 112.1
  vulva 112.1
  mouth 112.0
Necator americanus 126.1
nematode (intestinal) 127.9
  Ancylostoma (*see also* Ancylostoma) 126.9
  Ascaris lumbricoides 127.0
  conjunctiva NEC 128.9
  Dioctophyma 128.8
  Enterobius vermicularis 127.4
  Gnathostoma spinigerum 128.1
  Oesophagostomum (apiostomum) 127.7
  Physaloptera 127.4
  specified type NEC 127.7
  Strongyloides stercoralis 127.2
  Ternidens diminutus 127.7
  Trichinella spiralis 124
  Trichostrongylus 127.6
  Trichuris (trichiuria) 127.3
Oesophagostomum (apiostomum) 127.7
Oestrus ovis 134.0
Onchocerca (volvulus) 125.3
  eye 125.3 *[360.13]*
  eyelid 125.3 *[373.6]*
Opisthorchis (felineus) (tenuicollis) (viverrini)
    121.0
Oxyuris vermicularis 127.4
Paragonimus (westermani) 121.2
parasite, parasitic NEC 136.9
  eyelid 134.9 *[373.6]*
  intestinal 129
  mouth 112.0
  orbit 376.13
  skin 134.9
  tongue 112.0
pediculus 132.9
  capitis (humanus) (any site) 132.0
  corporis (humanus) (any site) 132.1
  eyelid 132.0 *[373.6]*
  mixed (classifiable to more than one
    category in 132.0-132.2) 132.3
  pubis (any site) 132.2
phthirus (pubis) (any site) 132.2
  with any infestation classifiable to 132.0,
    132.1 and 132.3
pinworm 127.4
pork tapeworm (adult) 123.0
protozoal NEC 136.8
pubic louse 132.2
rat tapeworm 123.6
red bug 133.8
roundworm (large) NEC 127.0
sand flea 134.1
saprophytic NEC 136.8
Sarcoptes scabiei 133.0
scabies 133.0
Schistosoma 120.9
  bovis 120.8
  cercariae 120.3
  hematobium 120.0
  intercalatum 120.8
  japonicum 120.2
  mansoni 120.1
  mattheii 120.8
  specified
    site — *see* Schistosomiasis

Infestation — *continued*
  Schistosoma — *continued*
    specified — *continued*
      type NEC 120.8
      spindale 120.8
  screw worms 134.0
  skin NEC 134.9
  Sparganum (mansoni) (proliferum) 123.5
    larval 123.5
  specified type NEC 134.8
  Spirometra larvae 123.5
  Sporozoa NEC 136.8
  Stellantchasmus falcatus 121.6
  Strongyloides 127.2
  Strongylus (gibsoni) 127.7
  Taenia 123.3
    diminuta 123.6
    Echinococcus (*see also* Echinococcus) 122.9
    mediocanellata 123.2
    nana 123.6
    saginata (mediocanellata) 123.2
    solium (intestinal form) 123.0
      larval form 123.1
  Taeniarhynchus saginatus 123.2
  tapeworm 123.9
    beef 123.2
    broad 123.4
      larval 123.5
    dog 123.8
    dwarf 123.6
    fish 123.4
      larval 123.5
    pork 123.0
    rat 123.6
  Ternidens diminutus 127.7
  Tetranychus molestissimus 133.8
  threadworm 127.4
  tongue 112.0
  Toxocara (cani) (cati) (felis) 128.0
  trematode(s) NEC 121.9
  Trichina spiralis 124
  Trichinella spiralis 124
  Trichocephalus 127.3
  Trichomonas 131.9
    bladder 131.09
    cervix 131.09
    intestine 007.3
    prostate 131.03
    specified site NEC 131.8
    urethra (female) (male) 131.02
    urogenital 131.00
    vagina 131.01
    vulva 131.01
  Trichophyton — *see* Dermatophytosis
  Trichostrongylus instabilis 127.6
  Trichuris (trichiuria) 127.3
  Trombicula (irritans) 133.8
  Trypanosoma — *see* Trypanosomiasis
  Tunga penetrans 134.1
  Uncinaria americana 126.1
  whipworm 127.3
  worms NEC 128.9
    intestinal 127.9
  Wuchereria 125.0
    bancrofti 125.0
    malayi 125.1
Infiltrate, infiltration
  with an iron compound 275.0
  amyloid (any site) (generalized) 277.3

Infiltrate, infiltration — *continued*
  calcareous (muscle) NEC 275.49
    localized — *see* Degeneration, by site
  calcium salt (muscle) 275.49
  corneal (*see also* Edema, cornea) 371.20
  eyelid 373.9
  fatty (diffuse) (generalized) 272.8
    localized — *see* Degeneration, by site, fatty
  glycogen, glycogenic (*see also* Disease, glycogen storage) 271.0
  heart, cardiac
    fatty (*see also* Degeneration, myocardial) 429.1
    glycogenic 271.0 [425.7]
  inflammatory in vitreous 379.29
  kidney (*see also* Disease, renal) 593.9
  leukemic (M9800/3) — *see* Leukemia
  liver 573.8
    fatty — *see* Fatty, liver
    glycogen (*see also* Disease, glycogen storage) 271.0
  lung (*see also* Infiltrate, pulmonary) 518.3
    eosinophilic 518.3
    x-ray finding only 793.1
  lymphatic (*see also* Leukemia, lymphatic) 204.9
    gland, pigmentary 289.3
  muscle, fatty 728.9
  myelogenous (*see also* Leukemia, myeloid) 205.9
  myocardium, myocardial
    fatty (*see also* Degeneration, myocardial) 429.1
    glycogenic 271.0 [425.7]
  pulmonary 518.3
    with
      eosinophilia 518.3
      pneumonia — *see* Pneumonia, by type
    x-ray finding only 793.1
  Ranke's primary (*see also* Tuberculosis) 010.0
  skin, lymphocytic (benign) 709.8
  thymus (gland) (fatty) 254.8
  urine 788.8
  vitreous humor 379.29
Infirmity 799.8
  senile 797
Inflammation, inflamed, inflammatory (with exudation)
  abducens (nerve) 378.54
  accessory sinus (chronic) (*see also* Sinusitis) 473.9
  adrenal (gland) 255.8
  alimentary canal — *see* Enteritis
  alveoli (teeth) 526.5
    scorbutic 267
  amnion — *see* Amnionitis
  anal canal 569.49
  antrum (chronic) (*see also* Sinusitis, maxillary) 473.0
  anus 569.49
  appendix (*see also* Appendicitis) 541
  arachnoid — *see* Meningitis
  areola 611.0
    puerperal, postpartum 675.0
  areolar tissue NEC 686.9
  artery — *see* Arteritis
  auditory meatus (external) (*see also* Otitis, externa) 380.10
  Bartholin's gland 616.8
  bile duct or passage 576.1

Index to Diseases

Inflammation, inflamed, inflammatory — *continued*
  bladder (*see also* Cystitis) 595.9
  bone — *see* Osteomyelitis
  bowel (*see also* Enteritis) 558.9
  brain (*see also* Encephalitis) 323.9
    late effect — *see* category 326
    membrane — *see* Meningitis
  breast 611.0
    puerperal, postpartum 675.2 ✓5ᵗʰ
  broad ligament (*see also* Disease, pelvis, inflammatory) 614.4
    acute 614.3
  bronchus — *see* Bronchitis
  bursa — *see* Bursitis
  capsule
    liver 573.3
    spleen 289.59
  catarrhal (*see also* Catarrh) 460
    vagina 616.10
  cecum (*see also* Appendicitis) 541
  cerebral (*see also* Encephalitis) 323.9
    late effect — *see* category 326
    membrane — *see* Meningitis
  cerebrospinal (*see also* Meningitis) 322.9
    late effect — *see* category 326
    meningococcal 036.0
    tuberculous (*see also* Tuberculosis) 013.6 ✓5ᵗʰ
  cervix (uteri) (*see also* Cervicitis) 616.0
  chest 519.9
  choroid NEC (*see also* Choroiditis) 363.20
  cicatrix (tissue) — *see* Cicatrix
  colon (*see also* Enteritis) 558.9
    granulomatous 555.1
    newborn 558.9
  connective tissue (diffuse) NEC 728.9
  cornea (*see also* Keratitis) 370.9
    with ulcer (*see also* Ulcer, cornea) 370.00
  corpora cavernosa (penis) 607.2
  cranial nerve — *see* Disorder, nerve, cranial
  diarrhea — *see* Diarrhea
  disc (intervertebral) (space) 722.90
    cervical, cervicothoracic 722.91
    lumbar, lumbosacral 722.93
    thoracic, thoracolumbar 722.92
  Douglas' cul-de-sac or pouch (chronic) (*see also* Disease, pelvis, inflammatory) 614.4
    acute 614.3
  due to (presence of) any device, implant, or graft classifiable to 996.0-996.5 — *see* Complications, infection and inflammation, due to (presence of) any device, implant, or graft classified to 996.0-996.5 NEC
  duodenum 535.6 ✓5ᵗʰ
  dura mater — *see* Meningitis
  ear — *see also* Otitis
    external (*see also* Otitis, externa) 380.10
    inner (*see also* Labyrinthitis) 386.30
    middle — *see* Otitis media
  esophagus 530.10
  ethmoidal (chronic) (sinus) (*see also* Sinusitis, ethmoidal) 473.2
  Eustachian tube (catarrhal) 381.50
    acute 381.51
    chronic 381.52
  extrarectal 569.49
  eye 379.99
  eyelid 373.9
    specified NEC 373.8

Inflammation, inflamed, inflammatory — *continued*
  fallopian tube (*see also* Salpingo-oophoritis) 614.2
  fascia 728.9
  fetal membranes (acute) 658.4 ✓5ᵗʰ
    affecting fetus or newborn 762.7
  follicular, pharynx 472.1
  frontal (chronic) (sinus) (*see also* Sinusitis, frontal) 473.1
  gallbladder (*see also* Cholecystitis, acute) 575.0
  gall duct (*see also* Cholecystitis) 575.10
  gastrointestinal (*see also* Enteritis) 558.9
  genital organ (diffuse) (internal)
    female 614.9
      with
        abortion — *see* Abortion, by type, with sepsis
        ectopic pregnancy (*see also* categories 633.0-633.9) 639.0
        molar pregnancy (*see also* categories 630-632) 639.0
      complicating pregnancy, childbirth, or puerperium 646.6 ✓5ᵗʰ
        affecting fetus or newborn 760.8
      following
        abortion 639.0
        ectopic or molar pregnancy 639.0
    male 608.4
  gland (lymph) (*see also* Lymphadenitis) 289.3
  glottis (*see also* Laryngitis) 464.00
    with obstruction 464.01
  granular, pharynx 472.1
  gum 523.1
  heart (*see also* Carditis) 429.89
  hepatic duct 576.8
  hernial sac — *see* Hernia, by site
  ileum (*see also* Enteritis) 558.9
    terminal or regional 555.0
    with large intestine 555.2
  intervertebral disc 722.90
    cervical, cervicothoracic 722.91
    lumbar, lumbosacral 722.93
    thoracic, thoracolumbar 722.92
  intestine (*see also* Enteritis) 558.9
  jaw (acute) (bone) (chronic) (lower) (suppurative) (upper) 526.4
  jejunum — *see* Enteritis
  joint NEC (*see also* Arthritis) 716.9 ✓5ᵗʰ
    sacroiliac 720.2
  kidney (*see also* Nephritis) 583.9
  knee (joint) 716.66
    tuberculous (active) (*see also* Tuberculosis) 015.2 ✓5ᵗʰ
  labium (majus) (minus) (*see also* Vulvitis) 616.10
  lacrimal
    gland (*see also* Dacryoadenitis) 375.00
    passages (duct) (sac) (*see also* Dacryocystitis) 375.30
  larynx (*see also* Laryngitis) 464.00
    with obstruction 464.01
    diphtheritic 032.3
  leg NEC 686.9
  lip 528.5
  liver (capsule) (*see also* Hepatitis) 573.3
    acute 570
    chronic 571.40
    suppurative 572.0
  lung (acute) (*see also* Pneumonia) 486
    chronic (interstitial) 518.89

**Inflammation, inflamed, inflammatory — **
continued
lymphatic vessel (*see also* Lymphangitis) 457.2
lymph node or gland (*see also* Lymphadenitis) 289.3
mammary gland 611.0
   puerperal, postpartum 675.2 ✓5ᵗʰ
maxilla, maxillary 526.4
   sinus (chronic) (*see also* Sinusitis, maxillary) 473.0
membranes of brain or spinal cord — *see* Meningitis
meninges — *see* Meningitis
mouth 528.0
muscle 728.9
myocardium (*see also* Myocarditis) 429.0
nasal sinus (chronic) (*see also* Sinusitis) 473.9
nasopharynx — *see* Nasopharyngitis
navel 686.9
   newborn NEC 771.4
nerve NEC 729.2
nipple 611.0
   puerperal, postpartum 675.0 ✓5ᵗʰ
nose 478.1
   suppurative 472.0
oculomotor nerve 378.51
optic nerve 377.30
orbit (chronic) 376.10
   acute 376.00
   chronic 376.10
ovary (*see also* Salpingo-oophoritis) 614.2
oviduct (*see also* Salpingo-oophoritis) 614.2
pancreas — *see* Pancreatitis
parametrium (chronic) (*see also* Disease, pelvis, inflammatory) 614.4
   acute 614.3
parotid region 686.9
   gland 527.2
pelvis, female (*see also* Disease, pelvis, inflammatory) 614.9
penis (corpora cavernosa) 607.2
perianal 569.49
pericardium (*see also* Pericarditis) 423.9
perineum (female) (male) 686.9
perirectal 569.49
peritoneum (*see also* Peritonitis) 567.9
periuterine (*see also* Disease, pelvis, inflammatory) 614.9
perivesical (*see also* Cystitis) 595.9
petrous bone (*see also* Petrositis) 383.20
pharynx (*see also* Pharyngitis) 462
   follicular 472.1
   granular 472.1
pia mater — *see* Meningitis
pleura — *see* Pleurisy
postmastoidectomy cavity 383.30
   chronic 383.33
prostate (*see also* Prostatitis) 601.9
rectosigmoid — *see* Rectosigmoiditis
rectum (*see also* Proctitis) 569.49
respiratory, upper (*see also* Infection, respiratory, upper) 465.9
   chronic, due to external agent — *see* Condition, respiratory, chronic, due to, external agent
   due to
      fumes or vapors (chemical) (inhalation) 506.2
      radiation 508.1
retina (*see also* Retinitis) 363.20
retrocecal (*see also* Appendicitis) 541

**Inflammation, inflamed, inflammatory — **
continued
retroperitoneal (*see also* Peritonitis) 567.9
salivary duct or gland (any) (suppurative) 527.2
scorbutic, alveoli, teeth 267
scrotum 608.4
sigmoid — *see* Enteritis
sinus (*see also* Sinusitis) 473.9
Skene's duct or gland (*see also* Urethritis) 597.89
skin 686.9
spermatic cord 608.4
sphenoidal (sinus) (*see also* Sinusitis, sphenoidal) 473.3
spinal
   cord (*see also* Encephalitis) 323.9
      late effect — *see* category 326
   membrane — *see* Meningitis
   nerve — *see* Disorder, nerve
spine (*see also* Spondylitis) 720.9
spleen (capsule) 289.59
stomach — *see* Gastritis
stricture, rectum 569.49
subcutaneous tissue NEC 686.9
suprarenal (gland) 255.8
synovial (fringe) (membrane) — *see* Bursitis
tendon (sheath) NEC 726.90
testis (*see also* Orchitis) 604.90
thigh 686.9
throat (*see also* Sore throat) 462
thymus (gland) 254.8
thyroid (gland) (*see also* Thyroiditis) 245.9
tongue 529.0
tonsil — *see* Tonsillitis
trachea — *see* Tracheitis
trochlear nerve 378.53
tubal (*see also* Salpingo-oophoritis) 614.2
tuberculous NEC (*see also* Tuberculosis) 011.9 ✓5ᵗʰ
tubo-ovarian (*see also* Salpingo-oophoritis) 614.2
tunica vaginalis 608.4
tympanic membrane — *see* Myringitis
umbilicus, umbilical 686.9
   newborn NEC 771.4
uterine ligament (*see also* Disease, pelvis, inflammatory) 614.4
   acute 614.3
uterus (catarrhal) (*see also* Endometritis) 615.9
uveal tract (anterior) (*see also* Iridocyclitis) 364.3
   posterior — *see* Chorioretinitis
   sympathetic 360.11
vagina (*see also* Vaginitis) 616.10
vas deferens 608.4
vein (*see also* Phlebitis) 451.9
   thrombotic 451.9
      cerebral (*see also* Thrombosis, brain) 434.0 ✓5ᵗʰ
      leg 451.2
         deep (vessels) NEC 451.19
         superficial (vessels) 451.0
      lower extremity 451.2
         deep (vessels) NEC 451.19
         superficial (vessels) 451.0
vocal cord 478.5
vulva (*see also* Vulvitis) 616.10
Inflation, lung imperfect (newborn) 770.5

Influenza, influenzal 487.1
 with
  bronchitis 487.1
  bronchopneumonia 487.0
  cold (any type) 487.1
  digestive manifestations 487.8
  hemoptysis 487.1
  involvement of
   gastrointestinal tract 487.8
   nervous system 487.8
  laryngitis 487.1
  manifestations NEC 487.8
   respiratory 487.1
    pneumonia 487.0
  pharyngitis 487.1
  pneumonia (any form classifiable to 480-483, 485-486) 487.0
  respiratory manifestations NEC 487.1
  sinusitis 487.1
  sore throat 487.1
  tonsillitis 487.1
  tracheitis 487.1
  upper respiratory infection (acute) 487.1
 abdominal 487.8
 Asian 487.1
 bronchial 487.1
 bronchopneumonia 487.0
 catarrhal 487.1
 epidemic 487.1
 gastric 487.8
 intestinal 487.8
 laryngitis 487.1
 maternal affecting fetus or newborn 760.2
  manifest influenza in infant 771.2
 pharyngitis 487.1
 pneumonia (any form) 487.0
 respiratory (upper) 487.1
 stomach 487.8
 vaccination, prophylactic (against) V04.8
Influenza-like disease 487.1
Infraction, Freiberg's (metatarsal head) 732.5
Infusion complication, misadventure, or reaction — see Complication, infusion
Ingestion
 chemical — see Table of Drugs and Chemicals
 drug or medicinal substance
  overdose or wrong substance given or taken 977.9
   specified drug — see Table of Drugs and Chemicals
 foreign body NEC (see also Foreign body) 938
Ingrowing
 hair 704.8
 nail (finger) (toe) (infected) 703.0
Inguinal — see also condition
 testis 752.51
Inhalation
 carbon monoxide 986
 flame
  mouth 947.0
  lung 947.1
 food or foreign body (see also Asphyxia, food or foreign body) 933.1
 gas, fumes, or vapor (noxious) 987.9
  specified agent — see Table of Drugs and Chemicals
 liquid or vomitus (see also Asphyxia, food or foreign body) 933.1
  lower respiratory tract NEC 934.9
 meconium (fetus or newborn) 770.1

Inhalation — continued
 mucus (see also Asphyxia, mucus) 933.1
 oil (causing suffocation) (see also Asphyxia, food or foreign body) 933.1
 pneumonia — see Pneumonia, aspiration
 smoke 987.9
 steam 987.9
 stomach contents or secretions (see also Asphyxia, food or foreign body) 933.1
  in labor and delivery 668.0 ✓5ᵗʰ
Inhibition, inhibited
 academic as adjustment reaction 309.23
 orgasm
  female 302.73
  male 302.74
 sexual
  desire 302.71
  excitement 302.72
 work as adjustment reaction 309.23
Inhibitor, systemic lupus erythematosus (presence of) 286.5
Iniencephalus, iniencephaly 740.2
Injected eye 372.74
Injury 959.9

> Note — For abrasion, insect bite (nonvenomous), blister, or scratch, see Injury, superficial.
>
> For laceration, traumatic rupture, tear, or penetrating wound of internal organs, such as heart, lung, liver, kidney, pelvic organs, whether or not accompanied by open wound in the same region, see Injury, internal.
>
> For nerve injury, see Injury, nerve.
>
> For late effect of injuries classifiable to 850-854, 860-869, 900-919, 950-959, see Late, effect, injury, by type.

 abdomen, abdominal (viscera) — see also Injury, internal, abdomen
  muscle or wall 959.1
 acoustic, resulting in deafness 951.5
 adenoid 959.09
 adrenal (gland) — see Injury, internal, adrenal
 alveolar (process) 959.09
 ankle (and foot) (and knee) (and leg, except thigh) 959.7
 anterior chamber, eye 921.3
 anus 959.1
 aorta (thoracic) 901.0
  abdominal 902.0
 appendix — see Injury, internal, appendix
 arm, upper (and shoulder) 959.2
 artery (complicating trauma) (see also Injury, blood vessel, by site) 904.9
  cerebral or meningeal (see also Hemorrhage, brain, traumatic, subarachnoid) 852.0 ✓5ᵗʰ
 auditory canal (external) (meatus) 959.09
 auricle, auris, ear 959.09
 axilla 959.2
 back 959.1
 bile duct — see Injury, internal, bile duct
 birth — see also Birth, injury
  canal NEC, complicating delivery 665.9 ✓5ᵗʰ
 bladder (sphincter) — see Injury, internal, bladder

Injury — *continued*
- blast (air) (hydraulic) (immersion) (underwater) NEC 869.0
  - with open wound into cavity NEC 869.1
  - abdomen or thorax — *see* Injury, internal, by site
  - brain — *see* Concussion, brain
  - ear (acoustic nerve trauma) 951.5
    - with perforation of tympanic membrane — *see* Wound, open, ear, drum
- blood vessel NEC 904.9
  - abdomen 902.9
    - multiple 902.87
    - specified NEC 902.89
  - aorta (thoracic) 901.0
    - abdominal 902.0
  - arm NEC 903.9
  - axillary 903.00
    - artery 903.01
    - vein 903.02
  - azygos vein 901.89
  - basilic vein 903.1
  - brachial (artery) (vein) 903.1
  - bronchial 901.89
  - carotid artery 900.00
    - common 900.01
    - external 900.02
    - internal 900.03
  - celiac artery 902.20
    - specified branch NEC 902.24
  - cephalic vein (arm) 903.1
  - colica dextra 902.26
  - cystic
    - artery 902.24
    - vein 902.39
  - deep plantar 904.6
  - digital (artery) (vein) 903.5
  - due to accidental puncture or laceration during procedure 998.2
  - extremity
    - lower 904.8
      - multiple 904.7
      - specified NEC 904.7
    - upper 903.9
      - multiple 903.8
      - specified NEC 903.8
  - femoral
    - artery (superficial) 904.1
      - above profunda origin 904.0
      - common 904.0
    - vein 904.2
  - gastric
    - artery 902.21
    - vein 902.39
  - head 900.9
    - intracranial — *see* Injury, intracranial
    - multiple 900.82
    - specified NEC 900.89
  - hemiazygos vein 901.89
  - hepatic
    - artery 902.22
    - vein 902.11
  - hypogastric 902.59
    - artery 902.51
    - vein 902.52
  - ileocolic
    - artery 902.26
    - vein 902.31
  - iliac 902.50
    - artery 902.53
    - specified branch NEC 902.59
    - vein 902.54

Injury — *continued*
- blood vessel NEC — *continued*
  - innominate
    - artery 901.1
    - vein 901.3
  - intercostal (artery) (vein) 901.81
  - jugular vein (external) 900.81
    - internal 900.1
  - leg NEC 904.8
  - mammary (artery) (vein) 901.82
  - mesenteric
    - artery 902.20
      - inferior 902.27
      - specified branch NEC 902.29
      - superior (trunk) 902.25
        - branches, primary 902.26
    - vein 902.39
      - inferior 902.32
      - superior (and primary subdivisions) 902.31
  - neck 900.9
    - multiple 900.82
    - specified NEC 900.89
  - ovarian 902.89
    - artery 902.81
    - vein 902.82
  - palmar artery 903.4
  - pelvis 902.9
    - multiple 902.87
    - specified NEC 902.89
  - plantar (deep) (artery) (vein) 904.6
  - popliteal 904.40
    - artery 904.41
    - vein 904.42
  - portal 902.33
  - pulmonary 901.40
    - artery 901.41
    - vein 901.42
  - radial (artery) (vein) 903.2
  - renal 902.40
    - artery 902.41
    - specified NEC 902.49
    - vein 902.42
  - saphenous
    - artery 904.7
    - vein (greater) (lesser) 904.3
  - splenic
    - artery 902.23
    - vein 902.34
  - subclavian
    - artery 901.1
    - vein 901.3
  - suprarenal 902.49
  - thoracic 901.9
    - multiple 901.83
    - specified NEC 901.89
  - tibial 904.50
    - artery 904.50
      - anterior 904.51
      - posterior 904.53
    - vein 904.50
      - anterior 904.52
      - posterior 904.54
  - ulnar (artery) (vein) 903.3
  - uterine 902.59
    - artery 902.55
    - vein 902.56
  - vena cava
    - inferior 902.10
      - specified branches NEC 902.19
    - superior 901.2

Index to Diseases

Injury — *continued*
- brachial plexus 953.4
  - newborn 767.6
- brain NEC (*see also* Injury, intracranial) 854.0 ✓5ᵗʰ
- breast 959.1
- broad ligament — *see* Injury, internal, broad ligament
- bronchus, bronchi — *see* Injury, internal, bronchus
- brow 959.09
- buttock 959.1
- canthus, eye 921.1
- cathode ray 990
- cauda equina 952.4
  - with fracture, vertebra — *see* Fracture, vertebra, sacrum
- cavernous sinus (*see also* Injury, intracranial) 854.0 ✓5ᵗʰ
- cecum — *see* Injury, internal, cecum
- celiac ganglion or plexus 954.1
- cerebellum (*see also* Injury, intracranial) 854.0 ✓5ᵗʰ
- cervix (uteri) — *see* Injury, internal, cervix
- cheek 959.09
- chest — *see also* Injury, internal, chest
  - wall 959.1
- childbirth — *see also* Birth, injury
  - maternal NEC 665.9 ✓5ᵗʰ
- chin 959.09
- choroid (eye) 921.3
- clitoris 959.1
- coccyx 959.1
  - complicating delivery 665.6 ✓5ᵗʰ
- colon — *see* Injury, internal, colon
- common duct — *see* Injury, internal, common duct
- conjunctiva 921.1
  - superficial 918.2
- cord
  - spermatic — *see* Injury, internal, spermatic cord
  - spinal — *see* Injury, spinal, by site
- cornea 921.3
  - abrasion 918.1
    - due to contact lens 371.82
  - penetrating — *see* Injury, eyeball, penetrating
  - superficial 918.1
    - due to contact lens 371.82
- cortex (cerebral) (*see also* Injury, intracranial) 854.0 ✓5ᵗʰ
  - visual 950.3
- costal region 959.1
- costochondral 959.1
- cranial
  - bones — *see* Fracture, skull, by site
  - cavity (*see also* Injury, intracranial) 854.0 ✓5ᵗʰ
  - nerve — *see* Injury, nerve, cranial
- crushing — *see* Crush
- cutaneous sensory nerve
  - lower limb 956.4
  - upper limb 955.5 ✓5ᵗʰ
- delivery — *see also* Birth, injury
  - maternal NEC 665.9 ✓5ᵗʰ
- Descemet's membrane — *see* Injury, eyeball, penetrating
- diaphragm — *see* Injury, internal, diaphragm
- duodenum — *see* Injury, internal, duodenum
- ear (auricle) (canal) (drum) (external) 959.09

Injury — *continued*
- elbow (and forearm) (and wrist) 959.3
- epididymis 959.1
- epigastric region 959.1
- epiglottis 959.09
- epiphyseal, current — *see* Fracture, by site
- esophagus — *see* Injury, internal, esophagus
- Eustachian tube 959.09
- extremity (lower) (upper) NEC 959.8
- eye 921.9
  - penetrating eyeball — *see* Injury, eyeball, penetrating
  - superficial 918.9
- eyeball 921.3
  - penetrating 871.7
    - with
      - partial loss (of intraocular tissue) 871.2
      - prolapse or exposure (of intraocular tissue) 871.1
    - without prolapse 871.0
    - foreign body (nonmagnetic) 871.6
      - magnetic 871.5
  - superficial 918.9
- eyebrow 959.09
- eyelid(s) 921.1
  - laceration — *see* Laceration, eyelid
  - superficial 918.0
- face (and neck) 959.09
- fallopian tube — *see* Injury, internal, fallopian tube
- finger(s) (nail) 959.5
- flank 959.1
- foot (and ankle) (and knee) (and leg except thigh) 959.7
- forceps NEC 767.9
  - scalp 767.1
- forearm (and elbow) (and wrist) 959.3
- forehead 959.09
- gallbladder — *see* Injury, internal, gallbladder
- gasserian ganglion 951.2
- gastrointestinal tract — *see* Injury, internal, gastrointestinal tract
- genital organ(s)
  - with
    - abortion — *see* Abortion, by type, with, damage to pelvic organs
    - ectopic pregnancy (*see also* categories 633.0-633.9) 639.2
    - molar pregnancy (*see also* categories 630-632) 639.2
  - external 959.1
  - following
    - abortion 639.2
    - ectopic or molar pregnancy 639.2
  - internal — *see* Injury, internal, genital organs
  - obstetrical trauma NEC 665.9 ✓5ᵗʰ
    - affecting fetus or newborn 763.89
- gland
  - lacrimal 921.1
    - laceration 870.8
  - parathyroid 959.09
  - salivary 959.09
  - thyroid 959.09
- globe (eye) (*see also* Injury, eyeball) 921.3
- grease gun — *see* Wound, open, by site, complicated
- groin 959.1
- gum 959.09
- hand(s) (except fingers) 959.4

Injury — *continued*
   head NEC 959.01
      with
         loss of consciousness 850.5
         skull fracture — *see* Fracture, skull, by site
      heart — *see* Injury, internal, heart
      heel 959.7
      hip (and thigh) 959.6
      hymen 959.1
      hyperextension (cervical) (vertebra) 847.0
      ileum — *see* Injury, internal, ileum
      iliac region 959.1
      infrared rays NEC 990
      instrumental (during surgery) 998.2
         birth injury — *see* Birth, injury
         nonsurgical (*see also* Injury, by site) 959.9
         obstetrical 665.9 ☒5☒
            affecting fetus or newborn 763.89
            bladder 665.5 ☒5☒
            cervix 665.3 ☒5☒
            high vaginal 665.4 ☒5☒
            perineal NEC 664.9 ☒5☒
            urethra 665.5 ☒5☒
            uterus 665.5 ☒5☒
      internal 869.0

> *Note* — For injury of internal organ(s) by foreign body entering through a natural orifice (e.g., inhaled, ingested, or swallowed) — *see* Foreign body, entering through orifice.
>
> For internal injury of any of the following sites with internal injury of any other of the sites — *see* Injury, internal, multiple.

         with
            fracture
               open wound into cavity 869.1
               pelvis — *see* Fracture, pelvis
               specified site, except pelvis — *see* Injury, internal, by site
         abdomen, abdominal (viscera) NEC 868.00
            with
               fracture, pelvis — *see* Fracture, pelvis
               open wound into cavity 868.10
               specified site NEC 868.09
                  with open wound into cavity 868.19
         adrenal (gland) 868.01
            with open wound into cavity 868.11
         aorta (thoracic) 901.0
            abdominal 902.0
         appendix 863.85
            with open wound into cavity 863.95
         bile duct 868.02
            with open wound into cavity 868.12
         bladder (sphincter) 867.0
            with
               abortion — *see* Abortion, by type, with damage to pelvic organs
               ectopic pregnancy (*see also* categories 633.0-633.9) 639.2
               molar pregnancy (*see also* categories 630-632) 639.2
               open wound into cavity 867.1
            following
               abortion 639.2
               ectopic or molar pregnancy 639.2
            obstetrical trauma 665.5 ☒5☒
               affecting fetus or newborn 763.89

Injury — *continued*
   internal — *continued*
      blood vessel — *see* Injury, blood vessel, by site
      broad ligament 867.6
         with open wound into cavity 867.7
      bronchus, bronchi 862.21
         with open wound into cavity 862.31
      cecum 863.89
         with open wound into cavity 863.99
      cervix (uteri) 867.4
         with
            abortion — *see* Abortion, by type, with damage to pelvic organs
            ectopic pregnancy (*see also* categories 633.0-633.9) 639.2
            molar pregnancy (*see also* categories 630-632) 639.2
            open wound into cavity 867.5
         following
            abortion 639.2
            ectopic or molar pregnancy 639.2
         obstetrical trauma 665.3 ☒5☒
            affecting fetus or newborn 763.89
      chest (*see also* Injury, internal, intrathoracic organs) 862.8
         with open wound into cavity 862.9
      colon 863.40
         with
            open wound into cavity 863.50
            rectum 863.46
               with open wound into cavity 863.56
         ascending (right) 863.41
            with open wound into cavity 863.51
         descending (left) 863.43
            with open wound into cavity 863.53
         multiple sites 863.46
            with open wound into cavity 863.56
         sigmoid 863.44
            with open wound into cavity 863.54
         specified site NEC 863.49
            with open wound into cavity 863.59
         transverse 863.42
            with open wound into cavity 863.52
      common duct 868.02
         with open wound into cavity 868.12
      complicating delivery 665.9 ☒5☒
         affecting fetus or newborn 763.89
      diaphragm 862.0
         with open wound into cavity 862.1
      duodenum 863.21
         with open wound into cavity 863.31
      esophagus (intrathoracic) 862.22
         with open wound into cavity 862.32
         cervical region 874.4
            complicated 874.5
      fallopian tube 867.6
         with open wound into cavity 867.7
      gallbladder 868.02
         with open wound into cavity 868.12
      gastrointestinal tract NEC 863.80
         with open wound into cavity 863.90
      genital organ NEC 867.6
         with open wound into cavity 867.7
      heart 861.00
         with open wound into thorax 861.10
      ileum 863.29
         with open wound into cavity 863.39

Index to Diseases

Injury — *continued*
  internal — *continued*
    intestine NEC 863.89
      with open wound into cavity 863.99
      large NEC 863.40
        with open wound into cavity 863.50
      small NEC 863.20
        with open wound into cavity 863.30
    intra-abdominal (organ) 868.00
      with open wound into cavity 868.10
      multiple sites 868.09
        with open wound into cavity 868.19
      specified site NEC 868.09
        with open wound into cavity 868.19
    intrathoracic organs (multiple) 862.8
      with open wound into cavity 862.9
      diaphragm (only) — *see* Injury, internal, diaphragm
      heart (only) — *see* Injury, internal, heart
      lung (only) — *see* Injury, internal, lung
      specified site NEC 862.29
        with open wound into cavity 862.39
    intrauterine (*see also* Injury, internal, uterus) 867.4
      with open wound into cavity 867.5
    jejunum 863.29
      with open wound into cavity 863.39
    kidney (subcapsular) 866.00
      with
        disruption of parenchyma (complete) 866.03
          with open wound into cavity 866.13
        hematoma (without rupture of capsule) 866.01
          with open wound into cavity 866.11
        laceration 866.02
          with open wound into cavity 866.12
        open wound into cavity 866.10
    liver 864.00
      with
        contusion 864.01
          with open wound into cavity 864.11
        hematoma 864.01
          with open wound into cavity 864.11
        laceration 864.05
          with open wound into cavity 864.15
          major (disruption of hepatic parenchyma) 864.04
            with open wound into cavity 864.14
          minor (capsule only) 864.02
            with open wound into cavity 864.12
          moderate (involving parenchyma) 864.03
            with open wound into cavity 864.13
          multiple 864.04
          stellate 864.04
            with open wound into cavity 864.14
        open wound into cavity 864.10

Injury — *continued*
  internal — *continued*
    lung 861.20
      with open wound into thorax 861.30
      hemopneumothorax — *see* Hemopneumothorax, traumatic
      hemothorax — *see* Hemothorax, traumatic
      pneumohemothorax — *see* Pneumohemothorax, traumatic
      pneumothorax — *see* Pneumothorax, traumatic
    mediastinum 862.29
      with open wound into cavity 862.39
    mesentery 863.89
      with open wound into cavity 863.99
    mesosalpinx 867.6
      with open wound into cavity 867.7
    multiple 869.0

> *Note* — *Multiple internal injuries of sites classifiable to the same three- or four-digit category should be classified to that category.*
>
> *Multiple injuries classifiable to different fourth-digit subdivisions of 861 (heart and lung injuries) should be dealt with according to coding rules.*

      internal
        with open wound into cavity 869.1
      intra-abdominal organ (sites classifiable to 863-868)
        with
          intrathoracic organ(s) (sites classifiable to 861-862) 869.0
            with open wound into cavity 869.1
          other intra-abdominal organ(s) (sites classifiable to 863-868, except where classifiable to the same three-digit category) 868.09
            with open wound into cavity 868.19
      intrathoracic organ (sites classifiable to 861-862)
        with
          intra-abdominal organ(s) (sites classifiable to 863-868) 869.0
            with open wound into cavity 869.1
          other intrathoracic organ(s) (sites classifiable to 861-862, except where classifiable to the same three-digit category) 862.8
            with open wound into cavity 862.9
    myocardium — *see* Injury, internal, heart
    ovary 867.6
      with open wound into cavity 867.7
    pancreas (multiple sites) 863.84
      with open wound into cavity 863.94
      body 863.82
        with open wound into cavity 863.92
      head 863.81
        with open wound into cavity 863.91

Injury — *continued*
   internal — *continued*
      pancreas — *continued*
         tail 863.83
            with open wound into cavity 863.93
      pelvis, pelvic (organs) (viscera) 867.8
         with
            fracture, pelvis — *see* Fracture, pelvis
            open wound into cavity 867.9
         specified site NEC 867.6
            with open wound into cavity 867.7
      peritoneum 868.03
         with open wound into cavity 868.13
      pleura 862.29
         with open wound into cavity 862.39
      prostate 867.6
         with open wound into cavity 867.7
      rectum 863.45
         with
            colon 863.46
               with open wound into cavity 863.56
            open wound into cavity 863.55
      retroperitoneum 868.04
         with open wound into cavity 868.14
      round ligament 867.6
         with open wound into cavity 867.7
      seminal vesicle 867.6
         with open wound into cavity 867.7
      spermatic cord 867.6
         with open wound into cavity 867.7
         scrotal — *see* Wound, open, spermatic cord
      spleen 865.00
         with
            disruption of parenchyma (massive) 865.04
               with open wound into cavity 865.14
            hematoma (without rupture of capsule) 865.01
               with open wound into cavity 865.11
            open wound into cavity 865.10
            tear, capsular 865.02
               with open wound into cavity 865.12
                  extending into parenchyma 865.03
                     with open wound into cavity 865.13
      stomach 863.0
         with open wound into cavity 863.1
      suprarenal gland (multiple) 868.01
         with open wound into cavity 868.11
      thorax, thoracic (cavity) (organs) (multiple) (*see also* Injury, internal, intrathoracic organs) 862.8
         with open wound into cavity 862.9
      thymus (gland) 862.29
         with open wound into cavity 862.39
      trachea (intrathoracic) 862.29
         with open wound into cavity 862.39
         cervical region (*see also* Wound, open, trachea) 874.02
      ureter 867.2
         with open wound into cavity 867.3
      urethra (sphincter) 867.0
         with
            abortion — *see* Abortion, by type, with damage to pelvic organs

Injury — *continued*
   internal — *continued*
      urethra — *continued*
         with — *continued*
            ectopic pregnancy (*see also* categories 633.0-633.9) 639.2
            molar pregnancy (*see also* categories 630-632) 639.2
            open wound into cavity 867.1
         following
            abortion 639.2
            ectopic or molar pregnancy 639.2
         obstetrical trauma 665.5 ✓5ᵗʰ
            affecting fetus or newborn 763.89
      uterus 867.4
         with
            abortion — *see* Abortion, by type, with damage to pelvic organs
            ectopic pregnancy (*see also* categories 633.0-633.9) 639.2
            molar pregnancy (*see also* categories 630-632) 639.2
            open wound into cavity 867.5
         following
            abortion 639.2
            ectopic or molar pregnancy 639.2
         obstetrical trauma NEC 665.5 ✓5ᵗʰ
            affecting fetus or newborn 763.89
      vas deferens 867.6
         with open wound into cavity 867.7
      vesical (sphincter) 867.0
         with open wound into cavity 867.1
      viscera (abdominal) (*see also* Injury, internal, multiple) 868.00
         with
            fracture, pelvis — *see* Fracture, pelvis
            open wound into cavity 868.10
         thoracic NEC (*see also* Injury, internal, intrathoracic organs) 862.8
            with open wound into cavity 862.9
   interscapular region 959.1
   intervertebral disc 959.1
   intestine — *see* Injury, internal, intestine
   intra-abdominal (organs) NEC — *see* Injury, internal, intra-abdominal
   intracranial 854.0 ✓5ᵗʰ

Note — Use the following fifth-digit subclassification with categories 851-854:

0   unspecified state of consciousness
1   with no loss of consciousness
2   with brief [less than one hour] loss of consciousness
3   with moderate [1-24 hours] loss of consciousness
4   with prolonged [more than 24 hours] loss of consciousness and return to pre-existing conscious level
5   with prolonged [more than 24 hours] loss of consciousness, without return to pre-existing conscious level

Use fifth-digit 5 to designate when a patient is unconscious and dies before regaining consciousness, regardless of the duration of the loss of consciousness

6   with loss of consciousness of unspecified duration
9   with concussion, unspecified

Index to Diseases — **Injury**

Injury — *continued*
  internal — *continued*
    with
      open intracranial wound 854.1 ✓5ᵗʰ
      skull fracture — *see* Fracture, skull, by site
    contusion 851.8 ✓5ᵗʰ
      with open intracranial wound 851.9 ✓5ᵗʰ
      brain stem 851.4 ✓5ᵗʰ
        with open intracranial wound 851.5 ✓5ᵗʰ
      cerebellum 851.4 ✓5ᵗʰ
        with open intracranial wound 851.5 ✓5ᵗʰ
      cortex (cerebral) 851.0 ✓5ᵗʰ
        with open intracranial wound 851.2 ✓5ᵗʰ
    hematoma — *see* Injury, intracranial, hemorrhage
    hemorrhage 853.0 ✓5ᵗʰ
      with
        laceration — *see* Injury, intracranial, laceration
        open intracranial wound 853.1 ✓5ᵗʰ
      extradural 852.4 ✓5ᵗʰ
        with open intracranial wound 852.5 ✓5ᵗʰ
      subarachnoid 852.0 ✓5ᵗʰ
        with open intracranial wound 852.1 ✓5ᵗʰ
      subdural 852.2 ✓5ᵗʰ
        with open intracranial wound 852.3 ✓5ᵗʰ
    laceration 851.8 ✓5ᵗʰ
      with open intracranial wound 851.9 ✓5ᵗʰ
      brain stem 851.6 ✓5ᵗʰ
        with open intracranial wound 851.7 ✓5ᵗʰ
      cerebellum 851.6 ✓5ᵗʰ
        with open intracranial wound 851.7 ✓5ᵗʰ
      cortex (cerebral) 851.2 ✓5ᵗʰ
        with open intracranial wound 851.3 ✓5ᵗʰ
  intraocular — *see* Injury, eyeball, penetrating
  intrathoracic organs (multiple) — *see* Injury, internal, intrathoracic organs
  intrauterine — *see* Injury, internal, intrauterine
  iris 921.3
    penetrating — *see* Injury, eyeball, penetrating
  jaw 959.09
  jejunum — *see* Injury, internal, jejunum
  joint NEC 959.9
    old or residual 718.80
      ankle 718.87
      elbow 718.82
      foot 718.87
      hand 718.84
      hip 718.85
      knee 718.86
      multiple sites 718.89
      pelvic region 718.85
      shoulder (region) 718.81
      specified site NEC 718.88
      wrist 718.83
  kidney — *see* Injury, internal, kidney
  knee (and ankle) (and foot) (and leg, except thigh) 959.7
  labium (majus) (minus) 959.1

Injury — *continued*
  labyrinth, ear 959.09
  lacrimal apparatus, gland, or sac 921.1
    laceration 870.8
  larynx 959.09
  late effect — *see* Late, effects (of), injury
  leg except thigh (and ankle) (and foot) (and knee) 959.7
    upper or thigh 959.6
  lens, eye 921.3
    penetrating — *see* Injury, eyeball, penetrating
  lid, eye — *see* Injury, eyelid
  lip 959.09
  liver — *see* Injury, internal, liver
  lobe, parietal — *see* Injury, intracranial
  lumbar (region) 959.1
    plexus 953.5
  lumbosacral (region) 959.1
    plexus 953.5
  lung — *see* Injury, internal, lung
  malar region 959.09
  mastoid region 959.09
  maternal, during pregnancy, affecting fetus or newborn 760.5
  maxilla 959.09
  mediastinum — *see* Injury, internal, mediastinum
  membrane
    brain (*see also* Injury, intracranial) 854.0 ✓5ᵗʰ
    tympanic 959.09
  meningeal artery — *see* Hemorrhage, brain, traumatic, subarachnoid
  meninges (cerebral) — *see* Injury, intracranial
  mesenteric
    artery — *see* Injury, blood vessel, mesenteric, artery
    plexus, inferior 954.1
    vein — *see* Injury, blood vessel, mesenteric, vein
  mesentery — *see* Injury, internal, mesentery
  mesosalpinx — *see* Injury, internal, mesosalpinx
  middle ear 959.09
  midthoracic region 959.1
  mouth 959.09
  multiple (sites not classifiable to the same four-digit category in 959.0-959.7) 959.8
    internal 869.0
      with open wound into cavity 869.1
  musculocutaneous nerve 955.4
  nail
    finger 959.5
    toe 959.7
  nasal (septum) (sinus) 959.09
  nasopharynx 959.09
  neck (and face) 959.09
  nerve 957.9
    abducens 951.3
    abducent 951.3
    accessory 951.6
    acoustic 951.5
    ankle and foot 956.9
    anterior crural, femoral 956.1
    arm (*see also* Injury, nerve, upper limb) 955.9
    auditory 951.5
    axillary 955.0
    brachial plexus 953.4
    cervical sympathetic 954.0

✓4ᵗʰ Fourth-digit Required   ✓5ᵗʰ Fifth-digit Required

Injury — *continued*
  nerve — *continued*
    cranial 951.9
      first or olfactory 951.8
      second or optic 950.0
      third or oculomotor 951.0
      fourth or trochlear 951.1
      fifth or trigeminal 951.2
      sixth or abducens 951.3
      seventh or facial 951.4
      eighth, acoustic, or auditory 951.5
      ninth or glossopharyngeal 951.8
      tenth, pneumogastric, or vagus 951.8
      eleventh or accessory 951.6
      twelfth or hypoglossal 951.7
      newborn 767.7
    cutaneous sensory
      lower limb 956.4
      upper limb 955.5 ✓5ᵗʰ
    digital (finger) 955.6
      toe 956.5
    facial 951.4
      newborn 767.5
    femoral 956.1
    finger 955.9
    foot and ankle 956.9
    forearm 955.9
    glossopharyngeal 951.8
    hand and wrist 955.9
    head and neck, superficial 957.0
    hypoglossal 951.7
    involving several parts of body 957.8
    leg (*see also* Injury, nerve, lower limb) 956.9
    lower limb 956.9
      multiple 956.8
      specified site NEC 956.5
    lumbar plexus 953.5
    lumbosacral plexus 953.5
    median 955.1
      forearm 955.1
      wrist and hand 955.1
    multiple (in several parts of body) (sites not classifiable to the same three-digit category) 957.8
    musculocutaneous 955.4
    musculospiral 955.3
      upper arm 955.3
    oculomotor 951.0
    olfactory 951.8
    optic 950.0
    pelvic girdle 956.9
      multiple sites 956.8
      specified site NEC 956.5
    peripheral 957.9
      multiple (in several regions) (sites not classifiable to the same three-digit category) 957.8
      specified site NEC 957.1
    peroneal 956.3
      ankle and foot 956.3
      lower leg 956.3
    plantar 956.5
    plexus 957.9
      celiac 954.1
      mesenteric, inferior 954.1
      spinal 953.9
    brachial 953.4
    lumbosacral 953.5
    multiple sites 953.8
      sympathetic NEC 954.1

Injury — *continued*
  nerve — *continued*
    pneumogastric 951.8
    radial 955.3
      wrist and hand 955.3
    sacral plexus 953.5
    sciatic 956.0
      thigh 956.0
    shoulder girdle 955.9
      multiple 955.8
      specified site NEC 955.7
    specified site NEC 957.1
    spinal 953.9
      plexus — *see* Injury, nerve, plexus, spinal
      root 953.9
        cervical 953.0
        dorsal 953.1
        lumbar 953.2
        multiple sites 953.8
        sacral 953.3
    splanchnic 954.1
    sympathetic NEC 954.1
      cervical 954.0
    thigh 956.9
    tibial 956.5
      ankle and foot 956.2
      lower leg 956.5
      posterior 956.2
    toe 956.9
    trigeminal 951.2
    trochlear 951.1
    trunk, excluding shoulder and pelvic girdles 954.9
      specified site NEC 954.8
      sympathetic NEC 954.1
    ulnar 955.2
      forearm 955.2
      wrist (and hand) 955.2
    upper limb 955.9
      multiple 955.8
      specified site NEC 955.7
    vagus 951.8
    wrist and hand 955.9
  nervous system, diffuse 957.8
  nose (septum) 959.09
  obstetrical NEC 665.9 ✓5ᵗʰ
    affecting fetus or newborn 763.89
  occipital (region) (scalp) 959.09
    lobe (*see also* Injury, intracranial) 854.0 ✓5ᵗʰ
  optic 950.9
    chiasm 950.1
    cortex 950.3
    nerve 950.0
    pathways 950.2
  orbit, orbital (region) 921.2
    penetrating 870.3
      with foreign body 870.4
  ovary — *see* Injury, internal, ovary
  paint-gun — *see* Wound, open, by site, complicated
  palate (soft) 959.09
  pancreas — *see* Injury, internal, pancreas
  parathyroid (gland) 959.09
  parietal (region) (scalp) 959.09
    lobe — *see* Injury, intracranial
  pelvic
    floor 959.1
      complicating delivery 664.1 ✓5ᵗʰ
        affecting fetus or newborn 763.89

Injury — *continued*
　pelvic — *continued*
　　joint or ligament, complicating delivery
　　　665.6 ☑5ᵗʰ
　　　　affecting fetus or newborn 763.89
　　organs — *see also* Injury, internal, pelvis
　　　with
　　　　abortion — *see* Abortion, by type,
　　　　　with damage to pelvic organs
　　　　ectopic pregnancy (*see also* categories
　　　　　633.0-633.9) 639.2
　　　　molar pregnancy (*see also* categories
　　　　　633.0-633.9) 639.2
　　　following
　　　　abortion 639.2
　　　　ectopic or molar pregnancy 639.2
　　　obstetrical trauma 665.5 ☑5ᵗʰ
　　　　affecting fetus or newborn 763.89
　pelvis 959.1
　penis 959.1
　perineum 959.1
　peritoneum — *see* Injury, internal, peritoneum
　periurethral tissue
　　with
　　　abortion — *see* Abortion, by type, with
　　　　damage to pelvic organs
　　　ectopic pregnancy (*see also* categories
　　　　633.0-633.9) 639.2
　　　molar pregnancy (*see also* categories
　　　　630-632) 639.2
　　complicating delivery 665.5 ☑5ᵗʰ
　　　affecting fetus or newborn 763.89
　　following
　　　abortion 639.2
　　　ectopic or molar pregnancy 639.2
　phalanges
　　foot 959.7
　　hand 959.5
　pharynx 959.09
　pleura — *see* Injury, internal, pleura
　popliteal space 959.7
　prepuce 959.1
　prostate — *see* Injury, internal, prostate
　pubic region 959.1
　pudenda 959.1
　radiation NEC 990
　radioactive substance or radium NEC 990
　rectovaginal septum 959.1
　rectum — *see* Injury, internal, rectum
　retina 921.3
　　penetrating — *see* Injury, eyeball,
　　　penetrating
　retroperitoneal — *see* Injury, internal,
　　retroperitoneum
　roentgen rays NEC 990
　round ligament — *see* Injury, internal, round
　　ligament
　sacral (region) 959.1
　　plexus 953.5
　sacroiliac ligament NEC 959.1
　sacrum 959.1
　salivary ducts or glands 959.09
　scalp 959.09
　　due to birth trauma 767.1
　　fetus or newborn 767.1
　scapular region 959.2
　sclera 921.3
　　penetrating — *see* Injury, eyeball,
　　　penetrating
　　superficial 918.2
　scrotum 959.1

Injury — *continued*
　seminal vesicle — *see* Injury, internal, seminal
　　vesicle
　shoulder (and upper arm) 959.2
　sinus
　　cavernous (*see also* Injury, intracranial)
　　　854.0 ☑5ᵗʰ
　　nasal 959.09
　skeleton NEC, birth injury 767.3
　skin NEC 959.9
　skull — *see* Fracture, skull, by site
　soft tissue (of external sites) (severe) — *see*
　　Wound, open, by site
　specified site NEC 959.8
　spermatic cord — *see* Injury, internal,
　　spermatic cord
　spinal (cord) 952.9
　　with fracture, vertebra — *see* Fracture,
　　　vertebra, by site, with spinal cord
　　　injury
　　cervical (C_1-C_4) 952.00
　　　with
　　　　anterior cord syndrome 952.02
　　　　central cord syndrome 952.03
　　　　complete lesion of cord 952.01
　　　　incomplete lesion NEC 952.04
　　　　posterior cord syndrome 952.04
　　C_5-C_7 level 952.05
　　　with
　　　　anterior cord syndrome 952.07
　　　　central cord syndrome 952.08
　　　　complete lesion of cord 952.06
　　　　incomplete lesion NEC 952.09
　　　　posterior cord syndrome 952.09
　　　specified type NEC 952.09
　　specified type NEC 952.04
　　dorsal (D_1-D_6) (T_1-T_6) (thoracic) 952.10
　　　with
　　　　anterior cord syndrome 952.12
　　　　central cord syndrome 952.13
　　　　complete lesion of cord 952.11
　　　　incomplete lesion NEC 952.14
　　　　posterior cord syndrome 952.14
　　D_7-D_{12} level (T_7-T_{12}) 952.15
　　　with
　　　　anterior cord syndrome 952.17
　　　　central cord syndrome 952.18
　　　　complete lesion of cord 952.16
　　　　incomplete lesion NEC 952.19
　　　　posterior cord syndrome 952.19
　　　specified type NEC 952.19
　　specified type NEC 952.14
　　lumbar 952.2
　　multiple sites 952.8
　　nerve (root) NEC — *see* Injury, nerve,
　　　spinal, root
　　plexus 953.9
　　　brachial 953.4
　　　lumbosacral 953.5
　　　multiple sites 953.8
　　sacral 952.3
　　thoracic (*see also* Injury, spinal, dorsal)
　　　952.10
　spleen — *see* Injury, internal, spleen
　stellate ganglion 954.1
　sternal region 959.1
　stomach — *see* Injury, internal, stomach
　subconjunctival 921.1
　subcutaneous 959.9
　subdural — *see* Injury, intracranial
　submaxillary region 959.09

☑4ᵗʰ Fourth-digit Required　　　☑5ᵗʰ Fifth-digit Required

Injury — *continued*
  submental region 959.09
  subungual
    fingers 959.5
    toes 959.7
  superficial 919 ✓4ᵗʰ

> Note — Use the following fourth-digit subdivisions with categories 910-919:
>
> 0 Abrasion or friction burn without mention of infection
> 1 Abrasion or friction burn, infected
> 2 Blister without mention of infection
> 3 Blister, infected
> 4 Insect bite, nonvenomous, without mention of infection
> 5 Insect bite, nonvenomous, infected
> 6 Superficial foreign body (splinter) without major open wound and without mention of infection
> 7 Superficial foreign body (splinter) without major open wound, infected
> 8 Other and unspecified superficial injury without mention of infection
> 9 Other and unspecified superficial injury, infected
>
> For late effects of superficial injury, see category 906.2.

  abdomen, abdominal (muscle) (wall) (and other part(s) of trunk) 911 ✓4ᵗʰ
  ankle (and hip, knee, leg, or thigh) 916 ✓4ᵗʰ
  anus (and other part(s) of trunk) 911 ✓4ᵗʰ
  arm 913 ✓4ᵗʰ
    upper (and shoulder) 912 ✓4ᵗʰ
  auditory canal (external) (meatus) (and other part(s) of face, neck, or scalp, except eye) 910 ✓4ᵗʰ
  axilla (and upper arm) 912 ✓4ᵗʰ
  back (and other part(s) of trunk) 911 ✓4ᵗʰ
  breast (and other part(s) of trunk) 911 ✓4ᵗʰ
  brow (and other part(s) of face, neck, or scalp, except eye) 910 ✓4ᵗʰ
  buttock (and other part(s) of trunk) 911 ✓4ᵗʰ
  canthus, eye 918.0
  cheek(s) (and other part(s) of face, neck, or scalp, except eye) 910 ✓4ᵗʰ
  chest wall (and other part(s) of trunk) 911 ✓4ᵗʰ
  chin (and other part(s) of face, neck, or scalp, except eye) 910 ✓4ᵗʰ
  clitoris (and other part(s) of trunk) 911 ✓4ᵗʰ
  conjunctiva 918.2
  cornea 918.1
    due to contact lens 371.82
  costal region (and other part(s) of trunk) 911 ✓4ᵗʰ
  ear(s) (auricle) (canal) (drum) (external) (and other part(s) of face, neck, or scalp, except eye) 910 ✓4ᵗʰ
  elbow (and forearm) (and wrist) 913 ✓4ᵗʰ
  epididymis (and other part(s) of trunk) 911 ✓4ᵗʰ
  epigastric region (and other part(s) of trunk) 911 ✓4ᵗʰ
  epiglottis (and other part(s) of face, neck, or scalp, except eye) 910 ✓4ᵗʰ
  eye(s) (and adnexa) NEC 918.9
  eyelid(s) (and periocular area) 918.0

Injury — *continued*
  superficial — *continued*
    face (any part(s), except eye) (and neck or scalp) 910 ✓4ᵗʰ
    finger(s) (nail) (any) 915 ✓4ᵗʰ
    flank (and other part(s) of trunk) 911 ✓4ᵗʰ
    foot (phalanges) (and toe(s)) 917 ✓4ᵗʰ
    forearm (and elbow) (and wrist) 913 ✓4ᵗʰ
    forehead (and other part(s) of face, neck, or scalp, except eye) 910 ✓4ᵗʰ
    globe (eye) 918.9
    groin (and other part(s) of trunk) 911 ✓4ᵗʰ
    gum(s) (and other part(s) of face, neck, or scalp, except eye) 910 ✓4ᵗʰ
    hand(s) (except fingers alone) 914 ✓4ᵗʰ
    head (and other part(s) of face, neck, or scalp, except eye) 910 ✓4ᵗʰ
    heel (and foot or toe) 917 ✓4ᵗʰ
    hip (and ankle, knee, leg, or thigh) 916 ✓4ᵗʰ
    iliac region (and other part(s) of trunk) 911 ✓4ᵗʰ
    interscapular region (and other part(s) of trunk) 911 ✓4ᵗʰ
    iris 918.9
    knee (and ankle, hip, leg, or thigh) 916 ✓4ᵗʰ
    labium (majus) (minus) (and other part(s) of trunk) 911 ✓4ᵗʰ
    lacrimal (apparatus) (gland) (sac) 918.0
    leg (lower) (upper) (and ankle, hip, knee, or thigh) 916 ✓4ᵗʰ
    lip(s) (and other part(s) of face, neck, or scalp, except eye) 910 ✓4ᵗʰ
    lower extremity (except foot) 916 ✓4ᵗʰ
    lumbar region (and other part(s) of trunk) 911 ✓4ᵗʰ
    malar region (and other part(s) of face, neck, or scalp, except eye) 910 ✓4ᵗʰ
    mastoid region (and other part(s) of face, neck, or scalp, except eye) 910 ✓4ᵗʰ
    midthoracic region (and other part(s) of trunk) 911 ✓4ᵗʰ
    mouth (and other part(s) of face, neck, or scalp, except eye) 910 ✓4ᵗʰ
    multiple sites (not classifiable to the same three-digit category) 919 ✓4ᵗʰ
    nasal (septum) (and other part(s) of face, neck, or scalp, except eye) 910 ✓4ᵗʰ
    neck (and face or scalp, any part(s), except eye) 910 ✓4ᵗʰ
    nose (septum) (and other part(s) of face, neck, or scalp, except eye) 910 ✓4ᵗʰ
    occipital region (and other part(s) of face, neck, or scalp, except eye) 910 ✓4ᵗʰ
    orbital region 918.0
    palate (soft) (and other part(s) of face, neck, or scalp, except eye) 910 ✓4ᵗʰ
    parietal region (and other part(s) of face, neck, or scalp, except eye) 910 ✓4ᵗʰ
    penis (and other part(s) of trunk) 911 ✓4ᵗʰ
    perineum (and other part(s) of trunk) 911 ✓4ᵗʰ
    periocular area 918.0
    pharynx (and other part(s) of face, neck, or scalp, except eye) 910 ✓4ᵗʰ
    popliteal space (and ankle, hip, leg, or thigh) 916 ✓4ᵗʰ
    prepuce (and other part(s) of trunk) 911 ✓4ᵗʰ
    pubic region (and other part(s) of trunk) 911 ✓4ᵗʰ

Index to Diseases — Insertion

Injury — *continued*
  superficial — *continued*
    pudenda (and other part(s) of trunk) 911 ✓4ᵗʰ
    sacral region (and other part(s) of trunk) 911 ✓4ᵗʰ
    salivary (ducts) (glands) (and other part(s) of face, neck, or scalp, except eye) 910 ✓4ᵗʰ
    scalp (and other part(s) of face or neck, except eye) 910 ✓4ᵗʰ
    scapular region (and upper arm) 912 ✓4ᵗʰ
    sclera 918.2
    scrotum (and other part(s) of trunk) 911 ✓4ᵗʰ
    shoulder (and upper arm) 912 ✓4ᵗʰ
    skin NEC 919 ✓4ᵗʰ
    specified site(s) NEC 919 ✓4ᵗʰ
    sternal region (and other part(s) of trunk) 911 ✓4ᵗʰ
    subconjunctival 918.2
    subcutaneous NEC 919 ✓4ᵗʰ
    submaxillary region (and other part(s) of face, neck, or scalp, except eye) 910 ✓4ᵗʰ
    submental region (and other part(s) of face, neck, or scalp, except eye) 910 ✓4ᵗʰ
    supraclavicular fossa (and other part(s) of face, neck or scalp, except eye) 910 ✓4ᵗʰ
    supraorbital 918.0
    temple (and other part(s) of face, neck, or scalp, except eye) 910 ✓4ᵗʰ
    temporal region (and other part(s) of face, neck, or scalp, except eye) 910 ✓4ᵗʰ
    testis (and other part(s) of trunk) 911 ✓4ᵗʰ
    thigh (and ankle, hip, knee, or leg) 916 ✓4ᵗʰ
    thorax, thoracic (external) (and other part(s) of trunk) 911 ✓4ᵗʰ
    throat (and other part(s) of face, neck, or scalp, except eye) 910 ✓4ᵗʰ
    thumb(s) (nail) 915 ✓4ᵗʰ
    toe(s) (nail) (subungual) (and foot) 917 ✓4ᵗʰ
    tongue (and other part(s) of face, neck, or scalp, except eye) 910 ✓4ᵗʰ
    tooth, teeth 521.2
    trunk (any part(s)) 911 ✓4ᵗʰ
    tunica vaginalis (and other part(s) of trunk) 911 ✓4ᵗʰ
    tympanum, tympanic membrane (and other part(s) of face, neck, or scalp, except eye) 910 ✓4ᵗʰ
    upper extremity NEC 913 ✓4ᵗʰ
    uvula (and other part(s) of face, neck, or scalp, except eye) 910 ✓4ᵗʰ
    vagina (and other part(s) of trunk) 911 ✓4ᵗʰ
    vulva (and other part(s) of trunk) 911 ✓4ᵗʰ
    wrist (and elbow) (and forearm) 913 ✓4ᵗʰ
  supraclavicular fossa 959.1
  supraorbital 959.09
  surgical complication (external or internal site) 998.2
  symphysis pubis 959.1
    complicating delivery 665.6 ✓5ᵗʰ
      affecting fetus or newborn 763.89
  temple 959.09
  temporal region 959.09
  testis 959.1
  thigh (and hip) 959.6
  thorax, thoracic (external) 959.1
    cavity — *see* Injury, internal, thorax

Injury — *continued*
  thorax, thoracic — *continued*
    internal — *see* Injury, internal, intrathoracic organs
  throat 959.09
  thumb(s) (nail) 959.5
  thymus — *see* Injury, internal, thymus
  thyroid (gland) 959.09
  toe (nail) (any) 959.7
  tongue 959.09
  tonsil 959.09
  tooth NEC 873.63
    complicated 873.73
  trachea — *see* Injury, internal, trachea
  trunk 959.1
  tunica vaginalis 959.1
  tympanum, tympanic membrane 959.09
  ultraviolet rays NEC 990
  ureter — *see* Injury, internal, ureter
  urethra (sphincter) — *see* Injury, internal, urethra
  uterus — *see* Injury, internal, uterus
  uvula 959.09
  vagina 959.1
  vascular — *see* Injury, blood vessel
  vas deferens — *see* Injury, internal, vas deferens
  vein (*see also* Injury, blood vessel, by site) 904.9
  vena cava
    inferior 902.10
    superior 901.2
  vesical (sphincter) — *see* Injury, internal, vesical
  viscera (abdominal) — *see also* Injury, internal, viscera
    with fracture, pelvis — *see* Fracture, pelvis
  visual 950.9
    cortex 950.3
  vitreous (humor) 871.2
  vulva 959.1
  whiplash (cervical spine) 847.0
  wringer — *see* Crush, by site
  wrist (and elbow) (and forearm) 959.3
  x-ray NEC 990

Inoculation — *see also* Vaccination
  complication or reaction — *see* Complication, vaccination

Insanity, insane (*see also* Psychosis) 298.9
  adolescent (*see also* Schizophrenia) 295.9 ✓5ᵗʰ
  alternating (*see also* Psychosis, affective, circular) 296.7
  confusional 298.9
    acute 293.0
    subacute 293.1
  delusional 298.9
  paralysis, general 094.1
    progressive 094.1
  paresis, general 094.1
  senile 290.20

Insect
  bite — *see* Injury, superficial, by site
  venomous, poisoning by 989.5

Insemination, artificial V26.1

Insertion
  cord (umbilical) lateral or velamentous 663.8 ✓5ᵗʰ
    affecting fetus or newborn 762.6
  intrauterine contraceptive device V25.1
  placenta, vicious — *see* Placenta, previa
  subdermal implantable contraceptive V25.5

Insertion — *continued*
  velamentous, umbilical cord 663.8 ✓5ᵗʰ
    affecting fetus or newborn 762.6
Insolation 992.0
  meaning sunstroke 992.0
Insomnia 780.52
  with sleep apnea 780.51
  nonorganic origin 307.41
    persistent (primary) 307.42
    transient 307.41
    subjective complaint 307.49
Inspiration
  food or foreign body (*see also* Asphyxia, food or foreign body) 933.1
  mucus (*see also* Asphyxia, mucus) 933.1
Inspissated bile syndrome, newborn 774.4
Instability
  detrusor 596.59
  emotional (excessive) 301.3
  joint (posttraumatic) 718.80
    ankle 718.87
    elbow 718.82
    foot 718.87
    hand 718.84
    hip 718.85
    knee 718.86
    lumbosacral 724.6
    multiple sites 718.89
    pelvic region 718.85
    sacroiliac 724.6
    shoulder (region) 718.81
    specified site NEC 718.88
    wrist 718.83
  lumbosacral 724.6
  nervous 301.89
  personality (emotional) 301.59
  thyroid, paroxysmal 242.9 ✓5ᵗʰ
  urethral 599.83
  vasomotor 780.2
Insufficiency, insufficient
  accommodation 367.4
  adrenal (gland) (acute) (chronic) 255.4
    medulla 255.5
    primary 255.4
    specified NEC 255.5
  adrenocortical 255.4
  anus 569.49
  aortic (valve) 424.1
    with
      mitral (valve) disease 396.1
        insufficiency, incompetence, or regurgitation 396.3
        stenosis or obstruction 396.1
      stenosis or obstruction 424.1
        with mitral (valve) disease 396.8
    congenital 746.4
    rheumatic 395.1
      with
        mitral (valve) disease 396.1
          insufficiency, incompetence, or regurgitation 396.3
          stenosis or obstruction 396.1
        stenosis or obstruction 395.2
          with mitral (valve) disease 396.8
    specified cause NEC 424.1
    syphilitic 093.22
  arterial 447.1
    basilar artery 435.0
    carotid artery 435.8
    cerebral 437.1

Insufficiency, insufficient — *continued*
  arterial — *continued*
    coronary (acute or subacute) 411.89
    mesenteric 557.1
    peripheral 443.9
    precerebral 435.9
    vertebral artery 435.1
    vertebrobasilar 435.3
  arteriovenous 459.9
  basilar artery 435.0
  biliary 575.8
  cardiac (*see also* Insufficiency, myocardial) 428.0
    complicating surgery 997.1
    due to presence of (cardiac) prosthesis 429.4
    postoperative 997.1
      long-term effect of cardiac surgery 429.4
    specified during or due to a procedure 997.1
      long-term effect of cardiac surgery 429.4
  cardiorenal (*see also* Hypertension, cardiorenal) 404.90
  cardiovascular (*see also* Disease, cardiovascular) 429.2
    renal (*see also* Hypertension, cardiorenal) 404.90
  carotid artery 435.8
  cerebral (vascular) 437.9
  cerebrovascular 437.9
    with transient focal neurological signs and symptoms 435.9
    acute 437.1
      with transient focal neurological signs and symptoms 435.9
  circulatory NEC 459.9
    fetus or newborn 779.89 ▲
  convergence 378.83
  coronary (acute or subacute) 411.89
    chronic or with a stated duration of over 8 weeks 414.8
  corticoadrenal 255.4
  dietary 269.9
  divergence 378.85
  food 994.2
  gastroesophageal 530.89
  gonadal
    ovary 256.39
    testis 257.2
  gonadotropic hormone secretion 253.4
  heart — *see also* Insufficiency, myocardial
    fetus or newborn 779.89 ▲
    valve (*see also* Endocarditis) 424.90
      congenital NEC 746.89
  hepatic 573.8
  idiopathic autonomic 333.0
  kidney ▶(acute) (chronic)◀ 593.9
  labyrinth, labyrinthine (function) 386.53
    bilateral 386.54
    unilateral 386.53
  lacrimal 375.15
  liver 573.8
  lung (acute) (*see also* Insufficiency, pulmonary) 518.82
    following trauma, surgery, or shock 518.5
    newborn 770.89 ▲
  mental (congenital) (*see also* Retardation, mental) 319
  mesenteric 557.1

Insufficiency, insufficient — *continued*
  mitral (valve) 424.0
    with
      aortic (valve) disease 396.3
        insufficiency, incompetence, or regurgitation 396.3
          stenosis or obstruction 396.2
        obstruction or stenosis 394.2
          with aortic valve disease 396.8
      congenital 746.6
      rheumatic 394.1
        with
          aortic (valve) disease 396.3
            insufficiency, incompetence, or regurgitation 396.3
              stenosis or obstruction 396.2
            obstruction or stenosis 394.2
              with aortic valve disease 396.8
          active or acute 391.1
            with chorea, rheumatic (Sydenham's) 392.0
      specified cause, except rheumatic 424.0
  muscle
    heart — *see* Insufficiency, myocardial
    ocular (*see also* Strabismus) 378.9
  myocardial, myocardium (with arteriosclerosis) 428.0
    with rheumatic fever (conditions classifiable to 390)
      active, acute, or subacute 391.2
        with chorea 392.0
      inactive or quiescent (with chorea) 398.0
    congenital 746.89
    due to presence of (cardiac) prosthesis 429.4
    fetus or newborn 779.89 ▲
    following cardiac surgery 429.4
    hypertensive (*see also* Hypertension, heart) 402.91
      benign 402.11
      malignant 402.01
    postoperative 997.1
      long-term effect of cardiac surgery 429.4
    rheumatic 398.0
      active, acute, or subacute 391.2
        with chorea (Sydenham's) 392.0
    syphilitic 093.82
  nourishment 994.2
  organic 799.8
  ovary 256.39
    postablative 256.2
  pancreatic 577.8
  parathyroid (gland) 252.1
  peripheral vascular (arterial) 443.9
  pituitary (anterior) 253.2
    posterior 253.5
  placental — *see* Placenta, insufficiency
  platelets 287.5
  prenatal care in current pregnancy V23.7
  progressive pluriglandular 258.9
  pseudocholinesterase 289.8
  pulmonary (acute) 518.82
    following
      shock 518.5
      surgery 518.5
      trauma 518.5
    newborn 770.89 ▲
    valve (*see also* Endocarditis, pulmonary) 424.3
      congenital 746.09
  pyloric 537.0

Insufficiency, insufficient — *continued*
  renal ▶(acute) (chronic)◀ 593.9
    due to a procedure 997.5
  respiratory 786.09
    acute 518.82
      following shock, surgery, or trauma 518.5
    newborn 770.89 ▲
  rotation — *see* Malrotation
  suprarenal 255.4
    medulla 255.5
  tarso-orbital fascia, congenital 743.66
  tear film 375.15
  testis 257.2
  thyroid (gland) (acquired) — *see also* Hypothyroidism
    congenital 243
  tricuspid (*see also* Endocarditis, tricuspid) 397.0
    congenital 746.89
    syphilitic 093.23
  urethral sphincter 599.84
  valve, valvular (heart) (*see also* Endocarditis) 424.90
  vascular 459.9
    intestine NEC 557.9
    mesenteric 557.1
    peripheral 443.9
    renal (*see also* Hypertension, kidney) 403.90
  velopharyngeal
    acquired 528.9
    congenital 750.29
  venous (peripheral) 459.81
  ventricular — *see* Insufficiency, myocardial
  vertebral artery 435.1
  vertebrobasilar artery 435.3
  weight gain during pregnancy 646.8 ✓5ᵗʰ
  zinc 269.3
Insufflation
  fallopian
    fertility testing V26.21
    following sterilization reversal V26.22
  meconium 770.1
Insular — *see* condition
Insulinoma (M8151/0)
  malignant (M8151/3)
    pancreas 157.4
    specified site — *see* Neoplasm, by site, malignant
    unspecified site 157.4
  pancreas 211.7
  specified site — *see* Neoplasm, by site, benign
  unspecified site 211.7
Insuloma — *see* Insulinoma
Insult
  brain 437.9
    acute 436
  cerebral 437.9
    acute 436
  cerebrovascular 437.9
    acute 436
  vascular NEC 437.9
    acute 436
Insurance examination (certification) V70.3
Intemperance (*see also* Alcoholism) 303.9 ✓5ᵗʰ
Interception of pregnancy (menstrual extraction) V25.3

Intermenstrual
bleeding 626.6
  irregular 626.6
  regular 626.5
hemorrhage 626.6
  irregular 626.6
  regular 626.5
pain(s) 625.2
Intermittent — see condition
Internal — see condition
Interproximal wear 521.1
Interruption
  aortic arch 747.11
  bundle of His 426.50
  fallopian tube (for sterilization) V25.2
  phase-shift, sleep cycle 307.45
  repeated REM-sleep 307.48
  sleep
    due to perceived environmental disturbances 307.48
    phase-shift, of 24-hour sleep-wake cycle 307.45
    repeated REM-sleep type 307.48
  vas deferens (for sterilization) V25.2
Intersexuality 752.7
Interstitial — see condition
Intertrigo 695.89
  labialis 528.5
Intervertebral disc — see condition
Intestine, intestinal — see also condition
  flu 487.8
Intolerance
  carbohydrate NEC 579.8
  cardiovascular exercise, with pain (at rest) (with less than ordinary activity) (with ordinary activity) V47.2
  cold 780.99 ▲
  dissacharide (hereditary) 271.3
  drug
    correct substance properly administered 995.2
    wrong substance given or taken in error 977.9
      specified drug — see Table of Drugs and Chemicals
  effort 306.2
  fat NEC 579.8
  foods NEC 579.8
  fructose (hereditary) 271.2
  glucose (-galactose) (congenital) 271.3
  gluten 579.0
  lactose (hereditary) (infantile) 271.3
  lysine (congenital) 270.7
  milk NEC 579.8
  protein (familial) 270.7
  starch NEC 579.8
  sucrose (-isomaltose) (congenital) 271.3
Intoxicated NEC (see also Alcoholism) 305.0
Intoxication
  acid 276.2
  acute
    alcoholic 305.0
      with alcoholism 303.0
      hangover effects 305.0
    caffeine 305.9
    hallucinogenic (see also Abuse, drugs, nondependent) 305.3
  alcohol (acute) 305.0
    with alcoholism 303.0

Intoxication — continued
  alcohol — continued
    hangover effects 305.0
    idiosyncratic 291.4
    pathological 291.4
  alimentary canal 558.2
  ammonia (hepatic) 572.2
  chemical — see also Table of Drugs and Chemicals
    via placenta or breast milk 760.70
      alcohol 760.71
      anti-infective agents 760.74
      cocaine 760.75
      "crack" 760.75
      hallucinogenic agents NEC 760.73
      medicinal agents NEC 760.79
      narcotics 760.72
      obstetric anesthetic or analgesic drug 763.5
      specified agent NEC 760.79
      suspected, affecting management of pregnancy 655.5
  cocaine, through placenta or breast milk 760.75
  delirium
    alcohol 291.0
    drug 292.81
  drug
    with delirium 292.81
    correct substance properly administered (see also Allergy, drug) 995.2
    newborn 779.4
    obstetric anesthetic or sedation 668.9
      affecting fetus or newborn 763.5
    overdose or wrong substance given or taken — see Table of Drugs and Chemicals
    pathologic 292.2
    specific to newborn 779.4
    via placenta or breast milk 760.70
      alcohol 760.71
      anti-infective agents 760.74
      cocaine 760.75
      "crack" 760.75
      hallucinogenic agents 760.73
      medicinal agents NEC 760.79
      narcotics 760.72
      obstetric anesthetic or analgesic drug 763.5
      specified agent NEC 760.79
      suspected, affecting management of pregnancy 655.5
  enteric — see Intoxication, intestinal
  fetus or newborn, via placenta or breast milk 760.70
    alcohol 760.71
    anti-infective agents 760.74
    cocaine 760.75
    "crack" 760.75
    hallucinogenic agents 760.73
    medicinal agents NEC 760.79
    narcotics 760.72
    obstetric anesthetic or analgesic drug 763.5
    specified agent NEC 760.79
    suspected, affecting management of pregnancy 655.5
  food — see Poisoning, food
  gastrointestinal 558.2
  hallucinogenic (acute) 305.3
  hepatocerebral 572.2
  idiosyncratic alcohol 291.4

Intoxication — continued
  intestinal 569.89
    due to putrefaction of food 005.9
    methyl alcohol (see also Alcoholism) 305.0 ✓5ᵗʰ
      with alcoholism 303.0 ✓5ᵗʰ
  pathologic 291.4
    drug 292.2
  potassium (K) 276.7
  septic
    with
      abortion — see Abortion, by type, with sepsis
      ectopic pregnancy (see also categories 633.0-633.9) 639.0
      molar pregnancy (see also categories 630-632) 639.0
    during labor 659.3 ✓5ᵗʰ
    following
      abortion 639.0
      ectopic or molar pregnancy 639.0
    generalized — see Septicemia
    puerperal, postpartum, childbirth 670 ✓4ᵗʰ
  serum (prophylactic) (therapeutic) 999.5
  uremic — see Uremia
  water 276.6
Intracranial — see condition
Intrahepatic gallbladder 751.69
Intraligamentous — see also condition
  pregnancy — see Pregnancy, cornual
Intraocular — see also condition
  sepsis 360.00
Intrathoracic — see also condition
  kidney 753.3
  stomach — see Hernia, diaphragm
Intrauterine contraceptive device
  checking V25.42
  insertion V25.1
  in situ V45.51
  management V25.42
  prescription V25.02
    repeat V25.42
  reinsertion V25.42
  removal V25.42
Intraventricular — see condition
Intrinsic deformity — see Deformity
Intrusion, repetitive, of sleep (due to environmental disturbances) (with atypical polysomnographic features) 307.48
Intumescent, lens (eye) NEC 366.9
  senile 366.12
Intussusception (colon) (enteric) (intestine) (rectum) 560.0
  appendix 543.9
  congenital 751.5
  fallopian tube 620.8
  ileocecal 560.0
  ileocolic 560.0
  ureter (with obstruction) 593.4
Invagination
  basilar 756.0
  colon or intestine 560.0
Invalid (since birth) 799.8
Invalidism (chronic) 799.8
Inversion
  albumin-globulin (A-G) ratio 273.8
  bladder 596.8
  cecum (see also Intussusception) 560.0
  cervix 622.8

Inversion — continued
  nipple 611.79
    congenital 757.6
    puerperal, postpartum 676.3 ✓5ᵗʰ
  optic papilla 743.57
  organ or site, congenital NEC — see Anomaly, specified type NEC
  sleep rhythm 780.55
    nonorganic origin 307.45
  testis (congenital) 752.51
  uterus (postinfectional) (postpartal, old) 621.7
    chronic 621.7
    complicating delivery 665.2 ✓5ᵗʰ
      affecting fetus or newborn 763.89
  vagina — see Prolapse, vagina
Investigation
  allergens V72.7
  clinical research (control) (normal comparison) (participant) V70.7
Inviability — see Immaturity
Involuntary movement, abnormal 781.0
Involution, involutional — see also condition
  breast, cystic or fibrocystic 610.1
  depression (see also Psychosis, affective) 296.2 ✓5ᵗʰ
    recurrent episode 296.3 ✓5ᵗʰ
    single episode 296.2 ✓5ᵗʰ
  melancholia (see also Psychosis, affective) 296.2 ✓5ᵗʰ
    recurrent episode 296.3 ✓5ᵗʰ
    single episode 296.2 ✓5ᵗʰ
  ovary, senile 620.3
  paranoid state (reaction) 297.2
  paraphrenia (climacteric) (menopause) 297.2
  psychosis 298.8
  thymus failure 254.8
IQ
  under 20 318.2
  20-34 318.1
  35-49 318.0
  50-70 317
IRDS 769
Irideremia 743.45
Iridis rubeosis 364.42
  diabetic 250.5 ✓5ᵗʰ [364.42]
Iridochoroiditis (panuveitis) 360.12
Iridocyclitis NEC 364.3
  acute 364.00
    primary 364.01
    recurrent 364.02
  chronic 364.10
    in
      lepromatous leprosy 030.0 [364.11]
      sarcoidosis 135 [364.11]
      tuberculosis (see also Tuberculosis) 017.3 ✓5ᵗʰ [364.11]
  due to allergy 364.04
  endogenous 364.01
  gonococcal 098.41
  granulomatous 364.10
  herpetic (simplex) 054.44
    zoster 053.22
  hypopyon 364.05
  lens induced 364.23
  nongranulomatous 364.00
  primary 364.01
  recurrent 364.02
  rheumatic 364.10
  secondary 364.04
    infectious 364.03

Iridocyclitis NEC — continued
  secondary — continued
    noninfectious 364.04
  subacute 364.00
    primary 364.01
    recurrent 364.02
  sympathetic 360.11
  syphilitic (secondary) 091.52
  tuberculous (chronic) (see also Tuberculosis) 017.3 ✓5ᵗʰ [364.11]
Iridocyclochoroiditis (panuveitis) 360.12
Iridodialysis 364.76
Iridodonesis 364.8
Iridoplegia (complete) (partial) (reflex) 379.49
Iridoschisis 364.52
Iris — see condition
Iritis 364.3
  acute 364.00
    primary 364.01
    recurrent 364.02
  chronic 364.10
    in
      sarcoidosis 135 [364.11]
      tuberculosis (see also Tuberculosis) 017.3 ✓5ᵗʰ [364.11]
  diabetic 250.5 ✓5ᵗʰ [364.42]
  due to
    allergy 364.04
    herpes simplex 054.44
    leprosy 030.0 [364.11]
  endogenous 364.01
  gonococcal 098.41
  gouty 274.89 [364.11]
  granulomatous 364.10
  hypopyon 364.05
  lens induced 364.23
  nongranulomatous 364.00
  papulosa 095.8 [364.11]
  primary 364.01
  recurrent 364.02
  rheumatic 364.10
  secondary 364.04
    infectious 364.03
    noninfectious 364.04
  subacute 364.00
    primary 364.01
    recurrent 364.02
  sympathetic 360.11
  syphilitic (secondary) 091.52
    congenital 090.0 [364.11]
    late 095.8 [364.11]
  tuberculous (see also Tuberculosis) 017.3 ✓5ᵗʰ [364.11]
  uratic 274.89 [364.11]
Iron
  deficiency anemia 280.9
  metabolism disease 275.0
  storage disease 275.0
Iron-miners' lung 503
Irradiated enamel (tooth, teeth) 521.8
Irradiation
  burn — see Burn, by site
  effects, adverse 990
Irreducible, irreducibility — see condition
Irregular, irregularity
  action, heart 427.9
  alveolar process 525.8
  bleeding NEC 626.4
  breathing 786.09

Irregular, irregularity — continued
  colon 569.89
  contour of cornea 743.41
    acquired 371.70
  dentin in pulp 522.3
  eye movements NEC 379.59
  menstruation (cause unknown) 626.4
  periods 626.4
  prostate 602.9
  pupil 364.75
  respiratory 786.09
  septum (nasal) 470
  shape, organ or site, congenital NEC — see Distortion
  sleep-wake rhythm (non-24-hour) 780.55
    nonorganic origin 307.45
  vertebra 733.99
Irritability (nervous) 799.2
  bladder 596.8
    neurogenic 596.54
      with cauda equina syndrome 344.61
  bowel (syndrome) 564.1
  bronchial (see also Bronchitis) 490
  cerebral, newborn 779.1
  colon 564.1
    psychogenic 306.4
  duodenum 564.89
  heart (psychogenic) 306.2
  ileum 564.89
  jejunum 564.89
  myocardium 306.2
  rectum 564.89
  stomach 536.9
    psychogenic 306.4
  sympathetic (nervous system) (see also Neuropathy, peripheral, autonomic) 337.9
  urethra 599.84
  ventricular (heart) (psychogenic) 306.2
Irritable — see Irritability
Irritation
  anus 569.49
  axillary nerve 353.0
  bladder 596.8
  brachial plexus 353.0
  brain (traumatic) (see also Injury, intracranial) 854.0 ✓5ᵗʰ
    nontraumatic — see Encephalitis
  bronchial (see also Bronchitis) 490
  cerebral (traumatic) (see also Injury, intracranial) 854.0 ✓5ᵗʰ
    nontraumatic — see Encephalitis
  cervical plexus 353.2
  cervix (see also Cervicitis) 616.0
  choroid, sympathetic 360.11
  cranial nerve — see Disorder, nerve, cranial
  digestive tract 536.9
    psychogenic 306.4
  gastric 536.9
    psychogenic 306.4
  gastrointestinal (tract) 536.9
    functional 536.9
    psychogenic 306.4
  globe, sympathetic 360.11
  intestinal (bowel) 564.9
  labyrinth 386.50
  lumbosacral plexus 353.1
  meninges (traumatic) (see also Injury, intracranial) 854.0 ✓5ᵗʰ
    nontraumatic — see Meningitis
  myocardium 306.2
  nerve — see Disorder, nerve

Irritation — *continued*
    nervous 799.2
    nose 478.1
    penis 607.89
    perineum 709.9
    peripheral
        autonomic nervous system (*see also*
            Neuropathy, peripheral, autonomic)
            337.9
        nerve — *see* Disorder, nerve
    peritoneum (*see also* Peritonitis) 567.9
    pharynx 478.29
    plantar nerve 355.6
    spinal (cord) (traumatic) — *see also* Injury,
            spinal, by site
        nerve — *see also* Disorder, nerve
            root NEC 724.9
        traumatic — *see* Injury, nerve, spinal
        nontraumatic — *see* Myelitis
    stomach 536.9
        psychogenic 306.4
    sympathetic nerve NEC (*see also* Neuropathy,
            peripheral, autonomic) 337.9
    ulnar nerve 354.2
    vagina 623.9
Isambert's disease 012.3 ✓5ᵗʰ
Ischemia, ischemic 459.9
    basilar artery (with transient neurologic
            deficit) 435.0
    bone NEC 733.40
    bowel (transient) 557.9
        acute 557.0
        chronic 557.1
        due to mesenteric artery insufficiency
            557.1
    brain — *see also* Ischemia, cerebral
        recurrent focal 435.9
    cardiac (*see also* Ischemia, heart) 414.9
    cardiomyopathy 414.8
    carotid artery (with transient neurologic
            deficit) 435.8
    cerebral (chronic) (generalized) 437.1
        arteriosclerotic 437.0
        intermittent (with transient neurologic
            deficit) 435.9
        puerperal, postpartum, childbirth 674.0
            ✓5ᵗʰ
        recurrent focal (with transient neurologic
            deficit) 435.9
        transient (with transient neurologic deficit)
            435.9
    colon 557.9
        acute 557.0
        chronic 557.1
        due to mesenteric artery insufficiency
            557.1
    coronary (chronic) (*see also* Ischemia, heart)
            414.9
    heart (chronic or with a stated duration of
            over 8 weeks) 414.9
        acute or with a stated duration of 8 weeks
            or less (*see also* Infarct, myocardium)
            410.9 ✓5ᵗʰ
        without myocardial infarction 411.89
            with coronary (artery) occlusion
                411.81
        subacute 411.89
    intestine (transient) 557.9
        acute 557.0
        chronic 557.1
        due to mesenteric artery insufficiency
            557.1

Ischemia, ischemic — *continued*
    kidney 593.81
    labyrinth 386.50
    muscles, leg 728.89
    myocardium, myocardial (chronic or with a
            stated duration of over 8 weeks) 414.8
        acute (*see also* Infarct, myocardium)
            410.9 ✓5ᵗʰ
        without myocardial infarction 411.89
            with coronary (artery) occlusion
                411.81
    renal 593.81
    retina, retinal 362.84
    small bowel 557.9
        acute 557.0
        chronic 557.1
        due to mesenteric artery insufficiency
            557.1
    spinal cord 336.1
    subendocardial (*see also* Insufficiency,
            coronary) 411.89
    vertebral artery (with transient neurologic
            deficit) 435.1
Ischialgia (*see also* Sciatica) 724.3
Ischiopagus 759.4
Ischium, ischial — *see* condition
Ischomenia 626.8
Ischuria 788.5
Iselin's disease or osteochondrosis 732.5
Islands of
    parotid tissue in
        lymph nodes 750.26
        neck structures 750.26
    submaxillary glands in
        fascia 750.26
        lymph nodes 750.26
        neck muscles 750.26
Islet cell tumor, pancreas (M8150/0) 211.7
Isoimmunization NEC (*see also* Incompatibility)
        656.2 ✓5ᵗʰ
    fetus or newborn 773.2
        ABO blood groups 773.1
        Rhesus (Rh) factor 773.0
Isolation V07.0
    social V62.4
Isosporosis 007.2
Issue
    medical certificate NEC V68.0
        cause of death V68.0
        fitness V68.0
        incapacity V68.0
    repeat prescription NEC V68.1
        appliance V68.1
        contraceptive V25.40
            device NEC V25.49
                intrauterine V25.42
                specified type NEC V25.49
            pill V25.41
        glasses V68.1
        medicinal substance V68.1
Itch (*see also* Pruritus) 698.9
    bakers' 692.89
    barbers' 110.0
    bricklayers' 692.89
    cheese 133.8
    clam diggers' 120.3
    coolie 126.9
    copra 133.8
    Cuban 050.1

Itch — *continued*
  dew 126.9
  dhobie 110.3
  eye 379.99
  filarial (*see also* Infestation, filarial) 125.9
  grain 133.8
  grocers' 133.8
  ground 126.9
  harvest 133.8
  jock 110.3
  Malabar 110.9
    beard 110.0
    foot 110.4
    scalp 110.0
  meaning scabies 133.0
  Norwegian 133.0
  perianal 698.0
  poultrymen's 133.8
  sarcoptic 133.0
  scrub 134.1
  seven year V61.10
    meaning scabies 133.0
  straw 133.8
  swimmers' 120.3
  washerwoman's 692.4
  water 120.3
  winter 698.8
Itsenko-Cushing syndrome (pituitary basophilism) 255.0
Ivemark's syndrome (asplenia with congenital heart disease) 759.0
Ivory bones 756.52
Ixodes 134.8
Ixodiasis 134.8

J

Jaccoud's nodular fibrositis, chronic (Jaccoud's syndrome) 714.4
Jackson's
  membrane 751.4
  paralysis or syndrome 344.89
  veil 751.4
Jacksonian
  epilepsy (*see also* Epilepsy) 345.5
  seizures (focal) (*see also* Epilepsy) 345.5
Jacob's ulcer (M8090/3) — *see* Neoplasm, skin, malignant, by site
Jacquet's dermatitis (diaper dermatitis) 691.0
Jadassohn's
  blue nevus (M8780/0) — *see* Neoplasm, skin, benign
  disease (maculopapular erythroderma) 696.2
  intraepidermal epithelioma (M8096/0) — *see* Neoplasm, skin, benign
Jadassohn-Lewandowski syndrome (pachyonychia congenita) 757.5
Jadassohn-Pellizari's disease (anetoderma) 701.3
Jadassohn-Tièche nevus (M8780/0) — *see* Neoplasm, skin, benign
Jaffe-Lichtenstein (-Uehlinger) syndrome 252.0
Jahnke's syndrome (encephalocutaneous angiomatosis) 759.6
Jakob-Creutzfeldt disease or syndrome 046.1
  with dementia
    with behavioral disturbance 046.1 [294.11]

Jakob-Creutzfeldt disease or syndrome — *continued*
  with dementia — *continued*
    without behavioral disturbance 046.1 [294.10]
Jaksch (-Luzet) disease or syndrome (pseudoleukemia infantum) 285.8
Jamaican
  neuropathy 349.82
  paraplegic tropical ataxic-spastic syndrome 349.82
Janet's disease (psychasthenia) 300.89
Janiceps 759.4
Jansky-Bielschowsky amaurotic familial idiocy 330.1
Japanese
  B type encephalitis 062.0
  river fever 081.2
  seven-day fever 100.89
Jaundice (yellow) 782.4
  acholuric (familial) (splenomegalic) (*see also* Spherocytosis) 282.0
    acquired 283.9
  breast milk 774.39
  catarrhal (acute) 070.1
    with hepatic coma 070.0
    chronic 571.9
    epidemic — *see* Jaundice, epidemic
  cholestatic (benign) 782.4
  chronic idiopathic 277.4
  epidemic (catarrhal) 070.1
    with hepatic coma 070.0
    leptospiral 100.0
    spirochetal 100.0
  febrile (acute) 070.1
    with hepatic coma 070.0
    leptospiral 100.0
    spirochetal 100.0
  fetus or newborn 774.6
    due to or associated with
      ABO
        antibodies 773.1
        incompatibility, maternal/fetal 773.1
        isoimmunization 773.1
      absence or deficiency of enzyme system for bilirubin conjugation (congenital) 774.39
      blood group incompatibility NEC 773.2
      breast milk inhibitors to conjugation 774.39
        associated with preterm delivery 774.2
      bruising 774.1
      Crigler-Najjar syndrome 277.4 [774.31]
      delayed conjugation 774.30
        associated with preterm delivery 774.2
        development 774.39
      drugs or toxins transmitted from mother 774.1
      G-6-PD deficiency 282.2 [774.0]
      galactosemia 271.1 [774.5]
      Gilbert's syndrome 277.4 [774.31]
      hepatocellular damage 774.4
      hereditary hemolytic anemia (*see also* Anemia, hemolytic) 282.9 [774.0]
      hypothyroidism, congenital 243 [774.31]
      incompatibility, maternal/fetal NEC 773.2
      infection 774.1

Jaundice — continued
  fetus or newborn — continued
    due to or associated with — continued
      inspissated bile syndrome 774.4
      isoimmunization NEC 773.2
      mucoviscidosis 277.01 *[774.5]*
      obliteration of bile duct, congenital 751.61 *[774.5]*
      polycythemia 774.1
      preterm delivery 774.2
      red cell defect 282.9 *[774.0]*
      Rh
        antibodies 773.0
        incompatibility, maternal/fetal 773.0
        isoimmunization 773.0
      spherocytosis (congenital) 282.0 *[774.0]*
      swallowed maternal blood 774.1
    physiological NEC 774.6
  from injection, inoculation, infusion, or transfusion (blood) (plasma) (serum) (other substance) (onset within 8 months after administration) — see Hepatitis, viral
  Gilbert's (familial nonhemolytic) 277.4
  hematogenous 283.9
  hemolytic (acquired) 283.9
    congenital (*see also* Spherocytosis) 282.0
  hemorrhagic (acute) 100.0
    leptospiral 100.0
    newborn 776.0
    spirochetal 100.0
  hepatocellular 573.8
  homologous (serum) — *see* Hepatitis, viral
  idiopathic, chronic 277.4
  infectious (acute) (subacute) 070.1
    with hepatic coma 070.0
    leptospiral 100.0
    spirochetal 100.0
  leptospiral 100.0
  malignant (*see also* Necrosis, liver) 570
  newborn (physiological) (*see also* Jaundice, fetus or newborn) 774.6
  nonhemolytic, congenital familial (Gilbert's) 277.4
  nuclear, newborn (*see also* Kernicterus of newborn) 774.7
  obstructive NEC (*see also* Obstruction, biliary) 576.8
  postimmunization — *see* Hepatitis, viral
  posttransfusion — *see* Hepatitis, viral
  regurgitation (*see also* Obstruction, biliary) 576.8
  serum (homologous) (prophylactic) (therapeutic) — *see* Hepatitis, viral
  spirochetal (hemorrhagic) 100.0
  symptomatic 782.4
    newborn 774.6

Jaw — *see* condition
Jaw-blinking 374.43
  congenital 742.8
Jaw-winking phenomenon or syndrome 742.8
Jealousy
  alcoholic 291.5
  childhood 313.3
  sibling 313.3
Jejunitis (*see also* Enteritis) 558.9
Jejunostomy status V44.4
Jejunum, jejunal — *see* condition
Jensen's disease 363.05
Jericho boil 085.1

Jerks, myoclonic 333.2
Jeune's disease or syndrome (asphyxiating thoracic dystrophy) 756.4
Jigger disease 134.1
Job's syndrome (chronic granulomatous disease) 288.1
Jod-Basedow phenomenon 242.8 ✓5ᵗʰ
Johnson-Stevens disease (erythema multiforme exudativum) 695.1
Joint — *see also* condition
  Charcôt's 094.0 *[713.5]*
  false 733.82
  flail — *see* Flail, joint
  mice — *see* Loose, body, joint, by site
  sinus to bone 730.9 ✓5ᵗʰ
  von Gies' 095.8
Jordan's anomaly or syndrome 288.2
Josephs-Diamond-Blackfan anemia (congenital hypoplastic) 284.0
Joubert syndrome 759.89
Jumpers' knee 727.2
Jungle yellow fever 060.0
Jüngling's disease (sarcoidosis) 135
Junin virus hemorrhagic fever 078.7
Juvenile — *see also* condition
  delinquent 312.9
    group (*see also* Disturbance, conduct) 312.2 ✓5ᵗʰ
  neurotic 312.4

K

Kahler (-Bozzolo) disease (multiple myeloma) (M9730/3) 203.0
Kakergasia 300.9
Kakke 265.0
Kala-azar (Indian) (infantile) (Mediterranean) (Sudanese) 085.0
Kalischer's syndrome (encephalocutaneous angiomatosis) 759.6
Kallmann's syndrome (hypogonadotropic hypogonadism with anosmia) 253.4
Kanner's syndrome (autism) (*see also* Psychosis, childhood) 299.0
Kaolinosis 502
Kaposi's
  disease 757.33
    lichen ruber 696.4
      acuminatus 696.4
      moniliformis 697.8
    xeroderma pigmentosum 757.33
  sarcoma (M9140/3) 176.9
    adipose tissue 176.1
    aponeurosis 176.1
    artery 176.1
    blood vessel 176.1
    bursa 176.1
    connective tissue 176.1
    external genitalia 176.8
    fascia 176.1
    fatty tissue 176.1
    fibrous tissue 176.1
    gastrointestinal tract NEC 176.3
    ligament 176.1
    lung 176.4
    lymph
      gland(s) 176.5
      node(s) 176.5
    lymphatic(s) NEC 176.1
    muscle (skeletal) 176.1
    oral cavity NEC 176.8
    palate 176.2
    scrotum 176.8
    skin 176.0
    soft tissue 176.1
    specified site NEC 176.8
    subcutaneous tissue 176.1
    synovia 176.1
    tendon (sheath) 176.1
    vein 176.1
    vessel 176.1
    viscera NEC 176.9
    vulva 176.8
  varicelliform eruption 054.0
    vaccinia 999.0
Kartagener's syndrome or triad (sinusitis, bronchiectasis, situs inversus) 759.3
Kasabach-Merritt syndrome (capillary hemangioma associated with thrombocytopenic purpura) 287.3
Kaschin-Beck disease (endemic polyarthritis) — *see* Disease, Kaschin-Beck
Kast's syndrome (dyschondroplasia with hemangiomas) 756.4
Katatonia (*see also* Schizophrenia) 295.2
Katayama disease or fever 120.2
Kathisophobia 781.0
Kawasaki disease 446.1
Kayser-Fleischer ring (cornea) (pseudosclerosis) 275.1 *[371.14]*
Kaznelson's syndrome (congenital hypoplastic anemia) 284.0
Kedani fever 081.2
Kelis 701.4
Kelly (-Patterson) syndrome (sideropenic dysphagia) 280.8
Keloid, cheloid 701.4
  Addison's (morphea) 701.0
  cornea 371.00
  Hawkins' 701.4
  scar 701.4
Keloma 701.4
Kenya fever 082.1
Keratectasia 371.71
  congenital 743.41
Keratitis (nodular) (nonulcerative) (simple) (zonular) NEC 370.9
  with ulceration (*see also* Ulcer, cornea) 370.00
  actinic 370.24
  arborescens 054.42
  areolar 370.22
  bullosa 370.8
  deep — *see* Keratitis, interstitial
  dendritic(a) 054.42
  desiccation 370.34
  diffuse interstitial 370.52
  disciform(is) 054.43
    varicella 052.7 *[370.44]*
  epithelialis vernalis 372.13 *[370.32]*
  exposure 370.34
  filamentary 370.23
  gonococcal (congenital) (prenatal) 098.43
  herpes, herpetic (simplex) NEC 054.43
    zoster 053.21
  hypopyon 370.04
  in
    chickenpox 052.7 *[370.44]*
    exanthema (*see also* Exanthem) 057.9 *[370.44]*
    paravaccinia (*see also* Paravaccinia) 051.9 *[370.44]*
    smallpox (*see also* Smallpox) 050.9 *[370.44]*
    vernal conjunctivitis 372.13 *[370.32]*
  interstitial (nonsyphilitic) 370.50
    with ulcer (*see also* Ulcer, cornea) 370.00
    diffuse 370.52
    herpes, herpetic (simplex) 054.43
      zoster 053.21
    syphilitic (congenital) (hereditary) 090.3
    tuberculous (*see also* Tuberculosis) 017.3 *[370.59]*
  lagophthalmic 370.34
  macular 370.22
  neuroparalytic 370.35
  neurotrophic 370.35
  nummular 370.22
  oyster-shuckers' 370.8
  parenchymatous — *see* Keratitis, interstitial
  petrificans 370.8
  phlyctenular 370.31
  postmeasles 055.71
  punctata, punctate 370.21
    leprosa 030.0 *[370.21]*
    profunda 090.3
    superficial (Thygeson's) 370.21
  purulent 370.8
  pustuliformis profunda 090.3
  rosacea 695.3 *[370.49]*

Index to Diseases

Keratitis — *continued*
  sclerosing 370.54
  specified type NEC 370.8
  stellate 370.22
  striate 370.22
  superficial 370.20
    with conjunctivitis (*see also*
      Keratoconjunctivitis) 370.40
    punctate (Thygeson's) 370.21
  suppurative 370.8
  syphilitic (congenital) (prenatal) 090.3
  trachomatous 076.1
    late effect 139.1
  tuberculous (phlyctenular) (*see also*
      Tuberculosis) 017.3 ✓5ᵗʰ *[370.31]*
  ulcerated (*see also* Ulcer, cornea) 370.00
  vesicular 370.8
  welders' 370.24
  xerotic (*see also* Keratomalacia) 371.45
    vitamin A deficiency 264.4
Keratoacanthoma 238.2
Keratocele 371.72
Keratoconjunctivitis (*see also* Keratitis) 370.40
  adenovirus type 8 077.1
  epidemic 077.1
  exposure 370.34
  gonococcal 098.43
  herpetic (simplex) 054.43
    zoster 053.21
  in
    chickenpox 052.7 *[370.44]*
    exanthema (*see also* Exanthem) 057.9
      [370.44]
    paravaccinia (*see also* Paravaccinia) 051.9
      [370.44]
    smallpox (*see also* Smallpox) 050.9 *[370.44]*
  infectious 077.1
  neurotrophic 370.35
  phlyctenular 370.31
  postmeasles 055.71
  shipyard 077.1
  sicca (Sjögren's syndrome) 710.2
    not in Sjögren's syndrome 370.33
  specified type NEC 370.49
  tuberculous (phlyctenular) (*see also*
      Tuberculosis) 017.3 ✓5ᵗʰ *[370.31]*
Keratoconus 371.60
  acute hydrops 371.62
  congenital 743.41
  stable 371.61
Keratocyst (dental) 526.0
Keratoderma, keratodermia (congenital)
    (palmaris et plantaris) (symmetrical) 757.39
  acquired 701.1
  blennorrhagica 701.1
    gonococcal 098.81
  climacterium 701.1
  eccentrica 757.39
  gonorrheal 098.81
  punctata 701.1
  tylodes, progressive 701.1
Keratodermatocele 371.72
Keratoglobus 371.70
  congenital 743.41
    associated with buphthalmos 743.22
Keratohemia 371.12
Keratoiritis (*see also* Iridocyclitis) 364.3
  syphilitic 090.3
  tuberculous (*see also* Tuberculosis) 017.3 ✓5ᵗʰ
    [364.11]

Keratolysis exfoliativa (congenital) 757.39
  acquired 695.89
  neonatorum 757.39
Keratoma 701.1
  congenital 757.39
  malignum congenitale 757.1
  palmaris et plantaris hereditarium 757.39
  senile 702.0
Keratomalacia 371.45
  vitamin A deficiency 264.4
Keratomegaly 743.41
Keratomycosis 111.1
  nigricans (palmaris) 111.1
Keratopathy 371.40
  band (*see also* Keratitis) 371.43
  bullous (*see also* Keratitis) 371.23
  degenerative (*see also* Degeneration, cornea)
    371.40
  hereditary (*see also* Dystrophy, cornea)
    371.50
  discrete colliquative 371.49
Keratoscleritis, tuberculous (*see also*
    Tuberculosis) 017.3 ✓5ᵗʰ *[370.31]*
Keratosis 701.1
  actinic 702.0
  arsenical 692.4
  blennorrhagica 701.1
    gonococcal 098.81
  congenital (any type) 757.39
  ear (middle) (*see also* Cholesteatoma) 385.30
  female genital (external) 629.8
  follicular, vitamin A deficiency 264.8
  follicularis 757.39
    acquired 701.1
    congenital (acneiformis) (Siemens') 757.39
    spinulosa (decalvans) 757.39
    vitamin A deficiency 264.8
  gonococcal 098.81
  larynx, laryngeal 478.79
  male genital (external) 608.89
  middle ear (*see also* Cholesteatoma) 385.30
  nigricans 701.2
    congenital 757.39
  obturans 380.21
  palmaris et plantaris (symmetrical) 757.39
  penile 607.89
  pharyngeus 478.29
  pilaris 757.39
    acquired 701.1
  punctata (palmaris et plantaris) 701.1
  scrotal 608.89
  seborrheic 702.19
    inflamed 702.11
  senilis 702.0
  solar 702.0
  suprafollicularis 757.39
  tonsillaris 478.29
  vagina 623.1
  vegetans 757.39
  vitamin A deficiency 264.8
Kerato-uveitis (*see also* Iridocyclitis) 364.3
Keraunoparalysis 994.0
Kerion (celsi) 110.0
Kernicterus of newborn (not due to
    isoimmunization) 774.7
  due to isoimmunization (conditions classifiable
    to 773.0-773.2) 773.4
Ketoacidosis 276.2
  diabetic 250.1 ✓5ᵗʰ

Ketonuria 791.6
 branched-chain, intermittent 270.3
Ketosis 276.2
 diabetic 250.1
Kidney — see condition
Kienböck's
 disease 732.3
  adult 732.8
  osteochondrosis 732.3
Kimmelstiel (-Wilson) disease or syndrome (intercapillary glomerulosclerosis) 250.4 [581.81]
Kink, kinking
 appendix 543.9
 artery 447.1
 cystic duct, congenital 751.61
 hair (acquired) 704.2
 ileum or intestine (see also Obstruction, intestine) 560.9
 Lane's (see also Obstruction, intestine) 560.9
 organ or site, congenital NEC — see Anomaly, specified type NEC, by site
 ureter (pelvic junction) 593.3
  congenital 753.20
 vein(s) 459.2
  caval 459.2
  peripheral 459.2
Kinnier Wilson's disease (hepatolenticular degeneration) 275.1
Kissing
 osteophytes 721.5
 spine 721.5
 vertebra 721.5
Klauder's syndrome (erythema multiforme, exudativum) 695.1
Klebs' disease (see also Nephritis) 583.9
Klein-Waardenburg syndrome (ptosisepicanthus) 270.2
Kleine-Levin syndrome 349.89
Kleptomania 312.32
Klinefelter's syndrome 758.7
Klinger's disease 446.4
Klippel's disease 723.8
Klippel-Feil disease or syndrome (brevicollis) 756.16
Klippel-Trenaunay syndrome 759.89
Klumpke (-Déjérine) palsy, paralysis (birth) (newborn) 767.6
Klüver-Bucy (-Terzian) syndrome 310.0
Knee — see condition
Knifegrinders' rot (see also Tuberculosis) 011.4
Knock-knee (acquired) 736.41
 congenital 755.64
Knot
 intestinal, syndrome (volvulus) 560.2
 umbilical cord (true) 663.2
  affecting fetus or newborn 762.5
Knots, surfer 919.8
 infected 919.9
Knotting (of)
 hair 704.2
 intestine 560.2
Knuckle pads (Garrod's) 728.79
Köbner's disease (epidermolysis bullosa) 757.39

Koch's
 infection (see also Tuberculosis, pulmonary) 011.9
 relapsing fever 087.9
Koch-Weeks conjunctivitis 372.03
Koenig-Wichman disease (pemphigus) 694.4
Köhler's disease (osteochondrosis) 732.5
 first (osteochondrosis juvenilis) 732.5
 second (Freiburg's infarction, metatarsal head) 732.5
 patellar 732.4
 tarsal navicular (bone) (osteoarthrosis juvenilis) 732.5
Köhler-Mouchet disease (osteoarthrosis juvenilis) 732.5
Köhler-Pellegrini-Stieda disease or syndrome (calcification, knee joint) 726.62
Koilonychia 703.8
 congenital 757.5
Kojevnikov's, Kojewnikoff's epilepsy (see also Epilepsy) 345.7
König's
 disease (osteochondritis dissecans) 732.7
 syndrome 564.89
Koniophthisis (see also Tuberculosis) 011.4
Koplik's spots 055.9
Kopp's asthma 254.8
Korean hemorrhagic fever 078.6
Korsakoff (-Wernicke) disease, psychosis, or syndrome (nonalcoholic) 294.0
 alcoholic 291.1
Korsakov's disease — see Korsakoff's disease
Korsakow's disease — see Korsakoff's disease
Kostmann's disease or syndrome (infantile genetic agranulocytosis) 288.0
Krabbe's
 disease (leukodystrophy) 330.0
 syndrome
  congenital muscle hypoplasia 756.89
  cutaneocerebral angioma 759.6
Kraepelin-Morel disease (see also Schizophrenia) 295.9
Kraft-Weber-Dimitri disease 759.6
Kraurosis
 ani 569.49
 penis 607.0
 vagina 623.8
 vulva 624.0
Kreotoxism 005.9
Krukenberg's
 spindle 371.13
 tumor (M8490/6) 198.6
Kufs' disease 330.1
Kugelberg-Welander disease 335.11
Kuhnt-Junius degeneration or disease 362.52
Kulchitsky's cell carcinoma (carcinoid tumor of intestine) 259.2
Kümmell's disease or spondylitis 721.7
Kundrat's disease (lymphosarcoma) 200.1
Kunekune — see Dermatophytosis
Kunkel syndrome (lupoid hepatitis) 571.49
Kupffer cell sarcoma (M9124/3) 155.0
Kuru 046.0
Kussmaul's
 coma (diabetic) 250.3
 disease (polyarteritis nodosa) 446.0

Kussmaul's — *continued*
  respiration (air hunger) 786.09
Kwashiorkor (marasmus type) 260
Kyasanur Forest disease 065.2
Kyphoscoliosis, kyphoscoliotic (acquired) (*see also* Scoliosis) 737.30
  congenital 756.19
  due to radiation 737.33
  heart (disease) 416.1
  idiopathic 737.30
    infantile
      progressive 737.32
      resolving 737.31
    late effect of rickets 268.1 *[737.43]*
    specified NEC 737.39
    thoracogenic 737.34
    tuberculous (*see also* Tuberculosis) 015.0 ✓5ᵗʰ *[737.43]*
Kyphosis, kyphotic (acquired) (postural) 737.10
  adolescent postural 737.0
  congenital 756.19
  dorsalis juvenilis 732.0
  due to or associated with
    Charcôt-Marie-Tooth disease 356.1 *[737.41]*
    mucopolysaccharidosis 277.5 *[737.41]*
    neurofibromatosis 237.71 *[737.41]*
    osteitis
      deformans 731.0 *[737.41]*
      fibrosa cystica 252.0 *[737.41]*
    osteoporosis (*see also* Osteoporosis) 733.0 ✓5ᵗʰ *[737.41]*
    poliomyelitis (*see also* Poliomyelitis) 138 *[737.41]*
    radiation 737.11
    tuberculosis (*see also* Tuberculosis) 015.0 ✓5ᵗʰ *[737.41]*
  Kümmell's 721.7
  late effect of rickets 268.1 *[737.41]*
  Morquio-Brailsford type (spinal) 277.5 *[737.41]*
  pelvis 738.6
  postlaminectomy 737.12
  specified cause NEC 737.19
  syphilitic, congenital 090.5 *[737.41]*
  tuberculous (*see also* Tuberculosis) 015.0 ✓5ᵗʰ *[737.41]*
Kyrle's disease (hyperkeratosis follicularis in cutem penetrans) 701.1

L

Labia, labium — *see* condition
Labiated hymen 752.49
Labile
  blood pressure 796.2
  emotions, emotionality 301.3
  vasomotor system 443.9
Labioglossal paralysis 335.22
Labium leporinum (*see also* Cleft, lip) 749.10
Labor (*see also* Delivery)
  with complications — *see* Delivery, complicated
  abnormal NEC 661.9 ✓5ᵗʰ
    affecting fetus or newborn 763.7
  arrested active phase 661.1 ✓5ᵗʰ
    affecting fetus or newborn 763.7
  desultory 661.2 ✓5ᵗʰ
    affecting fetus or newborn 763.7
  dyscoordinate 661.4 ✓5ᵗʰ
    affecting fetus or newborn 763.7
  early onset (22-36 weeks gestation) 644.2 ✓5ᵗʰ

Labor — *continued*
  failed
    induction 659.1 ✓5ᵗʰ
      mechanical 659.0 ✓5ᵗʰ
      medical 659.1 ✓5ᵗʰ
      surgical 659.0 ✓5ᵗʰ
    trial (vaginal delivery) 660.6 ✓5ᵗʰ
  false 644.1 ✓5ᵗʰ
  forced or induced, affecting fetus or newborn 763.89
  hypertonic 661.4 ✓5ᵗʰ
    affecting fetus or newborn 763.7
  hypotonic 661.2 ✓5ᵗʰ
    affecting fetus or newborn 763.7
    primary 661.0 ✓5ᵗʰ
      affecting fetus or newborn 763.7
    secondary 661.1 ✓5ᵗʰ
      affecting fetus or newborn 763.7
  incoordinate 661.4 ✓5ᵗʰ
    affecting fetus or newborn 763.7
  irregular 661.2 ✓5ᵗʰ
    affecting fetus or newborn 763.7
  long — *see* Labor, prolonged
  missed (at or near term) 656.4 ✓5ᵗʰ
  obstructed NEC 660.9 ✓5ᵗʰ
    affecting fetus or newborn 763.1
    specified cause NEC 660.8 ✓5ᵗʰ
      affecting fetus or newborn 763.1
  pains, spurious 644.1 ✓5ᵗʰ
  precipitate 661.3 ✓5ᵗʰ
    affecting fetus or newborn 763.6
  premature 644.2 ✓5ᵗʰ
    threatened 644.0 ✓5ᵗʰ
  prolonged or protracted 662.1 ✓5ᵗʰ
    affecting fetus or newborn 763.89
    first stage 662.0 ✓5ᵗʰ
      affecting fetus or newborn 763.89
    second stage 662.2 ✓5ᵗʰ
      affecting fetus or newborn 763.89
  threatened NEC 644.1 ✓5ᵗʰ
  undelivered 644.1 ✓5ᵗʰ
Labored breathing (*see also* Hyperventilation) 786.09
Labyrinthitis (inner ear) (destructive) (latent) 386.30
  circumscribed 386.32
  diffuse 386.31
  focal 386.32
  purulent 386.33
  serous 386.31
  suppurative 386.33
  syphilitic 095.8
  toxic 386.34
  viral 386.35
Laceration — *see also* Wound, open, by site
  accidental, complicating surgery 998.2
  Achilles tendon 845.09
    with open wound 892.2
  anus (sphincter) 863.89
    with
      abortion — *see* Abortion, by type, with damage to pelvic organs
      ectopic pregnancy (*see also* categories 633.0-633.9) 639.2
      molar pregnancy (*see also* categories 630-632) 639.2
    complicating delivery 664.2 ✓5ᵗʰ
      with laceration of anal or rectal mucosa 664.3 ✓5ᵗʰ

Laceration — *continued*
  anus — *continued*
    following
      abortion 639.2
      ectopic or molar pregnancy 639.2
    nontraumatic, nonpuerperal 565.0
  bladder (urinary)
    with
      abortion — *see* Abortion, by type, with damage to pelvic organs
      ectopic pregancy (*see also* categories 633.0-633.9) 639.2
      molar pregnancy (*see also* categories 630-632) 639.2
    following
      abortion 639.2
      ectopic or molar pregnancy 639.2
    obstetrical trauma 665.5 ✓5ᵗʰ
  blood vessel — *see* Injury, blood vessel, by site
  bowel
    with
      abortion — *see* Abortion, by type, with damage to pelvic organs
      ectopic pregnancy (*see also* categories 633.0-633.9) 639.2
      molar pregnancy (*see also* categories 630-632) 639.2
    following
      abortion 639.2
      ectopic or molar pregnancy 639.2
    obstetrical trauma 665.5 ✓5ᵗʰ
  brain (with hemorrhage) (cerebral) (membrane) 851.8 ✓5ᵗʰ
  brain (cerebral) (membrane) 851.8 ✓5ᵗʰ

> Note — Use the following fifth-digit subclassification with categories 851-854:
> 0   unspecified state of consciousness
> 1   with no loss of consciousness
> 2   with brief [less than one hour] loss of consciousness
> 3   with moderate [1-24 hours] loss of consciousness
> 4   with prolonged [more than 24 hours] loss of consciousness and return to pre-existing conscious level
> 5   with prolonged [more than 24 hours] loss of consciousness, without return to pre-existing conscious level
> Use fifth-digit 5 to designate when a patient is unconscious and dies before regaining consciousness, regardless of the duration of the loss of consciousness
> 6   with loss of consciousness of unspecified duration
> 9   with concussion, unspecified

    with
      open intracranial wound 851.9 ✓5ᵗʰ
      skull fracture — *see* Fracture, skull, by site
    cerebellum 851.6 ✓5ᵗʰ
      with open intracranial wound 851.7 ✓5ᵗʰ
    cortex 851.2 ✓5ᵗʰ
      with open intracranial wound 851.3 ✓5ᵗʰ
    during birth 767.0
    stem 851.6 ✓5ᵗʰ
      with open intracranial wound 851.7 ✓5ᵗʰ

Laceration — *continued*
  broad ligament
    with
      abortion — *see* Abortion, by type, with damage to pelvic organs
      ectopic pregnancy (*see also* categories 633.0-633.9) 639.2
      molar pregnancy (*see also* categories 630-632) 639.2
    following
      abortion 639.2
      ectopic or molar pregnancy 639.2
    nontraumatic 620.6
    obstetrical trauma 665.6 ✓5ᵗʰ
    syndrome (nontraumatic) 620.6
  capsule, joint — *see* Sprain, by site
  cardiac — *see* Laceration, heart
  causing eversion of cervix uteri (old) 622.0
  central, complicating delivery 664.4 ✓5ᵗʰ
  cerebellum — *see* Laceration, brain, cerebellum
  cerebral — *see also* Laceration, brain during birth 767.0
  cervix (uteri)
    with
      abortion — *see* Abortion, by type, with damage to pelvic organs
      ectopic pregnancy (*see also* categories 633.0-633.9) 639.2
      molar pregnancy (*see also* categories 630-632) 639.2
    following
      abortion 639.2
      ectopic or molar pregnancy 639.2
    nonpuerperal, nontraumatic 622.3
    obstetrical trauma (current) 665.3 ✓5ᵗʰ
    old (postpartal) 622.3
    traumatic — *see* Injury, internal, cervix
  chordae heart 429.5
  complicated 879.9
  cornea — *see* Laceration, eyeball
    superficial 918.1
  cortex (cerebral) — *see* Laceration, brain, cortex
  esophagus 530.89
  eye(s) — *see* Laceration, ocular
  eyeball NEC 871.4
    with prolapse or exposure of intraocular tissue 871.1
    penetrating — *see* Penetrating wound, eyeball
    specified as without prolapse of intraocular tissue 871.0
  eyelid NEC 870.8
    full thickness 870.1
      involving lacrimal passages 870.2
    skin (and periocular area) 870.0
    penetrating — *see* Penetrating wound, orbit
  fourchette
    with
      abortion — *see* Abortion, by type, with damage to pelvic organs
      ectopic pregnancy (*see also* categories 633.0-633.9) 639.2
      molar pregnancy (*see also* categories 630-632) 639.2
    complicating delivery 664.0 ✓5ᵗʰ
    following
      abortion 639.2
      ectopic or molar pregnancy 639.2

Laceration — continued
  heart (without penetration of heart chambers) 861.02
    with
      open wound into thorax 861.12
      penetration of heart chambers 861.03
        with open wound into thorax 861.13
  hernial sac — see Hernia, by site
  internal organ (abdomen) (chest) (pelvis) NEC — see Injury, internal, by site
  kidney (parenchyma) 866.02
    with
      complete disruption of parenchyma (rupture) 866.03
        with open wound into cavity 866.13
      open wound into cavity 866.12
  labia
    complicating delivery 664.0 ✓5ᵗʰ
  ligament — see also Sprain, by site
    with open wound — see Wound, open, by site
  liver 864.05
    with open wound into cavity 864.15
    major (disruption of hepatic parenchyma) 864.04
      with open wound into cavity 864.14
    minor (capsule only) 864.02
      with open wound into cavity 864.12
    moderate (involving parenchyma without major disruption) 864.03
      with open wound into cavity 864.13
    multiple 864.04
      with open wound into cavity 864.14
    stellate 864.04
      with open wound into cavity 864.14
  lung 861.22
    with open wound into thorax 861.32
  meninges — see Laceration, brain
  meniscus (knee) (see also Tear, meniscus) 836.2
    old 717.5
    site other than knee — see also Sprain, by site
      old NEC (see also Disorder, cartilage, articular) 718.0 ✓5ᵗʰ
  muscle — see also Sprain, by site
    with open wound — see Wound, open, by site
  myocardium — see Laceration, heart
  nerve — see Injury, nerve, by site
  ocular NEC (see also Laceration, eyeball) 871.4
    adnexa NEC 870.8
      penetrating 870.3
        with foreign body 870.4
  orbit (eye) 870.8
    penetrating 870.3
      with foreign body 870.4
  pelvic
    floor (muscles)
      with
        abortion — see Abortion, by type, with damage to pelvic organs
        ectopic pregnancy (see also categories 633.0-633.9) 639.2
        molar pregnancy (see also categories 630-632) 639.2
      complicating delivery 664.1 ✓5ᵗʰ
      following
        abortion 639.2
        ectopic or molar pregnancy 639.2
      nonpuerperal 618.7

Laceration — continued
  pelvic — continued
    floor — continued
      old (postpartal) 618.7
    organ NEC
      with
        abortion — see Abortion, by type, with damage to pelvic organs
        ectopic pregnancy (see also categories 633.0-633.9) 639.2
        molar pregnancy (see also categories 630-632) 639.2
      complicating delivery 665.5 ✓5ᵗʰ
        affecting fetus or newborn 763.89
      following
        abortion 639.2
        ectopic or molar pregnancy 639.2
      obstetrical trauma 665.5 ✓5ᵗʰ
  perineum, perineal (old) (postpartal) 618.7
    with
      abortion — see Abortion, by type, with damage to pelvic floor
      ectopic pregnancy (see also categories 633.0-633.9) 639.2
      molar pregnancy (see also categories 630-632) 639.2
    complicating delivery 664.4 ✓5ᵗʰ
      first degree 664.0 ✓5ᵗʰ
      second degree 664.1 ✓5ᵗʰ
      third degree 664.2 ✓5ᵗʰ
      fourth degree 664.3 ✓5ᵗʰ
    central 664.4 ✓5ᵗʰ
    involving
      anal sphincter 664.2 ✓5ᵗʰ
      fourchette 664.0 ✓5ᵗʰ
      hymen 664.0 ✓5ᵗʰ
      labia 664.0 ✓5ᵗʰ
      pelvic floor 664.1 ✓5ᵗʰ
      perineal muscles 664.1 ✓5ᵗʰ
      rectovaginal septum 664.2 ✓5ᵗʰ
        with anal mucosa 664.3 ✓5ᵗʰ
      skin 664.0 ✓5ᵗʰ
      sphincter (anal) 664.2 ✓5ᵗʰ
        with anal mucosa 664.3 ✓5ᵗʰ
      vagina 664.0 ✓5ᵗʰ
      vaginal muscles 664.1 ✓5ᵗʰ
      vulva 664.0 ✓5ᵗʰ
    secondary 674.2 ✓5ᵗʰ
    following
      abortion 639.2
      ectopic or molar pregnancy 639.2
    male 879.6
      complicated 879.7
    muscles, complicating delivery 664.1 ✓5ᵗʰ
    nonpuerperal, current injury 879.6
      complicated 879.7
    secondary (postpartal) 674.2 ✓5ᵗʰ
  peritoneum
    with
      abortion — see Abortion, by type, with damage to pelvic organs
      ectopic pregnancy (see also categories 633.0-633.9) 639.2
      molar pregnancy (see also categories 630-632) 639.2
    following
      abortion 639.2
      ectopic or molar pregnancy 639.2
    obstetrical trauma 665.5 ✓5ᵗʰ

Laceration — *continued*
  periurethral tissue
    with
      abortion — *see* Abortion, by type, with damage to pelvic organs
      ectopic pregnancy (*see also* categories 633.0-633.9) 639.2
      molar pregnancy (*see also* categories 630-632) 639.2
    following
      abortion 639.2
      ectopic or molar pregnancy 639.2
    obstetrical trauma 665.5 ✓5ᵗʰ
  rectovaginal (septum)
    with
      abortion — *see* Abortion, by type, with damage to pelvic organs
      ectopic pregnancy (*see also* categories 633.0-633.9) 639.2
      molar pregnancy (*see also* categories 630-632) 639.2
    complicating delivery 665.4 ✓5ᵗʰ
      with perineum 664.2 ✓5ᵗʰ
        involving anal or rectal mucosa 664.3 ✓5ᵗʰ
    following
      abortion 639.2
      ectopic or molar pregnancy 639.2
    nonpuerperal 623.4
    old (postpartal) 623.4
  spinal cord (meninges) — *see also* Injury, spinal, by site
    due to injury at birth 767.4
    fetus or newborn 767.4
  spleen 865.09
    with
      disruption of parenchyma (massive) 865.04
        with open wound into cavity 865.14
      open wound into cavity 865.19
      capsule (without disruption of parenchyma) 865.02
        with open wound into cavity 865.12
      parenchyma 865.03
        with open wound into cavity 865.13
        massive disruption (rupture) 865.04
          with open wound into cavity 865.14
  tendon 848.9
    with open wound — *see* Wound, open, by site
    Achilles 845.09
      with open wound 892.2
    lower limb NEC 844.9
      with open wound NEC 894.2
    upper limb NEC 840.9
      with open wound NEC 884.2
  tentorium cerebelli — *see* Laceration, brain, cerebellum
  tongue 873.64
    complicated 873.74
  urethra
    with
      abortion — *see* Abortion, by type, with damage to pelvic organs
      ectopic pregnancy (*see also* categories 633.0-633.9) 639.2
      molar pregnancy (*see also* categories 630-632) 639.2
    following
      abortion 639.2
      ectopic or molar pregnancy 639.2

Laceration — *continued*
  urethra — *continued*
    nonpuerperal, nontraumatic 599.84
    obstetrical trauma 665.5 ✓5ᵗʰ
  uterus
    with
      abortion — *see* Abortion, by type, with damage to pelvic organs
      ectopic pregnancy (*see also* categories 633.0-633.9) 639.2
      molar pregnancy (*see also* categories 630-632) 639.2
    following
      abortion 639.2
      ectopic or molar pregnancy 639.2
    nonpuerperal, nontraumatic 621.8
    obstetrical trauma NEC 665.8 ▲
    old (postpartal) 621.8
  vagina
    with
      abortion — *see* Abortion, by type, with damage to pelvic organs
      ectopic pregnancy (*see also* categories 633.0-633.9) 639.2
      molar pregnancy (*see also* categories 630-632) 639.2
      perineal involvement, complicating delivery 664.0 ✓5ᵗʰ
    complicating delivery 665.4 ✓5ᵗʰ
      first degree 664.0 ✓5ᵗʰ
      second degree 664.1 ✓5ᵗʰ
      third degree 664.2 ✓5ᵗʰ
      fourth degree 664.3 ✓5ᵗʰ
      high 665.4 ✓5ᵗʰ
      muscles 664.1 ✓5ᵗʰ
      sulcus 665.4 ✓5ᵗʰ
      wall 665.4 ✓5ᵗʰ
    following
      abortion 639.2
      ectopic or molar pregnancy 639.2
    nonpuerperal, nontraumatic 623.4
    old (postpartal) 623.4
  valve, heart — *see* Endocarditis
  vulva
    with
      abortion — *see* Abortion, by type, with damage to pelvic organs,
      ectopic pregnancy (*see also* categories 633.0-633.9) 639.2
      molar pregnancy (*see also* categories 630-632) 639.2
    complicating delivery 664.0 ✓5ᵗʰ
    following
      abortion 639.2
      ectopic or molar pregnancy 639.2
    nonpuerperal, nontraumatic 624.4
    old (postpartal) 624.4

Lachrymal — *see* condition
Lachrymonasal duct — *see* condition
Lack of
  appetite (*see also* Anorexia) 783.0
  care
    in home V60.4
    of adult 995.84
    of infant (at or after birth) 995.52
  coordination 781.3
  development — *see also* Hypoplasia
    physiological in childhood 783.40
  education V62.3
  energy 780.79
  financial resources V60.2

Lack of — *continued*
  food 994.2
    in environment V60.8
    growth in childhood 783.43
  heating V60.1
  housing (permanent) (temporary) V60.0
    adequate V60.1
  material resources V60.2
  medical attention 799.8
  memory (*see also* Amnesia) 780.99
    mild, following organic brain damage 310.1
  ovulation 628.0
  person able to render necessary care V60.4
  physical exercise V69.0
  physiologic development in childhood 783.40
  prenatal care in current pregnancy V23.7
  shelter V60.0
  water 994.3
Lacrimal — *see* condition
Lacrimation, abnormal (*see also* Epiphora) 375.20
Lacrimonasal duct — *see* condition
Lactation, lactating (breast) (puerperal) (postpartum)
  defective 676.4
  disorder 676.9
    specified type NEC 676.8
  excessive 676.6
  failed 676.4
  mastitis NEC 675.2
  mother (care and/or examination) V24.1
  nonpuerperal 611.6
  suppressed 676.5
Lacticemia 271.3
  excessive 276.2
Lactosuria 271.3
Lacunar skull 756.0
Laennec's cirrhosis (alcoholic) 571.2
  nonalcoholic 571.5
Lafora's disease 333.2
Lag, lid (nervous) 374.41
Lagleyze-von Hippel disease (retinocerebral angiomatosis) 759.6
Lagophthalmos (eyelid) (nervous) 374.20
  cicatricial 374.23
  keratitis (*see also* Keratitis) 370.34
  mechanical 374.22
  paralytic 374.21
La grippe — *see* Influenza
Lahore sore 085.1
Lakes, venous (cerebral) 437.8
Laki-Lorand factor deficiency (*see also* Defect, coagulation) 286.3
Lalling 307.9
Lambliasis 007.1
Lame back 724.5
Lancereaux's diabetes (diabetes mellitus with marked emaciation) 250.8 [261]
Landouzy-Déjérine dystrophy (fascioscapulohumeral atrophy) 359.1
Landry's disease or paralysis 357.0
Landry-Guillain-Barré syndrome 357.0
Lane's
  band 751.4
  disease 569.89
  kink (*see also* Obstruction, intestine) 560.9
Langdon Down's syndrome (mongolism) 758.0

Language abolition 784.69
Lanugo (persistent) 757.4
Laparoscopic surgical procedure converted to open procedure V64.4
Lardaceous
  degeneration (any site) 277.3
  disease 277.3
  kidney 277.3 [583.81]
  liver 277.3
Large
  baby (regardless of gestational age) 766.1
    exceptionally (weight of 4500 grams or more) 766.0
  of diabetic mother 775.0
  ear 744.22
  fetus — *see also* Oversize, fetus
    causing disproportion 653.5
      with obstructed labor 660.1
  for dates
    fetus or newborn (regardless of gestational age) 766.1
      affecting management of pregnancy 656.6
      exceptionally (weight of 4500 grams or more) 766.0
  physiological cup 743.57
  waxy liver 277.3
  white kidney — *see* Nephrosis
Larsen's syndrome (flattened facies and multiple congenital dislocations) 755.8
Larsen-Johansson disease (juvenile osteopathia patellae) 732.4
Larva migrans
  cutaneous NEC 126.9
    ancylostoma 126.9
  of Diptera in vitreous 128.0
  visceral NEC 128.0
Laryngeal — *see also* condition syncope 786.2
Laryngismus (acute) (infectious) (stridulous) 478.75
  congenital 748.3
  diphtheritic 032.3
Laryngitis (acute) (edematous) (fibrinous) (gangrenous) (infective) (infiltrative) (malignant) (membranous) (phlegmonous) (pneumococcal) (pseudomembranous) (septic) (subglottic) (suppurative) (ulcerative) (viral) 464.00
  with
    influenza, flu, or grippe 487.1
    obstruction 464.01
    tracheitis (*see also* Laryngotracheitis) 464.20
      with obstruction 464.21
      acute 464.20
        with obstruction 464.21
      chronic 476.1
  atrophic 476.0
  Borrelia vincentii 101
  catarrhal 476.0
  chronic 476.0
    with tracheitis (chronic) 476.1
    due to external agent — *see* Condition, respiratory, chronic, due to
  diphtheritic (membranous) 032.3
  due to external agent — *see* Inflammation, respiratory, upper, due to
  H. influenzae 464.00
    with obstruction 464.01

Laryngitis — continued
  Hemophilus influenzae 464.00
    wtih obstruction 464.01
  hypertrophic 476.0
  influenzal 487.1
  pachydermic 478.79
  sicca 476.0
  spasmodic 478.75
    acute 464.00
      with obstruction 464.01
  streptococcal 034.0
  stridulous 478.75
  syphilitic 095.8
    congenital 090.5
  tuberculous (see also Tuberculosis, larynx) 012.3 ✓5ᵗʰ
  Vincent's 101
Laryngocele (congenital) (ventricular) 748.3
Laryngofissure 478.79
  congenital 748.3
Laryngomalacia (congenital) 748.3
Laryngopharyngitis (acute) 465.0
  chronic 478.9
    due to external agent — see Condition, respiratory, chronic, due to
  due to external agent — see Inflammation, respiratory, upper, due to
  septic 034.0
Laryngoplegia (see also Paralysis, vocal cord) 478.30
Laryngoptosis 478.79
Laryngospasm 478.75
  due to external agent — see Condition, respiratory, acute, due to
Laryngostenosis 478.74
  congenital 748.3
Laryngotracheitis (acute) (infectional) (viral) (see also Laryngitis) 464.20
  with obstruction 464.21
  atrophic 476.1
  Borrelia vincenti 101
  catarrhal 476.1
  chronic 476.1
    due to external agent — see Condition, respiratory, chronic, due to
  diphtheritic (membranous) 032.3
  due to external agent — see Inflammation, respiratory, upper, due to
  H. influenzae 464.20
    with obstruction 464.21
  hypertrophic 476.1
  influenzal 487.1
  pachydermic 478.75
  sicca 476.1
  spasmodic 478.75
    acute 464.20
      with obstruction 464.21
  streptococcal 034.0
  stridulous 478.75
  syphilitic 095.8
    congenital 090.5
  tuberculous (see also Tuberculosis, larynx) 012.3 ✓5ᵗʰ
  Vincent's 101
Laryngotracheobronchitis (see also Bronchitis) 490
  acute 466.0
  chronic 491.8
  viral 466.0

Laryngotracheobronchopneumonitis — see Pneumonia, broncho-
Larynx, laryngeal — see condition
Lasègue's disease (persecution mania) 297.9
Lassa fever 078.89
Lassitude (see also Weakness) 780.79
Late — see also condition
  effect(s) (of) — see also condition
    abscess
      intracranial or intraspinal (conditions classifiable to 324) — see category 326
    adverse effect of drug, medicinal or biological substance 909.5
    amputation
      postoperative (late) 997.60
      traumatic (injury classifiable to 885-887 and 895-897) 905.9
    burn (injury classifiable to 948-949) 906.9
      extremities NEC (injury classifiable to 943 or 945) 906.7
      hand or wrist (injury classifiable to 944) 906.6
      eye (injury classifiable to 940) 906.5
      face, head, and neck (injury classifiable to 941) 906.5
      specified site NEC (injury classifiable to 942 and 946-947) 906.8
    cerebrovascular disease (conditions classifiable to 430-437) 438.9
      with
        alterations of sensations 438.6 •
        aphasia 438.11
        apraxia 438.81
        ataxia 438.84 •
        cognitive deficits 438.0
        disturbances of vision 438.7 •
        dysphagia 438.82
        dysphasia 438.12
        facial droop 438.83 •
        facial weakness 438.83 •
        hemiplegia/hemiparesis
          affecting
            dominant side 438.21
            nondominant side 438.22
            unspecified side 438.20
        monoplegia of lower limb
          affecting
            dominant side 438.41
            nondominant side 438.42
            unspecified side 438.40
        monoplegia of upper limb
          affecting
            dominant side 438.31
            nondominant side 438.32
            unspecified side 438.30
        paralytic syndrome NEC
          affecting
            bilateral 438.53
            dominant side 438.51
            nondominant side 438.52
            unspecified side 438.50
        speech and language deficit 438.10
        vertigo 438.85 •
      specified type NEC 438.89
    childbirth complication(s) 677
    complication(s) of
      childbirth 677
      delivery 677

Late — *continued*
  effect(s) (of) — continued
    complication(s) of — *continued*
      pregnancy 677
      puerperium 677
      surgical and medical care (conditions classifiable to 996-999) 909.3
      trauma (conditions classifiable to 958) 908.6
    contusion (injury classifiable to 920-924) 906.3
    crushing (injury classifiable to 925-929) 906.4
    delivery complication(s) 677
    dislocation (injury classifiable to 830-839) 905.6
    encephalitis or encephalomyelitis (conditions classifiable to 323) — *see* category 326
      in infectious diseases 139.8
      viral (conditions classifiable to 049.8, 049.9, 062-064) 139.0
    external cause NEC (conditions classifiable to 995) 909.9
      certain conditions classifiable to categories 991-994 909.4
    foreign body in orifice (injury classifiable to 930-939) 908.5
    fracture (multiple) (injury classifiable to 828-829) 905.5
      extremity
        lower (injury classifiable to 821-827) 905.4
          neck of femur (injury classifiable to 820) 905.3
          upper (injury classifiable to 810-819) 905.2
      face and skull (injury classifiable to 800-804) 905.0
      skull and face (injury classifiable to 800-804) 905.0
      spine and trunk (injury classifiable to 805 and 807-809) 905.1
        with spinal cord lesion (injury classifiable to 806) 907.2
    infection
      pyogenic, intracranial — *see* category 326
    infectious diseases (conditions classifiable to 001-136) NEC 139.8
    injury (injury classifiable to 959) 908.9
      blood vessel 908.3
        abdomen and pelvis (injury classifiable to 902) 908.4
        extremity (injury classifiable to 903-904) 908.3
        head and neck (injury classifiable to 900) 908.3
        intracranial (injury classifiable to 850-854) 907.0
          with skull fracture 905.0
        thorax (injury classifiable to 901) 908.4
      internal organ NEC (injury classifiable to 867 and 869) 908.2
        abdomen (injury classifiable to 863-866 and 868) 908.1
        thorax (injury classifiable to 860-862) 908.0
      intracranial (injury classifiable to 850-854) 907.0

Late — *continued*
  effect(s) (of) — continued
    injury — *continued*
      intracranial — *continued*
        with skull fracture (injury classifiable to 800-801 and 803-804) 905.0
      nerve NEC (injury classifiable to 957) 907.9
        cranial (injury classifiable to 950-951) 907.1
        peripheral NEC (injury classifiable to 957) 907.9
          lower limb and pelvic girdle (injury classifiable to 956) 907.5
          upper limb and shoulder girdle (injury classifiable to 955) 907.4
        roots and plexus(es), spinal (injury classifiable to 953) 907.3
        trunk (injury classifiable to 954) 907.3
      spinal
        cord (injury classifiable to 806 and 952) 907.2
        nerve root(s) and plexus(es) (injury classifiable to 953) 907.3
      superficial (injury classifiable to 910-919) 906.2
      tendon (tendon injury classifiable to 840-848, 880-884 with .2, and 890-894 with .2) 905.8
    meningitis
      bacterial (conditions classifiable to 320) — *see* category 326
      unspecified cause (conditions classifiable to 322) — *see* category 326
    myelitis (*see also* Late, effect(s) (of), encephalitis) — *see* category 326
    parasitic diseases (conditions classifiable to 001-136 NEC) 139.8
    phlebitis or thrombophlebitis of intracranial venous sinuses (conditions classifiable to 325) — *see* category 326
    poisoning due to drug, medicinal or biological substance (conditions classifiable to 960-979) 909.0
    poliomyelitis, acute (conditions classifiable to 045) 138
    pregnancy complication(s) 677
    puerperal complication(s) 677
    radiation (conditions classifiable to 990) 909.2
    rickets 268.1
    sprain and strain without mention of tendon injury (injury classifiable to 840-848, except tendon injury) 905.7
      tendon involvement 905.8
    toxic effect of
      drug, medicinal or biological substance (conditions classifiable to 960-979) 909.0
      nonmedical substance (conditions classifiable to 980-989) 909.1
    trachoma (conditions classifiable to 076) 139.1
    tuberculosis 137.0
      bones and joints (conditions classifiable to 015) 137.3
      central nervous system (conditions classifiable to 013) 137.1

Late — continued
  effect(s) (of) — continued
    tuberculosis — continued
      genitourinary (conditions classifiable to 016) 137.2
      pulmonary (conditions classifiable to 010-012) 137.0
      specified organs NEC (conditions classifiable to 014, 017-018) 137.4
      viral encephalitis (conditions classifiable to 049.8, 049.9, 062-064) 139.0
    wound, open
      extremity (injury classifiable to 880-884 and 890-894, except .2) 906.1
        tendon (injury classifiable to 880-884 with .2 and 890-894 with.2) 905.8
      head, neck, and trunk (injury classifiable to 870-879) 906.0
Latent — *see* condition
Lateral — *see* condition
Laterocession — *see* Lateroversion
Lateroflexion — *see* Lateroversion
Lateroversion
  cervix — *see* Lateroversion, uterus
  uterus, uterine (cervix) (postinfectional) (postpartal, old) 621.6
    congenital 752.3
    in pregnancy or childbirth 654.4 ✓5ᵗʰ
      affecting fetus or newborn 763.89
Lathyrism 988.2
Launois' syndrome (pituitary gigantism) 253.0
Launois-Bensaude's lipomatosis 272.8
Launois-Cléret syndrome (adiposogenital dystrophy) 253.8
Laurence-Moon-Biedl syndrome (obesity, polydactyly, and mental retardation) 759.89
LAV (disease) (illness) (infection) — *see* Human immunodeficiency virus (disease) (illness) (infection)
LAV/HTLV-III (disease) (illness) (infection) — *see* Human immunodeficiency virus (disease) (illness) (infection)
Lawford's syndrome (encephalocutaneous angiomatosis) 759.6
Lax, laxity — *see also* Relaxation
  ligament 728.4
  skin (acquired) 701.8
    congenital 756.83
Laxative habit (*see also* Abuse, drugs, nondependent) 305.9 ✓5ᵗʰ
Lazy leukocyte syndrome 288.0
Lead — *see also* condition
  exposure to V15.86
  incrustation of cornea 371.15
  poisoning 984.9
    specified type of lead — *see* Table of Drugs and Chemicals
Lead miners' lung 503
Leakage
  amniotic fluid 658.1 ✓5ᵗʰ
    with delayed delivery 658.2 ✓5ᵗʰ
    affecting fetus or newborn 761.1
  bile from drainage tube (T tube) 997.4
  blood (microscopic), fetal, into maternal circulation 656.0 ✓5ᵗʰ
    affecting management of pregnancy or puerperium 656.0 ✓5ᵗʰ

Leakage — *continued*
  device, implant, or graft — *see* Complications, mechanical
  spinal fluid at lumbar puncture site 997.09
  urine, continuous 788.37
Leaky heart — *see* Endocarditis
Learning defect, specific NEC (strephosymbolia) 315.2
Leather bottle stomach (M8142/3) 151.9
Leber's
  congenital amaurosis 362.76
  optic atrophy (hereditary) 377.16
Lederer's anemia or disease (acquired infectious hemolytic anemia) 283.19
Lederer-Brill syndrome (acquired infectious hemolytic anemia) 283.19
Leeches (aquatic) (land) 134.2
Left-sided neglect 781.8
Leg — *see* condition
Legal investigation V62.5
Legg (-Calvé) -Perthes disease or syndrome (osteochondrosis, femoral capital) 732.1
Legionnaires' disease 482.84
Leigh's disease 330.8
Leiner's disease (exfoliative dermatitis) 695.89
Leiofibromyoma (M8890/0) — *see also* Leiomyoma
  uterus (cervix) (corpus) (*see also* Leiomyoma, uterus) 218.9
Leiomyoblastoma (M8891/1) — *see* Neoplasm, connective tissue, uncertain behavior
Leiomyofibroma (M8890/0) — *see also* Neoplasm, connective tissue, benign
  uterus (cervix) (corpus) (*see also* Leiomyoma, uterus) 218.9
Leiomyoma (M8890/0) — *see also* Neoplasm, connective tissue, benign
  bizarre (M8893/0) — *see* Neoplasm, connective tissue, benign
  cellular (M8892/1) — *see* Neoplasm, connective tissue, uncertain behavior
  epithelioid (M8891/1) — *see* Neoplasm, connective tissue, uncertain behavior
  prostate (polypoid) 600.2
  uterus (cervix) (corpus) 218.9
    interstitial 218.1
    intramural 218.1
    submucous 218.0
    subperitoneal 218.2
    subserous 218.2
  vascular (M8894/0) — *see* Neoplasm, connective tissue, benign
Leiomyomatosis (intravascular) (M8890/1) — *see* Neoplasm, connective tissue, uncertain behavior
Leiomyosarcoma (M8890/3) — *see also* Neoplasm, connective tissue, malignant
  epithelioid (M8891/3) — *see* Neoplasm, connective tissue, malignant
Leishmaniasis 085.9
  American 085.5
    cutaneous 085.4
    mucocutaneous 085.5
  Asian desert 085.2
  Brazilian 085.5
  cutaneous 085.9
    acute necrotizing 085.2
    American 085.4

Leishmaniasis — *continued*
  cutaneous — *continued*
    Asian desert 085.2
    diffuse 085.3
    dry form 085.1
    Ethiopian 085.3
    eyelid 085.5 *[373.6]*
    late 085.1
    lepromatous 085.3
    recurrent 085.1
    rural 085.2
    ulcerating 085.1
    urban 085.1
    wet form 085.2
    zoonotic form 085.2
  dermal — *see also* Leishmaniasis, cutaneous
    post kala-azar 085.0
  eyelid 085.5 *[373.6]*
  infantile 085.0
  Mediterranean 085.0
  mucocutaneous (American) 085.5
  naso-oral 085.5
  nasopharyngeal 085.5
  Old World 085.1
  tegumentaria diffusa 085.4
  vaccination, prophylactic (against) V05.2
  visceral (Indian) 085.0
Leishmanoid, dermal — *see also* Leishmaniasis, cutaneous
  post kala-azar 085.0
Leloir's disease 695.4
Lenegre's disease 426.0
Lengthening, leg 736.81
Lennox's syndrome (*see also* Epilepsy) 345.0 ✓5ᵗʰ
Lens — *see* condition
Lenticonus (anterior) (posterior) (congenital) 743.36
Lenticular degeneration, progressive 275.1
Lentiglobus (posterior) (congenital) 743.36
Lentigo (congenital) 709.09
  juvenile 709.09
  Maligna (M8742/2) — *see also* Neoplasm, skin, in situ
    melanoma (M8742/3) — *see* Melanoma
  senile 709.09
Leonine leprosy 030.0
Leontiasis
  ossium 733.3
  syphilitic 095.8
    congenital 090.5
Léopold-Lévi's syndrome (paroxysmal thyroid instability) 242.9 ✓5ᵗʰ
Lepore hemoglobin syndrome 282.4
Lepothrix 039.0
Lepra 030.9
  Willan's 696.1
Leprechaunism 259.8
Lepromatous leprosy 030.0
Leprosy 030.9
  anesthetic 030.1
  beriberi 030.1
  borderline (group B) (infiltrated) (neuritic) 030.3
  cornea (*see also* Leprosy, by type) 030.9 *[371.89]*

Leprosy — *continued*
  dimorphous (group B) (infiltrated) (lepromatous) (neuritic) (tuberculoid) 030.3
  eyelid 030.0 *[373.4]*
  indeterminate (group I) (macular) (neuritic) (uncharacteristic) 030.2
  leonine 030.0
  lepromatous (diffuse) (infiltrated) (macular) (neuritic) (nodular) (type L) 030.0
  macular (early) (neuritic) (simple) 030.2
  maculoanesthetic 030.1
  mixed 030.0
  neuro 030.1
  nodular 030.0
  primary neuritic 030.3
  specified type or group NEC 030.8
  tubercular 030.1
  tuberculoid (macular) (maculoanesthetic) (major) (minor) (neuritic) (type T) 030.1
Leptocytosis, hereditary 282.4
Leptomeningitis (chronic) (circumscribed) (hemorrhagic) (nonsuppurative) (*see also* Meningitis) 322.9
  aseptic 047.9
    adenovirus 049.1
    Coxsackie virus 047.0
    ECHO virus 047.1
    enterovirus 047.9
    lymphocytic choriomeningitis 049.0
  epidemic 036.0
  late effect — *see* category 326
  meningococcal 036.0
  pneumococcal 320.1
  syphilitic 094.2
  tuberculous (*see also* Tuberculosis, meninges) 013.0 ✓5ᵗʰ
Leptomeningopathy (*see also* Meningitis) 322.9
Leptospiral — *see* condition
Leptospirochetal — *see* condition
Leptospirosis 100.9
  autumnalis 100.89
  canicula 100.89
  grippotyphosa 100.89
  hebdomidis 100.89
  icterohemorrhagica 100.0
  nanukayami 100.89
  pomona 100.89
  Weil's disease 100.0
Leptothricosis — *see* Actinomycosis
Leptothrix infestation — *see* Actinomycosis
Leptotricosis — *see* Actinomycosis
Leptus dermatitis 133.8
Léris pleonosteosis 756.89
Léri-Weill syndrome 756.59
Leriche's syndrome (aortic bifurcation occlusion) 444.0
Lermoyez's syndrome (*see also* Disease, Ménière's) 386.00
Lesbianism — *omit code*
  ego-dystonic 302.0
  problems with 302.0
Lesch-Nyhan syndrome (hypoxanthineguanine-phosphoribosyltransferase deficiency) 277.2
Lesion
  abducens nerve 378.54
  alveolar process 525.8
  anorectal 569.49
  aortic (valve) — *see* Endocarditis, aortic

Lesion — *continued*
  auditory nerve 388.5
  basal ganglion 333.90
  bile duct (*see also* Disease, biliary) 576.8
  bladder 596.9
  bone 733.90
  brachial plexus 353.0
  brain 348.8
    congenital 742.9
    vascular (*see also* Lesion, cerebrovascular) 437.9
      degenerative 437.1
      healed or old without residuals V12.59
      hypertensive 437.2
      late effect — *see* Late effect(s) (of) cerebrovascular disease
  buccal 528.9
  calcified — *see* Calcification
  canthus 373.9
  carate — *see* Pinta, lesions
  cardia 537.89
  cardiac — *see also* Disease, heart
    congenital 746.9
    valvular — *see* Endocarditis
  cauda equina 344.60
    with neurogenic bladder 344.61
  cecum 569.89
  cerebral — *see* Lesion, brain
  cerebrovascular (*see also* Disease, cerebrovascular NEC) 437.9
    degenerative 437.1
      healed or old without residuals V12.59
      hypertensive 437.2
      specified type NEC 437.8
  cervical root (nerve) NEC 353.2
  chiasmal 377.54
    associated with
      inflammatory disorders 377.54
      neoplasm NEC 377.52
        pituitary 377.51
      pituitary disorders 377.51
      vascular disorders 377.53
  chorda tympani 351.8
  coin, lung 793.1
  colon 569.89
  congenital — *see* Anomaly
  conjunctiva 372.9
  coronary artery (*see also* Ischemia, heart) 414.9
  cranial nerve 352.9
    first 352.0
    second 377.49
    third
      partial 378.51
      total 378.52
    fourth 378.53
    fifth 350.9
    sixth 378.54
    seventh 351.9
    eighth 388.5
    ninth 352.2
    tenth 352.3
    eleventh 352.4
    twelfth 352.5
  cystic — *see* Cyst
  degenerative — *see* Degeneration
  Dieulafoy (hemorrhagic)
    of
      duodenum 537.84
      intestine 569.86
      stomach 537.84
  dermal (skin) 709.9

Lesion — *continued*
  duodenum 537.89
    with obstruction 537.3
  eyelid 373.9
  gasserian ganglion 350.8
  gastric 537.89
  gastroduodenal 537.89
  gastrointestinal 569.89
  glossopharyngeal nerve 352.2
  heart (organic) — *see also* Disease, heart
    vascular — *see* Disease, cardiovascular
  helix (ear) 709.9
  hyperchromic, due to pinta (carate) 103.1
  hyperkeratotic (*see also* Hyperkeratosis) 701.1
  hypoglossal nerve 352.5
  hypopharynx 478.29
  hypothalamic 253.9
  ileocecal coil 569.89
  ileum 569.89
  iliohypogastric nerve 355.79
  ilioinguinal nerve 355.79
  in continuity — *see* Injury, nerve, by site
  inflammatory — *see* Inflammation
  intestine 569.89
  intracerebral — *see* Lesion, brain
  intrachiasmal (optic) (*see also* Lesion, chiasmal) 377.54
  intracranial, space-occupying NEC 784.2
  joint 719.90
    ankle 719.97
    elbow 719.92
    foot 719.97
    hand 719.94
    hip 719.95
    knee 719.96
    multiple sites 719.99
    pelvic region 719.95
    sacroiliac (old) 724.6
    shoulder (region) 719.91
    specified site NEC 719.98
    wrist 719.93
  keratotic (*see also* Keratosis) 701.1
  kidney (*see also* Disease, renal) 593.9
  laryngeal nerve (recurrent) 352.3
  leonine 030.0
  lip 528.5
  liver 573.8
  lumbosacral
    plexus 353.1
    root (nerve) NEC 353.4
  lung 518.89
    coin 793.1
  maxillary sinus 473.0
  mitral — *see* Endocarditis, mitral
  motor cortex 348.8
  nerve (*see also* Disorder, nerve) 355.9
  nervous system 349.9
    congenital 742.9
  nonallopathic NEC 739.9
    in region (of)
      abdomen 739.9
      acromioclavicular 739.7
      cervical, cervicothoracic 739.1
      costochondral 739.8
      costovertebral 739.8
      extremity
        lower 739.6
        upper 739.7
      head 739.0
      hip 739.5
      lower extremity 739.6

Lesion — continued
  nonallopathic — continued
    in region (of) — continued
      lumbar, lumbosacral 739.3
      occipitocervical 739.0
      pelvic 739.5
      pubic 739.5
      rib cage 739.8
      sacral, sacrococcygeal, sacroiliac 739.4
      sternochondral 739.8
      sternoclavicular 739.7
      thoracic, thoracolumbar 739.2
      upper extremity 739.7
  nose (internal) 478.1
  obstructive — see Obstruction
  obturator nerve 355.79
  occlusive
    artery — see Embolism, artery
  organ or site NEC — see Disease, by site
  osteolytic 733.90
  paramacular, of retina 363.32
  peptic 537.89
  periodontal, due to traumatic occlusion 523.8
  perirectal 569.49
  peritoneum (granulomatous) 568.89
  pigmented (skin) 709.00
  pinta — see Pinta, lesions
  polypoid — see Polyp
  prechiasmal (optic) (see also Lesion, chiasmal) 377.54
  primary — see also Syphilis, primary
    carate 103.0
    pinta 103.0
    yaws 102.0
  pulmonary 518.89
    valve (see also Endocarditis, pulmonary) 424.3
  pylorus 537.89
  radiation NEC 990
  radium NEC 990
  rectosigmoid 569.89
  retina, retinal — see also Retinopathy
    vascular 362.17
  retroperitoneal 568.89
  romanus 720.1
  sacroiliac (joint) 724.6
  salivary gland 527.8
    benign lymphoepithelial 527.8
  saphenous nerve 355.79
  secondary — see Syphilis, secondary
  sigmoid 569.89
  sinus (accessory) (nasal) (see also Sinusitis) 473.9
  skin 709.9
    suppurative 686.00
  SLAP (superior glenoid labrum) 840.7
  space-occupying, intracranial NEC 784.2
  spinal cord 336.9
    congenital 742.9
    traumatic (complete) (incomplete) (transverse) — see also Injury, spinal, by site
      with
        broken
          back — see Fracture, vertebra, by site, with spinal cord injury
          neck — see Fracture, vertebra, cervical, with spinal cord injury

Lesion — continued
  spinal cord — continued
    traumatic — continued
      with — continued
        fracture, vertebra — see Fracture, vertebra, by site, with spinal cord injury
  spleen 289.50
  stomach 537.89
  superior glenoid labrum (SLAP) 840.7
  syphilitic — see Syphilis
  tertiary — see Syphilis, tertiary
  thoracic root (nerve) 353.3
  tonsillar fossa 474.9
  tooth, teeth 525.8
    white spot 521.01
  traumatic NEC (see also nature and site of injury) 959.9
  tricuspid (valve) — see Endocarditis, tricuspid
  trigeminal nerve 350.9
  ulcerated or ulcerative — see Ulcer
  uterus NEC 621.9
  vagina 623.8
  vagus nerve 352.3
  valvular — see Endocarditis
  vascular 459.9
    affecting central nervous system (see also Lesion, cerebrovascular) 437.9
    following trauma (see also Injury, blood vessel, by site) 904.9
    retina 362.17
    traumatic — see Injury, blood vessel, by site
  umbilical cord 663.6 ✓5ᵗʰ
    affecting fetus or newborn 762.6
  visual
    cortex NEC (see also Disorder, visual, cortex) 377.73
    pathway NEC (see also Disorder, visual, pathway) 377.63
  warty — see Verruca
  white spot, on teeth 521.01
  x-ray NEC 990
Lethargic — see condition
Lethargy 780.79
Letterer-Siwe disease (acute histiocytosis X) (M9722/3) 202.5 ✓5ᵗʰ
Leucinosis 270.3
Leucocoria 360.44
Leucosarcoma (M9850/3) 207.8 ✓5ᵗʰ
Leukasmus 270.2
Leukemia, leukemic (congenital) (M9800/3) 208.9 ✓5ᵗʰ

> Note — Use the following fifth-digit subclassification for categories 203–208:
>
> 0   without mention of remission
> 1   with remission

  acute NEC (M9801/3) 208.0 ✓5ᵗʰ
  aleukemic NEC (M9804/3) 208.8 ✓5ᵗʰ
    granulocytic (M9864/3) 205.8 ✓5ᵗʰ
  basophilic (M9870/3) 205.1 ✓5ᵗʰ
  blast (cell) (M9801/3) 208.0 ✓5ᵗʰ
  blastic (M9801/3) 208.0 ✓5ᵗʰ
    granulocytic (M9861/3) 205.0 ✓5ᵗʰ
  chronic NEC (M9803/3) 208.1 ✓5ᵗʰ
  compound (M9810/3) 207.8 ✓5ᵗʰ
  eosinophilic (M9880/3) 205.1 ✓5ᵗʰ

Leukemia, leukemic — *continued*
  giant cell (M9910/3) 207.2
  granulocytic (M9860/3) 205.9
    acute (M9861/3) 205.0
    aleukemic (M9864/3) 205.8
    blastic (M9861/3) 205.0
    chronic (M9863/3) 205.1
    subacute (M9862/3) 205.2
    subleukemic (M9864/3) 205.8
  hairy cell (M9940/3) 202.4
  hemoblastic (M9801/3) 208.0
  histiocytic (M9890/3) 206.9
  lymphatic (M9820/3) 204.9
    acute (M9821/3) 204.0
    aleukemic (M9824/3) 204.8
    chronic (M9823/3) 204.1
    subacute (M9822/3) 204.2
    subleukemic (M9824/3) 204.8
  lymphoblastic (M9821/3) 204.0
  lymphocytic (M9820/3) 204.9
    acute (M9821/3) 204.0
    aleukemic (M9824/3) 204.8
    chronic (M9823/3) 204.1
    subacute (M9822/3) 204.2
    subleukemic (M9824/3) 204.8
  lymphogenous (M9820/3) — see Leukemia, lymphoid
  lymphoid (M9820/3) 204.9
    acute (M9821/3) 204.0
    aleukemic (M9824/3) 204.8
    blastic (M9821/3) 204.0
    chronic (M9823/3) 204.1
    subacute (M9822/3) 204.2
    subleukemic (M9824/3) 204.8
  lymphosarcoma cell (M9850/3) 207.8
  mast cell (M9900/3) 207.8
  megakaryocytic (M9910/3) 207.2
  megakaryocytoid (M9910/3) 207.2
  mixed (cell) (M9810/3) 207.8
  monoblastic (M9891/3) 206.0
  monocytic (Schilling-type) (M9890/3) 206.9
    acute (M9891/3) 206.0
    aleukemic (M9894/3) 206.8
    chronic (M9893/3) 206.1
    Naegeli-type (M9863/3) 205.1
    subacute (M9892/3) 206.2
    subleukemic (M9894/3) 206.8
  monocytoid (M9890/3) 206.9
    acute (M9891/3) 206.0
    aleukemic (M9894/3) 206.8
    chronic (M9893/3) 206.1
    myelogenous (M9863/3) 205.1
    subacute (M9892/3) 206.2
    subleukemic (M9894/3) 206.8
  monomyelocytic (M9860/3) — see Leukemia, myelomonocytic
  myeloblastic (M9861/3) 205.0
  myelocytic (M9863/3) 205.1
    acute (M9861/3) 205.0
  myelogenous (M9860/3) 205.9
    acute (M9861/3) 205.0
    aleukemic (M9864/3) 205.8
    chronic (M9863/3) 205.1
    monocytoid (M9863/3) 205.1
    subacute (M9862/3) 205.2
    subleukemic (M9864) 205.8
  myeloid (M9860/3) 205.9
    acute (M9861/3) 205.0
    aleukemic (M9864/3) 205.8
    chronic (M9863/3) 205.1

Leukemia, leukemic — *continued*
  myeloid — *continued*
    subacute (M9862/3) 205.2
    subleukemic (M9864/3) 205.8
  myelomonocytic (M9860/3) 205.9
    acute (M9861/3) 205.0
    chronic (M9863/3) 205.1
  Naegeli-type monocytic (M9863/3) 205.1
  neutrophilic (M9865/3) 205.1
  plasma cell (M9830/3) 203.1
  plasmacytic (M9830/3) 203.1
  prolymphocytic (M9825/3) — see Leukemia, lymphoid
  promyelocytic, acute (M9866/3) 205.0
  Schilling-type monocytic (M9890/3) — see Leukemia, monocytic
  stem cell (M9801/3) 208.0
  subacute NEC (M9802/3) 208.2
  subleukemic NEC (M9804/3) 208.8
  thrombocytic (M9910/3) 207.2
  undifferentiated (M9801/3) 208.0
Leukemoid reaction (lymphocytic) (monocytic) (myelocytic) 288.8
Leukoclastic vasculitis 446.29
Leukocoria 360.44
Leukocythemia — *see* Leukemia
Leukocytosis 288.8
  basophilic 288.8
  eosinophilic 288.3
  lymphocytic 288.8
  monocytic 288.8
  neutrophilic 288.8
Leukoderma 709.09
  syphilitic 091.3
    late 095.8
Leukodermia (*see also* Leukoderma) 709.09
Leukodystrophy (cerebral) (globoid cell) (metachromatic) (progressive) (sudanophilic) 330.0
Leukoedema, mouth or tongue 528.7
Leukoencephalitis
  acute hemorrhagic (postinfectious) NEC 136.9 [323.6]
    postimmunization or postvaccinal 323.5
  subacute sclerosing 046.2
    van Bogaert's 046.2
  van Bogaert's (sclerosing) 046.2
Leukoencephalopathy (*see also* Encephalitis) 323.9
  acute necrotizing hemorrhagic (postinfectious) 136.9 [323.6]
    postimmunization or postvaccinal 323.5
  metachromatic 330.0
  multifocal (progressive) 046.3
  progressive multifocal 046.3
Leukoerythroblastosis 289.0
Leukoerythrosis 289.0
Leukokeratosis (*see also* Leukoplakia) 702.8
  mouth 528.6
  nicotina palati 528.7
  tongue 528.6
Leukokoria 360.44
Leukokraurosis vulva, vulvae 624.0
Leukolymphosarcoma (M9850/3) 207.8
Leukoma (cornea) (interfering with central vision) 371.03
  adherent 371.04
Leukomalacia, periventricular 779.7

Leukomelanopathy, hereditary 288.2
Leukonychia (punctata) (striata) 703.8
 congenital 757.5
Leukopathia
 unguium 703.8
  congenital 757.5
Leukopenia 288.0
 cyclic 288.0
 familial 288.0
 malignant 288.0
 periodic 288.0
 transitory neonatal 776.7
Leukopenic — *see* condition
Leukoplakia 702.8
 anus 569.49
 bladder (postinfectional) 596.8
 buccal 528.6
 cervix (uteri) 622.2
 esophagus 530.83
 gingiva 528.6
 kidney (pelvis) 593.89
 larynx 478.79
 lip 528.6
 mouth 528.6
 oral soft tissue (including tongue) (mucosa) 528.6
 palate 528.6
 pelvis (kidney) 593.89
 penis (infectional) 607.0
 rectum 569.49
 syphilitic 095.8
 tongue 528.6
 tonsil 478.29
 ureter (postinfectional) 593.89
 urethra (postinfectional) 599.84
 uterus 621.8
 vagina 623.1
 vesical 596.8
 vocal cords 478.5
 vulva 624.0
Leukopolioencephalopathy 330.0
Leukorrhea (vagina) 623.5
 due to trichomonas (vaginalis) 131.00
 trichomonal (Trichomonas vaginalis) 131.00
Leukosarcoma (M9850/3) 207.8
Leukosis (M9800/3) — *see* Leukemia
Lev's disease or syndrome (acquired complete heart block) 426.0
Levi's syndrome (pituitary dwarfism) 253.3
Levocardia (isolated) 746.87
 with situs inversus 759.3
Levulosuria 271.2
Lewandowski's disease (primary) (*see also* Tuberculosis) 017.0
Lewandowski-Lutz disease (epidermodysplasia verruciformis) 078.19
Leyden's disease (periodic vomiting) 536.2
Leyden-Möbius dystrophy 359.1
Leydig cell
 carcinoma (M8650/3)
  specified site — *see* Neoplasm, by site, malignant
  unspecified site
   female 183.0
   male 186.9

Leydig cell — *continued*
 tumor (M8650/1)
  benign (M8650/0)
   specified site — *see* Neoplasm, by site, benign
   unspecified site
    female 220
    male 222.0
  malignant (M8650/3)
   specified site — *see* Neoplasm, by site, malignant
   unspecified site
    female 183.0
    male 186.9
  specified site — *see* Neoplasm, by site, uncertain behavior
  unspecified site
   female 236.2
   male 236.4
Leydig-Sertoli cell tumor (M8631/0)
 specified site — *see* Neoplasm, by site, benign
 unspecified site
  female 220
  male 222.0
LGSIL (low grade squamous intraepithelial dysplasia) 622.1
Liar, pathologic 301.7
Libman-Sacks disease or syndrome 710.0
 [424.91]
Lice (infestation) 132.9
 body (pediculus corporis) 132.1
 crab 132.2
 head (pediculus capitis) 132.0
 mixed (classifiable to more than one of the categories 132.0-132.2) 132.3
 pubic (pediculus pubis) 132.2
Lichen 697.9
 albus 701.0
 annularis 695.89
 atrophicus 701.0
 corneus obtusus 698.3
 myxedematous 701.8
 nitidus 697.1
 pilaris 757.39
  acquired 701.1
 planopilaris 697.0
 planus (acute) (chronicus) (hypertrophic) (verrucous) 697.0
  morphoeicus 701.0
  sclerosus (et atrophicus) 701.0
 ruber 696.4
  acuminatus 696.4
  moniliformis 697.8
  obtusus corneus 698.3
  of Wilson 697.0
  planus 697.0
 selerosus (et atrophicus) 701.0
 scrofulosus (primary) (*see also* Tuberculosis) 017.0
 simplex (Vidal's) 698.3
  chronicus 698.3
  circumscriptus 698.3
 spinulosus 757.39
  mycotic 117.9
 striata 697.8
 urticatus 698.2
Lichenification 698.3
 nodular 698.3
Lichenoides tuberculosis (primary) (*see also* Tuberculosis) 017.0

Lichtheim's disease or syndrome (subacute combined sclerosis with pernicious anemia) 281.0 [336.2]
Lien migrans 289.59
Lientery (see also Diarrhea) 787.91
  infectious 009.2
Life circumstance problem NEC V62.89
Li-Fraumeni cancer syndrome 758.3
Ligament — see condition
Light-for-dates (infant) 764.0 ✓5ᵗʰ
  with signs of fetal malnutrition 764.1 ✓5ᵗʰ
  affecting management of pregnancy 656.5 ✓5ᵗʰ
Light-headedness 780.4
Lightning (effects) (shock) (stroke) (struck by) 994.0
  burn — see Burn, by site
  foot 266.2
Lightwood's disease or syndrome (renal tubular acidosis) 588.8
Lignac's disease (cystinosis) 270.0
Lignac (-de Toni) (-Fanconi) (-Debré) syndrome (cystinosis) 270.0
Lignac (-Fanconi) syndrome (cystinosis) 270.0
Ligneous thyroiditis 245.3
Likoff's syndrome (angina in menopausal women) 413.9
Limb — see condition
Limitation of joint motion (see also Stiffness, joint) 719.5 ✓5ᵗʰ
  sacroiliac 724.6
Limit dextrinosis 271.0
Limited
  cardiac reserve — see Disease, heart
  duction, eye NEC 378.63
Lindau's disease (retinocerebral angiomatosis) 759.6
Lindau (-von Hippel) disease (angiomatosis retinocerebellosa) 759.6
Linea corneae senilis 371.41
Lines
  Beau's (transverse furrows on fingernails) 703.8
  Harris' 733.91
  Hudson-Stähli 371.11
  Stähli's 371.11
Lingua
  geographical 529.1
  nigra (villosa) 529.3
  plicata 529.5
    congenital 750.13
  tylosis 528.6
Lingual (tongue) — see also condition
  thyroid 759.2
Linitis (gastric) 535.4 ✓5ᵗʰ
  plastica (M8142/3) 151.9
Lioderma essentialis (cum melanosis et telangiectasia) 757.33
Lip — see also condition
  biting 528.9
Lipalgia 272.8
Lipedema — see Edema
Lipemia (see also Hyperlipidemia) 272.4
  retina, retinalis 272.3
Lipidosis 272.7
  cephalin 272.7
  cerebral (infantile) (juvenile) (late) 330.1
  cerebroretinal 330.1 [362.71]

Lipidosis — continued
  cerebroside 272.7
  cerebrospinal 272.7
  chemically-induced 272.7
  cholesterol 272.7
  diabetic 250.8 ✓5ᵗʰ [272.7]
  dystopic (hereditary) 272.7
  glycolipid 272.7
  hepatosplenomegalic 272.3
  hereditary, dystopic 272.7
  sulfatide 330.0
Lipoadenoma (M8324/0) — see Neoplasm, by site, benign
Lipoblastoma (M8881/0) — see Lipoma, by site
Lipoblastomatosis (M8881/0) — see Lipoma, by site
Lipochondrodystrophy 277.5
Lipochrome histiocytosis (familial) 288.1
Lipodystrophia progressiva 272.6
Lipodystrophy (progressive) 272.6
  insulin 272.6
  intestinal 040.2
Lipofibroma (M8851/0) — see Lipoma, by site
Lipoglycoproteinosis 272.8
Lipogranuloma, sclerosing 709.8
Lipogranulomatosis (disseminated) 272.8
  kidney 272.8
Lipoid — see also condition
  histiocytosis 272.7
    essential 272.7
  nephrosis (see also Nephrosis) 581.3
  proteinosis of Urbach 272.8
Lipoidemia (see also Hyperlipidemia) 272.4
Lipoidosis (see also Lipidosis) 272.7
Lipoma (M8850/0) 214.9
  breast (skin) 214.1
  face 214.0
  fetal (M8881/0) — see also Lipoma, by site
    fat cell (M8880/0) — see Lipoma, by site
  infiltrating (M8856/0) — see Lipoma, by site
  intra-abdominal 214.3
  intramuscular (M8856/0) — see Lipoma, by site
  intrathoracic 214.2
  kidney 214.3
  mediastinum 214.2
  muscle 214.8
  peritoneum 214.3
  retroperitoneum 214.3
  skin 214.1
    face 214.0
  spermatic cord 214.4
  spindle cell (M8857/0) — see Lipoma, by site
  stomach 214.3
  subcutaneous tissue 214.1
    face 214.0
  thymus 214.2
  thyroid gland 214.2
Lipomatosis (dolorosa) 272.8
  epidural 214.8
  fetal (M8881/0) — see Lipoma, by site
  Launois-Bensaude's 272.8
Lipomyohemangioma (M8860/0)
  specified site — see Neoplasm, connective tissue, benign
  unspecified site 223.0
Lipomyoma (M8860/0)
  specified site — see Neoplasm, connective tissue, benign

Lipomyoma — *continued*
  unspecified site 223.0
Lipomyxoma (M8852/0) — *see* Lipoma, by site
Lipomyxosarcoma (M8852/3) — *see* Neoplasm, connective tissue, malignant
Lipophagocytosis 289.8
Lipoproteinemia (alpha) 272.4
  broad-beta 272.2
  floating-beta 272.2
  hyper-pre-beta 272.1
Lipoproteinosis (Rössle-Urbach-Wiethe) 272.8
Liposarcoma (M8850/3) — *see also* Neoplasm, connective tissue, malignant
  differentiated type (M8851/3) — *see* Neoplasm, connective tissue, malignant
  embryonal (M8852/3) — *see* Neoplasm, connective tissue, malignant
  mixed type (M8855/3) — *see* Neoplasm, connective tissue, malignant
  myxoid (M8852/3) — *see* Neoplasm, connective tissue, malignant
  pleomorphic (M8854/3) — *see* Neoplasm, connective tissue, malignant
  round cell (M8853/3) — *see* Neoplasm, connective tissue, malignant
  well differentiated type (M8851/3) — *see* Neoplasm, connective tissue, malignant
Lipsynovitis prepatellaris 272.8
Lipping
  cervix 622.0
  spine (*see also* Spondylosis) 721.90
  vertebra (*see also* Spondylosis) 721.90
Lip pits (mucus), congenital 750.25
Lipschütz disease or ulcer 616.50
Lipuria 791.1
  bilharziasis 120.0
Liquefaction, vitreous humor 379.21
Lisping 307.9
Lissauer's paralysis 094.1
Lissencephalia, lissencephaly 742.2
Listerellose 027.0
Listeriose 027.0
Listeriosis 027.0
  congenital 771.2
  fetal 771.2
  suspected fetal damage affecting management of pregnancy 655.4 ✓5ᵗʰ
Listlessness 780.79
Lithemia 790.6
Lithiasis — *see also* Calculus
  hepatic (duct) — *see* Choledocholithiasis
  urinary 592.9
Lithopedion 779.9
  affecting management of pregnancy 656.8 ✓5ᵗʰ
Lithosis (occupational) 502
  with tuberculosis — *see* Tuberculosis, pulmonary
Lithuria 791.9
Litigation V62.5
Little
  league elbow 718.82
  stroke syndrome 435.9
Little's disease — *see* Palsy, cerebral
Littre's
  gland — *see* condition
  hernia — *see* Hernia, Littre's

Littritis (*see also* Urethritis) 597.89
Livedo 782.61
  annularis 782.61
  racemose 782.61
  reticularis 782.61
Live flesh 781.0
Liver — *see also* condition
  donor V59.6
Livida, asphyxia
  newborn 768.6
Living
  alone V60.3
  with handicapped person V60.4
Lloyd's syndrome 258.1
Loa loa 125.2
Loasis 125.2
Lobe, lobar — *see* condition
Lobo's disease or blastomycosis 116.2
Lobomycosis 116.2
Lobotomy syndrome 310.0
Lobstein's disease (brittle bones and blue sclera) 756.51
Lobster-claw hand 755.58
Lobulation (congenital) — *see also* Anomaly, specified type NEC, by site
  kidney, fetal 753.3
  liver, abnormal 751.69
  spleen 759.0
Lobule, lobular — *see* condition
Local, localized — *see* condition
Locked bowel or intestine (*see also* Obstruction, intestine) 560.9
Locked-in state 344.81
Locked twins 660.5 ✓5ᵗʰ
  affecting fetus or newborn 763.1
Locking
  joint (*see also* Derangement, joint) 718.90
  knee 717.9
Lockjaw (*see also* Tetanus) 037
Locomotor ataxia (progressive) 094.0
Löffler's
  endocarditis 421.0
  eosinophilia or syndrome 518.3
  pneumonia 518.3
  syndrome (eosinophilic pneumonitis) 518.3
Löfgren's syndrome (sarcoidosis) 135
Loiasis 125.2
  eyelid 125.2 [373.6]
Loneliness V62.89
Lone star fever 082.8
Long labor 662.1 ✓5ᵗʰ
  affecting fetus or newborn 763.89
  first stage 662.0 ✓5ᵗʰ
  second stage 662.2 ✓5ᵗʰ
Longitudinal stripes or grooves, nails 703.8
  congenital 757.5
Long-term (current) drug use V58.69
  antibiotics V58.62
  anticoagulants V58.61
Loop
  intestine (*see also* Volvulus) 560.2
  intrascleral nerve 379.29
  vascular on papilla (optic) 743.57

Loose — *see also* condition
  body
    in tendon sheath 727.82
    joint 718.10
      ankle 718.17
      elbow 718.12
      foot 718.17
      hand 718.14
      hip 718.15
      knee 717.6
      multiple sites 718.19
      pelvic region 718.15
      prosthetic implant — *see* Complications, mechanical
      shoulder (region) 718.11
      specified site NEC 718.18
      wrist 718.13
    cartilage (joint) (*see also* Loose, body, joint) 718.1 ✓5ᵗʰ
      knee 717.6
    facet (vertebral) 724.9
    prosthetic implant — *see* Complications, mechanical
    sesamoid, joint (*see also* Loose, body, joint) 718.1 ✓5ᵗʰ
    tooth, teeth 525.8
Loosening epiphysis 732.9
Looser (-Debray) -Milkman syndrome (osteomalacia with pseudofractures) 268.2
Lop ear (deformity) 744.29
Lorain's disease or syndrome (pituitary dwarfism) 253.3
Lorain-Levi syndrome (pituitary dwarfism) 253.3
Lordosis (acquired) (postural) 737.20
  congenital 754.2
  due to or associated with
    Charcôt-Marie-Tooth disease 356.1 [737.42]
    mucopolysaccharidosis 277.5 [737.42]
    neurofibromatosis 237.71 [737.42]
    osteitis
      deformans 731.0 [737.42]
      fibrosa cystica 252.0 [737.42]
    osteoporosis (*see also* Osteoporosis) 733.00 [737.42]
    poliomyelitis (*see also* Poliomyelitis) 138 [737.42]
    tuberculosis (*see also* Tuberculosis) 015.0 ✓5ᵗʰ [737.42]
  late effect of rickets 268.1 [737.42]
  postlaminectomy 737.21
  postsurgical NEC 737.22
  rachitic 268.1 [737.42]
  specified NEC 737.29
  tuberculous (*see also* Tuberculosis) 015.0 ✓5ᵗʰ [737.42]
Loss
  appetite 783.0
    hysterical 300.11
    nonorganic origin 307.59
    psychogenic 307.59
  blood — *see* Hemorrhage
  central vision 368.41
  consciousness 780.09
    transient 780.2
  control, sphincter, rectum 787.6
    nonorganic origin 307.7
  ear ossicle, partial 385.24
  elasticity, skin 782.8

Loss — *continued*
  extremity or member, traumatic, current — *see* Amputation, traumatic
  fluid (acute) 276.5
    with
      hypernatremia 276.0
      hyponatremia 276.1
    fetus or newborn 775.5
  hair 704.00
  hearing — *see also* Deafness
    central 389.14
    conductive (air) 389.00
      with sensorineural hearing loss 389.2
      combined types 389.08
      external ear 389.01
      inner ear 389.04
      middle ear 389.03
      multiple types 389.08
      tympanic membrane 389.02
    mixed type 389.2
    nerve 389.12
    neural 389.12
    noise-induced 388.12
    perceptive NEC (*see also* Loss, hearing, sensorineural) 389.10
    sensorineural 389.10
      with conductive hearing loss 389.2
      central 389.14
      combined types 389.18
      multiple types 389.18
      neural 389.12
      sensory 389.11
    sensory 389.11
    specified type NEC 389.8
    sudden NEC 388.2
  height 781.91
  labyrinthine reactivity (unilateral) 386.55
    bilateral 386.56
  memory (*see also* Amnesia) 780.99 ▲
    mild, following organic brain damage 310.1
  mind (*see also* Psychosis) 298.9
  organ or part — *see* Absence, by site, acquired
  sensation 782.0
  sense of
    smell (*see also* Disturbance, sensation) 781.1
    taste (*see also* Disturbance, sensation) 781.1
    touch (*see also* Disturbance, sensation) 781.1
  sight (acquired) (complete) (congenital) *see* Blindness
  spinal fluid
    headache 349.0
  substance of
    bone (*see also* Osteoporosis) 733.00
    cartilage 733.99
    ear 380.32
    vitreous (humor) 379.26
  tooth, teeth
    acquired 525.10
      due to
        caries 525.13
        extraction 525.10
        periodontal disease 525.12
        specified NEC 525.19
        trauma 525.11
  vision, visual (*see also* Blindness) 369.9
    both eyes (*see also* Blindness, both eyes) 369.3

Index to Diseases

Loss — *continued*
 vision, visual — *continued*
  complete (*see also* Blindness, both eyes) 369.00
  one eye 369.8
  sudden 368.11
  transient 368.12
 vitreous 379.26
 voice (*see also* Aphonia) 784.41
 weight (cause unknown) 783.21
Lou Gehrig's disease 335.20
Louis-Bar syndrome (ataxia-telangiectasia) 334.8
Louping ill 063.1
Lousiness — *see* Lice
Low
 back syndrome 724.2
 basal metabolic rate (BMR) 794.7
 birthweight 765.1
  extreme (less than 1000 grams) 765.0
  for gestational age 764.0
  status (*see also* Status, low birth weight) V21.30
 bladder compliance 596.52
 blood pressure (*see also* Hypotension) 458.9
  reading (incidental) (isolated) (nonspecific) 796.3
 cardiac reserve — *see* Disease, heart
 compliance bladder 596.52
 frequency deafness — *see* Disorder, hearing
 function — *see also* Hypofunction
  kidney (*see also* Disease, renal) 593.9
  liver 573.9
 hemoglobin 285.9
 implantation, placenta — *see* Placenta, previa
 insertion, placenta — *see* placenta, previa
 lying
  kidney 593.0
  organ or site, congenital — *see* Malposition, congenital
  placenta — *see* Placenta, previa
 output syndrome (cardiac) (*see also* Failure, heart) 428.9
 platelets (blood) (*see also* Thrombocytopenia) 287.5
 reserve, kidney (*see also* Disease, renal) 593.9
 salt syndrome 593.9
 tension glaucoma 365.12
 vision 369.9
  both eyes 369.20
  one eye 369.70
Lowe (-Terrey-MacLachlan) syndrome (oculocerebrorenal dystrophy) 270.8
Lower extremity — *see* condition
Lown (-Ganong) -Levine syndrome (short P-R interval, normal QRS complex, and paroxysmal supraventricular tachycardia) 426.81
LSD reaction (*see also* Abuse, drugs, nondependent) 305.3
L-shaped kidney 753.3
Lucas-Championnière disease (fibrinous bronchitis) 466.0
Lucey-Driscoll syndrome (jaundice due to delayed conjugation) 774.30
Ludwig's
 angina 528.3
 disease (submaxillary cellulitis) 528.3
Lues (venerea), luetic — *see* Syphilis
Luetscher's syndrome (dehydration) 276.5

Lumbago 724.2
 due to displacement, intervertebral disc 722.10
Lumbalgia 724.2
 due to displacement, intervertebral disc 722.10
Lumbar — *see* condition
Lumbarization, vertebra 756.15
Lumbermen's itch 133.8
Lump — *see also* Mass
 abdominal 789.3
 breast 611.72
 chest 786.6
 epigastric 789.3
 head 784.2
 kidney 753.3
 liver 789.1
 lung 786.6
 mediastinal 786.6
 neck 784.2
 nose or sinus 784.2
 pelvic 789.3
 skin 782.2
 substernal 786.6
 throat 784.2
 umbilicus 789.3
Lunacy (*see also* Psychosis) 298.9
Lunatomalacia 732.3
Lung — *see also* condition
 donor V59.8
 drug addict's 417.8
 mainliners' 417.8
 vanishing 492.0
Lupoid (miliary) **of Boeck** 135
Lupus 710.0
 Cazenave's (erythematosus) 695.4
 discoid (local) 695.4
 disseminated 710.0
 erythematosus (discoid) (local) 695.4
  disseminated 710.0
  eyelid 373.34
  systemic 710.0
   with
    encephalitis 710.0 *[323.8]*
    lung involvement 710.0 *[517.8]*
    inhibitor (presence of) 286.5
 exedens 017.0
 eyelid (*see also* Tuberculosis) 017.0 *[373.4]*
  Hilliard's 017.0
 hydralazine
  correct substance properly administered 695.4
  overdose or wrong substance given or taken 972.6
 miliaris disseminatus faciei 017.0
 nephritis 710.0 *[583.81]*
  acute 710.0 *[580.81]*
  chronic 710.0 *[582.81]*
 nontuberculous, not disseminated 695.4
 pernio (Besnier) 135
 tuberculous (*see also* Tuberculosis) 017.0
  eyelid (*see also* Tuberculosis) 017.0 *[373.4]*
 vulgaris 017.0
Luschka's joint disease 721.90
Luteinoma (M8610/0) 220
Lutembacher's disease or syndrome (atrial septal defect with mitral stenosis) 745.5
Luteoma (M8610/0) 220

Lutz-Miescher disease (elastosis perforans serpiginosa) 701.1
Lutz-Splendore-de Almeida disease (Brazilian blastomycosis) 116.1
Luxatio
  bulbi due to birth injury 767.8
  coxae congenita (see also Dislocation, hip, congenital) 754.30
  erecta — see Dislocation, shoulder
  imperfecta — see Sprain, by site
  perinealis — see Dislocation, hip
Luxation — see also Dislocation, by site
  eyeball 360.81
    due to birth injury 767.8
    lateral 376.36
  genital organs (external) NEC — see Wound, open, genital organs
  globe (eye) 360.81
    lateral 376.36
  lacrimal gland (postinfectional) 375.16
  lens (old) (partial) 379.32
    congenital 743.37
      syphilitic 090.49 [379.32]
    Marfan's disease 090.49
    spontaneous 379.32
  penis — see Wound, open, penis
  scrotum — see Wound, open, scrotum
  testis — see Wound, open, testis
L-xyloketosuria 271.8
Lycanthropy (see also Psychosis) 298.9
Lyell's disease or syndrome (toxic epidermal necrolysis) 695.1
  due to drug
    correct substance properly administered 695.1
    overdose or wrong substance given or taken 977.9
      specified drug — see Table of Drugs and Chemicals
Lyme disease 088.81
Lymph
  gland or node — see condition
  scrotum (see also Infestation, filarial) 125.9
Lymphadenitis 289.3
  with
    abortion — see Abortion, by type, with sepsis
    ectopic pregnancy (see also categories 633.0-633.9) 639.0
    molar pregnancy (see also categories 630-632) 639.0
  acute 683
    mesenteric 289.2
  any site, except mesenteric 289.3
    acute 683
    chronic 289.1
    mesenteric (acute) (chronic) (nonspecific) (subacute) 289.2
    subacute 289.1
      mesenteric 289.2
  breast, puerperal, postpartum 675.2
  chancroidal (congenital) 099.0
  chronic 289.1
    mesenteric 289.2
  dermatopathic 695.89
  due to
    anthracosis (occupational) 500
    Brugia (Wuchereria) malayi 125.1
    diphtheria (toxin) 032.89
    lymphogranuloma venereum 099.1

Lymphadenitis — continued
  due to — continued
    Wuchereria bancrofti 125.0
  following
    abortion 639.0
    ectopic or molar pregnancy 639.0
  generalized 289.3
  gonorrheal 098.89
  granulomatous 289.1
  infectional 683
  mesenteric (acute) (chronic) (nonspecific) (subacute) 289.2
    due to Bacillus typhi 002.0
    tuberculous (see also Tuberculosis) 014.8
  mycobacterial 031.8
  purulent 683
  pyogenic 683
  regional 078.3
  septic 683
  streptococcal 683
  subacute, unspecified site 289.1
  suppurative 683
  syphilitic (early) (secondary) 091.4
    late 095.8
  tuberculous — see Tuberculosis, lymph gland
  venereal 099.1
Lymphadenoid goiter 245.2
Lymphadenopathy (general) 785.6
  due to toxoplasmosis (acquired) 130.7
  congenital (active) 771.2
Lymphadenopathy-associated virus (disease) (illness) (infection) — see Human immunodeficiency virus (disease) (illness) (infection)
Lymphadenosis 785.6
  acute 075
Lymphangiectasis 457.1
  conjunctiva 372.89
  postinfectional 457.1
  scrotum 457.1
Lymphangiectatic elephantiasis, nonfilarial 457.1
Lymphangioendothelioma (M9170/0) 228.1
  malignant (M9170/3) — see Neoplasm, connective tissue, malignant
Lymphangioma (M9170/0) 228.1
  capillary (M9171/0) 228.1
  cavernous (M9172/0) 228.1
  cystic (M9173/0) 228.1
  malignant (M9170/3) — see Neoplasm, connective tissue, malignant
Lymphangiomyoma (M9174/0) 228.1
Lymphangiomyomatosis (M9174/1) — see Neoplasm, connective tissue, uncertain behavior
Lymphangiosarcoma (M9170/3) — see Neoplasm, connective tissue, malignant
Lymphangitis 457.2
  with
    abortion — see Abortion, by type, with sepsis
    abscess — see Abscess, by site
    cellulitis — see Abscess, by site
    ectopic pregnancy (see also categories 633.0-633.9) 639.0
    molar pregnancy (see also categories 630-632) 639.0

Index to Diseases

Lymphangitis — *continued*
  acute (with abscess or cellulitis) 682.9
    specified site — *see* Abscess, by site
  breast, puerperal, postpartum 675.2 ✓5ᵗʰ
  chancroidal 099.0
  chronic (any site) 457.2
  due to
    Brugia (Wuchereria) malayi 125.1
    Wuchereria bancrofti 125.0
  following
    abortion 639.0
    ectopic or molar pregnancy 639.0
  gangrenous 457.2
  penis
    acute 607.2
    gonococcal (acute) 098.0
      chronic or duration of 2 months or more 098.2
  puerperal, postpartum, childbirth 670 ✓4ᵗʰ
  strumous, tuberculous (*see also* Tuberculosis) 017.2 ✓5ᵗʰ
  subacute (any site) 457.2
  tuberculous — *see* Tuberculosis, lymph gland
Lymphatic (vessel) — *see* condition
Lymphatism 254.8
  scrofulous (*see also* Tuberculosis) 017.2 ✓5ᵗʰ
Lymphectasia 457.1
Lymphedema (*see also* Elephantiasis) 457.1
  acquired (chronic) 457.1
  chronic hereditary 757.0
  congenital 757.0
  idiopathic hereditary 757.0
  praecox 457.1
  secondary 457.1
  surgical NEC 997.99
    postmastectomy (syndrome) 457.0
Lymph-hemangioma (M9120/0) — *see* Hemangioma, by site
Lymphoblastic — *see* condition
Lymphoblastoma (diffuse) (M9630/3) 200.1 ✓5ᵗʰ
  giant follicular (M9690/3) 202.0 ✓5ᵗʰ
  macrofollicular (M9690/3) 202.0 ✓5ᵗʰ
Lymphoblastosis, acute benign 075
Lymphocele 457.8
Lymphocythemia 288.8
Lymphocytic — *see also* condition
  chorioencephalitis (acute) (serous) 049.0
  choriomeningitis (acute) (serous) 049.0
Lymphocytoma (diffuse) (malignant) (M9620/3) 200.1 ✓5ᵗʰ
Lymphocytomatosis (M9620/3) 200.1 ✓5ᵗʰ
Lymphocytopenia 288.8
Lymphocytosis (symptomatic) 288.8
  infectious (acute) 078.89
Lymphoepithelioma (M8082/3) — *see* Neoplasm, by site, malignant
Lymphogranuloma (malignant) (M9650/3) 201.9 ✓5ᵗʰ
  inguinale 099.1
  venereal (any site) 099.1
    with stricture of rectum 099.1
  venereum 099.1
Lymphogranulomatosis (malignant) (M9650/3) 201.9 ✓5ᵗʰ
  benign (Boeck's sarcoid) (Schaumann's) 135
  Hodgkin's (M9650/3) 201.9 ✓5ᵗʰ
Lymphoid — *see* condition
Lympholeukoblastoma (M9850/3) 207.8 ✓5ᵗʰ

Lympholeukosarcoma (M9850/3) 207.8 ✓5ᵗʰ
Lymphoma (malignant) (M9590/3) 202.8 ✓5ᵗʰ

> Note — Use the following fifth-digit subclassification with categories 200–202:
>
> 0   unspecified site
> 1   lymph nodes of head, face, and neck
> 2   intrathoracic lymph nodes
> 3   intra-abdominal lymph nodes
> 4   lymph nodes of axilla and upper limb
> 5   lymph nodes of inguinal region and lower limb
> 6   intrapelvic lymph nodes
> 7   spleen
> 8   lymph nodes of multiple sites

  benign (M9590/0) — *see* Neoplasm, by site, benign
  Burkitt's type (lymphoblastic) (undifferentiated) (M9750/3) 200.2 ✓5ᵗʰ
  Castleman's (mediastinal lymph node hyperplasia) 785.6
  centroblastic-centrocytic
    diffuse (M9614/3) 202.8 ✓5ᵗʰ
    follicular (M9692/3) 202.0 ✓5ᵗʰ
  centroblastic type (diffuse) (M9632/3) 202.8 ✓5ᵗʰ
    follicular (M9697/3) 202.0 ✓5ᵗʰ
  centrocytic (M9622/3) 202.8 ✓5ᵗʰ
  compound (M9613/3) 200.8 ✓5ᵗʰ
  convoluted cell type (lymphoblastic) (M9602/3) 202.8 ✓5ᵗʰ
  diffuse NEC (M9590/3) 202.8 ✓5ᵗʰ
  follicular (giant) (M9690/3) 202.0 ✓5ᵗʰ
    center cell (diffuse) (M9615/3) 202.8 ✓5ᵗʰ
    cleaved (diffuse) (M9623/3) 202.8 ✓5ᵗʰ
      follicular (M9695/3) 202.0 ✓5ᵗʰ
    non-cleaved (diffuse) (M9633/3) 202.8 ✓5ᵗʰ
      follicular (M9698/3) 202.0 ✓5ᵗʰ
  centroblastic-centrocytic (M9692/3) 202.0 ✓5ᵗʰ
  centroblastic type (M9697/3) 202.0 ✓5ᵗʰ
  lymphocytic
    intermediate differentiation (M9694/3) 202.0 ✓5ᵗʰ
    poorly differentiated (M9696/3) 202.0 ✓5ᵗʰ
    mixed (cell type) (lymphocytic-histiocytic) (small cell and large cell) (M9691/3) 202.0 ✓5ᵗʰ
  germinocytic (M9622/3) 202.8 ✓5ᵗʰ
  giant, follicular or follicle (M9690/3) 202.0 ✓5ᵗʰ
  histiocytic (diffuse) (M9640/3) 200.0 ✓5ᵗʰ
    nodular (M9642/3) 200.0 ✓5ᵗʰ
    pleomorphic cell type (M9641/3) 200.0 ✓5ᵗʰ
  Hodgkin's (M9650/3) (*see also* Disease, Hodgkin's) 201.9 ✓5ᵗʰ
  immunoblastic (type) (M9612/3) 200.8 ✓5ᵗʰ
  large cell (M9640/3) 200.0 ✓5ᵗʰ
    nodular (M9642/3) 200.0 ✓5ᵗʰ
    pleomorphic cell type (M9641/3) 200.0 ✓5ᵗʰ
  lymphoblastic (diffuse) (M9630/3) 200.1 ✓5ᵗʰ
    Burkitt's type (M9750/3) 200.2 ✓5ᵗʰ
    convoluted cell type (M9602/3) 202.8 ✓5ᵗʰ
  lymphocytic (cell type) (diffuse) (M9620/3) 200.1 ✓5ᵗʰ

Lymphoma — *continued*
  lymphocytic — *continued*
    with plasmacytoid differentiation, diffuse
      (M9611/3) 200.8
    intermediate differentiation (diffuse)
      (M9621/3) 200.1
      follicular (M9694/3) 202.0
      nodular (M9694/3) 202.0
    nodular (M9690/3) 202.0
    poorly differentiated (diffuse) (M9630/3)
      200.1
      follicular (M9696/3) 202.0
      nodular (M9696/3) 202.0
    well differentiated (diffuse) (M9620/3)
      200.1
      follicular (M9693/3) 202.0
      nodular (M9693/3) 202.0
  lymphocytic-histiocytic, mixed (diffuse)
    (M9613/3) 200.8
    follicular (M9691/3) 202.0
    nodular (M9691/3) 202.0
  lymphoplasmacytoid type (M9611/3)
    200.8
  lymphosarcoma type (M9610/3) 200.1
  macrofollicular (M9690/3) 202.0
  mixed cell type (diffuse) (M9613/3) 200.8
    follicular (M9691/3) 202.0
    nodular (M9691/3) 202.0
  nodular (M9690/3) 202.0
    histiocytic (M9642/3) 200.0
    lymphocytic (M9692/3) 202.0
      intermediate differentiation (M9694/3)
        202.0
      poorly differentiated (M9696/3)
        202.0
    mixed (cell type) (lymphocytic-histiocytic)
      (small cell and large cell) (M9691/3)
      202.0
  non-Hodgkin's type NEC (M9591/3) 202.8
  reticulum cell (type) (M9640/3) 200.0
  small cell and large cell, mixed (diffuse)
    (M9613/3) 200.8
    follicular (M9691/3) 202.0
    nodular (9691/3) 202.0
  stem cell (type) (M9601/3) 202.8
  T-cell 202.1
  undifferentiated (cell type) (non-Burkitt's)
    (M9600/3) 202.8
    Burkitt's type (M9750/3) 200.2

Lymphomatosis (M9590/3) — *see also*
  Lymphoma
  granulomatous 099.1

Lymphopathia
  venereum 099.1
  veneris 099.1

Lymphopenia 288.8
  familial 279.2

Lymphoreticulosis, benign (of inoculation)
  078.3

Lymphorrhea 457.8

Lymphosarcoma (M9610/3) 200.1
  diffuse (M9610/3) 200.1
    with plasmacytoid differentiation
      (M9611/3) 200.8
    lymphoplasmacytic (M9611/3) 200.8
  follicular (giant) (M9690/3) 202.0
    lymphoblastic (M9696/3) 202.0
    lymphocytic, intermediate differentiation
      (M9694/3) 202.0
    mixed cell type (M9691/3) 202.0

Lymphosarcoma — *continued*
  giant follicular (M9690/3) 202.0
  Hodgkin's (M9650/3) 201.9
  immunoblastic (M9612/3) 200.8
  lymphoblastic (diffuse) (M9630/3) 200.1
    follicular (M9696/3) 202.0
    nodular (M9696/3) 202.0
  lymphocytic (diffuse) (M9620/3) 200.1
    intermediate differentiation (diffuse)
      (M9621/3) 200.1
      follicular (M9694/3) 202.0
      nodular (M9694/3) 202.0
  mixed cell type (diffuse) (M9613/3) 200.8
    follicular (M9691/3) 202.0
    nodular (M9691/3) 202.0
  nodular (M9690/3) 202.0
    lymphoblastic (M9696/3) 202.0
    lymphocytic, intermediate differentiation
      (M9694/3) 202.0
    mixed cell type (M9691/3) 202.0
  prolymphocytic (M9631/3) 200.1
  reticulum cell (M9640/3) 200.0

Lymphostasis 457.8

Lypemania (*see also* Melancholia) 296.2

Lyssa 071

M

Macacus ear 744.29

Maceration
  fetus (cause not stated) 779.9
  wet feet, tropical (syndrome) 991.4

Machado-Joseph disease 334.8

Machupo virus hemorrhagic fever 078.7

Macleod's syndrome (abnormal transradiancy, one lung) 492.8

Macrocephalia, macrocephaly 756.0

Macrocheilia (congenital) 744.81

Macrochilia (congenital) 744.81

Macrocolon (congenital) 751.3

Macrocornea 743.41
  associated with buphthalmos 743.22

Macrocytic — *see* condition

Macrocytosis 289.8

Macrodactylia, macrodactylism (fingers)
  (thumbs) 755.57
  toes 755.65

Macrodontia 520.2

Macroencephaly 742.4

Macrogenia 524.05

Macrogenitosomia (female) (male) (praecox)
  255.2

Macrogingivae 523.8

Macroglobulinemia (essential) (idiopathic)
  (monoclonal) (primary) (syndrome)
  (Waldenström's) 273.3

Macroglossia (congenital) 750.15
  acquired 529.8

Macrognathia, macrognathism (congenital)
  524.00
  mandibular 524.02
    alveolar 524.72
  maxillary 524.01
    alveolar 524.71

Macrogyria (congenital) 742.4

Macrohydrocephalus (*see also* Hydrocephalus)
  331.4

Macromastia (see also Hypertrophy, breast) 611.1
Macropsia 368.14
Macrosigmoid 564.7
  congenital 751.3
Macrospondylitis, acromegalic 253.0
Macrostomia (congenital) 744.83
Macrotia (external ear) (congenital) 744.22
Macula
  cornea, corneal
    congenital 743.43
      interfering with vision 743.42
      interfering with central vision 371.03
      not interfering with central vision 371.02
    degeneration (see also Degeneration, macula) 362.50
    hereditary (see also Dystrophy, retina) 362.70
  edema, cystoid 362.53
Maculae ceruleae 132.1
Macules and papules 709.8
Maculopathy, toxic 362.55
Madarosis 374.55
Madelung's
  deformity (radius) 755.54
  disease (lipomatosis) 272.8
  lipomatosis 272.8
Madness (see also Psychosis) 298.9
  myxedema (acute) 293.0
    subacute 293.1
Madura
  disease (actinomycotic) 039.9
    mycotic 117.4
  foot (actinomycotic) 039.4
    mycotic 117.4
Maduromycosis (actinomycotic) 039.9
  mycotic 117.4
Maffucci's syndrome (dyschondroplasia with hemangiomas) 756.4
Magenblase syndrome 306.4
Main en griffe (acquired) 736.06
  congenital 755.59
Maintenance
  chemotherapy regimen or treatment V58.1
  dialysis regimen or treatment
    extracorporeal (renal) V56.0
    peritoneal V56.8
    renal V56.0
  drug therapy or regimen V58.1
  external fixation NEC V54.89 ▲
  radiotherapy V58.0
  traction NEC V54.89 ▲
Majocchi's
  disease (purpura annularis telangiectodes) 709.1
  granuloma 110.6
Major — see condition
Mal
  cerebral (idiopathic) (see also Epilepsy) 345.9 ✓5ᵗʰ
  comital (see also Epilepsy) 345.9 ✓5ᵗʰ
  de los pintos (see also Pinta) 103.9
  de Meleda 757.39
  de mer 994.6
  lie — see Presentation, fetal
  perforant (see also Ulcer, lower extremity) 707.15

Malabar itch 110.9
  beard 110.0
  foot 110.4
  scalp 110.0
Malabsorption 579.9
  calcium 579.8
  carbohydrate 579.8
  disaccharide 271.3
  drug-induced 579.8
  due to bacterial overgrowth 579.8
  fat 579.8
  folate, congenital 281.2
  galactose 271.1
  glucose-galactose (congenital) 271.3
  intestinal 579.9
  isomaltose 271.3
  lactose (hereditary) 271.3
  methionine 270.4
  monosaccharide 271.8
  postgastrectomy 579.3
  postsurgical 579.3
  protein 579.8
  sucrose (-isomaltose) (congenital) 271.3
  syndrome 579.9
    postgastrectomy 579.3
    postsurgical 579.3
Malacia, bone 268.2
  juvenile (see also Rickets) 268.0
  Kienböck's (juvenile) (lunate) (wrist) 732.3
    adult 732.8
Malacoplakia
  bladder 596.8
  colon 569.89
  pelvis (kidney) 593.89
  ureter 593.89
  urethra 599.84
Malacosteon 268.2
  juvenile (see also Rickets) 268.0
Maladaptation — see Maladjustment
Maladie de Roger 745.4
Maladjustment
  conjugal V61.10
    involving divorce or estrangement V61.0
  educational V62.3
  family V61.9
    specified circumstance NEC V61.8
  marital V61.10
    involving divorce or estrangement V61.0
  occupational V62.2
  simple, adult (see also Reaction, adjustment) 309.9
  situational acute (see also Reaction, adjustment) 309.9
  social V62.4
Malaise 780.79
Malakoplakia — see Malacoplakia
Malaria, malarial (fever) 084.6
  algid 084.9
  any type, with
    algid malaria 084.9
    blackwater fever 084.8
    fever
      blackwater 084.8
      hemoglobinuric (bilious) 084.8
    hemoglobinuria, malarial 084.8
    hepatitis 084.9 [573.2]
    nephrosis 084.9 [581.81]
    pernicious complication NEC 084.9
      cardiac 084.9
      cerebral 084.9

Malaria, malarial — *continued*
  cardiac 084.9
  carrier (suspected) of V02.9
  cerebral 084.9
  complicating pregnancy, childbirth, or puerperium 647.4 ✓5ᵗʰ
  congenital 771.2
  congestion, congestive 084.6
    brain 084.9
  continued 084.0
  estivo-autumnal 084.0
  falciparum (malignant tertian) 084.0
  hematinuria 084.8
  hematuria 084.8
  hemoglobinuria 084.8
  hemorrhagic 084.6
  induced (therapeutically) 084.7
    accidental — *see* Malaria, by type
  liver 084.9 [573.2]
  malariae (quartan) 084.2
  malignant (tertian) 084.0
  mixed infections 084.5
  monkey 084.4
  ovale 084.3
  pernicious, acute 084.0
  Plasmodium, P.
    falciparum 084.0
    malariae 084.2
    ovale 084.3
    vivax 084.1
  quartan 084.2
  quotidian 084.0
  recurrent 084.6
    induced (therapeutically) 084.7
      accidental — *see* Malaria, by type
  remittent 084.6
  specified types NEC 084.4
  spleen 084.6
  subtertian 084.0
  tertian (benign) 084.1
    malignant 084.0
  tropical 084.0
  typhoid 084.6
  vivax (benign tertian) 084.1
Malassez's disease (testicular cyst) 608.89
Malassimilation 579.9
Maldescent, testis 752.51
Maldevelopment — *see also* Anomaly, by site
  brain 742.9
  colon 751.5
  hip (joint) 755.63
    congenital dislocation (*see also* Dislocation, hip, congenital) 754.30
  mastoid process 756.0
  middle ear, except ossicles 744.03
    ossicles 744.04
  newborn (not malformation) 764.9 ✓5ᵗʰ
  ossicles, ear 744.04
  spine 756.10
  toe 755.66
Male type pelvis 755.69
  with disproportion (fetopelvic) 653.2 ✓5ᵗʰ
    affecting fetus or newborn 763.1
    causing obstructed labor 660.1 ✓5ᵗʰ
      affecting fetus or newborn 763.1
Malformation (congenital) — *see also* Anomaly
  bone 756.9
  bursa 756.9
  circulatory system NEC 747.9
    specified type NEC 747.89

Malformation — *continued*
  Chiari
    type I 348.4
    type II (*see also* Spina bifida) 741.0 ✓5ᵗʰ
    type III 742.0
    type IV 742.2
  cochlea 744.05
  digestive system NEC 751.9
    lower 751.5
    specified type NEC 751.8
    upper 750.9
  eye 743.9
  gum 750.9
  heart NEC 746.9
    specified type NEC 746.89
    valve 746.9
  internal ear 744.05
  joint NEC 755.9
    specified type NEC 755.8
  Mondini's (congenital) (malformation, cochlea) 744.05
  muscle 756.9
  nervous system (central) 742.9
  pelvic organs or tissues
    in pregnancy or childbirth 654.9 ✓5ᵗʰ
      affecting fetus or newborn 763.89
      causing obstructed labor 660.2 ✓5ᵗʰ
        affecting fetus or newborn 763.1
  placenta (*see also* Placenta, abnormal) 656.7 ✓5ᵗʰ
  respiratory organs 748.9
    specified type NEC 748.8
  Rieger's 743.44
  sense organs NEC 742.9
    specified type NEC 742.8
  skin 757.9
    specified type NEC 757.8
  spinal cord 742.9
  teeth, tooth NEC 520.9
  tendon 756.9
  throat 750.9
  umbilical cord (complicating delivery) 663.9 ✓5ᵗʰ
    affecting fetus or newborn 762.6
  umbilicus 759.9
  urinary system NEC 753.9
    specified type NEC 753.8
Malfunction — *see also* Dysfunction
  arterial graft 996.1
  cardiac pacemaker 996.01
  catheter device — *see* Complications, mechanical, catheter
  colostomy 569.62
  cystostomy 997.5
  device, implant, or graft NEC — *see* Complications, mechanical
  enteric stoma 569.62
  enterostomy 569.62
  gastroenteric 536.8
  gastrostomy 536.42
  nephrostomy 997.5
  pacemaker — *see* Complications, mechanical, pacemaker
  prosthetic device, internal — *see* Complications, mechanical
  tracheostomy 519.02
  vascular graft or shunt 996.1
Malgaigne's fracture (closed) 808.43
  open 808.53

Malherbe's
 calcifying epithelioma (M8110/0) — see
  Neoplasm, skin, benign
 tumor (M8110/0) — see Neoplasm, skin,
  benign
Malibu disease 919.8
 infected 919.9
Malignancy (M8000/3) — see Neoplasm, by site,
  malignant
Malignant — see condition
Malingerer, malingering V65.2
Mallet, finger (acquired) 736.1
 congenital 755.59
 late effect of rickets 268.1
Malleus 024
Mallory's bodies 034.1
Mallory-Weiss syndrome 530.7
Malnutrition (calorie) 263.9
 complicating pregnancy 648.9
 degree
  first 263.1
  second 263.0
  third 262
  mild 263.1
  moderate 263.0
  severe 261
   protein-calorie 262
 fetus 764.2
  "light-for-dates" 764.1
 following gastrointestinal surgery 579.3
 intrauterine or fetal 764.2
  fetus or infant "light-for-dates" 764.1
 lack of care, or neglect (child) (infant) 995.52
  adult 995.84
 malignant 260
 mild 263.1
 moderate 263.0
 protein 260
 protein-calorie 263.9
  severe 262
  specified type NEC 263.8
 severe 261
  protein-calorie NEC 262
Malocclusion (teeth) 524.4
 due to
  abnormal swallowing 524.5
  accessory teeth (causing crowding) 524.3
  dentofacial abnormality NEC 524.8
  impacted teeth (causing crowding) 524.3
  missing teeth 524.3
  mouth breathing 524.5
  supernumerary teeth (causing crowding)
   524.3
  thumb sucking 524.5
  tongue, lip, or finger habits 524.5
 temporomandibular (joint) 524.69
Malposition
 cardiac apex (congenital) 746.87
 cervix — see Malposition, uterus
 congenital
  adrenal (gland) 759.1
  alimentary tract 751.8
   lower 751.5
   upper 750.8
  aorta 747.21
  appendix 751.5
  arterial trunk 747.29

Malposition — continued
 congenital — continued
  artery (peripheral) NEC (see also
   Malposition, congenital, peripheral
   vascular system) 747.60
   coronary 746.85
   pulmonary 747.3
  auditory canal 744.29
   causing impairment of hearing 744.02
  auricle (ear) 744.29
   causing impairment of hearing 744.02
   cervical 744.43
  biliary duct or passage 751.69
  bladder (mucosa) 753.8
   exteriorized or extroverted 753.5
  brachial plexus 742.8
  brain tissue 742.4
  breast 757.6
  bronchus 748.3
  cardiac apex 746.87
  cecum 751.5
  clavicle 755.51
  colon 751.5
  digestive organ or tract NEC 751.8
   lower 751.5
   upper 750.8
  ear (auricle) (external) 744.29
   ossicles 744.04
  endocrine (gland) NEC 759.2
  epiglottis 748.3
  Eustachian tube 744.24
  eye 743.8
  facial features 744.89
  fallopian tube 752.19
  finger(s) 755.59
   supernumerary 755.01
  foot 755.67
  gallbladder 751.69
  gastrointestinal tract 751.8
  genitalia, genital organ(s) or tract
   female 752.8
    external 752.49
    internal NEC 752.8
   male 752.8
    penis 752.69
  glottis 748.3
  hand 755.59
  heart 746.87
   dextrocardia 746.87
    with complete transposition of viscera
     759.3
  hepatic duct 751.69
  hip (joint) (see also Dislocation, hip,
   congenital) 754.30
  intestine (large) (small) 751.5
   with anomalous adhesions, fixation, or
    malrotation 751.4
  joint NEC 755.8
  kidney 753.3
  larynx 748.3
  limb 755.8
   lower 755.69
   upper 755.59
  liver 751.69
  lung (lobe) 748.69
  nail(s) 757.5
  nerve 742.8
  nervous system NEC 742.8
  nose, nasal (septum) 748.1
  organ or site NEC — see Anomaly, specified
   type NEC, by site

Malposition — *continued*
  congenital — *continued*
    ovary 752.0
    pancreas 751.7
    parathyroid (gland) 759.2
    patella 755.64
    peripheral vascular system 747.60
      gastrointestinal 747.61
      lower limb 747.64
      renal 747.62
      specified NEC 747.69
      spinal 747.82
      upper limb 747.63
    pituitary (gland) 759.2
    respiratory organ or system NEC 748.9
    rib (cage) 756.3
      supernumerary in cervical region 756.2
    scapula 755.59
    shoulder 755.59
    spinal cord 742.59
    spine 756.19
    spleen 759.0
    sternum 756.3
    stomach 750.7
    symphysis pubis 755.69
    testis (undescended) 752.51
    thymus (gland) 759.2
    thyroid (gland) (tissue) 759.2
      cartilage 748.3
    toe(s) 755.66
      supernumerary 755.02
    tongue 750.19
    trachea 748.3
    uterus 752.3
    vein(s) (peripheral) NEC (*see also* Malposition, congenital, peripheral vascular system) 747.60
      great 747.49
      portal 747.49
      pulmonary 747.49
      vena cava (inferior) (superior) 747.49
  device, implant, or graft — *see* Complications, mechanical
  fetus NEC — (*see also* Presentation, fetal) 652.9
    with successful version 652.1
    affecting fetus or newborn 763.1
    before labor, affecting fetus or newborn 761.7
    causing obstructed labor 660.0
    in multiple gestation (one fetus or more) 652.6
      with locking 660.5
      causing obstructed labor 660.0
  gallbladder — (*see also* Disease, gallbladder) 575.8
  gastrointestinal tract 569.89
    congenital 751.8
  heart (*see also* Malposition, congenital, heart) 746.87
  intestine 569.89
    congenital 751.5
  pelvic organs or tissues
    in pregnancy or childbirth 654.4
      affecting fetus or newborn 763.89
      causing obstructed labor 660.2
      affecting fetus or newborn 763.1
  placenta — *see* Placenta, previa
  stomach 537.89
    congenital 750.7
  tooth, teeth (with impaction) 524.3

Malposition — *continued*
  uterus or cervix (acquired) (acute) (adherent) (any degree) (asymptomatic) (postinfectional) (postpartal, old) 621.6
    anteflexion or anteversion (*see also* Anteversion, uterus) 621.6
    congenital 752.3
    flexion 621.6
      lateral (*see also* Lateroversion, uterus) 621.6
    in pregnancy or childbirth 654.4
      affecting fetus or newborn 763.89
      causing obstructed labor 660.2
      affecting fetus or newborn 763.1
    inversion 621.6
    lateral (flexion) (version) (*see also* Lateroversion, uterus) 621.6
    lateroflexion (*see also* Lateroversion, uterus) 621.6
    lateroversion (*see also* Lateroversion, uterus) 621.6
    retroflexion or retroversion (*see also* Retroversion, uterus) 621.6

Malposture 729.9
Malpresentation, fetus — (*see also* Presentation, fetal) 652.9
Malrotation
  cecum 751.4
  colon 751.4
  intestine 751.4
  kidney 753.3
Malta fever (*see also* Brucellosis) 023.9
Maltosuria 271.3
Maltreatment (of)
  adult 995.80
    emotional 995.82
    multiple forms 995.85
    neglect (nutritional) 995.84
    physical 995.81
    psychological 995.82
    sexual 995.83
  child 995.50
    emotional 995.51
    multiple forms 995.59
    neglect (nutritional) 995.52
    physical 995.54
    shaken infant syndrome 995.55
    psychological 995.51
    sexual 995.53
  spouse 995.80 — (*see also* Maltreatment, adult)
Malt workers' lung 495.4
Malum coxae senilis 715.25
Malunion, fracture 733.81
Mammillitis (*see also* Mastitis) 611.0
  puerperal, postpartum 675.2
Mammitis (*see also* Mastitis) 611.0
  puerperal, postpartum 675.2
Mammographic microcalcification 793.81
Mammoplasia 611.1
Management
  contraceptive V25.9
    specified type NEC V25.8
  procreative V26.9
    specified type NEC V26.8
Mangled NEC (*see also* nature and site of injury) 959.9

Mania (monopolar) — (see also Psychosis, affective) 296.0 ✓5ᵗʰ
 alcoholic (acute) (chronic) 291.9
 Bell's — see Mania, chronic
 chronic 296.0 ✓5ᵗʰ
  recurrent episode 296.1 ✓5ᵗʰ
  single episode 296.0 ✓5ᵗʰ
 compulsive 300.3
 delirious (acute) 296.0 ✓5ᵗʰ
  recurrent episode 296.1 ✓5ᵗʰ
  single episode 296.0 ✓5ᵗʰ
 epileptic (see also Epilepsy) 345.4 ✓5ᵗʰ
 hysterical 300.10
 inhibited 296.89
 puerperal (after delivery) 296.0 ✓5ᵗʰ
  recurrent episode 296.1 ✓5ᵗʰ
  single episode 296.0 ✓5ᵗʰ
 recurrent episode 296.1 ✓5ᵗʰ
 senile 290.8
 single episode 296.0 ✓5ᵗʰ
 stupor 296.89
 stuporous 296.89
 unproductive 296.89
Manic-depressive insanity, psychosis, reaction, or syndrome (see also Psychosis, affective) 296.80
 circular (alternating) 296.7
  currently
   depressed 296.5 ✓5ᵗʰ
   episode unspecified 296.7
   hypomanic, previously depressed 296.4 ✓5ᵗʰ
   manic 296.4 ✓5ᵗʰ
   mixed 296.6 ✓5ᵗʰ
 depressed (type), depressive 296.2 ✓5ᵗʰ
  atypical 296.82
  recurrent episode 296.3 ✓5ᵗʰ
  single episode 296.2 ✓5ᵗʰ
 hypomanic 296.0 ✓5ᵗʰ
  recurrent episode 296.1 ✓5ᵗʰ
  single episode 296.0 ✓5ᵗʰ
 manic 296.0 ✓5ᵗʰ
  atypical 296.81
  recurrent episode 296.1 ✓5ᵗʰ
  single episode 296.0 ✓5ᵗʰ
 mixed NEC 296.89
 perplexed 296.89
 stuporous 296.89
Manifestations, rheumatoid
 lungs 714.81
 pannus — see Arthritis, rheumatoid
 subcutaneous nodules — see Arthritis, rheumatoid
Mankowsky's syndrome (familial dysplastic osteopathy) 731.2
Mannoheptulosuria 271.8
Mannosidosis 271.8
Manson's
 disease (schistosomiasis) 120.1
 pyosis (pemphigus contagiosus) 684
 schistosomiasis 120.1
Mansonellosis 125.5
Manual — see condition
Maple bark disease 495.6
Maple bark-strippers' lung 495.6
Maple syrup (urine) disease or syndrome 270.3
Marable's syndrome (celiac artery compression) 447.4

Marasmus 261
 brain 331.9
 due to malnutrition 261
 intestinal 569.89
 nutritional 261
 senile 797
 tuberculous NEC (see also Tuberculosis) 011.9 ✓5ᵗʰ
Marble
 bones 756.52
 skin 782.61
Marburg disease (virus) 078.89
March
 foot 733.94
 hemoglobinuria 283.2
Marchand multiple nodular hyperplasia (liver) 571.5
Marchesani (-Weill) syndrome (brachymorphism and ectopia lentis) 759.89
Marchiafava (-Bignami) disease or syndrome 341.8
Marchiafava-Micheli syndrome (paroxysmal nocturnal hemoglobinuria) 283.2
Marcus Gunn's syndrome (jaw-winking syndrome) 742.8
Marfan's
 congenital syphilis 090.49
 disease 090.49
 syndrome (arachnodactyly) 759.82
  meaning congenital syphilis 090.49
  with luxation of lens 090.49 [379.32]
Marginal
 implantation, placenta — see Placenta, previa
 placenta — see Placenta, previa
 sinus (hemorrhage) (rupture) 641.2 ✓5ᵗʰ
  affecting fetus or newborn 762.1
Marie's
 cerebellar ataxia 334.2
 syndrome (acromegaly) 253.0
Marie-Bamberger disease or syndrome (hypertrophic) (pulmonary) (secondary) 731.2
 idiopathic (acropachyderma) 757.39
 primary (acropachyderma) 757.39
Marie-Charcôt-Tooth neuropathic atrophy, muscle 356.1
Marie-Strümpell arthritis or disease (ankylosing spondylitis) 720.0
Marihuana, marijuana
 abuse (see also Abuse, drugs, nondependent) 305.2 ✓5ᵗʰ
 dependence (see also Dependence) 304.3 ✓5ᵗʰ
Marion's disease (bladder neck obstruction) 596.0
Marital conflict V61.10
Mark
 port wine 757.32
 raspberry 757.32
 strawberry 757.32
 stretch 701.3
 tattoo 709.09
Maroteaux-Lamy syndrome (mucopolysaccharidosis VI) 277.5
Marriage license examination V70.3
Marrow (bone)
 arrest 284.9
 megakaryocytic 287.3
 poor function 289.9

Marseilles fever 082.1
Marsh's disease (exophthalmic goiter) 242.0 ✓5ᵗʰ
Marshall's (hidrotic) **ectodermal dysplasia** 757.31
Marsh fever (see also Malaria) 084.6
Martin's disease 715.27
Martin-Albright syndrome (pseudohypoparathyroidism) 275.49
Martorell-Fabre syndrome (pulseless disease) 446.7
Masculinization, female, with adrenal hyperplasia 255.2
Masculinovoblastoma (M8670/0) 220
Masochism 302.83
Masons' lung 502
Mass
   abdominal 789.3 ✓5ᵗʰ
   anus 787.99
   bone 733.90
   breast 611.72
   cheek 784.2
   chest 786.6
   cystic — see Cyst
   ear 388.8
   epigastric 789.3 ✓5ᵗʰ
   eye 379.92
   female genital organ 625.8
   gum 784.2
   head 784.2
   intracranial 784.2
   joint 719.60
      ankle 719.67
      elbow 719.62
      foot 719.67
      hand 719.64
      hip 719.65
      knee 719.66
      multiple sites 719.69
      pelvic region 719.65
      shoulder (region) 719.61
      specified site NEC 719.68
      wrist 719.63
   kidney (see also Disease, kidney) 593.9
   lung 786.6
   lymph node 785.6
   malignant (M8000/3) — see Neoplasm, by site, malignant
   mediastinal 786.6
   mouth 784.2
   muscle (limb) 729.89
   neck 784.2
   nose or sinus 784.2
   palate 784.2
   pelvis, pelvic 789.3 ✓5ᵗʰ
   penis 607.89
   perineum 625.8
   rectum 787.99
   scrotum 608.89
   skin 782.2
   specified organ NEC — see Disease of specified organ or site
   splenic 789.2
   substernal 786.6
      thyroid (see also Goiter) 240.9
   superficial (localized) 782.2
   testes 608.89
   throat 784.2
   tongue 784.2
   umbilicus 789.3 ✓5ᵗʰ

Mass — continued
   uterus 625.8
   vagina 625.8
   vulva 625.8
Massive — see condition
Mastalgia 611.71
   psychogenic 307.89
Mast cell
   disease 757.33
      systemic (M9741/3) 202.6 ✓5ᵗʰ
   leukemia (M9900/3) 207.8 ✓5ᵗʰ
   sarcoma (M9742/3) 202.6 ✓5ᵗʰ
   tumor (M9740/1) 238.5
      malignant (M9740/3) 202.6 ✓5ᵗʰ
Masters-Allen syndrome 620.6
Mastitis (acute) (adolescent) (diffuse) (interstitial) (lobular) (nonpuerperal) (nonsuppurative) (parenchymatous) (phlegmonous) (simple) (subacute) (suppurative) 611.0
   chronic (cystic) (fibrocystic) 610.1
   cystic 610.1
      Schimmelbusch's type 610.1
   fibrocystic 610.1
   infective 611.0
   lactational 675.2 ✓5ᵗʰ
   lymphangitis 611.0
   neonatal (noninfective) 778.7
      infective 771.5
   periductal 610.4
   plasma cell 610.4
   puerperal, postpartum, (interstitial) (nonpurulent) (parenchymatous) 675.2 ✓5ᵗʰ
      purulent 675.1 ✓5ᵗʰ
      stagnation 676.2 ✓5ᵗʰ
   puerperalis 675.2 ✓5ᵗʰ
   retromammary 611.0
      puerperal, postpartum 675.1 ✓5ᵗʰ
   submammary 611.0
      puerperal, postpartum 675.1 ✓5ᵗʰ
Mastocytoma (M9740/1) 238.5
   malignant (M9740/3) 202.6 ✓5ᵗʰ
Mastocytosis 757.33
   malignant (M9741/3) 202.6 ✓5ᵗʰ
   systemic (M9741/3) 202.6 ✓5ᵗʰ
Mastodynia 611.71
   psychogenic 307.89
Mastoid — see condition
Mastoidalgia (see also Otalgia) 388.70
Mastoiditis (coalescent) (hemorrhagic) (pneumococcal) (streptococcal) (suppurative) 383.9
   acute or subacute 383.00
      with
         Gradenigo's syndrome 383.02
         petrositis 383.02
         specified complication NEC 383.02
         subperiosteal abscess 383.01
   chronic (necrotic) (recurrent) 383.1
   tuberculous (see also Tuberculosis) 015.6 ✓5ᵗʰ
Mastopathy, mastopathia 611.9
   chronica cystica 610.1
   diffuse cystic 610.1
   estrogenic 611.8
   ovarian origin 611.8
Mastoplasia 611.1
Masturbation 307.9

Maternal condition, affecting fetus or newborn
  acute yellow atrophy of liver 760.8
  albuminuria 760.1
  anesthesia or analgesia 763.5
  blood loss 762.1
  chorioamnionitis 762.7
  circulatory disease, chronic (conditions
      classifiable to 390-459, 745-747) 760.3
  congenital heart disease (conditions
      classifiable to 745-746) 760.3
  cortical necrosis of kidney 760.1
  death 761.6
  diabetes mellitus 775.0
    manifest diabetes in the infant 775.1
  disease NEC 760.9
    circulatory system, chronic (conditions
        classifiable to 390-459, 745-747)
        760.3
    genitourinary system (conditions
        classifiable to 580-599) 760.1
    respiratory (conditions classifiable to 490-
        519, 748) 760.3
  eclampsia 760.0
  hemorrhage NEC 762.1
  hepatitis acute, malignant, or subacute 760.8
  hyperemesis (gravidarum) 761.8
  hypertension (arising during pregnancy)
      (conditions classifiable to 642) 760.0
  infection
    disease classifiable to 001-136 760.2
    genital tract NEC 760.8
    urinary tract 760.1
  influenza 760.2
    manifest influenza in the infant 771.2
  injury (conditions classifiable to 800-996)
      760.5
  malaria 760.2
    manifest malaria in infant or fetus 771.2
  malnutrition 760.4
  necrosis of liver 760.8
  nephritis (conditions classifiable to 580-583)
      760.1
  nephrosis (conditions classifiable to 581)
      760.1
  noxious substance transmitted via breast milk
      or placenta 760.70
    alcohol 760.71
    anti-infective agents 760.74
    cocaine 760.75
    "crack" 760.75
    diethylstilbestrol [DES] 760.76
    hallucinogenic agents 760.73
    medicinal agents NEC 760.79
    narcotics 760.72
    obstetric anesthetic or analgesic drug
      760.72
    specified agent NEC 760.79
  nutritional disorder (conditions classifiable to
      260-269) 760.4
  operation unrelated to current delivery 760.6
  preeclampsia 760.0
  pyelitis or pyelonephritis, arising during
      pregnancy (conditions classifiable to
      590) 760.1
  renal disease or failure 760.1
  respiratory disease, chronic (conditions
      classifiable to 490-519, 748) 760.3
  rheumatic heart discase (chronic) (conditions
      classifiable to 393-398) 760.3
  rubella (conditions classifiable to 056) 760.2

Maternal condition, affecting fetus or newborn
  — *continued*
  rubella — *continued*
    manifest rubella in the infant or fetus
      771.0
  surgery unrelated to current delivery 760.6
    to uterus or pelvic organs 763.89
  syphilis (conditions classifiable to 090-097)
      760.2
    manifest syphilis in the infant or fetus
      090.0
  thrombophlebitis 760.3
  toxemia (of pregnancy) 760.0
    preeclamptic 760.0
  toxoplasmosis (conditions classifiable to 130)
      760.2
    manifest toxoplasmosis in the infant or
      fetus 771.2
  transmission of chemical substance through
      the placenta 760.70
    alcohol 760.71
    anti-infective 760.74
    cocaine 760.75
    "crack" 760.75
    diethylstilbestrol [DES] 760.76
    hallucinogenic agents 760.73
    narcotics 760.72
    specified substance NEC 760.79
  uremia 760.1
  urinary tract conditions (conditions
      classifiable to 580-599) 760.1
  vomiting (pernicious) (persistent) (vicious)
      761.8
Maternity — *see* Delivery
Matheiu's disease (leptospiral jaundice) 100.0
Mauclaire's disease or osteochondrosis 732.3
Maxcy's disease 081.0
Maxilla, maxillary — *see* condition
May (-Hegglin) anomaly or syndrome 288.2
Mayaro fever 066.3
Mazoplasia 610.8
MBD (minimal brain dysfunction), child (*see also*
    Hyperkinesia) 314.9
McArdle (-Schmid-Pearson) disease or
  syndrome (glycogenosis V) 271.0
McCune-Albright syndrome (osteitis fibrosa
  disseminata) 756.59
MCLS (mucocutaneous lymph node syndrome)
  446.1
McQuarrie's syndrome (idiopathic familial
  hypoglycemia) 251.2
Measles (black) (hemorrhagic) (suppressed) 055.9
  with
    encephalitis 055.0
    keratitis 055.71
    keratoconjunctivitis 055.71
    otitis media 055.2
    pneumonia 055.1
    complication 055.8
      specified type NEC 055.79
  encephalitis 055.0
  French 056.9
  German 056.9
  keratitis 055.71
  keratoconjunctivitis 055.71
  liberty 056.9
  otitis media 055.2
  pneumonia 055.1
  specified complications NEC 055.79

Measles — *continued*
  vaccination, prophylactic (against) V04.2
Meatitis, urethral (*see also* Urethritis) 597.89
Meat poisoning — *see* Poisoning, food
Meatus, meatal — *see* condition
Meat-wrappers' asthma 506.9
Meckel's
  diverticulitis 751.0
  diverticulum (displaced) (hypertrophic) 751.0
Meconium
  aspiration 770.1
  delayed passage in newborn 777.1
  ileus 777.1
    due to cystic fibrosis 277.01
  in liquor 792.3
    noted during delivery 656.8 ✓5ᵗʰ
  insufflation 770.1
  obstruction
    fetus or newborn 777.1
      in mucoviscidosis 277.01
  passage of 792.3
    noted during delivery — *omit code*
  peritonitis 777.6
  plug syndrome (newborn) NEC 777.1
Median — *see also* condition
  arcuate ligament syndrome 447.4
  bar (prostate) 600.9
    vesical orifice 600.9
  rhomboid glossitis 529.2
Mediastinal shift 793.2
Mediastinitis (acute) (chronic) 519.2
  actinomycotic 039.8
  syphilitic 095.8
  tuberculous (*see also* Tuberculosis) 012.8 ✓5ᵗʰ
Mediastinopericarditis (*see also* Pericarditis) 423.9
  acute 420.90
  chronic 423.8
    rheumatic 393
  rheumatic, chronic 393
Mediastinum, mediastinal — *see* condition
Medical services provided for — *see* Health, services provided because (of)
Medicine poisoning (by overdose) (wrong substance given or taken in error) 977.9
  specified drug or substance — *see* Table of Drugs and Chemicals
Medin's disease (poliomyelitis) 045.9 ✓5ᵗʰ
Mediterranean
  anemia (with other hemoglobinopathy) 282.4
  disease or syndrome (hemipathic) 282.4
  fever (*see also* Brucellosis) 023.9
    familial 277.3
  kala-azar 085.0
  leishmaniasis 085.0
  tick fever 082.1
Medulla — *see* condition
Medullary
  cystic kidney 753.16
  sponge kidney 753.17
Medullated fibers
  optic (nerve) 743.57
  retina 362.85
Medulloblastoma (M9470/3)
  desmoplastic (M9471/3) 191.6
  specified site — *see* Neoplasm, by site, malignant
  unspecified site 191.6

Medulloepithelioma (M9501/3) — *see also* Neoplasm, by site, malignant
  teratoid (M9502/3) — *see* Neoplasm, by site, malignant
Medullomyoblastoma (M9472/3)
  specified site — *see* Neoplasm, by site, malignant
  unspecified site 191.6
Meekeren-Ehlers-Danlos syndrome 756.83
Megacaryocytic — *see* condition
Megacolon (acquired) (functional) (not Hirschsprung's disease) 564.7
  aganglionic 751.3
  congenital, congenitum 751.3
  Hirschsprung's (disease) 751.3
  psychogenic 306.4
  toxic (*see also* Colitis, ulcerative) 556.9
Megaduodenum 537.3
Megaesophagus (functional) 530.0
  congenital 750.4
Megakaryocytic — *see* condition
Megalencephaly 742.4
Megalerythema (epidermicum) (infectiosum) 057.0
Megalia, cutis et ossium 757.39
Megaloappendix 751.5
Megalocephalus, megalocephaly NEC 756.0
Megalocornea 743.41
  associated with buphthalmos 743.22
Megalocytic anemia 281.9
Megalodactylia (fingers) (thumbs) 755.57
  toes 755.65
Megaloduodenum 751.5
Megaloesophagus (functional) 530.0
  congenital 750.4
Megalogastria (congenital) 750.7
Megalomania 307.9
Megalophthalmos 743.8
Megalopsia 368.14
Megalosplenia (*see also* Splenomegaly) 789.2
Megaloureter 593.89
  congenital 753.22
Megarectum 569.49
Megasigmoid 564.7
  congenital 751.3
Megaureter 593.89
  congenital 753.22
Megrim 346.9 ✓5ᵗʰ
Meibomian
  cyst 373.2
    infected 373.12
  gland — *see* condition
  infarct (eyelid) 374.85
  stye 373.11
Meibomitis 373.12
Meige
  -Milroy disease (chronic hereditary edema) 757.0
  syndrome (blepharospasm-oromandibular dystonia) 333.82
Melalgia, nutritional 266.2
Melancholia (*see also* Psychosis, affective) 296.90
  climacteric 296.2 ✓5ᵗʰ
  recurrent episode 296.3 ✓5ᵗʰ
  single episode 296.2 ✓5ᵗʰ

Index to Diseases

Melancholia — *continued*
　hypochondriac 300.7
　intermittent 296.2 ✓5ᵗʰ
　　recurrent episode 296.3 ✓5ᵗʰ
　　single episode 296.2 ✓5ᵗʰ
　involutional 296.2 ✓5ᵗʰ
　　recurrent episode 296.3 ✓5ᵗʰ
　　single episode 296.2 ✓5ᵗʰ
　menopausal 296.2 ✓5ᵗʰ
　　recurrent episode 296.3 ✓5ᵗʰ
　　single episode 296.2 ✓5ᵗʰ
　puerperal 296.2 ✓5ᵗʰ
　reactive (from emotional stress, psychological trauma) 298.0
　recurrent 296.3 ✓5ᵗʰ
　senile 290.21
　stuporous 296.2 ✓5ᵗʰ
　　recurrent episode 296.3 ✓5ᵗʰ
　　single episode 296.2 ✓5ᵗʰ

Melanemia 275.0

Melanoameloblastoma (M9363/0) — *see* Neoplasm, bone, benign

Melanoblastoma (M8720/3) — *see* Melanoma

Melanoblastosis
　Block-Sulzberger 757.33
　cutis linearis sive systematisata 757.33

Melanocarcinoma (M8720/3) — *see* Melanoma

Melanocytoma, eyeball (M8726/0) 224.0

Melanoderma, melanodermia 709.09
　Addison's (primary adrenal insufficiency) 255.4

Melanodontia, infantile 521.05

Melanodontoclasia 521.05

Melanoepithelioma (M8720/3) — *see* Melanoma

Melanoma (malignant) (M8720/3) 172.9

> Note — Except where otherwise indicated, the morphological varieties of melanoma in the list below should be coded by site as for "Melanoma (malignant)". Internal sites should be coded to malignant neoplasm of those sites.

　abdominal wall 172.5
　ala nasi 172.3
　amelanotic (M8730/3) — *see* Melanoma, by site
　ankle 172.7
　anus, anal 154.3
　　canal 154.2
　arm 172.6
　auditory canal (external) 172.2
　auricle (ear) 172.2
　auricular canal (external) 172.2
　axilla 172.5
　axillary fold 172.5
　back 172.5
　balloon cell (M8722/3) — *see* Melanoma, by site
　benign (M8720/0) — *see* Neoplasm, skin, benign
　breast (female) (male) 172.5
　brow 172.3
　buttock 172.5
　canthus (eye) 172.1
　cheek (external) 172.3
　chest wall 172.5
　chin 172.3
　choroid 190.6
　conjunctiva 190.3

Melanoma — *continued*
　ear (external) 172.2
　epithelioid cell (M8771/3) — *see also* Melanoma, by site
　　and spindle cell, mixed (M8775/3) — *see* Melanoma, by site
　external meatus (ear) 172.2
　eye 190.9
　eyebrow 172.3
　eyelid (lower) (upper) 172.1
　face NEC 172.3
　female genital organ (external) NEC 184.4
　finger 172.6
　flank 172.5
　foot 172.7
　forearm 172.6
　forehead 172.3
　foreskin 187.1
　gluteal region 172.5
　groin 172.5
　hand 172.6
　heel 172.7
　helix 172.2
　hip 172.7
　in
　　giant pigmented nevus (M8761/3) — *see* Melanoma, by site
　　Hutchinson's melanotic freckle (M8742/3) — *see* Melanoma, by site
　　junctional nevus (M8740/3) — *see* Melanoma, by site
　　precancerous melanosis (M8741/3) — *see* Melanoma, by site
　interscapular region 172.5
　iris 190.0
　jaw 172.3
　juvenile (M8770/0) — *see* Neoplasm, skin, benign
　knee 172.7
　labium
　　majus 184.1
　　minus 184.2
　lacrimal gland 190.2
　leg 172.7
　lip (lower) (upper) 172.0
　liver 197.7
　lower limb NEC 172.7
　male genital organ (external) NEC 187.9
　meatus, acoustic (external) 172.2
　meibomian gland 172.1
　metastatic
　　of or from specified site — *see* Melanoma, by site
　　site not of skin — *see* Neoplasm, by site, malignant, secondary
　　to specified site — *see* Neoplasm, by site, malignant, secondary
　　unspecified site 172.9
　nail 172.9
　　finger 172.6
　　toe 172.7
　neck 172.4
　nodular (M8721/3) — *see* Melanoma, by site
　nose, external 172.3
　orbit 190.1
　penis 187.4
　perianal skin 172.5
　perineum 172.5
　pinna 172.2
　popliteal (fossa) (space) 172.7
　prepuce 187.1

✓4ᵗʰ Fourth-digit Required　　✓5ᵗʰ Fifth-digit Required

Melanoma — continued
  pubes 172.5
  pudendum 184.4
  retina 190.5
  scalp 172.4
  scrotum 187.7
  septum nasal (skin) 172.3
  shoulder 172.6
  skin NEC 172.8
  spindle cell (M8772/3) — see also Melanoma, by site
    type A (M8773/3) 190.0
    type B (M8774/3) 190.0
  submammary fold 172.5
  superficial spreading (M8743/3) — see Melanoma, by site
  temple 172.3
  thigh 172.7
  toe 172.7
  trunk NEC 172.5
  umbilicus 172.5
  upper limb NEC 172.6
  vagina vault 184.0
  vulva 184.4
Melanoplakia 528.9
Melanosarcoma (M8720/3) — see also Melanoma
  epithelioid cell (M8771/3) — see Melanoma
Melanosis 709.09
  addisonian (primary adrenal insufficiency) 255.4
    tuberculous (see also Tuberculosis) 017.6
  adrenal 255.4
  colon 569.89
  conjunctiva 372.55
    congenital 743.49
  corii degenerativa 757.33
  cornea (presenile) (senile) 371.12
    congenital 743.43
      interfering with vision 743.42
    prenatal 743.43
      interfering with vision 743.42
  eye 372.55
    congenital 743.49
  jute spinners' 709.09
  lenticularis progressiva 757.33
  liver 573.8
  precancerous (M8741/2) — see also Neoplasm, skin, in situ
    malignant melanoma in (M8741/3) — see Melanoma
  Riehl's 709.09
  sclera 379.19
    congenital 743.47
  suprarenal 255.4
  tar 709.09
  toxic 709.09
Melanuria 791.9
MELAS 758.89
Melasma 709.09
  adrenal (gland) 255.4
  suprarenal (gland) 255.4
Melena 578.1
  due to
    swallowed maternal blood 777.3
    ulcer — see Ulcer, by site, with hemorrhage
  newborn 772.4
    due to swallowed maternal blood 777.3

Meleney's
  gangrene (cutaneous) 686.09
  ulcer (chronic undermining) 686.09
Melioidosis 025
Melitensis, febris 023.0
Melitococcosis 023.0
Melkersson (-Rosenthal) syndrome 351.8
Mellitus, diabetes — see Diabetes
Melorheostosis (bone) (leri) 733.99
Meloschisis 744.83
Melotia 744.29
Membrana
  capsularis lentis posterior 743.39
  epipapillaris 743.57
Membranacea placenta — see Placenta, abnormal
Membranaceous uterus 621.8
Membrane, membranous — see also condition
  folds, congenital — see Web
  Jackson's 751.4
  over face (causing asphyxia), fetus or newborn 768.9
  premature rupture — see Rupture, membranes, premature
  pupillary 364.74
    persistent 743.46
  retained (complicating delivery) (with hemorrhage) 666.2
    without hemorrhage 667.1
  secondary (eye) 366.50
  unruptured (causing asphyxia) 768.9
  vitreous humor 379.25
Membranitis, fetal 658.4
  affecting fetus or newborn 762.7
Memory disturbance, loss or lack (see also Amnesia) 780.99 ▲
  mild, following organic brain damage 310.1
Menadione (vitamin K) deficiency 269.0
Menarche, precocious 259.1
Mendacity, pathologic 301.7
Mende's syndrome (ptosis-epicanthus) 270.2
Mendelson's syndrome (resulting from a procedure) 997.3
  obstetric 668.0
Ménétrier's disease or syndrome (hypertrophic gastritis) 535.2
Ménière's disease, syndrome, or vertigo 386.00
  cochlear 386.02
  cochleovestibular 386.01
  inactive 386.04
  in remission 386.04
  vestibular 386.03
Meninges, meningeal — see condition
Meningioma (M9530/0) — see also Neoplasm, meninges, benign
  angioblastic (M9535/0) — see Neoplasm, meninges, benign
  angiomatous (M9534/0) — see Neoplasm, meninges, benign
  endotheliomatous (M9531/0) — see Neoplasm, meninges, benign
  fibroblastic (M9532/0) — see Neoplasm, meninges, benign
  fibrous (M9532/0) — see Neoplasm, meninges, benign

Meningioma — *continued*
- hemangioblastic (M9535/0) — *see* Neoplasm, meninges, benign
- hemangiopericytic (M9536/0) — *see* Neoplasm, meninges, benign
- malignant (M9530/3) — *see* Neoplasm, meninges, malignant
- meningiothelial (M9531/0) — *see* Neoplasm, meninges, benign
- meningotheliomatous (M9531/0) — *see* Neoplasm, meninges, benign
- mixed (M9537/0) — *see* Neoplasm, meninges, benign
- multiple (M9530/1) 237.6
- papillary (M9538/1) 237.6
- psammomatous (M9533/0) — *see* Neoplasm, meninges, benign
- syncytial (M9531/0) — *see* Neoplasm, meninges, benign
- transitional (M9537/0) — *see* Neoplasm, meninges, benign

Meningiomatosis (diffuse) (M9530/1) 237.6

Meningism (*see also* Meningismus) 781.6

Meningismus (infectional) (pneumococcal) 781.6
- due to serum or vaccine 997.09 *[321.8]*
- influenzal NEC 487.8

Meningitis (basal) (basic) (basilar) (brain) (cerebral) (cervical) (congestive) (diffuse) (hemorrhagic) (infantile) (membranous) (metastatic) (nonspecific) (pontine) (progressive) (simple) (spinal) (subacute) (sympathetica) (toxic) 322.9
- abacterial NEC (*see also* Meningitis, aseptic) 047.9
- actinomycotic 039.8 *[320.7]*
- adenoviral 049.1
- Aerobacter aerogenes 320.82
    - anaerobes (cocci) (gram-negative) (gram-positive) (mixed) (NEC) 320.81
- arbovirus NEC 066.9 *[321.2]*
    - specified type NEC 066.8 *[321.2]*
- aseptic (acute) NEC 047.9
    - adenovirus 049.1
    - Coxsackievirus 047.0
    - due to
        - adenovirus 049.1
        - Coxsackievirus 047.0
        - ECHO virus 047.1
        - enterovirus 047.9
        - mumps 072.1
        - poliovirus (*see also* Poliomyelitis) 045.2 ✓5ᵗʰ *[321.2]*
    - ECHO virus 047.1
    - herpes (simplex) virus 054.72
        - zoster 053.0
    - leptospiral 100.81
    - lymphocytic choriomeningitis 049.0
    - noninfective 322.0
- Bacillus pyocyaneus 320.89
- bacterial NEC 320.9
    - anaerobic 320.81
    - gram-negative 320.82
        - anaerobic 320.81
- Bacteroides (fragilis) (oralis) (melaninogenicus) 320.81
- cancerous (M8000/6) 198.4
- candidal 112.83
- carcinomatous (M8010/6) 198.4
- caseous (*see also* Tuberculosis, meninges) 013.0 ✓5ᵗʰ

Meningitis — *continued*
- cerebrospinal (acute) (chronic) (diplococcal) (endemic) (epidemic) (fulminant) (infectious) (malignant) (meningococcal) (sporadic) 036.0
    - carrier (suspected) of V02.59
- chronic NEC 322.2
- clear cerebrospinal fluid NEC 322.0
- Clostridium (haemolyticum) (novyi) NEC 320.81
- coccidioidomycosis 114.2
- Coxsackievirus 047.0
- cryptococcal 117.5 *[321.0]*
- diplococcal 036.0
    - gram-negative 036.0
    - gram-positive 320.1
- Diplococcus pneumoniae 320.1
- due to
    - actinomycosis 039.8 *[320.7]*
    - adenovirus 049.1
    - coccidiomycosis 114.2
    - enterovirus 047.9
        - specified NEC 047.8
    - histoplasmosis (*see also* Histoplasmosis) 115.91
    - Listerosis 027.0 *[320.7]*
    - Lyme disease 088.81 *[320.7]*
    - moniliasis 112.83
    - mumps 072.1
    - neurosyphilis 094.2
    - nonbacterial organisms NEC 321.8
    - oidiomycosis 112.83
    - poliovirus (*see also* Poliomyelitis) 045.2 ✓5ᵗʰ *[321.2]*
    - preventive immunization, inoculation, or vaccination 997.09 *[321.8]*
    - sarcoidosis 135 *[321.4]*
    - sporotrichosis 117.1 *[321.1]*
    - syphilis 094.2
        - acute 091.81
        - congenital 090.42
        - secondary 091.81
    - trypanosomiasis (*see also* Trypanosomiasis) 086.9 *[321.3]*
    - whooping cough 033.9 *[320.7]*
- E. coli 320.82
- ECHO virus 047.1
- endothelial-leukocytic, benign, recurrent 047.9
- Enterobacter aerogenes 320.82
- enteroviral 047.9
    - specified type NEC 047.8
- enterovirus 047.9
    - specified NEC 047.8
- eosinophilic 322.1
- epidemic NEC 036.0
- Escherichia coli (E. coli) 320.82
- Eubacterium 320.81
- fibrinopurulent NEC 320.9
    - specified type NEC 320.89
- Friedländer (bacillus) 320.82
- fungal NEC 117.9 *[321.1]*
- Fusobacterium 320.81
- gonococcal 098.82
- gram-negative bacteria NEC 320.82
    - anaerobic 320.81
    - cocci 036.0
        - specified NEC 320.82
- gram-negative cocci NEC 036.0
    - specified NEC 320.82
- gram-positive cocci NEC 320.9

Meningitis — continued
- H. influenzae 320.0
- herpes (simplex) virus 054.72
  - zoster 053.0
- infectious NEC 320.9
- influenzal 320.0
- Klebsiella pneumoniae 320.82
- late effect — see Late, effect, meningitis
- leptospiral (aseptic) 100.81
- Listerella (monocytogenes) 027.0 [320.7]
- Listeria monocytogenes 027.0 [320.7]
- lymphocytic (acute) (benign) (serous) 049.0
  - choriomeningitis virus 049.0
- meningococcal (chronic) 036.0
- Mima polymorpha 320.82
- Mollaret's 047.9
- monilial 112.83
- mumps (virus) 072.1
- mycotic NEC 117.9 [321.1]
- Neisseria 036.0
- neurosyphilis 094.2
- nonbacterial NEC (see also Meningitis, aseptic) 047.9
- nonpyogenic NEC 322.0
- oidiomycosis 112.83
- ossificans 349.2
- Peptococcus 320.81
- Peptostreptococcus 320.81
- pneumococcal 320.1
- poliovirus (see also Poliomyelitis) 045.2 ✓5ᵗʰ [321.2]
- Proprionibacterium 320.81
- Proteus morganii 320.82
- Pseudomonas (aeruginosa) (pyocyaneus) 320.82
- purulent NEC 320.9
  - specified organism NEC 320.89
- pyogenic NEC 320.9
  - specified organism NEC 320.89
- Salmonella 003.21
- septic NEC 320.9
  - specified organism NEC 320.89
- serosa circumscripta NEC 322.0
- serous NEC (see also Meningitis, aseptic) 047.9
  - lymphocytic 049.0
  - syndrome 348.2
- Serratia (marcescens) 320.82
- specified organism NEC 320.89
- sporadic cerebrospinal 036.0
- sporotrichosis 117.1 [321.1]
- staphylococcal 320.3
- sterile 997.09
- streptococcal (acute) 320.2
- suppurative 320.9
  - specified organism NEC 320.89
- syphilitic 094.2
  - acute 091.81
  - congenital 090.42
  - secondary 091.81
- torula 117.5 [321.0]
- traumatic (complication of injury) 958.8
- Treponema (denticola) (Macrodenticum) 320.81
- trypanosomiasis 086.1 [321.3]
- tuberculous (see also Tuberculosis, meninges) 013.0 ✓5ᵗʰ
- typhoid 002.0 [320.7]
- Veillonella 320.81
- Vibrio vulnificus 320.82

Meningitis — continued
- viral, virus NEC (see also Meningitis, aseptic) 047.9
- Wallgren's (see also Meningitis, aseptic) 047.9

Meningocele (congenital) (spinal) (see also Spina bifida) 741.9 ✓5ᵗʰ
- acquired (traumatic) 349.2
- cerebral 742.0
- cranial 742.0

Meningocerebritis — see Meningoencephalitis

Meningococcemia (acute) (chronic) 036.2

Meningococcus, meningococcal (see also condition) 036.9
- adrenalitis, hemorrhagic 036.3
- carditis 036.40
- carrier (suspected) of V02.59
- cerebrospinal fever 036.0
- encephalitis 036.1
- endocarditis 036.42
- infection NEC 036.9
- meningitis (cerebrospinal) 036.0
- myocarditis 036.43
- optic neuritis 036.81
- pericarditis 036.41
- septicemia (chronic) 036.2

Meningoencephalitis (see also Encephalitis) 323.9
- acute NEC 048
- bacterial, purulent, pyogenic, or septic — see Meningitis
- chronic NEC 094.1
- diffuse NEC 094.1
- diphasic 063.2
- due to
  - actinomycosis 039.8 [320.7]
  - blastomycosis NEC (see also Blastomycosis) 116.0 [323.4]
  - free-living amebae 136.2
  - Listeria monocytogenes 027.0 [320.7]
  - Lyme disease 088.81 [320.7]
  - mumps 072.2
  - Naegleria (amebae) (gruberi) (organisms) 136.2
  - rubella 056.01
  - sporotrichosis 117.1 [321.1]
  - toxoplasmosis (acquired) 130.0
    - congenital (active) 771.2 [323.4]
  - Trypanosoma 086.1 [323.2]
- epidemic 036.0
- herpes 054.3
- herpetic 054.3
- H. influenzae 320.0
- infectious (acute) 048
- influenzal 320.0
- late effect — see category 326
- Listeria monocytogenes 027.0 [320.7]
- lymphocytic (serous) 049.0
- mumps 072.2
- parasitic NEC 123.9 [323.4]
- pneumococcal 320.1
- primary amebic 136.2
- rubella 056.01
- serous 048
  - lymphocytic 049.0
- specific 094.2
- staphylococcal 320.3
- streptococcal 320.2
- syphilitic 094.2
- toxic NEC 989.9 [323.7]
  - due to
    - carbon tetrachloride 987.8 [323.7]

Meningoencephalitis — *continued*
  toxic NEC — *continued*
    due to — *continued*
      hydroxyquinoline derivatives poisoning 961.3 *[323.7]*
      lead 984.9 *[323.7]*
      mercury 985.0 *[323.7]*
      thallium 985.8 *[323.7]*
  toxoplasmosis (acquired) 130.0
  trypanosomic 086.1 *[323.2]*
  tuberculous (*see also* Tuberculosis, meninges) 013.0 ✓5ᵗʰ
  virus NEC 048
Meningoencephalocele 742.0
  syphilitic 094.89
  congenital 090.49
Meningoencephalomyelitis (*see also* Meningoencephalitis) 323.9
  acute NEC 048
    disseminated (postinfectious) 136.9 *[323.6]*
      postimmunization or postvaccination 323.5
  due to
    actinomycosis 039.8 *[320.7]*
    torula 117.5 *[323.4]*
    toxoplasma or toxoplasmosis (acquired) 130.0
    congenital (active) 771.2 *[323.4]*
  late effect — *see* category 326
Meningoencephalomyelopathy (*see also* Meningoencephalo-myelitis) 349.9
Meningoencephalopathy (*see also* Meningoencephalitis) 348.3
Meningoencephalopoliomyelitis (*see also* Poliomyelitis, bulbar) 045.0 ✓5ᵗʰ
  late effect 138
Meningomyelitis (*see also* Meningoencephalitis) 323.9
  blastomycotic NEC (*see also* Blastomycosis) 116.0 *[323.4]*
  due to
    actinomycosis 039.8 *[320.7]*
    blastomycosis (*see also* Blastomycosis) 116.0 *[323.4]*
    Meningococcus 036.0
    sporotrichosis 117.1 *[323.4]*
    torula 117.5 *[323.4]*
  late effect — *see* category 326
  lethargic 049.8
  meningococcal 036.0
  syphilitic 094.2
  tuberculous (*see also* Tuberculosis, meninges) 013.0 ✓5ᵗʰ
Meningomyelocele (*see also* Spina bifida) 741.9 ✓5ᵗʰ
  syphilitic 094.89
Meningomyeloneuritis — *see* Meningoencephalitis
Meningoradiculitis — *see* Meningitis
Meningovascular — *see* condition
Meniscocytosis 282.60
Menkes' syndrome — *see* Syndrome, Menkes'
Menolipsis 626.0
Menometrorrhagia 626.2
Menopause, menopausal (symptoms) (syndrome) 627.2
  arthritis (any site) NEC 716.3 ✓5ᵗʰ
  artificial 627.4
  bleeding 627.0

Menopause, menopausal — *continued*
  crisis 627.2
  depression (*see also* Psychosis, affective) 296.2 ✓5ᵗʰ
    agitated 296.2 ✓5ᵗʰ
      recurrent episode 296.3 ✓5ᵗʰ
      single episode 296.2 ✓5ᵗʰ
    psychotic 296.2 ✓5ᵗʰ
      recurrent episode 296.3 ✓5ᵗʰ
      single episode 296.2 ✓5ᵗʰ
    recurrent episode 296.3 ✓5ᵗʰ
    single episode 296.2 ✓5ᵗʰ
  melancholia (*see also* Psychosis, affective) 296.2 ✓5ᵗʰ
    recurrent episode 296.3 ✓5ᵗʰ
    single episode 296.2 ✓5ᵗʰ
  paranoid state 297.2
  paraphrenia 297.2
  postsurgical 627.4
  premature 256.31
    postirradiation 256.2
    postsurgical 256.2
  psychoneurosis 627.2
  psychosis NEC 298.8
  surgical 627.4
  toxic polyarthritis NEC 716.39
Menorrhagia (primary) 626.2
  climacteric 627.0
  menopausal 627.0
  postclimacteric 627.1
  postmenopausal 627.1
  preclimacteric 627.0
  premenopausal 627.0
  puberty (menses retained) 626.3
Menorrhalgia 625.3
Menoschesis 626.8
Menostaxis 626.2
Menses, retention 626.8
Menstrual — *see also* Menstruation
  cycle, irregular 626.4
  disorders NEC 626.9
  extraction V25.3
  fluid, retained 626.8
  molimen 625.4
  period, normal V65.5
  regulation V25.3
Menstruation
  absent 626.0
  anovulatory 628.0
  delayed 626.8
  difficult 625.3
  disorder 626.9
    psychogenic 306.52
    specified NEC 626.8
  during pregnancy 640.8 ✓5ᵗʰ
  excessive 626.2
  frequent 626.2
  infrequent 626.1
  irregular 626.4
  latent 626.8
  membranous 626.8
  painful (primary) (secondary) 625.3
    psychogenic 306.52
  passage of clots 626.2
  precocious 626.8
  protracted 626.8
  retained 626.8
  retrograde 626.8
  scanty 626.1
  suppression 626.8

Menstruation — *continued*
　vicarious (nasal) 625.8
Mentagra (*see also* Sycosis) 704.8
Mental — *see also* condition
　deficiency (*see also* Retardation, mental) 319
　deterioration (*see also* Psychosis) 298.9.
　disorder (*see also* Disorder, mental) 300.9
　exhaustion 300.5
　insufficiency (congenital) (*see also*
　　Retardation, mental) 319
　observation without need for further medical
　　care NEC V71.09
　retardation (*see also* Retardation, mental) 319
　subnormality (*see also* Retardation, mental)
　　319
　　mild 317
　　moderate 318.0
　　profound 318.2
　　severe 318.1
　upset (*see also* Disorder, mental) 300.9
Meralgia paresthetica 355.1
Mercurial — *see* condition
Mercurialism NEC 985.0
Merergasia 300.9
MERRF 758.89
Merkel cell tumor — *see* Neoplasm, by site,
　malignant
Merocele (*see also* Hernia, femoral) 553.00
Meromelia 755.4
　lower limb 755.30
　　intercalary 755.32
　　　femur 755.34
　　　　tibiofibular (complete) (incomplete)
　　　　　755.33
　　　fibula 755.37
　　　metatarsal(s) 755.38
　　　tarsal(s) 755.38
　　　tibia 755.36
　　　tibiofibular 755.35
　　terminal (complete) (partial) (transverse)
　　　755.31
　　　longitudinal 755.32
　　　　metatarsal(s) 755.38
　　　　phalange(s) 755.39
　　　　tarsal(s) 755.38
　　　transverse 755.31
　upper limb 755.20
　　intercalary 755.22
　　　carpal(s) 755.28
　　　humeral 755.24
　　　　radioulnar (complete) (incomplete)
　　　　　755.23
　　　metacarpal(s) 755.28
　　　phalange(s) 755.29
　　　radial 755.26
　　　radioulnar 755.25
　　　ulnar 755.27
　　terminal (complete) (partial) (transverse)
　　　755.21
　　　longitudinal 755.22
　　　　carpal(s) 755.28
　　　　metacarpal(s) 755.28
　　　　phalange(s) 755.29
　　　transverse 755.21
Merosmia 781.1
Merycism — *see also* Vomiting
　psychogenic 307.53
Merzbacher-Pelizaeus disease 330.0
Mesaortitis — *see* Aortitis

Mesarteritis — *see* Arteritis
Mesencephalitis (*see also* Encephalitis) 323.9
　late effect — *see* category 326
Mesenchymoma (M8990/1) — *see also*
　Neoplasm, connective tissue, uncertain
　behavior
　benign (M8990/0) — *see* Neoplasm,
　　connective tissue, benign
　malignant (M8990/3) — *see* Neoplasm,
　　connective tissue, malignant
Mesentery, mesenteric — *see* condition
Mesiodens, mesiodentes 520.1
　causing crowding 524.3
Mesio-occlusion 524.2
Mesocardia (with asplenia) 746.87
Mesocolon — *see* condition
Mesonephroma (malignant) (M9110/3) — *see
　also* Neoplasm, by site, malignant
　benign (M9110/0) — *see* Neoplasm, by site,
　　benign
Mesophlebitis — *see* Phlebitis
Mesostromal dysgenesis 743.51
Mesothelioma (malignant) (M9050/3) — *see also*
　Neoplasm, by site, malignant
　benign (M9050/0) — *see* Neoplasm, by site,
　　benign
　biphasic type (M9053/3) — *see also*
　　Neoplasm, by site, malignant
　　benign (M9053/0) — *see* Neoplasm, by site,
　　　benign
　epithelioid (M9052/3) — *see also* Neoplasm,
　　by site, malignant
　　benign (M9052/0) — *see* Neoplasm, by site,
　　　benign
　fibrous (M9051/3) — *see also* Neoplasm, by
　　site, malignant
　　benign (M9051/0) — *see* Neoplasm, by site,
　　　benign
Metabolism disorder 277.9
　specified type NEC 277.8
Metagonimiasis 121.5
Metagonimus infestation (small intestine) 121.5
Metal
　pigmentation (skin) 709.00
　polishers' disease 502
Metalliferous miners' lung 503
Metamorphopsia 368.14
Metaplasia
　bone, in skin 709.3
　breast 611.8
　cervix — *omit code*
　endometrium (squamous) 621.8
　intestinal, of gastric mucosa 537.89
　kidney (pelvis) (squamous) (*see also* Disease,
　　renal) 593.89
　myelogenous 289.8
　myeloid (agnogenic) (megakaryocytic) 289.8
　spleen 289.59
　squamous cell
　　amnion 658.8
　　bladder 596.8
　　cervix — *see* condition
　　trachea 519.1
　　tracheobronchial tree 519.1
　　uterus 621.8
　　　cervix — *see* condition

Metastasis, metastatic
  abscess — see Abscess
  calcification 275.40
  cancer, neoplasm, or disease
    from specified site (M8000/3) — see
      Neoplasm, by site, malignant
    to specified site (M8000/6) — see
      Neoplasm, by site, secondary
  deposits (in) (M8000/6) — see Neoplasm, by
    site, secondary
  pneumonia 038.8 [484.8]
  spread (to) (M8000/6) — see Neoplasm, by
    site, secondary
Metatarsalgia 726.70
  anterior 355.6
  due to Freiberg's disease 732.5
  Morton's 355.6
Metatarsus, metatarsal — see also condition
  abductus valgus (congenital) 754.60
  adductus varus (congenital) 754.53
  primus varus 754.52
  valgus (adductus) (congenital) 754.60
  varus (abductus) (congenital) 754.53
    primus 754.52
Methemoglobinemia 289.7
  acquired (with sulfhemoglobinemia) 289.7
  congenital 289.7
  enzymatic 289.7
  Hb-M disease 289.7
  hereditary 289.7
  toxic 289.7
Methemoglobinuria (see also Hemoglobinuria)
  791.2
Methioninemia 270.4
Metritis (catarrhal) (septic) (suppurative) (see
    also Endometritis) 615.9
  blennorrhagic 098.16
    chronic or duration of 2 months or over
      098.36
  cervical (see also Cervicitis) 616.0
  gonococcal 098.16
    chronic or duration of 2 months or over
      098.36
  hemorrhagic 626.8
  puerperal, postpartum, childbirth 670
  tuberculous (see also Tuberculosis) 016.7
Metropathia hemorrhagica 626.8
Metroperitonitis (see also Peritonitis, pelvic,
    female) 614.5
Metrorrhagia 626.6
  arising during pregnancy — see Hemorrhage,
    pregnancy
  postpartum NEC 666.2
  primary 626.6
  psychogenic 306.59
  puerperal 666.2
Metrorrhexis — see Rupture, uterus
Metrosalpingitis (see also Salpingo-oophoritis)
  614.2
Metrostaxis 626.6
Metrovaginitis (see also Endometritis) 615.9
  gonococcal (acute) 098.16
    chronic or duration of 2 months or over
      098.36
Mexican fever — see Typhus, Mexican
Meyenburg-Altherr-Uehlinger syndrome 733.99
Meyer-Schwickerath and Weyers syndrome
    (dysplasia oculodentodigitalis) 759.89

Meynert's amentia (nonalcoholic) 294.0
  alcoholic 291.1
Mibelli's disease 757.39
Mice, joint (see also Loose, body, joint)
    718.1
  knee 717.6
Micheli-Rietti syndrome (thalassemia minor)
  282.4
Michotte's syndrome 721.5
Micrencephalon, micrencephaly 742.1
Microaneurysm, retina 362.14
  diabetic 250.5 [362.01]
Microangiopathy 443.9
  diabetic (peripheral) 250.7 [443.81]
    retinal 250.5 [362.01]
  peripheral 443.9
    diabetic 250.7 [443.81]
  retinal 362.18
    diabetic 250.5 [362.01]
  thrombotic 446.6
    Moschcowitz's (thrombotic
      thrombocytopenic purpura) 446.6
Microcalcification, mammographic 793.81
Microcephalus, microcephalic, microcephaly
  742.1
  due to toxoplasmosis (congenital) 771.2
Microcheilia 744.82
Microcolon (congenital) 751.5
Microcornea (congenital) 743.41
Microcytic — see condition
Microdontia 520.2
Microdrepanocytosis (thalassemia-Hb-S disease)
  282.4
Microembolism
  atherothrombotic — see Atheroembolism
  retina 362.33
Microencephalon 742.1
Microfilaria streptocerca infestation 125.3
Microgastria (congenital) 750.7
Microgenia 524.0
Microgenitalia (congenital) 752.8
  penis 752.64
Microglioma (M9710/3)
  specified site — see Neoplasm, by site,
    malignant
  unspecified site 191.9
Microglossia (congenital) 750.16
Micrognathia, micrognathism (congenital)
  524.00
  mandibular 524.04
    alveolar 524.74
  maxillary 524.03
    alveolar 524.73
Microgyria (congenital) 742.2
Microinfarct, heart (see also Insufficiency,
    coronary) 411.89
Microlithiasis, alveolar, pulmonary 516.2
Micromyelia (congenital) 742.59
Micropenis 752.64
Microphakia (congenital) 743.36
Microphthalmia (congenital) (see also
    Microphthalmos) 743.10
Microphthalmos (congenital) 743.10
  associated with eye and adnexal anomalies
    NEC 743.12
  due to toxoplasmosis (congenital) 771.2
  isolated 743.11

Microphthalmos — continued
  simple 743.11
  syndrome 759.89
Micropsia 368.14
Microsporidiosis 136.8
Microsporon furfur infestation 111.0
Microsporosis (see also Dermatophytosis) 110.9
  nigra 111.1
Microstomia (congenital) 744.84
Microthelia 757.6
Microthromboembolism — see Embolism
Microtia (congenital) (external ear) 744.23
Microtropia 378.34
Micturition
  disorder NEC 788.69
    psychogenic 306.53
  frequency 788.41
    psychogenic 306.53
  nocturnal 788.43
  painful 788.1
    psychogenic 306.53
Middle
  ear — see condition
  lobe (right) syndrome 518.0
Midplane — see condition
Miescher's disease 709.3
  cheilitis 351.8
  granulomatosis disciformis 709.3
Miescher-Leder syndrome or granulomatosis 709.3
Mieten's syndrome 759.89
Migraine (idiopathic) 346.9
  with aura 346.0
  abdominal (syndrome) 346.2
  allergic (histamine) 346.2
  atypical 346.1
  basilar 346.2
  classical 346.0
  common 346.1
  hemiplegic 346.8
  lower-half 346.2
  menstrual 625.4
  ophthalmic 346.8
  ophthalmoplegic 346.8
  retinal 346.2
  variant 346.2
Migrant, social V60.0
Migratory, migrating — see also condition
  person V60.0
  testis, congenital 752.52
Mikulicz's disease or syndrome (dryness of mouth, absent or decreased lacrimation) 527.1
Milian atrophia blanche 701.3
Miliaria (crystallina) (rubra) (tropicalis) 705.1
  apocrine 705.82
Miliary — see condition
Milium (see also Cyst, sebaceous) 706.2
  colloid 709.3
  eyelid 374.84
Milk
  crust 690.11
  excess secretion 676.6
  fever, female 672
  poisoning 988.8
  retention 676.2
  sickness 988.8

Milk — continued
  spots 423.1
Milkers' nodes 051.1
Milk-leg (deep vessels) 671.4
  complicating pregnancy 671.3
  nonpuerperal 451.19
  puerperal, postpartum, childbirth 671.4
Milkman (-Looser) disease or syndrome (osteomalacia with pseudofractures) 268.2
Milky urine (see also Chyluria) 791.1
Millar's asthma (laryngismus stridulus) 478.75
Millard-Gubler paralysis or syndrome 344.89
Millard-Gubler-Foville paralysis 344.89
Miller's disease (osteomalacia) 268.2
Miller Fisher's syndrome 357.0
Milles' syndrome (encephalocutaneous angiomatosis) 759.6
Mills' disease 335.29
Millstone makers' asthma or lung 502
Milroy's disease (chronic hereditary edema) 757.0
Miners' — see also condition
  asthma 500
  elbow 727.2
  knee 727.2
  lung 500
  nystagmus 300.89
  phthisis (see also Tuberculosis) 011.4
  tuberculosis (see also Tuberculosis) 011.4
Minkowski-Chauffard syndrome (see also Spherocytosis) 282.0
Minor — see condition
Minor's disease 336.1
Minot's disease (hemorrhagic disease, newborn) 776.0
Minot-von Willebrand (-Jürgens) disease or syndrome (angiohemophilia) 286.4
Minus (and plus) hand (intrinsic) 736.09
Miosis (persistent) (pupil) 379.42
Mirizzi's syndrome (hepatic duct stenosis) (see also Obstruction, biliary) 576.2
  with calculus, cholelithiasis, or stones — see Choledocholithiasis
Mirror writing 315.09
  secondary to organic lesion 784.69
Misadventure (prophylactic) (therapeutic) (see also Complications) 999.9
  administration of insulin 962.3
  infusion — see Complications, infusion
  local applications (of fomentations, plasters, etc.) 999.9
    burn or scald — see Burn, by site
  medical care (early) (late) NEC 999.9
    adverse effect of drugs or chemicals — see Table of Drugs and Chemicals
    burn or scald — see Burn, by site
  radiation NEC 990
  radiotherapy NEC 990
  surgical procedure (early) (late) — see Complications, surgical procedure
  transfusion — see Complications, transfusion
  vaccination or other immunological procedure — see Complications, vaccination
Misanthropy 301.7
Miscarriage — see Abortion, spontaneous
Mischief, malicious, child (see also Disturbance, conduct) 312.0

Misdirection
  aqueous 365.83
Mismanagement, feeding 783.3
Misplaced, misplacement
  kidney (see also Disease, renal) 593.0
    congenital 753.3
  organ or site, congenital NEC — see
      Malposition, congenital
Missed
  abortion 632
  delivery (at or near term) 656.4
  labor (at or near term) 656.4
Missing — see also Absence
  teeth (acquired) 525.10
    congenital (see also Anodontia) 520.0
    due to
      caries 525.13
      extraction 525.10
      periodontal disease 525.12
      specified NEC 525.19
      trauma 525.11
  vertebrae (congenital) 756.13
Misuse of drugs NEC (see also Abuse, drug, nondependent) 305.9
Mitchell's disease (erythromelalgia) 443.89
Mite(s)
  diarrhea 133.8
  grain (itch) 133.8
  hair follicle (itch) 133.8
  in sputum 133.8
Mitral — see condition
Mittelschmerz 625.2
Mixed — see condition
Mljet disease (mal de Meleda) 757.39
Mobile, mobility
  cecum 751.4
  coccyx 733.99
  excessive — see Hypermobility
  gallbladder 751.69
  kidney 593.0
    congenital 753.3
  organ or site, congenital NEC — see
      Malposition, congenital
  spleen 289.59
Mobitz heart block (atrioventricular) 426.10
  type I (Wenckebach's) 426.13
  type II 426.12
Möbius'
  disease 346.8
  syndrome
    congenital oculofacial paralysis 352.6
    ophthalmoplegic migraine 346.8
Moeller (-Barlow) disease (infantile scurvy) 267
  glossitis 529.4
Mohr's syndrome (types I and II) 759.89
Mola destruens (M9100/1) 236.1
Molarization, premolars 520.2
Molar pregnancy 631
  hydatidiform (delivered) (undelivered) 630
Mold(s)
  in vitreous 117.9
Molding, head (during birth) 767.3
Mole (pigmented) (M8720/0) — see also
    Neoplasm, skin, benign
  blood 631
  Breus' 631
  cancerous (M8720/3) — see Melanoma

Mole — continued
  carneous 631
  destructive (M9100/1) 236.1
  ectopic — see Pregnancy, ectopic
  fleshy 631
  hemorrhagic 631
  hydatid, hydatidiform (benign) (complicating
      pregnancy) (delivered) (undelivered) (see
      also Hydatidiform mole) 630
    invasive (M9100/1) 236.1
    malignant (M9100/1) 236.1
    previous, affecting management of
        pregnancy V23.1
  invasive (hydatidiform) (M9100/1) 236.1
  malignant
    meaning
      malignant hydatidiform mole (9100/1)
          236.1
      melanoma (M8720/3) — see Melanoma
  nonpigmented (M8730/0) — see Neoplasm,
      skin, benign
  pregnancy NEC 631
  skin (M8720/0) — see Neoplasm, skin, benign
  tubal — see Pregnancy, tubal
  vesicular (see also Hydatidiform mole) 630
Molimen, molimina (menstrual) 625.4
Mollaret's meningitis 047.9
Mollities (cerebellar) (cerebral) 437.8
  ossium 268.2
Molluscum
  contagiosum 078.0
  epitheliale 078.0
  fibrosum (M8851/0) — see Lipoma, by site
  pendulum (M8851/0) — see Lipoma, by site
**Mönckeberg's arteriosclerosis, degeneration,
    disease, or sclerosis** (see also
    Arteriosclerosis, extremities) 440.20
Monday fever 504
Monday morning dyspnea or asthma 504
Mondini's malformation (cochlea) 744.05
Mondor's disease (thrombophlebitis of breast)
    451.89
**Mongolian, mongolianism, mongolism,
    mongoloid** 758.0
  spot 757.33
Monilethrix (congenital) 757.4
Monilia infestation — see Candidiasis
Moniliasis — see also Candidiasis
  neonatal 771.7
  vulvovaginitis 112.1
Monoarthritis 716.60
  ankle 716.67
  arm 716.62
    lower (and wrist) 716.63
    upper (and elbow) 716.62
  foot (and ankle) 716.67
  forearm (and wrist) 716.63
  hand 716.64
  leg 716.66
    lower 716.66
    upper 716.65
  pelvic region (hip) (thigh) 716.65
  shoulder (region) 716.61
  specified site NEC 716.68
Monoblastic — see condition
Monochromatism (cone) (rod) 368.54
Monocytic — see condition
Monocytosis (symptomatic) 288.8

Monofixation syndrome 378.34
Monomania (see also Psychosis) 298.9
Mononeuritis 355.9
 cranial nerve — see Disorder, nerve, cranial
 femoral nerve 355.2
 lateral
  cutaneous nerve of thigh 355.1
  popliteal nerve 355.3
 lower limb 355.8
  specified nerve NEC 355.79
 medial popliteal nerve 355.4
 median nerve 354.1
 multiplex 354.5
 plantar nerve 355.6
 posterior tibial nerve 355.5
 radial nerve 354.3
 sciatic nerve 355.0
 ulnar nerve 354.2
 upper limb 354.9
  specified nerve NEC 354.8
 vestibular 388.5
Mononeuropathy (see also Mononeuritis) 355.9
 diabetic NEC 250.6 [355.9]
  lower limb 250.6 [355.8]
  upper limb 250.6 [354.9]
 iliohypogastric 355.79
 ilioinguinal 355.79
 obturator 355.79
 saphenous 355.79
Mononucleosis, infectious 075
 with hepatitis 075 [573.1]
Monoplegia 344.5
 brain (current episode) (see also Paralysis, brain) 437.8
  fetus or newborn 767.8
 cerebral (current episode) (see also Paralysis, brain) 437.8
 congenital or infantile (cerebral) (spastic) (spinal) 343.3
 embolic (current) (see also Embolism, brain) 434.1
  late effect — see Late effect(s) (of) cerebrovascular disease
 infantile (cerebral) (spastic) (spinal) 343.3
 lower limb 344.30
  affecting
   dominant side 344.31
   nondominant side 344.32
  due to late effect of cerebrovascular accident — see Late effect(s) (of) cerebrovascular accident
 newborn 767.8
 psychogenic 306.0
  specified as conversion reaction 300.11
 thrombotic (current) (see also Thrombosis, brain) 434.0
  late effect — see Late effect(s) (of) cerebrovascular disease
 transient 781.4
 upper limb 344.40
  affecting
   dominant side 344.41
   nondominant side 344.42
  due to late effect of cerebrovascular accident — see Late effect(s) (of) cerebrovascular accident
Monorchism, monorchidism 752.8
Monster, monstrosity — see Anomaly
Monteggia's fracture (closed) 813.03
 open 813.13

Mood swings
 brief compensatory 296.99
 rebound 296.99
Moore's syndrome (see also Epilepsy) 345.5
Mooren's ulcer (cornea) 370.07
Mooser-Neill reaction 081.0
Mooser bodies 081.0
Moral
 deficiency 301.7
 imbecility 301.7
Morax-Axenfeld conjunctivitis 372.03
Morbilli (see also Measles) 055.9
Morbus
 anglicus, anglorum 268.0
 Beigel 111.2
 caducus (see also Epilepsy) 345.9
 caeruleus 746.89
 celiacus 579.0
 comitialis (see also Epilepsy) 345.9
 cordis — see also Disease, heart
  valvulorum — see Endocarditis
 coxae 719.95
  tuberculous (see also Tuberculosis) 015.1
 hemorrhagicus neonatorum 776.0
 maculosus neonatorum 772.6
 renum 593.0
 senilis (see also Osteoarthrosis) 715.9
Morel-Kraepelin disease (see also Schizophrenia) 295.9
Morel-Moore syndrome (hyperostosis frontalis interna) 733.3
Morel-Morgagni syndrome (hyperostosis frontalis interna) 733.3
Morgagni
 cyst, organ, hydatid, or appendage 752.8
  fallopian tube 752.11
 disease or syndrome (hyperostosis frontalis interna) 733.3
Morgagni-Adams-Stokes syndrome (syncope with heart block) 426.9
Morgagni-Stewart-Morel syndrome (hyperostosis frontalis interna) 733.3
Moria (see also Psychosis) 298.9
Morning sickness 643.0
Moron 317
Morphea (guttate) (linear) 701.0
Morphine dependence (see also Dependence) 304.0
Morphinism (see also Dependence) 304.0
Morphinomania (see also Dependence) 304.0
Morphoea 701.0
Morquio (-Brailsford) (-Ullrich) disease or syndrome (mucopolysaccharidosis IV) 277.5
 kyphosis 277.5
Morris syndrome (testicular feminization) 257.8
Morsus humanus (open wound) — see also Wound, open, by site
 skin surface intact — see Contusion
Mortification (dry) (moist) (see also Gangrene) 785.4
Morton's
 disease 355.6
 foot 355.6
 metatarsalgia (syndrome) 355.6
 neuralgia 355.6

Morton's — *continued*
  neuroma 355.6
  syndrome (metatarsalgia) (neuralgia) 355.6
  toe 355.6
Morvan's disease 336.0
Mosaicism, mosaic (chromosomal) 758.9
  autosomal 758.5
  sex 758.81
Moschcowitz's syndrome (thrombotic thrombocytopenic purpura) 446.6
Mother yaw 102.0
Motion sickness (from travel, any vehicle) (from roundabouts or swings) 994.6
Mottled teeth (enamel) (endemic) (nonendemic) 520.3
Mottling enamel (endemic) (nonendemic) (teeth) 520.3
Mouchet's disease 732.5
Mould(s) (in vitreous) 117.9
Moulders'
  bronchitis 502
  tuberculosis (*see also* Tuberculosis) 011.4 ✓5ᵗʰ
Mounier-Kuhn syndrome 494.0
  with acute exacerbation 494.1
Mountain
  fever — *see* Fever, mountain
  sickness 993.2
    with polycythemia, acquired 289.0
      acute 289.0
    tick fever 066.1
Mouse, joint (*see also* Loose, body, joint) 718.1 ✓5ᵗʰ
  knee 717.6
Mouth — *see* condition
Movable
  coccyx 724.71
  kidney (*see also* Disease, renal) 593.0
    congenital 753.3
  organ or site, congenital NEC — *see* Malposition, congenital
  spleen 289.59
Movement
  abnormal (dystonic) (involuntary) 781.0
  decreased fetal 655.7 ✓5ᵗʰ
  paradoxical facial 374.43
Moya Moya disease 437.5
Mozart's ear 744.29
Mucha's disease (acute parapsoriasis varioliformis) 696.2
Mucha-Haberman syndrome (acute parapsoriasis varioliformis) 696.2
Mu-chain disease 273.2
Mucinosis (cutaneous) (papular) 701.8
Mucocele
  appendix 543.9
  buccal cavity 528.9
  gallbladder (*see also* Disease, gallbladder) 575.3
  lacrimal sac 375.43
  orbit (eye) 376.81
  salivary gland (any) 527.6
  sinus (accessory) (nasal) 478.1
  turbinate (bone) (middle) (nasal) 478.1
  uterus 621.8
Mucocutaneous lymph node syndrome (acute) (febrile) (infantile) 446.1
Mucoenteritis 564.9

Mucolipidosis I, II, III 272.7
Mucopolysaccharidosis (types 1-6) 277.5
  cardiopathy 277.5 *[425.7]*
Mucormycosis (lung) 117.7
Mucositis — *see also* Inflammation by site
  necroticans agranulocytica 288.0
Mucous — *see also* condition
  patches (syphilitic) 091.3
    congenital 090.0
Mucoviscidosis 277.00
  with meconium obstruction 277.01
Mucus
  asphyxia or suffocation (*see also* Asphyxia, mucus) 933.1
    newborn 770.1
  in stool 792.1
  plug (*see also* Asphyxia, mucus) 933.1
    aspiration, of newborn 770.1
    tracheobronchial 519.1
      newborn 770.1
Muguet 112.0
Mulberry molars 090.5
Mullerian mixed tumor (M8950/3) — *see* Neoplasm, by site, malignant
Multicystic kidney 753.19
Multilobed placenta — *see* Placenta, abnormal
Multinodular prostate 600.1
Multiparity V61.5
  affecting
    fetus or newborn 763.89
    management of
      labor and delivery 659.4 ✓5ᵗʰ
      pregnancy V23.3
  requiring contraceptive management (*see also* Contraception) V25.9
Multipartita placenta — *see* Placenta, abnormal
Multiple, multiplex — *see also* condition
  birth
    affecting fetus or newborn 761.5
    healthy liveborn — *see* Newborn, multiple
  digits (congenital) 755.00
    fingers 755.01
    toes 755.02
  organ or site NEC — *see* Accessory
  personality 300.14
  renal arteries 747.62
Mumps 072.9
  with complication 072.8
    specified type NEC 072.79
  encephalitis 072.2
  hepatitis 072.71
  meningitis (aseptic) 072.1
  meningoencephalitis 072.2
  oophoritis 072.79
  orchitis 072.0
  pancreatitis 072.3
  polyneuropathy 072.72
  vaccination, prophylactic (against) V04.6
Mumu (*see also* Infestation, filarial) 125.9
Münchausen syndrome 301.51
Münchmeyer's disease or syndrome (exostosis luxurians) 728.11
Mural — *see* condition
Murmur (cardiac) (heart) (nonorganic) (organic) 785.2
  abdominal 787.5
  aortic (valve) (*see also* Endocarditis, aortic) 424.1

Murmur — continued
  benign — *omit code*
  cardiorespiratory 785.2
  diastolic — *see* condition
  Flint (*see also* Endocarditis, aortic) 424.1
  functional — *omit code*
  Graham Steell (pulmonic regurgitation) (*see also* Endocarditis, pulmonary) 424.3
  innocent — *omit code*
  insignificant — *omit code*
  midsystolic 785.2
  mitral (valve) — *see* Stenosis, mitral
  physiologic — *see* condition
  presystolic, mitral — *see* Insuficiency, mitral
  pulmonic (valve) (*see also* Endocarditis, pulmonary) 424.3
  Still's (vibratory) — *omit code*
  systolic (valvular) — *see* condition
  tricuspid (valve) — *see* Endocarditis, tricuspid
  undiagnosed 785.2
  valvular — *see* condition
  vibratory — *omit code*
Murri's disease (intermittent hemoglobinuria) 283.2
Muscae volitantes 379.24
Muscle, muscular — *see* condition
Musculoneuralgia 729.1
Mushrooming hip 718.95
Mushroom workers' (pickers') lung 495.5
Mutism (*see also* Aphasia) 784.3
  akinetic 784.3
  deaf (acquired) (congenital) 389.7
  elective (selective) 313.23
    adjustment reaction 309.83
  hysterical 300.11
Myà's disease (congenital dilation, colon) 751.3
Myalgia (intercostal) 729.1
  eosinophilia syndrome 710.5
  epidemic 074.1
    cervical 078.89
  psychogenic 307.89
  traumatic NEC 959.9
Myasthenia, myasthenic 358.0
  cordis — *see* Failure, heart
  gravis 358.0
    neonatal 775.2
    pseudoparalytica 358.0
  stomach 536.8
    psychogenic 306.4
  syndrome
    in
      botulism 005.1 *[358.1]*
      diabetes mellitus 250.6 *[358.1]*
      hypothyroidism (*see also* Hypothyroidism) 244.9 *[358.1]*
      malignant neoplasm NEC 199.1 *[358.1]*
      pernicious anemia 281.0 *[358.1]*
      thyrotoxicosis (*see also* Thyrotoxicosis) 242.9 *[358.1]*
Mycelium infection NEC 117.9
Mycetismus 988.1
Mycetoma (actinomycotic) 039.9
  bone 039.8
    mycotic 117.4
  foot 039.4
    mycotic 117.4
  madurae 039.9
    mycotic 117.4

Mycetoma — continued
  maduromycotic 039.9
    mycotic 117.4
  mycotic 117.4
  nocardial 039.9
Mycobacteriosis — *see* Mycobacterium
Mycobacterium, mycobacterial (infection) 031.9
  acid-fast (bacilli) 031.9
  anonymous (*see also* Mycobacterium, atypical) 031.9
  atypical (acid-fast bacilli) 031.9
    cutaneous 031.1
    pulmonary 031.0
      tuberculous (*see also* Tuberculosis, pulmonary) 011.9
    specified site NEC 031.8
  avium 031.0
    intracellulare complex bacteremia (MAC) 031.2
  balnei 031.1
  Battey 031.0
  cutaneous 031.1
  disseminated 031.2
    avium-intracellulare complex (DMAC) 031.2
  fortuitum 031.0
  intracellulare (battey bacillus) 031.0
  kakerifu 031.8
  kansasii 031.0
  kasongo 031.8
  leprae — *see* Leprosy
  luciflavum 031.0
  marinum 031.1
  pulmonary 031.0
    tuberculous (*see also* Tuberculosis, pulmonary) 011.9
  scrofulaceum 031.1
  tuberculosis (human, bovine) — *see also* Tuberculosis
    avian type 031.0
  ulcerans 031.1
  xenopi 031.0
Mycosis, mycotic 117.9
  cutaneous NEC 111.9
  ear 111.8 *[380.15]*
  fungoides (M9700/3) 202.1
  mouth 112.0
  pharynx 117.9
  skin NEC 111.9
  stomatitis 112.0
  systemic NEC 117.9
  tonsil 117.9
  vagina, vaginitis 112.1
Mydriasis (persistent) (pupil) 379.43
Myelatelia 742.59
Myelinoclasis, perivascular, acute (postinfectious) NEC 136.9 *[323.6]*
  postimmunization or postvaccinal 323.5
Myelinosis, central pontine 341.8
Myelitis (acute) (ascending) (cerebellar) (childhood) (chronic) (descending) (diffuse) (disseminated) (pressure) (progressive) (spinal cord) (subacute) (transverse) (*see also* Encephalitis) 323.9
  late effect — *see* category 326
  optic neuritis in 341.0
  postchickenpox 052.7
  postvaccinal 323.5
  syphilitic (transverse) 094.89
  tuberculous (*see also* Tuberculosis) 013.6
  virus 049.9

Myeloblastic — see condition
Myelocele (see also Spina bifida) 741.9 ✓5ᵗʰ
  with hydrocephalus 741.0 ✓5ᵗʰ
Myelocystocele (see also Spina bifida) 741.9 ✓5ᵗʰ
Myelocytic — see condition
Myelocytoma 205.1 ✓5ᵗʰ
Myelodysplasia (spinal cord) 742.59
  meaning myelodysplastic syndrome — see Syndrome, myelodysplastic
Myeloencephalitis — see Encephalitis
Myelofibrosis (osteosclerosis) 289.8
Myelogenous — see condition
Myeloid — see condition
Myelokathexis 288.0
Myeloleukodystrophy 330.0
Myelolipoma (M8870/0) — see Neoplasm, by site, benign
Myeloma (multiple) (plasma cell) (plasmacytic) (M9730/3) 203.0 ✓5ᵗʰ
  monostotic (M9731/1) 238.6
  solitary (M9731/1) 238.6
Myelomalacia 336.8
Myelomata, multiple (M9730/3) 203.0 ✓5ᵗʰ
Myelomatosis (M9730/3) 203.0 ✓5ᵗʰ
Myelomeningitis — see Meningoencephalitis
Myelomeningocele (spinal cord) (see also Spina bifida) 741.9 ✓5ᵗʰ
  fetal, causing fetopelvic disproportion 653.7 ✓5ᵗʰ
Myelo-osteo-musculodysplasia hereditaria 756.89
Myelopathic — see condition
Myelopathy (spinal cord) 336.9
  cervical 721.1
  diabetic 250.6 ✓5ᵗʰ [336.3]
  drug-induced 336.8
  due to or with
    carbon tetrachloride 987.8 [323.7]
    degeneration or displacement, intervertebral disc 722.70
      cervical, cervicothoracic 722.71
      lumbar, lumbosacral 722.73
      thoracic, thoracolumbar 722.72
    hydroxyquinoline derivatives 961.3 [323.7]
    infection — see Encephalitis
    intervertebral disc disorder 722.70
      cervical, cervicothoracic 722.71
      lumbar, lumbosacral 722.73
      thoracic, thoracolumbar 722.72
    lead 984.9 [323.7]
    mercury 985.0 [323.7]
    neoplastic disease (see also Neoplasm, by site) 239.9 [336.3]
    pernicious anemia 281.0 [336.3]
    spondylosis 721.91
      cervical 721.1
      lumbar, lumbosacral 721.42
      thoracic 721.41
    thallium 985.8 [323.7]
  lumbar, lumbosacral 721.42
  necrotic (subacute) 336.1
  radiation-induced 336.8
  spondylogenic NEC 721.91
    cervical 721.1
    lumbar, lumbosacral 721.42
    thoracic 721.41
  thoracic 721.41
  toxic NEC 989.9 [323.7]

Myelopathy — continued
  transverse (see also Encephalitis) 323.9
  vascular 336.1
Myeloproliferative disease (M9960/1) 238.7
Myeloradiculitis (see also Polyneuropathy) 357.0
Myeloradiculodysplasia (spinal) 742.59
Myelosarcoma (M9930/3) 205.3 ✓5ᵗʰ
Myelosclerosis 289.8
  with myeloid metaplasia (M9961/1) 238.7
  disseminated, of nervous system 340
  megakaryocytic (M9961/1) 238.7
Myelosis (M9860/3) (see also Leukemia, myeloid) 205.9 ✓5ᵗʰ
  acute (M9861/3) 205.0 ✓5ᵗʰ
  aleukemic (M9864/3) 205.8 ✓5ᵗʰ
  chronic (M9863/3) 205.1 ✓5ᵗʰ
  erythremic (M9840/3) 207.0 ✓5ᵗʰ
    acute (M9841/3) 207.0 ✓5ᵗʰ
  megakaryocytic (M9920/3) 207.2 ✓5ᵗʰ
  nonleukemic (chronic) 288.8
  subacute (M9862/3) 205.2 ✓5ᵗʰ
Myesthenia — see Myasthenia
Myiasis (cavernous) 134.0
  orbit 134.0 [376.13]
Myoadenoma, prostate 600.2
Myoblastoma
  granular cell (M9580/0) — see also Neoplasm, connective tissue, benign
    malignant (M9580/3) — see Neoplasm, connective tissue, malignant
  tongue (M9580/0) 210.1
Myocardial — see condition
Myocardiopathy (congestive) (constrictive) (familial) (hypertrophic nonobstructive) (idiopathic) (infiltrative) (obstructive) (primary) (restrictive) (sporadic) 425.4
  alcoholic 425.5
  amyloid 277.3 [425.7]
  beriberi 265.0 [425.7]
  cobalt-beer 425.5
  due to
    amyloidosis 277.3 [425.7]
    beriberi 265.0 [425.7]
    cardiac glycogenosis 271.0 [425.7]
    Chagas' disease 086.0
    Friedreich's ataxia 334.0 [425.8]
    influenza 487.8 [425.8]
    mucopolysaccharidosis 277.5 [425.7]
    myotonia atrophica 359.2 [425.8]
    progressive muscular dystrophy 359.1 [425.8]
    sarcoidosis 135 [425.8]
  glycogen storage 271.0 [425.7]
  hypertrophic obstructive 425.1
  metabolic NEC 277.9 [425.7]
  nutritional 269.9 [425.7]
  obscure (African) 425.2
  postpartum 674.8 ✓5ᵗʰ
  secondary 425.9
  thyrotoxic (see also Thyrotoxicosis) 242.9 ✓5ᵗʰ [425.7]
  toxic NEC 425.9
Myocarditis (fibroid) (interstitial) (old) (progressive) (senile) (with arteriosclerosis) 429.0
  with
    rheumatic fever (conditions classifiable to 390) 398.0

Myocarditis — continued
  with — continued
    rheumatic fever — continued
      active (see also Myocarditis, acute, rheumatic) 391.2
      inactive or quiescent (with chorea) 398.0
  active (nonrheumatic) 422.90
    rheumatic 391.2
      with chorea (acute) (rheumatic) (Sydenham's) 392.0
  acute or subacute (interstitial) 422.90
    due to Streptococcus (beta-hemolytic) 391.2
    idiopathic 422.91
    rheumatic 391.2
      with chorea (acute) (rheumatic) (Sydenham's) 392.0
    specified type NEC 422.99
  aseptic of newborn 074.23
  bacterial (acute) 422.92
  chagasic 086.0
  chronic (interstitial) 429.0
  congenital 746.89
  constrictive 425.4
  Coxsackie (virus) 074.23
  diphtheritic 032.82
  due to or in
    Coxsackie (virus) 074.23
    diphtheria 032.82
    epidemic louse-borne typhus 080 [422.0]
    influenza 487.8 [422.0]
    Lyme disease 088.81 [422.0]
    scarlet fever 034.1 [422.0]
    toxoplasmosis (acquired) 130.3
    tuberculosis (see also Tuberculosis) 017.9 ✔5ᵗʰ [422.0]
    typhoid 002.0 [422.0]
    typhus NEC 081.9 [422.0]
  eosinophilic 422.91
  epidemic of newborn 074.23
  Fiedler's (acute) (isolated) (subacute) 422.91
  giant cell (acute) (subacute) 422.91
  gonococcal 098.85
  granulomatous (idiopathic) (isolated) (nonspecific) 422.91
  hypertensive (see also Hypertension, heart) 402.90
  idiopathic 422.91
    granulomatous 422.91
  infective 422.92
  influenzal 487.8 [422.0]
  isolated (diffuse) (granulomatous) 422.91
  malignant 422.99
  meningococcal 036.43
  nonrheumatic, active 422.90
  parenchymatous 422.90
  pneumococcal (acute) (subacute) 422.92
  rheumatic (chronic) (inactive) (with chorea) 398.0
    active or acute 391.2
      with chorea (acute) (rheumatic) (Sydenham's) 392.0
  septic 422.92
  specific (giant cell) (productive) 422.91
  staphylococcal (acute) (subacute) 422.92
  suppurative 422.92
  syphilitic (chronic) 093.82
  toxic 422.93
    rheumatic (see also Myocarditis, acute rheumatic) 391.2
  tuberculous (see also Tuberculosis) 017.9 ✔5ᵗʰ [422.0]

Myocarditis — continued
  typhoid 002.0 [422.0]
  valvular — see Endocarditis
  viral, except Coxsackie 422.91
    Coxsackie 074.23
    of newborn (Coxsackie) 074.23
Myocardium, myocardial — see condition
Myocardosis (see also Cardiomyopathy) 425.4
Myoclonia (essential) 333.2
  epileptica 333.2
  Friedrich's 333.2
  massive 333.2
Myoclonic
  epilepsy, familial (progressive) 333.2
  jerks 333.2
Myoclonus (familial essential) (multifocal) (simplex) 333.2
  facial 351.8
  massive (infantile) 333.2
  pharyngeal 478.29
Myodiastasis 728.84
Myoendocarditis — see also Endocarditis
  acute or subacute 421.9
Myoepithelioma (M8982/0) — see Neoplasm, by site, benign
Myofascitis (acute) 729.1
  low back 724.2
Myofibroma (M8890/0) — see also Neoplasm, connective tissue, benign
  uterus (cervix) (corpus) (see also Leiomyoma) 218.9
Myofibrosis 728.2
  heart (see also Myocarditis) 429.0
  humeroscapular region 726.2
  scapulohumeral 726.2
Myofibrositis (see also Myositis) 729.1
  scapulohumeral 726.2
Myogelosis (occupational) 728.89
Myoglobinuria 791.3
Myoglobulinuria, primary 791.3
Myokymia — see also Myoclonus
  facial 351.8
Myolipoma (M8860/0)
  specified site — see Neoplasm, connective tissue, benign
  unspecified site 223.0
Myoma (M8895/0) — see also Neoplasm, connective tissue, benign
  cervix (stump) (uterus) (see also Leiomyoma) 218.9
  malignant (M8895/3) — see Neoplasm, connective tissue, malignant
  prostate 600.2
  uterus (cervix) (corpus) (see also Leiomyoma) 218.9
    in pregnancy or childbirth 654.1 ✔5ᵗʰ
      affecting fetus or newborn 763.89
      causing obstructed labor 660.2 ✔5ᵗʰ
        affecting fetus or newborn 763.1
Myomalacia 728.9
  cordis, heart (see also Degeneration, myocardial) 429.1
Myometritis (see also Endometritis) 615.9
Myometrium — see condition
Myonecrosis, clostridial 040.0
Myopathy 359.9
  alcoholic 359.4

Myopathy — continued
  amyloid 277.3 [359.6]
  benign congenital 359.0
  central core 359.0
  centronuclear 359.0
  congenital (benign) 359.0
  critical illness 359.81
  distal 359.1
  due to drugs 359.4
  endocrine 259.9 [359.5]
    specified type NEC 259.8 [359.5]
  extraocular muscles 376.82
  facioscapulohumeral 359.1
  in
    Addison's disease 255.4 [359.5]
    amyloidosis 277.3 [359.6]
    cretinism 243 [359.5]
    Cushing's syndrome 255.0 [359.5]
    disseminated lupus erythematosus 710.0 [359.6]
    giant cell arteritis 446.5 [359.6]
    hyperadrenocorticism NEC 255.3 [359.5]
    hyperparathyroidism 252.0 [359.5]
    hypopituitarism 253.2 [359.5]
    hypothyroidism (see also Hypothyroidism) 244.9 [359.5]
    malignant neoplasm NEC (M8000/3) 199.1 [359.6]
    myxedema (see also Myxedema) 244.9 [359.5]
    polyarteritis nodosa 446.0 [359.6]
    rheumatoid arthritis 714.0 [359.6]
    sarcoidosis 135 [359.6]
    scleroderma 710.1 [359.6]
    Sjögren's disease 710.2 [359.6]
    thyrotoxicosis (see also Thyrotoxicosis) 242.9 ☑5ᵗʰ [359.6]
  inflammatory 359.89
  intensive care (ICU) 359.81
  limb-girdle 359.1
  myotubular 359.0
  necrotizing, acute 359.81
  nemaline 359.0
  ocular 359.1
  oculopharyngeal 359.1
  of critical illness 359.81
  primary 359.89
  progressive NEC 359.89
  quadriplegic, acute 359.81
  rod body 359.0
  scapulohumeral 359.1
  specified type NEC 359.89
  toxic 359.4
Myopericarditis (see also Pericarditis) 423.9
Myopia (axial) (congenital) (increased curvature or refraction, nucleus of lens) 367.1
  degenerative, malignant 360.21
  malignant 360.21
  progressive high (degenerative) 360.21
Myosarcoma (M8895/3) — see Neoplasm, connective tissue, malignant
Myosis (persistent) 379.42
  stromal (endolymphatic) (M8931/1) 236.0
Myositis 729.1
  clostridial 040.0
  due to posture 729.1
  epidemic 074.1
  fibrosa or fibrous (chronic) 728.2
    Volkmann's (complicating trauma) 958.6
  infective 728.0
  interstitial 728.81

Myositis — continued
  multiple — see Polymyositis
  occupational 729.1
  orbital, chronic 376.12
  ossificans 728.12
    circumscribed 728.12
    progressive 728.11
    traumatic 728.12
  progressive fibrosing 728.11
  purulent 728.0
  rheumatic 729.1
  rheumatoid 729.1
  suppurative 728.0
  syphilitic 095.6
  traumatic (old) 729.1
Myospasia impulsiva 307.23
Myotonia (acquisita) (intermittens) 728.85
  atrophica 359.2
  congenita 359.2
  dystrophica 359.2
Myotonic pupil 379.46
Myriapodiasis 134.1
Myringitis
  with otitis media — see Otitis media
  acute 384.00
    specified type NEC 384.09
  bullosa hemorrhagica 384.01
  bullous 384.01
  chronic 384.1
Mysophobia 300.29
Mytilotoxism 988.0
Myxadenitis labialis 528.5
Myxedema (adult) (idiocy) (infantile) (juvenile) (thyroid gland) (see also Hypothyroidism) 244.9
  circumscribed 242.9 ☑5ᵗʰ
  congenital 243
  cutis 701.8
  localized (pretibial) 242.9 ☑5ᵗʰ
  madness (acute) 293.0
    subacute 293.1
  papular 701.8
  pituitary 244.8
  postpartum 674.8 ☑5ᵗʰ
  pretibial 242.9 ☑5ᵗʰ
  primary 244.9
Myxochondrosarcoma (M9220/3) — see Neoplasm, cartilage, malignant
Myxofibroma (M8811/0) — see also Neoplasm, connective tissue, benign
  odontogenic (M9320/0) 213.1
  upper jaw (bone) 213.0
Myxofibrosarcoma (M8811/3) — see Neoplasm, connective tissue, malignant
Myxolipoma (M8852/0) (see also Lipoma, by site) 214.9
Myxoliposarcoma (M8852/3) — see Neoplasm, connective tissue, malignant
Myxoma (M8840/0) — see also Neoplasm, connective tissue, benign
  odontogenic (M9320/0) 213.1
  upper jaw (bone) 213.0
Myxosarcoma (M8840/3) — see Neoplasm, connective tissue, malignant

N

Naegeli's
 disease (hereditary hemorrhagic thrombasthenia) 287.1
 leukemia, monocytic (M9863/3) 205.1 ✓5ᵗʰ
 syndrome (incontinentia pigmenti) 757.33
Naffziger's syndrome 353.0
Naga sore (*see also* Ulcer, skin) 707.9
Nägele's pelvis 738.6
 with disproportion (fetopelvic) 653.0 ✓5ᵗʰ
  affecting fetus or newborn 763.1
  causing obstructed labor 660.1 ✓5ᵗʰ
   affecting fetus or newborn 763.1
Nager-de Reynier syndrome (dysostosis mandibularis) 756.0
Nail — *see also* condition
 biting 307.9
 patella syndrome (hereditary osteoonychodysplasia) 756.89
Nanism, nonosomia (*see also* Dwarfism) 259.4
 hypophyseal 253.3
 pituitary 253.3
 renis, renalis 588.0
Nanukayami 100.89
Napkin rash 691.0
Narcissism 301.81
Narcolepsy 347
Narcosis
 carbon dioxide (respiratory) 786.09
 due to drug
  correct substance properly administered 780.09
  overdose or wrong substance given or taken 977.9
   specified drug — *see* Table of Drugs and Chemicals
Narcotism (chronic) (*see also* listing under Dependence) 304.9 ✓5ᵗʰ
 acute
  correct substance properly administered 349.82
  overdose or wrong substance given or taken 967.8
   specified drug — *see* Table of Drugs and Chemicals
Narrow
 anterior chamber angle 365.02
 pelvis (inlet) (outlet) — *see* Contraction, pelvis
Narrowing
 artery NEC 447.1
  auditory, internal 433.8 ✓5ᵗʰ
  basilar 433.0 ✓5ᵗʰ
   with other precerebral artery 433.3 ✓5ᵗʰ
    bilateral 433.3 ✓5ᵗʰ
  carotid 433.1 ✓5ᵗʰ
   with other precerebral artery 433.3 ✓5ᵗʰ
    bilateral 433.3 ✓5ᵗʰ
  cerebellar 433.8 ✓5ᵗʰ
  choroidal 433.8 ✓5ᵗʰ
  communicating posterior 433.8 ✓5ᵗʰ
  coronary — *see also* Arteriosclerosis, coronary
   congenital 746.85
    due to syphilis 090.5
  hypophyseal 433.8 ✓5ᵗʰ
  pontine 433.8 ✓5ᵗʰ
  precerebral NEC 433.9 ✓5ᵗʰ
   multiple or bilateral 433.3 ✓5ᵗʰ

Narrowing — *continued*
 artery NEC — *continued*
  precerebral NEC — *continued*
   specified NEC 433.8 ✓5ᵗʰ
  vertebral 433.2 ✓5ᵗʰ
   with other precerebral artery 433.3 ✓5ᵗʰ
    bilateral 433.3 ✓5ᵗʰ
 auditory canal (external) (*see also* Stricture, ear canal, acquired) 380.50
 cerebral arteries 437.0
 cicatricial — *see* Cicatrix
 congenital — *see* Anomaly, congenital
 coronary artery — *see* Narrowing, artery, coronary
 ear, middle 385.22
 Eustachian tube (*see also* Obstruction, Eustachian tube) 381.60
 eyelid 374.46
  congenital 743.62
 intervertebral disc or space NEC — *see* Degeneration, intervertebral disc
 joint space, hip 719.85
 larynx 478.74
 lids 374.46
  congenital 743.62
 mesenteric artery (with gangrene) 557.0
 palate 524.8
 palpebral fissure 374.46
 retinal artery 362.13
 ureter 593.3
 urethra (*see also* Stricture, urethra) 598.9
Narrowness, abnormal, eyelid 743.62
Nasal — *see* condition
Nasolacrimal — *see* condition
Nasopharyngeal — *see also* condition
 bursa 478.29
 pituitary gland 759.2
 torticollis 723.5
Nasopharyngitis (acute) (infective) (subacute) 460
 chronic 472.2
  due to external agent — *see* Condition, respiratory, chronic, due to
 due to external agent — *see* Condition, respiratory, due to
 septic 034.0
 streptococcal 034.0
 suppurative (chronic) 472.2
 ulcerative (chronic) 472.2
Nasopharynx, nasopharyngeal — *see* condition
Natal tooth, teeth 520.6
Nausea (*see also* Vomiting) 787.02
 with vomiting 787.01
 epidemic 078.82
 gravidarum — *see* Hyperemesis, gravidarum
 marina 994.6
Navel — *see* condition
Neapolitan fever (*see also* Brucellosis) 023.9
Nearsightedness 367.1
Near-syncope 780.2
Nebécourt's syndrome 253.3
Nebula, cornea (eye) 371.01
 congenital 743.43
  interfering with vision 743.42
Necator americanus infestation 126.1
Necatoriasis 126.1
Neck — *see* condition
Necrencephalus (*see also* Softening, brain) 437.8

Index to Diseases

Necrosis, necrotic

Necrobacillosis 040.3
Necrobiosis 799.8
   brain or cerebral (see also Softening, brain) 437.8
   lipoidica 709.3
      diabeticorum 250.8 [709.3]
Necrodermolysis 695.1
Necrolysis, toxic epidermal 695.1
   due to drug
      correct substance properly administered 695.1
      overdose or wrong substance given or taken 977.9
      specified drug — see Table of Drugs and Chemicals
Necrophilia 302.89
Necrosis, necrotic
   adrenal (capsule) (gland) 255.8
   antrum, nasal sinus 478.1
   aorta (hyaline) (see also Aneurysm, aorta) 441.9
      cystic medial 441.00
         abdominal 441.02
         thoracic 441.01
         thoracoabdominal 441.03
      ruptured 441.5
   arteritis 446.0
   artery 447.5
   aseptic, bone 733.40
      femur (head) (neck) 733.42
         medial condyle 733.43
      humoral head 733.41
      medial femoral condyle 733.43
      specific site NEC 733.49
      talus 733.44
   avascular, bone NEC (see also Necrosis, aseptic, bone) 733.40
   bladder (aseptic) (sphincter) 596.8
   bone (see also Osteomyelitis) 730.1
      acute 730.0
      aseptic or avascular 733.40
         femur (head) (neck) 733.42
            medial condyle 733.43
         humoral head 733.41
         medial femoral condyle 733.43
         specified site NEC 733.49
         talus 733.44
      ethmoid 478.1
      ischemic 733.40
      jaw 526.4
      marrow 289.8
      Paget's (osteitis deformans) 731.0
      tuberculous — see Tuberculosis, bone
   brain (softening) (see also Softening, brain) 437.8
   breast (aseptic) (fat) (segmental) 611.3
   bronchus, bronchi 519.1
   central nervous system NEC (see also Softening, brain) 437.8
   cerebellar (see also Softening, brain) 437.8
   cerebral (softening) (see also Softening, brain) 437.8
   cerebrospinal (softening) (see also Softening, brain) 437.8
   cornea (see also Keratitis) 371.40
   cortical, kidney 583.6
   cystic medial (aorta) 441.00
      abdominal 441.02
      thoracic 441.01
      thoracoabdominal 441.03

Necrosis, necrotic — continued
   dental 521.09
      pulp 522.1
   due to swallowing corrosive substance — see Burn, by site
   ear (ossicle) 385.24
   esophagus 530.89
   ethmoid (bone) 478.1
   eyelid 374.50
   fat, fatty (generalized) (see also Degeneration, fatty) 272.8
      breast (aseptic) (segmental) 611.3
      intestine 569.89
      localized — see Degeneration, by site, fatty
      mesentery 567.8
      omentum 567.8
      pancreas 577.8
      peritoneum 567.8
      skin (subcutaneous) 709.3
         newborn 778.1
   femur (aseptic) (avascular) 733.42
      head 733.42
      medial condyle 733.43
      neck 733.42
   gallbladder (see also Cholecystitis, acute) 575.0
   gangrenous 785.4
   gastric 537.89
   glottis 478.79
   heart (myocardium) — see Infarct, myocardium
   hepatic (see also Necrosis, liver) 570
   hip (aseptic) (avascular) 733.42
   intestine (acute) (hemorrhagic) (massive) 557.0
   ischemic 785.4
   jaw 526.4
   kidney (bilateral) 583.9
      acute 584.9
      cortical 583.6
         acute 584.6
            with
                abortion — see Abortion, by type, with renal failure
                ectopic pregnancy (see also categories 633.0-633.9) 639.3
                molar pregnancy (see also categories 630-632) 639.3
            complicating pregnancy 646.2
                affecting fetus or newborn 760.1
            following labor and delivery 669.3
      medullary (papillary) (see also Pyelitis) 590.80
         in
            acute renal failure 584.7
            nephritis, nephropathy 583.7
      papillary (see also Pyelitis) 590.80
         in
            acute renal failure 584.7
            nephritis, nephropathy 583.7
      tubular 584.5
         with
            abortion — see Abortion, by type, with renal failure
            ectopic pregnancy (see also categories 633.0-633.9) 639.3
            molar pregnancy (see also categories 630-632) 639.3
         complicating
            abortion 639.3
            ectopic or molar pregnancy 639.3

Necrosis, necrotic — *continued*
  kidney — *continued*
    tubular — *continued*
      complicating — *continued*
        pregnancy 646.2 ✓5ᵗʰ
          affecting fetus or newborn 760.1
          following labor and delivery 669.3 ✓5ᵗʰ
          traumatic 958.5
  larynx 478.79
  liver (acute) (congenital) (diffuse) (massive) (subacute) 570
    with
      abortion — *see* Abortion, by type, with specified complication NEC
      ectopic pregnancy (*see also* categories 633.0-633.9) 639.8
      molar pregnancy (*see also* categories 630-632) 639.8
    complicating pregnancy 646.7 ✓5ᵗʰ
      affecting fetus or newborn 760.8
    following
      abortion 639.8
      ectopic or molar pregnancy 639.8
    obstetrical 646.7 ✓5ᵗʰ
    postabortal 639.8
    puerperal, postpartum 674.8 ✓5ᵗʰ
    toxic 573.3
  lung 513.0
  lymphatic gland 683
  mammary gland 611.3
  mastoid (chronic) 383.1
  mesentery 557.0
    fat 567.8
  mitral valve — *see* Insufficiency, mitral
  myocardium, myocardial — *see* Infarct, myocardium
  nose (septum) 478.1
  omentum 557.0
    with mesenteric infarction 557.0
    fat 567.8
  orbit, orbital 376.10
  ossicles, ear (aseptic) 385.24
  ovary (*see also* Salpingo-oophoritis) 614.2
  pancreas (aseptic) (duct) (fat) 577.8
    acute 577.0
    infective 577.0
  papillary, kidney (*see also* Pyelitis) 590.80
  peritoneum 557.0
    with mesenteric infarction 557.0
    fat 567.8
  pharynx 462
    in granulocytopenia 288.0
  phosphorus 983.9
  pituitary (gland) (postpartum) (Sheehan) 253.2
  placenta (*see also* Placenta, abnormal) 656.7 ✓5ᵗʰ
  pneumonia 513.0
  pulmonary 513.0
  pulp (dental) 522.1
  pylorus 537.89
  radiation — *see* Necrosis, by site
  radium — *see* Necrosis, by site
  renal — *see* Necrosis, kidney
  sclera 379.19
  scrotum 608.89
  skin or subcutaneous tissue 709.8
    due to burn — *see* Burn, by site
    gangrenous 785.4
  spine, spinal (column) 730.18
    acute 730.18
    cord 336.1

Necrosis, necrotic — *continued*
  spleen 289.59
  stomach 537.89
  stomatitis 528.1
  subcutaneous fat 709.3
    fetus or newborn 778.1
  subendocardial — *see* Infarct, myocardium
  suprarenal (capsule) (gland) 255.8
  teeth, tooth 521.09
  testis 608.89
  thymus (gland) 254.8
  tonsil 474.8
  trachea 519.1
  tuberculous NEC — *see* Tuberculosis
  tubular (acute) (anoxic) (toxic) 584.5
    due to a procedure 997.5
  umbilical cord, affecting fetus or newborn 762.6
  vagina 623.8
  vertebra (lumbar) 730.18
    acute 730.18
    tuberculous (*see also* Tuberculosis) 015.0 ✓5ᵗʰ [730.8] ✓5ᵗʰ
  vesical (aseptic) (bladder) 596.8
  x-ray — *see* Necrosis, by site
Necrospermia 606.0
Necrotizing angiitis 446.0
Negativism 301.7
Neglect (child) (newborn) NEC 995.52
  adult 995.84
  after or at birth 995.52
  hemispatial 781.8
  left-sided 781.8
  sensory 781.8
  visuospatial 781.8
Negri bodies 071
Neill-Dingwall syndrome (microcephaly and dwarfism) 759.89
Neisserian infection NEC — *see* Gonococcus
Nematodiasis NEC (*see also* Infestation, Nematode) 127.9
  ancylostoma (*see also* Ancylostomiasis) 126.9
Neoformans cryptococcus infection 117.5
Neonatal — *see also* condition
  teeth, tooth 520.6
Neonatorum — *see* condition

	Malignant			Benign	Uncertain Behavior	Unspecified
	Primary	Secondary	Ca in situ			
Neoplasm, neoplastic	199.1	199.1	234.9	229.9	238.9	239.9

Notes — 1. The list below gives the code numbers for neoplasms by anatomical site. For each site there are six possible code numbers according to whether the neoplasm in question is malignant, benign, in situ, of uncertain behavior, or of unspecified nature. The description of the neoplasm will often indicate which of the six columns is appropriate; e.g., malignant melanoma of skin, benign fibroadenoma of breast, carcinoma in situ of cervix uteri.

Where such descriptors are not present, the remainder of the Index should be consulted where guidance is given to the appropriate column for each morphological (histological) variety listed; e.g., Mesonephroma — see Neoplasm, malignant; Embryoma — see also Neoplasm, uncertain behavior; Disease, Bowen's — see Neoplasm, skin, in situ. However, the guidance in the Index can be overridden if one of the descriptors mentioned above is present; e.g., malignant adenoma of colon is coded to 153.9 and not to 211.3 as the adjective "malignant" overrides the Index entry "Adenoma — see also Neoplasm, benign."

2. Sites marked with the sign * (e.g., face NEC*) should be classified to malignant neoplasm of skin of these sites if the variety of neoplasm is a squamous cell carcinoma or an epidermoid carcinoma, and to benign neoplasm of skin of these sites if the variety of neoplasm is a papilloma (any type).

	Primary	Secondary	Ca in situ	Benign	Uncertain Behavior	Unspecified
abdomen, abdominal	195.2	198.89	234.8	229.8	238.8	239.8
cavity	195.2	198.89	234.8	229.8	238.8	239.8
organ	195.2	198.89	234.8	229.8	238.8	239.8
viscera	195.2	198.89	234.8	229.8	238.8	239.8
wall	173.5	198.2	232.5	216.5	238.2	239.2
connective tissue	171.5	198.89	—	215.5	238.1	239.2
abdominopelvic	195.8	198.89	234.8	229.8	238.8	239.8
accessory sinus — see Neoplasm, sinus						
acoustic nerve	192.0	198.4	—	225.1	237.9	239.7
acromion (process)	170.4	198.5	—	213.4	238.0	239.2
adenoid (pharynx) (tissue)	147.1	198.89	230.0	210.7	235.1	239.0
adipose tissue (see also Neoplasm, connective tissue)	171.9	198.89	—	215.9	238.1	239.2
adnexa (uterine)	183.9	198.82	233.3	221.8	236.3	239.5
adrenal (cortex) (gland) (medulla)	194.0	198.7	234.8	227.0	237.2	239.7
ala nasi (external)	173.3	198.2	232.3	216.3	238.2	239.2
alimentary canal or tract NEC	159.9	197.8	230.9	211.9	235.5	239.0
alveolar	143.9	198.89	230.0	210.4	235.1	239.0
mucosa	143.9	198.89	230.0	210.4	235.1	239.0
lower	143.1	198.89	230.0	210.4	235.1	239.0
upper	143.0	198.89	230.0	210.4	235.1	239.0
ridge or process	170.1	198.5	—	213.1	238.0	239.2
carcinoma	143.9	—	—	—	—	—
lower	143.1	—	—	—	—	—
upper	143.0	—	—	—	—	—
lower	170.1	198.5	—	213.1	238.0	239.2
mucosa	143.9	198.89	230.0	210.4	235.1	239.0
lower	143.1	198.89	230.0	210.4	235.1	239.0
upper	143.0	198.89	230.0	210.4	235.1	239.0
upper	170.0	198.5	—	213.0	238.0	239.2
sulcus	145.1	198.89	230.0	210.4	235.1	239.0
alveolus	143.9	198.89	230.0	210.4	235.1	239.0
lower	143.1	198.89	230.0	210.4	235.1	239.0
upper	143.0	198.89	230.0	210.4	235.1	239.0
ampulla of Vater	156.2	197.8	230.8	211.5	235.3	239.0
ankle NEC*	195.5	198.89	232.7	229.8	238.8	239.8
anorectum, anorectal (junction)	154.8	197.5	230.7	211.4	235.2	239.0
antecubital fossa or space*	195.4	198.89	232.6	229.8	238.8	239.8
antrum (Highmore) (maxillary)	160.2	197.3	231.8	212.0	235.9	239.1
pyloric	151.2	197.8	230.2	211.1	235.2	239.0
tympanicum	160.1	197.3	231.8	212.0	235.9	239.1
anus, anal	154.3	197.5	230.6	211.4	235.5	239.0
canal	154.2	197.5	230.5	211.4	233.5	239.0

Neoplasm, anus, anal

	Malignant			Benign	Uncertain Behavior	Unspecified
	Primary	Secondary	Ca in situ			
Neoplasm, neoplastic — *continued*						
anus, anal — *continued*						
contiguous sites with rectosigmoid junction or rectum	154.8	—	—	—	—	—
margin	173.5	198.2	232.5	216.5	238.2	239.2
skin	173.5	198.2	232.5	216.5	238.2	239.2
sphincter	154.2	197.5	230.5	211.4	235.5	239.0
aorta (thoracic)	171.4	198.89	—	215.4	238.1	239.2
abdominal	171.5	198.89	—	215.5	238.1	239.2
aortic body	194.6	198.89	—	227.6	237.3	239.7
aponeurosis	171.9	198.89	—	215.9	238.1	239.2
palmar	171.2	198.89	—	215.2	238.1	239.2
plantar	171.3	198.89	—	215.3	238.1	239.2
appendix	153.5	197.5	230.3	211.3	235.2	239.0
arachnoid (cerebral)	192.1	198.4	—	225.2	237.6	239.7
spinal	192.3	198.4	—	225.4	237.6	239.7
areola (female)	174.0	198.81	233.0	217	238.3	239.3
male	175.0	198.81	233.0	217	238.3	239.3
arm NEC*	195.4	198.89	232.6	229.8	238.8	239.8
artery — *see* Neoplasm, connective tissue						
aryepiglottic fold	148.2	198.89	230.0	210.8	235.1	239.0
hypopharyngeal aspect	148.2	198.89	230.0	210.8	235.1	239.0
laryngeal aspect	161.1	197.3	231.0	212.1	235.6	239.1
marginal zone	148.2	198.89	230.0	210.8	235.1	239.0
arytenoid (cartilage)	161.3	197.3	231.0	212.1	235.6	239.1
fold — *see* Neoplasm, aryepiglottic						
atlas	170.2	198.5	—	213.2	238.0	239.2
atrium, cardiac	164.1	198.89	—	212.7	238.8	239.8
auditory						
canal (external) (skin)	173.2	198.2	232.2	216.2	238.2	239.2
internal	160.1	197.3	231.8	212.0	235.9	239.1
nerve	192.0	198.4	—	225.1	237.9	239.7
tube	160.1	197.3	231.8	212.0	235.9	239.1
opening	147.2	198.89	230.0	210.7	235.1	239.0
auricle, ear	173.2	198.2	232.2	216.2	238.2	239.2
cartilage	171.0	198.89	—	215.0	238.1	239.2
auricular canal (external)	173.2	198.2	232.2	216.2	238.2	239.2
internal	160.1	197.3	231.8	212.0	235.9	239.1
autonomic nerve or nervous system NEC	171.9	198.89	—	215.9	238.1	239.2
axilla, axillary	195.1	198.89	234.8	229.8	238.8	239.8
fold	173.5	198.2	232.5	216.5	238.2	239.2
back NEC*	195.8	198.89	232.5	229.8	238.8	239.8
Bartholin's gland	184.1	198.82	233.3	221.2	236.3	239.5
basal ganglia	191.0	198.3	—	225.0	237.5	239.6
basis pedunculi	191.7	198.3	—	225.0	237.5	239.6
bile or biliary (tract)	156.9	197.8	230.8	211.5	235.3	239.0
canaliculi (biliferi) (intrahepatic)	155.1	197.8	230.8	211.5	235.3	239.0
canals, interlobular	155.1	197.8	230.8	211.5	235.3	239.0
contiguous sites	156.8	—	—	—	—	—
duct or passage (common) (cystic) (extrahepatic)	156.1	197.8	230.8	211.5	235.3	239.0
contiguous sites with gallbladder	156.8	—	—	—	—	—
interlobular	155.1	197.8	230.8	211.5	235.3	239.0
intrahepatic	155.1	197.8	230.8	211.5	235.3	239.0
and extrahepatic	156.9	197.8	230.8	211.5	235.3	239.0
bladder (urinary)	188.9	198.1	233.7	223.3	236.7	239.4
contiguous sites	188.8	—	—	—	—	—
dome	188.1	198.1	233.7	223.3	236.7	239.4

Index to Diseases — Neoplasm, bone

	Malignant			Benign	Uncertain Behavior	Unspecified
	Primary	Secondary	Ca in situ			
Neoplasm, neoplastic — *continued*						
bladder — *continued*						
neck	188.5	198.1	233.7	223.3	236.7	239.4
orifice	188.9	198.1	233.7	223.3	236.7	239.4
ureteric	188.6	198.1	233.7	223.3	236.7	239.4
urethral	188.5	198.1	233.7	223.3	236.7	239.4
sphincter	188.8	198.1	233.7	223.3	236.7	239.4
trigone	188.0	198.1	233.7	223.3	236.7	239.4
urachus	188.7	—	233.7	223.3	236.7	239.4
wall	188.9	198.1	233.7	223.3	236.7	239.4
anterior	188.3	198.1	233.7	223.3	236.7	239.4
lateral	188.2	198.1	233.7	223.3	236.7	239.4
posterior	188.4	198.1	233.7	223.3	236.7	239.4
blood vessel — *see* Neoplasm, connective tissue						
bone (periosteum)	170.9	198.5	—	213.9	238.0	239.2

Note — Carcinomas and adenocarcinomas, of any type other than intraosseous or odontogenic, of the sites listed under "Neoplasm, bone" should be considered as constituting metastatic spread from an unspecified primary site and coded to 198.5 for morbidity coding and to 199.1 for underlying cause of death coding.

	Primary	Secondary	Ca in situ	Benign	Uncertain Behavior	Unspecified
acetabulum	170.6	198.5	—	213.6	238.0	239.2
acromion (process)	170.4	198.5	—	213.4	238.0	239.2
ankle	170.8	198.5	—	213.8	238.0	239.2
arm NEC	170.4	198.5	—	213.4	238.0	239.2
astragalus	170.8	198.5	—	213.8	238.0	239.2
atlas	170.2	198.5	—	213.2	238.0	239.2
axis	170.2	198.5	—	213.2	238.0	239.2
back NEC	170.2	198.5	—	213.2	238.0	239.2
calcaneus	170.8	198.5	—	213.8	238.0	239.2
calvarium	170.0	198.5	—	213.0	238.0	239.2
carpus (any)	170.5	198.5	—	213.5	238.0	239.2
cartilage NEC	170.9	198.5	—	213.9	238.0	239.2
clavicle	170.3	198.5	—	213.3	238.0	239.2
clivus	170.0	198.5	—	213.0	238.0	239.2
coccygeal vertebra	170.6	198.5	—	213.6	238.0	239.2
coccyx	170.6	198.5	—	213.6	238.0	239.2
costal cartilage	170.3	198.5	—	213.3	238.0	239.2
costovertebral joint	170.3	198.5	—	213.3	238.0	239.2
cranial	170.0	198.5	—	213.0	238.0	239.2
cuboid	170.8	198.5	—	213.8	238.0	239.2
cuneiform	170.9	198.5	—	213.9	238.0	239.2
ankle	170.8	198.5	—	213.8	238.0	239.2
wrist	170.5	198.5	—	213.5	238.0	239.2
digital	170.9	198.5	—	213.9	238.0	239.2
finger	170.5	198.5	—	213.5	238.0	239.2
toe	170.8	198.5	—	213.8	238.0	239.2
elbow	170.4	198.5	—	213.4	238.0	239.2
ethmoid (labyrinth)	170.0	198.5	—	213.0	238.0	239.2
face	170.0	198.5	—	213.0	238.0	239.2
lower jaw	170.1	198.5	—	213.1	238.0	239.2
femur (any part)	170.7	198.5	—	213.7	238.0	239.2
fibula (any part)	170.7	198.5	—	213.7	238.0	239.2
finger (any)	170.5	198.5	—	213.5	238.0	239.2
foot	170.8	198.5	—	213.8	238.0	239.2
forearm	170.4	198.5	—	213.4	238.0	239.2
frontal	170.0	198.5	—	213.0	238.0	239.2
hand	170.5	198.5	—	213.5	238.0	239.2
heel	170.8	198.5	—	213.8	238.0	239.2
hip	170.6	198.5	—	213.6	238.0	239.2
humerus (any part)	170.4	198.5	—	213.4	238.0	239.2
hyoid	170.0	198.5	—	213.0	238.0	239.2
ilium	170.6	198.5	—	213.6	238.0	239.2
innominate	170.6	198.5	—	213.6	238.0	239.2

✔4ᵗʰ Fourth-digit Required   ✔5ᵗʰ Fifth-digit Required

Neoplasm, bone

	Malignant			Benign	Uncertain Behavior	Unspecified
	Primary	Secondary	Ca in situ			
Neoplasm, neoplastic — *continued*						
bone — *continued*						
intervertebral cartilage or disc	170.2	198.5	—	213.2	238.0	239.2
ischium	170.6	198.5	—	213.6	238.0	239.2
jaw (lower)	170.1	198.5	—	213.1	238.0	239.2
upper	170.0	198.5	—	213.0	238.0	239.2
knee	170.7	198.5	—	213.7	238.0	239.2
leg NEC	170.7	198.5	—	213.7	238.0	239.2
limb NEC	170.9	198.5	—	213.9	238.0	239.2
lower (long bones)	170.7	198.5	—	213.7	238.0	239.2
short bones	170.8	198.5	—	213.8	238.0	239.2
upper (long bones)	170.4	198.5	—	213.4	238.0	239.2
short bones	170.5	198.5	—	213.5	238.0	239.2
long	170.9	198.5	—	213.9	238.0	239.2
lower limbs NEC	170.7	198.5	—	213.7	238.0	239.2
upper limbs NEC	170.4	198.5	—	213.4	238.0	239.2
malar	170.0	198.5	—	213.0	238.0	239.2
mandible	170.1	198.5	—	213.1	238.0	239.2
marrow NEC	202.9 ✓5ᵗʰ	198.5	—	—	—	238.7
mastoid	170.0	198.5	—	213.0	238.0	239.2
maxilla, maxillary (superior)	170.0	198.5	—	213.0	238.0	239.2
inferior	170.1	198.5	—	213.1	238.0	239.2
metacarpal (any)	170.5	198.5	—	213.5	238.0	239.2
metatarsus (any)	170.8	198.5	—	213.8	238.0	239.2
navicular (ankle)	170.8	198.5	—	213.8	238.0	239.2
hand	170.5	198.5	—	213.5	238.0	239.2
nose, nasal	170.0	198.5	—	213.0	238.0	239.2
occipital	170.0	198.5	—	213.0	238.0	239.2
orbit	170.0	198.5	—	213.0	238.0	239.2
parietal	170.0	198.5	—	213.0	238.0	239.2
patella	170.8	198.5	—	213.8	238.0	239.2
pelvic	170.6	198.5	—	213.6	238.0	239.2
phalanges	170.9	198.5	—	213.9	238.0	239.2
foot	170.8	198.5	—	213.8	238.0	239.2
hand	170.5	198.5	—	213.5	238.0	239.2
pubic	170.6	198.5	—	213.6	238.0	239.2
radius (any part)	170.4	198.5	—	213.4	238.0	239.2
rib	170.3	198.5	—	213.3	238.0	239.2
sacral vertebra	170.6	198.5	—	213.6	238.0	239.2
sacrum	170.6	198.5	—	213.6	238.0	239.2
scaphoid (of hand)	170.5	198.5	—	213.5	238.0	239.2
of ankle	170.8	198.5	—	213.8	238.0	239.2
scapula (any part)	170.4	198.5	—	213.4	238.0	239.2
sella turcica	170.0	198.5	—	213.0	238.0	239.2
short	170.9	198.5	—	213.9	238.0	239.2
lower limb	170.8	198.5	—	213.8	238.0	239.2
upper limb	170.5	198.5	—	213.5	238.0	239.2
shoulder	170.4	198.5	—	213.4	238.0	239.2
skeleton, skeletal NEC	170.9	198.5	—	213.9	238.0	239.2
skull	170.0	198.5	—	213.0	238.0	239.2
sphenoid	170.0	198.5	—	213.0	238.0	239.2
spine, spinal (column)	170.2	198.5	—	213.2	238.0	239.2
coccyx	170.6	198.5	—	213.6	238.0	239.2
sacrum	170.6	198.5	—	213.6	238.0	239.2
sternum	170.3	198.5	—	213.3	238.0	239.2
tarsus (any)	170.8	198.5	—	213.8	238.0	239.2
temporal	170.0	198.5	—	213.0	238.0	239.2
thumb	170.5	198.5	—	213.5	238.0	239.2
tibia (any part)	170.7	198.5	—	213.7	238.0	239.2
toe (any)	170.8	198.5	—	213.8	238.0	239.2
trapezium	170.5	198.5	—	213.5	238.0	239.2
trapezoid	170.5	198.5	—	213.5	238.0	239.2
turbinate	170.0	198.5	—	213.0	238.0	239.2

Index to Diseases — Neoplasm, breast

	Malignant			Benign	Uncertain Behavior	Unspecified
	Primary	Secondary	Ca in situ			
Neoplasm, neoplastic — *continued*						
bone — *continued*						
ulna (any part)	170.4	198.5	—	213.4	238.0	239.2
unciform	170.5	198.5	—	213.5	238.0	239.2
vertebra (column)	170.2	198.5	—	213.2	238.0	239.2
coccyx	170.6	198.5	—	213.6	238.0	239.2
sacrum	170.6	198.5	—	213.6	238.0	239.2
vomer	170.0	198.5	—	213.0	238.0	239.2
wrist	170.5	198.5	—	213.5	238.0	239.2
xiphoid process	170.3	198.5	—	213.3	238.0	239.2
zygomatic	170.0	198.5	—	213.0	238.0	239.2
book-leaf (mouth)	145.8	198.89	230.0	210.4	235.1	239.0
bowel — *see* Neoplasm, intestine						
brachial plexus	171.2	198.89	—	215.2	238.1	239.2
brain NEC	191.9	198.3	—	225.0	237.5	239.6
basal ganglia	191.0	198.3	—	225.0	237.5	239.6
cerebellopontine angle	191.6	198.3	—	225.0	237.5	239.6
cerebellum NOS	191.6	198.3	—	225.0	237.5	239.6
cerebrum	191.0	198.3	—	225.0	237.5	239.6
choroid plexus	191.5	198.3	—	225.0	237.5	239.6
contiguous sites	191.8	—	—	—	—	—
corpus callosum	191.8	198.3	—	225.0	237.5	239.6
corpus striatum	191.0	198.3	—	225.0	237.5	239.6
cortex (cerebral)	191.0	198.3	—	225.0	237.5	239.6
frontal lobe	191.1	198.3	—	225.0	237.5	239.6
globus pallidus	191.0	198.3	—	225.0	237.5	239.6
hippocampus	191.2	198.3	—	225.0	237.5	239.6
hypothalamus	191.0	198.3	—	225.0	237.5	239.6
internal capsule	191.0	198.3	—	225.0	237.5	239.6
medulla oblongata	191.7	198.3	—	225.0	237.5	239.6
meninges	192.1	198.4	—	225.2	237.6	239.7
midbrain	191.7	198.3	—	225.0	237.5	239.6
occipital lobe	191.4	198.3	—	225.0	237.5	239.6
parietal lobe	191.3	198.3	—	225.0	237.5	239.6
peduncle	191.7	198.3	—	225.0	237.5	239.6
pons	191.7	198.3	—	225.0	237.5	239.6
stem	191.7	198.3	—	225.0	237.5	239.6
tapetum	191.8	198.3	—	225.0	237.5	239.6
temporal lobe	191.2	198.3	—	225.0	237.5	239.6
thalamus	191.0	198.3	—	225.0	237.5	239.6
uncus	191.2	198.3	—	225.0	237.5	239.6
ventricle (floor)	191.5	198.3	—	225.0	237.5	239.6
branchial (cleft) (vestiges)	146.8	198.89	230.0	210.6	235.1	239.0
breast (connective tissue) (female) (glandular tissue) (soft parts)	174.9	198.81	233.0	217	238.3	239.3
areola	174.0	198.81	233.0	217	238.3	239.3
male	175.0	198.81	233.0	217	238.3	239.3
axillary tail	174.6	198.81	233.0	217	238.3	239.3
central portion	174.1	198.81	233.0	217	238.3	239.3
contiguous sites	174.8	—	—	—	—	—
ectopic sites	174.8	198.81	233.0	217	238.3	239.3
inner	174.8	198.81	233.0	217	238.3	239.3
lower	174.8	198.81	233.0	217	238.3	239.3
lower-inner quadrant	174.3	198.81	233.0	217	238.3	239.3
lower-outer quadrant	174.5	198.81	233.0	217	238.3	239.3
male	175.9	198.81	233.0	217	238.3	239.3
areola	175.0	198.81	233.0	217	238.3	239.3
ectopic tissue	175.9	198.81	233.0	217	238.3	239.3
nipple	175.0	198.81	233.0	217	238.3	239.3
mastectomy site (skin)	173.5	198.2	—	—	—	—
specified as breast tissue	174.8	198.81	—	—	—	—
midline	174.8	198.81	233.0	217	238.3	239.3

Fourth-digit Required   *Fifth-digit Required*

Neoplasm, breast **Index to Disease**

	Malignant			Benign	Uncertain Behavior	Unspecified
	Primary	Secondary	Ca in situ			
Neoplasm, neoplastic — *continued*						
breast — *continued*						
nipple	174.0	198.81	233.0	217	238.3	239.3
male	175.0	198.81	233.0	217	238.3	239.3
outer	174.8	198.81	233.0	217	238.3	239.3
skin	173.5	198.2	232.5	216.5	238.2	239.2
tail (axillary)	174.6	198.81	233.0	217	238.3	239.3
upper	174.8	198.81	233.0	217	238.3	239.3
upper-inner quadrant	174.2	198.81	233.0	217	238.3	239.3
upper-outer quadrant	174.4	198.81	233.0	217	238.3	239.3
broad ligament	183.3	198.82	233.3	221.0	236.3	239.5
bronchiogenic, bronchogenic (lung)	162.9	197.0	231.2	212.3	235.7	239.1
bronchiole	162.9	197.0	231.2	212.3	235.7	239.1
bronchus	162.9	197.0	231.2	212.3	235.7	239.1
carina	162.2	197.0	231.2	212.3	235.7	239.1
contiguous sites with lung or trachea	162.8	—	—	—	—	—
lower lobe of lung	162.5	197.0	231.2	212.3	235.7	239.1
main	162.2	197.0	231.2	212.3	235.7	239.1
middle lobe of lung	162.4	197.0	231.2	212.3	235.7	239.1
upper lobe of lung	162.3	197.0	231.2	212.3	235.7	239.1
brow	173.3	198.2	232.3	216.3	238.2	239.2
buccal (cavity)	145.9	198.89	230.0	210.4	235.1	239.0
commissure	145.0	198.89	230.0	210.4	235.1	239.0
groove (lower) (upper)	145.1	198.89	230.0	210.4	235.1	239.0
mucosa	145.0	198.89	230.0	210.4	235.1	239.0
sulcus (lower) (upper)	145.1	198.89	230.0	210.4	235.1	239.0
bulbourethral gland	189.3	198.1	233.9	223.81	236.99	239.5
bursa — *see* Neoplasm, connective tissue						
buttock NEC*	195.3	198.89	232.5	229.8	238.8	239.8
calf*	195.5	198.89	232.7	229.8	238.8	239.8
calvarium	170.0	198.5	—	213.0	238.0	239.2
calyx, renal	189.1	198.0	233.9	223.1	236.91	239.5
canal						
anal	154.2	197.5	230.5	211.4	235.5	239.0
auditory (external)	173.2	198.2	232.2	216.2	238.2	239.2
auricular (external)	173.2	198.2	232.2	216.2	238.2	239.2
canaliculi, biliary (biliferi) (intrahepatic)	155.1	197.8	230.8	211.5	235.3	239.0
canthus (eye) (inner) (outer)	173.1	198.2	232.1	216.1	238.2	239.2
capillary — *see* Neoplasm, connective tissue						
caput coli	153.4	197.5	230.3	211.3	235.2	239.0
cardia (gastric)	151.0	197.8	230.2	211.1	235.2	239.0
cardiac orifice (stomach)	151.0	197.8	230.2	211.1	235.2	239.0
cardio-esophageal junction	151.0	197.8	230.2	211.1	235.2	239.0
cardio-esophagus	151.0	197.8	230.2	211.1	235.2	239.0
carina (trachea) (bronchus)	162.2	197.0	231.2	212.3	235.7	239.1
carotid (artery)	171.0	198.89	—	215.0	238.1	239.2
body	194.5	198.89	—	227.5	237.3	239.7
carpus (any bone)	170.5	198.5	—	213.5	238.0	239.2
cartilage (articular) (joint) NEC — *see also* Neoplasm, bone	170.9	198.5	—	213.9	238.0	239.2
arytenoid	161.3	197.3	231.0	212.1	235.6	239.1
auricular	171.0	198.89	—	215.0	238.1	239.2
bronchi	162.2	197.3	—	212.3	235.7	239.1
connective tissue — *see* Neoplasm, connective tissue						
costal	170.3	198.5	—	213.3	238.0	239.2
cricoid	161.3	197.3	231.0	212.1	235.6	239.1
cuneiform	161.3	197.3	231.0	212.1	235.6	239.1

▶◀ Revised Text   ● New Line   ▲ Revised Code

Index to Diseases

	Malignant			Benign	Uncertain Behavior	Unspecified
	Primary	Secondary	Ca in situ			
Neoplasm, neoplastic — *continued*						
cartilage — *continued*						
ear (external)	171.0	198.89	—	215.0	238.1	239.2
ensiform	170.3	198.5	—	213.3	238.0	239.2
epiglottis	161.1	197.3	231.0	212.1	235.6	239.1
anterior surface	146.4	198.89	230.0	210.6	235.1	239.0
eyelid	171.0	198.89	—	215.0	238.1	239.2
intervertebral	170.2	198.5	—	213.2	238.0	239.2
larynx, laryngeal	161.3	197.3	231.0	212.1	235.6	239.1
nose, nasal	160.0	197.3	231.8	212.0	235.9	239.1
pinna	171.0	198.89	—	215.0	238.1	239.2
rib	170.3	198.5	—	213.3	238.0	239.2
semilunar (knee)	170.7	198.5	—	213.7	238.0	239.2
thyroid	161.3	197.3	231.0	212.1	235.6	239.1
trachea	162.0	197.3	231.1	212.2	235.7	239.1
cauda equina	192.2	198.3	—	225.3	237.5	239.7
cavity						
buccal	145.9	198.89	230.0	210.4	235.1	239.0
nasal	160.0	197.3	231.8	212.0	235.9	239.1
oral	145.9	198.89	230.0	210.4	235.1	239.0
peritoneal	158.9	197.6	—	211.8	235.4	239.0
tympanic	160.1	197.3	231.8	212.0	235.9	239.1
cecum	153.4	197.5	230.3	211.3	235.2	239.0
central						
nervous system — *see* Neoplasm, nervous system						
white matter	191.0	198.3	—	225.0	237.5	239.6
cerebellopontine (angle)	191.6	198.3	—	225.0	237.5	239.6
cerebellum, cerebellar	191.6	198.3	—	225.0	237.5	239.6
cerebrum, cerebral (cortex)						
(hemisphere) (white matter)	191.0	198.3	—	225.0	237.5	239.6
meninges	192.1	198.4	—	225.2	237.6	239.7
peduncle	191.7	198.3	—	225.0	237.5	239.6
ventricle (any)	191.5	198.3	—	225.0	237.5	239.6
cervical region	195.0	198.89	234.8	229.8	238.8	239.8
cervix (cervical) (uteri) (uterus)	180.9	198.82	233.1	219.0	236.0	239.5
canal	180.0	198.82	233.1	219.0	236.0	239.5
contiguous sites	180.8	—	—	—	—	—
endocervix (canal) (gland)	180.0	198.82	233.1	219.0	236.0	239.5
exocervix	180.1	198.82	233.1	219.0	236.0	239.5
external os	180.1	198.82	233.1	219.0	236.0	239.5
internal os	180.0	198.82	233.1	219.0	236.0	239.5
nabothian gland	180.0	198.82	233.1	219.0	236.0	239.5
squamocolumnar junction	180.8	198.82	233.1	219.0	236.0	239.5
stump	180.8	198.82	233.1	219.0	236.0	239.5
cheek	195.0	198.89	234.8	229.8	238.8	239.8
external	173.3	198.2	232.3	216.3	238.2	239.2
inner aspect	145.0	198.89	230.0	210.4	235.1	239.0
internal	145.0	198.89	230.0	210.4	235.1	239.0
mucosa	145.0	198.89	230.0	210.4	235.1	239.0
chest (wall) NEC	195.1	198.89	234.8	229.8	238.8	239.8
chiasma opticum	192.0	198.4	—	225.1	237.9	239.7
chin	173.3	198.2	232.3	216.3	238.2	239.2
choana	147.3	198.89	230.0	210.7	235.1	239.0
cholangiole	155.1	197.8	230.8	211.5	235.3	239.0
choledochal duct	156.1	197.8	230.8	211.5	235.3	239.0
choroid	190.6	198.4	234.0	224.6	238.8	239.8
plexus	191.5	198.3	—	225.0	237.5	239.6
ciliary body	190.0	198.4	234.0	224.0	238.8	239.8
clavicle	170.3	198.5	—	213.3	238.0	239.2
clitoris	184.3	198.82	233.3	221.2	236.3	239.5
clivus	170.0	198.5	—	213.0	238.0	239.2
cloacogenic zone	154.8	197.5	230.7	211.4	235.5	239.0

✓4ᵗʰ Fourth-digit Required   ✓5ᵗʰ Fifth-digit Required

	Malignant			Benign	Uncertain Behavior	Unspecified
	Primary	Secondary	Ca in situ			
Neoplasm, neoplastic — *continued*						
coccygeal						
body or glomus	194.6	198.89	—	227.6	237.3	239.7
vertebra	170.6	198.5	—	213.6	238.0	239.2
coccyx	170.6	198.5	—	213.6	238.0	239.2
colon — *see also* Neoplasm, intestine, large and rectum	154.0	197.5	230.4	211.4	235.2	239.0
column, spinal — *see* Neoplasm, spine						
columnella	173.3	198.2	232.3	216.3	238.2	239.2
commissure						
labial, lip	140.6	198.89	230.0	210.4	235.1	239.0
laryngeal	161.0	197.3	231.0	212.1	235.6	239.1
common (bile) duct	156.1	197.8	230.8	211.5	235.3	239.0
concha	173.2	198.2	232.2	216.2	238.2	239.2
nose	160.0	197.3	231.8	212.0	235.9	239.1
conjunctiva	190.3	198.4	234.0	224.3	238.8	239.8
connective tissue NEC	171.9	198.89	—	215.9	238.1	239.2

Note — For neoplasms of connective tissue (blood vessel, bursa, fascia, ligament, muscle, peripheral nerves, sympathetic and parasympathetic nerves and ganglia, synovia, tendon, etc.) or of morphological types that indicate connective tissue, code according to the list under "Neoplasm, connective tissue"; for sites that do not appear in this list, code to neoplasm of that site; e.g.,

    liposarcoma, shoulder 171.2
    leiomyosarcoma, stomach 151.9
    neurofibroma, chest wall 215.4

Morphological types that indicate connective tissue appear in the proper place in the alphabetic index with the instruction "see Neoplasm, connective tissue..."

	Primary	Secondary	Ca in situ	Benign	Uncertain Behavior	Unspecified
abdomen	171.5	198.89	—	215.5	238.1	239.2
abdominal wall	171.5	198.89	—	215.5	238.1	239.2
ankle	171.3	198.89	—	215.3	238.1	239.2
antecubital fossa or space	171.2	198.89	—	215.2	238.1	239.2
arm	171.2	198.89	—	215.2	238.1	239.2
auricle (ear)	171.0	198.89	—	215.0	238.1	239.2
axilla	171.4	198.89	—	215.4	238.1	239.2
back	171.7	198.89	—	215.7	238.1	239.2
breast (female) (*see also* Neoplasm, breast)	174.9	198.81	233.0	217	238.3	239.3
male	175.9	198.81	233.0	217	238.3	239.3
buttock	171.6	198.89	—	215.6	238.1	239.2
calf	171.3	198.89	—	215.3	238.1	239.2
cervical region	171.0	198.89	—	215.0	238.1	239.2
cheek	171.0	198.89	—	215.0	238.1	239.2
chest (wall)	171.4	198.89	—	215.4	238.1	239.2
chin	171.0	198.89	—	215.0	238.1	239.2
contiguous sites	171.8	—	—	—	—	—
diaphragm	171.4	198.89	—	215.4	238.1	239.2
ear (external)	171.0	198.89	—	215.0	238.1	239.2
elbow	171.2	198.89	—	215.2	238.1	239.2
extrarectal	171.6	198.89	—	215.6	238.1	239.2
extremity	171.8	198.89	—	215.8	238.1	239.2
lower	171.3	198.89	—	215.3	238.1	239.2
upper	171.2	198.89	—	215.2	238.1	239.2
eyelid	171.0	198.89	—	215.0	238.1	239.2
face	171.0	198.89	—	215.0	238.1	239.2
finger	171.2	198.89	—	215.2	238.1	239.2
flank	171.7	198.89	—	215.7	238.1	239.2
foot	171.3	198.89	—	215.3	238.1	239.2
forearm	171.2	198.89	—	215.2	238.1	239.2
forehead	171.0	198.89	—	215.0	238.1	239.2
gluteal region	171.6	198.89	—	215.6	238.1	239.2
great vessels NEC	171.4	198.89	—	215.4	238.1	239.2

Index to Diseases

	Malignant			Benign	Uncertain Behavior	Unspecified
	Primary	Secondary	Ca in situ			
Neoplasm, neoplastic — *continued*						
connective tissue NEC — *continued*						
groin	171.6	198.89	—	215.6	238.1	239.2
hand	171.2	198.89	—	215.2	238.1	239.2
head	171.0	198.89	—	215.0	238.1	239.2
heel	171.3	198.89	—	215.3	238.1	239.2
hip	171.3	198.89	—	215.3	238.1	239.2
hypochondrium	171.5	198.89	—	215.5	238.1	239.2
iliopsoas muscle	171.6	198.89	—	215.5	238.1	239.2
infraclavicular region	171.4	198.89	—	215.4	238.1	239.2
inguinal (canal) (region)	171.6	198.89	—	215.6	238.1	239.2
intrathoracic	171.4	198.89	—	215.4	238.1	239.2
ischorectal fossa	171.6	198.89	—	215.6	238.1	239.2
jaw	143.9	198.89	230.0	210.4	235.1	239.0
knee	171.3	198.89	—	215.3	238.1	239.2
leg	171.3	198.89	—	215.3	238.1	239.2
limb NEC	171.9	198.89	—	215.8	238.1	239.2
lower	171.3	198.89	—	215.3	238.1	239.2
upper	171.2	198.89	—	215.2	238.1	239.2
nates	171.6	198.89	—	215.6	238.1	239.2
neck	171.0	198.89	—	215.0	238.1	239.2
orbit	190.1	198.4	234.0	224.1	238.8	239.8
pararectal	171.6	198.89	—	215.6	238.1	239.2
para-urethral	171.6	198.89	—	215.6	238.1	239.2
paravaginal	171.6	198.89	—	215.6	238.1	239.2
pelvis (floor)	171.6	198.89	—	215.6	238.1	239.2
pelvo-abdominal	171.8	198.89	—	215.8	238.1	239.2
perineum	171.6	198.89	—	215.6	238.1	239.2
perirectal (tissue)	171.6	198.89	—	215.6	238.1	239.2
periurethral (tissue)	171.6	198.89	—	215.6	238.1	239.2
popliteal fossa or space	171.3	198.89	—	215.3	238.1	239.2
presacral	171.6	198.89	—	215.6	238.1	239.2
psoas muscle	171.5	198.89	—	215.5	238.1	239.2
pterygoid fossa	171.0	198.89	—	215.0	238.1	239.2
rectovaginal septum or wall	171.6	198.89	—	215.6	238.1	239.2
rectovesical	171.6	198.89	—	215.6	238.1	239.2
retroperitoneum	158.0	197.6	—	211.8	235.4	239.0
sacrococcygeal region	171.6	198.89	—	215.6	238.1	239.2
scalp	171.0	198.89	—	215.0	238.1	239.2
scapular region	171.4	198.89	—	215.4	238.1	239.2
shoulder	171.2	198.89	—	215.2	238.1	239.2
skin (dermis) NEC	173.9	198.2	232.9	216.9	238.2	239.2
submental	171.0	198.89	—	215.0	238.1	239.2
supraclavicular region	171.0	198.89	—	215.0	238.1	239.2
temple	171.0	198.89	—	215.0	238.1	239.2
temporal region	171.0	198.89	—	215.0	238.1	239.2
thigh	171.3	198.89	—	215.3	238.1	239.2
thoracic (duct) (wall)	171.4	198.89	—	215.4	238.1	239.2
thorax	171.4	198.89	—	215.4	238.1	239.2
thumb	171.2	198.89	—	215.2	238.1	239.2
toe	171.3	198.89	—	215.3	238.1	239.2
trunk	171.7	198.89	—	215.7	238.1	239.2
umbilicus	171.5	198.89	—	215.5	238.1	239.2
vesicorectal	171.6	198.89	—	215.6	238.1	239.2
wrist	171.2	198.89	—	215.2	238.1	239.2
conus medullaris	192.2	198.3	—	225.3	237.5	239.7
cord (true) (vocal)	161.0	197.3	231.0	212.1	235.6	239.1
false	161.1	197.3	231.0	212.1	235.6	239.1
spermatic	187.6	198.82	233.6	222.8	236.6	239.5
spinal (cervical) (lumbar) (thoracic)	192.2	198.3	—	225.3	237.5	239.7
cornea (limbus)	190.4	198.4	234.0	224.4	238.8	239.8
corpus						
albicans	183.0	198.6	233.3	220	236.2	239.5

Neoplasm, corpus — Index to Disease

	Malignant			Benign	Uncertain Behavior	Unspecified
	Primary	Secondary	Ca in situ			
Neoplasm, neoplastic — *continued*						
corpus — *continued*						
callosum, brain	191.8	198.3	—	225.0	237.5	239.6
cavernosum	187.3	198.82	233.5	222.1	236.6	239.5
gastric	151.4	197.8	230.2	211.1	235.2	239.0
penis	187.3	198.82	233.5	222.1	236.6	239.5
striatum, cerebrum	191.0	198.3	—	225.0	237.5	239.6
uteri	182.0	198.82	233.2	219.1	236.0	239.5
isthmus	182.1	198.82	233.2	219.1	236.0	239.5
cortex						
adrenal	194.0	198.7	234.8	227.0	237.2	239.7
cerebral	191.0	198.3	—	225.0	237.5	239.6
costal cartilage	170.3	198.5	—	213.3	238.0	239.2
costovertebral joint	170.3	198.5	—	213.3	238.0	239.2
Cowper's gland	189.3	198.1	233.9	223.81	236.99	239.5
cranial (fossa, any)	191.9	198.3	—	225.0	237.5	239.6
meninges	192.1	198.4	—	225.2	237.6	239.7
nerve (any)	192.0	198.4	—	225.1	237.9	239.7
craniobuccal pouch	194.3	198.89	234.8	227.3	237.0	239.7
craniopharyngeal (duct) (pouch)	194.3	198.89	234.8	227.3	237.0	239.7
cricoid	148.0	198.89	230.0	210.8	235.1	239.0
cartilage	161.3	197.3	231.0	212.1	235.6	239.1
cricopharynx	148.0	198.89	230.0	210.8	235.1	239.0
crypt of Morgagni	154.8	197.5	230.7	211.4	235.2	239.0
crystalline lens	190.0	198.4	234.0	224.0	238.8	239.8
cul-de-sac (Douglas')	158.8	197.6	—	211.8	235.4	239.0
cuneiform cartilage	161.3	197.3	231.0	212.1	235.6	239.1
cutaneous — *see* Neoplasm, skin						
cutis — *see* Neoplasm, skin						
cystic (bile) duct (common)	156.1	197.8	230.8	211.5	235.3	239.0
dermis — *see* Neoplasm, skin						
diaphragm	171.4	198.89	—	215.4	238.1	239.2
digestive organs, system, tube, or tract NEC	159.9	197.8	230.9	211.9	235.5	239.0
contiguous sites with peritoneum	159.8	—	—	—	—	—
disc, intervertebral	170.2	198.5	—	213.2	238.0	239.2
disease, generalized	199.0	199.0	234.9	229.9	238.9	199.0
disseminated	199.0	199.0	234.9	229.9	238.9	199.0
Douglas' cul-de-sac or pouch	158.8	197.6	—	211.8	235.4	239.0
duodenojejunal junction	152.8	197.4	230.7	211.2	235.2	239.0
duodenum	152.0	197.4	230.7	211.2	235.2	239.0
dura (cranial) (mater)	192.1	198.4	—	225.2	237.6	239.7
cerebral	192.1	198.4	—	225.2	237.6	239.7
spinal	192.3	198.4	—	225.4	237.6	239.7
ear (external)	173.2	198.2	232.2	216.2	238.2	239.2
auricle or auris	173.2	198.2	232.2	216.2	238.2	239.2
canal, external	173.2	198.2	232.2	216.2	238.2	239.2
cartilage	171.0	198.89	—	215.0	238.1	239.2
external meatus	173.2	198.2	232.2	216.2	238.2	239.2
inner	160.1	197.3	231.8	212.0	235.9	239.8 ▲
lobule	173.2	198.2	232.2	216.2	238.2	239.2
middle	160.1	197.3	231.8	212.0	235.9	239.8 ▲
contiguous sites with accessory sinuses or nasal cavities	160.8	—	—	—	—	—
skin	173.2	198.2	232.2	216.2	238.2	239.2
earlobe	173.2	198.2	232.2	216.2	238.2	239.2
ejaculatory duct	187.8	198.82	233.6	222.8	236.6	239.5
elbow NEC*	195.4	198.89	232.6	229.8	238.8	239.8
endocardium	164.1	198.89	—	212.7	238.8	239.8
endocervix (canal) (gland)	180.0	198.82	233.1	219.0	236.0	239.5

▶◀ Revised Text   ● New Line   ▲ Revised Code

Index to Diseases — Neoplasm, fauces, faucial

	Malignant			Benign	Uncertain Behavior	Unspecified
	Primary	Secondary	Ca in situ			
Neoplasm, neoplastic — *continued*						
endocrine gland NEC	194.9	198.89	—	227.9	237.4	239.7
pluriglandular NEC	194.8	198.89	234.8	227.8	237.4	239.7
endometrium (gland) (stroma)	182.0	198.82	233.2	219.1	236.0	239.5
ensiform cartilage	170.3	198.5	—	213.3	238.0	239.2
enteric — *see* Neoplasm, intestine						
ependyma (brain)	191.5	198.3	—	225.0	237.5	239.6
epicardium	164.1	198.89	—	212.7	238.8	239.8
epididymis	187.5	198.82	233.6	222.3	236.6	239.5
epidural	192.9	198.4	—	225.9	237.9	239.7
epiglottis	161.1	197.3	231.0	212.1	235.6	239.1
anterior aspect or surface	146.4	198.89	230.0	210.6	235.1	239.0
cartilage	161.3	197.3	231.0	212.1	235.6	239.1
free border (margin)	146.4	198.89	230.0	210.6	235.1	239.0
junctional region	146.5	198.89	230.0	210.6	235.1	239.0
posterior (laryngeal) surface	161.1	197.3	231.0	212.1	235.6	239.1
suprahyoid portion	161.1	197.3	231.0	212.1	235.6	239.1
esophagogastric junction	151.0	197.8	230.2	211.1	235.2	239.0
esophagus	150.9	197.8	230.1	211.0	235.5	239.0
abdominal	150.2	197.8	230.1	211.0	235.5	239.0
cervical	150.0	197.8	230.1	211.0	235.5	239.0
contiguous sites	150.8	—	—	—	—	—
distal (third)	150.5	197.8	230.1	211.0	235.5	239.0
lower (third)	150.5	197.8	230.1	211.0	235.5	239.0
middle (third)	150.4	197.8	230.1	211.0	235.5	239.0
proximal (third)	150.3	197.8	230.1	211.0	235.5	239.0
specified part NEC	150.8	197.8	230.1	211.0	235.5	239.0
thoracic	150.1	197.8	230.1	211.0	235.5	239.0
upper (third)	150.3	197.8	230.1	211.0	235.5	239.0
ethmoid (sinus)	160.3	197.3	231.8	212.0	235.9	239.1
bone or labyrinth	170.0	198.5	—	213.0	238.0	239.2
Eustachian tube	160.1	197.3	231.8	212.0	235.9	239.1
exocervix	180.1	198.82	233.1	219.0	236.0	239.5
external						
meatus (ear)	173.2	198.2	232.2	216.2	238.2	239.2
os, cervix uteri	180.1	198.82	233.1	219.0	236.0	239.5
extradural	192.9	198.4	—	225.9	237.9	239.7
extrahepatic (bile) duct	156.1	197.8	230.8	211.5	235.3	239.0
contiguous sites with gallbladder	156.8	—	—	—	—	—
extraocular muscle	190.1	198.4	234.0	224.1	238.8	239.8
extrarectal	195.3	198.89	234.8	229.8	238.8	239.8
extremity*	195.8	198.89	232.8	229.8	238.8	239.8
lower*	195.5	198.89	232.7	229.8	238.8	239.8
upper*	195.4	198.89	232.6	229.8	238.8	239.8
eye NEC	190.9	198.4	234.0	224.9	238.8	239.8
contiguous sites	190.8	—	—	—	—	—
specified sites NEC	190.8	198.4	234.0	224.8	238.8	239.8
eyeball	190.0	198.4	234.0	224.0	238.8	239.8
eyebrow	173.3	198.2	232.3	216.3	238.2	239.2
eyelid (lower) (skin) (upper)	173.1	198.2	232.1	216.1	238.2	239.2
cartilage	171.0	198.89	—	215.0	238.1	239.2
face NEC*	195.0	198.89	232.3	229.8	238.8	239.8
fallopian tube (accessory)	183.2	198.82	233.3	221.0	236.3	239.5
falx (cerebelli) (cerebri)	192.1	198.4	—	225.2	237.6	239.7
fascia — *see also* Neoplasm, connective tissue						
palmar	171.2	198.89	—	215.2	238.1	239.2
plantar	171.3	198.89	—	215.3	238.1	239.2
fatty tissue — *see* Neoplasm, connective tissue						
fauces, faucial NEC	146.9	198.89	230.0	210.6	235.1	239.0
pillars	146.2	198.89	230.0	210.6	235.1	239.0

Fourth-digit Required   Fifth-digit Required

Neoplasm, fauces, faucial — Index to Disease

	Malignant			Benign	Uncertain Behavior	Unspecified
	Primary	Secondary	Ca in situ			
Neoplasm, neoplastic — *continued*						
fauces, faucial NEC — *continued*						
tonsil	146.0	198.89	230.0	210.5	235.1	239.0
femur (any part)	170.7	198.5	—	213.7	238.0	239.2
fetal membrane	181	198.82	233.2	219.8	236.1	239.5
fibrous tissue — *see* Neoplasm, connective tissue						
fibula (any part)	170.7	198.5	—	213.7	238.0	239.2
filum terminale	192.2	198.3	—	225.3	237.5	239.7
finger NEC*	195.4	198.89	232.6	229.8	238.8	239.8
flank NEC*	195.8	198.89	232.5	229.8	238.8	239.8
follicle, nabothian	180.0	198.82	233.1	219.0	236.0	239.5
foot NEC*	195.5	198.89	232.7	229.8	238.8	239.8
forearm NEC*	195.4	198.89	232.6	229.8	238.8	239.8
forehead (skin)	173.3	198.2	232.3	216.3	238.2	239.2
foreskin	187.1	198.82	233.5	222.1	236.6	239.5
fornix						
pharyngeal	147.3	198.89	230.0	210.7	235.1	239.0
vagina	184.0	198.82	233.3	221.1	236.3	239.5
fossa (of)						
anterior (cranial)	191.9	198.3	—	225.0	237.5	239.6
cranial	191.9	198.3	—	225.0	237.5	239.6
ischiorectal	195.3	198.89	234.8	229.8	238.8	239.8
middle (cranial)	191.9	198.3	—	225.0	237.5	239.6
pituitary	194.3	198.89	234.8	227.3	237.0	239.7
posterior (cranial)	191.9	198.3	—	225.0	237.5	239.6
pterygoid	171.0	198.89	—	215.0	238.1	239.2
pyriform	148.1	198.89	230.0	210.8	235.1	239.0
Rosenmüller	147.2	198.89	230.0	210.7	235.1	239.0
tonsillar	146.1	198.89	230.0	210.6	235.1	239.0
fourchette	184.4	198.82	233.3	221.2	236.3	239.5
frenulum						
labii — *see* Neoplasm, lip, internal						
linguae	141.3	198.89	230.0	210.1	235.1	239.0
frontal						
bone	170.0	198.5	—	213.0	238.0	239.2
lobe, brain	191.1	198.3	—	225.0	237.5	239.6
meninges	192.1	198.4	—	225.2	237.6	239.7
pole	191.1	198.3	—	225.0	237.5	239.6
sinus	160.4	197.3	231.8	212.0	235.9	239.1
fundus						
stomach	151.3	197.8	230.2	211.1	235.2	239.0
uterus	182.0	198.82	233.2	219.1	236.0	239.5
gall duct (extrahepatic)	156.1	197.8	230.8	211.5	235.3	239.0
intrahepatic	155.1	197.8	230.8	211.5	235.3	239.0
gallbladder	156.0	197.8	230.8	211.5	235.3	239.0
contiguous sites with extrahepatic bile ducts	156.8	—	—	—	—	—
ganglia (*see also* Neoplasm, connective tissue)	171.9	198.89	—	215.9	238.1	239.2
basal	191.0	198.3	—	225.0	237.5	239.6
ganglion (*see also* Neoplasm, connective tissue)	171.9	198.89	—	215.9	238.1	239.2
cranial nerve	192.0	198.4	—	225.1	237.9	239.7
Gartner's duct	184.0	198.82	233.3	221.1	236.3	239.5
gastric — *see* Neoplasm, stomach						
gastrocolic	159.8	197.8	230.9	211.9	235.5	239.0
gastroesophageal junction	151.0	197.8	230.2	211.1	235.2	239.0
gastrointestinal (tract) NEC	159.9	197.8	230.9	211.9	235.5	239.0
generalized	199.0	199.0	234.9	229.9	238.9	199.0
genital organ or tract						
female NEC	184.9	198.82	233.3	221.9	236.3	239.5
contiguous sites	184.8	—	—	—	—	—

	Malignant			Benign	Uncertain Behavior	Unspecified
	Primary	Secondary	Ca in situ			
Neoplasm, neoplastic — continued						
genital organ or tract — continued						
female NEC — continued						
specified site NEC	184.8	198.82	233.3	221.8	236.3	239.5
male NEC	187.9	198.82	233.6	222.9	236.6	239.5
contiguous sites	187.8	—	—	—	—	—
specified site NEC	187.8	198.82	233.6	222.8	236.6	239.5
genitourinary tract						
female	184.9	198.82	233.3	221.9	236.3	239.5
male	187.9	198.82	233.6	222.9	236.6	239.5
gingiva (alveolar) (marginal)	143.9	198.89	230.0	210.4	235.1	239.0
lower	143.1	198.89	230.0	210.4	235.1	239.0
mandibular	143.1	198.89	230.0	210.4	235.1	239.0
maxillary	143.0	198.89	230.0	210.4	235.1	239.0
upper	143.0	198.89	230.0	210.4	235.1	239.0
gland, glandular (lymphatic) (system) — see also Neoplasm, lymph gland						
endocrine NEC	194.9	198.89	—	227.9	237.4	239.7
salivary — see Neoplasm, salivary, gland						
glans penis	187.2	198.82	233.5	222.1	236.6	239.5
globus pallidus	191.0	198.3	—	225.0	237.5	239.6
glomus						
coccygeal	194.6	198.89	—	227.6	237.3	239.7
jugularis	194.6	198.89	—	227.6	237.3	239.7
glosso-epiglottic fold(s)	146.4	198.89	230.0	210.6	235.1	239.0
glossopalatine fold	146.2	198.89	230.0	210.6	235.1	239.0
glossopharyngeal sulcus	146.1	198.89	230.0	210.6	235.1	239.0
glottis	161.0	197.3	231.0	212.1	235.6	239.1
gluteal region*	195.3	198.89	232.5	229.8	238.8	239.8
great vessels NEC	171.4	198.89	—	215.4	238.1	239.2
groin NEC*	195.3	198.89	232.5	229.8	238.8	239.8
gum	143.9	198.89	230.0	210.4	235.1	239.0
contiguous sites	143.8	—	—	—	—	—
lower	143.1	198.89	230.0	210.4	235.1	239.0
upper	143.0	198.89	230.0	210.4	235.1	239.0
hand NEC*	195.4	198.89	232.6	229.8	238.8	239.8
head NEC*	195.0	198.89	232.4	229.8	238.8	239.8
heart	164.1	198.89	—	212.7	238.8	239.8
contiguous sites with mediastinum or thymus	164.8	—	—	—	—	—
heel NEC*	195.5	198.89	232.7	229.8	238.8	239.8
helix	173.2	198.2	232.2	216.2	238.2	239.2
hematopoietic, hemopoietic tissue NEC	202.8 ✓5ᵗʰ	198.89	—	—	—	238.7
hemisphere, cerebral	191.0	198.3	—	225.0	237.5	239.6
hemorrhoidal zone	154.2	197.5	230.5	211.4	235.5	239.0
hepatic	155.2	197.7	230.8	211.5	235.3	239.0
duct (bile)	156.1	197.8	230.8	211.5	235.3	239.0
flexure (colon)	153.0	197.5	230.3	211.3	235.2	239.0
primary	155.0	—	—	—	—	—
hilus of lung	162.2	197.0	231.2	212.3	235.7	239.1
hip NEC*	195.5	198.89	232.7	229.8	238.8	239.8
hippocampus, brain	191.2	198.3	—	225.0	237.5	239.6
humerus (any part)	170.4	198.5	—	213.4	238.0	239.2
hymen	184.0	198.82	233.3	221.1	236.3	239.5
hypopharynx, hypopharyngeal NEC	148.9	198.89	230.0	210.8	235.1	239.0
contiguous sites	148.8	—	—	—	—	—
postcricoid region	148.0	198.89	230.0	210.8	235.1	239.0
posterior wall	148.3	198.89	230.0	210.8	235.1	239.0
pyriform fossa (sinus)	148.1	198.89	230.0	210.8	235.1	239.0
specified site NEC	148.8	198.89	230.0	210.8	235.1	239.0

✓4ᵗʰ Fourth-digit Required   ✓5ᵗʰ Fifth-digit Required

Neoplasm, hypopharynx, hypopharyngeal

	Malignant			Benign	Uncertain Behavior	Unspecified
	Primary	Secondary	Ca in situ			
Neoplasm, neoplastic — *continued*						
hypopharynx, hypopharyngeal NEC — *continued*						
wall	148.9	198.89	230.0	210.8	235.1	239.0
posterior	148.3	198.89	230.0	210.8	235.1	239.0
hypophysis	194.3	198.89	234.8	227.3	237.0	239.7
hypothalamus	191.0	198.3	—	225.0	237.5	239.6
ileocecum, ileocecal (coil) (junction) (valve)	153.4	197.5	230.3	211.3	235.2	239.0
ileum	152.2	197.4	230.7	211.2	235.2	239.0
ilium	170.6	198.5	—	213.6	238.0	239.2
immunoproliferative NEC	203.8 ▲5ᵗʰ	—	—	—	—	—
infraclavicular (region)*	195.1	198.89	232.5	229.8	238.8	239.8
inguinal (region)*	195.3	198.89	232.5	229.8	238.8	239.8
insula	191.0	198.3	—	225.0	237.5	239.6
insular tissue (pancreas)	157.4	197.8	230.9	211.7	235.5	239.0
brain	191.0	198.3	—	225.0	237.5	239.6
interarytenoid fold	148.2	198.89	230.0	210.8	235.1	239.0
hypopharyngeal aspect	148.2	198.89	230.0	210.8	235.1	239.0
laryngeal aspect	161.1	197.3	231.0	212.1	235.6	239.1
marginal zone	148.2	198.89	230.0	210.8	235.1	239.0
interdental papillae	143.9	198.89	230.0	210.4	235.1	239.0
lower	143.1	198.89	230.0	210.4	235.1	239.0
upper	143.0	198.89	230.0	210.4	235.1	239.0
internal						
capsule	191.0	198.3	—	225.0	237.5	239.6
os (cervix)	180.0	198.82	233.1	219.0	236.0	239.5
intervertebral cartilage or disc	170.2	198.5	—	213.2	238.0	239.2
intestine, intestinal	159.0	197.8	230.7	211.9	235.2	239.0
large	153.9	197.5	230.3	211.3	235.2	239.0
appendix	153.5	197.5	230.3	211.3	235.2	239.0
caput coli	153.4	197.5	230.3	211.3	235.2	239.0
cecum	153.4	197.5	230.3	211.3	235.2	239.0
colon	153.9	197.5	230.3	211.3	235.2	239.0
and rectum	154.0	197.5	230.4	211.4	235.2	239.0
ascending	153.6	197.5	230.3	211.3	235.2	239.0
caput	153.4	197.5	230.3	211.3	235.2	239.0
contiguous sites	153.8	—	—	—	—	—
descending	153.2	197.5	230.3	211.3	235.2	239.0
distal	153.2	197.5	230.3	211.3	235.2	239.0
left	153.2	197.5	230.3	211.3	235.2	239.0
pelvic	153.3	197.5	230.3	211.3	235.2	239.0
right	153.6	197.5	230.3	211.3	235.2	239.0
sigmoid (flexure)	153.3	197.5	230.3	211.3	235.2	239.0
transverse	153.1	197.5	230.3	211.3	235.2	239.0
contiguous sites	153.8	—	—	—	—	—
hepatic flexure	153.0	197.5	230.3	211.3	235.2	239.0
ileocecum, ileocecal (coil) (valve)	153.4	197.5	230.3	211.3	235.2	239.0
sigmoid flexure (lower) (upper)	153.3	197.5	230.3	211.3	235.2	239.0
splenic flexure	153.7	197.5	230.3	211.3	235.2	239.0
small	152.9	197.4	230.7	211.2	235.2	239.0
contiguous sites	152.8	—	—	—	—	—
duodenum	152.0	197.4	230.7	211.2	235.2	239.0
ileum	152.2	197.4	230.7	211.2	235.2	239.0
jejunum	152.1	197.4	230.7	211.2	235.2	239.0
tract NEC	159.0	197.8	230.7	211.9	235.2	239.0
intra-abdominal	195.2	198.89	234.8	229.8	238.8	239.8
intracranial NEC	191.9	198.3	—	225.0	237.5	239.6
intrahepatic (bile) duct	155.1	197.8	230.8	211.5	235.3	239.0
intraocular	190.0	198.4	234.0	224.0	238.8	239.8
intraorbital	190.1	198.4	234.0	224.1	238.8	239.8
intrasellar	194.3	198.89	234.8	227.3	237.0	239.7

	Malignant			Benign	Uncertain Behavior	Unspecified
	Primary	Secondary	Ca in situ			
Neoplasm, neoplastic — *continued*						
intrathoracic (cavity) (organs NEC)	195.1	198.89	234.8	229.8	238.8	239.8
contiguous sites with respiratory organs	165.8	—	—	—	—	—
iris	190.0	198.4	234.0	224.0	238.8	239.8
ischiorectal (fossa)	195.3	198.89	234.8	229.8	238.8	239.8
ischium	170.6	198.5	—	213.6	238.0	239.2
island of Reil	191.0	198.3	—	225.0	237.5	239.6
islands or islets of Langerhans	157.4	197.8	230.9	211.7	235.5	239.0
isthmus uteri	182.1	198.82	233.2	219.1	236.0	239.5
jaw	195.0	198.89	234.8	229.8	238.8	239.8
bone	170.1	198.5	—	213.1	238.0	239.2
carcinoma	143.9	—	—	—	—	—
lower	143.1	—	—	—	—	—
upper	143.0	—	—	—	—	—
lower	170.1	198.5	—	213.1	238.0	239.2
upper	170.0	198.5	—	213.0	238.0	239.2
carcinoma (any type) (lower) (upper)	195.0	—	—	—	—	—
skin	173.3	198.2	232.3	216.3	238.2	239.2
soft tissues	143.9	198.89	230.0	210.4	235.1	239.0
lower	143.1	198.89	230.0	210.4	235.1	239.0
upper	143.0	198.89	230.0	210.4	235.1	239.0
jejunum	152.1	197.4	230.7	211.2	235.2	239.0
joint NEC (*see also* Neoplasm, bone)	170.9	198.5	—	213.9	238.0	239.2
acromioclavicular	170.4	198.5	—	213.4	238.0	239.2
bursa or synovial membrane — *see* Neoplasm, connective tissue						
costovertebral	170.3	198.5	—	213.3	238.0	239.2
sternocostal	170.3	198.5	—	213.3	238.0	239.2
temporomandibular	170.1	198.5	—	213.1	238.0	239.2
junction						
anorectal	154.8	197.5	230.7	211.4	235.5	239.0
cardioesophageal	151.0	197.8	230.2	211.1	235.2	239.0
esophagogastric	151.0	197.8	230.2	211.1	235.2	239.0
gastroesophageal	151.0	197.8	230.2	211.1	235.2	239.0
hard and soft palate	145.5	198.89	230.0	210.4	235.1	239.0
ileocecal	153.4	197.5	230.3	211.3	235.2	239.0
pelvirectal	154.0	197.5	230.4	211.4	235.2	239.0
pelviureteric	189.1	198.0	233.9	223.1	236.91	239.5
rectosigmoid	154.0	197.5	230.4	211.4	235.2	239.0
squamocolumnar, of cervix	180.8	198.82	233.1	219.0	236.0	239.5
kidney (parenchyma)	189.0	198.0	233.9	223.0	236.91	239.5
calyx	189.1	198.0	233.9	223.1	236.91	239.5
hilus	189.1	198.0	233.9	223.1	236.91	239.5
pelvis	189.1	198.0	233.9	223.1	236.91	239.5
knee NEC*	195.5	198.89	232.7	229.8	238.8	239.8
labia (skin)	184.4	198.82	233.3	221.2	236.3	239.5
majora	184.1	198.82	233.3	221.2	236.3	239.5
minora	184.2	198.82	233.3	221.2	236.3	239.5
labial — *see also* Neoplasm, lip						
sulcus (lower) (upper)	145.1	198.89	230.0	210.4	235.1	239.0
labium (skin)	184.4	198.82	233.3	221.2	236.3	239.5
majus	184.1	198.82	233.3	221.2	236.3	239.5
minus	184.2	198.82	233.3	221.2	236.3	239.5
lacrimal						
canaliculi	190.7	198.4	234.0	224.7	238.8	239.8
duct (nasal)	190.7	198.4	234.0	224.7	238.8	239.8
gland	190.2	198.4	234.0	224.2	238.8	239.8
punctum	190.7	198.4	234.0	224.7	238.8	239.8
sac	190.7	198.4	234.0	224.7	238.8	239.8

	Malignant			Benign	Uncertain Behavior	Unspecified
	Primary	Secondary	Ca in situ			
Neoplasm, neoplastic — *continued*						
Langerhans, islands or islets	157.4	197.8	230.9	211.7	235.5	239.0
laryngopharynx	148.9	198.89	230.0	210.8	235.1	239.0
larynx, laryngeal NEC	161.9	197.3	231.0	212.1	235.6	239.1
aryepiglottic fold	161.1	197.3	231.0	212.1	235.6	239.1
cartilage (arytenoid) (cricoid) (cuneiform) (thyroid)	161.3	197.3	231.0	212.1	235.6	239.1
commissure (anterior) (posterior)	161.0	197.3	231.0	212.1	235.6	239.1
contiguous sites	161.8	—	—	—	—	—
extrinsic NEC	161.1	197.3	231.0	212.1	235.6	239.1
meaning hypopharynx	148.9	198.89	230.0	210.8	235.1	239.0
interarytenoid fold	161.1	197.3	231.0	212.1	235.6	239.1
intrinsic	161.0	197.3	231.0	212.1	235.6	239.1
ventricular band	161.1	197.3	231.0	212.1	235.6	239.1
leg NEC*	195.5	198.89	232.7	229.8	238.8	239.8
lens, crystalline	190.0	198.4	234.0	224.0	238.8	239.8
lid (lower) (upper)	173.1	198.2	232.1	216.1	238.2	239.2
ligament — *see also* Neoplasm, connective tissue						
broad	183.3	198.82	233.3	221.0	236.3	239.5
Mackenrodt's	183.8	198.82	233.3	221.8	236.3	239.5
non-uterine — *see* Neoplasm, connective tissue						
round	183.5	198.82	—	221.0	236.3	239.5
sacro-uterine	183.4	198.82	—	221.0	236.3	239.5
uterine	183.4	198.82	—	221.0	236.3	239.5
utero-ovarian	183.8	198.82	233.3	221.8	236.3	239.5
uterosacral	183.4	198.82	—	221.0	236.3	239.5
limb*	195.8	198.89	232.8	229.8	238.8	239.8
lower*	195.5	198.89	232.7	229.8	238.8	239.8
upper*	195.4	198.89	232.6	229.8	238.8	239.8
limbus of cornea	190.4	198.4	234.0	224.4	238.8	239.8
lingual NEC (*see also* Neoplasm, tongue)	141.9	198.89	230.0	210.1	235.1	239.0
lingula, lung	162.3	197.0	231.2	212.3	235.7	239.1
lip (external) (lipstick area) (vermillion border)	140.9	198.89	230.0	210.0	235.1	239.0
buccal aspect — *see* Neoplasm, lip, internal						
commissure	140.6	198.89	230.0	210.4	235.1	239.0
contiguous sites	140.8	—	—	—	—	—
with oral cavity or pharynx	149.8	—	—	—	—	—
frenulum — *see* Neoplasm, lip, internal						
inner aspect — *see* Neoplasm, lip, internal						
internal (buccal) (frenulum) (mucosa) (oral)	140.5	198.89	230.0	210.0	235.1	239.0
lower	140.4	198.89	230.0	210.0	235.1	239.0
upper	140.3	198.89	230.0	210.0	235.1	239.0
lower	140.1	198.89	230.0	210.0	235.1	239.0
internal (buccal)(frenulum) (mucosa) (oral)	140.4	198.89	230.0	210.0	235.1	239.0
mucosa — *see* Neoplasm, lip, internal						
oral aspect — *see* Neoplasm, lip, internal						
skin (commissure) (lower) (upper)	173.0	198.2	232.1	216.0	238.2	239.2
upper	140.0	198.89	230.0	210.0	235.1	239.0
internal (buccal) (frenulum) (mucosa) (oral)	140.3	198.89	230.0	210.0	235.1	239.0

Index to Diseases — Neoplasm, lymph, lymphatic

	Malignant			Benign	Uncertain Behavior	Unspecified
	Primary	Secondary	Ca in situ			
Neoplasm, neoplastic — *continued*						
liver	155.2	197.7	230.8	211.5	235.3	239.0
primary	155.0	—	—	—	—	—
lobe						
azygos	162.3	197.0	231.2	212.3	235.7	239.1
frontal	191.1	198.3	—	225.0	237.5	239.6
lower	162.5	197.0	231.2	212.3	235.7	239.1
middle	162.4	197.0	231.2	212.3	235.7	239.1
occipital	191.4	198.3	—	225.0	237.5	239.6
parietal	191.3	198.3	—	225.0	237.5	239.6
temporal	191.2	198.3	—	225.0	237.5	239.6
upper	162.3	197.0	231.2	212.3	235.7	239.1
lumbosacral plexus	171.6	198.4	—	215.6	238.1	239.2
lung	162.9	197.0	231.2	212.3	235.7	239.1
azgos lobe	162.3	197.0	231.2	212.3	235.7	239.1
carina	162.2	197.0	231.2	212.3	235.7	239.1
contiguous sites with bronchus or trachea	162.8	—	—	—	—	—
hilus	162.2	197.0	231.2	212.3	235.7	239.1
lingula	162.3	197.0	231.2	212.3	235.7	239.1
lobe NEC	162.9	197.0	231.2	212.3	235.7	239.1
lower lobe	162.5	197.0	231.2	212.3	235.7	239.1
main bronchus	162.2	197.0	231.2	212.3	235.7	239.1
middle lobe	162.4	197.0	231.2	212.3	235.7	239.1
upper lobe	162.3	197.0	231.2	212.3	235.7	239.1
lymph, lymphatic						
channel NEC (see also Neoplasm, connective tissue)	171.9	198.89	—	215.9	238.1	239.2
gland (secondary)	—	196.9	—	229.0	238.8	239.8
abdominal	—	196.2	—	229.0	238.8	239.
aortic	—	196.2	—	229.0	238.8	239.8
arm	—	196.3	—	229.0	238.8	239.8
auricular (anterior) (posterior)	—	196.0	—	229.0	238.8	239.8
axilla, axillary	—	196.3	—	229.0	238.8	239.8
brachial	—	196.3	—	229.0	238.8	239.8
bronchial	—	196.1	—	229.0	238.8	239.8
bronchopulmonary	—	196.1	—	229.0	238.8	239.8
celiac	—	196.2	—	229.0	238.8	239.8
cervical	—	196.0	—	229.0	238.8	239.8
cervicofacial	—	196.0	—	229.0	238.8	239.8
Cloquet	—	196.5	—	229.0	238.8	239.8
colic	—	196.2	—	229.0	238.8	239.8
common duct	—	196.2	—	229.0	238.8	239.8
cubital	—	196.3	—	229.0	238.8	239.8
diaphragmatic	—	196.1	—	229.0	238.8	239.8
epigastric, inferior	—	196.6	—	229.0	238.8	239.8
epitrochlear	—	196.3	—	229.0	238.8	239.8
esophageal	—	196.1	—	229.0	238.8	239.8
face	—	196.0	—	229.0	238.8	239.8
femoral	—	196.5	—	229.0	238.8	239.8
gastric	—	196.2	—	229.0	238.8	239.8
groin	—	196.5	—	229.0	238.8	239.8
head	—	196.0	—	229.0	238.8	239.8
hepatic	—	196.2	—	229.0	238.8	239.8
hilar (pulmonary)	—	196.1	—	229.0	238.8	239.8
splenic	—	196.2	—	229.0	238.8	239.8
hypogastric	—	196.6	—	229.0	238.8	239.8
ileocolic	—	196.2	—	229.0	238.8	239.8
iliac	—	196.6	—	229.0	238.8	239.8
infraclavicular	—	196.3	—	229.0	238.8	239.8
inguina, inguinal	—	196.5	—	229.0	238.8	239.8
innominate	—	196.1	—	229.0	238.8	239.8

✓4ᵗʰ Fourth-digit Required   ✓5ᵗʰ Fifth-digit Required

Neoplasm, lymph, lymphatic — Index to Disease

	Malignant			Benign	Uncertain Behavior	Unspecified
	Primary	Secondary	Ca in situ			
Neoplasm, neoplastic — *continued*						
lymph, lymphatic — *continued*						
gland — *continued*						
intercostal	—	196.1	—	229.0	238.8	239.8
intestinal	—	196.2	—	229.0	238.8	239.8
intra-abdominal	—	196.2	—	229.0	238.8	239.8
intrapelvic	—	196.6	—	229.0	238.8	239.8
intrathoracic	—	196.1	—	229.0	238.8	239.9
jugular	—	196.0	—	229.0	238.8	239.8
leg	—	196.5	—	229.0	238.8	239.8
limb						
lower	—	196.5	—	229.0	238.8	239.8
upper	—	196.3	—	229.0	238.8	239.8
lower limb	—	196.5	—	229.0	238.8	238.9
lumbar	—	196.2	—	229.0	238.8	239.8
mandibular	—	196.0	—	229.0	238.8	239.8
mediastinal	—	196.1	—	229.0	238.8	239.8
mesenteric (inferior) (superior)	—	196.2	—	229.0	238.8	239.8
midcolic	—	196.2	—	229.0	238.8	239.8
multiple sites in categories 196.0-196.6	—	196.8	—	229.0	238.8	239.8
neck	—	196.0	—	229.0	238.8	239.8
obturator	—	196.6	—	229.0	238.8	239.8
occipital	—	196.0	—	229.0	238.8	239.8
pancreatic	—	196.2	—	229.0	238.8	239.8
para-aortic	—	196.2	—	229.0	238.8	239.8
paracervical	—	196.6	—	229.0	238.8	239.8
parametrial	—	196.6	—	229.0	238.8	239.8
parasternal	—	196.1	—	229.0	238.8	239.8
parotid	—	196.0	—	229.0	238.8	239.8
pectoral	—	196.3	—	229.0	238.8	239.8
pelvic	—	196.6	—	229.0	238.8	239.8
peri-aortic	—	196.2	—	229.0	238.8	239.8
peripancreatic	—	196.2	—	229.0	238.8	239.8
popliteal	—	196.5	—	229.0	238.8	239.8
porta hepatis	—	196.2	—	229.0	238.8	239.8
portal	—	196.2	—	229.0	238.8	239.8
preauricular	—	196.0	—	229.0	238.8	239.8
prelaryngeal	—	196.0	—	229.0	238.8	239.8
presymphysial	—	196.6	—	229.0	238.8	239.8
pretracheal	—	196.0	—	229.0	238.8	239.8
primary (any site) NEC	202.9	—	—	—	—	—
pulmonary (hiler)	—	196.1	—	229.0	238.8	239.8
pyloric	—	196.2	—	229.0	238.8	239.8
retroperitoneal	—	196.2	—	229.0	238.8	239.8
retropharyngeal	—	196.0	—	229.0	238.8	239.8
Rosenmüller's	—	196.5	—	229.0	238.8	239.8
sacral	—	196.6	—	229.0	238.8	239.8
scalene	—	196.0	—	229.0	238.8	239.8
site NEC	—	196.9	—	229.0	238.8	239.8
splenic (hilar)	—	196.2	—	229.0	238.8	239.8
subclavicular	—	196.3	—	229.0	238.8	239.8
subinguinal	—	196.5	—	229.0	238.8	239.8
sublingual	—	196.0	—	229.0	238.8	239.8
submandibular	—	196.0	—	229.0	238.8	239.8
submaxillary	—	196.0	—	229.0	238.8	239.8
submental	—	196.0	—	229.0	238.8	239.8
subscapular	—	196.3	—	229.0	238.8	239.8
supraclavicular	—	196.0	—	229.0	238.8	239.8
thoracic	—	196.1	—	229.0	238.8	239.8
tibial	—	196.5	—	229.0	238.8	239.8
tracheal	—	196.1	—	229.0	238.8	239.8
tracheobronchial	—	196.1	—	229.0	238.8	239.8

Index to Diseases — Neoplasm, metacarpus

	Malignant			Benign	Uncertain Behavior	Unspecified
	Primary	Secondary	Ca in situ			
Neoplasm, neoplastic — continued						
lymph, lymphatic — continued						
gland — continued						
upper limb	—	196.3	—	229.0	238.8	239.8
Virchow's	—	196.0	—	229.0	238.8	239.8
node — see also Neoplasm, lymph gland						
primary NEC	202.9 ✓5	—	—	—	—	—
vessel (see also Neoplasm, connective tissue)	171.9	198.89	—	215.9	238.1	239.2
Nackenrodt's ligament	183.8	198.82	233.3	221.8	236.3	239.5
malar	170.0	198.5	—	213.0	238.0	239.2
region — see Neoplasm, cheek						
mammary gland — see Neoplasm, breast						
mandible	170.1	198.5	—	213.1	238.0	239.2
alveolar						
mucose	143.1	198.89	230.0	210.4	235.1	239.0
ridge or process	170.1	198.5	—	213.1	238.0	239.2
carcinoma	143.1	—	—	—	—	—
carcinoma	143.1	—	—	—	—	—
marrow (bone) NEC	202.9 ✓5	198.5	—	—	—	238.7
mastectomy site (skin)	173.5	198.2	—	—	—	—
specified as breast tissue	174.8	198.81	—	—	—	—
mastoid (air cells) (antrum) (cavity)	160.1	197.3	231.8	212.0	235.9	239.1
bone or process	170.0	198.5	—	213.0	238.0	239.2
maxilla, maxillary (superior)	170.0	198.5	—	213.0	238.0	239.2
alveolar						
mucosa	143.0	198.89	230.0	210.4	235.1	239.0
ridge or process	170.0	198.5	—	213.0	238.0	239.2
carcinoma	143.0	—	—	—	—	—
antrum	160.2	197.3	231.8	212.0	235.9	239.1
carcinoma	143.0	—	—	—	—	—
inferior — see Neoplasm, mandible						
sinus	160.2	197.3	231.8	212.0	235.9	239.1
meatus						
external (ear)	173.2	198.2	232.2	216.2	238.2	239.2
Meckel's diverticulum	152.3	197.4	230.7	211.2	235.2	239.0
mediastinum, mediastinal	164.9	197.1	—	212.5	235.8	239.8
anterior	164.2	197.1	—	212.5	235.8	239.8
contiguous sites with heart and thymus	164.8	—	—	—	—	—
posterior	164.3	197.1	—	212.5	235.8	239.8
medulla						
adrenal	194.0	198.7	234.8	227.0	237.2	239.7
oblongata	191.7	198.3	—	225.0	237.5	239.6
meibomian gland	173.1	198.2	232.1	216.1	238.2	239.2
melanoma — see Melanoma						
meninges (brain) (cerebral) (cranial) (intracranial)	192.1	198.4	—	225.2	237.6	239.7
spinal (cord)	192.3	198.4	—	225.4	237.6	239.7
meniscus, knee joint (lateral) (medial)	170.7	198.5	—	213.7	238.0	239.2
mesentery, mesenteric	158.8	197.6	—	211.8	235.4	239.0
mesoappendix	158.8	197.6	—	211.8	235.4	239.0
mesocolon	158.8	197.6	—	211.8	235.4	239.0
mesopharynx — see Neoplasm, oropharynx						
mesosalpinx	183.3	198.82	233.3	221.0	236.3	239.5
mesovarium	183.3	198.82	233.3	221.0	236.3	239.5
metacarpus (any bone)	170.5	198.5	—	213.5	238.0	239.2

✓4 Fourth-digit Required ✓5 Fifth-digit Required

Neoplasm, metastatic — Index to Disease

	Malignant			Benign	Uncertain Behavior	Unspecified
	Primary	Secondary	Ca in situ			
Neoplasm, neoplastic — continued						
metastatic NEC — see also Neoplasm, by site, secondary	—	199.1	—	—	—	—
metatarsus (any bone)	170.8	198.5	—	213.8	238.0	239.2
midbrain	191.7	198.3	—	225.0	237.5	239.6
milk duct — see Neoplasm, breast						
mons						
pubis	184.4	198.82	233.3	221.2	236.3	239.5
veneris	184.4	198.82	233.3	221.2	236.3	239.5
motor tract	192.9	198.4	—	225.9	237.9	239.7
brain	191.9	198.3	—	225.0	237.5	239.6
spinal	192.2	198.3	—	225.3	237.5	239.7
mouth	145.9	198.89	230.0	210.4	235.1	239.0
contiguous sites	145.8	—	—	—	—	—
floor	144.9	198.89	230.0	210.3	235.1	239.0
anterior portion	144.0	198.89	230.0	210.3	235.1	239.0
contiguous sites	144.8	—	—	—	—	—
lateral portion	144.1	198.89	230.0	210.3	235.1	239.0
roof	145.5	198.89	230.0	210.4	235.1	239.0
specified part NEC	145.8	198.89	230.0	210.4	235.1	239.0
vestibule	145.1	198.89	230.0	210.4	235.1	239.0
mucosa						
alveolar (ridge or process)	143.9	198.89	230.0	210.4	235.1	239.0
lower	143.1	198.89	230.0	210.4	235.1	239.0
upper	143.0	198.89	230.0	210.4	235.1	239.0
buccal	145.0	198.89	230.0	210.4	235.1	239.0
cheek	145.0	198.89	230.0	210.4	235.1	239.0
lip — see Neoplasm, lip, internal						
nasal	160.0	197.3	231.8	212.0	235.9	239.1
oral	145.0	198.89	230.0	210.4	235.1	239.0
Müllerian duct						
female	184.8	198.82	233.3	221.8	236.3	239.5
male	187.8	198.82	233.6	222.8	236.6	239.5
multiple sites NEC	199.0	199.0	234.9	229.9	238.9	199.0
muscle — see also Neoplasm, connective tissue						
extraocular	190.1	198.4	234.0	224.1	238.8	239.8
myocardium	164.1	198.89	—	212.7	238.8	239.8
myometrium	182.0	198.82	233.2	219.1	236.0	239.5
myopericardium	164.1	198.89	—	212.7	238.8	239.8
nabothian gland (follicle)	180.0	198.82	233.1	219.0	236.0	239.5
nail	173.9	198.2	232.9	216.9	238.2	239.2
finger	173.6	198.2	232.6	216.6	238.2	239.2
toe	173.7	198.2	232.7	216.7	238.2	239.2
nares, naris (anterior) (posterior)	160.0	197.3	231.8	212.0	235.9	239.1
nasal — see Neoplasm, nose						
nasolabial groove	173.3	198.2	232.3	216.3	238.2	239.2
nasolacrimal duct	190.7	198.4	234.0	224.7	238.8	239.8
nasopharynx, nasopharyngeal	147.9	198.89	230.0	210.7	235.1	239.0
contiguous sites	147.8	—	—	—	—	—
floor	147.3	198.89	230.0	210.7	235.1	239.0
roof	147.0	198.89	230.0	210.7	235.1	239.0
specified site NEC	147.8	198.89	230.0	210.7	235.1	239.0
wall	147.9	198.89	230.0	210.7	235.1	239.0
anterior	147.3	198.89	230.0	210.7	235.1	239.0
lateral	147.2	198.89	230.0	210.7	235.1	239.0
posterior	147.1	198.89	230.0	210.7	235.1	239.0
superior	147.0	198.89	230.0	210.7	235.1	239.0
nates	173.5	198.2	232.5	216.5	238.2	239.2
neck NEC*	195.0	198.89	234.8	229.8	238.8	239.8

Index to Diseases

	Malignant			Benign	Uncertain Behavior	Unspecified
	Primary	Secondary	Ca in situ			
Neoplasm, neoplastic — *continued*						
nerve (autonomic) (ganglion) (parasympathetic) (peripheral) (sympathetic) — *see also* Neoplasm, connective tissue						
abducens	192.0	198.4	—	225.1	237.9	239.7
accessory (spinal)	192.0	198.4	—	225.1	237.9	239.7
acoustic	192.0	198.4	—	225.1	237.9	239.7
auditory	192.0	198.4	—	225.1	237.9	239.7
brachial	171.2	198.89	—	215.2	238.1	239.2
cranial (any)	192.0	198.4	—	225.1	237.9	239.7
facial	192.0	198.4	—	225.1	237.9	239.7
femoral	171.3	198.89	—	215.3	238.1	239.2
glossopharyngeal	192.0	198.4	—	225.1	237.9	239.7
hypoglossal	192.0	198.4	—	225.1	237.9	239.7
intercostal	171.4	198.89	—	215.4	238.1	239.2
lumbar	171.7	198.89	—	215.7	238.1	239.2
median	171.2	198.89	—	215.2	238.1	239.2
obturator	171.3	198.89	—	215.3	238.1	239.2
oculomotor	192.0	198.4	—	225.1	237.9	239.7
olfactory	192.0	198.4	—	225.1	237.9	239.7
optic	192.0	198.4	—	225.1	237.9	239.7
peripheral NEC	171.9	198.89	—	215.9	238.1	239.2
radial	171.2	198.89	—	215.2	238.1	239.2
sacral	171.6	198.89	—	215.6	238.1	239.2
sciatic	171.3	198.89	—	215.3	238.1	239.2
spinal NEC	171.9	198.89	—	215.9	238.1	239.2
trigeminal	192.0	198.4	—	225.1	237.9	239.7
trochlear	192.0	198.4	—	225.1	237.9	239.7
ulnar	171.2	198.89	—	215.2	238.1	239.2
vagus	192.0	198.4	—	225.1	237.9	239.7
nervous system (central) NEC	192.9	198.4	—	225.9	237.9	239.7
autonomic NEC	171.9	198.89	—	215.9	238.1	239.2
brain — *see also* Neoplasm, brain						
membrane or meninges	192.1	198.4	—	225.2	237.6	239.7
contiguous sites	192.8	—	—	—	—	—
parasympathetic NEC	171.9	198.89	—	215.9	238.1	239.2
sympathetic NEC	171.9	198.89	—	215.9	238.1	239.2
nipple (female)	174.0	198.81	233.0	217	238.3	239.3
male	175.0	198.81	233.0	217	238.3	239.3
nose, nasal	195.0	198.89	234.8	229.8	238.8	239.8
ala (external)	173.3	198.2	232.3	216.3	238.2	239.2
bone	170.0	198.5	—	213.0	238.0	239.2
cartilage	160.0	197.3	231.8	212.0	235.9	239.1
cavity	160.0	197.3	231.8	212.0	235.9	239.1
contiguous sites with accessory sinuses or middle ear	160.8	—	—	—	—	—
choana	147.3	198.89	230.0	210.7	235.1	239.0
external (skin)	173.3	198.2	232.3	216.3	238.2	239.2
fossa	160.0	197.3	231.8	212.0	235.9	239.1
internal	160.0	197.3	231.8	212.0	235.9	239.1
mucosa	160.0	197.3	231.8	212.0	235.9	239.1
septum	160.0	197.3	231.8	212.0	235.9	239.1
posterior margin	147.3	198.89	230.0	210.7	235.1	239.0
sinus — *see* Neoplasm, sinus						
skin	173.3	198.2	232.3	216.3	238.2	239.2
turbinate (mucosa)	160.0	197.3	231.8	212.0	235.9	239.1
bone	170.0	198.5	—	213.0	238.0	239.2
vestibule	160.0	197.3	231.8	212.0	235.9	239.1
nostril	160.0	197.3	231.8	212.0	235.9	239.1
nucleus pulposus	170.2	198.5	—	213.2	238.0	239.2

Neoplasm, occipital   **Index to Disease**

	Malignant			Benign	Uncertain Behavior	Unspecified
	Primary	Secondary	Ca in situ			
Neoplasm, neoplastic — *continued*						
occipital						
bone	170.0	198.5	—	213.0	238.0	239.2
lobe or pole, brain	191.4	198.3	—	225.0	237.5	239.6
odontogenic — *see* Neoplasm, jaw bone						
oesophagus — *see* Neoplasm, esophagus						
olfactory nerve or bulb	192.0	198.4	—	225.1	237.9	239.7
olive (brain)	191.7	198.3	—	225.0	237.5	239.6
omentum	158.8	197.6	—	211.8	235.4	239.0
operculum (brain)	191.0	198.3	—	225.0	237.5	239.6
optic nerve, chiasm, or tract	192.0	198.4	—	225.1	237.9	239.7
oral (cavity)	145.9	198.89	230.0	210.4	235.1	239.0
contiguous sites with lip or pharynx	149.8	—	—	—	—	—
ill-defined	149.9	198.89	230.0	210.4	235.1	239.0
mucosa	145.9	198.89	230.0	210.4	235.1	239.0
orbit	190.1	198.4	234.0	224.1	238.8	239.8
bone	170.0	198.5	—	213.0	238.0	239.2
eye	190.1	198.4	234.0	224.1	238.8	239.8
soft parts	190.1	198.4	234.0	224.1	238.8	239.8
organ of Zuckerkandl	194.6	198.89	—	227.6	237.3	239.7
oropharynx	146.9	198.89	230.0	210.6	235.1	239.0
branchial cleft (vestige)	146.8	198.89	230.0	210.6	235.1	239.0
contiguous sites	146.8	—	—	—	—	—
junctional region	146.5	198.89	230.0	210.6	235.1	239.0
lateral wall	146.6	198.89	230.0	210.6	235.1	239.0
pillars of fauces	146.2	198.89	230.0	210.6	235.1	239.0
posterior wall	146.7	198.89	230.0	210.6	235.1	239.0
specified part NEC	146.8	198.89	230.0	210.6	235.1	239.0
vallecula	146.3	198.89	230.0	210.6	235.1	239.0
os						
external	180.1	198.82	233.1	219.0	236.0	239.5
internal	180.0	198.82	233.1	219.0	236.0	239.5
ovary	183.0	198.6	233.3	220	236.2	239.5
oviduct	183.2	198.82	233.3	221.0	236.3	239.5
palate	145.5	198.89	230.0	210.4	235.1	239.0
hard	145.2	198.89	230.0	210.4	235.1	239.0
junction of hard and soft palate	145.5	198.89	230.0	210.4	235.1	239.0
soft	145.3	198.89	230.0	210.4	235.1	239.0
nasopharyngeal surface	147.3	198.89	230.0	210.7	235.1	239.0
posterior surface	147.3	198.89	230.0	210.7	235.1	239.0
superior surface	147.3	198.89	230.0	210.7	235.1	239.0
palatoglossal arch	146.2	198.89	230.0	210.6	235.1	239.0
palatopharyngeal arch	146.2	198.89	230.0	210.6	235.1	239.0
pallium	191.0	198.3	—	225.0	237.5	239.6
palpebra	173.1	198.2	232.1	216.1	238.2	239.2
pancreas	157.9	197.8	230.9	211.6	235.5	239.0
body	157.1	197.8	230.9	211.6	235.5	239.0
contiguous sites	157.8	—	—	—	—	—
duct (of Santorini) (of Wirsung)	157.3	197.8	230.9	211.6	235.5	239.0
ectopic tissue	157.8	197.8	230.9	211.6	235.5	239.0
head	157.0	197.8	230.9	211.6	235.5	239.0
islet cells	157.4	197.8	230.9	211.7	235.5	239.0
neck	157.8	197.8	230.9	211.6	235.5	239.0
tail	157.2	197.8	230.9	211.6	235.5	239.0
para-aortic body	194.6	198.89	—	227.6	237.3	239.7
paraganglion NEC	194.6	198.89	—	227.6	237.3	239.7
parametrium	183.4	198.82	—	221.0	236.3	239.5
paranephric	158.0	197.6	—	211.8	235.4	239.0
pararectal	195.3	198.89	—	229.8	238.8	239.8

	Malignant			Benign	Uncertain Behavior	Unspecified
	Primary	Secondary	Ca in situ			
Neoplasm, neoplastic — *continued*						
parasagittal (region)	195.0	198.89	234.8	229.8	238.8	239.8
parasellar	192.9	198.4	—	225.9	237.9	239.7
parathyroid (gland)	194.1	198.89	234.8	227.1	237.4	239.7
paraurethral	195.3	198.89	—	229.8	238.8	239.8
gland	189.4	198.1	233.9	223.89	236.99	239.5
paravaginal	195.3	198.89	—	229.8	238.8	239.8
parenchyma, kidney	189.0	198.0	233.9	223.0	236.91	239.5
parietal						
bone	170.0	198.5	—	213.0	238.0	239.2
lobe, brain	191.3	198.3	—	225.0	237.5	239.6
paroophoron	183.3	198.82	233.3	221.0	236.3	239.5
parotid (duct) (gland)	142.0	198.89	230.0	210.2	235.0	239.0
parovarium	183.3	198.82	233.3	221.0	236.3	239.5
patella	170.8	198.5	—	213.8	238.0	239.2
peduncle, cerebral	191.7	198.3	—	225.0	237.5	239.6
pelvirectal junction	154.0	197.5	230.4	211.4	235.2	239.0
pelvis, pelvic	195.3	198.89	234.8	229.8	238.8	239.8
bone	170.6	198.5	—	213.6	238.0	239.2
floor	195.3	198.89	234.8	229.8	238.8	239.8
renal	189.1	198.0	233.9	223.1	236.91	239.5
viscera	195.3	198.89	234.8	229.8	238.8	239.8
wall	195.3	198.89	234.8	229.8	238.8	239.8
pelvo-abdominal	195.8	198.89	234.8	229.8	238.8	239.8
penis	187.4	198.82	233.5	222.1	236.6	239.5
body	187.3	198.82	233.5	222.1	236.6	239.5
corpus (cavernosum)	187.3	198.82	233.5	222.1	236.6	239.5
glans	187.2	198.82	233.5	222.1	236.6	239.5
skin NEC	187.4	198.82	233.5	222.1	236.6	239.5
periadrenal (tissue)	158.0	197.6	—	211.8	235.4	239.0
perianal (skin)	173.5	198.2	232.5	216.5	238.2	239.2
pericardium	164.1	198.89	—	212.7	238.8	239.8
perinephric	158.0	197.6	—	211.8	235.4	239.0
perineum	195.3	198.89	234.8	229.8	238.8	239.8
periodontal tissue NEC	143.9	198.89	230.0	210.4	235.1	239.0
periosteum — *see* Neoplasm, bone						
peripancreatic	158.0	197.6	—	211.8	235.4	239.0
peripheral nerve NEC	171.9	198.89	—	215.9	238.1	239.2
perirectal (tissue)	195.3	198.89	—	229.8	238.8	239.8
perirenal (tissue)	158.0	197.6	—	211.8	235.4	239.0
peritoneum, peritoneal (cavity)	158.9	197.6	—	211.8	235.4	239.0
contiguous sites	158.8	—	—	—	—	—
with digestive organs	159.8	—	—	—	—	—
parietal	158.8	197.6	—	211.8	235.4	239.0
pelvic	158.8	197.6	—	211.8	235.4	239.0
specified part NEC	158.8	197.6	—	211.8	235.4	239.0
peritonsillar (tissue)	195	198.89	234.8	229.8	238.8	239.8
periurethral tissue	195.3	198.89	—	229.8	238.8	239.8
phalanges	170.9	198.5	—	213.9	238.0	239.2
foot	170.8	198.5	—	213.8	238.0	239.2
hand	170.5	198.5	—	213.5	238.0	239.2
pharynx, pharyngeal	149.0	198.89	230.0	210.9	235.1	239.0
bursa	147.1	198.89	230.0	210.7	235.1	239.0
fornix	147.3	198.89	230.0	210.7	235.1	239.0
recess	147.2	198.89	230.0	210.7	235.1	239.0
region	149.0	198.89	230.0	210.9	235.1	239.0
tonsil	147.1	198.89	230.0	210.7	235.1	239.0
wall (lateral) (posterior)	149.0	198.89	230.0	210.9	235.1	239.0
pia mater (cerebral) (cranial)	192.1	198.4	—	225.2	237.6	239.7
spinal	192.3	198.4	—	225.4	237.6	239.7
pillars of fauces	146.2	198.89	230.0	210.6	235.1	239.0
pineal (body) (gland)	194.4	198.89	234.8	227.4	237.1	239.7

Neoplasm, pinna — Index to Disease

	Malignant			Benign	Uncertain Behavior	Unspecified
	Primary	**Secondary**	**Ca in situ**			
Neoplasm, neoplastic — *continued*						
pinna (ear) NEC	173.2	198.2	232.2	216.2	238.2	239.2
cartilage	171.0	198.89	—	215.0	238.1	239.2
piriform fossa or sinus	148.1	198.89	230.0	210.8	235.1	239.0
pituitary (body) (fossa) (gland) (lobe)	194.3	198.89	234.8	227.3	237.0	239.7
placenta	181	198.82	233.2	219.8	236.1	239.5
pleura, pleural (cavity)	163.9	197.2	—	212.4	235.8	239.1
contiguous sites	163.8	—	—	—	—	—
parietal	163.0	197.2	—	212.4	235.8	239.1
visceral	163.1	197.2	—	212.4	235.8	239.1
plexus						
brachial	171.2	198.89	—	215.2	238.1	239.2
cervical	171.0	198.89	—	215.0	238.1	239.2
choroid	191.5	198.3	—	225.0	237.5	239.6
lumbosacral	171.6	198.89	—	215.6	238.1	239.2
sacral	171.6	198.89	—	215.6	238.1	239.2
pluri-endocrine	194.8	198.89	234.8	227.8	237.4	239.7
pole						
frontal	191.1	198.3	—	225.0	237.5	239.6
occipital	191.4	198.3	—	225.0	237.5	239.6
pons (varolii)	191.7	198.3	—	225.0	237.5	239.6
popliteal fossa or space*	195.5	198.89	234.8	229.8	238.8	239.8
postcricoid (region)	148.0	198.89	230.0	210.8	235.1	239.0
posterior fossa (cranial)	191.6	198.3	—	225.0	237.5	239.6
postnasal space	147.9	198.89	230.0	210.7	235.1	239.0
prepuce	187.1	198.82	233.5	222.1	236.6	239.5
prepylorus	151.1	197.8	230.2	211.1	235.2	239.0
presacral (region)	195.3	198.89	—	229.8	238.8	239.8
prostate (gland)	185	198.82	233.4	222.2	236.5	239.5
utricle	189.3	198.1	233.9	223.81	236.99	239.5
pterygoid fossa	171.0	198.89	—	215.0	238.1	239.2
pubic bone	170.6	198.5	—	213.6	238.0	239.2
pudenda, pudendum (female)	184.4	198.82	233.3	221.2	236.3	239.5
pulmonary	162.9	197.0	231.2	212.3	235.7	239.1
putamen	191.0	198.3	—	225.0	237.5	239.6
pyloric						
antrum	151.2	197.8	230.2	211.1	235.2	239.0
canal	151.1	197.8	230.2	211.1	235.2	239.0
pylorus	151.1	197.8	230.2	211.1	235.2	239.0
pyramid (brain)	191.7	198.3	—	225.0	237.5	239.6
pyriform fossa or sinus	148.1	198.89	230.0	210.8	235.1	239.0
radius (any part)	170.4	198.5	—	213.4	238.0	239.2
Rathke's pouch	194.3	198.89	234.8	227.3	237.0	239.7
rectosigmoid (colon) (junction)	154.0	197.5	230.4	211.4	235.2	239.0
contiguous sites with anus or rectum	154.8	—	—	—	—	—
rectouterine pouch	158.8	197.6	—	211.8	235.4	239.0
rectovaginal septum or wall	195.3	198.89	234.8	229.8	238.8	239.8
rectovesical septum	195.3	198.89	234.8	229.8	238.8	239.8
rectum (ampulla)	154.1	197.5	230.4	211.4	235.2	239.0
and colon	154.0	197.5	230.4	211.4	235.2	239.0
contiguous sites with anus or rectosigmoid junction	154.8	—	—	—	—	—
renal	189.0	198.0	233.9	223.0	236.91	239.5
calyx	189.1	198.0	233.9	223.1	236.91	239.5
hilus	189.1	198.0	233.9	223.1	236.91	239.5
parenchyma	189.0	198.0	233.9	223.0	236.91	239.5
pelvis	189.1	198.0	233.9	223.1	236.91	239.5
respiratory						
organs or system NEC	165.9	197.3	231.9	212.9	235.9	239.1
contiguous sites with intrathoracic organs	165.8	—	—	—	—	—
specified sites NEC	165.8	197.3	231.8	212.8	235.9	239.1

Index to Diseases

Neoplasm, sinus

	Malignant			Benign	Uncertain Behavior	Unspecified
	Primary	Secondary	Ca in situ			
Neoplasm, neoplastic — *continued*						
respiratory — *continued*						
tract NEC	165.9	197.3	231.9	212.9	235.9	239.1
upper	165.0	197.3	231.9	212.9	235.9	239.1
retina	190.5	198.4	234.0	224.5	238.8	239.8
retrobulbar	190.1	198.4	—	224.1	238.8	239.8
retrocecal	158.0	197.6	—	211.8	235.4	239.0
retromolar (area) (triangle)						
(trigone)	145.6	198.89	230.0	210.4	235.1	239.0
retro-orbital	195.0	198.89	234.8	229.8	238.8	239.8
retroperitoneal (space) (tissue)	158.0	197.6	—	211.8	235.4	239.0
contiguous sites	158.8	—	—	—	—	—
retroperitoneum	158.0	197.6	—	211.8	235.4	239.0
contiguous sites	158.8	—	—	—	—	—
retropharyngeal	149.0	198.89	230.0	210.9	235.1	239.0
retrovesical (septum)	195.3	198.89	234.8	229.8	238.8	239.8
rhinencephalon	191.0	198.3	—	225.0	237.5	239.6
rib	170.3	198.5	—	213.3	238.0	239.2
Rosenmüller's fossa	147.2	198.89	230.0	210.7	235.1	239.0
round ligament	183.5	198.82	—	221.0	236.3	239.5
sacrococcyx, sacrococcygeal	170.6	198.5	—	213.6	238.0	239.2
region	195.3	198.89	234.8	229.8	238.8	239.8
sacrouterine ligament	183.4	198.82	—	221.0	236.3	239.5
sacrum, sacral (vertebra)	170.6	198.5	—	213.6	238.0	239.2
salivary gland or duct (major)	142.9	198.89	230.0	210.2	235.0	239.0
contiguous sites	142.8	—	—	—	—	—
minor NEC	145.9	198.89	230.0	210.4	235.1	239.0
parotid	142.0	198.89	230.0	210.2	235.0	239.0
pluriglandular	142.8	198.89	230.0	210.2	235.0	239.0
sublingual	142.2	198.89	230.0	210.2	235.0	239.0
submandibular	142.1	198.89	230.0	210.2	235.0	239.0
submaxillary	142.1	198.89	230.0	210.2	235.0	239.0
salpinx (uterine)	183.2	198.82	233.3	221.0	236.3	239.5
Santorini's duct	157.3	197.8	230.9	211.6	235.5	239.0
scalp	173.4	198.2	232.4	216.4	238.2	239.2
scapula (any part)	170.4	198.5	—	213.4	238.0	239.2
scapular region	195.1	198.89	234.8	229.8	238.8	239.8
scar NEC (*see also* Neoplasm,						
skin)	173.9	198.2	232.9	216.9	238.2	239.2
sciatic nerve	171.3	198.89	—	215.3	238.1	239.2
sclera	190.0	198.4	234.0	224.0	238.8	239.8
scrotum (skin)	187.7	198.82	233.6	222.4	236.6	239.5
sebaceous gland — *see*						
Neoplasm, skin						
sella turcica	194.3	198.89	234.8	227.3	237.0	239.7
bone	170.0	198.5	—	213.0	238.0	239.2
semilunar cartilage (knee)	170.7	198.5	—	213.7	238.0	239.2
seminal vesicle	187.8	198.82	233.6	222.8	236.6	239.5
septum						
nasal	160.0	197.3	231.8	212.0	235.9	239.1
posterior margin	147.3	198.89	230.0	210.7	235.1	239.0
rectovaginal	195.3	198.89	234.8	229.8	238.8	239.8
rectovesical	195.3	198.89	234.8	229.8	238.8	239.8
urethrovaginal	184.9	198.82	233.3	221.9	236.3	239.5
vesicovaginal	184.9	198.82	233.3	221.9	236.3	239.5
shoulder NEC*	195.4	198.89	232.6	229.8	238.8	239.8
sigmoid flexure (lower) (upper)	153.3	197.5	230.3	211.3	235.2	239.0
sinus (accessory)	160.9	197.3	231.8	212.0	235.9	239.1
bone (any)	170.0	198.5	—	213.0	238.0	239.2
contiguous sites with middle						
ear or nasal cavities	160.8	—	—	—	—	—
ethmoidal	160.3	197.3	231.8	212.0	235.9	239.1
frontal	160.4	197.3	231.8	212.0	235.9	239.1
maxillary	160.2	197.3	231.8	212.0	235.9	239.1

✓4ᵗʰ Fourth-digit Required   ✓5ᵗʰ Fifth-digit Required

Neoplasm, sinus   **Index to Disease**

	Malignant				Uncertain Behavior	Unspecified
	Primary	Secondary	Ca in situ	Benign		
Neoplasm, neoplastic — *continued*						
sinus — *continued*						
nasal, paranasal NEC	160.9	197.3	231.8	212.0	235.9	239.1
pyriform	148.1	198.89	230.0	210.8	235.1	239.0
sphenoidal	160.5	197.3	231.8	212.0	235.9	239.1
skeleton, skeletal NEC	170.9	198.5	—	213.9	238.0	239.2
Skene's gland	189.4	198.1	233.9	223.89	236.99	239.5
skin NEC	173.9	198.2	232.9	216.9	238.2	239.2
abdominal wall	173.5	198.2	232.5	216.5	238.2	239.2
ala nasi	173.3	198.2	232.3	216.3	238.2	239.2
ankle	173.7	198.2	232.7	216.7	238.2	239.2
antecubital space	173.6	198.2	232.6	216.6	238.2	239.2
anus	173.5	198.2	232.5	216.5	238.2	239.2
arm	173.6	198.2	232.6	216.6	238.2	239.2
auditory canal (external)	173.2	198.2	232.2	216.2	238.2	239.2
auricle (ear)	173.2	198.2	232.2	216.2	238.2	239.2
auricular canal (external)	173.2	198.2	232.2	216.2	238.2	239.2
axilla, axillary fold	173.5	198.2	232.5	216.5	238.2	239.2
back	173.5	198.2	232.5	216.5	238.2	239.2
breast	173.5	198.2	232.5	216.5	238.2	239.2
brow	173.3	198.2	232.3	216.3	238.2	239.2
buttock	173.5	198.2	232.5	216.5	238.2	239.2
calf	173.7	198.2	232.7	216.7	238.2	239.2
canthus (eye) (inner) (outer)	173.1	198.2	232.1	216.1	238.2	239.2
cervical region	173.4	198.2	232.4	216.4	238.2	239.2
cheek (external)	173.3	198.2	232.3	216.3	238.2	239.2
chest (wall)	173.5	198.2	232.5	216.5	238.2	239.2
chin	173.3	198.2	232.3	216.3	238.2	239.2
clavicular area	173.5	198.2	232.5	216.5	238.2	239.2
clitoris	184.3	198.82	233.3	221.2	236.3	239.5
columnella	173.3	198.2	232.3	216.3	238.2	239.2
concha	173.2	198.2	232.2	216.2	238.2	239.2
contiguous sites	173.8	—	—	—	—	—
ear (external)	173.2	198.2	232.2	216.2	238.2	239.2
elbow	173.6	198.2	232.6	216.6	238.2	239.2
eyebrow	173.3	198.2	232.3	216.3	238.2	239.2
eyelid	173.1	198.2	232.1	216.1	238.2	239.2
face NEC	173.3	198.2	232.3	216.3	238.2	239.2
female genital organs						
(external)	184.4	198.82	233.3	221.2	236.3	239.5
clitoris	184.3	198.82	233.3	221.2	236.3	239.5
labium NEC	184.4	198.82	233.3	221.2	236.3	239.5
majus	184.1	198.82	233.3	221.2	236.3	239.5
minus	184.2	198.82	233.3	221.2	236.3	239.5
pudendum	184.4	198.82	233.3	221.2	236.3	239.5
vulva	184.4	198.82	233.3	221.2	236.3	239.5
finger	173.6	198.2	232.6	216.6	238.2	239.2
flank	173.5	198.2	232.5	216.5	238.2	239.2
foot	173.7	198.2	232.7	216.7	238.2	239.2
forearm	173.6	198.2	232.6	216.6	238.2	239.2
forehead	173.3	198.2	232.3	216.3	238.2	239.2
glabella	173.3	198.2	232.3	216.3	238.2	239.2
gluteal region	173.5	198.2	232.5	216.5	238.2	239.2
groin	173.5	198.2	232.5	216.5	238.2	239.2
hand	173.6	198.2	232.6	216.6	238.2	239.2
head NEC	173.4	198.2	232.4	216.4	238.2	239.2
heel	173.7	198.2	232.7	216.7	238.2	239.2
helix	173.2	198.2	232.2	216.2	238.2	239.2
hip	173.7	198.2	232.7	216.7	238.2	239.2
infraclavicular region	173.5	198.2	232.5	216.5	238.2	239.2
inguinal region	173.5	198.2	232.5	216.5	238.2	239.2
jaw	173.3	198.2	232.3	216.3	238.2	239.2
knee	173.7	198.2	232.7	216.7	238.2	239.2

Index to Diseases

	Malignant			Benign	Uncertain Behavior	Unspecified
	Primary	Secondary	Ca in situ			
Neoplasm, neoplastic — *continued*						
skin NEC — *continued*						
labia						
majora	184.1	198.82	233.3	221.2	236.3	239.5
minora	184.2	198.82	233.3	221.2	236.3	239.5
leg	173.7	198.2	232.7	216.7	238.2	239.2
lid (lower) (upper)	173.1	198.2	232.1	216.1	238.2	239.2
limb NEC	173.9	198.2	232.9	216.9	238.2	239.5
lower	173.7	198.2	232.7	216.7	238.2	239.2
upper	173.6	198.2	232.6	216.6	238.2	239.2
lip (lower) (upper)	173.0	198.2	232.0	216.0	238.2	239.2
male genital organs	187.9	198.82	233.6	222.9	236.6	239.5
penis	187.4	198.82	233.5	222.1	236.6	239.5
prepuce	187.1	198.82	233.5	222.1	236.6	239.5
scrotum	187.7	198.82	233.6	222.4	236.6	239.5
mastectomy site	173.5	198.2	—	—	—	—
specified as breast tissue	174.8	198.81	—	—	—	—
meatus, acoustic (external)	173.2	198.2	232.2	216.2	238.2	239.2
melanoma — *see* Melanoma						
nates	173.5	198.2	232.5	216.5	238.2	239.0
neck	173.4	198.2	232.4	216.4	238.2	239.2
nose (external)	173.3	198.2	232.3	216.3	238.2	239.2
palm	173.6	198.2	232.6	216.6	238.2	239.2
palpebra	173.1	198.2	232.1	216.1	238.2	239.2
penis NEC	187.4	198.82	233.5	222.1	236.6	239.5
perianal	173.5	198.2	232.5	216.5	238.2	239.2
perineum	173.5	198.2	232.5	216.5	238.2	239.2
pinna	173.2	198.2	232.2	216.2	238.2	239.2
plantar	173.7	198.2	232.7	216.7	238.2	239.2
popliteal fossa or space	173.7	198.2	232.7	216.7	238.2	239.2
prepuce	187.1	198.82	233.5	222.1	236.6	239.5
pubes	173.5	198.2	232.5	216.5	238.2	239.2
sacrococcygeal region	173.5	198.2	232.5	216.5	238.2	239.2
scalp	173.4	198.2	232.4	216.4	238.2	239.2
scapular region	173.5	198.2	232.5	216.5	238.2	239.2
scrotum	187.7	198.82	233.6	222.4	236.6	239.5
shoulder	173.6	198.2	232.6	216.6	238.2	239.2
sole (foot)	173.7	198.2	232.7	216.7	238.2	239.2
specified sites NEC	173.8	198.2	232.8	216.8	232.8	239.2
submammary fold	173.5	198.2	232.5	216.5	238.2	239.2
supraclavicular region	173.4	198.2	232.4	216.4	238.2	239.2
temple	173.3	198.2	232.3	216.3	238.2	239.2
thigh	173.7	198.2	232.7	216.7	238.2	239.2
thoracic wall	173.5	198.2	232.5	216.5	238.2	239.2
thumb	173.6	198.2	232.6	216.6	238.2	239.2
toe	173.7	198.2	232.7	216.7	238.2	239.2
tragus	173.2	198.2	232.2	216.2	238.2	239.2
trunk	173.5	198.2	232.5	216.5	238.2	239.2
umbilicus	173.5	198.2	232.5	216.5	238.2	239.2
vulva	184.4	198.82	233.3	221.2	236.3	239.5
wrist	173.6	198.2	232.6	216.6	238.2	239.2
skull	170.0	198.5	—	213.0	238.0	239.2
soft parts or tissues — *see* Neoplasm, connective tissue						
specified site NEC	195.8	198.89	234.8	229.8	238.8	239.8
spermatic cord	187.6	198.82	233.6	222.8	236.6	239.5
sphenoid	160.5	197.3	231.8	212.0	235.9	239.1
bone	170.0	198.5	—	213.0	238.0	239.2
sinus	160.5	197.3	231.8	212.0	235.9	239.1
sphincter						
anal	154.2	197.5	230.5	211.4	235.5	239.0
of Oddi	156.1	197.8	230.8	211.5	235.3	239.0

Neoplasm, spine, spinal — Index to Disease

	Malignant			Benign	Uncertain Behavior	Unspecified
	Primary	Secondary	Ca in situ			
Neoplasm, neoplastic — *continued*						
spine, spinal (column)	170.2	198.5	—	213.2	238.0	239.2
bulb	191.7	198.3	—	225.0	237.5	239.6
coccyx	170.6	198.5	—	213.6	238.0	239.2
cord (cervical) (lumbar) (sacral) (thoracic)	192.2	198.3	—	225.3	237.5	239.7
dura mater	192.3	198.4	—	225.4	237.6	239.7
lumbosacral	170.2	198.5	—	213.2	238.0	239.2
membrane	192.3	198.4	—	225.4	237.6	239.7
meninges	192.3	198.4	—	225.4	237.6	239.7
nerve (root)	171.9	198.89	—	215.9	238.1	239.2
pia mater	192.3	198.4	—	225.4	237.6	239.7
root	171.9	198.89	—	215.9	238.1	239.2
sacrum	170.6	198.5	—	213.6	238.0	239.2
spleen, splenic NEC	159.1	197.8	230.9	211.9	235.5	239.0
flexure (colon)	153.7	197.5	230.3	211.3	235.2	239.0
stem, brain	191.7	198.3	—	225.0	237.5	239.6
Stensen's duct	142.0	198.89	230.0	210.2	235.0	239.0
sternum	170.3	198.5	—	213.3	238.0	239.2
stomach	151.9	197.8	230.2	211.1	235.2	239.0
antrum (pyloric)	151.2	197.8	230.2	211.1	235.2	239.0
body	151.4	197.8	230.2	211.1	235.2	239.0
cardia	151.0	197.8	230.2	211.1	235.2	239.0
cardiac orifice	151.0	197.8	230.2	211.1	235.2	239.0
contiguous sites	151.8	—	—	—	—	—
corpus	151.4	197.8	230.2	211.1	235.2	239.0
fundus	151.3	197.8	230.2	211.1	235.2	239.0
greater curvature NEC	151.6	197.8	230.2	211.1	235.2	239.0
lesser curvature NEC	151.5	197.8	230.2	211.1	235.2	239.0
prepylorus	151.1	197.8	230.2	211.1	235.2	239.0
pylorus	151.1	197.8	230.2	211.1	235.2	239.0
wall NEC	151.9	197.8	230.2	211.1	235.2	239.0
anterior NEC	151.8	197.8	230.2	211.1	235.2	239.0
posterior NEC	151.8	197.8	230.2	211.1	235.2	239.0
stroma, endometrial	182.0	198.82	233.2	219.1	236.0	239.5
stump, cervical	180.8	198.82	233.1	219.0	236.0	239.5
subcutaneous (nodule) (tissue) NEC — *see* Neoplasm, connective tissue						
subdural	192.1	198.4	—	225.2	237.6	239.7
subglottis, subglottic	161.2	197.3	231.0	212.1	235.6	239.1
sublingual	144.9	198.89	230.0	210.3	235.1	239.0
gland or duct	142.2	198.89	230.0	210.2	235.0	239.0
submandibular gland	142.1	198.89	230.0	210.2	235.0	239.0
submaxillary gland or duct	142.1	198.89	230.0	210.2	235.0	239.0
submental	195.0	198.89	234.8	229.8	238.8	239.8
subpleural	162.9	197.0	—	212.3	235.7	239.1
substernal	164.2	197.1	—	212.5	235.8	239.8
sudoriferous, sudoriparous gland, site unspecified specified site — *see* Neoplasm, skin	173.9	198.2	232.9	216.9	238.2	239.2
supraclavicular region	195.0	198.89	234.8	229.8	238.8	239.8
supraglottis	161.1	197.3	231.0	212.1	235.6	239.1
suprarenal (capsule) (cortex) (gland) (medulla)	194.0	198.7	234.8	227.0	237.2	239.7
suprasellar (region)	191.9	198.3	—	225.0	237.5	239.6
sweat gland (apocrine) (eccrine), site unspecified	173.9	198.2	232.9	216.9	238.2	239.2
specified site — *see* Neoplasm, skin						
sympathetic nerve or nervous system NEC	171.9	198.89	—	215.9	238.1	239.2
symphysis pubis	170.6	198.5	—	213.6	238.0	239.2

Index to Diseases — Neoplasm, tonsil

	Malignant			Benign	Uncertain Behavior	Unspecified
	Primary	Secondary	Ca in situ			
Neoplasm, neoplastic — *continued*						
synovial membrane — *see Neoplasm, connective tissue*						
tapetum, brain	191.8	198.3	—	225.0	237.5	239.6
tarsus (any bone)	170.8	198.5	—	213.8	238.0	239.2
temple (skin)	173.3	198.2	232.3	216.3	238.2	239.2
temporal						
bone	170.0	198.5	—	213.0	238.0	239.2
lobe or pole	191.2	198.3	—	225.0	237.5	239.6
region	195.0	198.89	234.8	229.8	238.8	239.8
skin	173.3	198.2	232.3	216.3	238.2	239.2
tendon (sheath) — *see Neoplasm, connective tissue*						
tentorium (cerebelli)	192.1	198.4	—	225.2	237.6	239.7
testis, testes (descended) (scrotal)	186.9	198.82	233.6	222.0	236.4	239.5
ectopic	186.0	198.82	233.6	222.0	236.4	239.5
retained	186.0	198.82	233.6	222.0	236.4	239.5
undescended	186.0	198.82	233.6	222.0	236.4	239.5
thalamus	191.0	198.3	—	225.0	237.5	239.6
thigh NEC*	195.5	198.89	234.8	229.8	238.8	239.8
thorax, thoracic (cavity) (organs NEC)	195.1	198.89	234.8	229.8	238.8	239.8
duct	171.4	198.89	—	215.4	238.1	239.2
wall NEC	195.1	198.89	234.8	229.8	238.8	239.8
throat	149.0	198.89	230.0	210.9	235.1	239.0
thumb NEC*	195.4	198.89	232.6	229.8	238.8	239.8
thymus (gland)	164.0	198.89	—	212.6	235.8	239.8
contiguous sites with heart and mediastinum	164.8	—	—	—	—	—
thyroglossal duct	193	198.89	234.8	226	237.4	239.7
thyroid (gland)	193	198.89	234.8	226	237.4	239.7
cartilage	161.3	197.3	231.0	212.1	235.6	239.1
tibia (any part)	170.7	198.5	—	213.7	238.0	239.2
toe NEC*	195.5	198.89	232.7	229.8	238.8	239.8
tongue	141.9	198.89	230.0	210.1	235.1	239.0
anterior (two-thirds) NEC	141.4	198.89	230.0	210.1	235.1	239.0
dorsal surface	141.1	198.89	230.0	210.1	235.1	239.0
ventral surface	141.3	198.89	230.0	210.1	235.1	239.0
base (dorsal surface)	141.0	198.89	230.0	210.1	235.1	239.0
border (lateral)	141.2	198.89	230.0	210.1	235.1	239.0
contiguous sites	141.8	—	—	—	—	—
dorsal surface NEC	141.1	198.89	230.0	210.1	235.1	239.0
fixed part NEC	141.0	198.89	230.0	210.1	235.1	239.0
foreamen cecum	141.1	198.89	230.0	210.1	235.1	239.0
frenulum linguae	141.3	198.89	230.0	210.1	235.1	239.0
junctional zone	141.5	198.89	230.0	210.1	235.1	239.0
margin (lateral)	141.2	198.89	230.0	210.1	235.1	239.0
midline NEC	141.1	198.89	230.0	210.1	235.1	239.0
mobile part NEC	141.4	198.89	230.0	210.1	235.1	239.0
posterior (third)	141.0	198.89	230.0	210.1	235.1	239.0
root	141.0	198.89	230.0	210.1	235.1	239.0
surface (dorsal)	141.1	198.89	230.0	210.1	235.1	239.0
base	141.0	198.89	230.0	210.1	235.1	239.0
ventral	141.3	198.89	230.0	210.1	235.1	239.0
tip	141.2	198.89	230.0	210.1	235.1	239.0
tonsil	141.6	198.89	230.0	210.1	235.1	239.0
tonsil	146.0	198.89	230.0	210.5	235.1	239.0
fauces, faucial	146.0	198.89	230.0	210.5	235.1	239.0
lingual	141.6	198.89	230.0	210.1	235.1	239.0
palatine	146.0	198.89	230.0	210.5	235.1	239.0
pharyngeal	147.1	198.89	230.0	210.7	235.1	239.0

✓4ᵗʰ Fourth-digit Required   ✓5ᵗʰ Fifth-digit Required

Neoplasm, tonsil

	Malignant			Benign	Uncertain Behavior	Unspecified
	Primary	Secondary	Ca in situ			
Neoplasm, neoplastic — *continued*						
tonsil — *continued*						
pillar (anterior) (posterior)	146.2	198.89	230.0	210.6	235.1	239.0
tonsillar fossa	146.1	198.89	230.0	210.6	235.1	239.0
tooth socket NEC	143.9	198.89	230.0	210.4	235.1	239.0
trachea (cartilage) (mucosa)	162.0	197.3	231.1	212.2	235.7	239.1
contiguous sites with						
bronchus or lung	162.8	—	—	—	—	—
tracheobronchial	162.8	197.3	231.1	212.2	235.7	239.1
contiguous sites with lung	162.8	—	—	—	—	—
tragus	173.2	198.2	232.2	216.2	238.2	239.2
trunk NEC*	195.8	198.89	232.5	229.8	238.8	239.8
tubo-ovarian	183.8	198.82	233.3	221.8	236.3	239.5
tunica vaginalis	187.8	198.82	233.6	222.8	236.6	239.5
turbinate (bone)	170.0	198.5	—	213.0	238.0	239.2
nasal	160.0	197.3	231.8	212.0	235.9	239.1
tympanic cavity	160.1	197.3	231.8	212.0	235.9	239.1
ulna (any part)	170.4	198.5	—	213.4	238.0	239.2
umbilicus, umbilical	173.5	198.2	232.5	216.5	238.2	239.2
uncus, brain	191.2	198.3	—	225.0	237.5	239.6
unknown site or unspecified	199.1	199.1	234.9	229.9	238.9	239.9
urachus	188.7	198.1	233.7	223.3	236.7	239.4
ureter, ureteral	189.2	198.1	233.9	223.2	236.91	239.5
orifice (bladder)	188.6	198.1	233.7	223.3	236.7	239.4
ureter-bladder junction	188.6	198.1	233.7	223.3	236.7	239.4
urethra, urethral (gland)	189.3	198.1	233.9	223.81	236.99	239.5
orifice, internal	188.5	198.1	233.7	223.3	236.7	239.4
urethrovaginal (septum)	184.9	198.82	233.3	221.9	236.3	239.5
urinary organ or system NEC	189.9	198.1	233.9	223.9	236.99	239.5
bladder — *see* Neoplasm, bladder						
contiguous sites	189.8	—	—	—	—	—
specified sites NEC	189.8	198.1	233.9	223.89	236.99	239.5
utero-ovarian	183.8	198.82	233.3	221.8	236.3	239.5
ligament	183.3	198.82	—	221.0	236.3	239.5
uterosacral ligament	183.4	198.82	—	221.0	236.3	239.5
uterus, uteri, uterine	179	198.82	233.2	219.9	236.0	239.5
adnexa NEC	183.9	198.82	233.3	221.8	236.3	239.5
contiguous sites	183.8	—	—	—	—	—
body	182.0	198.82	233.2	219.1	236.0	239.5
contiguous sites	182.8	—	—	—	—	—
cervix	180.9	198.82	233.1	219.0	236.0	239.5
tornu	182.0	198.82	233.2	219.1	236.0	239.5
corpus	182.0	198.82	233.2	219.1	236.0	239.5
endocervix (canal) (gland)	180.0	198.82	233.1	219.0	236.0	239.5
endometrium	182.0	198.82	233.2	219.1	236.0	239.5
exocervix	180.1	198.82	233.1	219.0	236.0	239.5
external os	180.1	198.82	233.1	219.0	236.0	239.5
fundus	182.0	198.82	233.2	219.1	236.0	239.5
internal os	180.0	198.82	233.1	219.0	236.0	239.5
isthmus	182.1	198.82	233.2	219.1	236.0	239.5
ligament	183.4	198.82	—	221.0	236.3	239.5
broad	183.3	198.82	233.3	221.0	236.3	239.5
round	183.5	198.82	—	221.0	236.3	239.5
lower segment	182.1	198.82	233.2	219.1	236.0	239.5
myometrium	182.0	198.82	233.2	219.1	236.0	239.5
squamocolumnar junction	180.8	198.82	233.1	219.0	236.0	239.5
tube	183.2	198.82	233.3	221.0	236.3	239.5
utricle, prostatic	189.3	198.1	233.9	223.81	236.99	239.5
uveal tract	190.0	198.4	234.0	224.0	238.8	239.8
uvula	145.4	198.89	230.0	210.4	235.1	239.0
vagina, vaginal (fornix) (vault) (wall)	184.0	198.82	233.3	221.1	236.3	239.5

Index to Diseases

Neoplasm, Zuckerkandl's organ

	Malignant			Benign	Uncertain Behavior	Unspecified
	Primary	Secondary	Ca in situ			
Neoplasm, neoplastic — *continued*						
vaginovesical	184.9	198.82	233.3	221.9	236.3	239.5
septum	194.9	198.82	233.3	221.9	236.3	239.5
vallecula (epiglottis)	146.3	198.89	230.0	210.6	235.1	239.0
vascular — *see* Neoplasm, connective tissue						
vas deferens	187.6	198.82	233.6	222.8	236.6	239.5
Vater's ampulla	156.2	197.8	230.8	211.5	235.3	239.0
vein, venous — *see* Neoplasm, connective tissue						
vena cava (abdominal) (inferior)	171.5	198.89	—	215.5	238.1	239.2
superior	171.4	198.89	—	215.4	238.1	239.2
ventricle (cerebral) (floor) (fourth) (lateral) (third)	191.5	198.3	—	225.0	237.5	239.6
cardiac (left) (right)	164.1	198.89	—	212.7	238.8	239.8
ventricular band of larynx	161.1	197.3	231.0	212.1	235.6	239.1
ventriculus — *see* Neoplasm, stomach						
vermillion border — *see* Neoplasm, lip						
vermis, cerebellum	191.6	198.3	—	225.0	237.5	239.6
vertebra (column)	170.2	198.5	—	213.2	238.0	239.2
coccyx	170.6	198.5	—	213.6	238.0	239.2
sacrum	170.6	198.5	—	213.6	238.0	239.2
vesical — *see* Neoplasm, bladder						
vesicle, seminal	187.8	198.82	233.6	222.8	236.6	239.5
vesicocervical tissue	184.9	198.82	233.3	221.9	236.3	239.5
vesicorectal	195.3	198.89	234.8	229.8	238.8	239.8
vesicovaginal	184.9	198.82	233.3	221.9	236.3	239.5
septum	184.9	198.82	233.3	221.9	236.3	239.5
vessel (blood) — *see* Neoplasm, connective tissue						
vestibular gland, greater	184.1	198.82	233.3	221.2	236.3	239.5
vestibule						
mouth	145.1	198.89	230.0	210.4	235.1	239.0
nose	160.0	197.3	231.8	212.0	235.9	239.1
Virchow's gland	—	196.0	—	229.0	238.8	239.8
viscera NEC	195.8	198.89	234.8	229.8	238.8	239.8
vocal cords (true)	161.0	197.3	231.0	212.1	235.6	239.1
false	161.1	197.3	231.0	212.1	235.6	239.1
vomer	170.0	198.5	—	213.0	238.0	239.2
vulva	184.4	198.82	233.3	221.2	236.3	239.5
vulvovaginal gland	184.4	198.82	233.3	221.2	236.3	239.5
Waldeyer's ring	149.1	198.89	230.0	210.9	235.1	239.0
Wharton's duct	142.1	198.89	230.0	210.2	235.0	239.0
white matter (central) (cerebral)	191.0	198.3	—	225.0	237.5	239.6
windpipe	162.0	197.3	231.1	212.2	235.7	239.1
Wirsung's duct	157.3	197.8	230.9	211.6	235.5	239.0
wolffian (body) (duct)						
female	184.8	198.82	233.3	221.8	236.3	239.5
male	187.8	198.82	233.6	222.8	236.6	239.5
womb — *see* Neoplasm, uterus						
wrist NEC*	195.4	198.89	232.6	229.8	238.8	239.8
xiphoid process	170.3	198.5	—	213.3	238.0	239.2
Zuckerkandl's organ	194.6	198.89	—	227.6	237.3	239.7

✓4ᵗʰ Fourth-digit Required   ✓5ᵗʰ Fifth-digit Required

Neovascularization
 choroid 362.16
 ciliary body 364.42
 cornea 370.60
  deep 370.63
  localized 370.61
 iris 364.42
 retina 362.16
 subretinal 362.16
Nephralgia 788.0
Nephritis, nephritic (albuminuric) (azotemic) (congenital) (degenerative) (diffuse) (disseminated) (epithelial) (familial) (focal) (granulomatous) (hemorrhagic) (infantile) (nonsuppurative, excretory) (uremic) 583.9
 with
  edema — see Nephrosis
  lesion of
   glomerulonephritis
    hypocomplementemic persistent 583.2
     with nephrotic syndrome 581.2
      chronic 582.2
    lobular 583.2
     with nephrotic syndrome 581.2
      chronic 582.2
    membranoproliferative 583.2
     with nephrotic syndrome 581.2
      chronic 582.2
    membranous 583.1
     with nephrotic syndrome 581.1
      chronic 582.1
    mesangiocapillary 583.2
     with nephrotic syndrome 581.2
      chronic 582.2
    mixed membranous and proliferative 583.2
     with nephrotic syndrome 581.2
      chronic 582.2
    proliferative (diffuse) 583.0
     with nephrotic syndrome 581.0
      acute 580.0
      chronic 582.0
    rapidly progressive 583.4
     acute 580.4
     chronic 582.4
   interstitial nephritis (diffuse) (focal) 583.89
    with nephrotic syndrome 581.89
    acute 580.89
    chronic 582.89
   necrotizing glomerulitis 583.4
    acute 580.4
    chronic 582.4
   renal necrosis 583.9
    cortical 583.6
    medullary 583.7
   specified pathology NEC 583.89
    with nephrotic syndrome 581.89
    acute 580.89
    chronic 582.89
  necrosis, renal 583.9
   cortical 583.6
   medullary (papillary) 583.7
  nephrotic syndrome (see also Nephrosis) 581.9
  papillary necrosis 583.7
  specified pathology NEC 583.89
 acute 580.9
  extracapillary with epithelial crescents 580.4

Nephritis, nephritic — continued
 acute — continued
  hypertensive (see also Hypertension, kidney) 403.90
  necrotizing 580.4
  poststreptococcal 580.0
  proliferative (diffuse) 580.0
  rapidly progressive 580.4
  specified pathology NEC 580.89
 amyloid 277.3 [583.81]
  chronic 277.3 [582.81]
 arteriolar (see also Hypertension, kidney) 403.90
 arteriosclerotic (see also Hypertension, kidney) 403.90
 ascending (see also Pyelitis) 590.80
 atrophic 582.9
 basement membrane NEC 583.89
  with
   pulmonary hemorrhage (Goodpasture's syndrome) 446.21 [583.81]
 calculous, calculus 592.0
 cardiac (see also Hypertension, kidney) 403.90
 cardiovascular (see also Hypertension, kidney) 403.90
 chronic 582.9
  arteriosclerotic (see also Hypertension, kidney) 403.90
  hypertensive (see also Hypertension, kidney) 403.90
 cirrhotic (see also Sclerosis, renal) 587
 complicating pregnancy, childbirth, or puerperium 646.2 ✓5ᵗʰ
  with hypertension 642.1 ✓5ᵗʰ
  affecting fetus or newborn 760.0
  affecting fetus or newborn 760.1
 croupous 580.9
 desquamative — see Nephrosis
 due to
  amyloidosis 277.3 [583.81]
   chronic 277.3 [582.81]
  arteriosclerosis (see also Hypertension, kidney) 403.90
  diabetes mellitus 250.4 ✓5ᵗʰ [583.81]
   with nephrotic syndrome 250.4 ✓5ᵗʰ [581.81]
  diphtheria 032.89 [580.81]
  gonococcal infection (acute) 098.19 [583.81]
   chronic or duration of 2 months or over 098.39 [583.81]
  gout 274.10
  infectious hepatitis 070.9 [580.81]
  mumps 072.79 [580.81]
  specified kidney pathology NEC 583.89
   acute 580.89
   chronic 582.89
  streptotrichosis 039.8 [583.81]
  subacute bacterial endocarditis 421.0
  systemic lupus erythematosus 710.0 [583.81]
   chronic 710.0 [582.81]
  typhoid fever 002.0 [580.81]
 endothelial 582.2
 end stage (chronic) (terminal) NEC 585
 epimembranous 581.1
 exudative 583.89
  with nephrotic syndrome 581.89
  acute 580.89
  chronic 582.89
 gonococcal (acute) 098.19 [583.81]
  chronic or duration of 2 months or over 098.39 [583.81]

Nephritis, nephritic — *continued*
  gouty 274.10
  hereditary (Alport's syndrome) 759.89
  hydremic — *see* Nephrosis
  hypertensive (*see also* Hypertension, kidney)
    403.90
  hypocomplementemic persistent 583.2
    with nephrotic syndrome 581.2
    chronic 582.2
  immune complex NEC 583.89
  infective (*see also* Pyelitis) 590.80
  interstitial (diffuse) (focal) 583.89
    with nephrotic syndrome 581.89
    acute 580.89
    chronic 582.89
  latent or quiescent — *see* Nephritis, chronic
  lead 984.9
    specified type of lead — *see* Table of Drugs
      and Chemicals
  lobular 583.2
    with nephrotic syndrome 581.2
    chronic 582.2
  lupus 710.0 [583.81]
    acute 710.0 [580.81]
    chronic 710.0 [582.81]
  membranoproliferative 583.2
    with nephrotic syndrome 581.2
    chronic 582.2
  membranous 583.1
    with nephrotic syndrome 581.1
    chronic 582.1
  mesangiocapillary 583.2
    with nephrotic syndrome 581.2
    chronic 582.2
  minimal change 581.3
  mixed membranous and proliferative 583.2
    with nephrotic syndrome 581.2
    chronic 582.2
  necrotic, necrotizing 583.4
    acute 580.4
    chronic 582.4
  nephrotic — *see* Nephrosis
  old — *see* Nephritis, chronic
  parenchymatous 581.89
  polycystic 753.12
    adult type (APKD) 753.13
    autosomal dominant 753.13
    autosomal recessive 753.14
    childhood type (CPKD) 753.14
    infantile type 753.14
  poststreptococcal 580.0
  pregnancy — *see* Nephritis, complicating
    pregnancy
  proliferative 583.0
    with nephrotic syndrome 581.0
    acute 580.0
    chronic 582.0
  purulent (*see also* Pyelitis) 590.80
  rapidly progressive 583.4
    acute 580.4
    chronic 582.4
  salt-losing or salt-wasting (*see also* Disease,
    renal) 593.9
  saturnine 984.9
    specified type of lead — *see* Table of Drugs
      and Chemicals
  septic (*see also* Pyelitis) 590.80
  specified pathology NEC 583.89
    acute 580.89
    chronic 582.89
  staphylococcal (*see also* Pyelitis) 590.80

Nephritis, nephritic — *continued*
  streptotrichosis 039.8 [583.81]
  subacute (*see also* Nephrosis) 581.9
  suppurative (*see also* Pyelitis) 590.80
  syphilitic (late) 095.4
    congenital 090.5 [583.81]
    early 091.69 [583.81]
  terminal (chronic) (end-stage) NEC 585
  toxic — *see* Nephritis, acute
  tubal, tubular — *see* Nephrosis, tubular
  tuberculous (*see also* Tuberculosis) 016.0 ✓5ᵗʰ
    [583.81]
  type II (Ellis) — *see* Nephrosis
  vascular — *see* Hypertension, kidney
  war 580.9
Nephroblastoma (M8960/3) 189.0
  epithelial (M8961/3) 189.0
  mesenchymal (M8962/3) 189.0
Nephrocalcinosis 275.49
Nephrocystitis, pustular (*see also* Pyelitis)
  590.80
Nephrolithiasis (congenital) (pelvis) (recurrent)
  592.0
  uric acid 274.11
Nephroma (M8960/3) 189.0
  mesoblastic (M8960/1) 236.9 ✓5ᵗʰ
Nephronephritis (*see also* Nephrosis) 581.9
Nephronopthisis 753.16
Nephropathy (*see also* Nephritis) 583.9
  with
    exudative nephritis 583.89
    interstitial nephritis (diffuse) (focal) 583.89
    medullary necrosis 583.7
    necrosis 583.9
      cortical 583.6
      medullary or papillary 583.7
    papillary necrosis 583.7
    specified lesion or cause NEC 583.89
  analgesic 583.89
    with medullary necrosis, acute 584.7
  arteriolar (*see also* Hypertension, kidney)
    403.90
  arteriosclerotic (*see also* Hypertension, kidney)
    403.90
  complicating pregnancy 646.2 ✓5ᵗʰ
  diabetic 250.4 ✓5ᵗʰ [583.81]
  gouty 274.10
    specified type NEC 274.19
  hypercalcemic 588.8
  hypertensive (*see also* Hypertension, kidney)
    403.90
  hypokalemic (vacuolar) 588.8
  obstructive 593.89
    congenital 753.20
  phenacetin 584.7
  phosphate-losing 588.0
  potassium depletion 588.8
  proliferative (*see also* Nephritis, proliferative)
    583.0
  protein-losing 588.8
  salt-losing or salt-wasting (*see also* Disease,
    renal) 593.9
  sickle-cell (*see also* Disease, sickle-cell) 282.60
    [583.81]
  toxic 584.5
  vasomotor 584.5
  water-losing 588.8
Nephroptosis (*see also* Disease, renal) 593.0
  congenital (displaced) 753.3
Nephropyosis (*see also* Abscess, kidney) 590.2

✓4ᵗʰ Fourth-digit Required   ✓5ᵗʰ Fifth-digit Required

Nephrorrhagia 593.81
Nephrosclerosis (arteriolar) (arteriosclerotic) (chronic) (hyaline) (see also Hypertension, kidney) 403.90
  gouty 274.10
  hyperplastic (arteriolar) (see also Hypertension, kidney) 403.90
  senile (see also Sclerosis, renal) 587
Nephrosis, nephrotic (Epstein's) (syndrome) 581.9
  with
    lesion of
      focal glomerulosclerosis 581.1
      glomerulonephritis
        endothelial 581.2
        hypocomplementemic persistent 581.2
        lobular 581.2
        membranoproliferative 581.2
        membranous 581.1
        mesangiocapillary 581.2
        minimal change 581.3
        mixed membranous and proliferative 581.2
        proliferative 581.0
      segmental hyalinosis 581.1
      specified pathology NEC 581.89
  acute — see Nephrosis, tubular
  anoxic — see Nephrosis, tubular
  arteriosclerotic (see also Hypertension, kidney) 403.90
  chemical — see Nephrosis, tubular
  cholemic 572.4
  complicating pregnancy, childbirth, or puerperium — see Nephritis, complicating pregnancy
  diabetic 250.4 ✓5ᵗʰ [581.81]
  hemoglobinuric — see Nephrosis, tubular
  in
    amyloidosis 277.3 [581.81]
    diabetes mellitus 250.4 ✓5ᵗʰ [581.81]
    epidemic hemorrhagic fever 078.6
    malaria 084.9 [581.81]
    polyarteritis 446.0 [581.81]
    systemic lupus erythematosus 710.0 [581.81]
  ischemic — see Nephrosis, tubular
  lipoid 581.3
  lower nephron — see Nephrosis, tubular
  lupoid 710.0 [581.81]
  lupus 710.0 [581.81]
  malarial 084.9 [581.81]
  minimal change 581.3
  necrotizing — see Nephrosis, tubular
  osmotic (sucrose) 588.8
  polyarteritic 446.0 [581.81]
  radiation 581.9
  specified lesion or cause NEC 581.89
  syphilitic 095.4
  toxic — see Nephrosis, tubular
  tubular (acute) 584.5
    due to a procedure 997.5
    radiation 581.9
Nephrosonephritis hemorrhagic (endemic) 078.6
Nephrostomy status V44.6
  with complication 997.5
Nerve — see condition
Nerves 799.2

Nervous (see also condition) 799.2
  breakdown 300.9
  heart 306.2
  stomach 306.4
  tension 799.2
Nervousness 799.2
Nesidioblastoma (M8150/0)
  pancreas 211.7
  specified site NEC — see Neoplasm, by site, benign
  unspecified site 211.7
Netherton's syndrome (ichthyosiform erythroderma) 757.1
Nettle rash 708.8
Nettleship's disease (urticaria pigmentosa) 757.33
Neumann's disease (pemphigus vegetans) 694.4
Neuralgia, neuralgic (acute) (see also Neuritis) 729.2
  accessory (nerve) 352.4
  acoustic (nerve) 388.5
  ankle 355.8
  anterior crural 355.8
  anus 787.99
  arm 723.4
  auditory (nerve) 388.5
  axilla 353.0
  bladder 788.1
  brachial 723.4
  brain — see Disorder, nerve, cranial
  broad ligament 625.9
  cerebral — see Disorder, nerve, cranial
  ciliary 346.2 ✓5ᵗʰ
  cranial nerve — see also Disorder, nerve, cranial
    fifth or trigeminal (see also Neuralgia, trigeminal) 350.1
  ear 388.71
    middle 352.1
  facial 351.8
  finger 354.9
  flank 355.8
  foot 355.8
  forearm 354.9
  Fothergill's (see also Neuralgia, trigeminal) 350.1
    postherpetic 053.12
  glossopharyngeal (nerve) 352.1
  groin 355.8
  hand 354.9
  heel 355.8
  Horton's 346.2 ✓5ᵗʰ
  Hunt's 053.11
  hypoglossal (nerve) 352.5
  iliac region 355.8
  infraorbital (see also Neuralgia, trigeminal) 350.1
  inguinal 355.8
  intercostal (nerve) 353.8
    postherpetic 053.19
  jaw 352.1
  kidney 788.0
  knee 355.8
  loin 355.8
  malarial (see also Malaria) 084.6
  mastoid 385.89
  maxilla 352.1
  median thenar 354.1
  metatarsal 355.6
  middle ear 352.1

Neuralgia, neuralgic — *continued*
  migrainous 346.2 ✓5ᵗʰ
  Morton's 355.6
  nerve, cranial — *see* Disorder, nerve, cranial
  nose 352.0
  occipital 723.8
  ophthalmic 377.30
    postherpetic 053.19
  optic (nerve) 377.30
  penis 607.9
  perineum 355.8
  pleura 511.0
  postherpetic NEC 053.19
    geniculate ganglion 053.11
    ophthalmic 053.19
    trifacial 053.12
    trigeminal 053.12
  pubic region 355.8
  radial (nerve) 723.4
  rectum 787.99
  sacroiliac joint 724.3
  sciatic (nerve) 724.3
  scrotum 608.9
  seminal vesicle 608.9
  shoulder 354.9
  Sluder's 337.0
  specified nerve NEC — *see* Disorder, nerve
  spermatic cord 608.9
  sphenopalatine (ganglion) 337.0
  subscapular (nerve) 723.4
  suprascapular (nerve) 723.4
  testis 608.89
  thenar (median) 354.1
  thigh 355.8
  tongue 352.5
  trifacial (nerve) (*see also* Neuralgia, trigeminal) 350.1
  trigeminal (nerve) 350.1
    postherpetic 053.12
  tympanic plexus 388.71
  ulnar (nerve) 723.4
  vagus (nerve) 352.3
  wrist 354.9
  writers' 300.89
    organic 333.84
Neurapraxia — *see* Injury, nerve, by site
Neurasthenia 300.5
  cardiac 306.2
  gastric 306.4
  heart 306.2
  postfebrile 780.79
  postviral 780.79
Neurilemmoma (M9560/0) — *see also* Neoplasm, connective tissue, benign
  acoustic (nerve) 225.1
  malignant (M9560/3) — *see also* Neoplasm, connective tissue, malignant
    acoustic (nerve) 192.0
Neurilemmosarcoma (M9560/3) — *see* Neoplasm, connective tissue, malignant
Neurilemoma — *see* Neurilemmoma
Neurinoma (M9560/0) — *see* Neurilemmoma
Neurinomatosis (M9560/1) — *see also* Neoplasm, connective tissue, uncertain behavior
  centralis 759.5
Neuritis (*see also* Neuralgia) 729.2
  abducens (nerve) 378.54
  accessory (nerve) 352.4

Neuritis — *continued*
  acoustic (nerve) 388.5
    syphilitic 094.86
  alcoholic 357.5
    with psychosis 291.1
  amyloid, any site 277.3 [357.4]
  anterior crural 355.8
  arising during pregnancy 646.4 ✓5ᵗʰ
  arm 723.4
  ascending 355.2
  auditory (nerve) 388.5
  brachial (nerve) NEC 723.4
    due to displacement, intervertebral disc 722.0
  cervical 723.4
  chest (wall) 353.8
  costal region 353.8
  cranial nerve — *see also* Disorder, nerve, cranial
    first or olfactory 352.0
    second or optic 377.30
    third or oculomotor 378.52
    fourth or trochlear 378.53
    fifth or trigeminal (*see also* Neuralgia, trigeminal) 350.1
    sixth or abducens 378.54
    seventh or facial 351.8
      newborn 767.5
    eighth or acoustic 388.5
    ninth or glossopharyngeal 352.1
    tenth or vagus 352.3
    eleventh or accessory 352.4
    twelfth or hypoglossal 352.5
  Déjérine-Sottas 356.0
  diabetic 250.6 ✓5ᵗʰ [357.2]
  diphtheritic 032.89 [357.4]
  due to
    beriberi 265.0 [357.4]
    displacement, prolapse, protrusion, or rupture of intervertebral disc 722.2
      cervical 722.0
      lumbar, lumbosacral 722.10
      thoracic, thoracolumbar 722.11
    herniation, nucleus pulposus 722.2
      cervical 722.0
      lumbar, lumbosacral 722.10
      thoracic, thoracolumbar 722.11
  endemic 265.0 [357.4]
  facial (nerve) 351.8
    newborn 767.5
  general — *see* Polyneuropathy
  geniculate ganglion 351.1
    due to herpes 053.11
  glossopharyngeal (nerve) 352.1
  gouty 274.89 [357.4]
  hypoglossal (nerve) 352.5
  ilioinguinal (nerve) 355.8
  in diseases classified elsewhere — *see* Polyneuropathy, in
  infectious (multiple) 357.0
  intercostal (nerve) 353.8
  interstitial hypertrophic progressive NEC 356.9
  leg 355.8
  lumbosacral NEC 724.4
  median (nerve) 354.1
    thenar 354.1
  multiple (acute) (infective) 356.9
    endemic 265.0 [357.4]
  multiplex endemica 265.0 [357.4]
  nerve root (*see also* Radiculitis) 729.2

Neuritis — *continued*
  oculomotor (nerve) 378.52
  olfactory (nerve) 352.0
  optic (nerve) 377.30
    in myelitis 341.0
    meningococcal 036.81
  pelvic 355.8
  peripheral (nerve) — *see also* Neuropathy, peripheral
    complicating pregnancy or puerperium 646.4 ☑5ᵗʰ
    specified nerve NEC — *see* Mononeuritis
  pneumogastric (nerve) 352.3
  postchickenpox 052.7
  postherpetic 053.19
  progressive hypertrophic interstitial NEC 356.9
  puerperal, postpartum 646.4 ☑5ᵗʰ
  radial (nerve) 723.4
  retrobulbar 377.32
    syphilitic 094.85
  rheumatic (chronic) 729.2
  sacral region 355.8
  sciatic (nerve) 724.3
    due to displacement of intervertebral disc 722.10
  serum 999.5
  specified nerve NEC — *see* Disorder, nerve
  spinal (nerve) 355.9
    root (*see also* Radiculitis) 729.2
  subscapular (nerve) 723.4
  suprascapular (nerve) 723.4
  syphilitic 095.8
  thenar (median) 354.1
  thoracic NEC 724.4
  toxic NEC 357.7
  trochlear (nerve) 378.53
  ulnar (nerve) 723.4
  vagus (nerve) 352.3
Neuroangiomatosis, encephalofacial 759.6
Neuroastrocytoma (M9505/1) — *see* Neoplasm, by site, uncertain behavior
Neuro-avitaminosis 269.2
Neuroblastoma (M9500/3)
  olfactory (M9522/3) 160.0
  specified site — *see* Neoplasm, by site, malignant
  unspecified site 194.0
Neurochorioretinitis (*see also* Chorioretinitis) 363.20
Neurocirculatory asthenia 306.2
Neurocytoma (M9506/0) — *see* Neoplasm, by site, benign
Neurodermatitis (circumscribed) (circumscripta) (local) 698.3
  atopic 691.8
  diffuse (Brocq) 691.8
  disseminated 691.8
  nodulosa 698.3
Neuroencephalomyelopathy, optic 341.0
Neuroepithelioma (M9503/3) — *see also* Neoplasm, by site, malignant
  olfactory (M9521/3) 160.0
Neurofibroma (M9540/0) — *see also* Neoplasm, connective tissue, benign
  melanotic (M9541/0) — *see* Neoplasm, connective tissue, benign
  multiple (M9540/1) 237.70
    type 1 237.71

Neurofibroma — *continued*
  multiple — *continued*
    type 2 237.72
    plexiform (M9550/0) — *see* Neoplasm, connective tissue, benign
Neurofibromatosis (multiple) (M9540/1) 237.70
  acoustic 237.72
  malignant (M9540/3) — *see* Neoplasm, connective tissue, malignant
  type 1 237.71
  type 2 237.72
  von Recklinghausen's 237.71
Neurofibrosarcoma (M9540/3) — *see* Neoplasm, connective tissue, malignant
Neurogenic — *see also* condition
  bladder (atonic) (automatic) (autonomic) (flaccid) (hypertonic) (hypotonic) (inertia) (infranuclear) (irritable) (motor) (nonreflex) (nuclear) (paralysis) (reflex) (sensory) (spastic) (supranuclear) (uninhibited) 596.54
    with cauda equina syndrome 344.61
  bowel 564.81
  heart 306.2
Neuroglioma (M9505/1) — *see* Neoplasm, by site, uncertain behavior
Neurolabyrinthitis (of Dix and Hallpike) 386.12
Neurolathyrism 988.2
Neuroleprosy 030.1
Neuroleptic malignant syndrome 333.92
Neurolipomatosis 272.8
Neuroma (M9570/0) — *see also* Neoplasm, connective tissue, benign
  acoustic (nerve) (M9560/0) 225.1
  amputation (traumatic) — *see also* Injury, nerve, by site
    surgical complication (late) 997.61
  appendix 211.3
  auditory nerve 225.1
  digital 355.6
  toe 355.6
  interdigital (toe) 355.6
  intermetatarsal 355.6
  Morton's 355.6
  multiple 237.70
    type 1 237.71
    type 2 237.72
  nonneoplastic 355.9
    arm NEC 354.9
    leg NEC 355.8
    lower extremity NEC 355.8
    specified site NEC — *see* Mononeuritis, by site
    upper extremity NEC 354.9
  optic (nerve) 225.1
  plantar 355.6
  plexiform (M9550/0) — *see* Neoplasm, connective tissue, benign
  surgical (nonneoplastic) 355.9
    arm NEC 354.9
    leg NEC 355.8
    lower extremity NEC 355.8
    upper extremity NEC 354.9
  traumatic — *see also* Injury, nerve, by site
    old — *see* Neuroma, nonneoplastic
Neuromyalgia 729.1
Neuromyasthenia (epidemic) 049.8
Neuromyelitis 341.8
  ascending 357.0
  optica 341.0

Neuromyopathy NEC 358.9
Neuromyositis 729.1
Neuronevus (M8725/0) — see Neoplasm, skin, benign
Neuronitis 357.0
  ascending (acute) 355.2
  vestibular 386.12
Neuroparalytic — see condition
Neuropathy, neuropathic (see also Disorder, nerve) 355.9
  acute motor 357.82
  alcoholic 357.5
    with psychosis 291.1
  arm NEC 354.9
  autonomic (peripheral) — see Neuropathy, peripheral, autonomic
  axillary nerve 353.0
  brachial plexus 353.0
  cervical plexus 353.2
  chronic
    progressive segmentally demyelinating 357.89 ▲
    relapsing demyelinating 357.89 ▲
  congenital sensory 356.2
  Déjérine-Sottas 356.0
  diabetic 250.6 [5ᵗʰ] [357.2]
  entrapment 355.9
    iliohypogastric nerve 355.79
    ilioinguinal nerve 355.79
    lateral cutaneous nerve of thigh 355.1
    median nerve 354.0
    obturator nerve 355.79
    peroneal nerve 355.3
    posterior tibial nerve 355.5
    saphenous nerve 355.79
    ulnar nerve 354.2
  facial nerve 351.9
  hereditary 356.9
    peripheral 356.0
    sensory (radicular) 356.2
  hypertrophic
    Charcôt-Marie-Tooth 356.1
    Déjérine-Sottas 356.0
    interstitial 356.9
    Refsum 356.3
  intercostal nerve 354.8
  ischemic — see Disorder, nerve
  Jamaican (ginger) 357.7
  leg NEC 355.8
  lower extremity NEC 355.8
  lumbar plexus 353.1
  median nerve 354.1
  motor
    acute 357.82
  multiple (acute) (chronic) (see also Polyneuropathy) 356.9
  optic 377.39
    ischemic 377.41
    nutritional 377.33
    toxic 377.34
  peripheral (nerve) (see also Polyneuropathy) 356.9
    arm NEC 354.9
    autonomic 337.9
      amyloid 277.3 [337.1]
      idiopathic 337.0
      in
        amyloidosis 277.3 [337.1]
        diabetes (mellitus) 250.6 [5ᵗʰ] [337.1]
        diseases classified elsewhere 337.1
        gout 274.89 [337.1]

Neuropathy, neuropathic — continued
  peripheral — continued
    autonomic — continued
      in — continued
        hyperthyroidism 242.9 [5ᵗʰ] [337.1]
      due to
        antitetanus serum 357.6
        arsenic 357.7
        drugs 357.6
        lead 357.7
        organophosphate compounds 357.7
        toxic agent NEC 357.7
      hereditary 356.0
      idiopathic 356.9
        progressive 356.4
        specified type NEC 356.8
      in diseases classified elsewhere — see Polyneuropathy, in
    leg NEC 355.8
    lower extremity NEC 355.8
    upper extremity NEC 354.9
  plantar nerves 355.6
  progressive hypertrophic interstitial 356.9
  radicular NEC 729.2
    brachial 723.4
    cervical NEC 723.4
    hereditary sensory 356.2
    lumbar 724.4
    lumbosacral 724.4
    thoracic NEC 724.4
  sacral plexus 353.1
  sciatic 355.0
  spinal nerve NEC 355.9
    root (see also Radiculitis) 729.2
  toxic 357.7
  trigeminal sensory 350.8
  ulnar nerve 354.2
  upper extremity NEC 354.9
  uremic 585 [357.4]
  vitamin B₁₂ 266.2 [357.4]
    with anemia (pernicious) 281.0 [357.4]
      due to dietary deficiency 281.1 [357.4]
Neurophthisis — (see also Disorder, nerve peripheral) 356.9
  diabetic 250.6 [5ᵗʰ] [357.2]
Neuropraxia — see Injury, nerve
Neuroretinitis 363.05
  syphilitic 094.85
Neurosarcoma (M9540/3) — see Neoplasm, connective tissue, malignant
Neurosclerosis — see Disorder, nerve
Neurosis, neurotic 300.9
  accident 300.16
  anancastic, anankastic 300.3
  anxiety (state) 300.00
    generalized 300.02
    panic type 300.01
  asthenic 300.5
  bladder 306.53
  cardiac (reflex) 306.2
  cardiovascular 306.2
  climacteric, unspecified type 627.2
  colon 306.4
  compensation 300.16
  compulsive, compulsion 300.3
  conversion 300.11
  craft 300.89
  cutaneous 306.3
  depersonalization 300.6
  depressive (reaction) (type) 300.4

Neurosis, neurotic

Neurosis, neurotic — *continued*
  endocrine 306.6
  environmental 300.89
  fatigue 300.5
  functional (*see also* Disorder, psychosomatic) 306.9
  gastric 306.4
  gastrointestinal 306.4
  genitourinary 306.50
  heart 306.2
  hypochondriacal 300.7
  hysterical 300.10
    conversion type 300.11
    dissociative type 300.15
  impulsive 300.3
  incoordination 306.0
    larynx 306.1
    vocal cord 306.1
  intestine 306.4
  larynx 306.1
    hysterical 300.11
    sensory 306.1
  menopause, unspecified type 627.2
  mixed NEC 300.89
  musculoskeletal 306.0
  obsessional 300.3
    phobia 300.3
  obsessive-compulsive 300.3
  occupational 300.89
  ocular 306.7
  oral 307.0
  organ (*see also* Disorder, psychosomatic) 306.9
  pharynx 306.1
  phobic 300.20
  posttraumatic (acute) (situational) 308.3
    chronic 309.81
  psychasthenic (type) 300.89
  railroad 300.16
  rectum 306.4
  respiratory 306.1
  rumination 306.4
  senile 300.89
  sexual 302.70
  situational 300.89
  specified type NEC 300.89
  state 300.9
    with depersonalization episode 300.6
  stomach 306.4
  vasomotor 306.2
  visceral 306.4
  war 300.16
Neurospongioblastosis diffusa 759.5
Neurosyphilis (arrested) (early) (inactive) (late) (latent) (recurrent) 094.9
  with ataxia (cerebellar) (locomotor) (spastic) (spinal) 094.0
  acute meningitis 094.2
  aneurysm 094.89
  arachnoid (adhesive) 094.2
  arteritis (any artery) 094.89
  asymptomatic 094.3
  congenital 090.40
  dura (mater) 094.89
  general paresis 094.1
  gumma 094.9
  hemorrhagic 094.9
  juvenile (asymptomatic) (meningeal) 090.40
  leptomeninges (aseptic) 094.2
  meningeal 094.2
  meninges (adhesive) 094.2

Neurosyphilis — *continued*
  meningovascular (diffuse) 094.2
  optic atrophy 094.84
  parenchymatous (degenerative) 094.1
  paresis (*see also* Paresis, general) 094.1
  paretic (*see also* Paresis, general) 094.1
  relapse 094.9
  remission in (sustained) 094.9
  serological 094.3
  specified nature or site NEC 094.89
  tabes (dorsalis) 094.0
    juvenile 090.40
  tabetic 094.0
    juvenile 090.40
  taboparesis 094.1
    juvenile 090.40
  thrombosis 094.89
  vascular 094.89
Neurotic (*see also* Neurosis) 300.9
  excoriation 698.4
    psychogenic 306.3
Neurotmesis — *see* Injury, nerve, by site
Neurotoxemia — *see* Toxemia
Neutroclusion 524.2
Neutropenia, neutropenic (chronic) (cyclic) (drug-induced) (genetic) (idiopathic) (immune) (infantile) (malignant) (periodic) (pernicious) (primary) (splenic) (splenomegaly) (toxic) 288.0
  chronic hypoplastic 288.0
  congenital (nontransient) 288.0
  fever 288.0
  neonatal, transitory (isoimmune) (maternal transfer) 776.7
Neutrophilia, hereditary giant 288.2
Nevocarcinoma (M8720/3) — *see* Melanoma
Nevus (M8720/0) — *see also* Neoplasm, skin, benign

> Note — Except where otherwise indicated, varieties of nevus in the list below that are followed by a morphology code number (M----/0) should be coded by site as for "Neoplasm, skin, benign."

  acanthotic 702.8
  achromic (M8730/0)
  amelanotic (M8730/0)
  anemic, anemicus 709.09
  angiomatous (M9120/0) (*see also* Hemangioma) 228.00
  araneus 448.1
  avasculosus 709.09
  balloon cell (M8722/0)
  bathing trunk (M8761/1) 238.2
  blue (M8780/0)
    cellular (M8790/0)
    giant (M8790/0)
    Jadassohn's (M8780/0)
    malignant (M8780/3) — *see* Melanoma
  capillary (M9131/0) (*see also* Hemangioma) 228.00
  cavernous (M9121/0) (*see also* Hemangioma) 228.00
  cellular (M8720/0)
    blue (M8790/0)
  comedonicus 757.33
  compound (M8760/0)
  conjunctiva (M8720/0) 224.3

Index to Diseases

Nevus — *continued*
  dermal (M8750/0)
    and epidermal (M8760/0)
  epithelioid cell (and spindle cell) (M8770/0)
  flammeus 757.32
    osteohypertrophic 759.89
  hairy (M8720/0)
  halo (M8723/0)
  hemangiomatous (M9120/0) (*see also* Hemangioma) 228.00
  intradermal (M8750/0)
  intraepidermal (M8740/0)
  involuting (M8724/0)
  Jadassohn's (blue) (M8780/0)
  junction, junctional (M8740/0)
    malignant melanoma in (M8740/3) — *see* Melanoma
  juvenile (M8770/0)
  lymphatic (M9170/0) 228.1
  magnocellular (M8726/0)
    specified site — *see* Neoplasm, by site, benign
    unspecified site 224.0
  malignant (M8720/3) — *see* Melanoma
  meaning hemangioma (M9120/0) (*see also* Hemangioma) 228.00
  melanotic (pigmented) (M8720/0)
  multiplex 759.5
  nonneoplastic 448.1
  nonpigmented (M8730/0)
  nonvascular (M8720/0)
  oral mucosa, white sponge 750.26
  osteohypertrophic, flammeus 759.89
  papillaris (M8720/0)
  papillomatosus (M8720/0)
  pigmented (M8720/0)
    giant (M8761/1) — *see also* Neoplasm, skin, uncertain behavior
      malignant melanoma in (M8761/3) — *see* Melanoma
    systematicus 757.33
  pilosus (M8720/0)
  port wine 757.32
  sanguineous 757.32
  sebaceous (senile) 702.8
  senile 448.1
  spider 448.1
  spindle cell (and epithelioid cell) (M8770/0)
  stellar 448.1
  strawberry 757.32
  syringocystadenomatous papilliferous (M8406/0)
  unius lateris 757.33
  Unna's 757.32
  vascular 757.32
  verrucous 757.33
  white sponge (oral mucosa) 750.26
Newborn (infant) (liveborn)
  gestation
    24 completed weeks 765.22
    25-26 completed weeks 765.23
    27-28 completed weeks 765.24
    29-30 completed weeks 765.25
    31-32 completed weeks 765.26
    33-34 completed weeks 765.27
    35-36 completed weeks 765.28
    37 or more completed weeks 765.29
    less than 24 completed weeks 765.21
    unspecified completed weeks 765.20

Newborn — *continued*
  multiple NEC
    born in hospital (without mention of cesarean delivery or section) V37.00
      with cesarean delivery or section V37.01
    born outside hospital
      hospitalized V37.1
      not hospitalized V37.2
    mates all liveborn
      born in hospital (without mention of cesarean delivery or section) V34.00
        with cesarean delivery or section V34.01
      born outside hospital
        hospitalized V34.1
        not hospitalized V34.2
    mates all stillborn
      born in hospital (without mention of cesarean delivery or section) V35.00
        with cesarean delivery or section V35.01
      born outside hospital
        hospitalized V35.1
        not hospitalized V35.2
    mates liveborn and stillborn
      born in hospital (without mention of cesarean delivery or section) V36.00
        with cesarean delivery or section V36.01
      born outside hospital
        hospitalized V36.1
        not hospitalized V36.2
  single
    born in hospital (without mention of cesarean delivery or section) V30.00
      with cesarean delivery or section V30.01
    born outside hospital
      hospitalized V30.1
      not hospitalized V30.2
  twin NEC
    born in hospital (without mention of cesarean delivery or section) V33.00
      with cesarean delivery or section V33.01
    born outside hospital
      hospitalized V33.1
      not hospitalized V33.2
    mate liveborn
      born in hospital V31.0
      born outside hospital
        hospitalized V31.1
        not hospitalized V31.2
    mate stillborn
      born in hospital V32.0
      born outside hospital
        hospitalized V32.1
        not hospitalized V32.2
  unspecified as to single or multiple birth
    born in hospital (without mention of cesarean delivery or section) V39.00
      with cesarean delivery or section V39.01
    born outside hospital
      hospitalized V39.1
      not hospitalized V39.2

Newcastle's conjunctivitis or disease 077.8

Nezelof's syndrome (pure alymphocytosis) 279.13

Niacin (amide) deficiency 265.2

Nicolas-Durand-Favre disease (climatic bubo) 099.1
Nicolas-Favre disease (climatic bubo) 099.1
Nicotinic acid (amide) deficiency 265.2
Niemann-Pick disease (lipid histiocytosis) (splenomegaly) 272.7
Night
   blindness (see also Blindness, night) 368.60
      congenital 368.61
      vitamin A deficiency 264.5
   cramps 729.82
   sweats 780.8
   terrors, child 307.46
Nightmare 307.47
   REM-sleep type 307.47
Nipple — see condition
Nisbet's chancre 099.0
Nishimoto (-Takeuchi) disease 437.5
Nitritoid crisis or reaction — see Crisis, nitritoid
Nitrogen retention, extrarenal 788.9
Nitrosohemoglobinemia 289.8
Njovera 104.0
No
   diagnosis 799.9
   disease (found) V71.9
   room at the inn V65.0
Nocardiasis — see Nocardiosis
Nocardiosis 039.9
   with pneumonia 039.1
   lung 039.1
   specified type NEC 039.8
Nocturia 788.43
   psychogenic 306.53
Nocturnal — see also condition
   dyspnea (paroxysmal) 786.09
   emissions 608.89
   enuresis 788.36
      psychogenic 307.6
   frequency (micturition) 788.43
      psychogenic 306.53
Nodal rhythm disorder 427.89
Nodding of head 781.0
Node(s) — see also Nodule
   Heberden's 715.04
   larynx 478.79
   lymph — see condition
   milkers' 051.1
   Osler's 421.0
   rheumatic 729.89
   Schmorl's 722.30
      lumbar, lumbosacral 722.32
      specified region NEC 722.39
      thoracic, thoracolumbar 722.31
   singers' 478.5
   skin NEC 782.2
   tuberculous — see Tuberculosis, lymph gland
   vocal cords 478.5
Nodosities, Haygarth's 715.04
Nodule(s), nodular
   actinomycotic (see also Actinomycosis) 039.9
   arthritic — see Arthritis, nodosa
   cutaneous 782.2
   Haygarth's 715.04
   inflammatory — see Inflammation
   juxta-articular 102.7
      syphilitic 095.7

Nodule(s), nodular — continued
   juxta-articular — continued
      yaws 102.7
   larynx 478.79
   lung, solitary 518.89
      emphysematous 492.8
   milkers' 051.1
   prostate 600.1
   rheumatic 729.89
   rheumatoid — see Arthritis, rheumatoid
   scrotum (inflammatory) 608.4
   singers' 478.5
   skin NEC 782.2
   solitary, lung 518.89
      emphysematous 492.8
   subcutaneous 782.2
   thyroid (gland) (nontoxic) (uninodular) 241.0
      with
         hyperthyroidism 242.1
         thyrotoxicosis 242.1
      toxic or with hyperthyroidism 242.1
   vocal cords 478.5
Noma (gangrenous) (hospital) (infective) 528.1
   auricle (see also Gangrene) 785.4
   mouth 528.1
   pudendi (see also Vulvitis) 616.10
   vulvae (see also Vulvitis) 616.10
Nomadism V60.0
Non-adherence
   artificial skin graft 996.55
   decellularized allodermis graft 996.55
Non-autoimmune hemolytic anemia NEC 283.10
Nonclosure — see also Imperfect, closure
   ductus
      arteriosus 747.0
      Botalli 747.0
   Eustachian valve 746.89
   foramen
      Botalli 745.5
      ovale 745.5
Noncompliance with medical treatment V15.81
Nondescent (congenital) — see also Malposition, congenital
   cecum 751.4
   colon 751.4
   testis 752.51
Nondevelopment
   brain 742.1
      specified part 742.2
   heart 746.89
   organ or site, congenital NEC — see Hypoplasia
Nonengagement
   head NEC 652.5
      in labor 660.1
         affecting fetus or newborn 763.1
Nonexanthematous tick fever 066.1
Nonexpansion, lung (newborn) NEC 770.4
Nonfunctioning
   cystic duct (see also Disease, gallbladder) 575.8
   gallbladder (see also Disease, gallbladder) 575.8
   kidney (see also Disease, renal) 593.9
   labyrinth 386.58
Nonhealing
   stump (surgical) 997.69

Nonhealing — *continued*
  wound, surgical 998.83
Nonimplantation of ovum, causing infertility 628.3
Noninsufflation, fallopian tube 628.2
Nonne-Milroy-Meige syndrome (chronic hereditary edema) 757.0
Nonovulation 628.0
Nonpatent fallopian tube 628.2
Nonpneumatization, lung NEC 770.4
Nonreflex bladder 596.54
  with cauda equina 344.61
Nonretention of food — *see* Vomiting
Nonrotation — *see* Malrotation
Nonsecretion, urine (*see also* Anuria) 788.5
  newborn 753.3
Nonunion
  fracture 733.82
  organ or site, congenital NEC — *see* Imperfect, closure
  symphysis pubis, congenital 755.69
  top sacrum, congenital 756.19
Nonviability 765.0
Nonvisualization, gallbladder 793.3
Nonvitalized tooth 522.9
Normal
  delivery — *see* category 650
  menses V65.5
  state (feared complaint unfounded) V65.5
Normoblastosis 289.8
Normocytic anemia (infectional) 285.9
  due to blood loss (chronic) 280.0
    acute 285.1
Norrie's disease (congenital) (progressive oculoacousticocerebral degeneration) 743.8
North American blastomycosis 116.0
Norwegian itch 133.0
Nose, nasal — *see* condition
Nosebleed 784.7
Nosomania 298.9
Nosophobia 300.29
Nostalgia 309.89
Notch of iris 743.46
Notched lip, congenital (*see also* Cleft, lip) 749.10
Notching nose, congenital (tip) 748.1
Nothnagel's
  syndrome 378.52
  vasomotor acroparesthesia 443.89
Novy's relapsing fever (American) 087.1
Noxious
  foodstuffs, poisoning by
    fish 988.0
    fungi 988.1
    mushrooms 988.1
    plants (food) 988.2
    shellfish 988.0
    specified type NEC 988.8
    toadstool 988.1
  substances transmitted through placenta or breast milk 760.70
    alcohol 760.71
    anti-infective agents 760.74
    cocaine 760.75
    "crack" 760.75
    diethylstilbestrol (DES) 760.76

Noxious — *continued*
  substances transmitted through placenta or breast milk — *continued*
    hallucinogenic agents NEC 760.73
    medicinal agents NEC 760.79
    narcotics 760.72
    obstetric anesthetic or analgesic 763.5
    specified agent NEC 760.79
    suspected, affecting management of pregnancy 655.5
Nuchal hitch (arm) 652.8
Nucleus pulposus — *see* condition
Numbness 782.0
Nuns' knee 727.2
Nursemaid's
  elbow 832.0
  shoulder 831.0
Nutmeg liver 573.8
Nutrition, deficient or insufficient (particular kind of food) 269.9
  due to
    insufficient food 994.2
    lack of
      care (child) (infant) 995.52
        adult 995.84
      food 994.2
Nyctalopia (*see also* Blindness, night) 368.60
  vitamin A deficiency 264.5
Nycturia 788.43
  psychogenic 306.53
Nymphomania 302.89
Nystagmus 379.50
  associated with vestibular system disorders 379.54
  benign paroxysmal positional 386.11
  central positional 386.2
  congenital 379.51
  deprivation 379.53
  dissociated 379.55
  latent 379.52
  miners' 300.89
  positional
    benign paroxysmal 386.11
    central 386.2
  specified NEC 379.56
  vestibular 379.54
  visual deprivation 379.53

Oasthouse urine disease 270.2
Obermeyer's relapsing fever (European) 087.0
Obesity (constitutional) (exogenous) (familial) (nutritional) (simple) 278.00
  adrenal 255.8
  due to hyperalimentation 278.00
  endocrine NEC 259.9
  endogenous 259.9
  Fröhlich's (adiposogenital dystrophy) 253.8
  glandular NEC 259.9
  hypothyroid (see also Hypothyroidism) 244.9
  morbid 278.01
  of pregnancy 646.1 ✓5ᵗʰ
  pituitary 253.8
  thyroid (see also Hypothyroidism) 244.9
Oblique — see also condition
  lie before labor, affecting fetus or newborn 761.7
Obliquity, pelvis 738.6
Obliteration
  abdominal aorta 446.7
  appendix (lumen) 543.9
  artery 447.1
  ascending aorta 446.7
  bile ducts 576.8
    with calculus, choledocholithiasis, or stones — see Choledocholithiasis
    congenital 751.61
      jaundice from 751.61 [774.5]
  common duct 576.8
    with calculus, choledocholithiasis, or stones — see Choledocholithiasis
    congenital 751.61
  cystic duct 575.8
    with calculus, choledocholithiasis, or stones — see Choledocholithiasis
  disease, arteriolar 447.1
  endometrium 621.8
  eye, anterior chamber 360.34
  fallopian tube 628.2
  lymphatic vessel 457.1
    postmastectomy 457.0
  organ or site, congenital NEC — see Atresia
  placental blood vessels — see Placenta, abnormal
  supra-aortic branches 446.7
  ureter 593.89
  urethra 599.84
  vein 459.9
  vestibule (oral) 525.8
Observation (for) V71.9
  without need for further medical care V71.9
  accident NEC V71.4
    at work V71.3
  criminal V71.6
  deleterious agent ingestion V71.89
  disease V71.9
    cardiovascular V71.7
    heart V71.7
    mental V71.09
    specified condition NEC V71.89
  foreign body ingestion V71.89
  growth and development variations V21.8
  injuries (accidental) V71.4
    inflicted NEC V71.6
      during alleged rape or seduction V71.5
  malignant neoplasm, suspected V71.1
  postpartum
    immediately after delivery V24.0

Observation (for) — continued
  postpartum — continued
    routine follow-up V24.2
  pregnancy
    high-risk V23.9
      specified problem NEC V23.8 ✓5ᵗʰ
    normal (without complication) V22.1
      with nonobstetric complication V22.2
      first V22.0
  rape or seduction, alleged V71.5
    injury during V71.5
  suicide attempt, alleged V71.89
  suspected (undiagnosed) (unproven)
    abuse V71.81
    cardiovascular disease V71.7
    child or wife battering victim V71.6
    concussion (cerebral) V71.6
    condition NEC V71.89
      infant — see Observation, suspected, condition, newborn
    newborn V29.9
      cardiovascular disease V29.8
      congenital anomaly V29.8
      genetic V29.3
      infectious V29.0
      ingestion foreign object V29.8
      injury V29.8
      metabolic V29.3
      neoplasm V29.8
      neurological V29.1
      poison, poisoning V29.8
      respiratory V29.2
      specified NEC V29.8
    exposure
      anthrax V71.82
      biologic agent NEC V71.83
    infectious disease not requiring isolation V71.89
    malignant neoplasm V71.1
    mental disorder V71.09
    neglect V71.81
    neoplasm
      benign V71.89
      malignant V71.1
    specified condition NEC V71.89
    tuberculosis V71.2
  tuberculosis, suspected V71.2
Obsession, obsessional 300.3
  ideas and mental images 300.3
  impulses 300.3
  neurosis 300.3
  phobia 300.3
  psychasthenia 300.3
  ruminations 300.3
  state 300.3
  syndrome 300.3
Obsessive-compulsive 300.3
  neurosis 300.3
  reaction 300.3
Obstetrical trauma NEC (complicating delivery) 665.9 ✓5ᵗʰ
  with
    abortion — see Abortion, by type, with damage to pelvic organs
    ectopic pregnancy (see also categories 633.0-633.9) 639.2
    molar pregnancy (see also categories 630-632) 639.2
  affecting fetus or newborn 763.89
  following
    abortion 639.2
    ectopic or molar pregnancy 639.2

Index to Diseases

Obstipation (see also Constipation) 564.00
  psychogenic 306.4
Obstruction, obstructed, obstructive
  airway NEC 519.8
    with
      allergic alveolitis NEC 495.9
      asthma NEC (see also Asthma) 493.9 ✓5ᵗʰ
        bronchiectasis 494.0
          with acute exacerbation 494.1
      bronchitis (chronic) (see also Bronchitis, with, obstruction) 491.20
      emphysema NEC 492.8
    chronic 496
      with
        allergic alveolitis NEC 495.5
        asthma NEC (see also Asthma) 493.2 ✓5ᵗʰ
          bronchiectasis 494.0
            with acute exacerbation 494.1
        bronchitis (chronic) (see also Bronchitis, with, obstruction) 491.20
        emphysema NEC 492.8
    due to
      bronchospasm 519.1
      foreign body 934.9
      inhalation of fumes or vapors 506.9
      laryngospasm 478.75
  alimentary canal (see also Obstruction, intestine) 560.9
  ampulla of Vater 576.2
    with calculus, cholelithiasis, or stones — see Choledocholithiasis
  aortic (heart) (valve) (see also Stenosis, aortic) 424.1
    rheumatic (see also Stenosis, aortic, rheumatic) 395.0
  aortoiliac 444.0
  aqueduct of Sylvius 331.4
    congenital 742.3
      with spina bifida (see also Spina bifida) 741.0 ✓5ᵗʰ
  Arnold-Chiari (see also Spina bifida) 741.0 ✓5ᵗʰ
  artery (see also Embolism, artery) 444.9
    basilar (complete) (partial) (see also Occlusion, artery, basilar) 433.0 ✓5ᵗʰ
    carotid (complete) (partial) (see also Occlusion, artery, carotid) 433.1 ✓5ᵗʰ
    precerebral — see Occlusion, artery, precerebral NEC
    retinal (central) (see also Occlusion, retina) 362.30
    vertebral (complete) (partial) (see also Occlusion, artery, vertebral) 433.2 ✓5ᵗʰ
  asthma (chronic) (with obstructive pulmonary disease) 493.2 ✓5ᵗʰ
  band (intestinal) 560.81
  bile duct or passage (see also Obstruction, biliary) 576.2
    congenital 751.61
      jaundice from 751.61 [774.5]
  biliary (duct) (tract) 576.2
    with calculus 574.51
      with cholecystitis (chronic) 574.41
        acute 574.31
    congenital 751.61
      jaundice from 751.61 [774.5]
  gallbladder 575.2
    with calculus 574.21
      with cholecystitis (chronic) 574.11
        acute 574.01

Obstruction, obstructed, obstructive — continued
  bladder neck (acquired) 596.0
    congenital 753.6
  bowel (see also Obstruction, intestine) 560.9
  bronchus 519.1
  canal, ear (see also Stricture, ear canal, acquired) 380.50
  cardia 537.89
  caval veins (inferior) (superior) 459.2
  cecum (see also Obstruction, intestine) 560.9
  circulatory 459.9
  colon (see also Obstruction, intestine) 560.9
    sympathicotonic 560.89
  common duct (see also Obstruction, biliary) 576.2
    congenital 751.61
  coronary (artery) (heart) — see also Arteriosclerosis, coronary
    acute (see also Infarct, myocardium) 410.9 ✓5ᵗʰ
      without myocardial infarction 411.81
  cystic duct (see also Obstruction, gallbladder) 575.2
    congenital 751.61
  device, implant, or graft — see Complications, due to (presence of) any device, implant, or graft classified to 996.0-996.5 NEC
  due to foreign body accidentally left in operation wound 998.4
  duodenum 537.3
    congenital 751.1
    due to
      compression NEC 537.3
      cyst 537.3
      intrinsic lesion or disease NEC 537.3
      scarring 537.3
      torsion 537.3
      ulcer 532.91
      volvulus 537.3
  ejaculatory duct 608.89
  endocardium 424.90
    arteriosclerotic 424.99
    specified cause, except rheumatic 424.99
  esophagus 530.3
  eustachian tube (complete) (partial) 381.60
    cartilaginous
      extrinsic 381.63
      intrinsic 381.62
    due to
      cholesteatoma 381.61
      osseous lesion NEC 381.61
      polyp 381.61
    osseous 381.61
  fallopian tube (bilateral) 628.2
  fecal 560.39
    with hernia — see also Hernia, by site, with obstruction
      gangrenous — see Hernia, by site, with gangrene
  foramen of Monro (congenital) 742.3
    with spina bifida (see also Spina bifida) 741.0 ✓5ᵗʰ
  foreign body — see Foreign body
  gallbladder 575.2
    with calculus, cholelithiasis, or stones 574.21
      with cholecystitis (chronic) 574.11
        acute 574.01
    congenital 751.69
      jaundice from 751.69 [774.5]
  gastric outlet 537.0

Obstruction, obstructed, obstructive —
   continued
   gastrointestinal (*see also* Obstruction,
      intestine) 560.9
   glottis 478.79
   hepatic 573.8
      duct (*see also* Obstruction, biliary) 576.2
         congenital 751.61
   icterus (*see also* Obstruction, biliary) 576.8
      congenital 751.61
   ileocecal coil (*see also* Obstruction, intestine)
      560.9
   ileum (*see also* Obstruction, intestine) 560.9
   iliofemoral (artery) 444.81
   internal anastomosis — *see* Complications,
      mechanical, graft
   intestine (mechanical) (neurogenic)
      (paroxysmal) (postinfectional) (reflex)
      560.9
      with
         adhesions (intestinal) (peritoneal) 560.81
         hernia — *see also* Hernia, by site, with
            obstruction
            gangrenous — *see* Hernia, by site,
               with gangrene
      adynamic (*see also* Ileus) 560.1
      by gallstone 560.31
      congenital or infantile (small) 751.1
         large 751.2
      due to
         Ascaris lumbricoides 127.0
         mural thickening 560.89
         procedure 997.4
            involving urinary tract 997.5
      impaction 560.39
      infantile — *see* Obstruction, intestine,
         congenital
      newborn
         due to
            fecaliths 777.1
            inspissated milk 777.2
            meconium (plug) 777.1
               in mucoviscidosis 277.01
            transitory 777.4
         specified cause NEC 560.89
         transitory, newborn 777.4
         volvulus 560.2
   intracardiac ball valve prosthesis 996.02
   jaundice (*see also* Obstruction, biliary) 576.8
      congenital 751.61
   jejunum (*see also* Obstruction, intestine)
      560.9
   kidney 593.89
   labor 660.9
      affecting fetus or newborn 763.1
      by
         bony pelvis (conditions classifiable to
            653.0-653.9) 660.1
         deep transverse arrest 660.3
         impacted shoulder 660.4
         locked twins 660.5
         malposition (fetus) (conditions
            classifiable to 652.0-652.9)
            660.0
         head during labor 660.3
         persistent occipitoposterior position
            660.3
         soft tissue, pelvic (conditions classifiable
            to 654.0-654.9) 660.2
   lacrimal
      canaliculi 375.53
      congenital 743.65

Obstruction, obstructed, obstructive —
   continued
   lacrimal — *continued*
      punctum 375.52
      sac 375.54
   lacrimonasal duct 375.56
      congenital 743.65
      neonatal 375.55
   lacteal, with steatorrhea 579.2
   laryngitis (*see also* Laryngitis) 464.01
   larynx 478.79
      congenital 748.3
   liver 573.8
      cirrhotic (*see also* Cirrhosis, liver) 571.5
   lung 518.89
      with
         asthma — *see* Asthma
         bronchitis (chronic) 491.2
         emphysema NEC 492.8
      airway, chronic 496
      chronic NEC 496
         with
            asthma (chronic) (obstructive)
               493.2
      disease, chronic 496
         with
            asthma (chronic) (obstructive)
               493.2
      emphysematous 492.8
   lymphatic 457.1
   meconium
      fetus or newborn 777.1
         in mucoviscidosis 277.01
      newborn due to fecaliths 777.1
   mediastinum 519.3
   mitral (rheumatic) — *see* Stenosis, mitral
   nasal 478.1
      duct 375.56
         neonatal 375.55
      sinus — *see* Sinusitis
   nasolacrimal duct 375.56
      congenital 743.65
      neonatal 375.55
   nasopharynx 478.29
   nose 478.1
   organ or site, congenital NEC — *see* Atresia
   pancreatic duct 577.8
   parotid gland 527.8
   pelviureteral junction (*see also* Obstruction,
      ureter) 593.4
   pharynx 478.29
   portal (circulation) (vein) 452
   prostate 600.9
      valve (urinary) 596.0
   pulmonary
      valve (heart) (*see also* Endocarditis,
         pulmonary) 424.3
      vein, isolated 747.49
   pyemic — *see* Septicemia
   pylorus (acquired) 537.0
      congenital 750.5
      infantile 750.5
   rectosigmoid (*see also* Obstruction, intestine)
      560.9
   rectum 569.49
   renal 593.89
   respiratory 519.8
      chronic 496
   retinal (artery) (vein) (central) (*see also*
      Occlusion, retina) 362.30
   salivary duct (any) 527.8
      with calculus 527.5

Index to Diseases — Occlusion

Obstruction, obstructed, obstructive — *continued*
  sigmoid (*see also* Obstruction, intestine) 560.9
  sinus (accessory) (nasal) (*see also* Sinusitis) 473.9
  Stensen's duct 527.8
  stomach 537.89
    acute 536.1
    congenital 750.7
  submaxillary gland 527.8
    with calculus 527.5
  thoracic duct 457.1
  thrombotic — *see* Thrombosis
  tooth eruption 520.6
  trachea 519.1
  tracheostomy airway 519.09
  tricuspid — *see* Endocarditis, tricuspid
  upper respiratory, congenital 748.8
  ureter (functional) 593.4
    congenital 753.20
    due to calculus 592.1
  ureteropelvic junction, congenital 753.21
  ureterovesical junction, congenital 753.22
  urethra 599.6
    congenital 753.6
  urinary (moderate) 599.6
    organ or tract (lower) 599.6
    prostatic valve 596.0
  uropathy 599.6
  uterus 621.8
  vagina 623.2
  valvular — *see* Endocarditis
  vascular graft or shunt 996.1
    atherosclerosis — *see* Arteriosclerosis, coronary
    embolism 996.74
    occlusion NEC 996.74
    thrombus 996.74
  vein, venous 459.2
    caval (inferior) (superior) 459.2
    thrombotic — *see* Thrombosis
  vena cava (inferior) (superior) 459.2
  ventricular shunt 996.2
  vesical 596.0
  vesicourethral orifice 596.0
  vessel NEC 459.9
Obturator — *see* condition
Occlusal wear, teeth 521.1
Occlusion
  anus 569.49
    congenital 751.2
    infantile 751.2
  aortoiliac (chronic) 444.0
  aqueduct of Sylvius 331.4
    congenital 742.3
      with spina bifida (*see also* Spina bifida) 741.0
  arteries of extremities, lower 444.22
    without thrombus or embolus (*see also* Arteriosclerosis, extremities) 440.20
    due to stricture or stenosis 447.1
    upper 444.21
      without thrombus or embolus (*see also* Arteriosclerosis, extremities) 440.20
      due to stricture or stenosis 447.1
  artery NEC (*see also* Embolism, artery) 444.9
    auditory, internal 433.8
    basilar 433.0
      with other precerebral artery 433.3
      bilateral 433.3

Occlusion — *continued*
  artery NEC — *continued*
    brain or cerebral (*see also* Infarct, brain) 434.9
    carotid 433.1
      with other precerebral artery 433.3
      bilateral 433.3
    cerebellar (anterior inferior) (posterior inferior) (superior) 433.8
    cerebral (*see also* Infarct, brain) 434.9
    choroidal (anterior) 433.8
    communicating posterior 433.8
    coronary (thrombotic) (*see also* Infarct, myocardium) 410.9
      acute 410.9
      without myocardial infarction 411.81
      healed or old 412
    hypophyseal 433.8
    iliac 444.81
    mesenteric (embolic) (thrombotic) (with gangrene) 557.0
    pontine 433.8
    precerebral NEC 433.9
      late effect — *see* Late effect(s) (of) cerebrovascular disease
      multiple or bilateral 433.3
      puerperal, postpartum, childbirth 674.0
      specified NEC 433.8
    renal 593.81
    retinal — *see* Occlusion, retina, artery
    spinal 433.8
    vertebral 433.2
      with other precerebral artery 433.3
      bilateral 433.3
  basilar (artery) — *see* Occlusion, artery, basilar
  bile duct (any) (*see also* Obstruction, biliary) 576.2
  bowel (*see also* Obstruction, intestine) 560.9
  brain (artery) (vascular) (*see also* Infarct, brain) 434.9
  breast (duct) 611.8
  carotid (artery) (common) (internal) — *see* Occlusion, artery, carotid
  cerebellar (anterior inferior) (artery) (posterior inferior) (superior) 433.8
  cerebral (artery) (*see also* Infarct, brain) 434.9
  cerebrovascular (*see also* Infarct, brain) 434.9
    diffuse 437.0
  cervical canal (*see also* Stricture, cervix) 622.4
    by falciparum malaria 084.0
  cervix (uteri) (*see also* Stricture, cervix) 622.4
  choanal 748.0
  choroidal (artery) 433.8
  colon (*see also* Obstruction, intestine) 560.9
  communicating posterior artery 433.8
  coronary (artery) (thrombotic) (*see also* Infarct, myocardium) 410.9
    acute 410.9
      without myocardial infarction 411.81
      healed or old 412
    without myocardial infarction 411.81
  cystic duct (*see also* Obstruction, gallbladder) 575.2
    congenital 751.69
  embolic — *see* Embolism

Occlusion — *continued*
  fallopian tube 628.2
    congenital 752.19
  gallbladder (*see also* Obstruction, gallbladder) 575.2
    congenital 751.69
      jaundice from 751.69 *[774.5]*
  gingiva, traumatic 523.8
  hymen 623.3
    congenital 752.42
  hypophyseal (artery) 433.8 ◢5ᵗʰ
  iliac artery 444.81
  intestine (*see also* Obstruction, intestine) 560.9
  kidney 593.89
  lacrimal apparatus — *see* Stenosis, lacrimal
  lung 518.89
  lymph or lymphatic channel 457.1
  mammary duct 611.8
  mesenteric artery (embolic) (thrombotic) (with gangrene) 557.0
  nose 478.1
    congenital 748.0
  organ or site, congenital NEC — *see* Atresia
  oviduct 628.2
    congenital 752.19
  periodontal, traumatic 523.8
  peripheral arteries (lower extremity) 444.22
    without thrombus or embolus (*see also* Arteriosclerosis, extremities) 440.20
    due to stricture or stenosis 447.1
    upper extremity 444.21
      without thrombus or embolus (*see also* Arteriosclerosis, extremities) 440.20
      due to stricture or stenosis 447.1
  pontine (artery) 433.8 ◢5ᵗʰ
  posterior lingual, of mandibular teeth 524.2
  precerebral artery — *see* Occlusion, artery, precerebral NEC
  puncta lacrimalia 375.52
  pupil 364.74
  pylorus (*see also* Stricture, pylorus) 537.0
  renal artery 593.81
  retina, retinal (vascular) 362.30
    artery, arterial 362.30
      branch 362.32
      central (total) 362.31
      partial 362.33
      transient 362.34
      tributary 362.32
    vein 362.30
      branch 362.36
      central (total) 362.35
      incipient 362.37
      partial 362.37
      tributary 362.36
  spinal artery 433.8 ◢5ᵗʰ
  stent
    coronary 996.72
  teeth (mandibular) (posterior lingual) 524.2
  thoracic duct 457.1
  tubal 628.2
  ureter (complete) (partial) 593.4
    congenital 753.29
  urethra (*see also* Stricture, urethra) 598.9
    congenital 753.6
  uterus 621.8
  vagina 623.2
  vascular NEC 459.9
  vein — *see* Thrombosis
  vena cava (inferior) (superior) 453.2
  ventricle (brain) NEC 331.4

Occlusion — *continued*
  vertebral (artery) — *see* Occlusion, artery, vertebral
  vessel (blood) NEC 459.9
  vulva 624.8
Occlusio pupillae 364.74
Occupational
  problems NEC V62.2
  therapy V57.21
Ochlophobia 300.29
Ochronosis (alkaptonuric) (congenital) (endogenous) 270.2
  with chloasma of eyelid 270.2
Ocular muscle — *see also* condition
  myopathy 359.1
  torticollis 781.93
Oculoauriculovertebral dysplasia 756.0
Oculogyric
  crisis or disturbance 378.87
    psychogenic 306.7
Oculomotor syndrome 378.81
Oddi's sphincter spasm 576.5
Odelberg's disease (juvenile osteochondrosis) 732.1
Odontalgia 525.9
Odontoameloblastoma (M9311/0) 213.1
  upper jaw (bone) 213.0
Odontoclasia 521.05
Odontoclasis 873.63
  complicated 873.73
Odontodysplasia, regional 520.4
Odontogenesis imperfecta 520.5
Odontoma (M9280/0) 213.1
  ameloblastic (M9311/0) 213.1
    upper jaw (bone) 213.0
  calcified (M9280/0) 213.1
    upper jaw (bone) 213.0
  complex (M9282/0) 213.1
    upper jaw (bone) 213.0
  compound (M9281/0) 213.1
    upper jaw (bone) 213.0
  fibroameloblastic (M9290/0) 213.1
    upper jaw (bone) 213.0
  follicular 526.0
  upper jaw (bone) 213.0
Odontomyelitis (closed) (open) 522.0
Odontonecrosis 521.09
Odontorrhagia 525.8
Odontosarcoma, ameloblastic (M9290/3) 170.1
  upper jaw (bone) 170.0
Odynophagia 787.2
Oesophagostomiasis 127.7
Oesophagostomum infestation 127.7
Oestriasis 134.0
Ogilvie's syndrome (sympathicotonic colon obstruction) 560.89
Oguchi's disease (retina) 368.61
Ohara's disease (*see also* Tularemia) 021.9
Oidiomycosis (*see also* Candidiasis) 112.9
Oidiomycotic meningitis 112.83
Oidium albicans infection (*see also* Candidiasis) 112.9
Old age 797
  dementia (of) 290.0
Olfactory — *see* condition
Oligemia 285.9

Oligergasia (see also Retardation, mental) 319
Oligoamnios 658.0
  affecting fetus or newborn 761.2
Oligoastrocytoma, mixed (M9382/3)
  specified site — see Neoplasm, by site, malignant
  unspecified site 191.9
Oligocythemia 285.9
Oligodendroblastoma (M9460/3)
  specified site — see Neoplasm, by site, malignant
  unspecified site 191.9
Oligodendroglioma (M9450/3)
  anaplastic type (M9451/3)
    specified site — see Neoplasm, by site, malignant
    unspecified site 191.9
  specified site — see Neoplasm, by site, malignant
  unspecified site 191.9
Oligodendroma — see Oligodendroglioma
Oligodontia (see also Anodontia) 520.0
Oligoencephalon 742.1
Oligohydramnios 658.0
  affecting fetus or newborn 761.2
  due to premature rupture of membranes 658.1
    affecting fetus or newborn 761.2
Oligohydrosis 705.0
Oligomenorrhea 626.1
Oligophrenia (see also Retardation, mental) 319
  phenylpyruvic 270.1
Oligospermia 606.1
Oligotrichia 704.09
  congenita 757.4
Oliguria 788.5
  with
    abortion — see Abortion, by type, with renal failure
    ectopic pregnancy (see also categories 633.0-633.9) 639.3
    molar pregnancy (see also categories 630-632) 639.3
  complicating
    abortion 639.3
    ectopic or molar pregnancy 639.3
    pregnancy 646.2
      with hypertension — see Toxemia, of pregnancy
  due to a procedure 997.5
  following labor and delivery 669.3
  heart or cardiac — see Failure, heart
  puerperal, postpartum 669.3
  specified due to a procedure 997.5
Ollier's disease (chondrodysplasia) 756.4
Omentitis (see also Peritonitis) 567.9
Omentocele (see also Hernia, omental) 553.8
Omentum, omental — see condition
Omphalitis (congenital) (newborn) 771.4
  not of newborn 686.9
  tetanus 771.3
Omphalocele 756.79
Omphalomesenteric duct, persistent 751.0
Omphalorrhagia, newborn 772.3
Omsk hemorrhagic fever 065.1
Onanism 307.9

Onchocerciasis 125.3
  eye 125.3 [360.13]
Onchocercosis 125.3
Oncocytoma (M8290/0) — see Neoplasm, by site, benign
Ondine's curse 348.8
Oneirophrenia (see also Schizophrenia) 295.4
Onychauxis 703.8
  congenital 757.5
Onychia (with lymphangitis) 681.9
  dermatophytic 110.1
  finger 681.02
  toe 681.11
Onychitis (with lymphangitis) 681.9
  finger 681.02
  toe 681.11
Onychocryptosis 703.0
Onychodystrophy 703.8
  congenital 757.5
Onychogryphosis 703.8
Onychogryposis 703.8
Onycholysis 703.8
Onychomadesis 703.8
Onychomalacia 703.8
Onychomycosis 110.1
  finger 110.1
  toe 110.1
Onycho-osteodysplasia 756.89
Onychophagy 307.9
Onychoptosis 703.8
Onychorrhexis 703.8
  congenital 757.5
Onychoschizia 703.8
Onychotrophia (see also Atrophy, nail) 703.8
O'nyong-nyong fever 066.3
Onyxis (finger) (toe) 703.0
Onyxitis (with lymphangitis) 681.9
  finger 681.02
  toe 681.11
Oophoritis (cystic) (infectional) (interstitial) (see also Salpingo-oophoritis) 614.2
  complicating pregnancy 646.6
  fetal (acute) 752.0
  gonococcal (acute) 098.19
    chronic or duration of 2 months or over 098.39
  tuberculous (see also Tuberculosis) 016.6
Opacity, opacities
  cornea 371.00
    central 371.03
    congenital 743.43
      interfering with vision 743.42
    degenerative (see also Degeneration, cornea) 371.40
    hereditary (see also Dystrophy, cornea) 371.50
    inflammatory (see also Keratitis) 370.9
    late effect of trachoma (healed) 139.1
    minor 371.01
    peripheral 371.02
  enamel (fluoride) (nonfluoride) (teeth) 520.3
  lens (see also Cataract) 366.9
  snowball 379.22
  vitreous (humor) 379.24
    congenital 743.51
Opalescent dentin (hereditary) 520.5

Open, opening
- abnormal, organ or site, congenital — *see* Imperfect, closure
- angle with
  - borderline intraocular pressure 365.01
  - cupping of discs 365.01
- bite (anterior) (posterior) 524.2
- false — *see* Imperfect, closure
- wound — *see* Wound, open, by site

Operation
- causing mutilation of fetus 763.89
- destructive, on live fetus, to facilitate birth 763.89
- for delivery, fetus or newborn 763.89
- maternal, unrelated to current delivery, affecting fetus or newborn 760.6

Operational fatigue 300.89
Operative — *see* condition
Operculitis (chronic) 523.4
- acute 523.3

Operculum, retina 361.32
- with detachment 361.01

Ophiasis 704.01
Ophthalmia (*see also* Conjunctivitis) 372.30
- actinic rays 370.24
- allergic (acute) 372.05
  - chronic 372.14
- blennorrhagic (neonatorum) 098.40
- catarrhal 372.03
- diphtheritic 032.81
- Egyptian 076.1
- electric, electrica 370.24
- gonococcal (neonatorum) 098.40
- metastatic 360.11
- migraine 346.8 ✓5ᵗʰ
- neonatorum, newborn 771.6
  - gonococcal 098.40
- nodosa 360.14
- phlyctenular 370.31
  - with ulcer (*see also* Ulcer, cornea) 370.00
- sympathetic 360.11

Ophthalmitis — *see* Ophthalmia
Ophthalmocele (congenital) 743.66
Ophthalmoneuromyelitis 341.0
Ophthalmopathy, infiltrative with thyrotoxicosis 242.0 ✓5ᵗʰ
Ophthalmoplegia (*see also* Strabismus) 378.9
- anterior internuclear 378.86
- ataxia-areflexia syndrome 357.0
- bilateral 378.9
- diabetic 250.5 ✓5ᵗʰ [378.86]
- exophthalmic 242.0 ✓5ᵗʰ [376.22]
- external 378.55
  - progressive 378.72
  - total 378.56
- internal(l) (complete) (total) 367.52
- internuclear 378.86
- migraine 346.8 ✓5ᵗʰ
- painful 378.55
- Parinaud's 378.81
- progressive external 378.72
- supranuclear, progressive 333.0
- total (external) 378.56
  - internal 367.52
- unilateral 378.9

Opisthognathism 524.00
Opisthorchiasis (felineus) (tenuicollis) (viverrini) 121.0
Opisthotonos, opisthotonus 781.0

Opitz's disease (congestive splenomegaly) 289.51
Opiumism (*see also* Dependence) 304.0 ✓5ᵗʰ
Oppenheim's disease 358.8
Oppenheim-Urbach disease or syndrome (necrobiosis lipoidica diabeticorum) 250.8 ✓5ᵗʰ [709.3]
Opsoclonia 379.59
Optic nerve — *see* condition
Orbit — *see* condition
Orchioblastoma (M9071/3) 186.9
Orchitis (nonspecific) (septic) 604.90
- with abscess 604.0
- blennorrhagic (acute) 098.13
  - chronic or duration of 2 months or over 098.33
- diphtheritic 032.89 [604.91]
- filarial 125.9 [604.91]
- gangrenous 604.99
- gonococcal (acute) 098.13
  - chronic or duration of 2 months or over 098.33
- mumps 072.0
- parotidea 072.0
- suppurative 604.99
- syphilitic 095.8 [604.91]
- tuberculous (*see also* Tuberculosis) 016.5 ✓5ᵗʰ [608.81]

Orf 051.2
Organic — *see also* condition
- heart — *see* Disease, heart
- insufficiency 799.8

Oriental
- bilharziasis 120.2
- schistosomiasis 120.2
- sore 085.1

Orifice — *see* condition
Origin, both great vessels from right ventricle 745.11
Ormond's disease or syndrome 593.4
Ornithosis 073.9
- with
  - complication 073.8
    - specified NEC 073.7
  - pneumonia 073.0
  - pneumonitis (lobular) 073.0

Orodigitofacial dysostosis 759.89
Oropouche fever 066.3
Orotaciduria, oroticaciduria (congenital) (hereditary) (pyrimidine deficiency) 281.4
Oroya fever 088.0
Orthodontics V58.5
- adjustment V53.4
- aftercare V58.5
- fitting V53.4

Orthopnea 786.02
Orthoptic training V57.4
Os, uterus — *see* condition
Osgood-Schlatter
- disease 732.4
- osteochondrosis 732.4

Osler's
- disease (M9950/1) (polycythemia vera) 238.4
- nodes 421.0

Osler-Rendu disease (familial hemorrhagic telangiectasia) 448.0
Osler-Vaquez disease (M9950/1) (polycythemia vera) 238.4

Index to Diseases

Osler-Weber-Rendu syndrome (familial hemorrhagic telangiectasia) 448.0
Osmidrosis 705.89
Osseous — *see* condition
Ossification
   artery — *see* Arteriosclerosis
   auricle (ear) 380.39
   bronchus 519.1
   cardiac (*see also* Degeneration, myocardial) 429.1
   cartilage (senile) 733.99
   coronary (artery) — *see* Arteriosclerosis, coronary
   diaphragm 728.10
   ear 380.39
      middle (*see also* Otosclerosis) 387.9
   falx cerebri 349.2
   fascia 728.10
   fontanel
      defective or delayed 756.0
      premature 756.0
   heart (*see also* Degeneration, myocardial) 429.1
      valve — *see* Endocarditis
   larynx 478.79
   ligament
      posterior longitudinal 724.8
         cervical 723.7
   meninges (cerebral) 349.2
      spinal 336.8
   multiple, eccentric centers 733.99
   muscle 728.10
      heterotopic, postoperative 728.13
   myocardium, myocardial (*see also* Degeneration, myocardial) 429.1
   penis 607.81
   periarticular 728.89
   sclera 379.16
   tendon 727.82
   trachea 519.1
   tympanic membrane (*see also* Tympanosclerosis) 385.00
   vitreous (humor) 360.44
Osteitis (*see also* Osteomyelitis) 730.2 ✓5ᵗʰ
   acute 730.0 ✓5ᵗʰ
   alveolar 526.5
   chronic 730.1 ✓5ᵗʰ
   condensans (ilii) 733.5
   deformans (Paget's) 731.0
      due to or associated with malignant neoplasm (*see also* Neoplasm, bone, malignant) 170.9 *[731.1]*
   due to yaws 102.6
   fibrosa NEC 733.29
      cystica (generalisata) 252.0
      disseminata 756.59
      osteoplastica 252.0
   fragilitans 756.51
   Garré's (sclerosing) 730.1 ✓5ᵗʰ
   infectious (acute) (subacute) 730.0 ✓5ᵗʰ
      chronic or old 730.1 ✓5ᵗʰ
   jaw (acute) (chronic) (lower) (neonatal) (suppurative) (upper) 526.4
   parathyroid 252.0
   petrous bone (*see also* Petrositis) 383.20
   pubis 733.5
   sclerotic, nonsuppurative 730.1 ✓5ᵗʰ
   syphilitic 095.5
   tuberculosa
      cystica (of Jüngling) 135
      multiplex cystoides 135

Osteochondromatosis

Osteoarthritica spondylitis (spine) (*see also* Spondylosis) 721.90
Osteoarthritis (*see also* Osteoarthrosis) 715.9 ✓5ᵗʰ
   distal interphalangeal 715.9 ✓5ᵗʰ
   hyperplastic 731.2
   interspinalis (*see also* Spondylosis) 721.90
   spine, spinal NEC (*see also* Spondylosis) 721.90
Osteoarthropathy (*see also* Osteoarthrosis) 715.9 ✓5ᵗʰ
   chronic idiopathic hypertrophic 757.39
   familial idiopathic 757.39
   hypertrophic pulmonary 731.2
      secondary 731.2
   idiopathic hypertrophic 757.39
   primary hypertrophic 731.2
   pulmonary hypertrophic 731.2
   secondary hypertrophic 731.2
Osteoarthrosis (degenerative) (hypertrophic) (rheumatoid) 715.9 ✓5ᵗʰ

> Note — Use the following fifth-digit subclassification with category 715:
>
> 0   site unspecified
> 1   shoulder region
> 2   upper arm
> 3   forearm
> 4   hand
> 5   pelvic region and thigh
> 6   lower leg
> 7   ankle and foot
> 8   other specified sites except spine
> 9   multiple sites

   Deformans alkaptonurica 270.2
   generalized 715.09
   juvenilis (Köhler's) 732.5
   localized 715.3 ✓5ᵗʰ
      idiopathic 715.1 ✓5ᵗʰ
      primary 715.1 ✓5ᵗʰ
      secondary 715.2 ✓5ᵗʰ
   multiple sites, not specified as generalized 715.89
   polyarticular 715.09
   spine (*see also* Spondylosis) 721.90
   temporomandibular joint 524.69
Osteoblastoma (M9200/0) — *see* Neoplasm, bone, benign
Osteochondritis (*see also* Osteochondrosis) 732.9
   dissecans 732.7
      hip 732.7
   ischiopubica 732.1
   multiple 756.59
   syphilitic (congenital) 090.0
Osteochondrodermodysplasia 756.59
Osteochondrodystrophy 277.5
   deformans 277.5
   familial 277.5
   fetalis 756.4
Osteochondrolysis 732.7
Osteochondroma (M9210/0) — *see* Neoplasm, bone, benign
   multiple, congenital 756.4
Osteochondromatosis (M9210/1) 238.0
   synovial 727.82

Osteochondromyxosarcoma (M9180/3) — see
  Neoplasm, bone, malignant
Osteochondropathy NEC 732.9
Osteochondrosarcoma (M9180/3) — see
  Neoplasm, bone, malignant
Osteochondrosis 732.9
  acetabulum 732.1
  adult spine 732.8
  astragalus 732.5
  Blount's 732.4
  Buchanan's (juvenile osteochondrosis of iliac
    crest) 732.1
  Buchman's (juvenile osteochondrosis) 732.1
  Burns' 732.3
  calcaneus 732.5
  capitular epiphysis (femur) 732.1
  carpal
    lunate (wrist) 732.3
    scaphoid 732.3
  coxae juvenilis 732.1
  deformans juvenilis (coxae) (hip) 732.1
    Scheuermann's 732.0
    spine 732.0
    tibia 732.4
    vertebra 732.0
  Diaz's (astragalus) 732.5
  dissecans (knee) (shoulder) 732.7
  femoral capital epiphysis 732.1
  femur (head) (juvenile) 732.1
  foot (juvenile) 732.5
  Freiberg's (disease) (second metatarsal) 732.5
  Haas' 732.3
  Haglund's (os tibiale externum) 732.5
  hand (juvenile) 732.3
  head of
    femur 732.1
    humerus (juvenile) 732.3
  hip (juvenile) 732.1
  humerus (juvenile) 732.3
  iliac crest (juvenile) 732.1
  ilium (juvenile) 732.1
  ischiopubic synchondrosis 732.1
  Iselin's (osteochondrosis fifth metatarsal)
    732.5
  juvenile, juvenilis 732.6
    arm 732.3
    capital femoral epiphysis 732.1
    capitellum humeri 732.3
    capitular epiphysis 732.1
    carpal scaphoid 732.3
    clavicle, sternal epiphysis 732.6
    coxae 732.1
    deformans 732.1
    foot 732.5
    hand 732.3
    hip and pelvis 732.1
    lower extremity, except foot 732.4
    lunate, wrist 732.3
    medial cuneiform bone 732.5
    metatarsal (head) 732.5
    metatarsophalangeal 732.5
    navicular, ankle 732.5
    patella 732.4
    primary patellar center (of Köhler) 732.4
    specified site NEC 732.6
    spine 732.0
    tarsal scaphoid 732.5
    tibia (epiphysis) (tuberosity) 732.4
    upper extremity 732.3
    vertebra (body) (Calvé) 732.0
      epiphyseal plates (of Scheuermann)
        732.0

Osteochondrosis — continued
  Kienböck's (disease) 732.3
  Köhler's (disease) (navicular, ankle) 732.5
    patellar 732.4
    tarsal navicular 732.5
  Legg-Calvé-Perthes (disease) 732.1
  lower extremity (juvenile) 732.4
  lunate bone 732.3
  Mauclaire's 732.3
  metacarpal heads (of Mauclaire) 732.3
  metatarsal (fifth) (head) (second) 732.5
  navicular, ankle 732.5
  os calcis 732.5
  Osgood-Schlatter 732.4
  os tibiale externum 732.5
  Panner's 732.3
  patella (juvenile) 732.4
  patellar center
    primary (of Köhler) 732.4
    secondary (of Sinding-Larsen) 732.4
  pelvis (juvenile) 732.1
  Pierson's 732.1
  radial head (juvenile) 732.3
  Scheuermann's 732.0
  Sever's (calcaneum) 732.5
  Sinding-Larsen (secondary patellar center)
    732.4
  spine (juvenile) 732.0
    adult 732.8
  symphysis pubis (of Pierson) (juvenile) 732.1
  syphilitic (congenital) 090.0
  tarsal (navicular) (scaphoid) 732.5
  tibia (proximal) (tubercle) 732.4
  tuberculous — see Tuberculosis, bone
  ulna 732.3
  upper extremity (juvenile) 732.3
  van Neck's (juvenile osteochondrosis) 732.1
  vertebral (juvenile) 732.0
    adult 732.8
Osteoclastoma (M9250/1) 238.0
  malignant (M9250/3) — see Neoplasm, bone,
    malignant
Osteocopic pain 733.90
Osteodynia 733.90
Osteodystrophy
  azotemic 588.0
  chronica deformans hypertrophica 731.0
  congenital 756.50
    specified type NEC 756.59
  deformans 731.0
  fibrosa localisata 731.0
  parathyroid 252.0
  renal 588.0
Osteofibroma (M9262/0) — see Neoplasm, bone,
  benign
Osteofibrosarcoma (M9182/3) — see Neoplasm,
  bone, malignant
Osteogenesis imperfecta 756.51
Osteogenic — see condition
Osteoma (M9180/0) — see also Neoplasm, bone,
  benign
  osteoid (M9191/0) — see also Neoplasm,
    bone, benign
    giant (M9200/0) — see Neoplasm, bone,
      benign
Osteomalacia 268.2
  chronica deformans hypertrophica 731.0
  due to vitamin D deficiency 268.2
  infantile (see also Rickets) 268.0
  juvenile (see also Rickets) 268.0

Index to Diseases

Osteomalacia — *continued*
   pelvis 268.2
   vitamin D-resistant 275.3
Osteomalacic bone 268.2
Osteomalacosis 268.2
Osteomyelitis (general) (infective) (localized) (neonatal) (purulent) (pyogenic) (septic) (staphylococcal) (streptococcal) (suppurative) (with periostitis) 730.2 ✓5ᵗʰ

> Note — Use the following fifth-digit subclassification with category 730:
>
> 0   site unspecified
> 1   shoulder region
> 2   upper arm
> 3   forearm
> 4   hand
> 5   pelvic region and thigh
> 6   lower leg
> 7   ankle and foot
> 8   other specified sites
> 9   multiple sites

   acute or subacute 730.0 ✓5ᵗʰ
   chronic or old 730.1 ✓5ᵗʰ
   due to or associated with
      diabetes mellitus 250.8 ✓5ᵗʰ [731.8]
      tuberculosis (*see also* Tuberculosis, bone) 015.9 ✓5ᵗʰ [730.8] ✓5ᵗʰ
         limb bones 015.5 ✓5ᵗʰ [730.8] ✓5ᵗʰ
         specified bones NEC 015.7 ✓5ᵗʰ [730.8] ✓5ᵗʰ
         spine 015.0 ✓5ᵗʰ [730.8] ✓5ᵗʰ
      typhoid 002.0 [730.8] ✓5ᵗʰ
   Garré's 730.1 ✓5ᵗʰ
   jaw (acute) (chronic) (lower) (neonatal) (suppurative) (upper) 526.4
   nonsuppurating 730.1 ✓5ᵗʰ
   orbital 376.03
   petrous bone (*see also* Petrositis) 383.20
   Salmonella 003.24
   sclerosing, nonsuppurative 730.1 ✓5ᵗʰ
   sicca 730.1 ✓5ᵗʰ
   syphilitic 095.5
      congenital 090.0 [730.8] ✓5ᵗʰ
   tuberculous — *see* Tuberculosis, bone
   typhoid 002.0 [730.8] ✓5ᵗʰ
Osteomyelofibrosis 289.8
Osteomyelosclerosis 289.8
Osteonecrosis 733.40
   meaning osteomyelitis 730.1 ✓5ᵗʰ
Osteo-onycho-arthro dysplasia 756.89
Osteo-onychodysplasia, hereditary 756.89
Osteopathia
   condensans disseminata 756.53
   hyperostotica multiplex infantilis 756.59
   hypertrophica toxica 731.2
   striata 756.4
Osteopathy resulting from poliomyelitis (*see also* Poliomyelitis) 045.9 ✓5ᵗʰ [730.7]
   familial dysplastic 731.2
Osteopecilia 756.53
Osteopenia 733.90
Osteoperiostitis (*see also* Osteomyelitis) 730.2 ✓5ᵗʰ
   ossificans toxica 731.2
   toxica ossificans 731.2
Osteopetrosis (familial) 756.52

Osteophyte — *see* Exostosis
Osteophytosis — *see* Exostosis
Osteopoikilosis 756.53
Osteoporosis (generalized) 733.00
   circumscripta 731.0
   disuse 733.03
   drug-induced 733.09
   idiopathic 733.02
   postmenopausal 733.01
   posttraumatic 733.7
   screening V82.81
   senile 733.01
   specified type NEC 733.09
Osteoporosis-osteomalacia syndrome 268.2
Osteopsathyrosis 756.51
Osteoradionecrosis, jaw 526.89
Osteosarcoma (M9180/3) — *see also* Neoplasm, bone, malignant
   chondroblastic (M9181/3) — *see* Neoplasm, bone, malignant
   fibroblastic (M9182/3) — *see* Neoplasm, bone, malignant
   in Paget's disease of bone (M9184/3) — *see* Neoplasm, bone, malignant
   juxtacortical (M9190/3) — *see* Neoplasm, bone, malignant
   parosteal (M9190/3) — *see* Neoplasm, bone, malignant
   telangiectatic (M9183/3) — *see* Neoplasm, bone, malignant
Osteosclerosis 756.52
   fragilis (generalisata) 756.52
   myelofibrosis 289.8
Osteosclerotic anemia 289.8
Osteosis
   acromegaloid 757.39
   cutis 709.3
   parathyroid 252.0
   renal fibrocystic 588.0
Österreicher-Turner syndrome 756.89
Ostium
   atrioventriculare commune 745.69
   primum (arteriosum) (defect) (persistent) 745.61
   secundum (arteriosum) (defect) (patent) (persistent) 745.5
Ostrum-Furst syndrome 756.59
Otalgia 388.70
   otogenic 388.71
   referred 388.72
Othematoma 380.31
Otitic hydrocephalus 348.2
Otitis 382.9
   with effusion 381.4
      purulent 382.4
      secretory 381.4
      serous 381.4
      suppurative 382.4
   acute 382.9
   adhesive (*see also* Adhesions, middle ear) 385.10
   chronic 382.9
      with effusion 381.3
      mucoid, mucous (simple) 381.20
      purulent 382.3
      secretory 381.3
      serous 381.10
      suppurative 382.3
   diffuse parasitic 136.8

Otitis — *continued*
  externa (acute) (diffuse) (hemorrhagica) 380.10
    actinic 380.22
    candidal 112.82
    chemical 380.22
    chronic 380.23
      mycotic — *see* Otitis, externa, mycotic
      specified type NEC 380.23
    circumscribed 380.10
    contact 380.22
    due to
      erysipelas 035 *[380.13]*
      impetigo 684 *[380.13]*
      seborrheic dermatitis 690.10 *[380.13]*
    eczematoid 380.22
    furuncular 680.0 *[380.13]*
    infective 380.10
      chronic 380.16
    malignant 380.14
    mycotic (chronic) 380.15
      due to
        aspergillosis 117.3 *[380.15]*
        moniliasis 112.82
        otomycosis 111.8 *[380.15]*
    reactive 380.22
    specified type NEC 380.22
    tropical 111.8 *[380.15]*
  insidiosa (*see also* Otosclerosis) 387.9
  interna (*see also* Labyrinthitis) 386.30
  media (hemorrhagic) (staphylococcal)
      (streptococcal) 382.9
    acute 382.9
      with effusion 381.00
      allergic 381.04
        mucoid 381.05
        sanguineous 381.06
        serous 381.04
      catarrhal 381.00
      exudative 381.00
      mucoid 381.02
        allergic 381.05
      necrotizing 382.00
        with spontaneous rupture of ear
            drum 382.01
        in
          influenza 487.8 *[382.02]*
          measles 055.2
          scarlet fever 034.1 *[382.02]*
      nonsuppurative 381.00
      purulent 382.00
        with spontaneous rupture of ear
            drum 382.01
      sanguineous 381.03
        allergic 381.06
      secretory 381.01
      seromucinous 381.02
      serous 381.01
        allergic 381.04
      suppurative 382.00
        with spontaneous rupture of ear
            drum 382.01
        due to
          influenza 487.8 *[382.02]*
          scarlet fever 034.1 *[382.02]*
      transudative 381.00
    adhesive (*see also* Adhesions, middle ear)
        385.10
    allergic 381.4
      acute 381.04
        mucoid 381.05
        sanguineous 381.06
        serous 381.04

Otitis — *continued*
  media — *continued*
    allergic — *continued*
      chronic 381.3
    catarrhal 381.4
      acute 381.00
      chronic (simple) 381.10
    chronic 382.9
      with effusion 381.3
      adhesive (*see also* Adhesions, middle
          ear) 385.10
      allergic 381.3
      atticoantral, suppurative (with posterior
          or superior marginal perforation of
          ear drum) 382.2
      benign suppurative (with anterior
          perforation of ear drum) 382.1
      catarrhal 381.10
      exudative 381.3
      mucinous 381.20
      mucoid, mucous (simple) 381.20
      mucosanguineous 381.29
      nonsuppurative 381.3
      purulent 382.3
      secretory 381.3
      seromucinous 381.3
      serosanguineous 381.19
      serous (simple) 381.10
      suppurative 382.3
        atticoantral (with posterior or
            superior marginal perforation of
            ear drum) 382.2
        benign (with anterior perforation of
            ear drum) 382.1
        tuberculous (*see also* Tuberculosis)
            017.4 ▲5▪
        tubotympanic 382.1
      transudative 381.3
    exudative 381.4
      acute 381.00
      chronic 381.3
    fibrotic (*see also* Adhesions, middle ear)
        385.10
    mucoid, mucous 381.4
      acute 381.02
      chronic (simple) 381.20
    mucosanguineous, chronic 381.29
    nonsuppurative 381.4
      acute 381.00
      chronic 381.3
    postmeasles 055.2
    purulent 382.4
      acute 382.00
        with spontaneous rupture of ear
            drum 382.01
      chronic 382.3
    sanguineous, acute 381.03
      allergic 381.06
    secretory 381.4
      acute or subacute 381.01
      chronic 381.3
    seromucinous 381.4
      acute or subacute 381.02
      chronic 381.3
    serosanguineous, chronic 381.19
    serous 381.4
      acute or subacute 381.01
      chronic (simple) 381.10
    subacute — *see* Otitis, media, acute

Index to Diseases

Otitis — continued
  media — continued
    suppurative 382.4
      acute 382.00
        with spontaneous rupture of ear drum 382.01
      chronic 382.3
        atticoantral 382.2
        benign 382.1
        tuberculous (see also Tuberculosis) 017.4 ✓5ᵗʰ
        tubotympanic 382.1
      transudative 381.4
        acute 381.00
        chronic 381.3
      tuberculous (see also Tuberculosis) 017.4 ✓5ᵗʰ
    postmeasles 055.2
Otoconia 386.8
Otolith syndrome 386.19
Otomycosis 111.8 [380.15]
  in
    aspergillosis 117.3 [380.15]
    moniliasis 112.82
Otopathy 388.9
Otoporosis (see also Otosclerosis) 387.9
Otorrhagia 388.69
  traumatic — see nature of injury
Otorrhea 388.60
  blood 388.69
  cerebrospinal (fluid) 388.61
Otosclerosis (general) 387.9
  cochlear (endosteal) 387.2
  involving
    otic capsule 387.2
    oval window
      nonobliterative 387.0
      obliterative 387.1
    round window 387.2
  nonobliterative 387.0
  obliterative 387.1
  specified type NEC 387.8
Otospongiosis (see also Otosclerosis) 387.9
Otto's disease or pelvis 715.35
Outburst, aggressive (see also Disturbance, conduct) 312.0 ✓5ᵗʰ
  in children and adolescents 313.9
Outcome of delivery
  multiple birth NEC V27.9
    all liveborn V27.5
    all stillborn V27.7
    some liveborn V27.6
    unspecified V27.9
  single V27.9
    liveborn V27.0
    stillborn V27.1
  twins V27.9
    both liveborn V27.2
    both stillborn V27.4
    one liveborn, one stillborn V27.3
Outlet — see also condition
  syndrome (thoracic) 353.0
Outstanding ears (bilateral) 744.29
Ovalocytosis (congenital) (hereditary) (see also Elliptocytosis) 282.1
Ovarian — see also condition
  pregnancy — see Pregnancy, ovarian
  remnant syndrome 620.8
  vein syndrome 593.4

Ovaritis (cystic) (see also Salpingo-oophoritis) 614.2
Ovary, ovarian — see condition
Overactive — see also Hyperfunction
  bladder 596.51
  eye muscle (see also Strabismus) 378.9
  hypothalamus 253.8
  thyroid (see also Thyrotoxicosis) 242.9 ✓5ᵗʰ
Overactivity, child 314.01
Overbite (deep) (excessive) (horizontal) (vertical) 524.2
Overbreathing (see also Hyperventilation) 786.01
Overconscientious personality 301.4
Overdevelopment — see also Hypertrophy
  breast (female) (male) 611.1
  nasal bones 738.0
  prostate, congenital 752.8
Overdistention — see Distention
Overdose, overdosage (drug) 977.9
  specified drug or substance — see Table of Drugs and Chemicals
Overeating 783.6
  with obesity 278.0 ✓5ᵗʰ
  nonorganic origin 307.51
Overexertion (effects) (exhaustion) 994.5
Overexposure (effects) 994.9
  exhaustion 994.4
Overfeeding (see also Overeating) 783.6
Overgrowth, bone NEC 733.99
Overheated (effects) (places) — see Heat
Overinhibited child 313.0
Overjet 524.2
Overlaid, overlying (suffocation) 994.7
Overlapping toe (acquired) 735.8
  congenital (fifth toe) 755.66
Overload
  fluid 276.6
  potassium (K) 276.7
  sodium (Na) 276.0
Overnutrition (see also Hyperalimentation) 783.6
Overproduction — see also Hypersecretion
  ACTH 255.3
  cortisol 255.0
  growth hormone 253.0
  thyroid-stimulating hormone (TSH) 242.8 ✓5ᵗʰ
Overriding
  aorta 747.21
  finger (acquired) 736.29
    congenital 755.59
  toe (acquired) 735.8
    congenital 755.66
Oversize
  fetus (weight of 4500 grams or more) 766.0
    affecting management of pregnancy 656.6 ✓5ᵗʰ
    causing disproportion 653.5 ✓5ᵗʰ
      with obstructed labor 660.1 ✓5ᵗʰ
    affecting fetus or newborn 763.1
Overstimulation, ovarian 256.1
Overstrained 780.79
  heart — see Hypertrophy, cardiac
Overweight (see also Obesity) 278.00
Overwork 780.79
Oviduct — see condition
Ovotestis 752.7

Ovulation (cycle)
  failure or lack of 628.0
  pain 625.2
Ovum
  blighted 631
  dropsical 631
  pathologic 631
Owren's disease or syndrome (parahemophilia)
  (see also Defect, coagulation) 286.3
Oxalosis 271.8
Oxaluria 271.8
Ox heart — see Hypertrophy, cardiac
OX syndrome 758.6
Oxycephaly, oxycephalic 756.0
  syphilitic, congenital 090.0
Oxyuriasis 127.4
Oxyuris vermicularis (infestation) 127.4
Ozena 472.0

P

Pacemaker syndrome 429.4
Pachyderma, pachydermia 701.8
  laryngis 478.5
  laryngitis 478.79
  larynx (verrucosa) 478.79
Pachydermatitis 701.8
Pachydermatocele (congenital) 757.39
  acquired 701.8
Pachydermatosis 701.8
Pachydermoperiostitis
  secondary 731.2
Pachydermoperiostosis
  primary idiopathic 757.39
  secondary 731.2
Pachymeningitis (adhesive) (basal) (brain)
    (cerebral) (cervical) (chronic)
    (circumscribed) (external) (fibrous)
    (hemorrhagic) (hypertrophic) (internal)
    (purulent) (spinal) (suppurative) (see also
    Meningitis) 322.9
  gonococcal 098.82
Pachyonychia (congenital) 757.5
  acquired 703.8
Pachyperiosteodermia
  primary or idiopathic 757.39
  secondary 731.2
Pachyperiostosis
  primary or idiopathic 757.39
  secondary 731.2
Pacinian tumor (M9507/0) — see Neoplasm,
    skin, benign
Pads, knuckle or Garrod's 728.79
Paget's disease (osteitis deformans) 731.0
  with infiltrating duct carcinoma of the breast
    (M8541/3) — see Neoplasm, breast,
    malignant
  bone 731.0
    osteosarcoma in (M9184/3) — see
      Neoplasm, bone, malignant
  breast (M8540/3) 174.0
  extramammary (M8542/3) — see also
    Neoplasm, skin, malignant
    anus 154.3
    skin 173.5
  malignant (M8540/3)
    breast 174.0

Paget's disease — continued
  malignant — continued
    specified site NEC (M8542/3) — see
      Neoplasm, skin, malignant
    unspecified site 174.0
  mammary (M8540/3) 174.0
  necrosis of bone 731.0
  nipple (M8540/3) 174.0
  osteitis deformans 731.0
Paget-Schroetter syndrome (intermittent
    venous claudication) 453.8
Pain(s)
  abdominal 789.0
  adnexa (uteri) 625.9
  alimentary, due to vascular insufficiency
      557.9
  anginoid (see also Pain, precordial)
      786.51 anus 569.42
  arch 729.5
  arm 729.5
  back (postural) 724.5
    low 724.2
    psychogenic 307.89
  bile duct 576.9
  bladder 788.9
  bone 733.90
  breast 611.71
    psychogenic 307.89
  broad ligament 625.9
  cartilage NEC 733.90
  cecum 789.0
  cervicobrachial 723.3
  chest (central) 786.50
    atypical 786.59
    midsternal 786.51
    musculoskeletal 786.59
    noncardiac 786.59
    substernal 786.51
    wall (anterior) 786.52
  coccyx 724.79
  colon 789.0
  common duct 576.9
  coronary — see Angina
  costochondral 786.52
  diaphragm 786.52
  due to (presence of) any device, implant, or
      graft classifiable to 996.0-996.5 — see
      Complications, due to (presence of) any
      device, implant, or graft classified to
      996.0-996.5 NEC
  ear (see also Otalgia) 388.70
  epigastric, epigastrium 789.0
  extremity (lower) (upper) 729.5
  eye 379.91
  face, facial 784.0
    atypical 350.2
    nerve 351.8
  false (labor) 644.1
  female genital organ NEC 625.9
    psychogenic 307.89
  finger 729.5
  flank 789.0
  foot 729.5
  gallbladder 575.9
  gas (intestinal) 787.3
  gastric 536.8
  generalized 780.99 ▲
  genital organ
    female 625.9
    male 608.9
    psychogenic 307.89

Index to Diseases — Painful

Pain(s) — *continued*
- groin 789.0 ✓5ᵗʰ
- growing 781.99
- hand 729.5
- head (*see also* Headache) 784.0
- heart (see also Pain, precordial) 786.51
- infraorbital (*see also* Neuralgia, trigeminal) 350.1
- intermenstrual 625.2
- jaw 526.9
- joint 719.40
  - ankle 719.47
  - elbow 719.42
  - foot 719.47
  - hand 719.44
  - hip 719.45
  - knee 719.46
  - multiple sites 719.49
  - pelvic region 719.45
  - psychogenic 307.89
  - shoulder (region) 719.41
  - specified site NEC 719.48
  - wrist 719.43
- kidney 788.0
- labor, false or spurious 644.1 ✓5ᵗʰ
- laryngeal 784.1
- leg 729.5
- limb 729.5
- low back 724.2
- lumbar region 724.2
- mastoid (*see also* Otalgia) 388.70
- maxilla 526.9
- metacarpophalangeal (joint) 719.44
- metatarsophalangeal (joint) 719.47
- mouth 528.9
- muscle 729.1
  - intercostal 786.59
- nasal 478.1
- nasopharynx 478.29
- neck NEC 723.1
  - psychogenic 307.89
- nerve NEC 729.2
- neuromuscular 729.1
- nose 478.1
- ocular 379.91
- ophthalmic 379.91
- orbital region 379.91
- osteocopic 733.90
- ovary 625.9
  - psychogenic 307.89
- over heart (*see also* Pain, precordial) 786.51
- ovulation 625.2
- pelvic (female) 625.9
  - male NEC 789.0 ✓5ᵗʰ
    - psychogenic 307.89
  - psychogenic 307.89
- penis 607.9
  - psychogenic 307.89
- pericardial (*see also* Pain, precordial) 786.51
- perineum
  - female 625.9
  - male 608.9
- pharynx 478.29
- pleura, pleural, pleuritic 786.52
- post-operative — *see* Pain, by site
- preauricular 388.70
- precordial (region) 786.51
  - psychogenic 307.89
- psychogenic 307.80
  - cardiovascular system 307.89
  - gastrointestinal system 307.89

Pain(s) — *continued*
- psychogenic — *continued*
  - genitourinary system 307.89
  - heart 307.89
  - musculoskeletal system 307.89
  - respiratory system 307.89
  - skin 306.3
- radicular (spinal) (*see also* Radiculitis) 729.2
- rectum 569.42
- respiration 786.52
- retrosternal 786.51
- rheumatic NEC 729.0
  - muscular 729.1
- rib 786.50
- root (spinal) (*see also* Radiculitis) 729.2
- round ligament (stretch) 625.9
- sacroiliac 724.6
- sciatic 724.3
- scrotum 608.9
  - psychogenic 307.89
- seminal vesicle 608.9
- sinus 478.1
- skin 782.0
- spermatic cord 608.9
- spinal root (*see also* Radiculitis) 729.2
- stomach 536.8
  - psychogenic 307.89
- substernal 786.51
- temporomandibular (joint) 524.62
- temporomaxillary joint 524.62
- testis 608.9
  - psychogenic 307.89
- thoracic spine 724.1
  - with radicular and visceral pain 724.4
- throat 784.1
- tibia 733.90
- toe 729.5
- tongue 529.6
- tooth 525.9
- trigeminal (*see also* Neuralgia, trigeminal) 350.1
- umbilicus 789.0 ✓5ᵗʰ
- ureter 788.0
- urinary (organ) (system) 788.0
- uterus 625.9
  - psychogenic 307.89
- vagina 625.9
- vertebrogenic (syndrome) 724.5
- vesical 788.9
- vulva 625.9
- xiphoid 733.90

Painful — *see also* Pain
- arc syndrome 726.19
- coitus
  - female 625.0
  - male 608.89
  - psychogenic 302.76
- ejaculation (semen) 608.89
  - psychogenic 302.79
- erection 607.3
- feet syndrome 266.2
- menstruation 625.3
  - psychogenic 306.52
- micturition 788.1
- ophthalmoplegia 378.55
- respiration 786.52
- scar NEC 709.2
- urination 788.1
- wire sutures 998.89

Painters' colic 984.9
  specified type of lead — see Table of Drugs and Chemicals
Palate — see condition
Palatoplegia 528.9
Palatoschisis (see also Cleft, palate) 749.00
Palilalia 784.69
Palindromic arthritis (see also Rheumatism, palindromic) 719.3
Palliative care V66.7
Pallor 782.61
  temporal, optic disc 377.15
Palmar — see also condition
  fascia — see condition
Palpable
  cecum 569.89
  kidney 593.89
  liver 573.9
  lymph nodes 785.6
  ovary 620.8
  prostate 602.9
  spleen (see also Splenomegaly) 789.2
  uterus 625.8
Palpitation (heart) 785.1
  psychogenic 306.2
Palsy (see also Paralysis) 344.9
  atrophic diffuse 335.20
  Bell's 351.0
    newborn 767.5
  birth 767.7
  brachial plexus 353.0
    fetus or newborn 767.6
  brain — see also Palsy, cerebral
    noncongenital or noninfantile 344.89
      due to vascular lesion — see category 438
      late effect — see Late effect(s) (of) cerebrovascular disease
    syphilitic 094.89
      congenital 090.49
  bulbar (chronic) (progressive) 335.22
    pseudo NEC 335.23
    supranuclear NEC 344.8
  cerebral (congenital) (infantile) (spastic) 343.9
    athetoid 333.7
    diplegic 343.0
      due to previous vascular lesion — see category 438
      late effect — see Late effect(s) (of) cerebrovascular disease
    hemiplegic 343.1
    monoplegic 343.3
    noncongenital or noninfantile 437.8
      due to previous vascular lesion — see category 438
      late effect — see Late effect(s) (of) cerebrovascular disease
    paraplegic 343.0
    quadriplegic 343.2
    spastic, not congenital or infantile 344.8
    syphilitic 094.89
      congenital 090.49
    tetraplegic 343.2
  cranial nerve — see also Disorder, nerve, cranial
    multiple 352.6
  creeping 335.21
  divers' 993.3

Palsy — continued
  Erb's (birth injury) 767.6
  facial 351.0
    newborn 767.5
  glossopharyngeal 352.2
  Klumpke (-Déjérine) 767.6
  lead 984.9
    specified type of lead — see Table of Drugs and Chemicals
  median nerve (tardy) 354.0
  peroneal nerve (acute) (tardy) 355.3
  progressive supranuclear 333.0
  pseudobulbar NEC 335.23
  radial nerve (acute) 354.3
  seventh nerve 351.0
    newborn 767.5
  shaking (see also Parkinsonism) 332.0
  spastic (cerebral) (spinal) 343.9
    hemiplegic 343.1
  specified nerve NEC — see Disorder, nerve
  supranuclear NEC 356.8
    progressive 333.0
  ulnar nerve (tardy) 354.2
  wasting 335.21
Paltauf-Sternberg disease 201.9
Paludism — see Malaria
Panama fever 084.0
Panaris (with lymphangitis) 681.9
  finger 681.02
  toe 681.11
Panaritium (with lymphangitis) 681.9
  finger 681.02
  toe 681.11
Panarteritis (nodosa) 446.0
  brain or cerebral 437.4
Pancake heart 793.2
  with cor pulmonale (chronic) 416.9
Pancarditis (acute) (chronic) 429.89
  with
    rheumatic
      fever (active) (acute) (chronic) (subacute) 391.8
        inactive or quiescent 398.99
    rheumatic, acute 391.8
      chronic or inactive 398.99
Pancoast's syndrome or tumor (carcinoma, pulmonary apex) (M8010/3) 162.3
Pancoast-Tobias syndrome (M8010/3) (carcinoma, pulmonary apex) 162.3
Pancolitis 556.6
Pancreas, pancreatic — see condition
Pancreatitis 577.0
  acute (edematous) (hemorrhagic) (recurrent) 577.0
  annular 577.0
  apoplectic 577.0
  calcercous 577.0
  chronic (infectious) 577.1
    recurrent 577.1
  cystic 577.2
  fibrous 577.8
  gangrenous 577.0
  hemorrhagic (acute) 577.0
  interstitial (chronic) 577.1
    acute 577.0
  malignant 577.0
  mumps 072.3
  painless 577.1
  recurrent 577.1

Pancreatitis — *continued*
　relapsing 577.1
　subacute 577.0
　suppurative 577.0
　syphilitic 095.8
Pancreatolithiasis 577.8
Pancytolysis 289.9
Pancytopenia (acquired) 284.8
　with malformations 284.0
　congenital 284.0
Panencephalitis — *see also* Encephalitis
　subacute, sclerosing 046.2
Panhematopenia 284.8
　congenital 284.0
　constitutional 284.0
　splenic, primary 289.4
Panhemocytopenia 284.8
　congenital 284.0
　constitutional 284.0
Panhypogonadism 257.2
Panhypopituitarism 253.2
　prepubertal 253.3
Panic (attack) (state) 300.01
　reaction to exceptional stress (transient) 308.0
Panmyelopathy, familial constitutional 284.0
Panmyelophthisis 284.9
　acquired (secondary) 284.8
　congenital 284.0
　idiopathic 284.9
Panmyelosis (acute) (M9951/1) 238.7
Panner's disease 732.3
　capitellum humeri 732.3
　head of humerus 732.3
　tarsal navicular (bone) (osteochondrosis) 732.5
Panneuritis endemica 265.0 [357.4]
Panniculitis 729.30
　back 724.8
　knee 729.31
　neck 723.6
　nodular, nonsuppurative 729.30
　sacral 724.8
　specified site NEC 729.39
Panniculus adiposus (abdominal) 278.1
Pannus 370.62
　allergic eczematous 370.62
　degenerativus 370.62
　keratic 370.62
　rheumatoid — *see* Arthritis, rheumatoid
　trachomatosus, trachomatous (active) 076.1
　　[370.62]
　　late effect 139.1
Panophthalmitis 360.02
Panotitis — *see* Otitis media
Pansinusitis (chronic) (hyperplastic) (nonpurulent) (purulent) 473.8
　acute 461.8
　due to fungus NEC 117.9
　tuberculous (*see also* Tuberculosis) 012.8
Panuveitis 360.12
　sympathetic 360.11
Panvalvular disease — *see* Endocarditis, mitral
Papageienkrankheit 073.9
Papanicolaou smear
　cervix (screening test) V76.2
　　as part of gynecological examination V72.3
　　for suspected malignant neoplasm V76.2
　　no disease found V71.1

Papanicolaou smear — *continued*
　cervix — *continued*
　　nonspecific abnormal finding 795.00
　　　atypical squamous cell changes of undetermined significance
　　　　favor benign (ASCUS favor benign) 795.01
　　　　favor dysplasia (ASCUS favor dysplasia) 795.02
　　　nonspecific finding NEC 795.09
　　　unsatisfactory 795.09
　　other specified site — *see also* Screening, malignant neoplasm
　　for suspected malignant neoplasm — *see also* Screening, malignant neoplasm
　　　no disease found V71.1
　　nonspecific abnormal finding 795.1
　vagina V76.47
　　following hysterectomy for malignant condition V67.01
Papilledema 377.00
　associated with
　　decreased ocular pressure 377.02
　　increased intracranial pressure 377.01
　　retinal disorder 377.03
　choked disc 377.00
　infectional 377.00
Papillitis 377.31
　anus 569.49
　chronic lingual 529.4
　necrotizing, kidney 584.7
　optic 377.31
　rectum 569.49
　renal, necrotizing 584.7
　tongue 529.0
Papilloma (M8050/0) — *see also* Neoplasm, by site, benign

> Note — Except where otherwise indicated, the morphological varieties of papilloma in the list below should be coded by site as for "Neoplasm, benign."

　acuminatum (female) (male) 078.1
　bladder (urinary) (transitional cell) (M8120/1) 236.7
　　benign (M8120/0) 223.3
　choroid plexus (M9390/0) 225.0
　　anaplastic type (M9390/3) 191.5
　　malignant (M9390/3) 191.5
　ductal (M8503/0)
　dyskeratotic (M8052/0)
　epidermoid (M8052/0)
　hyperkeratotic (M8052/0)
　intracystic (M8504/0)
　intraductal (M8503/0)
　inverted (M8053/0)
　keratotic (M8052/0)
　parakeratotic (M8052/0)
　pinta (primary) 103.0
　renal pelvis (transitional cell) (M8120/1) 236.99
　　benign (M8120/0) 223.1
　Schneiderian (M8121/0)
　　specified site — *see* Neoplasm, by site, benign
　　unspecified site 212.0
　serous surface (M8461/0)
　　borderline malignancy (M8461/1)
　　　specified site — *see* Neoplasm, by site, uncertain behavior

Papilloma — *continued*
  serous surface — *continued*
    borderline malignancy — *continued*
      unspecified site 236.2
    specified site — *see* Neoplasm, by site, benign
    unspecified site 220
  squamous (cell) (M8052/0)
  transitional (cell) (M8120/0)
    bladder (urinary) (M8120/1) 236.7
    inverted type (M8121/1) — *see* Neoplasm, by site, uncertain behavior
    renal pelvis (M8120/1) 236.91
    ureter (M8120/1) 236.91
  ureter (transitional cell) (M8120/1) 236.91
    benign (M8120/0) 223.2
  urothelial (M8120/1) — *see* Neoplasm, by site, uncertain behavior
  verrucous (M8051/0)
  villous (M8261/1) — *see* Neoplasm, by site, uncertain behavior
  yaws, plantar or palmar 102.1
Papillomata, multiple, of yaws 102.1
Papillomatosis (M8060/0) — *see also* Neoplasm, by site, benign
  confluent and reticulate 701.8
  cutaneous 701.8
  ductal, breast 610.1
  Gougerot-Carteaud (confluent reticulate) 701.8
  intraductal (diffuse) (M8505/0) — *see* Neoplasm, by site, benign
  subareolar duct (M8506/0) 217
Papillon-Léage and Psaume syndrome (orodigitofacial dysostosis) 759.89
Papule 709.8
  carate (primary) 103.0
  fibrous, of nose (M8724/0) 216.3
  pinta (primary) 103.0
Papulosis, malignant 447.8
Papyraceous fetus 779.89 ▲
  complicating pregnancy 646.0
Paracephalus 759.7
Parachute mitral valve 746.5
Paracoccidioidomycosis 116.1
  mucocutaneous-lymphangitic 116.1
  pulmonary 116.1
  visceral 116.1
Paracoccidiomycosis — *see* Paracoccidioidomycosis
Paracusis 388.40
Paradentosis 523.5
Paradoxical facial movements 374.43
Paraffinoma 999.9
Paraganglioma (M8680/1)
  adrenal (M8700/0) 227.0
    malignant (M8700/3) 194.0
  aortic body (M8691/1) 237.3
    malignant (M8691/3) 194.6
  carotid body (M8692/1) 237.3
    malignant (M8692/3) 194.5
  chromaffin (M8700/0) — *see also* Neoplasm, by site, benign
    malignant (M8700/3) — *see* Neoplasm, by site, malignant
  extra-adrenal (M8693/1)
    malignant (M8693/3)
      specified site — *see* Neoplasm, by site, malignant
      unspecified site 194.6

Paraganglioma — *continued*
  extra-adrenal — *continued*
    specified site — *see* Neoplasm, by site, uncertain behavior
    unspecified site 237.3
  glomus jugulare (M8690/1) 237.3
    malignant (M8690/3) 194.6
  jugular (M8690/1) 237.3
    malignant (M8680/3)
      specified site — *see* Neoplasm, by site, malignant
      unspecified site 194.6
  nonchromaffin (M8693/1)
    malignant (M8693/3)
      specified site — *see* Neoplasm, by site, malignant
      unspecified site 194.6
    specified site — *see* Neoplasm, by site, uncertain behavior
    unspecified site 237.3
  parasympathetic (M8682/1)
    specified site — *see* Neoplasm, by site, uncertain behavior
    unspecified site 237.3
  specified site — *see* Neoplasm, by site, uncertain behavior
  sympathetic (M8681/1)
    specified site — *see* Neoplasm, by site, uncertain behavior
    unspecified site 237.3
  unspecified site 237.3
Parageusia 781.1
  psychogenic 306.7
Paragonimiasis 121.2
Paragranuloma, Hodgkin's (M9660/3) 201.0
Parahemophilia (*see also* Defect, coagulation) 286.3
Parakeratosis 690.8
  psoriasiformis 696.2
  variegata 696.2
Paralysis, paralytic (complete) (incomplete) 344.9
  with
    broken
      back — *see* Fracture, vertebra, by site, with spinal cord injury
      neck — *see* Fracture, vertebra, cervical, with spinal cord injury
    fracture, vertebra — *see* Fracture, vertebra, by site, with spinal cord injury
    syphilis 094.89
  abdomen and back muscles 355.9
  abdominal muscles 355.9
  abducens (nerve) 378.54
  abductor 355.9
    lower extremity 355.8
    upper extremity 354.9
  accessory nerve 352.4
  accommodation 367.51
    hysterical 300.11
  acoustic nerve 388.5
  agitans 332.0
    arteriosclerotic 332.0
  alternating 344.89
    oculomotor 344.89
  amyotrophic 335.20
  ankle 355.8
  anterior serratus 355.9
  anus (sphincter) 569.49

Index to Diseases

Paralysis, paralytic

Paralysis, paralytic — *continued*
- apoplectic (current episode) (*see also* Disease, cerebrovascular, acute) 436
  - late effect — *see* Late effect(s) (of) cerebrovascular disease
- arm 344.40
  - affecting
    - dominant side 344.41
    - nondominant side 344.42
  - both 344.2
  - due to old CVA — *see* category 438 ✓4ᵗʰ
  - hysterical 300.11
  - late effect — *see* Late effect(s) (of) cerebrovascular disease
  - psychogenic 306.0 transient 781.4
    - traumatic NEC (*see also* Injury, nerve, upper limb) 955.9
- arteriosclerotic (current episode) 437.0
  - late effect — *see* Late effect(s) (of) cerebrovascular disease
- ascending (spinal), acute 357.0
- associated, nuclear 344.89
- asthenic bulbar 358.0
- ataxic NEC 334.9
  - general 094.1
- athetoid 333.7
- atrophic 356.9
  - infantile, acute (*see also* Poliomyelitis, with paralysis) 045.1 ✓5ᵗʰ
  - muscle NEC 355.9
  - progressive 335.21
  - spinal (acute) (*see also* Poliomyelitis, with paralysis) 045.1 ✓5ᵗʰ
- attack (*see also* Disease, cerebrovascular, acute) 436
- axillary 353.0
- Babinski-Nageotte's 344.89
- Bell's 351.0
  - newborn 767.5
- Benedikt's 344.89
- birth (injury) 767.7
  - brain 767.0
  - intracranial 767.0
  - spinal cord 767.4
- bladder (sphincter) 596.53
  - neurogenic 596.54
    - with cauda equina syndrome 344.61
  - puerperal, postpartum, childbirth 665.5 ✓5ᵗʰ
  - sensory 344.61
    - with cauda equina 344.61
  - spastic 344.61
    - with cauda equina 344.61
- bowel, colon, or intestine (*see also* Ileus) 560.1
- brachial plexus 353.0
  - due to birth injury 767.6
  - newborn 767.6
- brain
  - congenital — *see* Palsy, cerebral
  - current episode 437.8
  - diplegia 344.2
  - due to previous vascular lesion — *see* category 438 ✓4ᵗʰ
  - hemiplegia 342.9
    - due to previous vascular lesion — *see* category 438 ✓4ᵗʰ
    - late effect — *see* Late effect(s) (of) cerebrovascular disease
  - infantile — *see* Palsy, cerebral
  - late effect — *see* Late effect(s) (of) cerebrovascular disease

Paralysis, paralytic — *continued*
- brain — *continued*
  - monoplegia — *see also* Monoplegia
    - due to previous vascular lesion — *see* category 438 ✓4ᵗʰ
    - late effect — *see* Late effect(s) (of) cerebrovascular disease
  - paraplegia 344.1
  - quadriplegia — *see* Quadriplegia
  - syphilitic, congenital 090.49
  - triplegia 344.89
- bronchi 519.1
- Brown-Séquard's 344.89
- bulbar (chronic) (progressive) 335.22
  - infantile (*see also* Poliomyelitis, bulbar) 045.0 ✓5ᵗʰ
  - poliomyelitic (*see also* Poliomyelitis, bulbar) 045.0 ✓5ᵗʰ
  - pseudo 335.23
  - supranuclear 344.89
- bulbospinal 358.0
- cardiac (*see also* Failure, heart) 428.9
- cerebral
  - current episode 437.8
  - spastic, infantile — *see* Palsy, cerebral
- cerebrocerebellar 437.8
  - diplegic infantile 343.0
- cervical
  - plexus 353.2
  - sympathetic NEC 337.0
- Céstan-Chenais 344.89
- Charcôt-Marie-Tooth type 356.1
- childhood — *see* Palsy, cerebral
- Clark's 343.9
- colon (*see also* Ileus) 560.1
- compressed air 993.3
- compression
  - arm NEC 354.9
  - cerebral — *see* Paralysis, brain
  - leg NEC 355.8
  - lower extremity NEC 355.8
  - upper extremity NEC 354.9
- congenital (cerebral) (spastic) (spinal) — *see* Palsy, cerebral
- conjugate movement (of eye) 378.81
  - cortical (nuclear) (supranuclear) 378.81
- convergence 378.83
- cordis (*see also* Failure, heart) 428.9
- cortical (*see also* Paralysis, brain) 437.8
- cranial or cerebral nerve (*see also* Disorder, nerve, cranial) 352.9
- creeping 335.21
- crossed leg 344.89
- crutch 953.4
- deglutition 784.9
  - hysterical 300.11
- dementia 094.1
- descending (spinal) NEC 335.9
- diaphragm (flaccid) 519.4
  - due to accidental section of phrenic nerve during procedure 998.2
- digestive organs NEC 564.89
- diplegic — *see* Diplegia
- divergence (nuclear) 378.85
- divers' 993.3
- Duchenne's 335.22
  - due to intracranial or spinal birth injury — *see* Palsy, cerebral
- embolic (current episode) (*see also* Embolism, brain) 434.1 ✓5ᵗʰ
  - late effect — *see* Late effect(s) (of) cerebrovascular disease

Paralysis, paralytic — continued
 enteric (see also Ileus) 560.1
  with hernia — see Hernia, by site, with obstruction
 Erb's syphilitic spastic spinal 094.89
 Erb (-Duchenne) (birth) (newborn) 767.6
 esophagus 530.8
 essential, infancy (see also Poliomyelitis) 045.9
 extremity
  lower — see Paralysis, leg
  spastic (hereditary) 343.3
   noncongenital or noninfantile 344.1
  transient (cause unknown) 781.4
  upper — see Paralysis, arm
 eye muscle (extrinsic) 378.55
  intrinsic 367.51
 facial (nerve) 351.0
  birth injury 767.5
  congenital 767.5
  following operation NEC 998.2
  newborn 767.5
 familial 359.3
  periodic 359.3
  spastic 334.1
 fauces 478.29
 finger NEC 354.9
 foot NEC 355.8
 gait 781.2
 gastric nerve 352.3
 gaze 378.81
 general 094.1
  ataxic 094.1
  insane 094.1
  juvenile 090.40
  progressive 094.1
  tabetic 094.1
 glossopharyngeal (nerve) 352.2
 glottis (see also Paralysis, vocal cord) 478.30
 gluteal 353.4
 Gubler (-Millard) 344.89
 hand 354.9
  hysterical 300.11
  psychogenic 306.0
 heart (see also Failure, heart) 428.9
 hemifacial, progressive 349.89
 hemiplegic — see Hemiplegia
 hyperkalemic periodic (familial) 359.3
 hypertensive (current episode) 437.8
 hypoglossal (nerve) 352.5
 hypokalemic periodic 359.3
 Hyrtl's sphincter (rectum) 569.49
 hysterical 300.11
 ileus (see also Ileus) 560.1
 infantile (see also Poliomyelitis) 045.9
  atrophic acute 045.1
  bulbar 045.0
  cerebral — see Palsy, cerebral
  paralytic 045.1
  progressive acute 045.9
  spastic — see Palsy, cerebral
  spinal 045.9
 infective (see also Poliomyelitis) 045.9
 inferior nuclear 344.9
 insane, general or progressive 094.1
 internuclear 378.86
 interosseous 355.9
 intestine (see also Ileus) 560.1
 intracranial (current episode) (see also Paralysis, brain) 437.8
  due to birth injury 767.0

Paralysis, paralytic — continued
 iris 379.49
  due to diphtheria (toxin) 032.81 [379.49]
 ischemic, Volkmann's (complicating trauma) 958.6
 Jackson's 344.8
 jake 357.7
 Jamaica ginger (jake) 357.7
 juvenile general 090.40
 Klumpke (-Déjérine) (birth) (newborn) 767.6
 labioglossal (laryngeal) (pharyngeal) 335.22
 Landry's 357.0
 laryngeal nerve (recurrent) (superior) (see also Paralysis, vocal cord) 478.30
 larynx (see also Paralysis, vocal cord) 478.30
  due to diphtheria (toxin) 032.3
 late effect
  due to
   birth injury, brain or spinal (cord) — see Palsy, cerebral
   edema, brain or cerebral — see Paralysis, brain
   lesion
    cerebrovascular — see category 438
     late effect — see Late effect(s) (of) cerebrovascular disease
   spinal (cord) — see Paralysis, spinal
 lateral 335.24
 lead 984.9
  specified type of lead — see Table of Drugs and Chemicals
 left side — see Hemiplegia
 leg 344.30
  affecting
   dominant side 344.31
   nondominant side 344.32
  both (see also Paraplegia) 344.1
  crossed 344.89
  hysterical 300.11
  psychogenic 306.0
  transient or transitory 781.4
   traumatic NEC (see also Injury, nerve, lower limb) 956.9
 levator palpebrae superioris 374.31
 limb NEC 344.5
  all four — see Quadriplegia
  quadriplegia — see Quadriplegia
 lip 528.5
 Lissauer's 094.1
 local 355.9
 lower limb — see also Paralysis, leg
  both (see also Paraplegia) 344.1
 lung 518.89
  newborn 770.89
 median nerve 354.1
 medullary (tegmental) 344.89
 mesencephalic NEC 344.89
  tegmental 344.89
 middle alternating 344.89
 Millard-Gubler-Foville 344.89
 monoplegic — see Monoplegia
 motor NEC 344.9
  cerebral — see Paralysis, brain
  spinal — see Paralysis, spinal
 multiple
  cerebral — see Paralysis, brain
  spinal — see Paralysis, spinal
 muscle (flaccid) 359.9
  due to nerve lesion NEC 355.9
  eye (extrinsic) 378.55
   intrinsic 367.51

Paralysis, paralytic — *continued*
  muscle — *continued*
    eye — *continued*
      oblique 378.51
      iris sphincter 364.8
      ischemic (complicating trauma)
        (Volkmann's) 958.6
      pseudohypertrophic 359.1
  muscular (atrophic) 359.9
    progressive 335.21
  musculocutaneous nerve 354.9
  musculospiral 354.9
  nerve — *see also* Disorder, nerve
    third or oculomotor (partial) 378.51
      total 378.52
    fourth or trochlear 378.53
    sixth or abducens 378.54
    seventh or facial 351.0
      birth injury 767.5
      due to
        injection NEC 999.9
        operation NEC 997.09
      newborn 767.5
    accessory 352.4
    auditory 388.5
    birth injury 767.7
    cranial or cerebral (*see also* Disorder,
      nerve, cranial) 352.9
    facial 351.0
      birth injury 767.5
      newborn 767.5
    laryngeal (*see also* Paralysis, vocal cord)
      478.30
    newborn 767.7
    phrenic 354.8
      newborn 767.7
    radial 354.3
      birth injury 767.6
      newborn 767.6
    syphilitic 094.89
    traumatic NEC (*see also* Injury, nerve, by
      site) 957.9
    trigeminal 350.9
    ulnar 354.2
  newborn NEC 767.0
  normokalemic periodic 359.3
  obstetrical, newborn 767.7
  ocular 378.9
  oculofacial, congenital 352.6
  oculomotor (nerve) (partial) 378.51
    alternating 344.89
    external bilateral 378.55
    total 378.52
  olfactory nerve 352.0
  palate 528.9
  palatopharyngolaryngeal 352.6
  paratrigeminal 350.9
  periodic (familial) (hyperkalemic) (hypokalemic)
    (normokalemic) (secondary) 359.3
  peripheral
    autonomic nervous system — *see*
      Neuropathy, peripheral, autonomic
    nerve NEC 355.9
  peroneal (nerve) 355.3
  pharynx 478.29
  phrenic nerve 354.8
  plantar nerves 355.6
  pneumogastric nerve 352.3
  poliomyelitis (current) (*see also* Poliomyelitis,
    with paralysis) 045.1 ✓5ᵗʰ
    bulbar 045.0 ✓5ᵗʰ

Paralysis, paralytic — *continued*
  popliteal nerve 355.3
  pressure (*see also* Neuropathy, entrapment)
    355.9
  progressive 335.21
    atrophic 335.21
    bulbar 335.22
    general 094.1
    hemifacial 349.89
    infantile, acute (*see also* Poliomyelitis)
      045.9 ✓5ᵗʰ
    multiple 335.20
  pseudobulbar 335.23
  pseudohypertrophic 359.1
    muscle 359.1
  psychogenic 306.0
  pupil, pupillary 379.49
  quadriceps 355.8
  quadriplegic (*see also* Quadriplegia) 344.0
  radial nerve 354.3
    birth injury 767.6
  rectum (sphincter) 569.49
  rectus muscle (eye) 378.55
  recurrent laryngeal nerve (*see also* Paralysis,
    vocal cord) 478.30
  respiratory (muscle) (system) (tract) 786.09
    center NEC 344.89
      fetus or newborn 770.89
    congenital 768.9
    newborn 768.9
  right side — *see* Hemiplegia
  Saturday night 354.3
  saturnine 984.9
    specified type of lead — *see* Table of Drugs
      and Chemicals
  sciatic nerve 355.0
  secondary — *see* Paralysis, late effect
  seizure (cerebral) (current episode) (*see also*
    Disease, cerebrovascular, acute) 436
    late effect — *see* Late effect(s) (of)
      cerebrovascular disease
  senile NEC 344.9
  serratus magnus 355.9
  shaking (*see also* Parkinsonism) 332.0
  shock (*see also* Disease, cerebrovascular,
    acute) 436
    late effect — *see* Late effect(s) (of)
      cerebrovascular disease
  shoulder 354.9
  soft palate 528.9
  spasmodic — *see* Paralysis, spastic
  spastic 344.9
    cerebral infantile — *see* Palsy, cerebral
    congenital (cerebral) — *see* Palsy, cerebral
    familial 334.1
    hereditary 334.1
    infantile 343.9
    noncongenital or noninfantile, cerebral
      344.9
    syphilitic 094.0
      spinal 094.89
  sphincter, bladder (*see also* Paralysis, bladder)
    596.53
  spinal (cord) NEC 344.1
    accessory nerve 352.4
    acute (*see also* Poliomyelitis) 045.9 ✓5ᵗʰ
    ascending acute 357.0
    atrophic (acute) (*see also* Poliomyelitis, with
      paralysis) 045.1 ✓5ᵗʰ
      spastic, syphilitic 094.89
    congenital NEC 343.9

✓4ᵗʰ Fourth-digit Required   ✓5ᵗʰ Fifth-digit Required

Paralysis, paralytic — continued
  spinal (cord) NEC — continued
    hemiplegic — see Hemiplegia
    hereditary 336.8
    infantile (see also Poliomyelitis) 045.9 ✓5ᵗʰ
    late effect NEC 344.89
    monoplegic — see Monoplegia
    nerve 355.9
    progressive 335.10
    quadriplegic — see Quadriplegia
    spastic NEC 343.9
    traumatic — see Injury, spinal, by site
  sternomastoid 352.4
  stomach 536.3
    nerve 352.3
  stroke (current episode) (see also Disease, cerebrovascular, acute) 436
    late effect — see Late effect(s) (of) cerebrovascular disease
  subscapularis 354.8
  superior nuclear NEC 334.9
  supranuclear 356.8
  sympathetic
    cervical NEC 337.0
    nerve NEC (see also Neuropathy, peripheral, autonomic) 337.9
    nervous system — see Neuropathy, peripheral, autonomic
  syndrome 344.9
    specified NEC 344.89
  syphilitic spastic spinal (Erb's) 094.89
  tabetic general 094.1
  thigh 355.8
  throat 478.29
    diphtheritic 032.0
    muscle 478.29
  thrombotic (current episode) (see also Thrombosis, brain) 434.0 ✓5ᵗʰ
    late effect — see Late effect(s) (of) cerebrovascular disease
    old — see category 438 ✓4ᵗʰ
  thumb NEC 354.9
  tick (-bite) 989.5
  Todd's (postepileptic transitory paralysis) 344.89
  toe 355.6
  tongue 529.8
  transient
    arm or leg NEC 781.4
    traumatic NEC (see also Injury, nerve, by site) 957.9
  trapezius 352.4
  traumatic, transient NEC (see also Injury, nerve, by site) 957.9
  trembling (see also Parkinsonism) 332.0
  triceps brachii 354.9
  trigeminal nerve 350.9
  trochlear nerve 378.53
  ulnar nerve 354.2
  upper limb — see also Paralysis, arm
    both (see also Diplegia) 344.2
  uremic — see Uremia
  uveoparotitic 135
  uvula 528.9
    hysterical 300.11
    postdiphtheritic 032.0
  vagus nerve 352.3
  vasomotor NEC 337.9
  velum palati 528.9
  vesical (see also Paralysis, bladder) 596.53
  vestibular nerve 388.5

Paralysis, paralytic — continued
  visual field, psychic 368.16
  vocal cord 478.30
    bilateral (partial) 478.33
      complete 478.34
    complete (bilateral) 478.34
    unilateral (partial) 478.31
      complete 478.32
  Volkmann's (complicating trauma) 958.6
  wasting 335.21
  Weber's 344.89
  wrist NEC 354.9
Paramedial orifice, urethrovesical 753.8
Paramenia 626.9
Parametritis (chronic) (see also Disease, pelvis, inflammatory) 614.4
  acute 614.3
  puerperal, postpartum, childbirth 670 ✓4ᵗʰ
Parametrium, parametric — see condition
Paramnesia (see also Amnesia) 780.99 ▲
Paramolar 520.1
  causing crowding 524.3
Paramyloidosis 277.3
Paramyoclonus multiplex 333.2
Paramyotonia 359.2
  congenita 359.2
Paraneoplastic syndrome — see condition
Parangi (see also Yaws) 102.9
Paranoia 297.1
  alcoholic 291.5
  querulans 297.8
  senile 290.20
Paranoid
  dementia (see also Schizophrenia) 295.3 ✓5ᵗʰ
    praecox (acute) 295.3 ✓5ᵗʰ
    senile 290.20
  personality 301.0
  psychosis 297.9
    alcoholic 291.5
    climacteric 297.2
    drug-induced 292.11
    involutional 297.2
    menopausal 297.2
    protracted reactive 298.4
    psychogenic 298.4
      acute 298.3
    senile 290.20
  reaction (chronic) 297.9
    acute 298.3
  schizophrenia (acute) (see also Schizophrenia) 295.3 ✓5ᵗʰ
  state 297.9
    alcohol-induced 291.5
    climacteric 297.2
    drug-induced 292.11
    due to or associated with
      arteriosclerosis (cerebrovascular) 290.42
      presenile brain disease 290.12
      senile brain disease 290.20
    involutional 297.2
    menopausal 297.2
    senile 290.20
    simple 297.0
    specified type NEC 297.8
  tendencies 301.0
  traits 301.0
  trends 301.0
  type, psychopathic personality 301.0
Paraparesis (see also Paralysis) 344.9

Paraphasia 784.3
Paraphilia (*see also* Deviation, sexual) 302.9
Paraphimosis (congenital) 605
   chancroidal 099.0
Paraphrenia, paraphrenic (late) 297.2
   climacteric 297.2
   dementia (*see also* Schizophrenia) 295.3 ✓5ᵗʰ
   involutional 297.2
   menopausal 297.2
   schizophrenia (acute) (*see also* Schizophrenia) 295.3 ✓5ᵗʰ
Paraplegia 344.1
   with
      broken back — *see* Fracture, vertebra, by site, with spinal cord injury
      fracture, vertebra — *see* Fracture, vertebra, by site, with spinal cord injury
   ataxic — *see* Degeneration, combined, spinal cord
   brain (current episode) (*see also* Paralysis, brain) 437.8
   cerebral (current episode) (*see also* Paralysis, brain) 437.8
   congenital or infantile (cerebral) (spastic) (spinal) 343.0
   cortical — *see* Paralysis, brain
   familial spastic 334.1
   functional (hysterical) 300.11
   hysterical 300.11
   infantile 343.0
   late effect 344.1
   Pott's (*see also* Tuberculosis) 015.0 ✓5ᵗʰ [730.88]
   psychogenic 306.0
   spastic
      Erb's spinal 094.89
      hereditary 334.1
      not infantile or congenital 344.1
   spinal (cord)
      traumatic NEC — *see* Injury, spinal, by site
   syphilitic (spastic) 094.89
   traumatic NEC — *see* Injury, spinal, by site
Paraproteinemia 273.2
   benign (familial) 273.1
   monoclonal 273.1
   secondary to malignant or inflammatory disease 273.1
Parapsoriasis 696.2
   en plaques 696.2
   guttata 696.2
   lichenoides chronica 696.2
   retiformis 696.2
   varioliformis (acuta) 696.2
Parascarlatina 057.8
Parasitic — *see also* condition
   disease NEC (*see also* Infestation, parasitic) 136.9
      contact V01.89 ▲
      exposure to V01.89 ▲
      intestinal NEC 129
      skin NEC 134.9
   stomatitis 112.0
   sycosis 110.0
      beard 110.0
      scalp 110.0
   twin 759.4
Parasitism NEC 136.9
   intestinal NEC 129
   skin NEC 134.9
   specified — *see* Infestation

Parasitophobia 300.29
Parasomnia 780.59
   nonorganic origin 307.47
Paraspadias 752.69
Paraspasm facialis 351.8
Parathyroid gland — *see* condition
Parathyroiditis (autoimmune) 252.1
Parathyroprival tetany 252.1
Paratrachoma 077.0
Paratyphilitis (*see also* Appendicitis) 541
Paratyphoid (fever) — *see* Fever, paratyphoid
Paratyphus — *see* Fever, paratyphoid
Paraurethral duct 753.8
Para-urethritis 597.89
   gonococcal (acute) 098.0
      chronic or duration of 2 months or over 098.2
Paravaccinia NEC 051.9
   milkers' node 051.1
Paravaginitis (*see also* Vaginitis) 616.10
Parencephalitis (*see also* Encephalitis) 323.9
   late effect — *see* category 326
Parergasia 298.9
Paresis (*see also* Paralysis) 344.9
   accommodation 367.51
   bladder (spastic) (sphincter) (*see also* Paralysis, bladder) 596.53
      tabetic 094.0
   bowel, colon, or intestine (*see also* Ileus) 560.1
   brain or cerebral — *see* Paralysis, brain
   extrinsic muscle, eye 378.55
   general 094.1
      arrested 094.1
      brain 094.1
      cerebral 094.1
      insane 094.1
      juvenile 090.40
         remission 090.49
      progressive 094.1
      remission (sustained) 094.1
      tabetic 094.1
   heart (*see also* Failure, heart) 428.9
   infantile (*see also* Poliomyelitis) 045.9 ✓5ᵗʰ
   insane 094.1
   juvenile 090.40
   late effect — *see* Paralysis, late effect
   luetic (general) 094.1
   peripheral progressive 356.9
   pseudohypertrophic 359.1
   senile NEC 344.9
   stomach 536.3
   syphilitic (general) 094.1
      congenital 090.40
   transient, limb 781.4
   vesical (sphincter) NEC 596.53
Paresthesia (*see also* Disturbance, sensation) 782.0
   Berger's (paresthesia of lower limb) 782.0
   Bernhardt 355.1
   Magnan's 782.0
Paretic — *see* condition
Parinaud's
   conjunctivitis 372.02
   oculoglandular syndrome 372.02
   ophthalmoplegia 378.81
   syndrome (paralysis of conjugate upward gaze) 378.81

Parkes Weber and Dimitri syndrome
(encephalocutaneous angiomatosis) 759.6
Parkinson's disease, syndrome, or tremor —
see Parkinsonism
Parkinsonism (arteriosclerotic) (idiopathic)
(primary) 332.0
associated with orthostatic hypotension
(idiopathic) (symptomatic) 333.0
due to drugs 332.1
secondary 332.1
syphilitic 094.82
Parodontitis 523.4
Parodontosis 523.5
Paronychia (with lymphangitis) 681.9
candidal (chronic) 112.3
chronic 681.9
candidal 112.3
finger 681.02
toe 681.11
finger 681.02
toe 681.11
tuberculous (primary) (see also Tuberculosis)
017.0 ✓5ᵗʰ
Parorexia NEC 307.52
hysterical 300.11
Parosmia 781.1
psychogenic 306.7
Parotid gland — see condition
Parotiditis (see also Parotitis) 527.2
epidemic 072.9
infectious 072.9
Parotitis 527.2
allergic 527.2
chronic 527.2
epidemic (see also Mumps) 072.9
infectious (see also Mumps) 072.9
noninfectious 527.2
nonspecific toxic 527.2
not mumps 527.2
postoperative 527.2
purulent 527.2
septic 527.2
suppurative (acute) 527.2
surgical 527.2
toxic 527.2
Paroxysmal — see also condition
dyspnea (nocturnal) 786.09
Parrot's disease (syphilitic osteochondritis)
090.0
Parrot fever 073.9
Parry's disease or syndrome (exophthalmic
goiter) 242.0 ✓5ᵗʰ
Parry-Romberg syndrome 349.89
Parson's disease (exophthalmic goiter) 242.0 ✓5ᵗʰ
Parsonage-Aldren-Turner syndrome 353.5
Parsonage-Turner syndrome 353.5
Pars planitis 363.21
Particolored infant 757.39
Parturition — see Delivery
Passage
false, urethra 599.4
of sounds or bougies (see also Attention to
artificial opening) V55.9
Passive — see condition
Pasteurella septica 027.2
Pasteurellosis (see also Infection, Pasteurella)
027.2

PAT (paroxysmal atrial tachycardia) 427.0
Patau's syndrome (trisomy D) 758.1
Patch
herald 696.3
Patches
mucous (syphilitic) 091.3
congenital 090.0
smokers' (mouth) 528.6
Patellar — see condition
Patellofemoral syndrome 719.46
Patent — see also Imperfect closure
atrioventricular ostium 745.69
canal of Nuck 752.41
cervix 622.5
complicating pregnancy 654.5 ✓5ᵗʰ
affecting fetus or newborn 761.0
ductus arteriosus or Botalli 747.0
Eustachian
tube 381.7
valve 746.89
foramen
Botalli 745.5
ovale 745.5
interauricular septum 745.5
interventricular septum 745.4
omphalomesenteric duct 751.0
os (uteri) — see Patent, cervix
ostium secundum 745.5
urachus 753.7
vitelline duct 751.0
Paternity testing V70.4
Paterson's syndrome (sideropenic dysphagia)
280.8
Paterson (-Brown) (-Kelly) syndrome
(sideropenic dysphagia) 280.8
Paterson-Kelly syndrome or web (sideropenic
dysphagia) 280.8
Pathologic, pathological — see also condition
asphyxia 799.0
drunkenness 291.4
emotionality 301.3
liar 301.7
personality 301.9
resorption, tooth 521.4
sexuality (see also Deviation, sexual) 302.9
Pathology (of) — see Disease
Patterned motor discharge, idiopathic (see
also Epilepsy) 345.5 ✓5ᵗʰ
Patulous — see also Patent
anus 569.49
Eustachian tube 381.7
Pause, sinoatrial 427.81
Pavor nocturnus 307.46
Pavy's disease 593.6
Paxton's disease (white piedra) 111.2
Payr's disease or syndrome (splenic flexure
syndrome) 569.89
Pearls
Elschnig 366.51
enamel 520.2
Pearl-workers' disease (chronic osteomyelitis)
(see also Osteomyelitis) 730.1 ✓5ᵗʰ
Pectenitis 569.49
Pectenosis 569.49
Pectoral — see condition

Pectus
  carinatum (congenital) 754.82
    acquired 738.3
    rachitic (see also Rickets) 268.0
  excavatum (congenital) 754.81
    acquired 738.3
    rachitic (see also Rickets) 268.0
  recurvatum (congenital) 754.81
    acquired 738.3
Pedatrophia 261
Pederosis 302.2
Pediculosis (infestation) 132.9
  capitis (head louse) (any site) 132.0
  corporis (body louse) (any site) 132.1
  eyelid 132.0 [373.6]
  mixed (classifiable to more than one category in 132.0-132.2) 132.3
  pubis (pubic louse) (any site) 132.2
  vestimenti 132.1
  vulvae 132.2
Pediculus (infestation) — see Pediculosis
Pedophilia 302.2
Peg-shaped teeth 520.2
Pel's crisis 094.0
Pel-Ebstein disease — see Disease, Hodgkin's
Pelade 704.01
Pelger-Huât anomaly or syndrome (hereditary hyposegmentation) 288.2
Peliosis (rheumatica) 287.0
Pelizaeus-Merzbacher
  disease 330.0
  sclerosis, diffuse cerebral 330.0
Pellagra (alcoholic or with alcoholism) 265.2
  with polyneuropathy 265.2 [357.4]
Pellagra-cerebellar-ataxia-renal aminoaciduria syndrome 270.0
Pellegrini's disease (calcification, knee joint) 726.62
Pellegrini (-Stieda) disease or syndrome (calcification, knee joint) 726.62
Pellizzi's syndrome (pineal) 259.8
Pelvic — see also condition
  congestion-fibrosis syndrome 625.5
  kidney 753.3
Pelvioectasis 591
Pelviolithiasis 592.0
Pelviperitonitis
  female (see also Peritonitis, pelvic, female) 614.5
  male (see also Peritonitis) 567.2
Pelvis, pelvic — see also condition or type
  infantile 738.6
  Nägele's 738.6
  obliquity 738.6
  Robert's 755.69
Pemphigoid 694.5
  benign, mucous membrane 694.60
    with ocular involvement 694.61
  bullous 694.5
  cicatricial 694.60
    with ocular involvement 694.61
  juvenile 694.2
Pemphigus 694.4
  benign 694.5
    chronic familial 757.39
  Brazilian 694.4
  circinatus 694.0

Pemphigus — continued
  congenital, traumatic 757.39
  conjunctiva 694.61
  contagiosus 684
  erythematodes 694.4
  erythematosus 694.4
  foliaceus 694.4
  frambesiodes 694.4
  gangrenous (see also Gangrene) 785.4
  malignant 694.4
  neonatorum, newborn 684
  ocular 694.61
  papillaris 694.4
  seborrheic 694.4
  South American 694.4
  syphilitic (congenital) 090.0
  vegetans 694.4
  vulgaris 694.4
  wildfire 694.4
Pendred's syndrome (familial goiter with deaf-mutism) 243
Pendulous
  abdomen 701.9
    in pregnancy or childbirth 654.4 ✓5ᵗʰ
      affecting fetus or newborn 763.89
  breast 611.8
Penetrating wound — see also Wound, open, by site
  with internal injury — see Injury, internal, by site, with open wound
  eyeball 871.7
    with foreign body (nonmagnetic) 871.6
      magnetic 871.5
  ocular (see also Penetrating wound, eyeball) 871.7
  adnexa 870.3
    with foreign body 870.4
  orbit 870.3
    with foreign body 870.4
Penetration, pregnant uterus by instrument
  with
    abortion — see Abortion, by type, with damage to pelvic organs
    ectopic pregnancy (see also categories 633.0-633.9) 639.2
    molar pregnancy (see also categories 630-632) 639.2
  complication of delivery 665.1 ✓5ᵗʰ
    affecting fetus or newborn 763.89
  following
    abortion 639.2
    ectopic or molar pregnancy 639.2
Penfield's syndrome (see also Epilepsy) 345.5 ✓5ᵗʰ
Penicilliosis of lung 117.3
Penis — see condition
Penitis 607.2
Penta X syndrome 758.81
Pentalogy (of Fallot) 745.2
Pentosuria (benign) (essential) 271.8
Peptic acid disease 536.8
Peregrinating patient V65.2
Perforated — see Perforation
Perforation, perforative (nontraumatic)
  antrum (see also Sinusitis, maxillary) 473.0
  appendix 540.0
    with peritoneal abscess 540.1
  atrial septum, multiple 745.5

Perforation, perforative — *continued*
attic, ear 384.22
  healed 384.81
bile duct, except cystic (*see also* Disease, biliary) 576.3
  cystic 575.4
bladder (urinary) 596.6
  with
    abortion — *see* Abortion, by type, with damage to pelvic organs
    ectopic pregnancy (*see also* categories 633.0-633.9) 639.2
    molar pregnancy (*see also* categories 630-632) 639.2
  following
    abortion 639.2
    ectopic or molar pregnancy 639.2
  obstetrical trauma 665.5
bowel 569.83
  with
    abortion — *see* Abortion, by type, with damage to pelvic organs
    ectopic pregnancy (*see also* categories 633.0-633.9) 639.2
    molar pregnancy (*see also* categories 630-632) 639.2
  fetus or newborn 777.6
  following
    abortion 639.2
    ectopic or molar pregnancy 639.2
  obstetrical trauma 665.5
broad ligament
  with
    abortion — *see* Abortion, by type, with damage to pelvic organs
    ectopic pregnancy (*see also* categories 633.0-633.9) 639.2
    molar pregnancy (*see also* categories 630-632) 639.2
  following
    abortion 639.2
    ectopic or molar pregnancy 639.2
  obstetrical trauma 665.6
  by
    device, implant, or graft — *see* Complications, mechanical
    foreign body left accidentally in operation wound 998.4
    instrument (any) during a procedure, accidental 998.2
cecum 540.0
  with peritoneal abcess 540.1
cervix (uteri) — *see also* Injury, internal, cervix
  with
    abortion — *see* Abortion, by type, with damage to pelvic organs
    ectopic pregnancy (*see also* categories 633.0-633.9) 639.2
    molar pregnancy (*see also* categories 630-632) 639.2
  following
    abortion 639.2
    ectopic or molar pregnancy 639.2
  obstetrical trauma 665.3
colon 569.83
common duct (bile) 576.3
cornea (*see also* Ulcer, cornea) 370.00
  due to ulceration 370.06
cystic duct 575.4

Perforation, perforative — *continued*
diverticulum (*see also* Diverticula) 562.10
  small intestine 562.00
duodenum, duodenal (ulcer) — *see* Ulcer, duodenum, with perforation
ear drum — *see* Perforation, tympanum
enteritis — *see* Enteritis
esophagus 530.4
ethmoidal sinus (*see also* Sinusitis, ethmoidal) 473.2
foreign body (external site) — *see also* Wound, open, by site, complicated
  internal site, by ingested object — *see* Foreign body
frontal sinus (*see also* Sinusitis, frontal) 473.1
gallbladder or duct (*see also* Disease, gallbladder) 575.4
gastric (ulcer) — *see* Ulcer, stomach, with perforation
heart valve — *see* Endocarditis
ileum (*see also* Perforation, intestine) 569.83
instrumental
  external — *see* Wound, open, by site
  pregnant uterus, complicating delivery 665.9
  surgical (accidental) (blood vessel) (nerve) (organ) 998.2
intestine 569.83
  with
    abortion — *see* Abortion, by type, with damage to pelvic organs
    ectopic pregnancy (*see also* categories 633.0-633.9) 639.2
    molar pregnancy (*see also* categories 630-632) 639.2
  fetus or newborn 777.6
  obstetrical trauma 665.5
  ulcerative NEC 569.83
jejunum, jejunal 569.83
  ulcer — *see* Ulcer, gastrojejunal, with perforation
mastoid (antrum) (cell) 383.89
maxillary sinus (*see also* Sinusitis, maxillary) 473.0
membrana tympani — *see* Perforation, tympanum
nasal
  septum 478.1
    congenital 748.1
    syphilitic 095.8
  sinus (*see also* Sinusitis) 473.9
    congenital 748.1
palate (hard) 526.89
  soft 528.9
    syphilitic 095.8
    syphilitic 095.8
palatine vault 526.89
  syphilitic 095.8
    congenital 090.5
pelvic
  floor
    with
      abortion — *see* Abortion, by type, with damage to pelvic organs
      ectopic pregnancy (*see also* categories 633.0-633.9) 639.2
      molar pregnancy (*see also* categories 630-632) 639.2
      obstetrical trauma 664.1

Perforation, perforative — *continued*
  pelvic — *continued*
    organ
      with
        abortion — *see* Abortion, by type,
          with damage to pelvic organs
        ectopic pregnancy (*see also* categories
          633.0-633.9) 639.2
        molar pregnancy (*see also* categories
          630-632) 639.2
      following
        abortion 639.2
        ectopic or molar pregnancy 639.2
      obstetrical trauma 665.5 ✓5ᵗʰ
  perineum — *see* Laceration, perineum
  periurethral tissue
    with
      abortion — *see* Abortion, by type, with
        damage to pelvic organs
      ectopic pregnancy (*see also* categories
        630-632) 639.2
      molar pregnancy (*see also* categories
        630-632) 639.2
  pharynx 478.29
  pylorus, pyloric (ulcer) — *see* Ulcer, stomach,
    with perforation
  rectum 569.49
  sigmoid 569.83
  sinus (accessory) (chronic) (nasal) (*see also*
    Sinusitis) 473.9
  sphenoidal sinus (*see also* Sinusitis,
    sphenoidal) 473.3
  stomach (due to ulcer) — *see* Ulcer, stomach,
    with perforation
  surgical (accidental) (by instrument) (blood
    vessel) (nerve) (organ) 998.2
  traumatic
    external — *see* Wound, open, by site
    eye (*see also* Penetrating wound, ocular)
      871.7
    internal organ — *see* Injury, internal, by
      site
    tympanum (membrane) (persistent
      posttraumatic) (postinflammatory)
      384.20
      with
        otitis media — *see* Otitis media
      attic 384.22
      central 384.21
      healed 384.81
      marginal NEC 384.23
      multiple 384.24
      pars flaccida 384.22
      total 384.25
      traumatic — *see* Wound, open, ear, drum
  typhoid, gastrointestinal 002.0
  ulcer — *see* Ulcer, by site, with perforation
  ureter 593.89
  urethra
    with
      abortion — *see* Abortion, by type, with
        damage to pelvic organs
      ectopic pregnancy (*see also* categories
        633.0-633.9) 639.2
      molar pregnancy (*see also* categories
        630-632) 639.2
    following
      abortion 639.2
      ectopic or molar pregnancy 639.2
    obstetrical trauma 665.5 ✓5ᵗʰ

Perforation, perforative — *continued*
  uterus — *see also* Injury, internal, uterus
    with
      abortion — *see* Abortion, by type, with
        damage to pelvic organs
      ectopic pregnancy (*see also* categories
        633.0-633.9) 639.2
      molar pregnancy (*see also* categories
        630-632) 639.2
    by intrauterine contraceptive device 996.32
    following
      abortion 639.2
      ectopic or molar pregnancy 639.2
    obstetrical trauma — *see* Injury, internal,
      uterus, obstetrical trauma
  uvula 528.9
    syphilitic 095.8
  vagina — *see* Laceration, vagina
  viscus NEC 799.8
    traumatic 868.00
      with open wound into cavity 868.10
Periadenitis mucosa necrotica recurrens 528.2
Periangiitis 446.0
Periantritis 535.4 ✓5ᵗʰ
Periappendicitis (acute) (*see also* Appendicitis)
  541
Periarteritis (disseminated) (infectious)
  (necrotizing) (nodosa) 446.0
Periarthritis (joint) 726.90
  Duplay's 726.2
  gonococcal 098.50
  humeroscapularis 726.2
  scapulohumeral 726.2
  shoulder 726.2
  wrist 726.4
Periarthrosis (angioneural) — *see* Periarthritis
Peribronchitis 491.9
  tuberculous (*see also* Tuberculosis) 011.3 ✓5ᵗʰ
Pericapsulitis, adhesive (shoulder) 726.0
Pericarditis (granular) (with decompensation)
  (with effusion) 423.9
  with
    rheumatic fever (conditions classifiable to
      390)
      active (*see also* Pericarditis, rheumatic)
        391.0
      inactive or quiescent 393
  actinomycotic 039.8 *[420.0]*
  acute (nonrheumatic) 420.90
    with chorea (acute) (rheumatic)
      (Sydenham's) 392.0
    bacterial 420.99
    benign 420.91
    hemorrhagic 420.90
    idiopathic 420.91
    infective 420.90
    nonspecific 420.91
    rheumatic 391.0
      with chorea (acute) (rheumatic)
        (Sydenham's) 392.0
    sicca 420.90
    viral 420.91
  adhesive or adherent (external) (internal)
    423.1
    acute — *see* Pericarditis, acute
    rheumatic (external) (internal) 393
  amebic 006.8 *[420.0]*
  bacterial (acute) (subacute) (with serous or
    seropurulent effusion) 420.99
  calcareous 423.2

Pericarditis — continued
- cholesterol (chronic) 423.8
  - acute 420.90
- chronic (nonrheumatic) 423.8
  - rheumatic 393
- constrictive 423.2
- Coxsackie 074.21
- due to
  - actinomycosis 039.8 [420.0]
  - amebiasis 006.8 [420.0]
  - Coxsackie (virus) 074.21
  - histoplasmosis (see also Histoplasmosis) 115.93
  - nocardiosis 039.8 [420.0]
  - tuberculosis (see also Tuberculosis) 017.9 ✓5ᵗʰ [420.0]
- fibrinocaseous (see also Tuberculosis) 017.9 ✓5ᵗʰ [420.0]
- fibrinopurulent 420.99
- fibrinous — see Pericarditis, rheumatic
- fibropurulent 420.99
- fibrous 423.1
- gonococcal 098.83
- hemorrhagic 423.0
- idiopathic (acute) 420.91
- infective (acute) 420.90
- meningococcal 036.41
- neoplastic (chronic) 423.8
  - acute 420.90
- nonspecific 420.91
- obliterans, obliterating 423.1
- plastic 423.1
- pneumococcal (acute) 420.99
- postinfarction 411.0
- purulent (acute) 420.99
- rheumatic (active) (acute) (with effusion) (with pneumonia) 391.0
  - with chorea (acute) (rheumatic) (Sydenham's) 392.0
  - chronic or inactive (with chorea) 393
- septic (acute) 420.99
- serofibrinous — see Pericarditis, rheumatic
- staphylococcal (acute) 420.99
- streptococcal (acute) 420.99
- suppurative (acute) 420.99
- syphilitic 093.81
- tuberculous (acute) (chronic) (see also Tuberculosis) 017.9 ✓5ᵗʰ [420.0]
- uremic 585 [420.0]
- viral (acute) 420.91

Pericardium, pericardial — see condition
Pericellulitis (see also Cellulitis) 682.9
Pericementitis 523.4
- acute 523.3
- chronic (suppurative) 523.4

Pericholecystitis (see also Cholecystitis) 575.10
Perichondritis
- auricle 380.00
  - acute 380.01
  - chronic 380.02
- bronchus 491.9
- ear (external) 380.00
  - acute 380.01
  - chronic 380.02
- larynx 478.71
  - syphilitic 095.8
  - typhoid 002.0 [478.71]
- nose 478.1
- pinna 380.00
  - acute 380.01
  - chronic 380.02

Perichondritis — continued
- trachea 478.9
Periclasia 523.5
Pericolitis 569.89
Pericoronitis (chronic) 523.4
- acute 523.3
Pericystitis (see also Cystitis) 595.9
Pericytoma (M9150/1) — see also Neoplasm, connective tissue, uncertain behavior
- benign (M9150/0) — see Neoplasm, connective tissue, benign
- malignant (M9150/3) — see Neoplasm, connective tissue, malignant
Peridacryocystitis, acute 375.32
Peridiverticulitis (see also Diverticulitis) 562.11
Periduodenitis 535.6 ✓5ᵗʰ
Periendocarditis (see also Endocarditis) 424.90
- acute or subacute 421.9
Periepididymitis (see also Epididymitis) 604.90
Perifolliculitis (abscedens) 704.8
- capitis, abscedens et suffodiens 704.8
- dissecting, scalp 704.8
- scalp 704.8
- superficial pustular 704.8
Perigastritis (acute) 535.0 ✓5ᵗʰ
Perigastrojejunitis (acute) 535.0 ✓5ᵗʰ
Perihepatitis (acute) 573.3
- chlamydial 099.56
- gonococcal 098.86
Peri-ileitis (subacute) 569.89
Perilabyrinthitis (acute) — see Labyrinthitis
Perimeningitis — see Meningitis
Perimetritis (see also Endometritis) 615.9
Perimetrosalpingitis (see also Salpingo-oophoritis) 614.2
Perinephric — see condition
Perinephritic — see condition
Perinephritis (see also Infection, kidney) 590.9
- purulent (see also Abscess, kidney) 590.2
Perineum, perineal — see condition
Perineuritis NEC 729.2
Periodic — see also condition
- disease (familial) 277.3
- edema 995.1
  - hereditary 277.6
- fever 277.3
- paralysis (familial) 359.3
- peritonitis 277.3
- polyserositis 277.3
- somnolence 347
Periodontal
- cyst 522.8
- pocket 523.8
Periodontitis (chronic) (complex) (compound) (local) (simplex) 523.4
- acute 523.3
- apical 522.6
  - acute (pulpal origin) 522.4
Periodontoclasia 523.5
Periodontosis 523.5
Periods — see also Menstruation
- heavy 626.2
- irregular 626.4
Perionychia (with lymphangitis) 681.9
- finger 681.02
- toe 681.11

Perioophoritis (see also Salpingo-oophoritis) 614.2
Periorchitis (see also Orchitis) 604.90
Periosteum, periosteal — see condition
Periostitis (circumscribed) (diffuse) (infective) 730.3 ✓5ᵗʰ

> Note — Use the following fifth-digit subclassification with category 730:
>
> 0 site unspecified
> 1 shoulder region
> 2 upper arm
> 3 forearm
> 4 hand
> 5 pelvic region and thigh
> 6 lower leg
> 7 ankle and foot
> 8 other specified sites
> 9 multiple sites

    with osteomyelitis (see also Osteomyelitis) 730.2 ✓5ᵗʰ
      acute or subacute 730.0 ✓5ᵗʰ
      chronic or old 730.1 ✓5ᵗʰ
    albuminosa, albuminosus 730.3 ✓5ᵗʰ
    alveolar 526.5
    alveolodental 526.5
    dental 526.5
    gonorrheal 098.89
    hyperplastica, generalizada 731.2
    jaw (lower) (upper) 526.4
    monomelic 733.99
    orbital 376.02
    syphilitic 095.5
      congenital 090.0 [730.8] ✓5ᵗʰ
      secondary 091.61
    tuberculous (see also Tuberculosis, bone) 015.9 ✓5ᵗʰ [730.8] ✓5ᵗʰ
    yaws (early) (hypertrophic) (late) 102.6
Periostosis (see also Periostitis) 730.3 ✓5ᵗʰ
    with osteomyelitis (see also Osteomyelitis) 730.2 ✓5ᵗʰ
      acute or subacute 730.0 ✓5ᵗʰ
      chronic or old 730.1 ✓5ᵗʰ
    hyperplastic 756.59
Periphlebitis (see also Phlebitis) 451.9
    lower extremity 451.2
      deep (vessels) 451.19
      superficial (vessels) 451.0
    portal 572.1
    retina 362.18
    superficial (vessels) 451.0
    tuberculous (see also Tuberculosis) 017.9 ✓5ᵗʰ
      retina 017.3 ✓5ᵗʰ [362.18]
Peripneumonia — see Pneumonia
Periproctitis 569.49
Periprostatitis (see also Prostatitis) 601.9
Perirectal — see condition
Perirenal — see condition
Perisalpingitis (see also Salpingo-oophoritis) 614.2
Perisigmoiditis 569.89
Perisplenitis (infectional) 289.59
Perispondylitis — see Spondylitis
Peristalsis reversed or visible 787.4

Peritendinitis (see also Tenosynovitis) 726.90
    adhesive (shoulder) 726.0
Perithelioma (M9150/1) — see Pericytoma
Peritoneum, peritoneal — see also condition
    equilibration test V56.32
Peritonitis (acute) (adhesive) (fibrinous) (hemorrhagic) (idiopathic) (localized) (perforative) (primary) (with adhesions) (with effusion) 567.9
    with or following
      abortion — see Abortion, by type, with sepsis
      abscess 567.2
      appendicitis 540.0
        with peritoneal abcess 540.1
      ectopic pregnancy (see also categories 633.0-633.9) 639.0
      molar pregnancy (see also categories 630-632) 639.0
    aseptic 998.7
    bacterial 567.2
    bile, biliary 567.8
    chemical 998.7
    chlamydial 099.56
    chronic proliferative 567.8
    congenital NEC 777.6
    diaphragmatic 567.2
    diffuse NEC 567.2
    diphtheritic 032.83
    disseminated NEC 567.2
    due to
      bile 567.8
      foreign
        body or object accidentally left during a procedure (instrument) (sponge) (swab) 998.4
        substance accidentally left during a procedure (chemical) (powder) (talc) 998.7
      talc 998.7
      urine 567.8
    fibrinopurulent 567.2
    fibrinous 567.2
    fibrocaseous (see also Tuberculosis) 014.0 ✓5ᵗʰ
    fibropurulent 567.2
    general, generalized (acute) 567.2
    gonococcal 098.86
    in infective disease NEC 136.9 [567.0]
    meconium (newborn) 777.6
    pancreatic 577.8
    paroxysmal, benign 277.3
    pelvic
      female (acute) 614.5
        chronic NEC 614.7
          with adhesions 614.6
        puerperal, postpartum, childbirth 670 ✓4ᵗʰ
      male (acute) 567.2
    periodic (familial) 277.3
    phlegmonous 567.2
    pneumococcal 567.1
    postabortal 639.0
    proliferative, chronic 567.8
    puerperal, postpartum, childbirth 670 ✓4ᵗʰ
    purulent 567.2
    septic 567.2
    staphylococcal 567.2
    streptococcal 567.2
    subdiaphragmatic 567.2
    subphrenic 567.2
    suppurative 567.2

Peritonitis — *continued*
  syphilitic 095.2
    congenital 090.0 [567.0]
  talc 998.7
  tuberculous (*see also* Tuberculosis) 014.0 ✓5ᵗʰ
  urine 567.8
Peritonsillar — *see* condition
Peritonsillitis 475
Perityphlitis (*see also* Appendicitis) 541
Periureteritis 593.89
Periurethral — *see* condition
Periurethritis (gangrenous) 597.89
Periuterine — *see* condition
Perivaginitis (*see also* Vaginitis) 616.10
Perivasculitis, retinal 362.18
Perivasitis (chronic) 608.4
Periventricular leukomalacia 779.7
Perivesiculitis (seminal) (*see also* Vesiculitis) 608.0
Perlèche 686.8
  due to
    moniliasis 112.0
    riboflavin deficiency 266.0
Pernicious — *see* condition
Pernio, perniosis 991.5
Persecution
  delusion 297.9
  social V62.4
Perseveration (tonic) 784.69
Persistence, persistent (congenital) 759.89
  anal membrane 751.2
  arteria stapedia 744.04
  atrioventricular canal 745.69
  bloody ejaculate 792.2
  branchial cleft 744.41
  bulbus cordis in left ventricle 745.8
  canal of Cloquet 743.51
  capsule (opaque) 743.51
  cilioretinal artery or vein 743.51
  cloaca 751.5
  communication — *see* Fistula, congenital
  convolutions
    aortic arch 747.21
    fallopian tube 752.19
    oviduct 752.19
    uterine tube 752.19
  double aortic arch 747.21
  ductus
    arteriosus 747.0
    Botalli 747.0
  fetal
    circulation 747.83 ▲
    form of cervix (uteri) 752.49
    hemoglobin (hereditary) ("Swiss variety") 282.7
    pulmonary hypertension 747.83 ▲
  foramen
    Botalli 745.5
    ovale 745.5
  Gartner's duct 752.11
  hemoglobin, fetal (hereditary) (HPFH) 282.7
  hyaloid
    artery (generally incomplete) 743.51
    system 743.51
  hymen (tag)
    in pregnancy or childbirth 654.8 ✓5ᵗʰ
      causing obstructed labor 660.2 ✓5ᵗʰ
  lanugo 757.4

Persistence, persistent — *continued*
  left
    posterior cardinal vein 747.49
    root with right arch of aorta 747.21
    superior vena cava 747.49
  Meckel's diverticulum 751.0
  mesonephric duct 752.8
    fallopian tube 752.11
  mucosal disease (middle ear) (with posterior or superior marginal perforation of ear drum) 382.2
  nail(s), anomalous 757.5
  occiput, anterior or posterior 660.3 ✓5ᵗʰ
    fetus or newborn 763.1
  omphalomesenteric duct 751.0
  organ or site NEC — *see* Anomaly, specified type NEC
  ostium
    atrioventriculare commune 745.69
    primum 745.61
    secundum 745.5
  ovarian rests in fallopian tube 752.19
  pancreatic tissue in intestinal tract 751.5
  primary (deciduous)
    teeth 520.6
    vitreous hyperplasia 743.51
  pulmonary hypertension 747.83 ▲
  pupillary membrane 743.46
    iris 743.46
  Rhesus (Rh) titer 999.7
  right aortic arch 747.21
  sinus
    urogenitalis 752.8
    venosus with imperfect incorporation in right auricle 747.49
  thymus (gland) 254.8
    hyperplasia 254.0
  thyroglossal duct 759.2
  thyrolingual duct 759.2
  truncus arteriosus or communis 745.0
  tunica vasculosa lentis 743.39
  umbilical sinus 753.7
  urachus 753.7
  vegetative state 780.03
  vitelline duct 751.0
  wolffian duct 752.8
Person (with)
  admitted for clinical research, as participant or control subject V70.7
  awaiting admission to adequate facility elsewhere V63.2
    undergoing social agency investigation V63.8
  concern (normal) about sick person in family V61.49
  consulting on behalf of another V65.1
  feared
    complaint in whom no diagnosis was made V65.5
    condition not demonstrated V65.5
  feigning illness V65.2
  healthy, accompanying sick person V65.0
  living (in)
    alone V60.3
    boarding school V60.6
    residence remote from hospital or medical care facility V63.0
    residential institution V60.6
    without
      adequate
        financial resources V60.2

Persistence, persistent — *continued*
  living (in) — *continued*
    without — *continued*
      adequate — *continued*
        housing (heating) (space) V60.1
        housing (permanent) (temporary) V60.0
        material resources V60.2
        person able to render necessary care V60.4
        shelter V60.0
  medical services in home not available V63.1
  on waiting list V63.2
    undergoing social agency investigation V63.8
  sick or handicapped in family V61.49
  "worried well" V65.5

Personality
  affective 301.10
  aggressive 301.3
  amoral 301.7
  anancastic, anankastic 301.4
  antisocial 301.7
  asocial 301.7
  asthenic 301.6
  avoidant 301.82
  borderline 301.83
  change 310.1
  compulsive 301.4
  cycloid 301.13
  cyclothymic 301.13
  dependent 301.6
  depressive (chronic) 301.12
  disorder, disturbance NEC 301.9
    with
      antisocial disturbance 301.7
      pattern disturbance NEC 301.9
      sociopathic disturbance 301.7
      trait disturbance 301.9
  dual 300.14
  dyssocial 301.7
  eccentric 301.89
    "haltlose" type 301.89
  emotionally unstable 301.59
  epileptoid 301.3
  explosive 301.3
  fanatic 301.0
  histrionic 301.50
  hyperthymic 301.11
  hypomanic 301.11
  hypothymic 301.12
  hysterical 301.50
  immature 301.89
  inadequate 301.6
  labile 301.59
  masochistic 301.89
  morally defective 301.7
  multiple 300.14
  narcissistic 301.81
  obsessional 301.4
  obsessive (-compulsive) 301.4
  overconscientious 301.4
  paranoid 301.0
  passive (-dependent) 301.6
  passive-aggressive 301.84
  pathologic NEC 301.9
  pattern defect or disturbance 301.9
  pseudosocial 301.7
  psychoinfantile 301.59
  psychoneurotic NEC 301.89

Personality — *continued*
  psychopathic 301.9
    with
      amoral trend 301.7
      antisocial trend 301.7
      asocial trend 301.7
      pathologic sexuality (*see also* Deviation, sexual) 302.9
    mixed types 301.9
  schizoid 301.20
    introverted 301.21
    schizotypal 301.22
    with sexual deviation (*see also* Deviation, sexual) 302.9
    antisocial 301.7
    dyssocial 301.7
  type A 301.4
  unstable (emotional) 301.59

Perthes' disease (capital femoral osteochondrosis) 732.1

Pertussis (*see also* Whooping cough) 033.9
  vaccination, prophylactic (against) V03.6

Peruvian wart 088.0

Perversion, perverted
  appetite 307.52
    hysterical 300.11
  function
    pineal gland 259.8
    pituitary gland 253.9
      anterior lobe
        deficient 253.2
        excessive 253.1
      posterior lobe 253.6
  placenta — *see* Placenta, abnormal
  sense of smell or taste 781.1
    psychogenic 306.7
  sexual (*see also* Deviation, sexual) 302.9

Pervious, congenital — *see also* Imperfect, closure
  ductus arteriosus 747.0

Pes (congenital) (*see also* Talipes) 754.70
  abductus (congenital) 754.60
    acquired 736.79
  acquired NEC 736.79
    planus 734
  adductus (congenital) 754.79
    acquired 736.79
  cavus 754.71
    acquired 736.73
  planovalgus (congenital) 754.69
    acquired 736.79
  planus (acquired) (any degree) 734
    congenital 754.61
    rachitic 268.1
  valgus (congenital) 754.61
    acquired 736.79
  varus (congenital) 754.50
    acquired 736.79

Pest (*see also* Plague) 020.9

Pestis (*see also* Plague) 020.9
  bubonica 020.0
  fulminans 020.0
  minor 020.8
  pneumonica — *see* Plague, pneumonic

Petechia, petechiae 782.7
  fetus or newborn 772.6

Petechial
  fever 036.0
  typhus 081.9

Petges-Cléjat or Petges-Clégat syndrome
(poikilodermatomyositis) 710.3
Petit's
disease (*see also* Hernia, lumbar) 553.8
Petit mal (idiopathic) (*see also* Epilepsy) 345.0 ✓5ᵗʰ
status 345.2
Petrellidosis 117.6
Petrositis 383.20
acute 383.21
chronic 383.22
Peutz-Jeghers disease or syndrome 759.6
Peyronie's disease 607.89
Pfeiffer's disease 075
Phacentocele 379.32
traumatic 921.3
Phacoanaphylaxis 360.19
Phacocele (old) 379.32
traumatic 921.3
Phaehyphomycosis 117.8
Phagedena (dry) (moist) (*see also* Gangrene) 785.4
arteriosclerotic 440.2 ✓5ᵗʰ [785.4]
geometric 686.09
penis 607.89
senile 440.2 ✓5ᵗʰ [785.4]
sloughing 785.4
tropical (*see also* Ulcer, skin) 707.9
vulva 616.50
Phagedenic — *see also* condition
abscess — *see also* Abscess
chancroid 099.0
bubo NEC 099.8
chancre 099.0
ulcer (tropical) (*see also* Ulcer, skin) 707.9
Phagomania 307.52
Phakoma 362.89
Phantom limb (syndrome) 353.6
Pharyngeal — *see also* condition
arch remnant 744.41
pouch syndrome 279.11
Pharyngitis (acute) (catarrhal) (gangrenous) (infective) (malignant) (membranous) (phlegmonous) (pneumococcal) (pseudomembranous) (simple) (staphylococcal) (subacute) (suppurative) (ulcerative) (viral) 462
with influenza, flu, or grippe 487.1
aphthous 074.0
atrophic 472.1
chronic 472.1
chlamydial 099.51
coxsackie virus 074.0
diphtheritic (membranous) 032.0
follicular 472.1
fusospirochetal 101
gonococcal 098.6
granular (chronic) 472.1
herpetic 054.79
hypertrophic 472.1
infectional, chronic 472.1
influenzal 487.1
lymphonodular, acute 074.8
septic 034.0
streptococcal 034.0
tuberculous (*see also* Tuberculosis) 012.8 ✓5ᵗʰ
vesicular 074.0
Pharyngoconjunctival fever 077.2
Pharyngoconjunctivitis, viral 077.2

Pharyngolaryngitis (acute) 465.0
chronic 478.9
septic 034.0
Pharyngoplegia 478.29
Pharyngotonsillitis 465.8
tuberculous 012.8 ✓5ᵗʰ
Pharyngotracheitis (acute) 465.8
chronic 478.9
Pharynx, pharyngeal — *see* condition
Phase of life problem NEC V62.89
Phenomenon
Arthus' — *see* Arthus' phenomenon
flashback (drug) 292.89
jaw-winking 742.8
Jod-Basedow 242.8 ✓5ᵗʰ
L. E. cell 710.0
lupus erythematosus cell 710.0
Pelger-Huët (hereditary hyposegmentation) 288.2
Raynaud's (paroxysmal digital cyanosis) (secondary) 443.0
Reilly's (*see also* Neuropathy, peripheral, autonomic) 337.9
vasomotor 780.2
vasospastic 443.9
vasovagal 780.2
Wenckebach's, heart block (second degree) 426.13
Phenylketonuria (PKU) 270.1
Phenylpyruvicaciduria 270.1
Pheochromoblastoma (M8700/3)
specified site — *see* Neoplasm, by site, malignant
unspecified site 194.0
Pheochromocytoma (M8700/0)
malignant (M8700/3)
specified site — *see* Neoplasm, by site, malignant
unspecified site 194.0
specified site — *see* Neoplasm, by site, benign
unspecified site 227.0
Phimosis (congenital) 605
chancroidal 099.0
due to infection 605
Phlebectasia (*see also* Varicose, vein) 454.9
congenital 747.6 ✓5ᵗʰ
esophagus (*see also* Varix, esophagus) 456.1
with hemorrhage (*see also* Varix, esophagus, bleeding) 456.0
Phlebitis (infective) (pyemic) (septic) (suppurative) 451.9
antecubital vein 451.82
arm NEC 451.84
axillary vein 451.89
basilic vey 451.82
deep 451.83
superficial 451.82
basilic vein 451.82
blue 451.19
brachial vein 451.83
breast, superficial 451.89
cavernous (venous) sinus — *see* Phlebitis, intracranial sinus
cephalic vein 451.82
cerebral (venous) sinus — *see* Phlebitis, intracranial sinus
chest wall, superficial 451.89
complicating pregnancy or puerperium 671.9 ✓5ᵗʰ
affecting fetus or newborn 760.3

Phlebitis — *continued*
   cranial (venous) sinus — *see* Phlebitis,
      intracranial sinus
   deep (vessels) 451.19
      femoral vein 451.11
      specified vessel NEC 451.19
   due to implanted device — *see* Complications,
      due to (presence of) any device, implant
      or graft classified to 996.0-996.5 NEC
   during or resulting from a procedure 997.2
   femoral vein (deep) 451.11
   femoropopliteal 451.0
   following infusion, perfusion, or transfusion
      999.2
   gouty 274.89 *[451.9]*
   hepatic veins 451.89
   iliac vein 451.81
   iliofemoral 451.11
   intracranial sinus (any) (venous) 325
      late effect — *see* category 326
      nonpyogenic 437.6
         in pregnancy or puerperium 671.5 ✓5ᵗʰ
   jugular vein 451.89
   lateral (venous) sinus — *see* Phlebitis,
      intracranial sinus
   leg 451.2
      deep (vessels) 451.19
         femoral vein 451.11
         specified vessel NEC 451.19
      superficial (vessels) 451.0
         femoral vein 451.11
   longitudinal sinus — *see* Phlebitis,
      intracranial sinus
   lower extremity 451.2
      deep (vessels) 451.19
         femoral vein 451.11
         specified vessel NEC 451.19
      superficial (vessels) 451.0
         femoral vein 451.11
   migrans, migrating (superficial) 453.1
   pelvic
      with
         abortion — *see* Abortion, by type, with
            sepsis
         ectopic pregnancy (*see also* categories
            633.0-633.9) 639.0
         molar pregnancy (*see also* categories
            630-632) 639.0
      following
         abortion 639.0
         ectopic or molar pregnancy 639.0
      puerperal, postpartum 671.4 ✓5ᵗʰ
   popliteal vein 451.19
   portal (vein) 572.1
   postoperative 997.2
   pregnancy 671.9 ✓5ᵗʰ
      deep 671.3 ✓5ᵗʰ
         specified type NEC 671.5 ✓5ᵗʰ
      superficial 671.2 ✓5ᵗʰ
   puerperal, postpartum, childbirth 671.9 ✓5ᵗʰ
      deep 671.4 ✓5ᵗʰ
      lower extremities 671.2 ✓5ᵗʰ
      pelvis 671.4 ✓5ᵗʰ
      specified site NEC 671.5 ✓5ᵗʰ
      superficial 671.2 ✓5ᵗʰ
   radial vein 451.83
   retina 362.18
   saphenous (great) (long) 451.0
      accessory or small 451.0
   sinus (meninges) — *see* Phlebitis, intracranial
      sinus
   specified site NEC 451.89

Phlebitis — *continued*
   subclavian vein 451.89
   syphilitic 093.89
   tibial vein 451.19
   ulcer, ulcerative 451.9
      leg 451.2
         deep (vessels) 451.19
            femoral vein 451.11
            specified vessel NEC 451.19
         superficial (vessels) 451.0
            femoral vein 451.11
      lower extremity 451.2
         deep (vessels) 451.19
            femoral vein 451.11
            specified vessel NEC 451.19
         superficial (vessels) 451.0
   ulnar vein 451.83
   upper extremity — *see* Phlebitis, arm
   umbilicus 451.89
   uterus (septic) (*see also* Endometritis) 615.9
   varicose (leg) (lower extremity) (*see also*
      Varicose, vein) 454.1
Phlebofibrosis 459.89
Phleboliths 459.89
Phlebosclerosis 459.89
Phlebothrombosis — *see* Thrombosis
Phlebotomus fever 066.0
Phlegm, choked on 933.1
Phlegmasia
   alba dolens (deep vessels) 451.19
      complicating pregnancy 671.3 ✓5ᵗʰ
      nonpuerperal 451.19
      puerperal, postpartum, childbirth
         671.4 ✓5ᵗʰ
   cerulea dolens 451.19
Phlegmon (*see also* Abscess) 682.9
   erysipelatous (*see also* Erysipelas) 035
   iliac 682.2
      fossa 540.1
   throat 478.29
Phlegmonous — *see* condition
Phlyctenulosis (allergic) (keratoconjuctivitis)
   (nontuberculous) 370.31
   cornea 370.31
      with ulcer (*see also* Ulcer, cornea) 370.00
   tuberculous (*see also* Tuberculosis) 017.3 ✓5ᵗʰ
      [370.31]
Phobia, phobic (reaction) 300.20
   animal 300.29
   isolated NEC 300.29
   obsessional 300.3
   simple NEC 300.29
   social 300.23
   specified NEC 300.29
   state 300.20
Phocas' disease 610.1
Phocomelia 755.4
   lower limb 755.32
      complete 755.33
      distal 755.35
      proximal 755.34
   upper limb 755.22
      complete 755.23
      distal 755.25
      proximal 755.24
Phoria (*see also* Heterophoria) 378.40
Phosphate-losing tubular disorder 588.0
Phosphatemia 275.3
Phosphaturia 275.3
Photoallergic response 692.72
Photocoproporphyria 277.1

Photodermatitis

Photodermatitis (sun) 692.72
   light other than sun 692.82
Photokeratitis 370.24
Photo-ophthalmia 370.24
Photophobia 368.13
Photopsia 368.15
Photoretinitis 363.31
Photoretinopathy 363.31
Photosensitiveness (sun) 692.72
   light other than sun 692.82
Photosensitization (sun) skin 692.72
   light other than sun 692.82
Phototoxic response 692.72
Phrenitis 323.9
Phrynoderma 264.8
Phthiriasis (pubis) (any site) 132.2
   with any infestation classifiable to 132.0, 132.1 and 132.3
Phthirus infestation — see Phthiriasis
Phthisis (see also Tuberculosis) 011.9 ✓5ᵗʰ
   bulbi (infectional) 360.41
   colliers' 011.4 ✓5ᵗʰ
   cornea 371.05
   eyeball (due to infection) 360.41
   millstone makers' 011.4 ✓5ᵗʰ
   miners' 011.4 ✓5ᵗʰ
   potters' 011.4 ✓5ᵗʰ
   sandblasters' 011.4 ✓5ᵗʰ
   stonemasons' 011.4 ✓5ᵗʰ
Phycomycosis 117.7
Physalopteriasis 127.7
Physical therapy NEC V57.1
   breathing exercises V57.0
Physiological cup, optic papilla
   borderline, glaucoma suspect 365.00
   enlarged 377.14
   glaucomatous 377.14
Phytobezoar 938
   intestine 936
   stomach 935.2
Pian (see also Yaws) 102.9
Pianoma 102.1
Piarhemia, piarrhemia (see also Hyperlipemia) 272.4
   bilharziasis 120.9
Pica 307.52
   hysterical 300.11
Pick's
   cerebral atrophy 331.1
     with dementia
       with behavioral disturbance 331.1 [294.11]
       without behavioral disturbance 331.1 [294.10]
   disease
     brain 331.1
       dementia in
         with behavioral disturbance 331.1 [294.11]
         without behavioral disturbance 331.1 [294.10]
     lipid histiocytosis 272.7
     liver (pericardial pseudocirrhosis of liver) 423.2
     pericardium (pericardial pseudocirrhosis of liver) 423.2
     polyserositis (pericardial pseudocirrhosis of liver) 423.2

Pick's — continued
   syndrome
     heart (pericardial pseudocirrhosis of liver) 423.2
     liver (pericardial pseudocirrhosis of liver) 423.2
     tubular adenoma (M8640/0)
       specified site — see Neoplasm, by site, benign
       unspecified site
         female 220
         male 222.0
Pick-Herxheimer syndrome (diffuse idiopathic cutaneous atrophy) 701.8
Pick-Niemann disease (lipid histiocytosis) 272.7
Pickwickian syndrome (cardiopulmonary obesity) 278.8
Piebaldism, classic 709.09
Piedra 111.2
   beard 111.2
     black 111.3
     white 111.2
   black 111.3
   scalp 111.3
     black 111.3
     white 111.2
   white 111.2
Pierre Marie's syndrome (pulmonary hypertrophic osteoarthropathy) 731.2
Pierre Marie-Bamberger syndrome (hypertrophic pulmonary osteoarthropathy) 731.2
Pierre Mauriac's syndrome (diabetes-dwarfism-obesity) 258.1
Pierre Robin deformity or syndrome (congenital) 756.0
Pierson's disease or osteochondrosis 732.1
Pigeon
   breast or chest (acquired) 738.3
     congenital 754.82
     rachitic (see also Rickets) 268.0
   breeders' disease or lung 495.2
   fanciers' disease or lung 495.2
   toe 735.8
Pigmentation (abnormal) 709.00
   anomaly 709.00
     congenital 757.33
     specified NEC 709.09
   conjunctiva 372.55
   cornea 371.10
     anterior 371.11
     posterior 371.13
     stromal 371.12
   lids (congenital) 757.33
     acquired 374.52
   limbus corneae 371.10
   metals 709.00
   optic papilla, congenital 743.57
   retina (congenital) (grouped) (nevoid) 743.53
     acquired 362.74
   scrotum, congenital 757.33
Piles — see Hemorrhoids
Pili
   annulati or torti (congenital) 757.4
   incarnati 704.8
Pill roller hand (intrinsic) 736.09
Pilomatrixoma (M8110/0) — see Neoplasm, skin, benign

Pilonidal — *see* condition
Pimple 709.8
PIN I (prostatic intraepithelial neoplasia I) 602.3
PIN II (prostatic intraepithelial neoplasia II) 602.3
PIN III (prostatic intraepithelial neoplasia III) 233.4
Pinched nerve — *see* Neuropathy, entrapment
Pineal body or gland — *see* condition
Pinealoblastoma (M9362/3) 194.4
Pinealoma (M9360/1) 237.1
   malignant (M9360/3) 194.4
Pineoblastoma (M9362/3) 194.4
Pineocytoma (M9361/1) 237.1
Pinguecula 372.51
Pinhole meatus (*see also* Stricture, urethra) 598.9
Pink
   disease 985.0
   eye 372.03
   puffer 492.8
Pinkus' disease (lichen nitidus) 697.1
Pinpoint
   meatus (*see also* Stricture, urethra) 598.9
   os uteri (*see also* Stricture, cervix) 622.4
Pinselhaare (congenital) 757.4
Pinta 103.9
   cardiovascular lesions 103.2
   chancre (primary) 103.0
   erythematous plaques 103.1
   hyperchromic lesions 103.1
   hyperkeratosis 103.1
   lesions 103.9
      cardiovascular 103.2
      hyperchromic 103.1
      intermediate 103.1
      late 103.2
      mixed 103.3
      primary 103.0
      skin (achromic) (cicatricial) (dyschromic) 103.2
         hyperchromic 103.1
         mixed (achromic and hyperchromic) 103.3
   papule (primary) 103.0
   skin lesions (achromic) (cicatricial) (dyschromic) 103.2
      hyperchromic 103.1
      mixed (achromic and hyperchromic) 103.3
   vitiligo 103.2
Pintid 103.0
Pinworms (disease) (infection) (infestation) 127.4
Piry fever 066.8
Pistol wound — *see* Gunshot wound
Pit, lip (mucus), congenital 750.25
Pitchers' elbow 718.82
Pithecoid pelvis 755.69
   with disproportion (fetopelvic) 653.2
      affecting fetus or newborn 763.1
      causing obstructed labor 660.1
Pithiatism 300.11
Pitted — *see also* Pitting
   teeth 520.4
Pitting (edema) (*see also* Edema) 782.3
   lip 782.3
   nail 703.8
      congenital 757.5

Pituitary gland — *see* condition
Pituitary snuff-takers' disease 495.8
Pityriasis 696.5
   alba 696.5
   capitis 690.11
   circinata (et maculata) 696.3
   Hebra's (exfoliative dermatitis) 695.89
   lichenoides et varioliformis 696.2
   maculata (et circinata) 696.3
   nigra 111.1
   pilaris 757.39
      acquired 701.1
      Hebra's 696.4
   rosea 696.3
   rotunda 696.3
   rubra (Hebra) 695.89
      pilaris 696.4
   sicca 690.18
   simplex 690.18
   specified type NEC 696.5
   streptogenes 696.5
   versicolor 111.0
      scrotal 111.0
Placenta, placental
   ablatio 641.2
      affecting fetus or newborn 762.1
   abnormal, abnormality 656.7
      with hemorrhage 641.8
         affecting fetus or newborn 762.1
      affecting fetus or newborn 762.2
   abruptio 641.2
      affecting fetus or newborn 762.1
   accessory lobe — *see* Placenta, abnormal
   accreta (without hemorrhage) 667.0
      with hemorrhage 666.0
   adherent (without hemorrhage) 667.0
      with hemorrhage 666.0
   apoplexy — *see* Placenta, separation
   battledore — *see* Placenta, abnormal
   bilobate — *see* Placenta, abnormal
   bipartita — *see* Placenta, abnormal
   carneous mole 631
   centralis — *see* Placenta, previa
   circumvallata — *see* Placenta, abnormal
   cyst (amniotic) — *see* Placenta, abnormal
   deficiency — *see* Placenta, insufficiency
   degeneration — *see* Placenta, insufficiency
   detachment (partial) (premature) (with hemorrhage) 641.2
      affecting fetus or newborn 762.1
   dimidiata — *see* Placenta, abnormal
   disease 656.7
      affecting fetus or newborn 762.2
   duplex — *see* Placenta, abnormal
   dysfunction — *see* Placenta, insufficiency
   fenestrata — *see* Placenta, abnormal
   fibrosis — *see* Placenta, abnormal
   fleshy mole 631
   hematoma — *see* Placenta, abnormal
   hemorrhage NEC — *see* Placenta, separation
   hormone disturbance or malfunction — *see* Placenta, abnormal
   hyperplasia — *see* Placenta, abnormal
   increta (without hemorrhage) 667.0
      with hemorrhage 666.0
   infarction 656.7
      affecting fetus or newborn 762.2
   insertion, vicious — *see* Placenta, previa

Placenta, placental — *continued*
  insufficiency
    affecting
      fetus or newborn 762.2
      management of pregnancy 656.5 ✓5ᵗʰ
  lateral — *see* Placenta, previa
  low implantation or insertion — *see* Placenta, previa
  low-lying — *see* Placenta, previa
  malformation — *see* Placenta, abnormal
  malposition — *see* Placenta, previa
  marginalis, marginata — *see* Placenta, previa
  marginal sinus (hemorrhage) (rupture) 641.2 ✓5ᵗʰ
    affecting fetus or newborn 762.1
  membranacea — *see* Placenta, abnormal
  multilobed — *see* Placenta, abnormal
  multipartita — *see* Placenta, abnormal
  necrosis — *see* Placenta, abnormal
  percreta (without hemorrhage) 667.0 ✓5ᵗʰ
    with hemorrhage 666.0 ✓5ᵗʰ
  polyp 674.4 ✓5ᵗʰ
  previa (central) (centralis) (complete) (lateral) (marginal) (marginalis) (partial) (partialis) (total) (with hemorrhage) 641.1 ✓5ᵗʰ
    affecting fetus or newborn 762.0
    noted
      before labor, without hemorrhage (with cesarean delivery) 641.0 ✓5ᵗʰ
      during pregnancy (without hemorrhage) 641.0 ✓5ᵗʰ
    without hemorrhage (before labor and delivery) (during pregnancy) 641.0 ✓5ᵗʰ
  retention (with hemorrhage) 666.0 ✓5ᵗʰ
    fragments, complicating puerperium (delayed hemorrhage) 666.2 ✓5ᵗʰ
      without hemorrhage 667.1 ✓5ᵗʰ
    postpartum, puerperal 666.2 ✓5ᵗʰ
    without hemorrhage 667.0 ✓5ᵗʰ
  separation (normally implanted) (partial) (premature) (with hemorrhage) 641.2 ✓5ᵗʰ
    affecting fetus or newborn 762.1
  septuplex — *see* Placenta, abnormal
  small — *see* Placenta, insufficiency
  softening (premature) — *see* Placenta, abnormal
  spuria — *see* Placenta, abnormal
  succenturiata — *see* Placenta, abnormal
  syphilitic 095.8
  transfusion syndromes 762.3
  transmission of chemical substance — *see* Absorption, chemical, through placenta
  trapped (with hemorrhage) 666.0 ✓5ᵗʰ
    without hemorrhage 667.0 ✓5ᵗʰ
  trilobate — *see* Placenta, abnormal
  tripartita — *see* Placenta, abnormal
  triplex — *see* Placenta, abnormal
  varicose vessel — *see* Placenta, abnormal
  vicious insertion — *see* Placenta, previa

Placentitis
  affecting fetus or newborn 762.7
  complicating pregnancy 658.4 ✓5ᵗʰ

Plagiocephaly (skull) 754.0

Plague 020.9
  abortive 020.8
  ambulatory 020.8
  bubonic 020.0
  cellulocutaneous 020.1
  lymphatic gland 020.0
  pneumonic 020.5
    primary 020.3

Plague — *continued*
  pneumonic — *continued*
    secondary 020.4
  pulmonary — *see* Plague, pneumonic
  pulmonic — *see* Plague, pneumonic
  septicemic 020.2
  tonsillar 020.9
    septicemic 020.2
  vaccination, prophylactic (against) V03.3

Planning, family V25.09
  contraception V25.9
  procreation V26.4

Plaque
  artery, arterial — *see* Arteriosclerosis
  calcareous — *see* Calcification
  Hollenhorst's (retinal) 362.33
  tongue 528.6

Plasma cell myeloma 203.0 ✓5ᵗʰ

Plasmacytoma, plasmocytoma (solitary) (M9731/1) 238.6
  benign (M9731/0) — *see* Neoplasm, by site, benign
  malignant (M9731/3) 203.8 ✓5ᵗʰ

Plasmacytosis 288.8

Plaster ulcer (*see also* Decubitus) 707.0

Platybasia 756.0

Platyonychia (congenital) 757.5
  acquired 703.8

Platypelloid pelvis 738.6
  with disproportion (fetopelvic) 653.2 ✓5ᵗʰ
    affecting fetus or newborn 763.1
    causing obstructed labor 660.1 ✓5ᵗʰ
      affecting fetus or newborn 763.1
  congenital 755.69

Platyspondylia 756.19

Plethora 782.62
  newborn 776.4

Pleura, pleural — *see* condition

Pleuralgia 786.52

Pleurisy (acute) (adhesive) (chronic) (costal) (diaphragmatic) (double) (dry) (fetid) (fibrinous) (fibrous) (interlobar) (latent) (lung) (old) (plastic) (primary) (residual) (sicca) (sterile) (subacute) (unresolved) (with adherent pleura) 511.0
  with
    effusion (without mention of cause) 511.9
      bacterial, nontuberculous 511.1
      nontuberculous NEC 511.9
        bacterial 511.1
      pneumococcal 511.1
      specified type NEC 511.8
      staphylococcal 511.1
      streptococcal 511.1
      tuberculous (*see also* Tuberculosis, pleura) 012.0 ✓5ᵗʰ
        primary, progressive 010.1 ✓5ᵗʰ
    influenza, flu, or grippe 487.1
    tuberculosis — *see* Pleurisy, tuberculous
  encysted 511.8
  exudative (*see also* Pleurisy, with effusion) 511.9
    bacterial, nontuberculous 511.1
  fibrinopurulent 510.9
    with fistula 510.0
  fibropurulent 510.9
    with fistula 510.0
  hemorrhagic 511.8
  influenzal 487.1

Pleurisy — continued

pneumococcal 511.0
  with effusion 511.1
purulent 510.9
  with fistula 510.0
septic 510.9
  with fistula 510.0
serofibrinous (see also Pleurisy, with effusion) 511.9
  bacterial, nontuberculous 511.1
seropurulent 510.9
  with fistula 510.0
serous (see also Pleurisy, with effusion) 511.9
  bacterial, nontuberculous 511.1
staphylococcal 511.0
  with effusion 511.1
streptococcal 511.0
  with effusion 511.1
suppurative 510.9
  with fistula 510.0
traumatic (post) (current) 862.29
  with open wound into cavity 862.39
tuberculous (with effusion) (see also Tuberculosis, pleura) 012.0 ✓5ᵗʰ
  primary, progressive 010.1 ✓5ᵗʰ

Pleuritis sicca — see Pleurisy
Pleurobronchopneumonia (see also Pneumonia, broncho-) 485
Pleurodynia 786.52
  epidemic 074.1
  viral 074.1
Pleurohepatitis 573.8
Pleuropericarditis (see also Pericarditis) 423.9
  acute 420.90
Pleuropneumonia (acute) (bilateral) (double) (septic) (see also Pneumonia) 486
  chronic (see also Fibrosis, lung) 515
Pleurorrhea (see also Hydrothorax) 511.8
Plexitis, brachial 353.0
Plica
  knee 727.83
  polonica 132.0
  tonsil 474.8
Plicae dysphonia ventricularis 784.49
Plicated tongue 529.5
  congenital 750.13
Plug
  bronchus NEC 519.1
  meconium (newborn) NEC 777.1
  mucus — see Mucus, plug
Plumbism 984.9
  specified type of lead — see Table of Drugs and Chemicals
Plummer's disease (toxic nodular goiter) 242.3 ✓5ᵗʰ
Plummer-Vinson syndrome (sideropenic dysphagia) 280.8
Pluricarential syndrome of infancy 260
Plurideficiency syndrome of infancy 260
Plus (and minus) hand (intrinsic) 736.09
PMS 625.4
Pneumathemia — see Air, embolism, by type
Pneumatic drill or hammer disease 994.9
Pneumatocele (lung) 518.89
  intracranial 348.8
  tension 492.0

Pneumatosis
  cystoides intestinalis 569.89
  peritonei 568.89
  pulmonum 492.8
Pneumaturia 599.84
Pneumoblastoma (M8981/3) — see Neoplasm, lung, malignant
Pneumocephalus 348.8
Pneumococcemia 038.2
Pneumococcus, pneumococcal — see condition
Pneumoconiosis (due to) (inhalation of) 505
  aluminum 503
  asbestos 501
  bagasse 495.1
  bauxite 503
  beryllium 503
  carbon electrode makers' 503
  coal
    miners' (simple) 500
    workers' (simple) 500
  cotton dust 504
  diatomite fibrosis 502
  dust NEC 504
    inorganic 503
    lime 502
    marble 502
    organic NEC 504
  fumes or vapors (from silo) 506.9
  graphite 503
  hard metal 503
  mica 503
  moldy hay 495.0
  rheumatoid 714.81
  silica NEC 502
    and carbon 500
  silicate NEC 502
  talc 502
Pneumocystis carinii pneumonia 136.3
Pneumocystosis 136.3
  with pneumonia 136.3
Pneumoenteritis 025
Pneumohemopericardium (see also Pericarditis) 423.9
Pneumohemothorax (see also Hemothorax) 511.8
  traumatic 860.4
    with open wound into thorax 860.5
Pneumohydropericardium (see also Pericarditis) 423.9
Pneumohydrothorax (see also Hydrothorax) 511.8
Pneumomediastinum 518.1
  congenital 770.2
  fetus or newborn 770.2
Pneumomycosis 117.9
Pneumonia (acute) (Alpenstich) (benign) (bilateral) (brain) (cerebral) (circumscribed) (congestive) (creeping) (delayed resolution) (double) (epidemic) (fever) (flash) (fulminant) (fungoid) (granulomatous) (hemorrhagic) (incipient) (infantile) (infectious) (infiltration) (insular) (intermittent) (latent) (lobe) (migratory) (newborn) (organized) (overwhelming) (primary) (progressive) (pseudolobar) (purulent) (resolved) (secondary) (senile) (septic) (suppurative) (terminal) (true) (unresolved) (vesicular) 486
  with influenza, flu, or grippe 487.0
  adenoviral 480.0

Pneumonia — continued
- adynamic 514
- alba 090.0
- allergic 518.3
- alveolar — see Pneumonia, lobar
- anaerobes 482.81
- anthrax 022.1 *[484.5]*
- apex, apical — see Pneumonia, lobar
- ascaris 127.0 *[484.8]*
- aspiration 507.0
  - due to
    - aspiration of microorganisms
      - bacterial 482.9
        - specified type NEC 482.89
      - specified organism NEC 483.8
        - bacterial NEC 482.89
      - viral 480.9
        - specified type NEC 480.8
    - food (regurgitated) 507.0
    - gastric secretions 507.0
    - milk 507.0
    - oils, essences 507.1
    - solids, liquids NEC 507.8
    - vomitus 507.0
  - newborn 770.1
- asthenic 514
- atypical (disseminated, focal) (primary) 486
  - with influenza 487.0
- bacillus 482.9
  - specified type NEC 482.89
- bacterial 482.9
  - specified type NEC 482.89
- Bacteroides (fragilis) (oralis) (melaninogenicus) 482.81
- basal, basic, basilar — see Pneumonia, lobar
- broncho-, bronchial (confluent) (croupous) (diffuse) (disseminated) (hemorrhagic) (involving lobes) (lobar) (terminal) 485
  - with influenza 487.0
  - allergic 518.3
  - aspiration (*see also* Pneumonia, aspiration) 507.0
  - bacterial 482.9
    - specified type NEC 482.89
  - capillary 466.19
    - with bronchospasm or obstruction 466.19
  - chronic (*see also* Fibrosis, lung) 515
  - congenital (infective) 770.0
  - diplococcal 481
  - Eaton's agent 483.0
  - Escherichia coli (E. coli) 482.82
  - Friedländer's bacillus 482.0
  - Hemophilus influenzae 482.2
  - hiberno-vernal 083.0 *[484.8]*
  - hypostatic 514
  - influenzal 487.0
  - inhalation (*see also* Pneumonia, aspiration) 507.0
    - due to fumes or vapors (chemical) 506.0
  - Klebsiella 482.0
  - lipid 507.1
    - endogenous 516.8
  - Mycoplasma (pneumoniae) 483.0
  - ornithosis 073.0
  - pleuropneumonia-like organisms (PPLO) 483.0
  - pneumococcal 481
  - Proteus 482.83
  - pseudomonas 482.1

Pneumonia — continued
- broncho-, bronchial — *continued*
  - specified organism NEC 483.8
    - bacterial NEC 482.89
  - staphylococcal 482.40
    - aureus 482.41
    - specified type NEC 482.49
  - streptococcal — see Pneumonia, streptococcal
  - typhoid 002.0 *[484.8]*
  - viral, virus (*see also* Pneumonia, viral) 480.9
- butyrivibrio (fibriosolvens) 482.81
- Candida 112.4
- capillary 466.19
  - with bronchospasm or obstruction 466.19
- caseous (*see also* Tuberculosis) 011.6
- catarrhal — see Pneumonia, broncho-central
  - — see Pneumonia, lobar
- Chlamydia, chlamydial 483.1
  - pneumoniae 483.1
  - psittaci 073.0
  - specified type NEC 483.1
  - trachomatis 483.1
- cholesterol 516.8
- chronic (*see also* Fibrosis, lung) 515
- Clostridium (haemolyticum) (novyi) NEC 482.81
- confluent — see Pneumonia, broncho-
- congenital (infective) 770.0
  - aspiration 770.1
- croupous — see Pneumonia, lobar
- cytomegalic inclusion 078.5 *[484.1]*
- deglutition (*see also* Pneumonia, aspiration) 507.0
- desquamative interstitial 516.8
- diffuse — see Pneumonia, broncho-
- diplococcal, diplococcus (broncho-) (lobar) 481
- disseminated (focal) — see Pneumonia, broncho-
- due to
  - adenovirus 480.0
  - Bacterium anitratum 482.83
  - Chlamydia, chlamydial 483.1
    - pneumoniae 483.1
    - psittaci 073.0
    - specified type NEC 483.1
    - trachomatis 483.1
  - coccidioidomycosis 114.0
  - Diplococcus (pneumoniae) 481
  - Eaton's agent 483.0
  - Escherichia coli (E. coli) 482.82
  - Friedländer's bacillus 482.0
  - fumes or vapors (chemical) (inhalation) 506.0
  - fungus NEC 117.9 *[484.7]*
    - coccidioidomycosis 114.0
  - Hemophilus influenzae (H. influenzae) 482.2
  - Herellea 482.83
  - influenza 487.0
  - Klebsiella pneumoniae 482.0
  - Mycoplasma (pneumoniae) 483.0
  - parainfluenza virus 480.2
  - pleuropneumonia-like organism (PPLO) 483.0
  - Pneumococcus 481
  - Pneumocystis carinii 136.3
  - Proteus 482.83
  - pseudomonas 482.1
  - respiratory syncytial virus 480.1

Index to Diseases — Pneumonia

Pneumonia — *continued*
  due to — *continued*
    rickettsia 083.9 *[484.8]*
    specified
      bacteria NEC 482.89
      organism NEC 483.8
      virus NEC 480.8
    Staphylococcus 482.40
      aureus 482.41
      specified type NEC 482.49
    Streptococcus — *see also* Pneumonia, streptococcal
      pneumoniae 481
    virus (*see also* Pneumonia, viral) 480.9
  Eaton's agent 483.0
  embolic, embolism (*see also* Embolism, pulmonary) 415.1 ✓5th
  eosinophilic 518.3
  Escherichia coli (E. coli) 482.82
  Eubacterium 482.81
  fibrinous — *see* Pneumonia, lobar
  fibroid (chronic)(*see also* Fibrosis, lung) 515
  fibrous (*see also* Fibrosis, lung) 515
  Friedländer's bacillus 482.0
  Fusobacterium (nucleatum) 482.81
  gangrenous 513.0
  giant cell (*see also* Pneumonia, viral) 480.9
  gram-negative bacteria NEC 482.83
    anaerobic 482.81
  grippal 487.0
  Hemophilus influenzae (bronchial) (lobar) 482.2
  hypostatic (broncho-) (lobar) 514
  in
    actinomycosis 039.1
    anthrax 022.1 *[484.5]*
    aspergillosis 117.3 *[484.6]*
    candidiasis 112.4
    coccidioidomycosis 114.0
    cytomegalic inclusion disease 078.5 *[484.1]*
    histoplasmosis (*see also* Histoplasmosis) 115.95
    infectious disease NEC 136.9 *[484.8]*
    measles 055.1
    mycosis, systemic NEC 117.9 *[484.7]*
    nocardiasis, nocardiosis 039.1
    ornithosis 073.0
    pneumocystosis 136.3
    psittacosis 073.0
    Q fever 083.0 *[484.8]*
    salmonellosis 003.22
    toxoplasmosis 130.4
    tularemia 021.2
    typhoid (fever) 002.0 *[484.8]*
    varicella 052.1
    whooping cough (*see also* Whooping cough) 033.9 *[484.3]*
  infective, acquired prenatally 770.0
  influenzal (broncho) (lobar) (virus) 487.0
  inhalation (*see also* Pneumonia, aspiration) 507.0
    fumes or vapors (chemical) 506.0
  interstitial 516.8
    with influenzal 487.0
    acute 136.3
    chronic (*see also* Fibrosis, lung) 515
    desquamative 516.8
    hypostatic 514
    lipoid 507.1
    lymphoid 516.8
    plasma cell 136.3

Pneumonia — *continued*
  interstitial — *continued*
    pseudomonas 482.1
  intrauterine (infective) 770.0
    aspiration 770.1
  Klebsiella pneumoniae 482.0
  Legionnaires' 482.84
  lipid, lipoid (exogenous) (interstitial) 507.1
    endogenous 516.8
  lobar (diplococcal) (disseminated) (double) (interstitial) (pneumococcal, any type) 481
    with influenza 487.0
    bacterial 482.9
      specified type NEC 482.89
    chronic (*see also* Fibrosis, lung) 515
    Escherichia coli (E. coli) 482.82
    Friedländer's bacillus 482.0
    Hemophilus influenzae (H. influenzae) 482.2
    hypostatic 514
    influenzal 487.0
    Klebsiella 482.0
    ornithosis 073.0
    Proteus 482.83
    pseudomonas 482.1
    psittacosis 073.0
    specified organism NEC 483.8
      bacterial NEC 482.89
    staphylococcal 482.40
      aureus 482.41
      specified type NEC 482.49
    streptococcal — *see* Pneumonia, streptococcal
    viral, virus (*see also* Pneumonia, viral) 480.9
  lobular (confluent) — *see* Pneumonia, broncho-
  Löffler's 518.3
  massive — *see* Pneumonia, lobar
  meconium 770.1
  metastatic NEC 038.8 *[484.8]*
  Mycoplasma (pneumoniae) 483.0
  necrotic 513.0
  nitrogen dioxide 506.9
  orthostatic 514
  parainfluenza virus 480.2
  parenchymatous (*see also* Fibrosis, lung) 515
  passive 514
  patchy — *see* Pneumonia, broncho-
  Peptococcus 482.81
  Peptostreptococcus 482.81
  plasma cell 136.3
  pleurolobar — *see* Pneumonia, lobar
  pleuropneumonia-like organism (PPLO) 483.0
  pneumococcal (broncho) (lobar) 481
  Pneumocystis (carinii) 136.3
  postinfectional NEC 136.9 *[484.8]*
  postmeasles 055.1
  postoperative 997.3
  primary atypical 486
  Proprionibacterium 482.81
  Proteus 482.83
  pseudomonas 482.1
  psittacosis 073.0
  radiation 508.0
  respiratory syncytial virus 480.1
  resulting from a procedure 997.3
  rheumatic 390 *[517.1]*
  Salmonella 003.22

Pneumonia — continued
  segmented, segmental — *see* Pneumonia, broncho-
  Serratia (marcescens) 482.83
  specified
    bacteria NEC 482.89
    organism NEC 483.8
    virus NEC 480.8
  spirochetal 104.8 *[484.8]*
  staphylococcal (broncho) (lobar) 482.40
    aureus 482.41
    specified type NEC 482.49
  static, stasis 514
  streptococcal (broncho) (lobar) NEC 482.30
    Group
      A 482.31
      B 482.32
      specified NEC 482.39
    pneumoniae 481
    specified type NEC 482.39
  Streptococcus pneumoniae 481
  traumatic (complication) (early) (secondary) 958.8
  tuberculous (any) (*see also* Tuberculosis) 011.6 ✓5ᵗʰ
  tularemic 021.2
  TWAR agent 483.1
  varicella 052.1
  Veillonella 482.81
  viral, virus (broncho) (interstitial) (lobar) 480.9
    with influenza, flu, or grippe 487.0
    adenoviral 480.0
    parainfluenza 480.2
    respiratory syncytial 480.1
    specified type NEC 480.8
  white (congenital) 090.0
Pneumonic — *see* condition
Pneumonitis (acute) (primary) (*see also* Pneumonia) 486
  allergic 495.9
    specified type NEC 495.8
  aspiration 507.0
    due to fumes or gases 506.0
    newborn 770.1
    obstetric 668.0 ✓5ᵗʰ
  chemical 506.0
    due to fumes or gases 506.0
  cholesterol 516.8
  chronic (*see also* Fibrosis, lung) 515
  congenital rubella 771.0
  due to
    fumes or vapors 506.0
    inhalation
      food (regurgitated), milk, vomitus 507.0
      oils, essences 507.1
      saliva 507.0
      solids, liquids NEC 507.8
    toxoplasmosis (acquired) 130.4
      congenital (active) 771.2 *[484.8]*
  eosinophilic 518.3
  fetal aspiration 770.1
  hypersensitivity 495.9
  interstitial (chronic) (*see also* Fibrosis, lung) 515
    lymphoid 516.8
  lymphoid, interstitial 516.8
  meconium 770.1
  postanesthetic
    correct substance properly administered 507.0
    obstetric 668.0 ✓5ᵗʰ

Pneumonitis — *continued*
  postanesthetic — *continued*
    overdose or wrong substance given 968.4
    specified anesthetic — *see* Table of Drugs and Chemicals
  postoperative 997.3
    obstetric 668.0 ✓5ᵗʰ
  radiation 508.0
  rubella, congenital 771.0
  "ventilation" 495.7
  wood-dust 495.8
Pneumonoconiosis — *see* Pneumoconiosis
Pneumoparotid 527.8
Pneumopathy NEC 518.89
  alveolar 516.9
    specified NEC 516.8
  due to dust NEC 504
  parietoalveolar 516.9
  specified condition NEC 516.8
Pneumopericarditis (*see also* Pericarditis) 423.9
  acute 420.90
Pneumopericardium — *see also* Pericarditis
  congenital 770.2
  fetus or newborn 770.2
  traumatic (post) (*see also* Pneumothorax, traumatic) 860.0
    with open wound into thorax 860.1
Pneumoperitoneum 568.89
  fetus or newborn 770.2
Pneumophagia (psychogenic) 306.4
Pneumopleurisy, pneumopleuritis (*see also* Pneumonia) 486
Pneumopyopericardium 420.99
Pneumopyothorax (*see also* Pyopneumothorax) 510.9
  with fistula 510.0
Pneumorrhagia 786.3
  newborn 770.3
  tuberculous (*see also* Tuberculosis, pulmonary) 011.9 ✓5ᵗʰ
Pneumosiderosis (occupational) 503
Pneumothorax (acute) (chronic) 512.8
  congenital 770.2
  due to operative injury of chest wall or lung 512.1
    accidental puncture or laceration 512.1
  fetus or newborn 770.2
  iatrogenic 512.1
  postoperative 512.1
  spontaneous 512.8
    fetus or newborn 770.2
    tension 512.0
  sucking 512.8
    iatrogenic 512.1
    postoperative 512.1
  tense valvular, infectional 512.0
  tension 512.0
    iatrogenic 512.1
    postoperative 512.1
    spontaneous 512.0
  traumatic 860.0
    with
      hemothorax 860.4
        with open wound into thorax 860.5
      open wound into thorax 860.1
  tuberculous (*see also* Tuberculosis) 011.7 ✓5ᵗʰ
Pocket(s)
  endocardial (*see also* Endocarditis) 424.90
  periodontal 523.8

Podagra 274.9
Podencephalus 759.89
Poikilocytosis 790.09
Poikiloderma 709.09
   Civatte's 709.09
   congenital 757.33
   vasculare atrophicans 696.2
Poikilodermatomyositis 710.3
Pointed ear 744.29
Poise imperfect 729.9
Poisoned — see Poisoning
Poisoning (acute) — see also Table of Drugs and Chemicals
   Bacillus, B.
      aertrycke (see also Infection, Salmonella) 003.9
      botulinus 005.1
      cholerae (suis) (see also Infection, Salmonella) 003.9
      paratyphosus (see also Infection, Salmonella) 003.9
      suipestifer (see also Infection, Salmonella) 003.9
   bacterial toxins NEC 005.9
   berries, noxious 988.2
   blood (general) — see Septicemia
   botulism 005.1
   bread, moldy, mouldy — see Poisoning, food
   damaged meat — see Poisoning, food
   death-cap (Amanita phalloides) (Amanita verna) 988.1
   decomposed food — see Poisoning, food
   diseased food — see Poisoning, food
   drug — see Table of Drugs and Chemicals
   epidemic, fish, meat, or other food — see Poisoning, food
   fava bean 282.2
   fish (bacterial) — see also Poisoning, food
      noxious 988.0
   food (acute) (bacterial) (diseased) (infected) NEC 005.9
      due to
         bacillus
            aertrycke (see also Poisoning, food, due to Salmonella) 003.9
            botulinus 005.1
            cereus 005.89
            choleraesuis (see also Poisoning, food, due to Salmonella) 003.9
            paratyphosus (see also Poisoning, food, due to Salmonella) 003.9
            suipestifer (see also Poisoning, food, due to Salmonella) 003.9
         Clostridium 005.3
            botulinum 005.1
            perfringens 005.2
            welchii 005.2
         Salmonella (aertrycke) (callinarum) (choleraesuis) (enteritidis) (paratyphi) (suipestifer) 003.9
            with
               gastroenteritis 003.0
               localized infection(s) (see also Infection, Salmonella) 003.20
               septicemia 003.1
               specified manifestation NEC 003.8
         specified bacterium NEC 005.89
         Staphylococcus 005.0
         Streptococcus 005.8
         Vibrio parahaemolyticus 005.4

Poisoning — continued
   food — continued
      due to — continued
         Vibrio vulnificus 005.81
      noxious or naturally toxic 988.0
         berries 988.2
         fish 988.0
         mushroom 988.1
         plants NEC 988.2
   ice cream — see Poisoning, food
   ichthyotoxism (bacterial) 005.9
   kreotoxism, food 005.9
   malarial — see Malaria
   meat — see Poisoning, food
   mushroom (noxious) 988.1
   mussel — see also Poisoning, food
      noxious 988.0
   noxious foodstuffs (see also Poisoning, food, noxious) 988.9
      specified type NEC 988.8
   plants, noxious 988.2
   pork — see also Poisoning, food
      specified NEC 988.8
      Trichinosis 124
   ptomaine — see Poisoning, food
   putrefaction, food — see Poisoning, food
   radiation 508.0
   Salmonella (see also Infection, Salmonella) 003.9
   sausage — see also Poisoning, food
      Trichinosis 124
   saxitoxin 988.0
   shellfish — see also Poisoning, food
      noxious 988.0
   Staphylococcus, food 005.0
   toxic, from disease NEC 799.8
   truffles — see Poisoning, food
   uremic — see Uremia
   uric acid 274.9
Poison ivy, oak, sumac or other plant dermatitis 692.6
Poker spine 720.0
Policeman's disease 729.2
Polioencephalitis (acute) (bulbar) (see also Poliomyelitis, bulbar) 045.0
   inferior 335.22
   influenzal 487.8
   superior hemorrhagic (acute) (Wernicke's) 265.1
   Wernicke's (superior hemorrhagic) 265.1
Polioencephalomyelitis (acute) (anterior) (bulbar) (see also Polioencephalitis) 045.0
Polioencephalopathy, superior hemorrhagic 265.1
   with
      beriberi 265.0
      pellagra 265.2
Poliomeningoencephalitis — see Meningoencephalitis

Poliomyelitis (acute) (anterior) (epidemic) 045.9 ✓5ᵗʰ

> Note — Use the following fifth-digit subclassification with category 045:
>
> 0 poliovirus, unspecified type
> 1 poliovirus, type I
> 2 poliovirus, type II
> 3 poliovirus, type III

with
  paralysis 045.1 ✓5ᵗʰ
    bulbar 045.0 ✓5ᵗʰ
  abortive 045.2 ✓5ᵗʰ
  ascending 045.9 ✓5ᵗʰ
    progressive 045.9 ✓5ᵗʰ
  bulbar 045.0 ✓5ᵗʰ
  cerebral 045.0 ✓5ᵗʰ
  chronic 335.21
  congenital 771.2
  contact V01.2
  deformities 138
  exposure to V01.2
  late effect 138
  nonepidemic 045.9 ✓5ᵗʰ
  nonparalytic 045.2 ✓5ᵗʰ
  old with deformity 138
  posterior, acute 053.19
  residual 138
  sequelae 138
  spinal, acute 045.9 ✓5ᵗʰ
  syphilitic (chronic) 094.89
  vaccination, prophylactic (against) V04.0
Poliosis (eyebrow) (eyelashes) 704.3
  circumscripta (congenital) 757.4
    acquired 704.3
  congenital 757.4
Pollakiuria 788.4 ✓5ᵗʰ
  psychogenic 306.53
Pollinosis 477.0
Pollitzer's disease (hidradenitis suppurativa) 705.83
Polyadenitis (see also Adenitis) 289.3
  malignant 020.0
Polyalgia 729.9
Polyangiitis (essential) 446.0
Polyarteritis (nodosa) (renal) 446.0
Polyarthralgia 719.49
  psychogenic 306.0
Polyarthritis, polyarthropathy NEC 716.59
  due to or associated with other specified conditions — see Arthritis, due to or associated with
  endemic (see also Disease, Kaschin-Beck) 716.0 ✓5ᵗʰ
  inflammatory 714.9
    specified type NEC 714.89
  juvenile (chronic) 714.30
    acute 714.31
  migratory — see Fever, rheumatic
  rheumatic 714.0
    fever (acute) — see Fever, rheumatic
Polycarential syndrome of infancy 260
Polychondritis (atrophic) (chronic) (relapsing) 733.99
Polycoria 743.46

Polycystic (congenital) (disease) 759.89
  degeneration, kidney — see Polycystic, kidney
  kidney (congenital) 753.12
    adult type (APKD) 753.13
    autosomal dominant 753.13
    autosomal recessive 753.14
    childhood type (CPKD) 753.14
    infantile type 753.14
  liver 751.62
  lung 518.89
    congenital 748.4
  ovary, ovaries 256.4
  spleen 759.0
Polycythemia (primary) (rubra) (vera) (M9950/1) 238.4
  acquired 289.0
  benign 289.0
    familial 289.6
  due to
    donor twin 776.4
    fall in plasma volume 289.0
    high altitude 289.0
    maternal-fetal transfusion 776.4
    stress 289.0
  emotional 289.0
  erythropoietin 289.0
  familial (benign) 289.6
  Gaisböck's (hypertonica) 289.0
  high altitude 289.0
  hypertonica 289.0
  hypoxemic 289.0
  neonatorum 776.4
  nephrogenous 289.0
  relative 289.0
  secondary 289.0
  spurious 289.0
  stress 289.0
Polycytosis cryptogenica 289.0
Polydactylism, polydactyly 755.00
  fingers 755.01
  toes 755.02
Polydipsia 783.5
Polydystrophic oligophrenia 277.5
Polyembryoma (M9072/3) — see Neoplasm, by site, malignant
Polygalactia 676.6 ✓5ᵗʰ
Polyglandular
  deficiency 258.9
  dyscrasia 258.9
  dysfunction 258.9
  syndrome 258.8
Polyhydramnios (see also Hydramnios) 657 ✓5ᵗʰ
Polymastia 757.6
Polymenorrhea 626.2
Polymicrogyria 742.2
Polymyalgia 725
  arteritica 446.5
  rheumatica 725
Polymyositis (acute) (chronic) (hemorrhagic) 710.4
  with involvement of
    lung 710.4 [517.8]
    skin 710.3
  ossificans (generalisata) (progressiva) 728.19
  Wagner's (dermatomyositis) 710.3
Polyneuritis, polyneuritic (see also Polyneuropathy) 356.9
  alcoholic 357.5
    with psychosis 291.1

Polyneuritis, polyneuritic — *continued*
  cranialis 352.6
  diabetic 250.6 ✓5ᵗʰ *[357.2]*
  demyelinating, chronic inflammatory 357.81▲
  due to lack of vitamin NEC 269.2 *[357.4]*
  endemic 265.0 *[357.4]*
  erythredema 985.0
  febrile 357.0
  hereditary ataxic 356.3
  idiopathic, acute 357.0
  infective (acute) 357.0
  nutritional 269.9 *[357.4]*
  postinfectious 357.0
Polyneuropathy (peripheral) 356.9
  alcoholic 357.5
  amyloid 277.3 *[357.4]*
  arsenical 357.7
  critical illness 357.82
  diabetic 250.6 ✓5ᵗʰ *[357.2]*
  due to
    antitetanus serum 357.6
    arsenic 357.7
    drug or medicinal substance 357.6
      correct substance properly administered 357.6
      overdose or wrong substance given or taken 977.9
      specified drug — *see* Table of Drugs and Chemicals
    lack of vitamin NEC 269.2 *[357.4]*
    lead 357.7
    organophosphate compounds 357.7
    pellagra 265.2 *[357.4]*
    porphyria 277.1 *[357.4]*
    serum 357.6
    toxic agent NEC 357.7
  hereditary 356.0
  idiopathic 356.9
    progressive 356.4
  in
    amyloidosis 277.3 *[357.4]*
    avitaminosis 269.2 *[357.4]*
      specified NEC 269.1 *[357.4]*
    beriberi 265.0 *[357.4]*
    collagen vascular disease NEC 710.9 *[357.1]*
    deficiency
      B-complex NEC 266.2 *[357.4]*
      vitamin B 266.9 *[357.4]*
      vitamin B 266.1 *[357.4]*
    diabetes 250.6 ✓5ᵗʰ *[357.2]*
    diphtheria (*see also* Diphtheria) 032.89 *[357.4]*
    disseminated lupus erythematosus 710.0 *[357.1]*
    herpes zoster 053.13
    hypoglycemia 251.2 *[357.4]*
    malignant neoplasm (M8000/3) NEC 199.1 *[357.3]*
    mumps 072.72
    pellagra 265.2 *[357.4]*
    polyarteritis nodosa 446.0 *[357.1]*
    porphyria 277.1 *[357.4]*
    rheumatoid arthritis 714.0 *[357.1]*
    sarcoidosis 135 *[357.4]*
    uremia 585 *[357.4]*
  lead 357.7
  nutritional 269.9 *[357.4]*
    specified NEC 269.8 *[357.4]*
  postherpetic 053.13
  progressive 356.4

Polyneuropathy — *continued*
  sensory (hereditary) 356.2
Polyonychia 757.5
Polyopia 368.2
  refractive 368.15
Polyorchism, polyorchidism (three testes) 752.8
Polyorrhymenitis (peritoneal) (*see also* Polyserositis) 568.82
  pericardial 423.2
Polyostotic fibrous dysplasia 756.54
Polyotia 744.1
Polyp, polypus

> Note — *Polyps of organs or sites that do not appear in the list below should be coded to the residual category for diseases of the organ or site concerned.*

  accessory sinus 471.8
  adenoid tissue 471.0
  adenomatous (M8210/0) — *see also* Neoplasm, by site, benign
    adenocarcinoma in (M8210/3) — *see* Neoplasm, by site, malignant
    carcinoma in (M8210/3) — *see* Neoplasm, by site, malignant
    multiple (M8221/0) — *see* Neoplasm, by site, benign
  antrum 471.8
  anus, anal (canal) (nonadenomatous) 569.0
    adenomatous 211.4
  Bartholin's gland 624.6
  bladder (M8120/1) 236.7
  broad ligament 620.8
  cervix (uteri) 622.7
    adenomatous 219.0
    in pregnancy or childbirth 654.6 ✓5ᵗʰ
      affecting fetus or newborn 763.89
      causing obstructed labor 660.2 ✓5ᵗʰ
    mucous 622.7
    nonneoplastic 622.7
  choanal 471.0
  cholesterol 575.6
  clitoris 624.6
  colon (M8210/0) (*see also* Polyp, adenomatous) 211.3
  corpus uteri 621.0
  dental 522.0
  ear (middle) 385.30
  endometrium 621.0
  ethmoidal (sinus) 471.8
  fallopian tube 620.8
  female genital organs NEC 624.8
  frontal (sinus) 471.8
  gallbladder 575.6
  gingiva 523.8
  gum 523.8
  labia 624.6
  larynx (mucous) 478.4
  malignant (M8000/3) — *see* Neoplasm, by site, malignant
  maxillary (sinus) 471.8
  middle ear 385.30
  myometrium 621.0
  nares
    anterior 471.9
    posterior 471.0
  nasal (mucous) 471.9
    cavity 471.0
    septum 471.9

Polyp, polypus — continued
  nasopharyngeal 471.0
  neoplastic (M8210/0) — see Neoplasm, by site, benign
  nose (mucous) 471.9
  oviduct 620.8
  paratubal 620.8
  pharynx 478.29
    congenital 750.29
  placenta, placental 674.4 ✓5ᵗʰ
  prostate 600.2
  pudenda 624.6
  pulp (dental) 522.0
  rectosigmoid 211.4
  rectum (nonadenomatous) 569.0
    adenomatous 211.4
  septum (nasal) 471.9
  sinus (accessory) (ethmoidal) (frontal) (maxillary) (sphenoidal) 471.8
  sphenoidal (sinus) 471.8
  stomach (M8210/0) 211.1
  tube, fallopian 620.8
  turbinate, mucous membrane 471.8
  ureter 593.89
  urethra 599.3
  uterine
    ligament 620.8
    tube 620.8
  uterus (body) (corpus) (mucous) 621.0
    in pregnancy or childbirth 654.1 ✓5ᵗʰ
      affecting fetus or newborn 763.89
      causing obstructed labor 660.2 ✓5ᵗʰ
  vagina 623.7
  vocal cord (mucous) 478.4
  vulva 624.6
Polyphagia 783.6
Polypoid — see condition
Polyposis — see also Polyp
  coli (adenomatous) (M8220/0) 211.3
    adenocarcinoma in (M8220/3) 153.9
    carcinoma in (M8220/3) 153.9
  familial (M8220/0) 211.3
  intestinal (adenomatous) (M8220/0) 211.3
  multiple (M8221/0) — see Neoplasm, by site, benign
Polyradiculitis (acute) 357.0
Polyradiculoneuropathy (acute) (segmentally demyelinating) 357.0
Polysarcia 278.00
Polyserositis (peritoneal) 568.82
  due to pericarditis 423.2
  paroxysmal (familial) 277.3
  pericardial 423.2
  periodic 277.3
  pleural — see Pleurisy
  recurrent 277.3
  tuberculous (see also Tuberculosis, polyserositis) 018.9 ✓5ᵗʰ
Polysialia 527.7
Polysplenia syndrome 759.0
Polythelia 757.6
Polytrichia (see also Hypertrichosis) 704.1
Polyunguia (congenital) 757.5
  acquired 703.8
Polyuria 788.42
Pompe's disease (glycogenosis II) 271.0
Pompholyx 705.81
Poncet's disease (tuberculous rheumatism) (see also Tuberculosis) 015.9 ✓5ᵗʰ

Pond fracture — see Fracture, skull, vault
Ponos 085.0
Pons, pontine — see condition
Poor
  contractions, labor 661.2 ✓5ᵗʰ
    affecting fetus or newborn 763.7
  fetal growth NEC 764.9 ✓5ᵗʰ
    affecting management of pregnancy 656.5 ✓5ᵗʰ
  incorporation
    artificial skin graft 996.55
    decellularized allodermis graft 996.55
  obstetrical history V13.49 ▲
    affecting management of current
      pregnancy V23.49 ●
      pre-term labor V23.41 ●
    pre-term labor V13.41 ●
  sucking reflex (newborn) 796.1
  vision NEC 369.9
Poradenitis, nostras 099.1
Porencephaly (congenital) (developmental) (true) 742.4
  acquired 348.0
  nondevelopmental 348.0
  traumatic (post) 310.2
Porocephaliasis 134.1
Porokeratosis 757.39
  disseminated superficial actinic (DSAP) 692.75
Poroma, eccrine (M8402/0) — see Neoplasm, skin, benign
Porphyria (acute) (congenital) (constitutional) (erythropoietic) (familial) (hepatica) (idiopathic) (idiosyncratic) (intermittent) (latent) (mixed hepatic) (photosensitive) (South African genetic) (Swedish) 277.1
  acquired 277.1
  cutaneatarda
    hereditaria 277.1
    symptomatica 277.1
  due to drugs
    correct substance properly administered 277.1
    overdose or wrong substance given or taken 977.9
      specified drug — see Table of Drugs and Chemicals
  secondary 277.1
  toxic NEC 277.1
  variegata 277.1
Porphyrinuria (acquired) (congenital) (secondary) 277.1
Porphyruria (acquired) (congenital) 277.1
Portal — see condition
Port wine nevus or mark 757.32
Posadas-Wernicke disease 114.9
Position
  fetus, abnormal (see also Presentation, fetal) 652.9 ✓5ᵗʰ
  teeth, faulty 524.3
Positive
  culture (nonspecific) 795.39 ▲
    AIDS virus V08
    blood 790.7
    HIV V08
    human immunodeficiency virus V08
    nose 795.39 ▲
    skin lesion NEC 795.39 ▲
    spinal fluid 792.0
    sputum 795.39 ▲

Positive — *continued*
  culture — *continued*
    stool 792.1
    throat 795.39 ▲
    urine 791.9
    wound 795.39 ▲
  findings, anthrax 795.31 ●
  HIV V08
  human immunodeficiency virus (HIV) V08
  PPD 795.5
  serology
    AIDS virus V08
      inconclusive 795.71
    HIV V08
      inconclusive 795.71
    human immunodeficiency virus (HIV) V08
      inconclusive 795.71
    syphilis 097.1
      with signs or symptoms — *see* Syphilis, by site and stage
      false 795.6
  skin test 795.7
    tuberculin (without active tuberculosis) 795.5
  VDRL 097.1
    with signs or symptoms — *see* Syphilis, by site and stage
    false 795.6
  Wassermann reaction 097.1
    false 795.6
Postcardiotomy syndrome 429.4
Postcaval ureter 753.4
Postcholecystectomy syndrome 576.0
Postclimacteric bleeding 627.1
Postcommissurotomy syndrome 429.4
Postconcussional syndrome 310.2
Postcontusional syndrome 310.2
Postcricoid region — *see* condition
Post-dates (pregnancy) — *see* Pregnancy
Postencephalitic — *see also* condition
  syndrome 310.8
Posterior — *see* condition
Posterolateral sclerosis (spinal cord) — *see* Degeneration, combined
Postexanthematous — *see* condition
Postfebrile — *see* condition
Postgastrectomy dumping syndrome 564.2
Posthemiplegic chorea 344.89
Posthemorrhagic anemia (chronic) 280.0
  acute 285.1
  newborn 776.5
Posthepatitis syndrome 780.79
Postherpetic neuralgia (intercostal) (syndrome) (zoster) 053.19
  geniculate ganglion 053.11
  ophthalmica 053.19
  trigeminal 053.12
Posthitis 607.1
Postimmunization complication or reaction — *see* Complications, vaccination
Postinfectious — *see* condition
Postinfluenzal syndrome 780.79
Postlaminectomy syndrome 722.80
  cervical, cervicothoracic 722.81
  kyphosis 737.12
  lumbar, lumbosacral 722.83
  thoracic, thoracolumbar 722.82

Postleukotomy syndrome 310.0
Postlobectomy syndrome 310.0
Postmastectomy lymphedema (syndrome) 457.0
Postmaturity, postmature (fetus or newborn) 766.2
  affecting management of pregnancy
    post term pregnancy 645.1 ✓5ᵗʰ
    prolonged pregnancy 645.2 ✓5ᵗʰ
  syndrome 766.2
Postmeasles — *see also* condition
  complication 055.8
    specified NEC 055.79
Postmenopausal
  endometrium (atrophic) 627.8
    suppurative (see also Endometritis) 615.9
  hormone replacement V07.4
  status (age related) (natural) V49.81
Postnasal drip — *see* Sinusitis
Postnatal — *see* condition
Postoperative — *see also* condition
  confusion state 293.9
  psychosis 293.9
  status NEC (*see also* Status (post)) V45.89
Postpancreatectomy hyperglycemia 251.3
Postpartum — *see also* condition
  observation
    immediately after delivery V24.0
    routine follow-up V24.2
Postperfusion syndrome NEC 999.8
  bone marrow 996.85
Postpoliomyelitic — *see* condition
Postsurgery status NEC (*see also* Status (post)) V45.89
Post-term (pregnancy) 645.1 ✓5ᵗʰ
  infant (294 days or more gestation) 766.2
Posttraumatic — *see* condition
Posttraumatic brain syndrome, nonpsychotic 310.2
Post-typhoid abscess 002.0
Postures, hysterical 300.11
Postvaccinal reaction or complication — *see* Complications, vaccination
Postvagotomy syndrome 564.2
Postvalvulotomy syndrome 429.4
Postvasectomy sperm count V25.8
Potain's disease (pulmonary edema) 514
Potain's syndrome (gastrectasis with dyspepsia) 536.1
Pott's
  curvature (spinal) (*see also* Tuberculosis) 015.0 ✓5ᵗʰ [737.43]
  disease or paraplegia (*see also* Tuberculosis) 015.0 ✓5ᵗʰ [730.88]
  fracture (closed) 824.4
    open 824.5
  gangrene 440.24
  osteomyelitis (*see also* Tuberculosis) 015.0 ✓5ᵗʰ [730.88]
  spinal curvature (*see also* Tuberculosis) 015.0 ✓5ᵗʰ [737.43]
  tumor, puffy (*see also* Osteomyelitis) 730.2 ✓5ᵗʰ
Potter's
  asthma 502
  disease 753.0
  facies 754.0
  lung 502

Potter's — continued
  syndrome (with renal agenesis) 753.0
Pouch
  bronchus 748.3
  Douglas' — see condition
  esophagus, esophageal (congenital) 750.4
    acquired 530.6
  gastric 537.1
  Hartmann's (abnormal sacculation of gallbladder neck) 575.8
    of intestine V44.3
      attention to V55.3
  pharynx, pharyngeal (congenital) 750.27
Poulet's disease 714.2
Poultrymen's itch 133.8
Poverty V60.2
Prader-Labhart-Willi-Fanconi syndrome (hypogenital dystrophy with diabetic tendency) 759.81
Prader-Willi syndrome (hypogenital dystrophy with diabetic tendency) 759.81
Preachers' voice 784.49
Pre-AIDS — see Human immunodeficiency virus (disease) (illness) (infection)
Preauricular appendage 744.1
Prebetalipoproteinemia (acquired) (essential) (familial) (hereditary) (primary) (secondary) 272.1
  with chylomicronemia 272.3
Precipitate labor 661.3
  affecting fetus or newborn 763.6
Preclimacteric bleeding 627.0
  menorrhagia 627.0
Precocious
  adrenarche 259.1
  menarche 259.1
  menstruation 626.8
  pubarche 259.1
  puberty NEC 259.1
  sexual development NEC 259.1
  thelarche 259.1
Precocity, sexual (constitutional) (cryptogenic) (female) (idiopathic) (male) NEC 259.1
  with adrenal hyperplasia 255.2
Precordial pain 786.51
  psychogenic 307.89
Predeciduous teeth 520.2
Prediabetes, prediabetic 790.2
  complicating pregnancy, childbirth, or puerperium 648.8
  fetus or newborn 775.8
Predislocation status of hip, at birth (see also Subluxation, congenital, hip) 754.32
Preeclampsia (mild) 642.4
  with pre-existing hypertension 642.7
  affecting fetus or newborn 760.0
  severe 642.5
  superimposed on pre-existing hypertensive disease 642.7
Preeruptive color change, teeth, tooth 520.8
Preexcitation 426.7
  atrioventricular conduction 426.7
  ventricular 426.7
Preglaucoma 365.00

Pregnancy (single) (uterine) (without sickness) V22.2

> Note — Use the following fifth-digit subclassification with categories 640-648, 651-676:
>
> 0 unspecified as to episode of care
> 1 delivered, with or without mention of antepartum condition
> 2 delivered, with mention of postpartum complication
> 3 antepartum condition or complication
> 4 postpartum condition or complication

  abdominal (ectopic) 633.00
    with intrauterine pregnancy 633.01
    affecting fetus or newborn 761.4
  abnormal NEC 646.9
  ampullar — see Pregnancy, tubal
  broad ligament — see Pregnancy, cornual
  cervical — see Pregnancy, cornual
  combined (extrauterine and intrauterine) — see Pregnancy, cornual
  complicated (by)
    abnormal, abnormality NEC 646.9
      cervix 654.6
      cord (umbilical) 663.9
      glucose tolerance (conditions classifiable to 790.2) 648.8
      injury 648.9
        obstetrical NEC 665.9
      obstetrical trauma NEC 665.9
      pelvic organs or tissues NEC 654.9
      pelvis (bony) 653.0
      perineum or vulva 654.8
      placenta, placental (vessel) 656.7
      position
        cervix 654.4
        placenta 641.1
          without hemorrhage 641.0
        uterus 654.4
      size, fetus 653.5
      uterus (congenital) 654.0
    abscess or cellulitis
      bladder 646.6
      genitourinary tract (conditions classifiable to 590, 595, 597, 599.0, 614-616) 646.6
      kidney 646.6
      urinary tract NEC 646.6
    air embolism 673.0
    albuminuria 646.2
      with hypertension — see Toxemia, of pregnancy
    amnionitis 658.4
    amniotic fluid embolism 673.1
    anemia (conditions classifiable to 280-285) 648.2
    atrophy, yellow (acute) (liver) (subacute) 646.7
    bacilluria, asymptomatic 646.5
    bacteriuria, asymptomatic 646.5
    bicornis or bicornuate uterus 654.0
    bone and joint disorders (conditions classifiable to 720-724 or conditions affecting lower limbs classifiable to 711-719, 725-738) 648.7

Index to Diseases — Pregnancy

Pregnancy — *continued*
  complicated (by) — *continued*
    breech presentation 652.2
      with successful version 652.1
    cardiovascular disease (conditions classifiable to 390-398, 410-429) 648.6
      congenital (conditions classifiable to 745-747) 648.5
    cerebrovascular disorders (conditions classifiable to 430-434, 436-437) 674.0
    cervicitis (conditions classifiable to 616.0) 646.6
    chloasma (gravidarum) 646.8
    cholelithiasis 646.8
    chorea (gravidarum) — *see* Eclampsia, pregnancy
    contraction, pelvis (general) 653.1
      inlet 653.2
      outlet 653.3
    convulsions (eclamptic) (uremic) 642.6
      with pre-existing hypertension 642.7
    current disease or condition (nonobstetric)
      abnormal glucose tolerance 648.8
      anemia 648.2
      bone and joint (lower limb) 648.7
      cardiovascular 648.6
        congenital 648.5
      cerebrovascular 674.0
      diabetic 648.0
      drug dependence 648.3
      genital organ or tract 646.6
      gonorrheal 647.1
      hypertensive 642.2
        renal 642.1
      infectious 647.9
        specified type NEC 647.8
      liver 646.7
      malarial 647.4
      nutritional deficiency 648.9
      parasitic NEC 647.8
      renal 646.2
        hypertensive 642.1
      rubella 647.5
      specified condition NEC 648.9
      syphilitic 647.0
      thyroid 648.1
      tuberculous 647.3
      urinary 646.6
      venereal 647.2
      viral NEC 647.6
    cystitis 646.6
    cystocele 654.4
    death of fetus (near term) 656.4
      early pregnancy (before 22 completed weeks gestation) 632
    deciduitis 646.6
    decreased fetal movements 655.7
    diabetes (mellitus) (conditions classifiable to 250) 648.0
    disorders of liver 646.7
    displacement, uterus NEC 654.4
    disproportion — *see* Disproportion
    double uterus 654.0
    drug dependence (conditions classifiable to 304) 648.3
    dysplasia, cervix 654.6
    early onset of delivery (spontaneous) 644.2

Pregnancy — *continued*
  complicated (by) — *continued*
    eclampsia, eclamptic (coma) (convulsions) (delirium) (nephritis) (uremia) 642.6
      with pre-existing hypertension 642.7
    edema 646.1
      with hypertension — *see* Toxemia, of pregnancy
    effusion, amniotic fluid 658.1
      delayed delivery following 658.2
    embolism
      air 673.0
      amniotic fluid 673.1
      blood-clot 673.2
      cerebral 674.0
      pulmonary NEC 673.2
      pyemic 673.3
      septic 673.3
    emesis (gravidarum) — *see* Pregnancy, complicated, vomiting
    endometritis (conditions classifiable to 615.0-615.9) 646.6
      decidual 646.6
    excessive weight gain NEC 646.1
    face presentation 652.4
    failure, fetal head to enter pelvic brim 652.5
    false labor (pains) 644.1
    fatigue 646.8
    fatty metamorphosis of liver 646.7
    fetal
      death (near term) 656.4
        early (before 22 completed weeks gestation) 632
      deformity 653.7
      distress 656.8
    fibroid (tumor) (uterus) 654.1
    footling presentation 652.8
      with successful version 652.1
    gallbladder disease 646.8
    goiter 648.1
    gonococcal infection (conditions classifiable to 098) 647.1
    gonorrhea (conditions classifiable to 098) 647.1
    hemorrhage 641.9
      accidental 641.2
      before 22 completed weeks gestation NEC 640.9
      cerebrovascular 674.0
      due to
        afibrinogenemia or other coagulation defect (conditions classifiable to 286.0-286.9) 641.3
        leiomyoma, uterine 641.8
        marginal sinus (rupture) 641.2
        premature separation, placenta 641.2
        trauma 641.8
      early (before 22 completed weeks gestation) 640.9
      threatened abortion 640.0
      unavoidable 641.1
    hepatitis (acute) (malignant) (subacute) 646.7
      viral 647.6
    herniation of uterus 654.4
    high head at term 652.5
    hydatidiform mole (delivered) (undelivered) 630
    hydramnios 657

Pregnancy — continued
  complicated (by) — continued
    hydrocephalic fetus 653.6
    hydrops amnii 657
    hydrorrhea 658.1
    hyperemesis (gravidarum) — see Hyperemesis, gravidarum
    hypertension — see Hypertension, complicating pregnancy
    hypertensive
      heart and renal disease 642.2
      heart disease 642.2
      renal disease 642.2
    hyperthyroidism 648.1
    hypothyroidism 648.1
    hysteralgia 646.8
    icterus gravis 646.7
    incarceration, uterus 654.3
    incompetent cervix (os) 654.5
    infection 647.9
      amniotic fluid 658.4
      bladder 646.6
      genital organ (conditions classifiable to 614-616) 646.6
      kidney (conditions classifiable to 590.0-590.9) 646.6
      urinary (tract) 646.6
        asymptomatic 646.5
    infective and parasitic diseases NEC 647.8
    inflammation
      bladder 646.6
      genital organ (conditions classifiable to 614-616) 646.6
      urinary tract NEC 646.6
    insufficient weight gain 646.8
    intrauterine fetal death (near term) NEC 656.4
      early (before 22 completed weeks' gestation) 632
    malaria (conditions classifiable to 084) 647.4
    malformation, uterus (congenital) 654.0
    malnutrition (conditions classifiable to 260-269) 648.9
    malposition
      fetus — see Pregnancy, complicated, malpresentation
      uterus or cervix 654.4
    malpresentation 652.9
      with successful version 652.1
      in multiple gestation 652.6
      specified type NEC 652.8
    marginal sinus hemorrhage or rupture 641.2
    maternal obesity syndrome 646.1
    menstruation 640.8
    mental disorders (conditions classifiable to 290-303, 305-316, 317-319) 648.4
    mentum presentation 652.4
    missed
      abortion 632
      delivery (at or near term) 656.4
      labor (at or near term) 656.4
    necrosis
      genital organ or tract (conditions classifiable to 614-616) 646.6
      liver (conditions classifiable to 570) 646.7
      renal, cortical 646.2

Pregnancy — continued
  complicated (by) — continued
    nephritis or nephrosis (conditions classifiable to 580-589) 646.2
      with hypertension 642.1
    nephropathy NEC 646.2
    neuritis (peripheral) 646.4
    nutritional deficiency (conditions classifiable to 260-269) 648.9
    oblique lie or presentation 652.3
      with successful version 652.1
    obstetrical trauma NEC 665.9
    oligohydramnios NEC 658.0
    onset of contractions before 37 weeks 644.0
    oversize fetus 653.5
    papyraceous fetus 646.0
    patent cervix 654.5
    pelvic inflammatory disease (conditions classifiable to 614-616) 646.6
    placenta, placental
      abnormality 656.7
      abruptio or ablatio 641.2
      detachment 641.2
      disease 656.7
      infarct 656.7
      low implantation 641.1
        without hemorrhage 641.0
      malformation 656.7
      malposition 641.1
        without hemorrhage 641.0
      marginal sinus hemorrhage 641.2
      previa 641.1
        without hemorrhage 641.0
      separation (premature) (undelivered) 641.2
    placentitis 658.4
    polyhydramnios 657
    postmaturity
      post term 645.1
      prolonged 645.2
    prediabetes 648.8
    pre-eclampsia (mild) 642.4
      severe 642.5
      superimposed on pre-existing hypertensive disease 642.7
    premature rupture of membranes 658.1
      with delayed delivery 658.2
    previous
      infertility V23.0
      nonobstetric condition V23.8
      poor obstetrical history V23.49 ▲
      premature delivery V23.41 ▲
      trophoblastic disease (conditions classifiable to 630) V23.1
    prolapse, uterus 654.4
    proteinuria (gestational) 646.2
      with hypertension — see Toxemia, of pregnancy
    pruritus (neurogenic) 646.8
    psychosis or psychoneurosis 648.4
    ptyalism 646.8
    pyelitis (conditions classifiable to 590.0-590.9) 646.6
    renal disease or failure NEC 646.2
      with secondary hypertension 642.1
      hypertensive 642.2
    retention, retained dead ovum 631
    retroversion, uterus 654.3
    Rh immunization, incompatibility, or sensitization 656.1

Pregnancy — *continued*
  complicated (by) — *continued*
    rubella (conditions classifiable to 056) 647.5 ✓5ᵗʰ
    rupture
      amnion (premature) 658.1 ✓5ᵗʰ
        with delayed delivery 658.2 ✓5ᵗʰ
      marginal sinus (hemorrhage) 641.2 ✓5ᵗʰ
      membranes (premature) 658.1 ✓5ᵗʰ
        with delayed delivery 658.2 ✓5ᵗʰ
      uterus (before onset of labor) 665.0 ✓5ᵗʰ
    salivation (excessive) 646.8 ✓5ᵗʰ
    salpingo-oophoritis (conditions classifiable to 614.0-614.2) 646.6 ✓5ᵗʰ
    septicemia (conditions classifiable to 038.0-038.9) 647.8 ✓5ᵗʰ
      postpartum 670 ✓4ᵗʰ
      puerperal 670 ✓4ᵗʰ
    spasms, uterus (abnormal) 646.8 ✓5ᵗʰ
    specified condition NEC 646.8 ✓5ᵗʰ
    spurious labor pains 644.1 ✓5ᵗʰ
    superfecundation 651.9 ✓5ᵗʰ
    superfetation 651.9 ✓5ᵗʰ
    syphilis (conditions classifiable to 090-097) 647.0 ✓5ᵗʰ
    threatened
      abortion 640.0 ✓5ᵗʰ
      premature delivery 644.2 ✓5ᵗʰ
      premature labor 644.0 ✓5ᵗʰ
    thrombophlebitis (superficial) 671.2 ✓5ᵗʰ
      deep 671.3 ✓5ᵗʰ
    thrombosis 671.9 ✓5ᵗʰ
      venous (superficial) 671.2 ✓5ᵗʰ
        deep 671.3 ✓5ᵗʰ
    thyroid dysfunction (conditions classifiable to 240-246) 648.1 ✓5ᵗʰ
    thyroiditis 648.1 ✓5ᵗʰ
    thyrotoxicosis 648.1 ✓5ᵗʰ
    torsion of uterus 654.4 ✓5ᵗʰ
    toxemia — *see* Toxemia, of pregnancy
    transverse lie or presentation 652.3 ✓5ᵗʰ
      with successful version 652.1 ✓5ᵗʰ
    tuberculosis (conditions classifiable to 010-018) 647.3 ✓5ᵗʰ
    tumor
      cervix 654.6 ✓5ᵗʰ
      ovary 654.4 ✓5ᵗʰ
      pelvic organs or tissue NEC 654.4 ✓5ᵗʰ
      uterus (body) 654.1 ✓5ᵗʰ
        cervix 654.6 ✓5ᵗʰ
      vagina 654.7 ✓5ᵗʰ
      vulva 654.8 ✓5ᵗʰ
    unstable lie 652.0 ✓5ᵗʰ
    uremia — *see* Pregnancy, complicated, renal disease
    urethritis 646.6 ✓5ᵗʰ
    vaginitis or vulvitis (conditions classifiable to 616.1) 646.6 ✓5ᵗʰ
    varicose
      placental vessels 656.7 ✓5ᵗʰ
      veins (legs) 671.0 ✓5ᵗʰ
        perineum 671.1 ✓5ᵗʰ
        vulva 671.1 ✓5ᵗʰ
    varicosity, labia or vulva 671.1 ✓5ᵗʰ
    venereal disease NEC (conditions classifiable to 099) 647.2 ✓5ᵗʰ
    viral disease NEC (conditions classifiable to 042, 050-055, 057-079) 647.6 ✓5ᵗʰ
    vomiting (incoercible) (pernicious) (persistent) (uncontrollable) (vicious) 643.9 ✓5ᵗʰ

Pregnancy — *continued*
  complicated (by) — *continued*
    vomiting — *continued*
      due to organic disease or other cause 643.8 ✓5ᵗʰ
      early — *see* Hyperemesis, gravidarum
      late (after 22 completed weeks gestation) 643.2 ✓5ᵗʰ
    young maternal age 659.8 ✓5ᵗʰ
  complications NEC 646.9 ✓5ᵗʰ
  cornual 633.80 ▲
    with intrauterine pregnancy 633.81 ●
    affecting fetus or newborn 761.4
  death, maternal NEC 646.9 ✓5ᵗʰ
  delivered — *see* Delivery
  ectopic (ruptured) NEC 633.90 ▲
    with intrauterine pregnancy 633.91 ●
    abdominal — *see* Pregnancy, abdominal
    affecting fetus or newborn 761.4
    combined (extrauterine and intrauterine) — *see* Pregnancy, cornual
    ovarian — *see* Pregnancy, ovarian
    specified type NEC 633.80 ▲
      with intrauterine pregnancy 633.81 ●
      affecting fetus or newborn 761.4
    tubal — *see* Pregnancy, tubal
  examination, pregnancy not confirmed V72.4
  extrauterine — *see* Pregnancy, ectopic
  fallopian — *see* Pregnancy, tubal
  false 300.11
    labor (pains) 644.1 ✓5ᵗʰ
  fatigue 646.8 ✓5ᵗʰ
  illegitimate V61.6
  incidental finding V22.2
  in double uterus 654.0 ✓5ᵗʰ
  interstitial — *see* Pregnancy, cornual
  intraligamentous — *see* Pregnancy, cornual
  intramural — *see* Pregnancy, cornual
  intraperitoneal — *see* Pregnancy, abdominal
  isthmian — *see* Pregnancy, tubal
  management affected by
    abnormal, abnormality
      fetus (suspected) 655.9 ✓5ᵗʰ
        specified NEC 655.8 ✓5ᵗʰ
      placenta 656.7 ✓5ᵗʰ
    advanced maternal age NEC 659.6 ✓5ᵗʰ
      multigravida 659.6 ✓5ᵗʰ
      primigravida 659.5 ✓5ᵗʰ
    antibodies (maternal)
      anti-c 656.1 ✓5ᵗʰ
      anti-d 656.1 ✓5ᵗʰ
      anti-e 656.1 ✓5ᵗʰ
      blood group (ABO) 656.2 ✓5ᵗʰ
      Rh(esus) 656.1 ✓5ᵗʰ
    elderly multigravida 659.6 ✓5ᵗʰ
    elderly primigravida 659.5 ✓5ᵗʰ
    fetal (suspected)
      abnormality 655.9 ✓5ᵗʰ
        acid-base balance 656.8 ✓5ᵗʰ
        heart rate or rhythm 659.7 ✓5ᵗʰ
        specified NEC 655.8 ✓5ᵗʰ
      acidemia 656.3 ✓5ᵗʰ
      anencephaly 655.0 ✓5ᵗʰ
      bradycardia 659.7 ✓5ᵗʰ
      central nervous system malformation 655.0 ✓5ᵗʰ
      chromosomal abnormalities (conditions classifiable to 758.0-758.9) 655.1 ✓5ᵗʰ

Pregnancy — *continued*
　management affected by — *continued*
　　fetal — *continued*
　　　damage from
　　　　drugs 655.5 ✓5ᵗʰ
　　　　　obstetric, anesthetic, or sedative
　　　　　　655.5 ✓5ᵗʰ
　　　　　environmental toxins 655.8 ✓5ᵗʰ
　　　　　intrauterine contraceptive device
　　　　　　655.8 ✓5ᵗʰ
　　　　　maternal
　　　　　　alcohol addiction 655.4 ✓5ᵗʰ
　　　　　　disease NEC 655.4 ✓5ᵗʰ
　　　　　　drug use 655.5 ✓5ᵗʰ
　　　　　　listeriosis 655.4 ✓5ᵗʰ
　　　　　　rubella 655.3 ✓5ᵗʰ
　　　　　　toxoplasmosis 655.4 ✓5ᵗʰ
　　　　　　viral infection 655.3 ✓5ᵗʰ
　　　　　radiation 655.6 ✓5ᵗʰ
　　　death (near term) 656.4 ✓5ᵗʰ
　　　　early (before 22 completed weeks'
　　　　　gestation) 632
　　　distress 656.8 ✓5ᵗʰ
　　　excessive growth 656.6 ✓5ᵗʰ
　　　growth retardation 656.5 ✓5ᵗʰ
　　　hereditary disease 655.2 ✓5ᵗʰ
　　　hydrocephalus 655.0 ✓5ᵗʰ
　　　intrauterine death 656.4 ✓5ᵗʰ
　　　poor growth 656.5 ✓5ᵗʰ
　　　spina bifida (with myelomeningocele)
　　　　655.0 ✓5ᵗʰ
　　　fetal-maternal hemorrhage 656.0 ✓5ᵗʰ
　　　hereditary disease in family (possibly)
　　　　affecting fetus 655.2 ✓5ᵗʰ
　　　incompatibility, blood groups (ABO)
　　　　656.2 ✓5ᵗʰ
　　　　rh(esus) 656.1 ✓5ᵗʰ
　　　insufficient prenatal care V23.7
　　　intrauterine death 656.4 ✓5ᵗʰ
　　　isoimmunization (ABO) 656.2 ✓5ᵗʰ
　　　　rh(esus) 656.1 ✓5ᵗʰ
　　　large-for-dates fetus 656.6 ✓5ᵗʰ
　　　light-for-dates fetus 656.5 ✓5ᵗʰ
　　　meconium in liquor 656.8 ✓5ᵗʰ
　　　mental disorder (conditions classifiable to
　　　　290-303, 305-316, 317-319)
　　　　648.4 ✓5ᵗʰ
　　　multiparity (grand) 659.4 ✓5ᵗʰ
　　　poor obstetric history V23.49　▲
　　　　pre-term labor V23.41　●
　　　postmaturity
　　　　post term 645.1 ✓5ᵗʰ
　　　　prolonged 645.2 ✓5ᵗʰ
　　　post term pregnancy 645.1 ✓5ᵗʰ
　　　previous
　　　　abortion V23.2
　　　　　habitual 646.3 ✓5ᵗʰ
　　　　cesarean delivery 654.2 ✓5ᵗʰ
　　　　difficult delivery V23.49　▲
　　　　forceps delivery V23.49　▲
　　　　habitual abortions 646.3 ✓5ᵗʰ
　　　　hemorrhage, antepartum or postpartum
　　　　　V23.49　▲
　　　　hydatidiform mole V23.1
　　　　infertility V23.0
　　　　malignancy NEC V23.8 ✓5ᵗʰ
　　　　nonobstetrical conditions V23.8 ✓5ᵗʰ
　　　　premature delivery V23.41　▲
　　　　trophoblastic disease (conditions in 630)
　　　　　V23.1
　　　　vesicular mole V23.1

Pregnancy — *continued*
　management affected by — *continued*
　　prolonged pregnancy 645.2 ✓5ᵗʰ
　　small-for-dates fetus 656.5 ✓5ᵗʰ
　　young maternal age 659.8 ✓5ᵗʰ
　maternal death NEC 646.9 ✓5ᵗʰ
　mesometric (mural) — *see* Pregnancy, cornual
　molar 631
　　hydatidiform (*see also* Hydatidiform mole)
　　　630
　　　previous, affecting management of
　　　　pregnancy V23.1
　　previous, affecting management of
　　　pregnancy V23.49　▲
　multiple NEC 651.9 ✓5ᵗʰ
　　with fetal loss and retention of one or more
　　　fetus(es) 651.6 ✓5ᵗʰ
　　affecting fetus or newborn 761.5
　　specified type NEC 651.8 ✓5ᵗʰ
　　　with fetal loss and retention of one or
　　　　more fetus(es) 651.6 ✓5ᵗʰ
　mural — *see* Pregnancy, cornual
　observation NEC V22.1
　　first pregnancy V22.0
　　high-risk V23.9
　　　specified problem NEC V23.8 ✓5ᵗʰ
　ovarian 633.20　▲
　　with intrauterine pregnancy 633.21　●
　　affecting fetus or newborn 761.4
　postmature
　　post term 645.1 ✓5ᵗʰ
　　prolonged 645.2 ✓5ᵗʰ
　post term 645.1 ✓5ᵗʰ
　prenatal care only V22.1
　　first pregnancy V22.0
　　high-risk V23.9
　　　specified problem NEC V23.8 ✓5ᵗʰ
　prolonged 645.2 ✓5ᵗʰ
　quadruplet NEC 651.2 ✓5ᵗʰ
　　with fetal loss and retention of one or more
　　　fetus(es) 651.5 ✓5ᵗʰ
　　affecting fetus or newborn 761.5
　quintuplet NEC 651.8 ✓5ᵗʰ
　　with fetal loss and retention of one or more
　　　fetus(es) 651.6 ✓5ᵗʰ
　　affecting fetus or newborn 761.5
　sextuplet NEC 651.8 ✓5ᵗʰ
　　with fetal loss and retention of one or more
　　　fetus(es) 651.6 ✓5ᵗʰ
　　affecting fetus or newborn 761.5
　spurious 300.11
　superfecundation NEC 651.9 ✓5ᵗʰ
　　with fetal loss and retention of one or more
　　　fetus(es) 651.6 ✓5ᵗʰ
　superfetation NEC 651.9 ✓5ᵗʰ
　　with fetal loss and retention of one or more
　　　fetus(es) 651.6 ✓5ᵗʰ
　supervision (of) (for) — *see also* Pregnancy,
　　management affected by
　　elderly
　　　multigravida V23.82
　　　primigravida V23.81
　　high-risk V23.9
　　　insufficient prenatal care V23.7
　　　specified problem NEC V23.8 ✓5ᵗʰ
　　multiparity V23.3
　　normal NEC V22.1
　　　first V22.0
　　poor
　　　obstetric history V23.49　▲
　　　pre-term labor V23.41　●

Pregnancy — *continued*
　supervision — *continued*
　　poor — *continued*
　　　reproductive history V23.5
　　previous
　　　abortion V23.2
　　　hydatidiform mole V23.1
　　　infertility V23.0
　　　neonatal death V23.5
　　　stillbirth V23.5
　　　trophoblastic disease V23.1
　　　vesicular mole V23.1
　　specified problem NEC V23.8 ✓5ᵗʰ
　　young
　　　multigravida V23.84
　　　primigravida V23.83
　triplet NEC 651.1 ✓5ᵗʰ
　　with fetal loss and retention of one or more fetus(es) 651.4 ✓5ᵗʰ
　　affecting fetus or newborn 761.5
　tubal (with rupture) 633.10 ▲
　　with intrauterine pregnancy 633.11 ●
　　affecting fetus or newborn 761.4
　twin NEC 651.0 ✓5ᵗʰ
　　with fetal loss and retention of one fetus 651.3 ✓5ᵗʰ
　　affecting fetus or newborn 761.5
　unconfirmed V72.4
　undelivered (no other diagnosis) V22.2
　　with false labor 644.1 ✓5ᵗʰ
　　high-risk V23.9
　　　specified problem NEC V23.8 ✓5ᵗʰ
　unwanted NEC V61.7
Pregnant uterus — *see* condition
Preiser's disease (osteoporosis) 733.09
Prekwashiorkor 260
Preleukemia 238.7
Preluxation of hip, congenital (*see also* Subluxation, congenital, hip) 754.32
Premature — *see also* condition
　beats (nodal) 427.60
　　atrial 427.61
　　auricular 427.61
　　postoperative 997.1
　　specified type NEC 427.69
　　supraventricular 427.61
　　ventricular 427.69
　birth NEC 765.1 ✓5ᵗʰ
　closure
　　cranial suture 756.0
　　fontanel 756.0
　　foramen ovale 745.8
　contractions 427.60
　　atrial 427.61
　　auricular 427.61
　　auriculoventricular 427.61
　　heart (extrasystole) 427.60
　　junctional 427.60
　　nodal 427.60
　　postoperative 997.1
　　ventricular 427.69
　ejaculation 302.75
　infant NEC 765.1 ✓5ᵗʰ
　　excessive 765.0 ✓5ᵗʰ
　　light-for-dates — *see* Light-for-dates
　labor 644.2 ✓5ᵗʰ
　　threatened 644.0 ✓5ᵗʰ
　lungs 770.4
　menopause 256.31
　puberty 259.1

Premature — *continued*
　rupture of membranes or amnion 658.1 ✓5ᵗʰ
　　affecting fetus or newborn 761.1
　　delayed delivery following 658.2 ✓5ᵗʰ
　senility (syndrome) 259.8
　separation, placenta (partial) — *see* Placenta, separation
　ventricular systole 427.69
Prematurity NEC 765.1 ✓5ᵗʰ
　extreme 765.0 ✓5ᵗʰ
Premenstrual syndrome 625.4
Premenstrual tension 625.4
Premolarization, cuspids 520.2
Premyeloma 273.1
Prenatal
　care, normal pregnancy V22.1
　　first V22.0
　death, cause unknown — *see* Death, fetus
　screening — *see* Antenatal, screening
Prepartum — *see* condition
Preponderance, left or right ventricular 429.3
Prepuce — *see* condition
Presbycardia 797
　hypertensive (*see also* Hypertension, heart) 402.90
Presbycusis 388.01
Presbyesophagus 530.89
Presbyophrenia 310.1
Presbyopia 367.4
Prescription of contraceptives NEC V25.02
　diaphragm V25.02
　oral (pill) V25.01
　　repeat V25.41
　repeat V25.40
　　oral (pill) V25.41
Presenile — *see also* condition
　aging 259.8
　dementia (*see also* Dementia, presenile) 290.10
Presenility 259.8
Presentation, fetal
　abnormal 652.9 ✓5ᵗʰ
　　with successful version 652.1 ✓5ᵗʰ
　　before labor, affecting fetus or newborn 761.7
　　causing obstructed labor 660.0 ✓5ᵗʰ
　　　affecting fetus or newborn, any, except breech 763.1
　　in multiple gestation (one or more) 652.6 ✓5ᵗʰ
　　specified NEC 652.8 ✓5ᵗʰ
　arm 652.7 ✓5ᵗʰ
　　causing obstructed labor 660.0 ✓5ᵗʰ
　breech (buttocks) (complete) (frank) 652.2 ✓5ᵗʰ
　　with successful version 652.1 ✓5ᵗʰ
　　　before labor, affecting fetus or newborn 761.7
　　before labor, affecting fetus or newborn 761.7
　brow 652.4 ✓5ᵗʰ
　　causing obstructed labor 660.0 ✓5ᵗʰ
　buttocks 652.2 ✓5ᵗʰ
　chin 652.4 ✓5ᵗʰ
　complete 652.2 ✓5ᵗʰ
　compound 652.8 ✓5ᵗʰ
　cord 663.0 ✓5ᵗʰ
　extended head 652.4 ✓5ᵗʰ

Presentation, fetal — *continued*
    face 652.4 ✓5ᵗʰ
        to pubes 652.8 ✓5ᵗʰ
    footling 652.8 ✓5ᵗʰ
    frank 652.2 ✓5ᵗʰ
    hand, leg, or foot NEC 652.8 ✓5ᵗʰ
    incomplete 652.8 ✓5ᵗʰ
    mentum 652.4 ✓5ᵗʰ
    multiple gestation (one fetus or more) 652.6 ✓5ᵗʰ
    oblique 652.3 ✓5ᵗʰ
        with successful version 652.1 ✓5ᵗʰ
    shoulder 652.8 ✓5ᵗʰ
        affecting fetus or newborn 763.1
    transverse 652.3 ✓5ᵗʰ
        with successful version 652.1 ✓5ᵗʰ
    umbilical cord 663.0 ✓5ᵗʰ
    unstable 652.0 ✓5ᵗʰ
Prespondylolisthesis (congenital) (lumbosacral) 756.11
Pressure
    area, skin ulcer (*see also* Decubitus) 707.0
    atrophy, spine 733.99
    birth, fetus or newborn NEC 767.9
    brachial plexus 353.0
    brain 348.4
        injury at birth 767.0
    cerebral — *see* Pressure, brain
    chest 786.59
    cone, tentorial 348.4
        injury at birth 767.0
    funis — *see* Compression, umbilical cord
    hyposystolic (*see also* Hypotension) 458.9
    increased
        intracranial 781.99
            due to
                benign intracranial hypertension 348.2
                hydrocephalus — *see* hydrocephalus
        injury at birth 767.8
        intraocular 365.00
    lumbosacral plexus 353.1
    mediastinum 519.3
    necrosis (chronic) (skin) (*see also* Decubitus) 707.0
    nerve — *see* Compression, nerve
    paralysis (*see also* Neuropathy, entrapment) 355.9
    sore (chronic) (*see also* Decubitus) 707.0
    spinal cord 336.9
    ulcer (chronic) (*see also* Decubitus) 707.0
    umbilical cord — *see* Compression, umbilical cord
    venous, increased 459.89
Pre-syncope 780.2
Preterm infant NEC 765.1 ✓5ᵗʰ
    extreme 765.0 ✓5ᵗʰ
Priapism (penis) 607.3
Prickling sensation (*see also* Disturbance, sensation) 782.0
Prickly heat 705.1
Primary — *see* condition
Primigravida, elderly
    affecting
        fetus or newborn 763.89
        management of pregnancy, labor, and delivery 659.5 ✓5ᵗʰ

Primipara, old
    affecting
        fetus or newborn 763.89
        management of pregnancy, labor, and delivery 659.5 ✓5ᵗʰ
Primula dermatitis 692.6
Primus varus (bilateral) (metatarsus) 754.52
P.R.I.N.D. 436
Pringle's disease (tuberous sclerosis) 759.5
Prinzmetal's angina 413.1
Prinzmetal-Massumi syndrome (anterior chest wall) 786.52
Prizefighter ear 738.7
Problem (with) V49.9
    academic V62.3
    acculturation V62.4
    adopted child V61.29
    aged
        in-law V61.3
        parent V61.3
        person NEC V61.8
    alcoholism in family V61.41
    anger reaction (*see also* Disturbance, conduct) 312.0 ✓5ᵗʰ
    behavior, child 312.9
    behavioral V40.9
        specified NEC V40.3
    betting V69.3
    cardiorespiratory NEC V47.2
    care of sick or handicapped person in family or household V61.49
    career choice V62.2
    communication V40.1
    conscience regarding medical care V62.6
    delinquency (juvenile) 312.9
    diet, inappropriate V69.1
    digestive NEC V47.3
    ear NEC V41.3
    eating habits, inappropriate V69.1
    economic V60.2
        affecting care V60.9
        specified type NEC V60.8
    educational V62.3
    enuresis, child 307.6
    exercise, lack of V69.0
    eye NEC V41.1
    family V61.9
        specified circumstance NEC V61.8
    fear reaction, child 313.0
    feeding (elderly) (infant) 783.3
        newborn 779.3
        nonorganic 307.50
    fetal, affecting management of pregnancy 656.9 ✓5ᵗʰ
        specified type NEC 656.8 ✓5ᵗʰ
    financial V60.2
    foster child V61.29
        specified NEC V41.8
    functional V41.9
        specified type NEC V41.8
    gambling V69.3
    genital NEC V47.5
    head V48.9
        deficiency V48.0
        disfigurement V48.6
        mechanical V48.2
        motor V48.2
        movement of V48.2
        sensory V48.4
        specified condition NEC V48.8

Problem (with) — *continued*
  hearing V41.2
  high-risk sexual behavior V69.2
  influencing health status NEC V49.89
  internal organ NEC V47.9
    deficiency V47.0
    mechanical or motor V47.1
  interpersonal NEC V62.81
  jealousy, child 313.3
  learning V40.0
  legal V62.5
  life circumstance NEC V62.89
  lifestyle V69.9
    specified NEC V69.8
  limb V49.9
    deficiency V49.0
    disfigurement V49.4
    mechanical V49.1
    motor V49.2
    movement, involving
      musculoskeletal system V49.1
      nervous system V49.2
    sensory V49.3
    specified condition NEC V49.5
  litigation V62.5
  living alone V60.3
  loneliness NEC V62.89
  marital V61.10
    involving
      divorce V61.0
      estrangement V61.0
    psychosexual disorder 302.9
    sexual function V41.7
  mastication V41.6
  medical care, within family V61.49
  mental V40.9
    specified NEC V40.2
  mental hygiene, adult V40.9
  multiparity V61.5
  nail biting, child 307.9
  neck V48.9
    deficiency V48.1
    disfigurement V48.7
    mechanical V48.3
    motor V48.3
    movement V48.3
    sensory V48.5
    specified condition NEC V48.8
  neurological NEC 781.99
  none (feared complaint unfounded) V65.5
  occupational V62.2
  parent-child V61.20
  partner V61.10
  personal NEC V62.89
    interpersonal conflict NEC V62.81
  personality (*see also* Disorder, personality) 301.9
  phase of life V62.89
  placenta, affecting managment of pregnancy 656.9
    specified type NEC 656.8
  poverty V60.2
  presence of sick or handicapped person in family or household V61.49
  psychiatric 300.9
  psychosocial V62.9
    specified type NEC V62.89
  relational NEC V62.81
  relationship, childhood 313.3
  religious or spiritual belief
    other than medical care V62.89
    regarding medical care V62.6

Problem (with) — *continued*
  self-damaging behavior V69.8
  sexual
    behavior, high-risk V69.2
    function NEC V41.7
  sibling relational V61.8
  sight V41.0
  sleep disorder, child 307.40
  smell V41.5
  speech V40.1
  spite reaction, child (*see also* Disturbance, conduct) 312.0
  spoiled child reaction (*see also* Disturbance, conduct) 312.1
  swallowing V41.6
  tantrum, child (*see also* Disturbance, conduct) 312.1
  taste V41.5
  thumb sucking, child 307.9
  tic, child 307.21
  trunk V48.9
    deficiency V48.1
    disfigurement V48.7
    mechanical V48.3
    motor V48.3
    movement V48.3
    sensory V48.5
    specified condition NEC V48.8
  unemployment V62.0
  urinary NEC V47.4
  voice production V41.4
Procedure (surgical) not done NEC V64.3
  because of
    contraindication V64.1
    patient's decision V64.2
      for reasons of conscience or religion V62.6
    specified reason NEC V64.3
Procidentia
  anus (sphincter) 569.1
  rectum (sphincter) 569.1
  stomach 537.89
  uteri 618.1
Proctalgia 569.42
  fugax 564.6
  spasmodic 564.6
    psychogenic 307.89
Proctitis 569.49
  amebic 006.8
  chlamydial 099.52
  gonococcal 098.7
  granulomatous 555.1
  idiopathic 556.2
    with ulcerative sigmoiditis 556.3
  tuberculous (*see also* Tuberculosis) 014.8
  ulcerative (chronic) (nonspecific) 556.2
    with ulcerative sigmoiditis 556.3
Proctocele
  female (without uterine prolapse) 618.0
    with uterine prolapse 618.4
      complete 618.3
      incomplete 618.2
  male 569.49
Proctocolitis, idiopathic 556.2
  with ulcerative sigmoiditis 556.3
Proctoptosis 569.1
Proctosigmoiditis 569.89
  ulcerative (chronic) 556.3
Proctospasm 564.6
  psychogenic 306.4

Prodromal-AIDS — *see* Human immunodeficiency virus (disease) (illness) (infection)
Profichet's disease or syndrome 729.9
Progeria (adultorum) (syndrome) 259.8
Prognathism (mandibular) (maxillary) 524.00
Progonoma (melanotic) (M9363/0) — *see* Neoplasm, by site, benign
Progressive — *see* condition
Prolapse, prolapsed
  anus, anal (canal) (sphincter) 569.1
  arm or hand, complicating delivery 652.7
    causing obstructed labor 660.0
      affecting fetus or newborn 763.1
    fetus or newborn 763.1
  bladder (acquired) (mucosa) (sphincter)
    congenital (female) (male) 756.71
    female 618.0
    male 596.8
  breast implant (prosthetic) 996.54
  cecostomy 569.69
  cecum 569.89
  cervix, cervical (stump) (hypertrophied) 618.1
    anterior lip, obstructing labor 660.2
      affecting fetus or newborn 763.1
    congenital 752.49
    postpartal (old) 618.1
  ciliary body 871.1
  colon (pedunculated) 569.89
  colostomy 569.69
  conjunctiva 372.73
  cord — *see* Prolapse, umbilical cord
  disc (intervertebral) — *see* Displacement, intervertebral disc
  duodenum 537.89
  eye implant (orbital) 996.59
    lens (ocular) 996.53
  fallopian tube 620.4
  fetal extremity, complicating delivery 652.8
    causing obstructed labor 660.0
    fetus or newborn 763.1
  funis — *see* Prolapse, umbilical cord
  gastric (mucosa) 537.89
  genital, female 618.9
    specified NEC 618.8
  globe 360.81
  ileostomy bud 569.69
  intervertebral disc — *see* Displacement, intervertebral disc
  intestine (small) 569.89
  iris 364.8
    traumatic 871.1
  kidney (*see also* Disease, renal) 593.0
    congenital 753.3
  laryngeal muscles or ventricle 478.79
  leg, complicating delivery 652.8
    causing obstructed labor 660.0
    fetus or newborn 763.1
  liver 573.8
  meatus urinarius 599.5
  mitral valve 424.0
  ocular lens implant 996.53
  organ or site, congenital NEC — *see* Malposition, congenital
  ovary 620.4
  pelvic (floor), female 618.8
  perineum, female 618.8
  pregnant uterus 654.4

Prolapse, prolapsed — *continued*
  rectum (mucosa) (sphincter) 569.1
    due to Trichuris trichiuria 127.3
  spleen 289.59
  stomach 537.89
  umbilical cord
    affecting fetus or newborn 762.4
    complicating delivery 663.0
  ureter 593.89
    with obstruction 593.4
  ureterovesical orifice 593.89
  urethra (acquired) (infected) (mucosa) 599.5
    congenital 753.8
  uterovaginal 618.4
    complete 618.3
    incomplete 618.2
    specified NEC 618.8
  uterus (first degree) (second degree) (third degree) (complete) (without vaginal wall prolapse) 618.1
    with mention of vaginal wall prolapse — *see* Prolapse, uterovaginal
    congenital 752.3
    in pregnancy or childbirth 654.4
      affecting fetus or newborn 763.1
      causing obstructed labor 660.2
        affecting fetus or newborn 763.1
    postpartal (old) 618.1
  uveal 871.1
  vagina (anterior) (posterior) (vault) (wall) (without uterine prolapse) 618.0
    with uterine prolapse 618.4
      complete 618.3
      incomplete 618.2
    posthysterectomy 618.5
  vitreous (humor) 379.26
    traumatic 871.1
  womb — *see* Prolapse, uterus
Prolapsus, female 618.9
Proliferative — *see* condition
Prolinemia 270.8
Prolinuria 270.8
Prolonged, prolongation
  bleeding time (*see also* Defect, coagulation) 790.92
    "idiopathic" (in von Willebrand's disease) 286.4
  coagulation time (*see also* Defect, coagulation) 790.92
  gestation syndrome 766.2
  labor 662.1
    affecting fetus or newborn 763.89
    first stage 662.0
    second stage 662.2
  pregnancy 645.2
  PR interval 426.11
  prothrombin time (*see also* Defect, coagulation) 790.92
  rupture of membranes (24 hours or more prior to onset of labor) 658.2
  uterine contractions in labor 661.4
    affecting fetus or newborn 763.7
Prominauris 744.29
Prominence
  auricle (ear) (congenital) 744.29
    acquired 380.32
  ischial spine or sacral promontory
    with disproportion (fetopelvic) 653.3
      affecting fetus or newborn 763.1
      causing obstructed labor 660.1
        affecting fetus or newborn 763.1

Prominence — *continued*
  nose (congenital) 748.1
    acquired 738.0
Pronation
  ankle 736.79
  foot 736.79
    congenital 755.67
Prophylactic
  administration of
    antibiotics V07.39
    antitoxin, any V07.2
    antivenin V07.2
    chemotherapeutic agent NEC V07.39
      fluoride V07.31
    diphtheria antitoxin V07.2
    gamma globulin V07.2
    immune sera (gamma globulin) V07.2
    RhoGAM V07.2
    tetanus antitoxin V07.2
  chemotherapy NEC V07.39
    fluoride V07.31
  immunotherapy V07.2
  measure V07.9
    specified type NEC V07.8
  postmenopausal hormone replacement V07.4
  sterilization V25.2
Proptosis (ocular) (*see also* Exophthalmos) 376.30
  thyroid 242.0
Propulsion
  eyeball 360.81
Prosecution, anxiety concerning V62.5
Prostate, prostatic — *see* condition
Prostatism 600.9
Prostatitis (congestive) (suppurative) 601.9
  acute 601.0
  cavitary 601.8
  chlamydial 099.54
  chronic 601.1
  diverticular 601.8
  due to Trichomonas (vaginalis) 131.03
  fibrous 600.9
  gonococcal (acute) 098.12
    chronic or duration of 2 months or over 098.32
  granulomatous 601.8
  hypertrophic 600.0
  specified type NEC 601.8
  subacute 601.1
  trichomonal 131.03
  tuberculous (*see also* Tuberculosis) 016.5 [601.4]
Prostatocystitis 601.3
Prostatorrhea 602.8
Prostatoseminovesiculitis, trichomonal 131.03
Prostration 780.79
  heat 992.5
    anhydrotic 992.3
    due to
      salt (and water) depletion 992.4
      water depletion 992.3
  nervous 300.5
  newborn 779.89
  senile 797
Protanomaly 368.51
Protanopia (anomalous trichromat) (complete) (incomplete) 368.51
Protein
  deficiency 260

Protein — *continued*
  malnutrition 260
  sickness (prophylactic) (therapeutic) 999.5
Proteinemia 790.99
Proteinosis
  alveolar, lung or pulmonary 516.0
  lipid 272.8
  lipoid (of Urbach) 272.8
Proteinuria (*see also* Albuminuria) 791.0
  Bence-Jones NEC 791.0
  gestational 646.2
    with hypertension — *see* Toxemia, of pregnancy
  orthostatic 593.6
  postural 593.6
Proteolysis, pathologic 286.6
Protocoproporphyria 277.1
Protoporphyria (erythrohepatic) (erythropoietic) 277.1
Protrusio acetabuli 718.65
Protrusion
  acetabulum (into pelvis) 718.65
  device, implant, or graft — *see* Complications, mechanical
  ear, congenital 744.29
  intervertebral disc — *see* Displacement, intervertebral disc
  nucleus pulposus — *see* Displacement, intervertebral disc
Proud flesh 701.5
Prune belly (syndrome) 756.71
Prurigo (ferox) (gravis) (Hebra's) (hebrae) (mitis) (simplex) 698.2
  agria 698.3
  asthma syndrome 691.8
  Besnier's (atopic dermatitis) (infantile eczema) 691.8
  eczematodes allergicum 691.8
  estivalis (Hutchinson's) 692.72
  Hutchinson's 692.72
  nodularis 698.3
  psychogenic 306.3
Pruritus, pruritic 698.9
  ani 698.0
    psychogenic 306.3
  conditions NEC 698.9
    psychogenic 306.3
  due to Onchocerca volvulus 125.3
  ear 698.9
  essential 698.9
  genital organ(s) 698.1
    psychogenic 306.3
  gravidarum 646.8
  hiemalis 698.8
  neurogenic (any site) 306.3
  perianal 698.0
  psychogenic (any site) 306.3
  scrotum 698.1
    psychogenic 306.3
  senile, senilis 698.8
  Trichomonas 131.9
  vulva, vulvae 698.1
    psychogenic 306.3
Psammocarcinoma (M8140/3) — *see* Neoplasm, by site, malignant
Pseudarthrosis, pseudoarthrosis (bone) 733.82
  joint following fusion V45.4
Pseudoacanthosis
  nigricans 701.8

Pseudoaneurysm — Psilosis — Index to Disease

Pseudoaneurysm — see Aneurysm
Pseudoangina (pectoris) — see Angina
Pseudoangioma 452
Pseudo-Argyll-Robertson pupil 379.45
Pseudoarteriosus 747.89
Pseudoarthrosis — see Pseudarthrosis
Pseudoataxia 799.8
Pseudobursa 727.89
Pseudocholera 025
Pseudochromidrosis 705.89
Pseudocirrhosis, liver, pericardial 423.2
Pseudocoarctation 747.21
Pseudocowpox 051.1
Pseudocoxalgia 732.1
Pseudocroup 478.75
Pseudocyesis 300.11
Pseudocyst
   lung 518.89
   pancreas 577.2
   retina 361.19
Pseudodementia 300.16
Pseudoelephantiasis neuroarthritica 757.0
Pseudoemphysema 518.89
Pseudoencephalitis
   superior (acute) hemorrhagic 265.1
Pseudoerosion cervix, congenital 752.49
Pseudoexfoliation, lens capsule 366.11
Pseudofracture (idiopathic) (multiple) (spontaneous) (symmetrical) 268.2
Pseudoglanders 025
Pseudoglioma 360.44
Pseudogout — see Chondrocalcinosis
Pseudohallucination 780.1
Pseudohemianesthesia 782.0
Pseudohemophilia (Bernuth's) (hereditary) (type B) 286.4
   type A 287.8
   vascular 287.8
Pseudohermaphroditism 752.7
   with chromosomal anomaly — see Anomaly, chromosomal
   adrenal 255.2
   female (without adrenocortical disorder) 752.7
      with adrenocortical disorder 255.2
      adrenal 255.2
   male (without gonadal disorder) 752.7
      with
         adrenocortical disorder 255.2
         cleft scrotum 752.7
         feminizing testis 257.8
         gonadal disorder 257.9
      adrenal 255.2
Pseudohole, macula 362.54
Pseudo-Hurler's disease (mucolipidosis III) 272.7
Pseudohydrocephalus 348.2
Pseudohypertrophic muscular dystrophy (Erb's) 359.1
Pseudohypertrophy, muscle 359.1
Pseudohypoparathyroidism 275.49
Pseudoinfluenza 487.1
Pseudoinsomnia 307.49
Pseudoleukemia 288.8
   infantile 285.8
Pseudomembranous — see condition

Pseudomeningocele (cerebral) (infective) (surgical) 349.2
   spinal 349.2
Pseudomenstruation 626.8
Pseudomucinous
   cyst (ovary) (M8470/0) 220
   peritoneum 568.89
Pseudomyeloma 273.1
Pseudomyxoma peritonei (M8480/6) 197.6
Pseudoneuritis optic (nerve) 377.24
   papilla 377.24
      congenital 743.57
Pseudoneuroma — see Injury, nerve, by site
Pseudo-obstruction
   intestine 564.89
Pseudopapilledema 377.24.
Pseudoparalysis
   arm or leg 781.4
   atonic, congenital 358.8
Pseudopelade 704.09
Pseudophakia V43.1
Pseudopolycythemia 289.0
Pseudopolyposis, colon 556.4
Pseudoporencephaly 348.0
Pseudopseudohypoparathyroidism 275.49
Pseudopsychosis 300.16
Pseudopterygium 372.52
Pseudoptosis (eyelid) 374.34
Pseudorabies 078.89
Pseudoretinitis, pigmentosa 362.65
Pseudorickets 588.0
   senile (Pozzi's) 731.0
Pseudorubella 057.8
Pseudoscarlatina 057.8
Pseudosclerema 778.1
Pseudosclerosis (brain)
   Jakob's 046.1
   of Westphal (-Strümpell) (hepatolenticular degeneration) 275.1
   spastic 046.1
      with dementia
         with behavioral disturbance 046.1
         [294.11]
         without behavioral disturbance 046.1
         [294.10]
Pseudoseizure 780.39
   non-psychiatric 780.39
   psychiatric 300.11
Pseudotabes 799.8
   diabetic 250.6 [337.1]
Pseudotetanus (see also Convulsions) 780.39
Pseudotetany 781.7
   hysterical 300.11
Pseudothalassemia 285.0
Pseudotrichinosis 710.3
Pseudotruncus arteriosus 747.29
Pseudotuberculosis, pasteurella (infection) 027.2
Pseudotumor
   cerebri 348.2
   orbit (inflammatory) 376.11
Pseudo-Turner's syndrome 759.89
Pseudoxanthoma elasticum 757.39
Psilosis (sprue) (tropical) 579.1
   Monilia 112.89

Psilosis — continued
  nontropical 579.0
  not sprue 704.00
Psittacosis 073.9
Psoitis 728.89
Psora NEC 696.1
Psoriasis 696.1
  any type, except arthropathic 696.1
  arthritic, arthropathic 696.0
  buccal 528.6
  flexural 696.1
  follicularis 696.1
  guttate 696.1
  inverse 696.1
  mouth 528.6
  nummularis 696.1
  psychogenic 316 [696.1]
  punctata 696.1
  pustular 696.1
  rupioides 696.1
  vulgaris 696.1
Psorospermiasis 136.4
Psorospermosis 136.4
  follicularis (vegetans) 757.39
Psychalgia 307.80
Psychasthenia 300.89
  compulsive 300.3
  mixed compulsive states 300.3
  obsession 300.3
Psychiatric disorder or problem NEC 300.9
Psychogenic — *see also* condition
  factors associated with physical conditions 316
Psychoneurosis, psychoneurotic (*see also* Neurosis) 300.9
  anxiety (state) 300.00
  climacteric 627.2
  compensation 300.16
  compulsion 300.3
  conversion hysteria 300.11
  depersonalization 300.6
  depressive type 300.4
  dissociative hysteria 300.15
  hypochondriacal 300.7
  hysteria 300.10
    conversion type 300.11
    dissociative type 300.15
  mixed NEC 300.89
  neurasthenic 300.5
  obsessional 300.3
  obsessive-compulsive 300.3
  occupational 300.89
  personality NEC 301.89
  phobia 300.20
  senile NEC 300.89
Psychopathic — *see also* condition
  constitution, posttraumatic 310.2
    with psychosis 293.9
  personality 301.9
    amoral trends 301.7
    antisocial trends 301.7
    asocial trends 301.7
    mixed types 301.7
  state 301.9
Psychopathy, sexual (*see also* Deviation, sexual) 302.9
Psychophysiologic, psychophysiological condition — *see* Reaction, psychophysiologic

Psychose passionelle 297.8
Psychosexual identity disorder 302.6
  adult-life 302.85
  childhood 302.6
Psychosis 298.9
  acute hysterical 298.1
  affecting management of pregnancy, childbirth, or puerperium 648.4 ✓5ᵗʰ
  affective NEC 296.90

> Note — Use the following fifth-digit subclassification with categories 296.0-296.6:
>
> 0 unspecified
> 1 mild
> 2 moderate
> 3 severe, without mention of psychotic behavior
> 4 severe, specified as with psychotic behavior
> 5 in partial or unspecified remission
> 6 in full remission

  drug-induced 292.84
  due to or associated with physical condition 293.83
  involutional 296.2 ✓5ᵗʰ
    recurrent episode 296.3 ✓5ᵗʰ
    single episode 296.2 ✓5ᵗʰ
  manic-depressive 296.80
    circular (alternating) 296.7
      currently depressed 296.5 ✓5ᵗʰ
      currently manic 296.4 ✓5ᵗʰ
    depressed type 296.2 ✓5ᵗʰ
      atypical 296.82
      recurrent episode 296.3 ✓5ᵗʰ
      single episode 296.2 ✓5ᵗʰ
    manic 296.0 ✓5ᵗʰ
      atypical 296.81
      recurrent episode 296.1 ✓5ᵗʰ
      single episode 296.0 ✓5ᵗʰ
    mixed type NEC 296.89
    specified type NEC 296.89
  senile 290.21
  specified type NEC 296.99
  alcoholic 291.9
    with
      anxiety 291.89
      delirium tremens 291.0
      delusions 291.5
      dementia 291.2
      hallucinosis 291.3
      mood disturbance 291.89
      jealousy 291.5
      paranoia 291.5
      persisting amnesia 291.1
      sexual dysfunction 291.89
      sleep disturbance 291.89
    amnestic confabulatory 291.1
    delirium tremens 291.0
    hallucinosis 291.3
    Korsakoff's, Korsakov's, Korsakow's 291.1
    paranoid type 291.5
    pathological intoxication 291.4
    polyneuritic 291.1
    specified type NEC 291.89
  alternating (*see also* Psychosis, manic-depressive, circular) 296.7
  anergastic (*see also* Psychosis, organic) 294.9

Psychosis

Psychosis — *continued*
  arteriosclerotic 290.40
    with
      acute confusional state 290.41
      delirium 290.41
      delusional features 290.42
      depressive features 290.43
    depressed type 290.43
    paranoid type 290.42
    simple type 290.40
    uncomplicated 290.40
  atypical 298.9
    depressive 296.82
    manic 296.81
  borderline (schizophrenia) (see also
      Schizophrenia) 295.5 ✓5ᵗʰ
    of childhood (see also Psychosis, childhood)
      299.8 ✓5ᵗʰ
    prepubertal 299.8 ✓5ᵗʰ
  brief reactive 298.8
  childhood, with origin specific to 299.9 ✓5ᵗʰ

> Note — Use the following fifth-digit
> subclassification with category 299:
>
> 0   current or active state
> 1   residual state

    atypical 299.8 ✓5ᵗʰ
    specified type NEC 299.8 ✓5ᵗʰ
  circular (see also Psychosis, manic-depressive,
      circular) 296.7
  climacteric (see also Psychosis, involutional)
      298.8
  confusional 298.9
    acute 293.0
    reactive 298.2
    subacute 293.1
  depressive (see also Psychosis, affective)
      296.2 ✓5ᵗʰ
    atypical 296.82
    involutional 296.2 ✓5ᵗʰ
      recurrent episode 296.3 ✓5ᵗʰ
      single episode 296.2 ✓5ᵗʰ
    psychogenic 298.0
    reactive (emotional stress) (psychological
        trauma) 298.0
    recurrent episode 296.3 ✓5ᵗʰ
      with hypomania (bipolar II) 296.89
    single episode 296.2 ✓5ᵗʰ
  disintegrative (childhood) (see also Psychosis,
      childhood) 299.1 ✓5ᵗʰ
  drug 292.9
    with
      affective syndrome 292.84
      amnestic syndrome 292.83
      anxiety 292.89
      delirium 292.81
        withdrawal 292.0
      delusional syndrome 292.11
      dementia 292.82
      depressive state 292.84
      hallucinosis 292.12
      mood disturbance 292.84
      organic personality syndrome NEC
          292.89
      sexual dysfunction 292.89
      sleep disturbance 292.89
      withdrawal syndrome (and delirium)
          292.0
    affective syndrome 292.84
    delusional state 292.11

Psychosis — *continued*
  drug — *continued*
    hallucinatory state 292.12
    hallucinosis 292.12
    paranoid state 292.11
    specified type NEC 292.89
    withdrawal syndrome (and delirium) 292.0
  due to or associated with physical condition
      (see also Psychosis, organic) 293.9
  epileptic NEC 294.8
  excitation (psychogenic) (reactive) 298.1
  exhaustive (see also Reaction, stress, acute)
      308.9
  hypomanic (see also Psychosis, affective)
      296.0 ✓5ᵗʰ
    recurrent episode 296.1 ✓5ᵗʰ
    single episode 296.0 ✓5ᵗʰ
  hysterical 298.8
    acute 298.1
  incipient 298.8
    schizophrenic (see also Schizophrenia)
        295.5 ✓5ᵗʰ
  induced 297.3
  infantile (see also Psychosis, childhood)
      299.0 ✓5ᵗʰ
  infective 293.9
    acute 293.0
    subacute 293.1
  in pregnancy, childbirth, or puerperium
      648.4 ✓5ᵗʰ
  interactional (childhood) (see also Psychosis,
      childhood) 299.1 ✓5ᵗʰ
  involutional 298.8
    depressive (see also Psychosis, affective)
        296.2 ✓5ᵗʰ
      recurrent episode 296.3 ✓5ᵗʰ
      single episode 296.2 ✓5ᵗʰ
    melancholic 296.2 ✓5ᵗʰ
      recurrent episode 296.3 ✓5ᵗʰ
      single episode 296.2 ✓5ᵗʰ
    paranoid state 297.2
    paraphrenia 297.2
  Korsakoff's, Korakov's, Korsakow's
      (nonalcoholic) 294.0
    alcoholic 291.1
  mania (phase) (see also Psychosis, affective)
      296.0 ✓5ᵗʰ
    recurrent episode 296.1 ✓5ᵗʰ
    single episode 296.0 ✓5ᵗʰ
  manic (see also Psychosis, affective) 296.0 ✓5ᵗʰ
    atypical 296.81
    recurrent episode 296.1 ✓5ᵗʰ
    single episode 296.0 ✓5ᵗʰ
  manic-depressive 296.80
    circular 296.7
      currently
        depressed 296.5 ✓5ᵗʰ
        manic 296.4 ✓5ᵗʰ
      mixed 296.6 ✓5ᵗʰ
    depressive 296.2 ✓5ᵗʰ
      recurrent episode 296.3 ✓5ᵗʰ
        with hypomania (bipolar II) 296.89
      single episode 296.2 ✓5ᵗʰ
    hypomanic 296.0 ✓5ᵗʰ
      recurrent episode 296.1 ✓5ᵗʰ
      single episode 296.0 ✓5ᵗʰ
    manic 296.0 ✓5ᵗʰ
      atypical 296.81
      recurrent episode 296.1 ✓5ᵗʰ
      single episode 296.0 ✓5ᵗʰ
    mixed NEC 296.89

Index to Diseases

Psychosis

Psychosis — *continued*
  manic-depressive — *continued*
    perplexed 296.89
    stuporous 296.89
  menopausal (*see also* Psychosis, involutional) 298.8
  mixed schizophrenic and affective (*see also* Schizophrenia) 295.7 ✓5ᵗʰ
  multi-infarct (cerebrovascular) (*see also* Psychosis, arteriosclerotic) 290.40
  organic NEC 294.9
    due to or associated with
      addiction
        alcohol (*see also* Psychosis, alcoholic) 291.9
        drug (*see also* Psychosis, drug) 292.9
      alcohol intoxication, acute (*see also* Psychosis, alcoholic) 291.9
      alcoholism (*see also* Psychosis, alcoholic) 291.9
      arteriosclerosis (cerebral) (*see also* Psychosis, arteriosclerotic) 290.40
      cerebrovascular disease
        acute (psychosis) 293.0
        arteriosclerotic (*see also* Psychosis, arteriosclerotic) 290.40
      childbirth — *see* Psychosis, puerperal
      dependence
        alcohol (*see also* Psychosis, alcoholic) 291.9
        drug 292.9
      disease
        alcoholic liver (*see also* Psychosis, alcoholic) 291.9
        brain
          arteriosclerotic (*see also* Psychosis, arteriosclerotic) 290.40
          cerebrovascular
            acute (psychosis) 293.0
            arteriosclerotic (*see also* Psychosis, arteriosclerotic) 290.40
        endocrine or metabolic 293.9
          acute (psychosis) 293.0
          subacute (psychosis) 293.1
        Jakob-Creutzfeldt
          with behavioral disturbance 046.1 [294.11]
          without behavioral disturbance 046.1 [294.10]
        liver, alcoholic (*see also* Psychosis, alcoholic) 291.9
      disorder
        cerebrovascular
          acute (psychosis) 293.0
        endocrine or metabolic 293.9
          acute (psychosis) 293.0
          subacute (psychosis) 293.1
      epilepsy
        with behavioral disturbance 345.9 ✓5ᵗʰ [294.11]
        without behavioral disturbance 345.9 ✓5ᵗʰ [294.10]
        transient (acute) 293.0
      Huntington's chorea
        with behavioral disturbance 333.4 [294.11]
        without behavioral disturbance 333.4 [294.10]
      infection
        brain 293.9
          acute (psychosis) 293.0

Psychosis — *continued*
  organic NEC — *continued*
    due to or associated with — *continued*
      infection — *continued*
        brain — *continued*
          chronic 294.8
          subacute (psychosis) 293.1
        intracranial NEC 293.9
          acute (psychosis) 293.0
          chronic 294.8
          subacute (psychosis) 293.1
      intoxication
        alcoholic (acute) (*see also* Psychosis, alcoholic) 291.9
          pathological 291.4
        drug (*see also* Psychosis, drug) 292.2
      ischemia
        cerebrovascular (generalized) (*see also* Psychosis, arteriosclerotic) 290.40
      Jakob-Creutzfeldt disease or syndrome
        with behavioral disturbance 046.1 [294.11]
        without behavioral disturbance 046.1 [294.10]
      multiple sclerosis
        with behavioral disturbance 340 [294.11]
        without behavioral disturbance 340 [294.10]
      physical condition NEC 293.9
        with
          delusions 293.81
          hallucinations 293.82
      presenility 290.10
      puerperium — *see* Psychosis, puerperal
      sclerosis, multiple
        with behavioral disturbance 340 [294.11]
        without behavioral disturbance 340 [294.10]
      senility 290.20
      status epilepticus
        with behavioral disturbance 345.3 ✓5ᵗʰ [294.11]
        without behavioral disturbance 345.3 ✓5ᵗʰ [294.10]
      trauma
        brain (birth) (from electrical current) (surgical) 293.9
          acute (psychosis) 293.0
          chronic 294.8
          subacute (psychosis) 293.1
        unspecified physical condition 294.9
    infective 293.9
      acute (psychosis) 293.0
      subacute 293.1
    posttraumatic 293.9
      acute 293.0
      subacute 293.1
    specified type NEC 294.8
    transient 293.9
      with
        anxiety 293.84
        delusions 293.81
        depression 293.83
        hallucinations 293.82
      depressive type 293.83
      hallucinatory type 293.82
      paranoid type 293.81

✓4ᵗʰ Fourth-digit Required ✓5ᵗʰ Fifth-digit Required

Psychosis — continued
  organic NEC — continued
    transient — continued
      specified type NEC 293.89
  paranoic 297.1
  paranoid (chronic) 297.9
    alcoholic 291.5
    chronic 297.1
    climacteric 297.2
    involutional 297.2
    menopausal 297.2
    protracted reactive 298.4
    psychogenic 298.4
      acute 298.3
    schizophrenic (see also Schizophrenia) 295.3 ✓5ᵗʰ
    senile 290.20
  paroxysmal 298.9
    senile 290.20
  polyneuritic, alcoholic 291.1
  postoperative 293.9
  postpartum — see Psychosis, puerperal
  prepsychotic (see also Schizophrenia) 295.5 ✓5ᵗʰ
  presbyophrenic (type) 290.8
  presenile (see also Dementia, presenile) 290.10
  prison 300.16
  psychogenic 298.8
    depressive 298.0
    paranoid 298.4
      acute 298.3
  puerperal
    specified type — see categories 295-298 ✓5ᵗʰ
    unspecified type 293.89
      acute 293.0
      chronic 293.89
      subacute 293.1
  reactive (emotional stress) (psychological trauma) 298.8
    brief 298.8
    confusion 298.2
    depressive 298.0
    excitation 298.1
  schizo-affective (depressed) (excited) (see also Schizophrenia) 295.7 ✓5ᵗʰ
  schizophrenia, schizophrenic (see also Schizophrenia) 295.9 ✓5ᵗʰ
    borderline type 295.5 ✓5ᵗʰ
    of childhood (see also Psychosis, childhood) 299.8 ✓5ᵗʰ
    catatonic (excited) (withdrawn) 295.2 ✓5ᵗʰ
    childhood type (see also Psychosis, childhood) 299.9 ✓5ᵗʰ
    hebephrenic 295.1 ✓5ᵗʰ
    incipient 295.5 ✓5ᵗʰ
    latent 295.5 ✓5ᵗʰ
    paranoid 295.3 ✓5ᵗʰ
    prepsychotic 295.5 ✓5ᵗʰ
    prodromal 295.5 ✓5ᵗʰ
    pseudoneurotic 295.5 ✓5ᵗʰ
    pseudopsychopathic 295.5 ✓5ᵗʰ
    schizophreniform 295.4 ✓5ᵗʰ
    simple 295.0 ✓5ᵗʰ
  schizophreniform 295.4 ✓5ᵗʰ
  senile NEC 290.20
    with
      delusional features 290.20
      depressive features 290.21
    depressed type 290.21
    paranoid type 290.20

Psychosis — continued
  senile NEC — continued
    simple deterioration 290.20
    specified type — see categories 295-298 ✓5ᵗʰ
  shared 297.3
  situational (reactive) 298.8
  symbiotic (childhood) (see also Psychosis, childhood) 299.1 ✓5ᵗʰ
  toxic (acute) 293.9
Psychotic (see also condition) 298.9
  episode 298.9
    due to or associated with physical conditions (see also Psychosis, organic) 293.9
Pterygium (eye) 372.40
  central 372.43
  colli 744.5
  double 372.44
  peripheral (stationary) 372.41
    progressive 372.42
  recurrent 372.45
Ptilosis 374.55
Ptomaine (poisoning) (see also Poisoning, food) 005.9
Ptosis (adiposa) 374.30
  breast 611.8
  cecum 569.89
  colon 569.89
  congenital (eyelid) 743.61
    specified site NEC — see Anomaly, specified type NEC
  epicanthus syndrome 270.2
  eyelid 374.30
    congenital 743.61
    mechanical 374.33
    myogenic 374.32
    paralytic 374.31
  gastric 537.5
  intestine 569.89
  kidney (see also Disease, renal) 593.0
    congenital 753.3
  liver 573.8
  renal (see also Disease, renal) 593.0
    congenital 753.3
  splanchnic 569.89
  spleen 289.59
  stomach 537.5
  viscera 569.89
Ptyalism 527.7
  hysterical 300.11
  periodic 527.2
  pregnancy 646.8 ✓5ᵗʰ
  psychogenic 306.4
Ptyalolithiasis 527.5
Pubalgia 848.8
Pubarche, precocious 259.1
Pubertas praecox 259.1
Puberty V21.1
  abnormal 259.9
  bleeding 626.3
  delayed 259.0
  precocious (constitutional) (cryptogenic) (idiopathic) NEC 259.1
    due to
      adrenal
        cortical hyperfunction 255.2
        hyperplasia 255.2
        cortical hyperfunction 255.2

Puberty — *continued*
  precocious — *continued*
    due to — *continued*
      ovarian hyperfunction 256.1
        estrogen 256.0
      pineal tumor 259.8
      testicular hyperfunction 257.0
    premature 259.1
      due to
        adrenal cortical hyperfunction 255.2
        pineal tumor 259.8
        pituitary (anterior) hyperfunction 253.1
Puckering, macula 362.56
Pudenda, pudendum — *see* condition
Puente's disease (simple glandular cheilitis) 528.5
Puerperal
  abscess
    areola 675.1
    Bartholin's gland 646.6
    breast 675.1
    cervix (uteri) 670
    fallopian tube 670
    genital organ 670
    kidney 646.6
    mammary 675.1
    mesosalpinx 670
    nabothian 646.6
    nipple 675.0
    ovary, ovarian 670
    oviduct 670
    parametric 670
    para-uterine 670
    pelvic 670
    perimetric 670
    periuterine 670
    retro-uterine 670
    subareolar 675.1
    suprapelvic 670
    tubal (ruptured) 670
    tubo-ovarian 670
    urinary tract NEC 646.6
    uterine, uterus 670
    vagina (wall) 646.6
    vaginorectal 646.6
    vulvovaginal gland 646.6
  accident 674.9
  adnexitis 670
  afibrinogenemia, or other coagulation defect 666.3
  albuminuria (acute) (subacute) 646.2
    pre-eclamptic 642.4
  anemia (conditions classifiable to 280-285) 648.2
  anuria 669.3
  apoplexy 674.0
  asymptomatic bacteriuria 646.5
  atrophy, breast 676.3
  blood dyscrasia 666.3
  caked breast 676.2
  cardiomyopathy 674.8
  cellulitis — *see* Puerperal, abscess
  cerebrovascular disorder (conditions classifiable to 430-434, 436-437) 674.0
  cervicitis (conditions classifiable to 616.0) 646.6
  coagulopathy (any) 666.3
  complications 674.9
    specified type NEC 674.8

Puerperal — *continued*
  convulsions (eclamptic) (uremic) 642.6
    with pre-existing hypertension 642.7
  cracked nipple 676.1
  cystitis 646.6
  cystopyelitis 646.6
  deciduitis (acute) 670
  delirium NEC 293.9
  diabetes (mellitus) (conditions classifiable to 250) 648.0
  disease 674.9
    breast NEC 676.3
    cerebrovascular (acute) 674.0
    nonobstetric NEC (*see also* Pregnancy, complicated, current disease or condition) 648.9
    pelvis inflammatory 670
    renal NEC 646.2
    tubo-ovarian 670
    Valsuani's (progressive pernicious anemia) 648.2
  disorder
    lactation 676.9
      specified type NEC 676.8
    nonobstetric NEC (*see also* Pregnancy, complicated, current disease or condition) 648.9
  disruption
    cesarean wound 674.1
    episiotomy wound 674.2
    perineal laceration wound 674.2
  drug dependence (conditions classifiable to 304) 648.3
  eclampsia 642.6
    with pre-existing hypertension 642.7
  embolism (pulmonary) 673.2
    air 673.0
    amniotic fluid 673.1
    blood-clot 673.2
    brain or cerebral 674.0
    cardiac 674.8
    fat 673.8
    intracranial sinus (venous) 671.5
    pyemic 673.3
    septic 673.3
    spinal cord 671.5
  endometritis (conditions classifiable to 615.0-615.9) 670
  endophlebitis — *see* Puerperal, phlebitis
  endotrachelitis 646.6
  engorgement, breasts 676.2
  erysipelas 670
  failure
    lactation 676.4
    renal, acute 669.3
  fever 670
    meaning pyrexia (of unknown origin) 672
    meaning sepsis 670
  fissure, nipple 676.1
  fistula
    breast 675.1
    mammary gland 675.1
    nipple 675.0
  galactophoritis 675.2
  galactorrhea 676.6
  gangrene
    gas 670
    uterus 670
  gonorrhea (conditions classifiable to 098) 647.1

Puerperal — *continued*
  hematoma, subdural 674.0 ✓5ᵗʰ
  hematosalpinx, infectional 670 ✓4ᵗʰ
  hemiplegia, cerebral 674.0 ✓5ᵗʰ
  hemorrhage 666.1 ✓5ᵗʰ
    brain 674.0 ✓5ᵗʰ
    bulbar 674.0 ✓5ᵗʰ
    cerebellar 674.0 ✓5ᵗʰ
    cerebral 674.0 ✓5ᵗʰ
    cortical 674.0 ✓5ᵗʰ
    delayed (after 24 hours) (uterine) 666.2 ✓5ᵗʰ
    extradural 674.0 ✓5ᵗʰ
    internal capsule 674.0 ✓5ᵗʰ
    intracranial 674.0 ✓5ᵗʰ
    intrapontine 674.0 ✓5ᵗʰ
    meningeal 674.0 ✓5ᵗʰ
    pontine 674.0 ✓5ᵗʰ
    subarachnoid 674.0 ✓5ᵗʰ
    subcortical 674.0 ✓5ᵗʰ
    subdural 674.0 ✓5ᵗʰ
    uterine, delayed 666.2 ✓5ᵗʰ
    ventricular 674.0 ✓5ᵗʰ
  hemorrhoids 671.8 ✓5ᵗʰ
  hepatorenal syndrome 674.8 ✓5ᵗʰ
  hypertrophy
    breast 676.3 ✓5ᵗʰ
    mammary gland 676.3 ✓5ᵗʰ
  induration breast (fibrous) 676.3 ✓5ᵗʰ
  infarction
    lung — see Puerperal, embolism
    pulmonary — see Puerperal, embolism
  infection
    Bartholin's gland 646.6 ✓5ᵗʰ
    breast 675.2 ✓5ᵗʰ
      with nipple 675.9 ✓5ᵗʰ
        specified type NEC 675.8 ✓5ᵗʰ
    cervix 646.6 ✓5ᵗʰ
    endocervix 646.6 ✓5ᵗʰ
    fallopian tube 670 ✓4ᵗʰ
    generalized 670 ✓4ᵗʰ
    genital tract (major) 670 ✓4ᵗʰ
      minor or localized 646.6 ✓5ᵗʰ
    kidney (bacillus coli) 646.6 ✓5ᵗʰ
    mammary gland 675.2 ✓5ᵗʰ
      with nipple 675.9 ✓5ᵗʰ
        specified type NEC 675.8 ✓5ᵗʰ
    nipple 675.0 ✓5ᵗʰ
      with breast 675.9 ✓5ᵗʰ
        specified type NEC 675.8 ✓5ᵗʰ
    ovary 670 ✓4ᵗʰ
    pelvic 670 ✓4ᵗʰ
    peritoneum 670 ✓4ᵗʰ
    renal 646.6 ✓5ᵗʰ
    tubo-ovarian 670 ✓4ᵗʰ
    urinary (tract) NEC 646.6 ✓5ᵗʰ
      asymptomatic 646.5 ✓5ᵗʰ
    uterus, uterine 670 ✓4ᵗʰ
    vagina 646.6 ✓5ᵗʰ
  inflammation — see also Puerperal, infection
    areola 675.1 ✓5ᵗʰ
    Bartholin's gland 646.6 ✓5ᵗʰ
    breast 675.2 ✓5ᵗʰ
    broad ligament 670 ✓4ᵗʰ
    cervix (uteri) 646.6 ✓5ᵗʰ
    fallopian tube 670 ✓4ᵗʰ
    genital organs 670 ✓4ᵗʰ
      localized 646.6 ✓5ᵗʰ
    mammary gland 675.2 ✓5ᵗʰ
    nipple 675.0 ✓5ᵗʰ
    ovary 670 ✓4ᵗʰ
    oviduct 670 ✓4ᵗʰ

Puerperal — *continued*
  inflammation — *continued*
    pelvis 670 ✓4ᵗʰ
    periuterine 670 ✓4ᵗʰ
    tubal 670 ✓4ᵗʰ
    vagina 646.6 ✓5ᵗʰ
    vein — see Puerperal, phlebitis
  inversion, nipple 676.3 ✓5ᵗʰ
  ischemia, cerebral 674.0 ✓5ᵗʰ
  lymphangitis 670 ✓4ᵗʰ
    breast 675.2 ✓5ᵗʰ
  malaria (conditions classifiable to 084) 647.4 ✓5ᵗʰ
  malnutrition 648.9 ✓5ᵗʰ
  mammillitis 675.0 ✓5ᵗʰ
  mammitis 675.2 ✓5ᵗʰ
  mania 296.0 ✓5ᵗʰ
    recurrent episode 296.1 ✓5ᵗʰ
    single episode 296.0 ✓5ᵗʰ
  mastitis 675.2 ✓5ᵗʰ
    purulent 675.1 ✓5ᵗʰ
    retromammary 675.1 ✓5ᵗʰ
    submammary 675.1 ✓5ᵗʰ
  melancholia 296.2 ✓5ᵗʰ
    recurrent episode 296.3 ✓5ᵗʰ
    single episode 296.2 ✓5ᵗʰ
  mental disorder (conditions classifiable to 290-303, 305-316, 317-319) 648.4 ✓5ᵗʰ
  metritis (septic) (suppurative) 670 ✓4ᵗʰ
  metroperitonitis 670 ✓4ᵗʰ
  metrorrhagia 666.2 ✓5ᵗʰ
  metrosalpingitis 670 ✓4ᵗʰ
  metrovaginitis 670 ✓4ᵗʰ
  milk leg 671.4 ✓5ᵗʰ
  monoplegia, cerebral 674.0 ✓5ᵗʰ
  necrosis
    kidney, tubular 669.3 ✓5ᵗʰ
    liver (acute) (subacute) (conditions classifiable to 570) 674.8 ✓5ᵗʰ
    ovary 670 ✓4ᵗʰ
    renal cortex 669.3 ✓5ᵗʰ
  nephritis or nephrosis (conditions classifiable to 580-589) 646.2 ✓5ᵗʰ
    with hypertension 642.1 ✓5ᵗʰ
  nutritional deficiency (conditions classifiable to 260-269) 648.9 ✓5ᵗʰ
  occlusion, precerebral artery 674.0 ✓5ᵗʰ
  oliguria 669.3 ✓5ᵗʰ
  oophoritis 670 ✓4ᵗʰ
  ovaritis 670 ✓4ᵗʰ
  paralysis
    bladder (sphincter) 665.5 ✓5ᵗʰ
    cerebral 674.0 ✓5ᵗʰ
  paralytic stroke 674.0 ✓5ᵗʰ
  parametritis 670 ✓4ᵗʰ
  paravaginitis 646.6 ✓5ᵗʰ
  pelviperitonitis 670 ✓4ᵗʰ
  perimetritis 670 ✓4ᵗʰ
  perimetrosalpingitis 670 ✓4ᵗʰ
  perinephritis 646.6 ✓5ᵗʰ
  perioophoritis 670 ✓4ᵗʰ
  periphlebitis — see Puerperal, phlebitis
  perisalpingitis 670 ✓4ᵗʰ
  peritoneal infection 670 ✓4ᵗʰ
  peritonitis (pelvic) 670 ✓4ᵗʰ
  perivaginitis 646.6 ✓5ᵗʰ
  phlebitis 671.9 ✓5ᵗʰ
    deep 671.4 ✓5ᵗʰ
    intracranial sinus (venous) 671.5 ✓5ᵗʰ
    pelvic 671.4 ✓5ᵗʰ
    specified site NEC 671.5 ✓5ᵗʰ

Index to Diseases

Puerperal — *continued*
  phlebitis — *continued*
    superficial 671.2
  phlegmasia alba dolens 671.4
  placental polyp 674.4
  pneumonia, embolic — *see* Puerperal, embolism
  prediabetes 648.8
  pre-eclampsia (mild) 642.4
    with pre-existing hypertension 642.7
    severe 642.5
  psychosis, unspecified (*see also* Psychosis, puerperal) 293.89
  pyelitis 646.6
  pyelocystitis 646.6
  pyelohydronephrosis 646.6
  pyelonephritis 646.6
  pyelonephrosis 646.6
  pyemia 670
  pyocystitis 646.6
  pyohemia 670
  pyometra 670
  pyonephritis 646.6
  pyonephrosis 646.6
  pyo-oophoritis 670
  pyosalpingitis 670
  pyosalpinx 670
  pyrexia (of unknown origin) 672
  renal
    disease NEC 646.2
    failure, acute 669.3
  retention
    decidua (fragments) (with delayed hemorrhage) 666.2
      without hemorrhage 667.1
    placenta (fragments) (with delayed hemorrhage) 666.2
      without hemorrhage 667.1
    secundines (fragments) (with delayed hemorrhage) 666.2
      without hemorrhage 667.1
  retracted nipple 676.0
  rubella (conditions classifiable to 056) 647.5
  salpingitis 670
  salpingo-oophoritis 670
  salpingo-ovaritis 670
  salpingoperitonitis 670
  sapremia 670
  secondary perineal tear 674.2
  sepsis (pelvic) 670
  septicemia 670
  subinvolution (uterus) 674.8
  sudden death (cause unknown) 674.9
  suppuration — *see* Puerperal, abscess
  syphilis (conditions classifiable to 090-097) 647.0
  tetanus 670
  thelitis 675.0
  thrombocytopenia 666.3
  thrombophlebitis (superficial) 671.2
    deep 671.4
    pelvic 671.4
    specified site NEC 671.5
  thrombosis (venous) — *see* Thrombosis, puerperal
  thyroid dysfunction (conditions classifiable to 240-246) 648.1
  toxemia (*see also* Toxemia, of pregnancy) 642.4
    eclamptic 642.6

Puerperal — *continued*
  toxemia — *continued*
    eclamptic — *continued*
      with pre-existing hypertension 642.7
    pre-eclamptic (mild) 642.4
      with
        convulsions 642.6
        pre-existing hypertension 642.7
      severe 642.5
  tuberculosis (conditions classifiable to 010-018) 647.3
  uremia 669.3
  vaginitis (conditions classifiable to 616.1) 646.6
  varicose veins (legs) 671.0
    vulva or perineum 671.1
  vulvitis (conditions classifiable to 616.1) 646.6
  vulvovaginitis (conditions classifiable to 616.1) 646.6
  white leg 671.4
Pulled muscle — *see* Sprain, by site
Pulmolithiasis 518.89
Pulmonary — *see* condition
Pulmonitis (unknown etiology) 486
Pulpitis (acute) (anachoretic) (chronic) (hyperplastic) (putrescent) (suppurative) (ulcerative) 522.0
Pulpless tooth 522.9
Pulse
  alternating 427.89
    psychogenic 306.2
  bigeminal 427.89
  fast 785.0
  feeble, rapid, due to shock following injury 958.4
  rapid 785.0
  slow 427.89
  strong 785.9
  trigeminal 427.89
  water-hammer (*see also* Insufficiency, aortic) 424.1
  weak 785.9
Pulseless disease 446.7
Pulsus
  alternans or trigeminy 427.89
    psychogenic 306.2
Punch drunk 310.2
Puncta lacrimalia occlusion 375.52
Punctiform hymen 752.49
Puncture (traumatic) — *see also* Wound, open, by site
  accidental, complicating surgery 998.2
  bladder, nontraumatic 596.6
  by
    device, implant, or graft — *see* Complications, mechanical
    foreign body
      internal organs — *see also* Injury, internal, by site
        by ingested object — *see* Foreign body
      left accidentally in operation wound 998.4
    instrument (any) during a procedure, accidental 998.2
  internal organs, abdomen, chest, or pelvis — *see* Injury, internal, by site
  kidney, nontraumatic 593.89

Pupil — see condition
Pupillary membrane 364.74
  persistent 743.46
Pupillotonia 379.46
  pseudotabetic 379.46
Purpura 287.2
  abdominal 287.0
  allergic 287.0
  anaphylactoid 287.0
  annularis telangiectodes 709.1
  arthritic 287.0
  autoerythrocyte sensitization 287.2
  autoimmune 287.0
  bacterial 287.0
  Bateman's (senile) 287.2
  capillary fragility (hereditary) (idiopathic) 287.8
  cryoglobulinemic 273.2
  devil's pinches 287.2
  fibrinolytic (see also Fibrinolysis) 286.6
  fulminans, fulminous 286.6
  gangrenous 287.0
  hemorrhagic (see also Purpura, thrombocytopenic) 287.3
    nodular 272.7
    nonthrombocytopenic 287.0
    thrombocytopenic 287.3
  Henoch's (purpura nervosa) 287.0
  Henoch-Schönlein (allergic) 287.0
  hypergammaglobulinemic (benign primary) (Waldenström's) 273.0
  idiopathic 287.3
    nonthrombocytopenic 287.0
    thrombocytopenic 287.3
  infectious 287.0
  malignant 287.0
  neonatorum 772.6
  nervosa 287.0
  newborn NEC 772.6
  nonthrombocytopenic 287.2
    hemorrhagic 287.0
    idiopathic 287.0
  nonthrombopenic 287.2
  peliosis rheumatica 287.0
  pigmentaria, progressiva 709.09
  posttransfusion 287.4
  primary 287.0
  primitive 287.0
  red cell membrane sensitivity 287.2
  rheumatica 287.0
  Schönlein (-Henoch) (allergic) 287.0
  scorbutic 267
  senile 287.2
  simplex 287.2
  symptomatica 287.0
  telangiectasia annularis 709.1
  thrombocytopenic (congenital) (essential) (hereditary) (idiopathic) (primary) (see also Thrombocytopenia) 287.3
    neonatal, transitory (see also Thrombocytopenia, neonatal transitory) 776.1
    puerperal, postpartum 666.3 ✓5ᵗʰ
    thrombotic 446.6
  thrombohemolytic (see also Fibrinolysis) 286.6
  thrombopenic (congenital) (essential) (see also Thrombocytopenia) 287.3
    thrombotic 446.6
      thrombocytic 446.6
      thrombocytopenic 446.6
  toxic 287.0
  variolosa 050.0

Purpura — continued
  vascular 287.0
  visceral symptoms 287.0
  Werlhof's (see also Purpura, thrombocytopenic) 287.3
Purpuric spots 782.7
Purulent — see condition
Pus
  absorption, general — see Septicemia
  in
    stool 792.1
    urine 791.9
  tube (rupture) (see also Salpingo-oophoritis) 614.2
Pustular rash 782.1
Pustule 686.9
  malignant 022.0
  nonmalignant 686.9
Putnam's disease (subacute combined sclerosis with pernicious anemia) 281.0 [336.2]
Putnam-Dana syndrome (subacute combined sclerosis with pernicious anemia) 281.0 [336.2]
Putrefaction, intestinal 569.89
Putrescent pulp (dental) 522.1
Pyarthritis — see Pyarthrosis
Pyarthrosis (see also Arthritis, pyogenic) 711.0 ✓5ᵗʰ
  tuberculous — see Tuberculosis, joint
Pycnoepilepsy, pycnolepsy (idiopathic) (see also Epilepsy) 345.0 ✓5ᵗʰ
Pyelectasia 593.89
Pyelectasis 593.89
Pyelitis (congenital) (uremic) 590.80
  with
    abortion — see Abortion, by type, with specified complication NEC
    contracted kidney 590.00
    ectopic pregnancy (see also categories 633.0-633.9) 639.8
    molar pregnancy (see also categories 630-632) 639.8
  acute 590.10
    with renal medullary necrosis 590.11
  chronic 590.00
    with
      renal medullary necrosis 590.01
    complicating pregnancy, childbirth, or puerperium 646.6 ✓5ᵗʰ
    affecting fetus or newborn 760.1
  cystica 590.3
  following
    abortion 639.8
    ectopic or molar pregnancy 639.8
  gonococcal 098.19
    chronic or duration of 2 months or over 098.39
  tuberculous (see also Tuberculosis) 016.0 ✓5ᵗʰ [590.81]
Pyelocaliectasis 593.89
Pyelocystitis (see also Pyelitis) 590.80
Pyelohydronephrosis 591
Pyelonephritis (see also Pyelitis) 590.80
  acute 590.10
    with renal medullary necrosis 590.11
  chronic 590.00
  syphilitic (late) 095.4
  tuberculous (see also Tuberculosis) 016.0 ✓5ᵗʰ [590.81]

Index to Diseases

Pyelonephrosis (*see also* Pyelitis) 590.80
   chronic 590.00
Pyelophlebitis 451.89
Pyelo-ureteritis cystica 590.3
Pyemia, pyemic (purulent) (*see also* Septicemia) 038.9
   abscess — *see* Abscess
   arthritis (*see also* Arthritis, pyogenic) 711.0 ✓5ᵗʰ
   Bacillus coli 038.42
   embolism — *see* Embolism, pyemic
   fever 038.9
   infection 038.9
   joint (*see also* Arthritis, pyogenic) 711.0 ✓5ᵗʰ
   liver 572.1
   meningococcal 036.2
   newborn 771.81
   phlebitis — *see* Phlebitis
   pneumococcal 038.2
   portal 572.1
   postvaccinal 999.3
   specified organism NEC 038.8
   staphylococcal 038.10
      aureus 038.11
      specified organism NEC 038.19
   streptococcal 038.0
   tuberculous — *see* Tuberculosis, miliary
Pygopagus 759.4
Pykno-epilepsy, pyknolepsy (idiopathic) (*see also* Epilepsy) 345.0 ✓5ᵗʰ
Pyle (-Cohn) disease (craniometaphyseal dysplasia) 756.89
Pylephlebitis (suppurative) 572.1
Pylethrombophlebitis 572.1
Pylethrombosis 572.1
Pyloritis (*see also* Gastritis) 535.5 ✓5ᵗʰ
Pylorospasm (reflex) 537.81
   congenital or infantile 750.5
   neurotic 306.4
   newborn 750.5
   psychogenic 306.4
Pylorus, pyloric — *see* condition
Pyoarthrosis — *see* Pyarthrosis
Pyocele
   mastoid 383.00
   sinus (accessory) (nasal) (*see also* Sinusitis) 473.9
   turbinate (bone) 473.9
   urethra (*see also* Urethritis) 597.0
Pyococcal dermatitis 686.00
Pyococcide, skin 686.00
Pyocolpos (*see also* Vaginitis) 616.10
Pyocyaneus dermatitis 686.09
Pyocystitis (*see also* Cystitis) 595.9
Pyoderma, pyodermia 686.00
   gangrenosum 686.01
   specified type NEC 686.09
   vegetans 686.8
Pyodermatitis 686.00
   vegetans 686.8
Pyogenic — *see* condition
Pyohemia — *see* Septicemia
Pyohydronephrosis (*see also* Pyelitis) 590.80
Pyometra 615.9
Pyometritis (*see also* Endometritis) 615.9
Pyometrium (*see also* Endometritis) 615.9
Pyomyositis 728.0
   ossificans 728.19

Pyomyositis — *continued*
   tropical (bungpagga) 040.81
Pyonephritis (*see also* Pyelitis) 590.80
   chronic 590.00
Pyonephrosis (congenital) (*see also* Pyelitis) 590.80
   acute 590.10
Pyo-oophoritis (*see also* Salpingo-oophoritis) 614.2
Pyo-ovarium (*see also* Salpingo-oophoritis) 614.2
Pyopericarditis 420.99
Pyopericardium 420.99
Pyophlebitis — *see* Phlebitis
Pyopneumopericardium 420.99
Pyopneumothorax (infectional) 510.9
   with fistula 510.0
   subdiaphragmatic (*see also* Peritonitis) 567.2
   subphrenic (*see also* Peritonitis) 567.2
   tuberculous (*see also* Tuberculosis, pleura) 012.0 ✓5ᵗʰ
Pyorrhea (alveolar) (alveolaris) 523.4
   degenerative 523.5
Pyosalpingitis (*see also* Salpingo-oophoritis) 614.2
Pyosalpinx (*see also* Salpingo-oophoritis) 614.2
Pyosepticemia — *see* Septicemia
Pyosis
   Corlett's (impetigo) 684
   Manson's (pemphigus contagiosus) 684
Pyothorax 510.9
   with fistula 510.0
   tuberculous (*see also* Tuberculosis, pleura) 012.0 ✓5ᵗʰ
Pyoureter 593.89
   tuberculous (*see also* Tuberculosis) 016.2 ✓5ᵗʰ
Pyramidopallidonigral syndrome 332.0
Pyrexia (of unknown origin) (P.U.O.) 780.6
   atmospheric 992.0
   during labor 659.2 ✓5ᵗʰ
   environmentally-induced newborn 778.4
   heat 992.0
   newborn, environmentally-induced 778.4
   puerperal 672 ✓4ᵗʰ
Pyroglobulinemia 273.8
Pyromania 312.33
Pyrosis 787.1
Pyrroloporphyria 277.1
Pyuria (bacterial) 791.9

Q

Q fever 083.0
   with pneumonia 083.0 *[484.8]*
Quadricuspid aortic valve 746.89
Quadrilateral fever 083.0
Quadriparesis — *see* Quadriplegia
Quadriplegia 344.00
   with fracture, vertebra (process) — *see* Fracture, vertebra, cervical, with spinal cord injury
   brain (current episode) 437.8
   C1-C4
      complete 344.01
      incomplete 344.02
   C5-C7
      complete 344.03

Quadriplegia — continued
  C5-C7 — continued
    incomplete 344.04
  cerebral (current episode) 437.8
  congenital or infantile (cerebral) (spastic) (spinal) 343.2
  cortical 437.8
  embolic (current episode) (see also Embolism, brain) 434.1 ✓5ᵗʰ
  infantile (cerebral) (spastic) (spinal) 343.2
  newborn NEC 767.0
  specified NEC 344.09
  thrombotic (current episode) (see also Thrombosis, brain) 434.0 ✓5ᵗʰ
  traumatic — see Injury, spinal, cervical
Quadruplet
  affected by maternal complications of pregnancy 761.5
  healthy liveborn — see Newborn, multiple
  pregnancy (complicating delivery) NEC 651.8 ✓5ᵗʰ
    with fetal loss and retention of one or more fetus(es) 651.5 ✓5ᵗʰ
Quarrelsomeness 301.3
Quartan
  fever 084.2
  malaria (fever) 084.2
Queensland fever 083.0
  coastal 083.0
  seven-day 100.89
Quervain's disease 727.04
  thyroid (subacute granulomatous thyroiditis) 245.1
Queyrat's erythroplasia (M8080/2)
  specified site — see Neoplasm, skin, in situ
  unspecified site 233.5
Quincke's disease or edema — see Edema, angioneurotic
Quinquaud's disease (acne decalvans) 704.09
Quinsy (gangrenous) 475
Quintan fever 083.1
Quintuplet
  affected by maternal complications of pregnancy 761.5
  healthy liveborn — see Newborn, multiple
  pregnancy (complicating delivery) NEC 651.2 ✓5ᵗʰ
    with fetal loss and retention of one or more fetus(es) 651.6 ✓5ᵗʰ
Quotidian
  fever 084.0
  malaria (fever) 084.0

R

Rabbia 071
Rabbit fever (see also Tularemia) 021.9
Rabies 071
  contact V01.5
  exposure to V01.5
  inoculation V04.5
    reaction — see Complications, vaccination
  vaccination, prophylactic (against) V04.5
Rachischisis (see also Spina bifida) 741.9 ✓5ᵗʰ
Rachitic — see also condition
  deformities of spine 268.1

Rachitic — continued
  pelvis 268.1
    with disproportion (fetopelvic) 653.2 ✓5ᵗʰ
      affecting fetus or newborn 763.1
    causing obstructed labor 660.1 ✓5ᵗʰ
      affecting fetus or newborn 763.1
Rachitis, rachitism — see also Rickets
  acute 268.0
  fetalis 756.4
  renalis 588.0
  tarda 268.0
Racket nail 757.5
Radial nerve — see condition
Radiation effects or sickness — see also Effect, adverse, radiation
  cataract 366.46
  dermatitis 692.82
  sunburn (see also Sunburn) 692.71
Radiculitis (pressure) (vertebrogenic) 729.2
  accessory nerve 723.4
  anterior crural 724.4
  arm 723.4
  brachial 723.4
  cervical NEC 723.4
  due to displacement of intervertebral disc — see Neuritis, due to, displacement intervertebral disc
  leg 724.4
  lumbar NEC 724.4
  lumbosacral 724.4
  rheumatic 729.2
  syphilitic 094.89
  thoracic (with visceral pain) 724.4
Radiculomyelitis 357.0
  toxic, due to
    Clostridium tetani 037
    Corynebacterium diphtheriae 032.89
Radiculopathy (see also Radiculitis) 729.2
Radioactive substances, adverse effect — see Effect, adverse, radioactive substance
Radiodermal burns (acute) (chronic) (occupational) — see Burn, by site
Radiodermatitis 692.82
Radionecrosis — see Effect, adverse, radiation
Radiotherapy session V58.0
Radium, adverse effect — see Effect, adverse, radioactive substance
Raeder-Harbitz syndrome (pulseless disease) 446.7
Rage (see also Disturbance, conduct) 312.0 ✓5ᵗʰ
  meaning rabies 071
Rag sorters' disease 022.1
Raillietiniasis 123.8
Railroad neurosis 300.16
Railway spine 300.16
Raised — see Elevation
Raiva 071
Rake teeth, tooth 524.3
Rales 786.7
Ramifying renal pelvis 753.3
Ramsay Hunt syndrome (herpetic geniculate ganglionitis) 053.11
  meaning dyssynergia cerebellaris myoclonica 334.2
Ranke's primary infiltration (see also Tuberculosis) 010.0 ✓5ᵗʰ

Ranula 527.6
  congenital 750.26
Rape — see Injury, by site
  alleged, observation or examination V71.5
Rapid
  feeble pulse, due to shock, following injury 958.4
  heart (beat) 785.0
    psychogenic 306.2
  respiration 786.06
    psychogenic 306.1
  second stage (delivery) 661.3 ✓5ᵗʰ
    affecting fetus or newborn 763.6
  time-zone change syndrome 307.45
Rarefaction, bone 733.99
Rash 782.1
  canker 034.1
  diaper 691.0
  drug (internal use) 693.0
    contact 692.3
  ECHO 9 virus 078.89
  enema 692.89
  food (see also Allergy, food) 693.1
  heat 705.1
  napkin 691.0
  nettle 708.8
  pustular 782.1
  rose 782.1
    epidemic 056.9
    of infants 057.8
  scarlet 034.1
  serum (prophylactic) (therapeutic) 999.5
  toxic 782.1
  wandering tongue 529.1
Rasmussen's aneurysm (see also Tuberculosis) 011.2 ✓5ᵗʰ
Rat-bite fever 026.9
  due to Streptobacillus moniliformis 026.1 ✓5ᵗʰ
  spirochetal (morsus muris) 026.0 ✓5ᵗʰ
Rathke's pouch tumor (M9350/1) 237.0
Raymond (-Céstan) syndrome 433.8 ✓5ᵗʰ
Raynaud's
  disease or syndrome (paroxysmal digital cyanosis) 443.0
  gangrene (symmetric) 443.0 [785.4]
  phenomenon (paroxysmal digital cyanosis) (secondary) 443.0
RDS 769
Reaction
  acute situational maladjustment (see also Reaction, adjustment) 309.9
  adaptation (see also Reaction, adjustment) 309.9
  adjustment 309.9
    with
      anxious mood 309.24
        with depressed mood 309.28
      conduct disturbance 309.3
        combined with disturbance of emotions 309.4
      depressed mood 309.0
        brief 309.0
          with anxious mood 309.28
        prolonged 309.1
      elective mutism 309.83
      mixed emotions and conduct 309.4
      mutism, elective 309.83
      physical symptoms 309.82

Reaction — continued
  adjustment — continued
    with — continued
      predominant disturbance (of)
        conduct 309.3
        emotions NEC 309.29
          mixed 309.28
          mixed, emotions and conduct 309.4
          specified type NEC 309.89
      specific academic or work inhibition 309.23
      withdrawal 309.83
    depressive 309.0
      with conduct disturbance 309.4
      brief 309.0
      prolonged 309.1
    specified type NEC 309.89
  adverse food NEC 995.7
  affective (see also Psychosis, affective) 296.90
    specified type NEC 296.99
  aggressive 301.3
    unsocialized (see also Disturbance, conduct) 312.0 ✓5ᵗʰ
  allergic (see also Allergy) 995.3
    drug, medicinal substance, and biological — see Allergy, drug
    food — see Allergy, food
    serum 999.5
  anaphylactic — see Shock, anaphylactic
  anesthesia — see Anesthesia, complication
  anger 312.0 ✓5ᵗʰ
  antisocial 301.7
  antitoxin (prophylactic) (therapeutic) — see Complications, vaccination
  anxiety 300.00
  asthenic 300.5
  compulsive 300.3
  conversion (anesthetic) (autonomic) (hyperkinetic) (mixed paralytic) (paresthetic) 300.11
  deoxyribonuclease (DNA) (DNase) hypersensitivity NEC 287.2
  depressive 300.4
    acute 309.0
    affective (see also Psychosis, affective) 296.2 ✓5ᵗʰ
      recurrent episode 296.3 ✓5ᵗʰ
      single episode 296.2 ✓5ᵗʰ
    brief 309.0
    manic (see also Psychosis, affective) 296.80
    neurotic 300.4
    psychoneurotic 300.4
    psychotic 298.0
  dissociative 300.15
  drug NEC (see also Table of Drugs and Chemicals) 995.2
    allergic — see Allergy, drug
    correct substance properly administered 995.2
    obstetric anesthetic or analgesic NEC 668.9 ✓5ᵗʰ
      affecting fetus or newborn 763.5
      specified drug — see Table of Drugs and Chemicals
    overdose or poisoning 977.9
      specified drug — see Table of Drugs and Chemicals
    specific to newborn 779.4
    transmitted via placenta or breast milk — see Absorption, drug, through placenta

Reaction — *continued*
  drug NEC — *continued*
    withdrawal NEC 292.0
      infant of dependent mother 779.5
    wrong substance given or taken in error 977.9
      specified drug — *see* Table of Drugs and Chemicals
  dyssocial 301.7
  erysipeloid 027.1
  fear 300.20
    child 313.0
  fluid loss, cerebrospinal 349.0
  food — *see also* Allergy, food
    adverse NEC 995.7
    anaphylactic shock — *see* Anaphylactic shock, due to, food
  foreign
    body NEC 728.82
      in operative wound (inadvertently left) 998.4
        due to surgical material intentionally left — *see* Complications, due to (presence of) any device, implant, or graft classified to 996.0-996.5 NEC
    substance accidentally left during a procedure (chemical) (powder) (talc) 998.7
      body or object (instrument) (sponge) (swab) 998.4
  graft-versus-host (GVH) 996.85
  grief (acute) (brief) 309.0
    prolonged 309.1
  gross stress (*see also* Reaction, stress, acute) 308.9
  group delinquent (*see also* Disturbance, conduct) 312.2
  Herxheimer's 995.0
  hyperkinetic (*see also* Hyperkinesia) 314.9
  hypochondriacal 300.7
  hypoglycemic, due to insulin 251.0
    therapeutic misadventure 962.3
  hypomanic (*see also* Psychosis, affective) 296.0
    recurrent episode 296.1
    single episode 296.0
  hysterical 300.10
    conversion type 300.11
    dissociative 300.15
  id (bacterial cause) 692.89
  immaturity NEC 301.89
    aggressive 301.3
    emotional instability 301.59
  immunization — *see* Complications, vaccination
  incompatibility
    blood group (ABO) (infusion) (transfusion) 999.6
    Rh (factor) (infusion) (transfusion) 999.7
  inflammatory — *see* Infection
  infusion — *see* Complications, infusion
  inoculation (immune serum) — *see* Complications, vaccination
  insulin 995.2
  involutional
    paranoid 297.2
    psychotic (*see also* Psychosis, affective, depressive) 296.2
  leukemoid (lymphocytic) (monocytic) (myelocytic) 288.8

Reaction — *continued*
  LSD (*see also* Abuse, drugs, nondependent) 305.3
  lumbar puncture 349.0
  manic-depressive (*see also* Psychosis, affective) 296.80
    depressed 296.2
      recurrent episode 296.3
      single episode 296.2
    hypomanic 296.0
  neurasthenic 300.5
  neurogenic (*see also* Neurosis) 300.9
  neurotic NEC 300.9
  neurotic-depressive 300.4
  nitritoid — *see* Crisis, nitritoid
  obsessive (-compulsive) 300.3
  organic 293.9
    acute 293.0
    subacute 293.1
  overanxious, child or adolescent 313.0
  paranoid (chronic) 297.9
    acute 298.3
    climacteric 297.2
    involutional 297.2
    menopausal 297.2
    senile 290.20
    simple 297.0
  passive
    aggressive 301.84
    dependency 301.6
  personality (*see also* Disorder, personality) 301.9
  phobic 300.20
  postradiation — *see* Effect, adverse, radiation
  psychogenic NEC 300.9
  psychoneurotic (*see also* Neurosis) 300.9
    anxiety 300.00
    compulsive 300.3
    conversion 300.11
    depersonalization 300.6
    depressive 300.4
    dissociative 300.15
    hypochondriacal 300.7
    hysterical 300.10
      conversion type 300.11
      dissociative type 300.15
    neurasthenic 300.5
    obsessive 300.3
    obsessive-compulsive 300.3
    phobic 300.20
    tension state 300.9
  psychophysiologic NEC (*see also* Disorder, psychosomatic) 306.9
    cardiovascular 306.2
    digestive 306.4
    endocrine 306.6
    gastrointestinal 306.4
    genitourinary 306.50
    heart 306.2
    hemic 306.8
    intestinal (large) (small) 306.4
    laryngeal 306.1
    lymphatic 306.8
    musculoskeletal 306.0
    pharyngeal 306.1
    respiratory 306.1
    skin 306.3
    special sense organs 306.7
  psychosomatic (*see also* Disorder, psychosomatic) 306.9
  psychotic (*see also* Psychosis) 298.9

Reaction — continued
  psychotic — continued
    depressive 298.0
      due to or associated with physical condition (see also Psychosis, organic) 293.9
      involutional (see also Psychosis, affective) 296.2 ✓5th
        recurrent episode 296.3 ✓5th
        single episode 296.2 ✓5th
  pupillary (myotonic) (tonic) 379.46
  radiation — see Effect, adverse, radiation
  runaway — see also Disturbance, conduct
    socialized 312.2 ✓5th
    undersocialized, unsocialized 312.1 ✓5th
  scarlet fever toxin — see Complications, vaccination
  schizophrenic (see also Schizophrenia) 295.9 ✓5th
    latent 295.5 ✓5th
  serological for syphilis — see Serology for syphilis
  serum (prophylactic) (therapeutic) 999.5
    immediate 999.4
  situational (see also Reaction, adjustment) 309.9
    acute, to stress 308.3
    adjustment (see also Reaction, adjustment) 309.9
  somatization (see also Disorder, psychosomatic) 306.9
  spinal puncture 349.0
  spite, child (see also Disturbance, conduct) 312.0 ✓5th
  stress, acute 308.9
    with predominant disturbance (of)
      consciousness 308.1
      emotions 308.0
      mixed 308.4
      psychomotor 308.2
    specified type NEC 308.3
    bone or cartilage — see Fracture, stress
    surgical procedure — see Complications, surgical procedure
  tetanus antitoxin — see Complications, vaccination
  toxin-antitoxin — see Complications, vaccination
  transfusion (blood) (bone marrow) (lymphocytes) (allergic) — see Complications, transfusion
  tuberculin skin test, nonspecific (without active tuberculosis) 795.5
    positive (without active tuberculosis) 795.5
  ultraviolet — see Effect, adverse, ultraviolet
  undersocialized, unsocialized — see also Disturbance, conduct
    aggressive (type) 312.0 ✓5th
    unaggressive (type) 312.1 ✓5th
  vaccination (any) — see Complications, vaccination
  white graft (skin) 996.52
  withdrawing, child or adolescent 313.22
  x-ray — see Effect, adverse, x-rays
Reactive depression (see also Reaction, depressive) 300.4
  neurotic 300.4
  psychoneurotic 300.4
  psychotic 298.0
Rebound tenderness 789.6 ✓5th
Recalcitrant patient V15.81
Recanalization, thrombus — see Thrombosis

Recession, receding
  chamber angle (eye) 364.77
  chin 524.06
  gingival (generalized) (localized) (postinfective) (postoperative) 523.2
Recklinghausen's disease (M9540/1) 237.71
  bones (osteitis fibrosa cystica) 252.0
Recklinghausen-Applebaum disease (hemochromatosis) 275.0
Reclus' disease (cystic) 610.1
Recrudescent typhus (fever) 081.1
Recruitment, auditory 388.44
Rectalgia 569.42
Rectitis 569.49
Rectocele
  female (without uterine prolapse) 618.0
    with uterine prolapse 618.4
      complete 618.3
      incomplete 618.2
  in pregnancy or childbirth 654.4 ✓5th
    causing obstructed labor 660.2 ✓5th
      affecting fetus or newborn 763.1
  male 569.49
  vagina, vaginal (outlet) 618.0
Rectosigmoiditis 569.89
  ulcerative (chronic) 556.3
Rectosigmoid junction — see condition
Rectourethral — see condition
Rectovaginal — see condition
Rectovesical — see condition
Rectum, rectal — see condition
Recurrent — see condition
Red bugs 133.8
Red cedar asthma 495.8
Redness
  conjunctiva 379.93
  eye 379.93
  nose 478.1
Reduced ventilatory or vital capacity 794.2
Reduction
  function
    kidney (see also Disease, renal) 593.9
    liver 573.8
  ventilatory capacity 794.2
  vital capacity 794.2
Redundant, redundancy
  abdomen 701.9
  anus 751.5
  cardia 537.89
  clitoris 624.2
  colon (congenital) 751.5
  foreskin (congenital) 605
  intestine 751.5
  labia 624.3
  organ or site, congenital NEC — see Accessory
  panniculus (abdominal) 278.1
  prepuce (congenital) 605
  pylorus 537.89
  rectum 751.5
  scrotum 608.89
  sigmoid 751.5
  skin (of face) 701.9
    eyelids 374.30
  stomach 537.89
  uvula 528.9
  vagina 623.8
Reduplication — see Duplication

Referral
  adoption (agency) V68.89
  nursing care V63.8
  patient without examination or treatment V68.81
  social services V63.8
Reflex — *see also* condition
  blink, deficient 374.45
  hyperactive gag 478.29
  neurogenic bladder NEC 596.54
    atonic 596.54
      with cauda equina syndrome 344.61
  vasoconstriction 443.9
  vasovagal 780.2
Reflux
  esophageal 530.81
  esophagitis 530.11
  gastroesophageal 530.81
  mitral — *see* Insufficiency, mitral
  ureteral — *see* Reflux, vesicoureteral
  vesicoureteral 593.70
    with
      reflux nephropathy 593.73
        bilateral 593.72
        unilateral 593.71
Reformed gallbladder 576.0
Reforming, artificial openings (*see also* Attention to, artificial, opening) V55.9
Refractive error (*see also* Error, refractive) 367.9
Refsum's disease or syndrome (heredopathia atactica polyneuritiformis) 356.3
Refusal of
  food 307.59
    hysterical 300.11
  treatment because of, due to
    patient's decision NEC V64.2
    reason of conscience or religion V62.6
Regaud
  tumor (M8082/3) — *see* Neoplasm, nasopharynx, malignant
  type carcinoma (M8082/3) — *see* Neoplasm, nasopharynx, malignant
Regional — *see* condition
Regulation feeding (elderly) (infant) 783.3
  newborn 779.3
Regurgitated
  food, choked on 933.1
  stomach contents, choked on 933.1
Regurgitation
  aortic (valve) (*see also* Insufficiency, aortic) 424.1
    congenital 746.4
    syphilitic 093.22
  food — *see also* Vomiting
    with reswallowing — *see* Rumination
    newborn 779.3
  gastric contents — *see* Vomiting
  heart — *see* Endocarditis
  mitral (valve) — *see also* Insufficiency, mitral
    congenital 746.6
  myocardial — *see* Endocarditis
  pulmonary (heart) (valve) (*see also* Endocarditis, pulmonary) 424.3
  stomach — *see* Vomiting
  tricuspid — *see* Endocarditis, tricuspid
  valve, valvular — *see* Endocarditis
  vesicoureteral — *see* Reflux, vesicoureteral
Rehabilitation V57.9
  multiple types V57.89

Rehabilitation — *continued*
  occupational V57.21
  specified type NEC V57.89
  speech V57.3
  vocational V57.22
Reichmann's disease or syndrome (gastrosuccorrhea) 536.8
Reifenstein's syndrome (hereditary familial hypogonadism, male) 257.2
Reilly's syndrome or phenomenon (*see also* Neuropathy, peripheral, autonomic) 337.9
Reimann's periodic disease 277.3
Reinsertion, contraceptive device V25.42
Reiter's disease, syndrome, or urethritis 099.3 [711.1]
Rejection
  food, hysterical 300.11
  transplant 996.80
    bone marrow 996.85
    corneal 996.51
    organ (immune or nonimmune cause) 996.80
      bone marrow 996.85
      heart 996.83
      intestines 996.87
      kidney 996.81
      liver 996.82
      lung 996.84
      pancreas 996.86
      specified NEC 996.89
    skin 996.52
      artificial 996.55
      decellularized allodermis 996.55
Relapsing fever 087.9
  Carter's (Asiatic) 087.0
  Dutton's (West African) 087.1
  Koch's 087.9
  louse-borne (epidemic) 087.0
  Novy's (American) 087.1
  Obermeyer's (European) 087.0
  Spirillum 087.9
  tick-borne (endemic) 087.1
Relaxation
  anus (sphincter) 569.49
    due to hysteria 300.11
  arch (foot) 734
    congenital 754.61
  back ligaments 728.4
  bladder (sphincter) 596.59
  cardio-esophageal 530.89
  cervix (*see also* Incompetency, cervix) 622.5
  diaphragm 519.4
  inguinal rings — *see* Hernia, inguinal
  joint (capsule) (ligament) (paralytic) (*see also* Derangement, joint) 718.90
    congenital 755.8
  lumbosacral joint 724.6
  pelvic floor 618.8
  pelvis 618.8
  perineum 618.8
  posture 729.9
  rectum (sphincter) 569.49
  sacroiliac (joint) 724.6
  scrotum 608.89
  urethra (sphincter) 599.84
  uterus (outlet) 618.8
  vagina (outlet) 618.8
  vesical 596.59

Remains
  canal of Cloquet 743.51
  capsule (opaque) 743.51
Remittent fever (malarial) 084.6
Remnant
  canal of Cloquet 743.51
  capsule (opaque) 743.51
  cervix, cervical stump (acquired)
    (postoperative) 622.8
  cystic duct, postcholecystectomy 576.0
  fingernail 703.8
    congenital 757.5
  meniscus, knee 717.5
  thyroglossal duct 759.2
  tonsil 474.8
    infected 474.00
  urachus 753.7
Remote effect of cancer — see condition
Removal (of)
  catheter (urinary) (indwelling) V53.6
    from artificial opening — see Attention to,
      artificial, opening
    non-vascular V58.82
    vascular V58.81
  cerebral ventricle (communicating) shunt
    V53.01
  device — see also Fitting (of)
    contraceptive V25.42
    fixation
      external V54.89 ▲
      internal V54.0
      traction V54.89 ▲
  dressing V58.3
  ileostomy V55.2
  Kirschner wire V54.89 ▲
  nonvascular catheter V58.82
  pin V54.0
  plaster cast V54.89 ▲
  plate (fracture) V54.0
  rod V54.0
  screw V54.0
  splint, external V54.89 ▲
  subdermal implantable contraceptive V25.43
  suture V58.3
  traction device, external V54.89 ▲
  vascular catheter V58.81
Ren
  arcuatus 753.3
  mobile, mobilis (see also Disease, renal) 593.0
    congenital 753.3
  unguliformis 753.3
Renal — see also condition
  glomerulohyalinosis-diabetic syndrome
    250.4 [581.81]
Rendu-Osler-Weber disease or syndrome
    (familial hemorrhagic telangiectasia) 448.0
Reninoma (M8361/1) 236.91
Rénon-Delille syndrome 253.8
Repair
  pelvic floor, previous, in pregnancy or
    childbirth 654.4
    affecting fetus or newborn 763.89
  scarred tissue V51
Replacement by artificial or mechanical
  device or prosthesis of (see also Fitting
  (of))
    artificial skin V43.83
    bladder V43.5
    blood vessel V43.4
    breast V43.82

Replacement by artificial or mechanical
  device or prosthesis of — continued
    eye globe V43.0
    heart V43.2
      valve V43.3
    intestine V43.89
    joint V43.60
      ankle V43.66
      elbow V43.62
      finger V43.69
      hip (partial) (total) V43.64
      knee V43.65
      shoulder V43.61
      specified NEC V43.69
      wrist V43.63
    kidney V43.89
    larynx V43.81
    lens V43.1
    limb(s) V43.7
    liver V43.89
    lung V43.89
    organ NEC V43.89
    pancreas V43.89
    skin (artificial) V43.83
    tissue NEC V43.89
Reprogramming
  cardiac pacemaker V53.31
Request for expert evidence V68.2
Reserve, decreased or low
  cardiac — see Disease, heart
  kidney (see also Disease, renal) 593.9
Residual — see also condition
  bladder 596.8
  foreign body — see Retention, foreign body
  state, schizophrenic (see also Schizophrenia)
    295.6
  urine 788.69
Resistance, resistant (to)

Note — use the following subclassification for
categories V09.5, V09.7, V09.8, V09.9:

0	without mention of resistance to multiple drugs
1	with resistance to multiple drugs
V09.5	quinolones and fluoroquinolones
V09.7	antimycobacterial agents
V09.8	specified drugs NEC
V09.9	unspecified drugs
9	multiple sites

  drugs by microorganisms V09.9
    Amikacin V09.4
    aminoglycosides V09.4
    Amodiaquine V09.5
    Amoxicillin V09.0
    Ampicillin V09.0
    antimycobacterial agents V09.7 •
    Azithromycin V09.2
    Azlocillin V09.0
    Aztreonam V09.1
    B-lactam antibiotics V09.1
    bacampicillin V09.0
    Bacitracin V09.8
    Benznidazole V09.8
    Capreomycin V09.7
    Carbenicillin V09.0
    Cefaclor V09.1
    Cefadroxil V09.1

Resistance, resistant

Resistance, resistant (to) — *continued*
   drugs by microorganisms — *continued*
      Cefamandole V09.1
      Cefatetan V09.1
      Cefazolin V09.1
      Cefixime V09.1
      Cefonicid V09.1
      Cefoperazone V09.1
      Ceforanide V09.1
      Cefotaxime V09.1
      Cefoxitin V09.1
      Ceftazidime V09.1
      Ceftizoxime V09.1
      Ceftriaxone V09.1
      Cefuroxime V09.1
      Cephalexin V09.1
      Cephaloglycin V09.1
      Cephaloridine V09.1
      Cephalosporins V09.1
      Cephalothin V09.1
      Cephapirin V09.1
      Cephradine V09.1
      Chloramphenicol V09.8 ✓5ᵗʰ
      Chloraquine V09.5 ✓5ᵗʰ
      Chlorguanide V09.8 ✓5ᵗʰ
      Chlorproguanil V09.8 ✓5ᵗʰ
      Chlortetracycline V09.3
      Cinoxacin V09.5 ✓5ᵗʰ
      Ciprofloxacin V09.5 ✓5ᵗʰ
      Clarithromycin V09.2
      Clindamycin V09.8 ✓5ᵗʰ
      Clioquinol V09.5 ✓5ᵗʰ
      Clofazimine V09.7 ✓5ᵗʰ
      Cloxacillin V09.0
      Cyclacillin V09.0
      Cycloserine V09.7 ✓5ᵗʰ
      Dapsone [DZ] V09.7 ✓5ᵗʰ
      Demeclocycline V09.3
      Dicloxacillin V09.0
      Doxycycline V09.3
      Enoxacin V09.5 ✓5ᵗʰ
      Erythromycin V09.2
      Ethambutol [EMB] V09.7 ✓5ᵗʰ
      Ethionamide [ETA] V09.7 ✓5ᵗʰ
      fluoroquinolones V09.5 ✓5ᵗʰ
      Gentamicin V09.4
      Halofantrine V09.8 ✓5ᵗʰ
      Imipenem V09.1
      Iodoquinol V09.5 ✓5ᵗʰ
      Isoniazid [INH] V09.7 ✓5ᵗʰ
      Kanamycin V09.4
      macrolides V09.2
      Mafenide V09.6
      Mefloquine V09.8 ✓5ᵗʰ
      Melasoprol V09.8 ✓5ᵗʰ
      Methacycline V09.3
      Methenamine V09.8 ✓5ᵗʰ
      Methicillin V09.0
      Metronidazole V09.8 ✓5ᵗʰ
      Mezlocillin V09.0
      Minocycline V09.3
      Nafcillin V09.0
      Nalidixic acid V09.5 ✓5ᵗʰ
      Natamycin V09.2
      Neomycin V09.4
      Netilmicin V09.4
      Nifurtimox V09.8 ✓5ᵗʰ
      Nimorazole V09.8 ✓5ᵗʰ
      Nitrofurantoin V09.8 ✓5ᵗʰ
      Norfloxacin V09.5 ✓5ᵗʰ
      Nystatin V09.2

Resistance, resistant (to) — *continued*
   drugs by microorganisms — *continued*
      Ofloxacin V09.5 ✓5ᵗʰ
      Oleandomycin V09.2
      Oxacillin V09.0
      Oxytetracycline V09.3
      Para-amino salicylic acid [PAS] V09.7 ✓5ᵗʰ
      Paromomycin V09.4
      Penicillin (G) (V) (VK) V09.0
      penicillins V09.0
      Pentamidine V09.8 ✓5ᵗʰ
      Piperacillin V09.0
      Primaquine V09.5 ✓5ᵗʰ
      Proguanil V09.8 ✓5ᵗʰ
      Pyrazinamide [PZA] V09.7 ✓5ᵗʰ
      Pyrimethamine/sulfalene V09.8 ✓5ᵗʰ
      Pyrimethamine/sulfodoxine V09.8 ✓5ᵗʰ
      Quinacrine V09.5 ✓5ᵗʰ
      Quinidine V09.8 ✓5ᵗʰ
      Quinine V09.8 ✓5ᵗʰ
      quinolones V09.5 ✓5ᵗʰ
      Rifabutin V09.7 ✓5ᵗʰ
      Rifampin [RIF] V09.7 ✓5ᵗʰ
      Rifamycin V09.7 ✓5ᵗʰ
      Rolitetracycline V09.3
      Specified drugs NEC V09.8 ✓5ᵗʰ
      Spectinomycin V09.8 ✓5ᵗʰ
      Spiramycin V09.2
      Streptomycin [SM] V09.4
      Sulfacetamide V09.6
      Sulfacytine V09.6
      Sulfadiazine V09.6
      Sulfadoxine V09.6
      Sulfamethoxazole V09.6
      Sulfapyridine V09.6
      Sulfasalizine V09.6
      Sulfasoxazone V09.6
      sulfonamides V09.6
      Sulfoxone V09.7 ✓5ᵗʰ
      tetracycline V09.3
      tetracyclines V09.3
      Thiamphenicol V09.8 ✓5ᵗʰ
      Ticarcillin V09.0
      Tinidazole V09.8 ✓5ᵗʰ
      Tobramycin V09.4
      Triamphenicol V09.8 ✓5ᵗʰ
      Trimethoprim V09.8 ✓5ᵗʰ
      Vancomycin V09.8 ✓5ᵗʰ

Resorption
   biliary 576.8
      purulent or putrid (*see also* Cholecystitis) 576.8
   dental (roots) 521.4
      alveoli 525.8
   septic — *see* Septicemia
   teeth (external) (internal) (pathological) (roots) 521.4

Respiration
   asymmetrical 786.09
   bronchial 786.09
   Cheyne-Stokes (periodic respiration) 786.04
   decreased, due to shock following injury 958.4
   disorder of 786.00
      psychogenic 306.1
      specified NEC 786.09
   failure 518.81
      acute 518.81
      acute and chronic 518.84
      chronic 518.83
      newborn 770.84

Respiration — *continued*
  insufficiency 786.09
    acute 518.82
      newborn NEC 770.89 ▲
  Kussmaul (air hunger) 786.09
  painful 786.52
  periodic 786.09
  poor 786.09
    newborn NEC 770.89 ▲
  sighing 786.7
    psychogenic 306.1
  wheezing 786.07
Respiratory — *see also* condition
  distress 786.09
    acute 518.82
    fetus or newborn NEC 770.89 ▲
    syndrome (newborn) 769
      adult (following shock, surgery, or trauma) 518.5
        specified NEC 518.82
  failure 518.81
    acute 518.81
    acute and chronic 518.8
    chronic 518.83
Respiratory syncytial virus (RSV) 079.6
  bronchiolitis 466.11
  pneumonia 480.1
Response
  photoallergic 692.72
  phototoxic 692.72
Rest, rests
  mesonephric duct 752.8
    fallopian tube 752.11
  ovarian, in fallopian tubes 752.19
  wolffian duct 752.8
Restless leg (syndrome) 333.99
Restlessness 799.2
Restoration of organ continuity from previous sterilization (tuboplasty) (vasoplasty) V26.0
Restriction of housing space V60.1
Restzustand, schizophrenic (*see also* Schizophrenia) 295.6 ✓5ᵗʰ
Retained — *see* Retention
Retardation
  development, developmental, specific (*see also* Disorder, development, specific) 315.9
    learning, specific 315.2
      arithmetical 315.1
      language (skills) 315.31
        expressive 315.31
        mixed receptive-expressive 315.32
      mathematics 315.1
      reading 315.00
        phonological 315.39
      written expression 315.2
    motor 315.4
  endochondral bone growth 733.91
  growth (physical) in childhood 783.43
    due to malnutrition 263.2
    fetal (intrauterine) 764.9 ✓5ᵗʰ
      affecting management of pregnancy 656.5 ✓5ᵗʰ
    intrauterine growth 764.9 ✓5ᵗʰ
      affecting management of pregnancy 656.5 ✓5ᵗʰ
  mental 319
    borderline V62.89
    mild, IQ 50-70 317

Retardation — *continued*
  mental — *continued*
    moderate, IQ 35-49 318.0
    profound, IQ under 20 318.2
    severe, IQ 20-34 318.1
  motor, specific 315.4
  physical 783.43
    child 783.43
    due to malnutrition 263.2
    fetus (intrauterine) 764.9 ✓5ᵗʰ
      affecting management of pregnancy 656.5 ✓5ᵗʰ
  psychomotor NEC 307.9
  reading 315.00
Retching — *see* Vomiting
Retention, retained
  bladder NEC (*see also* Retention, urine) 788.20
    psychogenic 306.53
  carbon dioxide 276.2
  cyst — *see* Cyst
  dead
    fetus (after 22 completed weeks gestation) 656.4 ✓5ᵗʰ
    early fetal death (before 22 completed weeks gestation) 632
    ovum 631
  decidua (following delivery) (fragments) (with hemorrhage) 666.2 ✓5ᵗʰ
    without hemorrhage 667.1 ✓5ᵗʰ
  deciduous tooth 520.6
  dental root 525.3
  fecal (*see also* Constipation) 564.00
  fluid 276.6
  foreign body — *see also* Foreign body, retained
    bone 733.99
    current trauma — *see* Foreign body, by site or type
    middle ear 385.83
    muscle 729.6
    soft tissue NEC 729.6
  gastric 536.8
  membranes (following delivery) (with hemorrhage) 666.2 ✓5ᵗʰ
    with abortion — *see* Abortion, by type
    without hemorrhage 667.1 ✓5ᵗʰ
  menses 626.8
  milk (puerperal) 676.2 ✓5ᵗʰ
  nitrogen, extrarenal 788.9
  placenta (total) (with hemorrhage) 666.0 ✓5ᵗʰ
    with abortion — *see* Abortion, by type
    portions or fragments 666.2 ✓5ᵗʰ
      without hemorrhage 667.1 ✓5ᵗʰ
    without hemorrhage 667.0 ✓5ᵗʰ
  products of conception
    early pregnancy (fetal death before 22 completed weeks gestation) 632
    following
      abortion — *see* Abortion, by type
      delivery 666.2 ✓5ᵗʰ
        with hemorrhage 666.2 ✓5ᵗʰ
        without hemorrhage 667.1 ✓5ᵗʰ
  secundines (following delivery) (with hemorrhage) 666.2 ✓5ᵗʰ
    with abortion — *see* Abortion, by type
    complicating puerperium (delayed hemorrhage) 666.2 ✓5ᵗʰ
    without hemorrhage 667.1 ✓5ᵗʰ
  smegma, clitoris 624.8
  urine NEC 788.20
    bladder, incomplete emptying 788.21

Retention, retained — *continued*
  urine NEC — *continued*
    psychogenic 306.53
    specified NEC 788.29
  water (in tissue) (*see also* Edema) 782.3
Reticulation, dust (occupational) 504
Reticulocytosis NEC 790.99
Reticuloendotheliosis
  acute infantile (M9722/3) 202.5 ✓5ᵗʰ
  leukemic (M9940/3) 202.4 ✓5ᵗʰ
  malignant (M9720/3) 202.3 ✓5ᵗʰ
  nonlipid (M9722/3) 202.5 ✓5ᵗʰ
Reticulohistiocytoma (giant cell) 277.8
Reticulohistiocytosis, multicentric 272.8
Reticulolymphosarcoma (diffuse) (M9613/3) 200.8 ✓5ᵗʰ
  follicular (M9691/3) 202.0 ✓5ᵗʰ
  nodular (M9691/3) 202.0 ✓5ᵗʰ
Reticulosarcoma (M9640/3) 200.0 ✓5ᵗʰ
  nodular (M9642/3) 200.0 ✓5ᵗʰ
  pleomorphic cell type (M9641/3) 200.0 ✓5ᵗʰ
Reticulosis (skin)
  acute of infancy (M9722/3) 202.5 ✓5ᵗʰ
  histiocytic medullary (M9721/3) 202.3 ✓5ᵗʰ
  lipomelanotic 695.89
  malignant (M9720/3) 202.3 ✓5ᵗʰ
  Sézary's (M9701/3) 202.2 ✓5ᵗʰ
Retina, retinal — *see* condition
Retinitis (*see also* Chorioretinitis) 363.20
  albuminurica 585 *[363.10]*
  arteriosclerotic 440.8 *[362.13]*
  central angiospastic 362.41
  Coat's 362.12
  diabetic 250.5 ✓5ᵗʰ *[362.01]*
  disciformis 362.52
  disseminated 363.10
    metastatic 363.14
    neurosyphilitic 094.83
    pigment epitheliopathy 363.15
  exudative 362.12
  focal 363.00
    in histoplasmosis 115.92
      capsulatum 115.02
      duboisii 115.12
    juxtapapillary 363.05
    macular 363.06
    paramacular 363.06
    peripheral 363.08
    posterior pole NEC 363.07
  gravidarum 646.8 ✓5ᵗʰ
  hemorrhagica externa 362.12
  juxtapapillary (Jensen's) 363.05
  luetic — *see* Retinitis, syphilitic
  metastatic 363.14
  pigmentosa 362.74
  proliferans 362.29
  proliferating 362.29
  punctata albescens 362.76
  renal 585 *[363.13]*
  syphilitic (secondary) 091.51
    congenital 090.0 *[363.13]*
    early 091.51
    late 095.8 *[363.13]*
  syphilitica, central, recurrent 095.8 *[363.13]*
  tuberculous (*see also* Tuberculous) 017.3 ✓5ᵗʰ *[363.13]*
Retinoblastoma (M9510/3) 190.5
  differentiated type (M9511/3) 190.5
  undifferentiated type (M9512/3) 190.5

Retinochoroiditis (*see also* Chorioretinitis) 363.20
  central angiospastic 362.41
  disseminated 363.10
    metastatic 363.14
    neurosyphilitic 094.83
    pigment epitheliopathy 363.15
    syphilitic 094.83
  due to toxoplasmosis (acquired) (focal) 130.2
  focal 363.00
    in histoplasmosis 115.92
      capsulatum 115.02
      duboisii 115.12
    juxtapapillary (Jensen's) 363.05
    macular 363.06
    paramacular 363.06
    peripheral 363.08
    posterior pole NEC 363.07
  juxtapapillaris 363.05
  syphilitic (disseminated) 094.83
Retinopathy (background) 362.10
  arteriosclerotic 440.8 *[362.13]*
  atherosclerotic 440.8 *[362.13]*
  central serous 362.41
  circinate 362.10
  Coat's 362.12
  diabetic 250.5 ✓5ᵗʰ *[362.01]*
    proliferative 250.5 ✓5ᵗʰ *[362.02]*
  exudative 362.12
  hypertensive 362.11
  of prematurity 362.21
  pigmentary, congenital 362.74
  proliferative 362.29
    diabetic 250.5 *[362.02]*
    sickle-cell 282.60 *[362.29]*
  solar 363.31
Retinoschisis 361.10
  bullous 361.12
  congenital 743.56
  flat 361.11
  juvenile 362.73
Retractile testis 752.52
Retraction
  cervix (*see also* Retroversion, uterus) 621.6
  drum (membrane) 384.82
  eyelid 374.41
  finger 736.29
  head 781.0
  lid 374.41
  lung 518.89
  mediastinum 519.3
  nipple 611.79
    congenital 757.6
    puerperal, postpartum 676.0 ✓5ᵗʰ
  palmar fascia 728.6
  pleura (*see also* Pleurisy) 511.0
  ring, uterus (Bandl's) (pathological) 661.4 ✓5ᵗʰ
    affecting fetus or newborn 763.7
  sternum (congenital) 756.3
    acquired 738.3
    during respiration 786.9
  substernal 738.3
  supraclavicular 738.8
  syndrome (Duane's) 378.71
  uterus (*see also* Retroversion, uterus) 621.6
  valve (heart) — *see* Endocarditis
Retrobulbar — *see* condition
Retrocaval ureter 753.4
Retrocecal — *see also* condition
  appendix (congenital) 751.5

Retrocession — see Retroversion
Retrodisplacement — see Retroversion
Retroflection, retroflexion — see Retroversion
Retrognathia, retrognathism (mandibular) (maxillary) 524.06
Retrograde
 ejaculation 608.87
 menstruation 626.8
Retroiliac ureter 753.4
Retroperineal — see condition
Retroperitoneal — see condition
Retroperitonitis (see also Peritonitis) 567.9
Retropharyngeal — see condition
Retroplacental — see condition
Retroposition — see Retroversion
Retrosternal thyroid (congenital) 759.2
Retroversion, retroverted
 cervix (see also Retroversion, uterus) 621.6
 female NEC (see also Retroversion, uterus) 621.6
 iris 364.70
 testis (congenital) 752.51
 uterus, uterine (acquired) (acute) (adherent) (any degree) (asymptomatic) (cervix) (postinfectional) (postpartal, old) 621.6
  congenital 752.3
  in pregnancy or childbirth 654.3 ✓5ᵗʰ
   affecting fetus or newborn 763.89
   causing obstructed labor 660.2 ✓5ᵗʰ
    affecting fetus or newborn 763.1
Retrusion, premaxilla (developmental) 524.04
Rett's syndrome 330.8
Reverse, reversed
 peristalsis 787.4
Reye's syndrome 331.81
Reye-Sheehan syndrome (postpartum pituitary necrosis) 253.2
Rh (factor)
 hemolytic disease 773.0
 incompatibility, immunization, or sensitization
  affecting management of pregnancy 656.1 ✓5ᵗʰ
  fetus or newborn 773.0
  transfusion reaction 999.7
 negative mother, affecting fetus or newborn 773.0
 titer elevated 999.7
 transfusion reaction 999.7
Rhabdomyolysis (idiopathic) 728.89
Rhabdomyoma (M8900/0) — see also Neoplasm, connective tissue, benign
 adult (M8904/0) — see Neoplasm, connective tissue, benign
 fetal (M8903/0) — see Neoplasm, connective tissue, benign
 glycogenic (M8904/0) — see Neoplasm, connective tissue, benign
Rhabdomyosarcoma (M8900/3) — see also Neoplasm, connective tissue, malignant
 alveolar (M8920/3) — see Neoplasm, connective tissue, malignant
 embryonal (M8910/3) — see Neoplasm, connective tissue, malignant
 mixed type (M8902/3) — see Neoplasm, connective tissue, malignant
 pleomorphic (M8901/3) — see Neoplasm, connective tissue, malignant

Rhabdosarcoma (M8900/3) — see Rhabdomyosarcoma
Rhesus (factor) (Rh) incompatibility — see Rh, incompatibility
Rheumaticosis — see Rheumatism
Rheumatism, rheumatic (acute NEC) 729.0
 adherent pericardium 393
 arthritis
  acute or subacute — see Fever, rheumatic
  chronic 714.0
   spine 720.0
 articular (chronic) NEC (see also Arthritis) 716.9 ✓5ᵗʰ
  acute or subacute — see Fever, rheumatic
 back 724.9
 blennorrhagic 098.59
 carditis — see Disease, heart, rheumatic
 cerebral — see Fever, rheumatic
 chorea (acute) — see Chorea, rheumatic
 chronic NEC 729.0
 coronary arteritis 391.9
  chronic 398.99
 degeneration, myocardium (see also Degeneration, myocardium, with rheumatic fever) 398.0
 desert 114.0
 febrile — see Fever, rheumatic
 fever — see Fever, rheumatic
 gonococcal 098.59
 gout 274.0
 heart
  disease (see also Disease, heart, rheumatic) 398.90
  failure (chronic) (congestive) (inactive) 398.91
 hemopericardium — see Rheumatic, pericarditis
 hydropericardium — see Rheumatic, pericarditis
 inflammatory (acute) (chronic) (subacute) — see Fever, rheumatic
 intercostal 729.0
  meaning Tietze's disease 733.6
 joint (chronic) NEC (see also Arthritis) 716.9 ✓5ᵗʰ
  acute — see Fever, rheumatic
 mediastinopericarditis — see Rheumatic, pericarditis
 muscular 729.0
 myocardial degeneration (see also Degeneration, myocardium, with rheumatic fever) 398.0
 myocarditis (chronic) (inactive) (with chorea) 398.0
  active or acute 391.2
   with chorea (acute) (rheumatic) (Sydenham's) 392.0
 myositis 729.1
 neck 724.9
 neuralgic 729.0
 neuritis (acute) (chronic) 729.2
 neuromuscular 729.0
 nodose — see Arthritis, nodosa
 nonarticular 729.0
 palindromic 719.30
  ankle 719.37
  elbow 719.32
  foot 719.37
  hand 719.34
  hip 719.35
  knee 719.36

Rheumatism, rheumatic — *continued*
  palindromic — *continued*
    multiple sites 719.39
    pelvic region 719.35
    shoulder (region) 719.31
    specified site NEC 719.38
    wrist 719.33
  pancarditis, acute 391.8
    with chorea (acute) (rheumatic)
        (Sydenham's) 392.0
    chronic or inactive 398.99
  pericarditis (active) (acute) (with effusion) (with
      pneumonia) 391.0
    with chorea (acute) (rheumatic)
        (Sydenham's) 392.0
    chronic or inactive 393
  pericardium — *see* Rheumatic, pericarditis
  pleuropericarditis — *see* Rheumatic,
      pericarditis
  pneumonia 390 [517.1]
  pneumonitis 390 [517.1]
  pneumopericarditis — *see* Rheumatic,
      pericarditis
  polyarthritis
    acute or subacute — *see* Fever, rheumatic
    chronic 714.0
  polyarticular NEC (*see also* Arthritis)
      716.9 ✓5ᵗʰ
  psychogenic 306.0
  radiculitis 729.2
  sciatic 724.3
  septic — *see* Fever, rheumatic
  spine 724.9
  subacute NEC 729.0
  torticollis 723.5
  tuberculous NEC (*see also* Tuberculosis)
      015.9 ✓5ᵗʰ
  typhoid fever 002.0
Rheumatoid — *see also* condition
  lungs 714.81
Rhinitis (atrophic) (catarrhal) (chronic)
    (croupous) (fibrinous) (hyperplastic)
    (hypertrophic) (membranous) (purulent)
    (suppurative) (ulcerative) 472.0
  with
    hay fever (*see also* Fever, hay) 477.9
      with asthma (bronchial) 493.0 ✓5ᵗʰ
    sore throat — *see* Nasopharyngitis
  acute 460
  allergic (nonseasonal) (seasonal) (*see also*
      Fever, hay) 477.9
    with asthma (*see also* Asthma) 493.0 ✓5ᵗʰ
    due to food 477.1
  granulomatous 472.0
  infective 460
  obstructive 472.0
  pneumococcal 460
  syphilitic 095.8
    congenital 090.0
  tuberculous (*see also* Tuberculosis) 012.8 ✓5ᵗʰ
  vasomotor (*see also* Fever, hay) 477.9
Rhinoantritis (chronic) 473.0
  acute 461.0
Rhinodacryolith 375.57
Rhinolalia (aperta) (clausa) (open) 784.49
Rhinolith 478.1
  nasal sinus (*see also* Sinusitis) 473.9
Rhinomegaly 478.1
Rhinopharyngitis (acute) (subacute) (*see also*
    Nasopharyngitis) 460

Rhinopharyngitis — *continued*
  chronic 472.2
  destructive ulcerating 102.5
  mutilans 102.5
Rhinophyma 695.3
Rhinorrhea 478.1
  cerebrospinal (fluid) 349.81
  paroxysmal (*see also* Fever, hay) 477.9
  spasmodic (*see also* Fever, hay) 477.9
Rhinosalpingitis 381.50
  acute 381.51
  chronic 381.52
Rhinoscleroma 040.1
Rhinosporidiosis 117.0
Rhinovirus infection 079.3
Rhizomelique, pseudopolyarthritic 446.5
Rhoads and Bomford anemia (refractory) 284.9
Rhus
  diversiloba dermatitis 692.6
  radicans dermatitis 692.6
  toxicodendron dermatitis 692.6
  venenata dermatitis 692.6
  verniciflua dermatitis 692.6
Rhythm
  atrioventricular nodal 427.89
  disorder 427.9
    coronary sinus 427.89
    ectopic 427.89
    nodal 427.89
  escape 427.89
  heart, abnormal 427.9
    fetus or newborn — *see* Abnormal, heart
        rate
  idioventricular 426.89
    accelerated 427.89
  nodal 427.89
  sleep, inversion 780.55
    nonorganic origin 307.45
Rhytidosis facialis 701.8
Rib — *see also* condition
  cervical 756.2
Riboflavin deficiency 266.0
Rice bodies (*see also* Loose, body, joint)
    718.1 ✓5ᵗʰ
  knee 717.6
Richter's hernia — *see* Hernia, Richter's
Ricinism 988.2
Rickets (active) (acute) (adolescent) (adult) (chest
    wall) (congenital) (current) (infantile)
    (intestinal) 268.0
  celiac 579.0
  fetal 756.4
  hemorrhagic 267
  hypophosphatemic with nephroticglycosuric
      dwarfism 270.0
  kidney 588.0
  late effect 268.1
  renal 588.0
  scurvy 267
  vitamin D-resistant 275.3
Rickettsial disease 083.9
  specified type NEC 083.8
Rickettsialpox 083.2
Rickettsiosis NEC 083.9
  specified type NEC 083.8
  tick-borne 082.9
    specified type NEC 082.8
  vesicular 083.2

Ricord's chancre 091.0
Riddoch's syndrome (visual disorientation) 368.16
Rider's
  bone 733.99
  chancre 091.0
Ridge, alveolus — *see also* condition
  flabby 525.2
Ridged ear 744.29
Riedel's
  disease (ligneous thyroiditis) 245.3
  lobe, liver 751.69
  struma (ligneous thyroiditis) 245.3
  thyroiditis (ligneous) 245.3
Rieger's anomaly or syndrome (mesodermal dysgenesis, anterior ocular segment) 743.44
Riehl's melanosis 709.09
Rietti-Greppi-Micheli anemia or syndrome 282.4
Rieux's hernia — *see* Hernia, Rieux's
Rift Valley fever 066.3
Riga's disease (cachectic aphthae) 529.0
Riga-Fede disease (cachectic aphthae) 529.0
Riggs' disease (compound periodontitis) 523.4
Right middle lobe syndrome 518.0
Rigid, rigidity — *see also* condition
  abdominal 789.4
  articular, multiple congenital 754.89
  back 724.8
  cervix uteri
    in pregnancy or childbirth 654.6
      affecting fetus or newborn 763.89
      causing obstructed labor 660.2
        affecting fetus or newborn 763.1
  hymen (acquired) (congenital) 623.3
  nuchal 781.6
  pelvic floor
    in pregnancy or childbirth 654.4
      affecting fetus or newborn 763.89
      causing obstructed labor 660.2
        affecting fetus or newborn 763.1
  perineum or vulva
    in pregnancy or childbirth 654.8
      affecting fetus or newborn 763.89
      causing obstructed labor 660.2
        affecting fetus or newborn 763.1
  spine 724.8
  vagina
    in pregnancy or childbirth 654.7
      affecting fetus or newborn 763.89
      causing obstructed labor 660.2
        affecting fetus or newborn 763.1
Rigors 780.99
Riley-Day syndrome (familial dysautonomia) 742.8
Ring(s)
  aorta 747.21
  Bandl's, complicating delivery 661.4
    affecting fetus or newborn 763.7
  contraction, complicating delivery 661.4
    affecting fetus or newborn 763.7
  esophageal (congenital) 750.3
  Fleischer (-Kayser) (cornea) 275.1 [371.14]
  hymenal, tight (acquired) (congenital) 623.3
  Kayser-Fleischer (cornea) 275.1 [371.14]
  retraction, uterus, pathological 661.4
    affecting fetus or newborn 763.7

Ring(s) — *continued*
  Schatzki's (esophagus) (congenital) (lower) 750.3
    acquired 530.3
  Soemmering's 366.51
  trachea, abnormal 748.3
  vascular (congenital) 747.21
  Vossius' 921.3
    late effect 366.21
Ringed hair (congenital) 757.4
Ringing in the ear (*see also* Tinnitus) 388.30
Ringworm 110.9
  beard 110.0
  body 110.5
  Burmese 110.9
  corporeal 110.5
  foot 110.4
  groin 110.3
  hand 110.2
  honeycomb 110.0
  nails 110.1
  perianal (area) 110.3
  scalp 110.0
  specified site NEC 110.8
  Tokelau 110.5
Rise, venous pressure 459.89
Risk
  factor — *see* Problem
  suicidal 300.9
Ritter's disease (dermatitis exfoliativa neonatorum) 695.81
Rivalry, sibling 313.3
Rivalta's disease (cervicofacial actinomycosis) 039.3
River blindness 125.3 [360.13]
Robert's pelvis 755.69
  with disproportion (fetopelvic) 653.0
    affecting fetus or newborn 763.1
    causing obstructed labor 660.1
      affecting fetus or newborn 763.1
Robin's syndrome 756.0
Robinson's (hidrotic) ectodermal dysplasia 757.31
Robles' disease (onchocerciasis) 125.3 [360.13]
Rochalimea — *see* Rickettsial disease
Rocky Mountain fever (spotted) 082.0
Rodent ulcer (M8090/3) — *see also* Neoplasm, skin, malignant
  cornea 370.07
Roentgen ray, adverse effect — *see* Effect, adverse, x-ray
Roetheln 056.9
Roger's disease (congenital interventricular septal defect) 745.4
Rokitansky's
  disease (*see also* Necrosis, liver) 570
  tumor 620.2
Rokitansky-Aschoff sinuses (mucosal outpouching of gallbladder) (*see also* Disease, gallbladder) 575.8
Rokitansky-Kuster-Hauser syndrome (congenital absence vagina) 752.49
Rollet's chancre (syphilitic) 091.0
Rolling of head 781.0
Romano-Ward syndrome (prolonged Q-T interval) 794.31

Romanus lesion 720.1
Romberg's disease or syndrome 349.89
Roof, mouth — *see* condition
Rosacea 695.3
  acne 695.3
  keratitis 695.3 *[370.49]*
Rosary, rachitic 268.0
Rose
  cold 477.0
  fever 477.0
  rash 782.1
    epidemic 056.9
    of infants 057.8
Rosen-Castleman-Liebow syndrome (pulmonary proteinosis) 516.0
Rosenbach's erysipelatoid or erysipeloid 027.1
Rosenthal's disease (factor XI deficiency) 286.2
Roseola 057.8
  infantum, infantilis 057.8
Rossbach's disease (hyperchlorhydria) 536.8
  psychogenic 306.4
Rössle-Urbach-Wiethe lipoproteinosis 272.8
Ross river fever 066.3
Rostan's asthma (cardiac) (*see also* Failure, ventricular, left) 428.1
Rot
  Barcoo (*see also* Ulcer, skin) 707.9
  knife-grinders' (*see also* Tuberculosis) 011.4 ✓5ᵗʰ
Rot-Bernhardt disease 355.1
Rotation
  anomalous, incomplete or insufficient — *see* Malrotation
  cecum (congenital) 751.4
  colon (congenital) 751.4
  manual, affecting fetus or newborn 763.89
  spine, incomplete or insufficient 737.8
  tooth, teeth 524.3
  vertebra, incomplete or insufficient 737.8
Röteln 056.9
Roth's disease or meralgia 355.1
Roth-Bernhardt disease or syndrome 355.1
Rothmund (-Thomson) syndrome 757.33
Rotor's disease or syndrome (idiopathic hyperbilirubinemia) 277.4
Rotundum ulcus — *see* Ulcer, stomach
Round
  back (with wedging of vertebrae) 737.10
    late effect of rickets 268.1
  hole, retina 361.31
    with detachment 361.01
  ulcer (stomach) — *see* Ulcer, stomach
  worms (infestation) (large) NEC 127.0
Roussy-Lévy syndrome 334.3
Routine postpartum follow-up V24.2
Roy (-Jutras) syndrome (acropachyderma) 757.39
Rubella (German measles) 056.9
  complicating pregnancy, childbirth, or puerperium 647.5 ✓5ᵗʰ
  complication 056.8
    neurological 056.00
      encephalomyelitis 056.01
      specified type NEC 056.09
    specified type NEC 056.79
  congenital 771.0

Rubella — *continued*
  contact V01.4
  exposure to V01.4
  maternal
    with suspected fetal damage affecting management of pregnancy 655.3 ✓5ᵗʰ
    affecting fetus or newborn 760.2
      manifest rubella in infant 771.0
  specified complications NEC 056.79
  vaccination, prophylactic (against) V04.3
Rubeola (measles) (*see also* Measles) 055.9
  complicated 055.8
  meaning rubella (*see also* Rubella) 056.9
  scarlatinosis 057.8
Rubeosis iridis 364.42
  diabetica 250.5 ✓5ᵗʰ *[364.42]*
Rubinstein-Taybi's syndrome (brachydactylia, short stature, and mental retardation) 759.89
Rud's syndrome (mental deficiency, epilepsy, and infantilism) 759.89
Rudimentery (congenital) — *see also* Agenesis
  arm 755.22
  bone 756.9
  cervix uteri 752.49
  eye (*see also* Microphthalmos) 743.10
  fallopian tube 752.19
  leg 755.32
  lobule of ear 744.21
  patella 755.64
  respiratory organs in thoracopagus 759.4
  tracheal bronchus 748.3
  uterine horn 752.9
  uterus 752.3
    in male 752.7
    solid or with cavity 752.3
  vagina 752.49
Ruiter-Pompen (-Wyers) syndrome (angiokeratoma corporis diffusum) 272.7
Ruled out condition (*see also* Observation, suspected) V71.9
Rumination — *see also* Vomiting
  neurotic 300.3
  obsessional 300.3
  psychogenic 307.53
Runaway reaction — *see also* Disturbance, conduct
  socialized 312.2 ✓5ᵗʰ
  undersocialized, unsocialized 312.1 ✓5ᵗʰ
Runeberg's disease (progressive pernicious anemia) 281.0
Runge's syndrome (postmaturity) 766.2
Rupia 091.3
  congenital 090.0
  tertiary 095.9
Rupture, ruptured 553.9
  abdominal viscera NEC 799.8
    obstetrical trauma 665.5 ✓5ᵗʰ
  abscess (spontaneous) — *see* Abscess, by site
  amnion — *see* Rupture, membranes
  aneurysm — *see* Aneurysm
  anus (sphincter) — *see* Laceration, anus
  aorta, aortic 441.5
    abdominal 441.3
    arch 441.1
    ascending 441.1
    descending 441.5
      abdominal 441.3
      thoracic 441.1

Index to Diseases

Rupture, ruptured — *continued*
  aorta, aortic — *continued*
    syphilitic 093.0
    thoracoabdominal 441.6
    thorax, thoracic 441.1
    transverse 441.1
    traumatic (thoracic) 901.0
      abdominal 902.0
    valve or cusp (*see also* Endocarditis, aortic) 424.1
  appendix (with peritonitis) 540.0
    with peritoneal abscess 540.1
    traumatic — *see* Injury, internal, gastrointestinal tract
  arteriovenous fistula, brain (congenital) 430
  artery 447.2
    brain (*see also* Hemorrhage, brain) 431
    coronary (*see also* Infarct, myocardium) 410.9 ✓5ᵗʰ
    heart (*see also* Infarct, myocardium) 410.9 ✓5ᵗʰ
    pulmonary 417.8
    traumatic (complication) (*see also* Injury, blood vessel, by site) 904.9
  bile duct, except cystic (*see also* Disease, biliary) 576.3
    cystic 575.4
    traumatic — *see* Injury, internal, intra-abdominal
  bladder (sphincter) 596.6
    with
      abortion — *see* Abortion, by type, with damage to pelvic organs
      ectopic pregnancy (*see also* categories 633.0-633.9) 639.2
      molar pregnancy (*see also* categories 630-632) 639.2
    following
      abortion 639.2
      ectopic or molar pregnancy 639.2
    nontraumatic 596.6
    obstetrical trauma 665.5 ✓5ᵗʰ
    spontaneous 596.6
    traumatic — *see* Injury, internal, bladder
  blood vessel (*see also* Hemorrhage) 459.0
    brain (*see also* Hemorrhage, brain) 431
    heart (*see also* Infarct, myocardium) 410.9 ✓5ᵗʰ
    traumatic (complication) (*see also* Injury, blood vessel, by site) 904.9
  bone — *see* Fracture, by site
  bowel 569.89
    traumatic — *see* Injury, internal, intestine
  Bowman's membrane 371.31
  brain
    aneurysm (congenital) (*see also* Hemorrhage, subarachnoid) 430
      late effect — *see* Late effect(s) (of) cerebrovascular disease
      syphilitic 094.87
    hemorrhagic (*see also* Hemorrhage, brain) 431
    injury at birth 767.0
    syphilitic 094.89
  capillaries 448.9
  cardiac (*see also* Infarct, myocardium) 410.9 ✓5ᵗʰ
  cartilage (articular) (current) — *see also* Sprain, by site
    knee — *see* Tear, meniscus
    semilunar — *see* Tear, meniscus

Rupture, ruptured — *continued*
  cecum (with peritonitis) 540.0
    with peritoneal abscess 540.1
    traumatic 863.89
      with open wound into cavity 863.99
  cerebral aneurysm (congenital) (*see also* Hemorrhage, subarachnoid) 430
    late effect — *see* Late effect(s) (of) cerebrovascular disease
  cervix (uteri)
    with
      abortion — *see* Abortion, by type, with damage to pelvic organs
      ectopic pregnancy (*see also* categories 633.0-633.9) 639.2
      molar pregnancy (*see also* categories 630-632) 639.2
    following
      abortion 639.2
      ectopic or molar pregnancy 639.2
    obstetrical trauma 665.3 ✓5ᵗʰ
    traumatic — *see* Injury, internal, cervix
  chordae tendineae 429.5
  choroid (direct) (indirect) (traumatic) 363.63
  circle of Willis (*see also* Hemorrhage, subarachnoid) 430
    late effect — *see* Late effect(s) (of) cerebrovascular disease
  colon 569.89
    traumatic — *see* Injury, internal, colon
  cornea (traumatic) — *see also* Rupture, eye
    due to ulcer 370.00
  coronary (artery) (thrombotic) (*see also* Infarct, myocardium) 410.9 ✓5ᵗʰ
  corpus luteum (infected) (ovary) 620.1
  cyst — *see* Cyst
  cystic duct (*see also* Disease, gallbladder) 575.4
  Descemet's membrane 371.33
    traumatic — *see* Rupture, eye
  diaphragm — *see also* Hernia, diaphragm
    traumatic — *see* Injury, internal, diaphragm
  diverticulum
    bladder 596.3
    intestine (large) (*see also* Diverticula) 562.10
    small 562.00
  duodenal stump 537.89
  duodenum (ulcer) — *see* Ulcer, duodenum, with perforation
  ear drum (*see also* Perforation, tympanum) 384.20
    with otitis media — *see* Otitis media
    traumatic — *see* Wound, open, ear
  esophagus 530.4
    traumatic 862.22
      with open wound into cavity 862.32
      cervical region — *see* Wound, open, esophagus
  eye (without prolapse of intraocular tissue) 871.0
    with
      exposure of intraocular tissue 871.1
      partial loss of intraocular tissue 871.2
      prolapse of intraocular tissue 871.1
    due to burn 940.5
  fallopian tube 620.8
    due to pregnancy — *see* Pregnancy, tubal
    traumatic — *see* Injury, internal, fallopian tube

✓4ᵗʰ Fourth-digit Required   ✓5ᵗʰ Fifth-digit Required

Rupture, ruptured — *continued*
  fontanel 767.3
  free wall (ventricle) (*see also* Infarct,
    myocardium) 410.9 ✓5ᵗʰ
  gallbladder or duct (*see also* Disease,
    gallbladder) 575.4
    traumatic — *see* Injury, internal,
      gallbladder
  gastric (*see also* Rupture, stomach) 537.89
    vessel 459.0
  globe (eye) (traumatic) — *see* Rupture, eye
  graafian follicle (hematoma) 620.0
  heart (auricle) (ventricle) (*see also* Infarct,
    myocardium) 410.9 ✓5ᵗʰ
    infectional 422.90
    traumatic — *see* Rupture, myocardium,
      traumatic
  hymen 623.8
  internal
    organ, traumatic — *see also* Injury,
      internal, by site
      heart — *see* Rupture, myocardium,
        traumatic
      kidney — *see* Rupture, kidney
      liver — *see* Rupture, liver
      spleen — *see* Rupture, spleen, traumatic
    semilunar cartilage — *see* Tear, meniscus
  intervertebral disc — *see* Displacement,
    intervertebral disc
    traumatic (current) — *see* Dislocation,
      vertebra
  intestine 569.89
    traumatic — *see* Injury, internal, intestine
  intracranial, birth injury 767.0
  iris 364.76
    traumatic — *see* Rupture, eye
  joint capsule — *see* Sprain, by site
  kidney (traumatic) 866.03
    with open wound into cavity 866.13
    due to birth injury 767.8
    nontraumatic 593.89
  lacrimal apparatus (traumatic) 870.2
  lens (traumatic) 366.20
  ligament — *see also* Sprain, by site
    with open wound — *see* Wound, open, by
      site
    old (*see also* Disorder, cartilage, articular)
      718.0 ✓5ᵗʰ
  liver (traumatic) 864.04
    with open wound into cavity 864.14
    due to birth injury 767.8
    nontraumatic 573.8
  lymphatic (node) (vessel) 457.8
  marginal sinus (placental) (with hemorrhage)
    641.2 ✓5ᵗʰ
    affecting fetus or newborn 762.1
  meaning hernia — *see* Hernia
  membrana tympani (*see also* Perforation,
    tympanum) 384.20
    with otitis media — *see* Otitis media
    traumatic — *see* Wound, open, ear
  membranes (spontaneous)
    artificial
      delayed delivery following 658.3 ✓5ᵗʰ
        affecting fetus or newborn 761.1
        fetus or newborn 761.1
      delayed delivery following 658.2 ✓5ᵗʰ
        affecting fetus or newborn 761.1
      premature (less than 24 hours prior to
        onset of labor) 658.1 ✓5ᵗʰ
        affecting fetus or newborn 761.1

Rupture, ruptured — *continued*
  membranes — *continued*
    premature — *continued*
      delayed delivery following 658.2 ✓5ᵗʰ
        affecting fetus or newborn 761.1
  meningeal artery (*see also* Hemorrhage,
    subarachnoid) 430
    late effect — *see* Late effect(s) (of)
      cerebrovascular diseas
  meniscus (knee) — *see also* Tear, meniscus
    old (*see also* Derangement, meniscus)
      717.5
      site other than knee — *see* Disorder,
        cartilage, articular
      site other than knee — *see* Sprain, by site
  mesentery 568.89
    traumatic — *see* Injury, internal, mesentery
  mitral — *see* Insufficiency, mitral
  muscle (traumatic) NEC — *see also* Sprain, by
    site
    with open wound — *see* Wound, open, by
      site
    nontraumatic 728.83
  musculotendinous cuff (nontraumatic)
    (shoulder) 840.4
  mycotic aneurysm, causing cerebral
    hemorrhage (*see also* Hemorrhage,
      subarachnoid) 430
    late effect — *see* Late effect(s) (of)
      cerebrovascular disease
  myocardium, myocardial (*see also* Infarct,
    myocardium) 410.9 ✓5ᵗʰ
    traumatic 861.03
      with open wound into thorax 861.13
  nontraumatic (meaning hernia) (*see also*
    Hernia, by site) 553.9
  obstructed (*see also* Hernia, by site, with
    obstruction) 552.9
    gangrenous (*see also* Hernia, by site, with
      gangrene) 551.9
  operation wound 998.32   ▲
    internal 998.31   ●
  ovary, ovarian 620.8
    corpus luteum 620.1
    follicle (graafian) 620.0
  oviduct 620.8
    due to pregnancy — *see* Pregnancy, tubal
  pancreas 577.8
    traumatic — *see* Injury, internal, pancreas
  papillary muscle (ventricular) 429.6
  pelvic
    floor, complicating delivery 664.1 ✓5ᵗʰ
    organ NEC — *see* Injury, pelvic, organs
  penis (traumatic) — *see* Wound, open, penis
  perineum 624.8
    during delivery (*see also* Laceration,
      perineum, complicating delivery)
      664.4 ✓5ᵗʰ
  pharynx (nontraumatic) (spontaneous) 478.29
  pregnant uterus (before onset of labor)
    665.0 ✓5ᵗʰ
  prostate (traumatic) — *see* Injury, internal,
    prostate
  pulmonary
    artery 417.8
    valve (heart) (*see also* Endocarditis,
      pulmonary) 424.3
    vein 417.8
    vessel 417.8
  pupil, sphincter 364.75
  pus tube (*see also* Salpingo-oophoritis) 614.2

Index to Diseases

Rupture, ruptured — *continued*
  pyosalpinx (*see also* Salpingo-oophoritis)
    614.2
  rectum 569.49
    traumatic — *see* Injury, internal, rectum
  retina, retinal (traumatic) (without
    detachment) 361.30
    with detachment (*see also* Detachment,
      retina, with retinal defect) 361.00
  rotator cuff (capsule) (traumatic) 840.4
    nontraumatic, complete 727.61
  sclera 871.0
  semilunar cartilage, knee (*see also* Tear,
    meniscus) 836.2
    old (*see also* Derangement, meniscus)
      717.5
  septum (cardiac) 410.8
  sigmoid 569.89
    traumatic — *see* Injury, internal, colon,
      sigmoid
  sinus of Valsalva 747.29
  spinal cord — *see also* Injury, spinal, by site
    due to injury at birth 767.4
    fetus or newborn 767.4
    syphilitic 094.89
    traumatic — *see also* Injury, spinal, by site
      with fracture — *see* Fracture, vertebra,
        by site, with spinal cord injury
  spleen 289.59
    congenital 767.8
    due to injury at birth 767.8
    malarial 084.9
    nontraumatic 289.59
    spontaneous 289.59
    traumatic 865.04
      with open wound into cavity 865.14
  splenic vein 459.0
  stomach 537.89
    due to injury at birth 767.8
    traumatic — *see* Injury, internal, stomach
    ulcer — *see* Ulcer, stomach, with
      perforation
  synovium 727.50
    specified site NEC 727.59
  tendon (traumatic) — *see also* Sprain, by site
    with open wound — *see* Wound, open, by
      site
    Achilles 845.09
      nontraumatic 727.67
    ankle 845.09
      nontraumatic 727.68
    biceps (long bead) 840.8
      nontraumatic 727.62
    foot 845.10
      interphalangeal (joint) 845.13
      metatarsophalangeal (joint) 845.12
      nontraumatic 727.68
      specified site NEC 845.19
      tarsometatarsal (joint) 845.11
    hand 842.10
      carpometacarpal (joint) 842.11
      interphalangeal (joint) 842.13
      metacarpophalangeal (joint) 842.12
      nontraumatic 727.63
        extensors 727.63
        flexors 727.64
      specified site NEC 842.19
      nontraumatic 727.60
        specified site NEC 727.69
    patellar 844.8
      nontraumatic 727.66

Rupture, ruptured — *continued*
  tendon — *continued*
    quadriceps 844.8
      nontraumatic 727.65
    rotator cuff (capsule) 840.4
      nontraumatic, complete 727.61
    wrist 842.00
      carpal (joint) 842.01
      nontraumatic 727.63
        extensors 727.63
        flexors 727.64
      radiocarpal (joint) (ligament) 842.02
      radioulnar (joint), distal 842.09
      specified site NEC 842.09
  testis (traumatic) 878.2
    complicated 878.3
    due to syphilis 095.8
  thoracic duct 457.8
  tonsil 474.8
  traumatic
    with open wound — *see* Wound, open, by
      site
    aorta — *see* Rupture, aorta, traumatic
    ear drum — *see* Wound, open, ear, drum
    external site — *see* Wound, open, by site
    eye 871.2
    globe (eye) — *see* Wound, open, eyeball
    internal organ (abdomen, chest, or pelvis)
      — *see also* Injury, internal, by site
      heart — *see* Rupture, myocardium,
        traumatic
      kidney — *see* Rupture, kidney
      liver — *see* Rupture, liver
      spleen — *see* Rupture, spleen, traumatic
    ligament, muscle, or tendon — *see also*
      Sprain, by site
      with open wound — *see* Wound, open,
        by site
    meaning hernia — *see* Hernia
  tricuspid (heart) (valve) — *see* Endocarditis,
    tricuspid
  tube, tubal 620.8
    abscess (*see also* Salpingo-oophoritis) 614.2
    due to pregnancy — *see* Pregnancy, tubal
  tympanum, tympanic (membrane) (*see also*
    Perforation, tympanum) 384.20
    with otitis media — *see* Otitis media
    traumatic — *see* Wound, open, ear, drum
  umbilical cord 663.8
    fetus or newborn 772.0
  ureter (traumatic) (*see also* Injury, internal,
    ureter) 867.2
    nontraumatic 593.89
  urethra 599.84
    with
      abortion — *see* Abortion, by type, with
        damage to pelvic organs
      ectopic pregnancy (*see also* categories
        633.0-633.9) 639.2
      molar pregnancy (*see also* categories
        630-632) 639.2
    following
      abortion 639.2
      ectopic or molar pregnancy 639.2
    obstetrical trauma 665.5
    traumatic — *see* Injury, internal urethra
  uterosacral ligament 620.8
  uterus (traumatic) — *see also* Injury, internal
    uterus
    affecting fetus or newborn 763.89
    during labor 665.1

Rupture, ruptured — *continued*
  uterus — *continued*
    nonpuerperal, nontraumatic 621.8
    nontraumatic 621.8
    pregnant (during labor) 665.1 ✓5ᵗʰ
      before labor 665.0 ✓5ᵗʰ
  vagina 878.6
    complicated 878.7
    complicating delivery — *see* Laceration, vagina, complicating delivery
  valve, valvular (heart) — *see* Endocarditis
  varicose vein — *see* Varicose, vein
  varix — *see* Varix
  vena cava 459.0
  ventricle (free wall) (left) (*see also* Infarct, myocardium) 410.9 ✓5ᵗʰ
  vesical (urinary) 596.6
    traumatic — *see* Injury, internal, bladder
  vessel (blood) 459.0
    pulmonary 417.8
  viscus 799.8
  vulva 878.4
    complicated 878.5
    complicating delivery 664.0 ✓5ᵗʰ
Russell's dwarf (uterine dwarfism and craniofacial dysostosis) 759.89
Russell's dysentery 004.8
Russell (-Silver) syndrome (congenital hemihypertrophy and short stature) 759.89
Russian spring-summer type encephalitis 063.0
Rust's disease (tuberculous spondylitis) 015.0 ✓5ᵗʰ *[720.81]*
Rustitskii's disease (multiple myeloma) (M9730/3) 203.0 ✓5ᵗʰ
Ruysch's disease (Hirschsprung's disease) 751.3
Rytand-Lipsitch syndrome (complete atrioventricular bloc) 426.0

S

Saber
  shin 090.5
  tibia 090.5
Sac, lacrimal — *see* condition
Saccharomyces infection (*see also* Candidiasis) 112.9
Saccharopinuria 270.7
Saccular — *see* condition
Sacculation
  aorta (nonsyphilitic) (*see also* Aneurysm, aorta) 441.9
    ruptured 441.5
    syphilitic 093.0
  bladder 596.3
  colon 569.89
  intralaryngeal (congenital) (ventricular) 748.3
  larynx (congenital) (ventricular) 748.3
  organ or site, congenital — *see* Distortion
  pregnant uterus, complicating delivery 654.4 ✓5ᵗʰ
    affecting fetus or newborn 763.1
    causing obstructed labor 660.2 ✓5ᵗʰ
      affecting fetus or newborn 763.1
  rectosigmoid 569.89
  sigmoid 569.89
  ureter 593.89
  urethra 599.2
  vesical 596.3
Sachs (-Tay) disease (amaurotic familial idiocy) 330.1
Sacks-Libman disease 710.0 *[424.91]*
Sacralgia 724.6
Sacralization
  fifth lumbar vertebra 756.15
  incomplete (vertebra) 756.15
Sacrodynia 724.6
Sacroiliac joint — *see* condition
Sacroiliitis NEC 720.2
Sacrum — *see* condition
Saddle
  back 737.8
  embolus, aorta 444.0
  nose 738.0
    congenital 754.0
    due to syphilis 090.5
Sadism (sexual) 302.84
Saemisch's ulcer 370.04
Saenger's syndrome 379.46
Sago spleen 277.3
Sailors' skin 692.74
Saint
  Anthony's fire (*see also* Erysipelas) 035
  Guy's dance — *see* Chorea
  Louis-type encephalitis 062.3
  triad (*see also* Hernia, diaphragm) 553.3
  Vitus' dance — *see* Chorea
Salicylism
  correct substance properly administered 535.4 ✓5ᵗʰ
  overdose or wrong substance given or taken 965.1
Salivary duct or gland — *see also* condition
  virus disease 078.5
Salivation (excessive) (*see also* Ptyalism) 527.7

Salmonella (aertrycke) (choleraesuis) (enteritidis) (gallinarum) (suipestifer) (typhimurium) (*see also* Infection, Salmonella) 003.9
　arthritis 003.23
　carrier (suspected) of V02.3
　meningitis 003.21
　osteomyelitis 003.24
　pneumonia 003.22
　septicemia 003.1
　typhosa 002.0
　　carrier (suspected) of V02.1
Salmonellosis 003.0
　with pneumonia 003.22
Salpingitis (catarrhal) (fallopian tube) (nodular) (pseudofollicular) (purulent) (septic) (*see also* Salpingo-oophoritis) 614.2
　ear 381.50
　　acute 381.51
　　chronic 381.52
　Eustachian (tube) 381.50
　　acute 381.51
　　chronic 381.52
　follicularis 614.1
　gonococcal (chronic) 098.37
　　acute 098.17
　interstitial, chronic 614.1
　isthmica nodosa 614.1
　old — *see* Salpingo-oophoritis, chronic
　puerperal, postpartum, childbirth 670 ✓4ᵗʰ
　specific (chronic) 098.37
　　acute 098.17
　tuberculous (acute) (chronic) (*see also* Tuberculosis) 016.6 ✓5ᵗʰ
　venereal (chronic) 098.37
　　acute 098.17
Salpingocele 620.4
Salpingo-oophoritis (catarrhal) (purulent) (ruptured) (septic) (suppurative) 614.2
　acute 614.0
　　with
　　　abortion — *see* Abortion, by type, with sepsis
　　　ectopic pregnancy (*see also* categories 633.0-633.9) 639.0
　　　molar pregnancy (*see also* categories 630-632) 639.0
　　following
　　　abortion 639.0
　　　ectopic or molar pregnancy 639.0
　　gonococcal 098.17
　　puerperal, postpartum, childbirth 670 ✓4ᵗʰ
　　tuberculous (*see also* Tuberculosis) 016.6 ✓5ᵗʰ
　chronic 614.1
　　gonococcal 098.37
　　tuberculous (*see also* Tuberculosis) 016.6 ✓5ᵗʰ
　complicating pregnancy 646.6 ✓5ᵗʰ
　　affecting fetus or newborn 760.8
　gonococcal (chronic) 098.37
　　acute 098.17
　old — *see* Salpingo-oophoritis, chronic
　puerperal 670 ✓4ᵗʰ
　specific — *see* Salpingo-oophoritis, gonococcal
　subacute (*see also* Salpingo-oophoritis, acute) 614.0
　tuberculous (acute) (chronic) (*see also* Tuberculosis) 016.6 ✓5ᵗʰ
　venereal — *see* Salpingo-oophoritis, gonococcal

Salpingo-ovaritis (*see also* Salpingoooophoritis) 614.2
Salpingoperitonitis (*see also* Salpingo-oophoritis) 614.2
Salt-losing
　nephritis (*see also* Disease, renal) 593.9
　syndrome (*see also* Disease, renal) 593.9
Salt-rheum (*see also* Eczema) 692.9
Salzmann's nodular dystrophy 371.46
Sampson's cyst or tumor 617.1
Sandblasters'
　asthma 502
　lung 502
Sander's disease (paranoia) 297.1
Sandfly fever 066.0
Sandhoff's disease 330.1
Sanfilippo's syndrome (mucopolysaccharidosis III) 277.5
Sanger-Brown's ataxia 334.2
San Joaquin Valley fever 114.0
Sao Paulo fever or typhus 082.0
Saponification, mesenteric 567.8
Sapremia — *see* Septicemia
Sarcocele (benign)
　syphilitic 095.8
　　congenital 090.5
Sarcoepiplocele (*see also* Hernia) 553.9
Sarcoepiplomphalocele (*see also* Hernia, umbilicus) 553.1
Sarcoid (any site) 135
　with lung involvement 135 [517.8]
　Boeck's 135
　Darier-Roussy 135
　Spiegler-Fendt 686.8
Sarcoidosis 135
　cardiac 135 [425.8]
　lung 135 [517.8]
Sarcoma (M8800/3) — *see also* Neoplasm, connective tissue, malignant
　alveolar soft part (M9581/3) — *see* Neoplasm, connective tissue, malignant
　ameloblastic (M9330/3) 170.1
　　upper jaw (bone) 170.0
　botryoid (M8910/3) — *see* Neoplasm, connective tissue, malignant
　botryoides (M8910/3) — *see* Neoplasm, connective tissue, malignant
　cerebellar (M9480/3) 191.6
　　circumscribed (arachnoidal) (M9471/3) 191.6
　circumscribed (arachnoidal) cerebellar (M9471/3) 191.6
　clear cell, of tendons and aponeuroses (M9044/3) — *see* Neoplasm, connective tissue, malignant
　embryonal (M8991/3) — *see* Neoplasm, connective tissue, malignant
　endometrial (stromal) (M8930/3) 182.0
　　isthmus 182.1
　endothelial (M9130/3) — *see also* Neoplasm, connective tissue, malignant
　　bone (M9260/3) — *see* Neoplasm, bone, malignant
　epithelioid cell (M8804/3) — *see* Neoplasm, connective tissue, malignant
　Ewing's (M9260/3) — *see* Neoplasm, bone, malignant

Sarcoma — *continued*
 germinoblastic (diffuse) (M9632/3) 202.8 ☑5ᵗʰ
 follicular (M9697/3) 202.0 ☑5ᵗʰ
 giant cell (M8802/3) — *see also* Neoplasm, connective tissue, malignant
  bone (M9250/3) — *see* Neoplasm, bone, malignant
 glomoid (M8710/3) — *see* Neoplasm, connective tissue, malignant
 granulocytic (M9930/3) 205.3 ☑5ᵗʰ
 hemangioendothelial (M9130/3) — *see* Neoplasm, connective tissue, malignant
 hemorrhagic, multiple (M9140/3) — *see* Kaposi's, sarcoma
 Hodgkin's (M9662/3) 201.2 ☑5ᵗʰ
 immunoblastic (M9612/3) 200.8 ☑5ᵗʰ
 Kaposi's (M9140/3) — *see* Kaposi's, sarcoma
 Kupffer cell (M9124/3) 155.0
 leptomeningeal (M9530/3) — *see* Neoplasm, meninges, malignant
 lymphangioendothelial (M9170/3) — *see* Neoplasm, connective tissue, malignant
 lymphoblastic (M9630/3) 200.1 ☑5ᵗʰ
 lymphocytic (M9620/3) 200.1 ☑5ᵗʰ
 mast cell (M9740/3) 202.6 ☑5ᵗʰ
 melanotic (M8720/3) — *see* Melanoma
 meningeal (M9530/3) — *see* Neoplasm, meninges, malignant
 meningothelial (M9530/3) — *see* Neoplasm, meninges, malignant
 mesenchymal (M8800/3) — *see also* Neoplasm, connective tissue, malignant
  mixed (M8990/3) — *see* Neoplasm, connective tissue, malignant
 mesothelial (M9050/3) — *see* Neoplasm, by site, malignant
 monstrocellular (M9481/3)
  specified site — *see* Neoplasm, by site, malignant
  unspecified site 191.9
 myeloid (M9930/3) 205.3 ☑5ᵗʰ
 neurogenic (M9540/3) — *see* Neoplasm, connective tissue, malignant
 odontogenic (M9270/3) 170.1
  upper jaw (bone) 170.0
 osteoblastic (M9180/3) — *see* Neoplasm, bone, malignant
 osteogenic (M9180/3) — *see also* Neoplasm, bone, malignant
  juxtacortical (M9190/3) — *see* Neoplasm, bone, malignant
  periosteal (M9190/3) — *see* Neoplasm, bone, malignant
 periosteal (M8812/3) — *see also* Neoplasm, bone, malignant
  osteogenic (M9190/3) — *see* Neoplasm, bone, malignant
 plasma cell (M9731/3) 203.8 ☑5ᵗʰ
 pleomorphic cell (M8802/3) — *see* Neoplasm, connective tissue, malignant
 reticuloendothelial (M9720/3) 202.3 ☑5ᵗʰ
 reticulum cell (M9640/3) 200.0 ☑5ᵗʰ
  nodular (M9642/3) 200.0 ☑5ᵗʰ
  pleomorphic cell type (M9641/3) 200.0 ☑5ᵗʰ
 round cell (M8803/3) — *see* Neoplasm, connective tissue, malignant
 small cell (M8803/3) — *see* Neoplasm, connective tissue, malignant
 spindle cell (M8801/3) — *see* Neoplasm, connective tissue, malignant

Sarcoma — *continued*
 stromal (endometrial) (M8930/3) 182.0
  isthmus 182.1
 synovial (M9040/3) — *see also* Neoplasm, connective tissue, malignant
  biphasic type (M9043/3) — *see* Neoplasm, connective tissue, malignant
  epithelioid cell type (M9042/3) — *see* Neoplasm, connective tissue, malignant
  spindle cell type (M9041/3) — *see* Neoplasm, connective tissue, malignant

Sarcomatosis
 meningeal (M9539/3) — *see* Neoplasm, meninges, malignant
 specified site NEC (M8800/3) — *see* Neoplasm, connective tissue, malignant
 unspecified site (M8800/6) 171.9

Sarcosinemia 270.8
Sarcosporidiosis 136.5
Saturnine — *see* condition
Saturnism 984.9
 specified type of lead — *see* Table of Drugs and Chemicals
Satyriasis 302.89
Sauriasis — *see* Ichthyosis
Sauriderma 757.39
Sauriosis — *see* Ichthyosis
Savill's disease (epidemic exfoliative dermatitis) 695.89
SBE (subacute bacterial endocarditis) 421.0
Scabies (any site) 133.0
Scabs 782.8
Scaglietti-Dagnini syndrome (acromegalic macrospondylitis) 253.0
Scald, scalded — *see also* Burn, by site
 skin syndrome 695.1
Scalenus anticus (anterior) syndrome 353.0
Scales 782.8
Scalp — *see* condition
Scaphocephaly 756.0
Scaphoiditis, tarsal 732.5
Scapulalgia 733.90
Scapulohumeral myopathy 359.1
Scar, scarring (*see also* Cicatrix) 709.2
 adherent 709.2
 atrophic 709.2
 cervix
  in pregnancy or childbirth 654.6 ☑5ᵗʰ
   affecting fetus or newborn 763.89
   causing obstructed labor 660.2 ☑5ᵗʰ
    affecting fetus or newborn 763.1
 cheloid 701.4
 chorioretinal 363.30
  disseminated 363.35
  macular 363.32
  peripheral 363.34
  posterior pole NEC 363.33
 choroid (*see also* Scar, chorioretinal) 363.30
 compression, pericardial 423.9
 congenital 757.39
 conjunctiva 372.64
 cornea 371.00
  xerophthalmic 264.6

Index to Diseases

Scar, scarring — *continued*
  due to previous cesarean delivery,
    complicating pregnancy or childbirth
      654.2 ✓5ᵗʰ
    affecting fetus or newborn 763.89
  duodenal (bulb) (cap) 537.3
  hypertrophic 701.4
  keloid 701.4
  labia 624.4
  lung (base) 518.89
  macula 363.32
    disseminated 363.35
    peripheral 363.34
  muscle 728.89
  myocardium, myocardial 412
  painful 709.2
  papillary muscle 429.81
  posterior pole NEC 363.33
    macular — *see* Scar, macula
  postnecrotic (hepatic) (liver) 571.9
  psychic V15.49
  retina (*see also* Scar, chorioretinal) 363.30
  trachea 478.9
  uterus 621.8
    in pregnancy or childbirth NEC 654.9 ✓5ᵗʰ
      affecting fetus or newborn 763.89
      due to previous cesarean delivery
        654.2 ✓5ᵗʰ
  vulva 624.4
Scarabiasis 134.1
Scarlatina 034.1
  anginosa 034.1
  maligna 034.1
  myocarditis, acute 034.1 *[422.0]*
    old (*see also* Myocarditis) 429.0
  otitis media 034.1 *[382.02]*
  ulcerosa 034.1
Scarlatinella 057.8
Scarlet fever (albuminuria) (angina) (convulsions) (lesions of lid) (rash) 034.1
Schamberg's disease, dermatitis, or dermatosis (progressive pigmentary dermatosis) 709.09
Schatzki's ring (esophagus) (lower) (congenital) 750.3
  acquired 530.3
Schaufenster krankheit 413.9
Schaumann's
  benign lymphogranulomatosis 135
  disease (sarcoidosis) 135
  syndrome (sarcoidosis) 135
Scheie's syndrome (mucopolysaccharidosis IS) 277.5
Schenck's disease (sporotrichosis) 117.1
Scheuermann's disease or osteochondrosis 732.0
Scheuthauer-Marie-Sainton syndrome (cleidocranialis dysostosis) 755.59
Schilder (-Flatau) disease 341.1
Schilling-type monocytic leukemia (M9890/3) 206.9 ✓5ᵗʰ
Schimmelbusch's disease, cystic mastitis, or hyperplasia 610.1
Schirmer's syndrome (encephalocutaneous angiomatosis) 759.6
Schistocelia 756.79
Schistoglossia 750.13

Schizophrenia, schizophrenic

Schistosoma infestation — *see* Infestation, Schistosoma
Schistosomiasis 120.9
  Asiatic 120.2
  bladder 120.0
  chestermani 120.8
  colon 120.1
  cutaneous 120.3
  due to
    S. hematobium 120.0
    S. japonicum 120.2
    S. mansoni 120.1
    S. mattheii 120.8
  eastern 120.2
  genitourinary tract 120.0
  intestinal 120.1
  lung 120.2
  Manson's (intestinal) 120.1
  Oriental 120.2
  pulmonary 120.2
  specified type NEC 120.8
  vesical 120.0
Schizencephaly 742.4
Schizo-affective psychosis (*see also* Schizophrenia) 295.7 ✓5ᵗʰ
Schizodontia 520.2
Schizoid personality 301.20
  introverted 301.21
  schizotypal 301.22
Schizophrenia, schizophrenic (reaction) 295.9 ✓5ᵗʰ

> Note — Use the following fifth-digit subclassification with category 295:
>
> 0   unspecified
> 1   subchronic
> 2   chronic
> 3   subchronic with acute exacerbation
> 4   chronic with acute exacerbation
> 5   in remission

  acute (attack) NEC 295.8 ✓5ᵗʰ
    episode 295.4 ✓5ᵗʰ
  atypical form 295.8 ✓5ᵗʰ
  borderline 295.5 ✓5ᵗʰ
  catalepsy 295.2 ✓5ᵗʰ
  catatonic (type) (acute) (excited) (withdrawn) 295.2 ✓5ᵗʰ
  childhood (type) (*see also* Psychosis, childhood) 299.9 ✓5ᵗʰ
  chronic NEC 295.6 ✓5ᵗʰ
  coenesthesiopathic 295.8 ✓5ᵗʰ
  cyclic (type) 295.7 ✓5ᵗʰ
  disorganized (type) 295.1 ✓5ᵗʰ
  flexibilitas cerea 295.2 ✓5ᵗʰ
  hebephrenic (type) (acute) 295.1 ✓5ᵗʰ
  incipient 295.5 ✓5ᵗʰ
  latent 295.5 ✓5ᵗʰ
  paranoid (type) (acute) 295.3 ✓5ᵗʰ
  paraphrenic (acute) 295.3 ✓5ᵗʰ
  prepsychotic 295.5 ✓5ᵗʰ
  primary (acute) 295.0 ✓5ᵗʰ
  prodromal 295.5 ✓5ᵗʰ
  pseudoneurotic 295.5 ✓5ᵗʰ
  pseudopsychopathic 295.5 ✓5ᵗʰ
  reaction 295.9 ✓5ᵗʰ
  residual (state) (type) 295.6 ✓5ᵗʰ
  restzustand 295.6 ✓5ᵗʰ

Schizophrenia, schizophrenic — continued
 schizo-affective (type) (depressed) (excited) 295.7
 schizophreniform type 295.4
 simple (type) (acute) 295.0
 simplex (acute) 295.0
 specified type NEC 295.8
 syndrome of childhood NEC (see also Psychosis, childhood) 299.9
 undifferentiated 295.9
  acute 295.8
  chronic 295.6
Schizothymia 301.20
 introverted 301.21
 schizotypal 301.22
Schlafkrankheit 086.5
Schlatter's tibia (osteochondrosis) 732.4
Schlatter-Osgood disease (osteochondrosis, tibial tubercle) 732.4
Schloffer's tumor (see also Peritonitis) 567.2
Schmidt's syndrome
 sphallo-pharyngo-laryngeal hemiplegia 352.6
 thyroid-adrenocortical insufficiency 258.1
 vagoaccessory 352.6
Schmincke
 carcinoma (M8082/3) — see Neoplasm, nasopharynx, malignant
 tumor (M8082/3) — see Neoplasm, nasopharynx, malignant
Schmitz (-Stutzer) dysentery 004.0
Schmorl's disease or nodes 722.30
 lumbar, lumbosacral 722.32
 specified region NEC 722.39
 thoracic, thoracolumbar 722.31
Schneider's syndrome 047.9
Schneiderian
 carcinoma (M8121/3)
  specified site — see Neoplasm, by site, malignant
  unspecified site 160.0
 papilloma (M8121/0)
  specified site — see Neoplasm, by site, benign
  unspecified site 212.0
Schoffer's tumor (see also Peritonitis) 567.2
Scholte's syndrome (malignant carcinoid) 259.2
Scholz's disease 330.0
Scholz (-Bielschowsky-Henneberg) syndrome 330.0
Schönlein (-Henoch) disease (primary) (purpura) (rheumatic) 287.0
School examination V70.3
Schottmüller's disease (see also Fever, paratyphoid) 002.9
Schroeder's syndrome (endocrine-hypertensive) 255.3
Schüller-Christian disease or syndrome (chronic histiocytosis X) 277.8
Schultz's disease or syndrome (agranulocytosis) 288.0
Schultze's acroparesthesia, simple 443.89
Schwalbe-Ziehen-Oppenheimer disease 333.6
Schwannoma (M9560/0) — see also Neoplasm, connective tissue, benign
 malignant (M9560/3) — see Neoplasm, connective tissue, malignant
Schwartz (-Jampel) syndrome 756.89

Schwartz-Bartter syndrome (inappropriate secretion of antidiuretic hormone) 253.6
Schweninger-Buzzi disease (macular atrophy) 701.3
Sciatic — see condition
Sciatica (infectional) 724.3
 due to
  displacement of intervertebral disc 722.10
  herniation, nucleus pulposus 722.10
Scimitar syndrome (anomalous venous drainage, right lung to inferior vena cava) 747.49
Sclera — see condition
Sclerectasia 379.11
Scleredema
 adultorum 710.1
 Buschke's 710.1
 newborn 778.1
Sclerema
 adiposum (newborn) 778.1
 adultorum 710.1
 edematosum (newborn) 778.1
 neonatorum 778.1
 newborn 778.1
Scleriasis — see Scleroderma
Scleritis 379.00
 with corneal involvement 379.05
 anterior (annular) (localized) 379.03
 brawny 379.06
 granulomatous 379.09
 posterior 379.07
 specified NEC 379.09
 suppurative 379.09
 syphilitic 095.0
 tuberculous (nodular) (see also Tuberculosis) 017.3 [379.09]
Sclerochoroiditis (see also Scleritis) 379.00
Scleroconjunctivitis (see also Scleritis) 379.00
Sclerocystic ovary (syndrome) 256.4
Sclerodactylia 701.0
Scleroderma, sclerodermia (acrosclerotic) (diffuse) (generalized) (progressive) (pulmonary) 710.1
 circumscribed 701.0
 linear 701.0
 localized (linear) 701.0
 newborn 778.1
Sclerokeratitis 379.05
 meaning sclerosing keratitis 370.54
 tuberculous (see also Tuberculosis) 017.3 [379.09]
Scleroma, trachea 040.1
Scleromalacia
 multiple 731.0
 perforans 379.04
Scleromyxedema 701.8
Scleroperikeratitis 379.05
Sclerose en plaques 340
Sclerosis, sclerotic
 adrenal (gland) 255.8
 Alzheimer's 331.0
  with dementia — see Alzheimer's, dementia
 amyotrophic (lateral) 335.20
 annularis fibrosi
  aortic 424.1
  mitral 424.0

Sclerosis, sclerotic — *continued*
  aorta, aortic 440.0
    valve (*see also* Endocarditis, aortic) 424.1
  artery, arterial, arteriolar, arteriovascular —
      see Arteriosclerosis
  ascending multiple 340
  Baló's (concentric) 341.1
  basilar — *see* Sclerosis, brain
  bone (localized) NEC 733.99
  brain (general) (lobular) 341.9
    Alzheimer's — *see* Alzheimer's, dementia
    artery, arterial 437.0
    atrophic lobar 331.0
      with dementia
        with behavioral disturbance 331.0
            [294.11]
        without behavioral disturbance 331.0
            [294.10]
    diffuse 341.1
      familial (chronic) (infantile) 330.0
      infantile (chronic) (familial) 330.0
      Pelizaeus-Merzbacher type 330.0
    disseminated 340
    hereditary 334.2
    infantile, (degenerative) (diffuse) 330.0
    insular 340
    Krabbe's 330.0
    miliary 340
    multiple 340
    Pelizaeus-Merzbacher 330.0
    progressive familial 330.0
    senile 437.0
    tuberous 759.5
  bulbar, progressive 340
  bundle of His 426.50
    left 426.3
    right 426.4
  cardiac — *see* Arteriosclerosis, coronary
  cardiorenal (*see also* Hypertension,
      cardiorenal) 404.90
  cardiovascular (*see also* Disease,
      cardiovascular) 429.2
    renal (*see also* Hypertension, cardiorenal)
        404.90
  centrolobar, familial 330.0
  cerebellar — *see* Sclerosis, brain
  cerebral — *see* Sclerosis, brain
  cerebrospinal 340
    disseminated 340
    multiple 340
  cerebrovascular 437.0
  choroid 363.40
    diffuse 363.56
  combined (spinal cord) — *see also*
      Degeneration, combined
    multiple 340
  concentric, Baló's 341.1
  cornea 370.54
  coronary (artery) — *see* Arteriosclerosis,
      coronary
  corpus cavernosum
    female 624.8
    male 607.89
  Dewitzky's
    aortic 424.1
    mitral 424.0
  diffuse NEC 341.1
  disease, heart — *see* Arteriosclerosis, coronary
  disseminated 340
  dorsal 340

Sclerosis, sclerotic — *continued*
  dorsolateral (spinal cord) — *see* Degeneration,
      combined
  endometrium 621.8
  extrapyramidal 333.90
  eye, nuclear (senile) 366.16
  Friedreich's (spinal cord) 334.0
  funicular (spermatic cord) 608.89
  gastritis 535.4
  general (vascular) — *see* Arteriosclerosis
  gland (lymphatic) 457.8
  hepatic 571.9
  hereditary
    cerebellar 334.2
    spinal 334.0
  idiopathic cortical (Garré's) (*see also*
      Osteomyelitis) 730.1
  ilium, piriform 733.5
  insular 340
    pancreas 251.8
  Islands of Langerhans 251.8
  kidney — *see* Sclerosis, renal
  larynx 478.79
  lateral 335.24
    amyotrophic 335.20
    descending 335.24
    primary 335.24
    spinal 335.24
  liver 571.9
  lobar, atrophic (of brain) 331.0
    with dementia
      with behavioral disturbance 331.0
          [294.11]
      without behavioral disturbance 331.0
          [294.10]
  lung (*see also* Fibrosis, lung) 515
  mastoid 383.1
  mitral — *see* Endocarditis, mitral
  Mönckeberg's (medial) (*see also*
      Arteriosclerosis, extremities) 440.20
  multiple (brain stem) (cerebral) (generalized)
      (spinal cord) 340
  myocardium, myocardial — *see*
      Arteriosclerosis, coronary
  nuclear (senile), eye 366.16
  ovary 620.8
  pancreas 577.8
  penis 607.89
  peripheral arteries NEC (*see also*
      Arteriosclerosis, extremities) 440.20
  plaques 340
  pluriglandular 258.8
  polyglandular 258.8
  posterior (spinal cord) (syphilitic) 094.0
  posterolateral (spinal cord) — *see*
      Degeneration, combined
  prepuce 607.89
  primary lateral 335.24
  progressive systemic 710.1
  pulmonary (*see also* Fibrosis, lung) 515
    artery 416.0
    valve (heart) (*see also* Endocarditis,
        pulmonary) 424.3
  renal 587
    with
      cystine storage disease 270.0
      hypertension (*see also* Hypertension,
          kidney) 403.90
      hypertensive heart disease (conditions
          classifiable to 402) (*see also*
          Hypertension, cardiorenal) 404.90

Sclerosis, sclerotic — continued
  renal — continued
    arteriolar (hyaline) (see also Hypertension, kidney) 403.90
    hyperplastic (see also Hypertension, kidney) 403.90
  retina (senile) (vascular) 362.17
  rheumatic
    aortic valve 395.9
    mitral valve 394.9
  Schilder's 341.1
  senile — see Arteriosclerosis
  spinal (cord) (general) (progressive) (transverse) 336.8
    ascending 357.0
    combined — see also Degeneration, combined
    multiple 340
    syphilitic 094.89
    disseminated 340
    dorsolateral — see Degeneration, combined
    hereditary (Friedreich's) (mixed form) 334.0
    lateral (amyotrophic) 335.24
    multiple 340
    posterior (syphilitic) 094.0
  stomach 537.89
  subendocardial, congenital 425.3
  systemic (progressive) 710.1
    with lung involvement 710.1 [517.2]
  tricuspid (heart) (valve) — see Endocarditis, tricuspid
  tuberous (brain) 759.5
  tympanic membrane (see also Tympanosclerosis) 385.00
  valve, valvular (heart) — see Endocarditis
  vascular — see Arteriosclerosis
  vein 459.89

Sclerotenonitis 379.07

Sclerotitis (see also Scleritis) 379.00
  syphilitic 095.0
  tuberculous (see also Tuberculosis) 017.3 ✓5ᵗʰ [379.09]

Scoliosis (acquired) (postural) 737.30
  congenital 754.2
  due to or associated with
    Charcôt-Marie-Tooth disease 356.1 [737.43]
    mucopolysaccharidosis 277.5 [737.43]
    neurofibromatosis 237.71 [737.43]
    osteitis
      deformans 731.0 [737.43]
      fibrosa cystica 252.0 [737.43]
    osteoporosis (see also Osteoporosis) 733.00 [737.43]
    poliomyelitis 138 [737.43]
    radiation 737.33
    tuberculosis (see also Tuberculosis) 015.0 ✓5ᵗʰ [737.43]
  idiopathic 737.30
  infantile
    progressive 737.32
    resolving 737.31
  paralytic 737.39
  rachitic 268.1
  sciatic 724.3
  specified NEC 737.39
  thoracogenic 737.34
  tuberculous (see also Tuberculosis) 015.0 ✓5ᵗʰ [737.43]

Scoliotic pelvis 738.6
  with disproportion (fetopelvic) 653.0 ✓5ᵗʰ
    affecting fetus or newborn 763.1

Scoliotic pelvis — continued
  with disproportion — continued
    causing obstructed labor 660.1 ✓5ᵗʰ
      affecting fetus or newborn 763.1

Scorbutus, scorbutic 267
  anemia 281.8

Scotoma (ring) 368.44
  arcuate 368.43
  Bjerrum 368.43
  blind spot area 368.42
  central 368.41
  centrocecal 368.41
  paracecal 368.42
  paracentral 368.41
  scintillating 368.12
  Seidel 368.43

Scratch — see Injury, superficial, by site

Screening (for) V82.9
  alcoholism V79.1
  anemia, deficiency NEC V78.1
    iron V78.0
  anomaly, congenital V82.89
  antenatal V28.9
    alphafetoprotein levels, raised V28.1
    based on amniocentesis V28.2
      chromosomal anomalies V28.0
      raised alphafetoprotein levels V28.1
    fetal growth retardation using ultrasonics V28.4
    isoimmunization V28.5
    malformations using ultrasonics V28.3
    raised alphafetoprotein levels V28.1
    specified condition NEC V28.8
    Streptococcus B V28.6
  arterial hypertension V81.1
  arthropod-borne viral disease NEC V73.5
  asymptomatic bacteriuria V81.5
  bacterial
    conjunctivitis V74.4
    disease V74.9
      specified condition NEC V74.8
  bacteriuria, asymptomatic V81.5
  blood disorder NEC V78.9
    specified type NEC V78.8
  bronchitis, chronic V81.3
  brucellosis V74.8
  cancer — see Screening, malignant neoplasm
  cardiovascular disease NEC V81.2
  cataract V80.2
  Chagas' disease V75.3
  chemical poisoning V82.5
  cholera V74.0
  cholesterol level V77.91
  chromosomal
    anomalies
      by amniocentesis, antenatal V28.0
      maternal postnatal V82.4
  athletes V70.3
  condition
    cardiovascular NEC V81.2
    eye NEC V80.2
    genitourinary NEC V81.6
    neurological V80.0
    respiratory NEC V81.4
    skin V82.0
    specified NEC V82.89
  congenital
    anomaly V82.89
      eye V80.2
    dislocation of hip V82.3
    eye condition or disease V80.2

Screening — *continued*
- conjunctivitis, bacterial V74.4
- contamination NEC (*see also* Poisoning) V82.5
- coronary artery disease V81.0
- cystic fibrosis V77.6
- deficiency anemia NEC V78.1
  - iron V78.0
- dengue fever V73.5
- depression V79.0
- developmental handicap V79.9
  - in early childhood V79.3
  - specified type NEC V79.8
- diabetes mellitus V77.1
- diphtheria V74.3
- disease or disorder V82.9
  - bacterial V74.9
    - specified NEC V74.8
  - blood V78.9
    - specified type NEC V78.8
  - blood-forming organ V78.9
    - specified type NEC V78.8
  - cardiovascular NEC V81.2
    - hypertensive V81.1
    - ischemic V81.0
  - Chagas' V75.3
  - chlamydial V73.98
    - specified NEC V73.88
  - ear NEC V80.3
  - endocrine NEC V77.99
  - eye NEC V80.2
  - genitourinary NEC V81.6
  - heart NEC V81.2
    - hypertensive V81.1
    - ischemic V81.0
  - immunity NEC V77.99
  - infectious NEC V75.9
  - lipoid NEC V77.91
  - mental V79.9
    - specified type NEC V79.8
  - metabolic NEC V77.99
    - inborn NEC V77.7
  - neurological V80.0
  - nutritional NEC V77.99
  - rheumatic NEC V82.2
  - rickettsial V75.0
  - sickle-cell V78.2
    - trait V78.2
  - specified type NEC V82.89
  - thyroid V77.0
  - vascular NEC V81.2
    - ischemic V81.0
  - venereal V74.5
  - viral V73.99
    - arthropod-borne NEC V73.5
    - specified type NEC V73.89
- dislocation of hip, congenital V82.3
- drugs in athletes V70.3
- emphysema (chronic) V81.3
- encephalitis, viral (mosquito or tick borne) V73.5
- endocrine disorder NEC V77.99
- eye disorder NEC V80.2
  - congenital V80.2
- fever
  - dengue V73.5
  - hemorrhagic V73.5
  - yellow V73.4
- filariasis V75.6
- galactosemia V77.4
- genitourinary condition NEC V81.6
- glaucoma V80.1

Screening — *continued*
- gonorrhea V74.5
- gout V77.5
- Hansen's disease V74.2
- heart disease NEC V81.2
  - hypertensive V81.1
  - ischemic V81.0
- heavy metal poisoning V82.5
- helminthiasis, intestinal V75.7
- hematopoietic malignancy V76.89
- hemoglobinopathies NEC V78.3
- hemorrhagic fever V73.5
- Hodgkin's disease V76.89
- hormones in athletes V70.3
- hypercholesterolemia V77.91
- hyperlipidemia V77.91
- hypertension V81.1
- immunity disorder NEC V77.99
- inborn errors of metabolism NEC V77.7
- infection
  - bacterial V74.9
    - specified type NEC V74.8
  - mycotic V75.4
  - parasitic NEC V75.8
- infectious disease V75.9
  - specified type NEC V75.8
- ingestion of radioactive substance V82.5
- intestinal helminthiasis V75.7
- iron deficiency anemia V78.0
- ischemic heart disease V81.0
- lead poisoning V82.5
- leishmaniasis V75.2
- leprosy V74.2
- leptospirosis V74.8
- leukemia V76.89
- lipoid disorder NEC V77.91
- lymphoma V76.89
- malaria V75.1
- malignant neoplasm (of) V76.9
  - bladder V76.3
  - blood V76.89
  - breast V76.10
    - mammogram NEC V76.12
      - for high-risk patient V76.11
    - specified type NEC V76.19
  - cervix V76.2
  - colon V76.51
  - colorectal V76.51
  - hematopoietic system V76.89
  - intestine V76.50
    - colon V76.51
    - small V76.52
  - lymph (glands) V76.89
  - nervous system V76.81
  - oral cavity V76.42
  - other specified neoplasm NEC V76.89
  - ovary V76.46
  - prostate V76.44
  - rectum V76.41
  - respiratory organs V76.0
  - skin V76.43
  - specified sites NEC V76.49
  - testis V76.45
  - vagina V76.47
    - following hysterectomy for malignant condition V67.01
- maternal postnatal chromosomal anomalies V82.4
- malnutrition V77.2
- mammogram NEC V76.12
  - for high-risk patient V76.11

Screening — *continued*
  measles V73.2
  mental
    disorder V79.9
      specified type NEC V79.8
    retardation V79.2
  metabolic disorder NEC V77.99
  metabolic errors, inborn V77.7
  mucoviscidosis V77.6
  multiphasic V82.6
  mycosis V75.4
  mycotic infection V75.4
  nephropathy V81.5
  neurological condition V80.0
  nutritional disorder V77.99
  obesity V77.8
  osteoporosis V82.81
  parasitic infection NEC V75.8
  phenylketonuria V77.3
  plague V74.8
  poisoning
    chemical NEC V82.5
    contaminated water supply V82.5
      heavy metal V82.5
  poliomyelitis V73.0
  postnatal chromosomal anomalies, maternal V82.4
  prenatal — *see* Screening, antenatal
  pulmonary tuberculosis V74.1
  radiation exposure V82.5
  renal disease V81.5
  respiratory condition NEC V81.4
  rheumatic disorder NEC V82.2
  rheumatoid arthritis V82.1
  rickettsial disease V75.0
  rubella V73.3
  schistosomiasis V75.5
  senile macular lesions of eye V80.2
  sickle-cell anemia, disease, or trait V78.2
  skin condition V82.0
  sleeping sickness V75.3
  smallpox V73.1
  special V82.9
    specified condition NEC V82.89
  specified type NEC V82.89
  spirochetal disease V74.9
    specified type NEC V74.8
  stimulants in athletes V70.3
  syphilis V74.5
  tetanus V74.8
  thyroid disorder V77.0
  trachoma V73.6
  trypanosomiasis V75.3
  tuberculosis, pulmonary V74.1
  venereal disease V74.5
  viral encephalitis
    mosquito-borne V73.5
    tick-borne V73.5
  whooping cough V74.8
  worms, intestinal V75.7
  yaws V74.6
  yellow fever V73.3
Scrofula (*see also* Tuberculosis) 017.2
Scrofulide (primary) (*see also* Tuberculosis) 017.0
Scrofuloderma, scrofulodermia (any site) (primary) (*see also* Tuberculosis) 017.0
Scrofulosis (universal) (*see also* Tuberculosis) 017.2
Scrofulosis lichen (primary) (*see also* Tuberculosis) 017.0

Scrofulous — *see* condition
Scrotal tongue 529.5
  congenital 750.13
Scrotum — *see* condition
Scurvy (gum) (infantile) (rickets) (scorbutic) 267
Sea-blue histiocyte syndrome 272.7
Seabright-Bantam syndrome (pseudohypoparathyroidism) 275.49
Seasickness 994.6
Seatworm 127.4
Sebaceous
  cyst (*see also* Cyst, sebaceous) 706.2
  gland disease NEC 706.9
Sebocystomatosis 706.2
Seborrhea, seborrheic 706.3
  adiposa 706.3
  capitis 690.11
  congestiva 695.4
  corporis 706.3
  dermatitis 690.10
    infantile 690.12
  diathesis in infants 695.89
  eczema 690.18
    infantile 691.12
  keratosis 702.19
    inflamed 702.11
  nigricans 705.89
  sicca 690.18
  wart 702.19
    inflamed 702.11
Seckel's syndrome 759.89
Seclusion pupil 364.74
Seclusiveness, child 313.22
Secondary — *see also* condition
  neoplasm — *see* Neoplasm, by site, malignant, secondary
Secretan's disease or syndrome (posttraumatic edema) 782.3
Secretion
  antidiuretic hormone, inappropriate (syndrome) 253.6
  catecholamine, by pheochromocytoma 255.6
  hormone
    antidiuretic, inappropriate (syndrome) 253.6
    by
      carcinoid tumor 259.2
      pheochromocytoma 255.6
    ectopic NEC 259.3
  urinary
    excessive 788.42
    suppression 788.5
Section
  cesarean
    affecting fetus or newborn 763.4
    post mortem, affecting fetus or newborn 761.6
    previous, in pregnancy or childbirth 654.2
      affecting fetus or newborn 763.89
  nerve, traumatic — *see* Injury, nerve, by site
Seeligmann's syndrome (ichthyosis congenita) 757.1
Segmentation, incomplete (congenital) — *see also* Fusion
  bone NEC 756.9
    lumbosacral (joint) 756.15
  vertebra 756.15
    lumbosacral 756.15

Seizure 780.39
  akinetic (idiopathic) (see also Epilepsy) 345.0 ✓5ᵗʰ
    psychomotor 345.4 ✓5ᵗʰ
  apoplexy, apoplectic (see also Disease, cerebrovascular, acute) 436
  atonic (see also Epilepsy) 345.0 ✓5ᵗʰ
  autonomic 300.11
  brain or cerebral (see also Disease, cerebrovascular, acute) 436
  convulsive (see also Convulsions) 780.39
  cortical (focal) (motor) (see also Epilepsy) 345.5 ✓5ᵗʰ
  epilepsy, epileptic (cryptogenic) (see also Epilepsy) 345.9 ✓5ᵗʰ
  epileptiform, epileptoid 780.39
    focal (see also Epilepsy) 345.5 ✓5ᵗʰ
  febrile 780.31
  heart — see Disease, heart
  hysterical 300.11
  Jacksonian (focal) (see also Epilepsy) 345.5 ✓5ᵗʰ
    motor type 345.5 ✓5ᵗʰ
    sensory type 345.5 ✓5ᵗʰ
  newborn 779.0
  paralysis (see also Disease, cerebrovascular, acute) 436
  recurrent 780.39
    epileptic — see Epilepsy
  repetitive 780.39
    epileptic — see Epilepsy
  salaam (see also Epilepsy) 345.6 ✓5ᵗʰ
  uncinate (see also Epilepsy) 345.4 ✓5ᵗʰ
Self-mutilation 300.9
Semicoma 780.09
Semiconsciousness 780.09
Seminal
  vesicle — see condition
  vesiculitis (see also Vesiculitis) 608.0
Seminoma (M9061/3)
  anaplastic type (M9062/3)
    specified site — see Neoplasm, by site, malignant
    unspecified site 186.9
  specified site — see Neoplasm, by site, malignant
  spermatocytic (M9063/3)
    specified site — see Neoplasm, by site, malignant
    unspecified site 186.9
Semliki Forest encephalitis 062.8
Senear-Usher disease or syndrome (pemphigus erythematosus) 694.4
Senecio jacobae dermatitis 692.6
Senectus 797
Senescence 797
Senile (see also condition) 797
  cervix (atrophic) 622.8
  degenerative atrophy, skin 701.3
  endometrium (atrophic) 621.8
  fallopian tube (atrophic) 620.3
  heart (failure) 797
  lung 492.8
  ovary (atrophic) 620.3
  syndrome 259.8
  vagina, vaginitis (atrophic) 627.3
  wart 702.0

Senility 797
  with
    acute confusional state 290.3
    delirium 290.3
    mental changes 290.9
    psychosis NEC (see also Psychosis, senile) 290.20
  premature (syndrome) 259.8
Sensation
  burning (see also Disturbance, sensation) 782.0
    tongue 529.6
  choking 784.9
  loss of (see also Disturbance, sensation) 782.0
  prickling (see also Disturbance, sensation) 782.0
  tingling (see also Disturbance, sensation) 782.0
Sense loss (touch) (see also Disturbance, sensation) 782.0
  smell 781.1
  taste 781.1
Sensibility disturbance NEC (cortical) (deep) (vibratory) (see also Disturbance, sensation) 782.0
Sensitive dentine 521.8
Sensitiver Beziehungswahn 297.8
Sensitivity, sensitization — see also Allergy
  autoerythrocyte 287.2
  carotid sinus 337.0
  child (excessive) 313.21
  cold, autoimmune 283.0
  methemoglobin 289.7
  suxamethonium 289.8
  tuberculin, without clinical or radiological symptoms 795.5
Sensory
  extinction 781.8
  neglect 781.8
Separation
  acromioclavicular — see Dislocation, acromioclavicular
  anxiety, abnormal 309.21
  apophysis, traumatic — see Fracture, by site
  choroid 363.70
    hemorrhagic 363.72
    serous 363.71
  costochondral (simple) (traumatic) — see Dislocation, costochondral
  epiphysis, epiphyseal
    nontraumatic 732.9
      upper femoral 732.2
    traumatic — see Fracture, by site
  fracture — see Fracture, by site
  infundibulum cardiac from right ventricle by a partition 746.83
  joint (current) (traumatic) — see Dislocation, by site
  placenta (normally implanted) — see Placenta, separation
  pubic bone, obstetrical trauma 665.6 ✓5ᵗʰ
  retina, retinal (see also Detachment, retina) 361.9
    layers 362.40
      sensory (see also Retinoschisis) 361.10
    pigment epithelium (exudative) 362.42
      hemorrhagic 362.43
  sternoclavicular (traumatic) — see Dislocation, sternoclavicular

Separation — *continued*
  symphysis pubis, obstetrical trauma
    665.6
  tracheal ring, incomplete (congenital) 748.3
Sepsis (generalized) (*see also* Septicemia) 038.9
  with
    abortion — *see* Abortion, by type, with sepsis
    ectopic pregnancy (*see also* categories 633.0-633.9) 639.0
    molar pregnancy (*see also* categories 630-632) 639.0
  buccal 528.3
  complicating labor 659.3
  dental (pulpal origin) 522.4
  female genital organ NEC 614.9
  fetus (intrauterine) 771.81
  following
    abortion 639.0
    ectopic or molar pregnancy 639.0
    infusion, perfusion, or transfusion 999.3
  Friedländer's 038.49
  intraocular 360.00
  localized
    in operation wound 998.59
    skin (*see also* Abscess) 682.9
  malleus 024
  nadir 038.9
  newborn (umbilical) (organism unspecified) NEC 771.81
  oral 528.3
  puerperal, postpartum, childbirth (pelvic) 670
  resulting from infusion, injection, transfusion, or vaccination 999.3
  severe 995.92
  skin, localized (*see also* Abscess) 682.9
  umbilical (newborn) (organism unspecified) 771.89
    tetanus 771.3
  urinary 599.0
Septate — *see also* Septum
Septic — *see also* condition
  adenoids 474.01
    and tonsils 474.02
  arm (with lymphangitis) 682.3
  embolus — *see* Embolism
  finger (with lymphangitis) 681.00
  foot (with lymphangitis) 682.7
  gallbladder (*see also* Cholecystitis) 575.8
  hand (with lymphangitis) 682.4
  joint (*see also* Arthritis, septic) 711.0
  kidney (*see also* Infection, kidney) 590.9
  leg (with lymphangitis) 682.6
  mouth 528.3
  nail 681.9
    finger 681.02
    toe 681.11
  shock (endotoxic) 785.59
  sore (*see also* Abscess) 682.9
    throat 034.0
      milk-borne 034.0
      streptococcal 034.0
  spleen (acute) 289.59
  teeth (pulpal origin) 522.4
  throat 034.0
  thrombus — *see* Thrombosis
  toe (with lymphangitis) 681.0
  tonsils 474.00
    and adenoids 474.02

Septic — *continued*
  umbilical cord (newborn) (organism unspecified) 771.89
  uterus (*see also* Endometritis) 615.9
Septicemia, septicemic (generalized) (suppurative) 038.9
  with
    abortion — *see* Abortion, by type, with sepsis
    ectopic pregnancy (*see also* categories 633.0-633.9) 639.0
    molar pregnancy (*see also* categories 630-632) 639.0
  Aerobacter aerogenes 038.49
  anaerobic 038.3
  anthrax 022.3
  Bacillus coli 038.42
  Bacteroides 038.3
  Clostridium 038.3
  complicating labor 659.3
  cryptogenic 038.9
  enteric gram-negative bacilli 038.40
  Enterobacter aerogenes 038.49
  Erysipelothrix (insidiosa) (rhusiopathiae) 027.1
  Escherichia coli 038.42
  following
    abortion 639.0
    ectopic or molar pregnancy 639.0
    infusion, injection, transfusion, or vaccination 999.3
  Friedländer's (bacillus) 038.49
  gangrenous 038.9
  gonococcal 098.89
  gram-negative (organism) 038.40
    anaerobic 038.3
  Hemophilus influenzae 038.41
  herpes (simplex) 054.5
  herpetic 054.5
  Listeria monocytogenes 027.0
  meningeal — *see* Meningitis
  meningococcal (chronic) (fulminating) 036.2
  navel, newborn (organism unspecified) 771.89
  newborn (umbilical) (organism unspecified) 771.81
  plague 020.2
  pneumococcal 038.2
  postabortal 639.0
  postoperative 998.59
  Proteus vulgaris 038.49
  Pseudomonas (aeruginosa) 038.43
  puerperal, postpartum 670
  Salmonella (aertrycke) (callinarum) (choleraesuis) (enteritidis) (suipestifer) 003.1
  Serratia 038.44
  Shigella (*see also* Dysentery, bacillary) 004.9
  specified organism NEC 038.8
  staphylococcal 038.10
    aureus 038.11
    specified organism NEC 038.19
  streptococcal (anaerobic) 038.0
  suipestifer 003.1
  umbilicus, newborn (organism unspecified) 771.89
  viral 079.99
  Yersinia enterocolitica 038.49
Septum, septate (congenital) — *see also* Anomaly, specified type NEC
  anal 751.2

Index to Diseases

Septum, septate — *continued*
  aqueduct of Sylvius 742.3
    with spina bifida (*see also* Spina bifida) 741.0 ✓5ᵗʰ
  hymen 752.49
  uterus (*see also* Double, uterus) 752.2
  vagina 752.49
    in pregnancy or childbirth 654.7 ✓5ᵗʰ
      affecting fetus or newborn 763.89
      causing obstructed labor 660.2 ✓5ᵗʰ
        affecting fetus or newborn 763.1
Sequestration
  lung (congenital) (extralobar) (intralobar) 748.5
  orbit 376.10
  pulmonary artery (congenital) 747.3
Sequestrum
  bone (*see also* Osteomyelitis) 730.1 ✓5ᵗʰ
    jaw 526.4
  dental 525.8
  jaw bone 526.4
  sinus (accessory) (nasal) (*see also* Sinusitis) 473.9
    maxillary 473.0
Sequoiosis asthma 495.8
Serology for syphilis
  doubtful
    with signs or symptoms — *see* Syphilis, by site and stage
    follow-up of latent syphilis — *see* Syphilis, latent
  false positive 795.6
  negative, with signs or symptoms — *see* Syphilis, by site and stage
  positive 097.1
    with signs or symptoms — *see* Syphilis, by site and stage
    false 795.6
    follow-up of latent syphilis — *see* Syphilis, latent
    only finding — *see* Syphilis, latent
  reactivated 097.1
Seroma (postoperative) (non-infected) 998.13
  infected 998.51
Seropurulent — *see* condition
Serositis, multiple 569.89
  pericardial 423.2
  peritoneal 568.82
  pleural — *see* Pleurisy
Serotonin syndrome 333.99
Serous — *see* condition
Sertoli cell
  adenoma (M8640/0)
    specified site — *see* Neoplasm, by site, benign
    unspecified site
      female 220
      male 222.0
  carcinoma (M8640/3)
    specified site — *see* Neoplasm, by site, malignant
    unspecified site 186.9
  syndrome (germinal aplasia) 606.0
  tumor (M8640/0)
    with lipid storage (M8641/0)
      specified site — *see* Neoplasm, by site, benign
      unspecified site
        female 220
        male 222.0
    specified site — *see* Neoplasm, by site, benign

Sertoli cell — *continued*
  tumor — *continued*
    unspecified site
      female 220
      male 222.0
Sertoli-Leydig cell tumor (M8631/0)
  specified site — *see* Neoplasm, by site, benign
  unspecified site
    female 220
    male 222.0
Serum
  allergy, allergic reaction 999.5
    shock 999.4
  arthritis 999.5 *[713.6]*
  complication or reaction NEC 999.5
  disease NEC 999.5
  hepatitis 070.3 ✓5ᵗʰ
  intoxication 999.5
  jaundice (homologous) — *see* Hepatitis, viral
  neuritis 999.5
  poisoning NEC 999.5
  rash NEC 999.5
  reaction NEC 999.5
  sickness NEC 999.5
Sesamoiditis 733.99
Seven-day fever 061
  of
    Japan 100.89
    Queensland 100.89
Sever's disease or osteochondrosis (calcaneum) 732.5
Sex chromosome mosaics 758.81
Sextuplet
  affected by maternal complications of pregnancy 761.5
  healthy liveborn — *see* Newborn, multiple
  pregnancy (complicating delivery) NEC 651.8 ✓5ᵗʰ
    with fetal loss and retention of one or more fetus(es) 651.6 ✓5ᵗʰ
Sexual
  anesthesia 302.72
  deviation (*see also* Deviation, sexual) 302.9
  disorder (*see also* Deviation, sexual) 302.9
  frigidity (female) 302.72
  function, disorder of (psychogenic) 302.70
    specified type NEC 302.79
  immaturity (female) (male) 259.0
  impotence (psychogenic) 302.72
    organic origin NEC 607.84
  precocity (constitutional) (cryptogenic) (female) (idiopathic) (male) NEC 259.1
    with adrenal hyperplasia 255.2
  sadism 302.84
Sexuality, pathological (*see also* Deviation, sexual) 302.9
Sézary's disease, reticulosis, or syndrome (M9701/3) 202.2 ✓5ᵗʰ
Shadow, lung 793.1
Shaken infant syndrome 995.55
Shaking
  head (tremor) 781.0
  palsy or paralysis (*see also* Parkinsonism) 332.0
Shallowness, acetabulum 736.39
Shaver's disease or syndrome (bauxite pneumoconiosis) 503
Shearing
  artificial skin graft 996.55

Shearing — *continued*
  decellularized allodermis graft 996.55
Sheath (tendon) — *see* condition
Shedding
  nail 703.8
  teeth, premature, primary (deciduous) 520.6
Sheehan's disease or syndrome (postpartum pituitary necrosis) 253.2
Shelf, rectal 569.49
Shell
  shock (current) (*see also* Reaction, stress, acute) 308.9
    lasting state 300.16
  teeth 520.5
Shield kidney 753.3
Shift, mediastinal 793.2
Shifting
  pacemaker 427.89
  sleep-work schedule (affecting sleep) 307.45
Shiga's
  bacillus 004.0
  dysentery 004.0
Shigella (dysentery) (*see also* Dysentery, bacillary) 004.9
  carrier (suspected) of V02.3
Shigellosis (*see also* Dysentery, bacillary) 004.9
Shingles (*see also* Herpes, zoster) 053.9
  eye NEC 053.29
Shin splints 844.9
Shipyard eye or disease 077.1
Shirodkar suture, in pregnancy 654.5 ⚠
Shock 785.50
  with
    abortion — *see* Abortion, by type, with shock
    ectopic pregnancy (*see also* categories 633.0-633.9) 639.5
    molar pregnancy (*see also* categories 630-632) 639.5
  allergic — *see* Shock, anaphylactic
  anaclitic 309.21
  anaphylactic 995.0
    chemical — *see* Table of Drugs and Chemicals
    correct medicinal substance properly administered 995.0
    drug or medicinal substance
      correct substance properly administered 995.0
      overdose or wrong substance given or taken 977.9
        specified drug — *see* Table of Drugs and Chemicals
    following sting(s) 989.5
    food — *see* Anaphylactic shock, due to, food
    immunization 999.4
    serum 999.4
  anaphylactoid — *see* Shock, anaphylactic
  anesthetic
    correct substance properly administered 995.4
    overdose or wrong substance given 968.4
      specified anesthetic — *see* Table of Drugs and Chemicals
  birth, fetus or newborn NEC 779.89 ▲
  cardiogenic 785.51
  chemical substance — *see* Table of Drugs and Chemicals

Shock — *continued*
  circulatory 785.59
  complicating
    abortion — *see* Abortion, by type, with shock
    ectopic pregnancy (*see also* categories 633.0-633.9) 639.5
    labor and delivery 669.1 ⚠
    molar pregnancy (*see also* categories 630-632) 639.5
  culture 309.29
  due to
    drug 995.0
      correct substance properly administered 995.0
      overdose or wrong substance given or taken 977.9
        specified drug — *see* Table of Drugs and Chemicals
    food — *see* Anaphylactic shock, due to, food
  during labor and delivery 669.1 ⚠
  electric 994.8
  endotoxic 785.59
    due to surgical procedure 998.0
  following
    abortion 639.5
    ectopic or molar pregnancy 639.5
    injury (immediate) (delayed) 958.4
    labor and delivery 669.1 ⚠
  gram-negative 785.59
  hematogenic 785.59
  hemorrhagic
    due to
      disease 785.59
      surgery (intraoperative) (postoperative) 998.0
      trauma 958.4
  hypovolemic NEC 785.59
    surgical 998.0
    traumatic 958.4
  insulin 251.0
    therapeutic misadventure 962.3
  kidney 584.5
    traumatic (following crushing) 958.5
  lightning 994.0
  lung 518.5
  nervous (*see also* Reaction, stress, acute) 308.9
  obstetric 669.1 ⚠
    with
      abortion — *see* Abortion, by type, with shock
      ectopic pregnancy (*see also* categories 633.0-633.9) 639.5
      molar pregnancy (*see also* categories 630-632) 639.5
    following
      abortion 639.5
      ectopic or molar pregnancy 639.5
  paralysis, paralytic (*see also* Disease, cerebrovascular, acute) 436
    late effect — *see* Late effect(s) (of) cerebrovascular disease
  pleural (surgical) 998.0
    due to trauma 958.4
  postoperative 998.0
    with
      abortion — *see* Abortion, by type, with shock

Index to Diseases

Shock — continued
  postoperative — continued
    with — continued
      ectopic pregnancy (see also categories 633.0-633.9) 639.5
      molar pregnancy (see also categories 630-632) 639.5
      following
        abortion 639.5
        ectopic or molar pregnancy 639.5
  psychic (see also Reaction, stress, acute) 308.9
    past history (of) V15.49
  psychogenic (see also Reaction, stress, acute) 308.9
  septic 785.59
    with
      abortion — see Abortion, by type, with shock
      ectopic pregnancy (categories 633.0-633.9) 639.5
      molar pregnancy (see also categories 630-632) 639.5
    due to
      surgical procedure 998.0
      transfusion NEC 999.8
        bone marrow 996.85
    following
      abortion 639.5
      ectopic or molar pregnancy 639.5
      surgical procedure 998.0
      transfusion NEC 999.8
        bone marrow 996.85
  spinal — see also Injury, spinal, by site
    with spinal bone injury — see Fracture, vertebra, by site, with spinal cord injury
  surgical 998.0
  therapeutic misadventure NEC (see also Complications) 998.89
  thyroxin 962.7
  toxic 040.82
  transfusion — see Complications, transfusion
  traumatic (immediate) (delayed) 958.4
Shoemakers' chest 738.3
Short, shortening, shortness
  Achilles tendon (acquired) 727.81
  arm 736.89
    congenital 755.20
  back 737.9
  bowel syndrome 579.3
  breath 786.05
  common bile duct, congenital 751.69
  cord (umbilical) 663.4 ✓5ᵗʰ
    affecting fetus or newborn 762.6
  cystic duct, congenital 751.69
  esophagus (congenital) 750.4
  femur (acquired) 736.81
    congenital 755.34
  frenulum linguae 750.0
  frenum, lingual 750.0
  hamstrings 727.81
  hip (acquired) 736.39
    congenital 755.63
  leg (acquired) 736.81
    congenital 755.30
  metatarsus (congenital) 754.79
    acquired 736.79
  organ or site, congenital NEC — see Distortion
  palate (congenital) 750.26
  P-R interval syndrome 426.81

Short, shortening, shortness — continued
  radius (acquired) 736.09
    congenital 755.26
  round ligament 629.8
  sleeper 307.49
  stature, constitutional (hereditary) 783.43
  tendon 727.81
    Achilles (acquired) 727.81
      congenital 754.79
    congenital 756.89
  thigh (acquired) 736.81
    congenital 755.34
  tibialis anticus 727.81
  umbilical cord 663.4 ✓5ᵗʰ
    affecting fetus or newborn 762.6
  urethra 599.84
  uvula (congenital) 750.26
  vagina 623.8
Shortsightedness 367.1
Shoshin (acute fulminating beriberi) 265.0
Shoulder — see condition
Shovel-shaped incisors 520.2
Shower, thromboembolic — see Embolism
Shunt (status)
  aortocoronary bypass V45.81
  arterial-venous (dialysis) V45.1
  arteriovenous, pulmonary (acquired) 417.0
    congenital 747.3
    traumatic (complication) 901.40
  cerebral ventricle (communicating) in situ V45.2
  coronary artery bypass V45.81
  surgical, prosthetic, with complications — see Complications, shunt
  vascular NEC V45.89
Shutdown
  renal 586
    with
      abortion — see Abortion, by type, with renal failure
      ectopic pregnancy (see also categories 633.0-633.9) 639.3
      molar pregnancy (see also categories 630-632) 639.3
    complicating
      abortion 639.3
      ectopic or molar pregnancy 639.3
      following labor and delivery 669.3 ✓5ᵗʰ
Shwachman's syndrome 288.0
Shy-Drager syndrome (orthostatic hypotension with multisystem degeneration) 333.0
Sialadenitis (any gland) (chronic) (suppurative) 527.2
  epidemic — see Mumps
Sialadenosis, periodic 527.2
Sialaporia 527.7
Sialectasia 527.8
Sialitis 527.2
Sialoadenitis (see also Sialadenitis) 527.2
Sioloangitis 527.2
Sialodochitis (fibrinosa) 527.2
Sialodocholithiasis 527.5
Sialolithiasis 527.5
Sialorrhea (see also Ptyalism) 527.7
  periodic 527.2
Sialosis 527.8
  rheumatic 710.2

Siamese twin 759.4
Sicard's syndrome 352.6
Sicca syndrome (keratoconjunctivitis) 710.2
Sick 799.9
   cilia syndrome 759.89
   or handicapped person in family V61.49
Sickle-cell
   anemia (see also Disease, sickle-cell) 282.60
   disease (see also Disease, sickle-cell) 282.60
   hemoglobin
      C disease 282.63
      D disease 282.69
      E disease 282.69
   thalassemia 282.4
   trait 282.5
Sicklemia (see also Disease, sickle-cell) 282.60
   trait 282.5
Sickness
   air (travel) 994.6
   airplane 994.6
   alpine 993.2
   altitude 993.2
   Andes 993.2
   aviators' 993.2
   balloon 993.2
   car 994.6
   compressed air 993.3
   decompression 993.3
   green 280.9
   harvest 100.89
   milk 988.8
   morning 643.0
   motion 994.6
   mountain 993.2
      acute 289.0
   protein (see also Complications, vaccination) 999.5
   radiation NEC 990
   roundabout (motion) 994.6
   sea 994.6
   serum NEC 999.5
   sleeping (African) 086.5
      by Trypanosoma 086.5
         gambiense 086.3
         rhodesiense 086.4
      Gambian 086.3
      late effect 139.8
      Rhodesian 086.4
   sweating 078.2
   swing (motion) 994.6
   train (railway) (travel) 994.6
   travel (any vehicle) 994.6
Sick sinus syndrome 427.81
Sideropenia (see also Anemia, iron deficiency) 280.9
Siderosis (lung) (occupational) 503
   cornea 371.15
   eye (bulbi) (vitreous) 360.23
   lens 360.23
Siegal-Cattan-Mamou disease (periodic) 277.3
Siemens' syndrome
   ectodermal dysplasia 757.31
   keratosis follicularis spinulosa (decalvans) 757.39
Sighing respiration 786.7
Sigmoid
   flexure — see condition
   kidney 753.3
Sigmoiditis — see Enteritis

Silfverskiöld's syndrome 756.5
Silicosis, silicotic (complicated) (occupational) (simple) 502
   fibrosis, lung (confluent) (massive) (occupational) 502
   non-nodular 503
   pulmonum 502
Silicotuberculosis (see also Tuberculosis) 011.4
Silo fillers' disease 506.9
Silver's syndrome (congenital hemihypertrophy and short stature) 759.89
Silver wire arteries, retina 362.13
Silvestroni-Bianco syndrome (thalassemia minima) 282.4
Simian crease 757.2
Simmonds' cachexia or disease (pituitary cachexia) 253.2
Simons' disease or syndrome (progressive lipodystrophy) 272.6
Simple, simplex — see condition
Sinding-Larsen disease (juvenile osteopathia patellae) 732.4
Singapore hemorrhagic fever 065.4
Singers' node or nodule 478.5
Single
   atrium 745.69
   coronary artery 746.85
   umbilical artery 747.5
   ventricle 745.3
Singultus 786.8
   epidemicus 078.89
Sinus — see also Fistula
   abdominal 569.81
   arrest 426.6
   arrhythmia 427.89
   bradycardia 427.89
      chronic 427.81
   branchial cleft (external) (internal) 744.41
   coccygeal (infected) 685.1
      with abscess 685.0
   dental 522.7
   dermal (congenital) 685.1
      with abscess 685.0
   draining — see Fistula
   infected, skin NEC 686.9
   marginal, ruptured or bleeding 641.2
      affecting fetus or newborn 762.1
   pause 426.6
   pericranii 742.0
   pilonidal (infected) (rectum) 685.1
      with abscess 685.0
   preauricular 744.46
   rectovaginal 619.1
   sacrococcygeal (dermoid) (infected) 685.1
      with abscess 685.0
   skin
      infected NEC 686.9
      noninfected — see Ulcer, skin
   tachycardia 427.89
   tarsi syndrome 726.79
   testis 608.89
   tract (postinfectional) — see Fistula
   urachus 753.7
Sinuses, Rokitansky-Aschoff (see also Disease, gallbladder) 575.8
Sinusitis (accessory) (nasal) (hyperplastic) (nonpurulent) (purulent) (chronic) 473.9

Sinusitis — continued
    with influenza, flu, or grippe 487.1
    acute 461.9
        ethmoidal 461.2
        frontal 461.1
        maxillary 461.0
        specified type NEC 461.8
        sphenoidal 461.3
    allergic (see also Fever, hay) 477.9
    antrum — see Sinusitis, maxillary
    due to
        fungus, any sinus 117.9
        high altitude 993.1
    ethmoidal 473.2
        acute 461.2
    frontal 473.1
        acute 461.1
    influenzal 478.1
    maxillary 473.0
        acute 461.0
    specified site NEC 473.8
    sphenoidal 473.3
        acute 461.3
    syphilitic, any sinus 095.8
    tuberculous, any sinus (see also Tuberculosis) 012.8 ✓5ᵗʰ
Sinusitis-bronchiectasis-situs inversus (syndrome) (triad) 759.3
Sipple's syndrome (medullary thyroid carcinoma-pheochromocytoma) 193
Sirenomelia 759.89
Siriasis 992.0
Sirkari's disease 085.0
SIRS (systemic inflammatory response syndrome) 995.90
    due to
        infectious process 995.91
            with organ dysfunction 995.92
        non-infectious process 995.93
            with organ dysfunction 995.94
Siti 104.0
Sitophobia 300.29
Situation, psychiatric 300.9
Situational
    disturbance (transient) (see also Reaction, adjustment) 309.9
        acute 308.3
    maladjustment, acute (see also Reaction, adjustment) 309.9
    reaction (see also Reaction, adjustment) 309.9
        acute 308.3
Situs inversus or transversus 759.3
    abdominalis 759.3
    thoracis 759.3
Sixth disease 057.8
Sjögren (-Gougerot) syndrome or disease (keratoconjunctivitis sicca) 710.2
    with lung involvement 710.2 [517.8]
Sjögren-Larsson syndrome (ichthyosis congenita) 757.1
Skeletal — see condition
Skene's gland — see condition
Skenitis (see also Urethritis) 597.89
    gonorrheal (acute) 098.0
        chronic or duration of 2 months or over 098.2
Skerljevo 104.0
Skevas-Zerfus disease 989.5

Skin — see also condition
    donor V59.1
    hidebound 710.9
SLAP lesion (superior glenoid labrum) 840.7
Slate-dressers' lung 502
Slate-miners' lung 502
Sleep
    disorder 780.50
        with apnea — see Apnea, sleep
        child 307.40
        nonorganic origin 307.40
            specified type NEC 307.49
    disturbance 780.50
        with apnea — see Apnea, sleep
        nonorganic origin 307.40
            specified type NEC 307.49
    drunkenness 307.47
    paroxysmal 347
    rhythm inversion 780.55
        nonorganic origin 307.45
    walking 307.46
        hysterical 300.13
Sleeping sickness 086.5
    late effect 139.8
Sleeplessness (see also Insomnia) 780.52
    menopausal 627.2
    nonorganic origin 307.41
Slipped, slipping
    epiphysis (postinfectional) 732.9
        traumatic (old) 732.9
            current — see Fracture, by site
        upper femoral (nontraumatic) 732.2
    intervertebral disc — see Displacement, intervertebral disc
    ligature, umbilical 772.3
    patella 717.89
    rib 733.99
    sacroiliac joint 724.6
    tendon 727.9
    ulnar nerve, nontraumatic 354.2
    vertebra NEC (see also Spondylolisthesis) 756.12
Slocumb's syndrome 255.3
Sloughing (multiple) (skin) 686.9
    abscess — see Abscess, by site
    appendix 543.9
    bladder 596.8
    fascia 728.9
    graft — see Complications, graft
    phagedena (see also Gangrene) 785.4
    reattached extremity (see also Complications, reattached extremity) 996.90
    rectum 569.49
    scrotum 608.89
    tendon 727.9
    transplanted organ (see also Rejection, transplant, organ, by site) 996.80
    ulcer (see also Ulcer, skin) 707.9
Slow
    feeding newborn 779.3
    fetal, growth NEC 764.9 ✓5ᵗʰ
        affecting management of pregnancy 656.5 ✓5ᵗʰ
Slowing
    heart 427.89
    urinary stream 788.62
Sluder's neuralgia or syndrome 337.0
Slurred, slurring, speech 784.5

Small, smallness
cardiac reserve — *see* Disease, heart
for dates
  fetus or newborn 764.0 ✓5ᵗʰ
    with malnutrition 764.1 ✓5ᵗʰ
    affecting management of pregnancy
      656.5 ✓5ᵗʰ
  infant, term 764.0 ✓5ᵗʰ
    with malnutrition 764.1 ✓5ᵗʰ
    affecting management of pregnancy
      656.5 ✓5ᵗʰ
introitus, vagina 623.3
kidney, unknown cause 589.9
  bilateral 589.1
  unilateral 589.0
ovary 620.8
pelvis
  with disproportion (fetopelvic) 653.1 ✓5ᵗʰ
    affecting fetus or newborn 763.1
  causing obstructed labor 660.1 ✓5ᵗʰ
    affecting fetus or newborn 763.1
placenta — *see* Placenta, insufficiency
uterus 621.8
white kidney 582.9
Small-for-dates (*see also* Light-for-dates)
  764.0 ✓5ᵗʰ
  affecting management of pregnancy 656.5 ✓5ᵗʰ
Smallpox 050.9
  contact V01.3
  exposure to V01.3
  hemorrhagic (pustular) 050.0
  malignant 050.0
  modified 050.2
  vaccination
    complications — *see* Complications,
      vaccination
    prophylactic (against) V04.1
Smith's fracture (separation) (closed) 813.41
  open 813.51
Smith-Lemli Opitz syndrome
  (cerebrohepatorenal syndrome) 759.89
Smith-Strang disease (oasthouse urine) 270.2
Smokers'
  bronchitis 491.0
  cough 491.0
  syndrome (*see also* Abuse, drugs,
    nondependent) 305.1
  throat 472.1
  tongue 528.6
Smothering spells 786.09
Snaggle teeth, tooth 524.3
Snapping
  finger 727.05
  hip 719.65
  jaw 524.69
  knee 717.9
  thumb 727.05
Sneddon-Wilkinson disease or syndrome
  (subcorneal pustular dermatosis) 694.1
Sneezing 784.9
  intractable 478.1
Sniffing
  cocaine (*see also* Dependence) 304.2 ✓5ᵗʰ
  ether (*see also* Dependence) 304.6 ✓5ᵗʰ
  glue (airplane) (*see also* Dependence) 304.6
    ✓5ᵗʰ
Snoring 786.09
Snow blindness 370.24

Snuffles (nonsyphilitic) 460
  syphilitic (infant) 090.0
Social migrant V60.0
Sodoku 026.0
Soemmering's ring 366.51
Soft — *see also* condition
  enlarged prostate 600.0
  nails 703.8
Softening
  bone 268.2
  brain (necrotic) (progressive) 434.9 ✓5ᵗʰ
    arteriosclerotic 437.0
    congenital 742.4
    embolic (*see also* Embolism, brain)
      434.1 ✓5ᵗʰ
    hemorrhagic (*see also* Hemorrhage, brain)
      431
    occlusive 434.9 ✓5ᵗʰ
    thrombotic (*see also* Thrombosis, brain)
      434.0 ✓5ᵗʰ
  cartilage 733.92
  cerebellar — *see* Softening, brain
  cerebral — *see* Softening, brain
  cerebrospinal — *see* Softening, brain
  myocardial, heart (*see also* Degeneration,
    myocardial) 429.1
  nails 703.8
  spinal cord 336.8
  stomach 537.89
Solar fever 061
Soldier's
  heart 306.2
  patches 423.1
Solitary
  cyst
    bone 733.21
    kidney 593.2
  kidney (congenital) 753.0
  tubercle, brain (*see also* Tuberculosis, brain)
    013.2 ✓5ᵗʰ
  ulcer, bladder 596.8
Somatization reaction, somatic reaction (*see also* Disorder, psychosomatic) 306.9
  disorder 300.81
Somatoform disorder 300.82
  atypical 300.82
  severe 300.81
  undifferentiated 300.82
Somnambulism 307.46
  hysterical 300.13
Somnolence 780.09
  nonorganic origin 307.43
  periodic 349.89
Sonne dysentery 004.3
Soor 112.0
Sore
  Delhi 085.1
  desert (*see also* Ulcer, skin) 707.9
  eye 379.99
  Lahore 085.1
  mouth 528.9
    canker 528.2
    due to dentures 528.9
  muscle 729.1
  Naga (*see also* Ulcer, skin) 707.9
  oriental 085.1
  pressure 707.0
    with gangrene 707.0 [785.4]
  skin NEC 709.9

Index to Diseases

Sore — *continued*
  soft 099.0
  throat 462
    with influenza, flu, or grippe 487.1
    acute 462
    chronic 472.1
    clergyman's 784.49
    coxsackie (virus) 074.0
    diphtheritic 032.0
    epidemic 034.0
    gangrenous 462
    herpetic 054.79
    influenzal 487.1
    malignant 462
    purulent 462
    putrid 462
    septic 034.0
    streptococcal (ulcerative) 034.0
    ulcerated 462
    viral NEC 462
      Coxsackie 074.0
  tropical (*see also* Ulcer, skin) 707.9
  veldt (*see also* Ulcer, skin) 707.9
Sotos' syndrome (cerebral gigantism) 253.0
Sounds
  friction, pleural 786.7
  succussion, chest 786.7
South African cardiomyopathy syndrome 425.2
South American
  blastomycosis 116.1
  trypanosomiasis — *see* Trypanosomiasis
Southeast Asian hemorrhagic fever 065.4
Spacing, teeth, abnormal 524.3
Spade-like hand (congenital) 754.89
Spading nail 703.8
  congenital 757.5
Spanemia 285.9
Spanish collar 605
Sparganosis 123.5
Spasm, spastic, spasticity (*see also* condition) 781.0
  accommodation 367.53
  ampulla of Vater (*see also* Disease, gallbladder) 576.8
  anus, ani (sphincter) (reflex) 564.6
    psychogenic 306.4
  artery NEC 443.9
    basilar 435.0
    carotid 435.8
    cerebral 435.9
      specified artery NEC 435.8
    retinal (*see also* Occlusion, retinal, artery) 362.30
    vertebral 435.1
    vertebrobasilar 435.3
  Bell's 351.0
  bladder (sphincter, external or internal) 596.8
  bowel 564.9
    psychogenic 306.4
  bronchus, bronchiole 519.1
  cardia 530.0
  cardiac — *see* Angina
  carpopedal (*see also* Tetany) 781.7
  cecum 564.9
    psychogenic 306.4
  cerebral (arteries) (vascular) 435.9
    specified artery NEC 435.8
  cerebrovascular 435.9

Spasm, spastic, spasticity — *continued*
  cervix, complicating delivery 661.4 ✓5
    affecting fetus or newborn 763.7
  ciliary body (of accommodation) 367.53
  colon 564.1
    psychogenic 306.4
  common duct (*see also* Disease, biliary) 576.8
  compulsive 307.22
  conjugate 378.82
  convergence 378.84
  coronary (artery) — *see* Angina
  diaphragm (reflex) 786.8
    psychogenic 306.1
  duodenum, duodenal (bulb) 564.89
  esophagus (diffuse) 530.5
    psychogenic 306.4
  facial 351.8
  fallopian tube 620.8
  gait 781.2
  gastrointestinal (tract) 536.8
    psychogenic 306.4
  glottis 478.75
    hysterical 300.11
    psychogenic 306.1
      specified as conversion reaction 300.11
    reflex through recurrent laryngeal nerve 478.75
  habit 307.20
    chronic 307.22
    transient of childhood 307.21
  heart — *see* Angina
  hourglass — *see* Contraction, hourglass
  hysterical 300.11
  infantile (*see also* Epilepsy) 345.6 ✓5
  internal oblique, eye 378.51
  intestinal 564.9
    psychogenic 306.4
  larynx, laryngeal 478.75
    hysterical 300.11
    psychogenic 306.1
      specified as conversion reaction 300.11
  levator palpebrae superioris 333.81
  lightning (*see also* Epilepsy) 345.6 ✓5
  mobile 781.0
  muscle 728.85
    back 724.8
    psychogenic 306.0
  nerve, trigeminal 350.1
  nervous 306.0
  nodding 307.3
    infantile (*see also* Epilepsy) 345.6 ✓5
  occupational 300.89
  oculogyric 378.87
  ophthalmic artery 362.30
  orbicularis 781.0
  perineal 625.8
  peroneo-extensor (*see also* Flat, foot) 734
  pharynx (reflex) 478.29
    hysterical 300.11
    psychogenic 306.1
      specified as conversion reaction 300.11
  pregnant uterus, complicating delivery 661.4 ✓5
  psychogenic 306.0
  pylorus 537.81
    adult hypertrophic 537.0
    congenital or infantile 750.5
    psychogenic 306.4
  rectum (sphincter) 564.6
    psychogenic 306.4

✓4 Fourth-digit Required   ✓5 Fifth-digit Required

Spasm, spastic, spasticity — continued
  retinal artery NEC (see also Occlusion, retina, artery) 362.30
  sacroiliac 724.6
  salaam (infantile) (see also Epilepsy) 345.6
  saltatory 781.0
  sigmoid 564.9
    psychogenic 306.4
  sphincter of Oddi (see also Disease, gallbladder) 576.5
  stomach 536.8
    neurotic 306.4
  throat 478.29
    hysterical 300.11
    psychogenic 306.1
      specified as conversion reaction 300.11
  tic 307.20
    chronic 307.22
    transient of childhood 307.21
  tongue 529.8
  torsion 333.6
  trigeminal nerve 350.1
    postherpetic 053.12
  ureter 593.89
  urethra (sphincter) 599.84
  uterus 625.8
    complicating labor 661.4
      affecting fetus or newborn 763.7
  vagina 625.1
    psychogenic 306.51
  vascular NEC 443.9
  vasomotor NEC 443.9
  vein NEC 459.89
  vesical (sphincter, external or internal) 596.8
  viscera 789.0
Spasmodic — see condition
Spasmophilia (see also Tetany) 781.7
Spasmus nutans 307.3
Spastic — see also Spasm
  child 343.9
Spasticity — see also Spasm
  cerebral, child 343.9
Speakers' throat 784.49
Specific, specified — see condition
Speech
  defect, disorder, disturbance, impediment NEC 784.5
    psychogenic 307.9
  therapy V57.3
Spells 780.39
  breath-holding 786.9
Spencer's disease (epidemic vomiting) 078.82
Spens' syndrome (syncope with heart block) 426.9
Spermatic cord — see condition
Spermatocele 608.1
  congenital 752.8
Spermatocystitis 608.4
Spermatocytoma (M9063/3)
  specified site — see Neoplasm, by site, malignant
  unspecified site 186.9
Spermatorrhea 608.89
Sperm counts
  fertility testing V26.21
  following sterilization reversal V26.22
  postvasectomy V25.8
Sphacelus (see also Gangrene) 785.4

Sphenoidal — see condition
Sphenoiditis (chronic) (see also Sinusitis, sphenoidal) 473.3
Sphenopalatine ganglion neuralgia 337.0
Sphericity, increased, lens 743.36
Spherocytosis (congenital) (familial) (hereditary) 282.0
  hemoglobin disease 282.7
  sickle-cell (disease) 282.60
Spherophakia 743.36
Sphincter — see condition
Sphincteritis, sphincter of Oddi (see also Cholecystitis) 576.8
Sphingolipidosis 272.7
Sphingolipodystrophy 272.7
Sphingomyelinosis 272.7
Spicule tooth 520.2
Spider
  finger 755.59
  nevus 448.1
  vascular 448.1
Spiegler-Fendt sarcoid 686.8
Spielmeyer-Stock disease 330.1
Spielmeyer-Vogt disease 330.1
Spina bifida (aperta) 741.9

> Note — Use the following fifth-digit subclassification with category 741:
>
> 0 unspecified region
> 1 cervical region
> 2 dorsal [thoracic] region
> 3 lumbar region

  with hydrocephalus 741.0
    fetal (suspected), affecting management of pregnancy 655.0
  occulta 756.17
Spindle, Krukenberg's 371.13
Spine, spinal — see condition
Spiradenoma (eccrine) (M8403/0) — see Neoplasm, skin, benign
Spirillosis NEC (see also Fever, relapsing) 087.9
Spirillum minus 026.0
Spirillum obermeieri infection 087.0
Spirochetal — see condition
Spirochetosis 104.9
  arthritic, arthritica 104.9 [711.8]
  bronchopulmonary 104.8
  icterohemorrhagica 100.0
  lung 104.8
Spitting blood (see also Hemoptysis) 786.3
Splanchnomegaly 569.89
Splanchnoptosis 569.89
Spleen, splenic — see also condition
  agenesis 759.0
  flexure syndrome 569.89
  neutropenia syndrome 288.0
  sequestration syndrome 282.60
Splenectasis (see also Splenomegaly) 789.2
Splenitis (interstitial) (malignant) (nonspecific) 289.59
  malarial (see also Malaria) 084.6
  tuberculous (see also Tuberculosis) 017.7
Splenocele 289.59
Splenomegalia — see Splenomegaly

Index to Diseases

Splenomegalic — see condition
Splenomegaly 789.2
   Bengal 789.2
   cirrhotic 289.51
   congenital 759.0
   congestive, chronic 289.51
   cryptogenic 789.2
   Egyptian 120.1
   Gaucher's (cerebroside lipidosis) 272.7
   idiopathic 789.2
   malarial (see also Malaria) 084.6
   neutropenic 288.0
   Niemann-Pick (lipid histiocytosis) 272.7
   siderotic 289.51
   syphilitic 095.8
      congenital 090.0
   tropical (Bengal) (idiopathic) 789.2
Splenopathy 289.50
Splenopneumonia — see Pneumonia
Splenoptosis 289.59
Splinter — see Injury, superficial, by site
Split, splitting
   heart sounds 427.89
   lip, congenital (see also Cleft, lip) 749.10
   nails 703.8
   urinary stream 788.61
Spoiled child reaction (see also Disturbance, conduct) 312.1 ✓5ᵗʰ
Spondylarthritis (see also Spondylosis) 721.90
Spondylarthrosis (see also Spondylosis) 721.90
Spondylitis 720.9
   ankylopoietica 720.0
   ankylosing (chronic) 720.0
   atrophic 720.9
      ligamentous 720.9
   chronic (traumatic) (see also Spondylosis) 721.90
   deformans (chronic) (see also Spondylosis) 721.90
   gonococcal 098.53
   gouty 274.0
   hypertrophic (see also Spondylosis) 721.90
   infectious NEC 720.9
   juvenile (adolescent) 720.0
   Kümmell's 721.7
   Marie-Strümpell (ankylosing) 720.0
   muscularis 720.9
   ossificans ligamentosa 721.6
   osteoarthritica (see also Spondylosis) 721.90
   posttraumatic 721.7
   proliferative 720.0
   rheumatoid 720.0
   rhizomelica 720.0
   sacroiliac NEC 720.2
   senescent (see also Spondylosis) 721.90
   senile (see also Spondylosis) 721.90
   static (see also Spondylosis) 721.90
   traumatic (chronic) (see also Spondylosis) 721.90
   tuberculous (see also Tuberculosis) 015.0 ✓5ᵗʰ [720.81]
   typhosa 002.0 [720.81]
Spondyloarthrosis (see also Spondylosis) 721.90
Spondylolisthesis (congenital) (lumbosacral) 756.12
   with disproportion (fetopelvic) 653.3 ✓5ᵗʰ
      affecting fetus or newborn 763.1
      causing obstructed labor 660.1 ✓5ᵗʰ
         affecting fetus or newborn 763.1
   acquired 738.4
   degenerative 738.4
   traumatic 738.4

Spondylolisthesis — continued
   traumatic — continued
      acute (lumbar) — see Fracture, vertebra, lumbar
      site other than lumbosacral — see Fracture, vertebra, by site
Spondylolysis (congenital) 756.11
   acquired 738.4
   cervical 756.19
   lumbosacral region 756.11
   with disproportion (fetopelvic) 653.3 ✓5ᵗʰ
      affecting fetus or newborn 763.1
      causing obstructed labor 660.1 ✓5ᵗʰ
         affecting fetus or newborn 763.1
Spondylopathy
   inflammatory 720.9
      specified type NEC 720.89
   traumatic 721.7
Spondylose rhizomelique 720.0
Spondylosis 721.90
   with
      disproportion 653.3 ✓5ᵗʰ
         affecting fetus or newborn 763.1
         causing obstructed labor 660.1 ✓5ᵗʰ
            affecting fetus or newborn 763.1
      myelopathy NEC 721.91
   cervical, cervicodorsal 721.0
      with myelopathy 721.1
   inflammatory 720.9
   lumbar, lumbosacral 721.3
      with myelopathy 721.42
   sacral 721.3
      with myelopathy 721.42
   thoracic 721.2
      with myelopathy 721.41
   traumatic 721.7
Sponge
   divers' disease 989.5
   inadvertently left in operation wound 998.4
   kidney (medullary) 753.17
Spongioblastoma (M9422/3)
   multiforme (M9440/3)
      specified site — see Neoplasm, by site, malignant
      unspecified site 191.9
   polare (M9423/3)
      specified site — see Neoplasm, by site, malignant
      unspecified site 191.9
   primitive polar (M9443/3)
      specified site — see Neoplasm, by site, malignant
      unspecified site 191.9
   specified site — see Neoplasm, by site, malignant
   unspecified site 191.9
Spongiocytoma (M9400/3)
   specified site — see Neoplasm, by site, malignant
   unspecified site 191.9
Spongioneuroblastoma (M9504/3) — see Neoplasm, by site, malignant
Spontaneous — see also condition
   fracture — see Fracture, pathologic
Spoon nail 703.8
   congenital 757.5
Sporadic — see condition

Sporotrichosis (bones) (cutaneous) (disseminated) (epidermal) (lymphatic) (lymphocutaneous) (mucous membranes) (pulmonary) (skeletal) (visceral) 117.1
Sporotrichum schenckii infection 117.1
Spots, spotting
 atrophic (skin) 701.3
 Bitôt's (in the young child) 264.1
 café au lait 709.09
 cayenne pepper 448.1
 cotton wool (retina) 362.83
 de Morgan's (senile angiomas) 448.1
 Fúchs' black (myopic) 360.21
 intermenstrual
  irregular 626.6
  regular 626.5
 interpalpebral 372.53
 Koplik's 055.9
 liver 709.09
 Mongolian (pigmented) 757.33
 of pregnancy 641.9
 purpuric 782.7
 ruby 448.1
Spotted fever — see Fever, spotted
Sprain, strain (joint) (ligament) (muscle) (tendon) 848.9
 abdominal wall (muscle) 848.8
 Achilles tendon 845.09
 acromioclavicular 840.0
 ankle 845.00
  and foot 845.00
 anterior longitudinal, cervical 847.0
 arm 840.9
  upper 840.9
   and shoulder 840.9
 astragalus 845.00
 atlanto-axial 847.0
 atlanto-occipital 847.0
 atlas 847.0
 axis 847.0
 back (see also Sprain, spine) 847.9
 breast bone 848.40
 broad ligament — see Injury, internal, broad ligament
 calcaneofibular 845.02
 carpal 842.01
 carpometacarpal 842.11
 cartilage
  costal, without mention of injury to sternum 848.3
   involving sternum 848.42
  ear 848.8
  knee 844.9
   with current tear (see also Tear, meniscus) 836.2
  semilunar (knee) 844.8
   with current tear (see also Tear, meniscus) 836.2
  septal, nose 848.0
  thyroid region 848.2
  xiphoid 848.49
 cervical, cervicodorsal, cervicothoracic 847.0
 chondrocostal, without mention of injury to sternum 848.3
  involving sternum 848.42
 chondrosternal 848.42
 chronic (joint) — see Derangement, joint
 clavicle 840.9
 coccyx 847.4
 collar bone 840.9

Sprain, strain — continued
 collateral, knee (medial) (tibial) 844.1
  lateral (fibular) 844.0
  recurrent or old 717.89
   lateral 717.81
   medial 717.82
 coracoacromial 840.8
 coracoclavicular 840.1
 coracohumeral 840.2
 coracoid (process) 840.9
 coronary, knee 844.8
 costal cartilage, without mention of injury to sternum 848.3
  involving sternum 848.42
 cricoarytenoid articulation 848.2
 cricothyroid articulation 848.2
 cruciate
  knee 844.2
  old 717.89
   anterior 717.83
   posterior 717.84
 deltoid
  ankle 845.01
  shoulder 840.8
 dorsal (spine) 847.1
 ear cartilage 848.8
 elbow 841.9
  and forearm 841.9
  specified site NEC 841.8
 femur (proximal end) 843.9
  distal end 844.9
 fibula (proximal end) 844.9
  distal end 845.00
 fibulocalcaneal 845.02
 finger(s) 842.10
 foot 845.10
  and ankle 845.00
 forearm 841.9
  and elbow 841.9
  specified site NEC 841.8
 glenoid (shoulder) (see also SLAP lesion) 840.8
 hand 842.10
 hip 843.9
  and thigh 843.9
 humerus (proximal end) 840.9
  distal end 841.9
 iliofemoral 843.0
 infraspinatus 840.3
 innominate
  acetabulum 843.9
  pubic junction 848.5
  sacral junction 846.1
 internal
  collateral, ankle 845.01
  semilunar cartilage 844.8
   with current tear (see also Tear, meniscus) 836.2
   old 717.5
 interphalangeal
  finger 842.13
  toe 845.13
 ischiocapsular 843.1
 jaw (cartilage) (meniscus) 848.1
  old 524.69
 knee 844.9
  and leg 844.9
  old 717.5
   collateral
    lateral 717.81
    medial 717.82

Index to Diseases — Sprain, strain

Sprain, strain — *continued*
  knee — *continued*
    old — *continued*
      cruciate
        anterior 717.83
        posterior 717.84
  late effect — *see* Late, effects (of), sprain
  lateral collateral, knee 844.0
    old 717.81
  leg 844.9
    and knee 844.9
  ligamentum teres femoris 843.8
  low back 846.9
  lumbar (spine) 847.2
  lumbosacral 846.0
    chronic or old 724.6
  mandible 848.1
    old 524.69
  maxilla 848.1
  medial collateral, knee 844.1
    old 717.82
  meniscus
    jaw 848.1
      old 524.69
    knee 844.8
      with current tear (*see also* Tear, meniscus) 836.2
      old 717.5
    mandible 848.1
      old 524.69
    specified site NEC 848.8
  metacarpal 842.10
    distal 842.12
    proximal 842.11
  metacarpophalangeal 842.12
  metatarsal 845.10
  metatarsophalangeal 845.12
  midcarpal 842.19
  midtarsal 845.19
  multiple sites, except fingers alone or toes alone 848.8
  neck 847.0
  nose (septal cartilage) 848.0
  occiput from atlas 847.0
  old — *see* Derangement, joint
  orbicular, hip 843.8
  patella(r) 844.8
    old 717.89
  pelvis 848.5
  phalanx
    finger 842.10
    toe 845.10
  radiocarpal 842.02
  radiohumeral 841.2
  radioulnar 841.9
    distal 842.09
  radius, radial (proximal end) 841.9
    and ulna 841.9
      distal 842.09
    collateral 841.0
    distal end 842.00
  recurrent — *see* Sprain, by site
  rib (cage), without mention of injury to sternum 848.3
    involving sternum 848.42
  rotator cuff (capsule) 840.4
  round ligament — *see also* Injury, internal, round ligament
    femur 843.8
  sacral (spine) 847.3
  sacrococcygeal 847.3

Sprain, strain — *continued*
  sacroiliac (region) 846.9
    chronic or old 724.6
    ligament 846.1
    specified site NEC 846.8
  sacrospinatus 846.2
  sacrospinous 846.2
  sacrotuberous 846.3
  scaphoid bone, ankle 845.00
  scapula(r) 840.9
  semilunar cartilage (knee) 844.8
    with current tear (*see also* Tear, meniscus) 836.2
    old 717.5
  septal cartilage (nose) 848.0
  shoulder 840.9
    and arm, upper 840.9
    blade 840.9
  specified site NEC 848.8
  spine 847.9
    cervical 847.0
    coccyx 847.4
    dorsal 847.1
    lumbar 847.2
    lumbosacral 846.0
      chronic or old 724.6
    sacral 847.3
    sacroiliac (*see also* Sprain, sacroiliac) 846.9
      chronic or old 724.6
    thoracic 847.1
  sternoclavicular 848.41
  sternum 848.40
  subglenoid (*see also* SLAP lesion) 840.8
  subscapularis 840.5
  supraspinatus 840.6
  symphysis
    jaw 848.1
      old 524.69
    mandibular 848.1
      old 524.69
    pubis 848.5
  talofibular 845.09
  tarsal 845.10
  tarsometatarsal 845.11
  temporomandibular 848.1
    old 524.69
  teres
    ligamentum femoris 843.8
    major or minor 840.8
  thigh (proximal end) 843.9
    and hip 843.9
    distal end 844.9
  thoracic (spine) 847.1
  thorax 848.8
  thumb 842.10
  thyroid cartilage or region 848.2
  tibia (proximal end) 844.9
    distal end 845.00
  tibiofibular
    distal 845.03
    superior 844.3
  toe(s) 845.10
  trachea 848.8
  trapezoid 840.8
  ulna, ulnar (proximal end) 841.9
    collateral 841.1
    distal end 842.00
  ulnohumeral 841.3
  vertebrae (*see also* Sprain, spine) 847.9
    cervical, cervicodorsal, cervicothoracic 847.0

Sprain, strain — continued
  wrist (cuneiform) (scaphoid) (semilunar)
    842.00
  xiphoid cartilage 848.49
Sprengel's deformity (congenital) 755.52
Spring fever 309.23
Sprue 579.1
  celiac 579.0
  idiopathic 579.0
  meaning thrush 112.0
  nontropical 579.0
  tropical 579.1
Spur — see also Exostosis
  bone 726.91
    calcaneal 726.73
  calcaneal 726.73
  iliac crest 726.5
  nose (septum) 478.1
    bone 726.91
  septal 478.1
Spuria placenta — see Placenta, abnormal
Spurway's syndrome (brittle bones and blue sclera) 756.51
Sputum, abnormal (amount) (color) (excessive) (odor) (purulent) 786.4
  bloody 786.3
Squamous — see also condition
  cell metaplasia
    bladder 596.8
    cervix — see condition
  epithelium in
    cervical canal (congenital) 752.49
    uterine mucosa (congenital) 752.3
  metaplasia
    bladder 596.8
    cervix — see condition
Squashed nose 738.0
  congenital 754.0
Squeeze, divers' 993.3
Squint (see also Strabismus) 378.9
  accommodative (see also Esotropia) 378.00
  concomitant (see also Heterotropia) 378.30
Stab — see also Wound, open, by site
  internal organs — see Injury, internal, by site, with open wound
Staggering gait 781.2
  hysterical 300.11
Staghorn calculus 592.0
Stählh's
  ear 744.29
  pigment line (cornea) 371.11
Stälhi's pigment lines (cornea) 371.11
Stain
  port wine 757.32
  tooth, teeth (hard tissues) 521.7
    due to
      accretions 523.6
      deposits (betel) (black) (green) (materia alba) (orange) (tobacco) 523.6
      metals (copper) (silver) 521.7
      nicotine 523.6
      pulpal bleeding 521.7
      tobacco 523.6
Stammering 307.0
Standstill
  atrial 426.6
  auricular 426.6
  cardiac (see also Arrest, cardiac) 427.5

Standstill — continued
  sinoatrial 429.6
  sinus 426.6
  ventricular (see also Arrest, cardiac) 427.5
Stannosis 503
Stanton's disease (melioidosis) 025
Staphylitis (acute) (catarrhal) (chronic) (gangrenous) (membranous) (suppurative) (ulcerative) 528.3
Staphylococcemia 038.10
  aureus 038.11
  specified organism NEC 038.19
Staphylococcus, staphylococcal — see condition
Staphyloderma (skin) 686.00
Staphyloma 379.11
  anterior, localized 379.14
  ciliary 379.11
  cornea 371.73
  equatorial 379.13
  posterior 379.12
  posticum 379.12
  ring 379.15
  sclera NEC 379.11
Starch eating 307.52
Stargardt's disease 362.75
Starvation (inanition) (due to lack of food) 994.2
  edema 262
  voluntary NEC 307.1
Stasis
  bile (duct) (see also Disease, biliary) 576.8
  bronchus (see also Bronchitis) 490
  cardiac (see also Failure, heart) 428.0
  cecum 564.89
  colon 564.89
  dermatitis (see also Varix, with stasis dermatitis) 454.1
  duodenal 536.8
  eczema (see also Varix, with stasis dermatitis) 454.1
  edema (see also Hypertension, venous) 459.30
  foot 991.4
  gastric 536.3
  ileocecal coil 564.89
  ileum 564.89
  intestinal 564.89
  jejunum 564.89
  kidney 586
  liver 571.9
    cirrhotic — see Cirrhosis, liver
  lymphatic 457.8
  pneumonia 514
  portal 571.9
  pulmonary 514
  rectal 564.89
  renal 586
    tubular 584.5
  stomach 536.3
  ulcer
    with varicose veins 454.0
    without varicose veins 459.81
  urine NEC (see also Retention, urine) 788.20
  venous 459.81
State
  affective and paranoid, mixed, organic psychotic 294.8
  agitated 307.9
    acute reaction to stress 308.2

State — continued
  anxiety (neurotic) (see also Anxiety) 300.00
    specified type NEC 300.09
  apprehension (see also Anxiety) 300.00
    specified type NEC 300.09
  climacteric, female 627.2
    following induced menopause 627.4
  clouded
    epileptic (see also Epilepsy) 345.9 ✓5ᵗʰ
    paroxysmal (idiopathic) (see also Epilepsy) 345.9 ✓5ᵗʰ
  compulsive (mixed) (with obsession) 300.3
  confusional 298.9
    acute 293.0
      with
        arteriosclerotic dementia 290.41
        presenile brain disease 290.11
        senility 290.3
      alcoholic 291.0
      drug-induced 292.81
    epileptic 293.0
    postoperative 293.9
    reactive (emotional stress) (psychological trauma) 298.2
    subacute 293.1
  constitutional psychopathic 301.9
  convulsive (see also Convulsions) 780.39
  depressive NEC 311
    induced by drug 292.84
    neurotic 300.4
  dissociative 300.15
  hallucinatory 780.1
    induced by drug 292.12
  hyperdynamic beta-adrenergic circulatory 429.82
  locked-in 344.81
  menopausal 627.2
    artificial 627.4
    following induced menopause 627.4
  neurotic NEC 300.9
    with depersonalization episode 300.6
  obsessional 300.3
  oneiroid (see also Schizophrenia) 295.4 ✓5ᵗʰ
  panic 300.01
  paranoid 297.9
    alcohol-induced 291.5
    arteriosclerotic 290.42
    climacteric 297.2
    drug-induced 292.11
    in
      presenile brain disease 290.12
      senile brain disease 290.20
    involutional 297.2
    menopausal 297.2
    senile 290.20
    simple 297.0
  postleukotomy 310.0
  pregnant (see also Pregnancy) V22.2
  psychogenic, twilight 298.2
  psychotic, organic (see also Psychosis, organic) 294.9
    mixed paranoid and affective 294.8
    senile or presenile NEC 290.9
    transient NEC 293.9
      with
        anxiety 293.84
        delusions 293.81
        depression 293.83
        hallucinations 293.82
  residual schizophrenic (see also Schizophrenia) 295.6 ✓5ᵗʰ

State — continued
  tension (see also Anxiety) 300.9
  transient organic psychotic 293.9
    anxiety type 293.84
    depressive type 293.83
    hallucinatory type 293.83
    paranoid type 293.81
    specified type NEC 293.89
  twilight
    epileptic 293.0
    psychogenic 298.2
  vegetative (persistent) 780.03
Status (post)
  absence
    epileptic (see also Epilepsy) 345.2
    of organ, acquired (postsurgical) — see Absence, by site, acquired
  anastomosis of intestine (for bypass) V45.3
  angioplasty, percutaneous transluminal coronary V45.82
  anginosus 413.9
  ankle prosthesis V43.66
  aortocoronary bypass or shunt V45.81
  arthrodesis V45.4
  artificially induced condition NEC V45.89
  artificial opening (of) V44.9
    gastrointestinal tract NEC V44.4
    specified site NEC V44.8
    urinary tract NEC V44.6
    vagina V44.7
  aspirator V46.0
  asthmaticus (see also Asthma) 493.9 ✓5ᵗʰ
  breast implant removal V45.83
  cardiac
    device (in situ) V45.00
      carotid sinus V45.09
        fitting or adjustment V53.39
      defibrillator, automatic implantable V45.02
      pacemaker V45.01
        fitting or adjustmanet V53.31
  carotid sinus stimulator V45.09
  cataract extraction V45.61
  chemotherapy V66.2
    current V58.69
  colostomy V44.3
  contraceptive device V45.59
    intrauterine V45.51
    subdermal V45.52
  convulsivus idiopathicus (see also Epilepsy) 345.3
  coronary artery bypass or shunt V45.81
  cystostomy V44.50
    appendico-vesicostomy V44.52
    cutaneous-vesicostomy V44.51
    specified type NEC V44.59
  defibrillator, automatic implant-able cardiac V45.02
  dental crowns V45.84
  dental fillings V45.84
  dental restoration V45.84
  dental sealant V49.82
  dialysis V45.1
  donor V59.9
  drug therapy or regimen V67.59
    high-risk medication NEC V67.51
  elbow prosthesis V43.62
  enterostomy V44.4
  epileptic, epilepticus (absence) (grand mal) (see also Epilepsy) 345.3
    focal motor 345.7 ✓5ᵗʰ

Status — *continued*
  epileptic, epilepticus — *continued*
    partial 345.7 ✓5ᵗʰ
    petit mal 345.2
    psychomotor 345.7 ✓5ᵗʰ
    temporal lobe 345.7 ✓5ᵗʰ
  eye (adnexa) surgery V45.69
  filtering bleb (eye) (postglaucoma) V45.69
    with rupture or complication 997.99
    pastcataract extraction (complication) 997.99
  finger joint prosthesis V43.69
  gastrostomy V44.1
  grand mal 345.3
  heart valve prosthesis V43.3
  hip prosthesis (joint) (partial) (total) V43.64
  ileostomy V44.2
  intestinal bypass V45.3
  intrauterine contraceptive device V45.51
  jejunostomy V44.4
  knee joint prosthesis V43.65
  lacunaris 437.8
  lacunosis 437.8
  low birth weight V21.30
    less than 500 grams V21.31
    500-999 grams V21.32
    1000-1499 grams V21.33
    1500-1999 grams V21.34
    2000-2500 grams V21.35
  lymphaticus 254.8
  malignant neoplasm, ablated or excised — *see* History, malignant neoplasm
  marmoratus 333.7
  nephrostomy V44.6
  neuropacemaker NEC V45.89
    brain V45.89
    carotid sinus V45.09
    neurologic NEC V45.89
  organ replacement
    by artificial or mechanical device or prosthesis of
      artery V43.4
      artificial skin V43.83
      bladder V43.5
      blood vessel V43.4
      breast V43.82
      eye globe V43.0
      heart V43.2
        valve V43.3
      intestine V43.89
      joint V43.60
        ankle V43.66
        elbow V43.62
        finger V43.69
        hip (partial) (total) V43.64
        knee V43.65
        shoulder V43.61
        specified NEC V43.69
        wrist V43.63
      kidney V43.89
      larynx V43.81
      lens V43.1
      limb(s) V43.7
      liver V43.89
      lung V43.89
      organ NEC V43.89
      pancreas V43.89
      skin (artificial) V43.83
      tissue NEC V43.89
      vein V43.4

Status — *continued*
  organ replacement — *continued*
    by organ transplant (heterologous) (homologous) — *see* Status, transplant
  pacemaker
    brain V45.89
    cardiac V45.01
    carotid sinus V45.09
    neurologic NEC V45.89
    specified site NEC V45.89
  percutaneous transluminal coronary angioplasty V45.82
  petit mal 345.2
  postcommotio cerebri 310.2
  postmenopausal (age related) (natural) V49.81
  postoperative NEC V45.89
  postpartum NEC V24.2
    care immediately following delivery V24.0
    routine follow-up V24.2
  postsurgical NEC V45.89
  renal dialysis V45.1
  respirator V46.1
  reversed jejunal transposition (for bypass) V45.3
  shoulder prosthesis V43.61
  shunt
    aortocoronary bypass V45.81
    arteriovenous (for dialysis) V45.1
    cerebrospinal fluid V45.2
    vascular NEC V45.89
      aortocoronary (bypass) V45.81
    ventricular (communicating) (for drainage) V45.2
  sterilization
    tubal ligation V26.51
    vasectomy V26.52
  subdermal contraceptive device V45.52
  thymicolymphaticus 254.8
  thymicus 254.8
  thymolymphaticus 254.8
  tooth extraction 525.10
  tracheostomy V44.0
  transplant
    blood vessel V42.89
    bone V42.4
      marrow V42.81
    cornea V42.5
    heart V42.1
      valve V42.2
    intestine V42.84
    kidney V42.0
    liver V42.7
    lung V42.6
    organ V42.9
      specified site NEC V42.89
    pancreas V42.83
    peripheral stem cells V42.82
    skin V42.3
    stem cells, peripheral V42.82
    tissue V42.9
      specified type NEC V42.89
    vessel, blood V42.89
  tubal ligation V26.51
  ureterostomy V44.6
  urethrostomy V44.6
  vagina, artificial V44.7
  vascular shunt NEC V45.89
    aortocoronary (bypass) V45.81
  vasectomy V26.52
  ventilator V46.1
  wrist prosthesis V43.63

Index to Diseases

Stave fracture — *see* Fracture, metacarpus, metacarpal bone(s)
Steal
   subclavian artery 435.2
   vertebral artery 435.1
Stealing, solitary, child problem (*see also* Disturbance, conduct) 312.1 ✓5ᵗʰ
Steam burn — *see* Burn, by site
Steatocystoma multiplex 706.2
Steatoma (infected) 706.2
   eyelid (cystic) 374.84
   infected 373.13
Steatorrhea (chronic) 579.8
   with lacteal obstruction 579.2
   idiopathic 579.0
     adult 579.0
     infantile 579.0
   pancreatic 579.4
   primary 579.0
   secondary 579.8
   specified cause NEC 579.8
   tropical 579.1
Steatosis 272.8
   heart (*see also* Degeneration, myocardial) 429.1
   kidney 593.89
   liver 571.8
Steele-Richardson (-Olszewski) Syndrome 333.0
Stein's syndrome (polycystic ovary) 256.4
Stein-Leventhal syndrome (polycystic ovary) 256.4
Steinbrocker's syndrome (*see also* Neuropathy, peripheral, autonomic) 337.9
Steinert's disease 359.2
Stenocardia (*see also* Angina) 413.9
Stenocephaly 756.0
Stenosis (cicatricial) — *see also* Stricture
   ampulla of Vater 576.2
     with calculus, cholelithiasis, or stones — *see* Choledocholithiasis
   anus, anal (canal) (sphincter) 569.2
     congenital 751.2
   aorta (ascending) 747.22
     arch 747.10
     arteriosclerotic 440.0
     calcified 440.0
   aortic (valve) 424.1
     with
        mitral (valve)
           insufficiency or incompetence 396.2
           stenosis or obstruction 396.0
     atypical 396.0
     congenital 746.3
     rheumatic 395.0
        with
           insufficiency, incompetency or regurgitation 395.2
              with mitral (valve) disease 396.8
           mitral (valve)
              disease (stenosis) 396.0
              insufficiency or incompetence 396.2
              stenosis or obstruction 396.0
     specified cause, except rheumatic 424.1
     syphilitic 093.22
   aqueduct of Sylvius (congenital) 742.3
     with spina bifida (*see also* Spina bifida) 741.0 ✓5ᵗʰ
     acquired 331.4

Stenosis — *continued*
   artery NEC 447.1
     basilar — *see* Narrowing, artery, basilar
     carotid (common) (internal) — *see* Narrowing, artery, carotid
     celiac 447.4
     cerebral 437.0
        due to
           embolism (*see also* Embolism, brain) 434.1 ✓5ᵗʰ
           thrombus (*see also* Thrombosis, brain) 434.0 ✓5ᵗʰ
     precerebral — *see* Narrowing, artery, precerebral
     pulmonary (congenital) 747.3
        acquired 417.8
     renal 440.1
     vertebral — *see* Narrowing, artery, vertebral
   bile duct or biliary passage (*see also* Obstruction, biliary) 576.2
     congenital 751.61
   bladder neck (acquired) 596.0
     congenital 753.6
   brain 348.8
   bronchus 519.1
     syphilitic 095.8
   cardia (stomach) 537.89
     congenital 750.7
   cardiovascular (*see also* Disease, cardiovascular) 429.2
   carotid artery — *see* Narrowing, artery, carotid
   cervix, cervical (canal) 622.4
     congenital 752.49
     in pregnancy or childbirth 654.6 ✓5ᵗʰ
        affecting fetus or newborn 763.89
        causing obstructed labor 660.2 ✓5ᵗʰ
           affecting fetus or newborn 763.1
   colon (*see also* Obstruction, intestine) 560.9
     congenital 751.2
   colostomy 569.62
   common bile duct (*see also* Obstruction, biliary) 576.2
     congenital 751.61
   coronary (artery) — *see* Arteriosclerosis, coronary
   cystic duct (*see also* Obstruction, gallbladder) 575.2
     congenital 751.61
   due to (presence of) any device, implant, or graft classifiable to 996.0-996.5 — *see* Complications, due to (presence of) any device, implant, or graft classified to 996.0-996.5 NEC
   duodenum 537.3
     congenital 751.1
   ejaculatory duct NEC 608.89
   endocervical os — *see* Stenosis, cervix
   enterostomy 569.62
   esophagus 530.3
     congenital 750.3
     syphilitic 095.8
        congenital 090.5
   external ear canal 380.50
     secondary to
        inflammation 380.53
        surgery 380.52
        trauma 380.51
   gallbladder (*see also* Obstruction, gallbladder) 575.2
   glottis 478.74

✓4ᵗʰ Fourth-digit Required   ✓5ᵗʰ Fifth-digit Required

Stenosis — *continued*
  heart valve (acquired) — *see also* Endocarditis
    congenital NEC 746.89
      aortic 746.3
      mitral 746.5
      pulmonary 746.02
      tricuspid 746.1
  hepatic duct (*see also* Obstruction, biliary) 576.2
  hymen 623.3
  hypertrophic subaortic (idiopathic) 425.1
  infundibulum cardiac 746.83
  intestine (*see also* Obstruction, intestine) 560.9
    congenital (small) 751.1
      large 751.2
  lacrimal
    canaliculi 375.53
    duct 375.56
      congenital 743.65
    punctum 375.52
      congenital 743.65
    sac 375.54
      congenital 743.65
  lacrimonasal duct 375.56
    congenital 743.65
    neonatal 375.55
  larynx 478.74
    congenital 748.3
    syphilitic 095.8
      congenital 090.5
  mitral (valve) (chronic) (inactive) 394.0
    with
      aortic (valve)
        disease (insufficiency) 396.1
        insufficiency or incompetence 396.1
        stenosis or obstruction 396.0
      incompetency, insufficiency or regurgitation 394.2
        with aortic valve disease 396.8
    active or acute 391.1
      with chorea (acute) (rheumatic) (Sydenham's) 392.0
    congenital 746.5
    specified cause, except rheumatic 424.0
    syphilitic 093.21
  myocardium, myocardial (*see also* Degeneration, myocardial) 429.1
    hypertrophic subaortic (idiopathic) 425.1
  nares (anterior) (posterior) 478.1
    congenital 748.0
  nasal duct 375.56
    congenital 743.65
  nasolacrimal duct 375.56
    congenital 743.65
    neonatal 375.55
  organ or site, congenital NEC — *see* Atresia
  papilla of Vater 576.2
    with calculus, cholelithiasis, or stones — *see* Choledocholithiasis
  pulmonary (artery) (congenital) 747.3
    with ventricular septal defect, dextraposition of aorta and hypertrophy of right ventricle 745.2
    acquired 417.8
    infundibular 746.83
    in tetralogy of Fallot 745.2
    subvalvular 746.83
    valve (*see also* Endocarditis, pulmonary) 424.3
      congenital 746.02

Stenosis — *continued*
  pulmonary — *continued*
    vein 747.49
      acquired 417.8
    vessel NEC 417.8
  pulmonic (congenital) 746.02
    infundibular 746.83
    subvalvular 746.83
  pylorus (hypertrophic) 537.0
    adult 537.0
    congenital 750.5
    infantile 750.5
  rectum (sphincter) (*see also* Stricture, rectum) 569.2
  renal artery 440.1
  salivary duct (any) 527.8
  sphincter of Oddi (*see also* Obstruction, biliary) 576.2
  spinal 724.00
    cervical 723.0
    lumbar, lumbosacral 724.02
    nerve (root) NEC 724.9
    specified region NEC 724.09
    thoracic, thoracolumbar 724.01
  stomach, hourglass 537.6
  subaortic 746.81
    hypertrophic (idiopathic) 425.1
  supra (valvular)-aortic 747.22
  trachea 519.1
    congenital 748.3
    syphilitic 095.8
    tuberculous (*see also* Tuberculosis) 012.8
  tracheostomy 519.02
  tricuspid (valve) (*see also* Endocarditis, tricuspid) 397.0
    congenital 746.1
    nonrheumatic 424.2
  tubal 628.2
  ureter (*see also* Stricture, ureter) 593.3
    congenital 753.29
  urethra (*see also* Stricture, urethra) 598.9
  vagina 623.2
    congenital 752.49
    in pregnancy or childbirth 654.7
      affecting fetus or newborn 763.89
      causing obstructed labor 660.2
        affecting fetus or newborn 763.1
  valve (cardiac) (heart) (*see also* Endocarditis) 424.90
    congenital NEC 746.89
      aortic 746.3
      mitral 746.5
      pulmonary 746.02
      tricuspid 746.1
    urethra 753.6
  valvular (*see also* Endocarditis) 424.90
    congenital NEC 746.89
    urethra 753.6
  vascular graft or shunt 996.1
    atherosclerosis — *see* Arteriosclerosis, extremities
    embolism 996.74
    occlusion NEC 996.74
    thrombus 996.74
  vena cava (inferior) (superior) 459.2
    congenital 747.49
  ventricular shunt 996.2
  vulva 624.8

Stercolith (*see also* Fecalith) 560.39
  appendix 543.9

Stercoraceous, stercoral ulcer 569.82
  anus or rectum 569.41
Stereopsis, defective
  with fusion 368.33
  without fusion 368.32
Stereotypes NEC 307.3
Sterility
  female — see Infertility, female
  male (see also Infertility, male) 606.9
Sterilization, admission for V25.2
  status
    tubal ligation V26.51
    vasectomy V26.52
Sternalgia (see also Angina) 413.9
Sternopagus 759.4
Sternum bifidum 756.3
Sternutation 784.9
Steroid
  effects (adverse) (iatrogenic)
    cushingoid
      correct substance properly administered 255.0
      overdose or wrong substance given or taken 962.0
    diabetes
      correct substance properly administered 251.8
      overdose or wrong substance given or taken 962.0
    due to
      correct substance properly administered 255.8
      overdose or wrong substance given or taken 962.0
    fever
      correct substance properly administered 780.6
      overdose or wrong substance given or taken 962.0
    withdrawal
      correct substance properly administered 255.4
      overdose or wrong substance given or taken 962.0
  responder 365.03
Stevens-Johnson disease or syndrome (erythema multiforme exudativum) 695.1
Stewart-Morel syndrome (hyperostosis frontalis interna) 733.3
Sticker's disease (erythema infectiosum) 057.0
Sticky eye 372.03
Stieda's disease (calcification, knee joint) 726.62
Stiff
  back 724.8
  neck (see also Torticollis) 723.5
Stiff-man syndrome 333.91
Stiffness, joint NEC 719.50
  ankle 719.57
  back 724.8
  elbow 719.52
  finger 719.54
  hip 719.55
  knee 719.56
  multiple sites 719.59
  sacroiliac 724.6
  shoulder 719.51
  specified site NEC 719.58
  spine 724.9

Stiffness, joint — continued
  surgical fusion V45.4
  wrist 719.53
Stigmata, congenital syphilis 090.5
Still's disease or syndrome 714.30
Still-Felty syndrome (rheumatoid arthritis with splenomegaly and leukopenia) 714.1
Stillbirth, stillborn NEC 779.9
Stiller's disease (asthenia) 780.79
Stilling-Türk-Duane syndrome (ocular retraction syndrome) 378.71
Stimulation, ovary 256.1
Sting (animal) (bee) (fish) (insect) (jellyfish) (Portuguese man-o-war) (wasp) (venomous) 989.5
  anaphylactic shock or reaction 989.5
  plant 692.6
Stippled epiphyses 756.59
Stitch
  abscess 998.59
  burst (in operation wound) 998.32
    internal 998.31
  in back 724.5
Stojano's (subcostal) syndrome 098.86
Stokes' disease (exophthalmic goiter) 242.0
Stokes-Adams syndrome (syncope with heart block) 426.9
Stokvis' (-Talma) disease (enterogenous cyanosis) 289.7
Stomach — see condition
Stoma malfunction
  colostomy 569.62
  cystostomy 997.5
  enterostomy 569.62
  gastrostomy 536.42
  ileostomy 569.62
  nephrostomy 997.5
  tracheostomy 519.02
  ureterostomy 997.5
Stomatitis 528.0
  angular 528.5
    due to dietary or vitamin deficiency 266.0
  aphthous 528.2
  candidal 112.0
  catarrhal 528.0
  denture 528.9
  diphtheritic (membranous) 032.0
  due to
    dietary deficiency 266.0
    thrush 112.0
    vitamin deficiency 266.0
  epidemic 078.4
  epizootic 078.4
  follicular 528.0
  gangrenous 528.1
  herpetic 054.2
  herpetiformis 528.2
  malignant 528.0
  membranous acute 528.0
  monilial 112.0
  mycotic 112.0
  necrotic 528.1
    ulcerative 101
  necrotizing ulcerative 101
  parasitic 112.0
  septic 528.0
  spirochetal 101
  suppurative (acute) 528.0

Stomatitis — continued
  ulcerative 528.0
    necrotizing 101
  ulceromembranous 101
  vesicular 528.0
    with exanthem 074.3
  Vincent's 101
Stomatocytosis 282.8
Stomatomycosis 112.0
Stomatorrhagia 528.9
Stone(s) — see also Calculus
  bladder 594.1
    diverticulum 594.0
  cystine 270.0
  heart syndrome (see also Failure, ventricular, left) 428.1
  kidney 592.0
  prostate 602.0
  pulp (dental) 522.2
  renal 592.0
  salivary duct or gland (any) 527.5
  ureter 592.1
  urethra (impacted) 594.2
  urinary (duct) (impacted) (passage) 592.9
    bladder 594.1
      diverticulum 594.0
    lower tract NEC 594.9
    specified site 594.8
  xanthine 277.2
Stonecutters' lung 502
  tuberculous (see also Tuberculosis) 011.4 ✓5ᵗʰ
Stonemasons'
  asthma, disease, or lung 502
    tuberculous (see also Tuberculosis) 011.4 ✓5ᵗʰ
  phthisis (see also Tuberculosis) 011.4 ✓5ᵗʰ
Stoppage
  bowel (see also Obstruction, intestine) 560.9
  heart (see also Arrest, cardiac) 427.5
  intestine (see also Obstruction, intestine) 560.9
  urine NEC (see also Retention, urine) 788.20
Storm, thyroid (apathetic) (see also Thyrotoxicosis) 242.9 ✓5ᵗʰ
Strabismus (alternating) (congenital) (nonparalytic) 378.9
  concomitant (see also Heterotropia) 378.30
    convergent (see also Esotropia) 378.00
    divergent (see also Exotropia) 378.10
  convergent (see also Esotropia) 378.00
  divergent (see also Exotropia) 378.10
  due to adhesions, scars — see Strabismus, mechanical
  in neuromuscular disorder NEC 378.73
    intermittent 378.20
      vertical 378.31
    latent 378.40
      convergent (esophoria) 378.41
      divergent (exophoria) 378.42
      vertical 378.43
    mechanical 378.60
      due to
        Brown's tendon sheath syndrome 378.61
        specified musculofascial disorder NEC 378.62
    paralytic 378.50
      third or oculomotor nerve (partial) 378.51
        total 378.52
      fourth or trochlear nerve 378.53
      sixth or abducens nerve 378.54

Strabismus — continued
  specified type NEC 378.73
  vertical (hypertropia) 378.31
Strain — see also Sprain, by site
  eye NEC 368.13
  heart — see Disease, heart
  meaning gonorrhea — see Gonorrhea
  physical NEC V62.89
  postural 729.9
  psychological NEC V62.89
Strands
  conjunctiva 372.62
  vitreous humor 379.25
Strangulation, strangulated 994.7
  appendix 543.9
  asphyxiation or suffocation by 994.7
  bladder neck 596.0
  bowel — see Strangulation, intestine
  colon — see Strangulation, intestine
  cord (umbilical) — see Compression, umbilical cord
  due to birth injury 767.8
  food or foreign body (see also Asphyxia, food) 933.1
  hemorrhoids 455.8
    external 455.5
    internal 455.2
  hernia — see also Hernia, by site, with obstruction
    gangrenous — see Hernia, by site, with gangrene
  intestine (large) (small) 560.2
    with hernia — see also Hernia, by site, with obstruction
      gangrenous — see Hernia, by site, with gangrene
    congenital (small) 751.1
      large 751.2
  mesentery 560.2
  mucus (see also Asphyxia, mucus) 933.1
    newborn 770.1
  omentum 560.2
  organ or site, congenital NEC — see Atresia
  ovary 620.8
    due to hernia 620.4
  penis 607.89
    foreign body 939.3
  rupture (see also Hernia, by site, with obstruction) 552.9
    gangrenous (see also Hernia, by site, with gangrene) 551.9
  stomach, due to hernia (see also Hernia, by site, with obstruction) 552.9
    with gangrene (see also Hernia, by site, with gangrene) 551.9
  umbilical cord — see Compression, umbilical cord
  vesicourethral orifice 596.0
Strangury 788.1
Strawberry
  gallbladder (see also Disease, gallbladder) 575.6
  mark 757.32
  tongue (red) (white) 529.3
Straw itch 133.8
Streak, ovarian 752.0
Strephosymbolia 315.01
  secondary to organic lesion 784.69
Streptobacillary fever 026.1
Streptobacillus moniliformis 026.1

Index to Diseases

Streptococcemia 038.0
Streptococcicosis — *see* Infection, streptococcal
Streptococcus, streptococcal — *see* condition
Streptoderma 686.00
Streptomycosis — *see* Actinomycosis
Streptothricosis — *see* Actinomycosis
Streptothrix — *see* Actinomycosis
Streptotrichosis — *see* Actinomycosis
Stress
    fracture — *see* Fracture, stress
    polycythemia 289.0
    reaction (gross) (*see also* Reaction, stress, acute) 308.9
Stretching, nerve — *see* Injury, nerve, by site
Striae (albicantes) (atrophicae) (cutis distensae) (distensae) 701.3
Striations of nails 703.8
Stricture (*see also* Stenosis) 799.8
    ampulla of Vater 576.2
        with calculus, cholelithiasis, or stones — *see* Choledocholithiasis
    anus (sphincter) 569.2
        congenital 751.2
        infantile 751.2
    aorta (ascending) 747.22
        arch 747.10
        arteriosclerotic 440.0
        calcified 440.0
    aortic (valve) (*see also* Stenosis, aortic) 424.1
        congenital 746.3
    aqueduct of Sylvius (congenital) 742.3
        with spina bifida (*see also* Spina bifida) 741.0 ✓5ᵗʰ
        acquired 331.4
    artery 447.1
        basilar — *see* Narrowing, artery, basilar
        carotid (common) (internal) — *see* Narrowing, artery, carotid
        celiac 447.4
        cerebral 437.0
            congenital 747.81
            due to
                embolism (*see also* Embolism, brain) 434.1 ✓5ᵗʰ
                thrombus (*see also* Thrombosis, brain) 434.0 ✓5ᵗʰ
        congenital (peripheral) 747.60
            cerebral 747.81
            coronary 746.85
            gastrointestinal 747.61
            lower limb 747.64
            renal 747.62
            retinal 743.58
            specified NEC 747.69
            spinal 747.82
            umbilical 747.5
            upper limb 747.63
        coronary — *see* Arteriosclerosis, coronary
            congenital 746.85
        precerebral — *see* Narrowing, artery, precerebral NEC
        pulmonary (congenital) 747.3
            acquired 417.8
        renal 440.1
        vertebral — *see* Narrowing, artery, vertebral
    auditory canal (congenital) (external) 744.02
        acquired (*see also* Stricture, ear canal, acquired) 380.50
    bile duct or passage (any) (postoperative) (*see also* Obstruction, biliary) 576.2

Stricture — *continued*
    bile duct or passage — *continued*
        congenital 751.61
    bladder 596.8
        congenital 753.6
        neck 596.0
            congenital 753.6
    bowel (*see also* Obstruction, intestine) 560.9
    brain 348.8
    bronchus 519.1
        syphilitic 095.8
    cardia (stomach) 537.89
        congenital 750.7
    cardiac — *see also* Disease, heart
        orifice (stomach) 537.89
    cardiovascular (*see also* Disease, cardiovascular) 429.2
    carotid artery — *see* Narrowing, artery, carotid
    cecum (*see also* Obstruction, intestine) 560.9
    cervix, cervical (canal) 622.4
        congenital 752.49
        in pregnancy or childbirth 654.6 ✓5ᵗʰ
            affecting fetus or newborn 763.89
        causing obstructed labor 660.2 ✓5ᵗʰ
            affecting fetus or newborn 763.1
    colon (*see also* Obstruction, intestine) 560.9
        congenital 751.2
    colostomy 569.62
    common bile duct (*see also* Obstruction, biliary) 576.2
        congenital 751.61
    coronary (artery) — *see* Arteriosclerosis, coronary
        congenital 746.85
    cystic duct (*see also* Obstruction, gallbladder) 575.2
        congenital 751.61
    cystostomy 997.5
    digestive organs NEC, congenital 751.8
    duodenum 537.3
        congenital 751.1
    ear canal (external) (congenital) 744.02
        acquired 380.50
            secondary to
                inflammation 380.53
                surgery 380.52
                trauma 380.51
    ejaculatory duct 608.85
    enterostomy 569.62
    esophagus (corrosive) (peptic) 530.3
        congenital 750.3
        syphilitic 095.8
            congenital 090.5
    eustachian tube (*see also* Obstruction, Eustachian tube) 381.60
        congenital 744.24
    fallopian tube 628.2
        gonococcal (chronic) 098.37
            acute 098.17
        tuberculous (*see also* Tuberculosis) 016.6 ✓5ᵗʰ
    gallbladder (*see also* Obstruction, gallbladder) 575.2
        congenital 751.69
    glottis 478.74
    heart — *see also* Disease, heart
        congenital NEC 746.89
        valve — *see also* Endocarditis
            congenital NEC 746.89
                aortic 746.3
                mitral 746.5
                pulmonary 746.02

Stricture — *continued*
  heart — *continued*
    valve — *continued*
      congenital — *continued*
        tricuspid 746.1
  hepatic duct (*see also* Obstruction, biliary) 576.2
  hourglass, of stomach 537.6
  hymen 623.3
  hypopharynx 478.29
  intestine (*see also* Obstruction, intestine) 560.9
    congenital (small) 751.1
      large 751.2
    ischemic 557.1
  lacrimal
    canaliculi 375.53
      congenital 743.65
    punctum 375.52
      congenital 743.65
    sac 375.54
      congenital 743.65
  lacrimonasal duct 375.56
    congenital 743.65
    neonatal 375.55
  larynx 478.79
    congenital 748.3
    syphilitic 095.8
      congenital 090.5
  lung 518.89
  meatus
    ear (congenital) 744.02
      acquired (*see also* Stricture, ear canal, acquired) 380.50
    osseous (congenital) (ear) 744.03
      acquired (*see also* Stricture, ear canal, acquired) 380.50
    urinarius (*see also* Stricture, urethra) 598.9
      congenital 753.6
  mitral (valve) (*see also* Stenosis, mitral) 394.0
    congenital 746.5
    specified cause, except rheumatic 424.0
  myocardium, myocardial (*see also* Degeneration, myocardial) 429.1
    hypertrophic subaortic (idiopathic) 425.1
  nares (anterior) (posterior) 478.1
    congenital 748.0
  nasal duct 375.56
    congenital 743.65
    neonatal 375.55
  nasolacrimal duct 375.56
    congenital 743.65
    neonatal 375.55
  nasopharynx 478.29
    syphilitic 095.8
  nephrostomy 997.5
  nose 478.1
    congenital 748.0
  nostril (anterior) (posterior) 478.1
    congenital 748.0
  organ or site, congenital NEC — *see* Atresia
  osseous meatus (congenital) (ear) 744.03
    acquired (*see also* Stricture, ear canal, acquired) 380.50
  os uteri (*see also* Stricture, cervix) 622.4
  oviduct — *see* Stricture, fallopian tube
  pelviureteric junction 593.3
  pharynx (dilation) 478.29
  prostate 602.8

Stricture — *continued*
  pulmonary, pulmonic
    artery (congenital) 747.3
      acquired 417.8
      noncongenital 417.8
    infundibulum (congenital) 746.83
    valve (*see also* Endocarditis, pulmonary) 424.3
      congenital 746.02
    vein (congenital) 747.49
      acquired 417.8
    vessel NEC 417.8
  punctum lacrimale 375.52
    congenital 743.65
  pylorus (hypertrophic) 537.0
    adult 537.0
    congenital 750.5
    infantile 750.5
  rectosigmoid 569.89
  rectum (sphincter) 569.2
    congenital 751.2
    due to
      chemical burn 947.3
      irradiation 569.2
      lymphogranuloma venereum 099.1
    gonococcal 098.7
    inflammatory 099.1
    syphilitic 095.8
    tuberculous (*see also* Tuberculosis) 014.8 ✓5ᵗʰ
  renal artery 440.1
  salivary duct or gland (any) 527.8
  sigmoid (flexure) (*see also* Obstruction, intestine) 560.9
  spermatic cord 608.85
  stoma (following) (of)
    colostomy 569.62
    cystostomy 997.5
    enterostomy 569.62
    gastrostomy 536.42
    ileostomy 569.62
    nephrostomy 997.5
    tracheostomy 519.02
    ureterostomy 997.5
  stomach 537.89
    congenital 750.7
    hourglass 537.6
  subaortic 746.81
    hypertrophic (acquired) (idiopathic) 425.1
  subglottic 478.74
  syphilitic NEC 095.8
  tendon (sheath) 727.81
  trachea 519.1
    congenital 748.3
    syphilitic 095.8
    tuberculous (*see also* Tuberculosis) 012.8 ✓5ᵗʰ
  tracheostomy 519.02
  tricuspid (valve) (*see also* Endocarditis, tricuspid) 397.0
    congenital 746.1
    nonrheumatic 424.2
  tunica vaginalis 608.85
  ureter (postoperative) 593.3
    congenital 753.29
    tuberculous (*see also* Tuberculosis) 016.2 ✓5ᵗʰ
  ureteropelvic junction 593.3
    congenital 753.21
  ureterovesical orifice 593.3
    congenital 753.22

Stricture — *continued*
 urethra (anterior) (meatal) (organic) (posterior) (spasmodic) 598.9
  associated with schistosomiasis (*see also* Schistosomiasis) 120.9 *[598.01]*
  congenital (valvular) 753.6
  due to
   infection 598.00
    syphilis 095.8 *[598.01]*
   trauma 598.1
  gonococcal 098.2 *[598.01]*
  gonorrheal 098.2 *[598.01]*
  infective 598.00
  late effect of injury 598.1
  postcatheterization 598.2
  postobstetric 598.1
  postoperative 598.2
  specified cause NEC 598.8
  syphilitic 095.8 *[598.01]*
  traumatic 598.1
  valvular, congenital 753.6
 urinary meatus (*see also* Stricture, urethra) 598.9
  congenital 753.6
 uterus, uterine 621.5
  os (external) (internal) — *see* Stricture, cervix
 vagina (outlet) 623.2
  congenital 752.49
 valve (cardiac) (heart) (*see also* Endocarditis) 424.90
  congenital (cardiac) (heart) NEC 746.89
   aortic 746.3
   mitral 746.5
   pulmonary 746.02
   tricuspid 746.1
   urethra 753.6
 valvular (*see also* Endocarditis) 424.90
 vascular graft or shunt 996.1
  atherosclerosis — *see* Arteriosclersis, extremities
  embolism 996.74
  occlusion NEC 996.74
  thrombus 996.74
 vas deferens 608.85
  congenital 752.8
 vein 459.2
 vena cava (inferior) (superior) NEC 459.2
  congenital 747.49
 ventricular shunt 996.2
 vesicourethral orifice 596.0
  congenital 753.6
 vulva (acquired) 624.8
Stridor 786.1
 congenital (larynx) 748.3
Stridulous — *see* condition
Strippling of nails 703.8
Stroke (*see also* Disease, cerebrovascular, acute) 436
 apoplectic (*see also* Disease, cerebrovascular, acute) 436
 brain (*see also* Disease, cerebrovascular, acute) 436
 epileptic — *see* Epilepsy
 healed or old V12.59
 heart — *see* Disease, heart
 heat 992.0
 iatrogenic 997.02
 in evolution 435.9
 late effect — *see* Late effect(s) (of) cerebrovascular disease

Stroke — *continued*
 lightning 994.0
 paralytic (*see also* Disease, cerebrovascular, acute) 436
 postoperative 997.02
 progressive 435.9
Stromatosis, endometrial (M8931/1) 236.0
Strong pulse 785.9
Strongyloides stercoralis infestation 127.2
Strongyloidiasis 127.2
Strongyloidosis 127.2
Strongylus (gibsoni) infestation 127.7
Strophulus (newborn) 779.89
 pruriginosus 698.2
Struck by lightning 994.0
Struma (*see also* Goiter) 240.9
 fibrosa 245.3
 Hashimoto (struma lymphomatosa) 245.2
 lymphomatosa 245.2
 nodosa (simplex) 241.9
  endemic 241.9
  multinodular 241.1
  sporadic 241.9
  toxic or with hyperthyroidism 242.3 ✓5ᵗʰ
   multinodular 242.2 ✓5ᵗʰ
   uninodular 242.1 ✓5ᵗʰ
  toxicosa 242.3 ✓5ᵗʰ
   multinodular 242.2 ✓5ᵗʰ
   uninodular 242.1 ✓5ᵗʰ
  uninodular 241.0
 ovarii (M9090/0) 220
  and carcinoid (M9091/1) 236.2
  malignant (M9090/3) 183.0
 Riedel's (ligneous thyroiditis) 245.3
 scrofulous (*see also* Tuberculosis) 017.2 ✓5ᵗʰ
 tuberculous (*see also* Tuberculosis) 017.2 ✓5ᵗʰ
  abscess 017.2 ✓5ᵗʰ
  adenitis 017.2 ✓5ᵗʰ
  lymphangitis 017.2 ✓5ᵗʰ
  ulcer 017.2 ✓5ᵗʰ
Strumipriva cachexia (*see also* Hypothyroidism) 244.9
Strümpell-Marie disease or spine (ankylosing spondylitis) 720.0
Strümpell-Westphal pseudosclerosis (hepatolenticular degeneration) 275.1
Stuart's disease (congenital factor X deficiency) (*see also* Defect, coagulation) 286.3
Stuart-Prower factor deficiency (congenital factor X deficiency) (*see also* Defect, coagulation) 286.3
Students' elbow 727.2
Stuffy nose 478.1
Stump — *see also* Amputation
 cervix, cervical (healed) 622.8
Stupor 780.09
 catatonic (*see also* Schizophrenia) 295.2 ✓5ᵗʰ
 circular (*see also* Psychosis, manic-depressive, circular) 296.7
 manic 296.89
 manic-depressive (*see also* Psychosis, affective) 296.89
 mental (anergic) (delusional) 298.9
 psychogenic 298.8
 reaction to exceptional stress (transient) 308.2
 traumatic NEC — *see also* Injury, intracranial
  with spinal (cord)
   lesion — *see* Injury, spinal, by site
   shock — *see* Injury, spinal, by site

Sturge (-Weber) (-Dimitri) disease or syndrome — Index to Disease

Sturge (-Weber) (-Dimitri) disease or syndrome (encephalocutan-eous angiomatosis) 759.6
Sturge-Kalischer-Weber syndrome (encephalocutaneous angiomatosis) 759.6
Stuttering 307.0
Sty, stye 373.11
   external 373.11
   internal 373.12
   meibomian 373.12
Subacidity, gastric 536.8
   psychogenic 306.4
Subacute — see condition
Subarachnoid — see condition
Subclavian steal syndrome 435.2
Subcortical — see condition
Subcostal syndrome 098.86
   nerve compression 354.8
Subcutaneous, subcuticular — see condition
Subdelirium 293.1
Subdural — see condition
Subendocardium — see condition
Subependymoma (M9383/1) 237.5
Suberosis 495.3
Subglossitis — see Glossitis
Subhemophilia 286.0
Subinvolution (uterus) 621.1
   breast (postlactational) (postpartum) 611.8
   chronic 621.1
   puerperal, postpartum 674.8 ✓5ᵗʰ
Sublingual — see condition
Sublinguitis 527.2
Subluxation — see also Dislocation, by site
   congenital NEC — see also Malposition, congenital
   hip (unilateral) 754.32
     with dislocation of other hip 754.35
     bilateral 754.33
   joint
     lower limb 755.69
     shoulder 755.59
     upper limb 755.59
   lower limb (joint) 755.69
   shoulder (joint) 755.59
   upper limb (joint) 755.59
   lens 379.32
     anterior 379.33
     posterior 379.34
   rotary, cervical region of spine — see Fracture, vertebra, cervical
Submaxillary — see condition
Submersion (fatal) (nonfatal) 994.1
Submissiveness (undue), in child 313.0
Submucous — see condition
Subnormal, subnormality
   accommodation (see also Disorder, accommodation) 367.9
   mental (see also Retardation, mental) 319
     mild 317
     moderate 318.0
     profound 318.2
     severe 318.1
   temperature (accidental) 991.6
     not associated with low environmental temperature 780.99 ▲
Subphrenic — see condition
Subscapular nerve — see condition

Subseptus uterus 752.3
Subsiding appendicitis 542
Substernal thyroid (see also Goiter) 240.9
   congenital 759.2
Substitution disorder 300.11
Subtentorial — see condition
Subtertian
   fever 084.0
   malaria (fever) 084.0
Subthyroidism (acquired) (see also Hypothyroidism) 244.9
   congenital 243
Succenturiata placenta — see Placenta, abnormal
Succussion sounds, chest 786.7
Sucking thumb, child 307.9
Sudamen 705.1
Sudamina 705.1
Sudanese kala-azar 085.0
Sudden
   death, cause unknown (less than 24 hours) 798.1
     during childbirth 669.9 ✓5ᵗʰ
     infant 798.0
     puerperal, postpartum 674.9 ✓5ᵗʰ
   hearing loss NEC 388.2
   heart failure (see also Failure, heart) 428.9
   infant death syndrome 798.0
Sudeck's atrophy, disease, or syndrome 733.7
SUDS (Sudden unexplained death) 798.2
Suffocation (see also Asphyxia) 799.0
   by
     bed clothes 994.7
     bunny bag 994.7
     cave-in 994.7
     constriction 994.7
     drowning 994.1
     inhalation
       food or foreign body (see also Asphyxia, food or foreign body) 933.1
       oil or gasoline (see also Asphyxia, food or foreign body) 933.1
     overlying 994.7
     plastic bag 994.7
     pressure 994.7
     strangulation 994.7
   during birth 768.1
   mechanical 994.7
Sugar
   blood
     high 790.2
     low 251.2
   in urine 791.5
Suicide, suicidal (attempted)
   by poisoning — see Table of Drugs and Chemicals
   risk 300.9
   tendencies 300.9
   trauma NEC (see also nature and site of injury) 959.9
Suipestifer infection (see also Infection, Salmonella) 003.9
Sulfatidosis 330.0
Sulfhemoglobinemia, sulphemoglobinemia (acquired) (congenital) 289.7
Sumatran mite fever 081.2
Summer — see condition

Sunburn 692.71
  dermatitis 692.71
  due to
    other ultraviolet radiation 692.82
    tanning bed 692.82
  first degree 692.71
  second degree 692.76
  third degree 692.77
Sunken
  acetabulum 718.85
  fontanels 756.0
Sunstroke 992.0
Superfecundation 651.9 ✓5
  with fetal loss and retention of one or more fetus(es) 651.6 ✓5
Superfetation 651.9 ✓5
  with fetal loss and retention of one or more fetus(es) 651.6 ✓5
Superinvolution uterus 621.8
Supernumerary (congenital)
  aortic cusps 746.89
  auditory ossicles 744.04
  bone 756.9
  breast 757.6
  carpal bones 755.56
  cusps, heart valve NEC 746.89
    mitral 746.5
    pulmonary 746.09
  digit(s) 755.00
    finger 755.01
    toe 755.02
  ear (lobule) 744.1
  fallopian tube 752.19
  finger 755.01
  hymen 752.49
  kidney 753.3
  lacrimal glands 743.64
  lacrimonasal duct 743.65
  lobule (ear) 744.1
  mitral cusps 746.5
  muscle 756.82
  nipples 757.6
  organ or site NEC — see Accessory
  ossicles, auditory 744.04
  ovary 752.0
  oviduct 752.19
  pulmonic cusps 746.09
  rib 756.3
    cervical or first 756.2
      syndrome 756.2
  roots (of teeth) 520.2
  spinal vertebra 756.19
  spleen 759.0
  tarsal bones 755.67
  teeth 520.1
    causing crowding 524.3
  testis 752.8
  thumb 755.01
  toe 755.02
  uterus 752.2
  vagina 752.49
  vertebra 756.19
Supervision (of)
  contraceptive method previously prescribed V25.40
    intrauterine device V25.42
    oral contraceptive (pill) V25.41
    specified type NEC V25.49
    subdermal implantable contraceptive V25.43

Supervision (of) — *continued*
  dietary (for) V65.3
    allergy (food) V65.3
    colitis V65.3
    diabetes mellitus V65.3
    food allergy intolerance V65.3
    gastritis V65.3
    hypercholesterolemia V65.3
    hypoglycemia V65.3
    intolerance (food) V65.3
    obesity V65.3
    specified NEC V65.3
  lactation V24.1
  pregnancy — *see* Pregnancy, supervision of
Supplemental teeth 520.1
  causing crowding 524.3
Suppression
  binocular vision 368.31
  lactation 676.5 ✓5
  menstruation 626.8
  ovarian secretion 256.39
  renal 586
  urinary secretion 788.5
  urine 788.5
Suppuration, suppurative — *see also* condition
  accessory sinus (chronic) (*see also* Sinusitis) 473.9
  adrenal gland 255.8
  antrum (chronic) (*see also* Sinusitis, maxillary) 473.0
  bladder (*see also* Cystitis) 595.89
  bowel 569.89
  brain 324.0
    late effect 326
  breast 611.0
    puerperal, postpartum 675.1 ✓5
  dental periosteum 526.5
  diffuse (skin) 686.00
  ear (middle) (*see also* Otitis media) 382.4
    external (*see also* Otitis, externa) 380.10
    internal 386.33
  ethmoidal (sinus) (chronic) (*see also* Sinusitis, ethmoidal) 473.2
  fallopian tube (*see also* Salpingo-oophoritis) 614.2
  frontal (sinus) (chronic) (*see also* Sinusitis, frontal) 473.1
  gallbladder (*see also* Cholecystitis, acute) 575.0
  gum 523.3
  hernial sac — *see* Hernia, by site
  intestine 569.89
  joint (*see also* Arthritis, suppurative) 711.0 ✓5
  labyrinthine 386.33
  lung 513.0
  mammary gland 611.0
    puerperal, postpartum 675.1 ✓5
  maxilla, maxillary 526.4
    sinus (chronic) (*see also* Sinusitis, maxillary) 473.0
  muscle 728.0
  nasal sinus (chronic) (*see also* Sinusitis) 473.9
  pancreas 577.0
  parotid gland 527.2
  pelvis, pelvic
    female (*see also* Disease, pelvis, inflammatory) 614.4
      acute 614.3
    male (*see also* Peritonitis) 567.2
  pericranial (*see also* Osteomyelitis) 730.2 ✓5

Suppuration, suppurative — *continued*
  salivary duct or gland (any) 527.2
  sinus (nasal) (*see also* Sinusitis) 473.9
  sphenoidal (sinus) (chronic) (*see also*
      Sinusitis, sphenoidal) 473.3
  thymus (gland) 254.1
  thyroid (gland) 245.0
  tonsil 474.8
  uterus (*see also* Endometritis) 615.9
  vagina 616.10
  wound — *see also* Wound, open, by site,
      complicated
    dislocation — *see* Dislocation, by site,
        compound
    fracture — *see* Fracture, by site, open
    scratch or other superficial injury — *see*
        Injury, superficial, by site
Supraglottitis 464.50
  with obstruction 464.51
Suprapubic drainage 596.8
Suprarenal (gland) — *see* condition
Suprascapular nerve — *see* condition
Suprasellar — *see* condition
Supraspinatus syndrome 726.10
Surfer knots 919.8
  infected 919.9
Surgery
  cosmetic NEC V50.1
    following healed injury or operation V51
    hair transplant V50.0
  elective V50.9
    breast augmentation or reduction V50.1
    circumcision, ritual or routine (in absence
        of medical indication) V50.2
    cosmetic NEC V50.1
    ear piercing V50.3
    face-lift V50.1
    following healed injury or operation V51
    hair transplant V50.0
  not done because of
    contraindication V64.1
    patient's decision V64.2
    specified reason NEC V64.3
  plastic
    breast augmentation or reduction V50.1
    cosmetic V50.1
    face-lift V50.1
    following healed injury or operation V51
    repair of scarred tissue (following healed
        injury or operation) V51
    specified type NEC V50.8
  previous, in pregnancy or childbirth
    cervix 654.6 ✓5ᵗʰ
      affecting fetus or newborn 763.89
      causing obstructed labor 660.2 ✓5ᵗʰ
        affecting fetus or newborn 763.1
    pelvic soft tissues NEC 654.9 ✓5ᵗʰ
      affecting fetus or newborn 763.89
      causing obstructed labor 660.2 ✓5ᵗʰ
        affecting fetus or newborn 763.1
    perineum or vulva 654.8 ✓5ᵗʰ
    uterus NEC 654.9 ✓5ᵗʰ
      affecting fetus or newborn 763.89
      causing obstructed labor 660.2 ✓5ᵗʰ
        affecting fetus or newborn 763.1
      due to previous cesarean delivery
          654.2 ✓5ᵗʰ
    vagina 654.7 ✓5ᵗʰ

Surgical
  abortion — *see* Abortion, legal
  emphysema 998.81
  kidney (*see also* Pyelitis) 590.80
  operation NEC 799.9
  procedures, complication or misadventure —
      see Complications, surgical procedure
  shock 998.0
Suspected condition, ruled out (*see also*
      Observation, suspected) V71.9
  specified condition NEC V71.89
Suspended uterus, in pregnancy or childbirth
      654.4 ✓5ᵗʰ
  affecting fetus or newborn 763.89
  causing obstructed labor 660.2 ✓5ᵗʰ
    affecting fetus or newborn 763.1
Sutton's disease 709.09
Sutton and Gull's disease (arteriolar
      nephrosclerosis) (*see also* Hypertension,
      kidney) 403.90
Suture
  burst (in operation wound) 998.32 ▲
    internal 998.31 ●
  inadvertently left in operation wound 998.4
  removal V58.3
  Shirodkar, in pregnancy (with or without
      cervical incompetence) 654.5 ✓5ᵗʰ
Swab inadvertently left in operation wound
      998.4
Swallowed, swallowing
  difficulty (*see also* Dysphagia) 787.2
  foreign body NEC (*see also* Foreign body) 938
Swamp fever 100.89
Swan neck hand (intrinsic) 736.09
Sweat(s), sweating
  disease or sickness 078.2
  excessive 780.8
  fetid 705.89
  fever 078.2
  gland disease 705.9
    specified type NEC 705.89
  miliary 078.2
  night 780.8
Sweeley-Klionsky disease (angiokeratoma
      corporis diffusum) 272.7
Sweet's syndrome (acute febrile neutrophilic
      dermatosis) 695.89
Swelling
  abdominal (not referable to specific organ)
      789.3 ✓5ᵗʰ
  adrenal gland, cloudy 255.8
  ankle 719.07
  anus 787.99
  arm 729.81
  breast 611.72
  Calabar 125.2
  cervical gland 785.6
  cheek 784.2
  chest 786.6
  ear 388.8
  epigastric 789.3 ✓5ᵗʰ
  extremity (lower) (upper) 729.81
  eye 379.92
  female genital organ 625.8
  finger 729.81
  foot 729.81
  glands 785.6
  gum 784.2
  hand 729.81

Swelling — *continued*
  head 784.2
  inflammatory — *see* Inflammation
  joint (*see also* Effusion, joint) 719.0 ✓5ᵗʰ
    tuberculous — *see* Tuberculosis, joint
  kidney, cloudy 593.89
  leg 729.81
  limb 729.81
  liver 573.8
  lung 786.6
  lymph nodes 785.6
  mediastinal 786.6
  mouth 784.2
  muscle (limb) 729.81
  neck 784.2
  nose or sinus 784.2
  palate 784.2
  pelvis 789.3 ✓5ᵗʰ
  penis 607.83
  perineum 625.8
  rectum 787.99
  scrotum 608.86
  skin 782.2
  splenic (*see also* Splenomegaly) 789.2
  substernal 786.6
  superficial, localized (skin) 782.2
  testicle 608.86
  throat 784.2
  toe 729.81
  tongue 784.2
  tubular (*see also* Disease, renal) 593.9
  umbilicus 789.3 ✓5ᵗʰ
  uterus 625.8
  vagina 625.8
  vulva 625.8
  wandering, due to Gnathostoma (spinigerum) 128.1
  white — *see* Tuberculosis, arthritis
Swift's disease 985.0
Swimmers'
  ear (acute) 380.12
  itch 120.3
Swimming in the head 780.4
Swollen — *see also* Swelling
  glands 785.6
Swyer-James syndrome (unilateral hyperlucent lung) 492.8
Swyer's syndrome (XY pure gonadal dysgenesis) 752.7
Sycosis 704.8
  barbae (not parasitic) 704.8
  contagiosa 110.0
  lupoid 704.8
  mycotic 110.0
  parasitic 110.0
  vulgaris 704.8
Sydenham's chorea — *see* Chorea, Sydenham's
Sylvatic yellow fever 060.0
Sylvest's disease (epidemic pleurodynia) 074.1
Symblepharon 372.63
  congenital 743.62
Symonds' syndrome 348.2
Sympathetic — *see* condition
Sympatheticotonia (*see also* Neuropathy, peripheral, autonomic) 337.9
Sympathicoblastoma (M9500/3)
  specified site — *see* Neoplasm, by site, malignant
  unspecified site 194.0
Sympathicogonioma (M9500/3) — *see* Sympathicoblastoma
Sympathoblastoma (M9500/3) — *see* Sympathicoblastoma
Sympathogonioma (M9500/3) — *see* Sympathicoblastoma
Symphalangy (*see also* Syndactylism) 755.10
Symptoms, specified (general) NEC 780.99 ▲
  abdomen NEC 789.9
  bone NEC 733.90
  breast NEC 611.79
  cardiac NEC 785.9
  cardiovascular NEC 785.9
  chest NEC 786.9
  development NEC 783.9
  digestive system NEC 787.99
  eye NEC 379.99
  gastrointestinal tract NEC 787.99
  genital organs NEC
    female 625.9
    male 608.9
  head and neck NEC 784.9
  heart NEC 785.9
  joint NEC 719.60
    ankle 719.67
    elbow 719.62
    foot 719.67
    hand 719.64
    hip 719.65
    knee 719.66
    multiple sites 719.69
    pelvic region 719.65
    shoulder (region) 719.61
    specified site NEC 719.68
    wrist 719.63
  larynx NEC 784.9
  limbs NEC 729.89
  lymphatic system NEC 785.9
  menopausal 627.2
  metabolism NEC 783.9
  mouth NEC 528.9
  muscle NEC 728.9
  musculoskeletal NEC 781.99
    limbs NEC 729.89
  nervous system NEC 781.99
  neurotic NEC 300.9
  nutrition, metabolism, and development NEC 783.9
  pelvis NEC 789.9
    female 625.9
  peritoneum NEC 789.9
  respiratory system NEC 786.9
  skin and integument NEC 782.9
  subcutaneous tissue NEC 782.9
  throat NEC 784.9
  tonsil NEC 784.9
  urinary system NEC 788.9
  vascular NEC 785.9
Sympus 759.89
Synarthrosis 719.80
  ankle 719.87
  elbow 719.82
  foot 719.87
  hand 719.84
  hip 719.85
  knee 719.86
  multiple sites 719.89
  pelvic region 719.85
  shoulder (region) 719.81
  specified site NEC 719.88
  wrist 719.83

Syncephalus 759.4
Synchondrosis 756.9
   abnormal (congenital) 756.9
   ischiopubic (van Neck's) 732.1
Synchysis (senile) (vitreous humor) 379.21
   scintillans 379.22
Syncope (near) (pre-) 780.2
   anginosa 413.9
   bradycardia 427.89
   cardiac 780.2
   carotid sinus 337.0
   complicating delivery 669.2
   due to lumbar puncture 349.0
   fatal 798.1
   heart 780.2
   heat 992.1
   laryngeal 786.2
   tussive 786.2
   vasoconstriction 780.2
   vasodepressor 780.2
   vasomotor 780.2
   vasovagal 780.2
Syncytial infarct — see Placenta, abnormal
Syndactylism, syndactyly (multiple sites) 755.10
   fingers (without fusion of bone) 755.11
      with fusion of bone 755.12
   toes (without fusion of bone) 755.13
      with fusion of bone 755.14
Syndrome — see also Disease
   abdominal
      acute 789.0
      migraine 346.2
      muscle deficiency 756.79
   Abercrombie's (amyloid degeneration) 277.3
   abnormal innervation 374.43
   abstinence
      alcohol 291.81
      drug 292.0
   Abt-Letterer-Siwe (acute histiocytosis X) (M9722/3) 202.5
   Achard-Thiers (adrenogenital) 255.2
   acid pulmonary aspiration 997.3
      obstetric (Mendelson's) 668.0
   acquired immune deficiency 042
   acquired immunodeficiency 042
   acrocephalosyndactylism 755.55
   acute abdominal 789.0
   acute chest 282.62
   acute coronary 411.1
   Adair-Dighton (brittle bones and blue sclera, deafness) 756.51
   Adams-Stokes (-Morgagni) (syncope with heart block) 426.9
   addisonian 255.4
   Adie (-Holmes) (pupil) 379.46
   adiposogenital 253.8
   adrenal
      hemorrhage 036.3
      meningococcic 036.3
   adrenocortical 255.3
   adrenogenital (acquired) (congenital) 255.2
      feminizing 255.2
      iatrogenic 760.79
      virilism (acquired) (congenital) 255.2
   affective organic NEC 293.89
      drug-induced 292.84
   afferent loop NEC 537.89
   African macroglobulinemia 273.3

Syndrome — continued
   Ahumada-Del Castillo (nonpuerperal galactorrhea and amenorrhea) 253.1
   air blast concussion — see Injury, internal, by site
   Albright (-Martin) (pseudohypoparathyroidism) 275.49
   Albright-McCune-Sternberg (osteitis fibrosa disseminata) 756.59
   alcohol withdrawal 291.81
   Alder's (leukocyte granulation anomaly) 288.2
   Aldrich (-Wiskott) (eczema-thrombocytopenia) 279.12
   Alibert-Bazin (mycosis fungoides) (M9700/3) 202.1
   Alice in Wonderland 293.89
   Allen-Masters 620.6
   Alligator baby (ichthyosis congenita) 757.1
   Alport's (hereditary hematuria-nephropathy-deafness) 759.89
   Alvarez (transient cerebral ischemia) 435.9
   alveolar capillary block 516.3
   Alzheimer's 331.0
      with dementia — see Alzheimer's, dementia
   amnestic (confabulatory) 294.0
      alcoholic 291.1
      drug-induced 292.83
      posttraumatic 294.0
   amotivational 292.89
   amyostatic 275.1
   amyotrophic lateral sclerosis 335.20
   angina (see also Angina) 413.9
   ankyloglossia superior 750.0
   anterior
      chest wall 786.52
      compartment (tibial) 958.8
      spinal artery 433.8
         compression 721.1
      tibial (compartment) 958.8
   antibody deficiency 279.00
      agammaglobulinemic 279.00
      congenital 279.04
      hypogammaglobulinemic 279.00
   anticardiolipin antibody 795.79
   antimongolism 758.3
   antiphospholipid antibody 795.79
   Anton (-Babinski) (hemiasomatognosia) 307.9
   anxiety (see also Anxiety) 300.00
      organic 293.84
   aortic
      arch 446.7
      bifurcation (occlusion) 444.0
      ring 747.21
   Apert's (acrocephalosyndactyly) 755.55
   Apert-Gallais (adrenogenital) 255.2
   aphasia-apraxia-alexia 784.69
   "approximate answers" 300.16
   arcuate ligament (-celiac axis) 447.4
   arcus aortae 446.7
   arc-welders' 370.24
   argentaffin, argintaffinoma 259.2
   Argonz-Del Castillo (nonpuerperal galactorrhea and amenorrhea) 253.1
   Argyll Robertson's (syphilitic) 094.89
      nonsyphilitic 379.45
   arm-shoulder (see also Neuropathy, peripheral, autonomic) 337.9
   Arnold-Chiari (see also Spina bifida) 741.0
      type I 348.4
      type II 741.0
      type III 742.0
      type IV 742.2

Syndrome — continued
- Arrillaga-Ayerza (pulmonary artery sclerosis with pulmonary hypertension) 416.0
- arteriomesenteric duodenum occlusion 537.89
- arteriovenous steal 996.73
- arteritis, young female (obliterative brachiocephalic) 446.7
- aseptic meningitis — see Meningitis, aseptic
- Asherman's 621.5
- asphyctic (see also Anxiety) 300.00
- aspiration, of newborn, massive or meconium 770.1
- ataxia-telangiectasia 334.8
- Audry's (acropachyderma) 757.39
- auriculotemporal 350.8
- autosomal — see also Abnormal, autosomes NEC
  - deletion 758.3
- Avellis' 344.89
- Axenfeld's 743.44
- Ayerza (-Arrillaga) (pulmonary artery sclerosis with pulmonary hypertension) 416.0
- Baader's (erythema multiforme exudativum) 695.1
- Baastrup's 721.5
- Babinski (-Vaquez) (cardiovascular syphilis) 093.89
- Babinski-Fröhlich (adiposogenital dystrophy) 253.8
- Babinski-Nageotte 344.89
- Bagratuni's (temporal arteritis) 446.5
- Bakwin-Krida (craniometaphyseal dysplasia) 756.89
- Balint's (psychic paralysis of visual disorientation) 368.16
- Ballantyne (-Runge) (postmaturity) 766.2
- ballooning posterior leaflet 424.0
- Banti's — see Cirrhosis, liver
- Bard-Pic's (carcinoma, head of pancreas) 157.0
- Bardet-Biedl (obesity, polydactyly, and mental retardation) 759.89
- Barlow's (mitral valve prolapse) 424.0
- Barlow (-Möller) (infantile scurvy) 267
- Baron Munchausen's 301.51
- Barré-Guillain 357.0
- Barré-Liéou (posterior cervical sympathetic) 723.2
- Barrett's (chronic peptic ulcer of esophagus) 530.2
- Bársony-Polgár (corkscrew esophagus) 530.5
- Bársony-Teschendorf (corkscrew esophagus) 530.5
- Bartter's (secondary hyperaldosteronism with juxtaglomerular hyperplasia) 255.1
- Basedow's (exophthalmic goiter) 242.0
- basilar artery 435.0
- basofrontal 377.04
- Bassen-Kornzweig (abetalipoproteinemia) 272.5
- Batten-Steinert 359.2
- battered
  - adult 995.81
  - baby or child 995.54
  - spouse 995.81
- Baumgarten-Cruveilhier (cirrhosis of liver) 571.5
- Bearn-Kunkel (-Slater) (lupoid hepatitis) 571.49
- Beau's (see also Degeneration, myocardial) 429.1

Syndrome — continued
- Bechterew-Strümpell-Marie (ankylosing spondylitis) 720.0
- Beck's (anterior spinal artery occlusion) 433.8
- Beckwith (-Wiedemann) 759.89
- Behçet's 136.1
- Bekhterev-Strümpell-Marie (ankylosing spondylitis) 720.0
- Benedikt's 344.89
- Béquez César (-Steinbrinck-Chédiak- Higashi) (congenital gigantism of peroxidase granules) 288.2
- Bernard-Horner (see also Neuropathy, peripheral, autonomic) 337.9
- Bernard-Sergent (acute adrenocortical insufficiency) 255.4
- Bernhardt-Roth 355.1
- Bernheim's (see also Failure, heart) 428.0
- Bertolotti's (sacralization of fifth lumbar vertebra) 756.15
- Besnier-Boeck-Schaumann (sarcoidosis) 135
- Bianchi's (aphasia-apraxia-alexia syndrome) 784.69
- Biedl-Bardet (obesity, polydactyly, and mental retardation) 759.89
- Biemond's (obesity, polydactyly, and mental retardation) 759.89
- big spleen 289.4
- bilateral polycystic ovarian 256.4
- Bing-Horton's 346.2
- Biörck (-Thorson) (malignant carcinoid) 259.2
- Blackfan-Diamond (congenital hypoplastic anemia) 284.0
- black lung 500
- black widow spider bite 989.5
- bladder neck (see also Incontinence, urine) 788.30
- blast (concussion) — see Blast, injury
- blind loop (postoperative) 579.2
- Bloch-Siemens (incontinentia pigmenti) 757.33
- Bloch-Sulzberger (incontinentia pigmenti) 757.33
- Bloom (-Machacek) (-Torre) 757.39
- Blount-Barber (tibia vara) 732.4
- blue
  - bloater 491.2
  - diaper 270.0
  - drum 381.02
  - sclera 756.51
  - toe — see Atherosclerosis
- Boder-Sedgwick (ataxia-telangiectasia) 334.8
- Boerhaave's (spontaneous esophageal rupture) 530.4
- Bonnevie-Ullrich 758.6
- Bonnier's 386.19
- Bouillaud's (rheumatic heart disease) 391.9
- Bourneville (-Pringle) (tuberous sclerosis) 759.5
- Bouveret (-Hoffmann) (paroxysmal tachycardia) 427.2
- brachial plexus 353.0
- Brachman-de Lange (Amsterdam dwarf, mental retardation, and brachycephaly) 759.89
- bradycardia-tachycardia 427.81
- Brailsford-Morquio (dystrophy) (mucopolysaccharidosis IV) 277.5
- brain (acute) (chronic) (nonpsychotic) (organic) (with behavioral reaction) (with neurotic reaction) 310.9

Syndrome — *continued*
  brain — *continued*
    with
      presenile brain disease (*see also*
        Dementia, presenile) 290.10
      psychosis, psychotic reaction (*see also*
        Psychosis, organic) 294.9
    chronic alcoholic 291.2
    congenital (*see also* Retardation, mental)
      319
    postcontusional 310.2
    posttraumatic
      nonpsychotic 310.2
      psychotic 293.9
        acute 293.0
        chronic (*see also* Psychosis, organic)
          294.8
        subacute 293.1
    psycho-organic (*see also* Syndrome,
      psycho-organic) 310.9
    psychotic (*see also* Psychosis, organic)
      294.9
    senile (*see also* Dementia, senile) 290.0
  branchial arch 744.41
  Brandt's (acrodermatitis enteropathica) 686.8
  Brennemann's 289.2
  Briquet's 300.81
  Brissaud-Meige (infantile myxedema) 244.9
  broad ligament laceration 620.6
  Brock's (atelectasis due to enlarged lymph
    nodes) 518.0
  Brown's tendon sheath 378.61
  Brown-Séquard 344.89
  brown spot 756.59
  Brugada 746.89
  Brugsch's (acropachyderma) 757.39
  bubbly lung 770.7
  Buchem's (hyperostosis corticalis) 733.3
  Budd-Chiari (hepatic vein thrombosis) 453.0
  Büdinger-Ludloff-Läwen 717.89
  bulbar 335.22
    lateral (*see also* Disease, cerebrovascular,
      acute) 436
  Bullis fever 082.8
  bundle of Kent (anomalous atrioventricular
    excitation) 426.7
  Bürger-Grütz (essential familial hyperlipemia)
    272.3
  Burke's (pancreatic insufficiency and chronic
    neutropenia) 577.8
  Burnett's (milk-alkali) 999.9
  Burnier's (hypophyseal dwarfism) 253.3
  burning feet 266.2
  Bywaters' 958.5
  Caffey's (infantile cortical hyperostosis) 756.59
  Calvé-Legg-Perthes (osteochondrosis, femoral
    capital) 732.1
  Caplan (-Colinet) syndrome 714.81
  capsular thrombosis (*see also* Thrombosis,
    brain) 434.0
  carcinogenic thrombophlebitis 453.1
  carcinoid 259.2
  cardiac asthma (*see also* Failure, ventricular,
    left) 428.1
  cardiacos negros 416.0
  cardiopulmonary obesity 278.8
  cardiorenal (*see also* Hypertension,
    cardiorenal) 404.90
  cardiorespiratory distress (idiopathic),
    newborn 769

Syndrome — *continued*
  cardiovascular renal (*see also* Hypertension,
    cardiorenal) 404.90
  cardiovasorenal 272.7
  Carini's (ichthyosis congenita) 757.1
  carotid
    artery (internal) 435.8
    body or sinus 337.0
  carpal tunnel 354.0
  Carpenter's 759.89
  Cassidy (-Scholte) (malignant carcinoid) 259.2
  cat-cry 758.3
  cauda equina 344.60
  causalgia 355.9
    lower limb 355.71
    upper limb 354.4
  cavernous sinus 437.6
  celiac 579.0
    artery compression 447.4
    axis 447.4
  cerebellomedullary malformation (*see also*
    Spina bifida) 741.0
  cerebral gigantism 253.0
  cerebrohepatorenal 759.89
  cervical (root) (spine) NEC 723.8
    disc 722.71
    posterior, sympathetic 723.2
    rib 353.0
    sympathetic paralysis 337.0
    traumatic (acute) NEC 847.0
  cervicobrachial (diffuse) 723.3
  cervicocranial 723.2
  cervicodorsal outlet 353.2
  Céstan's 344.89
  Céstan (-Raymond) 433.8
  Céstan-Chenais 344.89
  chancriform 114.1
  Charcôt's (intermittent claudication) 443.9
    angina cruris 443.9
    due to atherosclerosis 440.21
  Charcôt-Marie-Tooth 356.1
  Charcôt-Weiss-Baker 337.0
  Cheadle (-Möller) (-Barlow) (infantile scurvy)
    267
  Chédiak-Higashi (-Steinbrinck) (congenital
    gigantism of peroxidase granules) 288.2
  chest wall 786.52
  Chiari's (hepatic vein thrombosis) 453.0
  Chiari-Frommel 676.6
  chiasmatic 368.41
  Chilaiditi's (subphrenic displacement, colon)
    751.4
  chondroectodermal dysplasia 756.55
  chorea-athetosis-agitans 275.1
  Christian's (chronic histiocytosis X) 277.8
  chromosome 4 short arm deletion 758.3
  Churg-Strauss 446.4
  Clarke-Hadfield (pancreatic infantilism) 577.8
  Claude's 352.6
  Claude Bernard-Horner (*see also* Neuropathy,
    peripheral, autonomic) 337.9
  Clérambault's
    automatism 348.8
    erotomania 297.8
  Clifford's (postmaturity) 766.2
  climacteric 627.2
  Clouston's (hidrotic ectodermal dysplasia)
    757.31
  clumsiness 315.4
  Cockayne's (microencephaly and dwarfism)
    759.89

Syndrome — *continued*
- Cockayne-Weber (epidermolysis bullosa) 757.39
- Cogan's (nonsyphilitic interstitial keratitis) 370.52
- cold injury (newborn) 778.2
- Collet (-Sicard) 352.6
- combined immunity deficiency 279.2
- compartment(al) (anterior) (deep) (posterior) (tibial) 958.8
  - nontraumatic 729.9
- compression 958.5
  - cauda equina 344.60
  - with neurogenic bladder 344.61
- concussion 310.2
- congenital
  - affecting more than one system 759.7
    - specified type NEC 759.89
  - facial diplegia 352.6
  - muscular hypertrophy-cerebral 759.89
- congestion-fibrosis (pelvic) 625.5
- conjunctivourethrosynovial 099.3
- Conn (-Louis) (primary aldosteronism) 255.1
- Conradi (-Hünermann) (chondrodysplasia calcificans congenita) 756.59
- conus medullaris 336.8
- Cooke-Apert-Gallais (adrenogenital) 255.2
- Cornelia de Lange's (Amsterdam dwarf, mental retardation, and brachycephaly) 759.8 ✓5ᵗʰ
- coronary insufficiency or intermediate 411.1
- cor pulmonale 416.9
- corticosexual 255.2
- Costen's (complex) 524.60
- costochondral junction 733.6
- costoclavicular 353.0
- costovertebral 253.0
- Cotard's (paranoia) 297.1
- craniovertebral 723.2
- Creutzfeldt-Jakob 046.1
  - with dementia
    - with behavioral disturbance 046.1 [294.11]
    - without behavioral disturbance 046.1 [294.10]
- crib death 798.0
- cricopharyngeal 787.2
- cri-du-chat 758.3
- Crigler-Najjar (congenital hyperbilirubinemia) 277.4
- crocodile tears 351.8
- Cronkhite-Canada 211.3
- croup 464.4
- CRST (cutaneous systemic sclerosis) 710.1
- crush 958.5
- crushed lung (*see also* Injury, internal, lung) 861.20
- Cruveilhier-Baumgarten (cirrhosis of liver) 571.5
- cubital tunnel 354.2
- Cuiffini-Pancoast (M8010/3) (carcinoma, pulmonary apex) 162.3
- Curschmann (-Batten) (-Steinert) 359.2
- Cushing's (iatrogenic) (idiopathic) (pituitary basophilism) (pituitary-dependent) 255.0
  - overdose or wrong substance given or taken 962.0
- Cyriax's (slipping rib) 733.99
- cystic duct stump 576.0
- Da Costa's (neurocirculatory asthenia) 306.2
- Dameshek's (erythroblastic anemia) 282.4

Syndrome — *continued*
- Dana-Putnam (subacute combined sclerosis with pernicious anemia) 281.0 *[336.2]*
- Danbolt (-Closs) (acrodermatitis enteropathica) 686.8
- Dandy-Walker (atresia, foramen of Magendie) 742.3
  - with spina bifida (*see also* Spina bifida) 741.0 ✓5ᵗʰ
- Danlos' 756.83
- Davies-Colley (slipping rib) 733.99
- dead fetus 641.3 ✓5ᵗʰ
- defeminization 255.2
- defibrination (*see also* Fibrinolysis) 286.6
- Degos' 447.8
- Deiters' nucleus 386.19
- Déjérine-Roussy 348.8
- Déjérine-Thomas 333.0
- de Lange's (Amsterdam dwarf, mental retardation, and brachycephaly) (Cornelia) 759.89
- Del Castillo's (germinal aplasia) 606.0
- deletion chromosomes 758.3
- delusional
  - induced by drug 292.11
- dementia-aphonia, of childhood (*see also* Psychosis, childhood) 299.1 ✓5ᵗʰ
- demyelinating NEC 341.9
- denial visual hallucination 307.9
- depersonalization 300.6
- Dercum's (adiposis dolorosa) 272.8
- de Toni-Fanconi (-Debré) (cystinosis) 270.0
- diabetes-dwarfism-obesity (juvenile) 258.1
- diabetes mellitus-hypertension-nephrosis 250.4 ✓5ᵗʰ *[581.81]*
- diabetes mellitus in newborn infant 775.1
- diabetes-nephrosis 250.4 ✓5ᵗʰ *[581.81]*
- diabetic amyotrophy 250.6 ✓5ᵗʰ *[358.1]*
- Diamond-Blackfan (congenital hypoplastic anemia) 284.0
- Diamond-Gardener (autoerythrocyte sensitization) 287.2
- DIC (diffuse or disseminated intravascular coagulopathy) (*see also* Fibrinolysis) 286.6
- diencephalohypophyseal NEC 253.8
- diffuse cervicobrachial 723.3
- diffuse obstructive pulmonary 496
- DiGeorge's (thymic hypoplasia) 279.11
- Dighton's 756.51
- Di Guglielmo's (erythremic myelosis) (M9841/3) 207.0 ✓5ᵗʰ
- disc — *see* Displacement, intervertebral disc
- discogenic — *see* Displacement, intervertebral disc
- disequilibrium 276.9
- disseminated platelet thrombosis 446.6
- Ditthomska 307.81
- Doan-Wiseman (primary splenic neutropenia) 288.0
- Döhle body-panmyelopathic 288.2
- Donohue's (leprechaunism) 259.8
- dorsolateral medullary (*see also* Disease, cerebrovascular, acute) 436
- double whammy 360.81
- Down's (mongolism) 758.0
- Dresbach's (elliptocytosis) 282.1
- Dressler's (postmyocardial infarction) 411.0
  - hemoglobinuria 283.2
- drug withdrawal, infant, of dependent mother 779.5

Syndrome — continued
dry skin 701.1
eye 375.15
DSAP (disseminated superficial actinic porokeratosis) 692.75
Duane's (retraction) 378.71
Duane-Stilling-Türk (ocular retraction syndrome) 378.71
Dubin-Johnson (constitutional hyperbilirubinemia) 277.4
Dubin-Sprinz (constitutional hyperbilirubinemia) 277.4
Duchenne's 335.22
due to abnormality
  autosomal NEC (see also Abnormal, autosomes NEC) 758.5
    13 758.1
    18 758.2
    21 or 22 758.0
    D 758.1
    E 758.2
    G 758.0
  chromosomal 758.89
    sex 758.81
dumping 564.2
  nonsurgical 536.8
Duplay's 726.2
Dupré's (meningism) 781.6
Dyke-Young (acquired macrocytic hemolytic anemia) 283.9
dyspraxia 315.4
dystocia, dystrophia 654.9 ✓5ᵗʰ
Eagle-Barret 756.71
Eales' 362.18
Eaton-Lambert (see also Neoplasm, by site, malignant) 199.1 [358.1]
Ebstein's (downward displacement, tricuspid valve into right ventricle) 746.2
ectopic ACTH secretion 255.0
eczema-thrombocytopenia 279.12
Eddowes' (brittle bones and blue sclera) 756.51
Edwards' 758.2
efferent loop 537.89
effort (aviators') (psychogenic) 306.2
Ehlers-Danlos 756.83
Eisenmenger's (ventricular septal defect) 745.4
Ekbom's (restless legs) 333.99
Ekman's (brittle bones and blue sclera) 756.51
electric feet 266.2
Elephant man 237.71
Ellison-Zollinger (gastric hypersecretion with pancreatic islet cell tumor) 251.5
Ellis-van Creveld (chondroectodermal dysplasia) 756.55
embryonic fixation 270.2
empty sella (turcica) 253.8
endocrine-hypertensive 255.3
Engel-von Recklinghausen (osteitis fibrosa cystica) 252.0
enteroarticular 099.3
entrapment — see Neuropathy, entrapment
eosinophilia myalgia 710.5
epidemic vomiting 078.82
Epstein's — see Nephrosis
Erb (-Oppenheim) — Goldflam 358.0
Erdheim's (acromegalic macrospondylitis) 253.0
Erlacher-Blount (tibia vara) 732.4
erythrocyte fragmentation 283.19
euthyroid sick 790.94

Syndrome — continued
Evans' (thrombocytopenic purpura) 287.3
excess cortisol, iatrogenic 255.0
exhaustion 300.5
extrapyramidal 333.90
eyelid-malar-mandible 756.0
eye retraction 378.71
Faber's (achlorhydric anemia) 280.9
Fabry (-Anderson) (angiokeratoma corporis diffusum) 272.7
facet 724.8
Fallot's 745.2
falx (see also Hemorrhage, brain) 431
familial eczema-thrombocytopenia 279.12
Fanconi's (anemia) (congenital pancytopenia) 284.0
Fanconi (-de Toni) (-Debré) (cystinosis) 270.0
Farber (-Uzman) (disseminated lipogranulomatosis) 272.8
fatigue NEC 300.5
  chronic 780.71
faulty bowel habit (idiopathic megacolon) 564.7
FDH (focal dermal hypoplasia) 757.39
fecal reservoir 560.39
Feil-Klippel (brevicollis) 756.16
Felty's (rheumatoid arthritis with splenomegaly and leukopenia) 714.1
fertile eunuch 257.2
fetal alcohol 760.71
  late effect 760.71
fibrillation-flutter 427.32
fibrositis (periarticular) 729.0
Fiedler's (acute isolated myocarditis) 422.91
Fiessinger-Leroy (-Reiter) 099.3
Fiessinger-Rendu (erythema multiforme exudativum) 695.1
first arch 756.0
Fisher's 357.0
Fitz's (acute hemorrhagic pancreatitis) 577.0
Fitz-Hugh and Curtis (gonococcal peritonitis) 098.86
Flajani (-Basedow) (exophthalmic goiter) 242.0 ✓5ᵗʰ
floppy
  infant 781.99
  valve (mitral) 424.0
flush 259.2
Foix-Alajouanine 336.1
Fong's (hereditary osteo-onychodysplasia) 756.89
foramen magnum 348.4
Forbes-Albright (nonpuerperal amenorrhea and lactation associated with pituitary tumor) 253.1
Foster-Kennedy 377.04
Foville's (peduncular) 344.89
fragile X 759.83
Franceschetti's (mandibulofacial dysostosis) 756.0
Fraser's 759.89
Freeman-Sheldon 759.89
Frey's (auriculotemporal) 350.8
Friderichsen-Waterhouse 036.3
Friedrich-Erb-Arnold (acropachyderma) 757.39
Fröhlich's (adiposogenital dystrophy) 253.8
Froin's 336.8
Frommel-Chiari 676.6 ✓5ᵗʰ
frontal lobe 310.0

Syndrome — continued
  Fuller Albright's (osteitis fibrosa disseminata) 756.59
  functional
    bowel 564.9
    prepubertal castrate 752.8
  Gaisböck's (polycythemia hypertonica) 289.0
  ganglion (basal, brain) 333.90
    geniculi 351.1
  Ganser's, hysterical 300.16
  Gardner-Diamond (autoerythrocyte sensitization) 287.2
  gastroesophageal junction 530.0
  gastroesophageal laceration-hemorrhage 530.7
  gastrojejunal loop obstruction 537.89
  Gayet-Wernicke's (superior hemorrhagic polioencephalitis) 265.1
  Gee-Herter-Heubner (nontropical sprue) 579.0
  Gélineau's 347
  genito-anorectal 099.1
  Gerhardt's (vocal cord paralysis) 478.30
  Gerstmann's (finger agnosia) 784.69
  Gilbert's 277.4
  Gilford (-Hutchinson) (progeria) 259.8
  Gilles de la Tourette's 307.23
  Gillespie's (dysplasia oculodentodigitalis) 759.89
  Glénard's (enteroptosis) 569.89
  Glinski-Simmonds (pituitary cachexia) 253.2
  glucuronyl transferase 277.4
  glue ear 381.20
  Goldberg (-Maxwell) (-Morris) (testicular feminization) 257.8
  Goldenhar's (oculoauriculovertebral dysplasia) 756.0
  Goldflam-Erb 358.0
  Goltz-Gorlin (dermal hypoplasia) 757.39
  Goodpasture's (pneumorenal) 446.21
  Gopalan's (burning feet) 266.2
  Gorlin-Chaudhry-Moss 759.89
  Gougerot (-Houwer) — Sjögren (keratoconjunctivitis sicca) 710.2
  Gougerot-Blum (pigmented purpuric lichenoid dermatitis) 709.1
  Gougerot-Carteaud (confluent reticulate papillomatosis) 701.8
  Gouley's (constrictive pericarditis) 423.2
  Gowers' (vasovagal attack) 780.2
  Gowers-Paton-Kennedy 377.04
  Gradenigo's 383.02
  gray or grey (chloramphenicol) (newborn) 779.4
  Greig's (hypertelorism) 756.0
  Gubler-Millard 344.89
  Guérin-Stern (arthrogryposis multiplex congenita) 754.89
  Guillain-Barré (-Strohl) 357.0
  Gunn's (jaw-winking syndrome) 742.8
  Günther's (congenital erythropoietic porphyria) 277.1
  gustatory sweating 350.8
  H₃O 759.81
  Hadfield-Clarke (pancreatic infantilism) 577.8
  Haglund-Läwen-Fründ 717.89
  hairless women 257.8
  Hallermann-Streiff 756.0
  Hallervorden-Spatz 333.0
  Hamman's (spontaneous mediastinal emphysema) 518.1
  Hamman-Rich (diffuse interstitial pulmonary fibrosis) 516.3

Syndrome — continued
  Hand-Schüller-Christian (chronic histiocytosis X) 277.8
  hand-foot 282.61
  Hanot-Chauffard (-Troisier) (bronze diabetes) 275.0
  Harada's 363.22
  Hare's (M8010/3) (carcinoma, pulmonary apex) 162.3
  Harkavy's 446.0
  harlequin color change 779.89 ▲
  Harris' (organic hyperinsulinism) 251.1
  Hart's (pellagra-cerebellar ataxia-renal aminoaciduria) 270.0
  Hayem-Faber (achlorhydric anemia) 280.9
  Hayem-Widal (acquired hemolytic jaundice) 283.9
  Heberden's (angina pectoris) 413.9
  Hedinger's (malignant carcinoid) 259.2
  Hegglin's 288.2
  Heller's (infantile psychosis) (see also Psychosis, childhood) 299.1 ✓5ᵗʰ
  H.E.L.L.P 642.5 ✓5ᵗʰ
  hemolytic-uremic (adult) (child) 283.11
  Hench-Rosenberg (palindromic arthritis) (see also Rheumatism, palindromic) 719.3 ✓5ᵗʰ
  Henoch-Schönlein (allergic purpura) 287.0
  hepatic flexure 569.89
  hepatorenal 572.4
    due to a procedure 997.4
    following delivery 674.8 ✓5ᵗʰ
  hepatourologic 572.4
  Herrick's (hemoglobin S disease) 282.61
  Herter (-Gee) (nontropical sprue) 579.0
  Heubner-Herter (nontropical sprue) 579.0
  Heyd's (hepatorenal) 572.4
  HHHO 759.81
  Hilger's 337.0
  Hoffa (-Kastert) (liposynovitis prepatellaris) 272.8
  Hoffmann's 244.9 [359.5]
  Hoffmann-Bouveret (paroxysmal tachycardia) 427.2
  Hoffmann-Werdnig 335.0
  Holländer-Simons (progressive lipodystrophy) 272.6
  Holmes' (visual disorientation) 368.16
  Holmes-Adie 379.46
  Hoppe-Goldflam 358.0
  Horner's (see also Neuropathy, peripheral, autonomic) 337.9
    traumatic — see Injury, nerve, cervical sympathetic
  hospital addiction 301.51
  Hunt's (herpetic geniculate ganglionitis) 053.11
    dyssynergia cerebellaris myoclonica 334.2
  Hunter (-Hurler) (mucopolysaccharidosis II) 277.5
  hunterian glossitis 529.4
  Hurler (-Hunter) (mucopolysaccharidosis II) 277.5
  Hutchinson's incisors or teeth 090.5
  Hutchinson-Boeck (sarcoidosis) 135
  Hutchinson-Gilford (progeria) 259.8
  hydralazine
    correct substance properly administered 695.4
    overdose or wrong substance given or taken 972.6

Syndrome — continued
- hydraulic concussion (abdomen) (*see also* Injury, internal, abdomen) 868.00
- hyperabduction 447.8
- hyperactive bowel 564.9
- hyperaldosteronism with hypokalemic alkalosis (Bartter's) 255.1
- hypercalcemic 275.42
- hypercoagulation NEC 289.8
- hypereosinophilic (idiopathic) 288.3
- hyperkalemic 276.7
- hyperkinetic — *see also* Hyperkinesia heart 429.82
- hyperlipemia-hemolytic anemia-icterus 571.1
- hypermobility 728.5
- hypernatremia 276.0
- hyperosmolarity 276.0
- hypersomnia-bulimia 349.89
- hypersplenic 289.4
- hypersympathetic (*see also* Neuropathy, peripheral, autonomic) 337.9
- hypertransfusion, newborn 776.4
- hyperventilation, psychogenic 306.1
- hyperviscosity (of serum) NEC 273.3
  - polycythemic 289.0
  - sclerothymic 282.8
- hypoglycemic (familial) (neonatal) 251.2
  - functional 251.1
- hypokalemic 276.8
- hypophyseal 253.8
- hypophyseothalamic 253.8
- hypopituitarism 253.2
- hypoplastic left heart 746.7
- hypopotassemia 276.8
- hyposmolality 276.1
- hypotension, maternal 669.2 ▪5▪
- hypotonia-hypomentia-hypogonadism-obesity 759.81
- ICF (intravascular coagulation-fibrinolysis) (*see also* Fibrinolysis) 286.6
- idiopathic cardiorespiratory distress, newborn 769
- idiopathic nephrotic (infantile) 581.9
- Imerslund (-Gräsbeck) (anemia due to familial selective vitamin B_{12} malabsorption) 281.1
- immobility (paraplegic) 728.3
- immunity deficiency, combined 279.2
- impending coronary 411.1
- impingement
  - shoulder 726.2
  - vertebral bodies 724.4
- inappropriate secretion of antidiuretic hormone (ADH) 253.6
- incomplete
  - mandibulofacial 756.0
- infant
  - death, sudden (SIDS) 798.0
  - Hercules 255.2
  - of diabetic mother 775.0
  - shaken 995.55
- infantilism 253.3
- inferior vena cava 459.2
- influenza-like 487.1
- inspissated bile, newborn 774.4
- intermediate coronary (artery) 411.1
- internal carotid artery (*see also* Occlusion, artery, carotid) 433.1 ▪5▪
- interspinous ligament 724.8
- intestinal
  - carcinoid 259.2

Syndrome — continued
- intestinal — *continued*
  - gas 787.3
  - knot 560.2
- intravascular
  - coagulation-fibrinolysis (ICF) (*see also* Fibrinolysis) 286.6
  - coagulopathy (*see also* Fibrinolysis) 286.6
- inverted Marfan's 759.89
- IRDS (idiopathic respiratory distress, newborn) 769
- irritable
  - bowel 564.1
  - heart 306.2
  - weakness 300.5
- ischemic bowel (transient) 557.9
  - chronic 557.1
  - due to mesenteric artery insufficiency 557.1
- Itsenko-Cushing (pituitary basophilism) 255.0
- IVC (intravascular coagulopathy) (*see also* Fibrinolysis) 286.6
- Ivemark's (asplenia with congenital heart disease) 759.0
- Jaccoud's 714.4
- Jackson's 344.89
- Jadassohn-Lewandowski (pachyonchia congenita) 757.5
- Jaffe-Lichtenstein (-Uehlinger) 252.0
- Jahnke's (encephalocutaneous angiomatosis) 759.6
- Jakob-Creutzfeldt 046.1
  - with dementia
    - with behavioral disturbance 046.1 [294.11]
    - without behavioral disturbance 046.1 [294.10]
- Jaksch's (pseudoleukemia infantum) 285.8
- Jaksch-Hayem (-Luzet) (pseudoleukemia infantum) 285.8
- jaw-winking 742.8
- jejunal 564.2
- jet lag 307.45
- Jeune's (asphyxiating thoracic dystrophy of newborn) 756.4
- Job's (chronic granulomatous disease) 288.1
- Jordan's 288.2
- Joseph-Diamond-Blackfan (congenital hypoplastic anemia) 284.0
- Joubert 759.89
- jugular foramen 352.6
- Kahler's (multiple myeloma) (M9730/3) 203.0 ▪5▪
- Kalischer's (encephalocutaneous angiomatosis) 759.6
- Kallmann's (hypogonadotropic hypogonadism with anosmia) 253.4
- Kanner's (autism) (*see also* Psychosis, childhood) 299.0 ▪5▪
- Kartagener's (sinusitis, bronchiectasis, situs inversus) 759.3
- Kasabach-Merritt (capillary hemangioma associated with thrombocytopenic purpura) 287.3
- Kast's (dyschondroplasia with hemangiomas) 756.4
- Kaznelson's (congenital hypoplastic anemia) 284.0
- Kelly's (sideropenic dysphagia) 280.8
- Kimmelstiel-Wilson (intercapillary glomerulosclerosis) 250.4 ▪5▪ *[581.81]*

Index to Diseases

Syndrome

Syndrome — *continued*
Klauder's (erythema multiforme exudativum) 695.1
Klein-Waardenburg (ptosis-epicanthus) 270.2
Kleine-Levin 349.89
Klinefelter's 758.7
Klippel-Feil (brevicollis) 756.16
Klippel-Trenaunay 759.89
Klumpke (-Déjérine) (injury to brachial plexus at birth) 767.6
Klüver-Bucy (-Terzian) 310.0
Köhler-Pellegrini-Stieda (calcification, knee joint) 726.62
König's 564.89
Korsakoff's (nonalcoholic) 294.0
   alcoholic 291.1
Korsakoff (-Wernicke) (nonalcoholic) 294.0
   alcoholic 291.1
Kostmann's (infantile genetic agranulocytosis) 288.0
Krabbe's
   congenital muscle hypoplasia 756.89
   cutaneocerebral angioma 759.6
Kunkel (lupoid hepatitis) 571.49
labyrinthine 386.50
laceration, broad ligament 620.6
Langdon Down (mongolism) 758.0
Larsen's (flattened facies and multiple congenital dislocations) 755.8
lateral
   cutaneous nerve of thigh 355.1
   medullary (*see also* Disease, cerebrovascular acute) 436
Launois' (pituitary gigantism) 253.0
Launois-Cléret (adiposogenital dystrophy) 253.8
Laurence-Moon (-Bardet) — Biedl (obesity, polydactyly, and mental retardation) 759.89
Lawford's (encephalocutaneous angiomatosis) 759.6
lazy
   leukocyte 288.0
   posture 728.3
Lederer-Brill (acquired infectious hemolytic anemia) 283.19
Legg-Calvé-Perthes (osteochondrosis capital femoral) 732.1
Lennox's (*see also* Epilepsy) 345.0 ✓5ᵗʰ
lenticular 275.1
Léopold-Lévi's (paroxysmal thyroid instability) 242.9 ✓5ᵗʰ
Lepore hemoglobin 282.4
Léri-Weill 756.59
Leriche's (aortic bifurcation occlusion) 444.0
Lermoyez's (*see also* Disease, Ménière's) 386.00
Lesch-Nyhan (hypoxanthine-guanine-phosphoribosyltransferase deficiency) 277.2
Lev's (acquired complete heart block) 426.0
Levi's (pituitary dwarfism) 253.3
Lévy-Roussy 334.3
Lichtheim's (subacute combined sclerosis with pernicious anemia) 281.0 [336.2]
Li-Fraumeni 758.3
Lightwood's (renal tubular acidosis) 588.8
Lignac (-de Toni) (-Fanconi) (-Debré) (cystinosis) 270.0
Likoff's (angina in menopausal women) 413.9
liver-kidney 572.4

Syndrome — *continued*
Lloyd's 258.1
lobotomy 310.0
Löffler's (eosinophilic pneumonitis) 518.3
Löfgren's (sarcoidosis) 135
long arm 18 or 21 deletion 758.3
Looser (-Debray) — Milkman (osteomalacia with pseudofractures) 268.2
Lorain-Levi (pituitary dwarfism) 253.3
Louis-Bar (ataxia-telangiectasia) 334.8
low
   atmospheric pressure 993.2
   back 724.2
      psychogenic 306.0
   output (cardiac) (*see also* Failure, heart) 428.9
Lowe's (oculocerebrorenal dystrophy) 270.8
Lowe-Terrey-MacLachlan (oculocerebrorenal dystrophy) 270.8
lower radicular, newborn 767.4
Lown (-Ganong)-Levine (short P-R interval, normal QRS complex, and supraventricular tachycardia) 426.81
Lucey-Driscoll (jaundice due to delayed conjugation) 774.30
Luetscher's (dehydration) 276.5
lumbar vertebral 724.4
Lutembacher's (atrial septal defect with mitral stenosis) 745.5
Lyell's (toxic epidermal necrolysis) 695.1
   due to drug
      correct substance properly administered 695.1
      overdose or wrong substance given or taken 977.9
      specified drug — *see* Table of Drugs and Chemicals
MacLeod's 492.8
macrogenitosomia praecox 259.8
macroglobulinemia 273.3
Maffucci's (dyschondroplasia with hemangiomas) 756.4
Magenblase 306.4
magnesium-deficiency 781.7
malabsorption 579.9
   postsurgical 579.3
   spinal fluid 331.3
malignant carcinoid 259.2
Mallory-Weiss 530.7
mandibulofacial dysostosis 756.0
manic-depressive (*see also* Psychosis, affective) 296.80
Mankowsky's (familial dysplastic osteopathy) 731.2
maple syrup (urine) 270.3
Marable's (celiac artery compression) 447.4
Marchesani (-Weill) (brachymorphism and ectopia lentis) 759.89
Marchiafava-Bignami 341.8
Marchiafava-Micheli (paroxysmal nocturnal hemoglobinuria) 283.2
Marcus Gunn's (jaw-winking syndrome) 742.8
Marfan's (arachnodactyly) 759.82
   meaning congenital syphilis 090.49
      with luxation of lens 090.49 [379.32]
Marie's (acromegaly) 253.0
   primary or idiopathic (acropachyderma) 757.39
   secondary (hypertrophic pulmonary osteoarthropathy) 731.2
Markus-Adie 379.46

Syndrome — *continued*
  Maroteaux-Lamy (mucopolysaccharidosis VI) 277.5
  Martin's 715.27
  Martin-Albright (pseudohypoparathyroidism) 275.49
  Martorell-Fabré (pulseless disease) 446.7
  massive aspiration of newborn 770.1
  Masters-Allen 620.6
  mastocytosis 757.33
  maternal hypotension 669.2 ✓5ᵗʰ
  maternal obesity 646.1 ✓5ᵗʰ
  May (-Hegglin) 288.2
  McArdle (-Schmid) (-Pearson) (glycogenosis V) 271.0
  McCune-Albright (osteitis fibrosa disseminata) 756.59
  McQuarrie's (idiopathic familial hypoglycemia) 251.2
  meconium
    aspiration 770.1
    plug (newborn) NEC 777.1
  median arcuate ligament 447.4
  mediastinal fibrosis 519.3
  Meekeren-Ehlers-Danlos 756.83
  Meige (blepharospasm-oromandibular dystonia) 333.82
    -Milroy (chronic hereditary edema) 757.0
  MELAS 758.89
  Melkersson (-Rosenthal) 351.8
  Mende's (ptosis-epicanthus) 270.2
  Mendelson's (resulting from a procedure) 997.3
    during labor 668.0 ✓5ᵗʰ
    obstetric 668.0 ✓5ᵗʰ
  Ménétrier's (hypertrophic gastritis) 535.2 ✓5ᵗʰ
  Ménière's (*see also* Disease, Ménière's) 386.00
  meningo-eruptive 047.1
  Menkes' 759.89
    glutamic acid 759.89
    maple syrup (urine) disease 270.3
  menopause 627.2
    postartificial 627.4
  menstruation 625.4
  MERFF 758.89
  mesenteric
    artery, superior 557.1
    vascular insufficiency (with gangrene) 557.1
  metastatic carcinoid 259.2
  Meyenburg-Altherr-Uehlinger 733.99
  Meyer-Schwickerath and Weyers (dysplasia oculodentodigitalis) 759.89
  Micheli-Rietti (thalassemia minor) 282.4
  Michotte's 721.5
  micrognathia-glossoptosis 756.0
  microphthalmos (congenital) 759.89
  midbrain 348.8
  middle
    lobe (lung) (right) 518.0
    radicular 353.0
  Miescher's
    familial acanthosis nigricans 701.2
    granulomatosis disciformis 709.3
  Mieten's 759.89
  migraine 346.0 ✓5ᵗʰ
  Mikity-Wilson (pulmonary dysmaturity) 770.7
  Mikulicz's (dryness of mouth, absent or decreased lacrimation) 527.1
  milk alkali (milk drinkers') 999.9

Syndrome — *continued*
  Milkman (-Looser) (osteomalacia with pseudofractures) 268.2
  Millard-Gubler 344.89
  Miller Fisher's 357.0
  Milles' (encephalocutaneous angiomatosis) 759.6
  Minkowski-Chauffard (*see also* Spherocytosis) 282.0
  Mirizzi's (hepatic duct stenosis) 576.2
    with calculus, cholelithiasis, or stones — *see* Choledocholithiasis
  mitral
    click (-murmur) 785.2
    valve prolapse 424.0
  Möbius'
    congenital oculofacial paralysis 352.6
    ophthalmoplegic migraine 346.8 ✓5ᵗʰ
  Mohr's (types I and II) 759.89
  monofixation 378.34
  Moore's (*see also* Epilepsy) 345.5 ✓5ᵗʰ
  Morel-Moore (hyperostosis frontalis interna) 733.3
  Morel-Morgagni (hyperostosis frontalis interna) 733.3
  Morgagni (-Stewart-Morel) (hyperostosis frontalis interna) 733.3
  Morgagni-Adams-Stokes (syncope with heart block) 426.9
  Morquio (-Brailsford) (-Ullrich) (mucopolysaccharidosis IV) 277.5
  Morris (testicular feminization) 257.8
  Morton's (foot) (metatarsalgia) (metatarsal neuralgia) (neuralgia) (neuroma) (toe) 355.6
  Moschcowitz (-Singer-Symmers) (thrombotic thrombocytopenic purpura) 446.6
  Mounier-Kuhn 494.0
    with acute exacerbation 494.1
  Mucha-Haberman (acute parapsoriasis varioliformis) 696.2
  mucocutaneous lymph node (acute) (febrile) (infantile) (MCLS) 446.1
  multiple
    deficiency 260
    operations 301.51
  Munchausen's 301.51
  Münchmeyer's (exostosis luxurians) 728.11
  Murchison-Sanderson — *see* Disease, Hodgkin's
  myasthenic — *see* Myasthenia, syndrome
  myelodysplastic 238.7
  myeloproliferative (chronic) (M9960/1) 238.7
  myofascial pain NEC 729.1
  Naffziger's 353.0
  Nager-de Reynier (dysostosis mandibularis) 756.0
  nail-patella (hereditary osteo-onychodysplasia) 756.89
  Nebécourt's 253.3
  Neill-Dingwall (microencephaly and dwarfism) 759.89
  nephrotic (*see also* Nephrosis) 581.9
    diabetic 250.4 ✓5ᵗʰ [581.81]
  Netherton's (ichthyosiform erythroderma) 757.1
  neurocutaneous 759.6
  neuroleptic malignant 333.92
  Nezelof's (pure alymphocytosis) 279.13
  Niemann-Pick (lipid histiocytosis) 272.7
  Nonne-Milroy-Meige (chronic hereditary edema) 757.0

Syndrome — *continued*
nonsense 300.16
Noonan's 759.89
Nothnagel's
 ophthalmoplegia-cerebellar ataxia 378.52
 vasomotor acroparesthesia 443.89
nucleus ambiguous-hypoglossal 352.6
OAV (oculoauriculovertebral dysplasia) 756.0
obsessional 300.3
oculocutaneous 364.24
oculomotor 378.81
oculourethroarticular 099.3
Ogilvie's (sympathicotonic colon obstruction) 560.89
ophthalmoplegia-cerebellar ataxia 378.52
Oppenheim-Urbach (necrobiosis lipoidica diabeticorum) 250.8 ✓5ᵗʰ *[709.3]*
oral-facial-digital 759.89
organic
 affective NEC 293.83
  drug-induced 292.84
 anxiety 293.84
 delusional 293.81
  alcohol-induced 291.5
  drug-induced 292.11
  due to or associated with
   arteriosclerosis 290.42
   presenile brain disease 290.12
   senility 290.20
 depressive 293.83
  drug-induced 292.84
  due to or associated with
   arteriosclerosis 290.43
   presenile brain disease 290.13
   senile brain disease 290.21
 hallucinosis 293.82
  drug-induced 292.84
organic affective 293.83
 induced by drug 292.84
organic personality 310.1
 induced by drug 292.89
Ormond's 593.4
orodigitofacial 759.89
orthostatic hypotensive-dysautonomic dyskinetic 333.0
Osler-Weber-Rendu (familial hemorrhagic telangiectasia) 448.0
osteodermopathic hyperostosis 757.39
osteoporosis-osteomalacia 268.2
Österreicher-Turner (hereditary osteo-onychodysplasia) 756.89
Ostrum-Furst 756.59
otolith 386.19
otopalatodigital 759.89
outlet (thoracic) 353.0
ovarian remant 620.8
ovarian vein 593.4
Owren's (*see also* Defect, coagulation) 286.3
OX 758.6
pacemaker 429.4
Paget-Schroetter (intermittent venous claudication) 453.8
pain — *see* Pain
painful
 apicocostal vertebral (M8010/3) 162.3
 arc 726.19
 bruising 287.2
 feet 266.2
Pancoast's (carcinoma, pulmonary apex) (M8010/3) 162.3
panhypopituitary (postpartum) 253.2

Syndrome — *continued*
papillary muscle 429.81
 with myocardial infarction 410.8 ✓5ᵗʰ
Papillon-Léage and Psaume (orodigitofacial dysostosis) 759.89
parabiotic (transfusion)
 donor (twin) 772.0
 recipient (twin) 776.4
paralysis agitans 332.0
paralytic 344.9
 specified type NEC 344.89
paraneoplastic — *see* condition
Parinaud's (paralysis of conjugate upward gaze) 378.81
 oculoglandular 372.02
Parkes Weber and Dimitri (encephalocutaneous angiomatosis) 759.6
Parkinson's (*see also* Parkinsonism) 332.0
parkinsonian (*see also* Parkinsonism) 332.0
Parry's (exophthalmic goiter) 242.0 ✓5ᵗʰ
Parry-Romberg 349.89
Parsonage-Aldren-Turner 353.5
Parsonage-Turner 353.5
Patau's (trisomy D) 758.1
patellofemoral 719.46
Paterson (-Brown) (-Kelly) (sideropenic dysphagia) 280.8
Payr's (splenic flexure syndrome) 569.89
pectoral girdle 447.8
pectoralis minor 447.8
Pelger-Huët (hereditary hyposegmentation) 288.2
pellagra-cerebellar ataxia-renal aminoaciduria 270.0
Pellegrini-Stieda 726.62
pellagroid 265.2
Pellizzi's (pineal) 259.8
pelvic congestion (-fibrosis) 625.5
Pendred's (familial goiter with deaf-mutism) 243
Penfield's (*see also* Epilepsy) 345.5 ✓5ᵗʰ
Penta X 758.81
peptic ulcer — *see* Ulcer, peptic 533.9 ✓5ᵗʰ
perabduction 447.8
periodic 277.3
periurethral fibrosis 593.4
persistent fetal circulation 747.83 ▲
Petges-Cléjat (poikilodermatomyositis) 710.3
Peutz-Jeghers 759.6
Pfeiffer (acrocephalosyndactyly) 755.55
phantom limb 353.6
pharyngeal pouch 279.11
Pick's (pericardial pseudocirrhosis of liver) 423.2
 heart 423.2
 liver 423.2
Pick-Herxheimer (diffuse idiopathic cutaneous atrophy) 701.8
Pickwickian (cardiopulmonary obesity) 278.8
PIE (pulmonary infiltration with eosinophilia) 518.3
Pierre Marie-Bamberger (hypertrophic pulmonary osteoarthropathy) 731.2
Pierre Mauriac's (diabetes-dwarfism-obesity) 258.1
Pierre Robin 756.0
pigment dispersion, iris 364.53
pineal 259.8
pink puffer 492.8
pituitary 253.0

Syndrome — continued
placental
dysfunction 762.2
insufficiency 762.2
transfusion 762.3
plantar fascia 728.71
plica knee 727.83
Plummer-Vinson (sideropenic dysphagia) 280.8
pluricarential of infancy 260
plurideficiency of infancy 260
pluriglandular (compensatory) 258.8
polycarential of infancy 260
polyglandular 258.8
polysplenia 759.0
pontine 433.8
popliteal
artery entrapment 447.8
web 756.89
postartificial menopause 627.4
postcardiotomy 429.4
postcholecystectomy 576.0
postcommissurotomy 429.4
postconcussional 310.2
postcontusional 310.2
postencephalitic 310.8
posterior
cervical sympathetic 723.2
fossa compression 348.4
inferior cerebellar artery (see also Disease, cerebrovascular, acute) 436
postgastrectomy (dumping) 564.2
post-gastric surgery 564.2
posthepatitis 780.79
postherpetic (neuralgia) (zoster) 053.19
geniculate ganglion 053.11
ophthalmica 053.19
postimmunization — see Complications, vaccination
postinfarction 411.0
postinfluenza (asthenia) 780.79
postirradiation 990
postlaminectomy 722.80
cervical, cervicothoracic 722.81
lumbar, lumbosacral 722.83
thoracic, thoracolumbar 722.82
postleukotomy 310.0
postlobotomy 310.0
postmastectomy lymphedema 457.0
postmature (of newborn) 766.2
postmyocardial infarction 411.0
postoperative NEC 998.9
blind loop 579.2
postpartum panhypopituitary 253.2
postperfusion NEC 999.8
bone marrow 996.85
postpericardiotomy 429.4
postphlebitic ▶(asymptomatic)◀ 459.10 ▲
with •
complications NEC 459.19 •
inflammation 459.12 •
and ulcer 459.13 •
stasis dermatitis 459.12 •
with ulcer 459.13 •
ulcer 459.11 •
with inflammation 459.13 •
postpolio (myelitis) 138
postvagotomy 564.2
postvalvulotomy 429.4
postviral (asthenia) NEC 780.79
Potain's (gastrectasis with dyspepsia) 536.1

Syndrome — continued
potassium intoxication 276.7
Potter's 753.0
Prader (-Labhart) -Willi (-Fanconi) 759.81
preinfarction 411.1
preleukemic 238.7
premature senility 259.8
premenstrual 625.4
premenstrual tension 625.4
pre ulcer 536.9
Prinzmetal-Massumi (anterior chest wall syndrome) 786.52
Profichet's 729.9
progeria 259.8
progressive pallidal degeneration 333.0
prolonged gestation 766.2
Proteus (dermal hypoplasia) 757.39
prune belly 756.71
prurigo-asthma 691.8
pseudocarpal tunnel (sublimis) 354.0
pseudohermaphroditism-virilism-hirsutism 255.2
pseudoparalytica 358.0
pseudo-Turner's 759.89
psycho-organic 293.9
acute 293.0
anxiety type 293.84
depressive type 293.83
hallucinatory type 293.82
nonpsychotic severity 310.1
specified focal (partial) NEC 310.8
paranoid type 293.81
specified type NEC 293.89
subacute 293.1
pterygolymphangiectasia 758.6
ptosis-epicanthus 270.2
pulmonary 660.1
arteriosclerosis 416.0
hypoperfusion (idiopathic) 769
renal (hemorrhagic) 446.21
pulseless 446.7
Putnam-Dana (subacute combined sclerosis with pernicious anemia) 281.0 [336.2]
pyloroduodenal 537.89
pyramidopallidonigral 332.0
pyriformis 355.0
Q-T interval prolongation 794.31
radicular NEC 729.2
lower limbs 724.4
upper limbs 723.4
newborn 767.4
Raeder-Harbitz (pulseless disease) 446.7
Ramsay Hunt's
dyssynergia cerebellaris myoclonica 334.2
herpetic geniculate ganglionitis 053.11
rapid time-zone change 307.45
Raymond (-Céstan) 433.8
Raynaud's (paroxysmal digital cyanosis) 443.0
RDS (respiratory distress syndrome, newborn) 769
Refsum's (heredopathia atactica polyneuritiformis) 356.3
Reichmann's (gastrosuccorrhea) 536.8
Reifenstein's (hereditary familial hypogonadism, male) 257.2
Reilly's (see also Neuropathy, peripheral, autonomic) 337.9
Reiter's 099.3
renal glomerulohyalinosis-diabetic 250.4 [581.81]

Syndrome — *continued*
- Rendu-Osler-Weber (familial hemorrhagic telangiectasia) 448.0
- renofacial (congenital biliary fibroangiomatosis) 753.0
- Rénon-Delille 253.8
- respiratory distress (idiopathic) (newborn) 769
  - adult (following shock, surgery, or trauma) 518.5
  - specified NEC 518.82
- restless leg 333.99
- retraction (Duane's) 378.71
- retroperitoneal fibrosis 593.4
- Rett's 330.8
- Reye's 331.81
- Reye-Sheehan (postpartum pituitary necrosis) 253.2
- Riddoch's (visual disorientation) 368.16
- Ridley's (*see also* Failure, ventricular, left) 428.1
- Rieger's (mesodermal dysgenesis, anterior ocular segment) 743.44
- Rietti-Greppi-Micheli (thalassemia minor) 282.4
- right ventricular obstruction — *see* Failure, heart
- Riley-Day (familial dysautonomia) 742.8
- Robin's 756.0
- Rokitansky-Kuster-Hauser (congenital absence, vagina) 752.49
- Romano-Ward (prolonged Q-T interval) 794.31
- Romberg's 349.89
- Rosen-Castleman-Liebow (pulmonary proteinosis) 516.0
- rotator cuff, shoulder 726.10
- Roth's 355.1
- Rothmund's (congenital poikiloderma) 757.33
- Rotor's (idiopathic hyperbilirubinemia) 277.4
- Roussy-Lévy 334.3
- Roy (-Jutras) (acropachyderma) 757.39
- rubella (congenital) 771.0
- Rubinstein-Taybi's (brachydactylia, short stature, and mental retardation) 759.89
- Rud's (mental deficiency, epilepsy, and infantilism) 759.89
- Ruiter-Pompen (-Wyers) (angiokeratoma corporis diffusum) 272.7
- Runge's (postmaturity) 766.2
- Russell (-Silver) (congenital hemihypertrophy and short stature) 759.89
- Rytand-Lipsitch (complete atrioventricular block) 426.0
- sacralization-scoliosis-sciatica 756.15
- sacroiliac 724.6
- Saenger's 379.46
- salt
  - depletion (*see also* Disease, renal) 593.9
    - due to heat NEC 992.8
      - causing heat exhaustion or prostration 992.4
  - low (*see also* Disease, renal) 593.9
- salt-losing (*see also* Disease, renal) 593.9
- Sanfilippo's (mucopolysaccharidosis III) 277.5
- Scaglietti-Dagnini (acromegalic macrospondylitis) 253.0
- scalded skin 695.1
- scalenus anticus (anterior) 353.0
- scapulocostal 354.8
- scapuloperoneal 359.1
- scapulovertebral 723.4
- Schaumann's (sarcoidosis) 135

Syndrome — *continued*
- Scheie's (mucopolysaccharidosis IS) 277.5
- Scheuthauer-Marie-Sainton (cleidocranialis dysostosis) 755.59
- Schirmer's (encephalocutaneous angiomatosis) 759.6
- schizophrenic, of childhood NEC (*see also* Psychosis, childhood) 299.9 [5]
- Schmidt's
  - sphallo-pharyngo-laryngeal hemiplegia 352.6
  - thyroid-adrenocortical insufficiency 258.1
  - vagoaccessory 352.6
- Schneider's 047.9
- Scholte's (malignant carcinoid) 259.2
- Scholz (-Bielschowsky-Henneberg) 330.0
- Schroeder's (endocrine-hypertensive) 255.3
- Schüller-Christian (chronic histiocytosis X) 277.8
- Schultz's (agranulocytosis) 288.0
- Schwartz (-Jampel) 756.89
- Schwartz-Bartter (inappropriate secretion of antidiuretic hormone) 253.6
- Scimitar (anomalous venous drainage, right lung to inferior vena cava) 747.49
- sclerocystic ovary 256.4
- sea-blue histiocyte 272.7
- Seabright-Bantam (pseudohypoparathyroidism) 275.49
- Seckel's 759.89
- Secretan's (posttraumatic edema) 782.3
- secretoinhibitor (keratoconjunctivitis sicca) 710.2
- Seeligmann's (ichthyosis congenita) 757.1
- Senear-Usher (pemphigus erythematosus) 694.4
- senilism 259.8
- serotonin 333.99
- serous meningitis 348.2
- Sertoli cell (germinal aplasia) 606.0
- sex chromosome mosaic 758.81
- Sézary's (reticulosis) (M9701/3) 202.2 [5]
- shaken infant 995.55
- Shaver's (bauxite pneumoconiosis) 503
- Sheehan's (postpartum pituitary necrosis) 253.2
- shock (traumatic) 958.4
  - kidney 584.5
    - following crush injury 958.5
  - lung 518.5
  - neurogenic 308.9
  - psychic 308.9
- short
  - bowel 579.3
  - P-R interval 426.81
- shoulder-arm (*see also* Neuropathy, peripheral, autonomic) 337.9
- shoulder-girdle 723.4
- shoulder-hand (*see also* Neuropathy, peripheral, autonomic) 337.9
- Shwachman's 288.0
- Shy-Drager (orthostatic hypotension with multisystem degeneration) 333.0
- Sicard's 352.6
- sicca (keratoconjunctivitis) 710.2
- sick
  - cell 276.1
  - cilia 759.89
  - sinus 427.81
- sideropenic 280.8

Syndrome — continued
  Siemens'
    ectodermal dysplasia 757.31
      keratosis follicularis spinulosa (decalvans) 757.39
  Silfverskiöld's (osteochondrodystrophy, extremities) 756.50
  Silver's (congenital hemihypertrophy and short stature) 759.89
  Silvestroni-Bianco (thalassemia minima) 282.4
  Simons' (progressive lipodystrophy) 272.6
  sinus tarsi 726.79
  sinusitis-bronchiectasis-situs inversus 759.3
  Sipple's (medullary thyroid carcinoma-pheochromocytoma) 193
  Sjögren (-Gougerot) (keratoconjunctivitis sicca) 710.2
    with lung involvement 710.2 [517.8]
  Sjögren-Larsson (ichthyosis congenita) 757.1
  Slocumb's 255.3
  Sluder's 337.0
  Smith-Lemli-Opitz (cerebrohepatorenal syndrome) 759.89
  smokers' 305.1
  Sneddon-Wilkinson (subcorneal pustular dermatosis) 694.1
  Sotos' (cerebral gigantism) 253.0
  South African cardiomyopathy 425.2
  spasmodic
    upward movement, eye(s) 378.82
    winking 307.20
  Spens' (syncope with heart block) 426.9
  spherophakia-brachymorphia 759.89
  spinal cord injury — see also Injury, spinal, by site
    with fracture, vertebra — see Fracture, vertebra, by site, with spinal cord injury
    cervical — see Injury, spinal, cervical
  fluid malabsorption (acquired) 331.3
  splenic
    agenesis 759.0
    flexure 569.89
    neutropenia 288.0
    sequestration 282.60
  Spurway's (brittle bones and blue sclera) 756.51
  staphylococcal scalded skin 695.1
  Stein's (polycystic ovary) 256.4
  Stein-Leventhal (polycystic ovary) 256.4
  Steinbrocker's (see also Neuropathy, peripheral, autonomic) 337.9
  Stevens-Johnson (erythema multiforme exudativum) 695.1
  Stewart-Morel (hyperostosis frontalis interna) 733.3
  stiff-man 333.91
  Still's (juvenile rheumatoid arthritis) 714.30
  Still-Felty (rheumatoid arthritis with splenomegaly and leukopenia) 714.1
  Stilling-Türk-Duane (ocular retraction syndrome) 378.71
  Stojano's (subcostal) 098.86
  Stokes (-Adams) (syncope with heart block) 426.9
  Stokvis-Talma (enterogenous cyanosis) 289.7
  stone heart (see also Failure, ventricular, left) 428.1
  straight-back 756.19
  stroke (see also Disease, cerebrovascular, acute) 436

Syndrome — continued
  stroke — continued
    little 435.9
  Sturge-Kalischer-Weber (encephalotrigeminal angiomatosis) 759.6
  Sturge-Weber (-Dimitri) (encephalocutaneous angiomatosis) 759.6
  subclavian-carotid obstruction (chronic) 446.7
  subclavian steal 435.2
  subcoracoid-pectoralis minor 447.8
  subcostal 098.86
    nerve compression 354.8
  subperiosteal hematoma 267
  subphrenic interposition 751.4
  sudden infant death (SIDS) 798.0
  Sudeck's 733.7
  Sudeck-Leriche 733.7
  superior
    cerebellar artery (see also Disease, cerebrovascular, acute) 436
    mesenteric artery 557.1
    pulmonary sulcus (tumor) (M8010/3) 162.3
    vena cava 459.2
  suprarenal cortical 255.3
  supraspinatus 726.10
  swallowed blood 777.3
  sweat retention 705.1
  Sweet's (acute febrile neutrophilic dermatosis) 695.89
  Swyer-James (unilateral hyperlucent lung) 492.8
  Swyer's (XY pure gonadal dysgenesis) 752.7
  Symonds' 348.2
  sympathetic
    cervical paralysis 337.0
    pelvic 625.5
  syndactylic oxycephaly 755.55
  syphilitic-cardiovascular 093.89
  systemic
    fibrosclerosing 710.8
    inflammatory response (SIRS) 995.90 ●
      due to
        infectious process 995.91 ●
          with organ dysfunction 995.92 ●
        non-infectious process 995.93 ●
          with organ dysfunction 995.94 ●
  systolic click (-murmur) 785.2
  Tabagism 305.1
  tachycardia-bradycardia 427.81
  Takayasu (-Onishi) (pulseless disease) 446.7
  Tapia's 352.6
  tarsal tunnel 355.5
  Taussig-Bing (transposition, aorta and overriding pulmonary artery) 745.11
  Taybi's (otopalatodigital) 759.89
  Taylor's 625.5
  teething 520.7
  tegmental 344.89
  telangiectasis-pigmentation-cataract 757.33
  temporal 383.02
    lobectomy behavior 310.0
  temporomandibular joint-pain-dysfunction [TMJ] NEC 524.60
    specified NEC 524.69
  Terry's 362.21
  testicular feminization 257.8
  testis, nonvirilizing 257.8
  tethered (spinal) cord 742.59
  thalamic 348.8
  Thibierge-Weissenbach (cutaneous systemic sclerosis) 710.1

Syndrome — continued
- Thiele 724.6
- thoracic outlet (compression) 353.0
- thoracogenous rheumatic (hypertrophic pulmonary osteoarthropathy) 731.2
- Thorn's (see also Disease, renal) 593.9
- Thorson-Biörck (malignant carcinoid) 259.2
- thrombopenia-hemangioma 287.3
- thyroid-adrenocortical insufficiency 258.1
- Tietze's 733.6
- time-zone (rapid) 307.45
- Tobias' (carcinoma, pulmonary apex) (M8010/3) 162.3
- toilet seat 926.0
- Tolosa-Hunt 378.55
- Toni-Fanconi (cystinosis) 270.0
- Touraine's (hereditary osteo-onychodysplasia) 756.89
- Touraine-Solente-Golé (acropachyderma) 757.39
- toxic
    - oil 710.5
    - shock 040.82 ▲
- transfusion
    - fetal-maternal 772.0
    - twin
        - donor (infant) 772.0
        - recipient (infant) 776.4
- Treacher Collins' (incomplete mandibulofacial dysostosis) 756.0
- trigeminal plate 259.8
- triple X female 758.81
- trisomy NEC 758.5
    - 13 or D$_1$ 758.1
    - 16-18 or E 758.2
    - 18 or E$_3$ 758.2
    - 20 758.5
    - 21 or G (mongolism) 758.0
    - 22 or G (mongolism) 758.0
    - G 758.0
- Troisier-Hanot-Chauffard (bronze diabetes) 275.0
- tropical wet feet 991.4
- Trousseau's (thrombophlebitis migrans visceral cancer) 453.1
- Türk's (ocular retraction syndrome) 378.71
- Turner's 758.6
- Turner-Varny 758.6
- twin-to-twin transfusion 762.3
    - recipient twin 776.4
- Uehlinger's (acropachyderma) 757.39
- Ullrich (-Bonnevie) (-Turner) 758.6
- Ullrich-Feichtiger 759.89
- underwater blast injury (abdominal) (see also Injury, internal, abdomen) 868.00
- universal joint, cervix 620.6
- Unverricht (-Lundborg) 333.2
- Unverricht-Wagner (dermatomyositis) 710.3
- upward gaze 378.81
- Urbach-Oppenheim (necrobiosis lipoidica diabeticorum) 250.8 ✓5th [709.3]
- Urbach-Wiethe (lipid proteinosis) 272.8
- uremia, chronic 585
- urethral 597.81
- urethro-oculoarticular 099.3
- urethro-oculosynovial 099.3
- urohepatic 572.4
- uveocutaneous 364.24
- uveomeningeal, uveomeningitis 363.22
- vagohypoglossal 352.6
- vagovagal 780.2

Syndrome — continued
- van Buchem's (hyperostosis corticalis) 733.3
- van der Hoeve's (brittle bones and blue sclera, deafness) 756.51
- van der Hoeve-Halbertsma-Waardenburg (ptosis-epicanthus) 270.2
- van der Hoeve-Waardenburg-Gualdi (ptosis-epicanthus) 270.2
- van Neck-Odelberg (juvenile osteochondrosis) 732.1
- vanishing twin 651.33
- vascular splanchnic 557.0
- vasomotor 443.9
- vasovagal 780.2
- VATER 759.89
- Velo-cardio-facial 759.89 ●
    - with chromosomal deletion 758.5 ●
- vena cava (inferior) (superior) (obstruction) 459.2
- Verbiest's (claudicatio intermittens spinalis) 435.1
- Vernet's 352.6
- vertebral
    - artery 435.1
        - compression 721.1
    - lumbar 724.4
    - steal 435.1
- vertebrogenic (pain) 724.5
- vertiginous NEC 386.9
- video display tube 723.8
- Villaret's 352.6
- Vinson-Plummer (sideropenic dysphagia) 280.8
- virilizing adrenocortical hyperplasia, congenital 255.2
- virus, viral 079.99
- visceral larval migrans 128.0
- visual disorientation 368.16
- vitamin B$_6$ deficiency 266.1
- vitreous touch 997.99
- Vogt's (corpus striatum) 333.7
- Vogt-Koyanagi 364.24
- Volkmann's 958.6
- von Bechterew-Strümpell (ankylosing spondylitis) 720.0
- von Graefe's 378.72
- von Hippel-Lindau (angiomatosis retinocerebellosa) 759.6
- von Schroetter's (intermittent venous claudication) 453.8
- von Willebrand (-Jürgens) (angiohemophilia) 286.4
- Waardenburg-Klein (ptosis epicanthus) 270.2
- Wagner (-Unverricht) (dermatomyositis) 710.3
- Waldenström's (macroglobulinemia) 273.3
- Waldenström-Kjellberg (sideropenic dysphagia) 280.8
- Wallenberg's (posterior inferior cerebellar artery) (see also Disease, cerebrovascular, acute) 436
- Waterhouse (-Friderichsen) 036.3
- water retention 276.6
- Weber's 344.89
- Weber-Christian (nodular nonsuppurative panniculitis) 729.30
- Weber-Cockayne (epidermolysis bullosa) 757.39
- Weber-Dimitri (encephalocutaneous angiomatosis) 759.6
- Weber-Gubler 344.89
- Weber-Leyden 344.89

Syndrome — continued
  Weber-Osler (familial hemorrhagic telangiectasia) 448.0
  Wegener's (necrotizing respiratory granulomatosis) 446.4
  Weill-Marchesani (brachymorphism and ectopia lentis) 759.89
  Weingarten's (tropical eosinophilia) 518.3
  Weiss-Baker (carotid sinus syncope) 337.0
  Weissenbach-Thibierge (cutaneous systemic sclerosis) 710.1
  Werdnig-Hoffmann 335.0
  Werlhof-Wichmann (see also Purpura, thrombocytopenic) 287.3
  Wermer's (polyendocrine adenomatosis) 258.0
  Werner's (progeria adultorum) 259.8
  Wernicke's (nonalcoholic) (superior hemorrhagic polioencephalitis) 265.1
  Wernicke-Korsakoff (nonalcoholic) 294.0
    alcoholic 291.1
  Westphal-Strümpell (hepatolenticular degeneration) 275.1
  wet
    brain (alcoholic) 303.9
    feet (maceration) (tropical) 991.4
    lung
      adult 518.5
      newborn 770.6
  whiplash 847.0
  Whipple's (intestinal lipodystrophy) 040.2
  "whistling face" (craniocarpotarsal dystrophy) 759.89
  Widal (-Abrami) (acquired hemolytic jaundice) 283.9
  Wilkie's 557.1
  Wilkinson-Sneddon (subcorneal pustular dermatosis) 694.1
  Willan-Plumbe (psoriasis) 696.1
  Willebrand (-Jürgens) (angiohemophilia) 286.4
  Willi-Prader (hypogenital dystrophy with diabetic tendency) 759.81
  Wilson's (hepatolenticular degeneration) 275.1
  Wilson-Mikity 770.7
  Wiskott-Aldrich (eczema-thrombocytopenia) 279.123
  withdrawal
    alcohol 291.81
    drug 292.0
      infant of dependent mother 779.5
  Woakes' (ethmoiditis) 471.1
  Wolff-Parkinson-White (anomalous atrioventricular excitation) 426.7
  Wright's (hyperabduction) 447.8
  X
    cardiac 413.9
    dysmetabolic 277.7
  xiphoidalgia 733.99
  XO 758.6
  XXX 758.81
  XXXXY 758.81
  XXY 758.7
  yellow vernix (placental dysfunction) 762.2
  Zahorsky's 074.0
  Zieve's (jaundice, hyperlipemia and hemolytic anemia) 571.1
  Zollinger-Ellison (gastric hypersecretion with pancreatic islet cell tumor) 251.5
  Zuelzer-Ogden (nutritional megaloblastic anemia) 281.2
Synechia (iris) (pupil) 364.70
  anterior 364.72
  peripheral 364.73

Synechia — continued
  intrauterine (traumatic) 621.5
  posterior 364.71
  vulvae, congenital 752.49
Synesthesia (see also Disturbance, sensation) 782.0
Synodontia 520.2
Synophthalmus 759.89
Synorchidism 752.8
Synorchism 752.8
Synostosis (congenital) 756.59
  astragaloscaphoid 755.67
  radioulnar 755.53
  talonavicular (bar) 755.67
  tarsal 755.67
Synovial — see condition
Synovioma (M9040/3) — see also Neoplasm, connective tissue, malignant
  benign (M9040/0) — see Neoplasm, connective tissue, benign
Synoviosarcoma (M9040/3) — see Neoplasm, connective tissue, malignant
Synovitis 727.00
  chronic crepitant, wrist 727.2
  due to crystals — see Arthritis, due to crystals
  gonococcal 098.51
  gouty 274.0
  syphilitic 095.7
    congenital 090.0
  traumatic, current — see Sprain, by site
  tuberculous — see Tuberculosis, synovitis
  villonodular 719.20
    ankle 719.27
    elbow 719.22
    foot 719.27
    hand 719.24
    hip 719.25
    knee 719.26
    multiple sites 719.29
    pelvic region 719.25
    shoulder (region) 719.21
    specified site NEC 719.28
    wrist 719.23
Syphilide 091.3
  congenital 090.0
  newborn 090.0
  tubercular 095.8
    congenital 090.0
Syphilis, syphilitic (acquired) 097.9
  with lung involvement 095.1
  abdomen (late) 095.2
  acoustic nerve 094.86
  adenopathy (secondary) 091.4
  adrenal (gland) 095.8
    with cortical hypofunction 095.8
  age under 2 years NEC (see also Syphilis, congenital) 090.9
    acquired 097.9
  alopecia (secondary) 091.82
  anemia 095.8
  aneurysm (artery) (ruptured) 093.89
    aorta 093.0
    central nervous system 094.89
    congenital 090.5
  anus 095.8
    primary 091.1
    secondary 091.3
  aorta, aortic (arch) (abdominal) (insufficiency) (pulmonary) (regurgitation) (stenosis) (thoracic) 093.89

Index to Diseases

Syphilis, syphilitic

Syphilis, syphilitic — *continued*
  aorta, aortic — *continued*
    aneurysm 093.0
  arachnoid (adhesive) 094.2
  artery 093.89
    cerebral 094.89
    spinal 094.89
  arthropathy (neurogenic) (tabetic) 094.0
    [713.5]
  asymptomatic — *see* Syphilis, latent
  ataxia, locomotor (progressive) 094.0
  atrophoderma maculatum 091.3
  auricular fibrillation 093.89
  Bell's palsy 094.89
  bladder 095.8
  bone 095.5
    secondary 091.61
  brain 094.89
  breast 095.8
  bronchus 095.8
  bubo 091.0
  bulbar palsy 094.89
  bursa (late) 095.7
  cardiac decompensation 093.89
  cardiovascular (early) (late) (primary)
    (secondary) (tertiary) 093.9
    specified type and site NEC 093.89
  causing death under 2 years of age (*see also*
    Syphilis, congenital) 090.9 ✓5ᵗʰ
    stated to be acquired NEC 097.9
  central nervous system (any site) (early) (late)
    (latent) (primary) (recurrent) (relapse)
    (secondary) (tertiary) 094.9
    with
      ataxia 094.0
      paralysis, general 094.1
        juvenile 090.40
      paresis (general) 094.1
        juvenile 090.40
      tabes (dorsalis) 094.0
        juvenile 090.40
      taboparesis 094.1
        juvenile 090.40
    aneurysm (ruptured) 094.87
    congenital 090.40
      juvenile 090.40
    remission in (sustained) 094.9
    serology doubtful, negative, or positive
      094.9
    specified nature or site NEC 094.89
    vascular 094.89
  cerebral 094.89
    meningovascular 094.2
    nerves 094.89
    sclerosis 094.89
    thrombosis 094.89
  cerebrospinal 094.89
    tabetic 094.0
  cerebrovascular 094.89
  cervix 095.8
  chancre (multiple) 091.0
    extragenital 091.2
    Rollet's 091.0
  Charcôt's joint 094.0 [713.5]
  choked disc 094.89 [377.00]
  chorioretinitis 091.51
    congenital 090.0 [363.13]
    late 094.83
  choroiditis 091.51
    congenital 090.0 [363.13]
    late 094.83

Syphilis, syphilitic — *continued*
  choroiditis — *continued*
    prenatal 090.0 [363.13]
  choroidoretinitis (secondary) 091.51
    congenital 090.0 [363.13]
    late 094.83
  ciliary body (secondary) 091.52
    late 095.8 [364.11]
  colon (late) 095.8
  combined sclerosis 094.89
  complicating pregnancy, childbirth or
    puerperium 647.0 ✓5ᵗʰ
    affecting fetus or newborn 760.2
  condyloma (latum) 091.3
  congenital 090.9 ✓5ᵗʰ
    with
      encephalitis 090.41
      paresis (general) 090.40
      tabes (dorsalis) 090.40
      taboparesis 090.40
    chorioretinitis, choroiditis 090.0 [363.13]
    early or less than 2 years after birth NEC
      090.2
      with manifestations 090.0
      latent (without manifestations) 090.1
        negative spinal fluid test 090.1
        serology, positive 090.1
      symptomatic 090.0
    interstitial keratitis 090.3
    juvenile neurosyphilis 090.40
    late or 2 years or more after birth NEC
      090.7 ✓5ᵗʰ
      chorioretinitis, choroiditis 090.5 [363.13]
      interstitial keratitis 090.3
      juvenile neurosyphilis NEC 090.40
      latent (without manifestations) 090.6 ✓5ᵗʰ
        negative spinal fluid test 090.6 ✓5ᵗʰ
        serology, positive 090.6 ✓5ᵗʰ
      symptomatic or with manifestations NEC
        090.5
        interstitial keratitis 090.3
  conjugal 097.9
    tabes 094.0
  conjunctiva 095.8 [372.10]
  contact V01.6
  cord, bladder 094.0
  cornea, late 095.8 [370.59]
  coronary (artery) 093.89
    sclerosis 093.89
  coryza 095.8
    congenital 090.0
  cranial nerve 094.89
  cutaneous — *see* Syphilis, skin
  dacryocystitis 095.8
  degeneration, spinal cord 094.89
  d'emblée 095.8
  dementia 094.1
    paralytica 094.1
      juvenilis 090.40
  destruction of bone 095.5
  dilatation, aorta 093.0
  due to blood transfusion 097.9
  dura mater 094.89
  ear 095.8
    inner 095.8
      nerve (eighth) 094.86
      neurorecurrence 094.86
  early NEC 091.0
    cardiovascular 093.9
    central nervous system 094.9
      paresis 094.1

Syphilis, syphilitic — continued
  early NEC — continued
    central nervous system — continued
      tabes 094.0
      latent (without manifestations) (less than 2 years after infection) 092.9
        negative spinal fluid test 092.9
        serological relapse following treatment 092.0
        serology positive 092.9
      paresis 094.1
      relapse (treated, untreated) 091.7
      skin 091.3
      symptomatic NEC 091.89
        extragenital chancre 091.2
        primary, except extragenital chancre 091.0
        secondary (see also Syphilis, secondary) 091.3
          relapse (treated, untreated) 091.7
      tabes 094.0
      ulcer 091.3
  eighth nerve 094.86
  endemic, nonvenereal 104.0
  endocarditis 093.20
    aortic 093.22
    mitral 093.21
    pulmonary 093.24
    tricuspid 093.23
  epididymis (late) 095.8
  epiglottis 095.8
  epiphysitis (congenital) 090.0
  esophagus 095.8
  Eustachian tube 095.8
  exposure to V01.6
  eye 095.8 [363.13]
    neuromuscular mechanism 094.85
  eyelid 095.8 [373.5]
    with gumma 095.8 [373.5]
    ptosis 094.89
  fallopian tube 095.8
  fracture 095.5
  gallbladder (late) 095.8
  gastric 095.8
    crisis 094.0
    polyposis 095.8
  general 097.9
    paralysis 094.1
      juvenile 090.40
  genital (primary) 091.0
  glaucoma 095.8
  gumma (late) NEC 095.9
    cardiovascular system 093.9
    central nervous system 094.9
    congenital 090.5
    heart or artery 093.89
  heart 093.89
    block 093.89
    decompensation 093.89
    disease 093.89
    failure 093.89
    valve (see also Syphilis, endocarditis) 093.20
  hemianesthesia 094.89
  hemianopsia 095.8
  hemiparesis 094.89
  hemiplegia 094.89
  hepatic artery 093.89
  hepatitis 095.3
  hepatomegaly 095.3
    congenital 090.0

Syphilis, syphilitic — continued
  hereditaria tarda (see also Syphilis, congenital, late) 090.7
  hereditary (see also Syphilis, congenital) 090.9
  interstitial keratitis 090.3
  Hutchinson's teeth 090.5
  hyalitis 095.8
  inactive — see Syphilis, latent
  infantum NEC (see also Syphilis, congenital) 090.9
  inherited — see Syphilis, congenital
  internal ear 095.8
  intestine (late) 095.8
  iris, iritis (secondary) 091.52
    late 095.8 [364.11]
  joint (late) 095.8
  keratitis (congenital) (early) (interstitial) (late) (parenchymatous) (punctata profunda) 090.3
  kidney 095.4
  lacrimal apparatus 095.8
  laryngeal paralysis 095.8
  larynx 095.8
  late 097.0
    cardiovascular 093.9
    central nervous system 094.9
    latent or 2 years or more after infection (without manifestations) 096
      negative spinal fluid test 096
      serology positive 096
    paresis 094.1
    specified site NEC 095.8
    symptomatic or with symptoms 095.9
    tabes 094.0
  latent 097.1
    central nervous system 094.9
    date of infection unspecified 097.1
    early or less than 2 years after infection 092.9
    late or 2 years or more after infection 096
    serology
      doubtful
        follow-up of latent syphilis 097.1
          central nervous system 094
          date of infection unspecified 097.1
          early or less than 2 years after infection 092
          late or 2 years or more after infection 096
      positive, only finding 097.1
        date of infection unspecified 097.1
        early or less than 2 years after infection 097.1
        late or 2 years or more after infection 097.1
  lens 095.8
  leukoderma 091.3
    late 095.8
  lienis 095.8
  lip 091.3
    chancre 091.2
    late 095.8
    primary 091.2
  Lissauer's paralysis 094.1
  liver 095.3
    secondary 091.62
  locomotor ataxia 094.0
  lung 095.1
  lymphadenitis (secondary) 091.4
  lymph gland (early) (secondary) 091.4
    late 095.8

Syphilis, syphilitic — *continued*
   macular atrophy of skin 091.3
      striated 095.8
   maternal, affecting fetus or newborn 760.2
      manifest syphilis in newborn — *see*
         Syphilis, congenital
   mediastinum (late) 095.8
   meninges (adhesive) (basilar) (brain) (spinal cord) 094.2
   meningitis 094.2
      acute 091.81
      congenital 090.42
   meningoencephalitis 094.2
   meningovascular 094.2
      congenital 090.49
   mesarteritis 093.89
      brain 094.89
      spine 094.89
   middle ear 095.8
   mitral stenosis 093.21
   monoplegia 094.89
   mouth (secondary) 091.3
      late 095.8
   mucocutaneous 091.3
      late 095.8
   mucous
      membrane 091.3
         late 095.8
      patches 091.3
         congenital 090.0
   mulberry molars 090.5
   muscle 095.6
   myocardium 093.82
   myositis 095.6
   nasal sinus 095.8
   neonatorum NEC (*see also* Syphilis, congenital) 090.9
   nerve palsy (any cranial nerve) 094.89
   nervous system, central 094.9
   neuritis 095.8
      acoustic nerve 094.86
   neurorecidive of retina 094.83
   neuroretinitis 094.85
   newborn (*see also* Syphilis, congenital) 090.9
   nodular superficial 095.8
   nonvenereal, endemic 104.0
   nose 095.8
      saddle back deformity 090.5
      septum 095.8
         perforated 095.8
   occlusive arterial disease 093.89
   ophthalmic 095.8 [363.13]
   ophthalmoplegia 094.89
   optic nerve (atrophy) (neuritis) (papilla) 094.84
   orbit (late) 095.8
   orchitis 095.8
   organic 097.9
   osseous (late) 095.5
   osteochondritis (congenital) 090.0
   osteoporosis 095.5
   ovary 095.8
   oviduct 095.8
   palate 095.8
      gumma 095.8
      perforated 090.5
   pancreas (late) 095.8
   pancreatitis 095.8
   paralysis 094.89
      general 094.1
      juvenile 090.40
   paraplegia 094.89

Syphilis, syphilitic — *continued*
   paresis (general) 094.1
      juvenile 090.40
   paresthesia 094.89
   Parkinson's disease or syndrome 094.82
   paroxysmal tachycardia 093.89
   pemphigus (congenital) 090.0
   penis 091.0
      chancre 091.0
      late 095.8
   pericardium 093.81
   perichondritis, larynx 095.8
   periosteum 095.5
      congenital 090.0
      early 091.61
      secondary 091.61
   peripheral nerve 095.8
   petrous bone (late) 095.5
   pharynx 095.8
      secondary 091.3
   pituitary (gland) 095.8
   placenta 095.8
   pleura (late) 095.8
   pneumonia, white 090.0
   pontine (lesion) 094.89
   portal vein 093.89
   primary NEC 091.2
      anal 091.1
      and secondary (*see also* Syphilis, secondary) 091.9
      cardiovascular 093.9
      central nervous system 094.9
      extragenital chancre NEC 091.2
      fingers 091.2
      genital 091.0
      lip 091.2
      specified site NEC 091.2
      tonsils 091.2
   prostate 095.8
   psychosis (intracranial gumma) 094.89
   ptosis (eyelid) 094.89
   pulmonary (late) 095.1
      artery 093.89
   pulmonum 095.1
   pyelonephritis 095.4
   recently acquired, symptomatic NEC 091.89
   rectum 095.8
   respiratory tract 095.8
   retina
      late 094.83
      neurorecidive 094.83
   retrobulbar neuritis 094.85
   salpingitis 095.8
   sclera (late) 095.0
   sclerosis
      cerebral 094.89
      coronary 093.89
      multiple 094.89
      subacute 094.89
   scotoma (central) 095.8
   scrotum 095.8
   secondary (and primary) 091.9
      adenopathy 091.4
      anus 091.3
      bone 091.61
      cardiovascular 093.9
      central nervous system 094.9
      chorioretinitis, choroiditis 091.51
      hepatitis 091.62
      liver 091.62
      lymphadenitis 091.4

Syphilis, syphilitic — continued
- secondary — continued
  - meningitis, acute 091.81
  - mouth 091.3
  - mucous membranes 091.3
  - periosteum 091.61
  - periostitis 091.61
  - pharynx 091.3
  - relapse (treated) (untreated) 091.7
  - skin 091.3
  - specified form NEC 091.89
  - tonsil 091.3
  - ulcer 091.3
  - viscera 091.69
  - vulva 091.3
- seminal vesicle (late) 095.8
- seronegative
  - with signs or symptoms — see Syphilis, by site and stage
- seropositive
  - with signs or symptoms — see Syphilis, by site and stage
  - follow-up of latent syphilis — see Syphilis, latent
  - only finding — see Syphilis, latent
- seventh nerve (paralysis) 094.89
- sinus 095.8
- sinusitis 095.8
- skeletal system 095.5
- skin (early) (secondary) (with ulceration) 091.3
  - late or tertiary 095.8
- small intestine 095.8
- spastic spinal paralysis 094.0
- spermatic cord (late) 095.8
- spinal (cord) 094.89
  - with
    - paresis 094.1
    - tabes 094.0
- spleen 095.8
- splenomegaly 095.8
- spondylitis 095.5
- staphyloma 095.8
- stigmata (congenital) 090.5
- stomach 095.8
- synovium (late) 095.7
- tabes dorsalis (early) (late) 094.0
  - juvenile 090.40
- tabetic type 094.0
  - juvenile 090.40
- taboparesis 094.1
  - juvenile 090.40
- tachycardia 093.89
- tendon (late) 095.7
- tertiary 097.0
  - with symptoms 095.8
  - cardiovascular 093.9
  - central nervous system 094.9
  - multiple NEC 095.8
  - specified site NEC 095.8
- testis 095.8
- thorax 095.8
- throat 095.8
- thymus (gland) 095.8
- thyroid (late) 095.8
- tongue 095.8
- tonsil (lingual) 095.8
  - primary 091.2
  - secondary 091.3
- trachea 095.8
- tricuspid valve 093.23
- tumor, brain 094.89

Syphilis, syphilitic — continued
- tunica vaginalis (late) 095.8
- ulcer (any site) (early) (secondary) 091.3
  - late 095.9
  - perforating 095.9
    - foot 094.0
- urethra (stricture) 095.8
- urogenital 095.8
- uterus 095.8
- uveal tract (secondary) 091.50
  - late 095.8 [363.13]
- uveitis (secondary) 091.50
  - late 095.8 [363.13]
- uvula (late) 095.8
  - perforated 095.8
- vagina 091.0
  - late 095.8
- valvulitis NEC 093.20
- vascular 093.89
  - brain or cerebral 094.89
- vein 093.89
  - cerebral 094.89
- ventriculi 095.8
- vesicae urinariae 095.8
- viscera (abdominal) 095.2
  - secondary 091.69
- vitreous (hemorrhage) (opacities) 095.8
- vulva 091.0
  - late 095.8
  - secondary 091.3

Syphiloma 095.9
- cardiovascular system 093.9
- central nervous system 094.9
- circulatory system 093.9
- congenital 090.5

Syphilophobia 300.29

Syringadenoma (M8400/0) — see also Neoplasm, skin, benign
- papillary (M8406/0) — see Neoplasm, skin, benign

Syringobulbia 336.0

Syringocarcinoma (M8400/3) — see Neoplasm, skin, malignant

Syringocystadenoma (M8400/0) — see also Neoplasm, skin, benign
- papillary (M8406/0) — see Neoplasm, skin, benign

Syringocystoma (M8407/0) — see Neoplasm, skin, benign

Syringoma (M8407/0) — see also Neoplasm, skin, benign
- chondroid (M8940/0) — see Neoplasm, by site, benign

Syringomyelia 336.0

Syringomyelitis 323.9
- late effect — see category 326

Syringomyelocele (see also Spina bifida) 741.9

Syringopontia 336.0

System, systemic — see also condition
- disease, combined — see Degeneration, combined
- fibrosclerosing syndrome 710.8
- inflammatory response syndrome (SIRS) 995.90
  - due to
    - infectious process 995.91
      - with organ dysfunction 995.92

System, systemic — *continued*
  inflammatory response syndrome — *continued*
    due to — *continued*
      non-infectious process 995.93 ●
        with organ dysfunction 995.94 ●
  lupus erythematosus 710.0
  inhibitor 286.5

T

Tab — *see* Tag
Tabacism 989.8
Tabacosis 989.8
Tabardillo 080
  flea-borne 081.0
  louse-borne 080
Tabes, tabetic
  with
    central nervous system syphilis 094.0
    Charcôt's joint 094.0 [713.5]
    cord bladder 094.0
    crisis, viscera (any) 094.0
    paralysis, general 094.1
    paresis (general) 094.1
    perforating ulcer 094.0
  arthropathy 094.0 [713.5]
  bladder 094.0
  bone 094.0
  cerebrospinal 094.0
  congenital 090.40
  conjugal 094.0
  dorsalis 094.0
    neurosyphilis 094.0
  early 094.0
  juvenile 090.40
  latent 094.0
  mesenterica (*see also* Tuberculosis) 014.8
  paralysis insane, general 094.1
  peripheral (nonsyphilitic) 799.8
  spasmodic 094.0
    not dorsal or dorsalis 343.9
  syphilis (cerebrospinal) 094.0
Taboparalysis 094.1
Taboparesis (remission) 094.1
  with
    Charcôt's joint 094.1 [713.5]
    cord bladder 094.1
    perforating ulcer 094.1
  juvenile 090.40
Tachyalimentation 579.3
Tachyarrhythmia, tachyrhythmia — *see also* Tachycardia
  paroxysmal with sinus bradycardia 427.81
Tachycardia 785.0
  atrial 427.89
  auricular 427.89
  newborn 779.82 ●
  nodal 427.89
    nonparoxysmal atrioventricular 426.89
    nonparoxysmal atrioventricular (nodal) 426.89
  paroxysmal 427.2
    with sinus bradycardia 427.81
    atrial (PAT) 427.0
      psychogenic 316 [427.0]
    atrioventricular (AV) 427.0
      psychogenic 316 [427.0]
    essential 427.2
    junctional 427.0
    nodal 427.0

Tachycardia — *continued*
  paroxysmal — *continued*
    psychogenic 316 [427.2]
      atrial 316 [427.0]
      supraventricular 316 [427.0]
      ventricular 316 [427.1]
    supraventricular 427.0
      psychogenic 316 [427.0]
    ventricular 427.1
      psychogenic 316 [427.1]
  postoperative 997.1
  psychogenic 306.2
  sick sinus 427.81
  sinoauricular 427.89
  sinus 427.89
  supraventricular 427.89
  ventricular (paroxysmal) 427.1
    psychogenic 316 [427.1]
Tachypnea 786.06
  hysterical 300.11
  newborn (idiopathic) (transitory) 770.6
  psychogenic 306.1
  transitory, of newborn 770.6
Taenia (infection) (infestation) (*see also* Infestation, taenia) 123.3
  diminuta 123.6
  echinococcal infestation (*see also* Echinococcus) 122.9
  nana 123.6
  saginata infestation 123.2
  solium (intestinal form) 123.0
    larval form 123.1
Taeniasis (intestine) (*see also* Infestation, Taenia) 123.3
  saginata 123.2
  solium 123.0
Taenzer's disease 757.4
Tag (hypertrophied skin) (infected) 701.9
  adenoid 474.8
  anus 455.9
  endocardial (*see also* Endocarditis) 424.90
  hemorrhoidal 455.9
  hymen 623.8
  perineal 624.8
  preauricular 744.1
  rectum 455.9
  sentinel 455.9
  skin 701.9
    accessory 757.39
    anus 455.9
    congenital 757.39
    preauricular 744.1
    rectum 455.9
  tonsil 474.8
  urethra, urethral 599.84
  vulva 624.8
Tahyna fever 062.5
Takayasu (-Onishi) disease or syndrome (pulseless disease) 446.7
Talc granuloma 728.82
Talcosis 502
Talipes (congenital) 754.70
  acquired NEC 736.79
    planus 734
  asymmetric 754.79
    acquired 736.79
  calcaneovalgus 754.62
    acquired 736.76
  calcaneovarus 754.59
    acquired 736.76

Talipes — *continued*
  calcaneus 754.79
    acquired 736.76
  cavovarus 754.59
    acquired 736.75
  cavus 754.71
    acquired 736.73
  equinovalgus 754.69
    acquired 736.72
  equinovarus 754.51
    acquired 736.71
  equinus 754.79
    acquired, NEC 736.72
  percavus 754.71
    acquired 736.73
  planovalgus 754.69
    acquired 736.79
  planus (acquired) (any degree) 734
    congenital 754.61
    due to rickets 268.1
  valgus 754.60
    acquired 736.79
  varus 754.50
    acquired 736.79
Talma's disease 728.85
Tamponade heart (Rose's) (*see also* Pericarditis) 423.9
Tanapox 078.89
Tangier disease (familial high-density lipoprotein deficiency) 272.5
Tank ear 380.12
Tantrum (childhood) (*see also* Disturbance, conduct) 312.1 ✓5ᵗʰ
Tapeworm (infection) (infestation) (*see also* Infestation, tapeworm) 123.9
Tapia's syndrome 352.6
Tarantism 297.8
Target-oval cell anemia 282.4
Tarlov's cyst 355.9
Tarral-Besnier disease (pityriasis rubra pilaris) 696.4
Tarsalgia 729.2
Tarsal tunnel syndrome 355.5
Tarsitis (eyelid) 373.00
  syphilitic 095.8 *[373.00]*
  tuberculous (*see also* Tuberculosis) 017.0 ✓5ᵗʰ *[373.4]*
Tartar (teeth) 523.6
Tattoo (mark) 709.09
Taurodontism 520.2
Taussig-Bing defect, heart, or syndrome (transposition, aorta and overriding pulmonary artery) 745.11
Tay's choroiditis 363.41
Tay-Sachs
  amaurotic familial idiocy 330.1
  disease 330.1
Taybi's syndrome (otopalatodigital) 759.89
Taylor's
  disease (diffuse idiopathic cutaneous atrophy) 701.8
  syndrome 625.5
Tear, torn (traumatic) — *see also* Wound, open, by site
  anus, anal (sphincter) 863.89
    with open wound in cavity 863.99

Tear, torn — *continued*
  anus, anal — *continued*
    complicating delivery 664.2 ✓5ᵗʰ
      with mucosa 664.3 ✓5ᵗʰ
    nontraumatic, nonpuerperal 565.0
  articular cartilage, old (*see also* Disorder, cartilage, articular) 718.0 ✓5ᵗʰ
  bladder
    with
      abortion — *see* Abortion, by type, with damage to pelvic organs
      ectopic pregnancy (*see also* categories 633.0-633.9) 639.2
      molar pregnancy (*see also* categories 630-632) 639.2
    following
      abortion 639.2
      ectopic or molar pregnancy 639.2
    obstetrical trauma 665.5 ✓5ᵗʰ
  bowel
    with
      abortion — *see* Abortion, by type, with damage to pelvic organs
      ectopic pregnancy (*see also* categories 633.0-633.9) 639.2
      molar pregnancy (*see also* categories 630-632) 639.2
    following
      abortion 639.2
      ectopic or molar pregnancy 639.2
    obstetrical trauma 665.5 ✓5ᵗʰ
  broad ligament
    with
      abortion — *see* Abortion, by type, with damage to pelvic organs
      ectopic pregnancy (*see also* categories 633.0-633.9) 639.2
      molar pregnancy (*see also* categories 630-632) 639.2
    following
      abortion 639.2
      ectopic or molar pregnancy 639.2
    obstetrical trauma 665.6 ✓5ᵗʰ
  bucket handle (knee) (meniscus) — *see* Tear, meniscus
  capsule
    joint — *see* Sprain, by site
    spleen — *see* Laceration, spleen, capsule
  cartilage — *see also* Sprain, by site
    articular, old (*see also* Disorder, cartilage, articular) 718.0 ✓5ᵗʰ
    knee — *see* Tear, meniscus
    semilunar (knee) (current injury) — *see* Tear, meniscus
  cervix
    with
      abortion — *see* Abortion, by type, with damage to pelvic organs
      ectopic pregnancy (*see also* categories 633.0-633.9) 639.2
      molar pregnancy (*see also* categories 630-632) 639.2
    following
      abortion 639.2
      ectopic or molar pregnancy 639.2
    obstetrical trauma (current) 665.3 ✓5ᵗʰ
    old 622.3
  internal organ (abdomen, chest, or pelvis) — *see* Injury, internal, by site

Tear, torn — *continued*
  ligament — *see also* Sprain, by site
    with open wound — *see* Wound, open by site
  meniscus (knee) (current injury) 836.2
    bucket handle 836.0
      old 717.0
    lateral 836.1
      anterior horn 836.1
        old 717.42
      bucket handle 836.1
        old 717.41
      old 717.40
      posterior horn 836.1
        old 717.43
      specified site NEC 836.1
        old 717.49
    medial 836.0
      anterior horn 836.0
        old 717.1
      bucket handle 836.0
        old 717.0
      old 717.3
      posterior horn 836.0
        old 717.2
    old NEC 717.5
    site other than knee — *see* Sprain, by site
  muscle — *see also* Sprain, by site
    with open wound — *see* Wound, open by site
  pelvic
    floor, complicating delivery 664.1 ✓5ᵗʰ
    organ NEC
      with
        abortion — *see* Abortion, by type, with damage to pelvic organs
        ectopic pregnancy (*see also* categories 633.0-633.9) 639.2
        molar pregnancy (*see also* categories 630-632) 639.2
      following
        abortion 639.2
        ectopic or molar pregnancy 639.2
      obstetrical trauma 665.5 ✓5ᵗʰ
  perineum — *see also* Laceration, perineum
    obstetrical trauma 665.5 ✓5ᵗʰ
  periurethral tissue
    with
      abortion — *see* Abortion, by type, with damage to pelvic organs
      ectopic pregnancy (*see also* categories 633.0-633.9) 639.2
      molar pregnancy (*see also* categories 630-632) 639.2
    following
      abortion 639.2
      ectopic or molar pregnancy 639.2
    obstetrical trauma 665.5 ✓5ᵗʰ
  rectovaginal septum — *see* Laceration, rectovaginal septum
  retina, retinal (recent) (with detachment) 361.00
    without detachment 361.30
    dialysis (juvenile) (with detachment) 361.04
    giant (with detachment) 361.03
    horseshoe (without detachment) 361.32
    multiple (with detachment) 361.02
      without detachment 361.33
    old
      delimited (partial) 361.06
      partial 361.06

Tear, torn — *continued*
  retina, retinal — *continued*
    old — *continued*
      total or subtotal 361.07
      partial (without detachment)
        giant 361.03
        multiple defects 361.02
        old (delimited) 361.06
        single defect 361.01
    round hole (without detachment) 361.31
    single defect (with detachment) 361.01
    total or subtotal (recent) 361.05
      old 361.07
  rotator cuff (traumatic) 840.4
    current injury 840.4
    degenerative 726.10
    nontraumatic 727.61
  semilunar cartilage, knee (*see also* Tear, meniscus) 836.2
    old 717.5
  tendon — *see also* Sprain, by site
    with open wound — *see* Wound, open by site
  tentorial, at birth 767.0
  umbilical cord
    affecting fetus or newborn 772.0
    complicating delivery 663.8 ✓5ᵗʰ
  urethra
    with
      abortion — *see* Abortion, by type, with damage to pelvic organs
      ectopic pregnancy (*see also* categories 633.0-633.9) 639.2
      molar pregnancy (*see also* categories 630-632) 639.2
    following
      abortion 639.2
      ectopic or molar pregnancy 639.2
    obstetrical trauma 665.5 ✓5ᵗʰ
  uterus — *see* Injury, internal, uterus
  vagina — *see* Laceration, vagina
  vessel, from catheter 998.2
  vulva, complicating delivery 664.0 ✓5ᵗʰ
Tear stone 375.57
Teeth, tooth — *see also* condition
  grinding 306.8
Teething 520.7
  syndrome 520.7
Tegmental syndrome 344.89
Telangiectasia, telangiectasis (verrucous) 448.9
  ataxic (cerebellar) 334.8
  familial 448.0
  hemorrhagic, hereditary (congenital) (senile) 448.0
  hereditary hemorrhagic 448.0
  retina 362.15
  spider 448.1
Telecanthus (congenital) 743.63
Telescoped bowel or intestine (*see also* Intussusception) 560.0
Teletherapy, adverse effect NEC 990
Telogen effluvium 704.02
Temperature
  body, high (of unknown origin) (*see also* Pyrexia) 780.6
  cold, trauma from 991.9
    newborn 778.2
    specified effect NEC 991.8

Temperature — continued
  high
    body (of unknown origin) (see also Pyrexia) 780.6
      trauma from — see Heat
Temper tantrum (childhood) (see also Disturbance, conduct) 312.1 ✓5ᵗʰ
Temple — see condition
Temporal — see also condition
  lobe syndrome 310.0
Temporomandibular joint-pain-dysfunction syndrome 524.60
Temporosphenoidal — see condition
Tendency
  bleeding (see also Defect, coagulation) 286.9
  homosexual, ego-dystonic 302.0
  paranoid 301.0
  suicide 300.9
Tenderness
  abdominal (generalized) (localized) 789.6 ✓5ᵗʰ
  rebound 789.6 ✓5ᵗʰ
  skin 782.0
Tendinitis, tendonitis (see also Tenosynovitis) 726.90
  Achilles 726.71
  adhesive 726.90
    shoulder 726.0
  calcific 727.82
    shoulder 726.11
  gluteal 726.5
  patellar 726.64
  peroneal 726.79
  pes anserinus 726.61
  psoas 726.5
  tibialis (anterior) (posterior) 726.72
  trochanteric 726.5
Tendon — see condition
Tendosynovitis — see Tenosynovitis
Tendovaginitis — see Tenosynovitis
Tenesmus 787.99
  rectal 787.99
  vesical 788.9
Tenia — see Taenia
Teniasis — see Taeniasis
Tennis elbow 726.32
Tenonitis — see also Tenosynovitis
  eye (capsule) 376.04
Tenontosynovitis — see Tenosynovitis
Tenontothecitis — see Tenosynovitis
Tenophyte 727.9
Tenosynovitis 727.00
  adhesive 726.90
    shoulder 726.0
  ankle 727.06
  bicipital (calcifying) 726.12
  buttock 727.09
  due to crystals — see Arthritis, due to crystals
  elbow 727.09
  finger 727.05
  foot 727.06
  gonococcal 098.51
  hand 727.05
  hip 727.09
  knee 727.09
  radial styloid 727.04
  shoulder 726.10
    adhesive 726.0
  spine 720.1

Tenosynovitis — continued
  supraspinatus 726.10
  toe 727.06
  tuberculous — see Tuberculosis, tenosynovitis
  wrist 727.05
Tenovaginitis — see Tenosynovitis
Tension
  arterial, high (see also Hypertension) 401.9
    without diagnosis of hypertension 796.2
  headache 307.81
  intraocular (elevated) 365.00
  nervous 799.2
  ocular (elevated) 365.00
  pneumothorax 512.0
    iatrogenic 512.1
    postoperative 512.1
    spontaneous 512.0
  premenstrual 625.4
  state 300.9
Tentorium — see condition
Teratencephalus 759.89
Teratism 759.7
Teratoblastoma (malignant) (M9080/3) — see Neoplasm, by site, malignant
Teratocarcinoma (M9081/3) — see also Neoplasm, by site, malignant
  liver 155.0
Teratoma (solid) (M9080/1) — see also Neoplasm, by site, uncertain behavior
  adult (cystic) (M9080/0) — see Neoplasm, by site, benign
  and embryonal carcinoma, mixed (M9081/3) — see Neoplasm, by site, malignant
  benign (M9080/0) — see Neoplasm, by site, benign
  combined with choriocarcinoma (M9101/3) — see Neoplasm, by site, malignant
  cystic (adult) (M9080/0) — see Neoplasm, by site, benign
  differentiated type (M9080/0) — see Neoplasm, by site, benign
  embryonal (M9080/3) — see also Neoplasm, by site, malignant
    liver 155.0
  fetal
    sacral, causing fetopelvic disproportion 653.7 ✓5ᵗʰ
  immature (M9080/3) — see Neoplasm, by site, malignant
  liver (M9080/3) 155.0
    adult, benign, cystic, differentiated type or mature (M9080/0) 211.5
  malignant (M9080/3) — see also Neoplasm, by site, malignant
    anaplastic type (M9082/3) — see Neoplasm, by site, malignant
    intermediate type (M9083/3) — see Neoplasm, by site, malignant
    liver (M9080/3) 155.0
    trophoblastic (M9102/3)
      specified site — see Neoplasm, by site, malignant
      unspecified site 186.9
    undifferentiated type (M9082/3) — see Neoplasm, by site, malignant
  mature (M9080/0) — see Neoplasm, by site, benign
  ovary (M9080/0) 220
    embryonal, immature, or malignant (M9080/3) 183.0

Index to Diseases

Teratoma — *continued*
  suprasellar (M9080/3) — *see* Neoplasm, by site, malignant
  testis (M9080/3) 186.9
    adult, benign, cystic, differentiated type or mature (M9080/0) 222.0
    undescended 186.0
Terminal care V66.7
Termination
  anomalous — *see also* Malposition, congenital
    portal vein 747.49
    right pulmonary vein 747.42
  pregnancy (legal) (therapeutic) (*see* Abortion, legal) 635.9 ✓5ᵗʰ
    fetus NEC 779.6
    illegal (*see also* Abortion, illegal) 636.9 ✓5ᵗʰ
Ternidens diminutus infestation 127.7
Terrors, night (child) 307.46
Terry's syndrome 362.21
Tertiary — *see* condition
Tessellated fundus, retina (tigroid) 362.89
Test(s)
  AIDS virus V72.6
  adequacy
    hemodialysis V56.31
    peritoneal dialysis V56.32
  allergen V72.7
  bacterial disease NEC (*see also* Screening, by name of disease) V74.9
  basal metabolic rate V72.6
  blood-alcohol V70.4
  blood-drug V70.4
    for therapeutic drug monitoring V58.83
  developmental, infant or child V20.2
  Dick V74.8
  fertility V26.21
  genetic V26.3
  hearing V72.1
  HIV V72.6
  human immunodeficiency virus V72.6
  Kveim V82.89
  laboratory V72.6
    for medicolegal reason V70.4
  Mantoux (for tuberculosis) V74.1
  mycotic organism V75.4
  parasitic agent NEC V75.8
  paternity V70.4
  peritoneal equilibration V56.32
  pregnancy
    positive V22.1
      first pregnancy V22.0
    unconfirmed V72.4
  preoperative V72.84
    cardiovascular V72.81
    respiratory V72.82
    specified NEC V72.83
  procreative management NEC V26.29
  sarcoidosis V82.89
  Schick V74.3
  Schultz-Charlton V74.8
  skin, diagnostic
    allergy V72.7
    bacterial agent NEC (*see also* Screening, by name of disease) V74.9
    Dick V74.8
    hypersensitivity V72.7
    Kveim V82.89
    Mantoux V74.1
    mycotic organism V75.4
    parasitic agent NEC V75.8

Test(s) — *continued*
  skin, diagnostic — *continued*
    sarcoidosis V82.89
    Schick V74.3
    Schultz-Charlton V74.8
    tuberculin V74.1
  specified type NEC V72.8 ✓5ᵗʰ
  tuberculin V74.1
  vision V72.0
  Wassermann
    positive (*see also* Serology for syphilis, positive) 097.1
    false 795.6
Testicle, testicular, testis — *see also* condition
  feminization (syndrome) 257.8
Tetanus, tetanic (cephalic) (convulsions) 037
  with
    abortion — *see* Abortion, by type, with sepsis
    ectopic pregnancy (*see also* categories 633.0-633.9) 639.0
    molar pregnancy (*see* categories 630-632) 639.0
  following
    abortion 639.0
    ectopic or molar pregnancy 639.0
  inoculation V03.7
    reaction (due to serum) — *see* Complications, vaccination
  neonatorum 771.3
  puerperal, postpartum, childbirth 670 ✓4ᵗʰ
Tetany, tetanic 781.7
  alkalosis 276.3
  associated with rickets 268.0
  convulsions 781.7
    hysterical 300.11
  functional (hysterical) 300.11
  hyperkinetic 781.7
    hysterical 300.11
  hyperpnea 786.01
    hysterical 300.11
    psychogenic 306.1
  hyperventilation 786.01
    hysterical 300.11
    psychogenic 306.1
  hypocalcemic, neonatal 775.4
  hysterical 300.11
  neonatal 775.4
  parathyroid (gland) 252.1
  parathyroprival 252.1
  postoperative 252.1
  postthyroidectomy 252.1
  pseudotetany 781.7
    hysterical 300.11
  psychogenic 306.1
    specified as conversion reaction 300.11
Tetralogy of Fallot 745.2
Tetraplegia — *see* Quadriplegia
Thailand hemorrhagic fever 065.4
Thalassanemia 282.4
Thalassemia (alpha) (beta) (disease) (Hb-C) (Hb-D) (Hb-E) (Hb-H) (Hb-I) (Hb-S) (high fetal gene) (high fetal hemoglobin) (intermedia) (major) (minima) (minor) (mixed) (sickle-cell) (trait) (with other hemoglobinopathy) 282.4
Thalassemic variants 282.4
Thaysen-Gee disease (nontropical sprue) 579.0
Thecoma (M8600/0) 220
  malignant (M8600/3) 183.0

✓4ᵗʰ Fourth-digit Required
✓5ᵗʰ Fifth-digit Required

Thelarche, precocious 259.1
Thelitis 611.0
   puerperal, postpartum 675.0 [5]
Therapeutic — *see* condition
Therapy V57.9
   blood transfusion, without reported diagnosis V58.2
   breathing V57.0
   chemotherapy V58.1
      fluoride V07.31
      prophylactic NEC V07.39
   dialysis (intermittent) (treatment)
      extracorporeal V56.0
      peritoneal V56.8
      renal V56.0
      specified type NEC V56.8
   exercise NEC V57.1
      breathing V57.0
   extracorporeal dialysis (renal) V56.0
   fluoride prophylaxis V07.31
   hemodialysis V56.0
   long term oxygen therapy V46.2 ●
   occupational V57.21
   orthoptic V57.4
   orthotic V57.81
   peritoneal dialysis V56.8
   physical NEC V57.1
   postmenopausal hormone replacement V07.4
   radiation V58.0
   speech V57.3
   vocational V57.22
Thermalgesia 782.0
Thermalgia 782.0
Thermanalgesia 782.0
Thermanesthesia 782.0
Thermic — *see* condition
Thermography (abnormal) 793.9
   breast 793.89
Thermoplegia 992.0
Thesaurismosis
   amyloid 277.3
   bilirubin 277.4
   calcium 275.40
   cystine 270.0
   glycogen (*see also* Disease, glycogen storage) 271.0
   kerasin 272.7
   lipoid 272.7
   melanin 255.4
   phosphatide 272.7
   urate 274.9
Thiaminic deficiency 265.1
   with beriberi 265.0
Thibierge-Weissenbach syndrome (cutaneous systemic sclerosis) 710.1
Thickened endometrium 793.5
Thickening
   bone 733.99
      extremity 733.99
   breast 611.79
   hymen 623.3
   larynx 478.79
   nail 703.8
      congenital 757.5
   periosteal 733.99
   pluera (*see also* Pleurisy) 511.0
   skin 782.8
   subepiglottic 478.79
   tongue 529.8
   valve, heart — *see* Endocarditis

Thiele syndrome 724.6
Thigh — *see* condition
Thinning vertebra (*see also* Osteoporosis) 733.00
Thirst, excessive 783.5
   due to deprivation of water 994.3
Thomsen's disease 359.2
Thomson's disease (congenital poikiloderma) 757.33
Thoracic — *see also* condition
   kidney 753.3
   outlet syndrome 353.0
   stomach — *see* Hernia, diaphragm
Thoracogastroschisis (congenital) 759.89
Thoracopagus 759.4
Thoracoschisis 756.3
Thorax — *see* condition
Thorn's syndrome (*see also* Disease, renal) 593.9
Thornwaldt's, Tornwaldt's
   bursitis (pharyngeal) 478.29
   cyst 478.26
   disease (pharyngeal bursitis) 478.29
Thorson-Biörck syndrome (malignant carcinoid) 259.2
Threadworm (infection) (infestation) 127.4
Threatened
   abortion or miscarriage 640.0 [5]
      with subsequent abortion (*see also* Abortion, spontaneous) 634.9 [5]
      affecting fetus 762.1
   labor 644.1 [5]
      affecting fetus or newborn 761.8
      premature 644.0 [5]
   miscarriage 640.0 [5]
      affecting fetus 762.1
   premature
      delivery 644.2 [5]
         affecting fetus or newborn 761.8
      labor 644.0 [5]
         before 22 completed weeks gestation 640.0 [5]
Three-day fever 066.0
Threshers' lung 495.0
Thrix annulata (congenital) 757.4
Throat — *see* condition
Thrombasthenia (Glanzmann's) (hemorrhagic) (hereditary) 287.1
Thromboangiitis 443.1
   obliterans (general) 443.1
      cerebral 437.1
   vessels
      brain 437.1
      spinal cord 437.1
Thromboarteritis — *see* Arteritis
Thromboasthenia (Glanzmann's) (hemorrhagic) (hereditary) 287.1
Thrombocytasthenia (Glanzmann's) 287.1
Thrombocythemia (essential) (hemorrhagic) (primary) (M9962/1) 238.7
   idiopathic (M9962/1) 238.7
Thrombocytopathy (dystrophic) (granulopenic) 287.1
Thrombocytopenia, thrombocytopenic 287.5
   with giant hemangioma 287.3
   amegakaryocytic, congenital 287.3
   congenital 287.3

Thrombocytopenia, thrombocytopenic — continued
  cyclic 287.3
  dilutional 287.4
  due to
    drugs 287.4
    extracorporeal circulation of blood 287.4
    massive blood transfusion 287.4
    platelet alloimmunization 287.4
  essential 287.3
  hereditary 287.3
  Kasabach-Merritt 287.3
  neonatal, transitory 776.1
    due to
      exchange transfusion 776.1
      idiopathic maternal thrombocytopenia 776.1
      isoimmunization 776.1
  primary 287.3
  puerperal, postpartum 666.3 ✓5ᵗʰ
  purpura (see also Purpura, thrombocytopenic) 287.3
    thrombotic 446.6
  secondary 287.4
  sex-linked 287.3
Thrombocytosis, essential 289.9
Thromboembolism — see Embolism
Thrombopathy (Bernard-Soulier) 287.1
  constitutional 286.4
  Willebrand-Jürgens (angiohemophilia) 286.4
Thrombopenia (see also Thrombocytopenia) 287.5
Thrombophlebitis 451.9
  antecubital vein 451.82
  antepartum (superficial) 671.2 ✓5ᵗʰ
    affecting fetus or newborn 760.3
    deep 671.3 ✓5ᵗʰ
  arm 451.89
    deep 451.83
    superficial 451.82
  breast, superficial 451.89
  cavernous (venous) sinus — see Thrombophlebitis, intracranial venous sinus
  cephalic vein 451.82
  cerebral (sinus) (vein) 325
    late effect — see category 326
    nonpyogenic 437.6
      in pregnancy or puerperium 671.5 ✓5ᵗʰ
      late effect — see Late effect(s) (of) cerebrovascular disease
  due to implanted device — see Complications, due to (presence of) any device, implant or graft classified to 996.0-996.5 NEC
  during or resulting from a procedure NEC 997.2
  femoral 451.11
  femoropopliteal 451.19
  following infusion, perfusion, or transfusion 999.2
  hepatic (vein) 451.89
  idiopathic, recurrent 453.1
  iliac vein 451.81
  iliofemoral 451.11
  intracranial venous sinus (any) 325
    late effect — see category 326
    nonpyogenic 437.6
      in pregnancy or puerperium 671.5 ✓5ᵗʰ
      late effect — see Late effect(s) (of) cerebrovascular disease
  jugular vein 451.89

Thrombophlebitis — continued
  lateral (venous) sinus — see Thrombophlebitis, intracranial venous sinus
  leg 451.2
    deep (vessels) 451.19
      femoral vein 451.11
      specified vessel NEC 451.19
    superficial (vessels) 451.0
      femoral vein 451.11
  longitudinal (venous) sinus — see Thrombophlebitis, intracranial venous sinus
  lower extremity 451.2
    deep (vessels) 451.19
      femoral vein 451.11
      specified vessel NEC 451.19
    superficial (vessels) 451.0
  migrans, migrating 453.1
  pelvic
    with
      abortion — see Abortion, by type, with sepsis
      ectopic pregnancy — (see also categories 633.0-633.9) 639.0
      molar pregnancy — (see also categories 630-632) 639.0
    following
      abortion 639.0
      ectopic or molar pregnancy 639.0
    puerperal 671.4 ✓5ᵗʰ
  popliteal vein 451.19
  portal (vein) 572.1
  postoperative 997.2
  pregnancy (superficial) 671.2 ✓5ᵗʰ
    affecting fetus or newborn 760.3
    deep 671.3 ✓5ᵗʰ
  puerperal, postpartum, childbirth (extremities) (superficial) 671.2 ✓5ᵗʰ
    deep 671.4 ✓5ᵗʰ
    pelvic 671.4 ✓5ᵗʰ
    specified site NEC 671.5 ✓5ᵗʰ
  radial vein 451.83
  saphenous (greater) (lesser) 451.0
  sinus (intracranial) — see Thrombophlebitis, intracranial venous sinus
    specified site NEC 451.89
  tibial vein 451.19
Thrombosis, thrombotic (marantic) (multiple) (progressive) (septic) (vein) (vessel) 453.9
  with childbirth or during the puerperium — see Thrombosis, puerperal, postpartum
  antepartum — see Thrombosis, pregnancy
  aorta, aortic 444.1
    abdominal 444.0
    bifurcation 444.0
    saddle 444.0
    terminal 444.0
    thoracic 444.1
    valve — see Endocarditis, aortic
  apoplexy (see also Thrombosis, brain) 434.0 ✓5ᵗʰ
    late effect — see Late effect(s) (of) cerebrovascular disease
  appendix, septic — see Appendicitis, acute
  arteriolar-capillary platelet, disseminated 446.6
  artery, arteries (postinfectional) 444.9
    auditory, internal 433.8 ✓5ᵗʰ
    basilar (see also Occlusion, artery, basilar) 433.0 ✓5ᵗʰ

Thrombosis, thrombotic — continued
  artery, arteries — continued
    carotid (common) (internal) (see also
      Occlusion, artery, carotid) 433.1 ✓5ᵗʰ
      with other precerebral artery 433.3 ✓5ᵗʰ
    cerebellar (anterior inferior) (posterior
      inferior) (superior) 433.8 ✓5ᵗʰ
    cerebral (see also Thrombosis, brain)
      434.0 ✓5ᵗʰ
    choroidal (anterior) 433.8 ✓5ᵗʰ
    communicating posterior 433.8 ✓5ᵗʰ
    coronary (see also Infarct, myocardium)
      410.9 ✓5ᵗʰ
      without myocardial infarction 411.81
      due to syphilis 093.89
      healed or specified as old 412
    extremities 444.22
      lower 444.22
      upper 444.21
    femoral 444.22
    hepatic 444.89
    hypophyseal 433.8 ✓5ᵗʰ
    meningeal, anterior or posterior 433.8 ✓5ᵗʰ
    mesenteric (with gangrene) 557.0
    ophthalmic (see also Occlusion, retina)
      362.30
    pontine 433.8 ✓5ᵗʰ
    popliteal 444.22
    precerebral — see Occlusion, artery,
      precerebral NEC
    pulmonary 415.19
      iatrogenic 415.11
      postoperative 415.11
    renal 593.81
    retinal (see also Occlusion, retina) 362.30
    specified site NEC 444.89
    spinal, anterior or posterior 433.8 ✓5ᵗʰ
    traumatic (complication) (early) (see also
      Injury, blood vessel, by site) 904.9
    vertebral (see also Occlusion, artery,
      vertebral) 433.2 ✓5ᵗʰ
      with other precerebral artery 433.3 ✓5ᵗʰ
  atrial (endocardial) 424.90
    due to syphilis 093.89
  auricular (see also Infarct, myocardium)
    410.9 ✓5ᵗʰ
  axillary (vein) 453.8
  basilar (artery) (see also Occlusion, artery,
    basilar) 433.0 ✓5ᵗʰ
  bland NEC 453.9
  brain (artery) (stem) 434.0 ✓5ᵗʰ
    due to syphilis 094.89
    iatrogenic 997.02
    late effect — see Late effect(s) (of)
      cerebrovascular disease
    postoperative 997.02
    puerperal, postpartum, childbirth 674.0
      ✓5ᵗʰ
    sinus (see also Thrombosis, intracranial
      venous sinus) 325
  capillary 448.9
    arteriolar, generalized 446.6
  cardiac (see also Infarct, myocardium)
    410.9 ✓5ᵗʰ
    due to syphilis 093.89
    healed or specified as old 412
    valve — see Endocarditis
  carotid (artery) (common) (internal) (see also
    Occlusion, artery, carotid) 433.1 ✓5ᵗʰ
    with other precerebral artery 433.3 ✓5ᵗʰ

Thrombosis, thrombotic — continued
  cavernous sinus (venous) — see Thrombosis,
    intracranial venous sinus
  cerebellar artery (anterior inferior) (posterior
    inferior) (superior) 433.8 ✓5ᵗʰ
    late effect — see Late effect(s) (of)
      cerebrovascular disease
  cerebral (arteries) (see also Thrombosis, brain)
    434.0 ✓5ᵗʰ
    late effect — see Late effect(s) (of)
      cerebrovascular disese
  coronary (artery) (see also Infarct,
    myocardium) 410.9 ✓5ᵗʰ
    without myocardial infarction 411.81
    due to syphilis 093.89
    healed or specified as old 412
  corpus cavernosum 607.82
  cortical (see also Thrombosis, brain) 434.0 ✓5ᵗʰ
  due to (presence of) any device, implant, or
    graft classifiable to 996.0-996.5— see
    Complications, due to (presence of) any
    device, implant, or graft classified to
    996.0-996.5 NEC
  effort 453.8
  endocardial — see Infarct, myocardium
  eye (see also Occlusion, retina) 362.30
  femoral (vein) (deep) 453.8
    with inflammation or phlebitis 451.11
    artery 444.22
  genital organ, male 608.83
  heart (chamber) (see also Infarct, myocardium)
    410.9 ✓5ᵗʰ
  hepatic (vein) 453.0
    artery 444.89
    infectional or septic 572.1
  iliac (vein) 453.8
    with inflammation or phlebitis 451.81
    artery (common) (external) (internal) 444.81
  inflammation, vein — see Thrombophlebitis
  internal carotid artery (see also Occlusion,
    artery, carotid) 433.1 ✓5ᵗʰ
    with other precerebral artery 433.3 ✓5ᵗʰ
  intestine (with gangrene) 557.0
  intracranial (see also Thrombosis, brain)
    434.0 ✓5ᵗʰ
    venous sinus (any) 325
      nonpyogenic origin 437.6
        in pregnancy or puerperium 671.5
          ✓5ᵗʰ
  intramural (see also Infarct, myocardium)
    410.9 ✓5ᵗʰ
    without
      cardiac condition 429.89
      coronary artery disease 429.89
      myocardial infarction 429.89
      healed or specified as old 412
  jugular (bulb) 453.8
  kidney 593.81
    artery 593.81
  lateral sinus (venous) — see Thrombosis,
    intracranial venous sinus
  leg 453.8
    with inflammation or phlebitis — see
      Thrombophlebitis
    deep (vessels) 453.8
    superficial (vessels) 453.8
  liver (venous) 453.0
    artery 444.89
    infectional or septic 572.1
    portal vein 452

Thrombosis, thrombotic — *continued*
   longitudinal sinus (venous) — *see* Thrombosis, intracranial venous sinus
   lower extremity — *see* Thrombosis, leg
   lung 415.19
      iatrogenic 415.11
      postoperative 415.11
   marantic, dural sinus 437.6
   meninges (brain) (*see also* Thrombosis, brain) 434.0
   mesenteric (artery) (with gangrene) 557.0
      vein (inferior) (superior) 557.0
   mitral — *see* Insufficiency, mitral
   mural (heart chamber) (*see also* Infarct, myocardium) 410.9
      without
         cardiac condition 429.89
         coronary artery disease 429.89
         myocardial infarction 429.89
      due to syphilis 093.89
      following myocardial infarction 429.79
      healed or specified as old 412
   omentum (with gangrene) 557.0
   ophthalmic (artery) (*see also* Occlusion, retina) 362.30
   pampiniform plexus (male) 608.83
      female 620.8
   parietal (*see also* Infarct, myocardium) 410.9
   penis, penile 607.82
   peripheral arteries 444.22
      lower 444.22
      upper 444.21
   platelet 446.6
   portal 452
      due to syphilis 093.89
      infectional or septic 572.1
   precerebral artery — *see also* Occlusion, artery, precerebral NEC
   pregnancy 671.9
      deep (vein) 671.3
      superficial (vein) 671.2
   puerperal, postpartum, childbirth 671.9
      brain (artery) 674.0
         venous 671.5
      cardiac 674.8
      cerebral (artery) 674.0
         venous 671.5
      deep (vein) 671.4
      intracranial sinus (nonpyogenic) (venous) 671.5
      pelvic 671.4
      pulmonary (artery) 673.2
      specified site NEC 671.5
      superficial 671.2
   pulmonary (artery) (vein) 415.19
      iatrogenic 415.11
      postoperative 415.11
   renal (artery) 593.81
      vein 453.3
   resulting from presence of shunt or other internal prosthetic device — *see* Complications, due to (presence of) any device, implant, or graft classified to 996.0-996.5 NEC
   retina, retinal (artery) 362.30
      arterial branch 362.32
      central 362.31
      partial 362.33
      vein
         central 362.35

Thrombosis, thrombotic — *continued*
   retina, retinal — *continued*
      vein — *continued*
         tributary (branch) 362.36
   scrotum 608.83
   seminal vesicle 608.83
   sigmoid (venous) sinus (*see* Thrombosis, intracranial venous sinus) 325
   silent NEC 453.9
   sinus, intracranial (venous) (any) (*see also* Thrombosis, intracranial venous sinus) 325
   softening, brain (*see also* Thrombosis, brain) 434.0
   specified site NEC 453.8
   spermatic cord 608.83
   spinal cord 336.1
      due to syphilis 094.89
      in pregnancy or puerperium 671.5
      pyogenic origin 324.1
         late effect — *see* category 326
   spleen, splenic 289.59
      artery 444.89
   testis 608.83
   traumatic (complication) (early) (*see also* Injury, blood vessel, by site) 904.9
   tricuspid — *see* Endocarditis, tricuspid
   tunica vaginalis 608.83
   umbilical cord (vessels) 663.6
      affecting fetus or newborn 762.6
   vas deferens 608.83
   vena cava (inferior) (superior) 453.2
Thrombus — *see* Thrombosis
Thrush 112.0
   newborn 771.7
Thumb — *see also* condition
   gamekeeper's 842.12
   sucking (child problem) 307.9
Thygeson's superficial punctate keratitis 370.21
Thymergasia (*see also* Psychosis, affective) 296.80
Thymitis 254.8
Thymoma (benign) (M8580/0) 212.6
   malignant (M8580/3) 164.0
Thymus, thymic (gland) — *see* condition
Thyrocele (*see also* Goiter) 240.9
Thyroglossal — *see also* condition
   cyst 759.2
   duct, persistent 759.2
Thyroid (body) (gland) — *see also* condition
   lingual 759.2
Thyroiditis 245.9
   acute (pyogenic) (suppurative) 245.0
      nonsuppurative 245.0
   autoimmune 245.2
   chronic (nonspecific) (sclerosing) 245.8
      fibrous 245.3
      lymphadenoid 245.2
      lymphocytic 245.2
      lymphoid 245.2
   complicating pregnancy, childbirth, or puerperium 648.1
   de Quervain's (subacute granulomatous) 245.1
   fibrous (chronic) 245.3
   giant (cell) (follicular) 245.1
   granulomatous (de Quervain's) (subacute) 245.1
   Hashimoto's (struma lymphomatosa) 245.2

Thyroiditis — continued
- iatrogenic 245.4
- invasive (fibrous) 245.3
- ligneous 245.3
- lymphocytic (chronic) 245.2
- lymphoid 245.2
- lymphomatous 245.2
- pseudotuberculous 245.1
- pyogenic 245.0
- radiation 245.4
- Riedel's (ligneous) 245.3
- subacute 245.1
- suppurative 245.0
- tuberculous (see also Tuberculosis) 017.5 ✓5ᵗʰ
- viral 245.1
- woody 245.3

Thyrolingual duct, persistent 759.2
Thyromegaly 240.9
Thyrotoxic
- crisis or storm (see also Thyrotoxicosis) 242.9 ✓5ᵗʰ
- heart failure (see also Thyrotoxicosis) 242.9 ✓5ᵗʰ [425.7]

Thyrotoxicosis 242.9 ✓5ᵗʰ

> Note — Use the following fifth-digit subclassification with category 242:
>
> 0   without mention of thyrotoxic crisis or storm
> 1   with mention of thyrotoxic crisis or storm

- with
    - goiter (diffuse) 242.0 ✓5ᵗʰ
        - adenomatous 242.3 ✓5ᵗʰ
            - multinodular 242.2 ✓5ᵗʰ
            - uninodular 242.1 ✓5ᵗʰ
        - nodular 242.3 ✓5ᵗʰ
            - multinodular 242.2 ✓5ᵗʰ
            - uninodular 242.1 ✓5ᵗʰ
    - infiltrative
        - dermopathy 242.0 ✓5ᵗʰ
        - ophthalmopathy 242.0 ✓5ᵗʰ
    - thyroid acropachy 242.0 ✓5ᵗʰ
- complicating pregnancy, childbirth, or puerperium 648.1 ✓5ᵗʰ
- due to
    - ectopic thyroid nodule 242.4 ✓5ᵗʰ
    - ingestion of (excessive) thyroid material 242.8 ✓5ᵗʰ
    - specified cause NEC 242.8 ✓5ᵗʰ
- factitia 242.8 ✓5ᵗʰ
- heart 242.9 ✓5ᵗʰ [425.7]
- neonatal (transient) 775.3

TIA (transient ischemic attack) 435.9
- with transient neurologic deficit 435.9
- late effect — see Late effect(s) (of) cerebrovascular disease

Tibia vara 732.4
Tic 307.20
- breathing 307.20
- child problem 307.21
- compulsive 307.22
- convulsive 307.20
- degenerative (generalized) (localized) 333.3
    - facial 351.8
- douloureux (see also Neuralgia, trigeminal) 350.1
    - atypical 350.2

Tic — continued
- habit 307.20
    - chronic (motor or vocal) 307.22
    - transient of childhood 307.21
- lid 307.20
    - transient of childhood 307.21
- motor-verbal 307.23
- occupational 300.89
- orbicularis 307.20
    - transient of childhood 307.21
- organic origin 333.3
- postchoreic — see Chorea
- psychogenic 307.20
    - compulsive 307.22
- salaam 781.0
- spasm 307.20
    - chronic (motor or vocal) 307.22
    - transient of childhood 307.21

Tick (-borne) fever NEC 066.1
- American mountain 066.1
- Colorado 066.1
- hemorrhagic NEC 065.3
    - Crimean 065.0
    - Kyasanur Forest 065.2
    - Omsk 065.1
- mountain 066.1
- nonexanthematous 066.1

Tick-bite fever NEC 066.1
- African 087.1
- Colorado (virus) 066.1
- Rocky Mountain 082.0

Tick paralysis 989.5
Tics and spasms, compulsive 307.22
Tietze's disease or syndrome 733.6
Tight, tightness
- anus 564.89
- chest 786.59
- fascia (lata) 728.9
- foreskin (congenital) 605
- hymen 623.3
- introitus (acquired) (congenital) 623.3
- rectal sphincter 564.89
- tendon 727.81
    - Achilles (heel) 727.81
- urethral sphincter 598.9

Tilting vertebra 737.9
Timidity, child 313.21
Tinea (intersecta) (tarsi) 110.9
- amiantacea 110.0
- asbestina 110.0
- barbae 110.0
- beard 110.0
- black dot 110.0
- blanca 111.2
- capitis 110.0
- corporis 110.5
- cruris 110.3
- decalvans 704.09
- flava 111.0
- foot 110.4
- furfuracea 111.0
- imbricata (Tokelau) 110.5
- lepothrix 039.0
- manuum 110.2
- microsporic (see also Dermatophytosis) 110.9
- nigra 111.1
- nodosa 111.2
- pedis 110.4
- scalp 110.0
- specified site NEC 110.8

Tinea — *continued*
  sycosis 110.0
  tonsurans 110.0
  trichophytic (*see also* Dermatophytosis) 110.9
  unguium 110.1
  versicolor 111.0
Tingling sensation (*see also* Disturbance, sensation) 782.0
Tin-miners' lung 503
Tinnitus (aurium) 388.30
  audible 388.32
  objective 388.32
  subjective 388.31
Tipping pelvis 738.6
  with disproportion (fetopelvic) 653.0 ✓5ᵗʰ
    affecting fetus or newborn 763.1
    causing obstructed labor 660.1 ✓5ᵗʰ
      affecting fetus or newborn 763.1
Tiredness 780.79
Tissue — *see* condition
Tobacco
  abuse (affecting health) NEC (*see also* Abuse, drugs, nondependent) 305.1
  heart 989.8 ✓5ᵗʰ
Tobias' syndrome (carcinoma, pulmonary apex) (M8010/3) 162.3
Tocopherol deficiency 269.1
Todd's
  cirrhosis — *see* Cirrhosis, biliary
  paralysis (postepileptic transitory paralysis) 344.8 ✓5ᵗʰ
Toe — *see* condition
Toilet, artificial opening (*see also* Attention to, artificial, opening) V55.9
Tokelau ringworm 110.5
Tollwut 071
Tolosa-Hunt syndrome 378.55
Tommaselli's disease
  correct substance properly administered 599.7
  overdose or wrong substance given or taken 961.4
Tongue — *see also* condition
  worms 134.1
Tongue tie 750.0
Toni-Fanconi syndrome (cystinosis) 270.0
Tonic pupil 379.46
Tonsil — *see* condition
Tonsillitis (acute) (catarrhal) (croupous) (follicular) (gangrenous) (infective) (lacunar) (lingual) (malignant) (membranous) (phlegmonous) (pneumococcal) (pseudomembranous) (purulent) (septic) (staphylococcal) (subacute) (suppurative) (toxic) (ulcerative) (vesicular) (viral) 463
  with influenza, flu, or grippe 487.1
  chronic 474.00
  diphtheritic (membranous) 032.0
  hypertrophic 474.00
  influenzal 487.1
  parenchymatous 475
  streptococcal 034.0
  tuberculous (*see also* Tuberculosis) 012.8 ✓5ᵗʰ
  Vincent's 101
Tonsillopharyngitis 465.8
Tooth, teeth — *see* condition
Toothache 525.9
Topagnosis 782.0

Tophi (gouty) 274.0
  ear 274.81
  heart 274.82
  specified site NEC 274.82
Torn — *see* Tear, torn
Tornwaldt's bursitis (disease) (pharyngeal bursitis) 478.29
  cyst 478.26
Torpid liver 573.9
Torsion
  accessory tube 620.5
  adnexa (female) 620.5
  aorta (congenital) 747.29
    acquired 447.1
  appendix epididymis 608.2
  bile duct 576.8
    with calculus, choledocholithiasis or stones — *see* Choledocholithiasis
    congenital 751.69
  bowel, colon, or intestine 560.2
  cervix (*see also* Malposition, uterus) 621.6
  duodenum 537.3
  dystonia — *see* Dystonia, torsion
  epididymis 608.2
    appendix 608.2
  fallopian tube 620.5
  gallbladder (*see also* Disease, gallbladder) 575.8
    congenital 751.69
  gastric 537.89
  hydatid of Morgagni (female) 620.5
  kidney (pedicle) 593.89
  Meckel's diverticulum (congenital) 751.0
  mesentery 560.2
  omentum 560.2
  organ or site, congenital NEC — *see* Anomaly, specified type NEC
  ovary (pedicle) 620.5
    congenital 752.0
  oviduct 620.5
  penis 607.89
    congenital 752.69
  renal 593.89
  spasm — *see* Dystonia, torsion
  spermatic cord 608.2
  spleen 289.59
  testicle, testis 608.2
  tibia 736.89
  umbilical cord — *see* Compression, umbilical cord
  uterus (*see also* Malposition, uterus) 621.6
Torticollis (intermittent) (spastic) 723.5
  congenital 754.1
    sternomastoid 754.1
  due to birth injury 767.8
  hysterical 300.11
  ocular 781.93
  psychogenic 306.0
    specified as conversion reaction 300.11
  rheumatic 723.5
  rheumatoid 714.0
  spasmodic 333.83
  traumatic, current NEC 847.0
Tortuous
  artery 447.1
  fallopian tube 752.19
  organ or site, congenital NEC — *see* Distortion
  renal vessel, congenital 747.62
  retina vessel (congenital) 743.58
    acquired 362.17

Tortuous — *continued*
  ureter 593.4
  urethra 599.84
  vein — *see* Varicose, vein
Torula, torular (infection) 117.5
  histolytica 117.5
  lung 117.5
Torulosis 117.5
Torus
  fracture
    fibula 823.41
      with tibia 823.42
    radius 813.45
    tibia 823.40
      with fibula 823.42
  mandibularis 526.81
  palatinus 526.81
Touch, vitreous 997.99
Touraine's syndrome (hereditary osteo-onychodysplasia) 756.89
Touraine-Solente-Golé syndrome (acropachyderma) 757.39
Tourette's disease (motor-verbal tic) 307.23
Tower skull 756.0
  with exophthalmos 756.0
Toxemia 799.8
  with
    abortion — *see* Abortion, by type, with toxemia
  bacterial — *see* Septicemia
  biliary (*see also* Disease, biliary) 576.8
  burn — *see* Burn, by site
  congenital NEC 779.89
  eclamptic 642.6
    with pre-existing hypertension 642.7
  erysipelatous (*see also* Erysipelas) 035
  fatigue 799.8
  fetus or newborn NEC 779.89
  food (*see also* Poisoning, food) 005.9
  gastric 537.89
  gastrointestinal 558.2
  intestinal 558.2
  kidney (*see also* Disease, renal) 593.9
  lung 518.89
  malarial NEC (*see also* Malaria) 084.6
  maternal (of pregnancy), affecting fetus or newborn 760.0
  myocardial — *see* Myocarditis, toxic
  of pregnancy (mild) (pre-eclamptic) 642.4
    with
      convulsions 642.6
      pre-existing hypertension 642.7
    affecting fetus or newborn 760.0
    severe 642.5
  pre-eclamptic — *see* Toxemia, of pregnancy
  puerperal, postpartum — *see* Toxemia, of pregnancy
  pulmonary 518.89
  renal (*see also* Disease, renal) 593.9
  septic (*see also* Septicemia) 038.9
  small intestine 558.2
  staphylococcal 038.10
    aureus 038.11
    due to food 005.0
    specified organism NEC 038.19
  stasis 799.8
  stomach 537.89
  uremic (*see also* Uremia) 586
  urinary 586

Toxemica cerebropathia psychica (nonalcoholic) 294.0
  alcoholic 291.1
Toxic (poisoning) — *see also* condition
  from drug or poison — *see* Table of Drugs and Chemicals
  oil syndrome 710.5
  shock syndrome 040.82
  thyroid (gland) (*see also* Thyrotoxicosis) 242.9
Toxicemia — *see* Toxemia
Toxicity
  dilantin
    asymptomatic 796.0
    symptomatic — *see* Table of Drugs and Chemicals
  drug
    asymptomatic 796.0
    symptomatic — *see* Table of Drugs and Chemicals
  fava bean 282.2
  from drug or poison
    asymptomatic 796.0
    symptomatic — *see* Table of Drugs and Chemicals
Toxicosis (*see also* Toxemia) 799.8
  capillary, hemorrhagic 287.0
Toxinfection 799.8
  gastrointestinal 558.2
Toxocariasis 128.0
Toxoplasma infection, generalized 130.9
Toxoplasmosis (acquired) 130.9
  with pneumonia 130.4
  congenital, active 771.2
  disseminated (multisystemic) 130.8
  maternal
    with suspected damage to fetus affecting management of pregnancy 655.4
    affecting fetus or newborn 760.2
      manifest toxoplasmosis in fetus or newborn 771.2
  multiple sites 130.8
  multisystemic disseminated 130.8
  specified site NEC 130.7
Trabeculation, bladder 596.8
Trachea — *see* condition
Tracheitis (acute) (catarrhal) (infantile) (membranous) (plastic) (pneumococcal) (septic) (suppurative) (viral) 464.10
  with
    bronchitis 490
      acute or subacute 466.0
      chronic 491.8
      tuberculosis — *see* Tuberculosis, pulmonary
    laryngitis (acute) 464.20
      with obstruction 464.21
      chronic 476.1
      tuberculous (*see also* Tuberculosis, larynx) 012.3
    obstruction 464.11
  chronic 491.8
    with
      bronchitis (chronic) 491.8
      laryngitis (chronic) 476.1
      due to external agent — *see* Condition, respiratory, chronic, due to

Tracheitis — *continued*
  diphtheritic (membranous) 032.3
    due to external agent — *see* Inflammation, respiratory, upper, due to
  edematous 464.11
  influenzal 487.1
  streptococcal 034.0
  syphilitic 095.8
  tuberculous (*see also* Tuberculosis) 012.8 ✓5ᵗʰ
Trachelitis (nonvenereal) (*see also* Cervicitis) 616.0
  trichomonal 131.09
Tracheobronchial — *see* condition
Tracheobronchitis (*see also* Bronchitis) 490
  acute or subacute 466.0
    with bronchospasm or obstruction 466.0
  chronic 491.8
  influenzal 487.1
  senile 491.8
Tracheobronchomegaly (congenital) 748.3
Tracheobronchopneumonitis — *see* Pneumonia, broncho
Tracheocele (external) (internal) 519.1
  congenital 748.3
Tracheomalacia 519.1
  congenital 748.3
Tracheopharyngitis (acute) 465.8
  chronic 478.9
    due to external agent — *see* Condition, respiratory, chronic, due to
    due to external agent — *see* Inflammation, respiratory, upper, due to
Tracheostenosis 519.1
  congenital 748.3
Tracheostomy
  attention to V55.0
  complication 519.00
  hemorrhage 519.09
  infection 519.01
  malfunctioning 519.02
  obstruction 519.09
  sepsis 519.01
  status V44.0
  stenosis 519.02
Trachoma, trachomatous 076.9
  active (stage) 076.1
  contraction of conjunctiva 076.1
  dubium 076.0
  healed or late effect 139.1
  initial (stage) 076.0
  Türck's (chronic catarrhal laryngitis) 476.0
Trachyphonia 784.49
Training
  orthoptic V57.4
  orthotic V57.81
Train sickness 994.6
Trait
  hemoglobin
    abnormal NEC 282.7
      with thalassemia 282.4
    C (*see also* Disease, hemoglobin, C) 282.7
      with elliptocytosis 282.7
    S (Hb-S) 282.5
  Lepore 282.4
    with other abnormal hemoglobin NEC 282.4
  paranoid 301.0

Trait — *continued*
  sickle-cell 282.5
    with
      elliptocytosis 282.5
      spherocytosis 282.5
Traits, paranoid 301.0
Tramp V60.0
Trance 780.09
  hysterical 300.13
Transaminasemia 790.4
Transfusion, blood
  donor V59.01
    stem cells V59.02
  incompatible 999.6
  reaction or complication — *see* Complications, transfusion
  syndrome
    fetomaternal 772.0
    twin-to-twin
      blood loss (donor twin) 772.0
      recipient twin 776.4
  without reported diagnosis V58.2
Transient — *see also* condition
  alteration of awareness 780.02
  blindness 368.12
  deafness (ischemic) 388.02
  global amnesia 437.7
  person (homeless) NEC V60.0
Transitional, lumbosacral joint of vertebra 756.19
Translocation
  autosomes NEC 758.5
    13-15 758.1
    16-18 758.2
    21 or 22 758.0
    balanced in normal individual 758.4
    D_1 758.1
    E_3 758.2
    G 758.0
  balanced autosomal in normal individual 758.4
  chromosomes NEC 758.89
  Down's syndrome 758.0
Translucency, iris 364.53
Transmission of chemical substances through the placenta (affecting fetus or newborn) 760.70
  alcohol 760.71
  anti-infective agents 760.74
  cocaine 760.75
  "crack" 760.75
  diethylstilbestrol [DES] 760.76
  hallucinogenic agents 760.73
  medicinal agents NEC 760.79
  narcotics 760.72
  obstetric anesthetic or analgesic drug 763.5
  specified agent NEC 760.79
  suspected, affecting management of pregnancy 655.5 ✓5ᵗʰ
Transplant(ed)
  bone V42.4
    marrow V42.81
  complication — *see also* Complications, due to (presence of) any device, implant, or graft classified to 996.0-996.5 NEC
    bone marrow 996.85
    corneal graft NEC 996.79
      infection or inflammation 996.69
      reaction 996.51

Transplant(ed) — *continued*
  complication — *continued*
    corneal graft NEC — *continued*
      rejection 996.51
    organ (failure) (immune or nonimmune cause) (infection) (rejection) 996.87
      bone marrow 996.85
      heart 996.83
      intestines 996.87
      kidney 996.81
      liver 996.82
      lung 996.84
      pancreas 996.86
      specified NEC 996.89
    skin NEC 996.79
      infection or inflammation 996.69
      rejection 996.52
        artificial 996.55
        decellularized allodermis 996.55
  cornea V42.5
  hair V50.0
  heart V42.1
    valve V42.2
  intestine V42.84
  kidney V42.0
  liver V42.7
  lung V42.6
  organ V42.9
    specified NEC V42.89
  pancreas V42.83
  peripheral stem cells V42.82
  skin V42.3
  stem cells, peripheral V42.82
  tissue V42.9
    specified NEC V42.89
Transplants, ovarian, endometrial 617.1
Transposed — *see* Transposition
Transposition (congenital) — *see also* Malposition, congenital
  abdominal viscera 759.3
  aorta (dextra) 745.11
  appendix 751.5
  arterial trunk 745.10
  colon 751.5
  great vessels (complete) 745.10
    both originating from right ventricle 745.11
    corrected 745.12
    double outlet right ventricle 745.11
    incomplete 745.11
    partial 745.11
    specified type NEC 745.19
  heart 746.87
    with complete transposition of viscera 759.3
  intestine (large) (small) 751.5
  pulmonary veins 747.49
  reversed jejunal (for bypass) (status) V45.3
  stomach 750.7
    with general transposition of viscera 759.3
  teeth, tooth 524.3
  vessels (complete) 745.10
    partial 745.11
  viscera (abdominal) (thoracic) 759.3
Trans-sexualism 302.50
  with
    asexual history 302.51
    heterosexual history 302.53
    homosexual history 302.52
Transverse — *see also* condition
  arrest (deep), in labor 660.3
    affecting fetus or newborn 763.1

Transverse — *continued*
  lie 652.3
    before labor, affecting fetus or newborn 761.7
    causing obstructed labor 660.0
      affecting fetus or newborn 763.1
    during labor, affecting fetus or newborn 763.1
Transvestism, transvestitism (transvestic fetishism) 302.3
Trapped placenta (with hemorrhage) 666.0
  without hemorrhage 667.0
Trauma, traumatism (*see also* Injury, by site) 959.9
  birth — *see* Birth, injury NEC
  causing hemorrhage of pregnancy or delivery 641.8
  complicating
    abortion — *see* Abortion, by type, with damage to pelvic organs
    ectopic pregnancy (*see also* categories 633.0-633.9) 639.2
    molar pregnancy (*see also* categories 630-632) 639.2
  during delivery NEC 665.9
  following
    abortion 639.2
    ectopic or molar pregnancy 639.2
  maternal, during pregnancy, affecting fetus or newborn 760.5
  neuroma — *see* Injury, nerve, by site
  previous major, affecting management of pregnancy, childbirth, or puerperium V23.8
  psychic (current) — *see also* Reaction, adjustment
    previous (history) V15.49
  psychologic, previous (affecting health) V15.49
  transient paralysis — *see* Injury, nerve, by site
Traumatic — *see* condition
Treacher Collins' syndrome (incomplete facial dysostosis) 756.0
Treitz's hernia — *see* Hernia, Treitz's
Trematode infestation NEC 121.9
Trematodiasis NEC 121.9
Trembles 988.8
Trembling paralysis (*see also* Parkinsonism) 332.0
Tremor 781.0
  essential (benign) 333.1
  familial 333.1
  flapping (liver) 572.8
  hereditary 333.1
  hysterical 300.11
  intention 333.1
  mercurial 985.0
  muscle 728.85
  Parkinson's (*see also* Parkinsonism) 332.0
  psychogenic 306.0
    specified as conversion reaction 300.11
  senilis 797
  specified type NEC 333.1
Trench
  fever 083.1
  foot 991.4
  mouth 101
  nephritis — *see* Nephritis, acute
Treponema pallidum infection (*see also* Syphilis) 097.9

Treponematosis 102.9
- due to
  - T. pallidum — see Syphilis
  - T. pertenue (yaws) (see also Yaws) 102.9

Triad
- Kartagener's 759.3
- Reiter's (complete) (incomplete) 099.3
- Saint's (see also Hernia, diaphragm) 553.3

Trichiasis 704.2
- cicatricial 704.2
- eyelid 374.05
  - with entropion (see also Entropion) 374.00

Trichinella spiralis (infection) (infestation) 124
Trichinelliasis 124
Trichinellosis 124
Trichiniasis 124
Trichinosis 124
Trichobezoar 938
- intestine 936
- stomach 935.2

Trichocephaliasis 127.3
Trichocephalosis 127.3
Trichocephalus infestation 127.3
Trichoclasis 704.2
Trichoepithelioma (M8100/0) — see also Neoplasm, skin, benign
- breast 217
- genital organ NEC — see Neoplasm, by site, benign
- malignant (M8100/3) — see Neoplasm, skin, malignant

Trichofolliculoma (M8101/0) — see Neoplasm, skin, benign
Tricholemmoma (M8102/0) — see Neoplasm, skin, benign
Trichomatosis 704.2
Trichomoniasis 131.9
- bladder 131.09
- cervix 131.09
- intestinal 007.3
- prostate 131.03
- seminal vesicle 131.09
- specified site NEC 131.8
- urethra 131.02
- urogenitalis 131.00
- vagina 131.01
- vulva 131.01
- vulvovaginal 131.01

Trichomycosis 039.0
- axillaris 039.0
- nodosa 111.2
- nodularis 111.2
- rubra 039.0

Trichonocardiosis (axillaris) (palmellina) 039.0
Trichonodosis 704.2
Trichophytid, trichophyton infection (see also Dermatophytosis) 110.9
Trichophytide — see Dermatophytosis
Trichophytobezoar 938
- intestine 936
- stomach 935.2

Trichophytosis — see Dermatophytosis
Trichoptilosis 704.2
Trichorrhexis (nodosa) 704.2
Trichosporosis nodosa 111.2
Trichostasis spinulosa (congenital) 757.4
Trichostrongyliasis (small intestine) 127.6

Trichostrongylosis 127.6
Trichostrongylus (instabilis) infection 127.6
Trichotillomania 312.39
Trichromat, anomalous (congenital) 368.59
Trichromatopsia, anomalous (congenital) 368.59
Trichuriasis 127.3
Trichuris trichiuria (any site) (infection) (infestation) 127.3
Tricuspid (valve) — see condition
Trifid — see also Accessory
- kidney (pelvis) 753.3
- tongue 750.13

Trigeminal neuralgia (see also Neuralgia, trigeminal) 350.1
Trigeminoencephaloangiomatosis 759.6
Trigeminy 427.89
- postoperative 997.1

Trigger finger (acquired) 727.03
- congenital 756.89

Trigonitis (bladder) (chronic) (pseudomembranous) 595.3
- tuberculous (see also Tuberculosis) 016.1

Trigonocephaly 756.0
Trihexosidosis 272.7
Trilobate placenta — see Placenta, abnormal
Trilocular heart 745.8
Tripartita placenta — see Placenta, abnormal
Triple — see also Accessory
- kidneys 753.3
- uteri 752.2
- X female 758.81

Triplegia 344.89
- congenital or infantile 343.8

Triplet
- affected by maternal complications of pregnancy 761.5
- healthy liveborn — see Newborn, multiple
- pregnancy (complicating delivery) NEC 651.1
  - with fetal loss and retention of one or more fetus(es) 651.4

Triplex placenta — see Placenta, abnormal
Triplication — see Accessory
Trismus 781.0
- neonatorum 771.3
- newborn 771.3

Trisomy (syndrome) NEC 758.5
- 13 (partial) 758.1
- 16-18 758.2
- 18 (partial) 758.2
- 21 (partial) 758.0
- 22 758.0
- autosomes NEC 758.5
- D_1 758.1
- E_3 758.2
- G (group) 758.0
- group D_1 758.1
- group E 758.2
- group G 758.0

Tritanomaly 368.53
Tritanopia 368.53
Troisier-Hanot-Chauffard syndrome (bronze diabetes) 275.0
Trombidiosis 133.8

Trophedema (hereditary) 757.0
  congenital 757.0
Trophoblastic disease (see also Hydatidiform mole) 630
  previous, affecting management of pregnancy V23.1
Tropholymphedema 757.0
Trophoneurosis NEC 356.9
  arm NEC 354.9
  disseminated 710.1
  facial 349.89
  leg NEC 355.8
  lower extremity NEC 355.8
  upper extremity NEC 354.9
Tropical — see also condition
  maceration feet (syndrome) 991.4
  wet foot (syndrome) 991.4
Trouble — see also Disease
  bowel 569.9
  heart — see Disease, heart
  intestine 569.9
  kidney (see also Disease, renal) 593.9
  nervous 799.2
  sinus (see also Sinusitis) 473.9
Trousseau's syndrome (thrombophlebitis migrans) 453.1
Truancy, childhood — see also Disturbance, conduct
  socialized 312.2 ✓5ᵗʰ
  undersocialized, unsocialized 312.1 ✓5ᵗʰ
Truncus
  arteriosus (persistent) 745.0
  common 745.0
  communis 745.0
Trunk — see condition
Trychophytide — see Dermatophytosis
Trypanosoma infestation — see Trypanosomiasis
Trypanosomiasis 086.9
  with meningoencephalitis 086.9 [323.2]
  African 086.5
    due to Trypanosoma 086.5
      gambiense 086.3
      rhodesiense 086.4
  American 086.2
    with
      heart involvement 086.0
      other organ involvement 086.1
    without mention of organ involvement 086.2
  Brazilian — see Trypanosomiasis, American
  Chagas' — see Trypanosomiasis, American
  due to Trypanosoma
    cruzi — see Trypanosomiasis, American
    gambiense 086.3
    rhodesiense 086.4
  gambiensis, Gambian 086.3
  North American — see Trypanosomiasis, American
  rhodesiensis, Rhodesian 086.4
  South American — see Trypanosomiasis, American
T-shaped incisors 520.2
Tsutsugamushi fever 081.2
Tube, tubal, tubular — see also condition
  ligation, admission for V25.2
Tubercle — see also Tuberculosis
  brain, solitary 013.2 ✓5ᵗʰ
  Darwin's 744.29

Tubercle — continued
  epithelioid noncaseating 135
  Ghon, primary infection 010.0 ✓5ᵗʰ
Tuberculid, tuberculide (indurating) (lichenoid) (miliary) (papulonecrotic) (primary) (skin) (subcutaneous) (see also Tuberculosis) 017.0 ✓5ᵗʰ
Tuberculoma — see also Tuberculosis
  brain (any part) 013.2 ✓5ᵗʰ
  meninges (cerebral) (spinal) 013.1 ✓5ᵗʰ
  spinal cord 013.4 ✓5ᵗʰ
Tuberculosis, tubercular, tuberculous (calcification) (calcified) (caseous) (chromogenic acid-fast bacilli) (congenital) (degeneration) (disease) (fibrocaseous) (fistula) (gangrene) (interstitial) (isolated circumscribed lesions) (necrosis) (parenchymatous) (ulcerative) 011.9

> Note — Use the following fifth-digit subclassification with categories 010-018:
>
> 0 unspecified
> 1 bacteriological or histological examination not done
> 2 bacteriological or histological examination unknown (at present)
> 3 tubercle bacilli found (in sputum) by microscopy
> 4 tubercle bacilli not found (in sputum) by microscopy, but found by bacterial culture
> 5 tubercle bacilli not found by bacteriological exam-ination, but tuberculosis confirmed histologically
> 6 tubercle bacilli not found by bacteriological or histological examination, but tuberculosis confirmed by other methods [inoculation of animals]
>
> For tuberculous conditions specified as late effects or sequelae, see category 137.

  abdomen 014.8 ✓5ᵗʰ
    lymph gland 014.8 ✓5ᵗʰ
  abscess 011.9 ✓5ᵗʰ
    arm 017.9 ✓5ᵗʰ
    bone (see also Osteomyelitis, due to, tuberculosis) 015.9 ✓5ᵗʰ [730.8] ✓5ᵗʰ
      hip 015.1 ✓5ᵗʰ [730.85]
      knee 015.2 ✓5ᵗʰ [730.96]
      sacrum 015.7 ✓5ᵗʰ [730.88]
      specified site NEC 015.7 ✓5ᵗʰ [730.88]
      spinal 015.0 ✓5ᵗʰ [730.88]
      vertebra 015.0 ✓5ᵗʰ [730.88]
    brain 013.3 ✓5ᵗʰ
    breast 017.9 ✓5ᵗʰ
    Cowper's gland 016.5 ✓5ᵗʰ
    dura (mater) 013.8 ✓5ᵗʰ
      brain 013.3 ✓5ᵗʰ
      spinal cord 013.5 ✓5ᵗʰ
    epidural 013.8 ✓5ᵗʰ
      brain 013.3 ✓5ᵗʰ
      spinal cord 013.5 ✓5ᵗʰ
    frontal sinus — see Tuberculosis, sinus
    genital organs NEC 016.9 ✓5ᵗʰ
      female 016.7 ✓5ᵗʰ
      male 016.5 ✓5ᵗʰ
    genitourinary NEC 016.9 ✓5ᵗʰ

Index to Diseases

Tuberculosis, tubercular, tuberculous

Tuberculosis, tubercular, tuberculous — *continued*
- abscess — *continued*
  - gland (lymphatic) — *see* Tuberculosis, lymph gland
  - hip 015.1 ✓5ᵗʰ
  - iliopsoas 015.0 ✓5ᵗʰ *[730.88]*
  - intestine 014.8 ✓5ᵗʰ
  - ischiorectal 014.8 ✓5ᵗʰ
  - joint 015.9 ✓5ᵗʰ
    - hip 015.1 ✓5ᵗʰ
    - knee 015.2 ✓5ᵗʰ
    - specified joint NEC 015.8 ✓5ᵗʰ
    - vertebral 015.0 ✓5ᵗʰ *[730.88]*
  - kidney 016.0 ✓5ᵗʰ *[590.81]*
  - knee 015.2 ✓5ᵗʰ
  - lumbar 015.0 ✓5ᵗʰ *[730.88]*
  - lung 011.2 ✓5ᵗʰ
    - primary, progressive 010.8 ✓5ᵗʰ
  - meninges (cerebral) (spinal) 013.0 ✓5ᵗʰ
  - pelvic 016.9 ✓5ᵗʰ
    - female 016.7 ✓5ᵗʰ
    - male 016.5 ✓5ᵗʰ
  - perianal 014.8 ✓5ᵗʰ
    - fistula 014.8 ✓5ᵗʰ
  - perinephritic 016.0 ✓5ᵗʰ *[590.81]*
  - perineum 017.9 ✓5ᵗʰ
  - perirectal 014.8 ✓5ᵗʰ
  - psoas 015.0 ✓5ᵗʰ *[730.88]*
  - rectum 014.8 ✓5ᵗʰ
  - retropharyngeal 012.8 ✓5ᵗʰ
  - sacrum 015.0 ✓5ᵗʰ *[730.88]*
  - scrofulous 017.2 ✓5ᵗʰ
  - scrotum 016.5 ✓5ᵗʰ
  - skin 017.0 ✓5ᵗʰ
    - primary 017.0 ✓5ᵗʰ
  - spinal cord 013.5 ✓5ᵗʰ
  - spine or vertebra (column) 015.0 ✓5ᵗʰ *[730.88]*
  - strumous 017.2 ✓5ᵗʰ
  - subdiaphragmatic 014.8 ✓5ᵗʰ
  - testis 016.5 ✓5ᵗʰ
  - thigh 017.9 ✓5ᵗʰ
  - urinary 016.3 ✓5ᵗʰ
    - kidney 016.0 ✓5ᵗʰ *[590.81]*
  - uterus 016.7 ✓5ᵗʰ
- accessory sinus — *see* Tuberculosis, sinus
- Addison's disease 017.6 ✓5ᵗʰ
- adenitis (*see also* Tuberculosis, lymph gland) 017.2 ✓5ᵗʰ
- adenoids 012.8 ✓5ᵗʰ
- adenopathy (*see also* Tuberculosis, lymph gland) 017.2 ✓5ᵗʰ
  - tracheobronchial 012.1 ✓5ᵗʰ
    - primary progressive 010.8 ✓5ᵗʰ
- adherent pericardium 017.9 ✓5ᵗʰ *[420.0]*
- adnexa (uteri) 016.7 ✓5ᵗʰ
- adrenal (capsule) (gland) 017.6 ✓5ᵗʰ
- air passage NEC 012.8 ✓5ᵗʰ
- alimentary canal 014.8 ✓5ᵗʰ
- anemia 017.9 ✓5ᵗʰ
- ankle (joint) 015.8 ✓5ᵗʰ
  - bone 015.5 ✓5ᵗʰ *[730.87]*
- anus 014.8 ✓5ᵗʰ
- apex (*see also* Tuberculosis, pulmonary) 011.9 ✓5ᵗʰ
- apical (*see also* Tuberculosis, pulmonary) 011.9 ✓5ᵗʰ
- appendicitis 014.8 ✓5ᵗʰ
- appendix 014.8 ✓5ᵗʰ
- arachnoid 013.0 ✓5ᵗʰ

Tuberculosis, tubercular, tuberculous — *continued*
- artery 017.9 ✓5ᵗʰ
- arthritis (chronic) (synovial) 015.9 ✓5ᵗʰ *[711.40]*
  - ankle 015.8 ✓5ᵗʰ *[730.87]*
  - hip 015.1 ✓5ᵗʰ *[711.45]*
  - knee 015.2 ✓5ᵗʰ *[711.46]*
  - specified site NEC 015.8 ✓5ᵗʰ *[711.48]*
  - spine or vertebra (column) 015.0 ✓5ᵗʰ *[720.81]*
  - wrist 015.8 ✓5ᵗʰ *[730.83]*
- articular — *see* Tuberculosis, joint
- ascites 014.0 ✓5ᵗʰ
- asthma (*see also* Tuberculosis, pulmonary) 011.9 ✓5ᵗʰ
- axilla, axillary 017.2 ✓5ᵗʰ
  - gland 017.2 ✓5ᵗʰ
- bilateral (*see also* Tuberculosis, pulmonary) 011.9 ✓5ᵗʰ
- bladder 016.1 ✓5ᵗʰ
- bone (*see also* Osteomyelitis, due to, tuberculosis) 015.9 ✓5ᵗʰ *[730.8]* ✓5ᵗʰ
  - hip 015.1 ✓5ᵗʰ *[730.85]*
  - knee 015.2 ✓5ᵗʰ *[730.86]*
  - limb NEC 015.5 ✓5ᵗʰ *[730.88]*
  - sacrum 015.0 ✓5ᵗʰ *[730.88]*
  - specified site NEC 015.7 ✓5ᵗʰ *[730.88]*
  - spinal or vertebral column 015.0 ✓5ᵗʰ *[730.88]*
- bowel 014.8 ✓5ᵗʰ
  - miliary 018.9 ✓5ᵗʰ
- brain 013.2 ✓5ᵗʰ
- breast 017.9 ✓5ᵗʰ
- broad ligament 016.7 ✓5ᵗʰ
- bronchi, bronchial, bronchus 011.3 ✓5ᵗʰ
  - ectasia, ectasis 011.5 ✓5ᵗʰ
  - fistula 011.3 ✓5ᵗʰ
    - primary, progressive 010.8 ✓5ᵗʰ
  - gland 012.1 ✓5ᵗʰ
    - primary, progressive 010.8 ✓5ᵗʰ
    - isolated 012.2 ✓5ᵗʰ
  - lymph gland or node 012.1 ✓5ᵗʰ
    - primary, progressive 010.8 ✓5ᵗʰ
- bronchiectasis 011.5 ✓5ᵗʰ
- bronchitis 011.3 ✓5ᵗʰ
- bronchopleural 012.0 ✓5ᵗʰ
- bronchopneumonia, bronchopneumonic 011.6 ✓5ᵗʰ
- bronchorrhagia 011.3 ✓5ᵗʰ
- bronchotracheal 011.3 ✓5ᵗʰ
  - isolated 012.2 ✓5ᵗʰ
- bronchus — *see* Tuberculosis, bronchi
- bronze disease (Addison's) 017.6 ✓5ᵗʰ
- buccal cavity 017.9 ✓5ᵗʰ
- bulbourethral gland 016.5 ✓5ᵗʰ
- bursa (*see also* Tuberculosis, joint) 015.9 ✓5ᵗʰ
- cachexia NEC (*see also* Tuberculosis, pulmonary) 011.9 ✓5ᵗʰ
- cardiomyopathy 017.9 ✓5ᵗʰ *[425.8]*
- caries (*see also* Tuberculosis, bone) 015.9 ✓5ᵗʰ *[730.8]* ✓5ᵗʰ
- cartilage (*see also* Tuberculosis, bone) 015.9 ✓5ᵗʰ *[730.8]* ✓5ᵗʰ
  - intervertebral 015.0 ✓5ᵗʰ *[730.88]*
- catarrhal (*see also* Tuberculosis, pulmonary) 011.9 ✓5ᵗʰ
- cecum 014.8 ✓5ᵗʰ
- cellular tissue (primary) 017.0 ✓5ᵗʰ
- cellulitis (primary) 017.0 ✓5ᵗʰ
- central nervous system 013.9 ✓5ᵗʰ
  - specified site NEC 013.8 ✓5ᵗʰ

Tuberculosis, tubercular, tuberculous — *continued*
- cerebellum (current) 013.2 ✓5ᵗʰ
- cerebral (current) 013.2 ✓5ᵗʰ
  - meninges 013.0 ✓5ᵗʰ
- cerebrospinal 013.6 ✓5ᵗʰ
  - meninges 013.0 ✓5ᵗʰ
- cerebrum (current) 013.2 ✓5ᵗʰ
- cervical 017.2 ✓5ᵗʰ
  - gland 017.2 ✓5ᵗʰ
  - lymph nodes 017.2 ✓5ᵗʰ
- cervicitis (uteri) 016.7 ✓5ᵗʰ
- cervix 016.7 ✓5ᵗʰ
- chest (*see also* Tuberculosis, pulmonary) 011.9 ✓5ᵗʰ
- childhood type or first infection 010.0 ✓5ᵗʰ
- choroid 017.3 ✓5ᵗʰ [363.13]
- choroiditis 017.3 ✓5ᵗʰ [363.13]
- ciliary body 017.3 ✓5ᵗʰ [364.11]
- colitis 014.8 ✓5ᵗʰ
- colliers' 011.4 ✓5ᵗʰ
- colliquativa (primary) 017.0 ✓5ᵗʰ
- colon 014.8 ✓5ᵗʰ
  - ulceration 014.8 ✓5ᵗʰ
- complex, primary 010.0 ✓5ᵗʰ
- complicating pregnancy, childbirth, or puerperium 647.3 ✓5ᵗʰ
  - affecting fetus or newborn 760.2
- congenital 771.2
- conjunctiva 017.3 ✓5ᵗʰ [370.31]
- connective tissue 017.9 ✓5ᵗʰ
  - bone — *see* Tuberculosis, bone
- contact V01.1
- converter (tuberculin test) (without disease) 795.5
- cornea (ulcer) 017.3 ✓5ᵗʰ [370.31]
- Cowper's gland 016.5 ✓5ᵗʰ
- coxae 015.1 ✓5ᵗʰ [730.85]
- coxalgia 015.1 ✓5ᵗʰ [730.85]
- cul-de-sac of Douglas 014.8 ✓5ᵗʰ
- curvature, spine 015.0 ✓5ᵗʰ [737.40]
- cutis (colliquativa) (primary) 017.0 ✓5ᵗʰ
- cyst, ovary 016.6 ✓5ᵗʰ
- cystitis 016.1 ✓5ᵗʰ
- dacryocystitis 017.3 ✓5ᵗʰ [375.32]
- dactylitis 015.5 ✓5ᵗʰ
- diarrhea 014.8 ✓5ᵗʰ
- diffuse (*see also* Tuberculosis, miliary) 018.9 ✓5ᵗʰ
  - lung — *see* Tuberculosis, pulmonary
  - meninges 013.0 ✓5ᵗʰ
- digestive tract 014.8 ✓5ᵗʰ
- disseminated (*see also* Tuberculosis, miliary) 018.9 ✓5ᵗʰ
  - meninges 013.0 ✓5ᵗʰ
- duodenum 014.8 ✓5ᵗʰ
- dura (mater) 013.9 ✓5ᵗʰ
  - abscess 013.8 ✓5ᵗʰ
    - cerebral 013.3 ✓5ᵗʰ
    - spinal 013.5 ✓5ᵗʰ
- dysentery 014.8 ✓5ᵗʰ
- ear (inner) (middle) 017.4 ✓5ᵗʰ
  - bone 015.6 ✓5ᵗʰ
  - external (primary) 017.0 ✓5ᵗʰ
  - skin (primary) 017.0 ✓5ᵗʰ
- elbow 015.8 ✓5ᵗʰ
- emphysema — *see* Tuberculosis, pulmonary
- empyema 012.0 ✓5ᵗʰ
- encephalitis 013.6 ✓5ᵗʰ
- endarteritis 017.9 ✓5ᵗʰ
- endocarditis (any valve) 017.9 ✓5ᵗʰ [424.91]

Tuberculosis, tubercular, tuberculous — *continued*
- endocardium (any valve) 017.9 ✓5ᵗʰ [424.91]
- endocrine glands NEC 017.9 ✓5ᵗʰ
- endometrium 016.7 ✓5ᵗʰ
- enteric, enterica 014.8 ✓5ᵗʰ
- enteritis 014.8 ✓5ᵗʰ
- enterocolitis 014.8 ✓5ᵗʰ
- epididymis 016.4 ✓5ᵗʰ
- epididymitis 016.4 ✓5ᵗʰ
- epidural abscess 013.8 ✓5ᵗʰ
  - brain 013.3 ✓5ᵗʰ
  - spinal cord 013.5 ✓5ᵗʰ
- epiglottis 012.3 ✓5ᵗʰ
- episcleritis 017.3 ✓5ᵗʰ [379.00]
- erythema (induratum) (nodosum) (primary) 017.1 ✓5ᵗʰ
- esophagus 017.8 ✓5ᵗʰ
- Eustachian tube 017.4 ✓5ᵗʰ
- exposure to V01.1
- exudative 012.0 ✓5ᵗʰ
  - primary, progressive 010.1 ✓5ᵗʰ
- eye 017.3 ✓5ᵗʰ
  - glaucoma 017.3 ✓5ᵗʰ [365.62]
- eyelid (primary) 017.0 ✓5ᵗʰ
  - lupus 017.0 ✓5ᵗʰ [373.4]
- fallopian tube 016.6 ✓5ᵗʰ
- fascia 017.9 ✓5ᵗʰ
- fauces 012.8 ✓5ᵗʰ
- finger 017.9 ✓5ᵗʰ
- first infection 010.0 ✓5ᵗʰ
- fistula, perirectal 014.8 ✓5ᵗʰ
- Florida 011.6 ✓5ᵗʰ
- foot 017.9 ✓6ᵗʰ
- funnel pelvis 137.3
- gallbladder 017.9 ✓5ᵗʰ
- galloping (*see also* Tuberculosis, pulmonary) 011.9 ✓5ᵗʰ
- ganglionic 015.9 ✓5ᵗʰ
- gastritis 017.9 ✓5ᵗʰ
- gastrocolic fistula 014.8 ✓5ᵗʰ
- gastroenteritis 014.8 ✓5ᵗʰ
- gastrointestinal tract 014.8 ✓5ᵗʰ
- general, generalized 018.9 ✓5ᵗʰ
  - acute 018.0 ✓5ᵗʰ
  - chronic 018.8 ✓5ᵗʰ
- genital organs NEC 016.9 ✓5ᵗʰ
  - female 016.7 ✓5ᵗʰ
  - male 016.5 ✓5ᵗʰ
- genitourinary NEC 016.9 ✓5ᵗʰ
- genu 015.2 ✓5ᵗʰ
- glandulae suprarenalis 017.6 ✓5ᵗʰ
- glandular, general 017.2 ✓5ᵗʰ
- glottis 012.3 ✓5ᵗʰ
- grinders' 011.4 ✓5ᵗʰ
- groin 017.2 ✓5ᵗʰ
- gum 017.9 ✓5ᵗʰ
- hand 017.9 ✓5ᵗʰ
- heart 017.9 ✓5ᵗʰ [425.8]
- hematogenous — *see* Tuberculosis, miliary
- hemoptysis (*see also* Tuberculosis, pulmonary) 011.9 ✓5ᵗʰ
- hemorrhage NEC (*see also* Tuberculosis, pulmonary) 011.9 ✓5ᵗʰ
- hemothorax 012.0 ✓5ᵗʰ
- hepatitis 017.9 ✓5ᵗʰ
- hilar lymph nodes 012.1 ✓5ᵗʰ
  - primary, progressive 010.8 ✓5ᵗʰ
- hip (disease) (joint) 015.1 ✓5ᵗʰ
  - bone 015.1 ✓5ᵗʰ [730.85]
- hydrocephalus 013.8 ✓5ᵗʰ

Index to Diseases

Tuberculosis, tubercular, tuberculous — continued

hydropneumothorax 012.0 ✓5ᵗʰ
hydrothorax 012.0 ✓5ᵗʰ
hypoadrenalism 017.6 ✓5ᵗʰ
hypopharynx 012.8 ✓5ᵗʰ
ileocecal (hyperplastic) 014.8 ✓5ᵗʰ
ileocolitis 014.8 ✓5ᵗʰ
ileum 014.8 ✓5ᵗʰ
iliac spine (superior) 015.0 ✓5ᵗʰ [730.88]
incipient NEC (see also Tuberculosis, pulmonary) 011.9 ✓5ᵗʰ
indurativa (primary) 017.1 ✓5ᵗʰ
infantile 010.0 ✓5ᵗʰ
infection NEC 011.9 ✓5ᵗʰ
 without clinical manifestation 010.0 ✓5ᵗʰ
infraclavicular gland 017.2 ✓5ᵗʰ
inguinal gland 017.2 ✓5ᵗʰ
inguinalis 017.2 ✓5ᵗʰ
intestine (any part) 014.8 ✓5ᵗʰ
iris 017.3 ✓5ᵗʰ [364.11]
iritis 017.3 ✓5ᵗʰ [364.11]
ischiorectal 014.8 ✓5ᵗʰ
jaw 015.7 ✓5ᵗʰ [730.88]
jejunum 014.8 ✓5ᵗʰ
joint 015.9 ✓5ᵗʰ
 hip 015.1 ✓5ᵗʰ
 knee 015.2 ✓5ᵗʰ
 specified site NEC 015.8 ✓5ᵗʰ
 vertebral 015.0 ✓5ᵗʰ [730.88]
keratitis 017.3 ✓5ᵗʰ [370.31]
 interstitial 017.3 ✓5ᵗʰ [370.59]
keratoconjunctivitis 017.3 ✓5ᵗʰ [370.31]
kidney 016.0 ✓5ᵗʰ
knee (joint) 015.2 ✓5ᵗʰ
kyphoscoliosis 015.0 ✓5ᵗʰ [737.43]
kyphosis 015.0 ✓5ᵗʰ [737.41]
lacrimal apparatus, gland 017.3 ✓5ᵗʰ
laryngitis 012.3 ✓5ᵗʰ
larynx 012.3 ✓5ᵗʰ
leptomeninges, leptomeningitis (cerebral) (spinal) 013.0 ✓5ᵗʰ
lichenoides (primary) 017.0 ✓5ᵗʰ
linguae 017.9 ✓5ᵗʰ
lip 017.9 ✓5ᵗʰ
liver 017.9 ✓5ᵗʰ
lordosis 015.0 ✓5ᵗʰ [737.42]
lung — see Tuberculosis, pulmonary
luposa 017.0 ✓5ᵗʰ
 eyelid 017.0 ✓5ᵗʰ [373.4]
lymphadenitis — see Tuberculosis, lymph gland
lymphangitis — see Tuberculosis, lymph gland
lymphatic (gland) (vessel) — see Tuberculosis, lymph gland
lymph gland or node (peripheral) 017.2 ✓5ᵗʰ
 abdomen 014.8 ✓5ᵗʰ
 bronchial 012.1 ✓5ᵗʰ
  primary, progressive 010.8 ✓5ᵗʰ
 cervical 017.2 ✓5ᵗʰ
 hilar 012.1 ✓5ᵗʰ
  primary, progressive 010.8 ✓5ᵗʰ
 intrathoracic 012.1 ✓5ᵗʰ
  primary, progressive 010.8 ✓5ᵗʰ
 mediastinal 012.1 ✓5ᵗʰ
  primary, progressive 010.8 ✓5ᵗʰ
 mesenteric 014.8 ✓5ᵗʰ
 peripheral 017.2 ✓5ᵗʰ
 retroperitoneal 014.8 ✓5ᵗʰ
 tracheobronchial 012.1 ✓5ᵗʰ
  primary, progressive 010.8 ✓5ᵗʰ

Tuberculosis, tubercular, tuberculous — continued

malignant NEC (see also Tuberculosis, pulmonary) 011.9 ✓5ᵗʰ
mammary gland 017.9 ✓5ᵗʰ
marasmus NEC (see also Tuberculosis, pulmonary) 011.9 ✓5ᵗʰ
mastoiditis 015.6 ✓5ᵗʰ
maternal, affecting fetus or newborn 760.2
mediastinal (lymph) gland or node 012.1 ✓5ᵗʰ
 primary, progressive 010.8 ✓5ᵗʰ
mediastinitis 012.8 ✓5ᵗʰ
 primary, progressive 010.8 ✓5ᵗʰ
mediastinopericarditis 017.9 ✓5ᵗʰ [420.0]
mediastinum 012.8 ✓5ᵗʰ
 primary, progressive 010.8 ✓5ᵗʰ
medulla 013.9 ✓5ᵗʰ
 brain 013.2 ✓5ᵗʰ
 spinal cord 013.4 ✓5ᵗʰ
melanosis, Addisonian 017.6 ✓5ᵗʰ
membrane, brain 013.0 ✓5ᵗʰ
meninges (cerebral) (spinal) 013.0 ✓5ᵗʰ
meningitis (basilar) (brain) (cerebral) (cerebrospinal) (spinal) 013.0 ✓5ᵗʰ
meningoencephalitis 013.0 ✓5ᵗʰ
mesentery, mesenteric 014.8 ✓5ᵗʰ
 lymph gland or node 014.8 ✓5ᵗʰ
miliary (any site) 018.9 ✓5ᵗʰ
 acute 018.0 ✓5ᵗʰ
 chronic 018.8 ✓5ᵗʰ
 specified type NEC 018.8 ✓5ᵗʰ
millstone makers' 011.4 ✓5ᵗʰ
miners' 011.4 ✓5ᵗʰ
moulders' 011.4 ✓5ᵗʰ
mouth 017.9 ✓5ᵗʰ
multiple 018.9 ✓5ᵗʰ
 acute 018.0 ✓5ᵗʰ
 chronic 018.8 ✓5ᵗʰ
muscle 017.9 ✓5ᵗʰ
myelitis 013.6 ✓5ᵗʰ
myocarditis 017.9 ✓5ᵗʰ [422.0]
myocardium 017.9 ✓5ᵗʰ [422.0]
nasal (passage) (sinus) 012.8 ✓5ᵗʰ
nasopharynx 012.8 ✓5ᵗʰ
neck gland 017.2 ✓5ᵗʰ
nephritis 016.0 ✓5ᵗʰ [583.81] ✓5ᵗʰ
nerve 017.9 ✓5ᵗʰ
nose (septum) 012.8 ✓5ᵗʰ
ocular 017.3 ✓5ᵗʰ
old NEC 137.0
 without residuals V12.01
omentum 014.8 ✓5ᵗʰ
oophoritis (acute) (chronic) 016.6 ✓5ᵗʰ
optic 017.3 ✓5ᵗʰ [377.39]
 nerve trunk 017.3 ✓5ᵗʰ [377.39]
 papilla, papillae 017.3 ✓5ᵗʰ [377.39]
orbit 017.3 ✓5ᵗʰ
orchitis 016.5 ✓5ᵗʰ [608.81]
organ, specified NEC 017.9 ✓5ᵗʰ
orificialis (primary) 017.0 ✓5ᵗʰ
osseous (see also Tuberculosis, bone) 015.9 ✓5ᵗʰ [730.8] ✓5ᵗʰ
osteitis (see also Tuberculosis, bone) 015.9 ✓5ᵗʰ [730.8] ✓5ᵗʰ
osteomyelitis (see also Tuberculosis, bone) 015.9 ✓5ᵗʰ [730.8] ✓5ᵗʰ
otitis (media) 017.4 ✓5ᵗʰ
ovaritis (acute) (chronic) 016.6 ✓5ᵗʰ
ovary (acute) (chronic) 016.6 ✓5ᵗʰ
oviducts (acute) (chronic) 016.6 ✓5ᵗʰ
pachymeningitis 013.0 ✓5ᵗʰ

Tuberculosis, tubercular, tuberculous — continued

palate (soft) 017.9
pancreas 017.9
papulonecrotic (primary) 017.0
parathyroid glands 017.9
paronychia (primary) 017.0
parotid gland or region 017.9
pelvic organ NEC 016.9
  female 016.7
  male 016.5
pelvis (bony) 015.7 [730.85]
penis 016.5
peribronchitis 011.3
pericarditis 017.9 [420.0]
pericardium 017.9 [420.0]
perichondritis, larynx 012.3
perineum 017.9
periostitis (see also Tuberculosis, bone) 015.9 [730.8]
periphlebitis 017.9
  eye vessel 017.3 [362.18]
  retina 017.3 [362.18]
perirectal fistula 014.8
peritoneal gland 014.8
peritoneum 014.0
peritonitis 014.0
pernicious NEC (see also Tuberculosis, pulmonary) 011.9
pharyngitis 012.8
pharynx 012.8
phlyctenulosis (conjunctiva) 017.3 [370.31]
phthisis NEC (see also Tuberculosis, pulmonary) 011.9
pituitary gland 017.9
placenta 016.7
pleura, pleural, pleurisy, pleuritis (fibrinous) (obliterative) (purulent) (simple plastic) (with effusion) 012.0
  primary, progressive 010.1
pneumonia, pneumonic 011.6
pneumothorax 011.7
polyserositis 018.9
  acute 018.0
  chronic 018.8
potters' 011.4
prepuce 016.5
primary 010.9
  complex 010.0
  complicated 010.8
    with pleurisy or effusion 010.1
  progressive 010.8
    with pleurisy or effusion 010.1
  skin 017.0
proctitis 014.8
prostate 016.5 [601.4]
prostatitis 016.5 [601.4]
pulmonaris (see also Tuberculosis, pulmonary) 011.9
pulmonary (artery) (incipient) (malignant) (multiple round foci) (pernicious) (reinfection stage) 011.9
  cavitated or with cavitation 011.2
    primary, progressive 010.8
  childhood type or first infection 010.0
  chromogenic acid-fast bacilli 795.39 ▲
  fibrosis or fibrotic 011.4
  infiltrative 011.0
    primary, progressive 010.9
  nodular 011.1

Tuberculosis, tubercular, tuberculous — continued

pulmonary — continued
  specified NEC 011.8
  sputum positive only 795.39 ▲
  status following surgical collapse of lung NEC 011.9
pyelitis 016.0 [590.81]
pyelonephritis 016.0 [590.81]
pyemia — see Tuberculosis, miliary
pyonephrosis 016.0
pyopneumothorax 012.0
pyothorax 012.0
rectum (with abscess) 014.8
  fistula 014.8
reinfection stage (see also Tuberculosis, pulmonary) 011.9
renal 016.0
renis 016.0
reproductive organ 016.7
respiratory NEC (see also Tuberculosis, pulmonary) 011.9
  specified site NEC 012.8
retina 017.3 [363.13]
retroperitoneal (lymph gland or node) 014.8
  gland 014.8
retropharyngeal abscess 012.8
rheumatism 015.9
rhinitis 012.8
sacroiliac (joint) 015.8
sacrum 015.0 [730.88]
salivary gland 017.9
salpingitis (acute) (chronic) 016.6
sandblasters' 011.4
sclera 017.3 [379.09]
scoliosis 015.0 [737.43]
scrofulous 017.2
scrotum 016.5
seminal tract or vesicle 016.5 [608.81]
senile NEC (see also Tuberculosis, pulmonary) 011.9
septic NEC (see also Tuberculosis, miliary) 018.9
shoulder 015.8
  blade 015.7 [730.8]
sigmoid 014.8
sinus (accessory) (nasal) 012.8
  bone 015.7 [730.88]
  epididymis 016.4
skeletal NEC (see also Osteomyelitis, due to tuberculosis) 015.9 [730.8]
skin (any site) (primary) 017.0
small intestine 014.8
soft palate 017.9
spermatic cord 016.5
spinal
  column 015.0 [730.88]
  cord 013.4
  disease 015.0 [730.88]
  medulla 013.4
  membrane 013.0
  meninges 013.0
spine 015.0 [730.88]
spleen 017.7
splenitis 017.7
spondylitis 015.0 [720.81]
spontaneous pneumothorax — see Tuberculosis, pulmonary
sternoclavicular joint 015.8
stomach 017.9
stonemasons' 011.4

Tuberculosis, tubercular, tuberculous — continued
  struma 017.2 ✓5
  subcutaneous tissue (cellular) (primary) 017.0 ✓5
  subcutis (primary) 017.0 ✓5
  subdeltoid bursa 017.9 ✓5
  submaxillary 017.9 ✓5
    region 017.9 ✓5
  supraclavicular gland 017.2 ✓5
  suprarenal (capsule) (gland) 017.6 ✓5
  swelling, joint (see also Tuberculosis, joint) 015.9 ✓5
  symphysis pubis 015.7 ✓5 [730.88]
  synovitis 015.9 ✓5 [727.01]
    hip 015.1 ✓5 [727.01]
    knee 015.2 ✓5 [727.01]
    specified site NEC 015.8 ✓5 [727.01]
    spine or vertebra 015.0 ✓5 [727.01]
  systemic — see Tuberculosis, miliary
  tarsitis (eyelid) 017.0 ✓5 [373.4]
    ankle (bone) 015.5 ✓5 [730.87]
  tendon (sheath) — see Tuberculosis, tenosynovitis
  tenosynovitis 015.9 ✓5 [727.01]
    hip 015.1 ✓5 [727.01]
    knee 015.2 ✓5 [727.01]
    specified site NEC 015.8 ✓5 [727.01]
    spine or vertebra 015.0 ✓5 [727.01]
  testis 016.5 ✓5 [608.81]
  throat 012.8 ✓5
  thymus gland 017.9 ✓5
  thyroid gland 017.5 ✓5
  toe 017.9 ✓5
  tongue 017.9 ✓5
  tonsil (lingual) 012.8 ✓5
  tonsillitis 012.8 ✓5
  trachea, tracheal 012.8 ✓5
    gland 012.1 ✓5
      primary, progressive 010.8 ✓5
      isolated 012.2 ✓5
  tracheobronchial 011.3 ✓5
    glandular 012.1 ✓5
      primary, progressive 010.8 ✓5
      isolated 012.2 ✓5
    lymph gland or node 012.1 ✓5
      primary, progressive 010.8 ✓5
  tubal 016.6 ✓5
  tunica vaginalis 016.5 ✓5
  typhlitis 014.8 ✓5
  ulcer (primary) (skin) 017.0 ✓5
    bowel or intestine 014.8 ✓5
    specified site NEC — see Tuberculosis, by site
  unspecified site — see Tuberculosis, pulmonary
  ureter 016.2 ✓5
  urethra, urethral 016.3 ✓5
  urinary organ or tract 016.3 ✓5
    kidney 016.0 ✓5
  uterus 016.7 ✓5
  uveal tract 017.3 ✓5 [363.13]
  uvula 017.9 ✓5
  vaccination, prophylactic (against) V03.2
  vagina 016.7 ✓5
  vas deferens 016.5 ✓5
  vein 017.9 ✓5
  verruca (primary) 017.0 ✓5
  verrucosa (cutis) (primary) 017.0 ✓5
  vertebra (column) 015.0 ✓5 [730.88]
  vesiculitis 016.5 ✓5 [608.81]
  viscera NEC 014.8 ✓5

Tuberculosis, tubercular, tuberculous — continued
  vulva 016.7 ✓5 [616.51]
  wrist (joint) 015.8 ✓5
    bone 015.5 ✓5 [730.83]
Tuberculum
  auriculae 744.29
  occlusal 520.2
  paramolare 520.2
Tuberous sclerosis (brain) 759.5
Tubo-ovarian — see condition
Tuboplasty, after previous sterilization V26.0
Tubotympanitis 381.10
Tularemia 021.9
  with
    conjunctivitis 021.3
    pneumonia 021.2
  bronchopneumonic 021.2
  conjunctivitis 021.3
  cryptogenic 021.1
  disseminated 021.8
  enteric 021.1
  generalized 021.8
  glandular 021.8
  intestinal 021.1
  oculoglandular 021.3
  ophthalmic 021.3
  pneumonia 021.2
  pulmonary 021.2
  specified NEC 021.8
  typhoidal 021.1
  ulceroglandular 021.0
  vaccination, prophylactic (against) V03.4
Tularensis conjunctivitis 021.3
Tumefaction — see also Swelling
  liver (see also Hypertrophy, liver) 789.1
Tumor (M8000/1) — see also Neoplasm, by site, unspecified nature
  Abrikossov's (M9580/0) — see also Neoplasm, connective tissue, benign
    malignant (M9580/3) — see Neoplasm, connective tissue, malignant
  acinar cell (M8550/1) — see Neoplasm, by site, uncertain behavior
  acinic cell (M8550/1) — see Neoplasm, by site, uncertain behavior
  adenomatoid (M9054/0) — see also Neoplasm, by site, benign
    odontogenic (M9300/0) 213.1
    upper jaw (bone) 213.0
  adnexal (skin) (M8390/0) — see Neoplasm, skin, benign
  adrenal
    cortical (benign) (M8370/0) 227.0
      malignant (M8370/3) 194.0
    rest (M8671/0) — see Neoplasm, by site, benign
  alpha cell (M8152/0)
    malignant (M8152/3)
      pancreas 157.4
      specified site NEC — see Neoplasm, by site, malignant
      unspecified site 157.4
    pancreas 211.7
    specified site NEC — see Neoplasm, by site, benign
    unspecified site 211.7
  aneurysmal (see also Aneurysm) 442.9
  aortic body (M8691/1) 237.3
    malignant (M8691/3) 194.6

✓4 Fourth-digit Required   ✓5 Fifth-digit Required

Tumor — *continued*
- argentaffin (M8241/1) — *see* Neoplasm, by site, uncertain behavior
- basal cell (M8090/1) — *see also* Neoplasm, skin, uncertain behavior
- benign (M8000/0) — *see* Neoplasm, by site, benign
- beta cell (M8151/0)
  - malignant (M8151/3)
    - pancreas 157.4
    - specified site — *see* Neoplasm, by site, malignant
    - unspecified site 157.4
  - pancreas 211.7
  - specified site NEC — *see* Neoplasm, by site, benign
  - unspecified site 211.7
- blood — *see* Hematoma
- Brenner (M9000/0) 220
  - borderline malignancy (M9000/1) 236.2
  - malignant (M9000/3) 183.0
  - proliferating (M9000/1) 236.2
- Brooke's (M8100/0) — *see* Neoplasm, skin, benign
- brown fat (M8880/0) — *see* Lipoma, by site
- Burkitt's (M9750/3) 200.2 ✓5ᵗʰ
- calcifying epithelial odontogenic (M9340/0) 213.1
  - upper jaw (bone) 213.0
- carcinoid (M8240/1) — *see* Carcinoid
- carotid body (M8692/1) 237.3
  - malignant (M8692/3) 194.5
- Castleman's (mediastinal lymph node hyperplasia) 785.6
- cells (M8001/1) — *see also* Neoplasm, by site, unspecified nature
  - benign (M8001/0) — *see* Neoplasm, by site, benign
  - malignant (M8001/3) — *see* Neoplasm, by site, malignant
  - uncertain whether benign or malignant (M8001/1) — *see* Neoplasm, by site, uncertain nature
- cervix
  - in pregnancy or childbirth 654.6 ✓5ᵗʰ
    - affecting fetus or newborn 763.89
    - causing obstructed labor 660.2 ✓5ᵗʰ
      - affecting fetus or newborn 763.1
- chondromatous giant cell (M9230/0) — *see* Neoplasm, bone, benign
- chromaffin (M8700/0) — *see also* Neoplasm, by site, benign
  - malignant (M8700/3) — *see* Neoplasm, by site, malignant
- Cock's peculiar 706.2
- Codman's (benign chondroblastoma) (M9230/0) — *see* Neoplasm, bone, benign
- dentigerous, mixed (M9282/0) 213.1
  - upper jaw (bone) 213.0
- dermoid (M9084/0) — *see* Neoplasm, by site, benign
  - with malignant transformation (M9084/3) 183.0
- desmoid (extra-abdominal) (M8821/1) — *see also* Neoplasm, connective tissue, uncertain behavior
  - abdominal (M8822/1) — *see* Neoplasm, connective tissue, uncertain behavior
- embryonal (mixed) (M9080/1) — *see also* Neoplasm, by site, uncertain behavior
  - liver (M9080/3) 155.0

Tumor — *continued*
- endodermal sinus (M9071/3)
  - specified site — *see* Neoplasm, by site, malignant
  - unspecified site
    - female 183.0
    - male 186.9
- epithelial
  - benign (M8010/0) — *see* Neoplasm, by site, benign
  - malignant (M8010/3) — *see* Neoplasm, by site, malignant
- Ewing's (M9260/3) — *see* Neoplasm, bone, malignant
- fatty — *see* Lipoma
- fetal, causing disproportion 653.7 ✓5ᵗʰ
  - causing obstructed labor 660.1 ✓5ᵗʰ
- fibroid (M8890/0) — *see* Leiomyoma
- G cell (M8153/1)
  - malignant (M8153/3)
    - pancreas 157.4
    - specified site NEC — *see* Neoplasm, site, malignant
    - unspecified site 157.4
  - specified site — *see* Neoplasm, by site, uncertain behavior
  - unspecified site 235.5
- giant cell (type) (M8003/1) — *see also* Neoplasm, by site, unspecified nature
  - bone (M9250/1) 238.0
    - malignant (M9250/3) — *see* Neoplasm, bone, malignant
  - chondromatous (M9230/0) — *see* Neoplasm, bone, benign
  - malignant (M8003/3) — *see* Neoplasm, by site, malignant
  - peripheral (gingiva) 523.8
  - soft parts (M9251/1) — *see also* Neoplasm, connective tissue, uncertain behavior
    - malignant (M9251/3) — *see* Neoplasm, connective tissue, malignant
  - tendon sheath 727.02
- glomus (M8711/0) — *see also* Hemangioma, by site
  - jugulare (M8690/1) 237.3
    - malignant (M8690/3) 194.6
- gonadal stromal (M8590/1) — *see* Neoplasm, by site, uncertain behavior
- granular cell (M9580/0) — *see also* Neoplasm, connective tissue, benign
  - malignant (M9580/3) — *see* Neoplasm, connective tissue, malignant
- granulosa cell (M8620/1) 236.2
  - malignant (M8620/3) 183.0
- granulosa cell-theca cell (M8621/1) 236.2
  - malignant (M8621/3) 183.0
- Grawitz's (hypernephroma) (M8312/3) 189.0
- hazard-crile (M8350/3) 193
- hemorrhoidal — *see* Hemorrhoids
- hilar cell (M8660/0) 220
- Hürthle cell (benign) (M8290/0) 226
  - malignant (M8290/3) 193
- hydatid (*see also* Echinococcus) 122.9
- hypernephroid (M8311/1) — *see also* Neoplasm, by site, uncertain behavior
- interstitial cell (M8650/1) — *see also* Neoplasm, by site, uncertain behavior
  - benign (M8650/0) — *see* Neoplasm, by site, benign
  - malignant (M8650/3) — *see* Neoplasm, by site, malignant

Tumor — *continued*
- islet cell (M8150/0)
  - malignant (M8150/3)
    - pancreas 157.4
    - specified site — *see* Neoplasm, by site, malignant
    - unspecified site 157.4
  - pancreas 211.7
  - specified site NEC — *see* Neoplasm, by site, benign
  - unspecified site 211.7
- juxtaglomerular (M8361/1) 236.91
- Krukenberg's (M8490/6) 198.6
- Leydig cell (M8650/1)
  - benign (M8650/0)
    - specified site — *see* Neoplasm, by site, benign
    - unspecified site
      - female 220
      - male 222.0
  - malignant (M8650/3)
    - specified site — *see* Neoplasm, by site, malignant
    - unspecified site
      - female 183.0
      - male 186.9
  - specified site — *see* Neoplasm, by site, uncertain behavior
  - unspecified site
    - female 236.2
    - male 236.4
- lipid cell, ovary (M8670/0) 220
- lipoid cell, ovary (M8670/0) 220
- lymphomatous, benign (M9590/0) — *see also* Neoplasm, by site, benign
- Malherbe's (M8110/0) — *see* Neoplasm, skin, benign
- malignant (M8000/3) — *see also* Neoplasm, by site, malignant
  - fusiform cell (type) (M8004/3) — *see* Neoplasm, by site, malignant
  - giant cell (type) (M8003/3) — *see* Neoplasm, by site, malignant
  - mixed NEC (M8940/3) — *see* Neoplasm, by site, malignant
  - small cell (type) (M8002/3) — *see* Neoplasm, by site, malignant
  - spindle cell (type) (M8004/3) — *see* Neoplasm, by site, malignant
- mast cell (M9740/1) 238.5
  - malignant (M9740/3) 202.6 ✓5ᵗʰ
- melanotic, neuroectodermal (M9363/0) — *see* Neoplasm, by site, benign
- Merkel cell — *see* Neoplasm, by site, malignant
- mesenchymal
  - malignant (M8800/3) — *see* Neoplasm, connective tissue, malignant
  - mixed (M8990/1) — *see* Neoplasm, connective tissue, uncertain behavior
- mesodermal, mixed (M8951/3) — *see also* Neoplasm, by site, malignant
  - liver 155.0
- mesonephric (M9110/1) — *see also* Neoplasm, by site, uncertain behavior
  - malignant (M9110/3) — *see also* Neoplasm, by site, malignant
- metastatic
  - from specified site (M8000/3) — *see* Neoplasm, by site, malignant

Tumor — *continued*
- metastatic — *continued*
  - to specified site (M8000/6) — *see* Neoplasm, by site, malignant, secondary
- mixed NEC (M8940/0) — *see also* Neoplasm, by site, benign
  - malignant (M8940/3) — *see* Neoplasm, by site, malignant
- mucocarcinoid, malignant (M8243/3) — *see* Neoplasm, by site, malignant
- mucoepidermoid (M8430/1) — *see* Neoplasm, by site, uncertain behavior
- Mullerian, mixed (M8950/3) — *see* Neoplasm, by site, malignant
- myoepithelial (M8982/0) — *see* Neoplasm, by site, benign
- neurogenic olfactory (M9520/3) 160.0
- nonencapsulated sclerosing (M8350/3) 193
- odontogenic (M9270/1) 238.0
  - adenomatoid (M9300/0) 213.1
    - upper jaw (bone) 213.0
  - benign (M9270/0) 213.1
    - upper jaw (bone) 213.0
  - calcifying epithelial (M9340/0) 213.1
    - upper jaw (bone) 213.0
  - malignant (M9270/3) 170.1
    - upper jaw (bone) 170.0
  - squamous (M9312/0) 213.1
    - upper jaw (bone) 213.0
- ovarian stromal (M8590/1) 236.2
- ovary
  - in pregnancy or childbirth 654.4 ✓5ᵗʰ
    - affecting fetus or newborn 763.89
  - causing obstructed labor 660.2 ✓5ᵗʰ
    - affecting fetus or newborn 763.1
- pacinian (M9507/0) — *see* Neoplasm, skin, benign
- Pancoast's (M8010/3) 162.3
- papillary — *see* Papilloma
- pelvic, in pregnancy or childbirth 654.9 ✓5ᵗʰ
  - affecting fetus or newborn 763.89
  - causing obstructed labor 660.2 ✓5ᵗʰ
    - affecting fetus or newborn 763.1
- phantom 300.11
- plasma cell (M9731/1) 238.6
  - benign (M9731/0) — *see* Neoplasm, by site, benign
  - malignant (M9731/3) 203.8 ✓5ᵗʰ
- polyvesicular vitelline (M9071/3)
  - specified site — *see* Neoplasm, by site, malignant
  - unspecified site
    - female 183.0
    - male 186.9
- Pott's puffy (*see also* Osteomyelitis) 730.2 ✓5ᵗʰ
- Rathke's pouch (M9350/1) 237.0
- regaud's (M8082/3) — *see* Neoplasm, nasopharynx, malignant
- rete cell (M8140/0) 222.0
- retinal anlage (M9363/0) — *see* Neoplasm, by site, benign
- Rokitansky's 620.2
- salivary gland type, mixed (M8940/0) — *see also* Neoplasm, by site, benign
  - malignant (M8940/3) — *see* Neoplasm, by site, malignant
- Sampson's 617.1
- Schloffer's (*see also* Peritonitis) 567.2
- Schmincke (M8082/3) — *see* Neoplasm, nasopharynx, malignant

Tumor — *continued*
  sebaceous (*see also* Cyst, sebaceous) 706.2
  secondary (M8000/6) — *see* Neoplasm, by site, secondary
  Sertoli cell (M8640/0)
    with lipid storage (M8641/0)
      specified site — *see* Neoplasm, by site, benign
      unspecified site
        female 220
        male 222.0
    specified site — *see* Neoplasm, by site, benign
    unspecified site
      female 220
      male 222.0
  Sertoli-Leydig cell (M8631/0)
    specified site, — *see* Neoplasm, by site, benign
    unspecified site
      female 220
      male 222.0
  sex cord (-stromal) (M8590/1) — *see* Neoplasm, by site, uncertain behavior
  skin appendage (M8390/0) — *see* Neoplasm, skin, benign
  soft tissue
    benign (M8800/0) — *see* Neoplasm, connective tissue, benign
    malignant (M8800/3) — *see* Neoplasm, connective tissue, malignant
  sternomastoid 754.1
  superior sulcus (lung) (pulmonary) (syndrome) (M8010/3) 162.3
  suprasulcus (M8010/3) 162.3
  sweat gland (M8400/1) — *see also* Neoplasm, skin, uncertain behavior
    benign (M8400/0) — *see* Neoplasm, skin, benign
    malignant (M8400/3) — *see* Neoplasm, skin, malignant
  syphilitic brain 094.89
    congenital 090.49
  testicular stromal (M8590/1) 236.4
  theca cell (M8600/0) 220
  theca cell-granulosa cell (M8621/1) 236.2
  theca-lutein (M8610/0) 220
  turban (M8200/0) 216.4
  uterus
    in pregnancy or childbirth 654.1 ✓5ᵗʰ
      affecting fetus or newborn 763.89
      causing obstructed labor 660.2 ✓5ᵗʰ
        affecting fetus or newborn 763.1
  vagina
    in pregnancy or childbirth 654.7 ✓5ᵗʰ
      affecting fetus or newborn 763.89
      causing obstructed labor 660.2 ✓5ᵗʰ
        affecting fetus or newborn 763.1
  varicose (*see also* Varicose, vein) 454.9
  von Recklinghausen's (M9540/1) 237.71
  vulva
    in pregnancy or childbirth 654.8 ✓5ᵗʰ
      affecting fetus or newborn 763.89
      causing obstructed labor 660.2 ✓5ᵗʰ
        affecting fetus or newborn 763.1
  Warthin's (salivary gland) (M8561/0) 210.2
  white — *see also* Tuberculosis, arthritis
  White-Darier 757.39
  Wilms' (nephroblastoma) (M8960/3) 189.0
  yolk sac (M9071/3)
    specified site — *see* Neoplasm, by site, malignant

Tumor — *continued*
  yolk sac — *continued*
    unspecified site
      female 183.0
      male 186.9
Tumorlet (M8040/1) — *see* Neoplasm, by site, uncertain behavior
Tungiasis 134.1
Tunica vasculosa lentis 743.39
Tunnel vision 368.45
Turban tumor (M8200/0) 216.4
Türck's trachoma (chronic catarrhal laryngitis) 476.0
Türk's syndrome (ocular retraction syndrome) 378.71
Turner's
  hypoplasia (tooth) 520.4
  syndrome 758.6
  tooth 520.4
Turner-Kieser syndrome (hereditary osteo-onychodysplasia) 756.89
Turner-Varny syndrome 758.6
Turricephaly 756.0
Tussis convulsiva (*see also* Whooping cough) 033.9
Twin
  affected by maternal complications of pregnancy 761.5
  conjoined 759.4
  healthy liveborn — *see* Newborn, twin
  pregnancy (complicating delivery) NEC 651.0 ✓5ᵗʰ
    with fetal loss and retention of one fetus 651.3 ✓5ᵗʰ
Twinning, teeth 520.2
Twist, twisted
  bowel, colon, or intestine 560.2
  hair (congenital) 757.4
  mesentery 560.2
  omentum 560.2
  organ or site, congenital NEC — *see* Anomaly, specified type NEC
  ovarian pedicle 620.5
    congenital 752.0
  umbilical cord — *see* Compression, umbilical cord
Twitch 781.0
Tylosis 700
  buccalis 528.6
  gingiva 523.8
  linguae 528.6
  palmaris et plantaris 757.39
Tympanism 787.3
Tympanites (abdominal) (intestine) 787.3
Tympanitis — *see* Myringitis
Tympanosclerosis 385.00
  involving
    combined sites NEC 385.09
      with tympanic membrane 385.03
    tympanic membrane 385.01
      with ossicles 385.02
        and middle ear 385.03
Tympanum — *see* condition
Tympany
  abdomen 787.3
  chest 786.7
Typhlitis (*see also* Appendicitis) 541

Index to Diseases

Ulcer, ulcerated, ulcerating, ulceration, ulcerative

Typhoenteritis 002.0
Typhogastric fever 002.0
Typhoid (abortive) (ambulant) (any site) (fever) (hemorrhagic) (infection) (intermittent) (malignant) (rheumatic) 002.0
   with pneumonia 002.0 *[484.8]*
   abdominal 002.0
   carrier (suspected) of V02.1
   cholecystitis (current) 002.0
   clinical (Widal and blood test negative) 002.0
   endocarditis 002.0 *[421.1]*
   inoculation reaction — *see* Complications, vaccination
   meningitis 002.0 *[320.7]*
   mesenteric lymph nodes 002.0
   myocarditis 002.0 *[422.0]*
   osteomyelitis (*see also* Osteomyelitis, due to, typhoid) 002.0 *[730.8]* ✓5ᵗʰ
   perichondritis, larynx 002.0 *[478.71]*
   pneumonia 002.0 *[484.8]*
   spine 002.0 *[720.81]*
   ulcer (perforating) 002.0
   vaccination, prophylactic (against) V03.1
   Widal negative 002.0
Typhomalaria (fever) (*see also* Malaria) 084.6
Typhomania 002.0
Typhoperitonitis 002.0
Typhus (fever) 081.9
   abdominal, abdominalis 002.0
   African tick 082.1
   amarillic (*see also* Fever, Yellow) 060.9
   brain 081.9
   cerebral 081.9
   classical 080
   endemic (flea-borne) 081.0
   epidemic (louse-borne) 080
   exanthematic NEC 080
   exanthematicus SAI 080
      brillii SAI 081.1
      Mexicanus SAI 081.0
      pediculo vestimenti causa 080
      typhus murinus 081.0
   flea-borne 081.0
   Indian tick 082.1
   Kenya tick 082.1
   louse-borne 080
   Mexican 081.0
      flea-borne 081.0
      louse-borne 080
      tabardillo 080
   mite-borne 081.2
   murine 081.0
   North Asian tick-borne 082.2
   petechial 081.9
   Queensland tick 082.3
   rat 081.0
   recrudescent 081.1
   recurrent (*see also* Fever, relapsing) 087.9
   São Paulo 082.0
   scrub (China) (India) (Malaya) (New Guinea) 081.2
   shop (of Malaya) 081.0
   Siberian tick 082.2
   tick-borne NEC 082.9
   tropical 081.2
   vaccination, prophylactic (against) V05.8
Tyrosinemia 270.2
   neonatal 775.8
Tyrosinosis (Medes) (Sakai) 270.2
Tyrosinuria 270.2
Tyrosyluria 270.2

U

Uehlinger's syndrome (acropachyderma) 757.39
Uhl's anomaly or disease (hypoplasia of myocardium, right ventricle) 746.84
Ulcer, ulcerated, ulcerating, ulceration, ulcerative 707.9
   with gangrene 707.9 *[785.4]*
   abdomen (wall) (*see also* Ulcer, skin) 707.8
   ala, nose 478.1
   alveolar process 526.5
   amebic (intestine) 006.9
      skin 006.6
   anastomotic — *see* Ulcer, gastrojejunal
   anorectal 569.41
   antral — *see* Ulcer, stomach
   anus (sphincter) (solitary) 569.41
      varicose — *see* Varicose, ulcer, anus
   aphthous (oral) (recurrent) 528.2
      genital organ(s)
         female 616.8
         male 608.89
      mouth 528.2
   arm (*see also* Ulcer, skin) 707.8
   arteriosclerotic plaque — *see* Arteriosclerosis, by site
   artery NEC 447.2
      without rupture 447.8
   atrophic NEC — *see* Ulcer, skin
   Barrett's (chronic peptic ulcer of esophagus) 530.2
   bile duct 576.8
   bladder (solitary) (sphincter) 596.8
      bilharzial (*see also* Schistosomiasis) 120.9 *[595.4]*
      submucosal (*see also* Cystitis) 595.1
      tuberculous (*see also* Tuberculosis) 016.1 ✓5ᵗʰ
   bleeding NEC — *see* Ulcer, peptic, with hemorrhage
   bone 730.9 ✓5ᵗʰ
   bowel (*see also* Ulcer, intestine) 569.82
   breast 611.0
   bronchitis 491.8
   bronchus 519.1
   buccal (cavity) (traumatic) 528.9
   burn (acute) — *see* Ulcer, duodenum
   Buruli 031.1
   buttock (*see also* Ulcer, skin) 707.8
      decubitus (*see also* Ulcer, decubitus) 707.0
   cancerous (M8000/3) — *see* Neoplasm, by site, malignant
   cardia — *see* Ulcer, stomach
   cardio-esophageal (peptic) 530.2
   cecum (*see also* Ulcer, intestine) 569.82
   cervix (uteri) (trophic) 622.0
      with mention of cervicitis 616.0
   chancroidal 099.0
   chest (wall) (*see also* Ulcer, skin) 707.8
   Chiclero 085.4
   chin (pyogenic) (*see also* Ulcer, skin) 707.8
   chronic (cause unknown) — *see also* Ulcer, skin
      penis 607.89
   Cochin-China 085.1
   colitis — *see* Colitis, ulcerative
   colon (*see also* Ulcer, intestine) 569.82
   conjunctiva (acute) (postinfectional) 372.00
   cornea (infectional) 370.00
      with perforation 370.06
      annular 370.02

Ulcer, ulcerated, ulcerating, ulceration, ulcerative — continued
  cornea — continued
    catarrhal 370.01
    central 370.03
    dendritic 054.42
    marginal 370.01
    mycotic 370.05
    phlyctenular, tuberculous (see also
      Tuberculosis) 017.3 ✓5ᵗʰ [370.31]
    ring 370.02
    rodent 370.07
    serpent, serpiginous 370.04
    superficial marginal 370.01
    tuberculous (see also Tuberculosis)
      017.3 ✓5ᵗʰ [370.31]
  corpus cavernosum (chronic) 607.89
  crural — see Ulcer, lower extremity
  Curling's — see Ulcer, duodenum
  Cushing's — see Ulcer, peptic
  cystitis (interstitial) 595.1
  decubitus (any site) 707.0
    with gangrene 707.0 [785.4]
  dendritic 054.42
  diabetes, diabetic (mellitus) 250.8 ✓5ᵗʰ [707.9]
    lower limb 250.8 ✓5ᵗʰ [707.10]
      ankle 250.8 ✓5ᵗʰ [707.13]
      calf 250.8 ✓5ᵗʰ [707.12]
      foot 250.8 ✓5ᵗʰ [707.15]
      heel 250.8 ✓5ᵗʰ [707.14]
      knee 250.8 ✓5ᵗʰ [707.19]
      specified site NEC 250.8 ✓5ᵗʰ [707.19]
      thigh 250.8 ✓5ᵗʰ [707.11]
      toes 250.8 ✓5ᵗʰ [707.15]
    specified site NEC 250.8 ✓5ᵗʰ [707.8]
  Dieulafoy — see ▶Lesion, Dieulafoy◀
  due to
    infection NEC — see Ulcer, skin
    radiation, radium — see Ulcer, by site
    trophic disturbance (any region) — see
      Ulcer, skin
    x-ray — see Ulcer, by site
  duodenum, duodenal (eroded) (peptic)
    532.9 ✓5ᵗʰ

  Note — Use the following fifth-digit
  subclassification with categories 531-534:

  0   without mention of obstruction
  1   with obstruction

    with
      hemorrhage (chronic) 532.4 ✓5ᵗʰ
        and perforation 532.6 ✓5ᵗʰ
      perforation (chronic) 532.5 ✓5ᵗʰ
        and hemorrhage 532.6 ✓5ᵗʰ
    acute 532.3 ✓5ᵗʰ
      with
        hemorrhage 532.0 ✓5ᵗʰ
          and perforation 532.2 ✓5ᵗʰ
        perforation 532.1 ✓5ᵗʰ
          and hemorrhage 532.2 ✓5ᵗʰ
    bleeding (recurrent) — see Ulcer,
      duodenum, with hemorrhage
    chronic 532.7 ✓5ᵗʰ
      with
        hemorrhage 532.4 ✓5ᵗʰ
          and perforation 532.6 ✓5ᵗʰ
        perforation 532.5 ✓5ᵗʰ
          and hemorrhage 532.6 ✓5ᵗʰ
    penetrating — see Ulcer, duodenum, with
      perforation

Ulcer, ulcerated, ulcerating, ulceration, ulcerative — continued
  duodenum, duodenal — continued
    perforating — see Ulcer, duodenum, with
      perforation
  dysenteric NEC 009.0
  elusive 595.1
  endocarditis (any valve) (acute) (chronic)
    (subacute) 421.0
  enteritis — see Colitis, ulcerative
  enterocolitis 556.0
  epiglottis 478.79
  esophagus (peptic) 530.2
    due to ingestion
      aspirin 530.2
      chemicals 530.2
      medicinal agents 530.2
    fungal 530.2
    infectional 530.2
    varicose (see also Varix, esophagus) 456.1
      bleeding (see also Varix, esophagus,
        bleeding) 456.0
  eye NEC 360.00
    dendritic 054.42
  eyelid (region) 373.01
  face (see also Ulcer, skin) 707.8
  fauces 478.29
  Fenwick (-Hunner) (solitary) (see also Cystitis)
    595.1
  fistulous NEC — see Ulcer, skin
  foot (indolent) (see also Ulcer, lower extremity)
    707.15
    perforating 707.15
      leprous 030.1
      syphilitic 094.0
    trophic 707.15
    varicose 454.0
      inflamed or infected 454.2
  frambesial, initial or primary 102.0
  gallbladder or duct 575.8
  gall duct 576.8
  gangrenous (see also Gangrene) 785.4
  gastric — see Ulcer, stomach
  gastrocolic — see Ulcer, gastrojejunal
  gastroduodenal — see Ulcer, peptic
  gastroesophageal — see Ulcer, stomach
  gastrohepatic — see Ulcer, stomach
  gastrointestinal — see Ulcer, gastrojejunal
  gastrojejunal (eroded) (peptic) 534.9

  Note — Use the following fifth-digit
  subclassification with categories 531-534:

  0   without mention of obstruction
  1   with obstruction

    with
      hemorrhage (chronic) 534.4 ✓5ᵗʰ
        and perforation 534.6 ✓5ᵗʰ
      perforation 534.5 ✓5ᵗʰ
        and hemorrhage 534.6 ✓5ᵗʰ
    acute 534.3 ✓5ᵗʰ
      with
        hemorrhage 534.0 ✓5ᵗʰ
          and perforation 534.2 ✓5ᵗʰ
        perforation 534.1 ✓5ᵗʰ
          and hemorrhage 534.2 ✓5ᵗʰ
    bleeding (recurrent) — see Ulcer,
      gastrojejunal, with hemorrhage

Ulcer, ulcerated, ulcerating, ulceration, ulcerative — *continued*
  gastrojejunal — *continued*
    chronic 534.7 ✓5ᵗʰ
      with
        hemorrhage 534.4 ✓5ᵗʰ
          and perforation 534.6 ✓5ᵗʰ
        perforation 534.5 ✓5ᵗʰ
          and hemorrhage 534.6 ✓5ᵗʰ
    penetrating — *see* Ulcer, gastrojejunal, with perforation
    perforating — *see* Ulcer, gastrojejunal, with perforation
  gastrojejunocolic — *see* Ulcer, gastrojejunal
  genital organ
    female 629.8
    male 608.89
  gingiva 523.8
  gingivitis 523.1
  glottis 478.79
  granuloma of pudenda 099.2
  groin (*see also* Ulcer, skin) 707.8
  gum 523.8
  gumma, due to yaws 102.4
  hand (*see also* Ulcer, skin) 707.8
  hard palate 528.9
  heel (*see also* Ulcer, lower extremity) 707.14
    decubitus (*see also* Ulcer, decubitus) 707.0
  hemorrhoids 455.8
    external 455.5
    internal 455.2
  hip (*see also* Ulcer, skin) 707.8
    decubitus (*see also* Ulcer, decubitus) 707.0
  Hunner's 595.1
  hypopharynx 478.29
  hypopyon (chronic) (subacute) 370.04
  hypostaticum — *see* Ulcer, varicose
  ileocolitis 556.1
  ileum (*see also* Ulcer, intestine) 569.82
  intestine, intestinal 569.82
    with perforation 569.83
    amebic 006.9
    duodenal — *see* Ulcer, duodenum
    granulocytopenic (with hemorrhage) 288.0
    marginal 569.82
    perforating 569.83
    small, primary 569.82
    stercoraceous 569.82
    stercoral 569.82
    tuberculous (*see also* Tuberculosis) 014.8 ✓5ᵗʰ
    typhoid (fever) 002.0
    varicose 456.8
  ischemic 707.9
    lower extremity (*see also* Ulcer, lower extremity) 707.10
      ankle 707.13
      calf 707.12
      foot 707.15
      heel 707.14
      knee 707.19
      specified site NEC 707.19
      thigh 707.11
      toes 707.15
  jejunum, jejunal — *see* Ulcer, gastrojejunal
  keratitis (*see also* Ulcer, cornea) 370.00
  knee — *see* Ulcer, lower extremity
  labium (majus) (minus) 616.50
  laryngitis (*see also* Laryngitis) 464.00
    with obstruction 464.01
  larynx (aphthous) (contact) 478.79

Ulcer, ulcerated, ulcerating, ulceration, ulcerative — *continued*
  larynx — *continued*
    diphtheritic 032.3
  leg — *see* Ulcer, lower extremity
  lip 528.5
  Lipschütz's 616.50
  lower extremity (atrophic) (chronic) (neurogenic) (perforating) (pyogenic) (trophic) (tropical) 707.10
    with gangrene (*see also* Ulcer, lower extremity) 707.10 *[785.4]*
    arteriosclerotic 440.24
    ankle 707.13
    arteriosclerotic 440.23
      with gangrene 440.24
    calf 707.12
    decubitus 707.0
      with gangrene 707.0 *[785.4]*
    foot 707.15
    heel 707.14
    knee 707.19
    specified site NEC 707.19
    thigh 707.11
    toes 707.15
    varicose 454.0
      inflamed or infected 454.2
  luetic — *see* Ulcer, syphilitic
  lung 518.89
    tuberculous (*see also* Tuberculosis) 011.2 ✓5ᵗʰ
  malignant (M8000/3) — *see* Neoplasm, by site, malignant
  marginal NEC — *see* Ulcer, gastrojejunal
  meatus (urinarius) 597.89
  Meckel's diverticulum 751.0
  Meleney's (chronic undermining) 686.09
  Mooren's (cornea) 370.07
  mouth (traumatic) 528.9
  mycobacterial (skin) 031.1
  nasopharynx 478.29
  navel cord (newborn) 771.4
  neck (*see also* Ulcer, skin) 707.8
    uterus 622.0
  neurogenic NEC — *see* Ulcer, skin
  nose, nasal (infectional) (passage) 478.1
    septum 478.1
      varicose 456.8
    skin — *see* Ulcer, skin
  spirochetal NEC 104.8
  oral mucosa (traumatic) 528.9
  palate (soft) 528.9
  penetrating NEC — *see* Ulcer, peptic, with perforation
  penis (chronic) 607.89
  peptic (site unspecified) 533.9

> *Note* — Use the following fifth-digit subclassification with categories 531-534:
>
> 0   without mention of obstruction
> 1   with obstruction

    with
      hemorrhage 533.4 ✓5ᵗʰ
        and perforation 533.6 ✓5ᵗʰ
      perforation (chronic) 533.5 ✓5ᵗʰ
        and hemorrhage 533.6 ✓5ᵗʰ
    acute 533.3 ✓5ᵗʰ
      with
        hemorrhage 533.0 ✓5ᵗʰ
          and perforation 533.2 ✓5ᵗʰ

Ulcer, ulcerated, ulcerating, ulceration, ulcerative   **Index to Disease**

Ulcer, ulcerated, ulcerating, ulceration,
   ulcerative — *continued*
  peptic — *continued*
    acute — *continued*
      with — *continued*
        perforation 533.1 ✓5ᵗʰ
          and hemorrhage 533.2 ✓5ᵗʰ
      bleeding (recurrent) — *see* Ulcer, peptic,
        with hemorrhage
    chronic 533.7 ✓5ᵗʰ
      with
        hemorrhage 533.4 ✓5ᵗʰ
          and perforation 533.6 ✓5ᵗʰ
        perforation 533.5 ✓5ᵗʰ
          and hemorrhage 533.6 ✓5ᵗʰ
    penetrating — *see* Ulcer, peptic, with
      perforation
    perforating NEC (*see also* Ulcer, peptic, with
      perforation) 533.5 ✓5ᵗʰ
    skin 707.9
  perineum (*see also* Ulcer, skin) 707.8
  peritonsillar 474.8
  phagedenic (tropical) NEC — *see* Ulcer, skin
  pharynx 478.29
  phlebitis — *see* Phlebitis
  plaster (*see also* Ulcer, decubitus) 707.0
  popliteal space — *see* Ulcer, lower extremity
  postpyloric — *see* Ulcer, duodenum
  prepuce 607.89
  prepyloric — *see* Ulcer, stomach
  pressure (*see also* Ulcer, decubitus) 707.0
  primary of intestine 569.82
    with perforation 569.83
  proctitis 556.2
    with ulcerative sigmoiditis 556.3
  prostate 601.8
  pseudopeptic — *see* Ulcer, peptic
  pyloric — *see* Ulcer, stomach
  rectosigmoid 569.82
    with perforation 569.83
  rectum (sphincter) (solitary) 569.41
    stercoraceous, stercoral 569.41
    varicose — *see* Varicose, ulcer, anus
  retina (*see also* Chorioretinitis) 363.20
  rodent (M8090/3) — *see also* Neoplasm, skin,
    malignant
    cornea 370.07
  round — *see* Ulcer, stomach
  sacrum (region) (*see also* Ulcer, skin) 707.8
  Saemisch's 370.04
  scalp (*see also* Ulcer, skin) 707.8
  sclera 379.09
  scrofulous (*see also* Tuberculosis) 017.2 ✓5ᵗʰ
  scrotum 608.89
    tuberculous (*see also* Tuberculosis)
      016.5 ✓5ᵗʰ
    varicose 456.4
  seminal vesicle 608.89
  sigmoid 569.82
    with perforation 569.83
  skin (atrophic) (chronic) (neurogenic) (non-
    healing) (perforating) (pyogenic) (trophic)
    707.9
    with gangrene 707.9 *[785.4]*
    amebic 006.6
    decubitus 707.0
      with gangrene 707.0 *[785.4]*
    in granulocytopenia 288.0
    lower extremity (*see also* Ulcer, lower
      extremity) 707.10
      with gangrene 707.10 *[785.4]*
        arteriosclerotic 440.24

Ulcer, ulcerated, ulcerating, ulceration,
   ulcerative — *continued*
  skin — *continued*
    lower extremity — *continued*
      ankle 707.13
      arteriosclerotic 440.23
        with gangrene 440.24
      calf 707.12
      foot 707.15
      heel 707.14
      knee 707.19
      specified site NEC 707.19
      thigh 707.11
      toes 707.15
    mycobacterial 031.1
    syphilitic (early) (secondary) 091.3
    tuberculous (primary) (*see also*
      Tuberculosis) 017.0 ✓5ᵗʰ
    varicose — *see* Ulcer, varicose
  sloughing NEC — *see* Ulcer, skin
  soft palate 528.9
  solitary, anus or rectum (sphincter) 569.41
  sore throat 462
    streptococcal 034.0
  spermatic cord 608.89
  spine (tuberculous) 015.0 ✓5ᵗʰ *[730.88]*
  stasis (leg) (venous) 454.0
    without varicose veins 459.81
    inflamed or infected 454.2
  stercoral, stercoraceous 569.82
    with perforation 569.83
    anus or rectum 569.41
  stoma, stomal — *see* Ulcer, gastrojejunal
  stomach (eroded) (peptic) (round) 531.9

> Note — Use the following fifth-digit
> subclassification with categories 531-534:
>
> 0   without mention of obstruction
> 1   with obstruction

    with
      hemorrhage 531.4 ✓5ᵗʰ
        and perforation 531.6 ✓5ᵗʰ
      perforation (chronic) 531.5 ✓5ᵗʰ
        and hemorrhage 531.6 ✓5ᵗʰ
    acute 531.3 ✓5ᵗʰ
      with
        hemorrhage 531.0 ✓5ᵗʰ
          and perforation 531.2 ✓5ᵗʰ
        perforation 531.1 ✓5ᵗʰ
          and hemorrhage 531.2 ✓5ᵗʰ
    bleeding (recurrent) — *see* Ulcer, stomach,
      with hemorrhage
    chronic 531.7 ✓5ᵗʰ
      with
        hemorrhage 531.4 ✓5ᵗʰ
          and perforation 531.6 ✓5ᵗʰ
        perforation 531.5 ✓5ᵗʰ
          and hemorrhage 531.6 ✓5ᵗʰ
    penetrating — *see* Ulcer, stomach, with
      perforation
    perforating — *see* Ulcer, stomach, with
      perforation
  stomatitis 528.00
  stress — *see* Ulcer, peptic
  strumous (tuberculous) (*see also* Tuberculosis)
    017.2 ✓5ᵗʰ
  submental (*see also* Ulcer, skin) 707.8
  submucosal, bladder 595.1
  syphilitic (any site) (early) (secondary) 091.3
    late 095.9

Ulcer, ulcerated, ulcerating, ulceration, ulcerative — *continued*
  syphilitic — *continued*
    perforating 095.9
      foot 094.0
  testis 608.89
  thigh — *see* Ulcer, lower extremity
  throat 478.29
    diphtheritic 032.0
  toe — *see* Ulcer, lower extremity
  tongue (traumatic) 529.0
  tonsil 474.8
    diphtheritic 032.0
  trachea 519.1
  trophic — *see* Ulcer, skin
  tropical NEC (*see also* Ulcer, skin) 707.9
  tuberculous — *see* Tuberculosis, ulcer
  tunica vaginalis 608.89
  turbinate 730.9
  typhoid (fever) 002.0
    perforating 002.0
  umbilicus (newborn) 771.4
  unspecified site NEC — *see* Ulcer, skin
  urethra (meatus) (*see also* Urethritis) 597.89
  uterus 621.8
  uterus 621.8
    cervix 622.0
      with mention of cervicitis 616.0
    neck 622.0
      with mention of cervicitis 616.0
  vagina 616.8
  valve, heart 421.0
  varicose (lower extremity, any part) 454.0
    anus — *see* Varicose, ulcer, anus
    broad ligament 456.5
    esophagus (*see also* Varix, esophagus) 456.1
      bleeding (*see also* Varix, esophagus, bleeding) 456.0
    inflamed or infected 454.2
    nasal septum 456.8
    perineum 456.6
    rectum — *see* Varicose, ulcer, anus
    scrotum 456.4
    specified site NEC 456.8
    sublingual 456.3
    vulva 456.6
  vas deferens 608.89
  vesical (*see also* Ulcer, bladder) 596.8
  vulva (acute) (infectional) 616.50
    Behçet's syndrome 136.1 *[616.51]*
    herpetic 054.12
    tuberculous 016.7 *[616.51]*
  vulvobuccal, recurring 616.50
  x-ray — *see* Ulcer, by site
  yaws 102.4
Ulcerosa scarlatina 034.1
Ulcus — *see also* Ulcer
  cutis tuberculosum (*see also* Tuberculosis) 017.0
  duodeni — *see* Ulcer, duodenum
  durum 091.0
    extragenital 091.2
  gastrojejunale — *see* Ulcer, gastrojejunal
  hypostaticum — *see* Ulcer, varicose
  molle (cutis) (skin) 099.0
  serpens corneae (pneumococcal) 370.04
  ventriculi — *see* Ulcer, stomach
Ulegyria 742.4
Ulerythema
  acneiforma 701.8

Ulerythema — *continued*
  centrifugum 695.4
  ophryogenes 757.4
Ullrich (-Bonnevie) (-Turner) syndrome 758.6
Ullrich-Feichtiger syndrome 759.89
Ulnar — *see* condition
Ulorrhagia 523.8
Ulorrhea 523.8
Umbilicus, umbilical — *see also* condition
  cord necrosis, affecting fetus or newborn 762.6
Unavailability of medical facilities (at) V63.9
  due to
    investigation by social service agency V63.8
    lack of services at home V63.1
    remoteness from facility V63.0
    waiting list V63.2
  home V63.1
  outpatient clinic V63.0
  specified reason NEC V63.8
Uncinaria americana infestion 126.1
Uncinariasis (*see also* Ancylostomiasis) 126.9
Unconscious, unconsciousness 780.09
Underdevelopment — *see also* Undeveloped
  sexual 259.0
Undernourishment 269.9
Undernutrition 269.9
Under observation — *see* Observation
Underweight 783.22
  for gestational age — *see* Light-for-dates
Underwood's disease (sclerema neonatorum) 778.1
Undescended — *see also* Malposition, congenital
  cecum 751.4
  colon 751.4
  testis 752.51
Undetermined diagnosis or cause 799.9
Undeveloped, undevelopment — *see also* Hypoplasia
  brain (congenital) 742.1
  cerebral (congenital) 742.1
  fetus or newborn 764.9
  heart 746.89
  lung 748.5
  testis 257.2
  uterus 259.0
Undiagnosed (disease) 799.9
Undulant fever (*see also* Brucellosis) 023.9
Unemployment, anxiety concerning V62.0
Unequal leg (acquired) (length) 736.81
  congenital 755.30
Unerupted teeth, tooth 520.6
Unextracted dental root 525.3
Unguis incarnatus 703.0
Unicornis uterus 752.3
Unicorporeus uterus 752.3
Uniformis uterus 752.3
Unilateral — *see also* condition
  development, breast 611.8
  organ or site, congenital NEC — *see* Agenesis
  vagina 752.49
Unilateralis uterus 752.3
Unilocular heart 745.8
Uninhibited bladder 596.54
  with cauda equina syndrome 344.61

Uninhibited bladder — *continued*
   neurogenic — *see* Neurogenic, bladder 596.54
Union, abnormal — *see also* Fusion
   divided tendon 727.89
   larynx and trachea 748.3
Universal
   joint, cervix 620.6
   mesentery 751.4
Unknown
   cause of death 799.9
   diagnosis 799.9
Unna's disease (seborrheic dermatitis) 690.10
Unresponsiveness, adrenocorticotropin (ACTH) 255.4
Unsoundness of mind (*see also* Psychosis) 298.9
Unspecified cause of death 799.9
Unstable
   back NEC 724.9
   colon 569.89
   joint — *see* Instability, joint
   lie 652.0
      affecting fetus or newborn (before labor) 761.7
      causing obstructed labor 660.0
         affecting fetus or newborn 763.1
   lumbosacral joint (congenital) 756.19
      acquired 724.6
   sacroiliac 724.6
   spine NEC 724.9
Untruthfulness, child problem (*see also* Disturbance, conduct) 312.0
Unverricht (-Lundborg) disease, syndrome, or epilepsy 333.2
Unverricht-Wagner syndrome (dermatomyositis) 710.3
Upper respiratory — *see* condition
Upset
   gastric 536.8
      psychogenic 306.4
   gastrointestinal 536.8
      psychogenic 306.4
      virus (*see also* Enteritis, viral) 008.8
   intestinal (large) (small) 564.9
      psychogenic 306.4
   menstruation 626.9
   mental 300.9
   stomach 536.8
      psychogenic 306.4
Urachus — *see also* condition
   patent 753.7
   persistent 753.7
Uratic arthritis 274.0
Urbach's lipoid proteinosis 272.8
Urbach-Oppenheim disease or syndrome (necrobiosis lipoidica diabeticorum) 250.8 [709.3]
Urbach-Wiethe disease or syndrome (lipoid proteinosis) 272.8
Urban yellow fever 060.1
Urea, blood, high — *see* Uremia
Uremia, uremic (absorption) (amaurosis) (amblyopia) (aphasia) (apoplexy) (coma) (delirium) (dementia) (dropsy) (dyspnea) (fever) (intoxication) (mania) (paralysis) (poisoning) (toxemia) (vomiting) 586
   with
      abortion — *see* Abortion, by type, with renal failure

Uremia, uremic — *continued*
   with — *continued*
      ectopic pregnancy (*see also* categories 633.0-633.9) 639.3
      hypertension (*see also* Hypertension, kidney) 403.91
      molar pregnancy (*see also* categories 630-632) 639.3
   chronic 585
   complicating
      abortion 639.3
      ectopic or molar pregnancy 639.3
      hypertension (*see also* Hypertension, kidney) 403.91
      labor and delivery 669.3
   congenital 779.89 ▲
   extrarenal 788.9
   hypertensive (chronic) (*see also* Hypertension, kidney) 403.91
   maternal NEC, affecting fetus or newborn 760.1
   neuropathy 585 [357.4]
   pericarditis 585 [420.0]
   prerenal 788.9
   pyelitic (*see also* Pyelitis) 590.80
Ureter, ureteral — *see* condition
Ureteralgia 788.0
Ureterectasis 593.89
Ureteritis 593.89
   cystica 590.3
   due to calculus 592.1
   gonococcal (acute) 098.19
      chronic or duration of 2 months or over 098.39
   nonspecific 593.89
Ureterocele (acquired) 593.89
   congenital 753.23
Ureterolith 592.1
Ureterolithiasis 592.1
Ureterostomy status V44.6
   with complication 997.5
Urethra, urethral — *see* condition
Urethralgia 788.9
Urethritis (abacterial) (acute) (allergic) (anterior) (chronic) (nonvenereal) (posterior) (recurrent) (simple) (subacute) (ulcerative) (undifferentiated) 597.80
   diplococcal (acute) 098.0
      chronic or duration of 2 months or over 098.2
   due to Trichomonas (vaginalis) 131.02
   gonococcal (acute) 098.0
      chronic or duration of 2 months or over 098.2
   nongonococcal (sexually transmitted) 099.40
      Chlamydia trachomatis 099.41
      Reiter's 099.3
      specified organism NEC 099.49
   nonspecific (sexually transmitted) (*see also* Urethritis, nongonococcal) 099.40
   not sexually transmitted 597.80
   Reiter's 099.3
   trichomonal or due to Trichomonas (vaginalis) 131.02
   tuberculous (*see also* Tuberculosis) 016.3
   venereal NEC (*see also* Urethritis, nongonococcal) 099.40

Index to Diseases

Urethrocele
  female 618.0
    with uterine prolapse 618.4
      complete 618.3
      incomplete 618.2
  male 599.5
Urethrolithiasis 594.2
Urethro-oculoarticular syndrome 099.3
Urethro-oculosynovial syndrome 099.3
Urethrorectal — *see* condition
Urethrorrhagia 599.84
Urethrorrhea 788.7
Urethrostomy status V44.6
  with complication 997.5
Urethrotrigonitis 595.3
Urethrovaginal — *see* condition
Urhidrosis, uridrosis 705.89
Uric acid
  diathesis 274.9
  in blood 790.6
Uricacidemia 790.6
Uricemia 790.6
Uricosuria 791.9
Urination
  frequent 788.41
  painful 788.1
Urine, urinary — *see also* condition
  abnormality NEC 788.69
  blood in (*see also* Hematuria) 599.7
  discharge, excessive 788.42
  enuresis 788.30
    nonorganic origin 307.6
  extravasation 788.8
  frequency 788.41
  incontinence 788.30
    active 788.30
    female 788.30
      stress 625.6
      and urge 788.33
    male 788.30
      stress 788.32
      and urge 788.33
    mixed (stress and urge) 788.33
    neurogenic 788.39
    nonorganic origin 307.6
    stress (female) 625.6
      male NEC 788.32
  intermittent stream 788.61
  pus in 791.9
  retention or stasis NEC 788.20
    bladder, incomplete emptying 788.21
    psychogenic 306.53
    specified NEC 788.29
  secretion
    deficient 788.5
    excessive 788.42
    frequency 788.41
  stream
    intermittent 788.61
    slowing 788.62
    splitting 788.61
    weak 788.62
Urinemia — *see* Uremia
Urinoma NEC 599.9
  bladder 596.8
  kidney 593.89
  renal 593.89
  ureter 593.89

Urinoma — *continued*
  urethra 599.84
Uroarthritis, infectious 099.3
Urodialysis 788.5
Urolithiasis 592.9
Uronephrosis 593.89
Uropathy 599.9
  obstructive 599.6
Urosepsis 599.0
  meaning sepsis 038.9
  meaning urinary tract infection 599.0
Urticaria 708.9
  with angioneurotic edema 995.1
    hereditary 277.6
  allergic 708.0
  cholinergic 708.5
  chronic 708.8
  cold, familial 708.2
  dermatographic 708.3
  due to
    cold or heat 708.2
    drugs 708.0
    food 708.0
    inhalants 708.0
    plants 708.8
    serum 999.5
  factitial 708.3
  giant 995.1
    hereditary 277.6
  gigantea 995.1
    hereditary 277.6
  idiopathic 708.1
  larynx 995.1
    hereditary 277.6
  neonatorum 778.8
  nonallergic 708.1
  papulosa (Hebra) 698.2
  perstans hemorrhagica 757.39
  pigmentosa 757.33
  recurrent periodic 708.8
  serum 999.5
  solare 692.72
  specified type NEC 708.8
  thermal (cold) (heat) 708.2
  vibratory 708.4
Urticarioides acarodermatitis 133.9
Use of
  nonprescribed drugs (*see also* Abuse, drugs, nondependent) 305.9
  patent medicines (*see also* Abuse, drugs, nondependent) 305.9
Usher-Senear disease (pemphigus erythematosus) 694.4
Uta 085.5
Uterine size-date discrepancy 646.8
Uteromegaly 621.2
Uterovaginal — *see* condition
Uterovesical — *see* condition
Uterus — *see* condition
Utriculitis (utriculus prostaticus) 597.89
Uveal — *see* condition
Uveitis (anterior) (*see also* Iridocyclitis) 364.3
  acute or subacute 364.00
    due to or associated with
      gonococcal infection 098.41
      herpes (simplex) 054.44
        zoster 053.22
    primary 364.01

Uveitis — *continued*
  acute or subacute — *continued*
    recurrent 364.02
    secondary (noninfectious) 364.04
      infectious 364.03
  allergic 360.11
  chronic 364.10
    due to or associated with
      sarcoidosis 135 *[364.11]*
      tuberculosis (*see also* Tuberculosis)
        017.3 ✓5ᵗʰ *[364.11]*
    due to
      operation 360.11
      toxoplasmosis (acquired) 130.2
        congenital (active) 771.2
  granulomatous 364.10
  heterochromic 364.21
  lens-induced 364.23
  nongranulomatous 364.00
  posterior 363.20
    disseminated — *see* Chorioretinitis, disseminated
    focal — *see* Chorioretinitis, focal
  recurrent 364.02
  sympathetic 360.11
  syphilitic (secondary) 091.50
    congenital 090.0 *[363.13]*
    late 095.8 *[363.13]*
  tuberculous (*see also* Tuberculosis) 017.3 ✓5ᵗʰ *[364.11]*
Uveoencephalitis 363.22
Uveokeratitis (*see also* Iridocyclitis) 364.3
Uveoparotid fever 135
Uveoparotitis 135
Uvula — *see* condition
Uvulitis (acute) (catarrhal) (chronic) (gangrenous) (membranous) (suppurative) (ulcerative) 528.3

V

Vaccination
  complication or reaction — *see* Complications, vaccination
  not done (contraindicated) V64.0
    because of patient's decision V64.2
  prophylactic (against) V05.9
    arthropod-borne viral
      disease NEC V05.1
      encephalitis V05.0
    chickenpox V05.4
    cholera (alone) V03.0
      with typhoid-paratyphoid (cholera + TAB) V06.0
    common cold V04.7
    diphtheria (alone) V03.5
      with
        poliomyelitis (DTP+ polio) V06.3
        tetanus V06.5
          pertussis combined (DTP) V06.1
            typhoid-paratyphoid (DTP + TAB) V06.2
    disease (single) NEC V05.9
      bacterial NEC V03.9
        specified type NEC V03.89
      combinations NEC V06.9
        specified type NEC V06.8
      specified type NEC V05.8
    encephalitis, viral, arthropod-borne V05.0
    Hemophilus influenzae, type B [Hib] V03.81

Vaccination — *continued*
  prophylactic — *continued*
    hepatitis, viral V05.3
    influenza V04.8
      with
        Streptococcus pneumoniae [pneumococcus] V06.6
    lileieishmaniasis V05.2
    measles (alone) V04.2
      with mumps-rubella (MMR) V06.4
    mumps (alone) V04.6
      with measles and rubella (MMR) V06.4
    pertussis alone V03.6
    plague V03.3
    poliomyelitis V04.0
      with diphtheria-tetanus-pertussis (DTP + polio) V06.3
    rabies V04.5
    rubella (alone) V04.3
      with measles and mumps (MMR) V06.4
    smallpox V04.1
    Streptococcus pneumoniae [pneumococcus] V03.82
      with
        influenza V06.6
    tetanus toxoid (alone) V03.7
      with diphtheria [Td] V06.5
        with
          pertussis (DTP) V06.1
            with poliomyelitis (DTP+polio) V06.3
    tuberculosis (BCG) V03.2
    tularemia V03.4
    typhoid-paratyphoid (TAB) (alone) V03.1
      with diphtheria-tetanus-pertussis (TAB + DTP) V06.2
    varicella V05.4
    viral
      encephalitis, arthropod-borne V05.0
      hepatitis V05.3
    yellow fever V04.4
Vaccinia (generalized) 999.0
  congenital 771.2
  conjunctiva 999.3
  eyelids 999.0 *[373.5]*
  localized 999.3
  nose 999.3
  not from vaccination 051.0
    eyelid 051.0 *[373.5]*
  sine vaccinatione 051.0
  without vaccination 051.0
Vacuum
  extraction of fetus or newborn 763.3
  in sinus (accessory) (nasal) (*see also* Sinusitis) 473.9
Vagabond V60.0
Vagabondage V60.0
Vagabonds' disease 132.1
Vagina, vaginal — *see* condition
Vaginalitis (tunica) 608.4
Vaginismus (reflex) 625.1
  functional 306.51
  hysterical 300.11
  psychogenic 306.51
Vaginitis (acute) (chronic) (circumscribed) (diffuse) (emphysematous) (Hemophilus vaginalis) (nonspecific) (nonvenereal) (ulcerative) 616.10

Index to Diseases

Vaginitis — continued
- with
  - abortion — see Abortion, by type, with sepsis
  - ectopic pregnancy (see also categories 633.0-633.9) 639.0
  - molar pregnancy (see also categories 630-632) 639.0
- adhesive, congenital 752.49
- atrophic, postmenopausal 627.3
- bacterial 616.10
- blennorrhagic (acute) 098.0
  - chronic or duration of 2 months or over 098.2
- candidal 112.1
- chlamydial 099.53
- complicating pregnancy or puerperium 646.6 ☑5ᵗʰ
  - affecting fetus or newborn 760.8
- congenital (adhesive) 752.49
- due to
  - C. albicans 112.1
  - Trichomonas (vaginalis) 131.01
- following
  - abortion 639.0
  - ectopic or molar pregnancy 639.0
- gonococcal (acute) 098.0
  - chronic or duration of 2 months or over 098.2
- granuloma 099.2
- Monilia 112.1
- mycotic 112.1
- pinworm 127.4 [616.11]
- postirradiation 616.10
- postmenopausal atrophic 627.3
- senile (atrophic) 627.3
- syphilitic (early) 091.0
  - late 095.8
- trichomonal 131.01
- tuberculous (see also Tuberculosis) 016.7 ☑5ᵗʰ
- venereal NEC 099.8

Vaginosis — see Vaginitis

Vagotonia 352.3

Vagrancy V60.0

Vallecula — see condition

Valley fever 114.0

Valsuani's disease (progressive pernicious anemia, puerperal) 648.2 ☑5ᵗʰ

Valve, valvular (formation) — see also condition
- cerebral ventricle (communicating) in situ V45.2
- cervix, internal os 752.49
- colon 751.5
- congenital NEC — see Atresia
- formation, congenital NEC — see Atresia
- heart defect — see Anomaly, heart, valve
- ureter 753.29
  - pelvic junction 753.21
  - vesical orifice 753.22
- urethra 753.6

Valvulitis (chronic) (see also Endocarditis) 424.90
- rheumatic (chronic) (inactive) (with chorea) 397.9
  - active or acute (aortic) (mitral) (pulmonary) (tricuspid) 391.1
- syphilitic NEC 093.20
  - aortic 093.22
  - mitral 093.21
  - pulmonary 093.24

Valvulitis — continued
- syphilitic — continued
  - tricuspid 093.23

Valvulopathy — see Endocarditis

van Bogaert's leukoencephalitis (sclerosing) (subacute) 046.2

van Bogaert-Nijssen (-Peiffer) disease 330.0

van Buchem's syndrome (hyperostosis corticalis) 733.3

van Creveld-von Gierke disease (glycogenosis I) 271.0

van den Bergh's disease (enterogenous cyanosis) 289.7

van der Hoeve's syndrome (brittle bones and blue sclera, deafness) 756.51

van der Hoeve-Halbertsma-Waardenburg syndrome (ptosis-epicanthus) 270.2

van der Hoeve-Waardenburg-Gualdi syndrome (ptosis epicanthus) 270.2

Vanillism 692.89

Vanishing lung 492.0

van Neck (-Odelberg) disease or syndrome (juvenile osteochondrosis) 732.1

Vanishing twin 651.33

Vapor asphyxia or suffocation NEC 987.9
- specified agent — see Table of Drugs and Chemicals

Vaquez's disease (M9950/1) 238.4

Vaquez-Osler disease (polycythemia vera) (M9950/1) 238.4

Variance, lethal ball, prosthetic heart valve 996.02

Variants, thalassemic 282.4

Variations in hair color 704.3

Varicella 052.9
- with
  - complication 052.8
    - specified NEC 052.7
  - pneumonia 052.1
  - vaccination and inoculation (prophylactic) V05.4

Varices — see Varix

Varicocele (scrotum) (thrombosed) 456.4
- ovary 456.5
- perineum 456.6
- spermatic cord (ulcerated) 456.4

Varicose
- aneurysm (ruptured) (see also Aneurysm) 442.9
- dermatitis (lower extremity) — see Varicose, vein, inflamed or infected
- eczema — see Varicose, vein
- phlebitis — see Varicose, vein, inflamed or infected
- placental vessel — see Placenta, abnormal
- tumor — see Varicose, vein
- ulcer (lower extremity, any part) 454.0
  - anus 455.8
    - external 455.5
    - internal 455.2
  - esophagus (see also Varix, esophagus) 456.1
    - bleeding (see also Varix, esophagus, bleeding) 456.0
  - inflamed or infected 454.2
  - nasal septum 456.8
  - perineum 456.6

☑4ᵗʰ Fourth-digit Required ☑5ᵗʰ Fifth-digit Required

Varicose — continued
  ulcer — continued
    rectum — see Varicose, ulcer, anus
    scrotum 456.4
    specified site NEC 456.8
  vein (lower extremity) (ruptured) (see also
      Varix) 454.9
    with
      complications NEC 454.8 •
      edema 454.8 •
      inflammation or infection 454.1
        ulcerated 454.2
      pain 454.8 •
      stasis dermatitis 454.1
        with ulcer 454.2
      swelling 454.8 •
    ulcer 454.0
      inflamed or infected 454.2
    anus — see Hemorrhoids
    broad ligament 456.5
    congenital (peripheral) NEC 747.60
      gastrointestinal 747.61
      lower limb 747.64
      renal 747.62
      specified NEC 747.69
      upper limb 747.63
    esophagus (ulcerated) (see also Varix,
        esophagus) 456.1
      bleeding (see also Varix, esophagus,
        bleeding) 456.0
    inflamed or infected 454.1
      with ulcer 454.2
    in pregnancy or puerperium 671.0 ✓5ᵗʰ
      vulva or perineum 671.1 ✓5ᵗʰ
    nasal septum (with ulcer) 456.8
    pelvis 456.5
    perineum 456.6
      in pregnancy, childbirth, or puerperium
        671.1 ✓5ᵗʰ
    rectum — see Hemorrhoids
    scrotum (ulcerated) 456.4
    specified site NEC 456.8
    sublingual 456.3
    ulcerated 454.0
      inflamed or infected 454.2
    umbilical cord, affecting fetus or newborn
        762.6
    urethra 456.8
    vulva 456.6
      in pregnancy, childbirth, or puerperium
        671.1 ✓5ᵗʰ
    vessel — see also Varix
      placenta — see Placenta, abnormal
Varicosis, varicosities, varicosity (see also
    Varix) 454.9
Variola 050.9
  hemorrhagic (pustular) 050.0
  major 050.0
  minor 050.1
  modified 050.2
Varioloid 050.2
Variolosa, purpura 050.0
Varix (lower extremity) (ruptured) 454.9
  with
    inflammation or infection 454.1
      with ulcer 454.2
    stasis dermatitis 454.1
      with ulcer 454.2
    ulcer 454.0
      with inflammation or infection 454.2

Varix — continued
  aneurysmal (see also Aneurysm) 442.9
  anus — see Hemorrhoids
  arteriovenous (congenital) (peripheral) NEC
      747.60
    gastrointestinal 747.61
    lower limb 747.64
    renal 747.62
    specified NEC 747.69
    spinal 747.82
    upper limb 747.63
  bladder 456.5
  broad ligament 456.5
  complications NEC 454.8 •
  congenital (peripheral) NEC 747.60
  edema 454.8 •
  esophagus (ulcerated) 456.1
    bleeding 456.0
      in
        cirrhosis of liver 571.5 [456.20]
        portal hypertension 572.3 [456.20]
    congenital 747.69
      in
        cirrhosis of liver 571.5 [456.21]
          with bleeding 571.5 [456.20]
        portal hypertension 572.3 [456.21]
          with bleeding 572.3 [456.20]
  gastric 456.8
  inflamed or infected 454.1
    ulcerated 454.2
  in pregnancy or puerperium 671.0 ✓5ᵗʰ
    perineum 671.1 ✓5ᵗʰ
    vulva 671.1 ✓5ᵗʰ
  labia (majora) 456.6
  orbit 456.8
    congenital 747.69
  ovary 456.5
  pain 454.8 •
  papillary 448.1
  pelvis 456.5
  perineum 456.6
    in pregnancy or puerperium 671.1 ✓5ᵗʰ
  pharynx 456.8
  placenta — see Placenta, abnormal
  prostate 456.8
  rectum — see Hemorrhoids
  renal papilla 456.8
  retina 362.17
  scrotum (ulcerated) 456.4
  sigmoid colon 456.8
  specified site NEC 456.8
  spinal (cord) (vessels) 456.8
  spleen, splenic (vein) (with phlebolith) 456.8
  sublingual 456.3
  swelling 454.8 •
  ulcerated 454.0
    inflamed or infected 454.2
  umbilical cord, affecting fetus or newborn
      762.6
  uterine ligament 456.5
  vocal cord 456.8
  vulva 456.6
    in pregnancy, childbirth, or puerperium
      671.1 ✓5ᵗʰ
Vasa previa 663.5 ✓5ᵗʰ
  affecting fetus or newborn 762.6
  hemorrhage from, affecting fetus or newborn
      772.0
Vascular — see also condition
  loop on papilla (optic) 743.57
  sheathing, retina 362.13

Index to Diseases

Vascular — *continued*
 spasm 443.9
 spider 448.1
Vascularity, pulmonary, congenital 747.3
Vascularization
 choroid 362.16
 cornea 370.60
  deep 370.63
  localized 370.61
 retina 362.16
 subretinal 362.16
Vasculitis 447.6
 allergic 287.0
 cryoglobulinemic 273.2
 disseminated 447.6
 kidney 447.8
 leukocytoclastic 446.29
 nodular 695.2
 retinal 362.18
 rheumatic — *see* Fever, rheumatic
Vas deferens — *see* condition
Vas deferentitis 608.4
Vasectomy, admission for V25.2
Vasitis 608.4
 nodosa 608.4
 scrotum 608.4
 spermatic cord 608.4
 testis 608.4
 tuberculous (*see also* Tuberculosis) 016.5
 tunica vaginalis 608.4
 vas deferens 608.4
Vasodilation 443.9
Vasomotor — *see* condition
Vasoplasty, after previous sterilization V26.0
Vasoplegia, splanchnic (*see also* Neuropathy, peripheral, autonomic) 337.9
Vasospasm 443.9
 cerebral (artery) 435.9
  with transient neurologic deficit 435.9
 nerve
  arm NEC 354.9
  autonomic 337.9
  brachial plexus 353.0
  cervical plexus 353.2
  leg NEC 355.8
  lower extremity NEC 355.8
  peripheral NEC 355.9
  spinal NEC 355.9
  sympathetic 337.9
  upper extremity NEC 354.9
 peripheral NEC 443.9
 retina (artery) (*see also* Occlusion, retinal, artery) 362.30
Vasospastic — *see* condition
Vasovagal attack (paroxysmal) 780.2
 psychogenic 306.2
Vater's ampulla — *see* condition
VATER syndrome 759.89
Vegetation, vegetative
 adenoid (nasal fossa) 474.2
 consciousness (persistent) 780.03
 endocarditis (acute) (any valve) (chronic) (subacute) 421.0
 heart (mycotic) (valve) 421.0
 state (persistent) 780.03
Veil
 Jackson's 751.4
 over face (causing asphyxia) 768.9

Vein, venous — *see* condition
Veldt sore (*see also* Ulcer, skin) 707.9
Velpeau's hernia — *see* Hernia, femoral
Venereal
 balanitis NEC 099.8
 bubo 099.1
 disease 099.9
  specified nature or type NEC 099.8
 granuloma inguinale 099.2
 lymphogranuloma (Durand-Nicolas-Favre), any site 099.1
 salpingitis 098.37
 urethritis (*see also* Urethritis, nongonococcal) 099.40
 vaginitis NEC 099.8
 warts 078.19
Vengefulness, in child (*see also* Disturbance, conduct) 312.0
Venofibrosis 459.89
Venom, venomous
 bite or sting (animal or insect) 989.5
 poisoning 989.5
Venous — *see* condition
Ventouse delivery NEC 669.5
 affecting fetus or newborn 763.3
Ventral — *see* condition
Ventricle, ventricular — *see also* condition
 escape 427.69
 standstill (*see also* Arrest, cardiac) 427.5
Ventriculitis, cerebral (*see also* Meningitis) 322.9
Ventriculostomy status V45.2
Verbiest's syndrome (claudicatio intermittens spinalis) 435.1
Vernet's syndrome 352.6
Verneuil's disease (syphilitic bursitis) 095.7
Verruca (filiformis) 078.10
 acuminata (any site) 078.11
 necrogenica (primary) (*see also* Tuberculosis) 017.0
 plana (juvenilis) 078.19
 peruana 088.0
 peruviana 088.0
 plantaris 078.19
 seborrheica 702.19
  inflamed 702.11
 senilis 702.0
 tuberculosa (primary) (*see also* Tuberculosis) 017.0
 venereal 078.19
 viral NEC 078.10
Verrucosities (*see also* Verruca) 078.10
Verrucous endocarditis (acute) (any valve) (chronic) (subacute) 710.0 *[424.91]*
 nonbacterial 710.0 *[424.91]*
Verruga
 peruana 088.0
 peruviana 088.0
Verse's disease (calcinosis intervertebralis) 275.49 *[722.90]*
Version
 before labor, affecting fetus or newborn 761.7
 cephalic (correcting previous malposition) 652.1
  affecting fetus or newborn 763.1
 cervix (*see also* Malposition, uterus) 621.6
 uterus (postinfectional) (postpartal, old) (*see also* Malposition, uterus) 621.6

Version — *continued*
    uterus — *continued*
        forward — *see* Anteversion, uterus
        lateral — *see* Lateroversion, uterus
Vertebra, vertebral — *see* condition
Vertigo 780.4
    auditory 386.19
    aural 386.19
    benign paroxysmal positional 386.11
    central origin 386.2
    cerebral 386.2
    Dix and Hallpike (epidemic) 386.12
    endemic paralytic 078.81
    epidemic 078.81
        Dix and Hallpike 386.12
        Gerlier's 078.81
        Pedersen's 386.12
        vestibular neuronitis 386.12
    epileptic — *see* Epilepsy
    Gerlier's (epidemic) 078.81
    hysterical 300.11
    labyrinthine 386.10
    laryngeal 786.2
    malignant positional 386.2
    Ménière's (*see also* Disease, Ménière's) 386.00
    menopausal 627.2
    otogenic 386.19
    paralytic 078.81
    paroxysmal positional, benign 386.11
    Pedersen's (epidemic) 386.12
    peripheral 386.10
        specified type NEC 386.19
    positional
        benign paroxysmal 386.11
        malignant 386.2
Verumontanitis (chronic) (*see also* Urethritis) 597.89
Vesania (*see also* Psychosis) 298.9
Vesical — *see* condition
Vesicle
    cutaneous 709.8
    seminal — *see* condition
    skin 709.8
Vesicocolic — *see* condition
Vesicoperineal — *see* condition
Vesicorectal — *see* condition
Vesicourethrorectal — *see* condition
Vesicovaginal — *see* condition
Vesicular — *see* condition
Vesiculitis (seminal) 608.0
    amebic 006.8
    gonorrheal (acute) 098.14
        chronic or duration of 2 months or over 098.34
    trichomonal 131.09
    tuberculous (*see also* Tuberculosis) 016.5 ✓5ᵗʰ [608.81]
Vestibulitis (ear) (*see also* Labyrinthitis) 386.30
    nose (external) 478.1
    vulvar 616.10
Vestibulopathy, acute peripheral (recurrent) 386.12
Vestige, vestigial — *see also* Persistence
    branchial 744.41
    structures in vitreous 743.51
Vibriosis NEC 027.9
Vidal's disease (lichen simplex chronicus) 698.3
Video display tube syndrome 723.8

Vienna type encephalitis 049.8
Villaret's syndrome 352.6
Villous — *see* condition
VIN I (vulvar intraepithelial neoplasia I) 624.8
VIN II (vulvar intraepithelial neoplasia II) 624.8
VIN III (vulvar intraepithelial neoplasia III) 233.3
Vincent's
    angina 101
    bronchitis 101
    disease 101
    gingivitis 101
    infection (any site) 101
    laryngitis 101
    stomatitis 101
    tonsillitis 101
Vinson-Plummer syndrome (sideropenic dysphagia) 280.8
Viosterol deficiency (*see also* Deficiency, calciferol) 268.9
Virchow's disease 733.99
Viremia 790.8
Virilism (adrenal) (female) NEC 255.2
    with
        3-beta-hydroxysteroid dehydrogenase defect 255.2
        11-hydroxylase defect 255.2
        21-hydroxylase defect 255.2
    adrenal
        hyperplasia 255.2
        insufficiency (congenital) 255.2
    cortical hyperfunction 255.2
Virilization (female) (suprarenal) (*see also* Virilism) 255.2
    isosexual 256.4
Virulent bubo 099.0
Virus, viral — *see also* condition
    infection NEC (*see also* Infection, viral) 079.99
    septicemia 079.99
Viscera, visceral — *see* condition
Visceroptosis 569.89
Visible peristalsis 787.4
Vision, visual
    binocular, suppression 368.31
    blurred, blurring 368.8
        hysterical 300.11
    defect, defective (*see also* Impaired, vision) 369.9
    disorientation (syndrome) 368.16
    disturbance NEC (*see also* Disturbance, vision) 368.9
        hysterical 300.11
    examination V72.0
    field, limitation 368.40
    fusion, with defective steropsis 368.33
    hallucinations 368.16
    halos 368.16
    loss 369.9
        both eyes (*see also* Blindness, both eyes) 369.3
        complete (*see also* Blindness, both eyes) 369.00
        one eye 369.8
        sudden 368.16
    low (both eyes) 369.20
        one eye (other eye normal) (*see also* Impaired, vision) 369.70
            blindness, other eye 369.10

Vision, visual — *continued*
  perception, simultaneous without fusion 368.32
  tunnel 368.45
Vitality, lack or want of 780.79
  newborn 779.89
Vitamin deficiency NEC (*see also* Deficiency, vitamin) 269.2
Vitelline duct, persistent 751.0
Vitiligo 709.01
  due to pinta (carate) 103.2
  eyelid 374.53
  vulva 624.8
Vitium cordis — *see* Disease, heart
Vitreous — *see also* condition
  touch syndrome 997.99
Vocal cord — *see* condition
Vocational rehabilitation V57.22
Vogt's (Cecile) disease or syndrome 333.7
Vogt-Koyanagi syndrome 364.24
Vogt-Spielmeyer disease (amaurotic familial idiocy) 330.1
Voice
  change (*see also* Dysphonia) 784.49
  loss (*see also* Aphonia) 784.41
Volhard-Fahr disease (malignant nephrosclerosis) 403.00
Volhynian fever 083.1
Volkmann's ischemic contracture or paralysis (complicating trauma) 958.6
Voluntary starvation 307.1
Volvulus (bowel) (colon) (intestine) 560.2
  with
    hernia — *see also* Hernia, by site, with obstruction
    gangrenous — *see* Hernia, by site, with gangrene
    perforation 560.2
  congenital 751.5
  duodenum 537.3
  fallopian tube 620.5
  oviduct 620.5
  stomach (due to absence of gastrocolic ligament) 537.89
Vomiting 787.03
  with nausea 787.01
  allergic 535.4 ✓5ᵗʰ
  asphyxia 933.1
  bilious (cause unknown) 787.0
    following gastrointestinal surgery 564.3
  blood (*see also* Hematemesis) 578.0
  causing asphyxia, choking, or suffocation (*see also* Asphyxia, food) 933.1
  cyclical 536.2
    psychogenic 306.4
  epidemic 078.82
  fecal matter 569.89
  following gastrointestinal surgery 564.3
  functional 536.8
    psychogenic 306.4
  habit 536.2
  hysterical 300.11
  nervous 306.4
  neurotic 306.4
  newborn 779.3
  of or complicating pregnancy 643.9 ✓5ᵗʰ
    due to
      organic disease 643.8 ✓5ᵗʰ

Vomiting — *continued*
  of or complicating pregnancy — *continued*
    due to — *continued*
      specific cause NEC 643.8 ✓5ᵗʰ
    early — *see* Hyperemesis, gravidarum
    late (after 22 completed weeks of gestation) 643.2 ✓5ᵗʰ
  pernicious or persistent 536.2
    complicating pregnancy — *see* Hyperemesis, gravidarum
    psychogenic 306.4
  physiological 787.0
  psychic 306.4
  psychogenic 307.54
  stercoral 569.89
  uncontrollable 536.2
    psychogenic 306.4
  uremic — *see* Uremia
  winter 078.82
von Bechterew (-Strumpell) disease or syndrome (ankylosing spondylitis) 720.0
von Bezold's abscess 383.01
von Economo's disease (encephalitis lethargica) 049.8
von Eulenburg's disease (congenital paramyotonia) 359.2
von Gierke's disease (glycogenosis I) 271.0
von Gies' joint 095.8
von Graefe's disease or syndrome 378.72
von Hippel (-Lindau) disease or syndrome (retinocerebral angiomatosis) 759.6
von Jaksch's anemia or disease (pseudoleukemia infantum) 285.8
von Recklinghausen's
  disease or syndrome (nerves) (skin) (M9540/1) 237.71
  bones (osteitis fibrosa cystica) 252.0
  tumor (M9540/1) 237.71
von Recklinghausen-Applebaum disease (hemochromatosis) 275.0
von Schroetter's syndrome (intermittent venous claudication) 453.8
von Willebrand (-Jürgens) (-Minot) disease or syndrome (angiohemophilia) 286.4
von Zambusch's disease (lichen sclerosus et atrophicus) 701.0
Voorhoeve's disease or dyschondroplasia 756.4
Vossius' ring 921.3
  late effect 366.21
Voyeurism 302.82
Vrolik's disease (osteogenesis imperfecta) 756.51
Vulva — *see* condition
Vulvismus 625.1
Vulvitis (acute) (allergic) (aphthous) (chronic) (gangrenous) (hypertrophic) (intertriginous) 616.10
  with
    abortion — *see* Abortion, by type, with sepsis
    ectopic pregnancy (*see also* categories 633.0-633.9) 639.0
    molar pregnancy (*see also* categories 630-632) 639.0
  adhesive, congenital 752.49
  blennorhagic (acute) 098.0
    chronic or duration of 2 months or over 098.2

Vulvitis — *continued*
chlamydial 099.53
complicating pregnancy or puerperium 646.6 ✓5ᵗʰ
due to Ducrey's bacillus 099.0
following
　abortion 639.0
　ectopic or molar pregnancy 639.0
gonococcal (acute) 098.0
　chronic or duration of 2 months or over 098.2
herpetic 054.11
leukoplakic 624.0
monilial 112.1
puerperal, postpartum, childbirth 646.6 ✓5ᵗʰ
syphilitic (early) 091.0
　late 095.8
trichomonal 131.01
Vulvodynia 625.9
Vulvorectal — *see* condition
Vulvovaginitis (*see also* Vulvitis) 616.10
amebic 006.8
chlamydial 099.53
gonococcal (acute) 098.0
　chronic or duration of 2 months or over 098.2
herpetic 054.11
monilial 112.1
trichomonal (Trichomonas vaginalis) 131.01

W

Waardenburg's syndrome 756.89
meaning ptosis-epicanthus 270.2
Waardenburg-Klein syndrome (ptosis-epicanthus) 270.2
Wagner's disease (colloid milium) 709.3
Wagner (-Unverricht) syndrome (dermatomyositis) 710.3
Waiting list, person on V63.2
undergoing social agency investigation V63.8
Wakefulness disorder (*see also* Hypersomnia) 780.54
nonorganic origin 307.43
Waldenström's
disease (osteochondrosis, capital femoral) 732.1
hepatitis (lupoid hepatitis) 571.49
hypergammaglobulinemia 273.0
macroglobulinemia 273.3
purpura, hypergammaglobulinemic 273.0
syndrome (macroglobulinemia) 273.3
Waldenström-Kjellberg syndrome (sideropenic dysphagia) 280.8
Walking
difficulty 719.7 ✓5ᵗʰ
　psychogenic 307.9
sleep 307.46
　hysterical 300.13
Wall, abdominal — *see* condition
Wallenberg's syndrome (posterior inferior cerebellar artery) (*see also* Disease, cerebrovascular, acute) 436
Wallgren's
disease (obstruction of splenic vein with collateral circulation) 459.89
meningitis (*see also* Meningitis, aseptic) 047.9

Wandering
acetabulum 736.39
gallbladder 751.69
kidney, congenital 753.3
organ or site, congenital NEC — *see* Malposition, congenital
pacemaker (atrial) (heart) 427.89
spleen 289.59
Wardrop's disease (with lymphangitis) 681.9
finger 681.02
toe 681.11
War neurosis 300.16
Wart (common) (digitate) (filiform) (infectious) (juvenile) (plantar) (viral) 078.10
external genital organs (venereal) 078.19
fig 078.19
Hassall-Henle's (of cornea) 371.41
Henle's (of cornea) 371.41
juvenile 078.19
moist 078.10
Peruvian 088.0
plantar 078.19
prosector (*see also* Tuberculosis) 017.0 ✓5ᵗʰ
seborrheic 702.19
　inflamed 702.11
senile 702.0
specified NEC 078.19
syphilitic 091.3
tuberculous (*see also* Tuberculosis) 017.0 ✓5ᵗʰ
venereal (female) (male) 078.19
Warthin's tumor (salivary gland) (M8561/0) 210.2
Washerwoman's itch 692.4
Wassilieff's disease (leptospiral jaundice) 100.0
Wasting
disease 799.4
　due to malnutrition 261
extreme (due to malnutrition) 261
muscular NEC 728.2
palsy, paralysis 335.21
Water
clefts 366.12
deprivation of 994.3
in joint (*see also* Effusion, joint) 719.0 ✓5ᵗʰ
intoxication 276.6
itch 120.3
lack of 994.3
loading 276.6
on
　brain — *see* Hydrocephalus
　chest 511.8
poisoning 276.6
Waterbrash 787.1
Water-hammer pulse (*see also* Insufficiency, aortic) 424.1
Waterhouse (-Friderichsen) disease or syndrome 036.3
Water-losing nephritis 588.8
Wax in ear 380.4
Waxy
degeneration, any site 277.3
disease 277.3
kidney 277.3 [583.81]
liver (large) 277.3
spleen 277.3
Weak, weakness (generalized) 780.79
arches (acquired) 734
　congenital 754.61
bladder sphincter 596.59

Index to Diseases

Weak, weakness — *continued*
congenital 779.89
eye muscle — *see* Strabismus
foot (double) — *see* Weak, arches
heart, cardiac (*see also* Failure, heart) 428.9
   congenital 746.9
mind 317
muscle 728.9
myocardium (*see also* Failure, heart) 428.9
newborn 779.89
pelvic fundus 618.8
pulse 785.9
senile 797
valvular — *see* Endocarditis
Wear, worn, tooth, teeth (approximal) (hard tissues) (interproximal) (occlusal) 521.1
Weather, weathered
effects of
   cold NEC 991.9
      specified effect NEC 991.8
   hot (*see also* Heat) 992.9
   skin 692.74
Web, webbed (congenital) — *see also* Anomaly, specified type NEC
canthus 743.63
digits (*see also* Syndactylism) 755.10
esophagus 750.3
fingers (*see also* Syndactylism, fingers) 755.11
larynx (glottic) (subglottic) 748.2
neck (pterygium colli) 744.5
Paterson-Kelly (sideropenic dysphagia) 280.8
popliteal syndrome 756.89
toes (*see also* Syndactylism, toes) 755.13
Weber's paralysis or syndrome 344.89
Weber-Christian disease or syndrome (nodular nonsuppurative panniculitis) 729.30
Weber-Cockayne syndrome (epidermolysis bullosa) 757.39
Weber-Dimitri syndrome 759.6
Weber-Gubler syndrome 344.89
Weber-Leyden syndrome 344.89
Weber-Osler syndrome (familial hemorrhagic telangiectasia) 448.0
Wedge-shaped or wedging vertebra (*see also* Osteoporosis) 733.00
Wegener's granulomatosis or syndrome 446.4
Wegner's disease (syphilitic osteochondritis) 090.0
Weight
gain (abnormal) (excessive) 783.1
   during pregnancy 646.1
      insufficient 646.8
less than 1000 grams at birth 765.0
loss (cause unknown) 783.21
Weightlessness 994.9
Weil's disease (leptospiral jaundice) 100.0
Weill-Marchesani syndrome (brachymorphism and ectopia lentis) 759.89
Weingarten's syndrome (tropical eosinophilia) 518.3
Weir Mitchell's disease (erythromelalgia) 443.89
Weiss-Baker syndrome (carotid sinus syncope) 337.0
Weissenbach-Thibierge syndrome (cutaneous systemic sclerosis) 710.1
Wen (*see also* Cyst, sebaceous) 706.2

Wenckebach's phenomenon, heart block (second degree) 426.13
Werdnig-Hoffmann syndrome (muscular atrophy) 335.0
Werlhof's disease (*see also* Purpura, thrombocytopenic) 287.3
Werlhof-Wichmann syndrome (*see also* Purpura, thrombocytopenic) 287.3
Wermer's syndrome or disease (polyendocrine adenomatosis) 258.0
Werner's disease or syndrome (progeria adultorum) 259.8
Werner-His disease (trench fever) 083.1
Werner-Schultz disease (agranulocytosis) 288.0
Wernicke's encephalopathy, disease, or syndrome (superior hemorrhagic polioencephalitis) 265.1
Wernicke-Korsakoff syndrome or psychosis (nonalcoholic) 294.0
   alcoholic 291.1
Wernicke-Posadas disease (*see also* Coccidioidomycosis) 114.9
Wesselsbron fever 066.3
West African fever 084.8
West Nile fever 066.4
West Nile virus 006.4
Westphal-Strümpell syndrome (hepatolenticular degeneration) 275.1
Wet
brain (alcoholic) (*see also* Alcoholism) 303.9
feet, tropical (syndrome) (maceration) 991.4
lung (syndrome)
   adult 518.5
   newborn 770.6
Wharton's duct — *see* condition
Wheal 709.8
Wheezing 786.07
Whiplash injury or syndrome 847.0
Whipple's disease or syndrome (intestinal lipodystrophy) 040.2
Whipworm 127.3
"Whistling face" syndrome (craniocarpotarsal dystrophy) 759.89
White — *see also* condition
kidney
   large — *see* Nephrosis
   small 582.9
leg, puerperal, postpartum, childbirth 671.4
   nonpuerperal 451.19
mouth 112.0
patches of mouth 528.6
sponge nevus of oral mucosa 750.26
spot lesions, teeth 521.01
White's disease (congenital) (keratosis follicularis) 757.39
Whitehead 706.2
Whitlow (with lymphangitis) 681.01
herpetic 054.6
Whitmore's disease or fever (melioidosis) 025
Whooping cough 033.9
with pneumonia 033.9 [484.3]
due to
   Bordetella
      bronchoseptica 033.8

Whooping cough — *continued*
  due to — *continued*
    Bordetella — *continued*
      bronchoseptica — *continued*
        with pneumonia 033.8 *[484.3]*
      parapertussis 033.1
        with pneumonia 033.1 *[484.3]*
      pertussis 033.0
        with pneumonia 033.0 *[484.3]*
      specified organism NEC 033.8
        with pneumonia 033.8 *[484.3]*
  vaccination, prophylactic (against) V03.6
Wichmann's asthma (laryngismus stridulus) 478.75
Widal (-Abrami) syndrome (acquired hemolytic jaundice) 283.9
Widening aorta (*see also* Aneurysm, aorta) 441.9
  ruptured 441.5
Wilkie's disease or syndrome 557.1
Wilkinson-Sneddon disease or syndrome (subcorneal pustular dermatosis) 694.1
Willan's lepra 696.1
Willan-Plumbe syndrome (psoriasis) 696.1
Willebrand (-Jürgens) syndrome or thrombopathy (angiohemophilia) 286.4
Willi-Prader syndrome (hypogenital dystrophy with diabetic tendency) 759.81
Willis' disease (diabetes mellitus) (*see also* Diabetes) 250.0 ✓5ᵗʰ
Wilms' tumor or neoplasm (nephroblastoma) (M8960/3) 189.0
Wilson's
  disease or syndrome (hepatolenticular degeneration) 275.1
  hepatolenticular degeneration 275.1
  lichen ruber 697.0
Wilson-Brocq disease (dermatitis exfoliativa) 695.89
Wilson-Mikity syndrome 770.7
Window — *see also* Imperfect, closure
  aorticopulmonary 745.0
Winged scapula 736.89
Winter — *see also* condition
  vomiting disease 078.82
Wise's disease 696.2
Wiskott-Aldrich syndrome (eczema-thrombocytopenia) 279.12
Withdrawal symptoms, syndrome
  alcohol 291.81
    delirium (acute) 291.0
      chronic 291.1
      newborn 760.71
  drug or narcotic 292.0
  newborn, infant of dependent mother 779.5
  steroid NEC
    correct substance properly administered 255.4
    overdose or wrong substance given or taken 962.0
Withdrawing reaction, child or adolescent 313.22
Witts' anemia (achlorhydric anemia) 280.9
Witzelsucht 301.9
Woakes' syndrome (ethmoiditis) 471.1
Wohlfart-Kugelberg-Welander disease 335.11
Woillez's disease (acute idiopathic pulmonary congestion) 518.5

Wolff-Parkinson-White syndrome (anomalous atrioventricular excitation) 426.7
Wolhynian fever 083.1
Wolman's disease (primary familial xanthomatosis) 272.7
Wood asthma 495.8
Woolly, wooly hair (congenital) (nevus) 757.4
Wool-sorters' disease 022.1
Word
  blindness (congenital) (developmental) 315.01
    secondary to organic lesion 784.61
  deafness (secondary to organic lesion) 784.69
    developmental 315.31
Worm(s) (colic) (fever) (infection) (infestation) (*see also* Infestation) 128.9
  guinea 125.7
  in intestine NEC 127.9
Worm-eaten soles 102.3
Worn out (*see also* Exhaustion) 780.79
"Worried well" V65.5
Wound, open (by cutting or piercing instrument) (by firearms) (cut) (dissection) (incised) (laceration) (penetration) (perforating) (puncture) (with initial hemorrhage, not internal) 879.8

> Note — For fracture with open wound, see Fracture.
>
> For laceration, traumatic rupture, tear or penetrating wound of internal organs, such as heart, lung, liver, kidney, pelvic organs, etc., whether or not accompanied by open wound or fracture in the same region, see Injury, internal.
>
> For contused wound, see Contusion. For crush injury, see Crush. For abrasion, insect bite (nonvenomous), blister, or scratch, see Injury, superficial.
>
> Complicated includes wounds with:
>   delayed healing
>   delayed treatment
>   foreign body
>   primary infection
>
> For late effect of open wound, see Late, effect, wound, open, by site.

  abdomen, abdominal (external) (muscle) 879.2
    complicated 879.3
    wall (anterior) 879.2
      complicated 879.3
      lateral 879.4
        complicated 879.5
  alveolar (process) 873.62
    complicated 873.72
  ankle 891.0
    with tendon involvement 891.2
    complicated 891.1
  anterior chamber, eye (*see also* Wound, open, intraocular) 871.9
  anus 879.6
    complicated 879.7
  arm 884.0
    with tendon involvement 884.2
    complicated 884.1
    forearm 881.00
      with tendon involvement 881.20
      complicated 881.10

Index to Diseases — **Wound, open**

Wound, open — continued
  arm — continued
    multiple sites — see Wound, open,
      multiple, upper limb
    upper 880.03
      with tendon involvement 880.23
      complicated 880.13
        multiple sites (with axillary or shoulder
          regions) 880.09
        with tendon involvement 880.29
        complicated 880.19
  artery — see Injury, blood vessel, by site
  auditory
    canal (external) (meatus) 872.02
      complicated 872.12
    ossicles (incus) (malleus) (stapes) 872.62
      complicated 872.72
  auricle, ear 872.01
    complicated 872.11
  axilla 880.02
    with tendon involvement 880.22
    complicated 880.12
      with tendon involvement 880.29
    involving other sites of upper arm 880.09
      complicated 880.19
  back 876.0
    complicated 876.1
  bladder — see Injury, internal, bladder
  blood vessel — see Injury, blood vessel, by site
  brain — see Injury, intracranial, with open
    intracranial wound
  breast 879.0
    complicated 879.1
  brow 873.42
    complicated 873.52
  buccal mucosa 873.61
    complicated 873.71
  buttock 877.0
    complicated 877.1
  calf 891.0
    with tendon involvement 891.2
    complicated 891.1
  canaliculus lacrimalis 870.8
    with laceration of eyelid 870.2
  canthus, eye 870.8
    laceration — see Laceration, eyelid
  cavernous sinus — see Injury, intracranial
  cerebellum — see Injury, intracranial
  cervical esophagus 874.4
    complicated 874.5
  cervix — see Injury, internal, cervix
  cheek(s) (external) 873.41
    complicated 873.51
    internal 873.61
      complicated 873.71
  chest (wall) (external) 875.0
    complicated 875.1
  chin 873.44
    complicated 873.54
  choroid 363.63
  ciliary body (eye) (see also Wound, open,
    intraocular) 871.9
  clitoris 878.8
    complicated 878.9
  cochlea 872.64
    complicated 872.74
  complicated 879.9
  conjunctiva — see Wound, open, intraocular
  cornea (nonpenetrating) (see also Wound,
    open, intraocular) 871.9

Wound, open — continued
  costal region 875.0
    complicated 875.1
  Descemet's membrane (see also Wound, open,
    intraocular) 871.9
  digit(s)
    foot 893.0
      with tendon involvement 893.2
      complicated 893.1
    hand 883.0
      with tendon involvement 883.2
      complicated 883.1
  drumhead, ear 872.61
    complicated 872.71
  ear 872.8
    canal 872.02
      complicated 872.12
    complicated 872.9
    drum 872.61
      complicated 872.71
    external 872.00
      complicated 872.10
    multiple sites 872.69
      complicated 872.79
    ossicles (incus) (malleus) (stapes) 872.62
      complicated 872.72
    specified part NEC 872.69
      complicated 872.79
  elbow 881.01
    with tendon involvement 881.21
    complicated 881.11
  epididymis 878.2
    complicated 878.3
  epigastric region 879.2
    complicated 879.3
  epiglottis 874.01
    complicated 874.11
  esophagus (cervical) 874.4
    complicated 874.5
    thoracic — see Injury, internal, esophagus
  Eustachian tube 872.63
    complicated 872.73
  extremity
    lower (multiple) NEC 894.0
      with tendon involvement 894.2
      complicated 894.1
    upper (multiple) NEC 884.0
      with tendon involvement 884.2
      complicated 884.1
  eye(s) (globe) — see Wound, open, intraocular
  eyeball NEC 871.9
    laceration (see also Laceration, eyeball)
      871.4
    penetrating (see also Penetrating wound,
      eyeball) 871.7
  eyebrow 873.42
    complicated 873.52
  eyelid NEC 870.8
    laceration — see Laceration, eyelid
  face 873.40
    complicated 873.50
    multiple sites 873.49
      complicated 873.59
    specified part NEC 873.49
      complicated 873.59
  fallopian tube — see Injury, internal, fallopian
    tube
  finger(s) (nail) (subungual) 883.0
    with tendon involvement 883.2
    complicated 883.1

Fourth-digit Required   Fifth-digit Required

Wound, open — *continued*
  flank 879.4
    complicated 879.5
  foot (any part except toe(s) alone) 892.0
    with tendon involvement 892.2
    complicated 892.1
  forearm 881.00
    with tendon involvement 881.20
    complicated 881.10
  forehead 873.42
    complicated 873.52
  genital organs (external) NEC 878.8
    complicated 878.9
    internal — *see* Injury, internal, by site
  globe (eye) (*see also* Wound, open, eyeball) 871.9
  groin 879.4
    complicated 879.5
  gum(s) 873.62
    complicated 873.72
  hand (except finger(s) alone) 882.0
    with tendon involvement 882.2
    complicated 882.1
  head NEC 873.8
    with intracranial injury — *see* Injury, intracranial
      due to or associated with skull fracture — *see* Fracture, skull
    complicated 873.9
    scalp — *see* Wound, open, scalp
  heel 892.0
    with tendon involvement 892.2
    complicated 892.1
  high-velocity (grease gun) — *see* Wound, open, complicated, by site
  hip 890.0
    with tendon involvement 890.2
    complicated 890.1
  hymen 878.6
    complicated 878.7
  hypochondrium 879.4
    complicated 879.5
  hypogastric region 879.2
    complicated 879.3
  iliac (region) 879.4
    complicated 879.5
  incidental to
    dislocation — *see* Dislocation, open, by site
    fracture — *see* Fracture, open, by site
    intracranial injury — *see* Injury, intracranial, with open intracranial wound
    nerve injury — *see* Injury, nerve, by site
  inguinal region 879.4
    complicated 879.5
  instep 892.0
    with tendon involvement 892.2
    complicated 892.1
  interscapular region 876.0
    complicated 876.1
  intracranial — *see* Injury, intracranial, with open intracranial wound
  intraocular 871.9
    with
      partial loss (of intraocular tissue) 871.2
      prolapse or exposure (of intraocular tissue) 871.1
    aceration (*see also* Laceration, eyeball) 871.4

Wound, open — *continued*
  intraocular — *continued*
    penetrating 871.7
      with foreign body (nonmagnetic) 871.6
        magnetic 871.5
      without prolapse (of intraocular tissue) 871.0
  iris (*see also* Wound, open, eyeball) 871.9
  jaw (fracture not involved) 873.44
    with fracture — *see* Fracture, jaw
    complicated 873.54
  knee 891.0
    with tendon involvement 891.2
    complicated 891.1
  labium (majus) (minus) 878.4
    complicated 878.5
  lacrimal apparatus, gland, or sac 870.8
    with laceration of eyelid 870.2
  larynx 874.01
    with trachea 874.00
      complicated 874.10
    complicated 874.11
  leg (multiple) 891.0
    with tendon involvement 891.2
    complicated 891.1
    lower 891.0
      with tendon involvement 891.2
      complicated 891.1
    thigh 890.0
      with tendon involvement 890.2
      complicated 890.1
    upper 890.0
      with tendon involvement 890.2
      complicated 890.1
  lens (eye) (alone) (*see also* Cataract, traumatic) 366.20
    with involvement of other eye structures — *see* Wound, open, eyeball
  limb
    lower (multiple) NEC 894.0
      with tendon involvement 894.2
      complicated 894.1
    upper (multiple) NEC 884.0
      with tendon involvement 884.2
      complicated 884.1
  lip 873.43
    complicated 873.53
  loin 876.0
    complicated 876.1
  lumbar region 876.0
    complicated 876.1
  malar region 873.41
    complicated 873.51
  mastoid region 873.49
    complicated 873.59
  mediastinum — *see* Injury, internal, mediastinum
  midthoracic region 875.0
    complicated 875.1
  mouth 873.60
    complicated 873.70
    floor 873.64
      complicated 873.74
    multiple sites 873.69
      complicated 873.79
    specified site NEC 873.69
      complicated 873.79

Index to Diseases

Wound, open

Wound, open — continued
multiple, unspecified site(s) 879.8

> Note — Multiple open wounds of sites classifiable to the same four-digit category should be classified to that category unless they are in different limbs.
>
> Multiple open wounds of sites classifiable to different four-digit categories, or to different limbs, should be coded separately.

 complicated 879.9
 lower limb(s) (one or both) (sites classifiable to more than one three-digit category in 890 to 893) 894.0
  with tendon involvement 894.2
  complicated 894.1
 upper limb(s) (one or both) (sites classifiable to more than one three-digit category in 880 to 883) 884.0
  with tendon involvement 884.2
  complicated 884.1
muscle — see Sprain, by site
nail
 finger(s) 883.0
  complicated 883.1
 thumb 883.0
  complicated 883.1
 toe(s) 893.0
  complicated 893.1
nape (neck) 874.8
 complicated 874.9
 specified part NEC 874.8
  complicated 874.9
nasal — see also Wound, open, nose
 cavity 873.22
  complicated 873.32
 septum 873.21
  complicated 873.31
 sinuses 873.23
  complicated 873.33
nasopharynx 873.22
 complicated 873.32
neck 874.8
 complicated 874.9
 nape 874.8
  complicated 874.9
 specified part NEC 874.8
  complicated 874.9
nerve — see Injury, nerve, by site
non-healing surgical 998.83
nose 873.20
 complicated 873.30
 multiple sites 873.29
  complicated 873.39
 septum 873.21
  complicated 873.31
 sinuses 873.23
  complicated 873.33
occipital region — see Wound, open, scalp
ocular NEC 871.9
 adnexa 870.9
  specified region NEC 870.8
 laceration (see also Laceration, ocular) 871.4
 muscle (extraocular) 870.3
  with foreign body 870.4
 eyelid 870.1
 intraocular — see Wound, open, eyeball
 penetrating (see also Penetrating wound, ocular) 871.7

Wound, open — continued
orbit 870.8
 penetrating 870.3
  with foreign body 870.4
orbital region 870.9
ovary — see Injury, internal, pelvic organs
palate 873.65
 complicated 873.75
palm 882.0
 with tendon involvement 882.2
 complicated 882.1
parathyroid (gland) 874.2
 complicated 874.3
parietal region — see Wound, open, scalp
pelvic floor or region 879.6
 complicated 879.7
penis 878.0
 complicated 878.1
perineum 879.6
 complicated 879.7
periocular area 870.8
 laceration of skin 870.0
pharynx 874.4
 complicated 874.5
pinna 872.01
 complicated 872.11
popliteal space 891.0
 with tendon involvement 891.2
 complicated 891.1
prepuce 878.0
 complicated 878.1
pubic region 879.2
 complicated 879.3
pudenda 878.8
 complicated 878.9
rectovaginal septum 878.8
 complicated 878.9
sacral region 877.0
 complicated 877.1
sacroiliac region 877.0
 complicated 877.1
salivary (ducts) (glands) 873.69
 complicated 873.79
scalp 873.0
 complicated 873.1
scalpel, fetus or newborn 767.8
scapular region 880.01
 with tendon involvement 880.21
 complicated 880.11
 involving other sites of upper arm 880.09
  with tendon involvement 880.29
  complicated 880.19
sclera — (see also Wound, open, intraocular) 871.9
scrotum 878.2
 complicated 878.3
seminal vesicle — see Injury, internal, pelvic organs
shin 891.0
 with tendon involvement 891.2
 complicated 891.1
shoulder 880.00
 with tendon involvement 880.20
 complicated 880.10
 involving other sites of upper arm 880.09
  with tendon involvement 880.29
  complicated 880.19
skin NEC 879.8
 complicated 879.9
skull — see also Injury, intracranial, with open intracranial wound

Wound, open — *continued*
  skull — *continued*
    with skull fracture — *see* Fracture, skull
  spermatic cord (scrotal) 878.2
    complicated 878.3
    pelvic region — *see* Injury, internal, spermatic cord
  spinal cord — *see* Injury, spinal
  sternal region 875.0
    complicated 875.1
  subconjunctival — *see* Wound, open, intraocular
  subcutaneous NEC 879.8
    complicated 879.9
  submaxillary region 873.44
    complicated 873.54
  submental region 873.44
    complicated 873.54
  subungual
    finger(s) (thumb) — *see* Wound, open, finger
    toe(s) — *see* Wound, open, toe
  supraclavicular region 874.8
    complicated 874.9
  supraorbital 873.42
    complicated 873.52
  surgical, non-healing 998.83
  temple 873.49
    complicated 873.59
  temporal region 873.49
    complicated 873.59
  testis 878.2
    complicated 878.3
  thigh 890.0
    with tendon involvement 890.2
    complicated 890.1
  thorax, thoracic (external) 875.0
    complicated 875.1
  throat 874.8
    complicated 874.9
  thumb (nail) (subungual) 883.0
    with tendon involvement 883.2
    complicated 883.1
  thyroid (gland) 874.2
    complicated 874.3
  toe(s) (nail) (subungual) 893.0
    with tendon involvement 893.2
    complicated 893.1
  tongue 873.64
    complicated 873.74
  tonsil — *see* Wound, open, neck
  trachea (cervical region) 874.02
    with larynx 874.00
      complicated 874.10
    complicated 874.12
    intrathoracic — *see* Injury, internal, trachea
  trunk (multiple) NEC 879.6
    complicated 879.7
    specified site NEC 879.6
      complicated 879.7
  tunica vaginalis 878.2
    complicated 878.3
  tympanic membrane 872.61
    complicated 872.71
  tympanum 872.61
    complicated 872.71
  umbilical region 879.2
    complicated 879.3
  ureter — *see* Injury, internal, ureter
  urethra — *see* Injury, internal, urethra
  uterus — *see* Injury, internal, uterus

Wound, open — *continued*
  uvula 873.69
    complicated 873.79
  vagina 878.6
    complicated 878.7
  vas deferens — *see* Injury, internal, vas deferens
  vitreous (humor) 871.2
  vulva 878.4
    complicated 878.5
  wrist 881.02
    with tendon involvement 881.22
    complicated 881.12
Wright's syndrome (hyperabduction) 447.8
  pneumonia 390 *[517.1]*
Wringer injury — *see* Crush injury, by site
Wrinkling of skin 701.8
Wrist — *see also* condition
  drop (acquired) 736.05
Wrong drug (given in error) NEC 977.9
  specified drug or substance — *see* Table of Drugs and Chemicals
Wry neck — *see also* Torticollis
  congenital 754.1
Wuchereria infestation 125.0
  bancrofti 125.0
  Brugia malayi 125.1
  malayi 125.1
Wuchereriasis 125.0
Wuchereriosis 125.0
Wuchernde struma langhans (M8332/3) 193

X

Xanthelasma 272.2
  eyelid 272.2 *[374.51]*
  palpebrarum 272.2 *[374.51]*
Xanthelasmatosis (essential) 272.2
Xanthelasmoidea 757.33
Xanthine stones 277.2
Xanthinuria 277.2
Xanthofibroma (M8831/0) — *see* Neoplasm, connective tissue, benign
Xanthoma(s), xanthomatosis 272.2
  with
    hyperlipoproteinemia
      type I 272.3
      type III 272.2
      type IV 272.1
      type V 272.3
  bone 272.7
  craniohypophyseal 277.8
  cutaneotendinous 272.7
  diabeticorum 250.8 ✓5th *[272.2]*
  disseminatum 272.7
  eruptive 272.2
  eyelid 272.2 *[374.51]*
  familial 272.7
  hereditary 272.7
  hypercholesterinemic 272.0
  hypercholesterolemic 272.0
  hyperlipemic 272.4
  hyperlipidemic 272.4
  infantile 272.7
  joint 272.7
  juvenile 272.7
  multiple 272.7
  multiplex 272.7

Xanthoma(s), xanthomatosis — *continued*
  primary familial 272.7
  tendon (sheath) 272.7
  tuberosum 272.2
  tuberous 272.2
  tubo-eruptive 272.2
Xanthosis 709.09
  surgical 998.81
Xenophobia 300.29
Xeroderma (congenital) 757.39
  acquired 701.1
    eyelid 373.33
  eyelid 373.33
  pigmentosum 757.33
  vitamin A deficiency 264.8
Xerophthalmia 372.53
  vitamin A deficiency 264.7
Xerosis
  conjunctiva 372.53
    with Bitôt's spot 372.53
      vitamin A deficiency 264.1
    vitamin A deficiency 264.0
  cornea 371.40
    with corneal ulceration 370.00
      vitamin A deficiency 264.3
    vitamin A deficiency 264.2
  cutis 706.8
  skin 706.8
Xerostomia 527.7
Xiphodynia 733.90
Xiphoidalgia 733.90
Xiphoiditis 733.99
Xiphopagus 759.4
XO syndrome 758.81
X-ray
  effects, adverse, NEC 990
  of chest
    for suspected tuberculosis V71.2
    routine V72.5
XXX syndrome 758.81
XXXXY syndrome 758.81
XXY syndrome 758.7
Xyloketosuria 271.8
Xylosuria 271.8
Xylulosuria 271.8
XYY syndrome 758.81

Y

Yawning 786.09
  psychogenic 306.1
Yaws 102.9
  bone or joint lesions 102.6
  butter 102.1
  chancre 102.0
  cutaneous, less than five years after infection 102.2
  early (cutaneous) (macular) (maculopapular) (micropapular) (papular) 102.2
    frambeside 102.2
    skin lesions NEC 102.2
  eyelid 102.9 *[373.4]*
  ganglion 102.6
  gangosis, gangosa 102.5
  gumma, gummata 102.4
    bone 102.6

Yaws — *continued*
  gummatous
    frambeside 102.4
    osteitis 102.6
    periostitis 102.6
  hydrarthrosis 102.6
  hyperkeratosis (early) (late) (palmar) (plantar) 102.3
  initial lesions 102.0
  joint lesions 102.6
  juxta-articular nodules 102.7
  late nodular (ulcerated) 102.4
  latent (without clinical manifestations) (with positive serology) 102.8
  mother 102.0
  mucosal 102.7
  multiple papillomata 102.1
  nodular, late (ulcerated) 102.4
  osteitis 102.6
  papilloma, papillomata (palmar) (plantar) 102.1
  periostitis (hypertrophic) 102.6
  ulcers 102.4
  wet crab 102.1
Yeast infection (*see also* Candidiasis) 112.9
Yellow
  atrophy (liver) 570
    chronic 571.8
    resulting from administration of blood, plasma, serum, or other biological substance (within 8 months of administration) — *see* Hepatitis, viral
  fever — *see* Fever, yellow
  jack (*see also* Fever, yellow) 060.9
  jaundice (*see also* Jaundice) 782.4
Yersinia septica 027.8

Z

Zagari's disease (xerostomia) 527.7
Zahorsky's disease (exanthema subitum) 057.8
  syndrome (herpangina) 074.0
Zenker's diverticulum (esophagus) 530.6
Ziehen-Oppenheim disease 333.6
Zieve's syndrome (jaundice, hyperlipemia, and hemolytic anemia) 571.1
Zika fever 066.3
Zollinger-Ellison syndrome (gastric hypersecretion with pancreatic islet cell tumor) 251.5
Zona (*see also* Herpes, zoster) 053.9
Zoophilia (erotica) 302.1
Zoophobia 300.29
Zoster (herpes) (*see also* Herpes, zoster) 053.9
Zuelzer (-Ogden) anemia or syndrome (nutritional megaloblastic anemia) 281.2
Zygodactyly (*see also* Syndactylism) 755.10
Zygomycosis 117.7
Zymotic — *see* condition

SECTION 2

Alphabetic Index to Poisoning and External Causes of Adverse Effects of Drugs and Other Chemical Substances

TABLE OF DRUGS AND CHEMICALS

This table contains a classification of drugs and other chemical substances to identify poisoning states and external causes of adverse effects.

Each of the listed substances in the table is assigned a code according to the poisoning classification (960-989). These codes are used when there is a statement of poisoning, overdose, wrong substance given or taken, or intoxication.

The table also contains a listing of external causes of adverse effects. An adverse effect is a pathologic manifestation due to ingestion or exposure to drugs or other chemical substances (e.g., dermatitis, hypersensitivity reaction, aspirin gastritis). The adverse effect is to be identified by the appropriate code found in Section 1, Index to Diseases and Injuries. An external cause code can then be used to identify the circumstances involved. The table headings pertaining to external causes are defined below:

> **Accidental poisoning (E850-E869)** — accidental overdose of drug, wrong substance given or taken, drug taken inadvertently, accidents in the usage of drugs and biologicals in medical and surgical procedures, and to show external causes of poisonings classifiable to 980-989.
>
> **Therapeutic use (E930-E949)** — a correct substance properly administered in therapeutic or prophylactic dosage as the external cause of adverse effects.
>
> **Suicide attempt (E950-E952)** — instances in which self-inflicted injuries or poisonings are involved.
>
> **Assault (E961-E962)** — injury or poisoning inflicted by another person with the intent to injure or kill.
>
> **Undetermined (E980-E982)** — to be used when the intent of the poisoning or injury cannot be determined whether it was intentional or accidental.

The American Hospital Formulary Service list numbers are included in the table to help classify new drugs not identified in the table by name. The AHFS list numbers are keyed to the continually revised American Hospital Formulary Service (AHFS).* These listings are found in the table under the main term **Drug.**

Excluded from the table are radium and other radioactive substances. The classification of adverse effects and complications pertaining to these substances will be found in Section 1, Index to Diseases and Injuries, and Section 3, Index to External Causes of Injuries.

Although certain substances are indexed with one or more subentries, the majority are listed according to one use or state. It is recognized that many substances may be used in various ways, in medicine and in industry, and may cause adverse effects whatever the state of the agent (solid, liquid, or fumes arising from a liquid). In cases in which the reported data indicates a use or state not in the table, or which is clearly different from the one listed, an attempt should be made to classify the substance in the form which most nearly expresses the reported facts.

*American Hospital Formulary Service, 2 vol. (Washington, D.C.: American Society of Hospital Pharmacists, 1959–)

Table of Drugs and Chemicals — Aconitum ferox

			External Cause (E-Code)			
	Poisoning	Accident	Therapeutic Use	Suicide Attempt	Assault	Undetermined
1-propanol	980.3	E860.4	—	E950.9	E962.1	E980.9
2-propanol	980.2	E860.3	—	E950.9	E962.1	E980.9
2, 4-D (dichlorophenoxyacetic acid)	989.4	E863.5	—	E950.6	E962.1	E980.7
2, 4-toluene diisocyanate	983.0	E864.0	—	E950.7	E962.1	E980.6
2, 4, 5-T (trichlorophenoxyacetic acid)	989.2	E863.5	—	E950.6	E962.1	E980.7
14-hydroxydihydromorphinone	965.09	E850.2	E935.2	E950.0	E962.0	E980.0
ABOB	961.7	E857	E931.7	E950.4	E962.0	E980.4
Abrus (seed)	988.2	E865.3	—	E950.9	E962.1	E980.9
Absinthe	980.0	E860.1	—	E950.9	E962.1	E980.9
beverage	980.0	E860.0	—	E950.9	E962.1	E980.9
Acenocoumarin, acenocoumarol	964.2	E858.2	E934.2	E950.4	E962.0	E980.4
Acepromazine	969.1	E853.0	E939.1	E950.3	E962.0	E980.3
Acetal	982.8	E862.4	—	E950.9	E962.1	E980.9
Acetaldehyde (vapor)	987.8	E869.8	—	E952.8	E962.2	E982.8
liquid	989.89	E866.8	—	E950.9	E962.1	E980.9
Acetaminophen	965.4	E850.4	E935.4	E950.0	E962.0	E980.0
Acetaminosalol	965.1	E850.3	E935.3	E950.0	E962.0	E980.0
Acetanilid(e)	965.4	E850.4	E935.4	E950.0	E962.0	E980.0
Acetarsol, acetarsone	961.1	E857	E931.1	E950.4	E962.0	E980.4
Acetazolamide	974.2	E858.5	E944.2	E950.4	E962.0	E980.4
Acetic						
acid	983.1	E864.1	—	E950.7	E962.1	E980.6
with sodium acetate (ointment)	976.3	E858.7	E946.3	E950.4	E962.0	E980.4
irrigating solution	974.5	E858.5	E944.5	E950.4	E962.0	E980.4
lotion	976.2	E858.7	E946.2	E950.4	E962.0	E980.4
anhydride	983.1	E864.1	—	E950.7	E962.1	E980.6
ether (vapor)	982.8	E862.4	—	E950.9	E962.1	E980.9
Acetohexamide	962.3	E858.0	E932.3	E950.4	E962.0	E980.4
Acetomenaphthone	964.3	E858.2	E934.3	E950.4	E962.0	E980.4
Acetomorphine	965.01	E850.0	E935.0	E950.0	E962.0	E980.0
Acetone (oils) (vapor)	982.8	E862.4	—	E950.9	E962.1	E980.9
Acetophenazine (maleate)	969.1	E853.0	E939.1	E950.3	E962.0	E980.3
Acetophenetidin	965.4	E850.4	E935.4	E950.0	E962.0	E980.0
Acetophenone	982.0	E862.4	—	E950.9	E962.1	E980.9
Acetorphine	965.09	E850.2	E935.2	E950.0	E962.0	E980.0
Acetosulfone (sodium)	961.8	E857	E931.8	E950.4	E962.0	E980.4
Acetrizoate (sodium)	977.8	E858.8	E947.8	E950.4	E962.0	E980.4
Acetylcarbromal	967.3	E852.2	E937.3	E950.2	E962.0	E980.2
Acetylcholine (chloride)	971.0	E855.3	E941.0	E950.4	E962.0	E980.4
Acetylcysteine	975.5	E858.6	E945.5	E950.4	E962.0	E980.4
Acetyldigitoxin	972.1	E858.3	E942.1	E950.4	E962.0	E980.4
Acetyldihydrocodeine	965.09	E850.2	E935.2	E950.0	E962.0	E980.0
Acetyldihydrocodeinone	965.09	E850.2	E935.2	E950.0	E962.0	E980.0
Acetylene (gas) (industrial)	987.1	E868.1	—	E951.8	E962.2	E981.8
incomplete combustion of — see Carbon monoxide, fuel, utility						
tetrachloride (vapor)	982.3	E862.4	—	E950.9	E962.1	E980.9
Acetyliodosalicylic acid	965.1	E850.3	E935.3	E950.0	E962.0	E980.0
Acetylphenylhydrazine	965.8	E850.8	E935.8	E950.0	E962.0	E980.0
Acetylsalicylic acid	965.1	E850.3	E935.3	E950.0	E962.0	E980.0
Achromycin	960.4	E856	E930.4	E950.4	E962.0	E980.4
ophthalmic preparation	976.5	E858.7	E946.5	E950.4	E962.0	E980.4
topical NEC	976.0	E858.7	E946.0	E950.4	E962.0	E980.4
Acidifying agents	963.2	E858.1	E933.2	E950.4	E962.0	E980.4
Acids (corrosive) NEC	983.1	E864.1	—	E950.7	E962.1	E980.6
Aconite (wild)	988.2	E865.4	—	E950.9	E962.1	E980.9
Aconitine (liniment)	976.8	E858.7	E946.8	E950.4	E962.0	E980.4
Aconitum ferox	988.2	E865.4	—	E950.9	E962.1	E980.9

Fourth-digit Required Fifth-digit Required

Table of Drugs and Chemicals

		External Cause (E-Code)				
	Poisoning	Accident	Therapeutic Use	Suicide Attempt	Assault	Undetermined
Acridine	983.0	E864.0	—	E950.7	E962.1	E980.6
vapor	987.8	E869.8	—	E952.8	E962.2	E982.8
Acriflavine	961.9	E857	E931.9	E950.4	E962.0	E980.4
Acrisorcin	976.0	E858.7	E946.0	E950.4	E962.0	E980.4
Acrolein (gas)	987.8	E869.8	—	E952.8	E962.2	E982.8
liquid	989.89	E866.8	—	E950.9	E962.1	E980.9
Actaea spicata	988.2	E865.4	—	E950.9	E962.1	E980.9
Acterol	961.5	E857	E931.5	E950.4	E962.0	E980.4
ACTH	962.4	E858.0	E932.4	E950.4	E962.0	E980.4
Acthar	962.4	E858.0	E932.4	E950.4	E962.0	E980.4
Actinomycin (C)(D)	960.7	E856	E930.7	E950.4	E962.0	E980.4
Adalin (acetyl)	967.3	E852.2	E937.3	E950.2	E962.0	E980.2
Adenosine (phosphate)	977.8	E858.8	E947.8	E950.4	E962.0	E980.4
Adhesives	989.89	E866.6	—	E950.9	E962.1	E980.9
ADH	962.5	E858.0	E932.5	E950.4	E962.0	E980.4
Adicillin	960.0	E856	E930.0	E950.4	E962.0	E980.4
Adiphenine	975.1	E855.6	E945.1	E950.4	E962.0	E980.4
Adjunct, pharmaceutical	977.4	E858.8	E947.4	E950.4	E962.0	E980.4
Adrenal (extract, cortex or medulla) (glucocorticoids) (hormones) (mineralocorticoids)	962.0	E858.0	E932.0	E950.4	E962.0	E980.4
ENT agent	976.6	E858.7	E946.6	E950.4	E962.0	E980.4
ophthalmic preparation	976.5	E858.7	E946.5	E950.4	E962.0	E980.4
topical NEC	976.0	E858.7	E946.0	E950.4	E962.0	E980.4
Adrenalin	971.2	E855.5	E941.2	E950.4	E962.0	E980.4
Adrenergic blocking agents	971.3	E855.6	E941.3	E950.4	E962.0	E980.4
Adrenergics	971.2	E855.5	E941.2	E950.4	E962.0	E980.4
Adrenochrome (derivatives)	972.8	E858.3	E942.8	E950.4	E962.0	E980.4
Adrenocorticotropic hormone	962.4	E858.0	E932.4	E950.4	E962.0	E980.4
Adrenocorticotropin	962.4	E858.0	E932.4	E950.4	E962.0	E980.4
Adriamycin	960.7	E856	E930.7	E950.4	E962.0	E980.4
Aerosol spray — see **Sprays**						
Aerosporin	960.8	E856	E930.8	E950.4	E962.0	E980.4
ENT agent	976.6	E858.7	E946.6	E950.4	E962.0	E980.4
ophthalmic preparation	976.5	E858.7	E946.5	E950.4	E962.0	E980.4
topical NEC	976.0	E858.7	E946.0	E950.4	E962.0	E980.4
Aethusa cynapium	988.2	E865.4	—	E950.9	E962.1	E980.9
Afghanistan black	969.6	E854.1	E939.6	E950.3	E962.0	E980.3
Aflatoxin	989.7	E865.9	—	E950.9	E962.1	E980.9
African boxwood	988.2	E865.4	—	E950.9	E962.1	E980.9
Agar (-agar)	973.3	E858.4	E943.3	E950.4	E962.0	E980.4
Agricultural agent NEC	989.89	E863.9	—	E950.6	E962.1	E980.7
Agrypnal	967.0	E851	E937.0	E950.1	E962.0	E980.1
Air contaminant(s), source or type not specified	987.9	E869.9	—	E952.9	E962.2	E982.9
specified type — see specific substance						
Akee	988.2	E865.4	—	E950.9	E962.1	E980.9
Akrinol	976.0	E858.7	E946.0	E950.4	E962.0	E980.4
Alantolactone	961.6	E857	E931.6	E950.4	E962.0	E980.4
Albamycin	960.8	E856	E930.8	E950.4	E962.0	E980.4
Albumin (normal human serum)	964.7	E858.2	E934.7	E950.4	E962.0	E980.4
Albuterol ●	975.7	E858.6	E945.7	E950.4	E962.0	E980.4
Alcohol	980.9	E860.9	—	E950.9	E962.1	E980.9
absolute	980.0	E860.1	—	E950.9	E962.1	E980.9
beverage	980.0	E860.0	E947.8	E950.9	E962.1	E980.9
amyl	980.3	E860.4	—	E950.9	E962.1	E980.9
antifreeze	980.1	E860.2	—	E950.9	E962.1	E980.9
butyl	980.3	E860.4	—	E950.9	E962.1	E980.9
dehydrated	980.0	E860.1	—	E950.9	E862.1	E980.9
beverage	980.0	E860.0	E947.8	E950.9	E962.1	E980.9
denatured	980.0	E860.1	—	E950.9	E962.1	E980.9

Table of Drugs and Chemicals

Aluminium, aluminum (gel) (hydroxide)

	Poisoning	External Cause (E-Code)				
		Accident	Therapeutic Use	Suicide Attempt	Assault	Undetermined
Alcohol — *continued*						
deterrents	977.3	E858.8	E947.3	E950.4	E962.0	E980.4
diagnostic (gastric function)	977.8	E858.8	E947.8	E950.4	E962.0	E980.4
ethyl	980.0	E860.1	—	E950.9	E962.1	E980.9
beverage	980.0	E860.0	E947.8	E950.9	E962.1	E980.9
grain	980.0	E860.1	—	E950.9	E962.1	E980.9
beverage	980.0	E860.0	E947.8	E950.9	E962.1	E980.9
industrial	980.9	E860.9	—	E950.9	E962.1	E980.9
isopropyl	980.2	E860.3	—	E950.9	E962.1	E980.9
methyl	980.1	E860.2	—	E950.9	E962.1	E980.9
preparation for consumption	980.0	E860.0	E947.8	E950.9	E962.1	E980.9
propyl	980.3	E860.4	—	E950.9	E962.1	E980.9
secondary	980.2	E860.3	—	E950.9	E962.1	E980.9
radiator	980.1	E860.2	—	E950.9	E962.1	E980.9
rubbing	980.2	E860.3	—	E950.9	E962.1	E980.9
specified type NEC	980.8	E860.8	—	E950.9	E962.1	E980.9
surgical	980.9	E860.9	—	E950.9	E962.1	E980.9
vapor (from any type of alcohol)	987.8	E869.8	—	E952.8	E962.2	E982.8
wood	980.1	E860.2	—	E950.9	E962.1	E980.9
Alcuronium chloride	975.2	E858.6	E945.2	E950.4	E962.0	E980.4
Aldactone	974.4	E858.5	E944.4	E950.4	E962.0	E980.4
Aldicarb	989.3	E863.2	—	E950.6	E962.1	E980.7
Aldomet	972.6	E858.3	E942.6	E950.4	E962.0	E980.4
Aldosterone	962.0	E858.0	E932.0	E950.4	E962.0	E980.4
Aldrin (dust)	989.2	E863.0	—	E950.6	E962.1	E980.7
Algeldrate	973.0	E858.4	E943.0	E950.4	E962.0	E980.4
Alidase	963.4	E858.1	E933.4	E950.4	E962.0	E980.4
Aliphatic thiocyanates	989.0	E866.8	—	E950.9	E962.1	E980.9
Alkaline antiseptic solution (aromatic)	976.6	E858.7	E946.6	E950.4	E962.0	E980.4
Alkalinizing agents (medicinal)	963.3	E858.1	E933.3	E950.4	E962.0	E980.4
Alkalis, caustic	983.2	E864.2	—	E950.7	E962.1	E980.6
Alkalizing agents (medicinal)	963.3	E858.1	E933.3	E950.4	E962.0	E980.4
Alka-seltzer	965.1	E850.3	E935.3	E950.0	E962.0	E980.0
Alkavervir	972.6	E858.3	E942.6	E950.4	E962.0	E980.4
Allegron	969.0	E854.0	E939.0	E950.3	E962.0	E980.3
Alleve — *see* **Naproxen**						
Allobarbital, allobarbitone	967.0	E851	E937.0	E950.1	E962.0	E980.1
Allopurinol	974.7	E858.5	E944.7	E950.4	E962.0	E980.4
Allylestrenol	962.2	E858.0	E932.2	E950.4	E962.0	E980.4
Allylisopropylacetylurea	967.8	E852.8	E937.8	E950.2	E962.0	E980.2
Allylisopropylmalonylurea	967.0	E851	E937.0	E950.1	E962.0	E980.1
Allyltribromide	967.3	E852.2	E937.3	E950.2	E962.0	E980.2
Aloe, aloes, aloin	973.1	E858.4	E943.1	E950.4	E962.0	E980.4
Alosetron	973.8	E858.4	E943.8	E950.4	E962.0	E980.4
Aloxidone	966.0	E855.0	E936.0	E950.4	E962.0	E980.4
Aloxiprin	965.1	E850.3	E935.3	E950.0	E962.0	E980.0
Alpha amylase	963.4	E858.1	E933.4	E950.4	E962.0	E980.4
Alphaprodine (hydrochloride)	965.09	E850.2	E935.2	E950.0	E962.0	E980.0
Alpha tocopherol	963.5	E858.1	E933.5	E950.4	E962.0	E980.4
Alseroxylon	972.6	E858.3	E942.6	E950.4	E962.0	E980.4
Alum (ammonium) (potassium)	983.2	E864.2	—	E950.7	E962.1	E980.6
medicinal (astringent) NEC	976.2	E858.7	E946.2	E950.4	E962.0	E980.4
Aluminium, aluminum (gel) (hydroxide)	973.0	E858.4	E943.0	E950.4	E962.0	E980.4
acetate solution	976.2	E858.7	E946.2	E950.4	E962.0	E980.4
aspirin	965.1	E850.3	E935.3	E950.0	E962.0	E980.0
carbonate	973.0	E858.4	E943.0	E950.4	E962.0	E980.4
glycinate	973.0	E858.4	E943.0	E950.4	E962.0	E980.4
nicotinate	972.2	E858.3	E942.2	E950.4	E962.0	E980.4
ointment (surgical) (topical)	976.3	E858.7	E946.3	E950.4	E962.0	E980.4
phosphate	973.0	E858.4	E943.0	E950.4	E962.0	E980.4

Aluminium — Table of Drugs and Chemicals

	Poisoning	External Cause (E-Code)				
		Accident	Therapeutic Use	Suicide Attempt	Assault	Undetermined
Aluminium — *continued*						
subacetate	976.2	E858.7	E946.2	E950.4	E962.0	E980.4
topical NEC	976.3	E858.7	E946.3	E950.4	E962.0	E980.4
Alurate	967.0	E851	E937.0	E950.1	E962.0	E980.1
Alverine (citrate)	975.1	E858.6	E945.1	E950.4	E962.0	E980.4
Alvodine	965.09	E850.2	E935.2	E950.0	E962.0	E980.0
Amanita phalloides	988.1	E865.5	—	E950.9	E962.1	E980.9
Amantadine (hydrochloride)	966.4	E855.0	E936.4	E950.4	E962.0	E980.4
Ambazone	961.9	E857	E931.9	E950.4	E962.0	E980.4
Ambenonium	971.0	E855.3	E941.0	E950.4	E962.0	E980.4
Ambutonium bromide	971.1	E855.4	E941.1	E950.4	E962.0	E980.4
Ametazole	977.8	E858.8	E947.8	E950.4	E962.0	E980.4
Amethocaine (infiltration)						
(topical)	968.5	E855.2	E938.5	E950.4	E962.0	E980.4
nerve block (peripheral)						
(plexus)	968.6	E855.2	E938.6	E950.4	E962.0	E980.4
spinal	968.7	E855.2	E938.7	E950.4	E962.0	E980.4
Amethopterin	963.1	E858.1	E933.1	E950.4	E962.0	E980.4
Amfepramone	977.0	E858.8	E947.0	E950.4	E962.0	E980.4
Amidon	965.02	E850.1	E935.1	E950.0	E962.0	E980.0
Amidopyrine	965.5	E850.5	E935.5	E950.0	E962.0	E980.0
Aminacrine	976.0	E858.7	E946.0	E950.4	E962.0	E980.4
Aminitrozole	961.5	E857	E931.5	E950.4	E962.0	E980.4
Aminoacetic acid	974.5	E858.5	E944.5	E950.4	E962.0	E980.4
Amino acids	974.5	E858.5	E944.5	E950.4	E962.0	E980.4
Aminocaproic acid	964.4	E858.2	E934.4	E950.4	E962.0	E980.4
Aminoethylisothiourium	963.8	E858.1	E933.8	E950.4	E962.0	E980.4
Aminoglutethimide	966.3	E855.0	E936.3	E950.4	E962.0	E980.4
Aminometradine	974.3	E858.5	E944.3	E950.4	E962.0	E980.4
Aminopentamide	971.1	E855.4	E941.1	E950.4	E962.0	E980.4
Aminophenazone	965.5	E850.5	E935.5	E950.0	E962.0	E980.0
Aminophenol	983.0	E864.0	—	E950.7	E962.1	E980.6
Aminophenylpyridone	969.5	E853.8	E939.5	E950.3	E962.0	E980.3
Aminophyllin	975.7	E858.6	E945.7	E950.4	E962.0	E980.4
Aminopterin	963.1	E858.1	E933.1	E950.4	E962.0	E980.4
Aminopyrine	965.5	E850.5	E935.5	E950.0	E962.0	E980.0
Aminosalicylic acid	961.8	E857	E931.8	E950.4	E962.0	E980.4
Amiphenazole	970.1	E854.3	E940.1	E950.4	E962.0	E980.4
Amiquinsin	972.6	E858.3	E942.6	E950.4	E962.0	E980.4
Amisometradine	974.3	E858.5	E944.3	E950.4	E962.0	E980.4
Amitriptyline	969.0	E854.0	E939.0	E950.3	E962.0	E980.3
Ammonia (fumes) (gas) (vapor)	987.8	E869.8	—	E952.8	E962.2	E982.8
liquid (household) NEC	983.2	E861.4	—	E950.7	E962.1	E980.6
spirit, aromatic	970.8	E854.3	E940.8	E950.4	E962.0	E980.4
Ammoniated mercury	976.0	E858.7	E946.0	E950.4	E962.0	E980.4
Ammonium						
carbonate	983.2	E864.2	—	E950.7	E962.1	E980.6
chloride (acidifying agent)	963.2	E858.1	E933.2	E950.4	E962.0	E980.4
expectorant	975.5	E858.6	E945.5	E950.4	E962.0	E980.4
compounds (household)						
NEC	983.2	E861.4	—	E950.7	E962.1	E980.6
fumes (any usage)	987.8	E869.8	—	E952.8	E962.2	E982.8
industrial	983.2	E864.2	—	E950.7	E962.1	E980.6
ichthyosulfonate	976.4	E858.7	E946.4	E950.4	E962.0	E980.4
mandelate	961.9	E857	E931.9	E950.4	E962.0	E980.4
Amobarbital	967.0	E851	E937.0	E950.1	E962.0	E980.1
Amodiaquin(e)	961.4	E857	E931.4	E950.4	E962.0	E980.4
Amopyroquin(e)	961.4	E857	E931.4	E950.4	E962.0	E980.4
Amphenidone	969.5	E853.8	E939.5	E950.3	E962.0	E980.3
Amphetamine	969.7	E854.2	E939.7	E950.3	E962.0	E980.3
Amphomycin	960.8	E856	E930.8	E950.4	E962.0	E980.4
Amphotericin B	960.1	E856	E930.1	E950.4	E962.0	E980.4
topical	976.0	E858.7	E946.0	E950.4	E962.0	E980.4
Ampicillin	960.0	E856	E930.0	E950.4	E962.0	E980.4

Table of Drugs and Chemicals — Anthelmintics

	Poisoning	External Cause (E-Code)				
		Accident	Therapeutic Use	Suicide Attempt	Assault	Undetermined
Amprotropine	971.1	E855.4	E941.1	E950.4	E962.0	E980.4
Amygdalin	977.8	E858.8	E947.8	E950.4	E962.0	E980.4
Amyl						
acetate (vapor)	982.8	E862.4	—	E950.9	E962.1	E980.9
alcohol	980.3	E860.4	—	E950.9	E962.1	E980.9
nitrite (medicinal)	972.4	E858.3	E942.4	E950.4	E962.0	E980.4
Amylase (alpha)	963.4	E858.1	E933.4	E950.4	E962.0	E980.4
Amylene hydrate	980.8	E860.8	—	E950.9	E962.1	E980.9
Amylobarbitone	967.0	E851	E937.0	E950.1	E962.0	E980.1
Amylocaine	968.9	E855.2	E938.9	E950.4	E962.0	E980.4
infiltration (subcutaneous)	968.5	E855.2	E938.5	E950.4	E962.0	E980.4
nerve block (peripheral) (plexus)	968.6	E855.2	E938.6	E950.4	E962.0	E980.4
spinal	968.7	E855.2	E938.7	E950.4	E962.0	E980.4
topical (surface)	968.5	E855.2	E938.5	E950.4	E962.0	E980.4
Amytal (sodium)	967.0	E851	E937.0	E950.1	E962.0	E980.1
Analeptics	970.0	E854.3	E940.0	E950.4	E962.0	E980.4
Analgesics	965.9	E850.9	E935.9	E950.0	E962.0	E980.0
aromatic NEC	965.4	E850.4	E935.4	E950.0	E962.0	E980.0
non-narcotic NEC	965.7	E850.7	E935.7	E950.0	E962.0	E980.0
specified NEC	965.8	E850.8	E935.8	E950.0	E962.0	E980.0
Anamirta cocculus	988.2	E865.3	—	E950.9	E962.1	E980.9
Ancillin	960.0	E856	E930.0	E950.4	E962.0	E980.4
Androgens (anabolic congeners)	962.1	E858.0	E932.1	E950.4	E962.0	E980.4
Androstalone	962.1	E858.0	E932.1	E950.4	E962.0	E980.4
Androsterone	962.1	E858.0	E932.1	E950.4	E962.0	E980.4
Anemone pulsatilla	988.2	E865.4	—	E950.9	E962.1	E980.9
Anesthesia, anesthetic						
(general) NEC	968.4	E855.1	E938.4	E950.4	E962.0	E980.4
block (nerve) (plexus)	968.6	E855.2	E938.6	E950.4	E962.0	E980.4
gaseous NEC	968.2	E855.1	E938.2	E950.4	E962.0	E980.4
halogenated hydrocarbon derivatives NEC	968.2	E855.1	E938.2	E950.4	E962.0	E980.4
infiltration (intradermal) (subcutaneous) (submucosal)	968.5	E855.2	E938.5	E950.4	E962.0	E980.4
intravenous	968.3	E855.1	E938.3	E950.4	E962.0	E980.4
local NEC	968.9	E855.2	E938.9	E950.4	E962.0	E980.4
nerve blocking (peripheral) (plexus)	968.6	E855.2	E938.6	E950.4	E962.0	E980.4
rectal NEC	968.3	E855.1	E938.3	E950.4	E962.0	E980.4
spinal	968.7	E855.2	E938.7	E950.4	E962.0	E980.4
surface	968.5	E855.2	E938.5	E950.4	E962.0	E980.4
topical	968.5	E855.2	E938.5	E950.4	E962.0	E980.4
Aneurine	963.5	E858.1	E933.5	E950.4	E962.0	E980.4
Angio-Conray	977.8	E858.8	E947.8	E950.4	E962.0	E980.4
Angiotensin	971.2	E855.5	E941.2	E950.4	E962.0	E980.4
Anhydrohydroxyprogesterone	962.2	E858.0	E932.2	E950.4	E962.0	E980.4
Anhydron	974.3	E858.5	E944.3	E950.4	E962.0	E980.4
Anileridine	965.09	E850.2	E935.2	E950.0	E962.0	E980.0
Aniline (dye) (liquid)	983.0	E864.0	—	E950.7	E962.1	E980.6
analgesic	965.4	E850.4	E935.4	E950.0	E962.0	E980.0
derivatives, therapeutic NEC	965.4	E850.4	E935.4	E950.0	E962.0	E980.0
vapor	987.8	E869.8	—	E952.8	E962.2	E982.8
Anisindione	964.2	E858.2	E934.2	E950.4	E962.0	E980.4
Aniscoropine	971.1	E855.4	E941.1	E950.4	E962.0	E980.4
Anorexic agents	977.0	E858.8	E947.0	E950.4	E962.0	E980.4
Ant (bite) (sting)	989.5	E905.5	—	E950.9	E962.1	E980.9
Antabuse	977.3	E858.8	E947.3	E950.4	E962.0	E980.4
Antacids	973.0	E858.4	E943.0	E950.4	E962.0	E980.4
Antazoline	963.0	E858.1	E933.0	E950.4	E962.0	E980.4
Anthelmintics	961.6	E857	E931.6	E950.4	E962.0	E980.4

Fourth-digit Required   Fifth-digit Required

Anthralin — Table of Drugs and Chemicals

	Poisoning	External Cause (E-Code)			
		Accident	Therapeutic Use	Suicide Attempt	Assault	Undetermined
Anthralin	976.4	E858.7	E946.4	E950.4	E962.0	E980.4
Anthramycin	960.7	E856	E930.7	E950.4	E962.0	E980.4
Antiadrenergics	971.3	E855.6	E941.3	E950.4	E962.0	E980.4
Antiallergic agents	963.0	E858.1	E933.0	E950.4	E962.0	E980.4
Antianemic agents NEC	964.1	E858.2	E934.1	E950.4	E962.0	E980.4
Antiaris toxicaria	988.2	E865.4	—	E950.9	E962.1	E980.9
Antiarteriosclerotic agents	972.2	E858.3	E942.2	E950.4	E962.0	E980.4
Antiasthmatics	975.7	E858.6	E945.7	E950.4	E962.0	E980.4
Antibiotics	960.9	E856	E930.9	E950.4	E962.0	E980.4
antifungal	960.1	E856	E930.1	E950.4	E962.0	E980.4
antimycobacterial	960.6	E856	E930.6	E950.4	E962.0	E980.4
antineoplastic	960.7	E856	E930.7	E950.4	E962.0	E980.4
cephalosporin (group)	960.5	E856	E930.5	E950.4	E962.0	E980.4
chloramphenicol (group)	960.2	E856	E930.2	E950.4	E962.0	E980.4
macrolides	960.3	E856	E930.3	E950.4	E962.0	E980.4
specified NEC	960.8	E856	E930.8	E950.4	E962.0	E980.4
tetracycline (group)	960.4	E856	E930.4	E950.4	E962.0	E980.4
Anticancer agents NEC	963.1	E858.1	E933.1	E950.4	E962.0	E980.4
antibiotics	960.7	E856	E930.7	E950.4	E962.0	E980.4
Anticholinergics	971.1	E855.4	E941.1	E950.4	E962.0	E980.4
Anticholinesterase (organophosphorus) (reversible)	971.0	E855.3	E941.0	E950.4	E962.0	E980.4
Anticoagulants	964.2	E858.2	E934.2	E950.4	E962.0	E980.4
antagonists	964.5	E858.2	E934.5	E950.4	E962.0	E980.4
Anti-common cold agents NEC	975.6	E858.6	E945.6	E950.4	E962.0	E980.4
Anticonvulsants NEC	966.3	E855.0	E936.3	E950.4	E962.0	E980.4
Antidepressants	969.0	E854.0	E939.0	E950.3	E962.0	E980.3
Antidiabetic agents	962.3	E858.0	E932.3	E950.4	E962.0	E980.4
Antidiarrheal agents	973.5	E858.4	E943.5	E950.4	E962.0	E980.4
Antidiuretic hormone	962.5	E858.0	E932.5	E950.4	E962.0	E980.4
Antidotes NEC	977.2	E858.8	E947.2	E950.4	E962.0	E980.4
Antiemetic agents	963.0	E858.1	E933.0	E950.4	E962.0	E980.4
Antiepilepsy agent NEC	966.3	E855.0	E936.3	E950.4	E962.0	E980.4
Antifertility pills	962.2	E858.0	E932.2	E950.4	E962.0	E980.4
Antiflatulents	973.8	E858.4	E943.8	E950.4	E962.0	E980.4
Antifreeze	989.89	E866.8	—	E950.9	E962.1	E980.9
alcohol	980.1	E860.2	—	E950.9	E962.1	E980.9
ethylene glycol	982.8	E862.4	—	E950.9	E962.1	E980.9
Antifungals (nonmedicinal) (sprays)	989.4	E863.6	—	E950.6	E962.1	E980.7
medicinal NEC	961.9	E857	E931.9	E950.4	E962.0	E980.4
antibiotic	960.1	E856	E930.1	E950.4	E962.0	E980.4
topical	976.0	E858.7	E946.0	E950.4	E962.0	E980.4
Antigastric secretion agents	973.0	E858.4	E943.0	E950.4	E962.0	E980.4
Anthelmintics	961.6	E857	E931.6	E950.4	E962.0	E980.4
Antihemophilic factor (human)	964.7	E858.2	E934.7	E950.4	E962.0	E980.4
Antihistamine	963.0	E858.1	E933.0	E950.4	E962.0	E980.4
Antihypertensive agents NEC	972.6	E858.3	E942.6	E950.4	E962.0	E980.4
Anti-infectives NEC	961.9	E857	E931.9	E950.4	E962.0	E980.4
antibiotics	960.9	E856	E930.9	E950.4	E962.0	E980.4
specified NEC	960.8	E856	E930.8	E950.4	E962.0	E980.4
anthelmintic	961.6	E857	E931.6	E950.4	E962.0	E980.4
antimalarial	961.4	E857	E931.4	E950.4	E962.0	E980.4
antimycobacterial NEC	961.8	E857	E931.8	E950.4	E962.0	E980.4
antibiotics	960.6	E856	E930.6	E950.4	E962.0	E980.4
antiprotozoal NEC	961.5	E857	E931.5	E950.4	E962.0	E980.4
blood	961.4	E857	E931.4	E950.4	E962.0	E980.4
antiviral	961.7	E857	E931.7	E950.4	E962.0	E980.4
arsenical	961.1	E857	E931.1	E950.4	E962.0	E980.4
ENT agents	976.6	E858.7	E946.6	E950.4	E962.0	E980.4
heavy metals NEC	961.2	E857	E931.2	E950.4	E962.0	E980.4
local	976.0	E858.7	E946.0	E950.4	E962.0	E980.4
ophthalmic preparation	976.5	E858.7	E946.5	E950.4	E962.0	E980.4

Table of Drugs and Chemicals — Aristocort

		External Cause (E-Code)				
	Poisoning	Accident	Therapeutic Use	Suicide Attempt	Assault	Undetermined
Anti-infectives — *continued*						
topical NEC	976.0	E858.7	E946.0	E950.4	E962.0	E980.4
Anti-inflammatory agents						
(topical)	976.0	E858.7	E946.0	E950.4	E962.0	E980.4
Antiknock (tetraethyl lead)	984.1	E862.1	—	E950.9	E962.1	E980.9
Antilipemics	972.2	E858.3	E942.2	E950.4	E962.0	E980.4
Antimalarials	961.4	E857	E931.4	E950.4	E962.0	E980.4
Antimony (compounds) (vapor) NEC	985.4	E866.2	—	E950.9	E962.1	E980.9
anti-infectives	961.2	E857	E931.2	E950.4	E962.0	E980.4
pesticides (vapor)	985.4	E863.4	—	E950.6	E962.2	E980.7
potassium tartrate	961.2	E857	E931.2	E950.4	E962.0	E980.4
tartrated	961.2	E857	E931.2	E950.4	E962.0	E980.4
Antimuscarinic agents	971.1	E855.4	E941.1	E950.4	E962.0	E980.4
Antimycobacterials NEC	961.8	E857	E931.8	E950.4	E962.0	E980.4
antibiotics	960.6	E856	E930.6	E950.4	E962.0	E980.4
Antineoplastic agents	963.1	E858.1	E933.1	E950.4	E962.0	E980.4
antibiotics	960.7	E856	E930.7	E950.4	E962.0	E980.4
Anti-Parkinsonism agents	966.4	E855.0	E936.4	E950.4	E962.0	E980.4
Antiphlogistics	965.69	E850.6	E935.6	E950.0	E962.0	E980.0
Antiprotozoals NEC	961.5	E857	E931.5	E950.4	E962.0	E980.4
blood	961.4	E857	E931.4	E950.4	E962.0	E980.4
Antipruritics (local)	976.1	E858.7	E946.1	E950.4	E962.0	E980.4
Antipsychotic agents NEC	969.3	E853.8	E939.3	E950.3	E962.0	E980.3
Antipyretics	965.9	E850.9	E935.9	E950.0	E962.0	E980.0
specified NEC	965.8	E850.8	E935.8	E950.0	E962.0	E980.0
Antipyrine	965.5	E850.5	E935.5	E950.0	E962.0	E980.0
Antirabies serum (equine)	979.9	E858.8	E949.9	E950.4	E962.0	E980.4
Antirheumatics	965.69	E850.6	E935.6	E950.0	E962.0	E980.0
Antiseborrheics	976.4	E858.7	E946.4	E950.4	E962.0	E980.4
Antiseptics (external) (medicinal)	976.0	E858.7	E946.0	E950.4	E962.0	E980.4
Antistine	963.0	E858.1	E933.0	E950.4	E962.0	E980.4
Antithyroid agents	962.8	E858.0	E932.8	E950.4	E962.0	E980.4
Antitoxin, any	979.9	E858.8	E949.9	E950.4	E962.0	E980.4
Antituberculars	961.8	E857	E931.8	E950.4	E962.0	E980.4
antibiotics	960.6	E856	E930.6	E950.4	E962.0	E980.4
Antitussives	975.4	E858.6	E945.4	E950.4	E962.0	E980.4
Antivaricose agents (sclerosing)	972.7	E858.3	E942.7	E950.4	E962.0	E980.4
Antivenin (crotaline) (spider-bite)	979.9	E858.8	E949.9	E950.4	E962.0	E980.4
Antivert	963.0	E858.1	E933.0	E950.4	E962.0	E980.4
Antivirals NEC	961.7	E857	E931.7	E950.4	E962.0	E980.4
Ant poisons — *see* Pesticides						
Antrol	989.4	E863.4	—	E950.6	E962.1	E980.7
fungicide	989.4	E863.6	—	E950.6	E962.1	E980.7
Apomorphine hydrochloride (emetic)	973.6	E858.4	E943.6	E950.4	E962.0	E980.4
Appetite depressants, central	977.0	E858.8	E947.0	E950.4	E962.0	E980.4
Apresoline	972.6	E858.3	E942.6	E950.4	E962.0	E980.4
Aprobarbital, aprobarbitone	967.0	E851	E937.0	E950.1	E962.0	E980.1
Apronalide	967.8	E852.8	E937.8	E950.2	E962.0	E980.2
Aqua fortis	983.1	E864.1	—	E950.7	E962.1	E980.6
Arachis oil (topical)	976.3	E858.7	E946.3	E950.4	E962.0	E980.4
cathartic	973.2	E858.4	E943.2	E950.4	E962.0	E980.4
Aralen	961.4	E857	E931.4	E950.4	E962.0	E980.4
Arginine salts	974.5	E858.5	E944.5	E950.4	E962.0	E980.4
Argyrol	976.0	E858.7	E946.0	E950.4	E962.0	E980.4
ENT agent	976.6	E858.7	E946.6	E950.4	E962.0	E980.4
ophthalmic preparation	976.5	E858.7	E946.5	E950.4	E962.0	E980.4
Aristocort	962.0	E858.0	E932.0	E950.4	E962.0	E980.4
ENT agent	976.6	E858.7	E946.6	E950.4	E962.0	E980.4
ophthalmic preparation	976.5	E858.7	E946.5	E950.4	E962.0	E980.4

✓4ᵗʰ Fourth-digit Required   ✓5ᵗʰ Fifth-digit Required

Table of Drugs and Chemicals

	External Cause (E-Code)					
	Poisoning	Accident	Therapeutic Use	Suicide Attempt	Assault	Undetermined
Aristocort — continued						
topical NEC	976.0	E858.7	E946.0	E950.4	E962.0	E980.4
Aromatics, corrosive	983.0	E864.0	—	E950.7	E962.1	E980.6
disinfectants	983.0	E861.4	—	E950.7	E962.1	E980.6
Arsenate of lead (insecticide)	985.1	E863.4	—	E950.8	E962.1	E980.8
herbicide	985.1	E863.5	—	E950.8	E962.1	E980.8
Arsenic, arsenicals (compounds) (dust) (fumes) (vapor) NEC	985.1	E866.3	—	E950.8	E962.1	E980.8
anti-infectives	961.1	E857	E931.1	E950.4	E962.0	E980.4
pesticide (dust) (fumes)	985.1	E863.4	—	E950.8	E962.1	E980.8
Arsine (gas)	985.1	E866.3	—	E950.8	E962.1	E980.8
Arsphenamine (silver)	961.1	E857	E931.1	E950.4	E962.0	E980.4
Arsthinol	961.1	E857	E931.1	E950.4	E962.0	E980.4
Artane	971.1	E855.4	E941.1	E950.4	E962.0	E980.4
Arthropod (venomous) NEC	989.5	E905.5	—	E950.9	E962.1	E980.9
Asbestos	989.81	E866.8	—	E950.9	E962.1	E980.9
Ascaridole	961.6	E857	E931.6	E950.4	E962.0	E980.4
Ascorbic acid	963.5	E858.1	E933.5	E950.4	E962.0	E980.4
Asiaticoside	976.0	E858.7	E946.0	E950.4	E962.0	E980.4
Aspidium (oleoresin)	961.6	E857	E931.6	E950.4	E962.0	E980.4
Aspirin	965.1	E850.3	E935.3	E950.0	E962.0	E980.0
Astringents (local)	976.2	E858.7	E946.2	E950.4	E962.0	E980.4
Atabrine	961.3	E857	E931.3	E950.4	E962.0	E980.4
Ataractics	969.5	E853.8	E939.5	E950.3	E962.0	E980.3
Atonia drug, intestinal	973.3	E858.4	E943.3	E950.4	E962.0	E980.4
Atophan	974.7	E858.5	E944.7	E950.4	E962.0	E980.4
Atropine	971.1	E855.4	E941.1	E950.4	E962.0	E980.4
Attapulgite	973.5	E858.4	E943.5	E950.4	E962.0	E980.4
Attenuvax	979.4	E858.8	E949.4	E950.4	E962.0	E980.4
Aureomycin	960.4	E856	E930.4	E950.4	E962.0	E980.4
ophthalmic preparation	976.5	E858.7	E946.5	E950.4	E962.0	E980.4
topical NEC	976.0	E858.7	E946.0	E950.4	E962.0	E980.4
Aurothioglucose	965.69	E850.6	E935.6	E950.0	E962.0	E980.0
Aurothioglycanide	965.69	E850.6	E935.6	E950.0	E962.0	E980.0
Aurothiomalate	965.69	E850.6	E935.6	E950.0	E962.0	E980.0
Automobile fuel	981	E862.1	—	E950.9	E962.1	E980.9
Autonomic nervous system agents NEC	971.9	E855.9	E941.9	E950.4	E962.0	E980.4
Avlosulfon	961.8	E857	E931.8	E950.4	E962.0	E980.4
Avomine	967.8	E852.8	E937.8	E950.2	E962.0	E980.2
Azacyclonol	969.5	E853.8	E939.5	E950.3	E962.0	E980.3
Azapetine	971.3	E855.6	E941.3	E950.4	E962.0	E980.4
Azaribine	963.1	E858.1	E933.1	E950.4	E962.0	E980.4
Azaserine	960.7	E856	E930.7	E950.4	E962.0	E980.4
Azathioprine	963.1	E858.1	E933.1	E950.4	E962.0	E980.4
Azosulfamide	961.0	E857	E931.0	E950.4	E962.0	E980.4
Azulfidine	961.0	E857	E931.0	E950.4	E962.0	E980.4
Azuresin	977.8	E858.8	E947.8	E950.4	E962.0	E980.4
Bacimycin	976.0	E858.7	E946.0	E950.4	E962.0	E980.4
ophthalmic preparation	976.5	E858.7	E946.5	E950.4	E962.0	E980.4
Bacitracin	960.8	E856	E930.8	E950.4	E962.0	E980.4
ENT agent	976.6	E858.7	E946.6	E950.4	E962.0	E980.4
ophthalmic preparation	976.5	E858.7	E946.5	E950.4	E962.0	E980.4
topical NEC	976.0	E858.7	E946.0	E950.4	E962.0	E980.4
Baking soda	963.3	E858.1	E933.3	E950.4	E962.0	E980.4
BAL	963.8	E858.1	E933.8	E950.4	E962.0	E980.4
Bamethan (sulfate)	972.5	E858.3	E942.5	E950.4	E962.0	E980.4
Bamipine	963.0	E858.1	E933.0	E950.4	E962.0	E980.4
Baneberry	988.2	E865.4	—	E950.9	E962.1	E980.9
Banewort	988.2	E865.4	—	E950.9	E962.1	E980.9
Barbenyl	967.0	E851	E937.0	E950.1	E962.0	E980.1
Barbital, barbitone	967.0	E851	E937.0	E950.1	E962.0	E980.1

Table of Drugs and Chemicals — Benzyl

	Poisoning	External Cause (E-Code)				
		Accident	Therapeutic Use	Suicide Attempt	Assault	Undetermined
Barbiturates, barbituric acid	967.0	E851	E937.0	E950.1	E962.0	E980.1
anesthetic (intravenous)	968.3	E855.1	E938.3	E950.4	E962.0	E980.4
Barium (carbonate) (chloride) (sulfate)	985.8	E866.4	—	E950.9	E962.1	E980.9
diagnostic agent	977.8	E858.8	E947.8	E950.4	E962.0	E980.4
pesticide	985.8	E863.4	—	E950.6	E962.1	E980.7
rodenticide	985.8	E863.7	—	E950.6	E962.1	E980.7
Barrier cream	976.3	E858.7	E946.3	E950.4	E962.0	E980.4
Battery acid or fluid	983.1	E864.1	—	E950.7	E962.1	E980.6
Bay rum	980.8	E860.8	—	E950.9	E962.1	E980.9
BCG vaccine	978.0	E858.8	E948.0	E950.4	E962.0	E980.4
Bearsfoot	988.2	E865.4	—	E950.9	E962.1	E980.9
Beclamide	966.3	E855.0	E936.3	E950.4	E962.0	E980.4
Bee (sting) (venom)	989.5	E905.3	—	E950.9	E962.1	E980.9
Belladonna (alkaloids)	971.1	E855.4	E941.1	E950.4	E962.0	E980.4
Bemegride	970	E854.3	E940.0	E950.4	E962.0	E980.4
Benactyzine	969.8	E855.8	E939.8	E950.3	E962.0	E980.3
Benadryl	963.0	E858.1	E933.0	E950.4	E962.0	E980.4
Bendrofluazide	974.3	E858.5	E944.3	E950.4	E962.0	E980.4
Bendroflumethiazide	974.3	E858.5	E944.3	E950.4	E962.0	E980.4
Benemid	974.7	E858.5	E944.7	E950.4	E962.0	E980.4
Benethamine penicillin G	960.0	E856	E930.0	E950.4	E962.0	E980.4
Benisone	976	E858.7	E946.0	E950.4	E962.0	E980.4
Benoquin	976.8	E858.7	E946.8	E950.4	E962.0	E980.4
Benoxinate	968.5	E855.2	E938.5	E950.4	E962.0	E980.4
Bentonite	976.3	E858.7	E946.3	E950.4	E962.0	E980.4
Benzalkonium (chloride)	976.0	E858.7	E946.0	E950.4	E962.0	E980.4
ophthalmic preparation	976.5	E858.7	E946.5	E950.4	E962.0	E980.4
Benzamidosalicylate (calcium)	961.8	E857	E931.8	E950.4	E962.0	E980.4
Benzathine penicillin	960.0	E856	E930.0	E950.4	E962.0	E980.4
Benzcarbimine	963.1	E858.1	E933.1	E950.4	E962.0	E980.4
Benzedrex	971.2	E855.5	E941.2	E950.4	E962.0	E980.4
Benzedrine (amphetamine)	969.7	E854.2	E939.7	E950.3	E962.0	E980.3
Benzene (acetyl) (dimethyl) (methyl) (solvent) (vapor)	982.0	E862.4	—	E950.9	E962.1	E980.9
hexachloride (gamma) (insecticide) (vapor)	989.2	E863.0	—	E950.6	E962.1	E980.7
Benzethonium	976.0	E858.7	E946.0	E950.4	E962.0	E980.4
Benzhexol (chloride)	966.4	E855.0	E936.4	E950.4	E962.0	E980.4
Benzilonium	971.1	E855.4	E941.1	E950.4	E962.0	E980.4
Benzin(e) — *see* Ligroin						
Benziodarone	972.4	E858.3	E942.4	E950.4	E962.0	E980.4
Benzocaine	968.5	E855.2	E938.5	E950.4	E962.0	E980.4
Benzodiapin	969.4	E853.2	E939.4	E950.3	E962.0	E980.3
Benzodiazepines (tranquilizers) NEC	969.4	E853.2	E939.4	E950.3	E962.0	E980.3
Benzoic acid (with salicylic acid) (anti-infective)	976.0	E858.7	E946.0	E950.4	E962.0	E980.4
Benzoin	976.3	E858.7	E946.3	E950.4	E962.0	E980.4
Benzol (vapor)	982.0	E862.4	—	E950.9	E962.1	E980.9
Benzomorphan	965.09	E850.2	E935.2	E950.0	E962.0	E980.0
Benzonatate	975.4	E858.6	E945.4	E950.4	E962.0	E980.4
Benzothiadiazides	974.3	E858.5	E944.3	E950.4	E962.0	E980.4
Benzoylpas	961.8	E857	E931.8	E950.4	E962.0	E980.4
Benzperidol	969.5	E853.8	E939.5	E950.3	E962.0	E980.3
Benzphetamine	977.0	E858.8	E947.0	E950.4	E962.0	E980.4
Benzpyrinium	971.0	E855.3	E941.0	E950.4	E962.0	E980.4
Benzquinamide	963.0	E858.1	E933.0	E950.4	E962.0	E980.4
Benzthiazide	974.3	E858.5	E944.3	E950.4	E962.0	E980.4
Benztropine	971.1	E855.4	E941.1	E950.4	E962.0	E980.4
Benzyl						
acetate	982.8	E862.4	—	E950.9	E962.1	E980.9
benzoate (anti-infective)	976.0	E858.7	E946.0	E950.4	E962.0	E980.4
morphine	965.09	E850.2	E935.2	E950.0	E962.0	E980.0

	External Cause (E-Code)					
	Poisoning	Accident	Therapeutic Use	Suicide Attempt	Assault	Undetermined
Benzyl — continued						
penicillin	960.0	E856	E930.0	E950.4	E962.0	E980.4
Bephenium hydroxynapthoate	961.6	E857	E931.6	E950.4	E962.0	E980.4
Bergamot oil	989.89	E866.8	—	E950.9	E962.1	E980.9
Berries, poisonous	988.2	E865.3	—	E950.9	E962.1	E980.9
Beryllium (compounds) (fumes)	985.3	E866.4	—	E950.9	E962.1	E980.9
Beta-carotene	976.3	E858.7	E946.3	E950.4	E962.0	E980.4
Beta-Chlor	967.1	E852.0	E937.1	E950.2	E962.0	E980.2
Betamethasone	962.0	E858.0	E932.0	E950.4	E962.0	E980.4
topical	976.0	E858.7	E946.0	E950.4	E962.0	E980.4
Betazole	977.8	E858.8	E947.8	E950.4	E962.0	E980.4
Bethanechol	971.0	E855.3	E941.0	E950.4	E962.0	E980.4
Bethanidine	972.6	E858.3	E942.6	E950.4	E962.0	E980.4
Betula oil	976.3	E858.7	E946.3	E950.4	E962.0	E980.4
Bhang	969.6	E854.1	E939.6	E950.3	E962.0	E980.3
Bialamicol	961.5	E857	E931.5	E950.4	E962.0	E980.4
Bichloride of mercury — see Mercury, chloride						
Bichromates (calcium) (crystals) (potassium)						
(sodium)	983.9	E864.3	—	E950.7	E962.1	E980.6
fumes	987.8	E869.8	—	E952.8	E962.2	E982.8
Biguanide derivatives, oral	962.3	E858.0	E932.3	E950.4	E962.0	E980.4
Biligrafin	977.8	E858.8	E947.8	E950.4	E962.0	E980.4
Bilopaque	977.8	E858.8	E947.8	E950.4	E962.0	E980.4
Bioflavonoids	972.8	E858.3	E942.8	E950.4	E962.0	E980.4
Biological substance NEC	979.9	E858.8	E949.9	E950.4	E962.0	E980.4
Biperiden	966.4	E855.0	E936.4	E950.4	E962.0	E980.4
Bisacodyl	973.1	E858.4	E943.1	E950.4	E962.0	E980.4
Bishydroxycoumarin	964.2	E858.2	E934.2	E950.4	E962.0	E980.4
Bismarsen	961.1	E857	E931.1	E950.4	E962.0	E980.4
Bismuth (compounds) NEC	985.8	E866.4	—	E950.9	E962.1	E980.9
anti-infectives	961.2	E857	E931.2	E950.4	E962.0	E980.4
subcarbonate	973.5	E858.4	E943.5	E950.4	E962.0	E980.4
sulfarsphenamine	961.1	E857	E931.1	E950.4	E962.0	E980.4
Bithionol	961.6	E857	E931.6	E950.4	E962.0	E980.4
Bitter almond oil	989.0	E866.8	—	E950.9	E962.1	E980.9
Bittersweet	988.2	E865.4	—	E950.9	E962.1	E930.9
Black						
flag	989.4	E863.4	—	E950.6	E962.1	E980.7
henbane	988.2	E865.4	—	E950.9	E962.1	E980.9
leaf (40)	989.4	E863.4	—	E950.6	E962.1	E980.7
widow spider (bite)	989.5	E905.1	—	E950.9	E962.1	E980.9
antivenin	979.9	E858.8	E949.9	E950.4	E962.0	E980.4
Blast furnace gas (carbon monoxide from)	986	E868.8	—	E952.1	E962.2	E982.1
Bleach NEC	983.9	E864.3	—	E950.7	E962.1	E980.6
Bleaching solutions	983.9	E864.3	—	E950.7	E962.1	E980.6
Bleomycin (sulfate)	960.7	E856	E930.7	E950.4	E962.0	E980.4
Blockain	968.9	E855.2	E938.9	E950.4	E962.0	E980.4
infiltration (subcutaneous)	968.5	E855.2	E938.5	E950.4	E962.0	E980.4
nerve block (peripheral) (plexus)	968.6	E855.2	E938.6	E950.4	E962.0	E980.4
topical (surface)	968.5	E855.2	E938.5	E950.4	E962.0	E980.4
Blood (derivatives) (natural) (plasma) (whole)	964.7	E858.2	E934.7	E950.4	E962.0	E980.4
affecting agent	964.9	E858.2	E934.9	E950.4	E962.0	E980.4
specified NEC	964.8	E858.2	E934.8	E950.4	E962.0	E980.4
substitute (macromolecular)	964.8	E858.2	E934.8	E950.4	E962.0	E980.4
Blue velvet	965.09	E850.2	E935.2	E950.0	E962.0	E980.0
Bone meal	989.89	E866.5	—	E950.9	E962.1	E980.9
Bonine	963.0	E858.1	E933.0	E950.4	E962.0	E980.4
Boracic acid	976.0	E858.7	E946.0	E950.4	E962.0	E980.4
ENT agent	976.6	E858.7	E946.6	E950.4	E962.0	E980.4

Table of Drugs and Chemicals — Butisol (sodium)

	Poisoning	Accident	Therapeutic Use	Suicide Attempt	Assault	Undetermined
Boracic acid — *continued*						
ophthalmic preparation	976.5	E858.7	E946.5	E950.4	E962.0	E980.4
Borate (cleanser) (sodium)	989.6	E861.3	—	E950.9	E962.1	E980.9
Borax (cleanser)	989.6	E861.3	—	E950.9	E962.1	E980.9
Boric acid	976.0	E858.7	E946.0	E950.4	E962.0	E980.4
ENT agent	976.6	E858.7	E946.6	E950.4	E962.0	E980.4
ophthalmic preparation	976.5	E858.7	E946.5	E950.4	E962.0	E980.4
Boron hydride NEC	989.89	E866.8	—	E950.9	E962.1	E980.9
fumes or gas	987.8	E869.8	—	E952.8	E962.2	E982.8
Brake fluid vapor	987.8	E869.8	—	E952.8	E962.2	E982.8
Brass (compounds) (fumes)	985.8	E866.4	—	E950.9	E962.1	E980.9
Brasso	981	E861.3	—	E950.9	E962.1	E980.9
Bretylium (tosylate)	972.6	E858.3	E942.6	E950.4	E962.0	E980.4
Brevital (sodium)	968.3	E855.1	E938.3	E950.4	E962.0	E980.4
British antilewisite	963.8	E858.1	E933.8	E950.4	E962.0	E980.4
Bromal (hydrate)	967.3	E852.2	E937.3	E950.2	E962.0	E980.2
Bromelains	963.4	E858.1	E933.4	E950.4	E962.0	E980.4
Bromides NEC	967.3	E852.2	E937.3	E950.2	E962.0	E980.2
Bromine (vapor)	987.8	E869.8	—	E952.8	E962.2	E982.8
compounds (medicinal)	967.3	E852.2	E937.3	E950.2	E962.0	E980.2
Bromisovalum	967.3	E852.2	E937.3	E950.2	E962.0	E980.2
Bromobenzyl cyanide	987.5	E869.3	—	E952.8	E962.2	E982.8
Bromodiphenhydramine	963.0	E858.1	E933.0	E950.4	E962.0	E980.4
Bromoform	967.3	E852.2	E937.3	E950.2	E962.0	E980.2
Bromophenol blue reagent	977.8	E858.8	E947.8	E950.4	E962.0	E980.4
Bromosalicylhydroxamic acid	961.8	E857	E931.8	E950.4	E962.0	E980.4
Bromo-seltzer	965.4	E850.4	E935.4	E950.0	E962.0	E980.0
Brompheniramine	963.0	E858.1	E933.0	E950.4	E962.0	E980.4
Bromural	967.3	E852.2	E937.3	E950.2	E962.0	E980.2
Brown spider (bite) (venom)	989.5	E905.1	—	E950.9	E962.1	E980.9
Brucia	988.2	E865.3	—	E950.9	E962.1	E980.9
Brucine	989.1	E863.7	—	E950.6	E962.1	E980.7
Brunswick green — *see* Copper						
Bruten — *see* Ibuprofen						
Bryonia (alba) (dioica)	988.2	E865.4	—	E950.9	E962.1	E980.9
Buclizine	969.5	E853.8	E939.5	E950.3	E962.0	E980.3
Bufferin	965.1	E850.3	E935.3	E950.0	E962.0	E980.0
Bufotenine	969.6	E854.1	E939.6	E950.3	E962.0	E980.3
Buphenine	971.2	E855.5	E941.2	E950.4	E962.0	E980.4
Bupivacaine	968.9	E855.2	E938.9	E950.4	E962.0	E980.4
infiltration (subcutaneous)	968.5	E855.2	E938.5	E950.4	E962.0	E980.4
nerve block (peripheral) (plexus)	968.6	E855.2	E938.6	E950.4	E962.0	E980.4
Busulfan	963.1	E858.1	E933.1	E950.4	E962.0	E980.4
Butabarbital (sodium)	967.0	E851	E937.0	E950.1	E962.0	E980.1
Butabarbitone	967.0	E851	E937.0	E950.1	E962.0	E980.1
Butabarpal	967.0	E851	E937.0	E950.1	E962.0	E980.1
Butacaine	968.5	E855.2	E938.5	E950.4	E962.0	E980.4
Butallylonal	967.0	E851	E937.0	E950.1	E962.0	E980.1
Butane (distributed in mobile container)	987.0	E868.0	—	E951.1	E962.2	E981.1
distributed through pipes	987.0	E867	—	E951.0	E962.2	E981.0
incomplete combustion of — *see* Carbon monoxide, butane						
Butanol	980.3	E860.4	—	E950.9	E962.1	E980.9
Butanone	982.8	E862.4	—	E950.9	E962.1	E980.9
Butaperazine	969.1	E853.0	E939.1	E950.3	E962.0	E980.3
Butazolidin	965.5	E850.5	E935.5	E950.0	E962.0	E980.0
Butethal	967.0	E851	E937.0	E950.1	E962.0	E980.1
Butethamate	971.1	E855.4	E941.1	E950.4	E962.0	E980.4
Buthalitone (sodium)	968.3	E855.1	E938.3	E950.4	E962.0	E980.4
Butisol (sodium)	967.0	E851	E937.0	E950.1	E962.0	E980.1

Table of Drugs and Chemicals

			External Cause (E-Code)			
	Poisoning	Accident	Therapeutic Use	Suicide Attempt	Assault	Undetermined
Butobarbital, butobarbitone	967.0	E851	E937.0	E950.1	E962.0	E980.1
Butriptyline	969.0	E854.0	E939.0	E950.3	E962.0	E980.3
Buttercups	988.2	E865.4	—	E950.9	E962.1	E980.9
Butter of antimony — *see* Antimony						
Butyl						
acetate (secondary)	982.8	E862.4	—	E950.9	E962.1	E980.9
alcohol	980.3	E860.4	—	E950.9	E962.1	E980.9
carbinol	980.8	E860.8	—	E950.9	E962.1	E980.9
carbitol	982.8	E862.4	—	E950.9	E962.1	E980.9
cellosolve	982.8	E862.4	—	E950.9	E962.1	E980.9
chloral (hydrate)	967.1	E852.0	E937.1	E950.2	E962.0	E980.2
formate	982.8	E862.4	—	E950.9	E962.1	E980.9
scopolammonium bromide	971.1	E855.4	E941.1	E950.4	E962.0	E980.4
Butyn	968.5	E855.2	E938.5	E950.4	E962.0	E980.4
Butyrophenone (-based tranquilizers)	969.2	E853.1	E939.2	E950.3	E962.0	E980.3
Cacodyl, cacodylic acid — *see* Arsenic						
Cactinomycin	960.7	E856	E930.7	E950.4	E962.0	E980.4
Cade oil	976.4	E858.7	E946.4	E950.4	E962.0	E980.4
Cadmium (chloride) (compounds) (dust) (fumes) (oxide)	985.5	E866.4	—	E950.9	E962.1	E980.9
sulfide (medicinal) NEC	976.4	E858.7	E946.4	E950.4	E962.0	E980.4
Caffeine	969.7	E854.2	E939.7	E950.3	E962.0	E980.3
Calabar bean	988.2	E865.4	—	E950.9	E962.1	E980.9
Caladium seguinium	988.2	E865.4	—	E950.9	E962.1	E980.9
Calamine (liniment) (lotion)	976.3	E858.7	E946.3	E950.4	E962.0	E980.4
Calciferol	963.5	E858.1	E933.5	E950.4	E962.0	E980.4
Calcium (salts) NEC	974.5	E858.5	E944.5	E950.4	E962.0	E980.4
acetylsalicylate	965.1	E850.3	E935.3	E950.0	E962.0	E980.0
benzamidosalicylate	961.8	E857	E931.8	E950.4	E962.0	E980.4
carbaspirin	965.1	E850.3	E935.3	E950.0	E962.0	E980.0
carbimide (citrated)	977.3	E858.8	E947.3	E950.4	E962.0	E980.4
carbonate (antacid)	973.0	E858.4	E943.0	E950.4	E962.0	E980.4
cyanide (citrated)	977.3	E858.8	E947.3	E950.4	E962.0	E980.4
dioctyl sulfosuccinate	973.2	E858.4	E943.2	E950.4	E962.0	E980.4
disodium edathamil	963.8	E858.1	E933.8	E950.4	E962.0	E980.4
disodium edetate	963.8	E858.1	E933.8	E950.4	E962.0	E980.4
EDTA	963.8	E858.1	E933.8	E950.4	E962.0	E980.4
hydrate, hydroxide	983.2	E864.2	—	E950.7	E962.1	E980.6
mandelate	961.9	E857	E931.9	E950.4	E962.0	E980.4
oxide	983.2	E864.2	—	E950.7	E962.1	E980.6
Calomel — *see* Mercury, chloride						
Caloric agents NEC	974.5	E858.5	E944.5	E950.4	E962.0	E980.4
Calusterone	963.1	E858.1	E933.1	E950.4	E962.0	E980.4
Camoquin	961.4	E857	E931.4	E950.4	E962.0	E980.4
Camphor (oil)	976.1	E858.7	E946.1	E950.4	E962.0	E980.4
Candeptin	976.0	E858.7	E946.0	E950.4	E962.0	E980.4
Candicidin	976.0	E858.7	E946.0	E950.4	E962.0	E980.4
Cannabinols	969.6	E854.1	E939.6	E950.3	E962.0	E980.3
Cannabis (derivatives) (indica) (sativa)	969.6	E854.1	E939.6	E950.3	E962.0	E980.3
Canned heat	980.1	E860.2	—	E950.9	E962.1	E980.9
Cantharides, cantharidin, cantharis	976.8	E858.7	E946.8	E950.4	E962.0	E980.4
Capillary agents	972.8	E858.3	E942.8	E950.4	E962.0	E980.4
Capreomycin	960.6	E856	E930.6	E950.4	E962.0	E980.4
Captodiame, captodiamine	969.5	E853.8	E939.5	E950.3	E962.0	E980.3
Caramiphen (hydrochloride)	971.1	E855.4	E941.1	E950.4	E962.0	E980.4
Carbachol	971.0	E855.3	E941.0	E950.4	E962.0	E980.4
Carbacrylamine resins	974.5	E858.5	E944.5	E950.4	E962.0	E980.4

Table of Drugs and Chemicals — Carbon

	Poisoning	External Cause (E-Code)				
		Accident	Therapeutic Use	Suicide Attempt	Assault	Undetermined
Carbamate (sedative)	967.8	E852.8	E937.8	E950.2	E962.0	E980.2
herbicide	989.3	E863.5	—	E950.6	E962.1	E980.7
insecticide	989.3	E863.2	—	E950.6	E962.1	E980.7
Carbamazepine	966.3	E855.0	E936.3	E950.4	E962.0	E980.4
Carbamic esters	967.8	E852.8	E937.8	E950.2	E962.0	E980.2
Carbamide	974.4	E858.5	E944.4	E950.4	E962.0	E980.4
topical	976.8	E858.7	E946.8	E950.4	E962.0	E980.4
Carbamylcholine chloride	971.0	E855.3	E941.0	E950.4	E962.0	E980.4
Carbarsone	961.1	E857	E931.1	E950.4	E962.0	E980.4
Carbaryl	989.3	E863.2	—	E950.6	E962.1	E980.7
Carbaspirin	965.1	E850.3	E935.3	E950.0	E962.0	E980.0
Carbazochrome	972.8	E858.3	E942.8	E950.4	E962.0	E980.4
Carbenicillin	960.0	E856	E930.0	E950.4	E962.0	E980.4
Carbenoxolone	973.8	E858.4	E943.8	E950.4	E962.0	E980.4
Carbetapentane	975.4	E858.6	E945.4	E950.4	E962.0	E980.4
Carbimazole	962.8	E858.0	E932.8	E950.4	E962.0	E980.4
Carbinol	980.1	E860.2	—	E950.9	E962.1	E980.9
Carbinoxamine	963.0	E858.1	E933.0	E950.4	E962.0	E980.4
Carbitol	982.8	E862.4	—	E950.9	E962.1	E980.9
Carbocaine	968.9	E855.2	E938.9	E950.4	E962.0	E980.4
infiltration (subcutaneous)	968.5	E855.2	E938.5	E950.4	E962.0	E980.4
nerve block (peripheral)						
(plexus)	968.6	E855.2	E938.6	E950.4	E962.0	E980.4
topical (surface)	968.5	E855.2	E938.5	E950.4	E962.0	E980.4
Carbol-fuchsin solution	976.0	E858.7	E946.0	E950.4	E962.0	E980.4
Carbolic acid (see also Phenol)	983.0	E864.0	—	E950.7	E962.1	E980.6
Carbomycin	960.8	E856	E930.8	E950.4	E962.0	E980.4
Carbon						
bisulfide (liquid) (vapor)	982.2	E862.4	—	E950.9	E962.1	E980.9
dioxide (gas)	987.8	E869.8	—	E952.8	E962.2	E982.8
disulfide (liquid) (vapor)	982.2	E862.4	—	E950.9	E962.1	E980.9
monoxide (from incomplete combustion of) (in)						
NEC	986	E868.9	—	E952.1	E962.2	E982.1
blast furnace gas	986	E868.8	—	E952.1	E962.2	E982.1
butane (distributed in mobile container)	986	E868.0	—	E951.1	E962.2	E981.1
distributed through pipes	986	E867	—	E951.0	E962.2	E981.0
charcoal fumes	986	E868.3	—	E952.1	E962.2	E982.1
coal						
gas (piped)	986	E867	—	E951.0	E962.2	E981.0
solid (in domestic stoves, fireplaces)	986	E868.3	—	E952.1	E962.2	E982.1
coke (in domestic stoves, fireplaces)	986	E868.3	—	E952.1	E962.2	E982.1
exhaust gas (motor) not in transit	986	E868.2	—	E952.0	E962.2	E982.0
combustion engine, any not in watercraft	986	E868.2	—	E952.0	E962.2	E982.0
farm tractor, not in transit	986	E868.2	—	E952.0	E962.2	E982.0
gas engine	986	E868.2	—	E952.0	E962.2	E982.0
motor pump	986	E868.2	—	E952.0	E962.2	E982.0
motor vehicle, not in transit	986	E868.2	—	E952.0	E962.2	E982.0
fuel (in domestic use)	986	E868.3	—	E952.1	E962.2	E982.1
gas (piped)	986	E867	—	E951.0	E962.2	E981.0
in mobile container	986	E868.0	—	E951.1	E962.2	E981.1
utility	986	E868.1	—	E951.8	E962.2	E981.1
in mobile container	986	E868.0	—	E951.1	E962.2	E981.1
piped (natural)	986	E867	—	E951.0	E962.2	E981.0

✓4ᵗʰ Fourth-digit Required   ✓5ᵗʰ Fifth-digit Required

Table of Drugs and Chemicals

	External Cause (E-Code)					
	Poisoning	Accident	Therapeutic Use	Suicide Attempt	Assault	Undetermined
Carbon — *continued*						
monoxide — *continued*						
illuminating gas	986	E868.1	—	E951.8	E962.2	E981.8
industrial fuels or gases, any	986	E868.8	—	E952.1	E962.2	E982.1
kerosene (in domestic stoves, fireplaces)	986	E868.3	—	E952.1	E962.2	E982.1
kiln gas or vapor	986	E868.8	—	E952.1	E962.2	E982.1
motor exhaust gas, not in transit	986	E868.2	—	E952.0	E962.2	E982.0
piped gas (manufactured) (natural)	986	E867	—	E951.0	E962.2	E981.0
producer gas	986	E868.8	—	E952.1	E962.2	E982.1
propane (distributed in mobile container)	986	E868.0	—	E951.1	E962.2	E981.1
distributed through pipes	986	E867	—	E951.0	E962.2	E981.0
specified source NEC	986	E868.8	—	E952.1	E962.2	E982.1
stove gas	986	E868.1	—	E951.8	E962.2	E981.8
piped	986	E867	—	E951.0	E962.2	E981.0
utility gas	986	E868.1	—	E951.8	E962.2	E981.8
piped	986	E867	—	E951.0	E962.2	E981.0
water gas	986	E868.1	—	E951.8	E962.2	E981.8
wood (in domestic stoves, fireplaces)	986	E868.3	—	E952.1	E962.2	E982.1
tetrachloride (vapor) NEC	987.8	E869.8	—	E952.8	E962.2	E982.8
liquid (cleansing agent) NEC	982.1	E861.3	—	E950.9	E962.1	E980.9
solvent	982.1	E862.4	—	E950.9	E962.1	E980.9
Carbonic acid (gas)	987.8	E869.8	—	E952.8	E962.2	E982.8
anhydrase inhibitors	974.2	E858.5	E944.2	E950.4	E962.0	E980.4
Carbowax	976.3	E858.7	E946.3	E950.4	E962.0	E980.4
Carbrital	967.0	E851	E937.0	E950.1	E962.0	E980.1
Carbromal (derivatives)	967.3	E852.2	E937.3	E950.2	E962.0	E980.2
Cardiac						
depressants	972.0	E858.3	E942.0	E950.4	E962.0	E980.4
rhythm regulators	972.0	E858.3	E942.0	E950.4	E962.0	E980.4
Cardiografin	977.8	E858.8	E947.8	E950.4	E962.0	E980.4
Cardio-green	977.8	E858.8	E947.8	E950.4	E962.0	E980.4
Cardiotonic glycosides	972.1	E858.3	E942.1	E950.4	E962.0	E980.4
Cardiovascular agents NEC	972.9	E858.3	E942.9	E950.4	E962.0	E980.4
Cardrase	974.2	E858.5	E944.2	E950.4	E962.0	E980.4
Carfusin	976.0	E858.7	E946.0	E950.4	E962.0	E980.4
Carisoprodol	968.0	E855.1	E938.0	E950.4	E962.0	E980.4
Carmustine	963.1	E858.1	E933.1	E950.4	E962.0	E980.4
Carotene	963.5	E858.1	E933.5	E950.4	E962.0	E980.4
Carphenazine (maleate)	969.1	E853.0	E939.1	E950.3	E962.0	E980.3
Carter's Little Pills	973.1	E858.4	E943.1	E950.4	E962.0	E980.4
Cascara (sagrada)	973.1	E858.4	E943.1	E950.4	E962.0	E980.4
Cassava	988.2	E865.4	—	E950.9	E962.1	E980.9
Castellani's paint	976.0	E858.7	E946.0	E950.4	E962.0	E980.4
Castor						
bean	988.2	E865.3	—	E950.9	E962.1	E980.9
oil	973.1	E858.4	E943.1	E950.4	E962.0	E980.4
Caterpillar (sting)	989.5	E905.5	—	E950.9	E962.1	E980.9
Catha (edulis)	970.8	E854.3	E940.8	E950.4	E962.0	E980.4
Cathartics NEC	973.3	E858.4	E943.3	E950.4	E962.0	E980.4
contact	973.1	E858.4	E943.1	E950.4	E962.0	E980.4
emollient	973.2	E858.4	E943.2	E950.4	E962.0	E980.4
intestinal irritants	973.1	E858.4	E943.1	E950.4	E962.0	E980.4
saline	973.3	E858.4	E943.3	E950.4	E962.0	E980.4
Cathomycin	960.8	E856	E930.8	E950.4	E962.0	E980.4

Table of Drugs and Chemicals

		External Cause (E-Code)				
	Poisoning	Accident	Therapeutic Use	Suicide Attempt	Assault	Undetermined
Caustic(s)	983.9	E864.4	—	E950.7	E962.1	E980.6
alkali	983.2	E864.2	—	E950.7	E962.1	E980.6
hydroxide	983.2	E864.2	—	E950.7	E962.1	E980.6
potash	983.2	E864.2	—	E950.7	E962.1	E980.6
soda	983.2	E864.2	—	E950.7	E962.1	E980.6
specified NEC	983.9	E864.3	—	E950.7	E962.1	E980.6
Ceepryn	976.0	E858.7	E946.0	E950.4	E962.0	E980.4
ENT agent	976.6	E858.7	E946.6	E950.4	E962.0	E980.4
lozenges	976.6	E858.7	E946.6	E950.4	E962.0	E980.4
Celestone	962.0	E858.0	E932.0	E950.4	E962.0	E980.4
topical	976.0	E858.7	E946.0	E950.4	E962.0	E980.4
Cellosolve	982.8	E862.4	—	E950.9	E962.1	E980.9
Cell stimulants and proliferants	976.8	E858.7	E946.8	E950.4	E962.0	E980.4
Cellulose derivatives, cathartic	973.3	E858.4	E943.3	E950.4	E962.0	E980.4
nitrates (topical)	976.3	E858.7	E946.3	E950.4	E962.0	E980.4
Centipede (bite)	989.5	E905.4	—	E950.9	E962.1	E980.9
Central nervous system						
depressants	968.4	E855.1	E938.4	E950.4	E962.0	E980.4
anesthetic (general) NEC	968.4	E855.1	E938.4	E950.4	E962.0	E980.4
gases NEC	968.2	E855.1	E938.2	E950.4	E962.0	E980.4
intravenous	968.3	E855.1	E938.3	E950.4	E962.0	E980.4
barbiturates	967.0	E851	E937.0	E950.1	E962.0	E980.1
bromides	967.3	E852.2	E937.3	E950.2	E962.0	E980.2
cannabis sativa	969.6	E854.1	E939.6	E950.3	E962.0	E980.3
chloral hydrate	967.1	E852.0	E937.1	E950.2	E962.0	E980.2
hallucinogenics	969.6	E854.1	E939.6	E950.3	E962.0	E980.3
hypnotics	967.9	E852.9	E937.9	E950.2	E962.0	E980.2
specified NEC	967.8	E852.8	E937.8	E950.2	E962.0	E980.2
muscle relaxants	968.0	E855.1	E938.0	E950.4	E962.0	E980.4
paraldehyde	967.2	E852.1	E937.2	E950.2	E962.0	E980.2
sedatives	967.9	E852.9	E937.9	E950.2	E962.0	E980.2
mixed NEC	967.6	E852.5	E937.6	E950.2	E962.0	E980.2
specified NEC	967.8	E852.8	E937.8	E950.2	E962.0	E980.2
muscle-tone depressants	968.0	E855.1	E938.0	E950.4	E962.0	E980.4
stimulants	970.9	E854.3	E940.9	E950.4	E962.0	E980.4
amphetamines	969.7	E854.2	E939.7	E950.3	E962.0	E980.3
analeptics	970.0	E854.3	E940.0	E950.4	E962.0	E980.4
antidepressants	969.0	E854.0	E939.0	E950.3	E962.0	E980.3
opiate antagonists	970.1	E854.3	E940.1	E950.4	E962.0	E980.4
specified NEC	970.8	E854.3	E940.8	E950.4	E962.0	E980.4
Cephalexin	960.5	E856	E930.5	E950.4	E962.0	E980.4
Cephaloglycin	960.5	E856	E930.5	E950.4	E962.0	E980.4
Cephaloridine	960.5	E856	E930.5	E950.4	E962.0	E980.4
Cephalosporins NEC	960.5	E856	E930.5	E950.4	E962.0	E980.4
N (adicillin)	960.0	E856	E930.0	E950.4	E962.0	E980.4
Cephalothin (sodium)	960.5	E856	E930.5	E950.4	E962.0	E980.4
Cerbera (odallam)	988.2	E865.4	—	E950.9	E962.1	E980.9
Cerberin	972.1	E858.3	E942.1	E950.4	E962.0	E980.4
Cerebral stimulants	970.9	E854.3	E940.9	E950.4	E962.0	E980.4
psychotherapeutic	969.7	E854.2	E939.7	E950.3	E962.0	E980.3
specified NEC	970.8	E854.3	E940.8	E950.4	E962.0	E980.4
Cetalkonium (chloride)	976.0	E858.7	E946.0	E950.4	E962.0	E980.4
Cetoxime	963.0	E858.1	E933.0	E950.4	E962.0	E980.4
Cetrimide	976.2	E858.7	E946.2	E950.4	E962.0	E980.4
Cetylpyridinium	976.0	E858.7	E946.0	E950.4	E962.0	E980.4
ENT agent	976.6	E858.7	E946.6	E950.4	E962.0	E980.4
lozenges	976.6	E858.7	E946.6	E950.4	E962.0	E980.4
Cevadilla — see Sabadilla						
Cevitamic acid	963.5	E858.1	E933.5	E950.4	E962.0	E980.4
Chalk, precipitated	973.0	E858.4	E943.0	E950.4	E962.0	E980.4
Charcoal						
fumes (carbon monoxide)	986	E868.3	—	E952.1	E962.2	E982.1
industrial	986	E868.8	—	E952.1	E962.2	E982.1

		External Cause (E-Code)				
	Poisoning	Accident	Therapeutic Use	Suicide Attempt	Assault	Undetermined
Charcoal — *continued*						
medicinal (activated)	973.0	E858.4	E943.0	E950.4	E962.0	E980.4
Chelating agents NEC	977.2	E858.8	E947.2	E950.4	E962.0	E980.4
Chelidonium majus	988.2	E865.4	—	E950.9	E962.1	E980.9
Chemical substance	989.9	E866.9	—	E950.9	E962.1	E980.9
specified NEC	989.89	E866.8	—	E950.9	E962.1	E980.9
Chemotherapy, antineoplastic	963.1	E858.1	E933.1	E950.4	E962.0	E980.4
Chenopodium (oil)	961.6	E857	E931.6	E950.4	E962.0	E980.4
Cherry laurel	988.2	E865.4	—	E950.9	E962.1	E980.9
Chiniofon	961.3	E857	E931.3	E950.4	E962.0	E980.4
Chlophedianol	975.4	E858.6	E945.4	E950.4	E962.0	E980.4
Chloral (betaine) (formamide)						
(hydrate)	967.1	E852.0	E937.1	E950.2	E962.0	E980.2
Chloralamide	967.1	E852.0	E937.1	E950.2	E962.0	E980.2
Chlorambucil	963.1	E858.1	E933.1	E950.4	E962.0	E980.4
Chloramphenicol	960.2	E856	E930.2	E950.4	E962.0	E980.4
ENT agent	976.6	E858.7	E946.6	E950.4	E962.0	E980.4
ophthalmic preparation	976.5	E858.7	E946.5	E950.4	E962.0	E980.4
topical NEC	976.0	E858.7	E946.0	E950.4	E962.0	E980.4
Chlorate(s) (potassium)						
(sodium) NEC	983.9	E864.3	—	E950.7	E962.1	E980.6
herbicides	989.4	E863.5	—	E950.6	E962.1	E980.7
Chlorcylizine	963.0	E858.1	E933.0	E950.4	E962.0	E980.4
Chlordan(e) (dust)	989.2	E863.0	—	E950.6	E962.1	E980.7
Chlordantoin	976.0	E858.7	E946.0	E950.4	E962.0	E980.4
Chlordiazepoxide	969.4	E853.2	E939.4	E950.3	E962.0	E980.3
Chloresium	976.8	E858.7	E946.8	E950.4	E962.0	E980.4
Chlorethiazol	967.1	E852.0	E937.1	E950.2	E962.0	E980.2
Chlorethyl — *see* **Ethyl, chloride**						
Chloretone	967.1	E852.0	E937.1	E950.2	E962.0	E980.2
Chlorex	982.3	E862.4	—	E950.9	E962.1	E980.9
Chlorhexadol	967.1	E852.0	E937.1	E950.2	E962.0	E980.2
Chlorhexidine (hydrochloride)	976.0	E858.7	E946.0	E950.4	E962.0	E980.4
Chlorhydroxyquinolin	976.0	E858.7	E946.0	E950.4	E962.0	E980.4
Chloride of lime (bleach)	983.9	E864.3	—	E950.7	E962.1	E980.6
Chlorinated						
camphene	989.2	E863.0	—	E950.6	E962.1	E980.7
diphenyl	989.89	E866.8	—	E950.9	E962.1	E980.9
hydrocarbons NEC	989.2	E863.0	—	E950.6	E962.1	E980.7
solvent	982.3	E862.4	—	E950.9	E962.1	E980.9
lime (bleach)	983.9	E864.3	—	E950.7	E962.1	E980.6
naphthalene — *see* Naphthalene						
pesticides NEC	989.2	E863.0	—	E950.6	E962.1	E980.7
soda — *see* Sodium, hypochlorite						
Chlorine (fumes) (gas)	987.6	E869.8	—	E952.8	E962.2	E982.8
bleach	983.9	E864.3	—	E950.7	E962.1	E980.6
compounds NEC	983.9	E864.3	—	E950.7	E962.1	E980.6
disinfectant	983.9	E861.4	—	E950.7	E962.1	E980.6
releasing agents NEC	983.9	E864.3	—	E950.7	E962.1	E980.6
Chlorisondamine	972.3	E858.3	E942.3	E950.4	E962.0	E980.4
Chlormadinone	962.2	E858.0	E932.2	E950.4	E962.0	E980.4
Chlormerodrin	974.0	E858.5	E944.0	E950.4	E962.0	E980.4
Chlormethiazole	967.1	E852.0	E937.1	E950.2	E962.0	E980.2
Chlormethylenecycline	960.4	E856	E930.4	E950.4	E962.0	E980.4
Chlormezanone	969.5	E853.8	E939.5	E950.3	E962.0	E980.3
Chloroacetophenone	987.5	E869.3	—	E952.8	E962.2	E982.8
Chloroaniline	983.0	E864.0	—	E950.7	E962.1	E980.6
Chlorobenzene, chlorobenzol	982.0	E862.4	—	E950.9	E962.1	E980.9
Chlorobutanol	967.1	E852.0	E937.1	E950.2	E962.0	E980.2
Chlorodinitrobenzene	983.0	E864.0	—	E950.7	E962.1	E980.6
dust or vapor	987.8	E869.8	—	E952.8	E962.2	E982.8

Table of Drugs and Chemicals — Chromates

	Poisoning	Accident	Therapeutic Use	Suicide Attempt	Assault	Undetermined
Chloroethane — see Ethyl, chloride						
Chloroform (fumes) (vapor)	987.8	E869.8	—	E952.8	E962.2	E982.8
anesthetic (gas)	968.2	E855.1	E938.2	E950.4	E962.0	E980.4
liquid NEC	968.4	E855.1	E938.4	E950.4	E962.0	E980.4
solvent	982.3	E862.4	—	E950.9	E962.1	E980.9
Chloroguanide	961.4	E857	E931.4	E950.4	E962.0	E980.4
Chloromycetin	960.2	E856	E930.2	E950.4	E962.0	E980.4
ENT agent	976.6	E858.7	E946.6	E950.4	E962.0	E980.4
ophthalmic preparation	976.5	E858.7	E946.5	E950.4	E962.0	E980.4
otic solution	976.6	E858.7	E946.6	E950.4	E962.0	E980.4
topical NEC	976.0	E858.7	E946.0	E950.4	E962.0	E980.4
Chloronitrobenzene	983.0	E864.0	—	E950.7	E962.1	E980.6
dust or vapor	987.8	E869.8	—	E952.8	E962.2	E982.8
Chlorophenol	983.0	E864.0	—	E950.7	E962.1	E980.6
Chlorophenothane	989.2	E863.0	—	E950.6	E962.1	E980.7
Chlorophyll (derivatives)	976.8	E858.7	E946.8	E950.4	E962.0	E980.4
Chloropicrin (fumes)	987.8	E869.8	—	E952.8	E962.2	E982.8
fumigant	989.4	E863.8	—	E950.6	E962.1	E980.7
fungicide	989.4	E863.6	—	E950.6	E962.1	E980.7
pesticide (fumes)	989.4	E863.4	—	E950.6	E962.1	E980.7
Chloroprocaine	968.9	E855.2	E938.9	E950.4	E962.0	E980.4
infiltration (subcutaneous)	968.5	E855.2	E938.5	E950.4	E962.0	E980.4
nerve block (peripheral) (plexus)	968.6	E855.2	E938.6	E950.4	E962.0	E980.4
Chloroptic	976.5	E858.7	E946.5	E950.4	E962.0	E980.4
Chloropurine	963.1	E858.1	E933.1	E950.4	E962.0	E980.4
Chloroquine (hydrochloride) (phosphate)	961.4	E857	E931.4	E950.4	E962.0	E980.4
Chlorothen	963.0	E858.1	E933.0	E950.4	E962.0	E980.4
Chlorothiazide	974.3	E858.5	E944.3	E950.4	E962.0	E980.4
Chlorotrianisene	962.2	E858.0	E932.2	E950.4	E962.0	E980.4
Chlorovinyldichloroarsine	985.1	E866.3	—	E950.8	E962.1	E980.8
Chloroxylenol	976.0	E858.7	E946.0	E950.4	E962.0	E980.4
Chlorphenesin (carbamate)	968.0	E855.1	E938.0	E950.4	E962.0	E980.4
topical (antifungal)	976.0	E858.7	E946.0	E950.4	E962.0	E980.4
Chlorpheniramine	963.0	E858.1	E933.0	E950.4	E962.0	E980.4
Chlorphenoxamine	966.4	E855.0	E936.4	E950.4	E962.0	E980.4
Chlorphentermine	977.0	E858.8	E947.0	E950.4	E962.0	E980.4
Chlorproguanil	961.4	E857	E931.4	E950.4	E962.0	E980.4
Chlorpromazine	969.1	E853.0	E939.1	E950.3	E962.0	E980.3
Chlorpropamide	962.3	E858.0	E932.3	E950.4	E962.0	E980.4
Chlorprothixene	969.3	E853.8	E939.3	E950.3	E962.0	E980.3
Chlorquinaldol	976.0	E858.7	E946.0	E950.4	E962.0	E980.4
Chlortetracycline	960.4	E856	E930.4	E950.4	E962.0	E980.4
Chlorthalidone	974.4	E858.5	E944.4	E950.4	E962.0	E980.4
Chlortrianisene	962.2	E858.0	E932.2	E950.4	E962.0	E980.4
Chlor-Trimeton	963.0	E858.1	E933.0	E950.4	E962.0	E980.4
Chlorzoxazone	968.0	E855.1	E938.0	E950.4	E962.0	E980.4
Choke damp	987.8	E869.8	—	E952.8	E962.2	E982.8
Cholebrine	977.8	E858.8	E947.8	E950.4	E962.0	E980.4
Cholera vaccine	978.2	E858.8	E948.2	E950.4	E962.0	E980.4
Cholesterol-lowering agents	972.2	E858.3	E942.2	E950.4	E962.0	E980.4
Cholestyramine (resin)	972.2	E858.3	E942.2	E950.4	E962.0	E980.4
Cholic acid	973.4	E858.4	E943.4	E950.4	E962.0	E980.4
Choline						
dihydrogen citrate	977.1	E858.8	E947.1	E950.4	E962.0	E980.4
salicylate	965.1	E850.3	E935.3	E950.0	E962.0	E980.0
theophyllinate	974.1	E858.5	E944.1	E950.4	E962.0	E980.4
Cholinergics	971.0	E855.3	E941.0	E950.4	E962.0	E980.4
Cholografin	977.8	E858.8	E947.8	E950.4	E962.0	E980.4
Chorionic gonadotropin	962.4	E858.0	E932.4	E950.4	E962.0	E980.4
Chromates	983.9	E864.3	—	E950.7	E962.1	E980.6
dust or mist	987.8	E869.8	—	E952.8	E962.2	E982.8

Chromates — Table of Drugs and Chemicals

	External Cause (E-Code)					
	Poisoning	Accident	Therapeutic Use	Suicide Attempt	Assault	Undetermined
Chromates — *continued*						
lead	984.0	E866.0	—	E950.9	E962.1	E980.9
paint	984.0	E861.5	—	E950.9	E962.1	E980.9
Chromic acid	983.9	E864.3	—	E950.7	E962.1	E980.6
dust or mist	987.8	E869.8	—	E952.8	E962.2	E982.8
Chromium	985.6	E866.4	—	E950.9	E962.1	E980.9
compounds — *see* Chromates						
Chromonar	972.4	E858.3	E942.4	E950.4	E962.0	E980.4
Chromyl chloride	983.9	E864.3	—	E950.7	E962.1	E980.6
Chrysarobin (ointment)	976.4	E858.7	E946.4	E950.4	E962.0	E980.4
Chrysazin	973.1	E858.4	E943.1	E950.4	E962.0	E980.4
Chymar	963.4	E858.1	E933.4	E950.4	E962.0	E980.4
ophthalmic preparation	976.5	E858.7	E946.5	E950.4	E962.0	E980.4
Chymotrypsin	963.4	E858.1	E933.4	E950.4	E962.0	E980.4
ophthalmic preparation	976.5	E858.7	E946.5	E950.4	E962.0	E980.4
Cicuta maculata or virosa	988.2	E865.4	—	E950.9	E962.1	E980.9
Cigarette lighter fluid	981	E862.1	—	E950.9	E962.1	E980.9
Cinchocaine (spinal)	968.7	E855.2	E938.7	E950.4	E962.0	E980.4
topical (surface)	968.5	E855.2	E938.5	E950.4	E962.0	E980.4
Cinchona	961.4	E857	E931.4	E950.4	E962.0	E980.4
Cinchonine alkaloids	961.4	E857	E931.4	E950.4	E962.0	E980.4
Cinchophen	974.7	E858.5	E944.7	E950.4	E962.0	E980.4
Cinnarizine	963.0	E858.1	E933.0	E950.4	E962.0	E980.4
Citanest	968.9	E855.2	E938.9	E950.4	E962.0	E980.4
infiltration (subcutaneous)	968.5	E855.2	E938.5	E950.4	E962.0	E980.4
nerve block (peripheral) (plexus)	968.6	E855.2	E938.6	E950.4	E962.0	E980.4
Citric acid	989.89	E866.8	—	E950.9	E962.1	E980.9
Citrovorum factor	964.1	E858.2	E934.1	E950.4	E962.0	E980.4
Claviceps purpurea	988.2	E865.4	—	E950.9	E962.1	E980.9
Cleaner, cleansing agent NEC	989.89	E861.1	—	E950.9	E962.1	E980.9
of paint or varnish	982.8	E862.9	—	E950.9	E962.1	E980.9
Clematis vitalba	988.2	E865.4	—	E950.9	E962.1	E980.9
Clemizole	963.0	E858.1	E933.0	E950.4	E962.0	E980.4
penicillin	960.0	E856	E930.0	E950.4	E962.0	E980.4
Clidinium	971.1	E855.4	E941.1	E950.4	E962.0	E980.4
Clindamycin	960.8	E856	E930.8	E950.4	E962.0	E980.4
Cliradon	965.09	E850.2	E935.2	E950.0	E962.0	E980.0
Clocortolone	962.0	E858.0	E932.0	E950.4	E962.0	E980.4
Clofedanol	975.4	E858.6	E945.4	E950.4	E962.0	E980.4
Clofibrate	972.2	E858.3	E942.2	E950.4	E962.0	E980.4
Clomethiazole	967.1	E852.0	E937.1	E950.2	E962.0	E980.2
Clomiphene	977.8	E858.8	E947.8	E950.4	E962.0	E980.4
Clonazepam	969.4	E853.2	E939.4	E950.3	E962.0	E980.3
Clonidine	972.6	E858.3	E942.6	E950.4	E962.0	E980.4
Clopamide	974.3	E858.5	E944.3	E950.4	E962.0	E980.4
Clorazepate	969.4	E853.2	E939.4	E950.3	E962.0	E980.3
Clorexolone	974.4	E858.5	E944.4	E950.4	E962.0	E980.4
Clorox (bleach)	983.9	E864.3	—	E950.7	E962.1	E980.6
Clortermine	977.0	E858.8	E947.0	E950.4	E962.0	E980.4
Clotrimazole	976.0	E858.7	E946.0	E950.4	E962.0	E980.4
Cloxacillin	960.0	E856	E930.0	E950.4	E962.0	E980.4
Coagulants NEC	964.5	E858.2	E934.5	E950.4	E962.0	E980.4
Coal (carbon monoxide from) — *see also* **Carbon, monoxide, coal**						
oil — *see* Kerosene						
tar NEC	983.0	E864.0	—	E950.7	E962.1	E980.6
fumes	987.8	E869.8	—	E952.8	E962.2	E982.8
medicinal (ointment)	976.4	E858.7	E946.4	E950.4	E962.0	E980.4
analgesics NEC	965.5	E850.5	E935.5	E950.0	E962.0	E980.0
naphtha (solvent)	981	E862.0	—	E950.9	E962.1	E980.9
Cobalt (fumes) (industrial)	985.8	E866.4	—	E950.9	E962.1	E980.9

Table of Drugs and Chemicals

Copper (dust) (fumes) (salts) NEC

		External Cause (E-Code)				
	Poisoning	Accident	Therapeutic Use	Suicide Attempt	Assault	Undetermined
Cobra (venom)	989.5	E905.0	—	E950.9	E962.1	E980.9
Coca (leaf)	970.8	E854.3	E940.8	E950.4	E962.0	E980.4
Cocaine (hydrochloride) (salt)	970.8 ▲	E854.3 ▲	E940.8 ▲	E950.4	E962.0	E980.4
topical anesthetic ●	968.5	E855.2	E938.5	E950.4	E962.0	E980.4
Coccidioidin	977.8	E858.8	E947.8	E950.4	E962.0	E980.4
Cocculus indicus	988.2	E865.3	—	E950.9	E962.1	E980.9
Cochineal	989.89	E866.8	—	E950.9	E962.1	E980.9
medicinal products	977.4	E858.8	E947.4	E950.4	E962.0	E980.4
Codeine	965.09	E850.2	E935.2	E950.0	E962.0	E980.0
Coffee	989.89	E866.8	—	E950.9	E962.1	E980.9
Cogentin	971.1	E855.4	E941.1	E950.4	E962.0	E980.4
Coke fumes or gas (carbon monoxide)	986	E868.3	—	E952.1	E962.2	E982.1
industrial use	986	E868.8	—	E952.1	E962.2	E982.1
Colace	973.2	E858.4	E943.2	E950.4	E962.0	E980.4
Colchicine	974.7	E858.5	E944.7	E950.4	E962.0	E980.4
Colchicum	988.2	E865.3	—	E950.9	E962.1	E980.9
Cold cream	976.3	E858.7	E946.3	E950.4	E962.0	E980.4
Colestipol	972.2	E858.3	E942.2	E950.4	E962.0	E980.4
Colistimethate	960.8	E856	E930.8	E950.4	E962.0	E980.4
Colistin	960.8	E856	E930.8	E950.4	E962.0	E980.4
Collagenase	976.8	E858.7	E946.8	E950.4	E962.0	E980.4
Collagen	977.8	E866.8	E947.8	E950.9	E962.1	E980.9
Collodion (flexible)	976.3	E858.7	E946.3	E950.4	E962.0	E980.4
Colocynth	973.1	E858.4	E943.1	E950.4	E962.0	E980.4
Coloring matter — see Dye(s)						
Combustion gas — see Carbon, monoxide						
Compazine	969.1	E853.0	E939.1	E950.3	E962.0	E980.3
Compound						
42 (warfarin)	989.4	E863.7	—	E950.6	E962.1	E980.7
269 (endrin)	989.2	E863.0	—	E950.6	E962.1	E980.7
497 (dieldrin)	989.2	E863.0	—	E950.6	E962.1	E980.7
1080 (sodium fluoroacetate)	989.4	E863.7	—	E950.6	E962.1	E980.7
3422 (parathion)	989.3	E863.1	—	E950.6	E962.1	E980.7
3911 (phorate)	989.3	E863.1	—	E950.6	E962.1	E980.7
3956 (toxaphene)	989.2	E863.0	—	E950.6	E962.1	E980.7
4049 (malathion)	989.3	E863.1	—	E950.6	E962.1	E980.7
4124 (dicapthon)	989.4	E863.4	—	E950.6	E962.1	E980.7
E (cortisone)	962.0	E858.0	E932.0	E950.4	E962.0	E980.4
F (hydrocortisone)	962.0	E858.0	E932.0	E950.4	E962.0	E980.4
Congo red	977.8	E858.8	E947.8	E950.4	E962.0	E980.4
Coniine, conine	965.7	E850.7	E935.7	E950.0	E962.0	E980.0
Conium (maculatum)	988.2	E865.4	—	E950.9	E962.1	E980.9
Conjugated estrogens (equine)	962.2	E858.0	E932.2	E950.4	E962.0	E980.4
Contac	975.6	E858.6	E945.6	E950.4	E962.0	E980.4
Contact lens solution	976.5	E858.7	E946.5	E950.4	E962.0	E980.4
Contraceptives (oral)	962.2	E858.0	E932.2	E950.4	E962.0	E980.4
vaginal	976.8	E858.7	E946.8	E950.4	E962.0	E980.4
Contrast media (roentgenographic)	977.8	E858.8	E947.8	E950.4	E962.0	E980.4
Convallaria majalis	988.2	E865.4	—	E950.9	E962.1	E980.9
Copper (dust) (fumes) (salts) NEC	985.8	E866.4	—	E950.9	E962.1	E980.9
arsenate, arsenite	985.1	E866.3	—	E950.8	E962.1	E980.8
insecticide	985.1	E863.4	—	E950.8	E962.1	E980.8
emetic	973.6	E858.4	E943.6	E950.4	E962.0	E980.4
fungicide	985.8	E863.6	—	E950.6	E962.1	E980.7
insecticide	985.8	E863.4	—	E950.6	E962.1	E980.7
oleate	976.0	E858.7	E946.0	E950.4	E962.0	E980.4
sulfate	983.9	E864.3	—	E950.7	E962.1	E980.6
fungicide	983.9	E863.6	—	E950.7	E962.1	E980.6
cupric	973.6	E858.4	E943.6	E950.4	E962.0	E980.4
cuprous	983.9	E864.3	—	E950.7	E962.1	E980.6

✓4ᵗʰ Fourth-digit Required   ✓5ᵗʰ Fifth-digit Required

Copperhead snake (bite) (venom) — Table of Drugs and Chemicals

	Poisoning	External Cause (E-Code)				
		Accident	Therapeutic Use	Suicide Attempt	Assault	Undetermined
Copperhead snake (bite) (venom)	989.5	E905.0	—	E950.9	E962.1	E980.9
Coral (sting)	989.5	E905.6	—	E950.9	E962.1	E980.9
snake (bite) (venom)	989.5	E905.0	—	E950.9	E962.1	E980.9
Cordran	976.0	E858.7	E946.0	E950.4	E962.0	E980.4
Corn cures	976.4	E858.7	E946.4	E950.4	E962.0	E980.4
Cornhusker's lotion	976.3	E858.7	E946.3	E950.4	E962.0	E980.4
Corn starch	976.3	E858.7	E946.3	E950.4	E962.0	E980.4
Corrosive	983.9	E864.4	—	E950.7	E962.1	E980.6
acids NEC	983.1	E864.1	—	E950.7	E962.1	E980.6
aromatics	983.0	E864.0	—	E950.7	E962.1	E980.6
disinfectant	983.0	E861.4	—	E950.7	E962.1	E980.6
fumes NEC	987.9	E869.9	—	E952.9	E962.2	E982.9
specified NEC	983.9	E864.3	—	E950.7	E962.1	E980.6
sublimate — see Mercury, chloride						
Cortate	962.0	E858.0	E932.0	E950.4	E962.0	E980.4
Cort-Dome	962.0	E858.0	E932.0	E950.4	E962.0	E980.4
ENT agent	976.6	E858.7	E946.6	E950.4	E962.0	E980.4
ophthalmic preparation	976.5	E858.7	E946.5	E950.4	E962.0	E980.4
topical NEC	976.0	E858.7	E946.0	E950.4	E962.0	E980.4
Cortef	962.0	E858.0	E932.0	E950.4	E962.0	E980.4
ENT agent	976.6	E858.7	E946.6	E950.4	E962.0	E980.4
ophthalmic preparation	976.5	E858.7	E946.5	E950.4	E962.0	E980.4
topical NEC	976.0	E858.7	E946.0	E950.4	E962.0	E980.4
Corticosteroids (fluorinated)	962.0	E858.0	E932.0	E950.4	E962.0	E980.4
ENT agent	976.6	E858.7	E946.6	E950.4	E962.0	E980.4
ophthalmic preparation	976.5	E858.7	E946.5	E950.4	E962.0	E980.4
topical NEC	976.0	E858.7	E946.0	E950.4	E962.0	E980.4
Corticotropin	962.4	E858.0	E932.4	E950.4	E962.0	E980.4
Cortisol	962.0	E858.0	E932.0	E950.4	E962.0	E980.4
ENT agent	976.6	E858.7	E946.6	E950.4	E962.0	E980.4
ophthalmic preparation	976.5	E858.7	E946.5	E950.4	E962.0	E980.4
topical NEC	976.0	E858.7	E946.0	E950.4	E962.0	E980.4
Cortisone derivatives (acetate)	962.0	E858.0	E932.0	E950.4	E962.0	E980.4
ENT agent	976.6	E858.7	E946.6	E950.4	E962.0	E980.4
ophthalmic preparation	976.5	E858.7	E946.5	E950.4	E962.0	E980.4
topical NEC	976.0	E858.7	E946.0	E950.4	E962.0	E980.4
Cortogen	962.0	E858.0	E932.0	E950.4	E962.0	E980.4
ENT agent	976.6	E858.7	E946.6	E950.4	E962.0	E980.4
ophthalmic preparation	976.5	E858.7	E946.5	E950.4	E962.0	E980.4
Cortone	962.0	E858.0	E932.0	E950.4	E962.0	E980.4
ENT agent	976.6	E858.7	E946.6	E950.4	E962.0	E980.4
ophthalmic preparation	976.5	E858.7	E946.5	E950.4	E962.0	E980.4
Cortril	962.0	E858.0	E932.0	E950.4	E962.0	E980.4
ENT agent	976.6	E858.7	E946.6	E950.4	E962.0	E980.4
ophthalmic preparation	976.5	E858.7	E946.5	E950.4	E962.0	E980.4
topical NEC	976.0	E858.7	E946.0	E950.4	E962.0	E980.4
Cosmetics	989.89	E866.7	—	E950.9	E962.1	E980.9
Cosyntropin	977.8	E858.8	E947.8	E950.4	E962.0	E980.4
Cotarnine	964.5	E858.2	E934.5	E950.4	E962.0	E980.4
Cottonseed oil	976.3	E858.7	E946.3	E950.4	E962.0	E980.4
Cough mixtures (antitussives)	975.4	E858.6	E945.4	E950.4	E962.0	E980.4
containing opiates	965.09	E850.2	E935.2	E950.0	E962.0	E980.0
expectorants	975.5	E858.6	E945.5	E950.4	E962.0	E980.4
Coumadin	964.2	E858.2	E934.2	E950.4	E962.0	E980.4
rodenticide	989.4	E863.7	—	E950.6	E962.1	E980.7
Coumarin	964.2	E858.2	E934.2	E950.4	E962.0	E980.4
Coumetarol	964.2	E858.2	E934.2	E950.4	E962.0	E980.4
Cowbane	988.2	E865.4	—	E950.9	E962.1	E980.9
Cozyme	963.5	E858.1	E933.5	E950.4	E962.0	E980.4
Crack ●	970.8	E854.3	E940.8	E950.4	E962.0	E980.4
Creolin	983.0	E864.0	—	E950.7	E962.1	E980.6
disinfectant	983.0	E861.4	—	E950.7	E962.1	E980.6

Table of Drugs and Chemicals

			External Cause (E-Code)			
	Poisoning	Accident	Therapeutic Use	Suicide Attempt	Assault	Undetermined
Creosol (compound)	983.0	E864.0	—	E950.7	E962.1	E980.6
Creosote (beechwood) (coal tar)	983.0	E864.0	—	E950.7	E962.1	E980.6
medicinal (expectorant)	975.5	E858.6	E945.5	E950.4	E962.0	E980.4
syrup	975.5	E858.6	E945.5	E950.4	E962.0	E980.4
Cresol	983.0	E864.0	—	E950.7	E962.1	E980.6
disinfectant	983.0	E861.4	—	E950.7	E962.1	E980.6
Cresylic acid	983.0	E864.0	—	E950.7	E962.1	E980.6
Cropropamide	965.7	E850.7	E935.7	E950.0	E962.0	E980.0
with crotethamide	970.0	E854.3	E940.0	E950.4	E962.0	E980.4
Crotamiton	976.0	E858.7	E946.0	E950.4	E962.0	E980.4
Crotethamide	965.7	E850.7	E935.7	E950.0	E962.0	E980.0
with cropropamide	970.0	E854.3	E940.0	E950.4	E962.0	E980.4
Croton (oil)	973.1	E858.4	E943.1	E950.4	E962.0	E980.4
chloral	967.1	E852.0	E937.1	E950.2	E962.0	E980.2
Crude oil	981	E862.1	—	E950.9	E962.1	E980.9
Cryogenine	965.8	E850.8	E935.8	E950.0	E962.0	E980.0
Cryolite (pesticide)	989.4	E863.4	—	E950.6	E962.1	E980.7
Cryptenamine	972.6	E858.3	E942.6	E950.4	E962.0	E980.4
Crystal violet	976.0	E858.7	E946.0	E950.4	E962.0	E980.4
Cuckoopint	988.2	E865.4	—	E950.9	E962.1	E980.9
Cumetharol	964.2	E858.2	E934.2	E950.4	E962.0	E980.4
Cupric sulfate	973.6	E858.4	E943.6	E950.4	E962.0	E980.4
Cuprous sulfate	983.9	E864.3	—	E950.7	E962.1	E980.6
Curare, curarine	975.2	E858.6	E945.2	E950.4	E962.0	E980.4
Cyanic acid — see **Cyanide(s)**						
Cyanide(s) (compounds) (hydrogen) (potassium) (sodium) NEC	989.0	E866.8	—	E950.9	E962.1	E980.9
dust or gas (inhalation) NEC	987.7	E869.8	—	E952.8	E962.2	E982.8
fumigant	989.0	E863.8	—	E950.6	E962.1	E980.7
mercuric — see Mercury						
pesticide (dust) (fumes)	989.0	E863.4	—	E950.6	E962.1	E980.7
Cyanocobalamin	964.1	E858.2	E934.1	E950.4	E962.0	E980.4
Cyanogen (chloride) (gas) NEC	987.8	E869.8	—	E952.8	E962.2	E982.8
Cyclaine	968.5	E855.2	E938.5	E950.4	E962.0	E980.4
Cyclamen europaeum	988.2	E865.4	—	E950.9	E962.1	E980.9
Cyclandelate	972.5	E858.3	E942.5	E950.4	E962.0	E980.4
Cyclazocine	965.09	E850.2	E935.2	E950.0	E962.0	E980.0
Cyclizine	963.0	E858.1	E933.0	E950.4	E962.0	E980.4
Cyclobarbital, cyclobarbitone	967.0	E851	E937.0	E950.1	E962.0	E980.1
Cycloguanil	961.4	E857	E931.4	E950.4	E962.0	E980.4
Cyclohexane	982.0	E862.4	—	E950.9	E962.1	E980.9
Cyclohexanol	980.8	E860.8	—	E950.9	E962.1	E980.9
Cyclohexanone	982.8	E862.4	—	E950.9	E962.1	E980.9
Cyclomethycaine	968.5	E855.2	E938.5	E950.4	E962.0	E980.4
Cyclopentamine	971.2	E855.5	E941.2	E950.4	E962.0	E980.4
Cyclopenthiazide	974.3	E858.5	E944.3	E950.4	E962.0	E980.4
Cyclopentolate	971.1	E855.4	E941.1	E950.4	E962.0	E980.4
Cyclophosphamide	963.1	E858.1	E933.1	E950.4	E962.0	E980.4
Cyclopropane	968.2	E855.1	E938.2	E950.4	E962.0	E980.4
Cycloserine	960.6	E856	E930.6	E950.4	E962.0	E980.4
Cyclothiazide	974.3	E858.5	E944.3	E950.4	E962.0	E980.4
Cycrimine	966.4	E855.0	E936.4	E950.4	E962.0	E980.4
Cymarin	972.1	E858.3	E942.1	E950.4	E962.0	E980.4
Cyproheptadine	963.0	E858.1	E933.0	E950.4	E962.0	E980.4
Cyprolidol	969.0	E854.0	E939.0	E950.3	E962.0	E980.3
Cytarabine	963.1	E858.1	E933.1	E950.4	E962.0	E980.4
Cytisus						
laburnum	988.2	E865.4	—	E950.9	E962.1	E980.9
scoparius	988.2	E865.4	—	E950.9	E962.1	E980.9
Cytomel	962.7	E858.0	E932.7	E950.4	E962.0	E980.4
Cytosine (antineoplastic)	963.1	E858.1	E933.1	E950.4	E962.0	E980.4
Cytoxan	963.1	E858.1	E933.1	E950.4	E962.0	E980.4

Fourth-digit Required   Fifth-digit Required

Dacarbazine — Table of Drugs and Chemicals

		External Cause (E-Code)				
	Poisoning	Accident	Therapeutic Use	Suicide Attempt	Assault	Undetermined
Dacarbazine	963.1	E858.1	E933.1	E950.4	E962.0	E980.4
Dactinomycin	960.7	E856	E930.7	E950.4	E962.0	E980.4
DADPS	961.8	E857	E931.8	E950.4	E962.0	E980.4
Dakin's solution (external)	976.0	E858.7	E946.0	E950.4	E962.0	E980.4
Dalmane	969.4	E853.2	E939.4	E950.3	E962.0	E980.3
DAM	977.2	E858.8	E947.2	E950.4	E962.0	E980.4
Danilone	964.2	E858.2	E934.2	E950.4	E962.0	E980.4
Danthron	973.1	E858.4	E943.1	E950.4	E962.0	E980.4
Dantrolene	975.2	E858.6	E945.2	E950.4	E962.0	E980.4
Daphne (gnidium) (mezereum)	988.2	E865.4	—	E950.9	E962.1	E980.9
berry	988.2	E865.3	—	E950.9	E962.1	E980.9
Dapsone	961.8	E857	E931.8	E950.4	E962.0	E980.4
Daraprim	961.4	E857	E931.4	E950.4	E962.0	E980.4
Darnel	988.2	E865.3	—	E950.9	E962.1	E980.9
Darvon	965.8	E850.8	E935.8	E950.0	E962.0	E980.0
Daunorubicin	960.7	E856	E930.7	E950.4	E962.0	E980.4
DBI	962.3	E858.0	E932.3	E950.4	E962.0	E980.4
D-Con (rodenticide)	989.4	E863.7	—	E950.6	E962.1	E980.7
DDS	961.8	E857	E931.8	E950.4	E962.0	E980.4
DDT	989.2	E863.0	—	E950.6	E962.1	E980.7
Deadly nightshade	988.2	E865.4	—	E950.9	E962.1	E980.9
berry	988.2	E865.3	—	E950.9	E962.1	E980.9
Deanol	969.7	E854.2	E939.7	E950.3	E962.0	E980.3
Debrisoquine	972.6	E858.3	E942.6	E950.4	E962.0	E980.4
Decaborane	989.89	E866.8	—	E950.9	E962.1	E980.9
fumes	987.8	E869.8	—	E952.8	E962.2	E982.8
Decadron	962.0	E858.0	E932.0	E950.4	E962.0	E980.4
ENT agent	976.6	E858.7	E946.6	E950.4	E962.0	E980.4
ophthalmic preparation	976.5	E858.7	E946.5	E950.4	E962.0	E980.4
topical NEC	976.0	E858.7	E946.0	E950.4	E962.0	E980.4
Decahydronaphthalene	982.0	E862.4	—	E950.9	E962.1	E980.9
Decalin	982.0	E862.4	—	E950.9	E962.1	E980.9
Decamethonium	975.2	E858.6	E945.2	E950.4	E962.0	E980.4
Decholin	973.4	E858.4	E943.4	E950.4	E962.0	E980.4
sodium (diagnostic)	977.8	E858.8	E947.8	E950.4	E962.0	E980.4
Declomycin	960.4	E856	E930.4	E950.4	E962.0	E980.4
Deferoxamine	963.8	E858.1	E933.8	E950.4	E962.0	E980.4
Dehydrocholic acid	973.4	E858.4	E943.4	E950.4	E962.0	E980.4
DeKalin	982.0	E862.4	—	E950.9	E962.1	E980.9
Delalutin	962.2	E858.0	E932.2	E950.4	E962.0	E980.4
Delphinium	988.2	E865.3	—	E950.9	E962.1	E980.9
Deltasone	962.0	E858.0	E932.0	E950.4	E962.0	E980.4
Deltra	962.0	E858.0	E932.0	E950.4	E962.0	E980.4
Delvinal	967.0	E851	E937.0	E950.1	E962.0	E980.1
Demecarium (bromide)	971.0	E855.3	E941.0	E950.4	E962.0	E980.4
Demeclocycline	960.4	E856	E930.4	E950.4	E962.0	E980.4
Demecolcine	963.1	E858.1	E933.1	E950.4	E962.0	E980.4
Demelanizing agents	976.8	E858.7	E946.8	E950.4	E962.0	E980.4
Demerol	965.09	E850.2	E935.2	E950.0	E962.0	E980.0
Demethylchlortetracycline	960.4	E856	E930.4	E950.4	E962.0	E980.4
Demethyltetracycline	960.4	E856	E930.4	E950.4	E962.0	E980.4
Demeton	989.3	E863.1	—	E950.6	E962.1	E980.7
Demulcents	976.3	E858.7	E946.3	E950.4	E962.0	E980.4
Demulen	962.2	E858.0	E932.2	E950.4	E962.0	E980.4
Denatured alcohol	980.0	E860.1	—	E950.9	E962.1	E980.9
Dendrid	976.5	E858.7	E946.5	E950.4	E962.0	E980.4
Dental agents, topical	976.7	E858.7	E946.7	E950.4	E962.0	E980.4
Deodorant spray (feminine hygiene)	976.8	E858.7	E946.8	E950.4	E962.0	E980.4
Deoxyribonuclease	963.4	E858.1	E933.4	E950.4	E962.0	E980.4
Depressants						
appetite, central	977.0	E858.8	E947.0	E950.4	E962.0	E980.4
cardiac	972.0	E858.3	E942.0	E950.4	E962.0	E980.4

▶◀ Revised Text   ● New Line   ▲ Revised Code

Table of Drugs and Chemicals — Dibenamine

	External Cause (E-Code)					
	Poisoning	Accident	Therapeutic Use	Suicide Attempt	Assault	Undetermined
Depressants — *continued*						
central nervous system						
(anesthetic)	968.4	E855.1	E938.4	E950.4	E962.0	E980.4
psychotherapeutic	969.5	E853.9	E939.5	E950.3	E962.0	E980.3
Dequalinium	976.0	E858.7	E946.0	E950.4	E962.0	E980.4
Dermolate	976.2	E858.7	E946.2	E950.4	E962.0	E980.4
DES	962.2	E858.0	E932.2	E950.4	E962.0	E980.4
Desenex	976.0	E858.7	E946.0	E950.4	E962.0	E980.4
Deserpidine	972.6	E858.3	E942.6	E950.4	E962.0	E980.4
Desipramine	969.0	E854.0	E939.0	E950.3	E962.0	E980.3
Deslanoside	972.1	E858.3	E942.1	E950.4	E962.0	E980.4
Desocodeine	965.09	E850.2	E935.2	E950.0	E962.0	E980.0
Desomorphine	965.09	E850.2	E935.2	E950.0	E962.0	E980.0
Desonide	976.0	E858.7	E946.0	E950.4	E962.0	E980.4
Desoxycorticosterone						
derivatives	962.0	E858.0	E932.0	E950.4	E962.0	E980.4
Desoxyephedrine	969.7	E854.2	E939.7	E950.3	E962.0	E980.3
DET	969.6	E854.1	E939.6	E950.3	E962.0	E980.3
Detergents (ingested)						
(synthetic)	989.6	E861.0	—	E950.9	E962.1	E980.9
external medication	976.2	E858.7	E946.2	E950.4	E962.0	E980.4
Deterrent, alcohol	977.3	E858.8	E947.3	E950.4	E962.0	E980.4
Detrothyronine	962.7	E858.0	E932.7	E950.4	E962.0	E980.4
Dettol (external medication)	976.0	E858.7	E946.0	E950.4	E962.0	E980.4
Dexamethasone	962.0	E858.0	E932.0	E950.4	E962.0	E980.4
ENT agent	976.6	E858.7	E946.6	E950.4	E962.0	E980.4
ophthalmic preparation	976.5	E858.7	E946.5	E950.4	E962.0	E980.4
topical NEC	976.0	E858.7	E946.0	E950.4	E962.0	E980.4
Dexamphetamine	969.7	E854.2	E939.7	E950.3	E962.0	E980.3
Dexedrine	969.7	E854.2	E939.7	E950.3	E962.0	E980.3
Dexpanthenol	963.5	E858.1	E933.5	E950.4	E962.0	E980.4
Dextran	964.8	E858.2	E934.8	E950.4	E962.0	E980.4
Dextriferron	964.0	E858.2	E934.0	E950.4	E962.0	E980.4
Dextroamphetamine	969.7	E854.2	E939.7	E950.3	E962.0	E980.3
Dextro calcium pantothenate	963.5	E858.1	E933.5	E950.4	E962.0	E980.4
Dextromethorphan	975.4	E858.6	E945.4	E950.4	E962.0	E980.4
Dextromoramide	965.09	E850.2	E935.2	E950.0	E962.0	E980.0
Dextro pantothenyl alcohol	963.5	E858.1	E933.5	E950.4	E962.0	E980.4
topical	976.8	E858.7	E946.8	E950.4	E962.0	E980.4
Dextropropoxyphene						
(hydrochloride)	965.8	E850.8	E935.8	E950.0	E962.0	E980.0
Dextrorphan	965.09	E850.2	E935.2	E950.0	E962.0	E980.0
Dextrose NEC	974.5	E858.5	E944.5	E950.4	E962.0	E980.4
Dextrothyroxin	962.7	E858.0	E932.7	E950.4	E962.0	E980.4
DFP	971.0	E855.3	E941.0	E950.4	E962.0	E980.4
DHE-45	972.9	E858.3	E942.9	E950.4	E962.0	E980.4
Diabinese	962.3	E858.0	E932.3	E950.4	E962.0	E980.4
Diacetyl monoxime	977.2	E858.8	E947.2	E950.4	E962.0	E980.4
Diacetylmorphine	965.01	E850.0	E935.0	E950.0	E962.0	E980.0
Diagnostic agents	977.8	E858.8	E947.8	E950.4	E962.0	E980.4
Dial (soap)	976.2	E858.7	E946.2	E950.4	E962.0	E980.4
sedative	967.0	E851	E937.0	E950.1	E962.0	E980.1
Diallylbarbituric acid	967.0	E851	E937.0	E950.1	E962.0	E980.1
Diaminodiphenylsulfone	961.8	E857	E931.8	E950.4	E962.0	E980.4
Diamorphine	965.01	E850.0	E935.0	E950.0	E962.0	E980.0
Diamox	974.2	E858.5	E944.2	E950.4	E962.0	E980.4
Diamthazole	976.0	E858.7	E946.0	E950.4	E962.0	E980.4
Diaphenylsulfone	961.8	E857	E931.8	E950.4	E962.0	E980.4
Diasone (sodium)	961.8	E857	E931.8	E950.4	E962.0	E980.4
Diazepam	969.4	E853.2	E939.4	E950.3	E962.0	E980.3
Diazinon	989.3	E863.1	—	E950.6	E962.1	E980.7
Diazomethane (gas)	987.8	E869.8	—	E952.8	E962.2	E982.8
Diazoxide	972.5	E858.3	E942.5	E950.4	E962.0	E980.4
Dibenamine	971.3	E855.6	E941.3	E950.4	E962.0	E980.4

		External Cause (E-Code)				
	Poisoning	Accident	Therapeutic Use	Suicide Attempt	Assault	Undetermined
Dibenzheptropine	963.0	E858.1	E933.0	E950.4	E962.0	E980.4
Dibenzyline	971.3	E855.6	E941.3	E950.4	E962.0	E980.4
Diborane (gas)	987.8	E869.8	—	E952.8	E962.2	E982.8
Dibromomannitol	963.1	E858.1	E933.1	E950.4	E962.0	E980.4
Dibucaine (spinal)	968.7	E855.2	E938.7	E950.4	E962.0	E980.4
topical (surface)	968.5	E855.2	E938.5	E950.4	E962.0	E980.4
Dibunate sodium	975.4	E858.6	E945.4	E950.4	E962.0	E980.4
Dibutoline	971.1	E855.4	E941.1	E950.4	E962.0	E980.4
Dicapthon	989.4	E863.4	—	E950.6	E962.1	E980.7
Dichloralphenazone	967.1	E852.0	E937.1	E950.2	E962.0	E980.2
Dichlorodifluoromethane	987.4	E869.2	—	E952.8	E962.2	E982.8
Dichloroethane	982.3	E862.4	—	E950.9	E962.1	E980.9
Dichloroethylene	982.3	E862.4	—	E950.9	E962.1	E980.9
Dichloroethyl sulfide	987.8	E869.8	—	E952.8	E962.2	E982.8
Dichlorohydrin	982.3	E862.4	—	E950.9	E962.1	E980.9
Dichloromethane (solvent)						
(vapor)	982.3	E862.4	—	E950.9	E962.1	E980.9
Dichlorophen(e)	961.6	E857	E931.6	E950.4	E962.0	E980.4
Dichlorphenamide	974.2	E858.5	E944.2	E950.4	E962.0	E980.4
Dichlorvos	989.3	E863.1	—	E950.6	E962.1	E980.7
Diclofenac sodium	965.69	E850.6	E935.6	E950.0	E962.0	E980.0
Dicoumarin, dicumarol	964.2	E858.2	E934.2	E950.4	E962.0	E980.4
Dicyanogen (gas)	987.8	E869.8	—	E952.8	E962.2	E982.8
Dicyclomine	971.1	E855.4	E941.1	E950.4	E962.0	E980.4
Dieldrin (vapor)	989.2	E863.0	—	E950.6	E962.1	E980.7
Dienestrol	962.2	E858.0	E932.2	E950.4	E962.0	E980.4
Dietetics	977.0	E858.8	E947.0	E950.4	E962.0	E980.4
Diethazine	966.4	E855.0	E936.4	E950.4	E962.0	E980.4
Diethyl						
barbituric acid	967.0	E851	E937.0	E950.1	E962.0	E980.1
carbamazine	961.6	E857	E931.6	E950.4	E962.0	E980.4
carbinol	980.8	E860.8	—	E950.9	E962.1	E980.9
carbonate	982.8	E862.4	—	E950.9	E962.1	E980.9
ether (vapor) — see Ether(s)						
propion	977.0	E858.8	E947.0	E950.4	E962.0	E980.4
stilbestrol	962.2	E858.0	E932.2	E950.4	E962.0	E980.4
Diethylene						
dioxide	982.8	E862.4	—	E950.9	E962.1	E980.9
glycol (monoacetate)						
(monoethyl ether)	982.8	E862.4	—	E950.9	E962.1	E980.9
Diethylsulfone-diethylmethane	967.8	E852.8	E937.8	E950.2	E962.0	E980.2
Difencloxazine	965.09	E850.2	E935.2	E950.0	E962.0	E980.0
Diffusin	963.4	E858.1	E933.4	E950.4	E962.0	E980.4
Diflos	971.0	E855.3	E941.0	E950.4	E962.0	E980.4
Digestants	973.4	E858.4	E943.4	E950.4	E962.0	E980.4
Digitalin(e)	972.1	E858.3	E942.1	E950.4	E962.0	E980.4
Digitalis glycosides	972.1	E858.3	E942.1	E950.4	E962.0	E980.4
Digitoxin	972.1	E858.3	E942.1	E950.4	E962.0	E980.4
Digoxin	972.1	E858.3	E942.1	E950.4	E962.0	E980.4
Dihydrocodeine	965.09	E850.2	E935.2	E950.0	E962.0	E980.0
Dihydrocodeinone	965.09	E850.2	E935.2	E950.0	E962.0	E980.0
Dihydroergocristine	972.9	E858.3	E942.9	E950.4	E962.0	E980.4
Dihydroergotamine	972.9	E858.3	E942.9	E950.4	E962.0	E980.4
Dihydroergotoxine	972.9	E858.3	E942.9	E950.4	E962.0	E980.4
Dihydrohydroxycodeinone	965.09	E850.2	E935.2	E950.0	E962.0	E980.0
Dihydrohydroxymorphinone	965.09	E850.2	E935.2	E950.0	E962.0	E980.0
Dihydroisocodeine	965.09	E850.2	E935.2	E950.0	E962.0	E980.0
Dihydromorphine	965.09	E850.2	E935.2	E950.0	E962.0	E980.0
Dihydromorphinone	965.09	E850.2	E935.2	E950.0	E962.0	E980.0
Dihydrostreptomycin	960.6	E856	E930.6	E950.4	E962.0	E980.4
Dihydrotachysterol	962.6	E858.0	E932.6	E950.4	E962.0	E980.4
Dihydroxyanthraquinone	973.1	E858.4	E943.1	E950.4	E962.0	E980.4
Dihydroxycodeinone	965.09	E850.2	E935.2	E950.0	E962.0	E980.0

Table of Drugs and Chemicals — Diphtheria

	Poisoning	External Cause (E-Code)				
		Accident	Therapeutic Use	Suicide Attempt	Assault	Undetermined
Diiodohydroxyquin	961.3	E857	E931.3	E950.4	E962.0	E980.4
topical	976.0	E858.7	E946.0	E950.4	E962.0	E980.4
Diiodohydroxyquinoline	961.3	E857	E931.3	E950.4	E962.0	E980.4
Dilantin	966.1	E855.0	E936.1	E950.4	E962.0	E980.4
Dilaudid	965.09	E850.2	E935.2	E950.0	E962.0	E980.0
Diloxanide	961.5	E857	E931.5	E950.4	E962.0	E980.4
Dimefline	970.	E854.3	E940.0	E950.4	E962.0	E980.4
Dimenhydrinate	963.0	E858.1	E933.0	E950.4	E962.0	E980.4
Dimercaprol	963.8	E858.1	E933.8	E950.4	E962.0	E980.4
Dimercaptopropanol	963.8	E858.1	E933.8	E950.4	E962.0	E980.4
Dimetane	963.0	E858.1	E933.0	E950.4	E962.0	E980.4
Dimethicone	976.3	E858.7	E946.3	E950.4	E962.0	E980.4
Dimethindene	963.0	E858.1	E933.0	E950.4	E962.0	E980.4
Dimethisoquin	968.5	E855.2	E938.5	E950.4	E962.0	E980.4
Dimethisterone	962.2	E858.0	E932.2	E950.4	E962.0	E980.4
Dimethoxanate	975.4	E858.6	E945.4	E950.4	E962.0	E980.4
Dimethyl						
arsine, arsinic acid — see Arsenic						
carbinol	980.2	E860.3	—	E950.9	E962.1	E980.9
diguanide	962.3	E858.0	E932.3	E950.4	E962.0	E980.4
ketone	982.8	E862.4	—	E950.9	E962.1	E980.9
vapor	987.8	E869.8	—	E952.8	E962.2	E982.8
meperidine	965.09	E850.2	E935.2	E950.0	E962.0	E980.0
parathion	989.3	E863.1	—	E950.6	E962.1	E980.7
polysiloxane	973.8	E858.4	E943.8	E950.4	E962.0	E980.4
sulfate (fumes)	987.8	E869.8	—	E952.8	E962.2	E982.8
liquid	983.9	E864.3	—	E950.7	E962.1	E980.6
sulfoxide NEC	982.8	E862.4	—	E950.9	E962.1	E980.9
medicinal	976.4	E858.7	E946.4	E950.4	E962.0	E980.4
triptamine	969.6	E854.1	E939.6	E950.3	E962.0	E980.3
tubocurarine	975.2	E858.6	E945.2	E950.4	E962.0	E980.4
Dindevan	964.2	E858.2	E934.2	E950.4	E962.0	E980.4
Dinitro (-ortho-) cresol						
(herbicide) (spray)	989.4	E863.5	—	E950.6	E962.1	E980.7
insecticide	989.4	E863.4	—	E950.6	E962.1	E980.7
Dinitrobenzene	983.0	E864.0	—	E950.7	E962.1	E980.6
vapor	987.8	E869.8	—	E952.8	E962.2	E982.8
Dinitro-orthocresol (herbicide)	989.4	E863.5	—	E950.6	E962.1	E980.7
insecticide	989.4	E863.4	—	E950.6	E962.1	E980.7
Dinitrophenol (herbicide)						
(spray)	989.4	E863.5	—	E950.6	E962.1	E980.7
insecticide	989.4	E863.4	—	E950.6	E962.1	E980.7
Dinoprost	975.0	E858.6	E945.0	E950.4	E962.0	E980.4
Dioctyl sulfosuccinate						
(calcium) (sodium)	973.2	E858.4	E943.2	E950.4	E962.0	E980.4
Diodoquin	961.3	E857	E931.3	E950.4	E962.0	E980.4
Dione derivatives NEC	966.3	E855.0	E936.3	E950.4	E962.0	E980.4
Dionin	965.09	E850.2	E935.2	E950.0	E962.0	E980.0
Dioxane	982.8	E862.4	—	E950.9	E962.1	E980.9
Dioxin — see Herbicide						
Dioxyline	972.5	E858.3	E942.5	E950.4	E962.0	E980.4
Dipentene	982.8	E862.4	—	E950.9	E962.1	E980.9
Diphemanil	971.1	E855.4	E941.1	E950.4	E962.0	E980.4
Diphenadione	964.2	E858.2	E934.2	E950.4	E962.0	E980.4
Diphenhydramine	963.0	E858.1	E933.0	E950.4	E962.0	E980.4
Diphenidol	963.0	E858.1	E933.0	E950.4	E962.0	E980.4
Diphenoxylate	973.5	E858.4	E943.5	E950.4	E962.0	E980.4
Diphenylchloroarsine	985.1	E866.3	—	E950.8	E962.1	E980.8
Diphenylhydantoin (sodium)	966.1	E855.0	E936.1	E950.4	E962.0	E980.4
Diphenylpyraline	963.0	E858.1	E933.0	E950.4	E962.0	E980.4
Diphtheria						
antitoxin	979.9	E858.8	E949.9	E950.4	E962.0	E980.4

🖪 Fourth-digit Required   🖪 Fifth-digit Required

Diphtheria — Table of Drugs and Chemicals

	Poisoning	Accident	Therapeutic Use	Suicide Attempt	Assault	Undetermined
Diphtheria — *continued*						
toxoid	978.5	E858.8	E948.5	E950.4	E962.0	E980.4
with tetanus toxoid	978.9	E858.8	E948.9	E950.4	E962.0	E980.4
with pertussis component	978.6	E858.8	E948.6	E950.4	E962.0	E980.4
vaccine	978.5	E858.8	E948.5	E950.4	E962.0	E980.4
Dipipanone	965.09	E850.2	E935.2	E950.0	E962.0	E980.0
Diplovax	979.5	E858.8	E949.5	E950.4	E962.0	E980.4
Diprophylline	975.1	E858.6	E945.1	E950.4	E962.0	E980.4
Dipyridamole	972.4	E858.3	E942.4	E950.4	E962.0	E980.4
Dipyrone	965.5	E850.5	E935.5	E950.0	E962.0	E980.0
Diquat	989.4	E863.5	—	E950.6	E962.1	E980.7
Disinfectant NEC	983.9	E861.4	—	E950.7	E962.1	E980.6
alkaline	983.2	E861.4	—	E950.7	E962.1	E980.6
aromatic	983.0	E861.4	—	E950.7	E962.1	E980.6
Disipal	966.4	E855.0	E936.4	E950.4	E962.0	E980.4
Disodium edetate	963.8	E858.1	E933.8	E950.4	E962.0	E980.4
Disulfamide	974.4	E858.5	E944.4	E950.4	E962.0	E980.4
Disulfanilamide	961.0	E857	E931.0	E950.4	E962.0	E980.4
Disulfiram	977.3	E858.8	E947.3	E950.4	E962.0	E980.4
Dithiazanine	961.6	E857	E931.6	E950.4	E962.0	E980.4
Dithioglycerol	963.8	E858.1	E933.8	E950.4	E962.0	E980.4
Dithranol	976.4	E858.7	E946.4	E950.4	E962.0	E980.4
Diucardin	974.3	E858.5	E944.3	E950.4	E962.0	E980.4
Diupres	974.3	E858.5	E944.3	E950.4	E962.0	E980.4
Diuretics NEC	974.4	E858.5	E944.4	E950.4	E962.0	E980.4
carbonic acid anhydrase inhibitors	974.2	E858.5	E944.2	E950.4	E962.0	E980.4
mercurial	974.0	E858.5	E944.0	E950.4	E962.0	E980.4
osmotic	974.4	E858.5	E944.4	E950.4	E962.0	E980.4
purine derivatives	974.1	E858.5	E944.1	E950.4	E962.0	E980.4
saluretic	974.3	E858.5	E944.3	E950.4	E962.0	E980.4
Diuril	974.3	E858.5	E944.3	E950.4	E962.0	E980.4
Divinyl ether	968.2	E855.1	E938.2	E950.4	E962.0	E980.4
D-lysergic acid diethylamide	969.6	E854.1	E939.6	E950.3	E962.0	E980.3
DMCT	960.4	E856	E930.4	E950.4	E962.0	E980.4
DMSO	982.8	E862.4	—	E950.9	E962.1	E980.9
DMT	969.6	E854.1	E939.6	E950.3	E962.0	E980.3
DNOC	989.4	E863.5	—	E950.6	E962.1	E980.7
DOCA	962.0	E858.0	E932.0	E950.4	E962.0	E980.4
Dolophine	965.02	E850.1	E935.1	E950.0	E962.0	E980.0
Doloxene	965.8	E850.8	E935.8	E950.0	E962.0	E980.0
DOM	969.6	E854.1	E939.6	E950.3	E962.0	E980.3
Domestic gas — *see* Gas, utility						
Domiphen (bromide) (lozenges)	976.6	E858.7	E946.6	E950.4	E962.0	E980.4
Dopa (levo)	966.4	E855.0	E936.4	E950.4	E962.0	E980.4
Dopamine	971.2	E855.5	E941.2	E950.4	E962.0	E980.4
Doriden	967.5	E852.4	E937.5	E950.2	E962.0	E980.2
Dormiral	967.0	E851	E937.0	E950.1	E962.0	E980.1
Dormison	967.8	E852.8	E937.8	E950.2	E962.0	E980.2
Dornase	963.4	E858.1	E933.4	E950.4	E962.0	E980.4
Dorsacaine	968.5	E855.2	E938.5	E950.4	E962.0	E980.4
Dothiepin hydrochloride	969.0	E854.0	E939.0	E950.3	E962.0	E980.3
Doxapram	970.0	E854.3	E940.0	E950.4	E962.0	E980.4
Doxepin	969.0	E854.0	E939.0	E950.3	E962.0	E980.3
Doxorubicin	960.7	E856	E930.7	E950.4	E962.0	E980.4
Doxycycline	960.4	E856	E930.4	E950.4	E962.0	E980.4
Doxylamine	963.0	E858.1	E933.0	E950.4	E962.0	E980.4
Dramamine	963.0	E858.1	E933.0	E950.4	E962.0	E980.4
Drano (drain cleaner)	983.2	E864.2	—	E950.7	E962.1	E980.6
Dromoran	965.09	E850.2	E935.2	E950.0	E962.0	E980.0
Dromostanolone	962.1	E858.0	E932.1	E950.4	E962.0	E980.4
Droperidol	969.2	E853.1	E939.2	E950.3	E962.0	E980.3

Table of Drugs and Chemicals

	Poisoning	\multicolumn{5}{c}{External Cause (E-Code)}			

	Poisoning	Accident	Therapeutic Use	Suicide Attempt	Assault	Undetermined
Drug	977.9	E858.9	E947.9	E950.5	E962.0	E980.5
specified NEC	977.8	E858.8	E947.8	E950.4	E962.0	E980.4
AHFS List						
4:00 antihistamine drugs	963.0	E858.1	E933.0	E950.4	E962.0	E980.4
8:04 amebacides	961.5	E857	E931.5	E950.4	E962.0	E980.4
arsenical anti-infectives	961.1	E857	E931.1	E950.4	E962.0	E980.4
quinoline derivatives	961.3	E857	E931.3	E950.4	E962.0	E980.4
8:08 anthelmintics	961.6	E857	E931.6	E950.4	E962.0	E980.4
quinoline derivatives	961.3	E857	E931.3	E950.4	E962.0	E980.4
8:12.04 antifungal antibiotics	960.1	E856	E930.1	E950.4	E962.0	E980.4
8:12.06 cephalosporins	960.5	E856	E930.5	E950.4	E962.0	E980.4
8:12.08 chloramphenicol	960.2	E856	E930.2	E950.4	E962.0	E980.4
8:12.12 erythromycins	960.3	E856	E930.3	E950.4	E962.0	E980.4
8:12.16 penicillins	960.0	E856	E930.0	E950.4	E962.0	E980.4
8:12.20 streptomycins	960.6	E856	E930.6	E950.4	E962.0	E980.4
8:12.24 tetracyclines	960.4	E856	E930.4	E950.4	E962.0	E980.4
8:12.28 other antibiotics	960.8	E856	E930.8	E950.4	E962.0	E980.4
antimycobacterial	960.6	E856	E930.6	E950.4	E962.0	E980.4
macrolides	960.3	E856	E930.3	E950.4	E962.0	E980.4
8:16 antituberculars	961.8	E857	E931.8	E950.4	E962.0	E980.4
antibiotics	960.6	E856	E930.6	E950.4	E962.0	E980.4
8:18 antivirals	961.7	E857	E931.7	E950.4	E962.0	E980.4
8:20 plasmodicides (antimalarials)	961.4	E857	E931.4	E950.4	E962.0	E980.4
8:24 sulfonamides	961.0	E857	E931.0	E950.4	E962.0	E980.4
8:26 sulfones	961.8	E857	E931.8	E950.4	E962.0	E980.4
8:28 treponemicides	961.2	E857	E931.2	E950.4	E962.0	E980.4
8:32 trichomonacides	961.5	E857	E931.5	E950.4	E962.0	E980.4
quinoline derivatives	961.3	E857	E931.3	E950.4	E962.0	E980.4
nitrofuran derivatives	961.9	E857	E931.9	E950.4	E962.0	E980.4
8:36 urinary germicides	961.9	E857	E931.9	E950.4	E962.0	E980.4
quinoline derivatives	961.3	E857	E931.3	E950.4	E962.0	E980.4
8:40 other anti-infectives	961.9	E857	E931.9	E950.4	E962.0	E980.4
10:00 antineoplastic agents	963.1	E858.1	E933.1	E950.4	E962.0	E980.4
antibiotics	960.7	E856	E930.7	E950.4	E962.0	E980.4
progestogens	962.2	E858.0	E932.2	E950.4	E962.0	E980.4
12:04 parasympathomimetic (cholinergic) agents	971.0	E855.3	E941.0	E950.4	E962.0	E980.4
12:08 parasympatholytic (cholinergic-blocking) agents	971.1	E855.4	E941.1	E950.4	E962.0	E980.4
12:12 Sympathomimetic (adrenergic) agents	971.2	E855.5	E941.2	E950.4	E962.0	E980.4
12:16 sympatholytic (adrenergic-blocking) agents	971.3	E855.6	E941.3	E950.4	E962.0	E980.4
12:20 skeletal muscle relaxants						
central nervous system muscle-tone depressants	968.0	E855.1	E938.0	E950.4	E962.0	E980.4
myoneural blocking agents	975.2	E858.6	E945.2	E950.4	E962.0	E980.4
16:00 blood derivatives	964.7	E858.2	E934.7	E950.4	E962.0	E980.4
20:04 antianemia drugs	964.1	E858.2	E934.1	E950.4	E962.0	E980.4
20:04.04 iron preparations	964.0	E858.2	E934.0	E950.4	E962.0	E980.4
20:04.08 liver and stomach preparations	964.1	E858.2	E934.1	E950.4	E962.0	E980.4
20:12.04 anticoagulants	964.2	E858.2	E934.2	E950.4	E962.0	E980.4
20:12.08 antiheparin agents	964.5	E858.2	E934.5	E950.4	E962.0	E980.4
20:12.12 coagulants	964.5	E858.2	E934.5	E950.4	E962.0	E980.4

✔4️⃣ Fourth-digit Required   ✔5️⃣ Fifth-digit Required

Table of Drugs and Chemicals

			External Cause (E-Code)			
	Poisoning	Accident	Therapeutic Use	Suicide Attempt	Assault	Undetermined
Drug — continued						
20:12.16 hemostatics NEC	964.5	E858.2	E934.5	E950.4	E962.0	E980.4
capillary active drugs	972.8	E858.3	E942.8	E950.4	E962.0	E980.4
24:04 cardiac drugs	972.9	E858.3	E942.9	E950.4	E962.0	E980.4
cardiotonic agents	972.1	E858.3	E942.1	E950.4	E962.0	E980.4
rhythm regulators	972.0	E858.3	E942.0	E950.4	E962.0	E980.4
24:06 antilipemic agents	972.2	E858.3	E942.2	E950.4	E962.0	E980.4
thyroid derivatives	962.7	E858.0	E932.7	E950.4	E962.0	E980.4
24:08 hypotensive agents	972.6	E858.3	E942.6	E950.4	E962.0	E980.4
adrenergic blocking agents	971.3	E855.6	E941.3	E950.4	E962.0	E980.4
ganglion blocking agents	972.3	E858.3	E942.3	E950.4	E962.0	E980.4
vasodilators	972.5	E858.3	E942.5	E950.4	E962.0	E980.4
24:12 vasodilating agents NEC	972.5	E858.3	E942.5	E950.4	E962.0	E980.4
coronary	972.4	E858.3	E942.4	E950.4	E962.0	E980.4
nicotinic acid derivatives	972.2	E858.3	E942.2	E950.4	E962.0	E980.4
24:16 sclerosing agents	972.7	E858.3	E942.7	E950.4	E962.0	E980.4
28:04 general anesthetics	968.4	E855.1	E938.4	E950.4	E962.0	E980.4
gaseous anesthetics	968.2	E855.1	E938.2	E950.4	E962.0	E980.4
halothane	968.1	E855.1	E938.1	E950.4	E962.0	E980.4
intravenous anesthetics	968.3	E855.1	E938.3	E950.4	E962.0	E980.4
28:08 analgesics and antipyretics	965.9	E850.9	E935.9	E950.0	E962.0	E980.0
antirheumatics	965.69	E850.6	E935.6	E950.0	E962.0	E980.0
aromatic analgesics	965.4	E850.4	E935.4	E950.0	E962.0	E980.0
non-narcotic NEC	965.7	E850.7	E935.7	E950.0	E962.0	E980.0
opium alkaloids	965.00	E850.2	E935.2	E950.0	E962.0	E980.0
heroin	965.01	E850.0	E935.0	E950.0	E962.0	E980.0
methadone	965.02	E850.1	E935.1	E950.0	E962.0	E980.0
specified type NEC	965.09	E850.2	E935.2	E950.0	E962.0	E980.0
pyrazole derivatives	965.5	E850.5	E935.5	E950.0	E962.0	E980.0
salicylates	965.1	E850.3	E935.3	E950.0	E962.0	E980.0
specified NEC	965.8	E850.8	E935.8	E950.0	E962.0	E980.0
28:10 narcotic antagonists	970.1	E854.3	E940.1	E950.4	E962.0	E980.4
28:12 anticonvulsants	966.3	E855.0	E936.3	E950.4	E962.0	E980.4
barbiturates	967.0	E851	E937.0	E950.1	E962.0	E980.1
benzodiazepine-based tranquilizers	969.4	E853.2	E939.4	E950.3	E962.0	E980.3
bromides	967.3	E852.2	E937.3	E950.2	E962.0	E980.2
hydantoin derivatives	966.1	E855.0	E936.1	E950.4	E962.0	E980.4
oxazolidine (derivatives)	966.0	E855.0	E936.0	E950.4	E962.0	E980.4
succinimides	966.2	E855.0	E936.2	E950.4	E962.0	E980.4
28:16.04 antidepressants	969.0	E854.0	E939.0	E950.3	E962.0	E980.3
28:16.08 tranquilizers	969.5	E853.9	E939.5	E950.3	E962.0	E980.3
benzodiazepine-based	969.4	E853.2	E939.4	E950.3	E962.0	E980.3
butyrophenone-based	969.2	E853.1	E939.2	E950.3	E962.0	E980.3
major NEC	969.3	E853.8	E939.3	E950.3	E962.0	E980.3
phenothiazine-based	969.1	E853.0	E939.1	E950.3	E962.0	E980.3
28:16.12 other psychotherapeutic agents	969.8	E855.8	E939.8	E950.3	E962.0	E980.3
28:20 respiratory and cerebral stimulants	970.9	E854.3	E940.9	E950.4	E962.0	E980.4
analeptics	970.0	E854.3	E940.0	E950.4	E962.0	E980.4
anorexigenic agents	977.0	E858.8	E947.0	E950.4	E962.0	E980.4
psychostimulants	969.7	E854.2	E939.7	E950.3	E962.0	E980.3
specified NEC	970.8	E854.3	E940.8	E950.4	E962.0	E980.4
28:24 sedatives and hypnotics	967.9	E852.9	E937.9	E950.2	E962.0	E980.2
barbiturates	967.0	E851	E937.0	E950.1	E962.0	E980.1
benzodiazepine-based tranquilizers	969.4	E853.2	E939.4	E950.3	E962.0	E980.3
chloral hydrate (group)	967.1	E852.0	E937.1	E950.2	E962.0	E980.2

Table of Drugs and Chemicals

		External Cause (E-Code)				
	Poisoning	Accident	Therapeutic Use	Suicide Attempt	Assault	Undetermined
Drug — *continued*						
28:24 sedatives and — continued						
glutethamide group	967.5	E852.4	E937.5	E950.2	E962.0	E980.2
intravenous anesthetics	968.3	E855.1	E938.3	E950.4	E962.0	E980.4
methaqualone (compounds)	967.4	E852.3	E937.4	E950.2	E962.0	E980.2
paraldehyde	967.2	E852.1	E937.2	E950.2	E962.0	E980.2
phenothiazine-based tranquilizers	969.1	E853.0	E939.1	E950.3	E962.0	E980.3
specified NEC	967.8	E852.8	E937.8	E950.2	E962.0	E980.2
thiobarbiturates	968.3	E855.1	E938.3	E950.4	E962.0	E980.4
tranquilizer NEC	969.5	E853.9	E939.5	E950.3	E962.0	E980.3
36:04 to 36:88 diagnostic agents	977.8	E858.8	E947.8	E950.4	E962.0	E980.4
40:00 electrolyte, caloric, and water balance agents NEC	974.5	E858.5	E944.5	E950.4	E962.0	E980.4
40:04 acidifying agents	963.2	E858.1	E933.2	E950.4	E962.0	E980.4
40:08 alkalinizing agents	963.3	E858.1	E933.3	E950.4	E962.0	E980.4
40:10 ammonia detoxicants	974.5	E858.5	E944.5	E950.4	E962.0	E980.4
40:12 replacement solutions	974.5	E858.5	E944.5	E950.4	E962.0	E980.4
plasma expanders	964.8	E858.2	E934.8	E950.4	E962.0	E980.4
40:16 sodium-removing resins	974.5	E858.5	E944.5	E950.4	E962.0	E980.4
40:18 potassium-removing resins	974.5	E858.5	E944.5	E950.4	E962.0	E980.4
40:20 caloric agents	974.5	E858.5	E944.5	E950.4	E962.0	E980.4
40:24 salt and sugar substitutes	974.5	E858.5	E944.5	E950.4	E962.0	E980.4
40:28 diuretics NEC	974.4	E858.5	E944.4	E950.4	E962.0	E980.4
carbonic acid anhydrase inhibitors	974.2	E858.5	E944.2	E950.4	E962.0	E980.4
mercurials	974.0	E858.5	E944.0	E950.4	E962.0	E980.4
purine derivatives	974.1	E858.5	E944.1	E950.4	E962.0	E980.4
saluretics	974.3	E858.5	E944.3	E950.4	E962.0	E980.4
thiazides	974.3	E858.5	E944.3	E950.4	E962.0	E980.4
40:36 irrigating solutions	974.5	E858.5	E944.5	E950.4	E962.0	E980.4
40:40 uricosuric agents	974.7	E858.5	E944.7	E950.4	E962.0	E980.4
44:00 enzymes	963.4	E858.1	E933.4	E950.4	E962.0	E980.4
fibrinolysis-affecting agents	964.4	E858.2	E934.4	E950.4	E962.0	E980.4
gastric agents	973.4	E858.4	E943.4	E950.4	E962.0	E980.4
48:00 expectorants and cough preparations						
antihistamine agents	963.0	E858.1	E933.0	E950.4	E962.0	E980.4
antitussives	975.4	E858.6	E945.4	E950.4	E962.0	E980.4
codeine derivatives	965.09	E850.2	E935.2	E950.0	E962.0	E980.0
expectorants	975.5	E858.6	E945.5	E950.4	E962.0	E980.4
narcotic agents NEC	965.09	E850.2	E935.2	E950.0	E962.0	E980.0
52:04 anti-infectives (EENT)						
ENT agent	976.6	E858.7	E946.6	E950.4	E962.0	E980.4
ophthalmic preparation	976.5	E858.7	E946.5	E950.4	E962.0	E980.4
52:04.04 antibiotics (EENT)						
ENT agent	976.6	E858.7	E946.6	E950.4	E962.0	E980.4
ophthalmic preparation	976.5	E858.7	E946.5	E950.4	E962.0	E980.4
52:04.06 antivirals (EENT)						
ENT agent	976.6	E858.7	E946.6	E950.4	E962.0	E980.4
ophthalmic preparation	976.5	E858.7	E946.5	E950.4	E962.0	E980.4
52:04.08 sulfonamides (EENT)						
ENT agent	976.6	E858.7	E946.6	E950.4	E962.0	E980.4
ophthalmic preparation	976.5	E858.7	E946.5	E950.4	E962.0	E980.4

✓4ᵗʰ Fourth-digit Required   ✓5ᵗʰ Fifth-digit Required

Table of Drugs and Chemicals

		External Cause (E-Code)				
	Poisoning	Accident	Therapeutic Use	Suicide Attempt	Assault	Undetermined
Drug — continued						
52:04.12 miscellaneous anti-infectives (EENT)						
ENT agent	976.6	E858.7	E946.6	E950.4	E962.0	E980.4
ophthalmic preparation	976.5	E858.7	E946.5	E950.4	E962.0	E980.4
52:08 anti-inflammatory agents (EENT)						
ENT agent	976.6	E858.7	E946.6	E950.4	E962.0	E980.4
ophthalmic preparation	976.5	E858.7	E946.5	E950.4	E962.0	E980.4
52:10 carbonic anhydrase inhibitors	974.2	E858.5	E944.2	E950.4	E962.0	E980.4
52:12 contact lens solutions	976.5	E858.7	E946.5	E950.4	E962.0	E980.4
52:16 local anesthetics (EENT)	968.5	E855.2	E938.5	E950.4	E962.0	E980.4
52:20 miotics	971.0	E855.3	E941.0	E950.4	E962.0	E980.4
52:24 mydriatics						
adrenergics	971.2	E855.5	E941.2	E950.4	E962.0	E980.4
anticholinergics	971.1	E855.4	E941.1	E950.4	E962.0	E980.4
antimuscarinics	971.1	E855.4	E941.1	E950.4	E962.0	E980.4
parasympatholytics	971.1	E855.4	E941.1	E950.4	E962.0	E980.4
spasmolytics	971.1	E855.4	E941.1	E950.4	E962.0	E980.4
sympathomimetics	971.2	E855.5	E941.2	E950.4	E962.0	E980.4
52:28 mouth washes and gargles	976.6	E858.7	E946.6	E950.4	E962.0	E980.4
52:32 vasoconstrictors (EENT)	971.2	E855.5	E941.2	E950.4	E962.0	E980.4
52:36 unclassified agents (EENT)						
ENT agent	976.6	E858.7	E946.6	E950.4	E962.0	E980.4
ophthalmic preparation	976.5	E858.7	E946.5	E950.4	E962.0	E980.4
56:04 antacids and adsorbents	973.0	E858.4	E943.0	E950.4	E962.0	E980.4
56:08 antidiarrhea agents	973.5	E858.4	E943.5	E950.4	E962.0	E980.4
56:10 antiflatulents	973.8	E858.4	E943.8	E950.4	E962.0	E980.4
56:12 cathartics NEC	973.3	E858.4	E943.3	E950.4	E962.0	E980.4
emollients	973.2	E858.4	E943.2	E950.4	E962.0	E980.4
irritants	973.1	E858.4	E943.1	E950.4	E962.0	E980.4
56:16 digestants	973.4	E858.4	E943.4	E950.4	E962.0	E980.4
56:20 emetics and antiemetics						
antiemetics	963.0	E858.1	E933.0	E950.4	E962.0	E980.4
emetics	973.6	E858.4	E943.6	E950.4	E962.0	E980.4
56:24 lipotropic agents	977.1	E858.8	E947.1	E950.4	E962.0	E980.4
56:40 miscellaneous G.I. drugs	973.8	E858.4	E943.8	E950.4	E962.0	E980.4
60:00 gold compounds	965.69	E850.6	E935.6	E950.0	E962.0	E980.0
64:00 heavy metal antagonists	963.8	E858.1	E933.8	E950.4	E962.0	E980.4
68:04 adrenals	962.0	E858.0	E932.0	E950.4	E962.0	E980.4
68:08 androgens	962.1	E858.0	E932.1	E950.4	E962.0	E980.4
68:12 contraceptives, oral	962.2	E858.0	E932.2	E950.4	E962.0	E980.4
68:16 estrogens	962.2	E858.0	E932.2	E950.4	E962.0	E980.4
68:18 gonadotropins	962.4	E858.0	E932.4	E950.4	E962.0	E980.4
68:20 insulins and antidiabetic agents	962.3	E858.0	E932.3	E950.4	E962.0	E980.4
68:20.08 insulins	962.3	E858.0	E932.3	E950.4	E962.0	E980.4
68:24 parathyroid	962.6	E858.0	E932.6	E950.4	E962.0	E980.4
68:28 pituitary (posterior) anterior	962.5 962.4	E858.0 E858.0	E932.5 E932.4	E950.4 E950.4	E962.0 E962.0	E980.4 E980.4
68:32 progestogens	962.2	E858.0	E932.2	E950.4	E962.0	E980.4
68:34 other corpus luteum hormones NEC	962.2	E858.0	E932.2	E950.4	E962.0	E980.4

Table of Drugs and Chemicals

		External Cause (E-Code)				
	Poisoning	Accident	Therapeutic Use	Suicide Attempt	Assault	Undetermined
Drug — continued						
68:36 thyroid and antithyroid						
antithyroid	962.8	E858.0	E932.8	E950.4	E962.0	E980.4
thyroid (derivatives)	962.7	E858.0	E932.7	E950.4	E962.0	E980.4
72:00 local anesthetics						
NEC	968.9	E855.2	E938.9	E950.4	E962.0	E980.4
topical (surface)	968.5	E855.2	E938.5	E950.4	E962.0	E980.4
infiltration (intradermal) (subcutaneous) (submucosal)	968.5	E855.2	E938.5	E950.4	E962.0	E980.4
nerve blocking (peripheral) (plexus) (regional)	968.6	E855.2	E938.6	E950.4	E962.0	E980.4
spinal	968.7	E855.2	E938.7	E950.4	E962.0	E980.4
76:00 oxytocics	975.0	E858.6	E945.0	E950.4	E962.0	E980.4
78:00 radioactive agents	990	—	—	—	—	—
80:04 serums NEC	979.9	E858.8	E949.9	E950.4	E962.0	E980.4
immune gamma globulin (human)	964.6	E858.2	E934.6	E950.4	E962.0	E980.4
80:08 toxoids NEC	978.8	E858.8	E948.8	E950.4	E962.0	E980.4
diphtheria	978.5	E858.8	E948.5	E950.4	E962.0	E980.4
and tetanus	978.9	E858.8	E948.9	E950.4	E962.0	E980.4
with pertussis component	978.6	E858.8	E948.6	E950.4	E962.0	E980.4
tetanus	978.4	E858.8	E948.4	E950.4	E962.0	E980.4
and diphtheria	978.9	E858.8	E948.9	E950.4	E962.0	E980.4
with pertussis component	978.6	E858.8	E948.6	E950.4	E962.0	E980.4
80:12 vaccines	979.9	E858.8	E949.9	E950.4	E962.0	E980.4
bacterial NEC	978.8	E858.8	E948.8	E950.4	E962.0	E980.4
with other bacterial components	978.9	E858.8	E948.9	E950.4	E962.0	E980.4
pertussis component	978.6	E858.8	E948.6	E950.4	E962.0	E980.4
viral and rickettsial components	979.7	E858.8	E949.7	E950.4	E962.0	E980.4
rickettsial NEC	979.6	E858.8	E949.6	E950.4	E962.0	E980.4
with bacterial component	979.7	E858.8	E949.7	E950.4	E962.0	E980.4
pertussis component	978.6	E858.8	E948.6	E950.4	E962.0	E980.4
viral component	979.7	E858.8	E949.7	E950.4	E962.0	E980.4
viral NEC	979.6	E858.8	E949.6	E950.4	E962.0	E980.4
with bacterial component	979.7	E858.8	E949.7	E950.4	E962.0	E980.4
pertussis component	978.6	E858.8	E948.6	E950.4	E962.0	E980.4
rickettsial component	979.7	E858.8	E949.7	E950.4	E962.0	E980.4
84:04.04 antibiotics (skin and mucous membrane)	976.0	E858.7	E946.0	E950.4	E962.0	E980.4
84:04.08 fungicides (skin and mucous membrane)	976.0	E858.7	E946.0	E950.4	E962.0	E980.4
84:04.12 scabicides and pediculicides (skin and mucous membrane)	976.0	E858.7	E946.0	E950.4	E962.0	E980.4

Fourth-digit Required   Fifth-digit Required

Table of Drugs and Chemicals

	Poisoning	External Cause (E-Code)				
		Accident	Therapeutic Use	Suicide Attempt	Assault	Undetermined
Drug — continued						
84:04.16 miscellaneous local anti-infectives (skin and mucous membrane)	976.0	E858.7	E946.0	E950.4	E962.0	E980.4
84:06 anti-inflammatory agents (skin and mucous membrane)	976.0	E858.7	E946.0	E950.4	E962.0	E980.4
84:08 antipruritics and local anesthetics						
antipruritics	976.1	E858.7	E946.1	E950.4	E962.0	E980.4
local anesthetics	968.5	E855.2	E938.5	E950.4	E962.0	E980.4
84:12 astringents	976.2	E858.7	E946.2	E950.4	E962.0	E980.4
84:16 cell stimulants and proliferants	976.8	E858.7	E946.8	E950.4	E962.0	E980.4
84:20 detergents	976.2	E858.7	E946.2	E950.4	E962.0	E980.4
84:24 emollients, demulcents, and protectants	976.3	E858.7	E946.3	E950.4	E962.0	E980.4
84:28 keratolytic agents	976.4	E858.7	E946.4	E950.4	E962.0	E980.4
84:32 keratoplastic agents	976.4	E858.7	E946.4	E950.4	E962.0	E980.4
84:36 miscellaneous agents (skin and mucous membrane)	976.8	E858.7	E946.8	E950.4	E962.0	E980.4
86:00 spasmolytic agents	975.1	E858.6	E945.1	E950.4	E962.0	E980.4
antiasthmatics	975.7	E858.6	E945.7	E950.4	E962.0	E980.4
papaverine	972.5	E858.3	E942.5	E950.4	E962.0	E980.4
theophylline	974.1	E858.5	E944.1	E950.4	E962.0	E980.4
88:04 vitamin A	963.5	E858.1	E933.5	E950.4	E962.0	E980.4
88:08 vitamin B complex	963.5	E858.1	E933.5	E950.4	E962.0	E980.4
hematopoietic vitamin	964.1	E858.2	E934.1	E950.4	E962.0	E980.4
nicotinic acid derivatives	972.2	E858.3	E942.2	E950.4	E962.0	E980.4
88:12 vitamin C	963.5	E858.1	E933.5	E950.4	E962.0	E980.4
88:16 vitamin D	963.5	E858.1	E933.5	E950.4	E962.0	E980.4
88:20 vitamin E	963.5	E858.1	E933.5	E950.4	E962.0	E980.4
88:24 vitamin K activity	964.3	E858.2	E934.3	E950.4	E962.0	E980.4
88:28 multivitamin preparations	963.5	E858.1	E933.5	E950.4	E962.0	E980.4
92:00 unclassified therapeutic agents	977.8	E858.8	E947.8	E950.4	E962.0	E980.4
Duboisine	971.1	E855.4	E941.1	E950.4	E962.0	E980.4
Dulcolax	973.1	E858.4	E943.1	E950.4	E962.0	E980.4
Duponol (C) (EP)	976.2	E858.7	E946.2	E950.4	E962.0	E980.4
Durabolin	962.1	E858.0	E932.1	E950.4	E962.0	E980.4
Dyclone	968.5	E855.2	E938.5	E950.4	E962.0	E980.4
Dyclonine	968.5	E855.2	E938.5	E950.4	E962.0	E980.4
Dydrogesterone	962.2	E858.0	E932.2	E950.4	E962.0	E980.4
Dyes NEC	989.89	E866.8	—	E950.9	E962.1	E980.9
diagnostic agents	977.8	E858.8	E947.8	E950.4	E962.0	E980.4
pharmaceutical NEC	977.4	E858.8	E947.4	E950.4	E962.0	E980.4
Dyfols	971.0	E855.3	E941.0	E950.4	E962.0	E980.4
Dymelor	962.3	E858.0	E932.3	E950.4	E962.0	E980.4
Dynamite	989.89	E866.8	—	E950.9	E962.1	E980.9
fumes	987.8	E869.8	—	E952.8	E962.2	E982.8
Dyphylline	975.1	E858.6	E945.1	E950.4	E962.0	E980.4
Ear preparations	976.6	E858.7	E946.6	E950.4	E962.0	E980.4
Echothiopate, ecothiopate	971.0	E855.3	E941.0	E950.4	E962.0	E980.4
Ectylurea	967.8	E852.8	E937.8	E950.2	E962.0	E980.2
Edathamil disodium	963.8	E858.1	E933.8	E950.4	E962.0	E980.4
Edecrin	974.4	E858.5	E944.4	E950.4	E962.0	E980.4
Edetate, disodium (calcium)	963.8	E858.1	E933.8	E950.4	E962.0	E980.4
Edrophonium	971.0	E855.3	E941.0	E950.4	E962.0	E980.4
Elase	976.8	E858.7	E946.8	E950.4	E962.0	E980.4
Elaterium	973.1	E858.4	E943.1	E950.4	E962.0	E980.4

Table of Drugs and Chemicals

Ether(s) (diethyl) (ethyl) (vapor)

			External Cause (E-Code)			
	Poisoning	Accident	Therapeutic Use	Suicide Attempt	Assault	Undetermined
Elder	988.2	E865.4	—	E950.9	E962.1	E980.9
berry (unripe)	988.2	E865.3	—	E950.9	E962.1	E980.9
Electrolytes NEC	974.5	E858.5	E944.5	E950.4	E962.0	E980.4
Electrolytic agent NEC	974.5	E858.5	E944.5	E950.4	E962.0	E980.4
Embramine	963.0	E858.1	E933.0	E950.4	E962.0	E980.4
Emetics	973.6	E858.4	E943.6	E950.4	E962.0	E980.4
Emetine (hydrochloride)	961.5	E857	E931.5	E950.4	E962.0	E980.4
Emollients	976.3	E858.7	E946.3	E950.4	E962.0	E980.4
Emylcamate	969.5	E853.8	E939.5	E950.3	E962.0	E980.3
Encyprate	969.0	E854.0	E939.0	E950.3	E962.0	E980.3
Endocaine	968.5	E855.2	E938.5	E950.4	E962.0	E980.4
Endrin	989.2	E863.0	—	E950.6	E962.1	E980.7
Enflurane	968.2	E855.1	E938.2	E950.4	E962.0	E980.4
Enovid	962.2	E858.0	E932.2	E950.4	E962.0	E980.4
ENT preparations						
(anti-infectives)	976.6	E858.7	E946.6	E950.4	E962.0	E980.4
Enzodase	963.4	E858.1	E933.4	E950.4	E962.0	E980.4
Enzymes NEC	963.4	E858.1	E933.4	E950.4	E962.0	E980.4
Epanutin	966.1	E855.0	E936.1	E950.4	E962.0	E980.4
Ephedra (tincture)	971.2	E855.5	E941.2	E950.4	E962.0	E980.4
Ephedrine	971.2	E855.5	E941.2	E950.4	E962.0	E980.4
Epiestriol	962.2	E858.0	E932.2	E950.4	E962.0	E980.4
Epilim — see Sodium Valproate						
Epinephrine	971.2	E855.5	E941.2	E950.4	E962.0	E980.4
Epsom sait	973.3	E858.4	E943.3	E950.4	E962.0	E980.4
Equanil	969.5	E853.8	E939.5	E950.3	E962.0	E980.3
Equisetum (diuretic)	974.4	E858.5	E944.4	E950.4	E962.0	E980.4
Ergometrine	975.0	E858.6	E945.0	E950.4	E962.0	E980.4
Ergonovine	975.0	E858.6	E945.0	E950.4	E962.0	E980.4
Ergot NEC	988.2	E865.4	—	E950.9	E962.1	E980.9
medicinal (alkaloids)	975.0	E858.6	E945.0	E950.4	E962.0	E980.4
Ergotamine (tartrate) (for migraine) NEC	972.9	E858.3	E942.9	E950.4	E962.0	E980.4
Ergotrate	975.0	E858.6	E945.0	E950.4	E962.0	E980.4
Erythrityl tetranitrate	972.4	E858.3	E942.4	E950.4	E962.0	E980.4
Erythrol tetranitrate	972.4	E858.3	E942.4	E950.4	E962.0	E980.4
Erythromycin	960.3	E856	E930.3	E950.4	E962.0	E980.4
ophthalmic preparation	976.5	E858.7	E946.5	E950.4	E962.0	E980.4
topical NEC	976.0	E858.7	E946.0	E950.4	E962.0	E980.4
Eserine	971.0	E855.3	E941.0	E950.4	E962.0	E980.4
Eskabarb	967.0	E851	E937.0	E950.1	E962.0	E980.1
Eskalith	969.8	E855.8	E939.8	E950.3	E962.0	E980.3
Estradiol (cypionate) (dipropionate) (valerate)	962.2	E858.0	E932.2	E950.4	E962.0	E980.4
Estriol	962.2	E858.0	E932.2	E950.4	E962.0	E980.4
Estrogens (with progestogens)	962.2	E858.0	E932.2	E950.4	E962.0	E980.4
Estrone	962.2	E858.0	E932.2	E950.4	E962.0	E980.4
Etafedrine	971.2	E855.5	E941.2	E950.4	E962.0	E980.4
Ethacrynate sodium	974.4	E858.5	E944.4	E950.4	E962.0	E980.4
Ethacrynic acid	974.4	E858.5	E944.4	E950.4	E962.0	E980.4
Ethambutol	961.8	E857	E931.8	E950.4	E962.0	E980.4
Ethamide	974.2	E858.5	E944.2	E950.4	E962.0	E980.4
Ethamivan	970.0	E854.3	E940.0	E950.4	E962.0	E980.4
Ethamsylate	964.5	E858.2	E934.5	E950.4	E962.0	E980.4
Ethanol	980.0	E860.1	—	E950.9	E962.1	E980.9
beverage	980.0	E860.0	—	E950.9	E962.1	E980.9
Ethchlorvynol	967.8	E852.8	E937.8	E950.2	E962.0	E980.2
Ethebenecid	974.7	E858.5	E944.7	E950.4	E962.0	E980.4
Ether(s) (diethyl) (ethyl) (vapor)	987.8	E869.8	—	E952.8	E962.2	E982.8
anesthetic	968.2	E855.1	E938.2	E950.4	E962.0	E980.4
petroleum — see Ligroin						
solvent	982.8	E862.4	—	E950.9	E962.1	E980.9

☑4ᵗʰ Fourth-digit Required   ☑5ᵗʰ Fifth-digit Required

Ethidine chloride (vapor) — Table of Drugs and Chemicals

	Poisoning	External Cause (E-Code)				
		Accident	Therapeutic Use	Suicide Attempt	Assault	Undetermined
Ethidine chloride (vapor)	987.8	E869.8	—	E952.8	E962.2	E982.8
liquid (solvent)	982.3	E862.4	—	E950.9	E962.1	E980.9
Ethinamate	967.8	E852.8	E937.8	E950.2	E962.0	E980.2
Ethinylestradiol	962.2	E858.0	E932.2	E950.4	E962.0	E980.4
Ethionamide	961.8	E857	E931.8	E950.4	E962.0	E980.4
Ethisterone	962.2	E858.0	E932.2	E950.4	E962.0	E980.4
Ethobral	967.0	E851	E937.0	E950.1	E962.0	E980.1
Ethocaine (infiltration) (topical)	968.5	E855.2	E938.5	E950.4	E962.0	E980.4
nerve block (peripheral) (plexus)	968.6	E855.2	E938.6	E950.4	E962.0	E980.4
spinal	968.7	E855.2	E938.7	E950.4	E962.0	E980.4
Ethoheptazine (citrate)	965.7	E850.7	E935.7	E950.0	E962.0	E980.0
Ethopropazine	966.4	E855.0	E936.4	E950.4	E962.0	E980.4
Ethosuximide	966.2	E855.0	E936.2	E950.4	E962.0	E980.4
Ethotoin	966.1	E855.0	E936.1	E950.4	E962.0	E980.4
Ethoxazene	961.9	E857	E931.9	E950.4	E962.0	E980.4
Ethoxzolamide	974.2	E858.5	E944.2	E950.4	E962.0	E980.4
Ethyl						
acetate (vapor)	982.8	E862.4	—	E950.9	E962.1	E980.9
alcohol	980.0	E860.1	—	E950.9	E962.1	E980.9
beverage	980.0	E860.0	—	E950.9	E962.1	E980.9
aldehyde (vapor)	987.8	E869.8	—	E952.8	E962.2	E982.8
liquid	989.89	E866.8	—	E950.9	E962.1	E980.9
aminobenzoate	968.5	E855.2	E938.5	E950.4	E962.0	E980.4
biscoumacetate	964.2	E858.2	E934.2	E950.4	E962.0	E980.4
bromide (anesthetic)	968.2	E855.1	E938.2	E950.4	E962.0	E980.4
carbamate (antineoplastic)	963.1	E858.1	E933.1	E950.4	E962.0	E980.4
carbinol	980.3	E860.4	—	E950.9	E962.1	E980.9
chaulmoogroff	961.8	E857	E931.8	E950.4	E962.0	E980.4
chloride (vapor)	987.8	E869.8	—	E952.8	E962.2	E982.8
anesthetic (local)	968.5	E855.2	E938.5	E950.4	E962.0	E980.4
inhaled	968.2	E855.1	E938.2	E950.4	E962.0	E980.4
solvent	982.3	E862.4	—	E950.9	E962.1	E980.9
estranol	962.1	E858.0	E932.1	E950.4	E962.0	E980.4
ether — see Ether(s)						
formate (solvent) NEC	982.8	E862.4	—	E950.9	E962.1	E980.9
iodoacetate	987.5	E869.3	—	E952.8	E962.2	E982.8
lactate (solvent) NEC	982.8	E862.4	—	E950.9	E962.1	E980.9
methylcarbinol	980.8	E860.8	—	E950.9	E962.1	E980.9
morphine	965.09	E850.2	E935.2	E950.0	E962.0	E980.0
Ethylene (gas)	987.1	E869.8	—	E952.8	E962.2	E982.8
anesthetic (general)	968.2	E855.1	E938.2	E950.4	E962.0	E980.4
chlorohydrin (vapor)	982.3	E862.4	—	E950.9	E962.1	E980.9
dichloride (vapor)	982.3	E862.4	—	E950.9	E962.1	E980.9
glycol(s) (any) (vapor)	982.8	E862.4	—	E950.9	E962.1	E980.9
Ethylidene						
chloride NEC	982.3	E862.4	—	E950.9	E962.1	E980.9
diethyl ether	982.8	E862.4	—	E950.9	E962.1	E980.9
Ethynodiol	962.2	E858.0	E932.2	E950.4	E962.0	E980.4
Etidocaine	968.9	E855.2	E938.9	E950.4	E962.0	E980.4
infiltration (subcutaneous)	968.5	E855.2	E938.5	E950.4	E962.0	E980.4
nerve (peripheral) (plexus)	968.6	E855.2	E938.6	E950.4	E962.0	E980.4
Etilfen	967.0	E851	E937.0	E950.1	E962.0	E980.1
Etomide	965.7	E850.7	E935.7	E950.0	E962.0	E980.0
Etorphine	965.09	E850.2	E935.2	E950.0	E962.0	E980.0
Etoval	967.0	E851	E937.0	E950.1	E962.0	E980.1
Etryptamine	969.0	E854.0	E939.0	E950.3	E962.0	E980.3
Eucaine	968.5	E855.2	E938.5	E950.4	E962.0	E980.4
Eucalyptus (oil) NEC	975.5	E858.6	E945.5	E950.4	E962.0	E980.4
Eucatropine	971.1	E855.4	E941.1	E950.4	E962.0	E980.4
Eucodal	965.09	E850.2	E935.2	E950.0	E962.0	E980.0
Euneryl	967.0	E851	E937.0	E950.1	E962.0	E980.1
Euphthalmine	971.1	E855.4	E941.1	E950.4	E962.0	E980.4
Eurax	976.0	E858.7	E946.0	E950.4	E962.0	E980.4

▶◀ Revised Text   ● New Line   ▲ Revised Code

Table of Drugs and Chemicals — Flumethasone

		External Cause (E-Code)				
	Poisoning	Accident	Therapeutic Use	Suicide Attempt	Assault	Undetermined
Euresol	976.4	E858.7	E946.4	E950.4	E962.0	E980.4
Euthroid	962.7	E858.0	E932.7	E950.4	E962.0	E980.4
Evans blue	977.8	E858.8	E947.8	E950.4	E962.0	E980.4
Evipal	967.0	E851	E937.0	E950.1	E962.0	E980.1
sodium	968.3	E855.1	E938.3	E950.4	E962.0	E980.4
Evipan	967.0	E851	E937.0	E950.1	E962.0	E980.1
sodium	968.3	E855.1	E938.3	E950.4	E962.0	E980.4
Exalgin	965.4	E850.4	E935.4	E950.0	E962.0	E980.0
Excipients, pharmaceutical	977.4	E858.8	E947.4	E950.4	E962.0	E980.4
Exhaust gas — see Carbon, monoxide						
Ex-Lax (phenolphthalein)	973.1	E858.4	E943.1	E950.4	E962.0	E980.4
Expectorants	975.5	E858.6	E945.5	E950.4	E962.0	E980.4
External medications (skin) (mucous membrane)	976.9	E858.7	E946.9	E950.4	E962.0	E980.4
dental agent	976.7	E858.7	E946.7	E950.4	E962.0	E980.4
ENT agent	976.6	E858.7	E946.6	E950.4	E962.0	E980.4
ophthalmic preparation	976.5	E858.7	E946.5	E950.4	E962.0	E980.4
specified NEC	976.8	E858.7	E946.8	E950.4	E962.0	E980.4
Eye agents (anti-infective)	976.5	E858.7	E946.5	E950.4	E962.0	E980.4
Factor IX complex (human)	964.5	E858.2	E934.5	E950.4	E962.0	E980.4
Fecal softeners	973.2	E858.4	E943.2	E950.4	E962.0	E980.4
Fenbutrazate	977.0	E858.8	E947.0	E950.4	E962.0	E980.4
Fencamfamin	970.8	E854.3	E940.8	E950.4	E962.0	E980.4
Fenfluramine	977.0	E858.8	E947.0	E950.4	E962.0	E980.4
Fenoprofen	965.61	E850.6	E935.6	E950.0	E962.0	E980.0
Fentanyl	965.09	E850.2	E935.2	E950.0	E962.0	E980.0
Fentazin	969.1	E853.0	E939.1	E950.3	E962.0	E980.3
Fenticlor, fentichlor	976.0	E858.7	E946.0	E950.4	E962.0	E980.4
Fer de lance (bite) (venom)	989.5	E905.0	—	E950.9	E962.1	E980.9
Ferric — see Iron						
Ferrocholinate	964.0	E858.2	E934.0	E950.4	E962.0	E980.4
Ferrous fumerate, gluconate, lactate, salt NEC, sulfate (medicinal)	964.0	E858.2	E934.0	E950.4	E962.0	E980.4
Ferrum — see Iron						
Fertilizers NEC	989.89	E866.5	—	E950.9	E962.1	E980.4
with herbicide mixture	989.4	E863.5	—	E950.6	E962.1	E980.7
Fibrinogen (human)	964.7	E858.2	E934.7	E950.4	E962.0	E980.4
Fibrinolysin	964.4	E858.2	E934.4	E950.4	E962.0	E980.4
Fibrinolysis-affecting agents	964.4	E858.2	E934.4	E950.4	E962.0	E980.4
Filix mas	961.6	E857	E931.6	E950.4	E962.0	E980.4
Fiorinal	965.1	E850.3	E935.3	E950.0	E962.0	E980.0
Fire damp	987.1	E869.8	—	E952.8	E962.2	E982.8
Fish, nonbacterial or noxious	988.0	E865.2	—	E950.9	E962.1	E980.9
shell	988.0	E865.1	—	E950.9	E962.1	E980.9
Flagyl	961.5	E857	E931.5	E950.4	E962.0	E980.4
Flavoxate	975.1	E858.6	E945.1	E950.4	E962.0	E980.4
Flaxedil	975.2	E858.6	E945.2	E950.4	E962.0	E980.4
Flaxseed (medicinal)	976.3	E858.7	E946.3	E950.4	E962.0	E980.4
Florantyrone	973.4	E858.4	E943.4	E950.4	E962.0	E980.4
Floraquin	961.3	E857	E931.3	E950.4	E962.0	E980.4
Florinef	962.0	E858.0	E932.0	E950.4	E962.0	E980.4
ENT agent	976.6	E858.7	E946.6	E950.4	E962.0	E980.4
ophthalmic preparation	976.5	E858.7	E946.5	E950.4	E962.0	E980.4
topical NEC	976.0	E858.7	E946.0	E950.4	E962.0	E980.4
Flowers of sulfur	976.4	E858.7	E946.4	E950.4	E962.0	E980.4
Floxuridine	963.1	E858.1	E933.1	E950.4	E962.0	E980.4
Flucytosine	961.9	E857	E931.9	E950.4	E962.0	E980.4
Fludrocortisone	962.0	E858.0	E932.0	E950.4	E962.0	E980.4
ENT agent	976.6	E858.7	E946.6	E950.4	E962.0	E980.4
ophthalmic preparation	976.5	E858.7	E946.5	E950.4	E962.0	E980.4
topical NEC	976.0	E858.7	E946.0	E950.4	E962.0	E980.4
Flumethasone	976.0	E858.7	E946.0	E950.4	E962.0	E980.4

✓4ᵗʰ Fourth-digit Required   ✓5ᵗʰ Fifth-digit Required

Flumethiazide

Table of Drugs and Chemicals

	Poisoning	External Cause (E-Code)					
		Accident	Therapeutic Use	Suicide Attempt	Assault	Undetermined
Flumethiazide	974.3	E858.5	E944.3	E950.4	E962.0	E980.4
Flumidin	961.7	E857	E931.7	E950.4	E962.0	E980.4
Flunitrazepam	969.4	E853.2	E939.4	E950.3	E962.0	E980.3 ▲
Fluocinolone	976.0	E858.7	E946.0	E950.4	E962.0	E980.4
Fluocortolone	962.0	E858.0	E932.0	E950.4	E962.0	E980.4
Fluohydrocortisone	962.0	E858.0	E932.0	E950.4	E962.0	E980.4
ENT agent	976.6	E858.7	E946.6	E950.4	E962.0	E980.4
ophthalmic preparation	976.5	E858.7	E946.5	E950.4	E962.0	E980.4
topical NEC	976.0	E858.7	E946.0	E950.4	E962.0	E980.4
Fluonid	976.0	E858.7	E946.0	E950.4	E962.0	E980.4
Fluopromazine	969.1	E853.0	E939.1	E950.3	E962.0	E980.3
Fluoracetate	989.4	E863.7	—	E950.6	E962.1	E980.7
Fluorescein (sodium)	977.8	E858.8	E947.8	E950.4	E962.0	E980.4
Fluoride(s) (pesticides) (sodium) NEC	989.4	E863.4	—	E950.6	E962.1	E980.7
hydrogen — see Hydrofluoric acid						
medicinal	976.7	E858.7	E946.7	E950.4	E962.0	E980.4
not pesticide NEC	983.9	E864.4	—	E950.7	E962.1	E980.6
stannous	976.7	E858.7	E946.7	E950.4	E962.0	E980.4
Fluorinated corticosteroids	962.0	E858.0	E932.0	E950.4	E962.0	E980.4
Fluorine (compounds) (gas)	987.8	E869.8	—	E952.8	E962.2	E982.8
salt — see Fluoride(s)						
Fluoristan	976.7	E858.7	E946.7	E950.4	E962.0	E980.4
Fluoroacetate	989.4	E863.7	—	E950.6	E962.1	E980.7
Fluorodeoxyuridine	963.1	E858.1	E933.1	E950.4	E962.0	E980.4
Fluorometholone (topical) NEC	976.0	E858.7	E946.0	E950.4	E962.0	E980.4
ophthalmic preparation	976.5	E858.7	E946.5	E950.4	E962.0	E980.4
Fluorouracil	963.1	E858.1	E933.1	E950.4	E962.0	E980.4
Fluothane	968.1	E855.1	E938.1	E950.4	E962.0	E980.4
Fluoxetine hydrochloride	969.0	E854.0	E939.0	E950.3	E962.0	E980.3
Fluoxymesterone	962.1	E858.0	E932.1	E950.4	E962.0	E980.4
Fluphenazine	969.1	E853.0	E939.1	E950.3	E962.0	E980.3
Fluprednisolone	962.0	E858.0	E932.0	E950.4	E962.0	E980.4
Flurandrenolide	976.0	E858.7	E946.0	E950.4	E962.0	E980.4
Flurazepam (hydrochloride)	969.4	E853.2	E939.4	E950.3	E962.0	E980.3
Flurbiprofen	965.61	E850.6	E935.6	E950.0	E962.0	E980.0
Flurobate	976.0	E858.7	E946.0	E950.4	E962.0	E980.4
Flurothyl	969.8	E855.8	E939.8	E950.3	E962.0	E980.3
Fluroxene	968.2	E855.1	E938.2	E950.4	E962.0	E980.4
Folacin	964.1	E858.2	E934.1	E950.4	E962.0	E980.4
Folic acid	964.1	E858.2	E934.1	E950.4	E962.0	E980.4
Follicle stimulating hormone	962.4	E858.0	E932.4	E950.4	E962.0	E980.4
Food, foodstuffs, nonbacterial or noxious	988.9	E865.9	—	E950.9	E962.1	E980.9
berries, seeds	988.2	E865.3	—	E950.9	E962.1	E980.9
fish	988.0	E865.2	—	E950.9	E962.1	E980.9
mushrooms	988.1	E865.5	—	E950.9	E962.1	E980.9
plants	988.2	E865.9	—	E950.9	E962.1	E980.9
specified type NEC	988.2	E865.4	—	E950.9	E962.1	E980.9
shellfish	988.0	E865.1	—	E950.9	E962.1	E980.9
specified NEC	988.8	E865.8	—	E950.9	E962.1	E980.9
Fool's parsley	988.2	E865.4	—	E950.9	E962.1	E980.9
Formaldehyde (solution)	989.89	E861.4	—	E950.9	E962.1	E980.9
fungicide	989.4	E863.6	—	E950.6	E962.1	E980.7
gas or vapor	987.8	E869.8	—	E952.8	E962.2	E982.8
Formalin	989.89	E861.4	—	E950.9	E962.1	E980.9
fungicide	989.4	E863.6	—	E950.6	E962.1	E980.7
vapor	987.8	E869.8	—	E952.8	E962.2	E982.8
Formic acid	983.1	E864.1	—	E950.7	E962.1	E980.6
vapor	987.8	E869.8	—	E952.8	E962.2	E982.8
Fowler's solution	985.1	E866.3	—	E950.8	E962.1	E980.8
Foxglove	988.2	E865.4	—	E950.9	E962.1	E980.9
Fox green	977.8	E858.8	E947.8	E950.4	E962.0	E980.4

▶◀ Revised Text   ● New Line   ▲ Revised Code

Table of Drugs and Chemicals — Fungicides

		External Cause (E-Code)				
	Poisoning	Accident	Therapeutic Use	Suicide Attempt	Assault	Undetermined
Framycetin	960.8	E856	E930.8	E950.4	E962.0	E980.4
Frangula (extract)	973.1	E858.4	E943.1	E950.4	E962.0	E980.4
Frei antigen	977.8	E858.8	E947.8	E950.4	E962.0	E980.4
Freons	987.4	E869.2	—	E952.8	E962.2	E982.8
Fructose	974.5	E858.5	E944.5	E950.4	E962.0	E980.4
Frusemide	974.4	E858.5	E944.4	E950.4	E962.0	E980.4
FSH	962.4	E858.0	E932.4	E950.4	E962.0	E980.4
Fuel						
automobile	981	E862.1	—	E950.9	E962.1	E980.9
exhaust gas, not in transit	986	E868.2	—	E952.0	E962.2	E982.0
vapor NEC	987.1	E869.8	—	E952.8	E962.2	E982.8
gas (domestic use) — see also Carbon, monoxide, fuel						
utility	987.1	E868.1	—	E951.8	E962.2	E981.8
incomplete combustion of — see Carbon, monoxide, fuel, utility						
in mobile container	987.0	E868.0	—	E951.1	E962.2	E981.1
piped (natural)	987.1	E867	—	E951.0	E962.2	E981.0
industrial, incomplete combustion	986	E868.3	—	E952.1	E962.2	E982.1
Fugillin	960.8	E856	E930.8	E950.4	E962.0	E980.4
Fulminate of mercury	985.0	E866.1	—	E950.9	E962.1	E980.9
Fulvicin	960.1	E856	E930.1	E950.4	E962.0	E980.4
Fumadil	960.8	E856	E930.8	E950.4	E962.0	E980.4
Fumagillin	960.8	E856	E930.8	E950.4	E962.0	E980.4
Fumes (from)	987.9	E869.9	—	E952.9	E962.2	E982.9
carbon monoxide — see Carbon, monoxide						
charcoal (domestic use)	986	E868.3	—	E952.1	E962.2	E982.1
chloroform — see Chloroform						
coke (in domestic stoves, fireplaces)	986	E868.3	—	E952.1	E962.2	E982.1
corrosive NEC	987.8	E869.8	—	E952.8	E962.2	E982.8
ether — see Ether(s)						
freons	987.4	E869.2	—	E952.8	E962.2	E982.8
hydrocarbons	987.1	E869.8	—	E952.8	E962.2	E982.8
petroleum (liquefied)	987.0	E868.0	—	E951.1	E962.2	E981.1
distributed through pipes (pure or mixed with air)	987.0	E867	—	E951.0	E962.2	E981.0
lead — see Lead						
metals — see specified metal						
nitrogen dioxide	987.2	E869.0	—	E952.8	E962.2	E982.8
pesticides — see Pesticides						
petroleum (liquefied)	987.0	E868.0	—	E951.1	E962.2	E981.1
distributed through pipes (pure or mixed with air)	987.0	E867	—	E951.0	E962.2	E981.0
polyester	987.8	E869.8	—	E952.8	E962.2	E982.8
specified source other (see also substance specified)	987.8	E869.8	—	E952.8	E962.2	E982.8
sulfur dioxide	987.3	E869.1	—	E952.8	E962.2	E982.8
Fumigants	989.4	E863.8	—	E950.6	E962.1	E980.7
Fungi, noxious, used as food	988.1	E865.5	—	E950.9	E962.1	E980.9
Fungicides (see also Antifungals)	989.4	E863.6	—	E950.6	E962.1	E980.7

Fourth-digit Required   Fifth-digit Required

Fungizone — Table of Drugs and Chemicals

			External Cause (E-Code)			
	Poisoning	Accident	Therapeutic Use	Suicide Attempt	Assault	Undetermined
Fungizone	960.1	E856	E930.1	E950.4	E962.0	E980.4
topical	976.0	E858.7	E946.0	E950.4	E962.0	E980.4
Furacin	976.0	E858.7	E946.0	E950.4	E962.0	E980.4
Furadantin	961.9	E857	E931.9	E950.4	E962.0	E980.4
Furazolidone	961.9	E857	E931.9	E950.4	E962.0	E980.4
Furnace (coal burning)						
(domestic), gas from	986	E868.3	—	E952.1	E962.2	E982.1
industrial	986	E868.8	—	E952.1	E962.2	E982.1
Furniture polish	989.89	E861.2	—	E950.9	E962.1	E980.9
Furosemide	974.4	E858.5	E944.4	E950.4	E962.0	E980.4
Furoxone	961.9	E857	E931.9	E950.4	E962.0	E980.4
Fusel oil (amyl) (butyl) (propyl)	980.3	E860.4	—	E950.9	E962.1	E980.9
Fusidic acid	960.8	E856	E930.8	E950.4	E962.0	E980.4
Gallamine	975.2	E858.6	E945.2	E950.4	E962.0	E980.4
Gallotannic acid	976.2	E858.7	E946.2	E950.4	E962.0	E980.4
Gamboge	973.1	E858.4	E943.1	E950.4	E962.0	E980.4
Gamimune	964.6	E858.2	E934.6	E950.4	E962.0	E980.4
Gamma-benzene hexachloride						
(vapor)	989.2	E863.0	—	E950.6	E962.1	E980.7
Gamma globulin	964.6	E858.2	E934.6	E950.4	E962.0	E980.4
Gamma Hydroxy Butyrate						
(GHB)	968.4	E855.1	E938.4	E950.4	E962.0	E980.4
Gamulin	964.6	E858.2	E934.6	E950.4	E962.0	E980.4
Ganglionic blocking agents	972.3	E858.3	E942.3	E950.4	E962.0	E980.4
Ganja	969.6	E854.1	E939.6	E950.3	E962.0	E980.3
Garamycin	960.8	E856	E930.8	E950.4	E962.0	E980.4
ophthalmic preparation	976.5	E858.7	E946.5	E950.4	E962.0	E980.4
topical NEC	976.0	E858.7	E946.0	E950.4	E962.0	E980.4
Gardenal	967.0	E851	E937.0	E950.1	E962.0	E980.1
Gardepanyl	967.0	E851	E937.0	E950.1	E962.0	E980.1
Gas	987.9	E869.9	—	E952.9	E962.2	E982.9
acetylene	987.1	E868.1	—	E951.8	E962.2	E981.8
incomplete combustion of — see Carbon, monoxide, fuel, utility						
air contaminants, source or type not specified	987.9	E869.9	—	E952.9	E962.2	E982.9
anesthetic (general) NEC	968.2	E855.1	E938.2	E950.4	E962.0	E980.4
blast furnace	986	E868.8	—	E952.1	E962.2	E982.1
butane — see Butane						
carbon monoxide — see Carbon, monoxide						
chlorine	987.6	E869.8	—	E952.8	E962.2	E982.8
coal — see Carbon, monoxide, coal						
cyanide	987.7	E869.8	—	E952.8	E962.2	E982.8
dicyanogen	987.8	E869.8	—	E952.8	E962.2	E982.8
domestic — see Gas, utility						
exhaust — see Carbon, monoxide, exhaust gas						
from wood- or coal-burning stove or fireplace	986	E868.3	—	E952.1	E962.2	E982.1
fuel (domestic use) — see also Carbon, monoxide, fuel						
industrial use	986	E868.8	—	E952.1	E962.2	E982.1
utility	987.1	E868.1	—	E951.8	E962.2	E981.8
incomplete combustion of — see Carbon, monoxide, fuel, utility						

Table of Drugs and Chemicals — Gasoline, gasolene

	Poisoning	External Cause (E-Code)				
		Accident	Therapeutic Use	Suicide Attempt	Assault	Undetermined
Gas — *continued*						
fuel — *continued*						
utility — *continued*						
in mobile container	987.0	E868.0	—	E951.1	E962.2	E981.1
piped (natural)	987.1	E867	—	E951.0	E962.2	E981.0
garage	986	E868.2	—	E952.0	E962.2	E982.0
hydrocarbon NEC	987.1	E869.8	—	E952.8	E962.2	E982.8
incomplete combustion of — *see* Carbon, monoxide, fuel, utility						
liquefied (mobile container)	987.0	E868.0	—	E951.1	E962.2	E981.1
piped	987.0	E867	—	E951.0	E962.2	E981.0
hydrocyanic acid	987.7	E869.8	—	E952.8	E962.2	E982.8
illuminating — *see* Gas, utility						
incomplete combustion, any — *see* Carbon, monoxide						
kiln	986	E868.8	—	E952.1	E962.2	E982.1
lacrimogenic	987.5	E869.3	—	E952.8	E962.2	E982.8
marsh	987.1	E869.8	—	E952.8	E962.2	E982.8
motor exhaust, not in transit	986	E868.8	—	E952.1	E962.2	E982.1
mustard — *see* Mustard, gas						
natural	987.1	E867	—	E951.0	E962.2	E981.0
nerve (war)	987.9	E869.9	—	E952.9	E962.2	E982.9
oils	981	E862.1	—	E950.9	E962.1	E980.9
petroleum (liquefied) (distributed in mobile containers)	987.0	E868.0	—	E951.1	E962.2	E981.1
piped (pure or mixed with air)	987.0	E867	—	E951.1	E962.2	E981.1
piped (manufactured) (natural) NEC	987.1	E867	—	E951.0	E962.2	E981.0
producer	986	E868.8	—	E952.1	E962.2	E982.1
propane — *see* Propane						
refrigerant (freon)	987.4	E869.2	—	E952.8	E962.2	E982.8
not freon	987.9	E869.9	—	E952.9	E962.2	E982.9
sewer	987.8	E869.8	—	E952.8	E962.2	E982.8
specified source NEC (*see also* substance specified)	987.8	E869.8	—	E952.8	E962.2	E982.8
stove — *see* Gas, utility						
tear	987.5	E869.3	—	E952.8	E962.2	E982.8
utility (for cooking, heating, or lighting) (piped) NEC	987.1	E868.1	—	E951.8	E962.2	E981.8
incomplete combustion of — *see* Carbon, monoxide, fuel, utility						
in mobile container	987.0	E868.0	—	E951.1	E962.2	E981.1
piped (natural)	987.1	E867	—	E951.0	E962.2	E981.0
water	987.1	E868.1	—	E951.8	E962.2	E981.8
incomplete combustion of — *see* Carbon, monoxide, fuel, utility						
Gaseous substance — *see* **Gas**						
Gasoline, gasolene	981	E862.1	—	E950.9	E962.1	E980.9
vapor	987.1	E869.8	—	E952.8	E962.2	E982.8

✓4ᵗʰ Fourth-digit Required   ✓5ᵗʰ Fifth-digit Required

Table of Drugs and Chemicals

		External Cause (E-Code)				
	Poisoning	Accident	Therapeutic Use	Suicide Attempt	Assault	Undetermined
Gastric enzymes	973.4	E858.4	E943.4	E950.4	E962.0	E980.4
Gastrografin	977.8	E858.8	E947.8	E950.4	E962.0	E980.4
Gastrointestinal agents	973.9	E858.4	E943.9	E950.4	E962.0	E980.4
specified NEC	973.8	E858.4	E943.8	E950.4	E962.0	E980.4
Gaultheria procumbens	988.2	E865.4	—	E950.9	E962.1	E980.9
Gelatin (intravenous)	964.8	E858.2	E934.8	E950.4	E962.0	E980.4
absorbable (sponge)	964.5	E858.2	E934.5	E950.4	E962.0	E980.4
Gelfilm	976.8	E858.7	E946.8	E950.4	E962.0	E980.4
Gelfoam	964.5	E858.2	E934.5	E950.4	E962.0	E980.4
Gelsemine	970.8	E854.3	E940.8	E950.4	E962.0	E980.4
Gelsemium (sempervirens)	988.2	E865.4	—	E950.9	E962.1	E980.9
Gemonil	967.0	E851	E937.0	E950.1	E962.0	E980.1
Gentamicin	960.8	E856	E930.8	E950.4	E962.0	E980.4
ophthalmic preparation	976.5	E858.7	E946.5	E950.4	E962.0	E980.4
topical NEC	976.0	E858.7	E946.0	E950.4	E962.0	E980.4
Gentian violet	976.0	E858.7	E946.0	E950.4	E962.0	E980.4
Gexane	976.0	E858.7	E946.0	E950.4	E962.0	E980.4
Gila monster (venom)	989.5	E905.0	—	E950.9	E962.1	E980.9
Ginger, Jamaica	989.89	E866.8	—	E950.9	E962.1	E980.9
Gitalin	972.1	E858.3	E942.1	E950.4	E962.0	E980.4
Gitoxin	972.1	E858.3	E942.1	E950.4	E962.0	E980.4
Glandular extract (medicinal) NEC	977.9	E858.9	E947.9	E950.5	E962.0	E980.5
Glaucarubin	961.5	E857	E931.5	E950.4	E962.0	E980.4
Globin zinc insulin	962.3	E858.0	E932.3	E950.4	E962.0	E980.4
Glucagon	962.3	E858.0	E932.3	E950.4	E962.0	E980.4
Glucochloral	967.1	E852.0	E937.1	E950.2	E962.0	E980.2
Glucocorticoids	962.0	E858.0	E932.0	E950.4	E962.0	E980.4
Glucose	974.5	E858.5	E944.5	E950.4	E962.0	E980.4
oxidase reagent	977.8	E858.8	E947.8	E950.4	E962.0	E980.4
Glucosulfone sodium	961.8	E857	E931.8	E950.4	E962.0	E980.4
Glue(s)	989.89	E866.6	—	E950.9	E962.1	E980.9
Glutamic acid (hydrochloride)	973.4	E858.4	E943.4	E950.4	E962.0	E980.4
Glutathione	963.8	E858.1	E933.8	E950.4	E962.0	E980.4
Glutethimide (group)	967.5	E852.4	E937.5	E950.2	E962.0	E980.2
Glycerin (lotion)	976.3	E858.7	E946.3	E950.4	E962.0	E980.4
Glycerol (topical)	976.3	E858.7	E946.3	E950.4	E962.0	E980.4
Glyceryl						
guaiacolate	975.5	E858.6	E945.5	E950.4	E962.0	E980.4
triacetate (topical)	976.0	E858.7	E946.0	E950.4	E962.0	E980.4
trinitrate	972.4	E858.3	E942.4	E950.4	E962.0	E980.4
Glycine	974.5	E858.5	E944.5	E950.4	E962.0	E980.4
Glycobiarsol	961.1	E857	E931.1	E950.4	E962.0	E980.4
Glycols (ether)	982.8	E862.4	—	E950.9	E962.1	E980.9
Glycopyrrolate	971.1	E855.4	E941.1	E950.4	E962.0	E980.4
Glymidine	962.3	E858.0	E932.3	E950.4	E962.0	E980.4
Gold (compounds) (salts)	965.69	E850.6	E935.6	E950.0	E962.0	E980.0
Golden sulfide of antimony	985.4	E866.2	—	E950.9	E962.1	E980.9
Goldylocks	988.2	E865.4	—	E950.9	E962.1	E980.9
Gonadal tissue extract	962.9	E858.0	E932.9	E950.4	E962.0	E980.4
female	962.2	E858.0	E932.2	E950.4	E962.0	E980.4
male	962.1	E858.0	E932.1	E950.4	E962.0	E980.4
Gonadotropin	962.4	E858.0	E932.4	E950.4	E962.0	E980.4
Grain alcohol	980.0	E860.1	—	E950.9	E962.1	E980.9
beverage	980.0	E860.0	—	E950.9	E962.1	E980.9
Gramicidin	960.8	E856	E930.8	E950.4	E962.0	E980.4
Gratiola officinalis	988.2	E865.4	—	E950.9	E962.1	E980.9
Grease	989.89	E866.8	—	E950.9	E962.1	E980.9
Green hellebore	988.2	E865.4	—	E950.9	E962.1	E980.9
Green soap	976.2	E858.7	E946.2	E950.4	E962.0	E980.4
Grifulvin	960.1	E856	E930.1	E950.4	E962.0	E980.4
Griseofulvin	960.1	E856	E930.1	E950.4	E962.0	E980.4
Growth hormone	962.4	E858.0	E932.4	E950.4	E962.0	E980.4
Guaiacol	975.5	E858.6	E945.5	E950.4	E962.0	E980.4

Table of Drugs and Chemicals

		External Cause (E-Code)				
	Poisoning	Accident	Therapeutic Use	Suicide Attempt	Assault	Undetermined
Guaiac reagent	977.8	E858.8	E947.8	E950.4	E962.0	E980.4
Guaifenesin	975.5	E858.6	E945.5	E950.4	E962.0	E980.4
Guaiphenesin	975.5	E858.6	E945.5	E950.4	E962.0	E980.4
Guanatol	961.4	E857	E931.4	E950.4	E962.0	E980.4
Guanethidine	972.6	E858.3	E942.6	E950.4	E962.0	E980.4
Guano	989.89	E866.5	—	E950.9	E962.1	E980.9
Guanochlor	972.6	E858.3	E942.6	E950.4	E962.0	E980.4
Guanoctine	972.6	E858.3	E942.6	E950.4	E962.0	E980.4
Guanoxan	972.6	E858.3	E942.6	E950.4	E962.0	E980.4
Hair treatment agent NEC	976.4	E858.7	E946.4	E950.4	E962.0	E980.4
Halcinonide	976.0	E858.7	E946.0	E950.4	E962.0	E980.4
Halethazole	976.0	E858.7	E946.0	E950.4	E962.0	E980.4
Hallucinogens	969.6	E854.1	E939.6	E950.3	E962.0	E980.3
Haloperidol	969.2	E853.1	E939.2	E950.3	E962.0	E980.3
Haloprogin	976.0	E858.7	E946.0	E950.4	E962.0	E980.4
Halotex	976.0	E858.7	E946.0	E950.4	E962.0	E980.4
Halothane	968.1	E855.1	E938.1	E950.4	E962.0	E980.4
Halquinols	976.0	E858.7	E946.0	E950.4	E962.0	E980.4
Harmonyl	972.6	E858.3	E942.6	E950.4	E962.0	E980.4
Hartmann's solution	974.5	E858.5	E944.5	E950.4	E962.0	E980.4
Hashish	969.6	E854.1	E939.6	E950.3	E962.0	E980.3
Hawaiian wood rose seeds	969.6	E854.1	E939.6	E950.3	E962.0	E980.3
Headache cures, drugs, powders NEC	977.9	E858.9	E947.9	E950.5	E962.0	E980.9
Heavenly Blue (morning glory)	969.6	E854.1	E939.6	E950.3	E962.0	E980.3
Heavy metal antagonists	963.8	E858.1	E933.8	E950.4	E962.0	E980.4
anti-infectives	961.2	E857	E931.2	E950.4	E962.0	E980.4
Hedaquinium	976.0	E858.7	E946.0	E950.4	E962.0	E980.4
Hedge hyssop	988.2	E865.4	—	E950.9	E962.1	E980.9
Heet	976.8	E858.7	E946.8	E950.4	E962.0	E980.4
Helenin	961.6	E857	E931.6	E950.4	E962.0	E980.4
Hellebore (black) (green) (white)	988.2	E865.4	—	E950.9	E962.1	E980.9
Hemlock	988.2	E865.4	—	E950.9	E962.1	E980.9
Hemostatics	964.5	E858.2	E934.5	E950.4	E962.0	E980.4
capillary active drugs	972.8	E858.3	E942.8	E950.4	E962.0	E980.4
Henbane	988.2	E865.4	—	E950.9	E962.1	E980.9
Heparin (sodium)	964.2	E858.2	E934.2	E950.4	E962.0	E980.4
Heptabarbital, heptabarbitone	967.0	E851	E937.0	E950.1	E962.0	E980.1
Heptachlor	989.2	E863.0	—	E950.6	E962.1	E980.7
Heptalgin	965.09	E850.2	E935.2	E950.0	E962.0	E980
Herbicides	989.4	E863.5	—	E950.6	E962.1	E980.7
Heroin	965.01	E850.0	E935.0	E950.0	E962.0	E980.0
Herplex	976.5	E858.7	E946.5	E950.4	E962.0	E980.4
HES	964.8	E858.2	E934.8	E950.4	E962.0	E980.4
Hetastarch	964.8	E858.2	E934.8	E950.4	E962.0	E980.4
Hexachlorocyclohexane	989.2	E863.0	—	E950.6	E962.1	E980.7
Hexachlorophene	976.2	E858.7	E946.2	E950.4	E962.0	E980.4
Hexadimethrine (bromide)	964.5	E858.2	E934.5	E950.4	E962.0	E980.4
Hexafluorenium	975.2	E858.6	E945.2	E950.4	E962.0	E980.4
Hexa-germ	976.2	E858.7	E946.2	E950.4	E962.0	E980.4
Hexahydrophenol	980.8	E860.8	—	E950.9	E962.1	E980.9
Hexalin	980.8	E860.8	—	E950.9	E962.1	E980.9
Hexamethonium	972.3	E858.3	E942.3	E950.4	E962.0	E980.4
Hexamethyleneamine	961.9	E857	E931.9	E950.4	E962.0	E980.4
Hexamine	961.9	E857	E931.9	E950.4	E962.0	E980.4
Hexanone	982.8	E862.4	—	E950.9	E962.1	E980.9
Hexapropymate	967.8	E852.8	E937.8	E950.2	E962.0	E980.2
Hexestrol	962.2	E858.0	E932.2	E950.4	E962.0	E980.4
Hexethal (sodium)	967.0	E851	E937.0	E950.1	E962.0	E980.1
Hexetidine	976.0	E858.7	E946.0	E950.4	E962.0	E980.4
Hexobarbital, hexobarbitone	967.0	E851	E937.0	E950.1	E962.0	E980.1
sodium (anesthetic)	968.3	E855.1	E938.3	E950.4	E962.0	E980.4
soluble	968.3	E855.1	E938.3	E950.4	E962.0	E980.4

Fourth-digit Required   Fifth-digit Required

Table of Drugs and Chemicals

	Poisoning	External Cause (E-Code)				
		Accident	Therapeutic Use	Suicide Attempt	Assault	Undetermined
Hexocyclium	971.1	E855.4	E941.1	E950.4	E962.0	E980.4
Hexoestrol	962.2	E858.0	E932.2	E950.4	E962.0	E980.4
Hexone	982.8	E862.4	—	E950.9	E962.1	E980.9
Hexylcaine	968.5	E855.2	E938.5	E950.4	E962.0	E980.4
Hexylresorcinol	961.6	E857	E931.6	E950.4	E962.0	E980.4
Hinkle's pills	973.1	E858.4	E943.1	E950.4	E962.0	E980.4
Histalog	977.8	E858.8	E947.8	E950.4	E962.0	E980.4
Histamine (phosphate)	972.5	E858.3	E942.5	E950.4	E962.0	E980.4
Histoplasmin	977.8	E858.8	E947.8	E950.4	E962.0	E980.4
Holly berries	988.2	E865.3	—	E950.9	E962.1	E980.9
Homatropine	971.1	E855.4	E941.1	E950.4	E962.0	E980.4
Homo-tet	964.6	E858.2	E934.6	E950.4	E962.0	E980.4
Hormones (synthetic substitute) NEC	962.9	E858.0	E932.9	E950.4	E962.0	E980.4
adrenal cortical steroids	962.0	E858.0	E932.0	E950.4	E962.0	E980.4
antidiabetic agents	962.3	E858.0	E932.3	E950.4	E962.0	E980.4
follicle stimulating	962.4	E858.0	E932.4	E950.4	E962.0	E980.4
gonadotropic	962.4	E858.0	E932.4	E950.4	E962.0	E980.4
growth	962.4	E858.0	E932.4	E950.4	E962.0	E980.4
ovarian (substitutes)	962.2	E858.0	E932.2	E950.4	E962.0	E980.4
parathyroid (derivatives)	962.6	E858.0	E932.6	E950.4	E962.0	E980.4
pituitary (posterior)	962.5	E858.0	E932.5	E950.4	E962.0	E980.4
anterior	962.4	E858.0	E932.4	E950.4	E962.0	E980.4
thyroid (derivative)	962.7	E858.0	E932.7	E950.4	E962.0	E980.4
Hornet (sting)	989.5	E905.3	—	E950.9	E962.1	E980.9
Horticulture agent NEC	989.4	E863.9	—	E950.6	E962.1	E980.7
Hyaluronidase	963.4	E858.1	E933.4	E950.4	E962.0	E980.4
Hyazyme	963.4	E858.1	E933.4	E950.4	E962.0	E980.4
Hycodan	965.09	E850.2	E935.2	E950.0	E962.0	E980.0
Hydantoin derivatives	966.1	E855.0	E936.1	E950.4	E962.0	E980.4
Hydeltra	962.0	E858.0	E932.0	E950.4	E962.0	E980.4
Hydergine	971.3	E855.6	E941.3	E950.4	E962.0	E980.4
Hydrabamine penicillin	960.0	E856	E930.0	E950.4	E962.0	E980.4
Hydralazine, hydrallazine	972.6	E858.3	E942.6	E950.4	E962.0	E980.4
Hydrargaphen	976.0	E858.7	E946.0	E950.4	E962.0	E980.4
Hydrazine	983.9	E864.3	—	E950.7	E962.1	E980.6
Hydriodic acid	975.5	E858.6	E945.5	E950.4	E962.0	E980.4
Hydrocarbon gas	987.1	E869.8	—	E952.8	E962.2	E982.8
incomplete combustion of — see Carbon, monoxide, fuel, utility						
liquefied (mobile container)	987.0	E868.0	—	E951.1	E962.2	E981.1
piped (natural)	987.0	E867	—	E951.0	E962.2	E981.0
Hydrochloric acid (liquid)	983.1	E864.1	—	E950.7	E962.1	E980.6
medicinal	973.4	E858.4	E943.4	E950.4	E962.0	E980.4
vapor	987.8	E869.8	—	E952.8	E962.2	E982.8
Hydrochlorothiazide	974.3	E858.5	E944.3	E950.4	E962.0	E980.4
Hydrocodone	965.09	E850.2	E935.2	E950.0	E962.0	E980.0
Hydrocortisone	962.0	E858.0	E932.0	E950.4	E962.0	E980.4
ENT agent	976.6	E858.7	E946.6	E950.4	E962.0	E980.4
ophthalmic preparation	976.5	E858.7	E946.5	E950.4	E962.0	E980.4
topical NEC	976.0	E858.7	E946.0	E950.4	E962.0	E980.4
Hydrocortone	962.0	E858.0	E932.0	E950.4	E962.0	E980.4
ENT agent	976.6	E858.7	E946.6	E950.4	E962.0	E980.4
ophthalmic preparation	976.5	E858.7	E946.5	E950.4	E962.0	E980.4
topical NEC	976.0	E858.7	E946.0	E950.4	E962.0	E980.4
Hydrocyanic acid — see Cyanide(s)						
Hydroflumethiazide	974.3	E858.5	E944.3	E950.4	E962.0	E980.4
Hydrofluoric acid (liquid)	983.1	E864.1	—	E950.7	E962.1	E980.6
vapor	987.8	E869.8	—	E952.8	E962.2	E982.8
Hydrogen	987.8	E869.8	—	E952.8	E962.2	E982.8
arsenide	985.1	E866.3	—	E950.8	E962.1	E980.8
arseniureted	985.1	E866.3	—	E950.8	E962.1	E980.8

Table of Drugs and Chemicals — Inderal

	Poisoning	External Cause (E-Code)				
		Accident	Therapeutic Use	Suicide Attempt	Assault	Undetermined
Hydrogen — *continued*						
cyanide (salts)	989.0	E866.8	—	E950.9	E962.1	E980.9
gas	987.7	E869.8	—	E952.8	E962.2	E982.8
fluoride (liquid)	983.1	E864.1	—	E950.7	E962.1	E980.6
vapor	987.8	E869.8	—	E952.8	E962.2	E982.8
peroxide (solution)	976.6	E858.7	E946.6	E950.4	E962.0	E980.4
phosphureted	987.8	E869.8	—	E952.8	E962.2	E982.8
sulfide (gas)	987.8	E869.8	—	E952.8	E962.2	E982.8
arseniureted	985.1	E866.3	—	E950.8	E962.1	E980.8
sulfureted	987.8	E869.8	—	E952.8	E962.2	E982.8
Hydromorphinol	965.09	E850.2	E935.2	E950.0	E962.0	E980.0
Hydromorphinone	965.09	E850.2	E935.2	E950.0	E962.0	E980.0
Hydromorphone	965.09	E850.2	E935.2	E950.0	E962.0	E980.0
Hydromox	974.3	E858.5	E944.3	E950.4	E962.0	E980.4
Hydrophilic lotion	976.3	E858.7	E946.3	E950.4	E962.0	E980.4
Hydroquinone	983.0	E864.0	—	E950.7	E962.1	E980.6
vapor	987.8	E869.8	—	E952.8	E962.2	E982.8
Hydrosulfuric acid (gas)	987.8	E869.8	—	E952.8	E962.2	E982.8
Hydrous wool fat (lotion)	976.3	E858.7	E946.3	E950.4	E962.0	E980.4
Hydroxide, caustic	983.2	E864.2	—	E950.7	E962.1	E980.6
Hydroxocobalamin	964.1	E858.2	E934.1	E950.4	E962.0	E980.4
Hydroxyamphetamine	971.2	E855.5	E941.2	E950.4	E962.0	E980.4
Hydroxychloroquine	961.4	E857	E931.4	E950.4	E962.0	E980.4
Hydroxydihydrocodeinone	965.09	E850.2	E935.2	E950.0	E962.0	E980.0
Hydroxyethyl starch	964.8	E858.2	E934.8	E950.4	E962.0	E980.4
Hydroxyphenamate	969.5	E853.8	E939.5	E950.3	E962.0	E980.3
Hydroxyphenylbutazone	965.5	E850.5	E935.5	E950.0	E962.0	E980.0
Hydroxyprogesterone	962.2	E858.0	E932.2	E950.4	E962.0	E980.4
Hydroxyquinoline derivatives	961.3	E857	E931.3	E950.4	E962.0	E980.4
Hydroxystilbamidine	961.5	E857	E931.5	E950.4	E962.0	E980.4
Hydroxyurea	963.1	E858.1	E933.1	E950.4	E962.0	E980.4
Hydroxyzine	969.5	E853.8	E939.5	E950.3	E962.0	E980.3
Hyoscine (hydrobromide)	971.1	E855.4	E941.1	E950.4	E962.0	E980.4
Hyoscyamine	971.1	E855.4	E941.1	E950.4	E962.0	E980.4
Hyoscyamus (albus) (niger)	988.2	E865.4	—	E950.9	E962.1	E980.9
Hypaque	977.8	E858.8	E947.8	E950.4	E962.0	E980.4
Hypertussis	964.6	E858.2	E934.6	E950.4	E962.0	E980.4
Hypnotics NEC	967.9	E852.9	E937.9	E950.2	E962.0	E980.2
Hypochlorites — *see* **Sodium, hypochlorite**						
Hypotensive agents NEC	972.6	E858.3	E942.6	E950.4	E962.0	E980.4
Ibufenac	965.69	E850.6	E935.6	E950.0	E962.0	E980.0
Ibuprofen	965.61	E850.6	E935.6	E950.0	E962.0	E980.0
ICG	977.8	E858.8	E947.8	E950.4	E962.0	E980.4
Ichthammol	976.4	E858.7	E946.4	E950.4	E962.0	E980.4
Ichthyol	976.4	E858.7	E946.4	E950.4	E962.0	E980.4
Idoxuridine	976.5	E858.7	E946.5	E950.4	E962.0	E980.4
IDU	976.5	E858.7	E946.5	E950.4	E962.0	E980.4
Iletin	962.3	E858.0	E932.3	E950.4	E962.0	E980.4
Ilex	988.2	E865.4	—	E950.9	E962.1	E980.9
Illuminating gas — *see* **Gas, utility**						
Ilopan	963.5	E858.1	E933.5	E950.4	E962.0	E980.4
Ilotycin	960.3	E856	E930.3	E950.4	E962.0	E980.4
ophthalmic preparation	976.5	E858.7	E946.5	E950.4	E962.0	E980.4
topical NEC	976.0	E858.7	E946.0	E950.4	E962.0	E980.4
Imipramine	969.0	E854.0	E939.0	E950.3	E962.0	E980.3
Immu-G	964.6	E858.2	E934.6	E950.4	E962.0	E980.4
Immuglobin	964.6	E858.2	E934.6	E950.4	E962.0	E980.4
Immune serum globulin	964.6	E858.2	E934.6	E950.4	E962.0	E980.4
Immunosuppressive agents	963.1	E858.1	E933.1	E950.4	E962.0	E980.4
Immu-tetanus	964.6	E858.2	E934.6	E950.4	E962.0	E980.4
Indandione (derivatives)	964.2	E858.2	E934.2	E950.4	E962.0	E980.4
Inderal	972.0	E858.3	E942.0	E950.4	E962.0	E980.4

Table of Drugs and Chemicals

		External Cause (E-Code)				
	Poisoning	Accident	Therapeutic Use	Suicide Attempt	Assault	Undetermined
Indian						
hemp	969.6	E854.1	E939.6	E950.3	E962.0	E980.3
tobacco	988.2	E865.4	—	E950.9	E962.1	E980.9
Indigo carmine	977.8	E858.8	E947.8	E950.4	E962.0	E980.4
Indocin	965.69	E850.6	E935.6	E950.0	E962.0	E980.0
Indocyanine green	977.8	E858.8	E947.8	E950.4	E962.0	E980.4
Indomethacin	965.69	E850.6	E935.6	E950.0	E962.0	E980.0
Industrial						
alcohol	980.9	E860.9	—	E950.9	E962.1	E980.9
fumes	987.8	E869.8	—	E952.8	E962.2	E982.8
solvents (fumes) (vapors)	982.8	E862.9	—	E950.9	E962.1	E980.9
Influenza vaccine	979.6	E858.8	E949.6	E950.4	E962.0	E982.8
Ingested substances NEC	989.9	E866.9	—	E950.9	E962.1	E980.9
INH (isoniazid)	961.8	E857	E931.8	E950.4	E962.0	E980.4
Inhalation, gas (noxious) —						
see Gas						
Ink	989.89	E866.8	—	E950.9	E962.1	E980.9
Innovar	967.6	E852.5	E937.6	E950.2	E962.0	E980.2
Inositol niacinate	972.2	E858.3	E942.2	E950.4	E962.0	E980.4
Inproquone	963.1	E858.1	E933.1	E950.4	E962.0	E980.4
Insect (sting), venomous	989.5	E905.5	—	E950.9	E962.1	E980.9
Insecticides (see also						
Pesticides)	989.4	E863.4	—	E950.6	E962.1	E980.7
chlorinated	989.2	E863.0	—	E950.6	E962.1	E980.7
mixtures	989.4	E863.3	—	E950.6	E962.1	E980.7
organochlorine (compounds)	989.2	E863.0	—	E950.6	E962.1	E980.7
organophosphorus						
(compounds)	989.3	E863.1	—	E950.6	E962.1	E980.7
Insular tissue extract	962.3	E858.0	E932.3	E950.4	E962.0	E980.4
Insulin (amorphous) (globin)						
(isophane) (Lente) (NPH)						
(protamine) (Semilente)						
(Ultralente) (zinc)	962.3	E858.0	E932.3	E950.4	E962.0	E980.4
Intranarcon	968.3	E855.1	E938.3	E950.4	E962.0	E980.4
Inulin	977.8	E858.8	E947.8	E950.4	E962.0	E980.4
Invert sugar	974.5	E858.5	E944.5	E950.4	E962.0	E980.4
Iodide NEC (see also Iodine)	976.0	E858.7	E946.0	E950.4	E962.0	E980.4
mercury (ointment)	976.0	E858.7	E946.0	E950.4	E962.0	E980.4
methylate	976.0	E858.7	E946.0	E950.4	E962.0	E980.4
potassium (expectorant)						
NEC	975.5	E858.6	E945.5	E950.4	E962.0	E980.4
Iodinated glycerol	975.5	E858.6	E945.5	E950.4	E962.0	E980.4
Iodine (antiseptic, external)						
(tincture) NEC	976.0	E858.7	E946.0	E950.4	E962.0	E980.4
diagnostic	977.8	E858.8	E947.8	E950.4	E962.0	E980.4
for thyroid conditions						
(antithyroid)	962.8	E858.0	E932.8	E950.4	E962.0	E980.4
vapor	987.8	E869.8	—	E952.8	E962.2	E982.8
Iodized oil	977.8	E858.8	E947.8	E950.4	E962.0	E980.4
Iodobismitol	961.2	E857	E931.2	E950.4	E962.0	E980.4
Iodochlorhydroxyquin	961.3	E857	E931.3	E950.4	E962.0	E980.4
topical	976.0	E858.7	E946.0	E950.4	E962.0	E980.4
Iodoform	976.0	E858.7	E946.0	E950.4	E962.0	E980.4
Iodopanoic acid	977.8	E858.8	E947.8	E950.4	E962.0	E980.4
Iodophthalein	977.8	E858.8	E947.8	E950.4	E962.0	E980.4
Ion exchange resins	974.5	E858.5	E944.5	E950.4	E962.0	E980.4
Iopanoic acid	977.8	E858.8	E947.8	E950.4	E962.0	E980.4
Iophendylate	977.8	E858.8	E947.8	E950.4	E962.0	E980.4
Iothiouracil	962.8	E858.0	E932.8	E950.4	E962.0	E980.4
Ipecac	973.6	E858.4	E943.6	E950.4	E962.0	E980.4
Ipecacuanha	973.6	E858.4	E943.6	E950.4	E962.0	E980.4
Ipodate	977.8	E858.8	E947.8	E950.4	E962.0	E980.4
Ipral	967.0	E851	E937.0	E950.1	E962.0	E980.1
Ipratropium ●	975.1	E858.6	E945.1	E950.4	E962.0	E980.4

▶◀ Revised Text   ● New Line   ▲ Revised Code

Table of Drugs and Chemicals

	Poisoning	External Cause (E-Code)				
		Accident	Therapeutic Use	Suicide Attempt	Assault	Undetermined
Iproniazid	969.0	E854.0	E939.0	E950.3	E962.0	E980.3
Iron (compounds) (medicinal)						
(preparations)	964.0	E858.2	E934.0	E950.4	E962.0	E980.4
dextran	964.0	E858.2	E934.0	E950.4	E962.0	E980.4
nonmedicinal (dust)						
(fumes) NEC	985.8	E866.4	—	E950.9	E962.1	E980.9
Irritant drug	977.9	E858.9	E947.9	E950.5	E962.0	E980.5
Ismelin	972.6	E858.3	E942.6	E950.4	E962.0	E980.4
Isoamyl nitrite	972.4	E858.3	E942.4	E950.4	E962.0	E980.4
Isobutyl acetate	982.8	E862.4	—	E950.9	E962.1	E980.9
Isocarboxazid	969.0	E854.0	E939.0	E950.3	E962.0	E980.3
Isoephedrine	971.2	E855.5	E941.2	E950.4	E962.0	E980.4
Isoetharine	971.2	E855.5	E941.2	E950.4	E962.0	E980.4
Isofluorophate	971.0	E855.3	E941.0	E950.4	E962.0	E980.4
Isoniazid (INH)	961.8	E857	E931.8	E950.4	E962.0	E980.4
Isopentaquine	961.4	E857	E931.4	E950.4	E962.0	E980.4
Isophane insulin	962.3	E858.0	E932.3	E950.4	E962.0	E980.4
Isopregnenone	962.2	E858.0	E932.2	E950.4	E962.0	E980.4
Isoprenaline	971.2	E855.5	E941.2	E950.4	E962.0	E980.4
Isopropamide	971.1	E855.4	E941.1	E950.4	E962.0	E980.4
Isopropanol	980.2	E860.3	—	E950.9	E962.1	E980.9
topical (germicide)	976.0	E858.7	E946.0	E950.4	E962.0	E980.4
Isopropyl						
acetate	982.8	E862.4	—	E950.9	E962.1	E980.9
alcohol	980.2	E860.3	—	E950.9	E962.1	E980.9
topical (germicide)	976.0	E858.7	E946.0	E950.4	E962.0	E980.4
ether	982.8	E862.4	—	E950.9	E962.1	E980.9
Isoproterenol	971.2	E855.5	E941.2	E950.4	E962.0	E980.4
Isosorbide dinitrate	972.4	E858.3	E942.4	E950.4	E962.0	E980.4
Isothipendyl	963.0	E858.1	E933.0	E950.4	E962.0	E980.4
Isoxazolyl penicillin	960.0	E856	E930.0	E950.4	E962.0	E980.4
Isoxsuprine hydrochloride	972.5	E858.3	E942.5	E950.4	E962.0	E980.4
l-thyroxine sodium	962.7	E858.0	E932.7	E950.4	E962.0	E980.4
Jaborandi (pilocarpus)						
(extract)	971.0	E855.3	E941.0	E950.4	E962.0	E980.4
Jalap	973.1	E858.4	E943.1	E950.4	E962.0	E980.4
Jamaica						
dogwood (bark)	965.7	E850.7	E935.7	E950.0	E962.0	E980.0
ginger	989.89	E866.8	—	E950.9	E962.1	E980.9
Jatropha	988.2	E865.4	—	E950.9	E962.1	E980.9
curcas	988.2	E865.3	—	E950.9	E962.1	E980.9
Jectofer	964.0	E858.2	E934.0	E950.4	E962.0	E980.4
Jellyfish (sting)	989.5	E905.6	—	E950.9	E962.1	E980.9
Jequirity (bean)	988.2	E865.3	—	E950.9	E962.1	E980.9
Jimson weed	988.2	E865.4	—	E950.9	E962.1	E980.9
seeds	988.2	E865.3	—	E950.9	E962.1	E980.9
Juniper tar (oil) (ointment)	976.4	E858.7	E946.4	E950.4	E962.0	E980.4
Kallikrein	972.5	E858.3	E942.5	E950.4	E962.0	E980.4
Kanamycin	960.6	E856	E930.6	E950.4	E962.0	E980.4
Kantrex	960.6	E856	E930.6	E950.4	E962.0	E980.4
Kaolin	973.5	E858.4	E943.5	E950.4	E962.0	E980.4
Karaya (gum)	973.3	E858.4	E943.3	E950.4	E962.0	E980.4
Kemithal	968.3	E855.1	E938.3	E950.4	E962.0	E980.4
Kenacort	962.0	E858.0	E932.0	E950.4	E962.0	E980.4
Keratolytics	976.4	E858.7	E946.4	E950.4	E962.0	E980.4
Keratoplastics	976.4	E858.7	E946.4	E950.4	E962.0	E980.4
Kerosene, kerosine (fuel)						
(solvent) NEC	981		—	E950.9	E962.1	E980.9
insecticide	981	E863.4	—	E950.6	E962.1	E980.7
vapor	987.1	E869.8	—	E952.8	E962.2	E982.8
Ketamine	968.3	E855.1	E938.3	E950.4	E962.0	E980.4
Ketobemidone	965.09	E850.2	E935.2	E950.0	E962.0	E980.0
Ketols	982.8	E862.4	—	E950.9	E962.1	E980.9
Ketone oils	982.8	E862.4	—	E950.9	E962.1	E980.9

Table of Drugs and Chemicals

	External Cause (E-Code)					
	Poisoning	Accident	Therapeutic Use	Suicide Attempt	Assault	Undetermined
Ketoprofen	965.61	E850.6	E935.6	E950.0	E962.0	E980.0
Kiln gas or vapor (carbon monoxide)	986	E868.8	—	E952.1	E962.2	E982.1
Konsyl	973.3	E858.4	E943.3	E950.4	E962.0	E980.4
Kosam seed	988.2	E865.3	—	E950.9	E962.1	E980.9
Krait (venom)	989.5	E905.0	—	E950.9	E962.1	E980.9
Kwell (insecticide)	989.2	E863.0	—	E950.6	E962.1	E980.7
anti-infective (topical)	976.0	E858.7	E946.0	E950.4	E962.0	E980.4
Laburnum (flowers) (seeds)	988.2	E865.3	—	E950.9	E962.1	E980.9
leaves	988.2	E865.4	—	E950.9	E962.1	E980.9
Lacquers	989.89	E861.6	—	E950.9	E962.1	E980.9
Lacrimogenic gas	987.5	E869.3	—	E952.8	E962.2	E982.8
Lactic acid	983.1	E864.1	—	E950.7	E962.1	E980.6
Lactobacillus acidophilus	973.5	E858.4	E943.5	E950.4	E962.0	E980.4
Lactoflavin	963.5	E858.1	E933.5	E950.4	E962.0	E980.4
Lactuca (virosa) (extract)	967.8	E852.8	E937.8	E950.2	E962.0	E980.2
Lactucarium	967.8	E852.8	E937.8	E950.2	E962.0	E980.2
Laevulose	974.5	E858.5	E944.5	E950.4	E962.0	E980.4
Lanatoside (C)	972.1	E858.3	E942.1	E950.4	E962.0	E980.4
Lanolin (lotion)	976.3	E858.7	E946.3	E950.4	E962.0	E980.4
Largactil	969.1	E853.0	E939.1	E950.3	E962.0	E980.3
Larkspur	988.2	E865.3	—	E950.9	E962.1	E980.9
Laroxyl	969.0	E854.0	E939.0	E950.3	E962.0	E980.3
Lasix	974.4	E858.5	E944.4	E950.4	E962.0	E980.4
Latex	989.82	E866.8	—	E950.9	E962.1	E980.9
Lathyrus (seed)	988.2	E865.3	—	E950.9	E962.1	E980.9
Laudanum	965.09	E850.2	E935.2	E950.0	E962.0	E980.0
Laudexium	975.2	E858.6	E945.2	E950.4	E962.0	E980.4
Laurel, black or cherry	988.2	E865.4	—	E950.9	E962.1	E980.9
Laurolinium	976.0	E858.7	E946.0	E950.4	E962.0	E980.4
Lauryl sulfoacetate	976.2	E858.7	E946.2	E950.4	E962.0	E980.4
Laxatives NEC	973.3	E858.4	E943.3	E950.4	E962.0	E980.4
emollient	973.2	E858.4	E943.2	E950.4	E962.0	E980.4
L-dopa	966.4	E855.0	E936.4	E950.4	E962.0	E980.4
Lead (dust) (fumes) (vapor)						
NEC	984.9	E866.0	—	E950.9	E962.1	E980.9
acetate (dust)	984.1	E866.0	—	E950.9	E962.1	E980.9
anti-infectives	961.2	E857	E931.2	E950.4	E962.0	E980.4
antiknock compound (tetraethyl)	984.1	E862.1	—	E950.9	E962.1	E980.9
arsenate, arsenite (dust) (insecticide) (vapor)	985.1	E863.4	—	E950.8	E962.1	E980.8
herbicide	985.1	E863.5	—	E950.8	E962.1	E980.8
carbonate	984.0	E866.0	—	E950.9	E962.1	E980.9
paint	984.0	E861.5	—	E950.9	E962.1	E980.9
chromate	984.0	E866.0	—	E950.9	E962.1	E980.9
paint	984.0	E861.5	—	E950.9	E962.1	E980.9
dioxide	984.0	E866.0	—	E950.9	E962.1	E980.9
inorganic (compound)	984.0	E866.0	—	E950.9	E962.1	E980.9
paint	984.0	E861.5	—	E950.9	E962.1	E980.9
iodide	984.0	E866.0	—	E950.9	E962.1	E980.9
pigment (paint)	984.0	E861.5	—	E950.9	E962.1	E980.9
monoxide (dust)	984.0	E866.0	—	E950.9	E962.1	E980.9
paint	984.0	E861.5	—	E950.9	E962.1	E980.9
organic	984.1	E866.0	—	E950.9	E962.1	E980.9
oxide	984.0	E866.0	—	E950.9	E962.1	E980.9
paint	984.0	E861.5	—	E950.9	E962.1	E980.9
paint	984.0	E861.5	—	E950.9	E962.1	E980.9
salts	984.0	E866.0	—	E950.9	E962.1	E980.9
specified compound NEC	984.8	E866.0	—	E950.9	E962.1	E980.9
tetra-ethyl	984.1	E862.1	—	E950.9	E962.1	E980.9
Lebanese red	969.6	E854.1	E939.6	E950.3	E962.0	E980.3
Lente Iletin (insulin)	962.3	E858.0	E932.3	E950.4	E962.0	E980.4
Leptazol	970.0	E854.3	E940.0	E950.4	E962.0	E980.4

Table of Drugs and Chemicals — Lizard (bite) (venom)

		External Cause (E-Code)				
	Poisoning	Accident	Therapeutic Use	Suicide Attempt	Assault	Undetermined
Leritine	965.09	E850.2	E935.2	E950.0	E962.0	E980.0
Letter	962.7	E858.0	E932.7	E950.4	E962.0	E980.4
Lettuce opium	967.8	E852.8	E937.8	E950.2	E962.0	E980.2
Leucovorin (factor)	964.1	E858.2	E934.1	E950.4	E962.0	E980.4
Leukeran	963.1	E858.1	E933.1	E950.4	E962.0	E980.4
Levalbuterol ●	975.7	E858.6	E945.7	E950.4	E962.0	E980.4
Levallorphan	970.1	E854.3	E940.1	E950.4	E962.0	E980.4
Levanil	967.8	E852.8	E937.8	E950.2	E962.0	E980.2
Levarterenol	971.2	E855.5	E941.2	E950.4	E962.0	E980.4
Levodopa	966.4	E855.0	E936.4	E950.4	E962.0	E980.4
Levo-dromoran	965.09	E850.2	E935.2	E950.0	E962.0	E980.0
Levoid	962.7	E858.0	E932.7	E950.4	E962.0	E980.4
Levo-iso-methadone	965.02	E850.1	E935.1	E950.0	E962.0	E980.0
Levomepromazine	967.8	E852.8	E937.8	E950.2	E962.0	E980.2
Levoprome	967.8	E852.8	E937.8	E950.2	E962.0	E980.2
Levopropoxyphene	975.4	E858.6	E945.4	E950.4	E962.0	E980.4
Levorphan, levophanol	965.09	E850.2	E935.2	E950.0	E962.0	E980.0
Levothyroxine (sodium)	962.7	E858.0	E932.7	E950.4	E962.0	E980.4
Levsin	971.1	E855.4	E941.1	E950.4	E962.0	E980.4
Levulose	974.5	E858.5	E944.5	E950.4	E962.0	E980.4
Lewisite (gas)	985.1	E866.3	—	E950.8	E962.1	E980.8
Librium	969.4	E853.2	E939.4	E950.3	E962.0	E980.3
Lidex	976.0	E858.7	E946.0	E950.4	E962.0	E980.4
Lidocaine (infiltration) (topical)	968.5	E855.2	E938.5	E950.4	E962.0	E980.4
nerve block (peripheral) (plexus)	968.6	E855.2	E938.6	E950.4	E962.0	E980.4
spinal	968.7	E855.2	E938.7	E950.4	E962.0	E980.4
Lighter fluid	981	E862.1	—	E950.9	E962.1	E980.9
Lignocaine (infiltration) (topical)	968.5	E855.2	E938.5	E950.4	E962.0	E980.4
nerve block (peripheral) (plexus)	968.6	E855.2	E938.6	E950.4	E962.0	E980.4
spinal	968.7	E855.2	E938.7	E950.4	E962.0	E980.4
Ligroin(e) (solvent)	981	E862.0	—	E950.9	E962.1	E980.9
vapor	987.1	E869.8	—	E952.8	E962.2	E982.8
Ligustrum vulgare	988.2	E865.3	—	E950.9	E962.1	E980.9
Lily of the valley	988.2	E865.4	—	E950.9	E962.1	E980.9
Lime (chloride)	983.2	E864.2	—	E950.7	E962.1	E980.6
solution, sulferated	976.4	E858.7	E946.4	E950.4	E962.0	E980.4
Limonene	982.8	E862.4	—	E950.9	E962.1	E980.9
Lincomycin	960.8	E856	E930.8	E950.4	E962.0	E980.4
Lindane (insecticide) (vapor)	989.2	E863.0	—	E950.6	E962.1	E980.7
anti-infective (topical)	976.0	E858.7	E946.0	E950.4	E962.0	E980.4
Liniments NEC	976.9	E858.7	E946.9	E950.4	E962.0	E980.4
Linoleic acid	972.2	E858.3	E942.2	E950.4	E962.0	E980.4
Liothyronine	962.7	E858.0	E932.7	E950.4	E962.0	E980.4
Liotrix	962.7	E858.0	E932.7	E950.4	E962.0	E980.4
Lipancreatin	973.4	E858.4	E943.4	E950.4	E962.0	E980.4
Lipo-Lutin	962.2	E858.0	E932.2	E950.4	E962.0	E980.4
Lipotropic agents	977.1	E858.8	E947.1	E950.4	E962.0	E980.4
Liquefied petroleum gases	987.0	E868.0	—	E951.1	E962.2	E981.1
piped (pure or mixed with air)	987.0	E867	—	E951.0	E962.2	E981.0
Liquid petrolatum	973.2	E858.4	E943.2	E950.4	E962.0	E980.4
substance	989.9	E866.9	—	E950.9	E962.1	E980.9
specified NEC	989.89	E866.8	—	E950.9	E962.1	E980.9
Lirugen	979.4	E858.8	E949.4	E950.4	E962.0	E980.4
Lithane	969.8	E855.8	E939.8	E950.3	E962.0	E980.3
Lithium	985.8	E866.4	—	E950.9	E962.1	E980.9
carbonate	969.8	E855.8	E939.8	E950.3	E962.0	E980.3
Lithonate	969.8	E855.8	E939.8	E950.3	E962.0	E980.3
Liver (extract) (injection) (preparations)	964.1	E858.2	E934.1	E950.4	E962.0	E980.4
Lizard (bite) (venom)	989.5	E905.0	—	E950.9	E962.1	E980.9

✓4ᵗʰ Fourth-digit Required ✓5ᵗʰ Fifth-digit Required

Table of Drugs and Chemicals

	Poisoning	External Cause (E-Code)				
		Accident	Therapeutic Use	Suicide Attempt	Assault	Undetermined
LMD	964.8	E858.2	E934.8	E950.4	E962.0	E980.4
Lobelia	988.2	E865.4	—	E950.9	E962.1	E980.9
Lobeline	970.0	E854.3	E940.0	E950.4	E962.0	E980.4
Locorten	976.0	E858.7	E946.0	E950.4	E962.0	E980.4
Lolium temulentum	988.2	E865.3	—	E950.9	E962.1	E980.9
Lomotil	973.5	E858.4	E943.5	E950.4	E962.0	E980.4
Lomustine	963.1	E858.1	E933.1	E950.4	E962.0	E980.4
Lophophora williamsii	969.6	E854.1	E939.6	E950.3	E962.0	E980.3
Lorazepam	969.4	E853.2	E939.4	E950.3	E962.0	E980.3
Lotions NEC	976.9	E858.7	E946.9	E950.4	E962.0	E980.4
Lotronex	973.8	E858.4	E943.8	E950.4	E962.0	E980.4
Lotusate	967.0	E851	E937.0	E950.1	E962.0	E980.1
Lowila	976.2	E858.7	E946.2	E950.4	E962.0	E980.4
Loxapine	969.3	E853.8	E939.3	E950.3	E962.0	E980.3
Lozenges (throat)	976.6	E858.7	E946.6	E950.4	E962.0	E980.4
LSD (25)	969.6	E854.1	E939.6	E950.3	E962.0	E980.3
Lubricating oil NEC	981	E862.2	—	E950.9	E962.1	E980.9
Lucanthone	961.6	E857	E931.6	E950.4	E962.0	E980.4
Luminal	967.0	E851	E937.0	E950.1	E962.0	E980.1
Lung irritant (gas) NEC	987.9	E869.9	—	E952.9	E962.2	E982.9
Lutocylol	962.2	E858.0	E932.2	E950.4	E962.0	E980.4
Lutromone	962.2	E858.0	E932.2	E950.4	E962.0	E980.4
Lututrin	975.0	E858.6	E945.0	E950.4	E962.0	E980.4
Lye (concentrated)	983.2	E864.2	—	E950.7	E962.1	E980.6
Lygranum (skin test)	977.8	E858.8	E947.8	E950.4	E962.0	E980.4
Lymecycline	960.4	E856	E930.4	E950.4	E962.0	E980.4
Lymphogranuloma venereum antigen	977.8	E858.8	E947.8	E950.4	E962.0	E980.4
Lynestrenol	962.2	E858.0	E932.2	E950.4	E962.0	E980.4
Lyovac Sodium Edecrin	974.4	E858.5	E944.4	E950.4	E962.0	E980.4
Lypressin	962.5	E858.0	E932.5	E950.4	E962.0	E980.4
Lysergic acid (amide) (diethylamide)	969.6	E854.1	E939.6	E950.3	E962.0	E980.3
Lysergide	969.6	E854.1	E939.6	E950.3	E962.0	E980.3
Lysine vasopressin	962.5	E858.0	E932.5	E950.4	E962.0	E980.4
Lysol	983.0	E864.0	—	E950.7	E962.1	E980.6
Lytta (vitatta)	976.8	E858.7	E946.8	E950.4	E962.0	E980.4
Mace	987.5	E869.3	—	E952.8	E962.2	E982.8
Macrolides (antibiotics)	960.3	E856	E930.3	E950.4	E962.0	E980.4
Mafenide	976.0	E858.7	E946.0	E950.4	E962.0	E980.4
Magaldrate	973.0	E858.4	E943.0	E950.4	E962.0	E980.4
Magic mushroom	969.6	E854.1	E939.6	E950.3	E962.0	E980.3
Magnamycin	960.8	E856	E930.8	E950.4	E962.0	E980.4
Magnesia magma	973.0	E858.4	E943.0	E950.4	E962.0	E980.4
Magnesium (compounds) (fumes) NEC	985.8	E866.4	—	E950.9	E962.1	E980.9
antacid	973.0	E858.4	E943.0	E950.4	E962.0	E980.4
carbonate	973.0	E858.4	E943.0	E950.4	E962.0	E980.4
cathartic	973.3	E858.4	E943.3	E950.4	E962.0	E980.4
citrate	973.3	E858.4	E943.3	E950.4	E962.0	E980.4
hydroxide	973.0	E858.4	E943.0	E950.4	E962.0	E980.4
oxide	973.0	E858.4	E943.0	E950.4	E962.0	E980.4
sulfate (oral)	973.3	E858.4	E943.3	E950.4	E962.0	E980.4
intravenous	966.2	E855.0	E936.3	E950.4	E962.0	E980.4
trisilicate	973.0	E858.4	E943.0	E950.4	E962.0	E980.4
Malathion (insecticide)	989.3	E863.1	—	E950.6	E962.1	E980.7
Male fern (oleoresin)	961.6	E857	E931.6	E950.4	E962.0	E980.4
Mandelic acid	961.9	E857	E931.9	E950.4	E962.0	E980.4
Manganese compounds (fumes) NEC	985.2	E866.4	—	E950.9	E962.1	E980.9
Mannitol (diuretic) (medicinal) NEC	974.4	E858.5	E944.4	E950.4	E962.0	E980.4
hexanitrate	972.4	E858.3	E942.4	E950.4	E962.0	E980.4
mustard	963.1	E858.1	E933.1	E950.4	E962.0	E980.4
Mannomustine	963.1	E858.1	E933.1	E950.4	E962.0	E980.4

Table of Drugs and Chemicals

	Poisoning	External Cause (E-Code)				
		Accident	Therapeutic Use	Suicide Attempt	Assault	Undetermined
MAO inhibitors	969.0	E854.0	E939.0	E950.3	E962.0	E980.3
Mapharsen	961.1	E857	E931.1	E950.4	E962.0	E980.4
Marcaine	968.9	E855.2	E938.9	E950.4	E962.0	E980.4
infiltration (subcutaneous)	968.5	E855.2	E938.5	E950.4	E962.0	E980.4
nerve block (peripheral) (plexus)	968.6	E855.2	E938.6	E950.4	E962.0	E980.4
Marezine	963.0	E858.1	E933.0	E950.4	E962.0	E980.4
Marihuana, marijuana (derivatives)	969.6	E854.1	E939.6	E950.3	E962.0	E980.3
Marine animals or plants (sting)	989.5	E905.6	—	E950.9	E962.1	E980.9
Marplan	969.0	E854.0	E939.0	E950.3	E962.0	E980.3
Marsh gas	987.1	E869.8	—	E952.8	E962.2	E982.8
Marsilid	969.0	E854.0	E939.0	E950.3	E962.0	E980.3
Matulane	963.1	E858.1	E933.1	E950.4	E962.0	E980.4
Mazindol	977.0	E858.8	E947.0	E950.4	E962.0	E980.4
Meadow saffron	988.2	E865.3	—	E950.9	E962.1	E980.9
Measles vaccine	979.4	E858.8	E949.4	E950.4	E962.0	E980.4
Meat, noxious or nonbacterial	988.8	E865.0	—	E950.9	E962.1	E980.9
Mebanazine	969.0	E854.0	E939.0	E950.3	E962.0	E980.3
Mebaral	967.0	E851	E937.0	E950.1	E962.0	E980.1
Mebendazole	961.6	E857	E931.6	E950.4	E962.0	E980.4
Mebeverine	975.1	E858.6	E945.1	E950.4	E962.0	E980.4
Mebhydroline	963.0	E858.1	E933.0	E950.4	E962.0	E980.4
Mebrophenhydramine	963.0	E858.1	E933.0	E950.4	E962.0	E980.4
Mebutamate	969.5	E853.8	E939.5	E950.3	E962.0	E980.3
Mecamylamine (chloride)	972.3	E858.3	E942.3	E950.4	E962.0	E980.4
Mechlorethamine hydrochloride	963.1	E858.1	E933.1	E950.4	E962.0	E980.4
Meclizene (hydrochloride)	963.0	E858.1	E933.0	E950.4	E962.0	E980.4
Meclofenoxate	970.0	E854.3	E940.0	E950.4	E962.0	E980.4
Meclozine (hydrochloride)	963.0	E858.1	E933.0	E950.4	E962.0	E980.4
Medazepam	969.4	E853.2	E939.4	E950.3	E962.0	E980.3
Medicine, medicinal substance	977.9	E858.9	E947.9	E950.5	E962.0	E980.5
specified NEC	977.8	E858.8	E947.8	E950.4	E962.0	E980.4
Medinal	967.0	E851	E937.0	E950.1	E962.0	E980.1
Medomin	967.0	E851	E937.0	E950.1	E962.0	E980.1
Medroxyprogesterone	962.2	E858.0	E932.2	E950.4	E962.0	E980.4
Medrysone	976.5	E858.7	E946.5	E950.4	E962.0	E980.4
Mefenamic acid	965.7	E850.7	E935.7	E950.0	E962.0	E980.0
Megahallucinogen	969.6	E854.1	E939.6	E950.3	E962.0	E980.3
Megestrol	962.2	E858.0	E932.2	E950.4	E962.0	E980.4
Meglumine	977.8	E858.8	E947.8	E950.4	E962.0	E980.4
Meladinin	976.3	E858.7	E946.3	E950.4	E962.0	E980.4
Melanizing agents	976.3	E858.7	E946.3	E950.4	E962.0	E980.4
Melarsoprol	961.1	E857	E931.1	E950.4	E962.0	E980.4
Melia azedarach	988.2	E865.3	—	E950.9	E962.1	E980.9
Mellaril	969.1	E853.0	E939.1	E950.3	E962.0	E980.3
Meloxine	976.3	E858.7	E946.3	E950.4	E962.0	E980.4
Melphalan	963.1	E858.1	E933.1	E950.4	E962.0	E980.4
Menadiol sodium diphosphate	964.3	E858.2	E934.3	E950.4	E962.0	E980.4
Menadione (sodium bisulfite)	964.3	E858.2	E934.3	E950.4	E962.0	E980.4
Menaphthone	964.3	E858.2	E934.3	E950.4	E962.0	E980.4
Meningococcal vaccine	978.8	E858.8	E948.8	E950.4	E962.0	E980.4
Menningovax-C	978.8	E858.8	E948.8	E950.4	E962.0	E980.4
Menotropins	962.4	E858.0	E932.4	E950.4	E962.0	E980.4
Menthol NEC	976.1	E858.7	E946.1	E950.4	E962.0	E980.4
Mepacrine	961.3	E857	E931.3	E950.4	E962.0	E980.4
Meparfynol	967.8	E852.8	E937.8	E950.2	E962.0	E980.2
Mepazine	969.1	E853.0	E939.1	E950.3	E962.0	E980.3
Mepenzolate	971.1	E855.4	E941.1	E950.4	E962.0	E980.4
Meperidine	965.09	E850.2	E935.2	E950.0	E962.0	E980.0
Mephenamin(e)	966.4	E855.0	E936.4	E950.4	E962.0	E980.4
Mephenesin (carbamate)	968.0	E855.1	E938.0	E950.4	E962.0	E980.4

Table of Drugs and Chemicals

	Poisoning	External Cause (E-Code)				
		Accident	Therapeutic Use	Suicide Attempt	Assault	Undetermined
Mephenoxalone	969.5	E853.8	E939.5	E950.3	E962.0	E980.3
Mephentermine	971.2	E855.5	E941.2	E950.4	E962.0	E980.4
Mephenytoin	966.1	E855.0	E936.1	E950.4	E962.0	E980.4
Mephobarbital	967.0	E851	E937.0	E950.1	E962.0	E980.1
Mepiperphenidol	971.1	E855.4	E941.1	E950.4	E962.0	E980.4
Mepivacaine	968.9	E855.2	E938.9	E950.4	E962.0	E980.4
infiltration (subcutaneous)	968.5	E855.2	E938.5	E950.4	E962.0	E980.4
nerve block (peripheral) (plexus)	968.6	E855.2	E938.6	E950.4	E962.0	E980.4
topical (surface)	968.5	E855.2	E938.5	E950.4	E962.0	E980.4
Meprednisone	962.0	E858.0	E932.0	E950.4	E962.0	E980.4
Meprobam	969.5	E853.8	E939.5	E950.3	E962.0	E980.3
Meprobamate	969.5	E853.8	E939.5	E950.3	E962.0	E980.3
Mepyramine (maleate)	963.0	E858.1	E933.0	E950.4	E962.0	E980.4
Meralluride	974.0	E858.5	E944.0	E950.4	E962.0	E980.4
Merbaphen	974.0	E858.5	E944.0	E950.4	E962.0	E980.4
Merbromin	976.0	E858.7	E946.0	E950.4	E962.0	E980.4
Mercaptomerin	974.0	E858.5	E944.0	E950.4	E962.0	E980.4
Mercaptopurine	963.1	E858.1	E933.1	E950.4	E962.0	E980.4
Mercumatilin	974.0	E858.5	E944.0	E950.4	E962.0	E980.4
Mercuramide	974.0	E858.5	E944.0	E950.4	E962.0	E980.4
Mercuranin	976.0	E858.7	E946.0	E950.4	E962.0	E980.4
Mercurochrome	976.0	E858.7	E946.0	E950.4	E962.0	E980.4
Mercury, mercuric, mercurous (compounds) (cyanide) (fumes) (nonmedicinal) (vapor) NEC	985.0	E866.1	—	E950.9	E962.1	E980.9
ammoniated	976.0	E858.7	E946.0	E950.4	E962.0	E980.4
anti-infective	961.2	E857	E931.2	E950.4	E962.0	E980.4
topical	976.0	E858.7	E946.0	E950.4	E962.0	E980.4
chloride (antiseptic) NEC	976.0	E858.7	E946.0	E950.4	E962.0	E980.4
fungicide	985.0	E863.6	—	E950.6	E962.1	E980.7
diuretic compounds	974.0	E858.5	E944.0	E950.4	E962.0	E980.4
fungicide	985.0	E863.6	—	E950.6	E962.1	E980.7
organic (fungicide)	985.0	E863.6	—	E950.6	E962.1	E980.7
Merethoxylline	974.0	E858.5	E944.0	E950.4	E962.0	E980.4
Mersalyl	974.0	E858.5	E944.0	E950.4	E962.0	E980.4
Merthiolate (topical)	976.0	E858.7	E946.0	E950.4	E962.0	E980.4
ophthalmic preparation	976.5	E858.7	E946.5	E950.4	E962.0	E980.4
Meruvax	979.4	E858.8	E949.4	E950.4	E962.0	E980.4
Mescal buttons	969.6	E854.1	E939.6	E950.3	E962.0	E980.3
Mescaline (salts)	969.6	E854.1	E939.6	E950.3	E962.0	E980.3
Mesoridazine besylate	969.1	E853.0	E939.1	E950.3	E962.0	E980.3
Mestanolone	962.1	E858.0	E932.1	E950.4	E962.0	E980.4
Mestranol	962.2	E858.0	E932.2	E950.4	E962.0	E980.4
Metacresylacetate	976.0	E858.7	E946.0	E950.4	E962.0	E980.4
Metaldehyde (snail killer) NEC	989.4	E863.4	—	E950.6	E962.1	E980.7
Metals (heavy) (nonmedicinal) NEC	985.9	E866.4	—	E950.9	E962.1	E980.9
dust, fumes, or vapor NEC	985.9	E866.4	—	E950.9	E962.1	E980.9
light NEC	985.9	E866.4	—	E950.9	E962.1	E980.9
dust, fumes, or vapor NEC	985.9	E866.4	—	E950.9	E962.1	E980.9
pesticides (dust) (vapor)	985.9	E863.4	—	E950.6	E962.1	E980.7
Metamucil	973.3	E858.4	E943.3	E950.4	E962.0	E980.4
Metaphen	976.0	E858.7	E946.0	E950.4	E962.0	E980.4
Metaproterenol	975.1	E858.6	E945.1	E950.4	E962.0	E980.4
Metaraminol	972.8	E858.3	E942.8	E950.4	E962.0	E980.4
Metaxalone	968.0	E855.1	E938.0	E950.4	E962.0	E980.4
Metformin	962.3	E858.0	E932.3	E950.4	E962.0	E980.4
Methacycline	960.4	E856	E930.4	E950.4	E962.0	E980.4
Methadone	965.02	E850.1	E935.1	E950.0	E962.0	E980.0
Methallenestril	962.2	E858.0	E932.2	E950.4	E962.0	E980.4
Methamphetamine	969.7	E854.2	E939.7	E950.3	E962.0	E980.3

Table of Drugs and Chemicals — Methyl

	Poisoning	External Cause (E-Code)				
		Accident	Therapeutic Use	Suicide Attempt	Assault	Undetermined
Methandienone	962.1	E858.0	E932.1	E950.4	E962.0	E980.4
Methandriol	962.1	E858.0	E932.1	E950.4	E962.0	E980.4
Methandrostenolone	962.1	E858.0	E932.1	E950.4	E962.0	E980.4
Methane gas	987.1	E869.8	—	E952.8	E962.2	E982.8
Methanol	980.1	E860.2	—	E950.9	E962.1	E980.9
vapor	987.8	E869.8	—	E952.8	E962.2	E982.8
Methantheline	971.1	E855.4	E941.1	E950.4	E962.0	E980.4
Methaphenilene	963.0	E858.1	E933.0	E950.4	E962.0	E980.4
Methapyrilene	963.0	E858.1	E933.0	E950.4	E962.0	E980.4
Methaqualone (compounds)	967.4	E852.3	E937.4	E950.2	E962.0	E980.2
Metharbital, metharbitone	967.0	E851	E937.0	E950.1	E962.0	E980.1
Methazolamide	974.2	E858.5	E944.2	E950.4	E962.0	E980.4
Methdilazine	963.0	E858.1	E933.0	E950.4	E962.0	E980.4
Methedrine	969.7	E854.2	E939.7	E950.3	E962.0	E980.3
Methenamine (mandelate)	961.9	E857	E931.9	E950.4	E962.0	E980.4
Methenolone	962.1	E858.0	E932.1	E950.4	E962.0	E980.4
Methergine	975.0	E858.6	E945.0	E950.4	E962.0	E980.4
Methiacil	962.8	E858.0	E932.8	E950.4	E962.0	E980.4
Methicillin (sodium)	960.0	E856	E930.0	E950.4	E962.0	E980.4
Methimazole	962.8	E858.0	E932.8	E950.4	E962.0	E980.4
Methionine	977.1	E858.8	E947.1	E950.4	E962.0	E980.4
Methisazone	961.7	E857	E931.7	E950.4	E962.0	E980.4
Methitural	967.0	E851	E937.0	E950.1	E962.0	E980.1
Methixene	971.1	E855.4	E941.1	E950.4	E962.0	E980.4
Methobarbital, methobarbitone	967.0	E851	E937.0	E950.1	E962.0	E980.1
Methocarbamol	968.0	E855.1	E938.0	E950.4	E962.0	E980.4
Methohexital, methohexitone (sodium)	968.3	E855.1	E938.3	E950.4	E962.0	E980.4
Methoin	966.1	E855.0	E936.1	E950.4	E962.0	E980.4
Methopholine	965.7	E850.7	E935.7	E950.0	E962.0	E980.0
Methorate	975.4	E858.6	E945.4	E950.4	E962.0	E980.4
Methoserpidine	972.6	E858.3	E942.6	E950.4	E962.0	E980.4
Methotrexate	963.1	E858.1	E933.1	E950.4	E962.0	E980.4
Methotrimeprazine	967.8	E852.8	E937.8	E950.2	E962.0	E980.2
Methoxa-Dome	976.3	E858.7	E946.3	E950.4	E962.0	E980.4
Methoxamine	971.2	E855.5	E941.2	E950.4	E962.0	E980.4
Methoxsalen	976.3	E858.7	E946.3	E950.4	E962.0	E980.4
Methoxybenzyl penicillin	960.0	E856	E930.0	E950.4	E962.0	E980.4
Methoxychlor	989.2	E863.0	—	E950.6	E962.1	E980.7
Methoxyflurane	968.2	E855.1	E938.2	E950.4	E962.0	E980.4
Methoxyphenamine	971.2	E855.5	E941.2	E950.4	E962.0	E980.4
Methoxypromazine	969.1	E853.0	E939.1	E950.3	E962.0	E980.3
Methoxypsoralen	976.3	E858.7	E946.3	E950.4	E962.0	E980.4
Methscopolamine (bromide)	971.1	E855.4	E941.1	E950.4	E962.0	E980.4
Methsuximide	966.2	E855.0	E936.2	E950.4	E962.0	E980.4
Methyclothiazide	974.3	E858.5	E944.3	E950.4	E962.0	E980.4
Methyl						
acetate	982.8	E862.4	—	E950.9	E962.1	E980.9
acetone	982.8	E862.4	—	E950.9	E962.1	E980.9
alcohol	980.1	E860.2	—	E950.9	E962.1	E980.9
amphetamine	969.7	E854.2	E939.7	E950.3	E962.0	E980.3
androstanolone	962.1	E858.0	E932.1	E950.4	E962.0	E980.4
atropine	971.1	E855.4	E941.1	E950.4	E962.0	E980.4
benzene	982.0	E862.4	—	E950.9	E962.1	E980.9
bromide (gas)	987.8	E869.8	—	E952.8	E962.2	E982.8
fumigant	987.8	E863.8	—	E950.6	E962.2	E980.7
butanol	980.8	E860.8	—	E950.9	E962.1	E980.9
carbinol	980.1	E860.2	—	E950.9	E962.1	E980.9
cellosolve	982.8	E862.4	—	E950.9	E962.1	E980.9
cellulose	973.3	E858.4	E943.3	E950.4	E962.0	E980.4
chloride (gas)	987.8	E869.8	—	E952.8	E962.2	E982.8
cyclohexane	982.8	E862.4	—	E950.9	E962.1	E980.9
cyclohexanone	982.8	E862.4	—	E950.9	E962.1	E980.9
dihydromorphinone	965.09	E850.2	E935.2	E950.0	E962.0	E980.0

✓4ᵗʰ Fourth-digit Required ✓5ᵗʰ Fifth-digit Required

Methyl — Table of Drugs and Chemicals

		External Cause (E-Code)				
	Poisoning	Accident	Therapeutic Use	Suicide Attempt	Assault	Undetermined
Methyl — *continued*						
ergometrine	975.0	E858.6	E945.0	E950.4	E962.0	E980.4
ergonovine	975.0	E858.6	E945.0	E950.4	E962.0	E980.4
ethyl ketone	982.8	E862.4	—	E950.9	E962.1	E980.9
hydrazine	983.9	E864.3	—	E950.7	E962.1	E980.6
isobutyl ketone	982.8	E862.4	—	E950.9	E962.1	E980.9
morphine NEC	965.09	E850.2	E935.2	E950.0	E962.0	E980.0
parafynol	967.8	E852.8	E937.8	E950.2	E962.0	E980.2
parathion	989.3	E863.1	—	E950.6	E962.1	E980.7
pentynol NEC	967.8	E852.8	E937.8	E950.2	E962.0	E980.2
peridol	969.2	E853.1	E939.2	E950.3	E962.0	E980.3
phenidate	969.7	E854.2	E939.7	E950.3	E962.0	E980.3
prednisolone	962.0	E858.0	E932.0	E950.4	E962.0	E980.4
ENT agent	976.6	E858.7	E946.6	E950.4	E962.0	E980.4
ophthalmic preparation	976.5	E858.7	E946.5	E950.4	E962.0	E980.4
topical NEC	976.0	E858.7	E946.0	E950.4	E962.0	E980.4
propylcarbinol	980.8	E860.8	—	E950.9	E962.1	E980.9
rosaniline NEC	976.0	E858.7	E946.0	E950.4	E962.0	E980.4
salicylate NEC	976.3	E858.7	E946.3	E950.4	E962.0	E980.4
sulfate (fumes)	987.8	E869.8	—	E952.8	E962.2	E982.8
liquid	983.9	E864.3	—	E950.7	E962.1	E980.6
sulfonal	967.8	E852.8	E937.8	E950.2	E962.0	E980.2
testosterone	962.1	E858.0	E932.1	E950.4	E962.0	E980.4
thiouracil	962.8	E858.0	E932.8	E950.4	E962.0	E980.4
Methylated spirit	980.0	E860.1	—	E950.9	E962.1	E980.9
Methyldopa	972.6	E858.3	E942.6	E950.4	E962.0	E980.4
Methylene						
blue	961.9	E857	E931.9	E950.4	E962.0	E980.4
chloride or dichloride (solvent) NEC	982.3	E862.4	—	E950.9	E962.1	E980.9
Methylhexabital	967.0	E851	E937.0	E950.1	E962.0	E980.1
Methylparaben (ophthalmic)	976.5	E858.7	E946.5	E950.4	E962.0	E980.4
Methyprylon	967.5	E852.4	E937.5	E950.2	E962.0	E980.2
Methysergide	971.3	E855.6	E941.3	E950.4	E962.0	E980.4
Metoclopramide	963.0	E858.1	E933.0	E950.4	E962.0	E980.4
Metofoline	965.7	E850.7	E935.7	E950.0	E962.0	E980.0
Metopon	965.09	E850.2	E935.2	E950.0	E962.0	E980.0
Metronidazole	961.5	E857	E931.5	E950.4	E962.0	E980.4
Metycaine	968.9	E855.2	E938.9	E950.4	E962.0	E980.4
infiltration (subcutaneous)	968.5	E855.2	E938.5	E950.4	E962.0	E980.4
nerve block (peripheral) (plexus)	968.6	E855.2	E938.6	E950.4	E962.0	E980.4
topical (surface)	968.5	E855.2	E938.5	E950.4	E962.0	E980.4
Metyrapone	977.8	E858.8	E947.8	E950.4	E962.0	E980.4
Mevinphos	989.3	E863.1	—	E950.6	E962.1	E980.7
Mezereon (berries)	988.2	E865.3	—	E950.9	E962.1	E980.9
Micatin	976.0	E858.7	E946.0	E950.4	E962.0	E980.4
Miconazole	976.0	E858.7	E946.0	E950.4	E962.0	E980.4
Midol	965.1	E850.3	E935.3	E950.0	E962.0	E980.0
Mifepristone	962.9	E858.0	E932.9	E950.4	E962.0	E980.4
Milk of magnesia	973.0	E858.4	E943.0	E950.4	E962.0	E980.4
Millipede (tropical) (venomous)	989.5	E905.4	—	E950.9	E962.1	E980.9
Miltown	969.5	E853.8	E939.5	E950.3	E962.0	E980.3
Mineral						
oil (medicinal)	973.2	E858.4	E943.2	E950.4	E962.0	E980.4
nonmedicinal	981	E862.1	—	E950.9	E962.1	E980.9
topical	976.3	E858.7	E946.3	E950.4	E962.0	E980.4
salts NEC	974.6	E858.5	E944.6	E950.4	E962.0	E980.4
spirits	981	E862.0	—	E950.9	E962.1	E980.9
Minocycline	960.4	E856	E930.4	E950.4	E962.0	E980.4
Mithramycin (antineoplastic)	960.7	E856	E930.7	E950.4	E962.0	E980.4
Mitobronitol	963.1	E858.1	E933.1	E950.4	E962.0	E980.4
Mitomycin (antineoplastic)	960.7	E856	E930.7	E950.4	E962.0	E980.4
Mitotane	963.1	E858.1	E933.1	E950.4	E962.0	E980.4

Table of Drugs and Chemicals

		External Cause (E-Code)				
	Poisoning	Accident	Therapeutic Use	Suicide Attempt	Assault	Undetermined
Moderil	972.6	E858.3	E942.6	E950.4	E962.0	E980.4
Mogadon — see **Nitrazepam**						
Molindone	969.3	E853.8	E939.3	E950.3	E962.0	E980.3
Monistat	976.0	E858.7	E946.0	E950.4	E962.0	E980.4
Monkshood	988.2	E865.4	—	E950.9	E962.1	E980.9
Monoamine oxidase inhibitors	969.0	E854.0	E939.0	E950.3	E962.0	E980.3
Monochlorobenzene	982.0	E862.4	—	E950.9	E962.1	E980.9
Monosodium glutamate	989.89	E866.8	—	E950.9	E962.1	E980.9
Monoxide, carbon — see **Carbon, monoxide**						
Moperone	969.2	E853.1	E939.2	E950.3	E962.0	E980.3
Morning glory seeds	969.6	E854.1	E939.6	E950.3	E962.0	E980.3
Moroxydine (hydrochloride)	961.7	E857	E931.7	E950.4	E962.0	E980.4
Morphazinamide	961.8	E857	E931.8	E950.4	E962.0	E980.4
Morphinans	965.09	E850.2	E935.2	E950.0	E962.0	E980.0
Morphine NEC	965.09	E850.2	E935.2	E950.0	E962.0	E980.0
antagonists	970.1	E854.3	E940.1	E950.4	E962.0	E980.4
Morpholinylethylmorphine	965.09	E850.2	E935.2	E950.0	E962.0	E980.0
Morrhuate sodium	972.7	E858.3	E942.7	E950.4	E962.0	E980.4
Moth balls (see also **Pesticides**)	989.4	E863.4	—	E950.6	E962.1	E980.7
naphthalene	983.0	E863.4	—	E950.7	E962.1	E980.6
Motor exhaust gas — see **Carbon, monoxide, exhaust gas**						
Mouth wash	976.6	E858.7	E946.6	E950.4	E962.0	E980.4
Mucolytic agent	975.5	E858.6	E945.5	E950.4	E962.0	E980.4
Mucomyst	975.5	E858.6	E945.5	E950.4	E962.0	E980.4
Mucous membrane agents (external)	976.9	E858.7	E946.9	E950.4	E962.0	E980.4
specified NEC	976.8	E858.7	E946.8	E950.4	E962.0	E980.4
Mumps						
immune globulin (human)	964.6	E858.2	E934.6	E950.4	E962.0	E980.4
skin test antigen	977.8	E858.8	E947.8	E950.4	E962.0	E980.4
vaccine	979.6	E858.8	E949.6	E950.4	E962.0	E980.4
Mumpsvax	979.6	E858.8	E949.6	E950.4	E962.0	E980.4
Muriatic acid — see **Hydrochloric acid**						
Muscarine	971.0	E855.3	E941.0	E950.4	E962.0	E980.4
Muscle affecting agents NEC	975.3	E858.6	E945.3	E950.4	E962.0	E980.4
oxytocic	975.0	E858.6	E945.0	E950.4	E962.0	E980.4
relaxants	975.3	E858.6	E945.3	E950.4	E962.0	E980.4
central nervous system	968.0	E855.1	E938.0	E950.4	E962.0	E980.4
skeletal	975.2	E858.6	E945.2	E950.4	E962.0	E980.4
smooth	975.1	E858.6	E945.1	E950.4	E962.0	E980.4
Mushrooms, noxious	988.1	E865.5	—	E950.9	E962.1	E980.9
Mussel, noxious	988.0	E865.1	—	E950.9	E962.1	E980.9
Mustard (emetic)	973.6	E858.4	E943.6	E950.4	E962.0	E980.4
gas	987.8	E869.8	—	E952.8	E962.2	E982.8
nitrogen	963.1	E858.1	E933.1	E950.4	E962.0	E980.4
Mustine	963.1	E858.1	E933.1	E950.4	E962.0	E980.4
M-vac	979.4	E858.8	E949.4	E950.4	E962.0	E980.4
Mycifradin	960.8	E856	E930.8	E950.4	E962.0	E980.4
topical	976.0	E858.7	E946.0	E950.4	E962.0	E980.4
Mycitracin	960.8	E856	E930.8	E950.4	E962.0	E980.4
ophthalmic preparation	976.5	E858.7	E946.5	E950.4	E962.0	E980.4
Mycostatin	960.1	E856	E930.1	E950.4	E962.0	E980.4
topical	976.0	E858.7	E946.0	E950.4	E962.0	E980.4
Mydriacyl	971.1	E855.4	E941.1	E950.4	E962.0	E980.4
Myelobromal	963.1	E858.1	E933.1	E950.4	E962.0	E980.4
Myleran	963.1	E858.1	E933.1	E950.4	E962.0	E980.4
Myochrysin(e)	965.69	E850.6	E935.6	E950.0	E962.0	E980.0
Myoneural blocking agents	975.2	E858.6	E945.2	E950.4	E962.0	E980.4
Myristica fragrans	988.2	E865.3	—	E950.9	E962.1	E980.9
Myristicin	988.2	E865.3	—	E950.9	E962.1	E980.9

Fourth-digit Required   Fifth-digit Required

Table of Drugs and Chemicals

		External Cause (E-Code)				
	Poisoning	Accident	Therapeutic Use	Suicide Attempt	Assault	Undetermined
Mysoline	966.3	E855.0	E936.3	E950.4	E962.0	E980.4
Nafcillin (sodium)	960.0	E856	E930.0	E950.4	E962.0	E980.4
Nail polish remover	982.8	E862.4	—	E950.9	E962.1	E908.9
Nalidixic acid	961.9	E857	E931.9	E950.4	E962.0	E980.4
Nalorphine	970.1	E854.3	E940.1	E950.4	E962.0	E980.4
Naloxone	970.1	E854.3	E940.1	E950.4	E962.0	E980.4
Nandrolone (decanoate) (phenproprioate)	962.1	E858.0	E932.1	E950.4	E962.0	E980.4
Naphazoline	971.2	E855.5	E941.2	E950.4	E962.0	E980.4
Naphtha (painter's) (petroleum)	981	E862.0	—	E950.9	E962.1	E980.9
solvent	981	E862.0	—	E950.9	E962.1	E980.9
vapor	987.1	E869.8	—	E952.8	E962.2	E982.8
Naphthalene (chlorinated)	983.0	E864.0	—	E950.7	E962.1	E980.6
insecticide or moth repellent	983.0	E863.4	—	E950.7	E962.1	E980.6
vapor	987.8	E869.8	—	E952.8	E962.2	E982.8
Naphthol	983.0	E864.0	—	E950.7	E962.1	E980.6
Naphthylamine	983.0	E864.0	—	E950.7	E962.1	E980.6
Naprosyn — see Naproxen						
Naproxen	965.61	E850.6	E935.6	E950.0	E962.0	E980.0
Narcotic (drug)	967.9	E852.9	E937.9	E950.2	E962.0	E980.2
analgesic NEC	965.8	E850.8	E935.8	E950.0	E962.0	E980.0
antagonist	970.1	E854.3	E940.1	E950.4	E962.0	E980.4
specified NEC	967.8	E852.8	E937.8	E950.2	E962.0	E980.2
Narcotine	975.4	E858.6	E945.4	E950.4	E962.0	E980.4
Nardil	969.0	E854.0	E939.0	E950.3	E962.0	E980.3
Natrium cyanide — see Cyanide(s)						
Natural						
blood (product)	964.7	E858.2	E934.7	E950.4	E962.0	E980.4
gas (piped)	987.1	E867	—	E951.0	E962.2	E981.0
incomplete combustion	986	E867	—	E951.0	E962.2	E981.0
Nealbarbital, nealbarbitone	967.0	E851	E937.0	E950.1	E962.0	E980.1
Nectadon	975.4	E858.6	E945.4	E950.4	E962.0	E980.4
Nematocyst (sting)	989.5	E905.6	—	E950.9	E962.1	E980.9
Nembutal	967.0	E851	E937.0	E950.1	E962.0	E980.1
Neoarsphenamine	961.1	E857	E931.1	E950.4	E962.0	E980.4
Neocinchophen	974.7	E858.5	E944.7	E950.4	E962.0	E980.4
Neomycin	960.8	E856	E930.8	E950.4	E962.0	E980.4
ENT agent	976.6	E858.7	E946.6	E950.4	E962.0	E980.4
ophthalmic preparation	976.5	E858.7	E946.5	E950.4	E962.0	E980.4
topical NEC	976.0	E858.7	E946.0	E950.4	E962.0	E980.4
Neonal	967.0	E851	E937.0	E950.1	E962.0	E980.1
Neoprontosil	961.0	E857	E931.0	E950.4	E962.0	E980.4
Neosalvarsan	961.1	E857	E931.1	E950.4	E962.0	E980.4
Neosilversalvarsan	961.1	E857	E931.1	E950.4	E962.0	E980.4
Neosporin	960.8	E856	E930.8	E950.4	E962.0	E980.4
ENT agent	976.6	E858.7	E946.6	E950.4	E962.0	E980.4
opthalmic preparation	976.5	E858.7	E946.5	E950.4	E962.0	E980.4
topical NEC	976.0	E858.7	E946.0	E950.4	E962.0	E980.4
Neostigmine	971.0	E855.3	E941.0	E950.4	E962.0	E980.4
Neraval	967.0	E851	E937.0	E950.1	E962.0	E980.1
Neravan	967.0	E851	E937.0	E950.1	E962.0	E980.1
Nerium oleander	988.2	E865.4	—	E950.9	E962.1	E980.9
Nerve gases (war)	987.9	E869.9	—	E952.9	E962.2	E982.9
Nesacaine	968.9	E855.2	E938.9	E950.4	E962.0	E980.4
infiltration (subcutaneous)	968.5	E855.2	E938.5	E950.4	E962.0	E980.4
nerve block (peripheral) (plexus)	968.6	E855.2	E938.6	E950.4	E962.0	E980.4
Neurobarb	967.0	E851	E937.0	E950.1	E962.0	E980.1
Neuroleptics NEC	969.3	E853.8	E939.3	E950.3	E962.0	E980.3
Neuroprotective agent	977.8	E858.8	E947.8	E950.4	E962.0	E980.4
Neutral spirits	980.0	E860.1	—	E950.9	E962.1	E980.9
beverage	980.0	E860.0	—	E950.9	E962.1	E980.9

Table of Drugs and Chemicals

		External Cause (E-Code)				
	Poisoning	Accident	Therapeutic Use	Suicide Attempt	Assault	Undetermined
Niacin, niacinamide	972.2	E858.3	E942.2	E950.4	E962.0	E980.4
Nialamide	969.0	E854.0	E939.0	E950.3	E962.0	E980.3
Nickle (carbonyl) (compounds) (fumes) (tetracarbonyl) (vapor)	985.8	E866.4	—	E950.9	E962.1	E980.9
Niclosamide	961.6	E857	E931.6	E950.4	E962.0	E980.4
Nicomorphine	965.09	E850.2	E935.2	E950.0	E962.0	E980.0
Nicotinamide	972.2	E858.3	E942.2	E950.4	E962.0	E980.4
Nicotine (insecticide) (spray) (sulfate) NEC	989.4	E863.4	—	E950.6	E962.1	E980.7
not insecticide	989.89	E866.8	—	E950.9	E962.1	E980.9
Nicotinic acid (derivatives)	972.2	E858.3	E942.2	E950.4	E962.0	E980.4
Nicotinyl alcohol	972.2	E858.3	E942.2	E950.4	E962.0	E980.4
Nicoumalone	964.2	E858.2	E934.2	E950.4	E962.0	E980.4
Nifenazone	965.5	E850.5	E935.5	E950.0	E962.0	E980.0
Nifuraldezone	961.9	E857	E931.9	E950.4	E962.0	E980.4
Nightshade (deadly)	988.2	E865.4	—	E950.9	E962.1	E980.9
Nikethamide	970.0	E854.3	E940.0	E950.4	E962.0	E980.4
Nilstat	960.1	E856	E930.1	E950.4	E962.0	E980.4
topical	976.0	E858.7	E946.0	E950.4	E962.0	E980.4
Nimodipine	977.8	E858.8	E947.8	E950.4	E962.0	E980.4
Niridazole	961.6	E857	E931.6	E950.4	E962.0	E980.4
Nisentil	965.09	E850.2	E935.2	E950.0	E962.0	E980.0
Nitrates	972.4	E858.3	E942.4	E950.4	E962.0	E980.4
Nitrazepam	969.4	E853.2	E939.4	E950.3	E962.0	E980.3
Nitric						
acid (liquid)	983.1	E864.1	—	E950.7	E962.1	E980.6
vapor	987.8	E869.8	—	E952.8	E962.2	E982.8
oxide (gas)	987.2	E869.0	—	E952.8	E962.2	E982.8
Nitrite, amyl (medicinal) (vapor)	972.4	E858.3	E942.4	E950.4	E962.0	E980.4
Nitroaniline	983.0	E864.0	—	E950.7	E962.1	E980.6
vapor	987.8	E869.8	—	E952.8	E962.2	E982.8
Nitrobenzene, nitrobenzol	983.0	E864.0	—	E950.7	E962.1	E980.6
vapor	987.8	E869.8	—	E952.8	E962.2	E982.8
Nitrocellulose	976.3	E858.7	E946.3	E950.4	E962.0	E980.4
Nitrofuran derivatives	961.9	E857	E931.9	E950.4	E962.0	E980.4
Nitrofurantoin	961.9	E857	E931.9	E950.4	E962.0	E980.4
Nitrofurazone	976.0	E858.7	E946.0	E950.4	E962.0	E980.4
Nitrogen (dioxide) (gas) (oxide)	987.2	E869.0	—	E952.8	E962.2	E982.8
mustard (antineoplastic)	963.1	E858.1	E933.1	E950.4	E962.0	E980.4
Nitroglycerin, nitroglycerol (medicinal)	972.4	E858.3	E942.4	E950.4	E962.0	E980.4
nonmedicinal	989.89	E866.8	—	E950.9	E962.1	E980.9
fumes	987.8	E869.8	—	E952.8	E962.2	E982.8
Nitrohydrochloric acid	983.1	E864.1	—	E950.7	E962.1	E980.6
Nitromersol	976.0	E858.7	E946.0	E950.4	E962.0	E980.4
Nitronaphthalene	983.0	E864.0	—	E950.7	E962.2	E980.6
Nitrophenol	983.0	E864.0	—	E950.7	E962.2	E980.6
Nitrothiazol	961.6	E857	E931.6	E950.4	E962.0	E980.4
Nitrotoluene, nitrotoluol	983.0	E864.0	—	E950.7	E962.1	E980.6
vapor	987.8	E869.8	—	E952.8	E962.2	E982.8
Nitrous	968.2	E855.1	E938.2	E950.4	E962.0	E980.4
acid (liquid)	983.1	E864.1	—	E950.7	E962.1	E980.6
fumes	987.2	E869.0	—	E952.8	E962.2	E982.8
oxide (anesthetic) NEC	968.2	E855.1	E938.2	E950.4	E962.0	E980.4
Nitrozone	976.0	E858.7	E946.0	E950.4	E962.0	E980.4
Noctec	967.1	E852.0	E937.1	E950.2	E962.0	E980.2
Noludar	967.5	E852.4	E937.5	E950.2	E962.0	E980.2
Noptil	967.0	E851	E937.0	E950.1	E962.0	E980.1
Noradrenalin	971.2	E855.5	E941.2	E950.4	E962.0	E980.4
Noramidopyrine	965.5	E850.5	E935.5	E950.0	E962.0	E980.0
Norepinephrine	971.2	E855.5	E941.2	E950.4	E962.0	E980.4
Norethandrolone	962.1	E858.0	E932.1	E950.4	E962.0	E980.4

	External Cause (E-Code)					
	Poisoning	Accident	Therapeutic Use	Suicide Attempt	Assault	Undetermined
Norethindrone	962.2	E858.0	E932.2	E950.4	E962.0	E980.4
Norethisterone	962.2	E858.0	E932.2	E950.4	E962.0	E980.4
Norethynodrel	962.2	E858.0	E932.2	E950.4	E962.0	E980.4
Norlestrin	962.2	E858.0	E932.2	E950.4	E962.0	E980.4
Norlutin	962.2	E858.0	E932.2	E950.4	E962.0	E980.4
Normison — see Benzodiazepines						
Normorphine	965.09	E850.2	E935.2	E950.0	E962.0	E980.0
Nortriptyline	969.0	E854.0	E939.0	E950.3	E962.0	E980.3
Noscapine	975.4	E858.6	E945.4	E950.4	E962.0	E980.4
Nose preparations	976.6	E858.7	E946.6	E950.4	E962.0	E980.4
Novobiocin	960.8	E856	E930.8	E950.4	E962.0	E980.4
Novocain (infiltration) (topical)	968.5	E855.2	E938.5	E950.4	E962.0	E980.4
nerve block (peripheral) (plexus)	968.6	E855.2	E938.6	E950.4	E962.0	E980.4
spinal	968.7	E855.2	E938.7	E950.4	E962.0	E980.4
Noxythiolin	961.9	E857	E931.9	E950.4	E962.0	E980.4
NPH Iletin (insulin)	962.3	E858.0	E932.3	E950.4	E962.0	E980.4
Numorphan	965.09	E850.2	E935.2	E950.0	E962.0	E980.0
Nunol	967.0	E851	E937.0	E950.1	E962.0	E980.1
Nupercaine (spinal anesthetic)	968.7	E855.2	E938.7	E950.4	E962.0	E980.4
topical (surface)	968.5	E855.2	E938.5	E950.4	E962.0	E980.4
Nutmeg oil (liniment)	976.3	E858.7	E946.3	E950.4	E962.0	E980.4
Nux vomica	989.1	E863.7	—	E950.6	E962.1	E980.7
Nydrazid	961.8	E857	E931.8	E950.4	E962.0	E980.4
Nylidrin	971.2	E855.5	E941.2	E950.4	E962.0	E980.4
Nystatin	960.1	E856	E930.1	E950.4	E962.0	E980.4
topical	976.0	E858.7	E946.0	E950.4	E962.0	E980.4
Nytol	963.0	E858.2	E934.2	E950.4	E962.0	E980.4
Oblivion	967.8	E852.8	E937.8	E950.2	E962.0	E980.2
Octyl nitrite	972.4	E858.3	E942.4	E950.4	E962.0	E980.4
Oestradiol (cypionate) (dipropionate) (valerate)	962.2	E858.0	E932.2	E950.4	E962.0	E980.4
Oestriol	962.2	E858.0	E932.2	E950.4	E962.0	E980.4
Oestrone	962.2	E858.0	E932.2	E950.4	E962.0	E980.4
Oil (of) NEC	989.89	E866.8	—	E950.9	E962.1	E980.9
bitter almond	989.0	E866.8	—	E950.9	E962.1	E980.9
camphor	976.1	E858.7	E946.1	E950.4	E962.0	E980.4
colors	989.89	E861.6	—	E950.9	E962.1	E980.9
fumes	987.8	E869.8	—	E952.8	E962.2	E982.8
lubricating	981	E862.2	—	E950.9	E962.1	E980.9
specified source, other — see substance specified						
vitriol (liquid)	983.1	E864.1	—	E950.7	E962.1	E980.6
fumes	987.8	E869.8	—	E952.8	E962.2	E982.8
wintergreen (bitter) NEC	976.3	E858.7	E946.3	E950.4	E962.0	E980.4
Ointments NEC	976.9	E858.7	E946.9	E950.4	E962.0	E980.4
Oleander	988.2	E865.4	—	E950.9	E962.1	E980.9
Oleandomycin	960.3	E856	E930.3	E950.4	E962.0	E980.4
Oleovitamin A	963.5	E858.1	E933.5	E950.4	E962.0	E980.4
Oleum ricini	973.1	E858.4	E943.1	E950.4	E962.0	E980.4
Olive oil (medicinal) NEC	973.2	E858.4	E943.2	E950.4	E962.0	E980.4
OMPA	989.3	E863.1	—	E950.6	E962.1	E980.7
Oncovin	963.1	E858.1	E933.1	E950.4	E962.0	E980.4
Ophthaine	968.5	E855.2	E938.5	E950.4	E962.0	E980.4
Ophthetic	968.5	E855.2	E938.5	E950.4	E962.0	E980.4
Opiates, opioids, opium NEC	965.00	E850.2	E935.2	E950.0	E962.0	E980.0
antagonists	970.1	E854.3	E940.1	E950.4	E962.0	E980.4
Oracon	962.2	E858.0	E932.2	E950.4	E962.0	E980.4
Oragrafin	977.8	E858.8	E947.8	E950.4	E962.0	E980.4
Oral contraceptives	962.2	E858.0	E932.2	E950.4	E962.0	E980.4
Orciprenaline	975.1	E858.6	E945.1	E950.4	E962.0	E980.4
Organidin	975.5	E858.6	E945.5	E950.4	E962.0	E980.4

Table of Drugs and Chemicals

	External Cause (E-Code)					
	Poisoning	Accident	Therapeutic Use	Suicide Attempt	Assault	Undetermined
Organophosphates	989.3	E863.1	—	E950.6	E962.1	E980.7
Orimune	979.5	E858.8	E949.5	E950.4	E962.0	E980.4
Orinase	962.3	E858.0	E932.3	E950.4	E962.0	E980.4
Orphenadrine	966.4	E855.0	E936.4	E950.4	E962.0	E980.4
Ortal (sodium)	967.0	E851	E937.0	E950.1	E962.0	E980.1
Orthoboric acid	976.0	E858.7	E946.0	E950.4	E962.0	E980.4
ENT agent	976.6	E858.7	E946.6	E950.4	E962.0	E980.4
ophthalmic preparation	976.5	E858.7	E946.5	E950.4	E962.0	E980.4
Orthocaine	968.5	E855.2	E938.5	E950.4	E962.0	E980.4
Ortho-Novum	962.2	E858.0	E932.2	E950.4	E962.0	E980.4
Orthotolidine (reagent)	977.8	E858.8	E947.8	E950.4	E962.0	E980.4
Osmic acid (liquid)	983.1	E864.1	—	E950.7	E962.1	E980.6
fumes	987.8	E869.8	—	E952.8	E962.2	E982.8
Osmotic diuretics	974.4	E858.5	E944.4	E950.4	E962.0	E980.4
Ouabain	972.1	E858.3	E942.1	E950.4	E962.0	E980.4
Ovarian hormones (synthetic substitutes)	962.2	E858.0	E932.2	E950.4	E962.0	E980.4
Ovral	962.2	E858.0	E932.2	E950.4	E962.0	E980.4
Ovulation suppressants	962.2	E858.0	E932.2	E950.4	E962.0	E980.4
Ovulen	962.2	E858.0	E932.2	E950.4	E962.0	E980.4
Oxacillin (sodium)	960.0	E856	E930.0	E950.4	E962.0	E980.4
Oxalic acid	983.1	E864.1	—	E950.7	E962.1	E980.6
Oxanamide	969.5	E853.8	E939.5	E950.3	E962.0	E980.3
Oxandrolone	962.1	E858.0	E932.1	E950.4	E962.0	E980.4
Oxaprozin	965.61	E850.6	E935.6	E950.0	E962.0	E980.0
Oxazepam	969.4	E853.2	E939.4	E950.3	E962.0	E980.3
Oxazolidine derivatives	966.0	E855.0	E936.0	E950.4	E962.0	E980.4
Ox bile extract	973.4	E858.4	E943.4	E950.4	E962.0	E980.4
Oxedrine	971.2	E855.5	E941.2	E950.4	E962.0	E980.4
Oxeladin	975.4	E858.6	E945.4	E950.4	E962.0	E980.4
Oxethazaine NEC	968.5	E855.2	E938.5	E950.4	E962.0	E980.4
Oxidizing agents NEC	983.9	E864.3	—	E950.7	E962.1	E980.6
Oxolinic acid	961.3	E857	E931.3	E950.4	E962.0	E980.4
Oxophenarsine	961.1	E857	E931.1	E950.4	E962.0	E980.4
Oxsoralen	976.3	E858.7	E946.3	E950.4	E962.0	E980.4
Oxtriphylline	975.7	E858.6	E945.7	E950.4	E962.0	E980.4
Oxybuprocaine	968.5	E855.2	E938.5	E950.4	E962.0	E980.4
Oxybutynin	975.1	E858.6	E945.1	E950.4	E962.0	E980.4
Oxycodone	965.09	E850.2	E935.2	E950.0	E962.0	E980.0
Oxygen	987.8	E869.8	—	E952.8	E962.2	E982.8
Oxylone	976.0	E858.7	E946.0	E950.4	E962.0	E980.4
ophthalmic preparation	976.5	E858.7	E946.5	E950.4	E962.0	E980.4
Oxymesterone	962.1	E858.0	E932.1	E950.4	E962.0	E980.4
Oxymetazoline	971.2	E855.5	E941.2	E950.4	E962.0	E980.4
Oxymetholone	962.1	E858.0	E932.1	E950.4	E962.0	E980.4
Oxymorphone	965.09	E850.2	E935.2	E950.0	E962.0	E980.0
Oxypertine	969.0	E854.0	E939.0	E950.3	E962.0	E980.3
Oxyphenbutazone	965.5	E850.5	E935.5	E950.0	E962.0	E980.0
Oxyphencyclimine	971.1	E855.4	E941.1	E950.4	E962.0	E980.4
Oxyphenisatin	973.1	E858.4	E943.1	E950.4	E962.0	E980.4
Oxyphenonium	971.1	E855.4	E941.1	E950.4	E962.0	E980.4
Oxyquinoline	961.3	E857	E931.3	E950.4	E962.0	E980.4
Oxytetracycline	960.4	E856	E930.4	E950.4	E962.0	E980.4
Oxytocics	975.0	E858.6	E945.0	E950.4	E962.0	E980.4
Oxytocin	975.0	E858.6	E945.0	E950.4	E962.0	E980.4
Ozone	987.8	E869.8	—	E952.8	E962.2	E982.8
PABA	976.3	E858.7	E946.3	E950.4	E962.0	E980.4
Packed red cells	964.7	E858.2	E934.7	E950.4	E962.0	E980.4
Paint NEC	989.89	E861.6	—	E950.9	E962.1	E980.9
cleaner	982.8	E862.9	—	E950.9	E962.1	E980.9
fumes NEC	987.8	E869.8	—	E952.8	E962.1	E982.8
lead (fumes)	984.0	E861.5	—	E950.9	E962.1	E980.9
solvent NEC	982.8	E862.9	—	E950.9	E962.1	E980.9
stripper	982.8	E862.9	—	E950.9	E962.1	E980.9

Fourth-digit Required   Fifth-digit Required

Table of Drugs and Chemicals

		External Cause (E-Code)				
	Poisoning	Accident	Therapeutic Use	Suicide Attempt	Assault	Undetermined
Palfium	965.09	E850.2	E935.2	E950.0	E962.0	E980.0
Palivizumab	979.9	E858.8	E949.6	E950.4	E962.0	E980.4
Paludrine	961.4	E857	E931.4	E950.4	E962.0	E980.4
PAM	977.2	E855.8	E947.2	E950.4	E962.0	E980.4
Pamaquine (naphthoate)	961.4	E857	E931.4	E950.4	E962.0	E980.4
Pamprin	965.1	E850.3	E935.3	E950.0	E962.0	E980.0
Panadol	965.4	E850.4	E935.4	E950.0	E962.0	E980.0
Pancreatic dornase (mucolytic)	963.4	E858.1	E933.4	E950.4	E962.0	E980.4
Pancreatin	973.4	E858.4	E943.4	E950.4	E962.0	E980.4
Pancrelipase	973.4	E858.4	E943.4	E950.4	E962.0	E980.4
Pangamic acid	963.5	E858.1	E933.5	E950.4	E962.0	E980.4
Panthenol	963.5	E858.1	E933.5	E950.4	E962.0	E980.4
topical	976.8	E858.7	E946.8	E950.4	E962.0	E980.4
Pantopaque	977.8	E858.8	E947.8	E950.4	E962.0	E980.4
Pantopon	965.00	E850.2	E935.2	E950.0	E962.0	E980.0
Pantothenic acid	963.5	E858.1	E933.5	E950.4	E962.0	E980.4
Panwarfin	964.2	E858.2	E934.2	E950.4	E962.0	E980.4
Papain	973.4	E858.4	E943.4	E950.4	E962.0	E980.4
Papaverine	972.5	E858.3	E942.5	E950.4	E962.0	E980.4
Para-aminobenzoic acid	976.3	E858.7	E946.3	E950.4	E962.0	E980.4
Para-aminophenol derivatives	965.4	E850.4	E935.4	E950.0	E962.0	E980.0
Para-aminosalicylic acid (derivatives)	961.8	E857	E931.8	E950.4	E962.0	E980.4
Paracetaldehyde (medicinal)	967.2	E852.1	E937.2	E950.2	E962.0	E980.2
Paracetamol	965.4	E850.4	E935.4	E950.0	E962.0	E980.0
Paracodin	965.09	E850.2	E935.2	E950.0	E962.0	E980.0
Paradione	966.0	E855.0	E936.0	E950.4	E962.0	E980.4
Paraffin(s) (wax)	981	E862.3	—	E950.9	E962.1	E980.9
liquid (medicinal)	973.2	E858.4	E943.2	E950.4	E962.0	E980.4
nonmedicinal (oil)	981	E962.1	—	E950.9	E962.1	E980.9
Paraldehyde (medicinal)	967.2	E852.1	E937.2	E950.2	E962.0	E980.2
Paramethadione	966.0	E855.0	E936.0	E950.4	E962.0	E980.4
Paramethasone	962.0	E858.0	E932.0	E950.4	E962.0	E980.4
Paraquat	989.4	E863.5	—	E950.6	E962.1	E980.7
Parasympatholytics	971.1	E855.4	E941.1	E950.4	E962.0	E980.4
Parasympathomimetics	971.0	E855.3	E941.0	E950.4	E962.0	E980.4
Parathion	989.3	E863.1	—	E950.6	E962.1	E980.7
Parathormone	962.6	E858.0	E932.6	E950.4	E962.0	E980.4
Parathyroid (derivatives)	962.6	E858.0	E932.6	E950.4	E962.0	E980.4
Paratyphoid vaccine	978.1	E858.8	E948.1	E950.4	E962.0	E980.4
Paredrine	971.2	E855.5	E941.2	E950.4	E962.0	E980.4
Paregoric	965.00	E850.2	E935.2	E950.0	E962.0	E980.0
Pargyline	972.3	E858.3	E942.3	E950.4	E962.0	E980.4
Paris green	985.1	E866.3	—	E950.8	E962.1	E980.8
insecticide	985.1	E863.4	—	E950.8	E962.1	E980.8
Parnate	969.0	E854.0	E939.0	E950.3	E962.0	E980.3
Paromomycin	960.8	E856	E930.8	E950.4	E962.0	E980.4
Paroxypropione	963.1	E858.1	E933.1	E950.4	E962.0	E980.4
Parzone	965.09	E850.2	E935.2	E950.0	E962.0	E980.0
PAS	961.8	E857	E931.8	E950.4	E962.0	E980.4
PCBs	981	E862.3	—	E950.9	E962.1	E980.9
PCP (pentachlorophenol)	989.4	E863.6	—	E950.6	E962.1	E980.7
herbicide	989.4	E863.5	—	E950.6	E962.1	E980.7
insecticide	989.4	E863.4	—	E950.6	E962.1	E980.7
phencyclidine	968.3	E855.1	E938.3	E950.4	E962.0	E980.4
Peach kernel oil (emulsion)	973.2	E858.4	E943.2	E950.4	E962.0	E980.4
Peanut oil (emulsion) NEC	973.2	E858.4	E943.2	E950.4	E962.0	E980.4
topical	976.3	E858.7	E946.3	E950.4	E962.0	E980.4
Pearly Gates (morning glory seeds)	969.6	E854.1	E939.6	E950.3	E962.0	E980.3
Pecazine	969.1	E853.0	E939.1	E950.3	E962.0	E980.3
Pecilocin	960.1	E856	E930.1	E950.4	E962.0	E980.4
Pectin (with kaolin) NEC	973.5	E858.4	E943.5	E950.4	E962.0	E980.4
Pelletierine tannate	961.6	E857	E931.6	E950.4	E962.0	E980.4

▶◀ Revised Text   ● New Line   ▲ Revised Code

Table of Drugs and Chemicals — Pesticides (dust) (fumes) (vapor)

	Poisoning	External Cause (E-Code)				
		Accident	Therapeutic Use	Suicide Attempt	Assault	Undetermined
Pemoline	969.7	E854.2	E939.7	E950.3	E962.0	E980.3
Pempidine	972.3	E858.3	E942.3	E950.4	E962.0	E980.4
Penamecillin	960.0	E856	E930.0	E950.4	E962.0	E980.4
Penethamate hydriodide	960.0	E856	E930.0	E950.4	E962.0	E980.4
Penicillamine	963.8	E858.1	E933.8	E950.4	E962.0	E980.4
Penicillin (any type)	960.0	E856	E930.0	E950.4	E962.0	E980.4
Penicillinase	963.4	E858.1	E933.4	E950.4	E962.0	E980.4
Pentachlorophenol (fungicide)	989.4	E863.6	—	E950.6	E962.1	E980.7
herbicide	989.4	E863.5	—	E950.6	E962.1	E980.7
insecticide	989.4	E863.4	—	E950.6	E962.1	E980.7
Pentaerythritol	972.4	E858.3	E942.4	E950.4	E962.0	E980.4
chloral	967.1	E852.0	E937.1	E950.2	E962.0	E980.2
tetranitrate NEC	972.4	E858.3	E942.4	E950.4	E962.0	E980.4
Pentagastrin	977.8	E858.8	E947.8	E950.4	E962.0	E980.4
Pentalin	982.3	E862.4	—	E950.9	E962.1	E980.9
Pentamethonium (bromide)	972.3	E858.3	E942.3	E950.4	E962.0	E980.4
Pentamidine	961.5	E857	E931.5	E950.4	E962.0	E980.4
Pentanol	980.8	E860.8	—	E950.9	E962.1	E980.9
Pentaquine	961.4	E857	E931.4	E950.4	E962.0	E980.4
Pentazocine	965.8	E850.8	E935.8	E950.0	E962.0	E980.0
Penthienate	971.1	E855.4	E941.1	E950.4	E962.0	E980.4
Pentobarbital, pentobarbitone (sodium)	967.0	E851	E937.0	E950.1	E962.0	E980.1
Pentolinium (tartrate)	972.3	E858.3	E942.3	E950.4	E962.0	E980.4
Pentothal	968.3	E855.1	E938.3	E950.4	E962.0	E980.4
Pentylenetetrazol	970.0	E854.3	E940.0	E950.4	E962.0	E980.4
Pentylsalicylamide	961.8	E857	E931.8	E950.4	E962.0	E980.4
Pepsin	973.4	E858.1	E943.4	E950.4	E962.0	E980.4
Peptavlon	977.8	E858.8	E947.8	E950.4	E962.0	E980.4
Percaine (spinal)	968.7	E855.2	E938.7	E950.4	E962.0	E980.4
topical (surface)	968.5	E855.2	E938.5	E950.4	E962.0	E980.4
Perchloroethylene (vapor)	982.3	E862.4	—	E950.9	E962.1	E980.9
medicinal	961.6	E857	E931.6	E950.4	E962.0	E980.4
Percodan	965.09	E850.2	E935.2	E950.0	E962.0	E980.0
Percogesic	965.09	E850.2	E935.2	E950.0	E962.0	E980.0
Percorten	962.0	E858.0	E932.0	E950.4	E962.0	E980.4
Pergonal	962.4	E858.0	E932.4	E950.4	E962.0	E980.4
Perhexiline	972.4	E858.3	E942.4	E950.4	E962.0	E980.4
Periactin	963.0	E858.1	E933.0	E950.4	E962.0	E980.4
Periclor	967.1	E852.0	E937.1	E950.2	E962.0	E980.2
Pericyazine	969.1	E853.0	E939.1	E950.3	E962.0	E980.3
Peritrate	972.4	E858.3	E942.4	E950.4	E962.0	E980.4
Permanganates NEC	983.9	E864.3	—	E950.7	E962.1	E980.6
potassium (topical)	976.0	E858.7	E946.0	E950.4	E962.0	E980.4
Pernocton	967.0	E851	E937.0	E950.1	E962.0	E980.1
Pernoston	967.0	E851	E937.0	E950.1	E962.0	E980.1
Peronin(e)	965.09	E850.2	E935.2	E950.0	E962.0	E980.0
Perphenazine	969.1	E853.0	E939.1	E950.3	E962.0	E980.3
Pertofrane	969.0	E854 ▸4ᵗʰ	E939.0	E950.3	E962.0	E980.3
Pertussis						
immune serum (human)	964.6	E858.2	E934.6	E950.4	E962.0	E980.4
vaccine (with diphtheria toxoid) (with tetanus toxoid)	978.6	E858.8	E948.6	E950.4	E962.0	E980.4
Peruvian balsam	976.8	E858.7	E946.8	E950.4	E962.0	E980.4
Pesticides (dust) (fumes) (vapor)	989.4	E863.4	—	E950.6	E962.1	E980.7
arsenic	985.1	E863.4	—	E950.8	E962.1	E980.8
chlorinated	989.2	E863.0	—	E950.6	E962.1	E980.7
cyanide	989.0	E863.4	—	E950.6	E962.1	E980.7
kerosene	981	E863.4	—	E950.6	E962.1	E980.7
mixture (of compounds)	989.4	E863.3	—	E950.6	E962.1	E980.7
naphthalene	983.0	E863.4	—	E950.7	E962.1	E980.6
organochlorine (compounds)	989.2	E863.0	—	E950.6	E962.1	E980.7

Pesticides | **Table of Drugs and Chemicals**

		External Cause (E-Code)				
	Poisoning	Accident	Therapeutic Use	Suicide Attempt	Assault	Undetermined
Pesticides — *continued*						
petroleum (distillate)						
(products) NEC	981	E863.4	—	E950.6	E962.1	E980.7
specified ingredient NEC	989.4	E863.4	—	E950.6	E962.1	E980.7
strychnine	989.1	E863.4	—	E950.6	E962.1	E980.7
thallium	985.8	E863.7	—	E950.6	E962.1	E980.7
Pethidine (hydrochloride)	965.09	E850.2	E935.2	E950.0	E962.0	E980.0
Petrichloral	967.1	E852.0	E937.1	E950.2	E962.0	E980.2
Petrol		981		—	E950.9	E962.1	E980.9
vapor	987.1	E869.8	—	E952.8	E962.2	E982.8
Petrolatum (jelly) (ointment)	976.3	E858.7	E946.3	E950.4	E962.0	E980.4
hydrophilic	976.3	E858.7	E946.3	E950.4	E962.0	E980.4
liquid	973.2	E858.4	E943.2	E950.4	E962.0	E980.4
topical	976.3	E858.7	E946.3	E950.4	E962.0	E980.4
nonmedicinal	981	E862.1	—	E950.9	E962.1	E980.9
Petroleum (cleaners) (fuels)						
(products) NEC	981	E862.1	—	E950.9	E962.1	E980.9
benzin(e) — *see* Ligroin						
ether — *see* Ligroin						
jelly — *see* Petrolatum						
naphtha — *see* Ligroin						
pesticide	981	E863.4	—	E950.6	E962.1	E980.7
solids	981	E862.3	—	E950.9	E962.1	E980.9
solvents	981	E862.0	—	E950.9	E962.1	E980.9
vapor	987.1	E869.8	—	E952.8	E962.2	E982.8
Peyote	969.6	E854.1	E939.6	E950.3	E962.0	E980.3
Phanodorm, phanodorn	967.0	E851	E937.0	E950.1	E962.0	E980.1
Phanquinone, phanquone	961.5	E857	E931.5	E950.4	E962.0	E980.4
Pharmaceutical excipient or						
adjunct	977.4	E858.8	E947.4	E950.4	E962.0	E980.4
Phenacemide	966.3	E855.0	E936.3	E950.4	E962.0	E980.4
Phenacetin	965.4	E850.4	E935.4	E950.0	E962.0	E980.0
Phenadoxone	965.09	E850.2	E935.2	E950.0	E962.0	E980.0
Phenaglycodol	969.5	E853.8	E939.5	E950.3	E962.0	E980.3
Phenantoin	966.1	E855.0	E936.1	E950.4	E962.0	E980.4
Phenaphthazine reagent	977.8	E858.8	E947.8	E950.4	E962.0	E980.4
Phenazocine	965.09	E850.2	E935.2	E950.0	E962.0	E980.0
Phenazone	965.5	E850.5	E935.5	E950.0	E962.0	E980.0
Phenazopyridine	976.1	E858.7	E946.1	E950.4	E962.0	E980.4
Phenbenicillin	960	E856	E930.0	E950.4	E962.0	E980.4
Phenbutrazate	977.0	E858.8	E947.0	E950.4	E962.0	E980.4
Phencyclidine	968.3	E855.1	E938.3	E950.4	E962.0	E980.4
Phendimetrazine	977.0	E858.8	E947.0	E950.4	E962.0	E980.4
Phenelzine	969.0	E854.0	E939.0	E950.3	E962.0	E980.3
Phenergan	967.8	E852.8	E937.8	E950.2	E962.0	E980.2
Phenethicillin (potassium)	960.0	E856	E930.0	E950.4	E962.0	E980.4
Phenetsal	965.1	E850.3	E935.3	E950.0	E962.0	E980.0
Pheneturide	966.3	E855.0	E936.3	E950.4	E962.0	E980.4
Phenformin	962.3	E858.0	E932.3	E950.4	E962.0	E980.4
Phenglutarimide	971.1	E855.4	E941.1	E950.4	E962.0	E980.4
Phenicarbazide	965.8	E850.8	E935.8	E950.0	E962.0	E980.0
Phenindamine (tartrate)	963.0	E858.1	E933.0	E950.4	E962.0	E980.4
Phenindione	964.2	E858.2	E934.2	E950.4	E962.0	E980.4
Pheniprazine	969.0	E854.0	E939.0	E950.3	E962.0	E980.3
Pheniramine (maleate)	963.0	E858.1	E933.0	E950.4	E962.0	E980.4
Phenmetrazine	977.0	E858.8	E947.0	E950.4	E962.0	E980.4
Phenobal	967.0	E851	E937.0	E950.1	E962.0	E980.1
Phenobarbital	967.0	E851	E937.0	E950.1	E962.0	E980.1
Phenobarbitone	967.0	E851	E937.0	E950.1	E962.0	E980.1
Phenoctide	976.0	E858.7	E946.0	E950.4	E962.0	E980.4
Phenol (derivatives) NEC	983.0	E864.0	—	E950.7	E962.1	E980.6
disinfectant	983.0	E864.0	—	E950.7	E962.1	E980.6
pesticide	989.4	E863.4	—	E950.6	E962.1	E980.7

▶◀ Revised Text   ● New Line   ▲ Revised Code

Table of Drugs and Chemicals — Pipamazine

		External Cause (E-Code)				
	Poisoning	Accident	Therapeutic Use	Suicide Attempt	Assault	Undetermined
Phenol — continued						
red	977.8	E858.8	E947.8	E950.4	E962.0	E980.4
Phenolphthalein	973.1	E858.4	E943.1	E950.4	E962.0	E980.4
Phenolsulfonphthalein	977.8	E858.8	E947.8	E950.4	E962.0	E980.4
Phenomorphan	965.09	E850.2	E935.2	E950.0	E962.0	E980.0
Phenonyl	967.0	E851	E937.0	E950.1	E962.0	E980.1
Phenoperidine	965.09	E850.2	E935.2	E950.0	E962.0	E980.0
Phenoquin	974.7	E858.5	E944.7	E950.4	E962.0	E980.4
Phenothiazines (tranquilizers)						
NEC	969.1	E853.0	E939.1	E950.3	E962.0	E980.3
insecticide	989.3	E863.4	—	E950.6	E962.1	E980.7
Phenoxybenzamine	971.3	E855.6	E941.3	E950.4	E962.0	E980.4
Phenoxymethyl penicillin	960.0	E856	E930.0	E950.4	E962.0	E980.4
Phenprocoumon	964.2	E858.2	E934.2	E950.4	E962.0	E980.4
Phensuximide	966.2	E855.0	E936.2	E950.4	E962.0	E980.4
Phentermine	977.0	E858.8	E947.0	E950.4	E962.0	E980.4
Phentolamine	971.3	E855.6	E941.3	E950.4	E962.0	E980.4
Phenyl						
butazone	965.5	E850.5	E935.5	E950.0	E962.0	E980.0
enediamine	983.0	E864.0	—	E950.7	E962.1	E980.6
hydrazine	983.0	E864.0	—	E950.7	E962.1	E980.6
antineoplastic	963.1	E858.1	E933.1	E950.4	E962.0	E980.4
mercuric compounds — see Mercury						
salicylate	976.3	E858.7	E946.3	E950.4	E962.0	E980.4
Phenylephrin	971.2	E855.5	E941.2	E950.4	E962.0	E980.4
Phenylethylbiguanide	962.3	E858.0	E932.3	E950.4	E962.0	E980.4
Phenylpropanolamine	971.2	E855.5	E941.2	E950.4	E962.0	E980.4
Phenylsulfthion	989.3	E863.1	—	E950.6	E962.1	E980.7
Phenyramidol, phenyramidon	965.7	E850.7	E935.7	E950.0	E962.0	E980.0
Phenytoin	966.1	E855.0	E936.1	E950.4	E962.0	E980.4
pHisoHex	976.2	E858.7	E946.2	E950.4	E962.0	E980.4
Pholcodine	965.09	E850.2	E935.2	E950.0	E962.0	E980.0
Phorate	989.3	E863.1	—	E950.6	E962.1	E980.7
Phosdrin	989.3	E863.1	—	E950.6	E962.1	E980.7
Phosgene (gas)	987.8	E869.8	—	E952.8	E962.2	E982.8
Phosphate (tricresyl)	989.89	E866.8	—	E950.9	E962.1	E980.9
organic	989.3	E863.1	—	E950.6	E962.1	E980.7
solvent	982.8	E862.4	—	E950.9	E926.1	E980.9
Phosphine	987.8	E869.8	—	E952.8	E962.2	E982.8
fumigant	987.8	E863.8	—	E950.6	E962.2	E980.7
Phosholine	971.0	E855.3	E941.0	E950.4	E962.0	E980.4
Phosphoric acid	983.1	E864.1	—	E950.7	E962.1	E980.6
Phosphorus (compounds) NEC	983.9	E864.3	—	E950.7	E962.1	E980.6
rodenticide	983.9	E863.7	—	E950.7	E962.1	E980.6
Phthalimidoglutarimide	967.8	E852.8	E937.8	E950.2	E962.0	P980.2
Phthalylsulfathiazole	961.0	E857	E931.0	E950.4	E962.0	E980.4
Phylloquinone	964.3	E858.2	E934.3	E950.4	E962.0	E980.4
Physeptone	965.02	E850.1	E935.1	E950.0	E962.0	E980.0
Physostigma venenosum	988.2	E865.4	—	E950.9	E962.1	E980.9
Physostigmine	971.0	E855.3	E941.0	E950.4	E962.0	E980.4
Phytolacca decandra	988.2	E865.4	—	E950.9	E962.1	E980.9
Phytomenadione	964.3	E858.2	E934.3	E950.4	E962.0	E980.4
Phytonadione	964.3	E858.2	E934.3	E950.4	E962.0	E980.4
Picric (acid)	983.0	E864.0	—	E950.7	E962.1	E980.6
Picrotoxin	970.0	E854.3	E940.0	E950.4	E962.0	E980.4
Pilocarpine	971.0	E855.3	E941.0	E950.4	E962.0	E980.4
Pilocarpus (jaborandi) extract	971.0	E855.3	E941.0	E950.4	E962.0	E980.4
Pimaricin	960.1	E856	E930.1	E950.4	E962.0	E980.4
Piminodine	965.09	E850.2	E935.2	E950.0	E962.0	E980.0
Pine oil, pinesol (disinfectant)	983.9	E861.4	—	E950.7	E962.1	E980.6
Pinkroot	961.6	E857	E931.6	E950.4	E962.0	E980.4
Pipadone	965.09	E850.2	E935.2	E950.0	E962.0	E980.0
Pipamazine	963.0	E858.1	E933.0	E950.4	E962.0	E980.4

Fourth-digit Required   Fifth-digit Required

Table of Drugs and Chemicals

			External Cause (E-Code)			
	Poisoning	Accident	Therapeutic Use	Suicide Attempt	Assault	Undetermined
Pipazethate	975.4	E858.6	E945.4	E950.4	E962.0	E980.4
Pipenzolate	971.1	E855.4	E941.1	E950.4	E962.0	E980.4
Piperacetazine	969.1	E853.0	E939.1	E950.3	E962.0	E980.3
Piperazine NEC	961.6	E857	E931.6	E950.4	E962.0	E980.4
estrone sulfate	962.2	E858.0	E932.2	E950.4	E962.0	E980.4
Piper cubeba	988.2	E865.4	—	E950.9	E962.1	E980.9
Piperidione	975.4	E858.6	E945.4	E950.4	E962.0	E980.4
Piperidolate	971.1	E855.4	E941.1	E950.4	E962.0	E980.4
Piperocaine	968.9	E855.2	E938.9	E950.4	E962.0	E980.4
infiltration (subcutaneous)	968.5	E855.2	E938.5	E950.4	E962.0	E980.4
nerve block (peripheral)						
(plexus)	968.6	E855.2	E938.6	E950.4	E962.0	E980.4
topical (surface)	968.5	E855.2	E938.5	E950.4	E962.0	E980.4
Pipobroman	963.1	E858.1	E933.1	E950.4	E962.0	E980.4
Pipradrol	970.8	E854.3	E940.8	E950.4	E962.0	E980.4
Piscidia (bark) (erythrina)	965.7	E850.7	E935.7	E950	E962.0	E980.0
Pitch	983.0	E864.0	—	E950.7	E962.1	E980.6
Pitkin's solution	968.7	E855.2	E938.7	E950.4	E962.0	E980.4
Pitocin	975.0	E858.6	E945.0	E950.4	E962.0	E980.4
Pitressin (tannate)	962.5	E858.0	E932.5	E950.4	E962.0	E980.4
Pituitary extracts (posterior)	962.5	E858.0	E932.5	E950.4	E962.0	E980.4
anterior	962.4	E858.0	E932.4	E950.4	E962.0	E980.4
Pituitrin	962.5	E858.0	E932.5	E950.4	E962.0	E980.4
Placental extract	962.9	E858.0	E932.9	E950.4	E962.0	E980.4
Placidyl	967.8	E852.8	E937.8	E950.2	E962.0	E980.2
Plague vaccine	978.3	E858.8	E948.3	E950.4	E962.0	E980.4
Plant foods or fertilizers NEC	989.89	E866.5	—	E950.9	E962.1	E980.9
mixed with herbicides	989.4	E863.5	—	E950.6	E962.1	E980.7
Plants, noxious, used as food	988.2	E865.9	—	E950.9	E962.1	E980.9
berries and seeds	988.2	E865.3	—	E950.9	E962.1	E980.9
specified type NEC	988.2	E865.4	—	E950.9	E962.1	E980.9
Plasma (blood)	964.7	E858.2	E934.7	E950.4	E962.0	E980.4
expanders	964.8	E858.2	E934.8	E950.4	E962.0	E980.4
Plasmanate	964.7	E858.2	E934.7	E950.4	E962.0	E980.4
Plegicil	969.1	E853.0	E939.1	E950.3	E962.0	E980.3
Podophyllin	976.4	E858.7	E946.4	E950.4	E962.0	E980.4
Podophyllum resin	976.4	E858.7	E946.4	E950.4	E962.0	E980.4
Poison NEC	989.9	E866.9	—	E950.9	E962.1	E980.9
Poisonous berries	988.2	E865.3	—	E950.9	E962.1	E980.9
Pokeweed (any part)	988.2	E865.4	—	E950.9	E962.1	E980.9
Poldine	971.1	E855.4	E941.1	E950.4	E962.0	E980.4
Poliomyelitis vaccine	979.5	E858.8	E949.5	E950.4	E962.0	E980.4
Poliovirus vaccine	979.5	E858.8	E949.5	E950.4	E962.0	E980.4
Polish (car) (floor) (furniture) (metal) (silver)	989.89	E861.2	—	E950.9	E962.1	E980.9
abrasive	989.89	E861.3	—	E950.9	E962.1	E980.9
porcelain	989.89	E861.3	—	E950.9	E962.1	E980.9
Poloxalkol	973.2	E858.4	E943.2	E950.4	E962.0	E980.4
Polyaminostyrene resins	974.5	E858.5	E944.5	E950.4	E962.0	E980.4
Polychlorinated biphenyl — see PCBs						
Polycycline	960.4	E856	E930.4	E950.4	E962.0	E980.4
Polyester resin hardener	982.8	E862.4	—	E950.9	E962.1	E980.9
fumes	987.8	E869.8	—	E952.8	E962.2	E982.8
Polyestradiol (phosphate)	962.2	E858.0	E932.2	E950.4	E962.0	E980.4
Polyethanolamine alkyl sulfate	976.2	E858.7	E946.2	E950.4	E962.0	E980.4
Polyethylene glycol	976.3	E858.7	E946.3	E950.4	E962.0	E980.4
Polyferose	964.0	E858.2	E934.0	E950.4	E962.0	E980.4
Polymyxin B	960.8	E856	E930.8	E950.4	E962.0	E980.4
ENT agent	976.6	E858.7	E946.6	E950.4	E962.0	E980.4
ophthalmic preparation	976.5	E858.7	E946.5	E950.4	E962.0	E980.4
topical NEC	976.0	E858.7	E946.0	E950.4	E962.0	E980.4
Polynoxylin(e)	976.0	E858.7	E946.0	E950.4	E962.0	E980.4
Polyoxymethyleneurea	976.0	E858.7	E946.0	E950.4	E962.0	E980.4

Table of Drugs and Chemicals — Procainamide (hydrochloride)

	Poisoning	External Cause (E-Code)				
		Accident	Therapeutic Use	Suicide Attempt	Assault	Undetermined
Polytetrafluoroethylene (inhaled)	987.8	E869.8	—	E952.8	E962.2	E982.8
Polythiazide	974.3	E858.5	E944.3	E950.4	E962.0	E980.4
Polyvinylpyrrolidone	964.8	E858.2	E934.8	E950.4	E962.0	E980.4
Pontocaine (hydrochloride) (infiltration) (topical)	968.5	E855.2	E938.5	E950.4	E962.0	E980.4
nerve block (peripheral) (plexus)	968.6	E855.2	E938.6	E950.4	E962.0	E980.4
spinal	968.7	E855.2	E938.7	E950.4	E962.0	E980.4
Pot	969.6	E854.1	E939.6	E950.3	E962.0	E980.3
Potash (caustic)	983.2	E864.2	—	E950.7	E962.1	E980.6
Potassic saline injection (lactated)	974.5	E858.5	E944.5	E950.4	E962.0	E980.4
Potassium (salts) NEC	974.5	E858.5	E944.5	E950.4	E962.0	E980.4
aminosalicylate	961.8	E857	E931.8	E950.4	E962.0	E980.4
arsenite (solution)	985.1	E866.3	—	E950.8	E962.1	E980.8
bichromate	983.9	E864.3	—	E950.7	E962.1	E980.6
bisulfate	983.9	E864.3	—	E950.7	E962.1	E980.6
bromide (medicinal) NEC	967.3	E852.2	E937.3	E950.2	E962.0	E980.2
carbonate	983.2	E864.2	—	E950.7	E962.1	E980.6
chlorate NEC	983.9	E864.3	—	E950.7	E962.1	E980.6
cyanide — see Cyanide						
hydroxide	983.2	E864.2	—	E950.7	E962.1	E980.6
iodide (expectorant) NEC	975.5	E858.6	E945.5	E950.4	E962.0	E980.4
nitrate	989.89	E866.8	—	E950.9	E962.1	E980.9
oxalate	983.9	E864.3	—	E950.7	E962.1	E980.6
perchlorate NEC	977.8	E858.8	E947.8	E950.4	E962.0	E980.4
antithyroid	962.8	E858.0	E932.8	E950.4	E962.0	E980.4
permanganate	976.0	E858.7	E946.0	E950.4	E962.0	E980.4
nonmedicinal	983.9	E864.3	—	E950.7	E962.1	E980.6
Povidone-iodine (anti-infective) NEC	976.0	E858.7	E946.0	E950.4	E962.0	E980.4
Practolol	972.0	E858.3	E942.0	E950.4	E962.0	E980.4
Pralidoxime (chloride)	977.2	E858.8	E947.2	E950.4	E962.0	E980.4
Pramoxine	968.5	E855.2	E938.5	E950.4	E962.0	E980.4
Prazosin	972.6	E858.3	E942.6	E950.4	E962.0	E980.4
Prednisolone	962.0	E858.0	E932.0	E950.4	E962.0	E980.4
ENT agent	976.6	E858.7	E946.6	E950.4	E962.0	E980.4
ophthalmic preparation	976.5	E858.7	E946.5	E950.4	E962.0	E980.4
topical NEC	976.0	E858.7	E946.0	E950.4	E962.0	E980.4
Prednisone	962.0	E858.0	E932.0	E950.4	E962.0	E980.4
Pregnanediol	962.2	E858.0	E932.2	E950.4	E962.0	E980.4
Pregneninolone	962.2	E858.0	E932.2	E950.4	E962.0	E980.4
Preludin	977.0	E858.8	E947.0	E950.4	E962.0	E980.4
Premarin	962.2	E858.0	E932.2	E950.4	E962.0	E980.4
Prenylamine	972.4	E858.3	E942.4	E950.4	E962.0	E980.4
Preparation H	976.8	E858.7	E946.8	E950.4	E962.0	E980.4
Preservatives	989.89	E866.8	—	E950.9	E962.1	E980.9
Pride of China	988.2	E865.3	—	E950.9	E962.1	E980.9
Prilocaine	968.9	E855.2	E938.9	E950.4	E962.0	E980.4
infiltration (subcutaneous)	968.5	E855.2	E938.5	E950.4	E962.0	E980.4
nerve block (peripheral) (plexus)	968.6	E855.2	E938.6	E950.4	E962.0	E980.4
Primaquine	961.4	E857	E931.4	E950.4	E962.0	E980.4
Primidone	966.3	E855.0	E936.3	E950.4	E962.0	E980.4
Primula (veris)	988.2	E865.4	—	E950.9	E962.1	E980.9
Prinadol	965.09	E850.2	E935.2	E950.0	E962.0	E980.0
Priscol, Priscoline	971.3	E855.6	E941.3	E950.4	E962.0	E980.4
Privet	988.2	E865.4	—	E950.9	E962.1	E980.9
Privine	971.2	E855.5	E941.2	E950.4	E962.0	E980.4
Pro-Banthine	971.1	E855.4	E941.1	E950.4	E962.0	E980.4
Probarbitol	967.0	E851	E937.0	E950.1	E962.0	E980.1
Probenecid	974.7	E858.5	E944.7	E950.4	E962.0	E980.4
Procainamide (hydrochloride)	972.0	E858.3	E942.0	E950.4	E962.0	E980.4

Fourth-digit Required   Fifth-digit Required

2002 Ingenix, Inc.

Procaine (hydrochloride) (infiltration) (topical) — Table of Drugs and Chemicals

		External Cause (E-Code)				
	Poisoning	Accident	Therapeutic Use	Suicide Attempt	Assault	Undetermined
Procaine (hydrochloride) (infiltration) (topical)	968.5	E855.2	E938.5	E950.4	E962.0	E980.4
nerve block (peripheral)						
(plexus)	968.6	E855.2	E938.6	E950.4	E962.0	E980.4
penicillin G	960.0	E856	E930.0	E950.4	E962.0	E980.4
spinal	968.7	E855.2	E938.7	E950.4	E962.0	E980.4
Procalmidol	969.5	E853.8	E939.5	E950.3	E962.0	E980.3
Procarbazine	963.1	E858.1	E933.1	E950.4	E962.0	E980.4
Prochlorperazine	969.1	E853.0	E939.1	E950.3	E962.0	E980.3
Procyclidine	966.4	E855.0	E936.4	E950.4	E962.0	E980.4
Producer gas	986	E868.8	—	E952.1	E962.2	E982.1
Profenamine	966.4	E855.0	E936.4	E950.4	E962.0	E980.4
Profenil	975.1	E858.6	E945.1	E950.4	E962.0	E980.4
Progesterones	962.2	E858.0	E932.2	E950.4	E962.0	E980.4
Progestin	962.2	E858.0	E932.2	E950.4	E962.0	E980.4
Progestogens (with estrogens)	962.2	E858.0	E932.2	E950.4	E962.0	E980.4
Progestone	962.2	E858.0	E932.2	E950.4	E962.0	E980.4
Proguanil	961.4	E857	E931.4	E950.4	E962.0	E980.4
Prolactin	962.4	E858.0	E932.4	E950.4	E962.0	E980.4
Proloid	962.7	E858.0	E932.7	E950.4	E962.0	E980.4
Proluton	962.2	E858.0	E932.2	E950.4	E962.0	E980.4
Promacetin	961.8	E857	E931.8	E950.4	E962.0	E980.4
Promazine	969.1	E853.0	E939.1	E950.3	E962.0	E980.3
Promedol	965.09	E850.2	E935.2	E950.0	E962.0	E980.0
Promethazine	967.8	E852.8	E937.8	E950.2	E962.0	E980.2
Promin	961.8	E857	E931.8	E950.4	E962.0	E980.4
Pronestyl (hydrochloride)	972.0	E858.3	E942.0	E950.4	E962.0	E980.4
Pronetalol, pronethalol	972.0	E858.3	E942.0	E950.4	E962.0	E980.4
Prontosil	961.0	E857	E931.0	E950.4	E962.0	E980.4
Propamidine isethionate	961.5	E857	E931.5	E950.4	E962.0	E980.4
Propanal (medicinal)	967.8	E862.1	E937.8	E950.2	E962.0	E980.2
Propane (gas) (distributed in mobile container)	987.0	E868.0	—	E951.1	E962.2	E981.1
distributed through pipes	987.0	E867	—	E951.0	E962.2	E981.0
incomplete combustion of — see Carbon monoxide, Propane						
Propanidid	968.3	E855.1	E938.3	E950.4	E962.0	E980.4
Propanol	980.3	E860.4	—	E950.9	E962.1	E980.9
Propantheline	971.1	E855.4	E941.1	E950.4	E962.0	E980.4
Proparacaine	968.5	E855.2	E938.5	E950.4	E962.0	E980.4
Propatyl nitrate	972.4	E858.3	E942.4	E950.4	E962.0	E980.4
Propicillin	960.0	E856	E930.0	E950.4	E962.0	E980.4
Propiolactone (vapor)	987.8	E869.8	—	E952.8	E962.2	E982.8
Propiomazine	967.8	E852.8	E937.8	E950.2	E962.0	E980.2
Propionaldehyde (medicinal)	967.8	E852.8	E937.8	E950.2	E962.0	E980.2
Propionate compound	976.0	E858.7	E946.0	E950.4	E962.0	E980.4
Propion gel	976.0	E858.7	E946.0	E950.4	E962.0	E980.4
Propitocaine	968.9	E855.2	E938.9	E950.4	E962.0	E980.4
infiltration (subcutaneous)	968.5	E855.2	E938.5	E950.4	E962.0	E980.4
nerve block (peripheral)						
(plexus)	968.6	E855.2	E938.6	E950.4	E962.0	E980.4
Propoxur	989.3	E863.2	—	E950.6	E962.1	E980.7
Propoxycaine	968.9	E855.2	E938.9	E950.4	E962.0	E980.4
infiltration (subcutaneous)	968.5	E855.2	E938.5	E950.4	E962.0	E980.4
nerve block (peripheral)						
(plexus)	968.6	E855.2	E938.6	E950.4	E962.0	E980.4
topical (surface)	968.5	E855.2	E938.5	E950.4	E962.0	E980.4
Propoxyphene (hydrochloride)	965.8	E850.8	E935.8	E950.0	E962.0	E980.0
Propranolol	972.0	E858.3	E942.0	E950.4	E962.0	E980.4
Propyl						
alcohol	980.3	E860.4	—	E950.9	E962.1	E980.9
carbinol	980.3	E860.4	—	E950.9	E962.1	E980.9
hexadrine	971.2	E855.5	E941.2	E950.4	E962.0	E980.4

▶◀ Revised Text ● New Line ▲ Revised Code

Table of Drugs and Chemicals — Pyribenzamine

	Poisoning	External Cause (E-Code)				
		Accident	Therapeutic Use	Suicide Attempt	Assault	Undetermined
Propyl — continued						
iodone	977.8	E858.8	E947.8	E950.4	E962.0	E980.4
thiouracil	962.8	E858.0	E932.8	E950.4	E962.0	E980.4
Propylene	987.1	E869.8	—	E952.8	E962.2	E982.8
Propylparaben (ophthalmic)	976.5	E858.7	E946.5	E950.4	E962.0	E980.4
Proscillaridin	972.1	E858.3	E942.1	E950.4	E962.0	E980.4
Prostaglandins	975.0	E858.6	E945.0	E950.4	E962.0	E980.4
Prostigmin	971.0	E855.3	E941.0	E950.4	E962.0	E980.4
Protamine (sulfate)	964.5	E858.2	E934.5	E950.4	E962.0	E980.4
zinc insulin	962.3	E858.0	E932.3	E950.4	E962.0	E980.4
Protectants (topical)	976.3	E858.7	E946.3	E950.4	E962.0	E980.4
Protein hydrolysate	974.5	E858.5	E944.5	E950.4	E962.0	E980.4
Prothiaden — see Dothiepin hydrochloride						
Prothionamide	961.8	E857	E931.8	E950.4	E962.0	E980.4
Prothipendyl	969.5	E853.8	E939.5	E950.3	E962.0	E980.3
Protokylol	971.2	E855.5	E941.2	E950.4	E962.0	E980.4
Protopam	977.2	E858.8	E947.2	E950.4	E962.0	E980.4
Protoveratrine(s) (A) (B)	972.6	E858.3	E942.6	E950.4	E962.0	E980.4
Protriptyline	969.0	E854.0	E939.0	E950.3	E962.0	E980.3
Provera	962.2	E858.0	E932.2	E950.4	E962.0	E980.4
Provitamin A	963.5	E858.1	E933.5	E950.4	E962.0	E980.4
Proxymetacaine	968.5	E855.2	E938.5	E950.4	E962.0	E980.4
Proxyphylline	975.1	E858.6	E945.1	E950.4	E962.0	E980.4
Prozac — see Fluoxetine hydrochloride						
Prunus						
laurocerasus	988.2	E865.4	—	E950.9	E962.1	E980.9
virginiana	988.2	E865.4	—	E950.9	E962.1	E980.9
Prussic acid	989.0	E866.8	—	E950.9	E962.1	E980.9
vapor	987.7	E869.8	—	E952.8	E962.2	E982.8
Pseudoephedrine	971.2	E855.5	E941.2	E950.4	E962.0	E980.4
Psilocin	969.6	E854.1	E939.6	E950.3	E962.0	E980.3
Psilocybin	969.6	E854.1	E939.6	E950.3	E962.0	E980.3
PSP	977.8	E858.8	E947.8	E950.4	E962.0	E980.4
Psychedelic agents	969.6	E854.1	E939.6	E950.3	E962.0	E980.3
Psychodysleptics	969.6	E854.1	E939.6	E950.3	E962.0	E980.3
Psychostimulants	969.7	E854.2	E939.7	E950.3	E962.0	E980.3
Psychotherapeutic agents	969.9	E855.9	E939.9	E950.3	E962.0	E980.3
antidepressants	969.0	E854.0	E939.0	E950.3	E962.0	E980.3
specified NEC	969.8	E855.8	E939.8	E950.3	E962.0	E980.3
tranquilizers NEC	969.5	E853.9	E939.5	E950.3	E962.0	E980.3
Psychotomimetic agents	969.6	E854.1	E939.6	E950.3	E962.0	E980.3
Psychotropic agents	969.9	E854.8	E939.9	E950.3	E962.0	E980.3
specified NEC	969.8	E854.8	E939.8	E950.3	E962.0	E980.3
Psyllium	973.3	E858.4	E943.3	E950.4	E962.0	E980.4
Pteroylglutamic acid	964.1	E858.2	E934.1	E950.4	E962.0	E980.4
Pteroyltriglutamate	963.1	E858.1	E933.1	E950.4	E962.0	E980.4
PTFE	987.8	E869.8	—	E952.8	E962.2	E982.8
Pulsatilla	988.2	E865.4	—	E950.9	E962.1	E980.9
Purex (bleach)	983.9	E864.3	—	E950.7	E962.1	E980.6
Purine diuretics	974.1	E858.5	E944.1	E950.4	E962.0	E980.4
Purinethol	963.1	E858.1	E933.1	E950.4	E962.0	E980.4
PVP	964.8	E858.2	E934.8	E950.4	E962.0	E980.4
Pyrabital	965.7	E850.7	E935.7	E950.0	E962.0	E980.0
Pyramidon	965.5	E850.5	E935.5	E950.0	E962.0	E980
Pyrantel (pamoate)	961.6	E857	E931.6	E950.4	E962.0	E980.4
Pyrathiazine	963.0	E858.1	E933.0	E950.4	E962.0	E980.4
Pyrazinamide	961.8	E857	E931.8	E950.4	E962.0	E980.4
Pyrazinoic acid (amide)	961.8	E857	E931.8	E950.4	E962.0	E980.4
Pyrazole (derivatives)	965.5	E850.5	E935.5	E950.0	E962.0	E980.0
Pyrazolone (analgesics)	965.5	E850.5	E935.5	E950.0	E962.0	E980.0
Pyrethrins, pyrethrum	989.4	E863.4	—	E950.6	E962.1	E980.7
Pyribenzamine	963.0	E858.1	E933.0	E950.4	E962.0	E980.4

Table of Drugs and Chemicals

	Poisoning	External Cause (E-Code)				
		Accident	Therapeutic Use	Suicide Attempt	Assault	Undetermined
Pyridine (liquid) (vapor)	982.0	E862.4	—	E950.9	E962.1	E980.9
aldoxime chloride	977.2	E858.8	E947.2	E950.4	E962.0	E980.4
Pyridium	976.1	E858.7	E946.1	E950.4	E962.0	E980.4
Pyridostigmine	971.0	E855.3	E941.0	E950.4	E962.0	E980.4
Pyridoxine	963.5	E858.1	E933.5	E950.4	E962.0	E980.4
Pyrilamine	963.0	E858.1	E933.0	E950.4	E962.0	E980.4
Pyrimethamine	961.4	E857	E931.4	E950.4	E962.0	E980.4
Pyrogallic acid	983.0	E864.0	—	E950.7	E962.1	E980.6
Pyroxylin	976.3	E858.7	E946.3	E950.4	E962.0	E980.4
Pyrrobutamine	963.0	E858.1	E933.0	E950.4	E962.0	E980.4
Pyrrocitine	968.5	E855.2	E938.5	E950.4	E962.0	E980.4
Pyrvinium (pamoate)	961.6	E857	E931.6	E950.4	E962.0	E980.4
PZI	962.3	E858.0	E932.3	E950.4	E962.0	E980.4
Quaalude	967.4	E852.3	E937.4	E950.2	E962.0	E980.2
Quaternary ammonium derivatives	971.1	E855.4	E941.1	E950.4	E962.0	E980.4
Quicklime	983.2	E864.2	—	E950.7	E962.1	E980.6
Quinacrine	961.3	E857	E931.3	E950.4	E962.0	E980.4
Quinaglute	972.0	E858.3	E942.0	E950.4	E962.0	E980.4
Quinalbarbitone	967.0	E851	E937.0	E950.1	E962.0	E980.1
Quinestradiol	962.2	E858.0	E932.2	E950.4	E962.0	E980.4
Quinethazone	974.3	E858.5	E944.3	E950.4	E962.0	E980.4
Quinidine (gluconate) (polygalacturonate) (salts) (sulfate)	972.0	E858.3	E942.0	E950.4	E962.0	E980.4
Quinine	961.4	E857	E931.4	E950.4	E962.0	E980.4
Quiniobine	961.3	E857	E931.3	E950.4	E962.0	E980.4
Quinolines	961.3	E857	E931.3	E950.4	E962.0	E980.4
Quotane	968.5	E855.2	E938.5	E950.4	E962.0	E980.4
Rabies						
immune globulin (human)	964.6	E858.2	E934.6	E950.4	E962.0	E980.4
vaccine	979.1	E858.8	E949.1	E950.4	E962.0	E980.4
Racemoramide	965.09	E850.2	E935.2	E950.0	E962.0	E980.0
Racemorphan	965.09	E850.2	E935.2	E950.0	E962.0	E980.0
Radiator alcohol	980.1	E860.2	—	E950.9	E962.1	E980.9
Radio-opaque (drugs) (materials)	977.8	E858.8	E947.8	E950.4	E962.0	E980.4
Ranunculus	988.2	E865.4	—	E950.9	E962.1	E980.9
Rat poison	989.4	E863.7	—	E950.6	E962.1	E980.7
Rattlesnake (venom)	989.5	E905.0	—	E950.9	E962.1	E980.9
Raudixin	972.6	E858.3	E942.6	E950.4	E962.0	E980.4
Rautensin	972.6	E858.3	E942.6	E950.4	E962.0	E980.4
Rautina	972.6	E858.3	E942.6	E950.4	E962.0	E980.4
Rautotal	972.6	E858.3	E942.6	E950.4	E962.0	E980.4
Rauwiloid	972.6	E858.3	E942.6	E950.4	E962.0	E980.4
Rauwoldin	972.6	E858.3	E942.6	E950.4	E962.0	E980.4
Rauwolfia (alkaloids)	972.6	E858.3	E942.6	E950.4	E962.0	E980.4
Realgar	985.1	E866.3	—	E950.8	E962.1	E980.8
Red cells, packed	964.7	E858.2	E934.7	E950.4	E962.0	E980.4
Reducing agents, industrial NEC	983.9	E864.3	—	E950.7	E962.1	E980.6
Refrigerant gas (freon)	987.4	E869.2	—	E952.8	E962.2	E982.8
not freon	987.9	E869.9	—	E952.9	E962.2	E982.9
Regroton	974.4	E858.5	E944.4	E950.4	E962.0	E980.4
Rela	968.0	E855.1	E938.0	E950.4	E962.0	E980.4
Relaxants, skeletal muscle						
(autonomic)	975.2	E858.6	E945.2	E950.4	E962.0	E980.4
central nervous system	968.0	E855.1	E938.0	E950.4	E962.0	E980.4
Renese	974.3	E858.5	E944.3	E950.4	E962.0	E980.4
Renografin	977.8	E858.8	E947.8	E950.4	E962.0	E980.4
Replacement solutions	974.5	E858.5	E944.5	E950.4	E962.0	E980.4
Rescinnamine	972.6	E858.3	E942.6	E950.4	E962.0	E980.4
Reserpine	972.6	E858.3	E942.6	E950.4	E962.0	E980.4
Resorcin, resorcinol	976.4	E858.7	E946.4	E950.4	E962.0	E980.4

Table of Drugs and Chemicals

		External Cause (E-Code)				
	Poisoning	Accident	Therapeutic Use	Suicide Attempt	Assault	Undetermined
Respaire	975.5	E858.6	E945.5	E950.4	E962.0	E980.4
Respiratory agents NEC	975.8	E858.6	E945.8	E950.4	E962.0	E980.4
Retinoic acid	976.8	E858.7	E946.8	E950.4	E962.0	E980.4
Retinol	963.5	E858.1	E933.5	E950.4	E962.0	E980.4
Rh (D) immune globulin (human)	964.6	E858.2	E934.6	E950.4	E962.0	E980.4
Rhodine	965.1	E850.3	E935.3	E950.0	E962.0	E980.0
RhoGAM	964.6	E858.2	E934.6	E950.4	E962.0	E980.4
Riboflavin	963.5	E858.1	E933.5	E950.4	E962.0	E980.4
Ricin	989.89	E866.8	—	E950.9	E962.1	E980.9
Ricinus communis	988.2	E865.3	—	E950.9	E962.1	E980.9
Rickettsial vaccine NEC	979.6	E858.8	E949.6	E950.4	E962.0	E980.4
with viral and bacterial vaccine	979.7	E858.8	E949.7	E950.4	E962.0	E980.4
Rifampin	960.6	E856	E930.6	E950.4	E962.0	E980.4
Rimifon	961.8	E857	E931.8	E950.4	E962.0	E980.4
Ringer's injection (lactated)	974.5	E858.5	E944.5	E950.4	E962.0	E980.4
Ristocetin	960.8	E856	E930.8	E950.4	E962.0	E980.4
Ritalin	969.7	E854.2	E939.7	E950.3	E962.0	E980.3
Roach killers — see Pesticides						
Rocky Mountain spotted fever vaccine	979.6	E858.8	E949.6	E950.4	E962.0	E980.4
Rodenticides	989.4	E863.7	—	E950.6	E962.1	E980.7
Rohypnol	969.4	E853.2	E939.4	E950.3	E962.0	E980.3 ▲
Rolaids	973.0	E858.4	E943.0	E950.4	E962.0	E980.4
Rolitetracycline	960.4	E856	E930.4	E950.4	E962.0	E980.4
Romilar	975.4	E858.6	E945.4	E950.4	E962.0	E980.4
Rose water ointment	976.3	E858.7	E946.3	E950.4	E962.0	E980.4
Rotenone	989.4	E863.7	—	E950.6	E962.1	E980.7
Rotoxamine	963.0	E858.1	E933.0	E950.4	E962.0	E980.4
Rough-on-rats	989.4	E863.7	—	E950.6	E962.1	E980.7
RU486	962.9	E858.0	E932.9	E950.4	E962.0	E980.4
Rubbing alcohol	980.2	E860.3	—	E950.9	E962.1	E980.9
Rubella virus vaccine	979.4	E858.8	E949.4	E950.4	E962.0	E980.4
Rubelogen	979.4	E858.8	E949.4	E950.4	E962.0	E980.4
Rubeovax	979.4	E858.8	E949.4	E950.4	E962.0	E980.4
Rubidomycin	960.7	E856	E930.7	E950.4	E962.0	E980.4
Rue	988.2	E865.4	—	E950.9	E962.1	E980.9
Ruta	988.2	E865.4	—	E950.9	E962.1	E980.9
Sabadilla (medicinal)	976.0	E858.7	E946.0	E950.4	E962.0	E980.4
pesticide	989.4	E863.4	—	E950.6	E962.1	E980.7
Sabin oral vaccine	979.5	E858.8	E949.5	E950.4	E962.0	E980.4
Saccharated iron oxide	964.0	E858.2	E934.0	E950.4	E962.0	E980.4
Saccharin	974.5	E858.5	E944.5	E950.4	E962.0	E980.4
Safflower oil	972.2	E858.3	E942.2	E950.4	E962.0	E980.4
Salbutamol sulfate	975.7	E858.6	E945.7	E950.4	E962.0	E980.4
Salicylamide	965.1	E850.3	E935.3	E950.0	E962.0	E980.0
Salicylate(s)	965.1	E850.3	E935.3	E950.0	E962.0	E980.0
methyl	976.3	E858.7	E946.3	E950.4	E962.0	E980.4
theobromine calcium	974.1	E858.5	E944.1	E950.4	E962.0	E980.4
Salicylazosulfapyridine	961.0	E857	E931.0	E950.4	E962.0	E980.4
Salicylhydroxamic acid	976.0	E858.7	E946.0	E950.4	E962.0	E980.4
Salicylic acid (keratolytic) NEC	976.4	E858.7	E946.4	E950.4	E962.0	E980.4
congeners	965.1	E850.3	E935.3	E950.0	E962.0	E980.0
salts	965.1	E850.3	E935.3	E950.0	E962.0	E980.0
Saliniazid	961.8	E857	E931.8	E950.4	E962.0	E980.4
Salol	976.3	E858.7	E946.3	E950.4	E962.0	E980.4
Salt (substitute) NEC	974.5	E858.5	E944.5	E950.4	E962.0	E980.4
Saluretics	974.3	E858.5	E944.3	E950.4	E962.0	E980.4
Saluron	974.3	E858.5	E944.3	E950.4	E962.0	E980.4
Salvarsan 606 (neosilver) (silver)	961.1	E857	E931.1	E950.4	E962.0	E980.4
Sambucus canadensis	988.2	E865.4	—	E950.9	E962.1	E980.9
berry	988.2	E865.3	—	E950.9	E962.1	E980.9

Fourth-digit Required   Fifth-digit Required

Sandril — Table of Drugs and Chemicals

	Poisoning	External Cause (E-Code)				
		Accident	Therapeutic Use	Suicide Attempt	Assault	Undetermined
Sandril	972.6	E858.3	E942.6	E950.4	E962.0	E980.4
Sanguinaria canadensis	988.2	E865.4	—	E950.9	E962.1	E980.9
Saniflush (cleaner)	983.9	E861.3	—	E950.7	E962.1	E980.6
Santonin	961.6	E857	E931.6	E950.4	E962.0	E980.4
Santyl	976.8	E858.7	E946.8	E950.4	E962.0	E980.4
Sarkomycin	960.7	E856	E930.7	E950.4	E962.0	E980.4
Saroten	969.0	E854.0	E939.0	E950.3	E962.0	E980.3
Saturnine — *see* Lead						
Savin (oil)	976.4	E858.7	E946.4	E950.4	E962.0	E980.4
Scammony	973.1	E858.4	E943.1	E950.4	E962.0	E980.4
Scarlet red	976.8	E858.7	E946.8	E950.4	E962.0	E980.4
Scheele's green	985.1	E866.3	—	E950.8	E962.1	E980.8
insecticide	985.1	E863.4	—	E950.8	E962.1	E980.8
Schradan	989.3	E863.1	—	E950.6	E962.1	E980.7
Schweinfurt(h) green	985.1	E866.3	—	E950.8	E962.1	E980.8
insecticide	985.1	E863.4	—	E950.8	E962.1	E980.8
Scilla — *see* Squill						
Sclerosing agents	972.7	E858.3	E942.7	E950.4	E962.0	E980.4
Scopolamine	971.1	E855.4	E941.1	E950.4	E962.0	E980.4
Scouring powder	989.89	E861.3	—	E950.9	E962.1	E980.9
Sea						
anemone (sting)	989.5	E905.6	—	E950.9	E962.1	E980.9
cucumber (sting)	989.5	E905.6	—	E950.9	E962.1	E980.9
snake (bite) (venom)	989.5	E905.0	—	E950.9	E962.1	E980.9
urchin spine (puncture)	989.5	E905.6	—	E950.9	E962.1	E980.9
Secbutabarbital	967.0	E851	E937.0	E950.1	E962.0	E980.1
Secbutabarbitone	967.0	E851	E937.0	E950.1	E962.0	E980.1
Secobarbital	967.0	E851	E937.0	E950.1	E962.0	E980.1
Seconal	967.0	E851	E937.0	E950.1	E962.0	E980.1
Secretin	977.8	E858.8	E947.8	E950.4	E962.0	E980.4
Sedatives, nonbarbiturate	967.9	E852.9	E937.9	E950.2	E962.0	E980.2
specified NEC	967.8	E852.8	E937.8	E950.2	E962.0	E980.2
Sedormid	967.8	E852.8	E937.8	E950.2	E962.0	E980.2
Seed (plant)	988.2	E865.3	—	E950.9	E962.1	E980.9
disinfectant or dressing	989.89	E866.5	—	E950.9	E962.1	E980.9
Selenium (fumes) NEC	985.8	E866.4	—	E950.9	E962.1	E980.9
disulfide or sulfide	976.4	E858.7	E946.4	E950.4	E962.0	E980.4
Selsun	976.4	E858.7	E946.4	E950.4	E962.0	E980.4
Senna	973.1	E858.4	E943.1	E950.4	E962.0	E980.4
Septisol	976.2	E858.7	E946.2	E950.4	E962.0	E980.4
Serax	969.4	E853.2	E939.4	E950.3	E962.0	E980.3
Serenesil	967.8	E852.8	E937.8	E950.2	E962.0	E980.2
Serenium (hydrochloride)	961.9	E857	E931.9	E950.4	E962.0	E980.4
Sernyl	968.3	E855.1	E938.3	E950.4	E962.0	E980.4
Serotonin	977.8	E858.8	E947.8	E950.4	E962.0	E980.4
Serpasil	972.6	E858.3	E942.6	E950.4	E962.0	E980.4
Sewer gas	987.8	E869.8	—	E952.8	E962.2	E982.8
Shampoo	989.6	E861.0	—	E950.9	E962.1	E980.9
Shellfish, nonbacterial or noxious	988.0	E865.1	—	E950.9	E962.1	E980.9
Silicones NEC	989.83	E866.8	E947.8	E950.9	E962.1	E980.9
Silvadene	976.0	E858.7	E946.0	E950.4	E962.0	E980.4
Silver (compound) (medicinal) NEC	976.0	E858.7	E946.0	E950.4	E962.0	E980.4
anti-infectives	976.0	E858.7	E946.0	E950.4	E962.0	E980.4
arsphenamine	961.1	E857	E931.1	E950.4	E962.0	E980.4
nitrate	976.0	E858.7	E946.0	E950.4	E962.0	E980.4
ophthalmic preparation	976.5	E858.7	E946.5	E950.4	E962.0	E980.4
toughened (keratolytic)	976.4	E858.7	E946.4	E950.4	E962.0	E980.4
nonmedicinal (dust)	985.8	E866.4	—	E950.9	E962.1	E980.9
protein (mild) (strong)	976.0	E858.7	E946.0	E950.4	E962.0	E980.4
salvarsan	961.1	E857	E931.1	E950.4	E962.0	E980.4
Simethicone	973.8	E858.4	E943.8	E950.4	E962.0	E980.4
Sinequan	969.0	E854.0	E939.0	E950.3	E962.0	E980.3

Table of Drugs and Chemicals — Sodium

		External Cause (E-Code)				
	Poisoning	Accident	Therapeutic Use	Suicide Attempt	Assault	Undetermined
Singoserp	972.6	E858.3	E942.6	E950.4	E962.0	E980.4
Sintrom	964.2	E858.2	E934.2	E950.4	E962.0	E980.4
Sitosterols	972.2	E858.3	E942.2	E950.4	E962.0	E980.4
Skeletal muscle relaxants	975.2	E858.6	E945.2	E950.4	E962.0	E980.4
Skin						
agents (external)	976.9	E858.7	E946.9	E950.4	E962.0	E980.4
specified NEC	976.8	E858.7	E946.8	E950.4	E962.0	E980.4
test antigen	977.8	E858.8	E947.8	E950.4	E962.0	E980.4
Sleep-eze	963.0	E858.1	E933.0	E950.4	E962.0	E980.4
Sleeping draught (drug) (pill) (tablet)	967.9	E852.9	E937.9	E950.2	E962.0	E980.2
Smallpox vaccine	979.0	E858.8	E949.0	E950.4	E962.0	E980.4
Smelter fumes NEC	985.9	E866.4	—	E950.9	E962.1	E980.9
Smog	987.3	E869.1	—	E952.8	E962.2	E982.8
Smoke NEC	987.9	E869.9	—	E952.9	E962.2	E982.9
Smooth muscle relaxant	975.1	E858.6	E945.1	E950.4	E962.0	E980.4
Snail killer	989.4	E863.4	—	E950.6	E962.1	E980.7
Snake (bite) (venom)	989.5	E905.0	—	E950.9	E962.1	E980.9
Snuff	989.89	E866.8	—	E950.9	E962.1	E980.9
Soap (powder) (product)	989.6	E861.1	—	E950.9	E962.1	E980.9
medicinal, soft	976.2	E858.7	E946.2	E950.4	E962.0	E980.4
Soda (caustic)	983.2	E864.2	—	E950.7	E962.1	E980.6
bicarb	963.3	E858.1	E933.3	E950.4	E962.0	E980.4
chlorinated — see Sodium, hypochlorite						
Sodium						
acetosulfone	961.8	E857	E931.8	E950.4	E962.0	E980.4
acetrizoate	977.8	E858.8	E947.8	E950.4	E962.0	E980.4
amytal	967.0	E851	E937.0	E950.1	E962.0	E980.1
arsenate — see Arsenic						
bicarbonate	963.3	E858.1	E933.3	E950.4	E962.0	E980.4
bichromate	983.9	E864.3	—	E950.7	E962.1	E980.6
biphosphate	963.2	E858.1	E933.2	E950.4	E962.0	E980.4
bisulfate	983.9	E864.3	—	E950.7	E962.1	E980.6
borate (cleanser)	989.6	E861.3	—	E950.9	E962.1	E980.9
bromide NEC	967.3	E852.2	E937.3	E950.2	E962.0	E980.2
cacodylate (nonmedicinal) NEC	978.8	E858.8	E948.8	E950.4	E962.0	E980.4
anti-infective	961.1	E857	E931.1	E950.4	E962.0	E980.4
herbicide	989.4	E863.5	—	E950.6	E962.1	E980.7
calcium edetate	963.8	E858.1	E933.8	E950.4	E962.0	E980.4
carbonate NEC	983.2	E864.2	—	E950.7	E962.1	E980.6
chlorate NEC	983.9	E864.3	—	E950.7	E962.1	E980.6
herbicide	983.9	E863.5	—	E950.7	E962.1	E980.6
chloride NEC	974.5	E858.5	E944.5	E950.4	E962.0	E980.4
chromate	983.9	E864.3	—	E950.7	E962.1	E980.6
citrate	963.3	E858.1	E933.3	E950.4	E962.0	E980.4
cyanide — see Cyanide(s)						
cyclamate	974.5	E858.5	E944.5	E950.4	E962.0	E980.4
diatrizoate	977.8	E858.8	E947.8	E950.4	E962.0	E980.4
dibunate	975.4	E858.6	E945.4	E950.4	E962.0	E980.4
dioctyl sulfosuccinate	973.2	E858.4	E943.2	E950.4	E962.0	E980.4
edetate	963.8	E858.1	E933.8	E950.4	E962.0	E980.4
ethacrynate	974.4	E858.5	E944.4	E950.4	E962.0	E980.4
fluoracetate (dust) (rodenticide)	989.4	E863.7	—	E950.6	E962.1	E980.7
fluoride — see Fluoride(s)						
free salt	974.5	E858.5	E944.5	E950.4	E962.0	E980.4
glucosulfone	961.8	E857	E931.8	E950.4	E962.0	E980.4
hydroxide	983.2	E864.2	—	E950.7	E962.1	E980.6
hypochlorite (bleach) NEC	983.9	E864.3	—	E950.7	E962.1	E980.6
disinfectant	983.9	E861.4	—	E950.7	E962.1	E980.6

Table of Drugs and Chemicals

	External Cause (E-Code)					
	Poisoning	Accident	Therapeutic Use	Suicide Attempt	Assault	Undetermined
Sodium — *continued*						
hypochlorite — *continued*						
medicinal (anti-infective) (external)	976.0	E858.7	E946.0	E950.4	E962.0	E980.4
vapor	987.8	E869.8	—	E952.8	E962.2	E982.8
hyposulfite	976.0	E858.7	E946.0	E950.4	E962.0	E980.4
indigotindisulfonate	977.8	E858.8	E947.8	E950.4	E962.0	E980.4
iodide	977.8	E858.8	E947.8	E950.4	E962.0	E980.4
iothalamate	977.8	E858.8	E947.8	E950.4	E962.0	E980.4
iron edetate	964.0	E858.2	E934.0	E950.4	E962.0	E980.4
lactate	963.3	E858.1	E933.3	E950.4	E962.0	E980.4
lauryl sulfate	976.2	E858.7	E946.2	E950.4	E962.0	E980.4
L-triiodothyronine	962.7	E858.0	E932.7	E950.4	E962.0	E980.4
metrizoate	977.8	E858.8	E947.8	E950.4	E962.0	E980.4
monofluoracetate (dust) (rodenticide)	989.4	E863.7	—	E950.6	E962.1	E980.7
morrhuate	972.7	E858.3	E942.7	E950.4	E962.0	E980.4
nafcillin	960.0	E856	E930.0	E950.4	E962.0	E980.4
nitrate (oxidizing agent)	983.9	E864.3	—	E950.7	E962.1	E980.6
nitrite (medicinal)	972.4	E858.3	E942.4	E950.4	E962.0	E980.4
nitroferricyanide	972.6	E858.3	E942.6	E950.4	E962.0	E980.4
nitroprusside	972.6	E858.3	E942.6	E950.4	E962.0	E980.4
para-aminohippurate	977.8	E858.8	E947.8	E950.4	E962.0	E980.4
perborate (nonmedicinal) NEC	989.89	E866.8	—	E950.9	E962.1	E980.9
medicinal	976.6	E858.7	E946.6	E950.4	E962.0	E980.4
soap	989.6	E861.1	—	E950.9	E962.1	E980.9
percarbonate — *see* Sodium, perborate						
phosphate	973.3	E858.4	E943.3	E950.4	E962.0	E980.4
polystyrene sulfonate	974.5	E858.5	E944.5	E950.4	E962.0	E980.4
propionate	976.0	E858.7	E946.0	E950.4	E962.0	E980.4
psylliate	972.7	E858.3	E942.7	E950.4	E962.0	E980.4
removing resins	974.5	E858.5	E944.5	E950.4	E962.0	E980.4
salicylate	965.1	E850.3	E935.3	E950.0	E962.0	E980.0
sulfate	973.3	E858.4	E943.3	E950.4	E962.0	E980.4
sulfoxone	961.8	E857	E931.8	E950.4	E962.0	E980.4
tetradecyl sulfate	972.7	E858.3	E942.7	E950.4	E962.0	E980.4
thiopental	968.3	E855.1	E938.3	E950.4	E962.0	E980.4
thiosalicylate	965.1	E850.3	E935.3	E950.0	E962.0	E980.0
thiosulfate	976.0	E858.7	E946.0	E950.4	E962.0	E980.4
tolbutamide	977.8	E858.8	E947.8	E950.4	E962.0	E980.4
tyropanoate	977.8	E858.8	E947.8	E950.4	E962.0	E980.4
valproate	966.3	E855.0	E936.3	E950.4	E962.0	E980.4
Solanine	977.8	E858.8	E947.8	E950.4	E962.0	E980.4
Solanum dulcamara	988.2	E865.4	—	E950.9	E962.1	E980.9
Solapsone	961.8	E857	E931.8	E950.4	E962.0	E980.4
Solasulfone	961.8	E857	E931.8	E950.4	E962.0	E980.4
Soldering fluid	983.1	E864.1	—	E950.7	E962.1	E980.6
Solid substance	989.9	E866.9	—	E950.9	E962.1	E980.9
specified NEC	989.9	E866.8	—	E950.9	E962.1	E980.9
Solvents, industrial	982.8	E862.9	—	E950.9	E962.1	E980.9
naphtha	981	E862.0	—	E950.9	E962.1	E980.9
petroleum	981	E862.0	—	E950.9	E962.1	E980.9
specified NEC	982.8	E862.4	—	E950.9	E962.1	E980.9
Soma	968.0	E855.1	E938.0	E950.4	E962.0	E980.4
Somatotropin	962.4	E858.0	E932.4	E950.4	E962.0	E980.4
Sominex	963.0	E858.1	E933.0	E950.4	E962.0	E980.4
Somnos	967.1	E852.0	E937.1	E950.2	E962.0	E980.2
Somonal	967.0	E851	E937.0	E950.1	E962.0	E980.1
Soneryl	967.0	E851	E937.0	E950.1	E962.0	E980.1
Soothing syrup	977.9	E858.9	E947.9	E950.5	E962.0	E980.5
Sopor	967.4	E852.3	E937.4	E950.2	E962.0	E980.2

Table of Drugs and Chemicals — Stimulants (central nervous system)

	External Cause (E-Code)					
	Poisoning	Accident	Therapeutic Use	Suicide Attempt	Assault	Undetermined
Soporific drug	967.9	E852.9	E937.9	E950.2	E962.0	E980.2
specified type NEC	967.8	E852.8	E937.8	E950.2	E962.0	E980.2
Sorbitol NEC	977.4	E858.8	E947.4	E950.4	E962.0	E980.4
Sotradecol	972.7	E858.3	E942.7	E950.4	E962.0	E980.4
Spacoline	975.1	E858.6	E945.1	E950.4	E962.0	E980.4
Spanish fly	976.8	E858.7	E946.8	E950.4	E962.0	E980.4
Sparine	969.1	E853.0	E939.1	E950.3	E962.0	E980.3
Sparteine	975.0	E858.6	E945.0	E950.4	E962.0	E980.4
Spasmolytics	975.1	E858.6	E945.1	E950.4	E962.0	E980.4
anticholinergics	971.1	E855.4	E941.1	E950.4	E962.0	E980.4
Spectinomycin	960.8	E856	E930.8	E950.4	E962.0	E980.4
Speed	969.7	E854.2	E939.7	E950.3	E962.0	E980.3
Spermicides	976.8	E858.7	E946.8	E950.4	E962.0	E980.4
Spider (bite) (venom)	989.5	E905.1	—	E950.9	E962.1	E980.9
antivenin	979.9	E858.8	E949.9	E950.4	E962.0	E980.4
Spigelia (root)	961.6	E857	E931.6	E950.4	E962.0	E980.4
Spiperone	969.2	E853.1	E939.2	E950.3	E962.0	E980.3
Spiramycin	960.3	E856	E930.3	E950.4	E962.0	E980.4
Spirilene	969.5	E853.8	E939.5	E950.3	E962.0	E980.3
Spirit(s) (neutral) NEC	980.0	E860.1	—	E950.9	E962.1	E980.9
beverage	980.0	E860.0	—	E950.9	E962.1	E980.9
industrial	980.9	E860.9	—	E950.9	E962.1	E980.9
mineral	981	E862.0	—	E950.9	E962.1	E980.9
of salt — see Hydrochloric acid						
surgical	980.9	E860.9	—	E950.9	E962.1	E980.9
Spironolactone	974.4	E858.5	E944.4	E950.4	E962.0	E980.4
Sponge, absorbable (gelatin)	964.5	E858.2	E934.5	E950.4	E962.0	E980.4
Sporostacin	976.0	E858.7	E946.0	E950.4	E962.0	E980.4
Sprays (aerosol)	989.89	E866.8	—	E950.9	E962.1	E980.9
cosmetic	989.89	E866.7	—	E950.9	E962.1	E980.9
medicinal NEC	977.9	E858.9	E947.9	E950.5	E962.0	E980.5
pesticides — see Pesticides						
specified content — see substance specified						
Spurge flax	988.2	E865.4	—	E950.9	E962.1	E980.9
Spurges	988.2	E865.4	—	E950.9	E962.1	E980.9
Squill (expectorant) NEC	975.5	E858.6	E945.5	E950.4	E962.0	E980.4
rat poison	989.4	E863.7	—	E950.6	E962.1	E980.7
Squirting cucumber (cathartic)	973.1	E858.4	E943.1	E950.4	E962.0	E980.4
Stains	989.89	E866.8	—	E950.9	E962.1	E980.9
Stannous — see also Tin						
fluoride	976.7	E858.7	E946.7	E950.4	E962.0	E980.4
Stanolone	962.1	E858.0	E932.1	E950.4	E962.0	E980.4
Stanozolol	962.1	E858.0	E932.1	E950.4	E962.0	E980.4
Staphisagria or stavesacre (pediculicide)	976.0	E858.7	E946.0	E950.4	E962.0	E980.4
Stelazine	969.1	E853.0	E939.1	E950.3	E962.0	E980.3
Stemetil	969.1	E853.0	E939.1	E950.3	E962.0	E980.3
Sterculia (cathartic) (gum)	973.3	E858.4	E943.3	E950.4	E962.0	E980.4
Sternutator gas	987.8	E869.8	—	E952.8	E962.2	E982.8
Steroids NEC	962.0	E858.0	E932.0	E950.4	E962.0	E980.4
ENT agent	976.6	E858.7	E946.6	E950.4	E962.0	E980.4
ophthalmic preparation	976.5	E858.7	E946.5	E950.4	E962.0	E980.4
topical NEC	976.0	E858.7	E946.0	E950.4	E962.0	E980.4
Stibine	985.8	E866.4	—	E950.9	E962.1	E980.9
Stibophen	961.2	E857	E931.2	E950.4	E962.0	E980.4
Stilbamide, stilbamidine	961.5	E857	E931.5	E950.4	E962.0	E980.4
Stilbestrol	962.2	E858.0	E932.2	E950.4	E962.0	E980.4
Stimulants (central nervous system)	970.9	E854.3	E940.9	E950.4	E962.0	E980.4
analeptics	970.0	E854.3	E940.0	E950.4	E962.0	E980.4
opiate antagonist	970.1	E854.3	E940.1	E950.4	E962.0	E980.4
psychotherapeutic NEC	969.0	E854.0	E939.0	E950.3	E962.0	E980.3

✓4ᵗʰ Fourth-digit Required   ✓5ᵗʰ Fifth-digit Required

Stimulants — Table of Drugs and Chemicals

	\multicolumn{6}{c}{External Cause (E-Code)}
	Poisoning	Accident	Therapeutic Use	Suicide Attempt	Assault	Undetermined
Stimulants — *continued*						
specified NEC	970.8	E854.3	E940.8	E950.4	E962.0	E980.4
Storage batteries (acid) (cells)	983.1	E864.1	—	E950.7	E962.1	E980.6
Stovaine	968.9	E855.2	E938.9	E950.4	E962.0	E980.4
infiltration (subcutaneous)	968.5	E855.2	E938.5	E950.4	E962.0	E980.4
nerve block (peripheral) (plexus)	968.6	E855.2	E938.6	E950.4	E962.0	E980.4
spinal	968.7	E855.2	E938.7	E950.4	E962.0	E980.4
topical (surface)	968.5	E855.2	E938.5	E950.4	E962.0	E980.4
Stovarsal	961.1	E857	E931.1	E950.4	E962.0	E980.4
Stove gas — *see* Gas, utility						
Stoxil	976.5	E858.7	E946.5	E950.4	E962.0	E980.4
STP	969.6	E854.1	E939.6	E950.3	E962.0	E980.3
Stramonium (medicinal) NEC	971.1	E855.4	E941.1	E950.4	E962.0	E980.4
natural state	988.2	E865.4	—	E950.9	E962.1	E980.9
Streptodornase	964.4	E858.2	E934.4	E950.4	E962.0	E980.4
Streptoduocin	960.6	E856	E930.6	E950.4	E962.0	E980.4
Streptokinase	964.4	E858.2	E934.4	E950.4	E962.0	E980.4
Streptomycin	960.6	E856	E930.6	E950.4	E962.0	E980.4
Streptozocin	960.7	E856	E930.7	E950.4	E962.0	E980.4
Stripper (paint) (solvent)	982.8	E862.9	—	E950.9	E962.1	E980.9
Strobane	989.2	E863.0	—	E950.6	E962.1	E980.7
Strophanthin	972.1	E858.3	E942.1	E950.4	E962.0	E980.4
Strophanthus hispidus or kombe	988.2	E865.4	—	E950.9	E962.1	E980.9
Strychnine (rodenticide) (salts)	989.1	E863.7	—	E950.6	E962.1	E980.7
medicinal NEC	970.8	E854.3	E940.8	E950.4	E962.0	E980.4
Strychnos (ignatii) — *see* Strychnine						
Styramate	968.0	E855.1	E938.0	E950.4	E962.0	E980.4
Styrene	983.0	E864.0	—	E950.7	E962.1	E980.6
Succinimide (anticonvulsant)	966.2	E855.0	E936.2	E950.4	E962.0	E980.4
mercuric — *see* Mercury						
Succinylcholine	975.2	E858.6	E945.2	E950.4	E962.0	E980.4
Succinylsulfathiazole	961.0	E857	E931.0	E950.4	E962.0	E980.4
Sucrose	974.5	E858.5	E944.5	E950.4	E962.0	E980.4
Sulfacetamide	961.0	E857	E931.0	E950.4	E962.0	E980.4
ophthalmic preparation	976.5	E858.7	E946.5	E950.4	E962.0	E980.4
Sulfachlorpyridazine	961.0	E857	E931.0	E950.4	E962.0	E980.4
Sulfacytine	961.0	E857	E931.0	E950.4	E962.0	E980.4
Sulfadiazine	961.0	E857	E931.0	E950.4	E962.0	E980.4
silver (topical)	976.0	E858.7	E946.0	E950.4	E962.0	E980.4
Sulfadimethoxine	961.0	E857	E931.0	E950.4	E962.0	E980.4
Sulfadimidine	961.0	E857	E931.0	E950.4	E962.0	E980.4
Sulfaethidole	961.0	E857	E931.0	E950.4	E962.0	E980.4
Sulfafurazole	961.0	E857	E931.0	E950.4	E962.0	E980.4
Sulfaguanidine	961.0	E857	E931.0	E950.4	E962.0	E980.4
Sulfamerazine	961.0	E857	E931.0	E950.4	E962.0	E980.4
Sulfameter	961.0	E857	E931.0	E950.4	E962.0	E980.4
Sulfamethizole	961.0	E857	E931.0	E950.4	E962.0	E980.4
Sulfamethoxazole	961.0	E857	E931.0	E950.4	E962.0	E980.4
Sulfamethoxydiazine	961.0	E857	E931.0	E950.4	E962.0	E980.4
Sulfamethoxypyridazine	961.0	E857	E931.0	E950.4	E962.0	E980.4
Sulfamethylthiazole	961.0	E857	E931.0	E950.4	E962.0	E980.4
Sulfamylon	976.0	E858.7	E946.0	E950.4	E962.0	E980.4
Sulfan blue (diagnostic dye)	977.8	E858.8	E947.8	E950.4	E962.0	E980.4
Sulfanilamide	961.0	E857	E931.0	E950.4	E962.0	E980.4
Sulfanilylguanidine	961.0	E857	E931.0	E950.4	E962.0	E980.4
Sulfaphenazole	961.0	E857	E931.0	E950.4	E962.0	E980.4
Sulfaphenylthiazole	961.0	E857	E931.0	E950.4	E962.0	E980.4
Sulfaproxyline	961.0	E857	E931.0	E950.4	E962.0	E980.4
Sulfapyridine	961.0	E857	E931.0	E950.4	E962.0	E980.4
Sulfapyrimidine	961.0	E857	E931.0	E950.4	E962.0	E980.4
Sulfarsphenamine	961.1	E857	E931.1	E950.4	E962.0	E980.4

Table of Drugs and Chemicals

		External Cause (E-Code)				
	Poisoning	Accident	Therapeutic Use	Suicide Attempt	Assault	Undetermined
Sulfasalazine	961.0	E857	E931.0	E950.4	E962.0	E980.4
Sulfasomizole	961.0	E857	E931.0	E950.4	E962.0	E980.4
Sulfasuxidine	961.0	E857	E931.0	E950.4	E962.0	E980.4
Sulfinpyrazone	974.7	E858.5	E944.7	E950.4	E962.0	E980.4
Sulfisoxazole	961.0	E857	E931.0	E950.4	E962.0	E980.4
ophthalmic preparation	976.5	E858.7	E946.5	E950.4	E962.0	E980.4
Sulfomyxin	960.8	E856	E930.8	E950.4	E962.0	E980.4
Sulfonal	967.8	E852.8	E937.8	E950.2	E962.0	E980.2
Sulfonamides (mixtures)	961.0	E857	E931.0	E950.4	E962.0	E980.4
Sulfones	961.8	E857	E931.8	E950.4	E962.0	E980.4
Sulfonethylmethane	967.8	E852.8	E937.8	E950.2	E962.0	E980.2
Sulfonmethane	967.8	E852.8	E937.8	E950.2	E962.0	E980.2
Sulfonphthal, sulfonphthol	977.8	E858.8	E947.8	E950.4	E962.0	E980.4
Sulfonylurea derivatives, oral	962.3	E858.0	E932.3	E950.4	E962.0	E980.4
Sulfoxone	961.8	E857	E931.8	E950.4	E962.0	E980.4
Sulfur, sulfureted, sulfuric, sulfurous, sulfuryl (compounds) NEC	989.89	E866.8	—	E950.9	E962.1	E980.9
acid	983.1	E864.1	—	E950.7	E962.1	E980.6
dioxide	987.3	E869.1	—	E952.8	E962.2	E982.8
ether — see Ether(s)						
hydrogen	987.8	E869.8	—	E952.8	E962.2	E982.8
medicinal (keratolytic) (ointment) NEC	976.4	E858.7	E946.4	E950.4	E962.0	E980.4
pesticide (vapor)	989.4	E863.4	—	E950.6	E962.1	E980.7
vapor NEC	987.8	E869.8	—	E952.8	E962.2	E982.8
Sulkowitch's reagent	977.8	E858.8	E947.8	E950.4	E962.0	E980.4
Sulph — see also Sulf-						
Sulphadione	961.8	E857	E931.8	E950.4	E962.0	E980.4
Sulthiame, sultiame	966.3	E855.0	E936.3	E950.4	E962.0	E980.4
Superinone	975.5	E858.6	E945.5	E950.4	E962.0	E980.4
Suramin	961.5	E857	E931.5	E950.4	E962.0	E980.4
Surfacaine	968.5	E855.2	E938.5	E950.4	E962.0	E980.4
Surital	968.3	E855.1	E938.3	E950.4	E962.0	E980.4
Sutilains	976.8	E858.7	E946.8	E950.4	E962.0	E980.4
Suxamethonium (bromide) (chloride) (iodide)	975.2	E858.6	E945.2	E950.4	E962.0	E980.4
Suxethonium (bromide)	975.2	E858.6	E945.2	E950.4	E962.0	E980.4
Sweet oil (birch)	976.3	E858.7	E946.3	E950.4	E962.0	E980.4
Sym-dichloroethyl ether	982.3	E862.4	—	E950.9	E962.1	E980.9
Sympatholytics	971.3	E855.6	E941.3	E950.4	E962.0	E980.4
Sympathomimetics	971.2	E855.5	E941.2	E950.4	E962.0	E980.4
Synagis	979.6 ▲	E858.8	E949.6	E950.4	E962.0	E980.4
Synalar	976.0	E858.7	E946.0	E950.4	E962.0	E980.4
Synthroid	962.7	E858.0	E932.7	E950.4	E962.0	E980.4
Syntocinon	975.0	E858.6	E945.0	E950.4	E962.0	E950.4
Syrosingopine	972.6	E858.3	E942.6	E950.4	E962.0	E980.4
Systemic agents (primarily)	963.9	E858.1	E933.9	E950.4	E962.0	E980.4
specified NEC	963.8	E858.1	E933.8	E950.4	E962.0	E980.4
Tablets (see also specified substance)	977.9	E858.9	E947.9	E950.5	E962.0	E980.5
Tace	962.2	E858.0	E932.2	E950.4	E962.0	E980.4
Tacrine	971.0	E855.3	E941.0	E950.4	E962.0	E980.4
Talbutal	967.0	E851	E937.0	E950.1	E962.0	E980.1
Talc	976.3	E858.7	E946.3	E950.4	E962.0	E980.4
Talcum	976.3	E858.7	E946.3	E950.4	E962.0	E980.4
Tandearil, tanderil	965.5	E850.5	E935.5	E950.0	E962.0	E980.0
Tannic acid	983.1	E864.1	—	E950.7	E962.1	E980.6
medicinal (astringent)	976.2	E858.7	E946.2	E950.4	E962.0	E980.4
Tannin — see Tannic acid						
Tansy	988.2	E865.4	—	E950.9	E962.1	E980.9
TAO	960.3	E856	E930.3	E950.4	E962.0	E980.4
Tapazole	962.8	E858.0	E932.8	E950.4	E962.0	E980.4

✓4ᵗʰ Fourth-digit Required   ✓5ᵗʰ Fifth-digit Required

Table of Drugs and Chemicals

			External Cause (E-Code)			
	Poisoning	Accident	Therapeutic Use	Suicide Attempt	Assault	Undetermined
Tar NEC	983.0	E864.0	—	E950.7	E962.1	E980.6
camphor — see Naphthalene						
fumes	987.8	E869.8	—	E952.8	E962.2	E982.8
Taractan	969.3	E853.8	E939.3	E950.3	E962.0	E980.3
Tarantula (venomous)	989.5	E905.1	—	E950.9	E962.1	E980.9
Tartar emetic (anti-infective)	961.2	E857	E931.2	E950.4	E962.0	E980.4
Tartaric acid	983.1	E864.1	—	E950.7	E962.1	E980.6
Tartrated antimony (anti-infective)	961.2	E857	E931.2	E950.4	E962.0	E980.4
TCA — see **Trichloroacetic acid**						
TDI	983.0	E864.0	—	E950.7	E962.1	E980.6
vapor	987.8	E869.8	—	E952.8	E962.2	E982.8
Tear gas	987.5	E869.3	—	E952.8	E962.2	E982.8
Teclothiazide	974.3	E858.5	E944.3	E950.4	E962.0	E980.4
Tegretol	966.3	E855.0	E936.3	E950.4	E962.0	E980.4
Telepaque	977.8	E858.8	E947.8	E950.4	E962.0	E980.4
Tellurium	985.8	E866.4	—	E950.9	E962.1	E980.9
fumes	985.8	E866.4	—	E950.9	E962.1	E980.9
TEM	963.1	E858.1	E933.1	E950.4	E962.0	E980.4
Temazepan — see **Benzodiazepines**						
TEPA	963.1	E858.1	E933.1	E950.4	E962.0	E980.4
TEPP	989.3	E863.1	—	E950.6	E962.1	E980.7
Terbutaline	971.2	E855.5	E941.2	E950.4	E962.0	E980.4
Teroxalene	961.6	E857	E931.6	E950.4	E962.0	E980.4
Terpin hydrate	975.5	E858.6	E945.5	E950.4	E962.0	E980.4
Terramycin	960.4	E856	E930.4	E950.4	E962.0	E980.4
Tessalon	975.4	E858.6	E945.4	E950.4	E962.0	E980.4
Testosterone	962.1	E858.0	E932.1	E950.4	E962.0	E980.4
Tetanus (vaccine)	978.4	E858.8	E948.4	E950.4	E962.0	E980.4
antitoxin	979.9	E858.8	E949.9	E950.4	E962.0	E980.4
immune globulin (human)	964.6	E858.2	E934.6	E950.4	E962.0	E980.4
toxoid	978.4	E858.8	E948.4	E950.4	E962.0	E980.4
with diphtheria toxoid	978.9	E858.8	E948.9	E950.4	E962.0	E980.4
with pertussis	978.6	E858.8	E948.6	E950.4	E962.0	E980.4
Tetrabenazine	969.5	E853.8	E939.5	E950.3	E962.0	E980.3
Tetracaine (infiltration) (topical)	968.5	E855.2	E938.5	E950.4	E962.0	E980.4
nerve block (peripheral) (plexus)	968.6	E855.2	E938.6	E950.4	E962.0	E980.4
spinal	968.7	E855.2	E938.7	E950.4	E962.0	E980.4
Tetrachlorethylene — see **Tetrachloroethylene**						
Tetrachlormethiazide	974.3	E858.5	E944.3	E950.4	E962.0	E980.4
Tetrachloroethane (liquid) (vapor)	982.3	E862.4	—	E950.9	E962.1	E980.9
paint or varnish	982.3	E861.6	—	E950.9	E962.1	E980.9
Tetrachloroethylene (liquid) (vapor)	982.3	E862.4	—	E950.9	E962.1	E980.9
medicinal	961.6	E857	E931.6	E950.4	E962.0	E980.4
Tetrachloromethane — see **Carbon, tetrachloride**						
Tetracycline	960.4	E856	E930.4	E950.4	E962.0	E980.4
ophthalmic preparation	976.5	E858.7	E946.5	E950.4	E962.0	E980.4
topical NEC	976.0	E858.7	E946.0	E950.4	E962.0	E980.4
Tetraethylammonium chloride	972.3	E858.3	E942.3	E950.4	E962.0	E980.4
Tetraethyl lead (antiknock compound)	984.1			E950.9	E962.1	E980.9
Tetraethyl pyrophosphate	989.3	E863.1	—	E950.6	E962.1	E980.7
Tetraethylthiuram disulfide	977.3	E858.8	E947.3	E950.4	E962.0	E980.4
Tetrahydroaminoacridine	971.0	E855.3	E941.0	E950.4	E962.0	E980.4
Tetrahydrocannabinol	969.6	E854.1	E939.6	E950.3	E962.0	E980.3
Tetrahydronaphthalene	982.0	E862.4	—	E950.9	E962.1	E980.9
Tetrahydrozoline	971.2	E855.5	E941.2	E950.4	E962.0	E980.4

Table of Drugs and Chemicals

	External Cause (E-Code)					
	Poisoning	Accident	Therapeutic Use	Suicide Attempt	Assault	Undetermined
Tetralin	982.0	E862.4	—	E950.9	E962.1	E980.9
Tetramethylthiuram (disulfide)						
NEC	989.4	E863.6	—	E950.6	E962.1	E980.7
medicinal	976.2	E858.7	E946.2	E950.4	E962.0	E980.4
Tetronal	967.8	E852.8	E937.8	E950.2	E962.0	E980.2
Tetryl	983.0	E864.0	—	E950.7	E962.1	E980.6
Thalidomide	967.8	E852.8	E937.8	E950.2	E962.0	E980.2
Thallium (compounds) (dust)						
NEC	985.8	E866.4	—	E950.9	E962.1	E980.9
pesticide (rodenticide)	985.8	E863.7	—	E950.6	E962.1	E980.7
THC	969.6	E854.1	E939.6	E950.3	E962.0	E980.3
Thebacon	965.09	E850.2	E935.2	E950.0	E962.0	E980.0
Thebaine	965.09	E850.2	E935.2	E950.0	E962.0	E980.0
Theobromine (calcium salicylate)	974.1	E858.5	E944.1	E950.4	E962.0	E980.4
Theophylline (diuretic)	974.1	E858.5	E944.1	E950.4	E962.0	E980.4
ethylenediamine	975.7	E858.6	E945.7	E950.4	E962.0	E980.4
Thiabendazole	961.6	E857	E931.6	E950.4	E962.0	E980.4
Thialbarbital, thialbarbitone	968.3	E855.1	E938.3	E950.4	E962.0	E980.4
Thiamine	963.5	E858.1	E933.5	E950.4	E962.0	E980.4
Thiamylal (sodium)	968.3	E855.1	E938.3	E950.4	E962.0	E980.4
Thiazesim	969.0	E854.0	E939.0	E950.3	E962.0	E980.3
Thiazides (diuretics)	974.3	E858.5	E944.3	E950.4	E962.0	E980.4
Thiethylperazine	963.0	E858.1	E933.0	E950.4	E962.0	E980.4
Thimerosal (topical)	976.0	E858.7	E946.0	E950.4	E962.0	E980.4
ophthalmic preparation	976.5	E858.7	E946.5	E950.4	E962.0	E980.4
Thioacetazone	961.8	E857	E931.8	E950.4	E962.0	E980.4
Thiobarbiturates	968.3	E855.1	E938.3	E950.4	E962.0	E980.4
Thiobismol	961.2	E857	E931.2	E950.4	E962.0	E980.4
Thiocarbamide	962.8	E858.0	E932.8	E950.4	E962.0	E980.4
Thiocarbarsone	961.1	E857	E931.1	E950.4	E962.0	E980.4
Thiocarlide	961.8	E857	E931.8	E950.4	E962.0	E980.4
Thioguanine	963.1	E858.1	E933.1	E950.4	E962.0	E980.4
Thiomercaptomerin	974.0	E858.5	E944.0	E950.4	E962.0	E980.4
Thiomerin	974.0	E858.5	E944.0	E950.4	E962.0	E980.4
Thiopental, thiopentone (sodium)	968.3	E855.1	E938.3	E950.4	E962.0	E980.4
Thiopropazate	969.1	E853.0	E939.1	E950.3	E962.0	E980.3
Thioproperazine	969.1	E853.0	E939.1	E950.3	E962.0	E980.3
Thioridazine	969.1	E853.0	E939.1	E950.3	E962.0	E980.3
Thio-TEPA, thiotepa	963.1	E858.1	E933.1	E950.4	E962.0	E980.4
Thiothixene	969.3	E853.8	E939.3	E950.3	E962.0	E980.3
Thiouracil	962.8	E858.0	E932.8	E950.4	E962.0	E980.4
Thiourea	962.8	E858.0	E932.8	E950.4	E962.0	E980.4
Thiphenamil	971.1	E855.4	E941.1	E950.4	E962.0	E980.4
Thiram NEC	989.4	E863.6	—	E950.6	E962.1	E980.7
medicinal	976.2	E858.7	E946.2	E950.4	E962.0	E980.4
Thonzylamine	963.0	E858.1	E933.0	E950.4	E962.0	E980.4
Thorazine	969.1	E853.0	E939.1	E950.3	E962.0	E980.3
Thornapple	988.2	E865.4	—	E950.9	E962.1	E980.9
Throat preparation (lozenges) NEC	976.6	E858.7	E946.6	E950.4	E962.0	E980.4
Thrombin	964.5	E858.2	E934.5	E950.4	E962.0	E980.4
Thrombolysin	964.4	E858.2	E934.4	E950.4	E962.0	E980.4
Thymol	983.0	E864.0	—	E950.7	E962.1	E980.6
Thymus extract	962.9	E858.0	E932.9	E950.4	E962.0	E980.4
Thyroglobulin	962.7	E858.0	E932.7	E950.4	E962.0	E980.4
Thyroid (derivatives) (extract)	962.7	E858.0	E932.7	E950.4	E962.0	E980.4
Thyrolar	962.7	E858.0	E932.7	E950.4	E962.0	E980.4
Thyrothrophin, thyrotropin	977.8	E858.8	E947.8	E950.4	E962.0	E980.4
Thyroxin(e)	962.7	E858.0	E932.7	E950.4	E962.0	E980.4
Tigan	963.0	E858.1	E933.0	E950.4	E962.0	E980.4
Tigloidine	968.0	E855.1	E938.0	E950.4	E962.0	E980.4

Fourth-digit Required   Fifth-digit Required

Table of Drugs and Chemicals

		External Cause (E-Code)				
	Poisoning	Accident	Therapeutic Use	Suicide Attempt	Assault	Undetermined
Tin (chloride) (dust) (oxide)						
NEC	985.8	E866.4	—	E950.9	E962.1	E980.9
anti-infectives	961.2	E857	E931.2	E950.4	E962.0	E980.4
Tinactin	976.0	E858.7	E946.0	E950.4	E962.0	E980.4
Tincture, iodine — *see* **Iodine**						
Tindal	969.1	E853.0	E939.1	E950.3	E962.0	E980.3
Titanium (compounds) (vapor)	985.8	E866.4	—	E950.9	E962.1	E980.9
ointment	976.3	E858.7	E946.3	E950.4	E962.0	E980.4
Titroid	962.7	E858.0	E932.7	E950.4	E962.0	E980.4
TMTD — *see* **Tetramethylthiuram disulfide**						
TNT	989.89	E866.8	—	E950.9	E962.1	E980.9
fumes	987.8	E869.8	—	E952.8	E962.2	E982.8
Toadstool	988.1	E865.5	—	E950.9	E962.1	E980.9
Tobacco NEC	989.84	E866.8	—	E950.9	E962.1	E980.9
Indian	988.2	E865.4	—	E950.9	E962.1	E980.9
smoke, second-hand	987.8	E869.4	—	—	—	—
Tocopherol	963.5	E858.1	E933.5	E950.4	E962.0	E980.4
Tocosamine	975.0	E858.6	E945.0	E950.4	E962.0	E980.4
Tofranil	969.0	E854.0	E939.0	E950.3	E962.0	E980.3
Toilet deodorizer	989.89	E866.8	—	E950.9	E962.1	E980.9
Tolazamide	962.3	E858.0	E932.3	E950.4	E962.0	E980.4
Tolazoline	971.3	E855.6	E941.3	E950.4	E962.0	E980.4
Tolbutamide	962.3	E858.0	E932.3	E950.4	E962.0	E980.4
sodium	977.8	E858.8	E947.8	E950.4	E962.0	E980.4
Tolmetin	965.69	E850.6	E935.6	E950.0	E962.0	E980.0
Tolnaftate	976.0	E858.7	E946.0	E950.4	E962.0	E980.4
Tolpropamine	976.1	E858.7	E946.1	E950.4	E962.0	E980.4
Tolserol	968.0	E855.1	E938.0	E950.4	E962.0	E980.4
Toluene (liquid) (vapor)	982.0	E862.4	—	E950.9	E962.1	E980.9
diisocyanate	983.0	E864.0	—	E950.7	E962.1	E980.6
Toluidine	983.0	E864.0	—	E950.7	E962.1	E980.6
vapor	987.8	E869.8	—	E952.8	E962.2	E982.8
Toluol (liquid) (vapor)	982.0	E862.4	—	E950.9	E962.1	E980.9
Tolylene-2, 4-diisocyanate	983.0	E864.0	—	E950.7	E962.1	E980.6
Tonics, cardiac	972.1	E858.3	E942.1	E950.4	E962.0	E980.4
Toxaphene (dust) (spray)	989.2	E863.0	—	E950.6	E962.1	E980.7
Toxoids NEC	978.8	E858.8	E948.8	E950.4	E962.0	E980.4
Tractor fuel NEC	981	E862.1	—	E950.9	E962.1	E980.9
Tragacanth	973.3	E858.4	E943.3	E950.4	E962.0	E980.4
Tramazoline	971.2	E855.5	E941.2	E950.4	E962.0	E980.4
Tranquilizers	969.5	E853.9	E939.5	E950.3	E962.0	E980.3
benzodiazepine-based	969.4	E853.2	E939.4	E950.3	E962.0	E980.3
butyrophenone-based	969.2	E853.1	E939.2	E950.3	E962.0	E980.3
major NEC	969.3	E853.8	E939.3	E950.3	E962.0	E980.3
phenothiazine-based	969.1	E853.0	E939.1	E950.3	E962.0	E980.3
specified NEC	969.5	E853.8	E939.5	E950.3	E962.0	E980.3
Trantoin	961.9	E857	E931.9	E950.4	E962.0	E980.4
Tranxene	969.4	E853.2	E939.4	E950.3	E962.0	E980.3
Tranylcypromine (sulfate)	969.0	E854.0	E939.0	E950.3	E962.0	E980.3
Trasentine	975.1	E858.6	E945.1	E950.4	E962.0	E980.4
Travert	974.5	E858.5	E944.5	E950.4	E962.0	E980.4
Trecator	961.8	E857	E931.8	E950.4	E962.0	E980.4
Tretinoin	976.8	E858.7	E946.8	E950.4	E962.0	E980.4
Triacetin	976.0	E858.7	E946.0	E950.4	E962.0	E980.4
Triacetyloleandomycin	960.3	E856	E930.3	E950.4	E962.0	E980.4
Triamcinolone	962.0	E858.0	E932.0	E950.4	E962.0	E980.4
ENT agent	976.6	E858.7	E946.6	E950.4	E962.0	E980.4
ophthalmic preparation	976.5	E858.7	E946.5	E950.4	E962.0	E980.4
topical NEC	976.0	E858.7	E946.0	E950.4	E962.0	E980.4
Triamterene	974.4	E858.5	E944.4	E950.4	E962.0	E980.4
Triaziquone	963.1	E858.1	E933.1	E950.4	E962.0	E980.4
Tribromacetaldehyde	967.3	E852.2	E937.3	E950.2	E962.0	E980.2

Table of Drugs and Chemicals — Tropicamide

		External Cause (E-Code)				
	Poisoning	Accident	Therapeutic Use	Suicide Attempt	Assault	Undetermined
Tribromoethanol	968.2	E855.1	E938.2	E950.4	E962.0	E980.4
Tribromomethane	967.3	E852.2	E937.3	E950.2	E962.0	E980.2
Trichlorethane	982.3	E862.4	—	E950.9	E962.1	E980.9
Trichlormethiazide	974.3	E858.5	E944.3	E950.4	E962.0	E980.4
Trichloroacetic acid	983.1	E864.1	—	E950.7	E962.1	E980.6
medicinal (keratolytic)	976.4	E858.7	E946.4	E950.4	E962.0	E980.4
Trichloroethanol	967.1	E852.0	E937.1	E950.2	E962.0	E980.2
Trichloroethylene (liquid)						
(vapor)	982.3	E862.4	—	E950.9	E962.1	E980.9
anesthetic (gas)	968.2	E855.1	E938.2	E950.4	E962.0	E980.4
Trichloroethyl phosphate	967.1	E852.0	E937.1	E950.2	E962.0	E980.2
Trichlorofluoromethane NEC	987.4	E869.2	—	E952.8	E962.2	E982.8
Trichlorotriethylamine	963.1	E858.1	E933.1	E950.4	E962.0	E980.4
Trichomonacides NEC	961.5	E857	E931.5	E950.4	E962.0	E980.4
Trichomycin	960.1	E856	E930.1	E950.4	E962.0	E980.4
Triclofos	967.1	E852.0	E937.1	E950.2	E962.0	E980.2
Tricresyl phosphate	989.89	E866.8	—	E950.9	E962.1	E980.9
solvent	982.8	E862.4	—	E950.9	E962.1	E980.9
Tricyclamol	966.4	E855.0	E936.4	E950.4	E962.0	E980.4
Tridesilon	976.0	E858.7	E946.0	E950.4	E962.0	E980.4
Tridihexethyl	971.1	E855.4	E941.1	E950.4	E962.0	E980.4
Tridione	966.0	E855.0	E936.0	E950.4	E962.0	E980.4
Triethanolamine NEC	983.2	E864.2	—	E950.7	E962.1	E980.6
detergent	983.2	E861.0	—	E950.7	E962.1	E980.6
trinitrate	972.4	E858.3	E942.4	E950.4	E962.0	E980.4
Triethanomelamine	963.1	E858.1	E933.1	E950.4	E962.0	E980.4
Triethylene melamine	963.1	E858.1	E933.1	E950.4	E962.0	E980.4
Triethylenephosphoramide	963.1	E858.1	E933.1	E950.4	E962.0	E980.4
Triethylenethiophosphoramide	963.1	E858.1	E933.1	E950.4	E962.0	E980.4
Trifluoperazine	969.1	E853.0	E939.1	E950.3	E962.0	E980.3
Trifluperidol	969.2	E853.1	E939.2	E950.3	E962.0	E980.3
Triflupromazine	969.1	E853.0	E939.1	E950.3	E962.0	E980.3
Trihexyphenidyl	971.1	E855.4	E941.1	E950.4	E962.0	E980.4
Triiodothyronine	962.7	E858.0	E932.7	E950.4	E962.0	E980.4
Trilene	968.2	E855.1	E938.2	E950.4	E962.0	E980.4
Trimeprazine	963.0	E858.1	E933.0	E950.4	E962.0	E980.4
Trimetazidine	972.4	E858.3	E942.4	E950.4	E962.0	E980.4
Trimethadione	966.0	E855.0	E936.0	E950.4	E962.0	E980.4
Trimethaphan	972.3	E858.3	E942.3	E950.4	E962.0	E980.4
Trimethidinium	972.3	E858.3	E942.3	E950.4	E962.0	E980.4
Trimethobenzamide	963.0	E858.1	E933.0	E950.4	E962.0	E980.4
Trimethylcarbinol	980.8	E860.8	—	E950.9	E962.1	E980.9
Trimethylpsoralen	976.3	E858.7	E946.3	E950.4	E962.0	E980.4
Trimeton	963.0	E858.1	E933.0	E950.4	E962.0	E980.4
Trimipramine	969.0	E854.0	E939.0	E950.3	E962.0	E980.3
Trimustine	963.1	E858.1	E933.1	E950.4	E962.0	E980.4
Trinitrin	972.4	E858.3	E942.4	E950.4	E962.0	E980.4
Trinitrophenol	983.0	E864.0	—	E950.7	E962.1	E980.6
Trinitrotoluene	989.89	E866.8	—	E950.9	E962.1	E980.9
fumes	987.8	E869.8	—	E952.8	E962.2	E982.8
Trional	967.8	E852.8	E937.8	E950.2	E962.0	E980.2
Trioxide of arsenic — see Arsenic						
Trioxsalen	976.3	E858.7	E946.3	E950.4	E962.0	E980.4
Tripelennamine	963.0	E858.1	E933.0	E950.4	E962.0	E980.4
Triperidol	969.2	E853.1	E939.2	E950.3	E962.0	E980.3
Triprolidine	963.0	E858.1	E933.0	E950.4	E962.0	E980.4
Trisoralen	976.3	E858.7	E946.3	E950.4	E962.0	E980.4
Troleandomycin	960.3	E856	E930.3	E950.4	E962.0	E980.4
Trolnitrate (phosphate)	972.4	E858.3	E942.4	E950.4	E962.0	E980.4
Trometamol	963.3	E858.1	E933.3	E950.4	E962.0	E980.4
Tromethamine	963.3	E858.1	E933.3	E950.4	E962.0	E980.4
Tronothane	968.5	E855.2	E938.5	E950.4	E962.0	E980.4
Tropicamide	971.1	E855.4	E941.1	E950.4	E962.0	E980.4

Fourth-digit Required   Fifth-digit Required

Troxidone — Table of Drugs and Chemicals

		External Cause (E-Code)				
	Poisoning	Accident	Therapeutic Use	Suicide Attempt	Assault	Undetermined
Troxidone	966.0	E855.0	E936.0	E950.4	E962.0	E980.4
Tryparsamide	961.1	E857	E931.1	E950.4	E962.0	E980.4
Trypsin	963.4	E858.1	E933.4	E950.4	E962.0	E980.4
Tryptizol	969.0	E854.0	E939.0	E950.3	E962.0	E980.3
Tuaminoheptane	971.2	E855.5	E941.2	E950.4	E962.0	E980.4
Tuberculin (old)	977.8	E858.8	E947.8	E950.4	E962.0	E980.4
Tubocurare	975.2	E858.6	E945.2	E950.4	E962.0	E980.4
Tubocurarine	975.2	E858.6	E945.2	E950.4	E962.0	E980.4
Turkish green	969.6	E854.1	E939.6	E950.3	E962.0	E980.3
Turpentine (spirits of) (liquid) (vapor)	982.8	E862.4	—	E950.9	E962.1	E980.9
Tybamate	969.5	E853.8	E939.5	E950.3	E962.0	E980.3
Tyloxapol	975.5	E858.6	E945.5	E950.4	E962.0	E980.4
Tymazoline	971.2	E855.5	E941.2	E950.4	E962.0	E980.4
Typhoid vaccine	978.1	E858.8	E948.1	E950.4	E962.0	E980.4
Typhus vaccine	979.2	E858.8	E949.2	E950.4	E962.0	E980.4
Tyrothricin	976.0	E858.7	E946.0	E950.4	E962.0	E980.4
ENT agent	976.6	E858.7	E946.6	E950.4	E962.0	E980.4
ophthalmic preparation	976.5	E858.7	E946.5	E950.4	E962.0	E980.4
Undecenoic acid	976.0	E858.7	E946.0	E950.4	E962.0	E980.4
Undecylenic acid	976.0	E858.7	E946.0	E950.4	E962.0	E980.4
Unna's boot	976.3	E858.7	E946.3	E950.4	E962.0	E980.4
Uracil mustard	963.1	E858.1	E933.1	E950.4	E962.0	E980.4
Uramustine	963.1	E858.1	E933.1	E950.4	E962.0	E980.4
Urari	975.2	E858.6	E945.2	E950.4	E962.0	E980.4
Urea	974.4	E858.5	E944.4	E950.4	E962.0	E980.4
topical	976.8	E858.7	E946.8	E950.4	E962.0	E980.4
Urethan(e) (antineoplastic)	963.1	E858.1	E933.1	E950.4	E962.0	E980.4
Urginea (maritima) (scilla) — see Squill						
Uric acid metabolism agents NEC	974.7	E858.5	E944.7	E950.4	E962.0	E980.4
Urokinase	964.4	E858.2	E934.4	E950.4	E962.0	E980.4
Urokon	977.8	E858.8	E947.8	E950.4	E962.0	E980.4
Urotropin	961.9	E857	E931.9	E950.4	E962.0	E980.4
Urtica	988.2	E865.4	—	E950.9	E962.1	E980.9
Utility gas — see Gas, utility						
Vaccine NEC	979.9	E858.8	E949.9	E950.4	E962.0	E980.4
bacterial NEC	978.8	E858.8	E948.8	E950.4	E962.0	E980.4
with other bacterial component	978.9	E858.8	E948.9	E950.4	E962.0	E980.4
pertussis component	978.6	E858.8	E948.6	E950.4	E962.0	E980.4
viral-rickettsial component	979.7	E858.8	E949.7	E950.4	E962.0	E980.4
mixed NEC	978.9	E858.8	E948.9	E950.4	E962.0	E980.4
BCG	978.0	E858.8	E948.0	E950.4	E962.0	E980.4
cholera	978.2	E858.8	E948.2	E950.4	E962.0	E980.4
diphtheria	978.5	E858.8	E948.5	E950.4	E962.0	E980.4
influenza	979.6	E858.8	E949.6	E950.4	E962.0	E980.4
measles	979.4	E858.8	E949.4	E950.4	E962.0	E980.4
meningococcal	978.8	E858.8	E948.8	E950.4	E962.0	E980.4
mumps	979.6	E858.8	E949.6	E950.4	E962.0	E980.4
paratyphoid	978.1	E858.8	E948.1	E950.4	E962.0	E980.4
pertussis (with diphtheria toxoid) (with tetanus toxoid)	978.6	E858.8	E948.6	E950.4	E962.0	E980.4
plague	978.3	E858.8	E948.3	E950.4	E962.0	E980.4
poliomyelitis	979.5	E858.8	E949.5	E950.4	E962.0	E980.4
poliovirus	979.5	E858.8	E949.5	E950.4	E962.0	E980.4
rabies	979.1	E858.8	E949.1	E950.4	E962.0	E980.4
respiratory syncytial virus	979.6 ▲	E858.8	E949.6	E950.4	E962.0	E980.4

Table of Drugs and Chemicals

	External Cause (E-Code)					
	Poisoning	Accident	Therapeutic Use	Suicide Attempt	Assault	Undetermined
Vaccine — *continued*						
rickettsial NEC	979.6	E858.8	E949.6	E950.4	E962.0	E980.4
with						
bacterial component	979.7	E858.8	E949.7	E950.4	E962.0	E980.4
pertussis component	978.6	E858.8	E948.6	E950.4	E962.0	E980.4
viral component	979.7	E858.8	E949.7	E950.4	E962.0	E980.4
Rocky mountain spotted fever	979.6	E858.8	E949.6	E950.4	E962.0	E980.4
rotavirus	979.6	E858.8	E949.6	E950.4	E962.0	E980.4
rubella virus	979.4	E858.8	E949.4	E950.4	E962.0	E980.4
sabin oral	979.5	E858.8	E949.5	E950.4	E962.0	E980.4
smallpox	979.0	E858.8	E949.0	E950.4	E962.0	E980.4
tetanus	978.4	E858.8	E948.4	E950.4	E962.0	E980.4
typhoid	978.1	E858.8	E948.1	E950.4	E962.0	E980.4
typhus	979.2	E858.8	E949.2	E950.4	E962.0	E980.4
viral NEC	979.6	E858.8	E949.6	E950.4	E962.0	E980.4
with						
bacterial component	979.7	E858.8	E949.7	E950.4	E962.0	E980.4
pertussis component	978.6	E858.8	E948.6	E950.4	E962.0	E980.4
rickettsial component	979.7	E858.8	E949.7	E950.4	E962.0	E980.4
yellow fever	979.3	E858.8	E949.3	E950.4	E962.0	E980.4
Vaccinia immune globulin (human)	964.6	E858.2	E934.6	E950.4	E962.0	E980.4
Vaginal contraceptives	976.8	E858.7	E946.8	E950.4	E962.0	E980.4
Valethamate	971.1	E855.4	E941.1	E950.4	E962.0	E980.4
Valisone	976.0	E858.7	E946.0	E950.4	E962.0	E980.4
Valium	969.4	E853.2	E939.4	E950.3	E962.0	E980.3
Valmid	967.8	E852.8	E937.8	E950.2	E962.0	E980.2
Vanadium	985.8	E866.4	—	E950.9	E962.1	E980.9
Vancomycin	960.8	E856	E930.8	E950.4	E962.0	E980.4
Vapor (*see also* **Gas**)	987.9	E869.9	—	E952.9	E962.2	E982.9
kiln (carbon monoxide)	986	E868.8	—	E952.1	E962.2	E982.1
lead — *see* Lead						
specified source NEC (*see also* specific substance)	987.8	E869.8	—	E952.8	E962.2	E982.8
Varidase	964.4	E858.2	E934.4	E950.4	E962.0	E980.4
Varnish	989.89	E861.6	—	E950.9	E962.1	E980.9
cleaner	982.8	E862.9	—	E950.9	E962.1	E980.9
Vaseline	976.3	E858.7	E946.3	E950.4	E962.0	E980.4
Vasodilan	972.5	E858.3	E942.5	E950.4	E962.0	E980.4
Vasodilators NEC	972.5	E858.3	E942.5	E950.4	E962.0	E980.4
coronary	972.4	E858.3	E942.4	E950.4	E962.0	E980.4
Vasopressin	962.5	E858.0	E932.5	E950.4	E962.0	E980.4
Vasopressor drugs	962.5	E858.0	E932.5	E950.4	E962.0	E980.4
Venom, venomous (bite) (sting)	989.5	E905.9	—	E950.9	E962.1	E980.9
arthropod NEC	989.5	E905.5	—	E950.9	E962.1	E980.9
bee	989.5	E905.3	—	E950.9	E962.1	E980.9
centipede	989.5	E905.4	—	E950.9	E962.1	E980.9
hornet	989.5	E905.3	—	E950.9	E962.1	E980.9
lizard	989.5	E905.0	—	E950.9	E962.1	E980.9
marine animals or plants	989.5	E905.6	—	E950.9	E962.1	E980.9
millipede (tropical)	989.5	E905.4	—	E950.9	E962.1	E980.9
plant NEC	989.5	E905.7	—	E950.9	E962.1	E980.9
marine	989.5	E905.6	—	E950.9	E962.1	E980.9
scorpion	989.5	E905.2	—	E950.9	E962.1	E980.9
snake	989.5	E905.0	—	E950.9	E962.1	E980.9
specified NEC	989.5	E905.8	—	E950.9	E962.1	E980.9
spider	989.5	E905.1	—	E950.9	E962.1	E980.9
wasp	989.5	E905.3	—	E950.9	E962.1	E980.9
Veramon	967.0	E851	E937.0	E950.1	E962.0	E980.1
Veratrum						
album	988.2	E865.4	—	E950.9	E962.1	E980.9
alkaloids	972.6	E858.3	E942.6	E950.4	E962.0	E980.4

▸4▪ Fourth-digit Required   ▸5▪ Fifth-digit Required

Table of Drugs and Chemicals

	Poisoning	\multicolumn{5}{c}{External Cause (E-Code)}

	Poisoning	Accident	Therapeutic Use	Suicide Attempt	Assault	Undetermined
Veratrum — *continued*						
viride	988.2	E865.4	—	E950.9	E962.1	E980.9
Verdigris (see also Copper)	985.8	E866.4	—	E950.9	E962.1	E980.9
Veronal	967.0	E851	E937.0	E950.1	E962.0	E980.1
Veroxil	961.6	E857	E931.6	E950.4	E962.0	E980.4
Versidyne	965.7	E850.7	E935.7	E950.0	E962.0	E980.0
Viagra	972.5	E858.3	E942.5	E950.4	E962.0	E980.4
Vienna						
green	985.1	E866.3	—	E950.8	E962.1	E980.8
insecticide	985.1	E863.4	—	E950.6	E962.1	E980.7
red	989.89	E866.8	—	E950.9	E962.1	E980.9
pharmaceutical dye	977.4	E858.8	E947.4	E950.4	E962.0	E980.4
Vinbarbital, vinbarbitone	967.0	E851	E937.0	E950.1	E962.0	E980.1
Vinblastine	963.1	E858.1	E933.1	E950.4	E962.0	E980.4
Vincristine	963.1	E858.1	E933.1	E950.4	E962.0	E980.4
Vinesthene, vinethene	968.2	E855.1	E938.2	E950.4	E962.0	E980.4
Vinyl						
bital	967.0	E851	E937.0	E950.1	E962.0	E980.1
ether	968.2	E855.1	E938.2	E950.4	E962.0	E980.4
Vioform	961.3	E857	E931.3	E950.4	E962.0	E980.4
topical	976.0	E858.7	E946.0	E950.4	E962.0	E980.4
Viomycin	960.6	E856	E930.6	E950.4	E962.0	E980.4
Viosterol	963.5	E858.1	E933.5	E950.4	E962.0	E980.4
Viper (venom)	989.5	E905.0	—	E950.9	E962.1	E980.9
Viprynium (embonate)	961.6	E857	E931.6	E950.4	E962.0	E980.4
Virugon	961.7	E857	E931.7	E950.4	E962.0	E980.4
Visine	976.5	E858.7	E946.5	E950.4	E962.0	E980.4
Vitamins NEC	963.5	E858.1	E933.5	E950.4	E962.0	E980.4
B_{12}	964.1	E858.2	E934.1	E950.4	E962.0	E980.4
hematopoietic	964.1	E858.2	E934.1	E950.4	E962.0	E980.4
K	964.3	E858.2	E934.3	E950.4	E962.0	E980.4
Vleminckx's solution	976.4	E858.7	E946.4	E950.4	E962.0	E980.4
Voltaren — *see* Diclofenac sodium						
Ventolin — *see* Salbutamol sulfate						
Warfarin (potassium) (sodium)	964.2	E858.2	E934.2	E950.4	E962.0	E980.4
rodenticide	989.4	E863.7	—	E950.6	E962.1	E980.7
Wasp (sting)	989.5	E905.3	—	E950.9	E962.1	E980.9
Water						
balance agents NEC	974.5	E858.5	E944.5	E950.4	E962.0	E980.4
gas	987.1	E868.1	—	E951.8	E962.2	E981.8
incomplete combustion of — *see* Carbon, monoxide, fuel, utility						
hemlock	988.2	E865.4	—	E950.9	E962.1	E980.9
moccasin (venom)	989.5	E905.0	—	E950.9	E962.1	E980.9
Wax (paraffin) (petroleum)	981	E862.3	—	E950.9	E962.1	E980.9
automobile	989.89	E861.2	—	E950.9	E962.1	E980.9
floor	981	E862.0	—	E950.9	E962.1	E980.9
Weed killers NEC	989.4	E863.5	—	E950.6	E962.1	E980.7
Welldorm	967.1	E852.0	E937.1	E950.2	E962.0	E980.2
White						
arsenic — *see* Arsenic						
hellebore	988.2	E865.4	—	E950.9	E962.1	E980.9
lotion (keratolytic)	976.4	E858.7	E946.4	E950.4	E962.0	E980.4
spirit	981	E862.0	—	E950.9	E962.1	E980.9
Whitewashes	989.89	E861.6	—	E950.9	E962.1	E980.9
Whole blood	964.7	E858.2	E934.7	E950.4	E962.0	E980.4
Wild						
black cherry	988.2	E865.4	—	E950.9	E962.1	E980.9
poisonous plants NEC	988.2	E865.4	—	E950.9	E962.1	E980.9
Window cleaning fluid	989.89	E861.3	—	E950.9	E962.1	E980.9

▶◀ Revised Text   ● New Line   ▲ Revised Code

Table of Drugs and Chemicals

		External Cause (E-Code)				
	Poisoning	Accident	Therapeutic Use	Suicide Attempt	Assault	Undetermined
Wintergreen (oil)	976.3	E858.7	E946.3	E950.4	E962.0	E980.4
Witch hazel	976.2	E858.7	E946.2	E950.4	E962.0	E980.4
Wood						
alcohol	980.1	E860.2	—	E950.9	E962.1	E980.9
spirit	980.1	E860.2	—	E950.9	E962.1	E980.9
Woorali	975.2	E858.6	E945.2	E950.4	E962.0	E980.4
Wormseed, American	961.6	E857	E931.6	E950.4	E962.0	E980.4
Xanthine diuretics	974.1	E858.5	E944.1	E950.4	E962.0	E980.4
Xanthocillin	960.0	E856	E930.0	E950.4	E962.0	E980.4
Xanthotoxin	976.3	E858.7	E946.3	E950.4	E962.0	E980.4
Xylene (liquid) (vapor)	982.0	E862.4	—	E950.9	E962.1	E980.9
Xylocaine (infiltration) (topical)	968.5	E855.2	E938.5	E950.4	E962.0	E980.4
nerve block (peripheral) (plexus)	968.6	E855.2	E938.6	E950.4	E962.0	E980.4
spinal	968.7	E855.2	E938.7	E950.4	E962.0	E980.4
Xylol (liquid) (vapor)	982.0	E862.4	—	E950.9	E962.1	E980.9
Xylometazoline	971.2	E855.5	E941.2	E950.4	E962.0	E980.4
Yellow						
fever vaccine	979.3	E858.8	E949.3	E950.4	E962.0	E980.4
jasmine	988.2	E865.4	—	E950.9	E962.1	E980.9
Yew	988.2	E865.4	—	E950.9	E962.1	E980.9
Zactane	965.7	E850.7	E935.7	E950.0	E962.0	E980.0
Zaroxolyn	974.3	E858.5	E944.3	E950.4	E962.0	E980.4
Zephiran (topical)	976.0	E858.7	E946.0	E950.4	E962.0	E980.4
ophthalmic preparation	976.5	E858.7	E946.5	E950.4	E962.0	E980.4
Zerone	980.1	E860.2	—	E950.9	E962.1	E980.9
Zinc (compounds) (fumes) (salts) (vapor) NEC	985.8	E866.4	—	E950.9	E962.1	E980.9
anti-infectives	976.0	E858.7	E946.0	E950.4	E962.0	E980.4
antivaricose	972.7	E858.3	E942.7	E950.4	E962.0	E980.4
bacitracin	976.0	E858.7	E946.0	E950.4	E962.0	E980.4
chloride	976.2	E858.7	E946.2	E950.4	E962.0	E980.4
gelatin	976.3	E858.7	E946.3	E950.4	E962.0	E980.4
oxide	976.3	E858.7	E946.3	E950.4	E962.0	E980.4
peroxide	976.0	E858.7	E946.0	E950.4	E962.0	E980.4
pesticides	985.8	E863.4	—	E950.6	E962.1	E980.7
phosphide (rodenticide)	985.8	E863.7	—	E950.6	E962.1	E980.7
stearate	976.3	E858.7	E946.3	E950.4	E962.0	E980.4
sulfate (antivaricose)	972.7	E858.3	E942.7	E950.4	E962.0	E980.4
ENT agent	976.6	E858.7	E946.6	E950.4	E962.0	E980.4
ophthalmic solution	976.5	E858.7	E946.5	E950.4	E962.0	E980.4
topical NEC	976.0	E858.7	E946.0	E950.4	E962.0	E980.4
undecylenate	976.0	E858.7	E946.0	E950.4	E962.0	E980.4
Zoxazolamine	968.0	E855.1	E938.0	E950.4	E962.0	E980.4
Zygadenus (venenosus)	988.2	E865.4	—	E950.9	E962.1	E980.9

SECTION 3
Alphabetic Index to External Causes of Injury and Poisoning (E Code)

This section contains the index to the codes which classify environmental events, circumstances, and other conditions as the cause of injury and other adverse effects. Where a code from the section Supplementary Classification of External Causes of Injury and Poisoning (E800-E998) is applicable, it is intended that the E code shall be used in addition to a code from the main body of the classification, Chapters 1 to 17.

The alphabetic index to the E codes is organized by main terms which describe the *accident, circumstance, event,* or *specific agent* which caused the injury or other adverse effect.

Note — Transport accidents (E800-E848) include accidents involving:
    aircraft and spacecraft (E840-E845)
    watercraft (E830-E838)
    motor vehicle (E810-E825)
    railway (E800-E807)
    other road vehicles (E826-E829)

For definitions and examples related to transport accidents — see Volume 1 code categories E800-E848.

The fourth-digit subdivisions for use with categories E800-E848 to identify the injured person are found at the end of this section.

For identifying the place in which an accident or poisoning occurred (circumstances classifiable to categories E850-E869 and E880-E928) — see the listing in this section under "Accident, occurring."

See the Table of Drugs and Chemicals (Section 2 of this volume) for identifying the specific agent involved in drug overdose or a wrong substance given or taken in error, and for intoxication or poisoning by a drug or other chemical substance.

The specific adverse effect, reaction, or localized toxic effect to a correct drug or substance properly administered in therapeutic or prophylactic dosage should be classified according to the nature of the adverse effect (e.g., allergy, dermatitis, tachycardia) listed in Section 1 of this volume.

Index to External Causes — **Accident (to)**

A

Abandonment
  causing exposure to weather conditions — see Exposure
  child, with intent to injure or kill E968.4
  helpless person, infant, newborn E904.0
    with intent to injure or kill E968.4
Abortion, criminal, injury to child E968.8
Abuse (alleged) (suspected)
  adult
    by
      child E967.4
      ex-partner E967.3
      ex-spouse E967.3
      father E967.0
      grandchild E967.7
      grandparent E967.6
      mother E967.2
      non-related caregiver E967.8
      other relative E967.7
      other specified person E967.1
      partner E967.3
      sibling E967.5
      spouse E967.3
      stepfather E967.0
      stepmother E967.2
      unspecified person E967.9
  child
    by
      boyfriend of parent or guardian E967.0
      child E967.4
      father E967.0
      female partner of parent or guardian E967.2
      girlfriend of parent or guardian E967.2
      grandchild E967.7
      grandparent E967.6
      male partner of parent or guardian E967.2
      mother E967.2
      non-related caregiver E967.8
      other relative E967.7
      other specified person(s) E967.1
      sibling E967.5
      stepfather E967.0
      stepmother E967.2
      unspecified person E967.9
Accident (to) E928.9
  aircraft (in transit) (powered) E841 ✓4th
    at landing, take-off E840 ✓4th
    due to, caused by cataclysm — see categories E908 ✓4th, E909 ✓4th
    late effect of E929.1
    unpowered (see also Collision, aircraft, unpowered) E842 ✓4th
    while alighting, boarding E843 ✓4th
  amphibious vehicle
    on
      land — see Accident, motor vehicle
      water — see Accident, watercraft
  animal, ridden NEC E828 ✓4th
  animal-drawn vehicle NEC E827 ✓4th
  balloon (see also Collision, aircraft, unpowered) E842 ✓4th
  caused by, due to
    abrasive wheel (metalworking) E919.3
    animal NEC E906.9
      being ridden (in sport or transport) E828 ✓4th

Accident (to) — *continued*
  caused by, due to — *continued*
    avalanche NEC E909.2
    band saw E919.4
    bench saw E919.4
    bore, earth-drilling or mining (land) (seabed) E919.1
    bulldozer E919.7
    cataclysmic
      earth surface movement or eruption E909.9
      storm E908.9
    chain
      hoist E919.2
        agricultural operations E919.0
        mining operations E919.1
      saw E920.1
    circular saw E919.4
    cold (excessive) (see also Cold, exposure to) E901.9
    combine E919.0
    conflagration — see Conflagration
    corrosive liquid, substance NEC E924.1
    cotton gin E919.8
    crane E919.2
      agricultural operations E919.0
      mining operations E919.1
    cutting or piercing instrument (see also Cut) E920.9
    dairy equipment E919.8
    derrick E919.2
      agricultural operations E919.0
      mining operations E919.1
    drill E920.1
      earth (land) (seabed) E919.1
      hand (powered) E920.1
        not powered E920.4
      metalworking E919.3
      woodworking E919.4
    earth(-)
      drilling machine E919.1
      moving machine E919.7
      scraping machine E919.7
    electric
      current (see also Electric shock) E925.9
      motor — see also Accident, machine, by type of machine
        current (of) — see Electric shock
    elevator (building) (grain) E919.2
      agricultural operations E919.0
      mining operations E919.1
    environmental factors NEC E928.9
    excavating machine E919.7
    explosive material (see also Explosion) E923.9
    farm machine E919.0
    fire, flames — see also Fire
      conflagration — see Conflagration
    firearm missile — see Shooting
    forging (metalworking) machine E919.3
    forklift (truck) E919.2
      agricultural operations E919.0
      mining operations E919.1
    gas turbine E919.5
    harvester E919.0
    hay derrick, mower, or rake E919.0
    heat (excessive) (see also Heat) E900.9
    hoist (see also Accident, caused by, due to, lift) E919.2

▶◀ Revised Text ● New Line ▲ Revised Code ✓4th Fourth-digit Required

Accident (to) — continued
  caused by, due to — continued
    hoist — continued
      chain — see Accident, caused by, due to, chain
      shaft E919.1
    hot
      liquid E924.0
        caustic or corrosive E924.1
      object (not producing fire or flames) E924.8
      substance E924.9
        caustic or corrosive E924.1
        liquid (metal) NEC E924.0
        specified type NEC E924.8
    human bite E928.3
    ignition — see Ignition
    internal combustion engine E919.5
    landslide NEC E909.2
    lathe (metalworking) E919.3
      turnings E920.8
      woodworking E919.4
    lift, lifting (appliances) E919.2
      agricultural operations E919.0
      mining operations E919.1
      shaft E919.1
    lightning NEC E907
    machine, machinery — see also Accident, machine
      drilling, metal E919.3
      manufacturing, for manufacture of
        beverages E919.8
        clothing E919.8
        foodstuffs E919.8
        paper E919.8
        textiles E919.8
      milling, metal E919.3
      moulding E919.4
      power press, metal E919.3
      printing E919.8
      rolling mill, metal E919.3
      sawing, metal E919.3
      specified type NEC E919.8
      spinning E919.8
      weaving E919.8
    natural factor NEC E928.9
    overhead plane E919.4
    plane E920.4
      overhead E919.4
    powered
      hand tool NEC E920.1
      saw E919.4
        hand E920.1
    printing machine E919.8
    pulley (block) E919.2
      agricultural operations E919.0
      mining operations E919.1
      transmission E919.6
    radial saw E919.4
    radiation — see Radiation
    reaper E919.0
    road scraper E919.7
      when in transport under its own power — see categories E810-E825 ✓4ᵗʰ
    roller coaster E919.8
    sander E919.4
    saw E920.4
      band E919.4
      bench E919.4
      chain E920.1

Accident (to) — continued
  caused by, due to — continued
    saw — continued
      circular E919.4
      hand E920.4
        powered E920.1
      powered, except hand E919.4
      radial E919.4
    sawing machine, metal E919.3
    shaft
      hoist E919.1
      lift E919.1
      transmission E919.6
    shears E920.4
      hand E920.4
        powered E920.1
      mechanical E919.3
    shovel E920.4
      steam E919.7
    spinning machine E919.8
    steam — see also Burning, steam
      engine E919.5
      shovel E919.7
    thresher E919.0
    thunderbolt NEC E907
    tractor E919.0
      when in transport under its own power — see categories E810-E825 ✓4ᵗʰ
    transmission belt, cable, chain, gear, pinion, pulley, shaft E919.6
    turbine (gas) (water driven) E919.5
    under-cutter E919.1
    weaving machine E919.8
    winch E919.2
      agricultural operations E919.0
      mining operations E919.1
  diving E883.0
    with insufficient air supply E913.2
  glider (hang) (see also Collision, aircraft, unpowered) E842 ✓4ᵗʰ
  hovercraft
    on
      land — see Accident, motor vehicle
      water — see Accident, watercraft
  ice yacht (see also Accident, vehicle NEC) E848
  in
    medical, surgical procedure
      as, or due to misadventure — see Misadventure
      causing an abnormal reaction or later complication without mention of misadventure — see Reaction, abnormal
  kite carrying a person (see also Collision, aircraft, unpowered) E842 ✓4ᵗʰ
  land yacht (see also Accident, vehicle NEC) E848
  late effect of — see Late effect
  launching pad E845 ✓4ᵗʰ
  machine, machinery (see also Accident, caused by, due to, by specific type of machine) E919.9
    agricultural including animal-powered E919.0
    earth-drilling E919.1
    earth moving or scraping E919.7
    excavating E919.7

Index to External Causes

Accident (to) — *continued*
  machine, machinery — *continued*
    involving transport under own power on highway or transport vehicle — *see* categories E810-E825 ✓4th, E840-E845 ✓4th
    lifting (appliances) E919.2
    metalworking E919.3
    mining E919.1
    prime movers, except electric motors E919.5
      electric motors — *see* Accident, machine, by specific type of machine
    recreational E919.8
    specified type NEC E919.8
    transmission E919.6
    watercraft (deck) (engine room) (galley) (laundry) (loading) E836 ✓4th
    woodworking or forming E919.4
  motor vehicle (on public highway) (traffic) E819 ✓4th
    due to cataclysm — *see* categories E908 ✓4th, E909 ✓4th
    involving
      collision (*see also* Collision, motor vehicle) E812 ✓4th
      nontraffic, not on public highway — *see* categories E820-E825 ✓4th
      not involving collision — *see* categories E816-E819 ✓4th
  nonmotor vehicle NEC E829 ✓4th
    nonroad — *see* Accident, vehicle NEC
    road, except pedal cycle, animal-drawn vehicle, or animal being ridden E829 ✓4th
  nonroad vehicle NEC — *see* Accident, vehicle NEC
  not elsewhere classifiable involving
    cable car (not on rails) E847
      on rails E829 ✓4th
    coal car in mine E846
    hand truck — *see* Accident, vehicle NEC
    logging car E846
    sled(ge), meaning snow or ice vehicle E848
    tram, mine or quarry E846
    truck
      mine or quarry E846
      self-propelled, industrial E846
      station baggage E846
    tub, mine or quarry E846
    vehicle NEC E848
      snow and ice E848
      used only on industrial premises E846
    wheelbarrow E848
  occurring (at) (in)
    apartment E849.0
    baseball field, diamond E849.4
    construction site, any E849.3
    dock E849.8
      yard E849.3
    dormitory E849.7
    factory (building) (premises) E849.3
    farm E849.1
      buildings E849.1
      house E849.0
    football field E849.4
    forest E849.8
    garage (place of work) E849.3
      private (home) E849.0

Accident (to) — *continued*
  occurring (at) (in) — *continued*
    gravel pit E849.2
    gymnasium E849.4
    highway E849.5
    home (private) (residential) E849.0
      institutional E849.7
    hospital E849.7
    hotel E849.6
    house (private) (residential) E849.0
      movie E849.6
      public E849.6
    institution, residential E849.7
    jail E849.7
    mine E849.2
    motel E849.6
    movie house E849.6
    office (building) E849.6
    orphanage E849.7
    park (public) E849.4
      mobile home E849.8
      trailer E849.8
    parking lot or place E849.8
    place
      industrial NEC E849.3
      parking E849.8
      public E849.8
        specified place NEC E849.5
      recreational NEC E849.4
      sport NEC E849.4
    playground (park) (school) E849.4
    prison E849.6
    public building NEC E849.6
    quarry E849.2
    railway
      line NEC E849.8
      yard E849.3
    residence
      home (private) E849.0
    resort (beach) (lake) (mountain) (seashore) (vacation) E849.4
    restaurant E849.6
    sand pit E849.2
    school (building) (private) (public) (state) E849.6
      reform E849.7
      riding E849.4
    seashore E849.8
      resort E849.4
    shop (place of work) E849.3
      commercial E849.6
    skating rink E849.4
    sports palace E849.4
    stadium E849.4
    store E849.6
    street E849.5
    swimming pool (public) E849.4
      private home or garden E849.0
    tennis court E849.4
    theatre, theater E849.6
    trailer court E849.8
    tunnel E849.8
      under construction E849.2
    warehouse E849.3
    yard
      dock E849.3
      industrial E849.3
      private (home) E849.0
      railway E849.3

Accident (to) — continued

- off-road type motor vehicle (not on public highway) NEC E821 ✓4ᵗʰ
- on public highway — see catagories E810-E819 ✓4ᵗʰ
- pedal cycle E826 ✓4ᵗʰ
- railway E807 ✓4ᵗʰ
  - due to cataclysm — see categories E908 ✓4ᵗʰ, E909 ✓4ᵗʰ
  - involving
    - avalanche E909.2
    - burning by engine, locomotive, train (see also Explosion, railway engine) E803 ✓4ᵗʰ
    - collision (see also Collision, railway) E800 ✓4ᵗʰ
    - derailment (see also Derailment, railway) E802 ✓4ᵗʰ
    - explosion (see also Explosion, railway engine) E803 ✓4ᵗʰ
    - fall (see also Fall, from, railway rolling stock) E804 ✓4ᵗʰ
    - fire (see also Explosion, railway engine) E803 ✓4ᵗʰ
    - hitting by, being struck by
      - object falling in, on, from, rolling stock, train, vehicle E806 ✓4ᵗʰ
      - rolling stock, train, vehicle E805 ✓4ᵗʰ
    - overturning, railway rolling stock, train, vehicle (see also Derailment, railway) E802 ✓4ᵗʰ
    - running off rails, railway (see also Derailment, railway) E802 ✓4ᵗʰ
    - specified circumstances NEC E806 ✓4ᵗʰ
    - train or vehicle hit by
      - avalanche E909 ✓4ᵗʰ
      - falling object (earth, rock, tree) E806 ✓4ᵗʰ
        - due to cataclysm — see categories E908 ✓4ᵗʰ, E909 ✓4ᵗʰ
      - landslide E909 ✓4ᵗʰ
- roller skate E885.1
- scooter (nonmotorized) E885.0
- skateboard E885.2
- ski(ing) E885.3
  - jump E884.9
  - lift or tow (with chair or gondola) E847
- snow vehicle, motor driven (not on public highway) E820 ✓4ᵗʰ
  - on public highway — see catagories E810-E819 ✓4ᵗʰ
- snowboard E885.4
- spacecraft E845 ✓4ᵗʰ
- specified cause NEC E928.8
- street car E829 ✓4ᵗʰ
- traffic NEC E819 ✓4ᵗʰ
- vehicle NEC (with pedestrian) E848
  - battery powered
    - airport passenger vehicle E846
    - truck (baggage) (mail) E846
  - powered commercial or industrial (with other vehicle or object within commercial or industrial premises) E846
- watercraft E838 ✓4ᵗʰ
  - with
    - drowning or submersion resulting from accident other than to watercraft E832 ✓4ᵗʰ
    - accident to watercraft E830 ✓4ᵗʰ

Accident (to) — continued

- watercraft — continued
  - with — continued
    - injury, except drowning or submersion, resulting from
      - accident other than to watercraft — see categories E833-E838 ✓4ᵗʰ
      - accident to watercraft E831 ✓4ᵗʰ
  - due to, caused by cataclysm — see categories E908 ✓4ᵗʰ, E909 ✓4ᵗʰ
- machinery E836 ✓4ᵗʰ

Acid throwing E961
Acosta syndrome E902.0
Aeroneurosis E902.1
Aero-otitis media — see Effects of, air pressure
Aerosinusitis — see Effects of, air pressure
After-effect, late — see Late effect
Air
- blast
  - in
    - terrorism E979.2
    - war operations E993
- embolism (traumatic) NEC E928.9
  - in
    - infusion or transfusion E874.1
    - perfusion E874.2
- sickness E903

Alpine sickness E902.0
Altitude sickness — see Effects of, air pressure
Anaphylactic shock, anaphylaxis (see also Table of Drugs and Chemicals) E947.9
- due to bite or sting (venomous) — see Bite, venomous

Andes disease E902.0
Apoplexy
- heat — see Heat

Arachnidism E905.1
Arson E968.0
Asphyxia, asphyxiation
- by
  - chemical
    - in
      - terrorism E979.7
      - war operations E997.2
  - explosion — see Explosion
  - food (bone) (regurgitated food) (seed) E911
  - foreign object, except food E912
  - fumes
    - in
      - terrorism (chemical weapons) E979.7
      - war operations E997.2
  - gas — see also Table of Drugs and Chemicals
    - in
      - terrorism E979.7
      - war operations E997.2
    - legal
      - execution E978
      - intervention (tear) E972
    - tear E972
  - mechanical means (see also Suffocation) E913.9
- from
  - conflagration — see Conflagration

Asphyxia, asphyxiation — *continued*
  from — *continued*
    fire — *see also* Fire E899
      in
        terrorism E979.3
        war operations E990.9
    ignition — *see* Ignition
Aspiration
  foreign body — *see* Foreign body, aspiration
  mucus, not of newborn (with asphyxia, obstruction respiratory passage, suffocation) E912
  phlegm (with asphyxia, obstruction respiratory passage, suffocation) E912
  vomitus (with asphyxia, obstruction respiratory passage, suffocation) (*see also* Foreign body, aspiration, food) E911
Assassination (attempt) (*see also* Assault) E968.9
Assault (homicidal) (by) (in) E968.9
  acid E961
    swallowed E962.1
  air gun E968.6
  BB gun E968.6
  bite NEC E968.8
    of human being E968.7
  bomb ((placed in) car or house) E965.8
    antipersonnel E965.5
    letter E965.7
    petrol E965.7
  brawl (hand) (fists) (foot) E960.0
  burning, burns (by fire) E968.0
    acid E961
      swallowed E962.1
    caustic, corrosive substance E961
      swallowed E962.1
    chemical from swallowing caustic, corrosive substance NEC E962.1
    hot liquid E968.3
    scalding E968.3
    vitriol E961
      swallowed E962.1
  caustic, corrosive substance E961
    swallowed E962.1
  cut, any part of body E966
  dagger E966
  drowning E964
  explosive(s) E965.9
    bomb (*see also* Assault, bomb) E965.8
    dynamite E965.8
  fight (hand) (fists) (foot) E960.0
    with weapon E968.9
      blunt or thrown E968.2
      cutting or piercing E966
      firearm — *see* Shooting, homicide
  fire E968.0
  firearm(s) — *see* Shooting, homicide
  garrotting E963
  gunshot (wound) — *see* Shooting, homicide
  hanging E963
  injury NEC E968.9
  knife E966
  late effect of E969
  ligature E963
  poisoning E962.9
    drugs or medicinals E962.0
    gas(es) or vapors, except drugs and medicinals E962.2

Assault — *continued*
  poisoning — *continued*
    solid or liquid substances, except drugs and medicinals E962.1
  puncture, any part of body E966
  pushing
    before moving object, train, vehicle E968.5
    from high place E968.1
  rape E960.1
  scalding E968.3
  shooting — *see* Shooting, homicide
  sodomy E960.1
  stab, any part of body E966
  strangulation E963
  submersion E964
  suffocation E963
  transport vehicle E968.5
  violence NEC E968.9
  vitriol E961
    swallowed E962.1
  weapon E968.9
    blunt or thrown E968.2
    cutting or piercing E966
    firearm — *see* Shooting, homicide
  wound E968.9
    cutting E966
    gunshot — *see* Shooting, homicide
    knife E966
    piercing E966
    puncture E966
    stab E966
Attack by animal NEC E906.9
Avalanche E909.2
  falling on or hitting
    motor vehicle (in motion) (on public highway) E909.2
    railway train E909.2
Aviators' disease E902.0

B

Barotitis, barodontalgia, barosinusitis, barotrauma (otitic) (sinus) — *see* Effects of, air pressure
Battered
  baby or child (syndrome) — *see* Abuse, child; category E967
  person other than baby or child — *see* Assault
Bayonet wound (*see also* Cut, by bayonet) E920.3
  in
    legal intervention E974
    terrorism E979.8
    war operations E995
Bean in nose E912
Bed set on fire NEC E898.0
Beheading (by guillotine)
  homicide E966
  legal execution E978
Bending, injury in E927
Bends E902.0
Bite
  animal (nonvenomous) NEC E906.5
    other specified (except arthropod) E906.3
    venomous NEC E905.9
  arthropod (nonvenomous) NEC E906.4
    venomous — *see* Sting
  black widow spider E905.1

Bite — *continued*
  cat E906.3
  centipede E905.4
  cobra E905.0
  copperhead snake E905.0
  coral snake E905.0
  dog E906.0
  fer de lance E905.0
  gila monster E905.0
  human being
    accidental E928.3
    assault E968.7
  insect (nonvenomous) E906.4
    venomous — *see* Sting
  krait E905.0
  late effect of — *see* Late effect
  lizard E906.2
    venomous E905.0
  mamba E905.0
  marine animal
    nonvenomous E906.3
      snake E906.2
    venomous E905.6
      snake E905.0
  millipede E906.4
    venomous E905.4
  moray eel E906.3
  rat E906.1
  rattlesnake E905.0
  rodent, except rat E906.3
  serpent — *see* Bite, snake
  shark E906.3
  snake (venomous) E905.0
    nonvenomous E906.2
    sea E905.0
  spider E905.1
    nonvenomous E906.4
  tarantula (venomous) E905.1
  venomous NEC E905.9
    by specific animal — *see category* E905 ✓4ᵗʰ
  viper E905.0
  water moccasin E905.0
Blast (air)
  from nuclear explosion E996
  in
    terrorism E979.2 •
      from nuclear explosion E979.5 •
      underwater E979.0 •
    war operations E993 •
      from nuclear explosion E996 •
      underwater E992 •
  underwater E992
Blizzard E908.3
Blow E928.9
  by law-enforcing agent, police (on duty) E975
    with blunt object (baton) (nightstick) (stave) (truncheon) E973
Blowing up (*see also* Explosion) E923.9
Brawl (hand) (fists) (foot) E960.0
Breakage (accidental)
  cable of cable car not on rails E847
  ladder (causing fall) E881.0
  part (any) of
    animal-drawn vehicle E827 ✓4ᵗʰ
    ladder (causing fall) E881.0
    motor vehicle
      in motion (on public highway) E818 ✓4ᵗʰ
      not on public highway E825 ✓4ᵗʰ

Breakage — *continued*
  part (any) of — *continued*
    nonmotor road vehicle, except animal-drawn vehicle or pedal cycle E829 ✓4ᵗʰ
    off-road type motor vehicle (not on public highway) NEC E821 ✓4ᵗʰ
      on public highway E818 ✓4ᵗʰ
    pedal cycle E826 ✓4ᵗʰ
    scaffolding (causing fall) E881.1
    snow vehicle, motor-driven (not on public highway) E820 ✓4ᵗʰ
      on public highway E818 ✓4ᵗʰ
    vehicle NEC — *see* Accident, vehicle
Broken
  glass
    fall on E888.0
    injury by E920.8
  power line (causing electric shock) E925.1
Bumping against, into (accidentally)
  object (moving) E917.9
    caused by crowd E917.1
      with subsequent fall E917.6
    furniture E917.3
      with subsequent fall E917.7
    in
      running water E917.2
      sports E917.0
        with subsequent fall E917.5
    stationary E917.4
      with subsequent fall E917.8
  person(s) E917.9
    with fall E886.9
      in sports E886.0
    as, or caused by, a crowd E917.1
      with subsequent fall E917.6
    in sports E917.0
      with fall E886.0
Burning, burns (accidental) (by) (from) (on) E899
  acid (any kind) E924.1
    swallowed — *see* Table of Drugs and Chemicals
  bedclothes (*see also* Fire, specified NEC) E898.0
  blowlamp (*see also* Fire, specified NEC) E898.1
  blowtorch (*see also* Fire, specified NEC) E898.1
  boat, ship, watercraft — *see categories* E830 ✓4ᵗʰ, E831 ✓4ᵗʰ, E837 ✓4ᵗʰ
  bonfire (controlled) E897
    uncontrolled E892
  candle (*see also* Fire, specified NEC) E898.1
  caustic liquid, substance E924.1
    swallowed — *see* Table of Drugs and Chemicals
  chemical E924.1
    from swallowing caustic, corrosive substance — *see* Table of Drugs and Chemicals
    in
      terrorism E979.7 •
      war operations E997.2
  cigar(s) or cigarette(s) (*see also* Fire, specified NEC) E898.1
  clothes, clothing, nightdress — *see* Ignition, clothes
    with conflagration — *see* Conflagration
  conflagration — *see* Conflagration

Burning, burns — *continued*
  corrosive liquid, substance E924.1
    swallowed — *see* Table of Drugs and
      Chemicals
  electric current (*see also* Electric shock)
    E925.9
  fire, flames (*see also* Fire) E899
  flare, Verey pistol E922.8
  heat
    from appliance (electrical) E924.8
    in local application, or packing during
      medical or surgical procedure E873.5
  homicide (attempt) (*see also* Assault, burning)
    E968.0
  hot
    liquid E924.0
      caustic or corrosive E924.1
    object (not producing fire or flames) E924.8
    substance E924.9
      caustic or corrosive E924.1
      liquid (metal) NEC E924.0
      specified type NEC E924.8
    tap water E924.2
  ignition — *see also* Ignition
    clothes, clothing, nightdress — *see also*
      Ignition, clothes
      with conflagration — *see* Conflagration
    highly inflammable material (benzine) (fat)
      (gasoline) (kerosene) (paraffin) (petrol)
      E894
  inflicted by other person
    stated as
      homicidal, intentional (*see also* Assault,
        burning) E968.0
      undetermined whether accidental or
        intentional (*see also* Burn, stated
        as undetermined whether
        accidental or intentional) E988.1
  internal, from swallowed caustic, corrosive
    liquid, substance — *see* Table of Drugs
    and Chemicals
  in
    terrorism E979.3
      from nuclear explosion E979.5
      petrol bomb E979.3
    war operations (from fire-producing
      device or conventional weapon)
      E990.9
      from nuclear explosion E996
      petrol bomb E990.0
  lamp (*see also* Fire, specified NEC) E898.1
  late effect of NEC E929.4
  lighter (cigar) (cigarette) (*see also* Fire,
    specified NEC) E898.1
  lightning E907
  liquid (boiling) (hot) (molten) E924.0
    caustic, corrosive (external) E924.1
      swallowed — *see* Table of Drugs and
        Chemicals
  local application of externally applied
    substance in medical or surgical care
    E873.5
  machinery — *see* Accident, machine
  matches (*see also* Fire, specified NEC) E898.1
  medicament, externally applied E873.5
  metal, molten E924.0
  object (hot) E924.8
    producing fire or flames — *see* Fire
  oven (electric) (gas) E924.8

Burning, burns — *continued*
  pipe (smoking) (*see also* Fire, specified NEC)
    E898.1
  radiation — *see* Radiation
  railway engine, locomotive, train (*see also*
    Explosion, railway engine) E803 ◢4ᵗʰ◣
  self-inflicted (unspecified whether accidental
    or intentional) E988.1
    caustic or corrosive substance NEC E988.7
    stated as intentional, purposeful E958.1
      caustic or corrosive substance NEC
        E958.7
    stated as undetermined whether accidental or
      intentional E988.1
    caustic or corrosive substance NEC E988.7
  steam E924.0
    pipe E924.8
  substance (hot) E924.9
    boiling or molten E924.0
    caustic, corrosive (external) E924.1
      swallowed — *see* Table of Drugs and
        Chemicals
  suicidal (attempt) NEC E958.1
    caustic substance E958.7
    late effect of E959
  tanning bed E926.2
  therapeutic misadventure
    overdose of radiation E873.2
  torch, welding (*see also* Fire, specified NEC)
    E898.1
  trash fire (*see also* Burning, bonfire) E897
  vapor E924.0
  vitriol E924.1
  x-rays E926.3
    in medical, surgical procedure — *see*
      Misadventure, failure, in dosage,
      radiation
Butted by animal E906.8

C

Cachexia, lead or saturnine E866.0
  from pesticide NEC (*see also* Table of Drugs
    and Chemicals) E863.4
Caisson disease E902.2
Capital punishment (any means) E978
Car sickness E903
Casualty (not due to war) NEC E928.9
  terrorism E979.8
  war (*see also* War operations) E995
Cat
  bite E906.3
  scratch E906.8
Cataclysmic (any injury)
  earth surface movement or eruption E909.9
    specified type NEC E909.8
  storm or flood resulting from storm E908.9
    specified type NEC E909.8
Catching fire — *see* Ignition
Caught
  between
    objects (moving) (stationary and moving)
      E918
    and machinery — *see* Accident, machine
  by cable car, not on rails E847
  in
    machinery (moving parts of) — *see*,
      Accident, machine

Caught — *continued*
　in — *continued*
　　object E918
Cave-in (causing asphyxia, suffocation (by pressure)) (*see also* Suffocation, due to, cave-in) E913.3
　with injury other than asphyxia or suffocation E916
　　with asphyxia or suffocation (*see also* Suffocation, due to, cave-in) E913.3
　struck or crushed by E916
　　with asphyxia or suffocation (*see also* Suffocation, due to, cave-in) E913.3
Change(s) in air pressure — *see also* Effects of, air pressure
　sudden, in aircraft (ascent) (descent) (causing aeroneurosis or aviators' disease) E902.1
Chilblains E901.0
　due to manmade conditions E901.1
Choking (on) (any object except food or vomitus) E912
　apple E911
　bone E911
　food, any type (regurgitated) E911
　mucus or phlegm E912
　seed E911
Civil insurrection — *see* War operations
Cloudburst E908.8
Cold, exposure to (accidental) (excessive) (extreme) (place) E901.9
　causing chilblains or immersion foot E901.0
　due to
　　manmade conditions E901.1
　　specified cause NEC E901.8
　　weather (conditions) E901.0
　late effect of NEC E929.5
　self-inflicted (undetermined whether accidental or intentional) E988.3
　　suicidal E958.3
　suicide E958.3
Colic, lead, painter's, or saturnine — *see* category E866 ▨
Collapse
　building (moveable) E916
　　burning ▶(uncontrolled fire)◀ E891.8 •
　　　in terrorism E979.3
　　　private E890.8
　dam E909.3
　due to heat — *see* Heat
　machinery — *see* Accident, machine
　man-made structure E909.3
　postoperative NEC E878.9
　structure, burning NEC E891.8
　　burning (uncontrolled fire) •
　　　in terrorism E979.3 •

Collision (accidental)

> Note — In the case of collisions between different types of vehicles, persons and objects, priority in classification is in the following order:
>
> 　Aircraft
> 　Watercraft
> 　Motor vehicle
> 　Railway vehicle
> 　Pedal cycle
> 　Animal-drawn vehicle
> 　Animal being ridden
> 　Streetcar or other nonmotor road vehicle
> 　Other vehicle
> 　Pedestrian or person using pedestrian conveyance
> 　Object (except where falling from or set in motion by vehicle etc. listed above)
>
> In the listing below, the combinations are listed only under the vehicle etc. having priority. For definitions, see Volume 1, page 247.

　aircraft (with object or vehicle) (fixed) (movable) (moving) E841 ▨
　　with
　　　person (while landing, taking off) (without accident to aircraft) E844 ▨
　　　powered (in transit) (with unpowered aircraft) E841 ▨
　　　　while landing, taking off E840 ▨
　　　unpowered E842 ▨
　　　　while landing, taking off E840 ▨
　animal being ridden (in sport or transport) E828 ▨
　　and
　　　animal (being ridden) (herded) (unattended) E828 ▨
　　　nonmotor road vehicle, except pedal cycle or animal-drawn vehicle E828 ▨
　　　object (fallen) (fixed) (movable) (moving) not falling from or set in motion by vehicle of higher priority E828 ▨
　　　pedestrian (conveyance or vehicle) E828 ▨
　animal-drawn vehicle E827 ▨
　　and
　　　animal (being ridden) (herded) (unattended) E827 ▨
　　　nonmotor road vehicle, except pedal cycle E827 ▨
　　　object (fallen) (fixed) (movable) (moving) not falling from or set in motion by vehicle of higher priority E827 ▨
　　　pedestrian (conveyance or vehicle) E827 ▨
　　　streetcar E827 ▨

Index to External Causes — Collision

Collision — *continued*
- motor vehicle (on public highway) (traffic accident) E812 ✓4th
  - after leaving, running off, public highway (without antecedent collision) (without re-entry) E816 ✓4th
  - with antecedent collision on public highway — *see* categories E810-E815 ✓4th
  - with re-entrance collision with another motor vehicle E811 ✓4th
  - and
    - abutment (bridge) (overpass) E815 ✓4th
    - animal (herded) (unattended) E815 ✓4th
    - carrying person, property E813 ✓4th
    - animal-drawn vehicle E813 ✓4th
    - another motor vehicle (abandoned) (disabled) (parked) (stalled) (stopped) E812 ✓4th
      - with, involving re-entrance (on same roadway) (across median strip) E811 ✓4th
    - any object, person, or vehicle off the public highway resulting from a noncollision motor vehicle nontraffic accident E816 ✓4th
    - avalanche, fallen or not moving E815 ✓4th
      - falling E909 ✓4th
    - boundary fence E815 ✓4th
    - culvert E815 ✓4th
    - fallen
      - stone E815 ✓4th
      - tree E815 ✓4th
    - falling E909.2
    - guard post or guard rail E815 ✓4th
    - inter-highway divider E815 ✓4th
    - landslide, fallen or not moving E815 ✓4th
      - moving E909 ✓4th
    - machinery (road) E815 ✓4th
      - moving E909.2
    - nonmotor road vehicle NEC E813 ✓4th
    - object (any object, person, or vehicle off the public highway resulting from a noncollision motor vehicle nontraffic accident) E815 ✓4th
      - off, normally not on, public highway resulting from a noncollision motor vehicle traffic accident E816 ✓4th
    - pedal cycle E813 ✓4th
    - pedestrian (conveyance) E814 ✓4th
    - person (using pedestrian conveyance) E814 ✓4th
    - post or pole (lamp) (light) (signal) (telephone) (utility) E815 ✓4th
    - railway rolling stock, train, vehicle E810 ✓4th
    - safety island E815 ✓4th
    - street car E813 ✓4th
    - traffic signal, sign, or marker (temporary) E815 ✓4th
    - tree E815 ✓4th
    - tricycle E813 ✓4th
    - wall of cut made for road E815 ✓4th
    - due to cataclysm — *see* categories E908 ✓4th, E909 ✓4th

Collision — *continued*
- motor vehicle — *continued*
  - not on public highway, nontraffic accident E822 ✓4th
  - and
    - animal (carrying person, property) (herded) (unattended) E822 ✓4th
    - animal-drawn vehicle E822 ✓4th
    - another motor vehicle (moving), except off-road motor vehicle E822 ✓4th
      - stationary E823 ✓4th
    - avalanche, fallen, not moving E823 ✓4th
      - moving E909 ✓4th
    - landslide, fallen, not moving E823 ✓4th
      - moving E909 ✓4th
    - nonmotor vehicle (moving) E822 ✓4th
      - stationary E823 ✓4th
    - object (fallen) (normally) (fixed) (movable but not in motion) (stationary) E823 ✓4th
      - moving, except when falling from, set in motion by, aircraft or cataclysm E822 ✓4th
    - pedal cycle (moving) E822 ✓4th
      - stationary E823 ✓4th
    - pedestrian (conveyance) E822 ✓4th
    - person (using pedestrian conveyance) E822 ✓4th
    - railway rolling stock, train, vehicle (moving) E822 ✓4th
      - stationary E823 ✓4th
    - road vehicle (any) (moving) E822 ✓4th
      - stationary E823 ✓4th
    - tricycle (moving) E822 ✓4th
      - stationary E823 ✓4th
    - moving E909.2
  - off-road type motor vehicle (not on public highway) E821 ✓4th
  - and
    - animal (being ridden) (-drawn vehicle) E821 ✓4th
    - another off-road motor vehicle, except snow vehicle E821 ✓4th
    - other motor vehicle, not on public highway E821 ✓4th
    - other object or vehicle NEC, fixed or movable, not set in motion by aircraft, motor vehicle on highway, or snow vehicle, motor driven E821 ✓4th
    - pedal cycle E821 ✓4th
    - pedestrian (conveyance) E821 ✓4th
    - railway train E821 ✓4th
    - on public highway — *see* Collision, motor vehicle
  - pedal cycle E826 ✓4th
  - and
    - animal (carrying person, property) (herded) (unherded) E826 ✓4th
    - animal-drawn vehicle E826 ✓4th
    - another pedal cycle E826 ✓4th
    - nonmotor road vehicle E826 ✓4th
    - object (fallen) (fixed) (movable) (moving) not falling from or set in motion by aircraft, motor vehicle, or railway train NEC E826 ✓4th
    - pedestrian (conveyance) E826 ✓4th

Collision — *continued*
  pedal cycle — *continued*
    and — *continued*
      person (using pedestrian conveyance) E826 ✓4ᵗʰ
      street car E826 ✓4ᵗʰ
  pedestrian(s) (conveyance) E917.9
    with fall E886.9
      in sports E886.0
    and
      crowd, human stampede E917.1
        with subsequent fall E917.6
      furniture E917.3
        with subsequent fall E917.7
      machinery — *see* Accident, machine
      object (fallen) (moving) not falling from NEC, fixed or set in motion by any vehicle classifiable to E800-E848 E917.9
        with subsequent fall E917.6
        caused by a crowd E917.1
          with subsequent fall E917.6
        furniture E917.3
          with subsequent fall E917.7
      in
        running water E917.2
          with drowning or submersion — *see* Submersion
        sports E917.0
          with subsequent fall E917.5
        stationary E917.4
          with subsequent fall E917.8
    vehicle, nonmotor, nonroad E848
      in
        running water E917.2
          with drowning or submersion — *see* Submersion
        sports E917.0
          with fall E886.0
  person(s) (using pedestrian conveyance) (*see also* Collision, pedestrian) E917.9
  railway (rolling stock) (train) (vehicle) (with (subsequent) derailment, explosion, fall or fire) E800 ✓4ᵗʰ
    with antecedent derailment E802 ✓4ᵗʰ
    and
      animal (carrying person) (herded) (unattended) E801 ✓4ᵗʰ
      another railway train or vehicle E800 ✓4ᵗʰ
      buffers E801 ✓4ᵗʰ
      fallen tree on railway E801 ✓4ᵗʰ
      farm machinery, nonmotor (in transport) (stationary) E801 ✓4ᵗʰ
      gates E801 ✓4ᵗʰ
      nonmotor vehicle E801 ✓4ᵗʰ
      object (fallen) (fixed) (movable) (moving) not falling from, set in motion by, aircraft or motor vehicle NEC E801 ✓4ᵗʰ
      pedal cycle E801 ✓4ᵗʰ
      pedestrian (conveyance) E805 ✓4ᵗʰ
      person (using pedestrian conveyance) E805 ✓4ᵗʰ
      platform E801 ✓4ᵗʰ
      rock on railway E801 ✓4ᵗʰ
      street car E801 ✓4ᵗʰ

Collision — *continued*
  snow vehicle, motor-driven (not on public highway) E820 ✓4ᵗʰ
    and
      animal (being ridden) (-drawn vehicle) E820 ✓4ᵗʰ
      another off-road motor vehicle E820 ✓4ᵗʰ
      other motor vehicle, not on public highway E820 ✓4ᵗʰ
      other object or vehicle NEC, fixed or movable, not set in motion by aircraft or motor vehicle on highway E820 ✓4ᵗʰ
      pedal cycle E820 ✓4ᵗʰ
      pedestrian (conveyance) E820 ✓4ᵗʰ
      railway train E820 ✓4ᵗʰ
    on public highway — *see* Collision, motor vehicle
  street car(s) E829 ✓4ᵗʰ
    and
      animal, herded, not being ridden, unattended E829 ✓4ᵗʰ
      nonmotor road vehicle NEC E829 ✓4ᵗʰ
      object (fallen) (fixed) (movable) (moving) not falling from or set in motion by aircraft, animal-drawn vehicle, animal being ridden, motor vehicle, pedal cycle, or railway train E829 ✓4ᵗʰ
      pedestrian (conveyance) E829 ✓4ᵗʰ
      person (using pedestrian conveyance) E829 ✓4ᵗʰ
  vehicle
    animal-drawn — *see* Collision, animal-drawn vehicle
    motor — *see* Collision, motor vehicle
    nonmotor
      nonroad E848
      and
        another nonmotor, nonroad vehicle E848
        object (fallen) (fixed) (movable) (moving) not falling from or set in motion by aircraft, animal-drawn vehicle, animal being ridden, motor vehicle, nonmotor road vehicle, pedal cycle, railway train, or streetcar E848
      road, except animal being ridden, animal-drawn vehicle, or pedal cycle E829 ✓4ᵗʰ
      and
        animal, herded, not being ridden, unattended E829 ✓4ᵗʰ
        another nonmotor road vehicle, except animal being ridden, animal-drawn vehicle, or pedal cycle E829 ✓4ᵗʰ
        object (fallen) (fixed) (movable) (moving) not falling from or set in motion by, aircraft, animal-drawn vehicle, animal being ridden, motor vehicle, pedal cycle, or railway train E829 ✓4ᵗʰ
        pedestrian (conveyance) E829 ✓4ᵗʰ

Index to External Causes

Collision — *continued*
  vehicle — *continued*
    nonmotor — *continued*
      road, except animal being ridden, animal-drawn vehicle, or pedal cycle — *continued*
        and — *continued*
          person (using pedestrian conveyance) E829 ✓4th
          vehicle, nonmotor, nonroad E829 ✓4th
    watercraft E838 ✓4th
      and
        person swimming or water skiing E838 ✓4th
      causing
        drowning, submersion E830 ✓4th
        injury except drowning, submersion E831 ✓4th

Combustion, spontaneous — *see* Ignition

Complication of medical or surgical procedure or treatment
  as an abnormal reaction — *see* Reaction, abnormal
  delayed, without mention of misadventure — *see* Reaction, abnormal
  due to misadventure — *see* Misadventure

Compression
  divers' squeeze E902.2
  trachea by
    food E911
    foreign body, except food E912

Conflagration
  building or structure, except private dwelling (barn) (church) (convalescent or residential home) (factory) (farm outbuilding) (hospital) (hotel) (institution (educational) (domitory) (residential)) (school) (shop) (store) (theatre) E891.9
    with or causing (injury due to)
      accident or injury NEC E891.9
        specified circumstance NEC E891.8
      burns, burning E891.3
      carbon monoxide E891.2
      fumes E891.2
        polyvinylchloride (PVC) or similar material E891.1
      smoke E891.2
    causing explosion E891.0
    in terrorism E979.3 •
  not in building or structure E892
  private dwelling (apartment) (boarding house) (camping place) (caravan) (farmhouse) (home (private)) (house) (lodging house) (private garage) (rooming house) (tenement) E890.9
    with or causing (injury due to)
      accident or injury NEC E890.9
        specified circumstance NEC E890.8
      burns, burning E890.3
      carbon monoxide E890.2
      fumes E890.2
        polyvinylchloride (PVC) or similar material E890.1
      smoke E890.2
    causing explosion E890.0

Contact with
  dry ice E901.1
  liquid air, hydrogen, nitrogen E901.1

Cramp(s)
  Heat — *see* Heat
  swimmers (*see also* category E910 ✓4th) E910.2
    not in recreation or sport E910.3

Cranking (car) (truck) (bus) (engine), injury by E917.9

Crash
  aircraft (in transit) (powered) E841 ✓4th
    at landing, take-off E840 ✓4th
    in
      terrorism E979.1 •
      war operations E994
    on runway NEC E840 ✓4th
    stated as
      homicidal E968.8
      suicidal E958.6
      undetermined whether accidental or intentional E988.6
    unpowered E842 ✓4th
  glider E842 ✓4th
  motor vehicle — *see also* Accident, motor vehicle
    homicidal E968.5
    suicidal E958.5
    undetermined whether accidental or intentional E988.5

Crushed (accidentally) E928.9
  between
    boat(s), ship(s), watercraft (and dock or pier) (without accident to watercraft) E838 ✓4th
      after accident to, or collision, watercraft E831 ✓4th
    objects (moving) (stationary and moving) E918
  by
    avalanche NEC E909.2
    boat, ship, watercraft after accident to, collision, watercraft E831 ✓4th
    cave-in E916
      with asphyxiation or suffocation (*see also* Suffocation, due to, cave-in) E913.3
    crowd, human stampede E917.1
    falling
      aircraft (*see also* Accident, aircraft) E841 ✓4th
      in
        terrorism E979.1 •
        war operations E994
      earth, material E916
        with asphyxiation or suffocation (*see also* Suffocation, due to, cave-in) E913.3
      object E916
        on ship, watercraft E838 ✓4th
        while loading, unloading watercraft E838 ✓4th
    landslide NEC E909.2
    lifeboat after abandoning ship E831 ✓4th
    machinery — *see* Accident, machine
    railway rolling stock, train, vehicle (part of) E805 ✓4th
    street car E829 ✓4th
    vehicle NEC — *see* Accident, vehicle NEC
  in
    machinery — *see* Accident, machine
    object E918

Crushed

Crushed — *continued*
  in — *continued*
    transport accident — *see* categories E800-E848 ✓4th
  late effect of NEC E929.9
Cut, cutting (any part of body) (accidental) E920.9
  by
    arrow E920.8
    axe E920.4
    bayonet (*see also* Bayonet wound) E920.3
    blender E920.2
    broken glass E920.8
      following fall E888.0
    can opener E920.4
      powered E920.2
    chisel E920.4
    circular saw E919.4
    cutting or piercing instrument — *see also* category E920 ✓4th
      following fall E888.0
      late effect of E929.8
    dagger E920.3
    dart E920.8
    drill — *see* Accident, caused by drill
    edge of stiff paper E920.8
    electric
      beater E920.2
      fan E920.2
      knife E920.2
      mixer E920.2
    fork E920.4
    garden fork E920.4
    hand saw or tool (not powered) E920.4
      powered E920.1
    hedge clipper E920.4
      powered E920.1
    hoe E920.4
    ice pick E920.4
    knife E920.3
      electric E920.2
    lathe turnings E920.8
    lawn mower E920.4
      powered E920.0
        riding E919.8
    machine — *see* Accident, machine
    meat
      grinder E919.8
      slicer E919.8
    nails E920.8
    needle E920.4
      hypodermic E920.5
    object, edged, pointed, sharp — *see* category E920 ✓4th
      following fall E888.0
    paper cutter E920.4
    piercing instrument — *see also* category E920 ✓4th
      late effect of E929.8
    pitchfork E920.4
    powered
      can opener E920.2
      garden cultivator E920.1
        riding E919.8
      hand saw E920.1
      hand tool NEC E920.1
      hedge clipper E920.1
      household appliance or implement E920.2

Cut, cutting — *continued*
  by — *continued*
    powered — *continued*
      lawn mower (hand) E920.0
        riding E919.8
      rivet gun E920.1
      staple gun E920.1
    rake E920.4
    saw
      circular E919.4
      hand E920.4
    scissors E920.4
    screwdriver E920.4
    sewing machine (electric) (powered) E920.2
      not powered E920.4
    shears E920.4
    shovel E920.4
    spade E920.4
    splinters E920.8
    sword E920.3
    tin can lid E920.8
    wood slivers E920.8
  homicide (attempt) E966
  inflicted by other person
    stated as
      intentional, homicidal E966
      undetermined whether accidental or intentional E986
  late effect of NEC E929.8
  legal
    execution E978
    intervention E974
  self-inflicted (unspecified whether accidental or intentional) E986
    stated as intentional, purposeful E956
  stated as undetermined whether accidental or intentional E986
  suicidal (attempt) E956
  terrorism E979.8
  war operations E995
Cyclone E908.1

D

Death due to injury occurring one year or more previous — *see* Late effect
Decapitation (accidental circumstances) NEC E928.9
  homicidal E966
  legal execution (by guillotine) E978
Deprivation — *see also* Privation
  homicidal intent E968.4
Derailment (accidental)
  railway (rolling stock) (train) (vehicle) (with subsequent collision) E802 ✓4th
  with
    collision (antecedent) (*see also* Collision, railway) E800 ✓4th
    explosion (subsequent) (without antecedent collision) E802 ✓4th
      antecedent collision E803 ✓4th
    fall (without collision (antecedent)) E802 ✓4th
    fire (without collision (antecedent)) E802 ✓4th
  street car E829 ✓4th

Index to External Causes — Execution, legal

Descent
  parachute (voluntary) (without accident to aircraft) E844 ✓4th
  due to accident to aircraft — see categories E840-E842 ✓4th

Desertion
  child, with intent to injure or kill E968.4
  helpless person, infant, newborn E904.0
  with intent to injure or kill E968.4

Destitution — see Privation

Disability, late effect or sequela of injury — see Late effect

Disease
  Andes E902.0
  aviators' E902.1
  caisson E902.2
  range E902.0

Divers' disease, palsy, paralysis, squeeze E902.0

Dog bite E906.0

Dragged by
  cable car (not on rails) E847
    on rails E829 ✓4th
  motor vehicle (on highway) E814 ✓4th
    not on highway, nontraffic accident E825 ✓4th
  street car E829 ✓4th

Drinking poison (accidental) — see Table of Drugs and Chemicals

Drowning — see Submersion

Dust in eye E914

E

Earth falling (on) (with asphyxia or suffocation (by pressure)) (see also Suffocation, due to, cave-in) E913.3
  as, or due to, a cataclysm (involving any transport vehicle) — see categories E908 ✓4th, E909 ✓4th
  not due to cataclysmic action E913.3
    motor vehicle (in motion) (on public highway) E810 ✓4th
      not on public highway E825 ✓4th
    nonmotor road vehicle NEC E829 ✓4th
    pedal cycle E826 ✓4th
    railway rolling stock, train, vehicle E806 ✓4th
    street car E829 ✓4th
  struck or crushed by E916
    with asphyxiation or suffocation E913.3
    with injury other than asphyxia, suffocation E916

Earthquake (any injury) E909.0

Effect(s) (adverse) of
  air pressure E902.9
    at high altitude E902.9
      in aircraft E902.1
      residence or prolonged visit (causing conditions classifiable to E902.0) E902.0
    due to
      diving E902.2
      specified cause NEC E902.8
    in aircraft E902.1
  cold, excessive (exposure to) (see also Cold, exposure to) E901.9
  heat (excessive) (see also Heat) E900.9

Effect(s) (adverse) of — continued
  hot
    place — see Heat
    weather E900.0
  insulation — see Heat
  late — see Late effect of
  motion E903
  nuclear explosion or weapon
    in
      terrorism E979.5 •
      war operations (blast) (fireball) (heat) (radiation) (direct) (secondary) E996
  radiation — see Radiation
  terrorism, secondary E979.9 •
  travel E903

Electric shock, electrocution (accidental) (from exposed wire, faulty appliance, high voltage cable, live rail, open socket) (by) (in) E925.9
  appliance or wiring
    domestic E925.0
    factory E925.2
    farm (building) E925.8
      house E925.0
    home E925.0
    industrial (conductor) (control apparatus) (transformer) E925.2
    outdoors E925.8
    public building E925.8
    residential institution E925.8
    school E925.8
    specified place NEC E925.8
  caused by other person
    stated as
      intentional, homicidal E968.8
      undetermined whether accidental or intentional E988.4
  electric power generating plant, distribution station E925.1
  homicidal (attempt) E968.8
  legal execution E978
  lightning E907
  machinery E925.9
    domestic E925.0
    factory E925.2
    farm E925.8
    home E925.0
  misadventure in medical or surgical procedure in electroshock therapy E873.4
  self-inflicted (undetermined whether accidental or intentional) E988.4
  stated as intentional E958.4
  stated as undetermined whether accidental or intentional E988.4
  suicidal (attempt) E958.4
  transmission line E925.1

Electrocution — see Electric shock

Embolism
  air (traumatic) NEC — see Air, embolism

Encephalitis
  lead or saturnine E866.0
    from pesticide NEC E863.4

Entanglement
  in
    bedclothes, causing suffocation E913.0
    wheel of pedal cycle E826 ✓4th

Entry of foreign body, material, any — see Foreign body

Execution, legal (any method) E978

Exhaustion
  cold — *see* Cold, exposure to
  due to excessive exertion E927
  heat — *see* Heat

Explosion (accidental) (in) (of) (on) E923.9
  acetylene E923.2
  aerosol can E921.8
  aircraft (in transit) (powered) E841 ✓4ᵗʰ
    at landing, take-off E840 ✓4ᵗʰ
    in
      terrorism E979.1 •
      war operations E994
    unpowered E842 ✓4ᵗʰ
  air tank (compressed) (in machinery) E921.1
  anesthetic gas in operating theatre E923.2
  automobile tire NEC E921.8
    causing transport accident — *see*
      categories E810-E825 ✓4ᵗʰ
  blasting (cap) (materials) E923.1
  boiler (machinery), not on transport vehicle E921.0
    steamship — *see* Explosion, watercraft
  bomb E923.8
    in
      terrorism E979.2 •
      war operations E993
        after cessation of hostilities E998
        atom, hydrogen or nuclear E996
        injury by fragments from E991.9
        antipersonnel bomb E991.3
  butane E923.2
  caused by
    other person
      stated as
        intentional, homicidal — *see* Assault, explosive
        undetermined whether accidental or homicidal E985.5
  coal gas E923.2
  detonator E923.1
  dyamite E923.1
  explosive (material) NEC E923.9
    gas(es) E923.2
    missile E923.8
      in
        terrorism E979.2 •
        war operations E993
          injury by fragments from E991.9
          antipersonnel bomb E991.3
    used in blasting operations E923.1
  fire-damp E923.2
  fireworks E923.0
  gas E923.2
    cylinder (in machinery) E921.1
    pressure tank (in machinery) E921.1
  gasoline (fumes) (tank) not in moving motor vehicle E923.2
  grain store (military) (munitions) E923.8
  grenade E923.8
    in
      terrorism E979.2 •
      war operations E993
        injury by fragments from E991.9
  homicide (attempt) — *see* Assault, explosive
  hot water heater, tank (in machinery) E921.0
  in mine (of explosive gases) NEC E923.2
  late effect of NEC E929.8
  machinery — *see also* Accident, machine
    pressure vessel — *see* Explosion, pressure vessel

Explosion — *continued*
  methane E923.2
  missile E923.8
    in
      terrorism E979.2 •
      war operations E993
        injury by fragments from E991.9
  motor vehicle (part of)
    in motion (on public highway) E818 ✓4ᵗʰ
    not on public highway E825 ✓4ᵗʰ
  munitions (dump) (factory) E923.8
    in
      terrorism E979.2 •
      war operations E993
  of mine E923.8
    in
      terrorism •
        at sea or in harbor E979.0 •
        land E979.2 •
        marine E979.0 •
      war operations
        after cessation of hostilities E998
        at sea or in harbor E992
        land E993
          after cessation of hostilities E998
          injury by fragments from E991.9
        marine E992
  own weapons
    in
      terrorism (*see also* Suicide) E979.2 •
      war operations E993
        injury by fragments from E991.9
        antipersonnel bomb E991.3
    injury by fragments from E991.9
      antipersonnel bomb E991.3
  pressure
    cooker E921.8
    gas tank (in machinery) E921.1
    vessel (in machinery) E921.9
      on transport vehicle — *see* categories E800-E848 ✓4ᵗʰ
    specified type NEC E921.8
  propane E923.2
  railway engine, locomotive, train (boiler) (with subsequent collision, derailment, fall) E803 ✓4ᵗʰ
    with
      collision (antecedent) (*see also* Collision, railway) E800 ✓4ᵗʰ
      derailment (antecedent) E802 ✓4ᵗʰ
      fire (without antecedent collision or derailment) E803 ✓4ᵗʰ
  secondary fire resulting from — *see* Fire
  self-inflicted (unspecified whether accidental or intentional) E985.5
    stated as intentional, purposeful E955.5
  shell (artillery) E923.8
    in
      terrorism E979.2 •
      war operations E993
        injury by fragments from E991.9
  stated as undetermined whether caused accidentally or purposely inflicted E985.5
  steam or water lines (in machinery) E921.0
  suicide (attempted) E955.5
  terrorism — *see* Terrorism, explosion •
  torpedo E923.8
    in
      terrorism E979.0 •

Index to External Causes

Explosion — *continued*
  torpedo — *continued*
    in — *continued*
      war operations E992
    transport accident — *see* categories
      E800-E848 ✓4ᵗʰ
  war operations — *see* War operations,
    explosion
  watercraft (boiler) E837 ✓4ᵗʰ
    causing drowning, submersion (after
      jumping from watercraft) E830 ✓4ᵗʰ
Exposure (weather) (conditions) (rain) (wind)
    E904.3
  with homicidal intent E968.4
  excessive E904.3
    cold (*see also* Cold, exposure to) E901.9
      self-inflicted — *see* Cold, exposure to,
        self-inflicted
    heat (*see also* Heat) E900.9
  fire — *see* Fire
  helpless person, infant, newborn due to
    abandonment or neglect E904.0
  noise E928.1
  prolonged in deep-freeze unit or refrigerator
    E901.1
  radiation — *see* Radiation
  resulting from transport accident — *see*
    categories E800-E848 ✓4ᵗʰ
  smoke from, due to
    fire — *see* Fire
  tobacco, second-hand E869.4
  vibration E928.2

F

Fall, falling (accidental) E888.9
  building E916
    burning E891.8
      private E890.8
  down
    escalator E880.0
    ladder E881.0
      in boat, ship, watercraft E833 ✓4ᵗʰ
    staircase E880.9
    stairs, steps — *see* Fall, from, stairs
  earth (with asphyxia or suffocation (by
    pressure)) (*see also* Earth, falling)
    E913.3
  from, off
    aircraft (at landing, take-off) (in-transit)
      (while alighting, boarding) E843 ✓4ᵗʰ
      resulting from accident to aircraft — *see*
        categories E840-E842 ✓4ᵗʰ
    animal (in sport or transport) E828 ✓4ᵗʰ
    animal-drawn vehicle E827 ✓4ᵗʰ
    balcony E882
    bed E884.4
    bicycle E826 ✓4ᵗʰ
    boat, ship, watercraft (into water) E832 ✓4ᵗʰ
      after accident to, collision, fire on
        E830 ✓4ᵗʰ
        and subsequently struck by (part of)
          boat E831 ✓4ᵗʰ
        and subsequently struck by (part of)
          boat E831 ✓4ᵗʰ
      burning, crushed, sinking E830 ✓4ᵗʰ
        and subsequently struck by (part of)
          boat E831 ✓4ᵗʰ
    bridge E882

Fall, falling — *continued*
  from, off — *continued*
    building E882
      burning ▶(uncontrolled fire)◀ E891.8
        in terrorism E979.3
      private E890.8
    bunk in boat, ship, watercraft E834 ✓4ᵗʰ
      due to accident to watercraft E831 ✓4ᵗʰ
    cable car (not on rails) E847
      on rails E829 ✓4ᵗʰ
    car — *see* Fall from motor vehicle
    chair E884.2
    cliff E884.1
    commode E884.6
    curb (sidewalk) E880.1
    elevation aboard ship E834 ✓4ᵗʰ
      due to accident to ship E831 ✓4ᵗʰ
    embankment E884.9
    escalator E880.0
    fire escape E882
    flagpole E882
    furniture NEC E884.5
    gangplank (into water) (*see also* Fall, from,
      boat) E832 ✓4ᵗʰ
      to deck, dock E834 ✓4ᵗʰ
    hammock on ship E834 ✓4ᵗʰ
      due to accident to watercraft E831 ✓4ᵗʰ
    haystack E884.9
    high place NEC E884.9
      stated as undetermined whether
        accidental or intentional — *see*
        Jumping, from, high place
    horse (in sport or transport) E828 ✓4ᵗʰ
    in-line skates E885.1
    ladder E881.0
      in boat, ship, watercraft E833 ✓4ᵗʰ
      due to accident to watercraft E831
        ✓4ᵗʰ
    machinery — *see also* Accident, machine
      not in operation E884.9
    motor vehicle (in motion) (on public
      highway) E818 ✓4ᵗʰ
      not on public highway E825 ✓4ᵗʰ
        stationary, except while alighting,
          boarding, entering, leaving
          E884.9
        while alighting, boarding, entering,
          leaving E824 ✓4ᵗʰ
      stationary, except while alighting,
        boarding, entering, leaving E884.9
      while alighting, boarding, entering,
        leaving, except off-road type motor
        vehicle E817 ✓4ᵗʰ
      off-road type — *see* Fall, from, off-
        road type motor vehicle
    nonmotor road vehicle (while alighting,
      boarding) NEC E829 ✓4ᵗʰ
      stationary, except while alighting,
        boarding, entering, leaving E884.9
    off road type motor vehicle (not on public
      highway) NEC E821 ✓4ᵗʰ
      on public highway E818 ✓4ᵗʰ
        while alighting, boarding, entering,
          leaving E817 ✓4ᵗʰ
    snow vehicle — *see* Fall from snow
      vehicle, motor-driven
    one
      deck to another on ship E834 ✓4ᵗʰ
        due to accident to ship E831 ✓4ᵗʰ
      level to another NEC E884.9

Fall, falling

Fall, falling — *continued*
  from, off — *continued*
    one — *continued*
      level to another — *continued*
        boat, ship, or watercraft E834 ✓4ᵗʰ
          due to accident to watercraft
            E831 ✓4ᵗʰ
    pedal cycle E826 ✓4ᵗʰ
    playground equipment E884.0
    railway rolling stock, train, vehicle, (while
      alighting, boarding) E804 ✓4ᵗʰ
      with
        collision (*see also* Collision, railway)
          E800 ✓4ᵗʰ
        derailment (*see also* Derailment,
          railway) E802 ✓4ᵗʰ
        explosion (*see also* Explosion, railway
          engine) E803 ✓4ᵗʰ
    rigging (aboard ship) E834 ✓4ᵗʰ
      due to accident to watercraft E831 ✓4ᵗʰ
    roller skates E885.1
    scaffolding E881.1
    scooter (nonmotorized) E885.0
    sidewalk (curb) E880.1
      moving E885.9
    skateboard E885.2
    skis E885.3
    snow vehicle, motor-driven (not on public
      highway) E820 ✓4ᵗʰ
      on public highway E818 ✓4ᵗʰ
        while alighting, boarding, entering,
          leaving E817 ✓4ᵗʰ
    snowboard E885.4
    stairs, step E880.9
      boat, ship, watercraft E833 ✓4ᵗʰ
        due to accident to watercraft E831
          ✓4ᵗʰ
      motor bus, motor vehicle — *see* Fall,
        from, motor vehicle, while
        alighting, boarding
      street car E829 ✓4ᵗʰ
    stationary vehicle NEC E884.9
    stepladder E881.0
    street car (while boarding, alighting)
      E829 ✓4ᵗʰ
      stationary, except while boarding or
        alighting F884.9 ✓4ᵗʰ
    structure NEC E882
      burning ▶(uncontrolled fire)◀ E891.8
      in terrorism E979.3
    table E884.9
    toilet E884.6
    tower E882
    tree E884.9
    turret E882
    vehicle NEC — *see also* Accident, vehicle
      NEC
      stationary E884.9
    viaduct E882
    wall E882
    wheelchair E884.3
    window E882
  in, on
    aircraft (at landing, take-off) (in-transit)
      E843 ✓4ᵗʰ
      resulting from accident to aircraft — *see*
        categories E840-E842 ✓4ᵗʰ
    boat, ship, watercraft E835 ✓4ᵗʰ
      due to accident to watercraft E831 ✓4ᵗʰ
      one level to another NEC E834 ✓4ᵗʰ

Fall, falling — *continued*
  in, on — *continued*
    boat, ship, watercraft — *continued*
      on ladder, stairs E833 ✓4ᵗʰ
    cutting or piercing instrument or machine
      E888.0
    deck (of boat, ship, watercraft) E835 ✓4ᵗʰ
      due to accident to watercraft E831 ✓4ᵗʰ
    escalator E880.0
    gangplank E835 ✓4ᵗʰ
    glass, broken E888.0
    knife E888.0
    ladder E881.0
      in boat, ship, watercraft E833 ✓4ᵗʰ
        due to accident to watercraft E831
          ✓4ᵗʰ
    object
      edged, pointed or sharp E888.0
      other E888.1
    pitchfork E888.0
    railway rolling stock, train, vehicle (while
      alighting, boarding) E804 ✓4ᵗʰ
      with
        collision (*see also* Collision, railway)
          E800 ✓4ᵗʰ
        derailment (*see also* Derailment,
          railway) E802 ✓4ᵗʰ
        explosion (see also Explosion, railway
          engine) E803 ✓4ᵗʰ
    scaffolding E881.1
    scissors E888.0
    staircase, stairs, steps (*see also* Fall, from,
      stairs) E880.9
    street car E829 ✓4ᵗʰ
    water transport (*see also* Fall, in, boat)
      E835 ✓4ᵗʰ
  into
    cavity E883.9
    dock E883.9
      from boat, ship, watercraft (*see also* Fall,
        from, boat) E832 ✓4ᵗʰ
    hold (of ship) E834 ✓4ᵗʰ
      due to accident to watercraft E831 ✓4ᵗʰ
    hole E883.9
    manhole E883.2
    moving part of machinery — *see* Accident,
      machine
    opening in surface NEC E883.9
    pit E883.9
    quarry E883.9
    shaft E883.9
    storm drain E883.2
    tank E883.9
    water (with drowning or submersion)
      E910.9
    well E883.1
  late effect of NEC E929.3
  object (*see also* Hit by, object, falling) E916
  other E888.8
  over
    animal E885.9
    cliff E884.1
    embankment E884.9
    small object E885
  overboard (*see also* Fall, from, boat) E832 ✓4ᵗʰ
  resulting in striking against object E888.1
    sharp E888.0
  rock E916
  same level NEC E888.9
    aircraft (any kind) E843 ✓4ᵗʰ

Index to External Causes — Fire

Fall, falling — *continued*
  same level — *continued*
    aircraft — *continued*
      resulting from accident to aircraft — *see* categories E840-E842 ✓4ᵗʰ
    boat, ship, watercraft E835 ✓4ᵗʰ
      due to accident to, collision, watercraft E831 ✓4ᵗʰ
    from
      collision, pushing, shoving, by or with other person(s) E886.9
        as, or caused by, a crowd E917.6
        in sports E886.0
        scooter (nonmotorized) E885.0
      slipping stumbling, tripping E885
  snowslide E916
    as avalanche E909.2
  stone E916
  through
    hatch (on ship) E834 ✓4ᵗʰ
      due to accident to watercraft E831 ✓4ᵗʰ
    roof E882
    window E882
  timber E916
  while alighting from, boarding, entering, leaving
    aircraft (any kind) E843 ✓4ᵗʰ
    motor bus, motor vehicle — *see* Fall, from, motor vehicle, while alighting, boarding
    nonmotor road vehicle NEC E829 ✓4ᵗʰ
    railway train E804 ✓4ᵗʰ
    street car E829 ✓4ᵗʰ

Fallen on by
  animal (horse) (not being ridden) E906.8
    being ridden (in sport or transport) E828 ✓4ᵗʰ

Fell or jumped from high place, so stated — *see* Jumping, from, high place

Felo-de-se (*see also* Suicide) E958.9

Fever
  heat — *see* Heat
  thermic — *see* Heat

Fight (hand) (fist) (foot) (*see also* Assault, fight) E960.0

Fire (accidental) (caused by great heat from appliance (electrical), hot object or hot substance) (secondary, resulting from explosion) E899
  conflagration — *see* Conflagration
  controlled, normal (in brazier, fireplace, furnace, or stove) (charcoal) (coal) (coke) (electric) (gas) (wood)
    bonfire E897
    brazier, not in building or structure E897
    in building or structure, except private dwelling (barn) (church) (convalescent or residential home) (factory) (farm outbuilding) (hospital) (hotel) (institution (educational) (dormitory) (residential)) (private garage) (school) (shop) (store) (theatre) E896
    in private dwelling (apartment) (boarding house) (camping place) (caravan) (farmhouse) (home (private)) (house) (lodging house) (rooming house) (tenement) E895
    not in building or structure E897
    trash E897

Fire — *continued*
  forest (uncontrolled) E892
  grass (uncontrolled) E892
  hay (uncontrolled) E892
  homicide (attempt) E968.0
    late effect of E969
  in, of, on, starting in E892
    aircraft (in transit) (powered) E841 ✓4ᵗʰ
      at landing, take-off E840 ✓4ᵗʰ
      stationary E892
      unpowered (balloon) (glider) E842 ✓4ᵗʰ
    balloon E842 ✓4ᵗʰ
    boat, ship, watercraft — *see* categories E830 ✓4ᵗʰ, E831 ✓4ᵗʰ, E837 ✓4ᵗʰ
    building or structure, except private dwelling (barn) (church) (convalescent or residential home) (factory) (farm outbuilding) (hospital) (hotel) (institution (educational) (dormitory) (residential)) (school) (shop) (store) (theatre) (*see also* Conflagration, building or structure, except private dwelling) E891.9
    forest (uncontrolled) E892
    glider E842 ✓4ᵗʰ
    grass (uncontrolled) E892
    hay (uncontrolled) E892
    lumber (uncontrolled) E892
    machinery — *see* Accident, machine
    mine (uncontrolled) E892
    motor vehicle (in motion) (on public highway) E818 ✓4ᵗʰ
      not on public highway E825 ✓4ᵗʰ
      stationary E892
    prairie (uncontrolled) E892
    private dwelling (apartment) (boarding house) (camping place) (caravan) (farmhouse) (home (private)) (house) (lodging house) (private garage) (rooming house) (tenement) (*see also* Conflagration, private dwelling) E890.9
    railway rolling stock, train, vehicle (*see also* Explosion, railway engine) E803 ✓4ᵗʰ
      stationary E892
    room NEC E898.1
    street car (in motion) E829 ✓4ᵗʰ
      stationary E892
    terrorism (by fire-producing device) E979.3
      fittings or furniture (burning building) (uncontrolled fire) E979.3
      from nuclear explosion E979.5
    transport vehicle, stationary NEC E892
    tunnel (uncontrolled) E892
    war operations (by fire-producing device or conventional weapon) E990.9
      from nuclear explosion E996
      petrol bomb E990.0
  late effect of NEC E929.4
  lumber (uncontrolled) E892
  mine (uncontrolled) E892
  prairie (uncontrolled) E892
  self-inflicted (unspecified whether accidental or intentional) E988.1
    stated as intentional, purposeful E958.1
  specified NEC E898.1
    with
      conflagration — *see* Conflagration

Fire — *continued*
  specified — *continued*
    with — *continued*
      ignition (of)
        clothing — *see* Ignition, clothes
        highly inflammable material (benzine) (fat) (gasoline) (kerosene) (paraffin) (petrol) E894
    started by other person
      stated as
        with intent to injure or kill E968.0
        undetermined whether or not with intent to injure or kill E988.1
    suicide (attempted) E958.1
      late effect of E959
    tunnel (uncontrolled) E892
Fireball effects from nuclear explosion
  in
    terrorism E979.5
    war operations E996
Fireworks (explosion) E923.0
Flash burns from explosion (*see also* Explosion) E923.9
Flood (any injury) (resulting from storm) E908.2
  caused by collapse of dam or manmade structure E909.3
Forced landing (aircraft) E840 ✓4ᵗʰ
Foreign body, object or material (entrance into (accidental))
  air passage (causing injury) E915
    with asphyxia, obstruction, suffocation E912
      food or vomitus E911
    nose (with asphyxia, obstruction, suffocation) E912
    causing injury without asphyxia, obstruction, suffocation E915
  alimentary canal (causing injury) (with obstruction) E915
    with asphyxia, obstruction respiratory passage, suffocation E912
      food E911
    mouth E915
      with asphyxia, obstruction, suffocation E912
        food E911
    pharynx E915
      with asphyxia, obstruction, suffocation E912
        food E911
  aspiration (with asphyxia, obstruction respiratory passage, suffocation) E912
    causing injury without asphyxia, obstruction respiratory passage, suffocation E915
    food (regurgitated) (vomited) E911
      causing injury without asphyxia, obstruction respiratory passage, suffocation E915
    mucus (not of newborn) E912
    phlegm E912
  bladder (causing injury or obstruction) E915
  bronchus, bronchi — *see* Foreign body, air passages
  conjunctival sac E914
  digestive system — *see* Foreign body, alimentary canal
  ear (causing injury or obstruction) E915

Foreign body, object or material — *continued*
  esophagus (causing injury or obstruction) (*see also* Foreign body, alimentary canal) E915
  eye (any part) E914
  eyelid E914
  hairball (stomach) (with obstruction) E915
  ingestion — *see* Foreign body, alimentary canal
  inhalation — *see* Foreign body, aspiration
  intestine (causing injury or obstruction) E915
  iris E914
  lacrimal apparatus E914
  larynx — *see* Foreign body, air passage
  late effect of NEC E929.8
  lung — *see* Foreign body, air passage
  mouth — *see* Foreign body, alimentary canal, mouth
  nasal passage — *see* Foreign body, air passage, nose
  nose — *see* Foreign body, air passage, nose
  ocular muscle E914
  operation wound (left in) — *see* Misadventure, foreign object
  orbit E914
  pharynx — *see* Foreign body, alimentary canal, pharynx
  rectum (causing injury or obstruction) E915
  stomach (hairball) (causing injury or obstruction) E915
  tear ducts or glands E914
  trachea — *see* Foreign body, air passage
  urethra (causing injury or obstruction) E915
  vagina (causing injury or obstruction) E915
Found dead, injured
  from exposure (to) — *see* Exposure
  on
    public highway E819 ✓4ᵗʰ
    railway right of way E807 ✓4ᵗʰ
Fracture (circumstances unknown or unspecified) E887
  due to specified external means — *see* manner of accident
  late effect of NEC E929.3
  occuring in water transport NEC E835 ✓4ᵗʰ
Freezing — *see* Cold, exposure to
Frostbite E901.0
  due to manmade conditions E901.1
Frozen — *see* Cold, exposure to

G

Garrotting, homicidal (attempted) E963
Gored E906.8
Gunshot wound (*see also* Shooting) E922.9

H

Hailstones, injury by E904.3
Hairball (stomach) (with obstruction) E915
Hanged himself (*see also* Hanging, self-inflicted) E983.0
Hang gliding E842 ✓4ᵗʰ
Hanging (accidental) E913.8
  caused by other person
    in accidental circumstances E913.8
    stated as
      intentional, homicidal E963

Hanging — *continued*
  caused by other person — *continued*
    stated as — *continued*
      undetermined whether accidental or intentional E983.0
  homicide (attempt) E963
  in bed or cradle E913.0
  legal execution E978
  self-inflicted (unspecified whether accidental or intentional) E983.0
    in accidental circumstances E913.8
    stated as intentional, purposeful E953.0
    stated as undetermined whether accidental or intentional E983.0
  suicidal (attempt) E953.0
Heat (apoplexy) (collapse) (cramps) (effects of) (excessive) (exhaustion) (fever) (prostration) (stroke) E900.9
  due to
    manmade conditions (as listed in E900.1, except boat, ship, watercraft) E900.1
    weather (conditions) E900.0
  from
    electric heating apparatus causing burning E924.8
    nuclear explosion
      in
        terrorism E979.5
        war operations E996
    generated in, boiler, engine, evaporator, fire room of boat, ship, watercraft E838 ✓4ᵗʰ
    inappropriate in local application or packing in medical or surgical procedure E873.5
  late effect of NEC E989
Hemorrhage
  delayed following medical or surgical treatment without mention of misadventure — *see* Reaction, abnormal
  during medical or surgical treatment as misadventure — *see* Misadventure, cut
High
  altitude, effects E902.9
  level of radioactivity, effects — *see* Radiation
  pressure effects — *see also* Effects of, air pressure
    from rapid descent in water (causing caisson or divers' disease, palsy, or paralysis) E902.2
  temperature, effects — *see* Heat
Hit, hitting (accidental) by
  aircraft (propeller) (without accident to aircraft) E844 ✓4ᵗʰ
    unpowered E842 ✓4ᵗʰ
  avalanche E909.2
  being thrown against object in or part of motor vehicle (in motion) (on public highway) E818 ✓4ᵗʰ
    not on public highway E825 ✓4ᵗʰ
    nonmotor road vehicle NEC E829 ✓4ᵗʰ
    street car E829 ✓4ᵗʰ
  boat, ship, watercraft
    after fall from watercraft E838 ✓4ᵗʰ
      damaged, involved in accident E831 ✓4ᵗʰ
    while swimming, water skiing E838 ✓4ᵗʰ
  bullet (*see also* Shooting) E922.9
    from air gun E922.4
    in
      terrorism E979.4
      war operations E991.2
        rubber E991.0

Hit, hitting — *continued*
  flare, Verey pistol (*see also* Shooting) E922.8
  hailstones E904.3
  landslide E909.2
  law-enforcing agent (on duty) E975
    with blunt object (baton) (night stick) (stave) (truncheon) E973
  machine — *see* Accident, machine
  missile
    firearm (*see also* Shooting) E922.9
    in
      terrorism — *see* Terrorism, mission
      war operations — *see* War operations, missile
  motor vehicle (on public highway) (traffic accident) E814 ✓4ᵗʰ
    not on public highway, nontraffic accident E822 ✓4ᵗʰ
  nonmotor road vehicle NEC E829 ✓4ᵗʰ
  object
    falling E916
      from, in, on
        aircraft E844 ✓4ᵗʰ
          due to accident to aircraft — *see* categories E840-E842 ✓4ᵗʰ
          unpowered E842 ✓4ᵗʰ
        boat, ship, watercraft E838 ✓4ᵗʰ
          due to accident to watercraft E831 ✓4ᵗʰ
        building E916
          burning (uncontrolled fire) E891.8
            in terrorism E979.3
            private E890.8
    cataclysmic
      earth surface movement or eruption E909.9
      storm E908.9
    cave-in E916
      with asphyxiation or suffocation (*see also* Suffocation, due to, cave-in) E913.3
    earthquake E909.0
    motor vehicle (in motion) (on public highway) E818 ✓4ᵗʰ
      not on public highway E825 ✓4ᵗʰ
      stationary E916
    nonmotor road vehicle NEC E829 ✓4ᵗʰ
    pedal cycle E826 ✓4ᵗʰ
    railway rolling stock, train, vehicle E806 ✓4ᵗʰ
    street car E829 ✓4ᵗʰ
    structure, burning NEC E891.8
    vehicle, stationary E916
  moving NEC — *see* Striking against, object
  projected NEC — *see* Striking against, object
  set in motion by
    compressed air or gas, spring, striking, throwing — *see* Striking against, object
  explosion — *see* Explosion
  thrown into, on, or towards
    motor vehicle (in motion) (on public highway) E818 ✓4ᵗʰ
    not on public highway E825 ✓4ᵗʰ
    nonmotor road vehicle NEC E829 ✓4ᵗʰ
    pedal cycle E826 ✓4ᵗʰ
    strect car E829 ✓4ᵗʰ
  off-road type motor vehicle (not on public highway) E821 ✓4ᵗʰ

Hit, hitting

Hit, hitting — *continued*
  off-road type motor vehicle — *continued*
    on public highway E814 ✓4th
  other person(s) E917.9
    with blunt or thrown object E917.9
      in sports E917.0
        with subsequent fall E917.5
      intentionally, homicidal E968.2
    as, or caused by, a crowd E917.1
      with subsequent fall E917.6
      in sports E917.0
  pedal cycle E826 ✓4th
  police (on duty) E975
    with blunt object (baton) (nightstick) (stave) (truncheon) E973
  railway, rolling stock, train, vehicle (part of) E805 ✓4th
  shot — *see* Shooting
  snow vehicle, motor-driven (not on public highway) E820 ✓4th
    on public highway E814 ✓4th
  street car E829 ✓4th
  vehicle NEC — *see* Accident, vehicle NEC
Homicide, homicidal (attempt) (justifiable) (*see also* Assault) E968.9
Hot
  liquid, object, substance, accident caused by — *see also* Accident, caused by, hot, by type of substance
    late effect of E929.8
  place, effects — *see* Heat
  weather, effects E900.0
Humidity, causing problem E904.3
Hunger E904.1
  resulting from
    abandonment or neglect E904.0
    transport accident — *see* categories E800-E848 ✓4th
Hurricane (any injury) E908.0
Hypobarism, hypobaropathy — *see* Effects of, air pressure
Hypothermia — *see* Cold, exposure to

I

Ictus
  caloris — *see* Heat
  solaris E900.0
Ignition (accidental)
  anesthetic gas in operating theatre E923.2
  bedclothes
    with
      conflagration — *see* Conflagration
      ignition (of)
        clothing — *see* Ignition, clothes
        highly inflammable material (benzine) (fat) (gasoline) (kerosene) (paraffin) (petrol) E894
  benzine E894
  clothes, clothing (from controlled fire) (in building) E893.9
    with conflagration — *see* Conflagration from
      bonfire E893.2
      highly inflammable material E894
      sources or material as listed in E893.8
      trash fire E893.2
    uncontrolled fire — *see* Conflagration

Ignition — *continued*
  clothes, clothing — *continued*
    in
      private dwelling E893.0
      specified building or structure, except private dwelling E893.1
    not in building or structure E893.2
  explosive material — *see* Explosion
  fat E894
  gasoline E894
  kerosene E894
  material
    explosive — *see* Explosion
    highly inflammable E894
      with conflagration — *see* Conflagration
      with explosion E923.2
  nightdress — *see* Ignition, clothes
  paraffin E894
  petrol E894
Immersion — *see* Submersion
Implantation of quills of porcupine E906.8
Inanition (from) E904.9
  hunger — *see* Lack of, food
  resulting from homicidal intent E968.4
  thirst — *see* Lack of, water
Inattention after, at birth E904.0
  homicidal, infanticidal intent E968.4
Infanticide (*see also* Assault)
Ingestion
  foreign body (causing injury) (with obstruction) — *see* Foreign body, alimentary canal
  poisonous substance NEC — *see* Table of Drugs and Chemicals
Inhalation
  excessively cold substance, manmade E901.1
  foreign body — *see* Foreign body, aspiration
  liquid air, hydrogen, nitrogen E901.1
  mucus, not of newborn (with asphyxia, obstruction respiratory passage, suffocation) E912
  phlegm (with asphyxia, obstruction respiratory passage, suffocation) E912
  poisonous gas — *see* Table of Drugs and Chemicals
  smoke from, due to
    fire — *see* Fire
    tobacco, second-hand E869.4
  vomitus (with asphyxia, obstruction respiratory passage, suffocation) E911
Injury, injured (accidental(ly)) NEC E928.9
  by, caused by, from
    air rifle (BB gun) E922.4
    animal (not being ridden) NEC E906.9
      being ridden (in sport or transport) E828 ✓4th
    assault (*see also* Assault) E968.9
    avalanche E909.2
    bayonet (*see also* Bayonet wound) E920.3
    being thrown against some part of, or object in
      motor vehicle (in motion) (on public highway) E818 ✓4th
        not on public highway E825 ✓4th
      nonmotor road vehicle NEC E829 ✓4th
      off-road motor vehicle NEC E821 ✓4th
      railway train E806 ✓4th
      snow vehicle, motor-driven E820 ✓4th
      street car E829 ✓4th
    bending E927

Index to External Causes

Injury, injured — *continued*
  by, caused by, from — *continued*
    broken glass E920.8
    bullet — *see* Shooting
    cave-in (*see also* Suffocation, due to, cave-in) E913.3
      earth surface movement or eruption E909.9
      earthquake E909.0
      flood E908.2
      hurricane E908.0
      landslide E909.2
      storm E908.9
      without asphyxiation or suffocation E916
    cloudburst E908.8
    cutting or piercing instrument (*see also* Cut) E920.9
    cyclone E908.1
    earth surface movement or eruption E909.9
    earthquake E909 ✓4ᵗʰ
    electric current (*see also* Electric shock) E925.9
    explosion (*see also* Explosion) E923.9
    fire — *see* Fire
    flare, Verey pistol E922.8
    flood E908
    foreign body — *see* Foreign body
    hailstones E904.3
    hurricane E908
    landslide E909 ✓4ᵗʰ
    law-enforcing agent, police, in course of legal intervention — *see* Legal intervention
    lightning E907
    live rail or live wire — *see* Electric shock
    machinery — *see also* Accident, machine
      aircraft, without accident to aircraft E844 ✓4ᵗʰ
      boat, ship, watercraft (deck) (engine room) (galley) (laundry) (loading) E836 ✓4ᵗʰ
    missile
      explosive E923.8
      firearm — *see* Shooting
      in
        terrorism — see Terrorism, missile •
        war operations — *see* War operations, missile
    moving part of motor vehicle (in motion) (on public highway) E818 ✓4ᵗʰ
      not on public highway, nontraffic accident E825 ✓4ᵗʰ
      while alighting, boarding, entering, leaving — *see* Fall, from, motor vehicle, while alighting, boarding
    nail E920.8
    needle (sewing) E920.4
      hypodermic E920.5
    noise E928.1
    object
      fallen on
        motor vehicle (in motion) (on public highway) E818 ✓4ᵗʰ
          not on public highway E825 ✓4ᵗʰ
      falling — *see* Hit by, object, falling
    paintball gun E922.5 •
    radiation — *see* Radiation
    railway rolling stock, train, vehicle (part of) E805 ✓4ᵗʰ

Injury, injured — *continued*
  by, caused by, from — *continued*
    railway rolling stock, train, vehicle — *continued*
      door or window E806 ✓4ᵗʰ
      rotating propeller, aircraft E844 ✓4ᵗʰ
      rough landing of off-road type motor vehicle (after leaving ground or rough terrain) E821 ✓4ᵗʰ
      snow vehicle E820 ✓4ᵗʰ
    saber (*see also* Wound, saber) E920.3
    shot — *see* Shooting
    sound waves E928.1
    splinter or sliver, wood E920.8
    straining E927
    street car (door) E829 ✓4ᵗʰ
    suicide (attempt) E958.9
    sword E920.3
    terrorism — *see* Terrorism •
    third rail — *see* Electric shock
    thunderbolt E907
    tidal wave E909.4
      caused by storm E908.0
    tornado E908.1
    torrential rain E908.2
    twisting E927
    vehicle NEC — *see* Accident, vehicle NEC
    vibration E928.2
    volcanic eruption E909.1
    weapon burst, in war operations E993
    weightlessness (in spacecraft, real or simulated) E928.0
    wood splinter or sliver E920.8
  due to
    civil insurrection — *see* War operations occurring after cessation of hostilities E998
    terrorism — *see* Terrorism •
    war operations — *see* War operations occurring after cessation of hostilities E998
  homicidal (*see also* Assault) E968.9
  in, on
    civil insurrection — *see* War operations
    fight E960.0
    parachute descent (voluntary) (without accident to aircraft) E844 ✓4ᵗʰ
      with accident to aircraft — *see* categories E840-E842 ✓4ᵗʰ
    public highway E819 ✓4ᵗʰ
    railway right of way E807 ✓4ᵗʰ
    terrorism — *see* Terrorism •
    war operations — *see* War operations
  inflicted (by)
    in course of arrest (attempted), suppression of disturbance, maintenance of order, by law enforcing agents — *see* Legal intervention
    law-enforcing agent (on duty) — *see* Legal intervention
    other person
      stated as
        accidental E928.9
        homicidal, intentional — *see* Assault
        undetermined whether accidental or intentional — *see* Injury, stated as undetermined
    police (on duty) — *see* Legal intervention
  late effect of E929.9
  purposely (inflicted) by other person(s) — *see* Assault

Injury, injured — continued
- self-inflicted (unspecified whether accidental or intentional) E988.9
  - stated as
    - accidental E928.9
    - intentionally, purposely E958.9
  - specified cause NEC E928.8
  - stated as
    - undetermined whether accidentally or purposely inflicted (by) E988.9
      - cut (any part of body) E986
      - cutting or piercing instrument (classifiable to E920) E986
      - drowning E984
      - explosive(s) (missile) E985.5
      - falling from high place E987.9
        - manmade structure, except residential E987.1
        - natural site E987.2
        - residential premises E987.0
      - hanging E983.0
      - knife E986
      - late effect of E989
      - puncture (any part of body) E986
      - shooting — see Shooting, stated as undetermined whether accidental or intentional
      - specified means NEC E988.8
      - stab (any part of body) E986
      - strangulation — see Suffocation, stated as undetermined whether accidental or intentional
      - submersion E984
      - suffocation — see Suffocation, stated as undetermined whether accidental or intentional
- to child due to criminal abortion E968.8

Insufficient nourishment — see also Lack of, food
- homicidal intent E968.4

Insulation, effects — see Heat

Interruption of respiration by
- food lodged in esophagus E911
- foreign body, except food, in esophagus E912

Intervention, legal — see Legal intervention

Intoxication, drug or poison — see Table of Drugs and Chemicals

Irradiation — see Radiation

J

Jammed (accidentally)
- between objects (moving) (stationary and moving) E918
- in object E918

Jumped or fell from high place, so stated — see Jumping, from, high place, stated as in undetermined circumstances

Jumping
- before train, vehicle or other moving object (unspecified whether accidental or intentional) E988.0
  - stated as
    - intentional, purposeful E958.0
    - suicidal (attempt) E958.0

Jumping — continued
- from
  - aircraft
    - by parachute (voluntarily) (without accident to aircraft) E844 ☑4th
    - due to accident to aircraft — see categories E840-E842 ☑4th
  - boat, ship, watercraft (into water)
    - after accident to, fire on, watercraft E830 ☑4th
      - and subsequently struck by (part of) boat E831 ☑4th
    - burning, crushed, sinking E830 ☑4th
      - and subsequently struck by (part of) boat E831 ☑4th
    - voluntarily, without accident (to boat)
      - with injury other than drowning or submersion E883.0
  - building ▶— see also Jumping, from, high place◀
    - burning ▶(uncontrolled fire)◀ E891.8
      - in terrorism E979.3
    - private E890.8
  - cable car (not on rails) E847
    - on rails E829 ☑4th
  - high place
    - in accidental circumstances or in sport — see categories E880-E884 ☑4th
    - stated as
      - with intent to injure self E957.9
        - man-made structures NEC E957.1
        - natural sites E957.2
        - residential premises E957.0
      - in undetermined circumstances E987.9
        - man-made structures NEC E987.1
        - natural sites E987.2
        - residential premises E987.0
      - suicidal (attempt) E957.9
        - man-made structures NEC E957.1
        - natural sites E957.1
        - residential premises E957.0
  - motor vehicle (in motion) (on public highway) — see Fall, from, motor vehicle
  - nonmotor road vehicle NEC E829 ☑4th
  - street car E829 ☑4th
  - structure ▶— see also Jumping, from, high place◀
    - burning NEC (uncontrolled fire) E891.8
    - in terrorism E979.3
- into water
  - with injury other than drowning or submersion E883.0
  - drowning or submersion — see Submersion
- from, off, watercraft — see Jumping, from, boat

Justifiable homicide — see Assault

K

Kicked by
- animal E906.8
- person(s) (accidentally) E917.9
  - with intent to injure or kill E960.0
  - as, or caused by a crowd E917.1
    - with subsequent fall E917.6

Kicked by — *continued*
  person(s) — *continued*
    in fight E960.0
    in sports E917.0
      with subsequent fall E917.5
Kicking against
  object (moving) E917.9
    in sports E917.0
      with subsequent fall E917.5
    stationary E917.4
      with subsequent fall E917.8
  person — *see* Striking against, person
Killed, killing (accidentally) NEC (*see also* Injury) E928.9
  in
    action — *see* War operations
    brawl, fight (hand) (fists) (foot) E960.0
      by weapon — *see also* Assault
        cutting, piercing E966
        firearm — *see* Shooting, homicide
  self
    stated as
      accident E928.9
      suicide — *see* Suicide
    unspecified whether accidental or suicidal E988.9
Knocked down (accidentally) (by) NEC E928.9
  animal (not being ridden) E906.8
  being ridden (in sport or transport) E828 ☑4ᵗʰ
  blast from explosion (*see also* Explosion) E923.9
  crowd, human stampede E917.6
  late effect of — *see* Late effect
  person (accidentally) E917.9
    in brawl, fight E960.0
    in sports E917.5
  transport vehicle — *see* vehicle involved under Hit by
  while boxing E917.5

L

Laceration NEC E928.9
Lack of
  air (refrigerator or closed place), suffocation by E913.2
  care (helpless person) (infant) (newborn) E904.0
    homicidal intent E968.4
  food except as result of transport accident E904.1
    helpless person, infant, newborn due to abandonment or neglect E904.0
  water except as result of transport accident E904.2
    helpless person, infant, newborn due to abandonment or neglect E904.0
Landslide E909.2
  falling on, hitting
    motor vehicle (any) (in motion) (on or off public highway) E909.2
    railway rolling stock, train, vehicle E909.2
Late effect of
  accident NEC (accident classifiable to E928.9) E929.9
  specified NEC (accident classifiable to E910-E928.8) E929.8
  assault E969

Late effect of — *continued*
  fall, accidental (accident classifiable to E880-E888) E929.3
  fire, accident caused by (accident classifiable to E890-E899) E929.4
  homicide, attempt (any means) E969
  injury due to terrorism E999.1 ●
  injury undetermined whether accidentally or purposely inflicted (injury classifiable to E980-E988) E989
  legal intervention (injury classifiable to E970-E976) E977
  medical or surgical procedure, test or therapy as, or resulting in, or from
    abnormal or delayed reaction or complication — *see* Reaction, abnormal
    misadventure — *see* Misadventure
  motor vehicle accident (accident classifiable to E810-E825) E929.0
  natural or environmental factor, accident due to (accident classifiable to E900-E909) E929.5
  poisoning, accidental (accident classifiable to E850-E858, E860-E869) E929.2
  suicide, attempt (any means) E959
  transport accident NEC (accident classifiable to E800-E807, E826-E838, E840-E848) E929.1
  war operations, injury due to (injury classifiable to E990-E998) E999.0 ▲
Launching pad accident E845 ☑4ᵗʰ
Legal
  execution, any method E978
  intervention (by) (injury from) E976
    baton E973
    bayonet E974
    blow E975
    blunt object (baton) (nightstick) (stave) (truncheon) E973
    cutting or piercing instrument E974
    dynamite E971
    execution, any method E973
    explosive(s) (shell) E971
    firearm(s) E970
    gas (asphyxiation) (poisoning) (tear) E972
    grenade E971
    late effect of E977
    machine gun E970
    manhandling E975
    mortar bomb E971
    nightstick E973
    revolver E970
    rifle E970
    specified means NEC E975
    stabbing E974
    stave E973
    truncheon E973
Lifting, injury in E927
Lightning (shock) (stroke) (struck by) E907
Liquid (noncorrosive) in eye E914
  corrosive E924.1
Loss of control
  motor vehicle (on public highway) (without antecedent collision) E816 ☑4ᵗʰ
    with
      antecedent collision on public highway — *see* Collision, motor vehicle
      involving any object, person or vehicle not on public highway E816 ☑4ᵗʰ

Loss of control — *continued*
  motor vehicle — *continued*
    with — *continued*
      antecedent collision on public highway
        — *continued*
        on public highway — *see* Collision,
          motor vehicle
        not on public highway, nontraffic
          accident E825 ◢4ᵗʰ
          with antecedent collision — *see*
            Collision, motor vehicle, not
            on public highway
      off-road type motor vehicle (not on public
        highway) E821 ◢4ᵗʰ
        on public highway — *see* Loss of control,
          motor vehicle
      snow vehicle, motor-driven (not on public
        highway) E820 ◢4ᵗʰ
        on public highway — *see* Loss of control,
          motor vehicle
Lost at sea E832 ◢4ᵗʰ
  with accident to watercraft E830 ◢4ᵗʰ
  in war operations E995
Low
  pressure, effects — *see* Effects of, air pressure
  temperature, effects — *see* Cold, exposure to
Lying before train, vehicle or other moving object (unspecified whether accidental or intentional) E988.0
  stated as intentional, purposeful, suicidal (attempt) E958.0
Lynching (*see also* Assault) E968.9

M

Malfunction, atomic power plant in water transport E838 ◢4ᵗʰ
Mangled (accidentally) NEC E928.9
Manhandling (in brawl, fight) E960.0
  legal intervention E975
Manslaughter (nonaccidental) — *see* Assault
Marble in nose E912
Mauled by animal E906.8
Medical procedure, complication of
  delayed or as an abnormal reaction without mention of misadventure — *see* Reaction, abnormal
  due to or as a result of misadventure — *see* Misadventure
Melting of fittings and furniture in burning ●
  in terrorism E979.3 ●
Minamata disease E865.2
Misadventure(s) to patient(s) during surgical or medical care E876.9
  contaminated blood, fluid, drug or biological substance (presence of agents and toxins as listed in E875) E875.9
    administered (by) NEC E875.9
      infusion E875.0
      injection E875.1
      specified means NEC E875.2
      transfusion E875.0
      vaccination E875.1
  cut, cutting, puncture, perforation or hemorrhage (accidental) (inadvertent) (inappropriate) (during) E870.9

Misadventure(s) to patient(s) during surgical or medical care — *continued*
  cut, cutting, puncture, perforation or hemorrhage — *continued*
    aspiration of fluid or tissue (by puncture or catheterization, except heart) E870.5
    biopsy E870.8
      needle (aspirating) E870.5
    blood sampling E870.5
    catheterization E870.5
      heart E870.6
    dialysis (kidney) E870.2
    endoscopic examination E870.4
    enema E870.7
    infusion E870.1
    injection E870.3
    lumbar puncture E870.5
    needle biopsy E870.5
    paracentesis, abdominal E870.5
    perfusion E870.2
    specified procedure NEC E870.8
    surgical operation E870.0
    thoracentesis E870.5
    transfusion E870.1
    vaccination E870.3
  excessive amount of blood or other fluid during transfusion or infusion E873.0
  failure
    in dosage E873.9
      electroshock therapy E873.4
      inappropriate temperature (too hot or too cold) in local application and packing E873.5
      infusion
        excessive amount of fluid E873.0
        incorrect dilution of fluid E873.1
      insulin-shock therapy E873.4
      nonadministration of necessary drug or medicinal E873.6
      overdose — *see also* Overdose
        radiation, in therapy E873.2
      radiation
        inadvertent exposure of patient (receiving radiation for test or therapy) E873.3
        not receiving radiation for test or therapy — *see* Radiation overdose E873.2
      specified procedure NEC E873.8
      transfusion
        excessive amount of blood E873.0
  mechanical, of instrument or apparatus (during procedure) E874.9
    aspiration of fluid or tissue (by puncture or catheterization, except of heart) E874.4
    biopsy E874.8
      needle (aspirating) E874.4
    blood sampling E874.4
    catheterization E874.4
      heart E874.5
    dialysis (kidney) E874.2
    endoscopic examination E874.3
    enema E874.8
    infusion E874.1
    injection E874.8
    lumbar puncture E874.4
    needle biopsy E874.4
    paracentesis, abdominal E874.4
    perfusion E874.2

Misadventure(s) to patient(s) during surgical or medical care — continued
  failure — continued
    mechanical, of instrument or apparatus — continued
      specified procedure NEC E874.8
      surgical operation E874.0
      thoracentesis E874.4
      transfusion E874.1
      vaccination E874.8
    sterile precautions (during procedure) E872.9
      aspiration of fluid or tissue (by puncture or catheterization, except heart) E872.5
      biopsy E872.8
        needle (aspirating) E872.5
      blood sampling E872.5
      catheterization E872.5
        heart E872.6
      dialysis (kidney) E872.2
      endoscopic examination E872.4
      enema E872.8
      infusion E872.1
      injection E872.3
      lumbar puncture E872.5
      needle biopsy E872.5
      paracentesis, abdominal E872.5
      perfusion E872.2
      removal of catheter or packing E872.8
      specified procedure NEC E872.8
      surgical operation E872.0
      thoracentesis E872.5
      transfusion E872.1
      vaccination E872.3
    suture or ligature during surgical procedure E876.2
    to introduce or to remove tube or instrument E876.4
      foreign object left in body — see Misadventure, foreign object
  foreign object left in body (during procedure) E871.9
    aspiration of fluid or tissue (by puncture or catheterization, except heart) E871.5
    biopsy E871.8
      needle (aspirating) E871.5
    blood sampling E871.5
    catheterization E871.5
      heart E871.6
    dialysis (kidney) E871.2
    endoscopic examination E871.4
    enema E871.8
    infusion E871.1
    injection E871.3
    lumbar puncture E871.5
    needle biopsy E871.5
    paracentesis, abdominal E871.5
    perfusion E871.2
    removal of catheter or packing E871.7
    specified procedure NEC E871.8
    surgical operation E871.0
    thoracentesis E871.5
    transfusion E871.1
    vaccination E871.3
  hemorrhage — see Misadventure, cut
  inadvertent exposure of patient to radiation (being received for test or therapy) E873.3

Misadventure(s) to patient(s) during surgical or medical care — continued
  inappropriate
    operation performed E876.5
    temperature (too hot or too cold) in local application or packing E873.5
  infusion — see also Misadventure, by specific type, infusion
    excessive amount of fluid E873.0
    incorrect dilution of fluid E873.1
    wrong fluid E876.1
  mismatched blood in transfusion E876.0
  nonadministration of necessary drug or medicinal E873.6
  overdose — see also Overdose
    radiation, in therapy E873.2
  perforation — see Misadventure, cut
  performance of inappropriate operation E876.5
  puncture — see Misadventure, cut
  specified type NEC E876.8
    failure
      suture or ligature during surgical operation E876.2
      to introduce or to remove tube or instrument E876.4
        foreign object left in body E871.9
    infusion of wrong fluid E876.1
    performance of inappropriate operation E876.5
    transfusion of mismatched blood E876.0
    wrong
      fluid in infusion E876.1
      placement of endotracheal tube during anesthetic procedure E876.3
  transfusion — see also Misadventure, by specific type, transfusion
    excessive amount of blood E873.0
    mismatched blood E876.0
  wrong
    drug given in error — see Table of Drugs and Chemicals
    fluid in infusion E876.1
    placement of endotracheal tube during anesthetic procedure E876.3
Motion (effects) E903
  sickness E903
Mountain sickness E902.0
Mucus aspiration or inhalation, not of newborn (with asphyxia, obstruction respiratory passage, suffocation) E912
Mudslide of cataclysmic nature E909.2
Murder (attempt) (see also Assault) E968.9

N

Nail, injury by E920.8
Needlestick (sewing needle) E920.4
  hypodermic E920.5
Neglect — see also Privation
  criminal E968.4
  homicidal intent E968.4
Noise (causing injury) (pollution) E928.1

Object — **Poisoning**

O

Object
 falling
  from, in, on, hitting
   aircraft E844 ✓4th
    due to accident to aircraft — see
      categories E840-E842 ✓4th
   machinery — see also Accident, machine
    not in operation E916
   motor vehicle (in motion) (on public
     highway) E818 ✓4th
    not on public highway E825 ✓4th
    stationary E916
   nonmotor road vehicle NEC E829 ✓4th
   pedal cycle E826 ✓4th
   person E916
   railway rolling stock, train, vehicle
     E806 ✓4th
   street car E829 ✓4th
   watercraft E838 ✓4th
    due to accident to watercraft
      E831 ✓4th
  set in motion by
   accidental explosion of pressure vessel —
     see category E921 ✓4th
   firearm — see category E922 ✓4th
   machine(ry) — see Accident, machine
   transport vehicle — see categories E800-
     E848 ✓4th
  thrown from, in, on, towards
   aircraft E844 ✓4th
   cable car (not on rails) E847
    on rails E829 ✓4th
   motor vehicle (in motion) (on public
     highway) E818 ✓4th
    not on public highway E825 ✓4th
   nonmotor road vehicle NEC E829 ✓4th
   pedal cycle E826 ✓4th
   street car E829 ✓4th
   vehicle NEC — see Accident, vehicle NEC
Obstruction
 air passages, larynx, respiratory passages
  by
   external means NEC — see Suffocation
   food, any type (regurgitated) (vomited)
     E911
   material or object, except food E912
   mucus E912
   phlegm E912
   vomitus E911
 digestive tract, except mouth or pharynx
  by
   food, any type E915
   foreign body (any) E915
 esophagus
  food E911
  foreign body, except food E912
  without asphyxia or obstruction of
    respiratory passage E915
 mouth or pharynx
  by
   food, any type E911
   material or object, except food E912
 respiration — see Obstruction, air passages
Oil in eye E914
Overdose
 anesthetic (drug) — see Table of Drugs and
   Chemicals
 drug — see Table of Drugs and Chemicals

Overexertion (lifting) (pulling) (pushing) E927
Overexposure (accidental) (to)
 cold (see also Cold, exposure to) E901.9
  due to manmade conditions E901.1
 heat (see also Heat) E900.9
 radiation — see Radiation
 radioactivity — see Radiation
 sun, except sunburn E900.0
 weather — see Exposure
 wind — see Exposure
Overheated (see also Heat) E900.9
Overlaid E913.0
Overturning (accidental)
 animal-drawn vehicle E827 ✓4th
 boat, ship, watercraft
  causing
   drowning, submersion E830 ✓4th
   injury except drowning, submersion
     E831 ✓4th
 machinery — see Accident, machine
 motor vehicle (see also Loss of control, motor
   vehicle) E816 ✓4th
  with antecedent collision on public highway
    — see Collision, motor vehicle
  not on public highway, nontraffic accident
    E825 ✓4th
   with antecedent collision — see
     Collision, motor vehicle, not on
     public highway
 nonmotor road vehicle NEC E829 ✓4th
 off-road type motor vehicle — see Loss of
   control, off-road type motor vehicle
 pedal cycle E826 ✓4th
 railway rolling stock, train, vehicle (see also
   Derailment, railway) E802 ✓4th
 street car E829 ✓4th
 vehicle NEC — see Accident, vehicle NEC

P

Palsy, divers' E902.2
Parachuting (voluntary) (without accident to
   aircraft) E844 ✓4th
 due to accident to aircraft — see categories
   E840-E842 ✓4th
Paralysis
 divers' E902.2
 lead or saturnine E866.0
  from pesticide NEC E863.4
Pecked by bird E906.8
Phlegm aspiration or inhalation (with asphyxia,
   obstruction respiratory passage,
   suffocation) E912
Piercing (see also Cut) E920.9
Pinched
 between objects (moving) (stationary and
   moving) E918
 in object E918
Pinned under
 machine(ry) — see Accident, machine
Place of occurrence of accident — see Accident
   (to), occurring (at) (in)
Plumbism E866.0
 from insecticide NEC E863.4
Poisoning (accidental) (by) — see also Table of
   Drugs and Chemicals

Index to External Causes — Radiation

Poisoning — *continued*
  carbon monoxide
    generated by
      aircraft in transit E844 ✓4th
      motor vehicle
        in motion (on public highway) E818 ✓4th
        not on public highway E825 ✓4th
      watercraft (in transit) (not in transit) E838 ✓4th
  caused by injection of poisons or toxins into or through skin by plant thorns, spines, or other mechanism E905.7
    marine or sea plants E905.6
  fumes or smoke due to
    conflagration — *see* Conflagration
    explosion or fire — *see* Fire
    ignition — *see* Ignition
  gas
    in legal intervention E972
    legal execution, by E978
    on watercraft E838 ✓4th
    used as anesthetic — *see* Table of Drugs and Chemicals
  in
    terrorism (chemical weapons) E979.7 •
    war operations E997.2
  late effect of — *see* Late effect
  legal
    execution E978
    intervention
      by gas E972
Pressure, external, causing asphyxia, suffocation (*see also* Suffocation) E913.9
Privation E904.9
  food (*see also* Lack of, food) E904.1
  helpless person, infant, newborn due to abandonment or neglect E904.0
  late effect of NEC E929.5
  resulting from transport accident — *see* categories E800-E848 ✓4th
  water (*see also* Lack of, water) E904.2
Projected objects, striking against or struck by — *see* Striking against, object
Prolonged stay in
  high altitude (causing conditions as listed in E902.0) E902.0
  weightless environment E928.0
Prostration
  heat — *see* Heat
Pulling, injury in E927
Puncture, puncturing (*see also* Cut) E920.9
  by
    plant thorns or spines E920.8
      toxic reaction E905.7
        marine or sea plants E905.6
    sea-urchin spine E905.6
Pushing (injury in) (overexertion) E927
  by other person(s) (accidental) E917.9
    as, or caused by, a crowd, human stampede E917.1
      with subsequent fall E917.6
    before moving vehicle or object
      stated as
        intentional, homicidal E968.5
        undetemined whether accidental or intentional E988.8

Pushing — *continued*
  by other person(s) — *continued*
    from
      high place
        in accidental circum-stances — *see* categories E880-E884 ✓4th
        stated as
          intentional, homicidal E968.1
          undetermined whether accidental or intentional E987.9
        man-made structure, except residential E987.1
        natural site E987.2
        residential E987.0
      motor vehicle (*see also* Fall, from, motor vehicle) E818 ✓4th
        stated as
          intentional, homicidal E968.5
          undetermined whether accidental or intentional E988.8
  in sports E917.0
    with fall E886.0
  with fall E886.9
    in sports E886.0

R

Radiation (exposure to) E926.9
  abnormal reaction to medical test or therapy E879.2
  arc lamps E926.2
  atomic power plant (malfunction) NEC E926.9
    in water transport E838 ✓4th
  electromagnetic, ionizing E926.3
  gamma rays E926.3
  in
    terrorism (from or following nuclear explosion) (direct) (secondary) E979.5 •••
    laser E979.8 •
    war operations (from or following nuclear explosion) (direct) (secondary) E996
      laser(s) E997.0
      water transport E838 ✓4th
  inadvertent exposure of patient (receiving test or therapy) E873.3
  infrared (heaters and lamps) E926.1
    excessive heat E900.1
  ionized, ionizing (particles, artificially accelerated) E926.8
    electromagnetic E926.3
  isotopes, radioactive — *see* Radiation, radioactive isotopes
  laser(s) E926.4
    in
      terrorism E979.8 •
      war operations E997.0
  misadventure in medical care — *see* Misadventure, failure, in dosage, radiation
  late effect of NEC E929.8
    excessive heat from — *see* Heat
  light sources (visible) (ultraviolet) E926.2
  misadventure in medical or surgical procedure — *see* Misadventure, failure, in dosage, radiation
  overdose (in medical or surgical procedure) E873.2
  radar E926.0

Radiation — *continued*
   radioactive isotopes E926.5
     atomic power plant malfunction E926.5
      in water transport E838 ▨4ᵗʰ
     misadventure in medical or surgical
      treatment — *see* Misadventure,
      failure, in dosage, radiation
   radiobiologicals — *see* Radiation, radioactive
     isotopes
   radiofrequency E926.0
   radiopharmaceuticals — *see* Radiation,
     radioactive isotopes
   radium NEC E926.9
   sun E926.2
     excessive heat from E900.0
   tanning bed E926.2
   welding arc or torch E926.2
     excessive heat from E900.1
   x-rays (hard) (soft) E926.3
     misadventure in medical or surgical
      treatment — *see* Misadventure,
      failure, in dosage, radiation
Rape E960.1
Reaction, abnormal to or following (medical or
   surgical procedure) E879.9
   amputation (of limbs) E878.5
   anastomosis (arteriovenous) (blood vessel)
     (gastrojejunal) (skin) (tendon) (natural,
     artificial material, tissue) E878.2
     external stoma, creation of E878.3
   aspiration (of fluid) E879.4
     tissue E879.8
   biopsy E879.8
   blood
     sampling E879.7
     transfusion
      procedure E879.8
   bypass — *see* Reaction, abnormal,
     anastomosis
   catheterization
     cardiac E879.0
     urinary E879.6
   colostomy E878.3
   cystostomy E878.3
   dialysis (kidney) E879.1
   drugs or biologicals — *see* Table of Drugs and
     Chemicals
   duodenostomy E878.3
   electroshock therapy E879.3
   formation of external stoma E878.3
   gastrostomy E878.3
   graft — *see* Reaction, abnormal, anastomosis
   hypothermia E879.8
   implant, implantation (of)
     artificial
      internal device (cardiac pacemaker)
       (electrodes in brain) (heart valve
       prosthesis) (orthopedic) E878.1
      material or tissue (for anastomosis or
       bypass) E878.2
       with creation of external stoma
        E878.3
      natural tissues (for anastomosis or bypass)
       E878.2
       as transplantation — *see* Reaction,
        abnormal, transplant
       with creation of external stoma E878.3
   infusion
     procedure E879.8

Reaction, abnormal to or following —
   continued
   injection
     procedure E879.8
   insertion of gastric or duodenal sound E879.5
   insulin-shock therapy E879.3
   lumbar puncture E879.4
   perfusion E879.1
   procedures other than surgical operation (*see*
     also Reaction, abnormal, by
     specific type of procedure) E879.9
     specified procedure NEC E879.8
   radiological procedure or therapy E879.2
   removal of organ (partial) (total) NEC E878.6
     with
      anastomosis, bypass or graft E878.2
      formation of external stoma E878.3
      impiant of artificial internal device
       E878.1
      transplant(ation)
       partial organ E878.4
       whole organ E878.0
   sampling
     blood E879.7
     fluid NEC E879.4
     tissue E879.8
   shock therapy E879.3
   surgical operation (*see also* Reaction,
     abnormal, by specified type of operation)
     E878.9
     restorative NEC E878.4
      with
       anastomosis, bypass or graft E878.2
       fomation of external stoma E878.3
       implant(ation) — *see* Reaction,
        abnormal, implant
       transplant(ation) — *see* Reaction,
        abnormal, transplant
     specified operation NEC E878.8
   thoracentesis E879.4
   transfusion
     procedure E879.8
   transplant, transplantation (heart) (kidney)
     (liver) E878.0
     partial organ E878.4
   ureterostomy E878.3
   vaccination E879.8
Reduction in
   atmospheric pressure — *see also* Effects of,
     air pressure
     while surfacing from
      deep water diving causing caisson or
       divers' disease, palsy or paralysis
       E902.2
      underground E902.8
Residual (effect) — *see* Late effect
Rock falling on or hitting (accidentally)
   motor vehicle (in motion) (on public highway)
     E818 ▨4ᵗʰ
     not on public highway E825 ▨4ᵗʰ
   nonmotor road vehicle NEC E829 ▨4ᵗʰ
   pedal cycle E826 ▨4ᵗʰ
   person E916
   railway rolling stock, train, vehicle E806 ▨4ᵗʰ
Running off, away
   animal (being ridden) (in sport or transport)
     E829 ▨4ᵗʰ
     not being ridden E906.8
   animal-drawn vehicle E827 ▨4ᵗʰ
   rails, railway (*see also* Derailment) E802 ▨4ᵗʰ

Running off, away — *continued*
  roadway
    motor vehicle (without antecedent collision) E816 ✓4th
      nontraffic accident E825 ✓4th
        with antecedent collision — *see* Collision, motor vehicle, not on public highway
      with
        antecedent collision — *see* Collision motor vehicle
        subsequent collision
          involving any object, person or vehicle not on public highway E816 ✓4th
          on public highway E811 ✓4th
    nonmotor road vehicle NEC E829 ✓4th
    pedal cycle E826 ✓4th
Run over (accidentally) (by)
  animal (not being ridden) E906.8
    being ridden (in sport or transport) E828 ✓4th
  animal-drawn vehicle E827 ✓4th
  machinery — *see* Accident, machine
  motor vehicle (on public highway) — *see* Hit by, motor vehicle
  nonmotor road vehicle NEC E829 ✓4th
  railway train E805 ✓4th
  street car E829 ✓4th
  vehicle NEC E848

S

Saturnism E866.0
  from insecticide NEC E863.4
Scald, scalding (accidental) (by) (from) (in) E924.0
  acid — *see* Scald, caustic
  boiling tap water E924.2
  caustic or corrosive liquid, substance E924.1
    swallowed — *see* Table of Drugs and Chemicals
  homicide (attempt) — *see* Assault, burning
  inflicted by other person
    stated as
      intentional or homicidal E968.3
      undetermined whether accidental or intentional E988.2
  late effect of NEC E929.8
  liquid (boiling) (hot) E924.0
  local application of externally applied substance in medical or surgical care E873.5
  molten metal E924.0
  self-inflicted (unspecified whether accidental or intentional) E988.2
    stated as intentional, purposeful E958.2
  stated as undetermined whether accidental or intentional E988.2
  steam E924.0
  tap water (boiling) E924.2
  transport accident — *see* catagories E800-E848
  vapor E924.0
Scratch, cat E906.8
Sea
  sickness E903
Self-mutilation — *see* Suicide

Sequelae (of)
  in
    terrorism E999.1
    war operations E999.0
Shock
  anaphylactic (*see also* Table of Drugs and Chemicals) E947.9
  due to
    bite (venomous) — *see* Bite, venomous NEC
    sting — *see* Sting
  electric (*see also* Electric shock) E925.9
  from electric appliance or current (*see also* Electric shock) E925.9
Shooting, shot (accidental(ly)) E922.9
  air gun E922.4
  BB gun E922.4
  hand gun (pistol) (revolver) E922.0
  himself (*see also* Shooting, self-inflicted) E985.4
    hand gun (pistol) (revolver) E985.0
    military firearm, except hand gun E985.3
      hand gun (pistol) (revolver) E985.0
    rifle (hunting) E985.2
      military E985.3
    shotgun (automatic) E985.1
    specified firearm NEC E985.4
    Verey pistol E985.4
  homicide (attempt) E965.4
    air gun E968.6
    BB gun E968.6
    hand gun (pistol) (revolver) E965.0
    military firearm, except hand gun E965.3
      hand gun (pistol) (revolver) E965.0
    paintball gun E965.4
    rifle (hunting) E965.2
      military E965.3
    shotgun (automatic) E965.1
    specified firearm NEC E965.4
    Verey pistol E965.4
  inflicted by other person
    in accidental circumstances E922.9
      hand gun (pistol) (revolver) E922.0
      military firearm, except hand gun E922.3
        hand gun (pistol) (revolver) E922.0
      rifle (hunting) E922.2
        military E922.3
      shotgun (automatic) E922.1
      specified firearm NEC E922.8
      Verey pistol E922.8
    stated as
      intentional, homicidal E965.4
        hand gun (pistol) (revolver) E965.0
        military firearm, except hand gun E965.3
          hand gun (pistol) (revolver) E965.0
        paintball gun E965.4
        rifle (hunting) E965.2
          military E965.3
        shotgun (automatic) E965.1
        specified firearm NEC E965.4
        Verey pistol E965.4
      undetermined whether accidental or intentional E985.4
        air gun E985.6
        BB gun E985.6
        hand gun (pistol) (revolver) E985.0
        military firearm, except hand gun E985.3

Shooting, shot — *continued*
  inflicted by other person — *continued*
    stated as — *continued*
      undetermined whether accidental or
        intentional — *continued*
        military firearm, except hand gun —
          continued
          hand gun (pistol) (revolver) E985.0
        paintball gun E985.7
        rifle (hunting) E985.2
        shotgun (automatic) E985.1
        specified firearm NEC E985.4
        Verey pistol E985.4
  in
    terrorism — *see* Terrorism, shooting
    war operations — *see* War operations,
      shooting
  legal
    execution E978
    intervention E970
  military firearm, except hand gun E922.3
    hand gun (pistol) (revolver) E922.0
  paintball gun E922.5
  rifle (hunting) E922.2
    military E922.3
  self-inflicted (unspecified whether accidental
    or intentional) E985.4
    air gun E985.6
    BB gun E985.6
    hand gun (pistol) (revolver) E985.0
    military firearm, except hand gun E985.3
      hand gun (pistol) (revolver) E985.0
    paintball gun E985.7
    rifle (hunting) E985.2
      military E985.3
    shotgun (automatic) E985.1
    specified firearm NEC E985.4
    stated as
      accidental E922.9
        hand gun (pistol) (revolver) E922.0
        military firearm, except hand gun
          E922.3
          hand gun (pistol) (revolver) E922.0
        paintball gun E922.5
        rifle (hunting) E922.2
          military E922.3
        shotgun (automatic) E922.1
        specified firearm NEC E922.8
        Verey pistol E922.8
      intentional, purposeful E955.4
        hand gun (pistol) (revolver) E955.0
        military firearm, except hand gun
          E955.3
          hand gun (pistol) (revolver) E955.0
        paintball gun E955.7
        rifle (hunting) E955.2
          military E955.3
        shotgun (automatic) E955.1
        specified firearm NEC E955.4
        Verey pistol E955.4
      shotgun (automatic) E922.1
      specified firearm NEC E922.8
      stated as undetermined whether accidental or
        intentional E985.4
        hand gun (pistol) (revolver) E985.0
        military firearm, except hand gun E985.3
          hand gun (pistol) (revolver) E985.0
        paintball gun E985.7
        rifle (hunting) E985.2
          military E985.3

Shooting, shot — *continued*
  stated as undetermined whether accidental or
    intentional — *continued*
    shotgun (automatic) E985.1
    specified firearm NEC E985.4
    Verey pistol E985.4
  suicidal (attempt) E955.4
    air gun E955.6
    BB gun E955.6
    hand gun (pistol) (revolver) E955.0
    military firearm, except hand gun E955.3
      hand gun (pistol) (revolver) E955.0
    paintball gun E955.7
    rifle (hunting) E955.2
      military E955.3
    shotgun (automatic) E955.1
    specified firearm NEC E955.4
    Verey pistol E955.4
  Verey pistol E922.8
Shoving (accidentally) by other person (*see also*
  Pushing by other person) E917.9
Sickness
  air E903
  alpine E902.0
  car E903
  motion E903
  mountain E902.0
  sea E903
  travel E903
Sinking (accidental)
  boat, ship, watercraft (causing drowning,
    submersion) E830 ✓4ᵗʰ
    causing injury except drowning,
      submersion E831 ✓4ᵗʰ
Siriasis E900.0
Skydiving E844 ✓4ᵗʰ
Slashed wrists (*see also* Cut, self-inflicted) E986
Slipping (accidental)
  on
    deck (of boat, ship, watercraft) (icy) (oily)
      (wet) E835 ✓4ᵗʰ
    ice E885
    ladder of ship E833 ✓4ᵗʰ
      due to accident to watercraft E831 ✓4ᵗʰ
    mud E885
    oil E885
    snow E885
    stairs of ship E833 ✓4ᵗʰ
      due to accident to watercraft E831 ✓4ᵗʰ
    surface
      slippery E885
      wet E885
Sliver, wood, injury by E920.8
Smouldering building or structure in
  terrorism E979.3
Smothering, smothered (*see also* Suffocation)
  E913.9
Sodomy (assault) E960.1
Solid substance in eye (any part) or adnexa
  E914
Sound waves (causing injury) E928.1
Splinter, injury by E920.8
Stab, stabbing E966
  accidental — *see* Cut
Starvation E904.1
  helpless person, infant, newborn — *see* Lack
    of food
  homicidal intent E968.4

Starvation — *continued*
  late effect of NEC E929.5
  resulting from accident connected with
    transport — *see* catagories E800-E848
Stepped on
  by
    animal (not being ridden) E906.8
      being ridden (in sport or transport)
        E828 ✓4ᵗʰ
    crowd E917.1
    person E917.9
      in sports E917.0
  in sports E917.0
Stepping on
  object (moving) E917.9
    in sports E917.0
    with subsequent fall E917.5
    stationary E917.4
      with subsequent fall E917.8
  person E917.9
    as, or caused by a crowd E917.1
      with subsequent fall E917.6
    in sports E917.0
Sting E905.9
  ant E905.5
  bee E905.3
  caterpillar E905.5
  coral E905.6
  hornet E905.3
  insect NEC E905.5
  jellyfish E905.6
  marine animal or plant E905.6
  nematocysts E905.6
  scorpion E905.2
  sea anemone E905.6
  sea cucumber E905.6
  wasp E905.3
  yellow jacket E905.3
Storm E908.9
  specified type NEC E908.8
Straining, injury in E927
Strangling — *see* Suffocation
Strangulation — *see* Suffocation
Strenuous movements (in recreational or other
    activities) E927
Striking against
  bottom (when jumping or diving into water)
    E883.0
  object (moving) E917.9
    caused by crowd E917.1
      with subsequent fall E917.6
    furniture E917.3
      with subsequent fall E917.7
    in
      running water E917.2
        with drowning or submersion — *see*
          Submersion
      sports E917.0
        with subsequent fall E917.5
      stationary E917.4
        with subsequent fall E917.8
  person(s) E917.9
    with fall E886.9
      in sports E886.0
    as, or caused by, a crowd E917.1
      with subsequent fall E917.6
      in sports E917.0
        with fall E886.0

Stroke
  heat — *see* Heat
  lightning E907
Struck by — *see also* Hit by
  bullet
    in
      terrorism E979.4
      war operations E991.2
        rubber E991.0
  lightning E907
  missile
    in terrorism — *see* Terrorism, missile
  object
    falling
      from, in, on
        building
          burning (uncontrolled fire)
            in terrorism E979.3
  thunderbolt E907
**Stumbling over animal, carpet, curb, rug or
  (small) object (with fall)** E885
  without fall — *see* Striking against, object
Submersion (accidental) E910.8
  boat, ship, watercraft (causing drowning,
    submersion) E830 ✓4ᵗʰ
    causing injury except drowning,
      submersion E831 ✓4ᵗʰ
  by other person
    in accidental circumstances — *see* category
      E910 ✓4ᵗʰ
    intentional, homicidal E964
    stated as undetermined whether due to
      accidental or intentional E984
  due to
    accident
      machinery — *see* Accident, machine
      to boat, ship, watercraft E830 ✓4ᵗʰ
      transport — *see* categories
        E800-E848 ✓4ᵗʰ
    avalanche E909.2
    cataclysmic
      earth surface movement or eruption E909.9
      storm E908.9
    cloudburst E908.8
    cyclone E908.1
    fall
      from
        boat, ship, watercraft (not involved in
          accident) E832 ✓4ᵗʰ
          burning, crushed E830 ✓4ᵗʰ
          involved in accident, collision
            E830 ✓4ᵗʰ
          gangplank (into water) E832 ✓4ᵗʰ
        overboard NEC E832 ✓4ᵗʰ
    flood E908.2
    hurricane E908.0
    jumping into water E910.8
      from boat, ship, watercraft
        burning, crushed, sinking E830 ✓4ᵗʰ
        involved in accident, collision
          E830 ✓4ᵗʰ
        not involved in accident, for swim
          E910.2
      in recreational activity (without diving
        equipment) E910.2
        with or using diving equipment E910.1
      to rescue another person E910.3
  homicide (attempt) E964

Submersion

Submersion — continued
 in
  bathtub E910.4
  specified activity, not sport, transport or recreational E910.3
  sport or recreational activity (without diving equipment) E910.2
   with or using diving equipment E910.1
   water skiing E910.0
  swimming pool NEC E910.8
  terrorism E979.8
  war operations E995
  water transport E832 ✓4th
   due to accident to boat, ship, watercraft E830 ✓4th
 landslide E909.2
 overturning boat, ship, watercraft E909.2
 sinking boat, ship, watercraft E909.2
 submersion boat, ship, watercraft E909.2
 tidal wave E909.4
  caused by storm E908.0
 torrential rain E908.2
 late effect of NEC E929.8
 quenching tank E910.8
 self-inflicted (unspecified whether accidental or intentional) E984
  in accidental circumstances — see category E910 ✓4th
  stated as intentional, purposeful E954
 stated as undetermined whether accidental or intentional E984
 suicidal (attempted) E954
 while
  attempting rescue of another person E910.3
  engaged in
   marine salvage E910.3
   underwater construction or repairs E910.3
  fishing, not from boat E910.2
  hunting, not from boat E910.2
  ice skating E910.2
  pearl diving E910.3
  placing fishing nets E910.3
  playing in water E910.2
  scuba diving E910.1
   nonrecreational E910.3
  skin diving E910.1
  snorkel diving E910.2
  spear fishing underwater E910.1
  surfboarding E910.2
  swimming (swimming pool) E910.2
  wading (in water) E910.2
  water skiing E910.0

Sucked
 into
  jet (aircraft) E844 ✓4th

Suffocation (accidental) (by external means) (by pressure) (mechanical) E913.9
 caused by other person
  in accidental circumstances — see category E913 ✓4th
  stated as
   intentional, homicidal E963
   undetermined whether accidental or intentional E983.9
  by, in
   hanging E983.0
   plastic bag E983.1
   specified means NEC E983.8

Suffocation — continued
 due to, by
  avalanche E909.2
  bedclothes E913.0
  bib E913.0
  blanket E913.0
  cave-in E913.3
   caused by cataclysmic earth surface movement or eruption E909.9
  conflagration — see Conflagration
  explosion — see Explosion
  falling earth, other substance E913.3
  fire — see Fire
  food, any type (ingestion) (inhalation) (regurgitated) (vomited) E911
  foreign body, except food (ingestion) (inhalation) E912
  ignition — see Ignition
  landslide E909.2
  machine(ry) — see Accident, machine
  material, object except food entering by nose or mouth, ingested, inhaled E912
  mucus (aspiration) (inhalation), not of newborn E912
  phlegm (aspiration) (inhalation) E912
  pillow E913.0
  plastic bag — see Suffocation, in, plastic bag
  sheet (plastic) E913.0
  specified means NEC E913.8
  vomitus (aspiration) (inhalation) E911
 homicidal (attempt) E963
 in
  airtight enclosed place E913.2
  baby carriage E913.0
  bed E913.0
  closed place E913.2
  cot, cradle E913.0
  perambulator E913.0
  plastic bag (in accidental circumstances) E913.1
   homicidal, purposely inflicted by other person E963
   self-inflicted (unspecified whether accidental or intentional) E983.1
    in accidental circumstances E913.1
    intentional, suicidal E953.1
   stated as undetermined whether accidentally or purposely inflicted E983.1
   suicidal, purposely self-inflicted E953.1
  refrigerator E913.2
 self-inflicted — see also Suffocation, stated as undetermined whether accidental or intentional E953.9
  in accidental circumstances — see category E913 ✓4th
  stated as intentional, purposeful — see Suicide, suffocation
 stated as undetermined whether accidental or intentional E983.9
  by, in
   hanging E983.0
   plastic bag E983.1
   specified means NEC E983.8
 suicidal — see Suicide, suffocation

Suicide, suicidal (attempted) (by) E958.9
 burning, burns E958.1

Suicide, suicidal — *continued*
  caustic substance E958.7
    poisoning E950.7
    swallowed E950.7
  cold, extreme E958.3
  cut (any part of body) E956
  cutting or piercing instrument (classifiable to E920) E956
  drowning E954
  electrocution E958.4
  explosive(s) (classifiable to E923) E955.5
  fire E958.1
  firearm (classifiable to E922) — *see* Shooting, suicidal
  hanging E953.0
  jumping
    before moving object, train, vehicle E958.0
    from high place — *see* Jumping, from, high place, stated as, suicidal
  knife E956
  late effect of E959
  motor vehicle, crashing of E958.5
  poisoning — *see* Table of Drugs and Chemicals
  puncture (any part of body) E956
  scald E958.2
  shooting — *see* Shooting, suicidal
  specified means NEC E958.8
  stab (any part of body) E956
  strangulation — *see* Suicide, suffocation
  submersion E954
  suffocation E953.9
    by, in
      hanging E953.0
      plastic bag E953.1
      specified means NEC E953.8
  wound NEC E958.9
Sunburn E926.2
Sunstroke E900.0
Supersonic waves (causing injury) E928.1
Surgical procedure, complication of
  delayed or as an abnormal reaction without mention of misadventure — *see* Reaction, abnormal
  due to or as a result of misadventure — *see* Misadventure
Swallowed, swallowing
  foreign body — *see* Foreign body, alimentary canal
  poison — *see* Table of Drugs and Chemicals
  substance
    caustic — *see* Table of Drugs and Chemicals
    corrosive — *see* Table or drugs and chemicals
    poisonous — *see* Table of Drugs and Chemicals
Swimmers cramp (*see also* category E910 ✓4ᵗʰ) E910.2
  not in recreation or sport E910.3
Syndrome, battered
  baby or child — *see* Abuse, child
  wife — *see* Assault

T

Tackle in sport E886.0
Terrorism (injury) (by) (in) E979.8
  air blast E979.2

Terrorism — *continued*
  aircraft burned, destroyed, exploded, shot down E979.1
    used as a weapon E979.1
  anthrax E979.6
  asphyxia from
    chemical (weapons) E979.7
    fire, conflagration (caused by fire-producing device) E979.3
    from nuclear explosion E979.5
    gas or fumes E979.7
  bayonet E979.8
  biological agents E979.6
  blast (air) (effects) E979.2
    from nuclear explosion E979.5
    underwater E979.0
  bomb (antipersonnel) (mortar) (explosion) (fragments) E979.2
  bullet(s) (from carbine, machine gun, pistol, rifle, shotgun) E979.4
  burn from
    chemical E979.7
    fire, conflagration (caused by fire-producing device) E979.3
    from nuclear explosion E979.5
    gas E979.7
  burning aircraft E979.1
  chemical E9797.7
  cholera E979.6
  conflagration E9779.3
  crushed by falling aircraft E979.1
  depth-charge E979.0
  destruction of aircraft E979.1
  disability, as sequelae one year or more after injury E999.1
  drowning E979.8
  effect
    of nuclear weapon (direct) (secondary) E979.5
    secondary NEC E979.9
    sequelae E999.1
  explosion (artillery shell) (breech-block) (cannon block) E979.2
    aircraft E979.1
    bomb (antipersonnel) (mortar) E979.2
    nuclear (atom) (hydrogen) E979.5
    depth-charge E979.0
  grenade E979.2
  injury by fragments from E979.2
  land-mine E979.2
  marine weapon E979.0
  mine (land) E979.2
    at sea or in harbor E979.0
    marine E979.0
  missile (explosive) NEC E979.2
  munitions (dump) (factory) E979.2
  nuclear (weapon) E979.5
    other direct and secondary effects of E979.5
  sea-based artillery shell E979.5
  torpedo E979.0
  exposure to ionizing radiation from nuclear explosion E979.5
  falling aircraft E979.1
  fire or fire-producing device E979.3
  firearms E979.4
  fireball effects from nuclear explosion E979.5
  fragments from artillery shell, bomb NEC, grenade, guided missile, land-mine, rocket, shell, shrapnel E979.2

Terrorism

Terrorism — *continued*
- gas or fumes E979.7
- grenade (explosion) (fragments) E979.2
- guided missile (explosion) (fragments) E979.2
- nuclear E979.5
- heat from nuclear explosion E979.5
- hot substances E979.3
- hydrogen cyanide E979.7
- land-mine (explosion) (fragments) E979.2
- laser(s) E979.8
- late effect of E999.1
- lewisite E979.7
- lung irritant (chemical) (fumes) (gas) E979.7
- marine mine E979.0
- mine E979.2
  - at sea E979.0
  - in harbor E979.0
  - land (explosion) (fragments) E979.2
  - marine E979.0
- missile (explosion) (fragments) (guided) E979.2
  - marine E979.0
  - nuclear E979.5
- mortar bomb (explosion) (fragments) E979.2
- mustard gas E979.7
- nerve gas E979.7
- nuclear weapons E979.5
- pellets (shotgun) E979.4
- petrol bomb E979.3
- piercing object E979.8
- phosgene E979.7
- poisoning (chemical) (fumes) (gas) E979.7
- radiation, ioninizing from nuclear explosion E979.5
- rocket (explosion) (fragments) E979.2
- saber, sabre E979.8
- sarin E979.7
- screening smoke E979.7
- sequelae effect (of) E999.1
- shell (aircraft) (artillery) (cannon) (land-based) (explosion) (fragments) E979.2
  - sea-based E979.0
- shooting E979.4
  - bullet(s) E979.4
  - pellet(s) (rifle) (shotgun) E979.4
- shrapnel E979.2
- smallpox E979.7
- stabbing object(s) E979.8
- submersion E979.8
- torpedo E979.0
- underwater blast E979.0
- vesicant (chemical) (fumes) (gas) E979.7
- weapon burst E979.2

Thermic fever E900.9
Thermoplegia E900.9
Thirst — *see also* Lack of water
- resulting from accident connected with transport — *see* categories E800-E848

Thrown (accidentally)
- against object in or part of vehicle
  - by motion of vehicle
    - aircraft E844
    - boat, ship, watercraft E838
    - motor vehicle (on public highway) E818
      - not on public highway E825

Thrown — *continued*
- against object in or part of vehicle — *continued*
  - by motion of vehicle — *continued*
    - motor vehicle — *continued*
      - off-road type (not on public highway) E821
      - on public highway E818
      - snow vehicle E820
        - on public high-way E818
      - nonmotor road vehicle NEC E829
      - railway rolling stock, train, vehicle E806
      - street car E829
- from
  - animal (being ridden) (in sport or transport) E828
  - high place, homicide (attempt) E968.1
  - machinery — *see* Accident, machine
  - vehicle NEC — *see* Accident, vehicle NEC
- off — *see* Thrown, from
- overboard (by motion of boat, ship, watercraft) E832
  - by accident to boat, ship, watercraft E830

Thunderbolt NEC E907
Tidal wave (any injury) E909.4
- caused by storm E908.0
Took
- overdose of drug — *see* Table of Drugs and Chemicals
- poison — *see* Table of Drugs and Chemicals
Tornado (any injury) E908.1
Torrential rain (any injury) E908.2
Traffic accident NEC E819
Trampled by animal E906.8
- being ridden (in sport or transport) E828
Trapped (accidentally)
- between
  - objects (moving) (stationary and moving) E918
- by
  - door of
    - elevator E918
    - motor vehicle (on public highway) (while alighting, boarding) — *see* Fall, from, motor vehicle, while alighting
    - railway train (underground) E806
    - street car E829
    - subway train E806
- in object E918
Travel (effects) E903
- sickness E903
Tree
- falling on or hitting E916
  - motor vehicle (in motion) (on public highway) E818
    - not on public highway E825
  - nonmotor road vehicle NEC E829
  - pedal cycle E826
  - person E916
  - railway rolling stock, train, vehicle E806
  - street car E829
Trench foot E901.0
Tripping over animal, carpet, curb, rug, or small object (with fall) E885
- without fall — *see* Striking against, object

Tsunami E909.4
Twisting, injury in E927

V

Violence, nonaccidental (see also Assault) E968.9
Volcanic eruption (any injury) E909.1
Vomitus in air passages (with asphyxia, obstruction or suffocation) E911

W

War operations (during hostilities) (injury) (by) (in) E995
  after cessation of hostilities, injury due to E998
  air blast E993
  aircraft burned, destroyed, exploded, shot down E994
  asphyxia from
    chemical E997.2
    fire, conflagration (caused by fire producing device or conventional weapon) E990.9
      from nuclear explosion E996
      petrol bomb E990.0
    fumes E997.2
    gas E997.2
  battle wound NEC E995
  bayonet E995
  biological warfare agents E997.1
  blast (air) (effects) E993
    from nuclear explosion E996
    underwater E992
  bomb (mortar) (explosion) E993
    after cessation of hostilities E998
    fragments, injury by E991.9
      antipersonnel E991.3
  bullet(s) (from carbine, machine gun, pistol, rifle, shotgun) E991.2
    rubber E991.0
  burn from
    chemical E997.2
    fire, conflagration (caused by fire-producing device or conventional weapon) E990.9
      from nuclear explosion E996
      petrol bomb E990.0
    gas E997.2
  burning aircraft E994
  chemical E997.2
  chlorine E997.2
  conventional warfare, specified from NEC E995
  crushing by falling aircraft E994
  depth charge E992
  destruction of aircraft E994
  disability as sequela one year or more after injury E999.0 ▲
  drowning E995
  effect (direct) (secondary) nuclear weapon E996
  explosion (artillery shell) (breech block) (cannon shell) E993
    after cessation of hostilities of bomb, mine placed in war E998
    aircraft E994

War operations — continued
  explosion — continued
    bomb (mortar) E993
      atom E996
      hydrogen E996
      injury by fragments from E991.9
        antipersonnel E991.3
      nuclear E996
    depth charge E992
    injury by fragments from E991.9
      antipersonnel E991.3
    marine weapon E992
    mine
      at sea or in harbor E992
      land E993
        injury by fragments from E991.9
      marine E992
    munitions (accidental) (being used in war) (dump) (factory) E993
    nuclear (weapon) E996
    own weapons (accidental) E993
      injury by fragments from E991.9
        antipersonnel E991.3
    sea-based artillery shell E992
    torpedo E992
  exposure to ionizing radiation from nuclear explosion E996
  falling aircraft E994
  fire or fire-producing device E990.9
    petrol bomb E990.0
  fireball effects from nuclear explosion E996
  fragments from
    antipersonnel bomb E991.3
    artillery shell, bomb NEC, grenade, guided missile, land mine, rocket, shell, shrapnel E991.9
  fumes E997.2
  gas E997.2
  grenade (explosion) E993
    fragments, injury by E991.9
  guided missile (explosion) E993
    fragments, injury by E991.9
    nuclear E996
  heat from nuclear explosion E996
  injury due to, but occurring after cessation of hostilities E998
  lacrimator (gas) (chemical) E997.2
  land mine (explosion) E993
    after cessation of hostilities E998
    fragments, injury by E991.9
  laser(s) E997.0
  late effect of E999.0 ▲
  lewisite E997.2
  lung irritant (chemical) (fumes) (gas) E997.2
  marine mine E992
  mine
    after cessation of hostilities E998
    at sea E992
    in harbor E992
    land (explosion) E993
      fragments, injury by E991.9
    marine E992
  missile (guided) (explosion) E993
    fragments, injury by E991.9
    marine E992
    nuclear E996
  mortar bomb (explosion) E993
    fragments, injury by E991.9
  mustard gas E997.2
  nerve gas E997.2
  phosgene E997.2

War operations — *continued*
  poisoning (chemical) (fumes) (gas) E997.2
  radiation, ionizing from nuclear explosion
      E996
  rocket (explosion) E993
    fragments, injury by E991.9
  saber, sabre E995
  screening smoke E997.8
  shell (aircraft) (artillery) (cannon) (land based)
      (explosion) E993
    fragments, injury by E991.9
    sea-based E992
  shooting E991.2
    after cessation of hostilities E998
    bullet(s) E991.2
      rubber E991.0
    pellet(s) (rifle) E991.1
    shrapnel E991.9
    submersion E995
    torpedo E992
  unconventional warfare, except by nuclear
      weapon E997.9
    biological (warfare) E997.1
    gas, fumes, chemicals E997.2
    laser(s) E997.0
    specified type NEC E997.8
  underwater blast E992
  vesicant (chemical) (fumes) (gas) E997.2
  weapon burst E993

Washed
  away by flood — *see* Flood
  away by tidal wave — *see* Tidal wave
  off road by storm (transport vehicle) E908.9
  overboard E832

Weather exposure — *see also* Exposure
  cold E901.0
  hot E900.0

Weightlessness (causing injury) (effects of) (in
    spacecraft, real or simulated) E928.0

Wound (accidental) NEC (*see also* Injury) E928.9
  battle (*see also* War operations) E995
  bayonet E920.3
    in
      legal intervention E974
      war operations E995
  gunshot — *see* Shooting
  incised — *see* Cut
  saber, sabre E920.3
    in war operations E995

Index to External Causes

Railway Accidents (E800-E807)

The following fourth-digit subdivisions are for use with categories E800-E807 to identify the injured person:

.0 **Railway employee**
Any person who by virtue of his employment in connection with a railway, whether by the railway company or not, is at increased risk of involvement in a railway accident, such as:
>catering staff on train
>postal staff on train
>driver
>railway fireman
>guard
>shunter
>porter

>sleeping car attendant

.1 **Passenger on railway**
Any authorized person traveling on a train, except a railway employee
>**EXCLUDES** *intending passenger waiting at station (.8)*
>*unauthorized rider on railway vehicle (.8)*

.2 **Pedestrian**
See definition (r), Vol. 1, page E Codes–4

.3 **Pedal cyclist**
See definition (p), Vol. 1, page E Codes–4

.8 **Other specified person**
Intending passenger waiting at station
Unauthorized rider on railway vehicle

.9 **Unspecified person**

Motor Vehicle Traffic and Nontraffic Accidents (E810-E825)

The following fourth-digit subdivisions are for use with categories E810-E819 and E820-E825 to identify the injured person:

.0 **Driver of motor vehicle other than motorcycle**
See definition (1), Vol. 1, page E Codes–3

.1 **Passenger in motor vehicle other than motorcycle**
See definition (1), Vol. 1, page E Codes–3

.2 **Motorcyclist**
See definition (1), Vol. 1, page E Codes–3

.3 **Passenger on motorcycle**
See definition (1), Vol. 1, page E Codes–3

.4 **Occupant of streetcar**

.5 **Rider of animal; occupant of animal-drawn vehicle**

.6 **Pedal cyclist**
See definition (p), Vol. 1, page E Codes–3

Index to External Causes

- **.7** **Pedestrian**
  See definition (r), Vol. 1, page E Codes–3

- **.8** **Other specified person**
  Occupant of vehicle other than above
  Person in railway train involved in accident
  Unauthorized rider of motor vehicle

- **.9** **Unspecified person**

Other Road Vehicle Accidents (E826-E829)

(animal-drawn vehicle, streetcar, pedal cycle, and other nonmotor road vehicle accidents)

The following fourth-digit subdivisions are for use with categories E826-E829 to identify the injured person:

- **.0** **Pedestrian**
  See definition (r), Vol. 1, page E Codes–4

- **.1** **Pedal cyclist** (does not apply to codes E827, E828, E829)
  See definition (p), Vol. 1, page E Codes–4

- **.2** **Rider of animal** (does not apply to code E829)

- **.3** **Occupant of animal-drawn vehicle** (does not apply to codes E828, E829)

- **.4** **Occupant of streetcar**

- **.8** **Other specified person**

- **.9** **Unspecified person**

Water Transport Accidents (E830-E838)

The following fourth-digit subdivisions are for use with categories E830-E838 to identify the injured person:

- **.0** **Occupant of small boat, unpowered**

- **.1** **Occupant of small boat, powered**
  See definition (t), Vol. 1, page E Codes–4
  EXCLUDES *water skier (.4)*

- **.2** **Occupant of other watercraft — crew**
  Persons:

  > engaged in operation of watercraft

  > providing passenger services [cabin attendants, ship's physician, catering personnel]

  > working on ship during voyage in other capacity [musician in band, operators of shops and beauty parlors]

- **.3** **Occupant of other watercraft — other than crew**
  Passenger
  Occupant of lifeboat, other than crew, after abandoning ship

Index to External Causes

.4 **Water skier**

.5 **Swimmer**

.6 **Dockers, stevedores**
Longshoreman employed on the dock in loading and unloading ships

.8 **Other specified person**
Immigration and custom officials on board ship
Persons:

    accompanying passenger or member of crew visiting boat

Pilot (guiding ship into port)

.9 **Unspecified person**

Air and Space Transport Accidents (E840-E845)

The following fourth-digit subdivisions are for use with categories E840-E845 to identify the injured person:

.0 **Occupant of spacecraft**

.1 **Occupant of military aircraft, any**

    Crew
    Passenger (civilian) (military)
    Troops
        in military aircraft [air force] [army] [national guard] [navy]

    EXCLUDES *occupants of aircraft operated under jurisdiction of police departments (.5)*
parachutist (.7)

.2 **Crew of commercial aircraft (powered) in surface to surface transport**

.3 **Other occupant of commercial aircraft (powered) in surface to surface transport**

    Flight personnel:
        not part of crew
        on familiarization flight

    Passenger on aircraft

.4 **Occupant of commercial aircraft (powered) in surface to air transport**

    Occupant [crew] [passenger] of aircraft (powered) engaged in activities, such as:

        air drops of emergency supplies
        air drops of parachutists, except from military craft
        crop dusting
        lowering of construction material [bridge or telephone pole]
        sky writing

Index to External Causes

.5 **Occupant of other powered aircraft**

Occupant [crew] [passenger] of aircraft (powered) engaged in activities, such as:

- aerial spraying (crops) (fire retardants)
- aerobatic flying
- aircraft racing
- rescue operation
- storm surveillance
- traffic suveillance

Occupant of private plane NOS

.6 **Occupant of unpowered aircraft, except parachutist**
Occupant of aircraft classifiable to E842

.7 **Parachutist (military) (other)**
Person making voluntary descent

EXCLUDES *person making descent after accident to aircraft (.1-.6)*

.8 **Ground crew, airline employee**
Persons employed at airfields (civil) (military) or launching pads, not occupants of aircraft

.9 **Other person**

INFECTIOUS AND PARASITIC DISEASES 001–003.9

1. INFECTIOUS AND PARASITIC DISEASES (001-139)

Note: Categories for "late effects" of infectious and parasitic diseases are to be found at 137-139.

INCLUDES diseases generally recognized as communicable or transmissible as well as a few diseases of unknown but possibly infectious origin

EXCLUDES acute respiratory infections (460-466)
carrier or suspected carrier of infectious organism (V02.0-V02.9)
certain localized infections
influenza (487.0-487.8)

INTESTINAL INFECTIOUS DISEASES (001-009)

EXCLUDES helminthiases (120.0-129)

✓4th **001 Cholera**

DEF: An acute infectious enteritis caused by a potent enterotoxin elaborated by *Vibrio cholerae*; the vibrio produces a toxin in the intestinal tract that changes the permeability of the mucosa leading to diarrhea and dehydration.

- 001.0 Due to Vibrio cholerae
- 001.1 Due to Vibrio cholerae el tor
- 001.9 Cholera, unspecified

✓4th **002 Typhoid and paratyphoid fevers**

DEF: Typhoid fever: an acute generalized illness caused by *Salmonella typhi*; notable clinical features are fever, headache, abdominal pain, cough, toxemia, leukopenia, abnormal pulse, rose spots on the skin, bacteremia, hyperplasia of intestinal lymph nodes, mesenteric lymphadenopathy, and Peyer's patches in the intestines.

DEF: Paratyphoid fever: a prolonged febrile illness, much like typhoid but usually less severe; caused by salmonella serotypes other than *S. typhi*, especially *S. enteritidis* serotypes paratyphi A and B and *S. choleraesuis*.

- 002.0 Typhoid fever
    Typhoid (fever) (infection) [any site]
- 002.1 Paratyphoid fever A
- 002.2 Paratyphoid fever B
- 002.3 Paratyphoid fever C
- 002.9 Paratyphoid fever, unspecified

✓4th **003 Other salmonella infections**

INCLUDES infection or food poisoning by Salmonella [any serotype]

DEF: Infections caused by a genus of gram-negative, anaerobic bacteria of the family *Enterobacteriaceae*; affecting warm-blooded animals, like humans; major symptoms are enteric fevers, acute gastroenteritis and septicemia.

- 003.0 Salmonella gastroenteritis
    Salmonellosis
- 003.1 Salmonella septicemia
- ✓5th 003.2 Localized salmonella infections
    - 003.20 Localized salmonella infection, unspecified
    - 003.21 Salmonella meningitis
    - 003.22 Salmonella pneumonia
    - 003.23 Salmonella arthritis
    - 003.24 Salmonella osteomyelitis
    - 003.29 Other
- 003.8 Other specified salmonella infections
- 003.9 Salmonella infection, unspecified

✓4th / ✓5th Additional Digit Required | Unspecified Code | Other Specified Code | Manifestation Code
MSP Medicare Secondary Payer | ▶◀ Revised Text | ● New Code | ▲ Revised Code Title

2002 Ingenix, Inc.　　　　　　　　　　　　　　　　　　Volume 1 — 1

✓4th 004 Shigellosis

INCLUDES bacillary dysentery

DEF: Acute infectious dysentery caused by the genus *Shigella*, of the family *Enterobacteriaceae*; affecting the colon causing the release of blood-stained stools with accompanying tenesmus, abdominal cramps and fever.

004.0 Shigella dysenteriae
Infection by group A Shigella (Schmitz) (Shiga)

004.1 Shigella flexneri
Infection by group B Shigella

004.2 Shigella boydii
Infection by group C Shigella

004.3 Shigella sonnei
Infection by group D Shigella

004.8 Other specified Shigella infections

004.9 Shigellosis, unspecified

✓4th 005 Other food poisoning (bacterial)

EXCLUDES salmonella infections (003.0-003.9)
toxic effect of:
  food contaminants (989.7)
  noxious foodstuffs (988.0-988.9)

DEF: Enteritis caused by ingesting contaminated foods and characterized by diarrhea, abdominal pain, vomiting; symptoms may be mild or life threatening.

005.0 Staphylococcal food poisoning
Staphylococcal toxemia specified as due to food

005.1 Botulism
Food poisoning due to Clostridium botulinum

005.2 Food poisoning due to Clostridium perfringens [C. welchii]
Enteritis necroticans

005.3 Food poisoning due to other Clostridia

005.4 Food poisoning due to Vibrio parahaemolyticus

✓5th 005.8 Other bacterial food poisoning
EXCLUDES salmonella food poisoning (003.0-003.9)

 005.81 Food poisoning due to Vibrio vulnificus

 005.89 Other bacterial food poisoning
Food poisoning due to Bacillus cereus

005.9 Food poisoning, unspecified

✓4th 006 Amebiasis

INCLUDES infection due to Entamoeba histolytica
EXCLUDES amebiasis due to organisms other than Entamoeba histolytica (007.8)

DEF: Infection of the large intestine caused by *Entamoeba histolytica*; usually asymptomatic but symptoms may range from mild diarrhea to profound life-threatening dysentery. Extraintestinal complications include hepatic abscess, which may rupture into the lung, pericardium or abdomen, causing life-threatening infections.

006.0 Acute amebic dysentery without mention of abscess
Acute amebiasis

006.1 Chronic intestinal amebiasis without mention of abscess
Chronic: Chronic:
 amebiasis   amebic dysentery

006.2 Amebic nondysenteric colitis
DEF: *Entamoeba histolytica* infection with inflamed colon but no dysentery.

006.3 Amebic liver abscess
Hepatic amebiasis

INFECTIOUS AND PARASITIC DISEASES

006.4 Amebic lung abscess
Amebic abscess of lung (and liver)

006.5 Amebic brain abscess
Amebic abscess of brain (and liver) (and lung)

006.6 Amebic skin ulceration
Cutaneous amebiasis

006.8 Amebic infection of other sites
Amebic: Ameboma
  appendicitis
  balanitis
  EXCLUDES specific infections by free-living amebae (136.2)

006.9 Amebiasis, unspecified
Amebiasis NOS

✓4th **007 Other protozoal intestinal diseases**
  INCLUDES protozoal: protozoal:
              colitis   dysentery
              diarrhea

007.0 Balantidiasis
Infection by Balantidium coli

007.1 Giardiasis
Infection by Giardia lamblia   Lambliasis

007.2 Coccidiosis
Infection by Isospora belli and Isospora hominis
Isosporiasis

007.3 Intestinal trichomoniasis
DEF: Colitis, diarrhea, or dysentery caused by the protozoa *Trichomonas*.

007.4 Cryptosporidiosis
DEF: An intestinal infection by protozoan parasites causing intractable diarrhea in patients with AIDS and other immunosuppressed individuals.

007.5 Cyclosporiasis
DEF: An infection of the small intestine by the protozoal organism, *Cyclospora caytenanesis*, spread to humans though ingestion of contaminated water or food. Symptoms include watery diarrhea with frequent explosive bowel movements, loss of appetite, loss of weight, bloating, increased gas, stomach cramps, nausea, vomiting, muscle aches, low grade fever, and fatigue.

007.8 Other specified protozoal intestinal diseases
Amebiasis due to organisms other than Entamoeba histolytica

007.9 Unspecified protozoal intestinal disease
Flagellate diarrhea
Protozoal dysentery NOS

✓4th **008 Intestinal infections due to other organisms**
  INCLUDES any condition classifiable to 009.0-009.3 with mention of the responsible organisms
  EXCLUDES food poisoning by these organisms (005.0-005.9)

✓5th **008.0 Escherichia coli [E. coli]**

008.00 E. coli, unspecified
E. coli enteritis NOS

008.01 Enteropathogenic E. coli
DEF: E. coli causing inflammation of intestines.

008.02 Enterotoxigenic E. coli
DEF: A toxic reaction to E. coli of the intestinal mucosa, causing voluminous watery secretions.

008.03 Enteroinvasive E. coli
DEF: E. coli infection penetrating intestinal mucosa.

008.04 Enterohemorrhagic E. coli
DEF: E. coli infection penetrating the intestinal mucosa, producing microscopic ulceration and bleeding.

008.09 Other intestinal E. coli infections

008.1 Arizona group of paracolon bacilli

008.2 Aerobacter aerogenes
Enterobacter aeogenes

008.3 Proteus (mirabilis) (morganii)

√5th **008.4 Other specified bacteria**

008.41 Staphylococcus
Staphylococcal enterocolitis

008.42 Pseudomonas

008.43 Campylobacter

008.44 Yersinia enterocolitica

008.45 Clostridium difficile
Pseudomembranous colitis

DEF: An overgrowth of a species of bacterium that is a part of the normal colon flora in human infants and sometimes in adults; produces a toxin that causes pseudomembranous enterocolitis; typically is seen in patients undergoing antibiotic therapy.

008.46 Other anaerobes
Anaerobic enteritis NOS
Bacteroides (fragilis)
Gram-negative anaerobes

008.47 Other gram-negative bacteria
Gram-negative enteritis NOS
EXCLUDES   gram-negative anaerobes (008.46)

008.49 Other

008.5 Bacterial enteritis, unspecified

√5th **008.6 Enteritis due to specified virus**

008.61 Rotavirus

008.62 Adenovirus

008.63 Norwalk virus
Norwalk-like agent

008.64 Other small round viruses [SRVs]
Small round virus NOS

008.65 Calicivirus
DEF: Enteritis due to a subgroup of *Picornaviruses*.

008.66 Astrovirus

008.67 Enterovirus NEC
Coxsackie virus   Echovirus
EXCLUDES   poliovirus (045.0-045.9)

008.69 Other viral enteritis
Torovirus

008.8 Other organism, not elsewhere classified
Viral:
  enteritis NOS
  gastroenteritis
EXCLUDES   influenza with involvement of gastrointestinal tract (487.8)

INFECTIOUS AND PARASITIC DISEASES

✓4th **009 Ill-defined intestinal infections**

> **EXCLUDES** diarrheal disease or intestinal infection due to specified organism (001.0-008.8)
> diarrhea following gastrointestinal surgery (564.4)
> intestinal malabsorption (579.0-579.9)
> ischemic enteritis (557.0-557.9)
> other noninfectious gastroenteritis and colitis (558.1-558.9)
> regional enteritis (555.0-555.9)
> ulcerative colitis (556)

009.0 Infectious colitis, enteritis, and gastroenteritis

Colitis
Enteritis } septic
Gastroenteritis

Dysentery:
 NOS
 catarrhal
 hemorrhagic

DEF: Colitis: An inflammation of mucous membranes of the colon.

DEF: Enteritis: An inflammation of mucous membranes of the small intestine.

DEF: Gastroenteritis: An inflammation of mucous membranes of stomach and intestines.

009.1 Colitis, enteritis, and gastroenteritis of presumed infectious origin

> **EXCLUDES** colitis NOS (558.9)
> enteritis NOS (558.9)
> gastroenteritis NOS (558.9)

009.2 Infectious diarrhea

Diarrhea:
 dysenteric
 epidemic
Infectious diarrheal disease NOS

009.3 Diarrhea of presumed infectious origin

> **EXCLUDES** diarrhea NOS (787.91)

TUBERCULOSIS (010-018)

> **INCLUDES** infection by Mycobacterium tuberculosis (human) (bovine)
> **EXCLUDES** congenital tuberculosis (771.2)
> late effects of tuberculosis (137.0-137.4)

The following fifth-digit subclassification is for use with categories 010-018:

 0 unspecified
 1 bacteriological or histological examination not done
 2 bacteriological or histological examination unknown (at present)
 3 tubercle bacilli found (in sputum) by microscopy
 4 tubercle bacilli not found (in sputum) by microscopy, but found by bacterial culture
 5 tubercle bacilli not found by bacteriological examination, but tuberculosis confirmed histologically
 6 tubercle bacilli not found by bacteriological or histological examination but tuberculosis confirmed by other methods [inoculation of animals]

DEF: An infection by *Mycobacterium tuberculosis* causes the formation of small, rounded nodules, called tubercles, that can disseminate throughout the body via lymph and blood vessels. Localized tuberculosis is most often seen in the lungs.

INFECTIOUS AND PARASITIC DISEASES

✓4th **010 Primary tuberculous infection**
DEF: Tuberculosis of the lungs occurring when the patient is first infected.

§ ✓5th **010.0 Primary tuberculous infection**
EXCLUDES nonspecific reaction to tuberculin skin test without active tuberculosis (795.5)
positive PPD (795.5)
positive tuberculin skin test without active tuberculosis (795.5)
DEF: Hilar or paratracheal lymph node enlargement in pulmonary tuberculosis.

§ ✓5th **010.1 Tuberculous pleurisy in primary progressive tuberculosis**
DEF: Inflammation and exudation in the lining of the tubercular lung.

§ ✓5th **010.8 Other primary progressive tuberculosis**
EXCLUDES tuberculous erythema nodosum (017.1)

§ ✓5th **010.9 Primary tuberculous infection, unspecified**

✓4th **011 Pulmonary tuberculosis**
Use additional code to identify any associated silicosis (502)

§ ✓5th **011.0 Tuberculosis of lung, infiltrative**
§ ✓5th **011.1 Tuberculosis of lung, nodular**
§ ✓5th **011.2 Tuberculosis of lung with cavitation**
§ ✓5th **011.3 Tuberculosis of bronchus**
EXCLUDES isolated bronchial tuberculosis (012.2)

§ ✓5th **011.4 Tuberculous fibrosis of lung**
§ ✓5th **011.5 Tuberculous bronchiectasis**
§ ✓5th **011.6 Tuberculous pneumonia [any form]**
DEF: Inflammatory pulmonary reaction to tuberculous cells.

§ ✓5th **011.7 Tuberculous pneumothorax**
DEF: Spontaneous rupture of damaged tuberculous pulmonary tissue.

§ ✓5th **011.8 Other specified pulmonary tuberculosis**
§ ✓5th **011.9 Pulmonary tuberculosis, unspecified**
Respiratory tuberculosis NOS
Tuberculosis of lung NOS

✓4th **012 Other respiratory tuberculosis**
EXCLUDES respiratory tuberculosis, unspecified (011.9)

§ ✓5th **012.0 Tuberculous pleurisy**
Tuberculosis of pleura   Tuberculous hydrothorax
Tuberculous empyema
EXCLUDES pleurisy with effusion without mention of cause (511.9)
tuberculous pleurisy in primary progressive tuberculosis (010.1)
DEF: Inflammation and exudation in the lining of the tubercular lung.

§ ✓5th **012.1 Tuberculosis of intrathoracic lymph nodes**
Tuberculosis of lymph nodes:
    hilar
    mediastinal
    tracheobronchial
Tuberculous tracheobronchial adenopathy
EXCLUDES that specified as primary (010.0-010.9)

§ ✓5th **012.2 Isolated tracheal or bronchial tuberculosis**
§ ✓5th **012.3 Tuberculous laryngitis**
Tuberculosis of glottis

§ Requires fifth-digit. See beginning of section 010–018 for codes and definitions.

N Newborn Age: 0   **P** Pediatric Age: 0-17   **M** Maternity Age: 12-55   **A** Adult Age: 15-124

INFECTIOUS AND PARASITIC DISEASES

§ ✓5ᵗʰ 012.8 Other specified respiratory tuberculosis
   Tuberculosis of:
      mediastinum
      nasopharynx
      nose (septum)
      sinus [any nasal]

✓4ᵗʰ 013 Tuberculosis of meninges and central nervous system

§ ✓5ᵗʰ 013.0 Tuberculous meningitis
   Tuberculosis of meninges (cerebral) (spinal)
   Tuberculous:
      leptomeningitis
      meningoencephalitis
   EXCLUDES tuberculoma of meninges (013.1)

§ ✓5ᵗʰ 013.1 Tuberculoma of meninges

§ ✓5ᵗʰ 013.2 Tuberculoma of brain
   Tuberculosis of brain (current disease)

§ ✓5ᵗʰ 013.3 Tuberculous abscess of brain

§ ✓5ᵗʰ 013.4 Tuberculoma of spinal cord

§ ✓5ᵗʰ 013.5 Tuberculous abscess of spinal cord

§ ✓5ᵗʰ 013.6 Tuberculous encephalitis or myelitis

§ ✓5ᵗʰ 013.8 Other specified tuberculosis of central nervous system

§ ✓5ᵗʰ 013.9 Unspecified tuberculosis of central nervous system
   Tuberculosis of central nervous system NOS

✓4ᵗʰ 014 Tuberculosis of intestines, peritoneum, and mesenteric glands

§ ✓5ᵗʰ 014.0 Tuberculous peritonitis
   Tuberculous ascites
   DEF: Tuberculous inflammation of the membrane lining the abdomen.

§ ✓5ᵗʰ 014.8 Other
   Tuberculosis (of):
      anus
      intestine (large) (small)
      mesenteric glands
      rectum
      retroperitoneal (lymph nodes)
   Tuberculous enteritis

✓4ᵗʰ 015 Tuberculosis of bones and joints
   Use additional code to identify manifestation, as:
      tuberculous:
         arthropathy (711.4)
         necrosis of bone (730.8)
         osteitis (730.8)
         osteomyelitis (730.8)
         synovitis (727.01)
         tenosynovitis (727.01)

§ ✓5ᵗʰ 015.0 Vertebral column
   Pott's disease
   Use additional code to identify manifestation, as:
      curvature of spine [Pott's] (737.4)
      kyphosis (737.4)
      spondylitis (720.81)

§ ✓5ᵗʰ 015.1 Hip

§ ✓5ᵗʰ 015.2 Knee

§ Requires fifth-digit. See beginning of section 010–018 for codes and definitions.

INFECTIOUS AND PARASITIC DISEASES

§ ✓5ᵗʰ **015.5 Limb bones**
Tuberculous dactylitis

§ ✓5ᵗʰ **015.6 Mastoid**
Tuberculous mastoiditis

§ ✓5ᵗʰ **015.7 Other specified bone**

§ ✓5ᵗʰ **015.8 Other specified joint**

§ ✓5ᵗʰ **015.9 Tuberculosis of unspecified bones and joints**

✓4ᵗʰ **016 Tuberculosis of genitourinary system**

§ ✓5ᵗʰ **016.0 Kidney**
Renal tuberculosis
Use additional code to identify manifestation, as:
tuberculous:
nephropathy (583.81)
pyelitis (590.81)
pyelonephritis (590.81)

§ ✓5ᵗʰ **016.1 Bladder**

§ ✓5ᵗʰ **016.2 Ureter**

§ ✓5ᵗʰ **016.3 Other urinary organs**

§ ✓5ᵗʰ **016.4 Epididymis** ♂

§ ✓5ᵗʰ **016.5 Other male genital organs** ♂
Use additional code to identify manifestation, as:
tuberculosis of:
prostate (601.4)
seminal vesicle (608.81)
testis (608.81)

§ ✓5ᵗʰ **016.6 Tuberculous oophoritis and salpingitis** ♀

§ ✓5ᵗʰ **016.7 Other female genital organs** ♀
Tuberculous: Tuberculous:
cervicitis   endometritis

§ ✓5ᵗʰ **016.9 Genitourinary tuberculosis, unspecified**

✓4ᵗʰ **017 Tuberculosis of other organs**

§ ✓5ᵗʰ **017.0 Skin and subcutaneous cellular tissue**
Lupus: Tuberculosis:
exedens   cutis
vulgaris   lichenoides
Scrofuloderma   papulonecrotica
Tuberculosis: verrucosa cutis
colliquativa
> **EXCLUDES** lupus erythematosus (695.4)
> disseminated (710.0)
> lupus NOS (710.0)
> nonspecific reaction to tuberculin skin test without active tuberculosis (795.5)
> positive PPD (795.5)
> positive tuberculin skin test without active tuberculosis (795.5)

§ ✓5ᵗʰ **017.1 Erythema nodosum with hypersensitivity reaction in tuberculosis**
Bazin's disease
Erythema:
induratum
nodosum, tuberculous
Tuberculosis indurativa
> **EXCLUDES** erythema nodosum NOS (695.2)

DEF: Tender, inflammatory, bilateral nodules appearing on the shins and thought to be an allergic reaction to tuberculotoxin.

§ Requires fifth-digit. See beginning of section 010–018 for codes and definitions.

INFECTIOUS AND PARASITIC DISEASES 017.2–020.0

§ ✓5ᵗʰ **017.2 Peripheral lymph nodes**
Scrofula
Scrofulous abscess
Tuberculous adenitis
> EXCLUDES tuberculosis of lymph nodes:
> bronchial and mediastinal (012.1)
> mesenteric and retroperitoneal (014.8)
> tuberculous tracheobronchial adenopathy (012.1)

DEF: Scrofula: Old name for tuberculous cervical lymphadenitis.

§ ✓5ᵗʰ **017.3 Eye**
Use additional code to identify manifestation, as:
tuberculous:
chorioretinitis, disseminated (363.13)
episcleritis (379.09)
interstitial keratitis (370.59)
iridocyclitis, chronic (364.11)
keratoconjunctivitis (phlyctenular) (370.31)

§ ✓5ᵗʰ **017.4 Ear**
Tuberculosis of ear
Tuberculous otitis media
> EXCLUDES tuberculous mastoiditis (015.6)

§ ✓5ᵗʰ **017.5 Thyroid gland**

§ ✓5ᵗʰ **017.6 Adrenal glands**
Addison's disease, tuberculous

§ ✓5ᵗʰ **017.7 Spleen**

§ ✓5ᵗʰ **017.8 Esophagus**

§ ✓5ᵗʰ **017.9 Other specified organs**
Use additional code to identify manifestation, as:
tuberculosis of:
endocardium [any valve] (424.91)
myocardium (422.0)
pericardium (420.0)

✓4ᵗʰ **018 Miliary tuberculosis**
> INCLUDES tuberculosis:
> disseminated
> generalized
> miliary, whether of a single specified site, multiple sites, or unspecified site
> polyserositis

DEF: A form of tuberculosis caused by caseous material carried through the bloodstream planting seedlike tubercles in various body organs.

§ ✓5ᵗʰ **018.0 Acute miliary tuberculosis**

§ ✓5ᵗʰ **018.8 Other specified miliary tuberculosis**

§ ✓5ᵗʰ **018.9 Miliary tuberculosis, unspecified**

ZOONOTIC BACTERIAL DISEASES (020–027)

✓4ᵗʰ **020 Plague**
> INCLUDES infection by Yersinia [Pasteurella] pestis

020.0 Bubonic
DEF: Most common acute and severe form of plague characterized by lymphadenopathy (buboes), chills, fever and headache.

---

§ Requires fifth-digit. See beginning of section 010–018 for codes and definitions.

- ✓4ᵗʰ / ✓5ᵗʰ Additional Digit Required
- MSP Medicare Secondary Payer
- Unspecified Code
- ►◄ Revised Text
- Other Specified Code
- ● New Code
- Manifestation Code
- ▲ Revised Code Title

2002 Ingenix, Inc.

020.1 Cellulocutaneous
DEF: Plague characterized by inflammation and necrosis of skin.

020.2 Septicemic
DEF: Plague characterized by massive infection in the bloodstream.

020.3 Primary pneumonic
DEF: Plague characterized by massive pulmonary infection.

020.4 Secondary pneumonic
DEF: Lung infection as a secondary complication of plague.

020.5 Pneumonic, unspecified

020.8 Other specified types of plague
Abortive plague
Ambulatory plague
Pestis minor

020.9 Plague, unspecified

√4th **021 Tularemia**

INCLUDES   deerfly fever
infection by Francisella [Pasteurella] tularensis
rabbit fever

DEF: A febrile disease transmitted by the bites of deer flies, fleas and ticks, by inhalations of aerosolized *F. tuarensis* or by ingestion of contaminated food or water; patients quickly develop fever, chills, weakness, headache, backache and malaise.

021.0 Ulceroglandular tularemia
DEF: Lesions occur at the site *Francisella tularensis*; organism enters body, usually the fingers or hands.

021.1 Enteric tularemia
Tularemia:
cryptogenic
intestinal
typhoidal

021.2 Pulmonary tularemia
Bronchopneumonic tularemia

021.3 Oculoglandular tularemia
DEF: Painful conjunctival infection by *Francisella tularensis* organism with possible corneal, preauricular lymph, or lacrimal involvement.

021.8 Other specified tularemia
Tularemia:
generalized or disseminated
glandular

021.9 Unspecified tularemia

√4th **022 Anthrax**
DEF: An infectious bacterial disease usually transmitted by contact with infected animals or their discharges or products; it is classified by primary routes of inoculation as cutaneous, gastrointestinal and by inhalation.

022.0 Cutaneous anthrax
Malignant pustule

022.1 Pulmonary anthrax
Respiratory anthrax
Wool-sorters' disease

INFECTIOUS AND PARASITIC DISEASES 022.2–026.9

022.2 Gastrointestinal anthrax
022.3 Anthrax septicemia
022.8 Other specified manifestations of anthrax
022.9 Anthrax, unspecified

√4th **023 Brucellosis**
  INCLUDES   fever:
                Malta
                Mediterranean
                undulant

DEF: An infectious disease caused by gram-negative, *aerobic coccobacilli* organisms; it is transmitted to humans through contact with infected tissue or dairy products; fever, sweating, weakness and aching are symptoms of the disease.

  023.0 Brucella melitensis
    DEF: Infection from direct or indirect contact with infected sheep or goats.

  023.1 Brucella abortus
    DEF: Infection from direct or indirect contact with infected cattle.

  023.2 Brucella suis
    DEF: Infection from direct or indirect contact with infected swine.

  023.3 Brucella canis
    DEF: Infection from direct or indirect contact with infected dogs.

  023.8 Other brucellosis
    Infection by more than one organism

  023.9 Brucellosis, unspecified

024 Glanders
  Infection by:
    Actinobacillus mallei
    Malleomyces mallei
    Pseudomonas mallei
  Farcy
  Malleus
  DEF: Equine infection causing mucosal inflammation and skin ulcers in humans.

025 Melioidosis
  Infection by:
    Malleomyces pseudomallei
    Pseudomonas pseudomallei
    Whitmore's bacillus
    Pseudoglanders
  DEF: Rare infection caused by *Pseudomonas pseudomallei*; clinical symptoms range from localized infection to fatal septicemia.

√4th **026 Rat-bite fever**
  026.0 Spirillary fever
    Rat-bite fever due to Spirillum minor [S. minus]
    Sodoku
  026.1 Streptobacillary fever
    Epidemic arthritic erythema
    Haverhill fever
    Rat-bite fever due to Streptobacillus moniliformis
  026.9 Unspecified rat-bite fever

INFECTIOUS AND PARASITIC DISEASES

✓4th **027 Other zoonotic bacterial diseases**

027.0 Listeriosis
Infection } by Listeria monocytogenes
Septicemia

Use additional code to identify manifestation, as meningitis (320.7)
EXCLUDES congenital listeriosis (771.2)

027.1 Erysipelothrix infection
Erysipeloid (of Rosenbach)
Infection } by Erysipelothrix insidiosa
Septicemia   [E. rhusiopathiae]

DEF: Usually associated with handling of fish, meat, or poultry; symptoms range from localized inflammation to septicemia.

027.2 Pasteurellosis
Pasteurella pseudotuberculosis infection
Mesenteric adenitis
Septic infection (cat bite) } by Pasteurella multocida [P. septica]
    (dog bite)

EXCLUDES infection by:
Francisella [Pasteurella] tularensis (021.0-021.9)
Yersinia [Pasteurella] pestis (020.0-020.9)

DEF: Swelling, abscesses, or septicemia from *Pasteurella multocida*, commonly transmitted to humans by a dog or cat scratch.

027.8 Other specified zoonotic bacterial diseases
027.9 Unspecified zoonotic bacterial disease

OTHER BACTERIAL DISEASES (030-041)

EXCLUDES bacterial venereal diseases (098.0-099.9)
bartonellosis (088.0)

✓4th **030 Leprosy**
INCLUDES Hansen's disease
infection by Mycobacterium leprae

030.0 Lepromatous [type L]
Lepromatous leprosy (macular) (diffuse) (infiltrated) (nodular) (neuritic)
DEF: Infectious disseminated leprosy bacilli with lesions and deformities.

030.1 Tuberculoid [type T]
Tuberculoid leprosy (macular) (maculoanesthetic) (major) (minor) (neuritic)
DEF: Relatively benign, self-limiting leprosy with neuralgia and scales.

030.2 Indeterminate [group I]
Indeterminate [uncharacteristic] leprosy (macular) (neuritic)
DEF: Uncharacteristic leprosy, frequently an early manifestation.

030.3 Borderline [group B]
Borderline or dimorphous leprosy (infiltrated) (neuritic)
DEF: Transitional form of leprosy, neither lepromatous nor tuberculoid.

030.8 Other specified leprosy
030.9 Leprosy, unspecified

INFECTIOUS AND PARASITIC DISEASES 031–033.9

✓4th **031 Diseases due to other mycobacteria**

031.0 Pulmonary
Battey disease
Infection by Mycobacterium:
avium
intracellulare [Battey bacillus]
kansasii

031.1 Cutaneous
Buruli ulcer
Infection by Mycobacterium:
marinum [M. balnei]
ulcerans

031.2 Disseminated
Disseminated mycobacterium avium-intracellulare complex (DMAC)
Mycobacterium avium-intracellulare complex (MAC) bacteremia

DEF: Disseminated mycobacterium avium-intracellulare complex (DMAC): A serious systemic form of MAC commonly observed in patients in the late course of AIDS.

DEF: Mycobacterium avium-intracellulare complex (MAC) bacterium: Human pulmonary disease, lymphadenitis in children and systemic disease in immunocompromised individuals caused by a slow growing, gram-positive, aerobic organism.

031.8 Other specified mycobacterial diseases

031.9 Unspecified diseases due to mycobacteria
Atypical mycobacterium infection NOS

✓4th **032 Diphtheria**
INCLUDES   infection by Corynebacterium diphtheriae

032.0 Faucial diphtheria
Membranous angina, diphtheritic
DEF: Diphtheria of the throat.

032.1 Nasopharyngeal diphtheria

032.2 Anterior nasal diphtheria

032.3 Laryngeal diphtheria
Laryngotracheitis, diphtheritic

✓5th **032.8 Other specified diphtheria**
032.81 Conjunctival diphtheria
Pseudomembranous diphtheritic conjunctivitis
032.82 Diphtheritic myocarditis
032.83 Diphtheritic peritonitis
032.84 Diphtheritic cystitis
032.85 Cutaneous diphtheria
032.89 Other

032.9 Diphtheria, unspecified

✓4th **033 Whooping cough**
INCLUDES   pertussis
Use additional code to identify any associated pneumonia (484.3)

DEF: An acute, highly contagious respiratory tract infection caused by *Bordetella pertussis* and *B. bronchiseptica*; characteristic paroxysmal cough.

033.0 Bordetella pertussis [B. pertussis]

033.1 Bordetella parapertussis [B. parapertussis]

033.8 Whooping cough due to other specified organism
Bordetella bronchiseptica [B. bronchiseptica]

033.9 Whooping cough, unspecified organism

✓4th
✓5th Additional Digit Required   Unspecified Code   Other Specified Code   Manifestation Code
 Medicare Secondary Payer   ▶◀ Revised Text   ● New Code   ▲ Revised Code Title

2002 Ingenix, Inc.   Volume 1 — 13

INFECTIOUS AND PARASITIC DISEASES

✓4th 034 Streptococcal sore throat and scarlet fever

034.0 Streptococcal sore throat
Septic:
 angina
 sore throat
Streptococcal:
 angina
Streptococcal:
 laryngitis
 pharyngitis
 tonsillitis

034.1 Scarlet fever
Scarlatina

EXCLUDES parascarlatina (057.8)

DEF: Streptococcal infection and fever with red rash spreading from trunk.

035 Erysipelas

EXCLUDES postpartum or puerperal erysipelas (670)

DEF: An acute superficial cellulitis involving the dermal lymphatics; it is often caused by group A streptococci.

✓4th 036 Meningococcal infection

036.0 Meningococcal meningitis
Cerebrospinal fever (meningococcal)
Meningitis:
 cerebrospinal
 epidemic

036.1 Meningococcal encephalitis

036.2 Meningococcemia
Meningococcal septicemia

036.3 Waterhouse-Friderichsen syndrome, meningococcal
Meningococcal hemorrhagic adrenalitis
Meningococcic adrenal syndrome
Waterhouse-Friderichsen syndrome NOS

✓5th 036.4 Meningococcal carditis

036.40 Meningococcal carditis, unspecified

036.41 Meningococcal pericarditis
DEF: Meningococcal infection of the outer membrane of the heart.

036.42 Meningococcal endocarditis
DEF: Meningococcal infection of the membranes lining the cavities of the heart.

036.43 Meningococcal myocarditis
DEF: Meningococcal infection of the muscle of the heart.

✓5th 036.8 Other specified meningococcal infections

036.81 Meningococcal optic neuritis

036.82 Meningococcal arthropathy

036.89 Other

036.9 Meningococcal infection, unspecified
Meningococcal infection NOS

037 Tetanus

EXCLUDES tetanus:
 complicating:
  abortion (634-638 with .0, 639.0)
  ectopic or molar pregnancy (639.0)
 neonatorum (771.3)
 puerperal (670)

DEF: An acute, often fatal, infectious disease caused by the anaerobic, spore-forming bacillus *Clostridium tetani*; the bacillus most often enters the body through a contaminated wound, burns, surgical wounds, or cutaneous ulcers. Symptoms include lockjaw, spasms, seizures, and paralysis.

INFECTIOUS AND PARASITIC DISEASES

✓4th 038 Septicemia
  EXCLUDES bacteremia (790.7)
  during labor (659.3)
  following ectopic or molar pregnancy (639.0)
  following infusion, injection, transfusion, or vaccination (999.3)
  postpartum, puerperal (670)
  ▶septicemia (sepsis) of newborn (771.81)◀
  that complicating abortion (634-638 with .0, 639.0)

  DEF: A systemic disease associated with the presence and persistence of pathogenic microorganisms or their toxins in the blood.

  038.0 Streptococcal septicemia
  ✓5th 038.1 Staphylococcal septicemia
      038.10 Staphylococcal septicemia, unspecified
      038.11 Staphylococcus aureus septicemia
      038.19 Other staphylococcal septicemia
  038.2 Pneumococcal septicemia [Streptococcus pneumoniae septicemia]
  038.3 Septicemia due to anaerobes
      Septicemia due to bacteroides
      EXCLUDES gas gangrene (040.0)
           that due to anaerobic streptococci (038.0)

  DEF: Infection of blood by microorganisms that thrive without oxygen.

  ✓5th 038.4 Septicemia due to other gram-negative organisms
  DEF: Infection of blood by microorganisms categorized as gram-negative by Gram's method of staining for identification of bacteria.

      038.40 Gram-negative organism, unspecified
          Gram-negative septicemia NOS
      038.41 Hemophilus influenzae [H. influenzae]
      038.42 Escherichia coli [E. coli]
      038.43 Pseudomonas
      038.44 Serratia
      038.49 Other

  038.8 Other specified septicemias
      EXCLUDES septicemia (due to):
           anthrax (022.3)
           gonococcal (098.89)
           herpetic (054.5)
           meningococcal (036.2)
           septicemic plague (020.2)

  038.9 Unspecified septicemia
      Septicemia NOS
      EXCLUDES bacteremia NOS (790.7)

✓4th 039 Actinomycotic infections
  INCLUDES actinomycotic mycetoma
  infection by Actinomycetales, such as species of Actinomyces, Actinomadura, Nocardia, Streptomyces
  maduromycosis (actinomycotic)
  schizomycetoma (actinomycotic)

  DEF: Inflammatory lesions and abscesses at site of infection by *Actinomyces israelii*.

INFECTIOUS AND PARASITIC DISEASES

039.0 Cutaneous
Erythrasma
Trichomycosis axillaris

039.1 Pulmonary
Thoracic actinomycosis

039.2 Abdominal

039.3 Cervicofacial

039.4 Madura foot
> EXCLUDES madura foot due to mycotic infection (117.4)

039.8 Of other specified sites

039.9 Of unspecified site
Actinomycosis NOS   Nocardiosis NOS
Maduromycosis NOS

√4th **040 Other bacterial diseases**
> EXCLUDES bacteremia NOS (790.7)
> bacterial infection NOS (041.9)

040.0 Gas gangrene
Gas bacillus infection or gangrene
Infection by Clostridium:
   histolyticum
   oedematiens
   perfringens [welchii]
   septicum
   sordellii
Malignant edema
Myonecrosis, clostridial
Myositis, clostridial

040.1 Rhinoscleroma
DEF: Growths on the nose and nasopharynx caused by *Klebsiella rhinoscleromatis*.

040.2 Whipple's disease
Intestinal lipodystrophy

040.3 Necrobacillosis
DEF: Infection with *Fusobacterium necrophorum* causing abscess or necrosis.

√5th **040.8 Other specified bacterial diseases**
  040.81 Tropical pyomyositis
  040.82 Toxic shock syndrome
     Use additional code to identify the organism
  040.89 Other

√4th **041 Bacterial infection in conditions classified elsewhere and of unspecified site**
Note: This category is provided to be used as an additional code to identify the bacterial agent in diseases classified elsewhere. This category will also be used to classify bacterial infections of unspecified nature or site.
> EXCLUDES bacteremia NOS (790.7)
> septicemia (038.0-038.9)

√5th **041.0 Streptococcus**
  041.00 Streptococcus, unspecified
  041.01 Group A
  041.02 Group B
  041.03 Group C
  041.04 Group D [Enterococcus]
  041.05 Group G
  041.09 Other Streptococcus

INFECTIOUS AND PARASITIC DISEASES

√5ᵗʰ 041.1 Staphylococcus
- 041.10 Staphylococcus, unspecified
- 041.11 Staphylococcus aureus
- 041.19 Other Staphylococcus

041.2 Pneumococcus

041.3 Friedländer's bacillus
Infection by Klebsiella pneumoniae

041.4 Escherichia coli [E. coli]

041.5 Hemophilus influenzae [H. influenzae]

041.6 Proteus (mirabilis) (morganii)

041.7 Pseudomonas

√5ᵗʰ 041.8 Other specified bacterial infections
- 041.81 Mycoplasma
  - Eaton's agent
  - Pleuropneumonia-like organisms [PPLO]
- 041.82 Bacillus fragilis
- 041.83 Clostridium perfringens
- 041.84 Other anaerobes
  - Bacteroides (fragilis)
  - Gram-negative anaerobes
  - **EXCLUDES** Helicobacter pylori (041.86)
- 041.85 Other gram-negative organisms
  - Aerobacter aerogenes
  - Gram-negative bacteria NOS
  - Mima polymorpha
  - Serratia
  - **EXCLUDES** gram-negative anaerobes (041.84)
- 041.86 Helicobacter pylori (H. pylori)
- 041.89 Other specified bacteria

041.9 Bacterial infection, unspecified

HUMAN IMMUNODEFICIENCY VIRUS (HIV) INFECTION (042)

042 Human immunodeficiency virus [HIV] disease
Acquired immune deficiency syndrome
Acquired immunodeficiency syndrome
AIDS
AIDS-like syndrome
AIDS-related complex
ARC
HIV infection, symptomatic
Use additional code(s) to identify all manifestations of HIV.
Use additional code to identify HIV-2 infection (079.53)
EXCLUDES asymptomatic HIV infection status (V08)
exposure to HIV virus (V01.7)
nonspecific serologic evidence of HIV (795.71)

√4ᵗʰ / √5ᵗʰ Additional Digit Required | Unspecified Code | Other Specified Code | Manifestation Code
MSP Medicare Secondary Payer | ▶◀ Revised Text | ● New Code | ▲ Revised Code Title

2002 Ingenix, Inc.

Volume 1 — 17

INFECTIOUS AND PARASITIC DISEASES

POLIOMYELITIS AND OTHER NON-ARTHROPOD-BORNE VIRAL DISEASES OF CENTRAL NERVOUS SYSTEM (045-049)

✓4th 045 Acute poliomyelitis

> **EXCLUDES** *late effects of acute poliomyelitis (138)*

The following fifth-digit subclassification is for use with category 045:
- 0 poliovirus, unspecified type
- 1 poliovirus type I
- 2 poliovirus type II
- 3 poliovirus type III

✓5th 045.0 Acute paralytic poliomyelitis specified as bulbar
  Infantile paralysis (acute) ⎫
  Poliomyelitis (acute)   ⎬ specified as bulbar
    (anterior)   ⎭

  Polioencephalitis (acute) (bulbar)
  Polioencephalomyelitis (acute) (anterior) (bulbar)

  DEF: Acute paralytic infection occurring where the brain merges with the spinal cord; affecting breathing, swallowing, and heart rate.

✓5th 045.1 Acute poliomyelitis with other paralysis
  Paralysis: Paralysis:
    acute atrophic, spinal infantile, paralytic
  Poliomyelitis (acute) ⎫
    anterior   ⎬ with paralysis except
    epidemic   ⎭   bulbar

  DEF: Paralytic infection affecting peripheral or spinal nerves.

✓5th 045.2 Acute nonparalytic poliomyelitis
  Poliomyelitis (acute) ⎫
    anterior   ⎬ specified as nonparalytic
    epidemic   ⎭

  DEF: Nonparalytic infection causing pain, stiffness, and paresthesias.

✓5th 045.9 Acute poliomyelitis, unspecified
  Infantile paralysis
  Poliomyelitis (acute) ⎫
    anterior   ⎬ unspecified whether paralytic or nonparalytic
    epidemic   ⎭

✓4th 046 Slow virus infection of central nervous system

  046.0 Kuru
  DEF: A chronic, progressive, fatal nervous system disorder; clinical symptoms include cerebellar ataxia, trembling, spasticity and progressive dementia.

  046.1 Jakob-Creutzfeldt disease
  Subacute spongiform encephalopathy
  DEF: Communicable, progressive spongiform encephalopathy thought to be caused by an infectious particle known as a "prion" (proteinaceous infection particle). This is a progressive, fatal disease manifested principally by mental deterioration.

  046.2 Subacute sclerosing panencephalitis
  Dawson's inclusion body encephalitis
  Van Bogaert's sclerosing leukoencephalitis
  DEF: Progressive viral infection causing cerebral dysfunction, blindness, dementia, and death (SSPE).

  046.3 Progressive multifocal leukoencephalopathy
  Multifocal leukoencephalopathy NOS
  DEF: Infection affecting cerebral cortex in patients with weakened immune systems.

INFECTIOUS AND PARASITIC DISEASES 046.8–049.9

046.8 **Other specified slow virus infection of central nervous system**

046.9 **Unspecified slow virus infection of central nervous system**

4th 047 Meningitis due to enterovirus

INCLUDES meningitis:
 abacterial
 aseptic
 viral

EXCLUDES meningitis due to:
 adenovirus (049.1)
 arthropod-borne virus (060.0-066.9)
 leptospira (100.81)
 virus of:
  herpes simplex (054.72)
  herpes zoster (053.0)
  lymphocytic choriomeningitis (049.0)
  mumps (072.1)
  poliomyelitis (045.0-045.9)
 any other infection specifically classified elsewhere

047.0 **Coxsackie virus**

047.1 **ECHO virus**
 Meningo-eruptive syndrome

047.8 **Other specified viral meningitis**

047.9 **Unspecified viral meningitis**
 Viral meningitis NOS

048 **Other enterovirus diseases of central nervous system**
 Boston exanthem

4th 049 Other non-arthropod-borne viral diseases of central nervous system

EXCLUDES late effects of viral encephalitis (139.0)

049.0 **Lymphocytic choriomeningitis**
 Lymphocytic:
  meningitis (serous) (benign)
  meningoencephalitis (serous) (benign)

049.1 **Meningitis due to adenovirus**
 DEF: Inflammation of lining of brain caused by Arenaviruses and usually occurring in adults in fall and winter months.

049.8 **Other specified non-arthropod-borne viral diseases of central nervous system**
 Encephalitis: Encephalitis:
  acute: lethargica
   inclusion body Rio Bravo
   necrotizing von Economo's disease
   epidemic

049.9 **Unspecified non-arthropod-borne viral diseases of central nervous system**
 Viral encephalitis NOS

VIRAL DISEASES ACCOMPANIED BY EXANTHEM (050-057)

EXCLUDES arthropod-borne viral diseases (060.0-066.9)
Boston exanthem (048)

✓4th **050 Smallpox**

050.0 Variola major
Hemorrhagic (pustular) smallpox
Malignant smallpox
Purpura variolosa
DEF: Form of smallpox known for its high mortality; exists only in laboratories.

050.1 Alastrim
Variola minor
DEF: Mild form of smallpox known for its low mortality rate.

050.2 Modified smallpox
Varioloid
DEF: Mild form occurring in patients with history of infection or vaccination.

050.9 Smallpox, unspecified

✓4th **051 Cowpox and paravaccinia**

051.0 Cowpox
Vaccinia not from vaccination
EXCLUDES vaccinia (generalized) (from vaccination) (999.0)
DEF: A disease contracted by milking infected cows; vesicles usually appear on the fingers, may spread to hands and adjacent areas and usually disappear without scarring; other associated features of the disease may include local edema, lymphangitis and regional lymphadenitis with or without fever.

051.1 Pseudocowpox
Milkers' node
DEF: Hand lesions and mild fever in dairy workers caused by exposure to paravaccinia.

051.2 Contagious pustular dermatitis
Ecthyma contagiosum
Orf
DEF: Skin eruptions caused by exposure to poxvirus-infected sheep or goats.

051.9 Paravaccinia, unspecified

✓4th **052 Chickenpox**
DEF: Contagious infection by varicella-zoster virus causing rash with pustules and fever.

052.0 Postvaricella encephalitis
Postchickenpox encephalitis

052.1 Varicella (hemorrhagic) pneumonitis

052.7 With other specified complications

052.8 With unspecified complication

052.9 Varicella without mention of complication
Chickenpox NOS
Varicella NOS

✓4th **053 Herpes zoster**
INCLUDES shingles
zona
DEF: Self-limiting infection by varicella-zoster virus causing unilateral eruptions and neuralgia along affected nerves.

053.0 With meningitis
DEF: Varicella-zoster virus infection causing inflammation of the lining of the brain and/or spinal cord.

INFECTIOUS AND PARASITIC DISEASES 053.1–054.5

- √5th **053.1** **With other nervous system complications**
  - **053.10** With unspecified nervous system complication
  - **053.11** Geniculate herpes zoster
    Herpetic geniculate ganglionitis
    DEF: Unilateral eruptions and neuralgia along the facial nerve geniculum affecting face and outer and middle ear.
  - **053.12** Postherpetic trigeminal neuralgia
    DEF: Severe oral or nasal pain following a herpes zoster infection.
  - **053.13** Postherpetic polyneuropathy
    DEF: Multiple areas of pain following a herpes zoster infection.
  - **053.19** Other
- √5th **053.2** **With ophthalmic complications**
  - **053.20** Herpes zoster dermatitis of eyelid
    Herpes zoster ophthalmicus
  - **053.21** Herpes zoster keratoconjunctivitis
  - **053.22** Herpes zoster iridocyclitis
  - **053.29** Other
- √5th **053.7** **With other specified complications**
  - **053.71** Otitis externa due to herpes zoster
  - **053.79** Other
- **053.8** **With unspecified complication**
- **053.9** **Herpes zoster without mention of complication**
  Herpes zoster NOS

- √4th **054** **Herpes simplex**
  - EXCLUDES   congenital herpes simplex (771.2)
  - **054.0** Eczema herpeticum
    Kaposi's varicelliform eruption
    DEF: Herpes simplex virus invading site of preexisting skin inflammation.
  - √5th **054.1** Genital herpes
    - **054.10** Genital herpes, unspecified
      Herpes progenitalis
    - **054.11** Herpetic vulvovaginitis
    - **054.12** Herpetic ulceration of vulva
    - **054.13** Herpetic infection of penis
    - **054.19** Other
  - **054.2** Herpetic gingivostomatitis
  - **054.3** Herpetic meningoencephalitis
    Herpes encephalitis
    Simian B disease
    DEF: Inflammation of the brain and its lining; caused by infection of herpes simplex 1 in adults and simplex 2 in newborns.
  - √5th **054.4** With ophthalmic complications
    - **054.40** With unspecified ophthalmic complication
    - **054.41** Herpes simplex dermatitis of eyelid
    - **054.42** Dendritic keratitis
    - **054.43** Herpes simplex disciform keratitis
    - **054.44** Herpes simplex iridocyclitis
    - **054.49** Other
  - **054.5** Herpetic septicemia

| √4th Additional Digit Required | Unspecified Code | Other Specified Code | Manifestation Code |
| MSP Medicare Secondary Payer | ▶◀ Revised Text | ● New Code | ▲ Revised Code Title |

2002 Ingenix, Inc.

054.6 **Herpetic whitlow**
Herpetic felon
DEF: A primary infection of the terminal segment of a finger by herpes simplex; intense itching and pain start the disease, vesicles form, and tissue ultimately is destroyed.

√5th **054.7** **With other specified complications**
054.71 Visceral herpes simplex
054.72 Herpes simplex meningitis
054.73 Herpes simplex otitis externa
054.79 Other

054.8 With unspecified complication
054.9 Herpes simplex without mention of complication

√4th **055 Measles**
INCLUDES morbilli
rubeola

055.0 Postmeasles encephalitis
055.1 Postmeasles pneumonia
055.2 Postmeasles otitis media

√5th **055.7** **With other specified complications**
055.71 Measles keratoconjunctivitis
Measles keratitis
055.79 Other

055.8 With unspecified complication
055.9 Measles without mention of complication

√4th **056 Rubella**
INCLUDES German measles
EXCLUDES congenital rubella (771.0)
DEF: Acute but usually benign togavirus infection causing fever, sore throat, and rash; associated with complications to fetus as a result of maternal infection.

√5th **056.0** **With neurological complications**
056.00 With unspecified neurological complication
056.01 Encephalomyelitis due to rubella
Encephalitis } due to rubella
Meningoencephalitis
056.09 Other

√5th **056.7** **With other specified complications**
056.71 Arthritis due to rubella
056.79 Other

056.8 With unspecified complications
056.9 Rubella without mention of complication

√4th **057 Other viral exanthemata**
DEF: Skin eruptions or rashes and fever caused by viruses, including poxviruses.

057.0 **Erythema infectiosum [fifth disease]**
DEF: A moderately contagious, benign, epidemic disease, usually seen in children, and of probable viral etiology; a red macular rash appears on the face and may spread to the limbs and trunk.

057.8 Other specified viral exanthemata
Dukes (-Filatow) disease
Exanthema subitum [sixth disease]
Fourth disease
Parascarlatina
Pseudoscarlatina
Roseola infantum

INFECTIOUS AND PARASITIC DISEASES 057.9–062.9

057.9 <mark>Viral exanthem, unspecified</mark>

ARTHROPOD-BORNE VIRAL DISEASES (060-066)
Use additional code to identify any associated meningitis (321.2)

EXCLUDES *late effects of viral encephalitis (139.0)*

✓4th 060 Yellow fever
DEF: Fever and jaundice from infection by mosquito-borne virus of genus Flavivirus.

060.0 **Sylvatic**
Yellow fever:
jungle
sylvan

DEF: Yellow fever transmitted from animal to man, via mosquito.

060.1 **Urban**
DEF: Yellow fever transmitted from man to man, via mosquito.

060.9 <mark>Yellow fever, unspecified</mark>

061 Dengue
Breakbone fever

EXCLUDES *hemorrhagic fever caused by dengue virus (065.4)*

DEF: Acute, self-limiting infection by mosquito-borne virus characterized by fever and generalized aches

✓4th 062 Mosquito-borne viral encephalitis

062.0 **Japanese encephalitis**
Japanese B encephalitis

DEF: Flavivirus causing inflammation of the brain, and Russia, with a wide range of clinical manifestations

062.1 **Western equine encephalitis**
DEF: Alphavirus WEE infection causing inflammation of the brain, found in areas west of the Mississippi; transmitted horse to mosquito to man.

062.2 **Eastern equine encephalitis**

EXCLUDES *Venezuelan equine encephalitis (066.2)*

DEF: Alphavirus EEE causing inflammation of the brain and spinal cord, found as far north as Canada and south into South America and Mexico; transmitted horse to mosquito to man.

062.3 **St. Louis encephalitis**
DEF: Epidemic form caused by Flavivirus and transmitted by mosquito, and characterized by fever, difficulty in speech, and headache.

062.4 **Australian encephalitis**
Australian arboencephalitis
Australian X disease
Murray Valley encephalitis

DEF: Flavivirus causing inflammation of the brain, occurring in Australia and New Guinea.

062.5 **California virus encephalitis**
Encephalitis: Tahyna fever
California
La Crosse

DEF: Bunya virus causing inflammation of the brain.

062.8 <mark>Other specified mosquito-borne viral encephalitis</mark>
Encephalitis by Ilheus virus

EXCLUDES ▶*West Nile virus (066.4)*◀

062.9 <mark>Mosquito-borne viral encephalitis, unspecified</mark>

✓4th / ✓5th Additional Digit Required | <mark>Unspecified Code</mark> | Other Specified Code | Manifestation Code
MSP Medicare Secondary Payer | ▶◀ Revised Text | ● New Code | ▲ Revised Code Title

INFECTIOUS AND PARASITIC DISEASES

√4th 063 Tick-borne viral encephalitis
  INCLUDES diphasic meningoencephalitis
- **063.0** Russian spring-summer [taiga] encephalitis
- **063.1** Louping ill
  DEF: Inflammation of brain caused by virus transmitted sheep to tick to man; incidence usually limited to British Isles.
- **063.2** Central European encephalitis
  DEF: Inflammation of brain caused by virus transmitted by tick; limited to central Europe and presenting with two distinct phases.
- **063.8** Other specified tick-borne viral encephalitis
  Langat encephalitis
  Powassan encephalitis
- **063.9** Tick-borne viral encephalitis, unspecified

064 Viral encephalitis transmitted by other and unspecified arthropods
  Arthropod-borne viral encephalitis, vector unknown
  Negishi virus encephalitis
  EXCLUDES viral encephalitis NOS (049.9)

√4th 065 Arthropod-borne hemorrhagic fever
- **065.0** Crimean hemorrhagic fever [CHF Congo virus]
  Central Asian hemorrhagic fever
- **065.1** Omsk hemorrhagic fever
- **065.2** Kyasanur Forest disease
- **065.3** Other tick-borne hemorrhagic fever
- **065.4** Mosquito-borne hemorrhagic fever
  Chikungunya hemorrhagic fever
  Dengue hemorrhagic fever
  EXCLUDES Chikungunya fever (066.3)
  dengue (061)
  yellow fever (060.0-060.9)
- **065.8** Other specified arthropod-borne hemorrhagic fever
  Mite-borne hemorrhagic fever
- **065.9** Arthropod-borne hemorrhagic fever, unspecified
  Arbovirus hemorrhagic fever NOS

√4th 066 Other arthropod-borne viral diseases
- **066.0** Phlebotomus fever
  Changuinola fever
  Sandfly fever
  DEF: Sandfly-borne viral infection occurring in Asia, Middle East and South America.
- **066.1** Tick-borne fever
  Nairobi sheep disease   Tick fever:
  Tick fever: Kemerovo
      American mountain   Quaranfil
      Colorado
- **066.2** Venezuelan equine fever
  Venezuelan equine encephalitis
  DEF: Alphavirus VEE infection causing inflammation of the brain, usually limited to South America, Mexico, and Florida; transmitted horse to mosquito to man.

INFECTIOUS AND PARASITIC DISEASES

066.3 **Other mosquito-borne fever**
Fever (viral):
- Bunyamwera
- Bwamba
- Chikungunya
- Guama
- Mayaro
- Mucambo
- O'Nyong-Nyong

Fever (viral):
- Oropouche
- Pixuna
- Rift valley
- Ross river
- Wesselsbron
- Zika

EXCLUDES dengue (061)
yellow fever (060.0-060.9)

066.4 **West Nile fever**
West Nile encephalitis
West Nile encephalomyelitis
West Nile virus

066.8 **Other specified arthropod-borne viral diseases**
Chandipura fever
Piry fever

066.9 **Arthropod-borne viral disease, unspecified**
Arbovirus infection NOS

OTHER DISEASES DUE TO VIRUSES AND CHLAMYDIAE (070-079)

√4th **070 Viral hepatitis**
INCLUDES viral hepatitis (acute) (chronic)
EXCLUDES cytomegalic inclusion virus hepatitis (078.5)

DEF: Hepatitis A: HAV infection is self-limiting with flu like symptoms; transmission, fecal-oral.

DEF: Hepatitis B: HBV infection can be chronic and systemic; transmission, bodily fluids.

DEF: Hepatitis C: HCV infection can be chronic and systemic; transmission, blood transfusion and unidentified agents.

DEF: Hepatitis D (delta): HDV occurs only in the presence of hepatitis B virus.

DEF: Hepatitis E: HEV is epidemic form; transmission and nature under investigation.

070.0 Viral hepatitis A with hepatic coma
070.1 Viral hepatitis A without mention of hepatic coma
Infectious hepatitis

The following fifth-digit subclassification is for use with categories 070.2 and 070.3:
- 0 acute or unspecified, without mention of hepatitis delta
- 1 acute or unspecified, with hepatitis delta
- 2 chronic, without mention of hepatitis delta
- 3 chronic, with hepatitis delta

√5th **070.2** Viral hepatitis B with hepatic coma
√5th **070.3** Viral hepatitis B without mention of hepatic coma
Serum hepatitis

√5th **070.4** Other specified viral hepatitis with hepatic coma
- **070.41** Acute or unspecified hepatitis C with hepatic coma
- **070.42** Hepatitis delta without mention of active hepatitis B disease with hepatic coma
  Hepatitis delta with hepatitis B carrier state
- **070.43** Hepatitis E with hepatic coma
- **070.44** Chronic hepatitis C with hepatic coma
- **070.49** Other specified viral hepatitis with hepatic coma

INFECTIOUS AND PARASITIC DISEASES

✓5th **070.5** Other specified viral hepatitis without mention of hepatic coma
  070.51 Acute or unspecified hepatitis C without mention of hepatic coma
  070.52 Hepatitis delta without mention of active hepatititis B disease or hepatic coma
  070.53 Hepatitis E without mention of hepatic coma
  070.54 Chronic hepatitis C without mention of hepatic coma
  070.59 Other specified viral hepatitis without mention of hepatic coma
070.6 Unspecified viral hepatitis with hepatic coma
070.9 Unspecified viral hepatitis without mention of hepatic coma
  Viral hepatitis NOS

071 Rabies
  Hydrophobia
  Lyssa
  DEF: Acute infectious disease of the CNS caused by a rhabdovirus; usually spread by virus-laden saliva from bites by infected animals; it progresses from fever, restlessness, and extreme excitability, to hydrophobia, seizures, confusion and death.

✓4th **072 Mumps**
  DEF: Acute infectious disease caused by paramyxovirus; usually seen in children less than 15 years of age; salivary glands are typically enlarged, and other organs, such as testes, pancreas and meninges, are often involved.

  072.0 Mumps orchitis ♂
  072.1 Mumps meningitis
  072.2 Mumps encephalitis
    Mumps meningoencephalitis
  072.3 Mumps pancreatitis
✓5th **072.7** Mumps with other specified complications
    072.71 Mumps hepatitis
    072.72 Mumps polyneuropathy
    072.79 Other
  072.8 Mumps with unspecified complication
  072.9 Mumps without mention of complication
    Epidemic parotitis
    Infectious parotitis

073 Ornithosis
  INCLUDES parrot fever
    psittacosis
  DEF: *Chlamydia psittaci* infection often transmitted from birds to humans.

  073.0 With pneumonia
    Lobular pneumonitis due to ornithosis
  073.7 With other specified complications
  073.8 With unspecified complication
  073.9 Ornithosis, unspecified

✓4th **074 Specific diseases due to Coxsackie virus**
    EXCLUDES *Coxsackie virus:*
      infection NOS (079.2)
      meningitis (047.0)
  074.0 Herpangina
    Vesicular pharyngitis
    DEF: Acute infectious coxsackie virus infection causing throat lesions, fever, and vomiting; generally affects children in summer.

INFECTIOUS AND PARASITIC DISEASES 074.1–077.1

074.1 Epidemic pleurodynia
Bornholm disease
Devil's grip
Epidemic:
   myalgia
   myositis
DEF: Paroxysmal pain in chest, accompanied by fever and usually limited to children and young adults; caused by coxsackie virus.

✓5th **074.2 Coxsackie carditis**
   074.20 Coxsackie carditis, unspecified
   074.21 Coxsackie pericarditis
      DEF: Coxsackie infection of the outer lining of the heart.
   074.22 Coxsackie endocarditis
      DEF: Coxsackie infection within the heart's cavities.
   074.23 Coxsackie myocarditis
      Aseptic myocarditis of newborn
      DEF: Coxsackie infection of the muscle of the heart.

074.3 Hand, foot, and mouth disease
Vesicular stomatitis and exanthem
DEF: Mild coxsackie infection causing lesions on hands, feet and oral mucosa; most commonly seen in preschool children.

074.8 Other specified diseases due to Coxsackie virus
Acute lymphonodular pharyngitis

075 Infectious mononucleosis
Glandular fever   Pfeiffer's disease
Monocytic angina
DEF: Acute infection by Epstein-Barr virus causing fever, sore throat, enlarged lymph glands and spleen, and fatigue; usually seen in teens and young adults.

✓4th **076 Trachoma**
   EXCLUDES late effect of trachoma (139.1)
DEF: A chronic infectious disease of the cornea and conjunctiva caused by a strain of the bacteria *Chlamydia trachomatis*; the infection can cause photophobia, pain, excessive tearing and sometimes blindness.

   076.0 Initial stage
      Trachoma dubium
   076.1 Active stage
      Granular conjunctivitis (trachomatous)
      Trachomatous
         follicular conjunctivitis
         pannus
   076.9 Trachoma, unspecified
      Trachoma NOS

✓4th **077 Other diseases of conjunctiva due to viruses and Chlamydiae**
   EXCLUDES ophthalmic complications of viral diseases classified elsewhere

   077.0 Inclusion conjunctivitis
      Paratrachoma
      Swimming pool conjunctivitis
      EXCLUDES inclusion blennorrhea (neonatal) (771.6)
      DEF: Pus in conjunctiva caused by *Chlamydiae trachomatis* infection.

   077.1 Epidemic keratoconjunctivitis
      Shipyard eye
      DEF: Highly contagious corneal or conjunctival infection caused by adenovirus type 8; symptoms include inflammation and corneal infiltrates.

 Additional Digit Required   **Unspecified Code**   **Other Specified Code**   **Manifestation Code**
MSP Medicare Secondary Payer   ▶◀ Revised Text   ● New Code   ▲ Revised Code Title

077.2 Pharyngoconjunctival fever
Viral pharyngoconjunctivitis

077.3 Other adenoviral conjunctivitis
Acute adenoviral follicular conjunctivitis

077.4 Epidemic hemorrhagic conjunctivitis
Apollo:
 conjunctivitis
 disease
Conjunctivitis due to enterovirus type 70
Hemorrhagic conjunctivitis (acute) (epidemic)

077.8 Other viral conjunctivitis
Newcastle conjunctivitis

√5th **077.9 Unspecified diseases of conjunctiva due to viruses and Chlamydiae**

DEF: A genus of the family *Chlamydiaceae; C. psittaci* causes psittacosis in man and ornithosis in birds, and *C. trachomatis* causes trachoma, conjunctivitis, lymphogranuloma venereum, pneumonitis and pneumonia.

077.98 Due to Chlamydiae
077.99 Due to viruses
Viral conjunctivitis NOS

√4th **078 Other diseases due to viruses and Chlamydiae**

EXCLUDES viral infection NOS (079.0-079.9)
 viremia NOS (790.8)

078.0 Molluscum contagiosum

DEF: Benign poxvirus infection causing small bumps on the skin or conjunctiva; transmitted by close contact.

√5th **078.1 Viral warts**
Viral warts due to human papilloma virus

DEF: A keratotic papilloma of the epidermis caused by the human papilloma virus; the superficial vegetative lesions last for varying durations and eventually regress spontaneously.

078.10 Viral warts, unspecified
Condyloma NOS Verruca:
Verruca: Vulgaris
 NOS   Warts (infectious)

078.11 Condyloma acuminatum

DEF: Clusters of mucosa or epidermal lesions on external genitalia; viral infection is sexually transmitted.

078.19 Other specified viral warts
Genital warts NOS
Verruca:
 plana
 plantaris

078.2 Sweating fever
Miliary fever
Sweating disease

DEF: A viral infection characterized by profuse sweating; various papular, vesicular and other eruptions cause the blockage of sweat glands.

078.3 Cat-scratch disease
Benign lymphoreticulosis (of inoculation)
Cat-scratch fever

078.4 Foot and mouth disease
Aphthous fever
Epizootic:
 aphthae
 stomatitis

DEF: Ulcers on oral mucosa, legs, and feet after exposure to infected animal.

INFECTIOUS AND PARASITIC DISEASES

078.5 Cytomegaloviral disease
Cytomegalic inclusion disease
Salivary gland virus disease
Use additional code to identify manifestation, as:
  cytomegalic inclusion virus:
    hepatitis (573.1)
    pneumonia (484.1)

EXCLUDES *congenital cytomegalovirus infection (771.1)*

DEF: A herpes virus inclusion associated with serious disease morbidity including fever, leukopenia, pneumonia, retinitis, hepatitis and organ transplant; often leads to syndromes such as hepatomegaly, splenomegaly and thrombocytopenia; a common post-transplant complication for organ transplant recipients.

078.6 Hemorrhagic nephrosonephritis
Hemorrhagic fever:
  epidemic
  Korean
  Russian
  with renal syndrome

DEF: Viral infection causing kidney dysfunction and bleeding disorders.

078.7 Arenaviral hemorrhagic fever
Hemorrhagic fever:
  Argentine
  Bolivian
  Junin virus
  Machupo virus

√5th 078.8 Other specified diseases due to viruses and Chlamydiae
EXCLUDES *epidemic diarrhea (009.2)*
lymphogranuloma venereum (099.1)

078.81 Epidemic vertigo

078.82 Epidemic vomiting syndrome
Winter vomiting disease

078.88 Other specified diseases due to Chlamydiae

078.89 Other specified diseases due to viruses
Epidemic cervical myalgia
Marburg disease
Tanapox

√4th 079 Viral and chlamydial infection in conditions classified elsewhere and of unspecified site

Note: This category is provided to be used as an additional code to identify the viral agent in diseases classifiable elsewhere. This category will also be used to classify virus infection of unspecified nature or site.

079.0 Adenovirus

079.1 ECHO virus
DEF: An "orphan" enteric RNA virus, certain serotypes of which are associated with human disease, especially aseptic meningitis.

079.2 Coxsackie virus
DEF: A heterogenous group of viruses associated with aseptic meningitis, myocarditis, pericarditis, and acute onset juvenile diabetes.

079.3 Rhinovirus
DEF: Rhinoviruses affect primarily the upper respiratory tract. Over 100 distinct types infect humans.

079.4 **Human papillomavirus**
DEF: Viral infection caused by the genus *Papillomavirus* causing cutaneous and genital warts, including verruca vulgaris and condyloma acuminatum; certain types are associated with cervical dysplasia, cancer and other genital malignancies.

√5th **079.5** **Retrovirus**
EXCLUDES human immunodeficiency virus, type 1 [HIV-1] (042)
human T-cell lymphotrophic virus, type III [HTLV-III] (042)
lymphadenopathy-associated virus [LAV] (042)

DEF: A large group of RNA viruses that carry reverse transcriptase and include the leukoviruses and lentiviruses.

079.50 Retrovirus, unspecified
079.51 Human T-cell lymphotrophic virus, type I [HTLV-I]
079.52 Human T-cell lymphotrophic virus, type II [HTLV-II]
079.53 Human immunodeficiency virus, type 2 [HIV-2]
079.59 Other specified retrovirus

079.6 **Respiratory syncytial virus (RSV)**
DEF: The major respiratory pathogen of young children, causing severe bronchitis and bronchopneumonia, and minor infection in adults.

√5th **079.8** **Other specified viral and chlamydial infections**
079.81 Hantavirus
DEF: An infection caused by the Muerto Canyon virus whose primary rodent reservoir is the deer mouse Peromyscus maniculatus; commonly characterized by fever, myalgias, headache, cough and rapid respiratory failure.

079.88 Other specified chlamydial infection
079.89 Other specified viral infection

√5th **079.9** **Unspecified viral and chlamydial infections**
EXCLUDES viremia NOS (790.8)

079.98 Unspecified chlamydial infection
Chlamydial infections NOS
079.99 Unspecified viral infection
Viral infections NOS

RICKETTSIOSES AND OTHER ARTHROPOD-BORNE DISEASES (080-088)
EXCLUDES arthropod-borne viral diseases (060.0-066.9)

080 **Louse-borne [epidemic] typhus**
Typhus (fever):   Typhus (fever):
  classical   exanthematic NOS
  epidemic   louse-borne
DEF: *Rickettsia prowazekii*; causes severe headache, rash, high fever.

√4th **081** **Other typhus**
081.0 Murine [endemic] typhus
Typhus (fever):   Typhus (fever):
  endemic   flea-borne
DEF: Milder typhus caused by *Rickettsia typhi (mooseri)*; transmitted by rat flea.

081.1 Brill's disease
Brill-Zinsser disease
Recrudescent typhus (fever)

081.2 Scrub typhus
Japanese river fever   Mite-borne typhus
Kedani fever   Tsutsugamushi
DEF: Typhus caused by *Rickettsia tsutsugamushi* transmitted by chigger.

INFECTIOUS AND PARASITIC DISEASES

081.9 **Typhus, unspecified**
Typhus (fever) NOS

✓4th **082 Tick-borne rickettsioses**

082.0 **Spotted fevers**
Rocky mountain spotted fever
Sao Paulo fever

082.1 **Boutonneuse fever**
African tick typhus   Marseilles fever
India tick typhus   Mediterranean tick fever
Kenya tick typhus

082.2 **North Asian tick fever**
Siberian tick typhus

082.3 **Queensland tick typhus**

✓5th **082.4** **Ehrlichiosis**

082.40 **Ehrlichiosis, unspecified**

082.41 **Ehrlichiosis chaffeensis [E. chaffeensis]**
DEF: A febrile illness caused by bacterial infection, also called human monocytic ehrlichiosis (HME). Causal organism is *Ehrlichia chaffeensis*, transmitted by the Lone Star tick, *Amblyomma americanum*. Symptoms include fever, chills, myalgia, nausea, vomiting, diarrhea, confusion, and severe headache occurring one week after a tick bite. Clinical findings are lymphadenopathy, rash, thrombocytopenia, leukopenia, and abnormal liver function tests

082.49 **Other ehrlichiosis**

082.8 **Other specified tick-borne rickettsioses**
Lone star fever

082.9 **Tick-borne rickettsiosis, unspecified**
Tick-borne typhus NOS

✓4th **083 Other rickettsioses**

083.0 **Q fever**
DEF: Infection of *Coxiella burnetii* usually acquired through airborne organisms.

083.1 **Trench fever**
Quintan fever   Wolhynian fever

083.2 **Rickettsialpox**
Vesicular rickettsiosis
DEF: Infection of *Rickettsia akari* usually acquired through a mite bite.

083.8 **Other specified rickettsioses**

083.9 **Rickettsiosis, unspecified**

✓4th **084 Malaria**
Note: Subcategories 084.0-084.6 exclude the listed conditions with mention of pernicious complications (084.8-084.9).

EXCLUDES congenital malaria (771.2)

DEF: Mosquito-borne disease causing high fever and prostration and cataloged by species of *Plasmodium: P. falciparum, P. malariae, P. ovale,* and *P. vivax.*

084.0 **Falciparum malaria [malignant tertian]**
Malaria (fever):
by Plasmodium falciparum
subtertian

084.1 **Vivax malaria [benign tertian]**
Malaria (fever) by Plasmodium vivax

084.2 **Quartan malaria**
Malaria (fever) by Plasmodium malariae
Malariae malaria

✓4th ✓5th Additional Digit Required | Unspecified Code | Other Specified Code | Manifestation Code

 Medicare Secondary Payer | ▶◀ Revised Text | ● New Code | ▲ Revised Code Title

INFECTIOUS AND PARASITIC DISEASES

084.3 Ovale malaria
Malaria (fever) by Plasmodium ovale

084.4 Other malaria
Monkey malaria

084.5 Mixed malaria
Malaria (fever) by more than one parasite

084.6 Malaria, unspecified
Malaria (fever) NOS

084.7 Induced malaria
Therapeutically induced malaria
> **EXCLUDES** accidental infection from syringe, blood transfusion, etc.
> (084.0-084.6, above, according to parasite species)
> transmission from mother to child during delivery (771.2)

084.8 Blackwater fever
Hemoglobinuric: Malarial hemoglobinuria
  fever (bilious)
  malaria

DEF: Severe hemic and renal complication of *Plasmodium falciparum* infection.

084.9 Other pernicious complications of malaria
Algid malaria
Cerebral malaria
Use additional code to identify complication, as:
  malarial:
    hepatitis (573.2)
    nephrosis (581.81)

✓4th 085 Leishmaniasis

085.0 Visceral [kala-azar]
Dumdum fever
Infection by Leishmania:
  donovani
  infantum
Leishmaniasis:
  dermal, post-kala-azar
  Mediterranean
  visceral (Indian)

085.1 Cutaneous, urban
Aleppo boil
Baghdad boil
Delhi boil
Infection by Leishmania tropica (minor)
Leishmaniasis, cutaneous:
  dry form
  late
  recurrent
  ulcerating
Oriental sore

085.2 Cutaneous, Asian desert
Infection by Leishmania tropica major
Leishmaniasis, cutaneous:
  acute necrotizing
  rural
  wet form
  zoonotic form

085.3 Cutaneous, Ethiopian
Infection by Leishmania ethiopica
Leishmaniasis, cutaneous:
  diffuse
  lepromatous

085.4 Cutaneous, American
Chiclero ulcer
Infection by Leishmania mexicana
Leishmaniasis tegumentaria diffusa

INFECTIOUS AND PARASITIC DISEASES

085.5 Mucocutaneous (American)
Espundia
Infection by Leishmania braziliensis
Uta

085.9 Leishmaniasis, unspecified

√4th **086 Trypanosomiasis**
Use additional code to identify manifestations, as:
trypanosomiasis:
encephalitis (323.2)
meningitis (321.3)

086.0 Chagas' disease with heart involvement
American trypanosomiasis ⎫
Infection by Trypanosoma ⎬ with heart involvement
cruzi ⎭
Any condition classifiable to 086.2 with heart involvement

086.1 Chagas' disease with other organ involvement
American trypanosomiasis ⎫
Infection by Trypanosoma ⎬ with involvement of organ other
cruzi ⎭ than heart
Any condition classifiable to 086.2 with involvement of organ other than heart

086.2 Chagas' disease without mention of organ involvement
American trypanosomiasis
Infection by Trypanosoma cruzi

086.3 Gambian trypanosomiasis
Gambian sleeping sickness
Infection by Trypanosoma gambiense

086.4 Rhodesian trypanosomiasis
Infection by Trypanosoma rhodesiense
Rhodesian sleeping sickness

086.5 African trypanosomiasis, unspecified
Sleeping sickness NOS

086.9 Trypanosomiasis, unspecified

√4th **087 Relapsing fever**
[INCLUDES] recurrent fever
DEF: Infection by *Borrelia*; symptoms are episodic and include fever and arthralgia.

087.0 Louse-borne
087.1 Tick-borne
087.9 Relapsing fever, unspecified

√4th **088 Other arthropod-borne diseases**

088.0 Bartonellosis
Carrión's disease   Verruga peruana
Oroya fever

√5th **088.8** Other specified arthropod-borne diseases
088.81 Lyme disease
Erythema chronicum migrans
DEF: A recurrent multisystem disorder caused by the spirochete *Borrelia burgdorferi* with the carrier being the tick *Ixodes dammini*; the disease begins with lesions of erythema chronicum migrans; it is followed by arthritis of the large joints, myalgia, malaise, and neurological and cardiac manifestations.

INFECTIOUS AND PARASITIC DISEASES

088.82 Babesiosis
Babesiasis
DEF: A tick-borne disease caused by infection of *Babesia*, characterized by fever, malaise, listlessness, severe anemia and hemoglobinuria.

088.89 Other

088.9 Arthropod-borne disease, unspecified

SYPHILIS AND OTHER VENEREAL DISEASES (090-099)

EXCLUDES nonvenereal endemic syphilis (104.0)
urogenital trichomoniasis (131.0)

√4th **090 Congenital syphilis**
DEF: Infection by spirochete *Treponema pallidum* acquired in utero from the infected mother.

090.0 Early congenital syphilis, symptomatic
Congenital syphilitic: Congenital syphilitic:
  choroiditis   splenomegaly
  coryza (chronic)   Syphilitic (congenital):
  hepatomegaly   epiphysitis
  mucous patches   osteochondritis
  periostitis   pemphigus
Any congenital syphilitic condition specified as early or manifest less than two years after birth

090.1 Early congenital syphilis, latent
Congenital syphilis without clinical manifestations, with positive serological reaction and negative spinal fluid test, less than two years after birth

090.2 Early congenital syphilis, unspecified
Congenital syphilis NOS, less than two years after birth

090.3 Syphilitic interstitial keratitis
Syphilitic keratitis: Syphilitic keratitis:
  parenchymatous   punctata profunda
EXCLUDES interstitial keratitis NOS (370.50)

√5th **090.4 Juvenile neurosyphilis**
Use additional code to identify any associated mental disorder
DEF: *Treponema pallidum* infection involving the nervous system.

090.40 Juvenile neurosyphilis, unspecified
Congenital neurosyphilis
Dementia paralytica juvenilis
Juvenile:
  general paresis
  tabes
  taboparesis

090.41 Congenital syphilitic encephalitis
DEF: Congenital *Treponema pallidum* infection involving the brain.

090.42 Congenital syphilitic meningitis
DEF: Congenital *Treponema pallidum* infection involving the lining of the brain and/or spinal cord.

090.49 Other

090.5 Other late congenital syphilis, symptomatic
Gumma due to congenital syphilis
Hutchinson's teeth
Syphilitic saddle nose
Any congenital syphilitic condition specified as late or manifest two years or more after birth

090.6 Late congenital syphilis, latent
Congenital syphilis without clinical manifestations, with positive serological reaction and negative spinal fluid test, two years or more after birth

INFECTIOUS AND PARASITIC DISEASES

090.7 Late congenital syphilis, unspecified
Congenital syphilis NOS, two years or more after birth

090.9 Congenital syphilis, unspecified

√4th **091** Early syphilis, symptomatic
EXCLUDES early cardiovascular syphilis (093.0-093.9)
early neurosyphilis (094.0-094.9)

091.0 Genital syphilis (primary)
Genital chancre
DEF: Genital lesion at the site of initial infection by *Treponema pallidum*.

091.1 Primary anal syphilis
DEF: Anal lesion at the site of initial infection by *Treponema pallidum*.

091.2 Other primary syphilis
Primary syphilis of: Primary syphilis of:
  breast   lip
  fingers   tonsils
DEF: Lesion at the site of initial infection by *Treponema pallidum*.

091.3 Secondary syphilis of skin or mucous membranes
Condyloma latum   Secondary syphilis of:
Secondary syphilis of: skin
  anus   tonsils
  mouth   vulva
  pharynx
DEF: Transitory or chronic lesions following initial syphilis infection.

091.4 Adenopathy due to secondary syphilis
Syphilitic adenopathy (secondary)
Syphilitic lymphadenitis (secondary)

√5th **091.5** Uveitis due to secondary syphilis
  091.50 Syphilitic uveitis, unspecified
  091.51 Syphilitic chorioretinitis (secondary)
    DEF: Inflammation of choroid and retina as a secondary infection.
  091.52 Syphilitic iridocyclitis (secondary)
    DEF: Inflammation of iris and ciliary body as a secondary infection.

√5th **091.6** Secondary syphilis of viscera and bone
  091.61 Secondary syphilitic periostitis
    DEF: Inflammation of outer layers of bone as a secondary infection.
  091.62 Secondary syphilitic hepatitis
    Secondary syphilis of liver
  091.69 Other viscera

091.7 Secondary syphilis, relapse
Secondary syphilis, relapse (treated) (untreated)

√5th **091.8** Other forms of secondary syphilis
  091.81 Acute syphilitic meningitis (secondary)
    DEF: Sudden, severe inflammation of the lining of the brain and/or spinal cord as a secondary infection.
  091.82 Syphilitic alopecia
    DEF: Hair loss following initial syphilis infection.
  091.89 Other

091.9 Unspecified secondary syphilis

INFECTIOUS AND PARASITIC DISEASES

√4th **092 Early syphilis, latent**
   INCLUDES syphilis (acquired) without clinical manifestations, with positive serological reaction and negative spinal fluid test, less than two years after infection
   092.0 Early syphilis, latent, serological relapse after treatment
   092.9 Early syphilis, latent, unspecified

√4th **093 Cardiovascular syphilis**
   093.0 Aneurysm of aorta, specified as syphilitic
       Dilatation of aorta, specified as syphilitic
   093.1 Syphilitic aortitis
       DEF: Inflammation of the aorta - the main artery leading from the heart.

   √5th **093.2 Syphilitic endocarditis**
       DEF: Inflammation of the tissues lining the cavities of the heart.
       093.20 Valve, unspecified
           Syphilitic ostial coronary disease
       093.21 Mitral valve
       093.22 Aortic valve
           Syphilitic aortic incompetence or stenosis
       093.23 Tricuspid valve
       093.24 Pulmonary valve

   √5th **093.8 Other specified cardiovascular syphilis**
       093.81 Syphilitic pericarditis
           DEF: Inflammation of the outer lining of the heart.
       093.82 Syphilitic myocarditis
           DEF: Inflammation of the muscle of the heart.
       093.89 Other
   093.9 Cardiovascular syphilis, unspecified

√4th **094 Neurosyphilis**
   Use additional code to identify any associated mental disorder
   094.0 Tabes dorsalis
       Locomotor ataxia (progressive)
       Posterior spinal sclerosis (syphilitic)
       Tabetic neurosyphilis
       Use additional code to identify manifestation, as:
           neurogenic arthropathy [Charcot's joint disease] (713.5)
       DEF: Progressive degeneration of nerves associated with long-term syphilis; causing pain, wasting away, incontinence, and ataxia.

   094.1 General paresis
       Dementia paralytica
       General paralysis (of the insane) (progressive)
       Paretic neurosyphilis
       Taboparesis
       DEF: Degeneration of brain associated with long-term syphilis, causing loss of brain function, progressive dementia, and paralysis.

   094.2 Syphilitic meningitis
       Meningovascular syphilis
           EXCLUDES acute syphilitic meningitis (secondary) (091.81)
       DEF: Inflammation of the lining of the brain and/or spinal cord.

   094.3 Asymptomatic neurosyphilis

   √5th **094.8 Other specified neurosyphilis**
       094.81 Syphilitic encephalitis

INFECTIOUS AND PARASITIC DISEASES

094.82 Syphilitic Parkinsonism
DEF: Decreased motor function, tremors, and muscular rigidity.

094.83 Syphilitic disseminated retinochoroiditis
DEF: Inflammation of retina and choroid due to neurosyphilis.

094.84 Syphilitic optic atrophy
DEF: Degeneration of the eye and its nerves due to neurosyphilis.

094.85 Syphilitic retrobulbar neuritis
DEF: Inflammation of the posterior optic nerve due to neurosyphilis.

094.86 Syphilitic acoustic neuritis
DEF: Inflammation of acoustic nerve due to neurosyphilis.

094.87 Syphilitic ruptured cerebral aneurysm

094.89 Other

094.9 Neurosyphilis, unspecified
Gumma (syphilitic)
Syphilis (early) (late) } of central nervous system NOS
Syphiloma

095 Other forms of late syphilis, with symptoms
INCLUDES: gumma (syphilitic)
syphilis, late, tertiary, or unspecified stage

095.0 Syphilitic episcleritis
095.1 Syphilis of lung
095.2 Syphilitic peritonitis
095.3 Syphilis of liver
095.4 Syphilis of kidney
095.5 Syphilis of bone
095.6 Syphilis of muscle
Syphilitic myositis
095.7 Syphilis of synovium, tendon, and bursa
Syphilitic: Syphilitic:
  bursitis   synovitis
095.8 Other specified forms of late symptomatic syphilis
EXCLUDES: cardiovascular syphilis (093.0-093.9)
neurosyphilis (094.0-094.9)
095.9 Late symptomatic syphilis, unspecified

096 Late syphilis, latent
Syphilis (acquired) without clinical manifestations, with positive serological reaction and negative spinal fluid test, two years or more after infection

097 Other and unspecified syphilis
097.0 Late syphilis, unspecified
097.1 Latent syphilis, unspecified
Positive serological reaction for syphilis
097.9 Syphilis, unspecified
Syphilis (acquired) NOS
EXCLUDES: syphilis NOS causing death under two years of age (090.9)

098 Gonococcal infections
DEF: *Neisseria gonorrhoeae* infection generally acquired in utero or in sexual congress.

INFECTIOUS AND PARASITIC DISEASES

098.0 **Acute, of lower genitourinary tract**
Gonococcal: Gonorrhea (acute):
  Bartholinitis (acute)   NOS
  urethritis (acute)   genitourinary (tract) NOS
  vulvovaginitis (acute)

√5ᵗʰ **098.1** **Acute, of upper genitourinary tract**

098.10 **Gonococcal infection (acute) of upper genitourinary tract, site unspecified**

098.11 **Gonococcal cystitis (acute)**
Gonorrhea (acute) of bladder

098.12 **Gonococcal prostatitis (acute)** ♂

098.13 **Gonococcal epididymo-orchitis (acute)** ♂
Gonococcal orchitis (acute)
DEF: Acute inflammation of the testes.

098.14 **Gonococcal seminal vesiculitis (acute)** ♂
Gonorrhea (acute) of seminal vesicle

098.15 **Gonococcal cervicitis (acute)** ♀
Gonorrhea (acute) of cervix

098.16 **Gonococcal endometritis (acute)** ♀
Gonorrhea (acute) of uterus

098.17 **Gonococcal salpingitis, specified as acute** ♀
DEF: Acute inflammation of the fallopian tubes.

098.19 **Other**

098.2 **Chronic, of lower genitourinary tract**
Gonococcal:
  Bartholinitis
  urethritis   } specified as chronic or with duration of
  vulvovaginitis   two months or more
Gonorrhea:
  NOS
  genitourinary (tract)

Any condition classifiable to 098.0 specified as chronic or with duration of two months or more

√5ᵗʰ **098.3** **Chronic, of upper genitourinary tract**
[INCLUDES] any condition classifiable to 098.1 stated as chronic or with a duration of two months or more

098.30 **Chronic gonococcal infection of upper genitourinary tract, site unspecified**

098.31 **Gonococcal cystitis, chronic**
Any condition classifiable to 098.11, specified as chronic
Gonorrhea of bladder, chronic

098.32 **Gonococcal prostatitis, chronic** ♂
Any condition classifiable to 098.12, specified as chronic

098.33 **Gonococcal epididymo-orchitis, chronic** ♂
Any condition classifiable to 098.13, specified as chronic
Chronic gonococcal orchitis
DEF: Chronic inflammation of the testes.

098.34 **Gonococcal seminal vesiculitis, chronic** ♂
Any condition classifiable to 098.14, specified as chronic
Gonorrhea of seminal vesicle, chronic

098.35 **Gonococcal cervicitis, chronic** ♀
Any condition classifiable to 098.15, specified as chronic
Gonorrhea of cervix, chronic

INFECTIOUS AND PARASITIC DISEASES

098.36 Gonococcal endometritis, chronic ♀
Any condition classifiable to 098.16, specified as chronic
DEF: Chronic inflammation of the uterus.

098.37 Gonococcal salpingitis (chronic) ♀
DEF: Chronic inflammation of the fallopian tubes.

098.39 Other

√5ᵗʰ **098.4 Gonococcal infection of eye**

098.40 Gonococcal conjunctivitis (neonatorum)
Gonococcal ophthalmia (neonatorum)
DEF: Inflammation and infection of conjunctiva present at birth.

098.41 Gonococcal iridocyclitis
DEF: Inflammation and infection of iris and ciliary body.

098.42 Gonococcal endophthalmia
DEF: Inflammation and infection of the contents of the eyeball.

098.43 Gonococcal keratitis
DEF: Inflammation and infection of the cornea.

098.49 Other

√5ᵗʰ **098.5 Gonococcal infection of joint**

098.50 Gonococcal arthritis
Gonococcal infection of joint NOS

098.51 Gonococcal synovitis and tenosynovitis

098.52 Gonococcal bursitis
DEF: Inflammation of the sac-like cavities in a joint.

098.53 Gonococcal spondylitis

098.59 Other
Gonococcal rheumatism

098.6 Gonococcal infection of pharynx

098.7 Gonococcal infection of anus and rectum
Gonococcal proctitis

√5ᵗʰ **098.8 Gonococcal infection of other specified sites**

098.81 Gonococcal keratosis (blennorrhagica)
DEF: Pustular skin lesions caused by *Neisseria gonorrhoeae*.

098.82 Gonococcal meningitis
DEF: Inflammation of the lining of the brain and/or spinal cord.

098.83 Gonococcal pericarditis
DEF: Inflammation of the outer lining of the heart.

098.84 Gonococcal endocarditis
DEF: Inflammation of the tissues lining the cavities of the heart.

098.85 Other gonococcal heart disease

098.86 Gonococcal peritonitis
DEF: Inflammation of the membrane lining the abdomen.

098.89 Other
Gonococcemia

INFECTIOUS AND PARASITIC DISEASES

✓4th **099 Other venereal diseases**

099.0 Chancroid
- Bubo (inguinal):
  - chancroidal
  - due to Hemophilus ducreyi
- Chancre:
  - Ducrey's
  - simple
  - soft
- Ulcus molle (cutis) (skin)

DEF: A sexually transmitted disease caused by *Haemophilus ducreyi*; it is identified by a painful primary ulcer at the site of inoculation (usually on the external genitalia) with related lymphadenitis.

099.1 Lymphogranuloma venereum
- Climatic or tropical bubo
- (Durand-) Nicolas-Favre disease
- Esthiomene
- Lymphogranuloma inguinale

DEF: Sexually transmitted infection of *Chlamydia trachomatis* causing skin lesions.

099.2 Granuloma inguinale
- Donovanosis
- Granuloma pudendi (ulcerating)
- Granuloma venereum
- Pudendal ulcer

DEF: Chronic, sexually transmitted infection of *Calymmatobacterium granulomatis*, resulting in progressive, anogenital skin ulcers.

099.3 Reiter's disease
- Reiter's syndrome
- Use additional code for associated:
  - arthropathy (711.1)
  - conjunctivitis (372.33)

DEF: A symptom complex of unknown etiology consisting of urethritis, conjunctivitis, arthritis and myocutaneous lesions. It occurs most commonly in young men and patients with HIV and may precede or follow AIDS. Also a form of reactive arthritis.

✓5th **099.4 Other nongonococcal urethritis [NGU]**

099.40 Unspecified
- Nonspecific urethritis

099.41 Chlamydia trachomatis

099.49 Other specified organism

✓5th **099.5 Other venereal diseases due to Chlamydia trachomatis**

> EXCLUDES   Chlamydia trachomatis infection of conjunctiva (076.0-076.9, 077.0, 077.9)
> Lymphogranuloma venereum (099.1)

DEF: Venereal diseases caused by *Chlamydia trachomatis* at other sites besides the urethra (e.g., pharynx, anus and rectum, conjunctiva and peritoneum).

099.50 Unspecified site

099.51 Pharynx

099.52 Anus and rectum

099.53 Lower genitourinary sites
> EXCLUDES   urethra (099.41)

Use additional code to specify site of infection, such as:
- bladder (595.4)
- cervix (616.0)
- vagina and vulva (616.11)

099.54 Other genitourinary sites

Use additional code to specify site of infection, such as:
- pelvic inflammatory disease NOS (614.9)
- testis and epididymis (604.91)

099.55 Unspecified genitourinary site

INFECTIOUS AND PARASITIC DISEASES 099.56–102.2

        099.56 Peritoneum
            Perihepatitis
        099.59 Other specified site
   099.8 Other specified venereal diseases
   099.9 Venereal disease, unspecified

OTHER SPIROCHETAL DISEASES (100-104)

√4th 100 Leptospirosis

DEF: An infection of any spirochete of the genus Leptospire in blood. This zoonosis is transmitted to humans most often by exposure with contaminated animal tissues or water and less often by contact with urine. Patients present with flulike symptoms, the most common being muscle aches involving the thighs and low back. Treatment is with hydration and antibiotics.

    100.0 Leptospirosis icterohemorrhagica
        Leptospiral or spirochetal jaundice (hemorrhagic)
        Weil's disease

√5th 100.8 Other specified leptospiral infections

      100.81 Leptospiral meningitis (aseptic)
      100.89 Other
          Fever: Infection by Leptospira:
            Fort Bragg   australis
            pretibial   bataviae
            swamp   pyrogenes

    100.9 Leptospirosis, unspecified

101 Vincent's angina

      Acute necrotizing ulcerative: Trench mouth
        gingivitis   Vincent's:
        stomatitis   gingivitis
      Fusospirochetal pharyngitis   infection [any site]
      Spirochetal stomatitis

DEF: Painful ulceration with edema and hypermic patches of the oropharyngeal and throat membranes; it is caused by spreading of acute ulcerative gingivitis.

√4th 102 Yaws

    INCLUDES   frambesia
                   pian

DEF: An infectious, endemic, tropical disease caused by *Treponema pertenue;* it usually affects persons 15 years old or younger; a primary cutaneous lesion develops, then a granulomatous skin eruption, and occasionally lesions that destroy skin and bone.

    102.0 Initial lesions
        Chancre of yaws
        Frambesia, initial or primary
        Initial frambesial ulcer
        Mother yaw

    102.1 Multiple papillomata and wet crab yaws
        Butter yaws
        Frambesioma
        Pianoma
        Plantar or palmar papilloma of yaws

    102.2 Other early skin lesions
        Cutaneous yaws, less than five years after infection
        Early yaws (cutaneous) (macular) (papular) (maculopapular) (micropapular)
        Frambeside of early yaws

INFECTIOUS AND PARASITIC DISEASES

102.3 Hyperkeratosis
　　Ghoul hand
　　Hyperkeratosis, palmar or plantar (early) (late) due to yaws
　　Worm-eaten soles
　DEF: Overgrowth of the skin of the palms or bottoms of the feet, due to yaws.

102.4 Gummata and ulcers
　　Gummatous frambeside
　　Nodular late yaws (ulcerated)
　DEF: Rubbery lesions and areas of dead skin caused by yaws.

102.5 Gangosa
　　Rhinopharyngitis mutilans
　DEF: Massive, mutilating lesions of the nose and oral cavity caused by yaws.

102.6 Bone and joint lesions
　　Goundou　　　　　　　　　　　⎫
　　Gumma, bone　　　　　　　　　⎬ of yaws (late)
　　Gummatous osteitis or periostitis ⎭

　　Hydrarthrosis　　　　　　　　⎫
　　Osteitis　　　　　　　　　　　⎬ of yaws (early) (late)
　　Periostitis (hypertrophic)　　　⎭

102.7 Other manifestations
　　Juxta-articular nodules of yaws
　　Mucosal yaws

102.8 Latent yaws
　　Yaws without clinical manifestations, with positive serology

102.9 Yaws, unspecified

✓4th 103 Pinta
DEF: A chronic form of treponematosis, endemic in areas of tropical America; it is identified by the presence of red, violet, blue, coffee-colored or white spots on the skin.

103.0 Primary lesions
　　Chancre (primary)　⎫
　　Papule (primary)　　⎬ of pinta [carate]
　　Pintid　　　　　　　⎭

103.1 Intermediate lesions
　　Erythematous plaques　⎫
　　Hyperchromic lesions　⎬ of pinta [carate]
　　Hyperkeratosis　　　　⎭

103.2 Late lesions
　　Cardiovascular lesions
　　Skin lesions:　　　　⎫
　　　achromic　　　　　 ⎪
　　　cicatricial　　　　　 ⎬ of pinta [carate]
　　　dyschromic　　　　 ⎪
　　Vitiligo　　　　　　　⎭

103.3 Mixed lesions
　　Achromic and hyperchromic skin lesions of pinta [carate]

103.9 Pinta, unspecified

✓4th 104 Other spirochetal infection
104.0 Nonvenereal endemic syphilis
　　Bejel　　　　　　Njovera
　DEF: *Treponema pallidum*, *T. pertenue*, or *T. carateum* infection transmitted non-sexually, causing lesions on mucosa and skin.

INFECTIOUS AND PARASITIC DISEASES

104.8 **Other specified spirochetal infections**
    EXCLUDES   *relapsing fever (087.0-087.9)*
                             syphilis (090.0-097.9)

104.9 **Spirochetal infection, unspecified**

MYCOSES (110-118)

Use additional code to identify manifestation as:
    arthropathy (711.6)
    meningitis (321.0-321.1)
    otitis externa (380.15)

    EXCLUDES   *infection by Actinomycetales, such as species of Actinomyces, Actinomadura, Nocardia, Streptomyces (039.0-039.9)*

✓4th **110 Dermatophytosis**
    INCLUDES   infection by species of Epidermophyton, Microsporum, and Trichophyton
                    tinea, any type except those in 111

DEF: Superficial infection of the skin caused by a parasitic fungus.

110.0 **Of scalp and beard**
    Kerion   Trichophytic tinea
    Sycosis, mycotic   [black dot tinea], scalp

110.1 **Of nail**
    Dermatophytic onychia   Tinea unguium
    Onychomycosis

110.2 **Of hand**
    Tinea manuum

110.3 **Of groin and perianal area**
    Dhobie itch   Tinea cruris
    Eczema marginatum

110.4 **Of foot**
    Athlete's foot   Tinea pedis

110.5 **Of the body**
    Herpes circinatus   Tinea imbricata [Tokelau]

110.6 **Deep seated dermatophytosis**
    Granuloma trichophyticum
    Majocchi's granuloma

110.8 **Of other specified sites**

110.9 **Of unspecified site**
    Favus NOS   Ringworm NOS
    Microsporic tinea NOS

✓4th **111 Dermatomycosis, other and unspecified**

111.0 **Pityriasis versicolor**
    Infection by Malassezia [Pityrosporum] furfur
    Tinea flava
    Tinea versicolor

111.1 **Tinea nigra**
    Infection by Cladosporium species
    Keratomycosis nigricans
    Microsporosis nigra
    Pityriasis nigra
    Tinea palmaris nigra

111.2 **Tinea blanca**
    Infection by Trichosporon (beigelii) cutaneum
    White piedra

111.3 **Black piedra**
    Infection by Piedraia hortai

✓4th ✓5th   Additional Digit Required   Unspecified Code   Other Specified Code   Manifestation Code

 Medicare Secondary Payer   ▶◀ Revised Text   ● New Code   ▲ Revised Code Title

2002 Ingenix, Inc.   Volume 1 — 43

INFECTIOUS AND PARASITIC DISEASES

111.8 Other specified dermatomycoses
111.9 Dermatomycosis, unspecified

√4th **112 Candidiasis**
  INCLUDES   infection by Candida species
                  moniliasis
  EXCLUDES   neonatal monilial infection (771.7)

  DEF: Fungal infection caused by *Candida*; usually seen in mucous membranes or skin.

  112.0 Of mouth
      Thrush (oral)
  112.1 Of vulva and vagina ♀
      Candidal vulvovaginitis
      Monilial vulvovaginitis
  112.2 Of other urogenital sites
      Candidal balanitis
  112.3 Of skin and nails
      Candidal intertrigo
      Candidal onychia
      Candidal perionyxis [paronychia]
  112.4 Of lung
      Candidal pneumonia
  112.5 Disseminated
      Systemic candidiasis
  √5th **112.8** Of other specified sites
      112.81 Candidal endocarditis
      112.82 Candidal otitis externa
          Otomycosis in moniliasis
      112.83 Candidal meningitis
      112.84 Candidal esophagitis
      112.85 Candidal enteritis
      112.89 Other
  112.9 Of unspecified site

√4th **114 Coccidioidomycosis**
  INCLUDES   infection by Coccidioides (immitis)
                  Posada-Wernicke disease

  DEF: A fungal disease caused by inhalation of dust particles containing arthrospores of *Coccidiodes immitis*; a self-limited respiratory infection; the primary form is known as San Joaquin fever, desert fever or valley fever.

  114.0 Primary coccidioidomycosis (pulmonary)
      Acute pulmonary coccidioidomycosis
      Coccidioidomycotic pneumonitis
      Desert rheumatism
      Pulmonary coccidioidomycosis
      San Joaquin Valley fever
      DEF: Acute, self-limiting *Coccidioides immitis* infection of the lung.
  114.1 Primary extrapulmonary coccidioidomycosis
      Chancriform syndrome
      Primary cutaneous coccidioidomycosis
      DEF: Acute, self-limiting *Coccidioides immitis* infection in non-pulmonary site.
  114.2 Coccidioidal meningitis
      DEF: *Coccidioides immitis* infection of the lining of the brain and/or spinal cord.
  114.3 Other forms of progressive coccidioidomycosis
      Coccidioidal granuloma
      Disseminated coccidioidomycosis

INFECTIOUS AND PARASITIC DISEASES 114.4–117.0

114.4 Chronic pulmonary coccidioidomycosis
114.5 Pulmonary coccidioidomycosis, unspecified
114.9 Coccidioidomycosis, unspecified

✓4th 115 Histoplasmosis

The following fifth-digit subclassification is for use with category 115:
- 0 without mention of manifestation
- 1 meningitis
- 2 retinitis
- 3 pericarditis
- 4 endocarditis
- 5 pneumonia
- 9 other

✓5th 115.0 Infection by Histoplasma capsulatum
American histoplasmosis
Darling's disease
Reticuloendothelial cytomycosis
Small form histoplasmosis

DEF: Infection resulting from inhalation of fungal spores, causing acute pneumonia, an influenza-like illness, or a disseminated disease of the reticuloendothelial system. In immunocompromised patients it can reactivate, affecting lungs, meninges, heart, peritoneum and adrenals.

✓5th 115.1 Infection by Histoplasma duboisii
African histoplasmosis
Large form histoplasmosis

✓5th 115.9 Histoplasmosis, unspecified
Histoplasmosis NOS

✓4th 116 Blastomycotic infection

116.0 Blastomycosis
Blastomycotic dermatitis
Chicago disease
Cutaneous blastomycosis
Disseminated blastomycosis
Gilchrist's disease
Infection by Blastomyces [Ajellomyces] dermatitidis
North American blastomycosis
Primary pulmonary blastomycosis

116.1 Paracoccidioidomycosis
Brazilian blastomycosis
Infection by Paracoccidioides [Blastomyces] brasiliensis
Lutz-Splendore-Almeida disease
Mucocutaneous-lymphangitic paracoccidioidomycosis
Pulmonary paracoccidioidomycosis
South American blastomycosis
Visceral paracoccidioidomycosis

116.2 Lobomycosis
Infections by Loboa [Blastomyces] loboi
Keloidal blastomycosis
Lobo's disease

✓4th 117 Other mycoses

117.0 Rhinosporidiosis
Infection by Rhinosporidium seeberi

INFECTIOUS AND PARASITIC DISEASES

117.1 Sporotrichosis
Cutaneous sporotrichosis
Disseminated sporotrichosis
Infection by Sporothrix [Sporotrichum] schenckii
Lymphocutaneous sporotrichosis
Pulmonary sporotrichosis
Sporotrichosis of the bones

117.2 Chromoblastomycosis
Chromomycosis
Infection by Cladosporidium carrionii, Fonsecaea compactum, Fonsecaea pedrosoi, Phialophora verrucosa

117.3 Aspergillosis
Infection by Aspergillus species, mainly A. fumigatus, A. flavus group, A. terreus group

117.4 Mycotic mycetomas
Infection by various genera and species of Ascomycetes and Deuteromycetes, such as Acremonium [Cephalosporium] falciforme, Neotestudina rosatii, Madurella grisea, Madurella mycetomii, Pyrenochaeta romeroi, Zopfia [Leptosphaeria] senegalensis
Madura foot, mycotic
Maduromycosis, mycotic
> **EXCLUDES** actinomycotic mycetomas (039.0-039.9)

117.5 Cryptococcosis
Busse-Buschke's disease
European cryptococcosis
Infection by Cryptococcus neoformans
Pulmonary cryptococcosis
Systemic cryptococcosis
Torula

117.6 Allescheriosis [Petriellidosis]
Infections by Allescheria [Petriellidium] boydii [Monosporium apiospermum]
> **EXCLUDES** mycotic mycetoma (117.4)

117.7 Zygomycosis [Phycomycosis or Mucormycosis]
Infection by species of Absidia, Basidiobolus, Conidiobolus, Cunninghamella, Entomophthora, Mucor, Rhizopus, Saksenaea

117.8 Infection by dematiacious fungi, [Phaehyphomycosis]
Infection by dematiacious fungi, such as Cladosporium trichoides [bantianum], Dreschlera hawaiiensis, Phialophora gougerotii, Phialophora jeanselmi

117.9 Other and unspecified mycoses

118 Opportunistic mycoses
Infection of skin, subcutaneous tissues, and/or organs by a wide variety of fungi generally considered to be pathogenic to compromised hosts only (e.g., infection by species of Alternaria, Dreschlera, Fusarium)

HELMINTHIASES (120-129)

✓4th 120 Schistosomiasis [bilharziasis]
DEF: Infection caused by *Schistosoma*, a genus of flukes or trematode parasites.

120.0 Schistosoma haematobium
Vesical schistosomiasis NOS

120.1 Schistosoma mansoni
Intestinal schistosomiasis NOS

120.2 Schistosoma japonicum
Asiatic schistosomiasis NOS
Katayama disease or fever

INFECTIOUS AND PARASITIC DISEASES

120.3 **Cutaneous**
Cercarial dermatitis
Infection by cercariae of Schistosoma
Schistosome dermatitis
Swimmers' itch

120.8 **Other specified schistosomiasis**
Infection by Schistosoma:
  bovis
  intercalatum
  mattheii
  spindale
Schistosomiasis chestermani

120.9 **Schistosomiasis, unspecified**
Blood flukes NOS
Hemic distomiasis

✓4th 121 Other trematode infections

121.0 **Opisthorchiasis**
Infection by:
  cat liver fluke
  Opisthorchis (felineus) (tenuicollis) (viverrini)

121.1 **Clonorchiasis**
Biliary cirrhosis due to clonorchiasis
Chinese liver fluke disease
Hepatic distomiasis due to Clonorchis sinensis
Oriental liver fluke disease

121.2 **Paragonimiasis**
Infection by Paragonimus
Lung fluke disease (oriental)
Pulmonary distomiasis

121.3 **Fascioliasis**
Infection by Fasciola:
  gigantica
  hepatica
Liver flukes NOS
Sheep liver fluke infection

121.4 **Fasciolopsiasis**
Infection by Fasciolopsis (buski)
Intestinal distomiasis

121.5 **Metagonimiasis**
Infection by Metagonimus yokogawai

121.6 **Heterophyiasis**
Infection by:
  Heterophyes heterophyes
  Stellantchasmus falcatus

121.8 **Other specified trematode infections**
Infection by:
  Dicrocoelium dendriticum
  Echinostoma ilocanum
  Gastrodiscoides hominis

121.9 **Trematode infection, unspecified**
Distomiasis NOS
Fluke disease NOS

✓4th 122 Echinococcosis

INCLUDES   echinococciasis
hydatid disease
hydatidosis

DEF: Infection caused by larval forms of tapeworms of the genus *Echinococcus*.

- **122.0** Echinococcus granulosus infection of liver
- **122.1** Echinococcus granulosus infection of lung
- **122.2** Echinococcus granulosus infection of thyroid
- **122.3** Echinococcus granulosus infection, other
- **122.4** Echinococcus granulosus infection, unspecified
- **122.5** Echinococcus multilocularis infection of liver
- **122.6** Echinococcus multilocularis infection, other
- **122.7** Echinococcus multilocularis infection, unspecified
- **122.8** Echinococcosis, unspecified, of liver
- **122.9** Echinococcosis, other and unspecified

✓4th 123 Other cestode infection

- **123.0** Taenia solium infection, intestinal form
  Pork tapeworm (adult) (infection)
- **123.1** Cysticercosis
  Cysticerciasis
  Infection by Cysticercus cellulosae [larval form of Taenia solium]
- **123.2** Taenia saginata infection
  Beef tapeworm (infection)
  Infection by Taeniarhynchus saginatus
- **123.3** Taeniasis, unspecified
- **123.4** Diphyllobothriasis, intestinal
  Diphyllobothrium (adult) (latum) (pacificum) infection
  Fish tapeworm (infection)
- **123.5** Sparganosis [larval diphyllobothriasis]
  Infection by:
    Diphyllobothrium larvae
    Sparganum (mansoni) (proliferum)
    Spirometra larvae
- **123.6** Hymenolepiasis
  Dwarf tapeworm (infection)
  Hymenolepis (diminuta) (nana) infection
  Rat tapeworm (infection)
- **123.8** Other specified cestode infection
  Diplogonoporus (grandis)
  Dipylidium (caninum) } infection
  Dog tapeworm (infection)
- **123.9** Cestode infection, unspecified
  Tapeworm (infection) NOS

124 Trichinosis

Trichinella spiralis infection
Trichinellosis
Trichiniasis

DEF: Infection by *Trichinella spiralis*, the smallest of the parasitic nematodes.

INFECTIOUS AND PARASITIC DISEASES   125–127.1

√4th 125 Filarial infection and dracontiasis

    125.0 Bancroftian filariasis
        Chyluria
        Elephantiasis
        Infection   } due to Wuchereria bancrofti
        Lymphadenitis
        Lymphangitis

        Wuchereriasis

    125.1 Malayan filariasis
        Brugia filariasis
        Chyluria
        Elephantiasis
        Infection   } due to Brugia [Wuchereria] malayi
        Lymphadenitis
        Lymphangitis

    125.2 Loiasis
        Eyeworm disease of Africa   Loa loa infection

    125.3 Onchocerciasis
        Onchocerca volvulus infection
        Onchocercais

    125.4 Dipetalonemiasis
        Infection by:
            Acanthocheilonema perstans
            Dipetalonema perstans

    125.5 Mansonella ozzardi infection
        Filariasis ozzardi

    125.6 Other specified filariasis
        Dirofilaria infection
        Infection by:
            Acanthocheilonema streptocerca
            Dipetalonema streptocerca

    125.7 Dracontiasis
        Guinea-worm infection
        Infection by Dracunculus medinensis

    125.9 Unspecified filariasis

√4th 126 Ancylostomiasis and necatoriasis

        [INCLUDES]   cutaneous larva migrans due to Ancylostoma
                        hookworm (disease) (infection)
                        uncinariasis

    126.0 Ancylostoma duodenale
    126.1 Necator americanus
    126.2 Ancylostoma braziliense
    126.3 Ancylostoma ceylanicum
    126.8 Other specified Ancylostoma
    126.9 Ancylostomiasis and necatoriasis, unspecified
        Creeping eruption NOS
        Cutaneous larva migrans NOS

√4th 127 Other intestinal helminthiases

    127.0 Ascariasis
        Ascaridiasis
        Infection by Ascaris lumbricoides
        Roundworm infection

    127.1 Anisakiasis
        Infection by Anisakis larva

√4th / √5th   Additional Digit Required   Unspecified Code   Other Specified Code   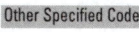 Manifestation Code

MSP   Medicare Secondary Payer   ▶◀ Revised Text   ● New Code   ▲ Revised Code Title

2002 Ingenix, Inc.   Volume 1 — 49

INFECTIOUS AND PARASITIC DISEASES

127.2 Strongyloidiasis
Infection by Strongyloides stercoralis
EXCLUDES trichostrongyliasis (127.6)

127.3 Trichuriasis
Infection by Trichuris trichiuria
Trichocephaliasis
Whipworm (disease) (infection)

127.4 Enterobiasis
Infection by Enterobius vermicularis
Oxyuriasis
Oxyuris vermicularis infection
Pinworm (disease) (infection)
Threadworm infection

127.5 Capillariasis
Infection by Capillaria philippinensis
EXCLUDES infection by Capillaria hepatica (128.8)

127.6 Trichostrongyliasis
Infection by Trichostrongylus species

127.7 Other specified intestinal helminthiasis
Infection by:
Oesophagostomum apiostomum and related species
Ternidens diminutus
other specified intestinal helminth
Physalopteriasis

127.8 Mixed intestinal helminthiasis
Infection by intestinal helminths classified to more than one of the categories 120.0-127.7
Mixed helminthiasis NOS

127.9 Intestinal helminthiasis, unspecified

✓4th **128 Other and unspecified helminthiases**

128.0 Toxocariasis
Larva migrans visceralis
Toxocara (canis) (cati) infection
Visceral larva migrans syndrome

128.1 Gnathostomiasis
Infection by Gnathostoma spinigerum and related species

128.8 Other specified helminthiasis
Infection by:
Angiostrongylus cantonensis
Capillaria hepatica
other specified helminth

128.9 Helminth infection, unspecified
Helminthiasis NOS
Worms NOS

129 Intestinal parasitism, unspecified

OTHER INFECTIOUS AND PARASITIC DISEASES (130–136)

✓4th **130 Toxoplasmosis**
INCLUDES   infection by toxoplasma gondii
toxoplasmosis (acquired)
EXCLUDES   congenital toxoplasmosis (771.2)

130.0 Meningoencephalitis due to toxoplasmosis
Encephalitis due to acquired toxoplasmosis

130.1 Conjunctivitis due to toxoplasmosis

130.2 Chorioretinitis due to toxoplasmosis
Focal retinochoroiditis due to acquired toxoplasmosis

130.3 Myocarditis due to toxoplasmosis

INFECTIOUS AND PARASITIC DISEASES   130.4–133.9

- **130.4** Pneumonitis due to toxoplasmosis
- **130.5** Hepatitis due to toxoplasmosis
- **130.7** Toxoplasmosis of other specified sites
- **130.8** Multisystemic disseminated toxoplasmosis
  - Toxoplasmosis of multiple sites
- **130.9** Toxoplasmosis, unspecified

√4th **131 Trichomoniasis**
  INCLUDES   infection due to Trichomonas (vaginalis)

  √5th **131.0 Urogenital trichomoniasis**
  - **131.00** Urogenital trichomoniasis, unspecified
    - Fluor (vaginalis) } trichomonal or due
    - Leukorrhea   } to Trichomonas
    - (vaginalis)   } (vaginalis)
    - DEF: *Trichomonas vaginalis* infection of reproductive and urinary organs, transmitted through coitus.
  - **131.01** Trichomonal vulvovaginitis ♀
    - Vaginitis, trichomonal or due to Trichomonas (vaginalis)
    - DEF: *Trichomonas vaginalis* infection of vulva and vagina; often asymptomatic, transmitted through coitus.
  - **131.02** Trichomonal urethritis
    - DEF: *Trichomonas vaginalis* infection of the urethra.
  - **131.03** Trichomonal prostatitis ♂
    - DEF: *Trichomonas vaginalis* infection of the prostate.
  - **131.09** Other

  131.8 Other specified sites
  EXCLUDES   intestinal (007.3)

  131.9 Trichomoniasis, unspecified

√4th **132 Pediculosis and phthirus infestation**
  - **132.0** Pediculus capitis [head louse]
  - **132.1** Pediculus corporis [body louse]
  - **132.2** Phthirus pubis [pubic louse]
    - Pediculus pubis
  - **132.3** Mixed infestation
    - Infestation classifiable to more than one of the categories 132.0-132.2
  - **132.9** Pediculosis, unspecified

√4th **133 Acariasis**
  - **133.0** Scabies
    - Infestation by Sarcoptes scabiei
    - Norwegian scabies
    - Sarcoptic itch
  - **133.8** Other acariasis
    - Chiggers
    - Infestation by:
      - Demodex folliculorum
      - Trombicula
  - **133.9** Acariasis, unspecified
    - Infestation by mites NOS

√4th √5th Additional Digit Required | Unspecified Code | Other Specified Code | Manifestation Code
MSP Medicare Secondary Payer | ▶◀ Revised Text | ● New Code | ▲ Revised Code Title

2002 Ingenix, Inc.   Volume 1 — 51

INFECTIOUS AND PARASITIC DISEASES

✓4th **134 Other infestation**

134.0 Myiasis
Infestation by:
Dermatobia (hominis)
fly larvae
Gasterophilus (intestinalis)
maggots
Oestrus ovis

134.1 Other arthropod infestation
Infestation by:
chigoe
sand flea
Tunga penetrans
Jigger disease
Tungiasis
Scarabiasis

134.2 Hirudiniasis
Hirudiniasis (external) (internal)
Leeches (aquatic) (land)

134.8 Other specified infestations

134.9 Infestation, unspecified
Infestation (skin) NOS
Skin parasites NOS

135 Sarcoidosis
Besnier-Boeck-Schaumann disease
Lupoid (miliary) of Boeck
Lupus pernio (Besnier)
Lymphogranulomatosis, benign (Schaumann's)
Sarcoid (any site):
  NOS
  Boeck
  Darier-Roussy
Uveoparotid fever

DEF: A chronic, granulomatous reticulosis (abnormal increase in cells), affecting any organ or tissue; acute form has high rate of remission; chronic form is progressive.

✓4th **136 Other and unspecified infectious and parasitic diseases**

136.0 Ainhum
Dactylolysis spontanea

DEF: A disease affecting the toes, especially the fifth digit, and sometimes the fingers, especially seen in black adult males; it is characterized by a linear constriction around the affected digit leading to spontaneous amputation of the distal part of the digit.

136.1 Behçet's syndrome

DEF: A chronic inflammatory disorder of unknown etiology involving the small blood vessels; it is characterized by recurrent aphthous ulceration of the oral and pharyngeal mucous membranes and the genitalia, skin lesions, severe uvetis, retinal vascularitis and optic atrophy.

136.2 Specific infections by free-living amebae
Meningoencephalitis due to Naegleria

136.3 Pneumocystosis
Pneumonia due to Pneumocystis carinii

DEF: *Pneumocystis carinii* fungus causing pneumonia in immunocompromised patients; a leading cause of death among AIDS patients.

136.4 Psorospermiasis

136.5 Sarcosporidiosis
Infection by Sarcocystis lindemanni

DEF: Sarcocystis infection causing muscle cysts of intestinal inflammation.

NEOPLASMS

136.8 Other specified infectious and parasitic diseases
Candiru infestation

136.9 Unspecified infectious and parasitic diseases
Infectious disease NOS
Parasitic disease NOS

LATE EFFECTS OF INFECTIOUS AND PARASITIC DISEASES (137-139)

✓4th **137 Late effects of tuberculosis**
Note: This category is to be used to indicate conditions classifiable to 010-018 as the cause of late effects, which are themselves classified elsewhere. The "late effects" include those specified as such, as sequelae, or as due to old or inactive tuberculosis, without evidence of active disease.

137.0 Late effects of respiratory or unspecified tuberculosis
137.1 Late effects of central nervous system tuberculosis
137.2 Late effects of genitourinary tuberculosis
137.3 Late effects of tuberculosis of bones and joints
137.4 Late effects of tuberculosis of other specified organs

138 Late effects of acute poliomyelitis
Note: This category is to be used to indicate conditions classifiable to 045 as the cause of late effects, which are themselves classified elsewhere. The "late effects" include conditions specified as such, or as sequelae, or as due to old or inactive poliomyelitis, without evidence of active disease.

✓4th **139 Late effects of other infectious and parasitic diseases**
Note: This category is to be used to indicate conditions classifiable to categories 001-009, 020-041, 046-136 as the cause of late effects, which are themselves classified elsewhere. The "late effects" include conditions specified as such; they also include sequela of diseases classifiable to the above categories if there is evidence that the disease itself is no longer present.

139.0 Late effects of viral encephalitis
Late effects of conditions classifiable to 049.8-049.9, 062-064

139.1 Late effects of trachoma
Late effects of conditions classifiable to 076

139.8 Late effects of other and unspecified infectious and parasitic diseases

2. NEOPLASMS (140-239)

Notes:

1. Content

This chapter contains the following broad groups:

140-195	Malignant neoplasms, stated or presumed to be primary, of specified sites, except of lymphatic and hematopoietic tissue
196-198	Malignant neoplasms, stated or presumed to be secondary, of specified sites
199	Malignant neoplasms, without specification of site
200-208	Malignant neoplasms, stated or presumed to be primary, of lymphatic and hematopoietic tissue
210-229	Benign neoplasms
230-234	Carcinoma in situ
235-238	Neoplasms of uncertain behavior [see Note at beginning of section]
239	Neoplasms of unspecified nature

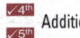 Additional Digit Required   Unspecified Code   Other Specified Code   Manifestation Code
MSP Medicare Secondary Payer   ▶◀ Revised Text   ● New Code   ▲ Revised Code Title

2002 Ingenix, Inc.   Volume 1 — 53

2. Functional activity

All neoplasms are classified in this chapter, whether or not functionally active. An additional code from Chapter 3 may be used to identify such functional activity associated with any neoplasm, e.g.:

> catecholamine-producing malignant pheochromocytoma of adrenal:
>> code 194.0, additional code 255.6
>
> basophil adenoma of pituitary with Cushing's syndrome:
>> code 227.3, additional code 255.0

3. Morphology [Histology]

For those wishing to identify the histological type of neoplasms, a comprehensive coded nomenclature, which comprises the morphology rubrics of the ICD-Oncology, is given in Appendix A.

4. Malignant neoplasms overlapping site boundaries

Categories 140-195 are for the classification of primary malignant neoplasms according to their point of origin. A malignant neoplasm that overlaps two or more subcategories within a three-digit rubric and whose point of origin cannot be determined should be classified to the subcategory .8 "Other."

For example, "carcinoma involving tip and ventral surface of tongue" should be assigned to 141.8. On the other hand, "carcinoma of tip of tongue, extending to involve the ventral surface" should be coded to 141.2, as the point of origin, the tip, is known. Three subcategories (149.8, 159.8, 165.8) have been provided for malignant neoplasms that overlap the boundaries of three-digit rubrics within certain systems.

Overlapping malignant neoplasms that cannot be classified as indicated above should be assigned to the appropriate subdivision of category 195 (Malignant neoplasm of other and ill-defined sites).

DEF: An abnormal growth, such as a tumor. Morphology determines behavior, i.e., whether it will remain intact (benign) or spread to adjacent tissue (malignant). The term mass is not synonymous with neoplasm, as it is often used to describe cysts and thickenings such as those occurring with hematoma or infection.

MALIGNANT NEOPLASM OF LIP, ORAL CAVITY, AND PHARYNX (140-149)

EXCLUDES carcinoma in situ (230.0)

✓4th **140 Malignant neoplasm of lip**

EXCLUDES skin of lip (173.0)

140.0 Upper lip, vermilion border
Upper lip: Upper lip:
  NOS   lipstick area
  external

140.1 Lower lip, vermilion border
Lower lip: Lower lip:
  NOS   lipstick area
  external

140.3 Upper lip, inner aspect
Upper lip: Upper lip:
  buccal aspect   mucosa
  frenulum   oral aspect

140.4 Lower lip, inner aspect
Lower lip: Lower lip:
  buccal aspect   mucosa
  frenulum   oral aspect

140.5 Lip, unspecified, inner aspect
Lip, not specified whether upper or lower:
  buccal aspect
  frenulum
  mucosa
  oral aspect

NEOPLASMS

140.6 Commissure of lip
Labial commissure

140.8 Other sites of lip
Malignant neoplasm of contiguous or overlapping sites of lip whose point of origin cannot be determined

140.9 Lip, unspecified, vermilion border
Lip, not specified as upper or lower:
NOS
external
lipstick area

√4ᵗʰ **141 Malignant neoplasm of tongue**

141.0 Base of tongue
Dorsal surface of base of tongue
Fixed part of tongue NOS

141.1 Dorsal surface of tongue
Anterior two-thirds of tongue, dorsal surface
Dorsal tongue NOS
Midline of tongue
EXCLUDES dorsal surface of base of tongue (141.0)

141.2 Tip and lateral border of tongue

141.3 Ventral surface of tongue
Anterior two-thirds of tongue, ventral surface
Frenulum linguae

141.4 Anterior two-thirds of tongue, part unspecified
Mobile part of tongue NOS

141.5 Junctional zone
Border of tongue at junction of fixed and mobile parts at insertion of anterior tonsillar pillar

141.6 Lingual tonsil

141.8 Other sites of tongue
Malignant neoplasm of contiguous or overlapping sites of tongue whose point of origin cannot be determined

141.9 Tongue, unspecified
Tongue NOS

√4ᵗʰ
√5ᵗʰ Additional Digit Required
MSP Medicare Secondary Payer

Unspecified Code
▶◀ Revised Text

Other Specified Code
● New Code

Manifestation Code
▲ Revised Code Title

2002 Ingenix, Inc.

Volume 1 — 55

Tongue

142 Malignant neoplasm of major salivary glands
INCLUDES salivary ducts
EXCLUDES malignant neoplasm of minor salivary glands:
  NOS (145.9)
  buccal mucosa (145.0)
  soft palate (145.3)
  tongue (141.0-141.9)
  tonsil, palatine (146.0)

- 142.0 Parotid gland
- 142.1 Submandibular gland
  Submaxillary gland
- 142.2 Sublingual gland
- 142.8 Other major salivary glands
  Malignant neoplasm of contiguous or overlapping sites of salivary glands and ducts whose point of origin cannot be determined
- 142.9 Salivary gland, unspecified
  Salivary gland (major) NOS

143 Malignant neoplasm of gum
INCLUDES alveolar (ridge) mucosa
  gingiva (alveolar) (marginal)
  interdental papillae
EXCLUDES malignant odontogenic neoplasms (170.0-170.1)

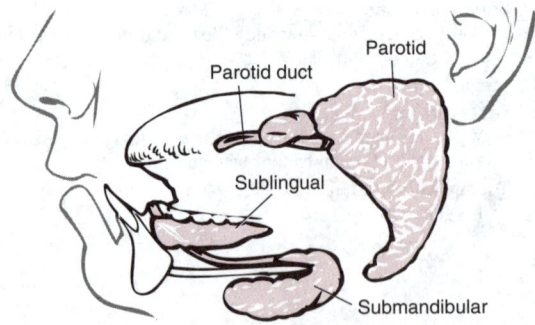

Main Salivary Glands

NEOPLASMS 143.0–145.9

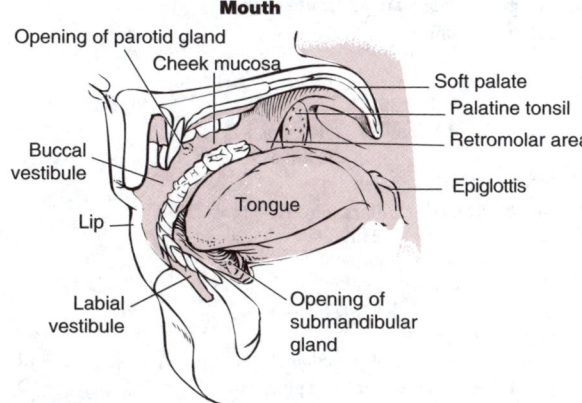

- **143.0** Upper gum
- **143.1** Lower gum
- **143.8** Other sites of gum
  Malignant neoplasm of contiguous or overlapping sites of gum whose point of origin cannot be determined
- **143.9** Gum, unspecified

√4th **144 Malignant neoplasm of floor of mouth**
- **144.0** Anterior portion
  Anterior to the premolar-canine junction
- **144.1** Lateral portion
- **144.8** Other sites of floor of mouth
  Malignant neoplasm of contiguous or overlapping sites of floor of mouth whose point of origin cannot be determined
- **144.9** Floor of mouth, part unspecified

√4th **145 Malignant neoplasm of other and unspecified parts of mouth**
  EXCLUDES   mucosa of lips (140.0-140.9)
- **145.0** Cheek mucosa
  Buccal mucosa
  Cheek, inner aspect
- **145.1** Vestibule of mouth
  Buccal sulcus (upper) (lower)
  Labial sulcus (upper) (lower)
- **145.2** Hard palate
- **145.3** Soft palate
  EXCLUDES   nasopharyngeal [posterior] [superior] surface of soft palate (147.3)
- **145.4** Uvula
- **145.5** Palate, unspecified
  Junction of hard and soft palate
  Roof of mouth
- **145.6** Retromolar area
- **145.8** Other specified parts of mouth
  Malignant neoplasm of contiguous or overlapping sites of mouth whose point of origin cannot be determined
- **145.9** Mouth, unspecified
  Buccal cavity NOS
  Minor salivary gland, unspecified site
  Oral cavity NOS

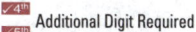

√4th √5th Additional Digit Required	Unspecified Code	Other Specified Code	Manifestation Code
MSP Medicare Secondary Payer	▶◀ Revised Text	● New Code	▲ Revised Code Title

2002 Ingenix, Inc.

NEOPLASMS

✓4ᵗʰ 146 Malignant neoplasm of oropharynx
- **146.0 Tonsil**
  - Tonsil: NOS
  - faucial
  - Tonsil: palatine
  - **EXCLUDES** lingual tonsil (141.6)
    pharyngeal tonsil (147.1)
- **146.1 Tonsillar fossa**
- **146.2 Tonsillar pillars (anterior) (posterior)**
  - Faucial pillar
  - Glossopalatine fold
  - Palatoglossal arch
  - Palatopharyngeal arch
- **146.3 Vallecula**
  - Anterior and medial surface of the pharyngoepiglottic fold
- **146.4 Anterior aspect of epiglottis**
  - Epiglottis, free border [margin]
  - Glossoepiglottic fold(s)
  - **EXCLUDES** epiglottis:
    NOS (161.1)
    suprahyoid portion (161.1)
- **146.5 Junctional region**
  - Junction of the free margin of the epiglottis, the aryepiglottic fold, and the pharyngoepiglottic fold
- **146.6 Lateral wall of oropharynx**
- **146.7 Posterior wall of oropharynx**
- **146.8 Other specified sites of oropharynx**
  - Branchial cleft
  - Malignant neoplasm of contiguous or overlapping sites of oropharynx whose point of origin cannot be determined
- **146.9 Oropharynx, unspecified**

✓4ᵗʰ 147 Malignant neoplasm of nasopharynx
- **147.0 Superior wall**
  - Roof of nasopharynx
- **147.1 Posterior wall**
  - Adenoid
  - Pharyngeal tonsil
- **147.2 Lateral wall**
  - Fossa of Rosenmüller
  - Opening of auditory tube
  - Pharyngeal recess

Nasopharynx

NEOPLASMS

147.3 **Anterior wall**
Floor of nasopharynx
Nasopharyngeal [posterior] [superior] surface of soft palate
Posterior margin of nasal septum and choanae

147.8 **Other specified sites of nasopharynx**
Malignant neoplasm of contiguous or overlapping sites of nasopharynx whose point of origin cannot be determined

147.9 **Nasopharynx, unspecified**
Nasopharyngeal wall NOS

√4th **148 Malignant neoplasm of hypopharynx**

148.0 Postcricoid region

148.1 Pyriform sinus
Pyriform fossa

148.2 Aryepiglottic fold, hypopharyngeal aspect
Aryepiglottic fold or interarytenoid fold:
  NOS
  marginal zone
  EXCLUDES aryepiglottic fold or interarytenoid fold, laryngeal aspect (161.1)

148.3 Posterior hypopharyngeal wall

148.8 **Other specified sites of hypopharynx**
Malignant neoplasm of contiguous or overlapping sites of hypopharynx whose point of origin cannot be determined

148.9 **Hypopharynx, unspecified**
Hypopharyngeal wall NOS
Hypopharynx NOS

√4th **149 Malignant neoplasm of other and ill-defined sites within the lip, oral cavity, and pharynx**

149.0 **Pharynx, unspecified**

149.1 Waldeyer's ring

149.8 **Other**
Malignant neoplasms of lip, oral cavity, and pharynx whose point of origin cannot be assigned to any one of the categories 140-148
  EXCLUDES "book leaf" neoplasm [ventral surface of tongue and floor of mouth] (145.8)

149.9 Ill-defined

Hypopharynx

√4th √5th Additional Digit Required   Unspecified Code   Other Specified Code   Manifestation Code
MSP Medicare Secondary Payer   ▶◀ Revised Text   ● New Code   ▲ Revised Code Title

2002 Ingenix, Inc.   Volume 1 — 59

Waldeyer's (Tonsillar) Ring

MALIGNANT NEOPLASM OF DIGESTIVE ORGANS AND PERITONEUM (150-159)

EXCLUDES carcinoma in situ (230.1-230.9)

√4th **150 Malignant neoplasm of esophagus**

- **150.0 Cervical esophagus**
- **150.1 Thoracic esophagus**
- **150.2 Abdominal esophagus**
  EXCLUDES adenocarcinoma (151.0)
  cardio-esophageal junction (151.0)
- **150.3 Upper third of esophagus**
  Proximal third of esophagus
- **150.4 Middle third of esophagus**
- **150.5 Lower third of esophagus**
  Distal third of esophagus
  EXCLUDES adenocarcinoma (151.0)
  cardio-esophageal junction (151.0)
- **150.8 Other specified part**
  Malignant neoplasm of contiguous or overlapping sites of esophagus whose point of origin cannot be determined
- **150.9 Esophagus, unspecified**

√4th **151 Malignant neoplasm of stomach**

- **151.0 Cardia**
  Cardiac orifice   Cardio-esophageal junction
  EXCLUDES squamous cell carcinoma (150.2, 150.5)
- **151.1 Pylorus**
  Prepylorus
  Pyloric canal
- **151.2 Pyloric antrum**
  Antrum of stomach NOS
- **151.3 Fundus of stomach**
- **151.4 Body of stomach**
- **151.5 Lesser curvature, unspecified**
  Lesser curvature, not classifiable to 151.1-151.4
- **151.6 Greater curvature, unspecified**
  Greater curvature, not classifiable to 151.0-151.4
- **151.8 Other specified sites of stomach**
  Anterior wall, not classifiable to 151.0-151.4
  Posterior wall, not classifiable to 151.0-151.4
  Malignant neoplasm of contiguous or overlapping sites of stomach whose point of origin cannot be determined

NEOPLASMS

151.9 **Stomach, unspecified**
Carcinoma ventriculi Gastric cancer

√4th **152 Malignant neoplasm of small intestine, including duodenum**
152.0 Duodenum
152.1 Jejunum
152.2 Ileum
  EXCLUDES ileocecal valve (153.4)
152.3 Meckel's diverticulum
152.8 **Other specified sites of small intestine**
Duodenojejunal junction
Malignant neoplasm of contiguous or overlapping sites of small intestine whose point of origin cannot be determined
152.9 **Small intestine, unspecified**

√4th **153 Malignant neoplasm of colon**
153.0 Hepatic flexure
153.1 Transverse colon
153.2 Descending colon
Left colon
153.3 Sigmoid colon
Sigmoid (flexure)
  EXCLUDES rectosigmoid junction (154.0)
153.4 Cecum
Ileocecal valve
153.5 Appendix
153.6 Ascending colon
Right colon
153.7 Splenic flexure
153.8 **Other specified sites of large intestine**
Malignant neoplasm of contiguous or overlapping sites of colon whose point of origin cannot be determined
  EXCLUDES ileocecal valve (153.4)
rectosigmoid junction (154.0)
153.9 **Colon, unspecified**
Large intestine NOS

√4th **154 Malignant neoplasm of rectum, rectosigmoid junction, and anus**
154.0 Rectosigmoid junction
Colon with rectum   Rectosigmoid (colon)

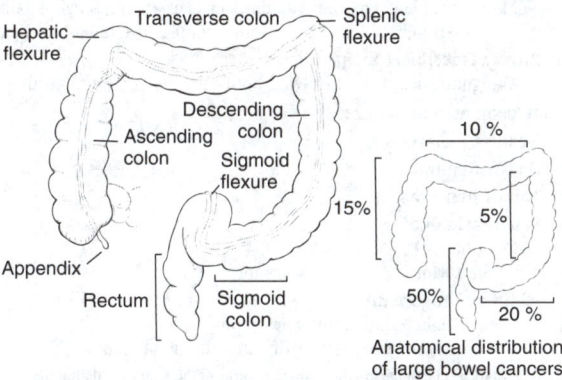

√4th √5th Additional Digit Required   Unspecified Code   Other Specified Code   Manifestation Code
MSP Medicare Secondary Payer   ▶◀ Revised Text   ● New Code   ▲ Revised Code Title

2002 Ingenix, Inc.

154.1–157.4 NEOPLASMS

- **154.1 Rectum**
  - Rectal ampulla
- **154.2 Anal canal**
  - Anal sphincter
  - **EXCLUDES** skin of anus (172.5, 173.5)
- **154.3 Anus, unspecified**
  - **EXCLUDES** anus:
    - margin (172.5, 173.5)
    - skin (172.5, 173.5)
    - perianal skin (172.5, 173.5)
- **154.8 Other**
  - Anorectum
  - Cloacogenic zone
  - Malignant neoplasm of contiguous or overlapping sites of rectum, rectosigmoid junction, and anus whose point of origin cannot be determined

✓4th 155 Malignant neoplasm of liver and intrahepatic bile ducts

- **155.0 Liver, primary**
  - Carcinoma:
    - hepatocellular
    - liver cell
  - Carcinoma:
    - liver, specified as primary
    - Hepatoblastoma
- **155.1 Intrahepatic bile ducts**
  - Canaliculi biliferi
  - Interlobular:
    - bile ducts
    - biliary canals
  - Intrahepatic:
    - biliary passages
    - canaliculi
    - gall duct
  - **EXCLUDES** hepatic duct (156.1)
- **155.2 Liver, not specified as primary or secondary**

✓4th 156 Malignant neoplasm of gallbladder and extrahepatic bile ducts

- **156.0 Gallbladder**
- **156.1 Extrahepatic bile ducts**
  - Biliary duct or passage NOS
  - Common bile duct
  - Cystic duct
  - Hepatic duct
  - Sphincter of Oddi
- **156.2 Ampulla of Vater**
  - DEF: Malignant neoplasm in the area of dilation at the juncture of the common bile and pancreatic ducts near the opening into the lumen of the duodenum.
- **156.8 Other specified sites of gallbladder and extrahepatic bile ducts**
  - Malignant neoplasm of contiguous or overlapping sites of gallbladder and extrahepatic bile ducts whose point of origin cannot be determined
- **156.9 Biliary tract, part unspecified**
  - Malignant neoplasm involving both intrahepatic and extrahepatic bile ducts

✓4th 157 Malignant neoplasm of pancreas

- **157.0 Head of pancreas**
- **157.1 Body of pancreas**
- **157.2 Tail of pancreas**
- **157.3 Pancreatic duct**
  - Duct of:
    - Santorini
  - Duct of:
    - Wirsung
- **157.4 Islets of Langerhans**
  - Islets of Langerhans, any part of pancreas
  - Use additional code to identify any functional activity
  - DEF: Malignant neoplasm within the structures of the pancreas that produce insulin, somatostatin and glucagon.

NEOPLASMS 157.8–159.8

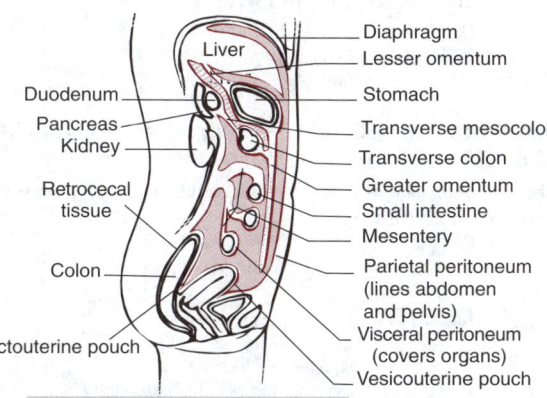

Retroperitoneum and Peritoneum

157.8 Other specified sites of pancreas
Ectopic pancreatic tissue
Malignant neoplasm of contiguous or overlapping sites of pancreas whose point of origin cannot be determined

157.9 Pancreas, part unspecified

158 Malignant neoplasm of retroperitoneum and peritoneum

158.0 Retroperitoneum
Periadrenal tissue   Perirenal tissue
Perinephric tissue   Retrocecal tissue

158.8 Specified parts of peritoneum
Cul-de-sac (of Douglas)
Mesentery
Mesocolon
Omentum
Peritoneum:
 parietal
 pelvic
Rectouterine pouch
Malignant neoplasm of contiguous or overlapping sites of retroperitoneum and peritoneum whose point of origin cannot be determined

158.9 Peritoneum, unspecified

159 Malignant neoplasm of other and ill-defined sites within the digestive organs and peritoneum

159.0 Intestinal tract, part unspecified
Intestine NOS

159.1 Spleen, not elsewhere classified
Angiosarcoma } of spleen
Fibrosarcoma

EXCLUDES Hodgkin's disease (201.0-201.9)
 lymphosarcoma (200.1)
 reticulosarcoma (200.0)

159.8 Other sites of digestive system and intra-abdominal organs
Malignant neoplasm of digestive organs and peritoneum whose point of origin cannot be assigned to any one of the categories 150-158

EXCLUDES anus and rectum (154.8)
 cardio-esophageal junction (151.0)
 colon and rectum (154.0)

159.9 Ill-defined
Alimentary canal or tract NOS
Gastrointestinal tract NOS
> **EXCLUDES** abdominal NOS (195.2)
> intra-abdominal NOS (195.2)

MALIGNANT NEOPLASM OF RESPIRATORY AND INTRATHORACIC ORGANS (160-165)
> **EXCLUDES** carcinoma in situ (231.0-231.9)

✓4th **160 Malignant neoplasm of nasal cavities, middle ear, and accessory sinuses**

160.0 Nasal cavities
Cartilage of nose   Septum of nose
Conchae, nasal   Vestibule of nose
Internal nose
> **EXCLUDES** nasal bone (170.0)
> nose NOS (195.0)
> olfactory bulb (192.0)
> posterior margin of septum and choanae (147.3)
> skin of nose (172.3, 173.3)
> turbinates (170.0)

160.1 Auditory tube, middle ear, and mastoid air cells
Antrum tympanicum   Tympanic cavity
Eustachian tube
> **EXCLUDES** auditory canal (external) (172.2, 173.2)
> bone of ear (meatus) (170.0)
> cartilage of ear (171.0)
> ear (external) (skin) (172.2, 173.2)

160.2 Maxillary sinus
Antrum (Highmore) (maxillary)

160.3 Ethmoidal sinus

160.4 Frontal sinus

160.5 Sphenoidal sinus

160.8 Other
Malignant neoplasm of contiguous or overlapping sites of nasal cavities, middle ear, and accessory sinuses whose point of origin cannot be determined

160.9 Accessory sinus, unspecified

✓4th **161 Malignant neoplasm of larynx**

161.0 Glottis
Intrinsic larynx   True vocal cord
Laryngeal commissure   Vocal cord NOS
  (anterior) (posterior)

161.1 Supraglottis
Aryepiglottic fold or interarytenoid fold, laryngeal aspect
Epiglottis (suprahyoid portion) NOS
Extrinsic larynx
False vocal cords
Posterior (laryngeal) surface of epiglottis
Ventricular bands
> **EXCLUDES** anterior aspect of epiglottis (146.4)
> aryepiglottic fold or interarytenoid fold:
>   NOS (148.2)
>   hypopharyngeal aspect (148.2)
>   marginal zone (148.2)

161.2 Subglottis

NEOPLASMS   161.3–165.9

- **161.3 Laryngeal cartilages**
  - Cartilage: arytenoid
  - Cartilage: cricoid
  - Cartilage: cuneiform
  - Cartilage: thyroid
- **161.8 Other specified sites of larynx**
  - Malignant neoplasm of contiguous or overlapping sites of larynx whose point of origin cannot be determined
- **161.9 Larynx, unspecified**

✓4th **162 Malignant neoplasm of trachea, bronchus, and lung**
- **162.0 Trachea**
  - Cartilage } of trachea
  - Mucosa
- **162.2 Main bronchus**
  - Carina
  - Hilus of lung
- **162.3 Upper lobe, bronchus or lung**
- **162.4 Middle lobe, bronchus or lung**
- **162.5 Lower lobe, bronchus or lung**
- **162.8 Other parts of bronchus or lung**
  - Malignant neoplasm of contiguous or overlapping sites of bronchus or lung whose point of origin cannot be determined
- **162.9 Bronchus and lung, unspecified**

✓4th **163 Malignant neoplasm of pleura**
- **163.0 Parietal pleura**
- **163.1 Visceral pleura**
- **163.8 Other specified sites of pleura**
  - Malignant neoplasm of contiguous or overlapping sites of pleura whose point of origin cannot be determined
- **163.9 Pleura, unspecified**

✓4th **164 Malignant neoplasm of thymus, heart, and mediastinum**
- **164.0 Thymus**
- **164.1 Heart**
  - Endocardium
  - Epicardium
  - Myocardium
  - Pericardium
  - **EXCLUDES** great vessels (171.4)
- **164.2 Anterior mediastinum**
- **164.3 Posterior mediastinum**
- **164.8 Other**
  - Malignant neoplasm of contiguous or overlapping sites of thymus, heart, and mediastinum whose point of origin cannot be determined
- **164.9 Mediastinum, part unspecified**

✓4th **165 Malignant neoplasm of other and ill-defined sites within the respiratory system and intrathoracic organs**
- **165.0 Upper respiratory tract, part unspecified**
- **165.8 Other**
  - Malignant neoplasm of respiratory and intrathoracic organs whose point of origin cannot be assigned to any one of the categories 160-164
- **165.9 Ill-defined sites within the respiratory system**
  - Respiratory tract NOS
  - **EXCLUDES** intrathoracic NOS (195.1)
  - thoracic NOS (195.1)

| ✓4th ✓5th Additional Digit Required | Unspecified Code | Other Specified Code | Manifestation Code |
| MSP Medicare Secondary Payer | ▶◀ Revised Text | ● New Code | ▲ Revised Code Title |

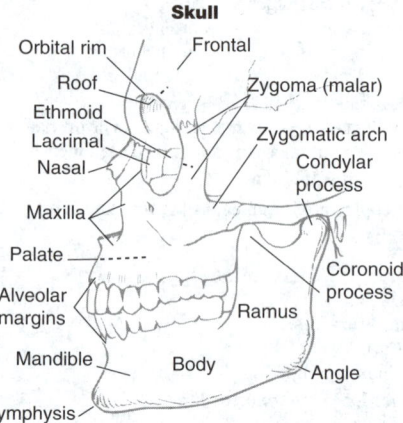

MALIGNANT NEOPLASM OF BONE, CONNECTIVE TISSUE, SKIN, AND BREAST (170-176)

EXCLUDES carcinoma in situ:
    breast (233.0)
    skin (232.0-232.9)

✓4th 170 Malignant neoplasm of bone and articular cartilage

INCLUDES cartilage (articular) (joint)
    periosteum

EXCLUDES bone marrow NOS (202.9)
    cartilage:
      ear (171.0)
      eyelid (171.0)
      larynx (161.3)
      nose (160.0)
    synovia (171.0-171.9)

170.0 Bones of skull and face, except mandible

Bone:
- ethmoid
- frontal
- malar
- nasal
- occipital
- orbital
- parietal

Bone:
- sphenoid
- temporal
- zygomatic
- Maxilla (superior)
- Turbinate
- Upper jaw bone
- Vomer

EXCLUDES carcinoma, any type except intraosseous or odontogenic:
    maxilla, maxillary (sinus) (160.2)
    upper jaw bone (143.0)
    jaw bone (lower) (170.1)

170.1 Mandible
Inferior maxilla
Jaw bone NOS
Lower jaw bone

EXCLUDES carcinoma, any type except intraosseous or odontogenic:
    jaw bone NOS (143.9)
    lower (143.1)
    upper jaw bone (170.0)

170.2 Vertebral column, excluding sacrum and coccyx
Spinal column   Vertebra
Spine

EXCLUDES sacrum and coccyx (170.6)

NEOPLASMS

170.3 **Ribs, sternum, and clavicle**
  Costal cartilage
  Costovertebral joint
  Xiphoid process

170.4 **Scapula and long bones of upper limb**
  Acromion
  Bones NOS of upper limb
  Humerus
  Radius
  Ulna

170.5 **Short bones of upper limb**
  Carpal
  Cuneiform, wrist
  Metacarpal
  Navicular, of hand
  Phalanges of hand
  Pisiform
  Scaphoid (of hand)
  Semilunar or lunate
  Trapezium
  Trapezoid
  Unciform

170.6 **Pelvic bones, sacrum, and coccyx**
  Coccygeal vertebra
  Ilium
  Ischium
  Pubic bone
  Sacral vertebra

170.7 **Long bones of lower limb**
  Bones NOS of lower limb
  Femur
  Fibula
  Tibia

170.8 **Short bones of lower limb**
  Astragalus [talus]
  Calcaneus
  Cuboid
  Cuneiform, ankle
  Metatarsal
  Navicular (of ankle)
  Patella
  Phalanges of foot
  Tarsal

170.9 **Bone and articular cartilage, site unspecified**

√4th **171** **Malignant neoplasm of connective and other soft tissue**

  INCLUDES
  blood vessel
  bursa
  fascia
  fat
  ligament, except uterine
  muscle
  peripheral, sympathetic, and parasympathetic nerves and ganglia
  synovia
  tendon (sheath)

  EXCLUDES
  cartilage (of):
    articular (170.0-170.9)
    larynx (161.3)
    nose (160.0)
  connective tissue:
    breast (174.0-175.9)
    internal organs—code to malignant neoplasm of the site [e.g., leiomyosarcoma of stomach, 151.9]
  heart (164.1)
  uterine ligament (183.4)

171.0 **Head, face, and neck**
  Cartilage of:
    ear
    eyelid

171.2 Upper limb, including shoulder
  Arm
  Finger
  Forearm
  Hand

171.3 Lower limb, including hip
  Foot
  Leg
  Popliteal space
  Thigh
  Toe

171.4 Thorax
  Axilla
  Diaphragm
  Great vessels
  EXCLUDES *heart (164.1)*
  mediastinum (164.2-164.9)
  thymus (164.0)

171.5 Abdomen
  Abdominal wall
  Hypochondrium
  EXCLUDES *peritoneum (158.8)*
  retroperitoneum (158.0)

171.6 Pelvis
  Buttock
  Groin
  Inguinal region
  Perineum
  EXCLUDES *pelvic peritoneum (158.8)*
  retroperitoneum (158.0)
  uterine ligament, any (183.3-183.5)

171.7 Trunk, unspecified
  Back NOS
  Flank NOS

171.8 Other specified sites of connective and other soft tissue
  Malignant neoplasm of contiguous or overlapping sites of connective tissue whose point of origin cannot be determined

171.9 Connective and other soft tissue, site unspecified

✓4th **172 Malignant melanoma of skin**
  INCLUDES melanocarcinoma
  melanoma (skin) NOS
  EXCLUDES *skin of genital organs (184.0-184.9, 187.1-187.9)*
  sites other than skin—code to malignant neoplasm of the site

DEF: Malignant neoplasm of melanocytes; most common in skin, may involve oral cavity, esophagus, anal canal, vagina, leptomeninges or conjunctiva.

172.0 Lip
  EXCLUDES *vermilion border of lip (140.0-140.1, 140.9)*

172.1 Eyelid, including canthus

172.2 Ear and external auditory canal
  Auricle (ear)
  Auricular canal, external
  External [acoustic] meatus
  Pinna

172.3 Other and unspecified parts of face
  Cheek (external)
  Chin
  Eyebrow
  Forehead
  Nose, external
  Temple

172.4 Scalp and neck

NEOPLASMS

172.5 **Trunk, except scrotum**
    Axilla   Perianal skin
    Breast   Perineum
    Buttock   Umbilicus
    Groin

    EXCLUDES anal canal (154.2)
                          anus NOS (154.3)
                          scrotum (187.7)

172.6 **Upper limb, including shoulder**
    Arm   Forearm
    Finger   Hand

172.7 **Lower limb, including hip**
    Ankle   Leg
    Foot   Popliteal area
    Heel   Thigh
    Knee   Toe

172.8 **Other specified sites of skin**
    Malignant melanoma of contiguous or overlapping sites of skin whose point of origin cannot be determined

172.9 **Melanoma of skin, site unspecified**

 173 Other malignant neoplasm of skin

    INCLUDES malignant neoplasm of:
                         sebaceous glands
                         sudoriferous, sudoriparous glands
                         sweat glands

    EXCLUDES Kaposi's sarcoma (176.0-176.9)
                          malignant melanoma of skin (172.0-172.9)
                          skin of genital organs (184.0-184.9, 187.1-187.9)

173.0 **Skin of lip**
    EXCLUDES vermilion border of lip (140.0-140.1, 140.9)

173.1 **Eyelid, including canthus**
    EXCLUDES cartilage of eyelid (171.0)

173.2 **Skin of ear and external auditory canal**
    Auricle (ear)
    Auricular canal, external
    External meatus
    Pinna
    EXCLUDES cartilage of ear (171.0)

173.3 **Skin of other and unspecified parts of face**
    Cheek, external   Forehead
    Chin   Nose, external
    Eyebrow   Temple

173.4 **Scalp and skin of neck**

173.5 **Skin of trunk, except scrotum**
    Axillary fold   Skin of:
    Perianal skin   buttock
    Skin of: chest wall
        abdominal wall   groin
        anus   perineum
        back   Umbilicus
        breast

    EXCLUDES anal canal (154.2)
                          anus NOS (154.3)
                          skin of scrotum (187.7)

✓4th / ✓5th Additional Digit Required	Unspecified Code	Other Specified Code	Manifestation Code
MSP Medicare Secondary Payer	▶◀ Revised Text	● New Code	▲ Revised Code Title

2002 Ingenix, Inc.

NEOPLASMS

173.6 Skin of upper limb, including shoulder
- Arm
- Finger
- Forearm
- Hand

173.7 Skin of lower limb, including hip
- Ankle
- Foot
- Heel
- Knee
- Leg
- Popliteal area
- Thigh
- Toe

173.8 Other specified sites of skin
Malignant neoplasm of contiguous or overlapping sites of skin whose point of origin cannot be determined

173.9 Skin, site unspecified

✓4th **174 Malignant neoplasm of female breast**

INCLUDES
- breast (female)
- connective tissue
- soft parts
- Paget's disease of:
  - breast
  - nipple

EXCLUDES skin of breast (172.5, 173.5)

174.0 Nipple and areola ♀
174.1 Central portion ♀
174.2 Upper-inner quadrant ♀
174.3 Lower-inner quadrant ♀
174.4 Upper-outer quadrant ♀
174.5 Lower-outer quadrant ♀
174.6 Axillary tail ♀
174.8 Other specified sites of female breast
- Ectopic sites
- Inner breast
- Lower breast
- Malignant neoplasm of contiguous or overlapping sites of breast whose point of origin cannot be determined
- Midline of breast
- Outer breast
- Upper breast

174.9 Breast (female), unspecified ♀

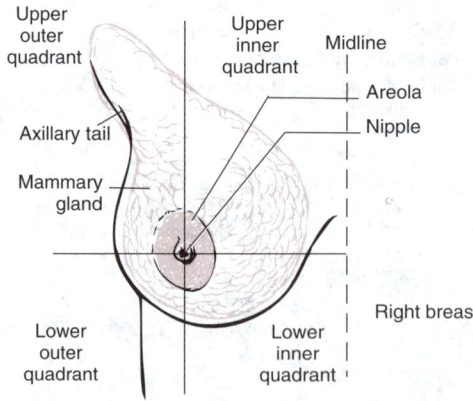

Female Breast

N Newborn Age: 0   P Pediatric Age: 0-17   M Maternity Age: 12-55   A Adult Age: 15-124

NEOPLASMS

√4ʰ 175 Malignant neoplasm of male breast
  EXCLUDES skin of breast (172.5, 173.5)
  - **175.0 Nipple and areola** ♂
  - **175.9 Other and unspecified sites of male breast** ♂
    Ectopic breast tissue, male

√4ʰ 176 Kaposi's sarcoma
  - **176.0 Skin**
  - **176.1 Soft tissue**
    INCLUDES
    blood vessel
    connective tissue
    fascia
    ligament
    lymphatic(s) NEC
    muscle
    EXCLUDES lymph glands and nodes (176.5)
  - **176.2 Palate**
  - **176.3 Gastrointestinal sites**
  - **176.4 Lung**
  - **176.5 Lymph nodes**
  - **176.8 Other specified sites**
    INCLUDES oral cavity NEC
  - **176.9 Unspecified**
    Viscera NOS

MALIGNANT NEOPLASM OF GENITOURINARY ORGANS (179-189)
  EXCLUDES carcinoma in situ (233.1-233.9)

179 Malignant neoplasm of uterus, part unspecified ♀

√4ʰ 180 Malignant neoplasm of cervix uteri
  √5ʰ
  INCLUDES invasive malignancy [carcinoma]
  EXCLUDES carcinoma in situ (233.1)
  - **180.0 Endocervix** ♀
    Cervical canal NOS   Endocervical gland
    Endocervical canal
  - **180.1 Exocervix** ♀
  - **180.8 Other specified sites of cervix** ♀
    Cervical stump
    Squamocolumnar junction of cervix
    Malignant neoplasm of contiguous or overlapping sites of cervix uteri whose point of origin cannot be determined
  - **180.9 Cervix uteri, unspecified** ♀

181 Malignant neoplasm of placenta ♀
    Choriocarcinoma NOS
    Chorioepithelioma NOS
    EXCLUDES chorioadenoma (destruens) (236.1)
    hydatidiform mole (630)
      malignant (236.1)
    invasive mole (236.1)
    male choriocarcinoma NOS (186.0-186.9)

182–186.9 NEOPLASMS

✓4th 182 Malignant neoplasm of body of uterus
  EXCLUDES carcinoma in situ (233.2)

- **182.0 Corpus uteri, except isthmus** ♀
  - Cornu
  - Endometrium
  - Fundus
  - Myometrium
- **182.1 Isthmus** ♀
  - Lower uterine segment
- **182.8 Other specified sites of body of uterus** ♀
  - Malignant neoplasm of contiguous or overlapping sites of body of uterus whose point of origin cannot be determined
  - *EXCLUDES* uterus NOS (179)

✓4th 183 Malignant neoplasm of ovary and other uterine adnexa
  EXCLUDES Douglas' cul-de-sac (158.8)

- **183.0 Ovary** ♀
  - Use additional code to identify any functional activity
- **183.2 Fallopian tube** ♀
  - Oviduct
  - Uterine tube
- **183.3 Broad ligament** ♀
  - Mesovarium
  - Parovarian region
- **183.4 Parametrium** ♀
  - Uterine ligament NOS
  - Uterosacral ligament
- **183.5 Round ligament** ♀
- **183.8 Other specified sites of uterine adnexa** ♀
  - Tubo-ovarian
  - Utero-ovarian
  - Malignant neoplasm of contiguous or overlapping sites of ovary and other uterine adnexa whose point of origin cannot be determined
- **183.9 Uterine adnexa, unspecified** ♀

✓4th 184 Malignant neoplasm of other and unspecified female genital organs
  EXCLUDES carcinoma in situ (233.3)

- **184.0 Vagina** ♀
  - Gartner's duct
  - Vaginal vault
- **184.1 Labia majora** ♀
  - Greater vestibular [Bartholin's] gland
- **184.2 Labia minora** ♀
- **184.3 Clitoris** ♀
- **184.4 Vulva, unspecified** ♀
  - External female genitalia NOS
  - Pudendum
- **184.8 Other specified sites of female genital organs** ♀
  - Malignant neoplasm of contiguous or overlapping sites of female genital organs whose point of origin cannot be determined
- **184.9 Female genital organ, site unspecified** ♀
  - Female genitourinary tract NOS

185 Malignant neoplasm of prostate ♂
  EXCLUDES seminal vesicles (187.8)

✓4th 186 Malignant neoplasm of testis
  Use additional code to identify any functional activity

- **186.0 Undescended testis** ♂
  - Ectopic testis
  - Retained testis
- **186.9 Other and unspecified testis** ♂
  - Testis:
    - NOS
    - descended
  - Testis:
    - scrotal

NEOPLASMS 187–189.9

✓4ᵗʰ 187 Malignant neoplasm of penis and other male genital organs
- **187.1 Prepuce** ♂
  Foreskin
- **187.2 Glans penis** ♂
- **187.3 Body of penis** ♂
  Corpus cavernosum
- **187.4 Penis, part unspecified** ♂
  Skin of penis NOS
- **187.5 Epididymis** ♂
- **187.6 Spermatic cord** ♂
  Vas deferens
- **187.7 Scrotum** ♂
  Skin of scrotum
- **187.8 Other specified sites of male genital organs** ♂
  Seminal vesicle
  Tunica vaginalis
  Malignant neoplasm of contiguous or overlapping sites of penis and other male genital organs whose point of origin cannot be determined
- **187.9 Male genital organ, site unspecified** ♂
  Male genital organ or tract NOS

✓4ᵗʰ 188 Malignant neoplasm of bladder
  EXCLUDES carcinoma in situ (233.7)
- **188.0 Trigone of urinary bladder**
- **188.1 Dome of urinary bladder**
- **188.2 Lateral wall of urinary bladder**
- **188.3 Anterior wall of urinary bladder**
- **188.4 Posterior wall of urinary bladder**
- **188.5 Bladder neck**
  Internal urethral orifice
- **188.6 Ureteric orifice**
- **188.7 Urachus**
- **188.8 Other specified sites of bladder**
  Malignant neoplasm of contiguous or overlapping sites of bladder whose point of origin cannot be determined
- **188.9 Bladder, part unspecified**
  Bladder wall NOS

✓4ᵗʰ 189 Malignant neoplasm of kidney and other and unspecified urinary organs
- **189.0 Kidney, except pelvis**
  Kidney NOS   Kidney parenchyma
- **189.1 Renal pelvis**
  Renal calyces
  Ureteropelvic junction
- **189.2 Ureter**
  EXCLUDES ureteric orifice of bladder (188.6)
- **189.3 Urethra**
  EXCLUDES urethral orifice of bladder (188.5)
- **189.4 Paraurethral glands**
- **189.8 Other specified sites of urinary organs**
  Malignant neoplasm of contiguous or overlapping sites of kidney and other urinary organs whose point of origin cannot be determined
- **189.9 Urinary organ, site unspecified**
  Urinary system NOS

✓4ᵗʰ Additional Digit Required | Unspecified Code | Other Specified Code | Manifestation Code
✓5ᵗʰ
MSP Medicare Secondary Payer | ▶◀ Revised Text | ● New Code | ▲ Revised Code Title

MALIGNANT NEOPLASM OF OTHER AND UNSPECIFIED SITES (190-199)

EXCLUDES carcinoma in situ (234.0-234.9)

✓4th 190 Malignant neoplasm of eye

EXCLUDES carcinoma in situ (234.0)
eyelid (skin) (172.1, 173.1)
  cartilage (171.0)
optic nerve (192.0)
orbital bone (170.0)

190.0 Eyeball, except conjunctiva, cornea, retina, and choroid
Ciliary body   Sclera
Crystalline lens   Uveal tract
Iris

190.1 Orbit
Connective tissue of orbit Retrobulbar
Extraocular muscle

EXCLUDES bone of orbit (170.0)

190.2 Lacrimal gland

190.3 Conjunctiva

190.4 Cornea

190.5 Retina

190.6 Choroid

190.7 Lacrimal duct
Lacrimal sac
Nasolacrimal duct

190.8 Other specified sites of eye
Malignant neoplasm of contiguous or overlapping sites of eye whose point of origin cannot be determined

190.9 Eye, part unspecified

✓4th 191 Malignant neoplasm of brain

EXCLUDES cranial nerves (192.0)
retrobulbar area (190.1)

191.0 Cerebrum, except lobes and ventricles
Basal ganglia   Globus pallidus
Cerebral cortex   Hypothalamus
Corpus striatum   Thalamus

191.1 Frontal lobe

191.2 Temporal lobe
Hippocampus   Uncus

191.3 Parietal lobe

191.4 Occipital lobe

191.5 Ventricles
Choroid plexus   Floor of ventricle

191.6 Cerebellum NOS
Cerebellopontine angle

191.7 Brain stem
Cerebral peduncle   Midbrain
Medulla oblongata   Pons

191.8 Other parts of brain
Corpus callosum
Tapetum
Malignant neoplasm of contiguous or overlapping sites of brain whose point of origin cannot be determined

191.9 Brain, unspecified
Cranial fossa NOS

NEOPLASMS

✓4th 192 Malignant neoplasm of other and unspecified parts of nervous system
> EXCLUDES peripheral, sympathetic, and parasympathetic nerves and ganglia (171.0-171.9)

192.0 Cranial nerves
Olfactory bulb

192.1 Cerebral meninges
Dura (mater)   Meninges NOS
Falx (cerebelli) (cerebri)   Tentorium

192.2 Spinal cord
Cauda equina

192.3 Spinal meninges

192.8 Other specified sites of nervous system
Malignant neoplasm of contiguous or overlapping sites of other parts of nervous system whose point of origin cannot be determined

192.9 Nervous system, part unspecified
Nervous system (central) NOS
> EXCLUDES meninges NOS (192.1)

193 Malignant neoplasm of thyroid gland
Sipple's syndrome
Thyroglossal duct
Use additional code to identify any functional activity

✓4th 194 Malignant neoplasm of other endocrine glands and related structures
Use additional code to identify any functional activity
> EXCLUDES islets of Langerhans (157.4)
> ovary (183.0)
> testis (186.0-186.9)
> thymus (164.0)

194.0 Adrenal gland
Adrenal cortex
Adrenal medulla
Suprarenal gland

194.1 Parathyroid gland

194.3 Pituitary gland and craniopharyngeal duct
Craniobuccal pouch
Hypophysis
Rathke's pouch
Sella turcica

194.4 Pineal gland

194.5 **Carotid body**
194.6 **Aortic body and other paraganglia**
Coccygeal body   Para-aortic body
Glomus jugulare
194.8 **Other**
Pluriglandular involvement NOS
Note: If the sites of multiple involvements are known, they should be coded separately.
194.9 **Endocrine gland, site unspecified**

✓4th 195 **Malignant neoplasm of other and ill-defined sites**
   INCLUDES   malignant neoplasms of contiguous sites, not elsewhere classified, whose point of origin cannot be determined
   EXCLUDES   malignant neoplasm:
      lymphatic and hematopoietic tissue (200.0-208.9)
      secondary sites (196.0-198.8)
      unspecified site (199.0-199.1)

195.0 **Head, face, and neck**
Cheek NOS
Jaw NOS
Nose NOS
Supraclavicular region NOS

195.1 **Thorax**
Axilla
Chest (wall) NOS
Intrathoracic NOS

195.2 **Abdomen**
Intra-abdominal NOS

195.3 **Pelvis**
Groin
Inguinal region NOS
Presacral region
Sacrococcygeal region
Sites overlapping systems within pelvis, as:
   rectovaginal (septum)
   rectovesical (septum)

195.4 **Upper limb**
195.5 **Lower limb**
195.8 **Other specified sites**
Back NOS   Trunk NOS
Flank NOS

✓4th 196 **Secondary and unspecified malignant neoplasm of lymph nodes**
   EXCLUDES   any malignant neoplasm of lymph nodes, specified as primary (200.0-202.9)
      Hodgkin's disease (201.0-201.9)
      lymphosarcoma (200.1)
      reticulosarcoma (200.0)
      other forms of lymphoma (202.0-202.9)

196.0 **Lymph nodes of head, face, and neck**
Cervical   Scalene
Cervicofacial   Supraclavicular

196.1 **Intrathoracic lymph nodes**
Bronchopulmonary   Mediastinal
Intercostal   Tracheobronchial

196.2 **Intra-abdominal lymph nodes**
Intestinal   Retroperitoneal
Mesenteric

NEOPLASMS

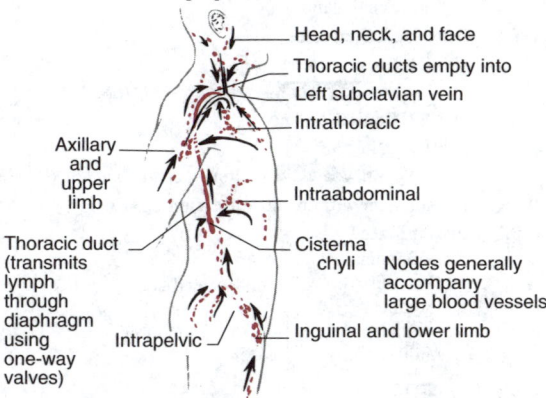

Lymph Nodes

- Head, neck, and face
- Thoracic ducts empty into
- Left subclavian vein
- Intrathoracic
- Axillary and upper limb
- Intraabdominal
- Thoracic duct (transmits lymph through diaphragm using one-way valves)
- Cisterna chyli
- Nodes generally accompany large blood vessels
- Intrapelvic
- Inguinal and lower limb

196.3 Lymph nodes of axilla and upper limb
  Brachial   Infraclavicular
  Epitrochlear   Pectoral

196.5 Lymph nodes of inguinal region and lower limb
  Femoral   Popliteal
  Groin   Tibial

196.6 Intrapelvic lymph nodes
  Hypogastric   Obturator
  Iliac   Parametrial

196.8 Lymph nodes of multiple sites

196.9 Site unspecified
  Lymph nodes NOS

✓4th **197 Secondary malignant neoplasm of respiratory and digestive systems**
  EXCLUDES lymph node metastasis (196.0-196.9)

  197.0 Lung
    Bronchus
  197.1 Mediastinum
  197.2 Pleura
  197.3 Other respiratory organs
    Trachea
  197.4 Small intestine, including duodenum
  197.5 Large intestine and rectum
  197.6 Retroperitoneum and peritoneum
  197.7 Liver, specified as secondary
  197.8 Other digestive organs and spleen

✓4th **198 Secondary malignant neoplasm of other specified sites**
  EXCLUDES lymph node metastasis (196.0-196.9)

  198.0 Kidney
  198.1 Other urinary organs
  198.2 Skin
    Skin of breast
  198.3 Brain and spinal cord
  198.4 Other parts of nervous system
    Meninges (cerebral) (spinal)
  198.5 Bone and bone marrow
  198.6 Ovary   ♀

 Additional Digit Required | Unspecified Code | Other Specified Code | Manifestation Code
MSP Medicare Secondary Payer | ▶◀ Revised Text | ● New Code | ▲ Revised Code Title

198.7 **Adrenal gland**
Suprarenal gland

√5th 198.8 **Other specified sites**
198.81 Breast
EXCLUDES *skin of breast (198.2)*
198.82 Genital organs
198.89 Other
EXCLUDES *retroperitoneal lymph nodes (196.2)*

√4th 199 **Malignant neoplasm without specification of site**
199.0 **Disseminated**
Carcinomatosis
Generalized: } unspecified site
  cancer   (primary)
  malignancy   (secondary)
Multiple cancer

199.1 **Other**
Cancer } unspecified site
Carcinoma   (primary)
Malignancy   (secondary)

MALIGNANT NEOPLASM OF LYMPHATIC AND HEMATOPOIETIC TISSUE (200-208)

EXCLUDES *secondary neoplasm of:*
  bone marrow (198.5)
  spleen (197.8)
secondary and unspecified neoplasm of lymph nodes (196.0-196.9)

The following fifth-digit subclassification is for use with categories 200-202:
0 unspecified site, extranodal and solid organ sites
1 lymph nodes of head, face, and neck
2 intrathoracic lymph nodes
3 intra-abdominal lymph nodes
4 lymph nodes of axilla and upper limb
5 lymph nodes of inguinal region and lower limb
6 intrapelvic lymph nodes
7 spleen
8 lymph nodes of multiple sites

√4th 200 **Lymphosarcoma and reticulosarcoma**
§ √5th 200.0 **Reticulosarcoma**
Lymphoma (malignant):
  histiocytic (diffuse):
    nodular
    pleomorphic cell type
    reticulum cell type
Reticulum cell sarcoma:
  NOS
  pleomorphic cell type

DEF: Malignant lymphoma of primarily histolytic cells; commonly originates in reticuloendothelium of lymph nodes.

§ Requires fifth-digit. See beginning of section 200-208 for codes and definitions.

NEOPLASMS 200.1–201.9

§ ✓5ᵗʰ 200.1 Lymphosarcoma
  Lymphoblastoma (diffuse)
  Lymphoma (malignant):
    lymphoblastic (diffuse)
    lymphocytic (cell type) (diffuse)
    lymphosarcoma type
  Lymphosarcoma:
    NOS
    diffuse NOS
    lymphoblastic (diffuse)
    lymphocytic (diffuse)
    prolymphocytic
  EXCLUDES *lymphosarcoma:*
    follicular or nodular (202.0)
    mixed cell type (200.8)
    lymphosarcoma cell leukemia (207.8)
  DEF: Malignant lymphoma created from anaplastic lymphoid cells resembling lymphocytes or lymphoblasts.

§ ✓5ᵗʰ 200.2 Burkitt's tumor or lymphoma
  Malignant lymphoma, Burkitt's type
  DEF: Large osteolytic lesion most common in jaw or as abdominal mass; usually found in central Africa but reported elsewhere.

§ ✓5ᵗʰ 200.8 Other named variants
  Lymphoma (malignant):
    lymphoplasmacytoid type
    mixed lymphocytic-histiocytic (diffuse)
  Lymphosarcoma, mixed cell type (diffuse)
  Reticulolymphosarcoma (diffuse)

✓4ᵗʰ 201 Hodgkin's disease
✓5ᵗʰ
  DEF: Painless, progressive enlargement of lymph nodes, spleen and general lymph tissue; symptoms include anorexia, lassitude, weight loss, fever, pruritis, night sweats, anemia.

§ ✓5ᵗʰ 201.0 Hodgkin's paragranuloma
§ ✓5ᵗʰ 201.1 Hodgkin's granuloma
§ ✓5ᵗʰ 201.2 Hodgkin's sarcoma
§ ✓5ᵗʰ 201.4 Lymphocytic-histiocytic predominance
§ ✓5ᵗʰ 201.5 Nodular sclerosis
  Hodgkin's disease, nodular sclerosis:
    NOS
    cellular phase
§ ✓5ᵗʰ 201.6 Mixed cellularity
§ ✓5ᵗʰ 201.7 Lymphocytic depletion
  Hodgkin's disease, lymphocytic depletion:
    NOS
    diffuse fibrosis
    reticular type
§ ✓5ᵗʰ 201.9 Hodgkin's disease, unspecified
  Hodgkin's: Malignant:
    disease NOS   lymphogranuloma
    lymphoma NOS   lymphogranulomatosis

---

§ Requires fifth-digit. See beginning of section 200–208 for codes and definitions.

202 Other malignant neoplasms of lymphoid and histiocytic tissue

202.0 Nodular lymphoma
Brill-Symmers disease
Lymphoma:
    follicular (giant)
    lymphocytic, nodular
Lymphosarcoma:
    follicular (giant)
    nodular
Reticulosarcoma, follicular or nodular

DEF: Lymphomatous cells clustered into nodules within the lymph node; usually occurs in older adults and may involve all nodes and possibly extranodal sites.

202.1 Mycosis fungoides
DEF: Type of cutaneous T-cell lymphoma; may evolve into generalized lymphoma; formerly thought to be of fungoid origin.

202.2 Sézary's disease
DEF: Type of cutaneous T-cell lymphoma with erythroderma, intense pruritus, peripheral lymphadenopathy, abnormal hyperchromatic mononuclear cells in skin, lymph nodes and peripheral blood.

202.3 Malignant histiocytosis
Histiocytic medullary reticulosis
Malignant:
    reticuloendotheliosis
    reticulosis

202.4 Leukemic reticuloendotheliosis
Hairy-cell leukemia

DEF: Chronic leukemia with large, mononuclear cells with "hairy" appearance in marrow, spleen, liver, blood.

202.5 Letterer-Siwe disease
Acute:
    differentiated progressive histiocytosis
    histiocytosis X (progressive)
    infantile reticuloendotheliosis
    reticulosis of infancy

EXCLUDES   Hand-Schüller-Christian disease (277.8)
                   histiocytosis (acute) (chronic) (277.8)
                   histiocytosis X (chronic) (277.8)

DEF: A recessive reticuloendotheliosis of early childhood, with a hemorrhagic tendency, eczema-like skin eruption, hepato-splenomegaly, including lymph node enlargement, and progressive anemia; it is often a fatal disease with no established cause.

202.6 Malignant mast cell tumors
Malignant: Mast cell sarcoma
    mastocytoma   Systemic tissue mast
    mastocytosis   cell disease

EXCLUDES   mast cell leukemia (207.8)

202.8 Other lymphomas
Lymphoma (malignant):
    NOS
    diffuse

EXCLUDES   benign lymphoma (229.0)

202.9 Other and unspecified malignant neoplasms of lymphoid and histiocytic tissue
Malignant neoplasm of bone marrow NOS

---

§ Requires fifth-digit. See beginning of section 200–208 for codes and definitions.

NEOPLASMS

✓4ᵗʰ 203 Multiple myeloma and immunoproliferative neoplasms

The following fifth-digit subclassification is for use with category 203:
0 without mention of remission
1 in remission

✓5ᵗʰ 203.0 Multiple myeloma
Kahler's disease   Myelomatosis
EXCLUDES solitary myeloma (238.6)

✓5ᵗʰ 203.1 Plasma cell leukemia
Plasmacytic leukemia

✓5ᵗʰ 203.8 Other immunoproliferative neoplasms

✓4ᵗʰ 204 Lymphoid leukemia
INCLUDES leukemia:
lymphatic
lymphoblastic
lymphocytic
lymphogenous

The following fifth-digit subclassification is for use with category 204:
0 without mention of remission
1 in remission

✓5ᵗʰ 204.0 Acute
EXCLUDES acute exacerbation of chronic lymphoid leukemia (204.1)

✓5ᵗʰ 204.1 Chronic

✓5ᵗʰ 204.2 Subacute

✓5ᵗʰ 204.8 Other lymphoid leukemia
Aleukemic leukemia: Aleukemic leukemia:
  lymphatic   lymphoid
  lymphocytic

✓5ᵗʰ 204.9 Unspecified lymphoid leukemia

✓4ᵗʰ 205 Myeloid leukemia
INCLUDES leukemia:
granulocytic
myeloblastic
myelocytic
myelogenous
myelomonocytic
myelosclerotic
myelosis

The following fifth-digit subclassification is for use with category 205:
0 without mention of remission
1 in remission

✓5ᵗʰ 205.0 Acute
Acute promyelocytic leukemia
EXCLUDES acute exacerbation of chronic myeloid leukemia (205.1)

✓5ᵗʰ 205.1 Chronic
Eosinophilic leukemia
Neutrophilic leukemia

✓5ᵗʰ 205.2 Subacute

✓4ᵗʰ / ✓5ᵗʰ Additional Digit Required   Unspecified Code   Other Specified Code   Manifestation Code
MSP Medicare Secondary Payer   ▶◀ Revised Text   ● New Code   ▲ Revised Code Title

§ ✓5ᵗʰ **205.3 Myeloid sarcoma**
Chloroma
Granulocytic sarcoma

§ ✓5ᵗʰ **205.8 Other myeloid leukemia**
Aleukemic leukemia:
  granulocytic
  myelogenous
  myeloid
Aleukemic myelosis

§ ✓5ᵗʰ **205.9 Unspecified myeloid leukemia**

✓4ᵗʰ **206 Monocytic leukemia**
  INCLUDES leukemia:
    histiocytic
    monoblastic
    monocytoid

The following fifth-digit subclassification is for use with category 206:
  0 without mention of remission
  1 in remission

✓5ᵗʰ **206.0 Acute**
  EXCLUDES acute exacerbation of chronic monocytic leukemia (206.1)

✓5ᵗʰ **206.1 Chronic**

✓5ᵗʰ **206.2 Subacute**

✓5ᵗʰ **206.8 Other monocytic leukemia**
Aleukemic:
  monocytic leukemia
  monocytoid leukemia

✓5ᵗʰ **206.9 Unspecified monocytic leukemia**

✓4ᵗʰ **207 Other specified leukemia**
  EXCLUDES leukemic reticuloendotheliosis (202.4)
    plasma cell leukemia (203.1)

The following fifth-digit subclassification is for use with category 207:
  0 without mention of remission
  1 in remission

✓5ᵗʰ **207.0 Acute erythremia and erythroleukemia**
Acute erythremic myelosis   Erythremic myelosis
Di Guglielmo's disease

DEF: Erythremia: polycythemia vera.

DEF: Erythroleukemia: a malignant blood dyscrasia (a myeloproliferative disorder).

✓5ᵗʰ **207.1 Chronic erythremia**
Heilmeyer-Schöner disease

✓5ᵗʰ **207.2 Megakaryocytic leukemia**
Megakaryocytic myelosis Thrombocytic leukemia

✓5ᵗʰ **207.8 Other specified leukemia**
Lymphosarcoma cell leukemia

✓4ᵗʰ **208 Leukemia of unspecified cell type**

The following fifth-digit subclassification is for use with category 208:
  0 without mention of remission
  1 in remission

---

§ Requires fifth-digit. See beginning of category 205 for codes and definitions.

N Newborn Age: 0   **P** Pediatric Age: 0-17   **M** Maternity Age: 12-55   **A** Adult Age: 15-124

NEOPLASMS

✓5th 208.0 Acute
Acute leukemia NOS   Stem cell leukemia
Blast cell leukemia
EXCLUDES acute exacerbation of chronic unspecified leukemia (208.1)

✓5th 208.1 Chronic
Chronic leukemia NOS

✓5th 208.2 Subacute
Subacute leukemia NOS

✓5th 208.8 Other leukemia of unspecified cell type

✓5th 208.9 Unspecified leukemia
Leukemia NOS

BENIGN NEOPLASMS (210-229)

✓4th 210 Benign neoplasm of lip, oral cavity, and pharynx
EXCLUDES cyst (of):
jaw (526.0-526.2, 526.89)
oral soft tissue (528.4)
radicular (522.8)

210.0 Lip
Frenulum labii
Lip (inner aspect) (mucosa) (vermilion border)
EXCLUDES labial commissure (210.4)
skin of lip (216.0)

210.1 Tongue
Lingual tonsil

210.2 Major salivary glands
Gland:
 parotid
 sublingual
 submandibular
EXCLUDES benign neoplasms of minor salivary glands:
NOS (210.4)
buccal mucosa (210.4)
lips (210.0)
palate (hard) (soft) (210.4)
tongue (210.1)
tonsil, palatine (210.5)

210.3 Floor of mouth

210.4 Other and unspecified parts of mouth
Gingiva   Oral mucosa
Gum (upper) (lower) Palate (hard) (soft)
Labial commissure   Uvula
Oral cavity NOS
EXCLUDES benign odontogenic neoplasms of bone (213.0-213.1)
developmental odontogenic cysts (526.0)
mucosa of lips (210.0)
nasopharyngeal [posterior] [superior] surface of soft palate (210.7)

210.5 Tonsil
Tonsil (faucial) (palatine)
EXCLUDES lingual tonsil (210.1)
pharyngeal tonsil (210.7)
tonsillar:
 fossa (210.6)
 pillars (210.6)

 Medicare Secondary Payer

210.6 Other parts of oropharynx
- Branchial cleft or vestiges
- Epiglottis, anterior aspect
- Fauces NOS
- Mesopharynx NOS
- Tonsillar:
  - fossa
  - pillars
- Vallecula

EXCLUDES epiglottis:
- NOS(212.1)
- suprahyoid portion (212.1)

210.7 Nasopharynx
- Adenoid tissue
- Lymphadenoid tissue
- Pharyngeal tonsil
- Posterior nasal septum

210.8 Hypopharynx
- Arytenoid fold
- Laryngopharynx
- Postcricoidregion
- Pyriform fossa

210.9 Pharynx, unspecified
- Throat NOS

✓4th 211 Benign neoplasm of other parts of digestive system

211.0 Esophagus

211.1 Stomach
- Body
- Cardia } of stomach
- Fundus
- Cardiac orifice
- Pylorus

211.2 Duodenum, jejunum, and ileum
- Small intestine NOS

EXCLUDES
- ampulla of Vater (211.5)
- ileocecal valve (211.3)

211.3 Colon
- Appendix
- Cecum
- Ileocecal valve
- Large intestine NOS

EXCLUDES rectosigmoid junction (211.4)

211.4 Rectum and anal canal
- Anal canal or sphincter
- Anus NOS
- Rectosigmoid junction

EXCLUDES anus:
- margin (216.5)
- skin (216.5)
- perianal skin (216.5)

211.5 Liver and biliary passages
- Ampulla of Vater
- Common bile duct
- Cystic duct
- Gallbladder
- Hepatic duct
- Sphincter of Oddi

211.6 Pancreas, except islets of Langerhans

211.7 Islets of Langerhans
- Islet cell tumor
- Use additional code to identify any functional activity

211.8 Retroperitoneum and peritoneum
- Mesentery
- Mesocolon
- Omentum
- Retroperitoneal tissue

211.9 Other and unspecified site
- Alimentary tract NOS
- Digestive system NOS
- Gastrointestinal tract NOS
- Intestinal tract NOS
- Intestine NOS
- Spleen, not elsewhere classified

NEOPLASMS

✓4th **212 Benign neoplasm of respiratory and intrathoracic organs**

212.0 Nasal cavities, middle ear, and accessory sinuses

Cartilage of nose
Eustachian tube
Nares
Septum of nose
Sinus
 ethomoidal
 frontal
 maxillary
 sphenoidal

EXCLUDES auditory canal (external) (216.2)
 bone of:
  ear (213.0)
  nose [turbinates] (213.0)
 cartilage of ear (215.0)
 ear (external) (skin) (216.2)
 nose NOS (229.8)
  skin (216.3)
 olfactory bulb (225.1)
 polyp of:
  accessory sinus (471.8)
  ear (385.30-385.35)
  nasal cavity (471.0)
 posterior margin of septum and choanae (210.7)

212.1 Larynx

Cartilage:
 arytenoid
 cricoid
 cuneiform
 thyroid
Epiglottis (suprahyoid portion) NOS
Glottis
Vocal cords (false) (true)

EXCLUDES epiglottis, anterior aspect (210.6)
 polyp of vocal cord or larynx (478.4)

212.2 Trachea

212.3 Bronchus and lung

Carina   Hilus of lung

212.4 Pleura

212.5 Mediastinum

212.6 Thymus

212.7 Heart

EXCLUDES great vessels (215.4)

212.8 Other specified sites

212.9 Site unspecified

Respiratory organ NOS
Upper respiratory tract NOS

EXCLUDES intrathoracic NOS (229.8)
 thoracic NOS (229.8)

✓4th **213 Benign neoplasm of bone and articular cartilage**

INCLUDES cartilage (articular) (joint)
 periosteum

EXCLUDES cartilage of:
  ear (215.0)
  eyelid (215.0)
  larynx (212.1)
  nose (212.0)
 exostosis NOS (726.91)
 synovia (215.0-215.9)

 Additional Digit Required   Unspecified Code   Other Specified Code   Manifestation Code
 Medicare Secondary Payer   ▶◀ Revised Text   ● New Code   ▲ Revised Code Title

2002 Ingenix, Inc.

213.0 Bones of skull and face
 EXCLUDES   lower jaw bone (213.1)
213.1 Lower jaw bone
213.2 Vertebral column, excluding sacrum and coccyx
213.3 Ribs, sternum, and clavicle
213.4 Scapula and long bones of upper limb
213.5 Short bones of upper limb
213.6 Pelvic bones, sacrum, and coccyx
213.7 Long bones of lower limb
213.8 Short bones of lower limb
213.9 Bone and articular cartilage, site unspecified

✓4th **214 Lipoma**
 INCLUDES   angiolipoma
fibrolipoma
hibernoma
lipoma (fetal) (infiltrating) (intramuscular)
myelolipoma
myxolipoma

DEF: Benign tumor frequently composed of mature fat cells; may occasionally be composed of fetal fat cells.

214.0 Skin and subcutaneous tissue of face
214.1 Other skin and subcutaneous tissue
214.2 Intrathoracic organs
214.3 Intra-abdominal organs
214.4 Spermatic cord ♂
214.8 Other specified sites
214.9 Lipoma, unspecified site

✓4th **215 Other benign neoplasm of connective and other soft tissue**
 INCLUDES   blood vessel
bursa
fascia
ligament
muscle
peripheral, sympathetic, and parasympathetic nerves and ganglia
synovia
tendon (sheath)
 EXCLUDES   cartilage:
   articular (213.0-213.9)
   larynx (212.1)
   nose (212.0)
connective tissue of:
   breast (217)
   internal organ, except lipoma and hemangioma—code to benign neoplasm of the site
lipoma (214.0-214.9)

215.0 Head, face, and neck
215.2 Upper limb, including shoulder
215.3 Lower limb, including hip
215.4 Thorax
 EXCLUDES   heart (212.7)
mediastinum (212.5)
thymus (212.6)
215.5 Abdomen
Abdominal wall   Hypochondrium

NEOPLASMS

215.6 Pelvis
- Buttock
- Groin
- Inguinal region
- Perineum

EXCLUDES uterine:
leiomyoma (218.0-218.9)
ligament, any (221.0)

215.7 Trunk, unspecified
- Back NOS
- Flank NOS

215.8 Other specified sites

215.9 Site unspecified

4th 216 Benign neoplasm of skin

INCLUDES
- blue nevus
- dermatofibroma
- hydrocystoma
- pigmented nevus
- syringoadenoma
- syringoma

EXCLUDES skin of genital organs (221.0-222.9)

216.0 Skin of lip

EXCLUDES vermilion border of lip (210.0)

216.1 Eyelid, including canthus

EXCLUDES cartilage of eyelid (215.0)

216.2 Ear and external auditory canal
- Auricle (ear)
- Auricular canal, external
- External meatus
- Pinna

EXCLUDES cartilage of ear (215.0)

216.3 Skin of other and unspecified parts of face
- Cheek, external
- Eyebrow
- Nose, external
- Temple

216.4 Scalp and skin of neck

216.5 Skin of trunk, except scrotum
- Axillary fold
- Perianal skin
- Skin of:
  - abdominal wall
  - anus
  - back
  - breast
- Skin of:
  - buttock
  - chest wall
  - groin
  - perineum
  - Umbilicus

EXCLUDES anal canal (211.4)
anus NOS (211.4)
skin of scrotum (222.4)

216.6 Skin of upper limb, including shoulder

216.7 Skin of lower limb, including hip

216.8 Other specified sites of skin

216.9 Skin, site unspecified

217 Benign neoplasm of breast

Breast (male) (female):
- connective tissue
- glandular tissue

Breast (male) (female):
- soft parts

EXCLUDES adenofibrosis (610.2)
benign cyst of breast (610.0)
fibrocystic disease (610.1)
skin of breast (216.5)

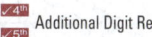 Additional Digit Required
MSP Medicare Secondary Payer
 Unspecified Code
▶◀ Revised Text
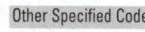 Other Specified Code
● New Code
Manifestation Code
▲ Revised Code Title

2002 Ingenix, Inc.

NEOPLASMS

✓4th 218 Uterine leiomyoma
  INCLUDES fibroid (bleeding) (uterine)
    uterine:
     fibromyoma
     myoma

DEF: Benign tumor primarily derived from uterine smooth muscle tissue; may contain fibrous, fatty, or epithelial tissue; also called uterine fibroid or myoma.

 218.0 Submucous leiomyoma of uterus ♀
 218.1 Intramural leiomyoma of uterus ♀
    Interstitial leiomyoma of uterus
 218.2 Subserous leiomyoma of uterus ♀
 218.9 Leiomyoma of uterus, unspecified ♀

✓4th 219 Other benign neoplasm of uterus
 219.0 Cervix uteri ♀
 219.1 Corpus uteri ♀
    Endometrium
    Fundus
    Myometrium
 219.8 Other specified parts of uterus ♀
 219.9 Uterus, part unspecified ♀

220 Benign neoplasm of ovary ♀
 Use additional code to identify any functional activity (256.0-256.1)
  EXCLUDES cyst:
    corpus albicans (620.2)
    corpus luteum (620.1)
    endometrial (617.1)
    follicular (atretic) (620.0)
    graafian follicle (620.0)
    ovarian NOS (620.2)
    retention (620.2)

✓4th 221 Benign neoplasm of other female genital organs
  INCLUDES adenomatous polyp
    benign teratoma
  EXCLUDES cyst:
    epoophoron (752.11)
    fimbrial (752.11)
    Gartner's duct (752.11)
    parovarian (752.11)

 221.0 Fallopian tube and uterine ligaments ♀
    Oviduct
    Parametruim
    Uterine ligament (broad) (round) (uterosacral)
    Uterine tube
 221.1 Vagina ♀
 221.2 Vulva ♀
    Clitoris
    External female genitalia NOS
    Greater vestibular [Bartholin's] gland
    Labia (majora) (minora)
    Pudendum
    EXCLUDES Bartholin's (duct) (gland) cyst (616.2)
 221.8 Other specified sites of female genital organs ♀
 221.9 Female genital organ, site unspecified ♀
    Female genitourinary tract NOS

NEOPLASMS

✓4th 222 Benign neoplasm of male genital organs
    222.0 Testis ♂
        Use additional code to identify any functional activity
    222.1 Penis ♂
        Corpus cavernosum
        Glans penis
        Prepuce
    222.2 Prostate ♂
        EXCLUDES adenomatous hyperplasia of prostate (600.2)
                         prostatic:
                                adenoma (600.2)
                                enlargement (600.0)
                                hypertrophy (600.0)
    222.3 Epididymis ♂
    222.4 Scrotum ♂
        Skin of scrotum
    222.8 Other specified sites of male genital organs ♂
        Seminal vesicle
        Spermatic cord
    222.9 Male genital organ, site unspecified ♂
        Male genitourinary tract NOS

✓4th 223 Benign neoplasm of kidney and other urinary organs
    223.0 Kidney, except pelvis
        Kidney NOS
        EXCLUDES renal:
                            calyces (223.1)
                            pelvis (223.1)
    223.1 Renal pelvis
    223.2 Ureter
        EXCLUDES ureteric orifice of bladder (223.3)
    223.3 Bladder
    ✓5th 223.8 Other specified sites of urinary organs
        223.81 Urethra
            EXCLUDES urethral orifice of bladder (223.3)
        223.89 Other
            Paraurethral glands
    223.9 Urinary organ, site unspecified
        Urinary system NOS

✓4th 224 Benign neoplasm of eye
    EXCLUDES cartilage of eyelid (215.0)
                    eyelid (skin) (216.1)
                  optic nerve (225.1)
                  orbital bone (213.0)
    224.0 Eyeball, except conjunctiva, cornea, retina, and choroid
        Ciliary body   Sclera
        Iris   Uveal tract
    224.1 Orbit
        EXCLUDES bone of orbit (213.0)
    224.2 Lacrimal gland
    224.3 Conjunctiva
    224.4 Cornea
    224.5 Retina
        EXCLUDES hemangioma of retina (228.03)

✓4th / ✓5th Additional Digit Required   Unspecified Code   Other Specified Code   Manifestation Code
MSP Medicare Secondary Payer   Revised Text   New Code   Revised Code Title

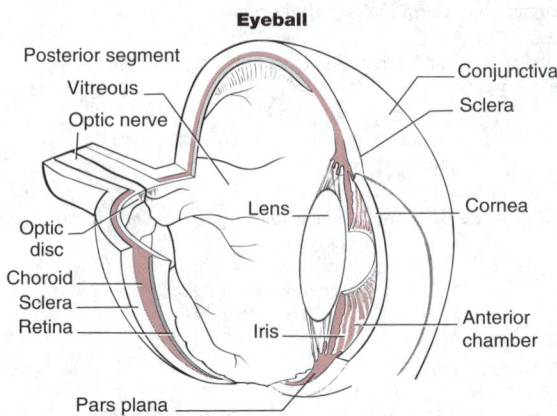

Eyeball

- 224.6 **Choroid**
- 224.7 **Lacrimal duct**
  - Lacrimal sac
  - Nasolacrimal duct
- 224.8 **Other specified parts of eye**
- 224.9 **Eye, part unspecified**

✓4th 225 **Benign neoplasm of brain and other parts of nervous system**

EXCLUDES hemangioma (228.02)
  neurofibromatosis (237.7)
  peripheral, sympathetic, and parasympathetic nerves and ganglia (215.0-215.9)
  retrobulbar (224.1)

- 225.0 **Brain**
- 225.1 **Cranial nerves**
- 225.2 **Cerebral meninges**
  - Meninges NOS
  - Meningioma (cerebral)
- 225.3 **Spinal cord**
  - Cauda equina
- 225.4 **Spinal meninges**
  - Spinal meningioma
- 225.8 **Other specified sites of nervous system**
- 225.9 **Nervous system, part unspecified**
  - Nervous system (central) NOS
  - EXCLUDES meninges NOS (225.2)

226 **Benign neoplasm of thyroid glands**
  Use additional code to identify any functional activity

✓4th 227 **Benign neoplasm of other endocrine glands and related structures**
  Use additional code to identify any functional activity
  EXCLUDES ovary (220)
    pancreas (211.6)
    testis (222.0)

- 227.0 **Adrenal gland**
  - Suprarenal gland
- 227.1 **Parathyroid gland**
- 227.3 **Pituitary gland and craniopharyngeal duct (pouch)**
  - Craniobuccal pouch
  - Rathke's pouch
  - Hypophysis
  - Sella turcica
- 227.4 **Pineal gland**
  - Pineal body
- 227.5 **Carotid body**

NEOPLASMS

227.6 Aortic body and other paraganglia
  Coccygeal body   Para-aortic body
  Glomus jugulare

227.8 Other

227.9 Endocrine gland, site unspecified

√4th **228 Hemangioma and lymphangioma, any site**
  INCLUDES angioma (benign) (cavernous) (congenital) NOS
    cavernous nevus
    glomus tumor
    hemangioma (benign) (congenital)
  EXCLUDES benign neoplasm of spleen, except hemangioma and lymphangioma (211.9)
    glomus jugulare (227.6)
    nevus:
      NOS (216.0-216.9)
      blue or pigmented (216.0-216.9)
      vascular (757.32)

√5th **228.0 Hemangioma, any site**
  DEF: A common benign tumor usually occurring in infancy; composed of newly formed blood vessels due to malformation of angioblastic tissue.

  228.00 Of unspecified site
  228.01 Of skin and subcutaneous tissue
  228.02 Of intracranial structures
  228.03 Of retina
  228.04 Of intra-abdominal structures
    Peritoneum
    Retroperitoneal tissue
  228.09 Of other sites
    Systemic angiomatosis

228.1 Lymphangioma, any site
  Congenital lymphangioma
  Lymphatic nevus

√4th **229 Benign neoplasm of other and unspecified sites**

229.0 Lymph nodes
  EXCLUDES lymphangioma (228.1)

229.8 Other specified sites
  Intrathoracic NOS   Thoracic NOS

229.9 Site unspecified

CARCINOMA IN SITU (230-234)

INCLUDES Bowen's disease
  erythroplasia
  Queyrat's erythroplasia

EXCLUDES leukoplakia—see Alphabetic Index

DEF: A neoplastic type; with tumor cells confined to epithelium of origin; without further invasion.

230 Carcinoma in situ of digestive organs

230.0 Lip, oral cavity, and pharynx
Gingiva
Hypopharynx
Mouth [any part]
Nasopharynx
Oropharynx
Salivary gland or duct
Tongue

EXCLUDES aryepiglottic fold or interarytenoid fold, laryngeal aspect (231.0)
epiglottis:
NOS (231.0)
suprahyoid portion (231.0)
skin of lip (232.0)

230.1 Esophagus

230.2 Stomach
Body
Cardia } of stomach
Fundus
Cardiac orifice
Pylorus

230.3 Colon
Appendix
Cecum
Ileocecal valve
Large intestine NOS

EXCLUDES rectosigmoid junction (230.4)

230.4 Rectum
Rectosigmoid junction

230.5 Anal canal
Anal sphincter

230.6 Anus, unspecified
EXCLUDES anus:
margin (232.5)
skin (232.5)
perianal skin (232.5)

230.7 Other and unspecified parts of intestine
Duodenum
Ileum
Jejunum
Small intestine NOS

EXCLUDES ampulla of Vater (230.8)

230.8 Liver and biliary system
Ampulla of Vater
Common bile duct
Cystic duct
Gallbladder
Hepatic duct
Sphincter of Oddi

230.9 Other and unspecified digestive organs
Digestive organ NOS
Gastrointestinal tract NOS
Pancreas
Spleen

231 Carcinoma in situ of respiratory system

231.0 Larynx
Cartilage:
  arytenoid
  cricoid
  cuneiform
  thyroid
Epiglottis:
  NOS
  posterior surface
  suprahyoid portion
Vocal cords (false) (true)

EXCLUDES aryepiglottic fold or interarytenoid fold:
NOS (230.0)
hypopharyngeal aspect (230.0)
marginal zone (230.0)

231.1 Trachea

NEOPLASMS

231.2 **Bronchus and lung**
Carina
Hilus of lung

231.8 **Other specified parts of respiratory system**
Accessory sinuses   Nasal cavities
Middle ear   Pleura
> EXCLUDES ear (external) (skin) (232.2)
>   nose NOS (234.8)
>   skin (232.3)

231.9 **Respiratory system, part unspecified**
Respiratory organ NOS

4th 232 Carcinoma in situ of skin
> INCLUDES pigment cells

232.0 **Skin of lip**
> EXCLUDES vermilion border of lip (230.0)

232.1 Eyelid, including canthus

232.2 Ear and external auditory canal

232.3 **Skin of other and unspecified parts of face**

232.4 Scalp and skin of neck

232.5 Skin of trunk, except scrotum
Anus, margin   Skin of:
Axillary fold   breast
Perianal skin   buttock
Skin of: chest wall
  abdominal wall   groin
  anus   perineum
  back   Umbilicus
> EXCLUDES anal canal (230.5)
>   anus NOS (230.6)
>   skin of genital organs (233.3, 233.5-233.6)

232.6 Skin of upper limb, including shoulder

232.7 Skin of lower limb, including hip

232.8 **Other specified sites of skin**

232.9 **Skin, site unspecified**

4th 233 Carcinoma in situ of breast and genitourinary system

233.0 **Breast**
> EXCLUDES Paget's disease (174.0-174.9)
>   skin of breast (232.5)

233.1 Cervix uteri

233.2 **Other and unspecified parts of uterus**

233.3 **Other and unspecified female genital organs**

233.4 Prostate

233.5 Penis

233.6 **Other and unspecified male genital organs**

233.7 Bladder

233.9 **Other and unspecified urinary organs**

4th 234 Carcinoma in situ of other and unspecified sites

234.0 **Eye**
> EXCLUDES cartilage of eyelid (234.8)
>   eyelid (skin) (232.1)
>   optic nerve (234.8)
>   orbital bone (234.8)

234.8 Other specified sites
Endocrine gland [any]

234.9 Site unspecified
Carcinoma in situ NOS

NEOPLASMS OF UNCERTAIN BEHAVIOR (235-238)

Note: Categories 235–238 classify by site certain histomorphologically well-defined neoplasms, the subsequent behavior of which cannot be predicted from the present appearance.

✓4ᵗʰ **235 Neoplasm of uncertain behavior of digestive and respiratory systems**

235.0 Major salivary glands
Gland:
  parotid
  sublingual
Gland:
  submandibular

EXCLUDES minor salivary glands (235.1)

235.1 Lip, oral cavity, and pharynx
Gingiva
Hypopharynx
Minor salivary glands
Mouth
Nasopharynx
Oropharynx
Tongue

EXCLUDES aryepiglottic fold or interarytenoid fold, laryngeal aspect (235.6)
epiglottis:
  NOS (235.6)
  suprahyoid portion (235.6)
skin of lip (238.2)

235.2 Stomach, intestines, and rectum

235.3 Liver and biliary passages
Ampulla of Vater
Bile ducts [any]
Gallbladder
Liver

235.4 Retroperitoneum and peritoneum

235.5 Other and unspecified digestive organs
Anal:
  canal
  sphincter
Anus NOS
Esophagus
Pancreas
Spleen

EXCLUDES anus:
  margin (238.2)
  skin (238.2)
perianal skin (238.2)

235.6 Larynx

EXCLUDES aryepiglottic fold or interarytenoid fold:
  NOS (235.1)
  hypopharyngeal aspect (235.1)
  marginal zone (235.1)

235.7 Trachea, bronchus, and lung

235.8 Pleura, thymus, and mediastinum

NEOPLASMS

235.9 Other and unspecified respiratory organs
Accessory sinuses
Middle ear
Nasal cavities
Respiratory organ NOS
EXCLUDES ear (external) (skin) (238.2)
nose (238.8)
skin (238.2)

√4th **236** Neoplasm of uncertain behavior of genitourinary organs
236.0 Uterus ♀
236.1 Placenta ♀
Chorioadenoma (destruens)
Invasive mole
Malignant hydatid(iform) mole
236.2 Ovary ♀
Use additional code to identify any functional activity
236.3 Other and unspecified female genital organs ♀
236.4 Testis ♂
Use additional code to identify any functional activity
236.5 Prostate ♂
236.6 Other and unspecified male genital organs ♂
236.7 Bladder
√5th **236.9** Other and unspecified urinary organs
236.90 Urinary organ, unspecified
236.91 Kidney and ureter
236.99 Other

√4th **237** Neoplasm of uncertain behavior of endocrine glands and nervous system
237.0 Pituitary gland and craniopharyngeal duct
Use additional code to identify any functional activity
237.1 Pineal gland
237.2 Adrenal gland
Suprarenal gland
Use additional code to identify any functional activity
237.3 Paraganglia
Aortic body
Carotid body
Coccygeal body
Glomus jugulare
237.4 Other and unspecified endocrine glands
Parathyroid gland
Thyroid gland
237.5 Brain and spinal cord
237.6 Meninges
Meninges:
  NOS
  cerebral
  spinal
√5th **237.7** Neurofibromatosis
von Recklinghausen's disease
DEF: An inherited condition with developmental changes in the nervous system, muscles, bones and skin; multiple soft tumors (neurofibromas) distributed over the entire body.

237.70 Neurofibromatosis, unspecified
237.71 Neurofibromatosis, type 1 [von Recklinghausen's disease]

√4th
√5th   Additional Digit Required   Unspecified Code   Other Specified Code   Manifestation Code
 Medicare Secondary Payer   Revised Text   ● New Code   ▲ Revised Code Title

2002 Ingenix, Inc.   Volume 1 — 95

237.72 Neurofibromatosis, type 2 [acoustic neurofibromatosis]
DEF: Inherited condition with cutaneous lesions, benign tumors of peripheral nerves and bilateral 8th nerve masses.

237.9 Other and unspecified parts of nervous system
Cranial nerves
> EXCLUDES peripheral, sympathetic, and parasympathetic nerves and ganglia (238.1)

4th 238 Neoplasm of uncertain behavior of other and unspecified sites and tissues

238.0 Bone and articular cartilage
> EXCLUDES cartilage:
> ear (238.1)
> eyelid (238.1)
> larynx (235.6)
> nose (235.9)
> synovia (238.1)

238.1 Connective and other soft tissue
Peripheral, sympathetic, and parasympathetic nerves and ganglia
> EXCLUDES cartilage (of):
> articular (238.0)
> larynx (235.6)
> nose (235.9)
> connective tissue of breast (238.3)

238.2 Skin
> EXCLUDES anus NOS (235.5)
> skin of genital organs (236.3, 236.6)
> vermilion border of lip (235.1)

238.3 Breast
> EXCLUDES skin of breast (238.2)

238.4 Polycythemia vera
DEF: Abnormal proliferation of all bone marrow elements, increased red cell mass and total blood volume; unknown etiology, frequently associated with splenomegaly, leukocytosis, and thrombocythemia.

238.5 Histiocytic and mast cells
Mast cell tumor NOS   Mastocytoma NOS

238.6 Plasma cells
Plasmacytoma NOS
Solitary myeloma

238.7 Other lymphatic and hematopoietic tissues
Disease:
  lymphoproliferative (chronic) NOS
  myeloproliferative (chronic) NOS
Idiopathic thrombocythemia
Megakaryocytic myelosclerosis
Myelodysplastic syndrome
Myelosclerosis with myeloid metaplasia
Panmyelosis (acute)
> EXCLUDES myelfibrosis (289.8)
> myelosclerosis NOS (289.8)
> myelosis:
> NOS (205.9)
> megakaryocytic (207.2)

238.8 Other specified sites
Eye
Heart
> EXCLUDES eyelid (skin) (238.2)
> cartilage (238.1)

238.9 Site unspecified

NEOPLASMS

NEOPLASMS OF UNSPECIFIED NATURE (239)

✓4th 239 Neoplasms of unspecified nature

Note: Category 239 classifies by site neoplasms of unspecified morphology and behavior. The term "mass," unless otherwise stated, is not to be regarded as a neoplastic growth.

INCLUDES "growth" NOS
neoplasm NOS
new growth NOS
tumor NOS

239.0 Digestive system

EXCLUDES anus:
margin (239.2)
skin (239.2)
perianal skin (239.2)

239.1 Respiratory system

239.2 Bone, soft tissue, and skin

EXCLUDES anal canal (239.0)
anus NOS (239.0)
bone marrow (202.9)
cartilage:
larynx (239.1)
nose (239.1)
connective tissue of breast (239.3)
skin of genital organs (239.5)
vermilion border of lip (239.0)

239.3 Breast

EXCLUDES skin of breast (239.2)

239.4 Bladder

239.5 Other genitourinary organs

239.6 Brain

EXCLUDES cerebral meninges (239.7)
cranial nerves (239.7)

239.7 Endocrine glands and other parts of nervous system

EXCLUDES peripheral, sympathetic, and parasympathetic nerves and ganglia (239.2)

239.8 Other specified sites

EXCLUDES eyelid (skin) (239.2)
cartilage (239.2)
great vessels (239.2)
optic nerve (239.7)

239.9 Site unspecified

3. ENDOCRINE, NUTRITIONAL AND METABOLIC DISEASES, AND IMMUNITY DISORDERS (240-279)

EXCLUDES endocrine and metabolic disturbances specific to the fetus and newborn (775.0-775.9)

Note: All neoplasms, whether functionally active or not, are classified in Chapter 2. Codes in Chapter 3 (i.e., 242.8, 246.0, 251-253, 255-259) may be used to identify such functional activity associated with any neoplasm, or by ectopic endocrine tissue.

ENDOCRINE, NUTRITIONAL, METABOLIC, IMMUNITY

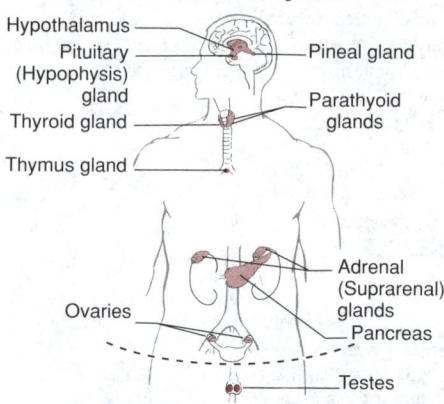

Endocrine System

DISORDERS OF THYROID GLAND (240-246)

✓4th 240 Simple and unspecified goiter
DEF: An enlarged thyroid gland often caused by an inadequate dietary intake of iodine.

240.0 Goiter, specified as simple
Any condition classifiable to 240.9, specified as simple

240.9 Goiter, unspecified
Enlargement of thyroid
Goiter or struma:
　NOS
　diffuse colloid
　endemic
Goiter or struma:
　hyperplastic
　nontoxic (diffuse)
　parenchymatous
　sporadic
EXCLUDES congenital (dyshormonogenic) goiter (246.1)

✓4th 241 Nontoxic nodular goiter
EXCLUDES adenoma of thyroid (226)
　　cystadenoma of thyroid (226)

241.0 Nontoxic uninodular goiter
Thyroid nodule
Uninodular goiter (nontoxic)
DEF: Enlarged thyroid, commonly due to decreased thyroid production, with single nodule; no clinical hypothyroidism.

241.1 Nontoxic multinodular goiter
Multinodular goiter (nontoxic)
DEF: Enlarged thyroid, commonly due to decreased thyroid production with multiple nodules; no clinical hypothyroidism.

241.9 Unspecified nontoxic nodular goiter
Adenomatous goiter
Nodular goiter (nontoxic) NOS
Struma nodosa (simplex)

✓4th 242 Thyrotoxicosis with or without goiter
EXCLUDES neonatal thyrotoxicosis (775.3)

The following fifth-digit subclassification is for use with category 242:
　0 without mention of thyrotoxic crisis or storm
　1 with mention of thyrotoxic crisis or storm

DEF: A condition caused by excess quantities of thyroid hormones being introduced into the tissues.

ENDOCRINE, NUTRITIONAL, METABOLIC, IMMUNITY

242.0 Toxic diffuse goiter
Basedow's disease
Exophthalmic or toxic goiter NOS
Graves' disease
Primary thyroid hyperplasia
DEF: Diffuse thyroid enlargement accompanied by hyperthyroidism, bulging eyes, and dermopathy.

242.1 Toxic uninodular goiter
Thyroid nodule } toxic or with
Uninodular goiter } hyperthyroidism
DEF: Symptomatic hyperthyroidism with a single nodule on the enlarged thyroid gland. Abrupt onset of symptoms; including extreme nervousness, insomnia, weight loss, tremors, and psychosis or coma.

242.2 Toxic multinodular goiter
Secondary thyroid hyperplasia
DEF: Symptomatic hyperthyroidism with multiple nodules on the enlarged thyroid gland. Abrupt onset of symptoms; including extreme nervousness, insomnia, weight loss, tremors, and psychosis or coma.

242.3 Toxic nodular goiter, unspecified
Adenomatous goiter }
Nodular goiter } toxic or with
Struma nodosa } hyperthyroidism
Any condition classifiable to 241.9 specified as toxic or with hyperthyroidism

242.4 Thyrotoxicosis from ectopic thyroid nodule

242.8 Thyrotoxicosis of other specified origin
Overproduction of thyroid-stimulating hormone [TSH]
Thyrotoxicosis:
    factitia from ingestion of excessive thyroid material
Use additional E code to identify cause, if drug-induced

242.9 Thyrotoxicosis without mention of goiter or other cause
Hyperthyroidism NOS
Thyrotoxicosis NOS

243 Congenital hypothyroidism
Congenital thyroid insufficiency
Cretinism (athyrotic) (endemic)
Use additional code to identify associated mental retardation
EXCLUDES congenital (dyshormonogenic) goiter (246.1)
DEF: Underproduction of thyroid hormone present from birth.

244 Acquired hypothyroidism
INCLUDES athyroidism (acquired)
hypothyroidism (acquired)
myxedema (adult) (juvenile)
thyroid (gland) insufficiency (acquired)

244.0 Postsurgical hypothyroidism
DEF: Underproduction of thyroid hormone due to surgical removal of all or part of the thyroid gland.

244.1 Other postablative hypothyroidism
Hypothyroidism following therapy, such as irradiation

244.2 Iodine hypothyroidism
Hypothyroidism resulting from administration or ingestion of iodide
Use additional E code to identify drug

244.3 Other iatrogenic hypothyroidism
Hypothyroidism resulting from:
- P-aminosalicylic acid [PAS]
- Phenylbutazone
- Resorcinol

Iatrogenic hypothyroidism NOS
Use additional E code to identify drug

244.8 Other specified acquired hypothyroidism
Secondary hypothyroidism NEC

244.9 Unspecified hypothyroidism
Hypothyroidism } primary or NOS
Myxedema

√4th 245 Thyroiditis

245.0 Acute thyroiditis
Abscess of thyroid
Thyroiditis:
- nonsuppurative, acute
- pyogenic
- suppurative

Use additional code to identify organism

DEF: Inflamed thyroid caused by infection, with abscess and liquid puris.

245.1 Subacute thyroiditis
Thyroiditis:
- de Quervain's
- giant cell
- granulomatous
- viral

DEF: Inflammation of the thyroid, characterized by fever and painful enlargement of the thyroid gland, with granulomas in the gland.

245.2 Chronic lymphocytic thyroiditis
Hashimoto's disease
Struma lymphomatosa
Thyroiditis:
- autoimmune
- lymphocytic (chronic)

DEF: Autoimmune disease of thyroid; lymphocytes infiltrate the gland and thyroid antibodies are produced; women more often affected.

245.3 Chronic fibrous thyroiditis
Struma fibrosa
Thyroiditis:
- invasive (fibrous)
- ligneous
- Riedel's

DEF: Persistent fibrosing inflammation of thyroid with adhesions to nearby structures; rare condition.

245.4 Iatrogenic thyroiditis
Use additional code to identify cause

DEF: Thyroiditis resulting from treatment or intervention by physician or in a patient intervention setting.

245.8 Other and unspecified chronic thyroiditis
Chronic thyroiditis:
- NOS
- nonspecific

ENDOCRINE, NUTRITIONAL, METABOLIC, IMMUNITY

245.9 **Thyroiditis, unspecified**
Thyroiditis NOS

✓4th **246 Other disorders of thyroid**

246.0 Disorders of thyrocalcitonin secretion
Hypersecretion of calcitonin or thyrocalcitonin

246.1 Dyshormonogenic goiter
Congenital (dyshormonogenic) goiter
Goiter due to enzyme defect in synthesis of thyroid hormone
Goitrous cretinism (sporadic)

246.2 Cyst of thyroid
EXCLUDES *cystadenoma of thyroid (226)*

246.3 Hemorrhage and infarction of thyroid

246.8 Other specified disorders of thyroid
Abnormality of thyroid-binding globulin
Atrophy of thyroid
Hyper-TBG-nemia
Hypo-TBG-nemia

246.9 **Unspecified disorder of thyroid**

DISEASES OF OTHER ENDOCRINE GLANDS (250-259)

✓4th **250 Diabetes mellitus**
EXCLUDES *gestational diabetes (648.8)*
hyperglycemia NOS (790.6)
neonatal diabetes mellitus (775.1)
nonclinical diabetes (790.2)

The following fifth-digit subclassification is for use with category 250:

0 **type II [non-insulin dependent type] [NIDDM type] [adult-onset type] or unspecified type, not stated as uncontrolled**
Fifth-digit 0 is for use for type II, adult-onset diabetic patients, even if the patient requires insulin

1 **type I [insulin dependent type] [IDDM] [juvenile type], not stated as uncontrolled**

2 **type II [non-insulin dependent type] [NIDDM type] [adult-onset type] or unspecified type, uncontrolled**
Fifth-digit 2 is for use for type II, adult-onset diabetic patients, even if the patient requires insulin

3 **type I [insulin dependent type] [IDDM] [juvenile type], uncontrolled**

DEF: Inability to metabolize carbohydrates, proteins, and fats with insufficient secretion of insulin. Symptoms may be unremarkable, with long-term complications, involving kidneys, nerves, blood vessels, and eyes.

✓5th **250.0** Diabetes mellitus without mention of complication
Diabetes mellitus without mention of complication or manifestation classifiable to 250.1-250.9
Diabetes (mellitus) NOS

✓5th **250.1** Diabetes with ketoacidosis
Diabetic:
acidosis } without mention
ketosis } of coma

DEF: Diabetic hyperglycemic crisis causing ketone presence in body fluids.

✓5th **250.2** Diabetes with hyperosmolarity
Hyperosmolar (nonketotic) coma

ENDOCRINE, NUTRITIONAL, METABOLIC, IMMUNITY

§ √5ᵗʰ **250.3 Diabetes with other coma**
    Diabetic coma (with ketoacidosis)
    Diabetic hypoglycemic coma
    Insulin coma NOS
        EXCLUDES *diabetes with hyperosmolar coma (250.2)*
    DEF: Coma (not hyperosmolar) caused by hyperglycemia or hypoglycemia as complication of diabetes.

§ √5ᵗʰ **250.4 Diabetes with renal manifestations**
    Use additional code to identify manifestation, as:
        diabetic:
            nephropathy NOS (583.81)
            nephrosis (581.81)
            intercapillary glomerulosclerosis (581.81)
            Kimmelstiel-Wilson syndrome (581.81)

§ √5ᵗʰ **250.5 Diabetes with ophthalmic manifestations**
    Use additional code to identify manifestation, as:
        diabetic:
            blindness (369.00-369.9)
            cataract (366.41)
            glaucoma (365.44)
            retinal edema (362.83)
            retinopathy (362.01-362.02)

§ √5ᵗʰ **250.6 Diabetes with neurological manifestations**
    Use additional code to identify manifestation, as:
        diabetic:
            amyotrophy (358.1)
            mononeuropathy (354.0-355.9)
            neurogenic arthropathy (713.5)
            peripheral autonomic neuropathy (337.1)
            polyneuropathy (357.2)

§ √5ᵗʰ **250.7 Diabetes with peripheral circulatory disorders**
    Use additional code to identify manifestation, as:
        diabetic:
            gangrene (785.4)
            peripheral angiopathy (443.81)
    DEF: Blood vessel damage or disease, usually in the feet, legs, or hands, as a complication of diabetes.

§ √5ᵗʰ **250.8 Diabetes with other specified manifestations**
    Diabetic hypoglycemia
    Hypoglycemic shock
    Use additional code to identify manifestation, as:
        any associated ulceration (707.10-707.9)
        diabetic bone changes (731.8)
    Use additional E code to identify cause, if drug-induced

§ √5ᵗʰ **250.9 Diabetes with unspecified complication**

√4ᵗʰ **251 Other disorders of pancreatic internal secretion**
    251.0 Hypoglycemic coma
        Iatrogenic hyperinsulinism
        Non-diabetic insulin coma
        Use additional E code to identify cause, if drug-induced
            EXCLUDES *hypoglycemic coma in diabetes mellitus (250.3)*
        DEF: Coma induced by low blood sugar in non-diabetic patient.

---

§ Requires fifth-digit. See beginning of category 250 for codes and definitions.

ENDOCRINE, NUTRITIONAL, METABOLIC, IMMUNITY 251.1–251.9

251.1 Other specified hypoglycemia
Hyperinsulinism:
  NOS
  ectopic
  functional
Hyperplasia of pancreatic
  islet beta cells NOS
  EXCLUDES hypoglycemia:
    in diabetes mellitus (250.8)
    in infant of diabetic mother (775.0)
    neonatal hypoglycemia (775.6)
    hypoglycemic coma (251.0)
Use additional E code to identify cause, if drug-induced.
DEF: Excessive production of insulin by the pancreas; associated with obesity and insulin-producing tumors.

251.2 Hypoglycemia, unspecified
Hypoglycemia:
  NOS
  reactive
  spontaneous
  EXCLUDES hypoglycemia:
    with coma (251.0)
    in diabetes mellitus (250.8)
    leucine-induced (270.3)

251.3 Postsurgical hypoinsulinemia
Hypoinsulinemia following complete or partial pancreatectomy
Postpancreatectomy hyperglycemia

251.4 Abnormality of secretion of glucagon
Hyperplasia of pancreatic islet alpha cells with glucagon excess
DEF: Production malfunction of a pancreatic hormone secreted by cells of the islets of Langerhans

251.5 Abnormality of secretion of gastrin
Hyperplasia of pancreatic alpha cells with gastrin excess
Zollinger-Ellison syndrome

251.8 Other specified disorders of pancreatic internal secretion

251.9 Unspecified disorder of pancreatic internal secretion
Islet cell hyperplasia NOS

Dorsal View of Parathyroid Glands

ENDOCRINE, NUTRITIONAL, METABOLIC, IMMUNITY

✓4th 252 Disorders of parathyroid gland

252.0 Hyperparathyroidism
Hyperplasia of parathyroid
Osteitis fibrosa cystica generalisata
von Recklinghausen's disease of bone
EXCLUDES ectopic hyperparathyroidism (259.3)
secondary hyperparathyroidism (of renal origin) (588.8)

DEF: Abnormally high secretion of parathyroid hormones causing bone deterioration, reduced renal function, kidney stones.

252.1 Hypoparathyroidism
Parathyroiditis (autoimmune)   Tetany:
Tetany: parathyroprival
  parathyroid
EXCLUDES pseudohypoparathyroidism (275.4)
pseudopseudohypoparathyroidism (275.4)
tetany NOS (781.7)
transitory neonatal hypoparathyroidism (775.4)

DEF: Abnormally low secretion of parathyroid hormones which causes decreased calcium and increased phosphorus in the blood. Resulting in muscle cramps, tetany, urinary frequency and cataracts.

252.8 Other specified disorders of parathyroid gland
Cyst   } of parathyroid gland
Hemorrhage

252.9 Unspecified disorder of parathyroid gland

✓4th 253 Disorders of the pituitary gland and its hypothalamic control
INCLUDES the listed conditions whether the disorder is in the pituitary or the hypothalamus
EXCLUDES Cushing's syndrome (255.0)

253.0 Acromegaly and gigantism
Overproduction of growth hormone

DEF: Acromegaly: chronic, beginning in middle age; caused by hypersecretion of the pituitary growth hormone; produces enlarged parts of skeleton, especially the nose, ears, jaws, fingers and toes.

DEF: Gigantism: pituitary gigantism caused by excess growth of short flat bones; men may grow 78 to 80 inches tall.

253.1 Other and unspecified anterior pituitary hyperfunction
Forbes-Albright syndrome
EXCLUDES overproduction of:
ACTH (255.3)
thyroid-stimulating hormone [TSH] (242.8)

DEF: Spontaneous galactorrhea-amenorrhea syndrome unrelated to pregnancy; usually related to presence of pituitary tumor.

253.2 Panhypopituitarism
Cachexia, pituitary
Necrosis of pituitary (postpartum)
Pituitary insufficiency NOS
Sheehan's syndrome
Simmonds' disease
EXCLUDES iatrogenic hypopituitarism (253.7)

DEF: Damage to or absence of pituitary gland leading to impaired sexual function, weight loss, fatigue, bradycardia, hypotension, pallor, depression, and impaired growth in children; called Simmonds' disease if cachexia is prominent.

ENDOCRINE, NUTRITIONAL, METABOLIC, IMMUNITY

253.3 Pituitary dwarfism
Isolated deficiency of (human) growth hormone [HGH]
Lorain-Levi dwarfism
DEF: Dwarfism with infantile physical characteristics due to abnormally low secretion of growth hormone and gonadotropin deficiency.

253.4 Other anterior pituitary disorders
Isolated or partial deficiency of an anterior pituitary hormone, other than growth hormone
Prolactin deficiency

253.5 Diabetes insipidus
Vasopressin deficiency
EXCLUDES   nephrogenic diabetes insipidus (588.1)
DEF: Metabolic disorder causing insufficient antidiuretic hormone release; symptoms include frequent urination, thirst, ravenous hunger, loss of weight, fatigue.

253.6 Other disorders of neurohypophysis
Syndrome of inappropriate secretion of antidiuretic hormone [ADH]
EXCLUDES   ectopic antidiuretic hormone secretion (259.3)
DEF: Pituitary dysfunction that results from drug therapy, radiation therapy, or surgery, causing mild to severe symptoms.

253.7 Iatrogenic pituitary disorders
Hypopituitarism:
  hormone-induced
  hypophysectomy-induced
  postablative
  radiotherapy-induced
Use additional E code to identify cause

253.8 Other disorders of the pituitary and other syndromes of diencephalohypophyseal origin
Abscess of pituitary
Adiposogenital dystrophy
Cyst of Rathke's pouch
Fröhlich's syndrome
EXCLUDES   craniopharyngioma (237.0)

253.9 Unspecified
Dyspituitarism

254 Diseases of thymus gland
EXCLUDES   aplasia or dysplasia with immunodeficiency (279.2)
hypoplasia with immunodeficiency (279.2)
myasthenia gravis (358.0)

254.0 Persistent hyperplasia of thymus
Hypertrophy of thymus
DEF: Continued abnormal growth of the twin lymphoid lobes that produce T lymphocytes.

254.1 Abscess of thymus

254.8 Other specified diseases of thymus gland
Atrophy } of thymus
Cyst
EXCLUDES   thymoma (212.6)

254.9 Unspecified disease of thymus gland

255 Disorders of adrenal glands
INCLUDES   the listed conditions whether the basic disorder is in the adrenals or is pituitary-induced

255.0 Cushing's syndrome
Adrenal hyperplasia due to excess ACTH
Cushing's syndrome:
- NOS
- iatrogenic
- idiopathic
- pituitary-dependent

Ectopic ACTH syndrome
Iatrogenic syndrome of excess cortisol
Overproduction of cortisol
Use additional E code to identify cause, if drug-induced

EXCLUDES congenital adrenal hyperplasia (255.2)

DEF: Due to adrenal cortisol oversecretion or glucocorticoid medications; may cause fatty tissue of the face, neck and body, osteoporosis and curvature of spine, hypertension, diabetes mellitus, female genitourinary problems, male impotence, degeneration of muscle tissues, weakness.

255.1 Hyperaldosteronism
Aldosteronism (primary) (secondary)
Bartter's syndrome
Conn's syndrome

DEF: Oversecretion of aldosterone causing fluid retention, hypertension.

255.2 Adrenogenital disorders
Achard-Thiers syndrome
Adrenogenital syndromes, virilizing or feminizing, whether acquired or associated with congenital adrenal hyperplasia consequent on inborn enzyme defects in hormone synthesis
Congenital adrenal hyperplasia
Female adrenal pseudohermaphroditism
Male:
- macrogenitosomia praecox
- sexual precocity with adrenal hyperplasia

Virilization (female) (suprarenal)

EXCLUDES adrenal hyperplasia due to excess ACTH (255.0)
isosexual virilization (256.4)

255.3 Other corticoadrenal overactivity
Acquired benign adrenal androgenic overactivity
Overproduction of ACTH

255.4 Corticoadrenal insufficiency
Addisonian crisis
Addison's disease NOS
Adrenal:
- atrophy (autoimmune)
- calcification
- crisis
- hemorrhage
- infarction
- insufficiency NOS

EXCLUDES tuberculous Addison's disease (017.6)

DEF: Underproduction of adrenal hormones causing low blood pressure.

255.5 Other adrenal hypofunction
Adrenal medullary insufficiency

EXCLUDES Waterhouse-Friderichsen syndrome (meningococcal) (036.3)

255.6 Medulloadrenal hyperfunction
Catecholamine secretion by pheochromocytoma

255.8 Other specified disorders of adrenal glands
Abnormality of cortisol-binding globulin

255.9 Unspecified disorder of adrenal glands

ENDOCRINE, NUTRITIONAL, METABOLIC, IMMUNITY

✓4th 256 Ovarian dysfunction

256.0 Hyperestrogenism ♀
DEF: Excess secretion of estrogen by the ovaries; characterized by ovaries containing multiple follicular cysts filled with serous fluid.

256.1 Other ovarian hyperfunction ♀
Hypersecretion of ovarian androgens

256.2 Postablative ovarian failure ♀
Ovarian failure: Ovarian failure:
  iatrogenic   postsurgical
  postirradiation
▶Use additional code for states associated with artificial menopause (627.4)◀
> **EXCLUDES**   acquired absence of ovary (V45.77)
>   asymptomatic age-related (natural) postmenopausal status (V49.81)

DEF: Failed ovarian function after medical or surgical intervention.

✓5th 256.3 Other ovarian failure
Use additional code for states associated with ▶natural menopause (627.2)◀
> **EXCLUDES**   asymptomatic age-related (natural) postmenopausal status (V49.81)

256.31 Premature menopause ♀
DEF: Permanent cessation of ovarian function before the age of 40 occuring naturally of unknown cause.

256.39 Other ovarian failure ♀
Delayed menarche   Primary ovarian failure NOS
Ovarian hypofunction

256.4 Polycystic ovaries ♀
Isosexual virilization   Stein-Leventhal syndrome
DEF: Multiple serous filled cysts of ovary; symptoms of infertility, hirsutism, oligomenorrhea or amenorrhea.

256.8 Other ovarian dysfunction ♀

256.9 Unspecified ovarian dysfunction ♀

✓4th 257 Testicular dysfunction

257.0 Testicular hyperfunction ♂
Hypersecretion of testicular hormones

257.1 Postablative testicular hypofunction ♂
Testicular hypofunction:
  iatrogenic
  postirradiation
  postsurgical

257.2 Other testicular hypofunction ♂
Defective biosynthesis of testicular androgen
Eunuchoidism:
  NOS
  hypogonadotropic
Failure:
  Leydig's cell, adult
  seminiferous tubule, adult
Testicular hypogonadism
> **EXCLUDES**   azoospermia (606.0)

257.8 Other testicular dysfunction ♂
Goldberg-Maxwell syndrome
Male pseudohermaphroditism with testicular feminization
Testicular feminization

✓4th ✓5th Additional Digit Required   Unspecified Code   Other Specified Code   Manifestation Code
MSP Medicare Secondary Payer   ▶◀ Revised Text   ● New Code   ▲ Revised Code Title

ENDOCRINE, NUTRITIONAL, METABOLIC, IMMUNITY

- **257.9** **Unspecified testicular dysfunction** ♂

- ✓4th **258 Polyglandular dysfunction and related disorders**
  - **258.0** **Polyglandular activity in multiple endocrine adenomatosis**
    - Wermer's syndrome
    - DEF: Wermer's syndrome: A rare hereditary condition characterized by the presence of adenomas or hyperplasia in more than one endocrine gland causing premature aging.
  - **258.1** **Other combinations of endocrine dysfunction**
    - Lloyd's syndrome
    - Schmidt's syndrome
  - **258.8** **Other specified polyglandular dysfunction**
  - **258.9** **Polyglandular dysfunction, unspecified**

- ✓4th **259 Other endocrine disorders**
  - **259.0** **Delay in sexual development and puberty, not elsewhere classified**
    - Delayed puberty
  - **259.1** **Precocious sexual development and puberty, not elsewhere classified** P
    - Sexual precocity: NOS
    - Sexual precocity: constitutional
    - Sexual precocity: cryptogenic
    - Sexual precocity: idiopathic
  - **259.2** **Carcinoid syndrome**
    - Hormone secretion by carcinoid tumors
    - DEF: Presence of carcinoid tumors that spread to liver; characterized by cyanotic flushing of skin, diarrhea, bronchospasm, acquired tricuspid and pulmonary stenosis, sudden drops in blood pressure, edema, ascites.
  - **259.3** **Ectopic hormone secretion, not elsewhere classified**
    - Ectopic:
      - antidiuretic hormone secretion [ADH]
      - hyperparathyroidism
    - EXCLUDES ectopic ACTH syndrome (255.0)
  - **259.4** **Dwarfism, not elsewhere classified**
    - Dwarfism:
      - NOS
      - constitutional
    - EXCLUDES dwarfism:
      - achondroplastic (756.4)
      - intrauterine (759.7)
      - nutritional (263.2)
      - pituitary (253.3)
      - renal (588.0)
      - progeria (259.8)
  - **259.8** **Other specified endocrine disorders**
    - Pineal gland dysfunction   Werner's syndrome
    - Progeria
  - **259.9** **Unspecified endocrine disorder**
    - Disturbance:
      - endocrine NOS
      - hormone NOS
    - Infantilism NOS

NUTRITIONAL DEFICIENCIES (260-269)

EXCLUDES deficiency anemias (280.0-281.9)

- **260 Kwashiorkor**
  - Nutritional edema with dyspigmentation of skin and hair
  - DEF: Syndrome, particularly of children; excessive carbohydrate with inadequate protein intake, inhibited growth potential, anomalies in skin and hair pigmentation, edema and liver disease.

ENDOCRINE, NUTRITIONAL, METABOLIC, IMMUNITY

261 Nutritional marasmus
Nutritional atrophy
Severe calorie deficiency
Severe malnutrition NOS

DEF: Protein-calorie malabsorption or malnutrition of children; characterized by tissue wasting, dehydration, and subcutaneous fat depletion; may occur with infectious disease; also called infantile atrophy.

262 Other severe, protein-calorie malnutrition
Nutritional edema without mention of dyspigmentation of skin and hair

√4th **263 Other and unspecified protein-calorie malnutrition**

263.0 Malnutrition of moderate degree
DEF: Malnutrition characterized by biochemical changes in electrolytes, lipids, blood plasma.

263.1 Malnutrition of mild degree

263.2 Arrested development following protein-calorie malnutrition
Nutritional dwarfism
Physical retardation due to malnutrition

263.8 Other protein-calorie malnutrition

263.9 Unspecified protein-calorie malnutrition
Dystrophy due to malnutrition
Malnutrition (calorie) NOS
EXCLUDES   nutritional deficiency NOS (269.9)

√4th **264 Vitamin A deficiency**

264.0 With conjunctival xerosis
DEF: Vitamin A deficiency with conjunctival dryness.

264.1 With conjunctival xerosis and Bitot's spot
Bitot's spot in the young child
DEF: Vitamin A deficiency with conjunctival dryness, superficial spots of keratinized epithelium.

264.2 With corneal xerosis
DEF: Vitamin A deficiency with corneal dryness.

264.3 With corneal ulceration and xerosis
DEF: Vitamin A deficiency with corneal dryness, epithelial ulceration.

264.4 With keratomalacia
DEF: Vitamin A deficiency creating corneal dryness; progresses to corneal insensitivity, softness, necrosis; usually bilateral.

264.5 With night blindness
DEF: Vitamin A deficiency causing vision failure in dim light.

264.6 With xerophthalmic scars of cornea
DEF: Vitamin A deficiency with corneal scars from dryness.

264.7 Other ocular manifestations of vitamin A deficiency
Xerophthalmia due to vitamin A deficiency

264.8 Other manifestations of vitamin A deficiency
Follicular keratosis   } due to vitamin A
Xeroderma   } deficiency

264.9 Unspecified vitamin A deficiency
Hypovitaminosis A NOS

ENDOCRINE, NUTRITIONAL, METABOLIC, IMMUNITY

✓4th **265 Thiamine and niacin deficiency states**

265.0 Beriberi

DEF: Inadequate vitamin B_1 (thiamine) intake, affects heart and peripheral nerves; individual may become edematous and develop cardiac disease due to the excess fluid; alcoholics and people with a diet of excessive polished rice prone to the disease.

265.1 Other and unspecified manifestations of thiamine deficiency

Other vitamin B_1 deficiency states

265.2 Pellagra

Deficiency:
  niacin (-tryptophan)
  nicotinamide
  nicotinic acid

Deficiency:
  vitamin PP
  Pellagra (alcoholic)

DEF: Niacin deficiency causing dermatitis, inflammation of mucous membranes, diarrhea, and psychic disturbances.

✓4th **266 Deficiency of B-complex components**

266.0 Ariboflavinosis

Riboflavin [vitamin B_2] deficiency

DEF: Vitamin B_2 (riboflavin) deficiency marked by swollen lips and tongue fissures, corneal vascularization, scaling lesions, and anemia.

266.1 Vitamin B_6 deficiency

Deficiency:
  pyridoxal
  pyridoxamine

Deficiency:
  pyridoxine
  Vitamin B_6 deficiency syndrome

EXCLUDES vitamin B_6-responsive sideroblastic anemia (285.0)

DEF: Vitamin B_6 deficiency causing skin, lip, and tongue disturbances, peripheral neuropathy; and convulsions in infants.

266.2 Other B-complex deficiencies

Deficiency:
  cyanocobalamin
  folic acid

Deficiency:
  vitamin B_{12}

EXCLUDES combined system disease with anemia (281.0-281.1)
deficiency anemias (281.0-281.9)
subacute degeneration of spinal cord with anemia (281.0-281.1)

266.9 Unspecified vitamin B deficiency

267 Ascorbic acid deficiency

Deficiency of vitamin C   Scurvy

EXCLUDES scorbutic anemia (281.8)

DEF: Vitamin C deficiency causing swollen gums, myalgia, weight loss, and weakness.

✓4th **268 Vitamin D deficiency**

EXCLUDES vitamin D-resistant:
osteomalacia (275.3)
rickets (275.3)

268.0 Rickets, active

EXCLUDES celiac rickets (579.0)
renal rickets (588.0)

DEF: Inadequate vitamin D intake, usually in pediatrics, that affects bones most involved with muscular action; may cause nodules on ends and sides of bones; delayed closure of fontanels in infants; symptoms may include muscle soreness, and profuse sweating.

268.1 Rickets, late effect

Any condition specified as due to rickets and stated to be a late effect or sequela of rickets
Use additional code to identify the nature of late effect

DEF: Distorted or demineralized bones as a result of vitamin D deficiency.

ENDOCRINE, NUTRITIONAL, METABOLIC, IMMUNITY 268.2–270.1

268.2 **Osteomalacia, unspecified**
DEF: Softening of bones due to decrease in calcium; marked by pain, tenderness, muscular weakness, anorexia, and weight loss.

268.9 **Unspecified vitamin D deficiency**
Avitaminosis D

√4th **269 Other nutritional deficiencies**

269.0 **Deficiency of vitamin K**
EXCLUDES deficiency of coagulation factor due to vitamin K deficiency (286.7)
vitamin K deficiency of newborn (776.0)

269.1 **Deficiency of other vitamins**
Deficiency:
vitamin E
vitamin P

269.2 **Unspecified vitamin deficiency**
Multiple vitamin deficiency NOS

269.3 **Mineral deficiency, not elsewhere classified**
Deficiency:
calcium, dietary
iodine
EXCLUDES deficiency:
calcium NOS (275.4)
potassium (276.8)
sodium (276.1)

269.8 **Other nutritional deficiency**
EXCLUDES adult failure to thrive (783.7)
failure to thrive in childhood (783.41)
feeding problems (783.3)
newborn (779.3)

269.9 **Unspecified nutritional deficiency**

OTHER METABOLIC AND IMMUNITY DISORDERS (270-279)
Use additional code to identify any associated mental retardation

√4th **270 Disorders of amino-acid transport and metabolism**
EXCLUDES abnormal findings without manifest disease (790.0-796.9)
disorders of purine and pyrimidine metabolism (277.1-277.2)
gout (274.0-274.9)

270.0 **Disturbances of amino-acid transport**
Cystinosis
Cystinuria
Fanconi (-de Toni) (-Debré) syndrome
Glycinuria (renal)
Hartnup disease

270.1 **Phenylketonuria [PKU]**
Hyperphenylalaninemia
DEF: Inherited metabolic condition causing excess phenylpyruvic and other acids in urine; results in mental retardation, neurological manifestations, including spasticity and tremors, light pigmentation, eczema, and mousy odor.

270.2 Other disturbances of aromatic amino-acid metabolism
Albinism
Alkaptonuria
Alkaptonuric ochronosis
Disturbances of metabolism of tyrosine and tryptophan
Homogentisic acid defects
Hydroxykynureninuria
Hypertyrosinemia
Indicanuria
Kynureninase defects
Oasthouse urine disease
Ochronosis
Tyrosinosis
Tyrosinuria
Waardenburg syndrome

EXCLUDES *vitamin B_6-deficiency syndrome (266.1)*

270.3 Disturbances of branched-chain amino-acid metabolism
Disturbances of metabolism of leucine, isoleucine, and valine
Hypervalinemia
Intermittent branched-chain ketonuria
Leucine-induced hypoglycemia
Leucinosis
Maple syrup urine disease

270.4 Disturbances of sulphur-bearing amino-acid metabolism
Cystathioninemia
Cystathioninuria
Disturbances of metabolism of methionine, homocystine, and cystathionine
Homocystinuria
Hypermethioninemia
Methioninemia

270.5 Disturbances of histidine metabolism
Carnosinemia
Histidinemia
Hyperhistidinemia
Imidazole aminoaciduria

270.6 Disorders of urea cycle metabolism
Argininosuccinic aciduria
Citrullinemia
Disorders of metabolism of ornithine, citrulline, argininosuccinic acid, arginine, and ammonia
Hyperammonemia
Hyperomithinemia

270.7 Other disturbances of straight-chain amino-acid metabolism
Glucoglycinuria
Glycinemia (with methyl-malonic acidemia)
Hyperglycinemia
Hyperlysinemia
Other disturbances of metabolism of glycine, threonine, serine, glutamine, and lysine
Pipecolic acidemia
Saccharopinuria

270.8 Other specified disorders of amino-acid metabolism
Alaninemia
Ethanolaminuria
Glycoprolinuria
Hydroxyprolinemia
Hyperprolinemia
Iminoacidopathy
Prolinemia
Prolinuria
Sarcosinemia

270.9 Unspecified disorder of amino-acid metabolism

ENDOCRINE, NUTRITIONAL, METABOLIC, IMMUNITY

✓4th 271 Disorders of carbohydrate transport and metabolism

EXCLUDES abnormality of secretion of glucagon (251.4)
diabetes mellitus (250.0-250.9)
hypoglycemia NOS (251.2)
mucopolysaccharidosis (277.5)

271.0 Glycogenosis
Amylopectinosis
Glucose-6-phosphatase deficiency
Glycogen storage disease
McArdle's disease
Pompe's disease
von Gierke's disease

DEF: Excess glycogen storage; rare inherited trait affects liver, kidneys; causes various symptoms depending on type, though often weakness, and muscle cramps.

271.1 Galactosemia
Galactose-1-phosphate uridyl transferase deficiency
Galactosuria

DEF: Any of three genetic disorders due to defective galactose metabolism; symptoms include failure to thrive in infancy, jaundice, liver and spleen damage, cataracts, and mental retardation.

271.2 Hereditary fructose intolerance
Essential benign fructosuria
Fructosemia

DEF: Chromosome recessive disorder of carbohydrate metabolism; in infants, occurs after dietary sugar introduced; characterized by enlarged spleen, yellowish cast to skin, and progressive inability to thrive.

271.3 Intestinal disaccharidase deficiencies and disaccharide malabsorption
Intolerance or malabsorption (congenital) (of):
  glucose-galactose
  lactose
  sucrose-isomaltose

271.4 Renal glycosuria
Renal diabetes

DEF: Persistent abnormal levels of glucose in urine, with normal blood glucose levels; caused by failure of the renal tubules to reabsorb glucose.

271.8 Other specified disorders of carbohydrate transport and metabolism
Essential benign pentosuria
Fucosidosis
Glycolic aciduria
Hyperoxaluria (primary)
Mannosidosis
Oxalosis
Xylosuria
Xylulosuria

271.9 Unspecified disorder of carbohydrate transport and metabolism

✓4th 272 Disorders of lipoid metabolism

EXCLUDES localized cerebral lipidoses (330.1)

272.0 Pure hypercholesterolemia
Familial hypercholesterolemia
Fredrickson Type IIa hyperlipoproteinemia
Hyperbetalipoproteinemia
Hyperlipidemia, Group A
Low-density-lipoid-type [LDL] hyperlipoproteinemia

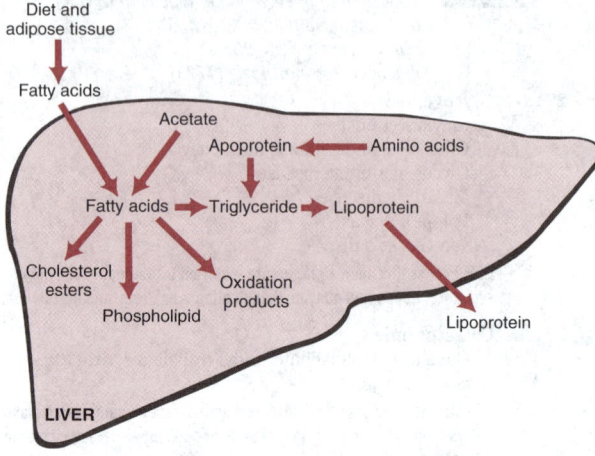

Lipid Metabolism

272.1 Pure hyperglyceridemia
Endogenous hyperglyceridemia
Fredrickson Type IV hyperlipoproteinemia
Hyperlipidemia, Group B
Hyperprebetalipoproteinemia
Hypertriglyceridemia, essential
Very-low-density-lipoid-type [VLDL] hyperlipoproteinemia

272.2 Mixed hyperlipidemia
Broad- or floating-betalipoproteinemia
Fredrickson Type IIb or III hyperlipoproteinemia
Hypercholesterolemia with endogenous hyperglyceridemia
Hyperbetalipoproteinemia with prebetalipoproteinemia
Tubo-eruptive xanthoma
Xanthoma tuberosum

DEF: Elevated levels of lipoprotein, a complex of fats and proteins, in blood due to inherited metabolic disorder.

272.3 Hyperchylomicronemia
Bürger-Grütz syndrome
Fredrickson type I or V hyperlipoproteinemia
Hyperlipidemia, Group D
Mixed hyperglyceridemia

272.4 Other and unspecified hyperlipidemia
Alpha-lipoproteinemia
Combined hyperlipidemia
Hyperlipidemia NOS
Hyperlipoproteinemia NOS

DEF: Hyperlipoproteinemia: elevated levels of transient chylomicrons in the blood which are a form of lipoproteins which transport dietary cholesterol and triglycerides from the small intestine to the blood.

272.5 Lipoprotein deficiencies
Abetalipoproteinemia
Bassen-Kornzweig syndrome
High-density lipoid deficiency (familial)
Hypoalphalipoproteinemia
Hypobetalipoproteinemia

DEF: Abnormally low levels of lipoprotein, a complex of fats and protein, in the blood.

ENDOCRINE, NUTRITIONAL, METABOLIC, IMMUNITY

272.6 Lipodystrophy
Barraquer-Simons disease
Progressive lipodystrophy
Use additional E code to identify cause, if iatrogenic
   EXCLUDES   intestinal lipodystrophy (040.2)
DEF: Disturbance of fat metabolism resulting in loss of fatty tissue in some areas of the body.

272.7 Lipidoses
Chemically-induced lipidosis
Disease:
   Anderson's
   Fabry's
   Gaucher's
   I cell [mucolipidosis I]
   lipoid storage NOS
   Niemann-Pick
   pseudo-Hurler's or mucolipdosis III
   triglyceride storage, Type I or II
   Wolman's or triglyceride storage, Type III
Mucolipidosis II
Primary familial xanthomatosis
   EXCLUDES   cerebral lipidoses (330.1)
                  Tay-Sachs disease (330.1)
DEF: Lysosomal storage diseases marked by an abnormal amount of lipids in reticuloendothelial cells.

272.8 Other disorders of lipoid metabolism
Hoffa's disease or liposynovitis prepatellaris
Launois-Bensaude's lipomatosis
Lipoid dermatoarthritis

272.9 Unspecified disorder of lipoid metabolism

✓4ᵗʰ 273 Disorders of plasma protein metabolism
   EXCLUDES   agammaglobulinemia and hypogammaglobulinemia (279.0-279.2)
                  coagulation defects (286.0-286.9)
                  hereditary hemolytic anemias (282.0-282.9)

273.0 Polyclonal hypergammaglobulinemia
Hypergammaglobulinemic purpura:
   benign primary
   Waldenström's
DEF: Elevated blood levels of gamma globulins, frequently found in patients with chronic infectious diseases.

273.1 Monoclonal paraproteinemia
Benign monoclonal hypergammaglobulinemia [BMH]
Monoclonal gammopathy:
   NOS
   associated with lymphoplasmacytic dyscrasias
   benign
Paraproteinemia:
   benign (familial)
   secondary to malignant or inflammatory disease
DEF: Elevated blood levels of macroglobulins (plasma globulins of high weight); characterized by malignant neoplasms of bone marrow, spleen, liver, or lymph nodes; symptoms include weakness, fatigue, bleeding disorders, and vision problems.

ENDOCRINE, NUTRITIONAL, METABOLIC, IMMUNITY

273.2 Other paraproteinemias
Cryoglobulinemic:
  purpura
  vasculitis
Mixed cryoglobulinemia

273.3 Macroglobulinemia
Macroglobulinemia (idiopathic) (primary)
Waldenström's macroglobulinemia

273.8 Other disorders of plasma protein metabolism
Abnormality of transport protein
Bisalbuminemia

273.9 Unspecified disorder of plasma protein metabolism

√4th **274 Gout**

> EXCLUDES lead gout (984.0-984.9)

DEF: Purine and pyrimidine metabolic disorders; manifested by hyperuricemia and recurrent acute inflammatory arthritis; monosodium urate or monohydrate crystals may be deposited in and around the joints, leading to joint destruction, and severe crippling.

274.0 Gouty arthropathy

√5th **274.1 Gouty nephropathy**

274.10 Gouty nephropathy, unspecified

274.11 Uric acid nephrolithiasis
DEF: Sodium urate stones in the kidney.

274.19 Other

√5th **274.8 Gout with other specified manifestations**

274.81 Gouty tophi of ear
DEF: Chalky sodium urate deposit in the ear due to gout; produces chronic inflammation of external ear.

274.82 Gouty tophi of other sites
Gouty tophi of heart

274.89 Other
Use additional code to identify manifestations, as:
  gouty:
    iritis (364.11)
    neuritis (357.4)

274.9 Gout, unspecified

√4th **275 Disorders of mineral metabolism**

> EXCLUDES abnormal findings without manifest disease (790.0-796.9)

275.0 Disorders of iron metabolism
Bronzed diabetes
Hemochromatosis
Pigmentary cirrhosis (of liver)
> EXCLUDES anemia:
>   iron deficiency (280.0-280.9)
>   sideroblastic (285.0)

275.1 Disorders of copper metabolism
Hepatolenticular degeneration
Wilson's disease

275.2 Disorders of magnesium metabolism
Hypermagnesemia
Hypomagnesemia

275.3 Disorders of phosphorus metabolism
Familial hypophosphatemia
Hypophosphatasia
Vitamin D-resistant:
  osteomalacia
  rickets

ENDOCRINE, NUTRITIONAL, METABOLIC, IMMUNITY

275.4 Disorders of calcium metabolism
  EXCLUDES parathyroid disorders (252.0-252.9)
          vitamin D deficiency (268.0-268.9)

275.40 Unspecified disorder of calcium metabolism

275.41 Hypocalcemia
  DEF: Abnormally decreased blood calcium level; symptoms include hyperactive deep tendon reflexes, muscle, abdominal cramps, and carpopedal spasm.

275.42 Hypercalcemia
  DEF: Abnormally increased blood calcium level; symptoms include muscle weakness, fatigue, nausea, depression, and constipation.

275.49 Other disorders of calcium metabolism
  Nephrocalcinosis
  Pseudohypoparathyroidism
  Pseudopseudohypoparathryoidism

  DEF: Nephrocalcinosis: calcium phosphate deposits in the tubules of the kidney with resultant renal insufficiency.

  DEF: Pseudohypoparathyroidism: inherited disorder with signs and symptoms of hypoparathyroidism; caused by inadequate response to parathyroid hormone, not hormonal deficiency. Symptoms include muscle cramps, tetany, urinary frequency, blurred vision due to cataracts, and dry scaly skin.

  DEF: Pseudopseudohypoparathyroidism: clinical manifestations of hypoparathyroidism without affecting blood calcium levels.

275.8 Other specified disorders of mineral metabolism
275.9 Unspecified disorder of mineral metabolism

276 Disorders of fluid, electrolyte, and acid-base balance
  EXCLUDES diabetes insipidus (253.5)
          familial periodic paralysis (359.3)

276.0 Hyperosmolality and/or hypernatremia
  Sodium [Na] excess   Sodium [Na] overload

276.1 Hyposmolality and/or hyponatremia
  Sodium [Na] deficiency

276.2 Acidosis
  Acidosis: Acidosis:
    NOS   metabolic
    lactic   respiratory
  EXCLUDES diabetic acidosis (250.1)

  DEF: Disorder involves decrease of pH (hydrogen ion) concentration in blood and cellular tissues; caused by increase in acid and decrease in bicarbonate.

276.3 Alkalosis
  Alkalosis: Alkalosis:
    NOS   respiratory
    metabolic

  DEF: Accumulation of base (non-acid part of salt), or loss of acid without relative loss of base in body fluids; caused by increased arterial plasma bicarbonate concentration or loss of carbon dioxide due to hyperventilation.

276.4 Mixed acid-base balance disorder
  Hypercapnia with mixed acid-base disorder

276.5 Volume depletion
Dehydration
Depletion of volume of plasma or extracellular fluid
Hypovolemia
EXCLUDES hypovolemic shock:
     postoperative (998.0)
     traumatic (958.4)

276.6 Fluid overload
Fluid retention
EXCLUDES ascites (789.5)
     localized edema (782.3)

276.7 Hyperpotassemia
Hyperkalemia   Potassium [K]:
Potassium [K]:   intoxication
   excess   overload

DEF: Elevated blood levels of potassium; symptoms include abnormal EKG readings, weakness; related to defective renal excretion.

276.8 Hypopotassemia
Hypokalemia
Potassium [K] deficiency

DEF: Decreased blood levels of potassium; symptoms include neuromuscular disorders.

276.9 Electrolyte and fluid disorders not elsewhere classified
Electrolyte imbalance Hypochloremia
Hyperchloremia
EXCLUDES electrolyte imbalance:
     associated with hyperemesis gravidarum (643.1)
     complicating labor and delivery (669.0)
     following abortion and ectopic or molar pregnancy (634-638 with .4, 639.4)

√4ᵗʰ **277 Other and unspecified disorders of metabolism**

√5ᵗʰ **277.0 Cystic fibrosis**
Fibrocystic disease of the pancreas
Mucoviscidosis

DEF: Generalized, genetic disorder of infants, children, and young adults marked by exocrine gland dysfunction; characterized by chronic pulmonary disease with excess mucus production, pancreatic deficiency, high levels of electrolytes in the sweat.

277.00 Without mention of meconium ileus
▶Cystic fibrosis NOS◀

277.01 With meconium ileus
Meconium:
   ileus (of newborn)
   obstruction of intestine in mucoviscidosis

277.02 With pulmonary manifestations
Cystic fibrosis with pulmonary exacerbation
Use additional code to identify any infectious organism present, such as:
   pseudomonas (041.7)

277.03 With gastrointestinal manifestations
EXCLUDES with meconium ileus (277.01)

277.09 With other manifestations

ENDOCRINE, NUTRITIONAL, METABOLIC, IMMUNITY 277.1–277.6

277.1 Disorders of porphyrin metabolism
Hematoporphyria
Hematoporphyrinuria
Hereditary coproporphyria
Porphyria
Porphyrinuria
Protocoproporphyria
Protoporphyria
Pyrroloporphyria

277.2 Other disorders of purine and pyrimidine metabolism
Hypoxanthine-guanine-phosphoribosyltransferase deficiency [HG-PRT deficiency]
Lesch-Nyhan syndrome
Xanthinuria
EXCLUDES gout (274.0-274.9)
orotic aciduric anemia (281.4)

277.3 Amyloidosis
Amyloidosis:
NOS
inherited systemic
nephropathic
neuropathic (Portuguese) (Swiss)
secondary
Benign paroxysmal peritonitis
Familial Mediterranean fever
Hereditary cardiac amyloidosis
DEF: Conditions of diverse etiologies characterized by the accumulation of insoluble fibrillar proteins (amyloid) in various organs and tissues of the body, compromising vital functions.

277.4 Disorders of bilirubin excretion
Hyperbilirubinemia: Syndrome:
  congenital   Dubin-Johnson
  constitutional   Gilbert's
Syndrome: Rotor's
  Crigler-Najjar
EXCLUDES hyperbilirubinemias specific to the perinatal period (774.0-774.7)

277.5 Mucopolysaccharidosis
Gargoylism
Hunter's syndrome
Hurler's syndrome
Lipochondrodystrophy
Maroteaux-Lamy syndrome
Morquio-Brailsford disease
Osteochondrodystrophy
Sanfilippo's syndrome
Scheie's syndrome
DEF: Metabolism disorders evidenced by excretion of various mucopolysaccharides in urine and infiltration of these substances into connective tissue, with resulting various defects of bone, cartilage and connective tissue.

277.6 Other deficiencies of circulating enzymes
Alpha 1-antitrypsin deficiency
Hereditary angioedema

277.7–279.04 ENDOCRINE, NUTRITIONAL, METABOLIC, IMMUNITY

277.7 Dysmetabolic syndrome X **A**
Use additional code for associated manifestations, such as:
cardiovascular disease ▶(414.00-414.06)◀
obesity (278.00-278.01)

DEF: A specific group of metabolic disorders that are related to the state of insulin resistance (decreased cellular response to insulin) without elevated blood sugars; often related to elevated cholesterol and triglycerides, obesity, cardiovascular disease, and high blood pressure.

277.8 Other specified disorders of metabolism
Hand-Schüller-Christian disease
Histiocytosis (acute) (chronic)
Histiocytosis X (chronic)
EXCLUDES histiocytosis:
acute differentiated progressive (202.5)
X, acute (progressive) (202.5)

277.9 Unspecified disorder of metabolism
Enzymopathy NOS

✓4th **278 Obesity and other hyperalimentation**
EXCLUDES hyperalimentation NOS (783.6)
poisoning by vitamins NOS (963.5)
polyphagia (783.6)

✓5th **278.0 Obesity**
EXCLUDES adiposogenital dystrophy (253.8)
obesity of endocrine origin NOS (259.9)

278.00 Obesity, unspecified
Obesity NOS

278.01 Morbid obesity
DEF: Increased weight beyond limits of skeletal and physical requirements (125 percent or more over ideal body weight), as a result of excess fat in subcutaneous connective tissues.

278.1 Localized adiposity
Fat pad

278.2 Hypervitaminosis A

278.3 Hypercarotinemia
DEF: Elevated blood carotene level due to ingesting excess carotenoids or the inability to convert carotenoids to vitamin A.

278.4 Hypervitaminosis D
DEF: Weakness, fatigue, loss of weight, and other symptoms resulting from ingesting excessive amounts of vitamin D.

278.8 Other hyperalimentation

✓4th **279 Disorders involving the immune mechanism**

✓5th **279.0 Deficiency of humoral immunity**
DEF: Inadequate immune response to bacterial infections with potential reinfection by viruses due to lack of circulating immunoglobulins (acquired antibodies).

279.00 Hypogammaglobulinemia, unspecified◀
Agammaglobulinemia NOS

279.01 Selective IgA immunodeficiency

279.02 Selective IgM immunodeficiency

279.03 Other selective immunoglobulin deficiencies
Selective deficiency of IgG

279.04 Congenital hypogammaglobulinemia
Agammaglobulinemia:
Bruton's type
X-linked

ENDOCRINE, NUTRITIONAL, METABOLIC, IMMUNITY 279.05–279.9

279.05 Immunodeficiency with increased IgM
Immunodeficiency with hyper-IgM:
autosomal recessive
X-linked

279.06 Common variable immunodeficiency
Dysgammaglobulinemia (acquired) (congenital) (primary)
Hypogammaglobulinemia:
acquired primary
congenital non-sex-linked
sporadic

279.09 Other
Transient hypogammaglobulinemia of infancy

√5ᵗʰ **279.1 Deficiency of cell-mediated immunity**

279.10 Immunodeficiency with predominant T-cell defect, unspecified

279.11 DiGeorge's syndrome
Pharyngeal pouch syndrome
Thymic hypoplasia

DEF: Congenital disorder due to defective development of the third and fourth pharyngeal pouches; results in hypoplasia or aplasia of the thymus, parathyroid glands; related to congenital heart defects, anomalies of the great vessels, esophageal atresia, and abnormalities of facial structures.

279.12 Wiskott-Aldrich syndrome

DEF: A disease characterized by chronic conditions, such as eczema, suppurative otitis media and anemia; it results from an X-linked recessive gene and is classified as an immune deficiency syndrome.

279.13 Nezelof's syndrome
Cellular immunodeficiency with abnormal immunoglobulin deficiency

DEF: Immune system disorder characterized by a pathological deficiency in cellular immunity and humoral antibodies resulting in inability to fight infectious diseases.

279.19 Other
EXCLUDES ataxia-telangiectasia (334.8)

279.2 Combined immunity deficiency
Agammaglobulinemia:
autosomal recessive
Swiss-type
x-linked recessive
Severe combined immunodeficiency [SCID]
Thymic:
alymophoplasia
aplasia or dysplasia with immunodeficiency
EXCLUDES thymic hypoplasia (279.11)

DEF: Agammaglobulinemia: no immunoglobulins in the blood.

DEF: Thymic alymphoplasia: severe combined immunodeficiency; result of failed lymphoid tissue development.

279.3 Unspecified immunity deficiency

279.4 Autoimmune disease, not elsewhere classified
Autoimmune disease NOS
EXCLUDES transplant failure or rejection (996.80-996.89)

279.8 Other specified disorders involving the immune mechanism
Single complement [C1-C9] deficiency or dysfunction

279.9 Unspecified disorder of immune mechanism

√4ᵗʰ
√5ᵗʰ Additional Digit Required
 Medicare Secondary Payer

▶◀ Revised Text

● New Code

Unspecified Code

Other Specified Code

Manifestation Code

▲ Revised Code Title

2002 Ingenix, Inc.

Volume 1 — 121

4. DISEASES OF THE BLOOD AND BLOOD-FORMING ORGANS (280-289)

> **EXCLUDES** *anemia complicating pregnancy or the puerperium (648.2)*

✓4ᵗʰ 280 Iron deficiency anemias

> **INCLUDES** anemia:
> asiderotic
> hypochromic-microcytic
> sideropenic
>
> **EXCLUDES** *familial microcytic anemia (282.4)*

280.0 Secondary to blood loss (chronic)
Normocytic anemia due to blood loss
> **EXCLUDES** *acute posthemorrhagic anemia (285.1)*

280.1 Secondary to inadequate dietary iron intake

280.8 Other specified iron deficiency anemias
Paterson-Kelly syndrome
Plummer-Vinson syndrome
Sideropenic dysphagia

280.9 Iron deficiency anemia, unspecified
Anemia: Anemia:
achlorhydric   idiopathic hypochromic
chlorotic   iron [Fe] deficiency NOS

✓4ᵗʰ 281 Other deficiency anemias

281.0 Pernicious anemia
Anemia:
Addison's
Biermer's
congenital pernicious
Congenital intrinsic factor [Castle's] deficiency
> **EXCLUDES** *combined system disease without mention of anemia (266.2)*
> *subacute degeneration of spinal cord without mention of anemia (266.2)*

DEF: Chronic progressive anemia due to Vitamin B_{12} malabsorption; caused by lack of a secretion known as intrinsic factor, which is produced by the gastric mucosa of the stomach.

281.1 Other vitamin B_{12} deficiency anemia
Anemia:
vegan's
vitamin B_{12} deficiency (dietary)
due to selective vitamin B_{12} malabsorption with proteinuria
Syndrome:
Imerslund's
Imerslund-Gräsbeck
> **EXCLUDES** *combined system disease without mention of anemia (266.2)*
> *subacute degeneration of spinal cord without mention of anemia (266.2)*

281.2 Folate-deficiency anemia
Congenital folate malabsorption
Folate or folic acid deficiency anemia:
NOS
dietary
drug-induced
Goat's milk anemia
Nutritional megaloblastic anemia (of infancy)
Use additional E code to identify drug

DEF: Macrocytic anemia resembles pernicious anemia but without absence of hydrochloric acid secretions; responsive to folic acid therapy.

BLOOD AND BLOOD-FORMING ORGANS

281.3 Other specified megaloblastic anemias not elsewhere classified
   Combined B$_{12}$ and folate-deficiency anemia
   Refractory megaloblastic anemia

   DEF: Megaloblasts predominant in bone marrow with few normoblasts; rare familial type associated with proteinuria and genitourinary tract anomalies.

281.4 Protein-deficiency anemia
   Amino-acid-deficiency anemia

281.8 Anemia associated with other specified nutritional deficiency
   Scorbutic anemia

281.9 Unspecified deficiency anemia
   Anemia:
      dimorphic
      macrocytic
      megaloblastic NOS
      nutritional NOS
      simple chronic

✓4th 282 Hereditary hemolytic anemias

DEF: Escalated rate of erythrocyte destruction; similar to all anemias, occurs when imbalance exists between blood loss and blood production.

282.0 Hereditary spherocytosis
   Acholuric (familial) jaundice
   Congenital hemolytic anemia (spherocytic)
   Congenital spherocytosis
   Minkowski-Chauffard syndrome
   Spherocytosis (familial)
      EXCLUDES *hemolytic anemia of newborn (773.0-773.5)*

   DEF: Hereditary, chronic illness marked by abnormal red blood cell membrane; symptoms include enlarged spleen, jaundice; and anemia in severe cases.

282.1 Hereditary elliptocytosis
   Elliptocytosis (congenital)
   Ovalocytosis (congenital) (hereditary)

   DEF: Genetic hemolytic anemia characterized by malformed, elliptical erythrocytes; there is increased destruction of red cells with resulting anemia.

282.2 Anemias due to disorders of glutathione metabolism
   Anemia:
      6-phosphogluconic dehydrogenase deficiency
      enzyme deficiency, drug-induced
      erythrocytic glutathione deficiency
      glucose-6-phosphate dehydrogenase [G-6-PD] deficiency
      glutathione-reductase deficiency
      hemolytic nonspherocytic (hereditary), type I
   Disorder of pentose phosphate pathway
   Favism

282.3 Other hemolytic anemias due to enzyme deficiency
   Anemia:
      hemolytic nonspherocytic (hereditary), type II
      hexokinase deficiency
      pyruvate kinase [PK] deficiency
      triosephosphate isomerase deficiencyz

282.4 Thalassemias
Cooley's anemia
Hereditary leptocytosis
Mediterranean anemia (with other hemoglobinopathy)
Microdrepanocytosis
Sickle-cell thalassemia
Thalassemia (alpha) (beta) (intermedia) (major) (minima) (minor) (mixed) (trait) (with other hemoglobinopathy)
Thalassemia-Hb-S disease

EXCLUDES sickle-cell:
anemia (282.60-282.69)
trait (282.5)

DEF: Group of hereditary anemias occurring in the Mediterranean and Southeast Asia; characterized by impaired hemoglobin synthesis; homozygous form may cause death in utero; mild red blood cell anomalies in heterozygous.

282.5 Sickle-cell trait
Hb-AS genotype
Hemoglobin S [Hb-S] trait
Heterozygous:
  hemoglobin S
  Hb-S

EXCLUDES that with other hemoglobinopathy (282.60-282.69)
that with thalassemia (282.4)

DEF: Heterozygous genetic makeup characterized by one gene for normal hemoglobin and one for sickle-cell hemoglobin; clinical disease rarely present.

√5th 282.6 Sickle-cell anemia
EXCLUDES sickle-cell thalassemia (282.4)
sickle-cell trait (282.5)

DEF: Inherited blood disorder; sickle-shaped red blood cells are hard and pointed, clogging blood flow; anemia characterized by, periodic episodes of pain, acute abdominal discomfort, skin ulcerations of the legs, increased infections; occurs primarily in persons of African descent.

282.60 Sickle-cell anemia, unspecified
282.61 Hb-S disease without mention of crisis
282.62 Hb-S disease with mention of crisis
Sickle-cell crisis NOS
282.63 Sickle-cell/Hb-C disease
Hb-S/Hb-C disease
282.69 Other
Disease:
  Hb-S/Hb-D
  Hb-S/Hb-E
Disease:
  sickle-cell/Hb-D
  sickle-cell/Hb-E

282.7 Other hemoglobinopathies
Abnormal hemoglobin NOS
Congenital Heinz-body anemia
Disease:
  Hb-Bart's
  hemoglobin C [Hb-C]
  hemoglobin D [Hb-D]
  hemoglobin E [Hb-E]
  hemoglobin Zurich [Hb-Zurich]
Hemoglobinopathy NOS
Hereditary persistence of fetal hemoglobin [HPFH]
Unstable hemoglobin hemolytic disease

EXCLUDES familial polycythemia (289.6)
hemoglobin M [Hb-M] disease (289.7)
high-oxygen-affinity hemoglobin (289.0)

DEF: Any disorder of hemoglobin due to alteration of molecular structure; may include overt anemia.

BLOOD AND BLOOD-FORMING ORGANS 282.8–284.0

282.8 Other specified hereditary hemolytic anemias
Stomatocytosis

282.9 Hereditary hemolytic anemia, unspecified
Hereditary hemolytic anemia NOS

√4th **283 Acquired hemolytic anemias**
DEF: Non-hereditary anemia characterized by premature destruction of red blood cells; caused by infectious organisms, poisons, and physical agents.

283.0 Autoimmune hemolytic anemias
Autoimmune hemolytic disease (cold type) (warm type)
Chronic cold hemagglutinin disease
Cold agglutinin disease or hemoglobinuria
Hemolytic anemia:
    cold type (secondary) (symptomatic)
    drug-induced
    warm type (secondary) (symptomatic)
Use additional E code to identify cause, if drug-induced
EXCLUDES Evans' syndrome (287.3)
    hemolytic disease of newborn (773.0-773.5)

√5th **283.1 Non-autoimmune hemolytic anemias**
Use additional E code to identify cause

DEF: Hemolytic anemia and thrombocytopenia with acute renal failure; relatively rare condition; 50 percent of patients require renal dialysis.

283.10 Non-autoimmune hemolytic anemia, unspecified

283.11 Hemolytic-uremic syndrome

283.19 Other non-autoimmune hemolytic anemias
Hemolytic anemia:
    mechanical
    microangiopathic
    toxic

283.2 Hemoglobinuria due to hemolysis from external causes
Acute intravascular hemolysis
Hemoglobinuria:
    from exertion
    march
    paroxysmal (cold) (nocturnal)
    due to other hemolysis
Marchiafava-Micheli syndrome
Use additional E code to identify cause

283.9 Acquired hemolytic anemia, unspecified
Acquired hemolytic anemia NOS
Chronic idiopathic hemolytic anemia

√4th **284 Aplastic anemia**
DEF: Bone marrow failure to produce the normal amount of blood components; generally non-responsive to usual therapy.

284.0 Constitutional aplastic anemia
Aplasia, (pure) red cell:
    congenital
    of infants
    primary
Blackfan-Diamond syndrome
Familial hypoplastic anemia
Fanconi's anemia
Pancytopenia with malformations

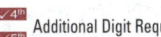 Additional Digit Required   Unspecified Code   Other Specified Code   Manifestation Code

MSP Medicare Secondary Payer   ▶◀ Revised Text   ● New Code   ▲ Revised Code Title

2002 Ingenix, Inc.   Volume 1 — 125

284.8 Other specified aplastic anemias
　　Aplastic anemia (due to):
　　　chronic systemic disease
　　　drugs
　　　infection
　　　radiation
　　　toxic (paralytic)
　　Pancytopenia (acquired)
　　Red cell aplasia (acquired) (adult) (pure) (with thymoma)
　　Use additional E code to identify cause

284.9 Aplastic anemia, unspecified
　　Anemia:　　　　　　　　　　Anemia:
　　　aplastic (idiopathic) NOS　　nonregenerative
　　　aregenerative　　　　　　　refractory
　　　hypoplastic NOS　　　　　　Medullary hypoplasia

✓4th **285 Other and unspecified anemias**

　285.0 Sideroblastic anemia
　　Anemia:
　　　hypochromic with iron loading
　　　sideroachrestic
　　　sideroblastic
　　　　acquired
　　　　congenital
　　　　hereditary
　　　　primary
　　　　refractory
　　　　secondary (drug-induced) (due to disease)
　　　　sex-linked hypochromic
　　　　vitamin B_6-responsive
　　Pyridoxine-responsive (hypochromic) anemia
　　Use additional E code to identify cause, if drug induced

　　DEF: Characterized by a disruption of final heme synthesis; results in iron overload of reticuloendothelial tissues.

　285.1 Acute posthemorrhagic anemia
　　Anemia due to acute blood loss
　　　EXCLUDES　anemia due to chronic blood loss (280.0)
　　　　　　　　blood loss anemia NOS (280.0)

✓5th **285.2 Anemia in chronic illness**
　　285.21 Anemia in end-stage renal disease
　　285.22 Anemia in neoplastic disease
　　285.29 Anemia of other chronic illness

　285.8 Other specified anemias
　　Anemia:　　　　　　　　　　Anemia:
　　　dyserythropoietic　　　　　leukoerythroblastic
　　　　(congenital)　　　　　　von Jaksch's
　　　dyshematopoietic　　　　Infantile pseudoleukemia
　　　　(congenital)

　285.9 Anemia, unspecified
　　Anemia:　　　　　　　　　　Anemia:
　　　NOS　　　　　　　　　　　profound
　　　essential　　　　　　　　　progressive
　　　normocytic, not　　　　　　secondary
　　　　due to blood loss　　　　Oligocythemia
　　　EXCLUDES　anemia (due to):
　　　　　　　　　blood loss:
　　　　　　　　　　acute (285.1)
　　　　　　　　　　chronic or unspecified (280.0)
　　　　　　　　　iron deficiency (280.0-280.9)

BLOOD AND BLOOD-FORMING ORGANS

✓4th 286 Coagulation defects

286.0 Congenital factor VIII disorder
Antihemophilic globulin [AHG] deficiency
Factor VIII (functional) deficiency
Hemophilia:
- NOS
- A
- classical
- familial
- hereditary

Subhemophilia

> **EXCLUDES** *factor VIII deficiency with vascular defect (286.4)*

DEF: Hereditary, sex-linked, results in missing antihemophilic globulin (AHG) (factor VIII); causes abnormal coagulation characterized by increased tendency to bleeding, large bruises of skin, soft tissue; may also be bleeding in mouth, nose, gastrointestinal tract; after childhood, hemorrhages in joints, resulting in swelling and impaired function.

286.1 Congenital factor IX disorder
Christmas disease
Deficiency:
- factor IX (functional)
- plasma thromboplastin component [PTC]

Hemophilia B

DEF: Deficiency of plasma thromboplastin component (PTC) (factor IX) and plasma thromboplastin antecedent (PTA); PTC deficiency clinically indistinguishable from classical hemophilia; PTA deficiency found in both sexes.

286.2 Congenital factor XI deficiency
Hemophilia C
Plasma thromboplastin antecedent [PTA] deficiency
Rosenthal's disease

286.3 Congenital deficiency of other clotting factors
Congenital afibrinogenemia
Deficiency:
- AC globulin factor:
  - I [fibrinogen]
  - II [prothrombin]
  - V [labile]
  - VII [stable]
  - X [Stuart-Prower]
  - XII [Hageman]
  - XIII [fibrin stabilizing]
- Laki-Lorand factor
- proaccelerin

Disease
- Owren's
- Stuart-Prower

Dysfibrinogenemia (congenital)
Dysprothrombinemia (constitutional)
Hypoproconvertinemia
Hypoprothrmbinemia (hereditary)
Parahemophilia

BLOOD AND BLOOD-FORMING ORGANS

286.4 von Willebrand's disease
Angiohemophilia (A) (B)
Constitutional thrombopathy
Factor VIII deficiency with vascular defect
Pseudohemophilia type B
Vascular hemophilia
von Willebrand's (-Jürgens') disease
> EXCLUDES factor VIII deficiency:
> NOS (286.0)
> with functional defect (286.0)
> hereditary capillary fragility (287.8)

DEF: Abnormal blood coagulation caused by deficient blood Factor VII; congenital; symptoms include excess or prolonged bleeding, such as hemorrhage during menstruation, following birthing, or after surgical procedure.

286.5 Hemorrhagic disorder due to circulating anticoagulants
Antithrombinemia
Antithromboplastinemia
Antithromboplastino-genemia
Hyperheparinemia
Increase in:
  anti-VIIIa
  anti-IXa
  anti-Xa
  anti-XIa
  antithrombin
Systemic lupus erythematosus [SLE] inhibitor
Use additional E code to identify cause, if drug induced

286.6 Defibrination syndrome
Afibrinogenemia, acquired
Consumption coagulopathy
Diffuse or disseminated intravascular coagulation [DIC syndrome]
Fibrinolytic hemorrhage, acquired
Hemorrhagic fibrinogenolysis
Pathologic fibrinolysis
Purpura:
  fibrinolytic
  fulminans
> EXCLUDES that complicating:
> abortion (634-638 with .1, 639.1)
> pregnancy or the puerperium (641.3, 666.3)
> disseminated intravascular coagulation in newborn (776.2)

DEF: Characterized by destruction of circulating fibrinogen; often precipitated by other conditions, such as injury, causing release of thromboplastic particles in blood stream.

286.7 Acquired coagulation factor deficiency
Deficiency of coagulation factor due to:
  liver disease
  vitamin K deficiency
Hypoprothrombinemia, acquired
Use additional E code to identify cause, if drug induced
> EXCLUDES vitamin K deficiency of newborn (776.0)

BLOOD AND BLOOD-FORMING ORGANS

286.9 Other and unspecified coagulation defects
Defective coagulation NOS
Deficiency, coagulation factor NOS
Delay, coagulation
Disorder:
  coagulation
  hemostasis
  EXCLUDES abnormal coagulation profile (790.92)
            hemorrhagic disease of newborn (776.0)
            that complicating:
              abortion (634-638 with .1, 639.1)
              pregnancy or the puerperium (641.3, 666.3)

√4th **287 Purpura and other hemorrhagic conditions**
  EXCLUDES hemorrhagic thrombocythemia (238.7)
            purpura fulminans (286.6)

287.0 Allergic purpura
Peliosis rheumatica   Purpura:
Purpura: rheumatica
  anaphylactoid   Schönlein-Henoch
  autoimmune   vascular
  Henoch's   Vasculitis, allergic
  nonthrombocytopenic:
    hemorrhagic
    idiopathic
  EXCLUDES hemorrhagic purpura (287.3)
            purpura annularis telangiectodes (709.1)

DEF: Any hemorrhagic condition, thrombocytic or nonthrombocytopenic in origin, caused by a presumed allergic reaction.

287.1 Qualitative platelet defects
Thrombasthenia (hemorrhagic) (hereditary)
Thrombocytasthenia
Thrombocytopathy (dystrophic)
Thrombopathy (Bernard-Soulier)
  EXCLUDES von Willebrand's disease (286.4)

287.2 Other nonthrombocytopenic purpuras
Purpura:
  NOS
  senile
  simplex

287.3 Primary thrombocytopenia
Evans' syndrome
Megakaryocytic hypoplasia
Purpura, thrombocytopenic
  congenital
  hereditary
  idiopathic
Throbocytopenia:
  congenital
  hereditary
  primary
Tidal platelet dysgenesis
  EXCLUDES thrombotic thrombocytopenic purpura (446.6)
            transient thrombocytopenia of newborn (776.1)

DEF: Decrease in number of blood platelets in circulating blood and purpural skin hemorrhages.

287.4 Secondary thrombocytopenia
　　Posttransfusion purpura
　　Thrombocytopenia (due to):
　　　dilutional
　　　drugs
　　　extracorporeal circulation of blood
　　　platelet alloimmunization
　　Use additional E code to identify cause
　　　EXCLUDES　transient thrombocytopenia of newborn (776.1)
DEF: Reduced number of platelets in circulating blood as consequence of an underlying disease or condition.

287.5 Thrombocytopenia, unspecified
287.8 Other specified hemorrhagic conditions
　　Capillary fragility (hereditary)
　　Vascular pseudohemophilia
287.9 Unspecified hemorrhagic conditions
　　Hemorrhagic diathesis (familial)

✓4th 288 Diseases of white blood cells
　　EXCLUDES　leukemia (204.0-208.9)

288.0 Agranulocytosis
　　Infantile genetic agranulocytosis
　　Kostmann's syndrome
　　Neutropenia:
　　　NOS
　　　cyclic
　　　drug-induced
　　　immune
　　　periodic
　　　toxic
　　Neutropenic splenomegaly
　　Use additional E code to identify drug or other cause
　　　EXCLUDES　transitory neonatal neutropenia (776.7)
DEF: Sudden, severe condition characterized by reduced number of white blood cells; results in sores in the throat, stomach or skin; symptoms include chills, fever; some drugs can bring on condition.

288.1 Functional disorders of polymorphonuclear neutrophils
　　Chronic (childhood) granulomatous disease
　　Congenital dysphagocytosis
　　Job's syndrome
　　Lipochrome histiocytosis (familial)
　　Progressive septic granulomatosis

288.2 Genetic anomalies of leukocytes
　　Anomaly (granulation) (granulocyte) or syndrome:
　　　Alder's (-Reilly)
　　　Chédiak-Steinbrinck (-Higashi)
　　　Jordan's
　　　May-Hegglin
　　　Pelger-Huet
　　Hereditary:
　　　hypersegmentation
　　　hyposegmentation
　　　leukomelanopathy

BLOOD AND BLOOD-FORMING ORGANS

288.3 Eosinophilia
Eosinophilia:
　allergic
　hereditary
　idiopathic
　secondary
Eosinophilic leukocytosis
> **EXCLUDES** Löffler's syndrome (518.3)
> pulmonary eosinophilia (518.3)

DEF: Elevated number of eosinophils in the blood; characteristic of allergic states and various parasitic infections.

288.8 Other specified disease of white blood cells
Leukemoid reaction
　lymphocytic
　monocytic
　myelocytic
Leukocytosis
Lymphocytopenia
Lymphocytosis (symptomatic)
Lymphopenia
Monocytosis (symptomatic)
Plasmacytosis
> **EXCLUDES** immunity disorders (279.0-279.9)

288.9 Unspecified disease of white blood cells

289 Other diseases of blood and blood-forming organs

289.0 Polycythemia, secondary
High-oxygen-affinity hemoglobin
Polycythemia:
　acquired
　benign
　due to:
　　fall in plasma volume
　　high altitude
　emotional
　erythropoietin
　hypoxemic
　nephrogenous
　relative
　spurious
　stress
> **EXCLUDES** polycythemia:
> 　neonatal (776.4)
> 　primary (238.4)
> 　vera (238.4)

DEF: Elevated number of red blood cells in circulating blood as result of reduced oxygen supply to the tissues.

289.1 Chronic lymphadenitis
Chronic:
　adenitis　　} any lymph node, except
　lymphadenitis}　mesenteric
> **EXCLUDES** acute lymphadenitis (683)
> mesenteric (289.2)
> enlarged glands NOS (785.6)

DEF: Persistent inflammation of lymph node tissue; origin of infection is usually elsewhere.

289.2 Nonspecific mesenteric lymphadenitis
Mesenteric lymphadenitis (acute) (chronic)
DEF: Inflammation of the lymph nodes in peritoneal fold that encases abdominal organs; disease resembles acute appendicitis; unknown etiology.

289.3 Lymphadenitis, unspecified, except mesenteric

289.4 Hypersplenism
"Big spleen" syndrome   Hypersplenia
Dyssplenism
> EXCLUDES   *primary splenic neutropenia (288.0)*

DEF: An overactive spleen; it causes a deficiency of the peripheral blood components, an increase in bone marrow cells and sometimes a notable increase in the size of the spleen.

√5th **289.5 Other diseases of spleen**

289.50 Disease of spleen, unspecified

289.51 Chronic congestive splenomegaly

289.59 Other
Lien migrans
Perisplenitis
Splenic:
   abscess
   atrophy
   cyst
Splenic:
   fibrosis
   infarction
   rupture, nontraumatic
Splenitis
Wandering spleen
> EXCLUDES   *bilharzial splenic fibrosis (120.0-120.9)*
> *hepatolienal fibrosis (571.5)*
> *splenomegaly NOS (789.2)*

289.6 Familial polycythemia
Familial:
   benign polycythemia
   erythrocytosis
DEF: Elevated number of red blood cells.

289.7 Methemoglobinemia
Congenital NADH [DPNH]-methemoglobin-reductase deficiency
Hemoglobin M [Hb-M] disease
Methemoglobinemia:
   NOS
   acquired (with sulfhemoglobinemia)
   hereditary
   toxic
Stokvis' disease
Sulfhemoglobinemia
Use additional E code to identify cause

DEF: Presence in the blood of methemoglobin, a chemically altered form of hemoglobin; causes cyanosis, headache, dizziness, ataxia dyspnea, tachycardia, nausea, stupor, coma, and, rarely, death.

289.8 Other specified diseases of blood and blood-forming organs
Hypergammaglobulinemia
Myelofibrosis
Pseudocholinesterase deficiency

289.9 Unspecified diseases of blood and blood-forming organs
Blood dyscrasia NOS
Erythroid hyperplasia

MENTAL DISORDERS

5. MENTAL DISORDERS (290-319)

In the *International Classification of Diseases, 9th Revision* (ICD-9), the corresponding Chapter V, "Mental Disorders," includes a glossary which defines the contents of each category. The introduction to Chapter V in ICD-9 indicates that the glossary is intended so that psychiatrists can make the diagnosis based on the descriptions provided rather than from the category titles. Lay coders are instructed to code whatever diagnosis the physician records.

Chapter 5, "Mental Disorders," in ICD-9-CM uses the standard classification format with inclusion and exclusion terms, omitting the glossary as part of the main text.

The mental disorders section of ICD-9-CM has been expanded to incorporate additional psychiatric disorders not listed in ICD-9. The glossary from ICD-9 does not contain all these terms. It now appears in Appendix B, which also contains descriptions and definitions for the terms added in ICD-9-CM. Some of these were provided by the American Psychiatric Association's Task Force on Nomenclature and Statistics who are preparing the Diagnostic and Statistical Manual, Third Edition (DSM-III), and others from A Psychiatric Glossary.

The American Psychiatric Association provided invaluable assistance in modifying Chapter 5 of ICD-9-CM to incorporate detail useful to American clinicians and gave permission to use material from the aforementioned sources.

1. Manual of the *International Statistical Classification of Diseases, Injuries, and Causes of Death*, 9th Revision, World Health Organization, Geneva, Switzerland, 1975.
2. American Psychiatric Association, Task Force on Nomenclature and Statistics, Robert L. Spitzer, M.D., Chairman.
3. *A Psychiatric Glossary*, Fourth Edition, American Psychiatric Association, Washington, D.C., 1975.

PSYCHOSES (290-299)

> **EXCLUDES** mental retardation (317-319)

ORGANIC PSYCHOTIC CONDITIONS (290-294)

> **INCLUDES** psychotic organic brain syndrome
>
> **EXCLUDES** nonpsychotic syndromes of organic etiology (310.0-310.9)
> psychoses classifiable to 295-298 and without impairment of orientation, comprehension, calculation, learning capacity, and judgment, but associated with physical disease, injury, or condition affecting the brain [eg., following childbirth] (295.0-298.8)

√4th 290 Senile and presenile organic psychotic conditions
Code first the associated neurological condition

> **EXCLUDES** dementia not classified as senile, presenile, or arteriosclerotic (294.10-294.11)
> psychoses classifiable to 295-298 occurring in the senium without dementia or delirium (295.0-298.8)
> senility with mental changes of nonpsychotic severity (310.1)
> transient organic psychotic conditions (293.0-293.9)

290.0 Senile dementia, uncomplicated ▲

Senile dementia: NOS
Senile dementia: simple type

> **EXCLUDES** mild memory disturbances, not amounting to dementia, associated with senile brain disease (310.1)
> senile dementia with:
> delirium or confusion (290.3)
> delusional [paranoid] features (290.20)
> depressive features (290.21)

MENTAL DISORDERS

√5th 290.1 Presenile dementia
Brain syndrome with presenile brain disease
EXCLUDES arteriosclerotic dementia (290.40-290.43)
dementia associated with other cerebral conditions (294.10-294.11)

290.10 Presenile dementia, uncomplicated Ⓐ
Presenile dementia:
NOS
simple type

290.11 Presenile dementia with delirium Ⓐ
Presenile dementia with acute confusional state

290.12 Presenile dementia with delusional features Ⓐ
Presenile dementia, paranoid type

290.13 Presenile dementia with depressive features Ⓐ
Presenile dementia, depressed type

√5th 290.2 Senile dementia with delusional or depressive features
EXCLUDES senile dementia:
NOS (290.0)
with delirium and/or confusion (290.3)

290.20 Senile dementia with delusional features Ⓐ
Senile dementia, paranoid type
Senile psychosis NOS

290.21 Senile dementia with depressive features Ⓐ

290.3 Senile dementia with delirium Ⓐ
Senile dementia with acute confusional state
EXCLUDES senile:
dementia NOS (290.0)
psychosis NOS (290.20)

√5th 290.4 Arteriosclerotic dementia
Multi-infarct dementia or psychosis
Use additional code to identify cerebral atherosclerosis (437.0)
EXCLUDES suspected cases with no clear evidence of arteriosclerosis (290.9)

290.40 Arteriosclerotic dementia, uncomplicated Ⓐ
Arteriosclerotic dementia:
NOS
simple type

290.41 Arteriosclerotic dementia with delirium Ⓐ
Arteriosclerotic dementia with acute confusional state

290.42 Arteriosclerotic dementia with delusional features Ⓐ
Arteriosclerotic dementia, paranoid type

290.43 Arteriosclerotic dementia with depressive features Ⓐ
Arteriosclerotic dementia, depressed type

290.8 Other specified senile psychotic conditions
Presbyophrenic psychosis

290.9 Unspecified senile psychotic condition Ⓐ

√4th 291 Alcoholic psychoses
EXCLUDES alcoholism without psychosis (303.0-303.9)

291.0 Alcohol withdrawal delirium
Alcoholic delirium   Delirium tremens
EXCLUDES alcohol withdrawal (291.81)

291.1 Alcohol amnestic syndrome
Alcoholic polyneuritic psychosis
Korsakoff's psychosis, alcoholic
Wernicke-Korsakoff syndrome (alcoholic)
DEF: Prominent and lasting reduced memory span, disordered time appreciation and confabulation, occurring in alcoholics, as sequel to acute alcoholic psychosis.

Ⓝ Newborn Age: 0   Ⓟ Pediatric Age: 0-17   Ⓜ Maternity Age: 12-55   Ⓐ Adult Age: 15-124

MENTAL DISORDERS 291.2–292.11

291.2 Other alcoholic dementia
    Alcoholic dementia NOS
    Alcoholism associated with dementia NOS
    Chronic alcoholic brain syndrome

291.3 Alcohol withdrawal hallucinosis
    Alcoholic: Alcoholic:
      hallucinosis (acute)   psychosis with hallucinosis
    EXCLUDES alcohol withdrawal with delirium (291.0)
          schizophrenia (295.0-295.9) and paranoid states (297.0-297.9) taking the form of chronic hallucinosis with clear consciousness in an alcoholic

DEF: Psychosis lasting less than six months with slight or no clouding of consciousness in which auditory hallucinations predominate.

291.4 Idiosyncratic alcohol intoxication
    Pathologic:
      alcohol intoxication
      drunkenness
    EXCLUDES acute alcohol intoxication (305.0)
          in alcoholism (303.0)
          simple drunkenness (305.0)

DEF: Unique behavioral patterns, like belligerence, after intake of relatively small amounts of alcohol; behavior not due to excess consumption.

291.5 Alcoholic jealousy
    Alcoholic:
      paranoia
      psychosis, paranoid type
    EXCLUDES nonalcoholic paranoid states (297.0-297.9)
          schizophrenia, paranoid type (295.3)

√5th **291.8 Other specified alcoholic psychosis**
    291.81 Alcohol withdrawal
      Alcohol:
        abstinence syndrome or symptoms
        withdrawal syndrome or symptoms
      EXCLUDES alcohol withdrawal:
            delirium (291.0)
            hallucinosis (291.3)
            delirium tremens (291.0)
    291.89 Other

291.9 Unspecified alcoholic psychosis
    Alcoholic:
      mania NOS
      psychosis NOS
    Alcoholism (chronic) with psychosis

√4th **292 Drug psychoses**
    INCLUDES drug-induced mental disorders
          organic brain syndrome associated with consumption of drugs
    Use additional code for any associated drug dependence (304.0-304.9)
    Use additional E code to identify drug

    292.0 Drug withdrawal syndrome
      Drug:
        abstinence syndrome or symptoms
        withdrawal syndrome or symptoms

√5th **292.1 Paranoid and/or hallucinatory states induced by drugs**
    292.11 Drug-induced organic delusional syndrome
      Paranoid state induced by drugs

√4th / √5th Additional Digit Required   Unspecified Code   Other Specified Code   Manifestation Code
MSP Medicare Secondary Payer   ▶◀ Revised Text   ● New Code   ▲ Revised Code Title

2002 Ingenix, Inc.

292.12 Drug-induced hallucinosis
Hallucinatory state induced by drugs
> **EXCLUDES** states following LSD or other hallucinogens, lasting only a few days or less ["bad trips"] (305.3)

292.2 Pathological drug intoxication
Drug reaction:
- NOS
- idiosyncratic
- pathologic

} resulting in brief psychotic states

> **EXCLUDES** expected brief psychotic reactions to hallucinogens ["bad trips"] (305.3)
> physiological side-effects of drugs (e.g., dystonias)

√5th **292.8 Other specified drug-induced mental disorders**
292.81 Drug-induced delirium
292.82 Drug-induced dementia
292.83 Drug-induced amnestic syndrome
292.84 Drug-induced organic affective syndrome
Depressive state induced by drugs
292.89 Other
Drug-induced organic personality syndrome
292.9 Unspecified drug-induced mental disorder
Organic psychosis NOS due to or associated with drugs

√4th **293 Transient organic psychotic conditions**
> **INCLUDES** transient organic mental disorders not associated with alcohol or drugs

Code first the associated physical or neurological condition
> **EXCLUDES** confusional state or delirium superimposed on senile dementia (290.3)
> dementia due to:
>   alcohol (291.0-291.9)
>   arteriosclerosis (290.40-290.43)
>   drugs (292.82)
>   senility (290.0)

293.0 Acute delirium
Acute:
- confusional state
- infective psychosis
- organic reaction
- posttraumatic organic psychosis
- psycho-organic syndrome

Acute psychosis associated with endocrine, metabolic, or cerebrovascular disorder
Epileptic:
- confusional state
- twilight state

293.1 Subacute delirium
Subacute:
- confusional state
- infective psychosis
- organic reaction
- posttraumatic organic psychosis
- psycho-organic syndrome

psychosis associated with endocrine or metabolic disorder

√5th **293.8 Other specified transient organic mental disorders**
293.81 Organic delusional syndrome
Transient organic psychotic condition, paranoid type
293.82 Organic hallucinosis syndrome
Transient organic psychotic condition, hallucinatory type

MENTAL DISORDERS 293.83–294.9

- **293.83 Organic affective syndrome**
  Transient organic psychotic condition, depressive type
- **293.84 Organic anxiety syndrome**
- **293.89 Other**
- **293.9 Unspecified transient organic mental disorder**
  Organic psychosis:
    infective NOS
    posttraumatic NOS
    transient NOS
  Psycho-organic syndrome

✓4th **294 Other organic psychotic conditions (chronic)**
  INCLUDES organic psychotic brain syndromes (chronic), not elsewhere classified

- **294.0 Amnestic syndrome**
  Korsakoff's psychosis or syndrome (nonalcoholic)
  EXCLUDES alcoholic:
      amnestic syndrome (291.1)
      Korsakoff's psychosis (291.1)

✓5th **294.1 Dementia in conditions classified elsewhere**
  Code first any underlying physical condition, as:
  dementia in:
    Alzheimer's disease (331.0)
    cerebral lipidoses (330.1)
    epilepsy (345.0-345.9)
    general paresis [syphilis] (094.1)
    hepatolenticular degeneration (275.1)
    Huntington's chorea (333.4)
    Jakob-Creutzfeldt disease (046.1)
    multiple sclerosis (340)
    Pick's disease of the brain (331.1)
    polyarteritis nodosa (446.0)
    syphilis (094.1)
  EXCLUDES *dementia:*
      arteriosclerotic (290.40-290.43)
      presenile (290.10-290.13)
      senile (290.0)
      epileptic psychosis NOS (294.8)

- **294.10 Dementia in conditions classified elsewhere without behavioral disturbance**
  Dementia in conditions classified elsewhere NOS
- **294.11 Dementia in conditions classified elsewhere with behavioral disturbance**
  Aggressive behavior   Violent behavior
  Combative behavior   Wandering off

- **294.8 Other specified organic brain syndromes (chronic)**
  Epileptic psychosis NOS
  Mixed paranoid and affective organic psychotic states
  Use additional code for associated epilepsy (345.0-345.9)
  EXCLUDES *mild memory disturbances, not amounting to dementia (310.1)*

- **294.9 Unspecified organic brain syndrome (chronic)**
  Organic psychosis (chronic)

MENTAL DISORDERS

OTHER PSYCHOSES (295-299)

Use additional code to identify any associated physical disease, injury, or condition affecting the brain with psychoses classifiable to 295-298

295 Schizophrenic disorders

INCLUDES: schizophrenia of the types described in 295.0-295.9 occurring in children

EXCLUDES: childhood type schizophrenia (299.9)
infantile autism (299.0)

The following fifth-digit subclassification is for use with category 295:
- 0 unspecified
- 1 subchronic
- 2 chronic
- 3 subchronic with acute exacerbation
- 4 chronic with acute exacerbation
- 5 in remission

DEF: Group of disorders with disturbances in thought (delusions, hallucinations), mood (blunted, flattened, inappropriate affect), sense of self, relationship to world; also bizarre, purposeless behavior, repetitious activity, or inactivity.

295.0 Simple type
Schizophrenia simplex

EXCLUDES: latent schizophrenia (295.5)

295.1 Disorganized type
Hebephrenia   Hebephrenic type schizophrenia

DEF: Inappropriate behavior; results in extreme incoherence and disorganization of time, place and sense of social appropriateness; withdrawal from routine social interaction may occur.

295.2 Catatonic type
Catatonic (schizophrenia):   Schizophrenic:
  agitation   catalepsy
  excitation   catatonia
  excited type   flexibilitas cerea
  stupor
  withdrawn type

DEF: Extreme changes in motor activity; one extreme is decreased response or reaction to the environment and the other is spontaneous activity.

295.3 Paranoid type
Paraphrenic schizophrenia

EXCLUDES: involutional paranoid state (297.2)
paranoia (297.1)
paraphrenia (297.2)

DEF: Preoccupied with delusional suspicions and auditory hallucinations related to single theme; usually hostile, grandiose, overly religious, occasionally hypochondriacal.

295.4 Acute schizophrenic episode
Oneirophrenia   Schizophreniform:
Schizophreniform: disorder
  attack   psychosis, confusional type

EXCLUDES: acute forms of schizophrenia of:
catatonic type (295.2)
hebephrenic type (295.1)
paranoid type (295.3)
simple type (295.0)
undifferentiated type (295.8)

MENTAL DISORDERS

√5ᵗʰ 295.5 Latent schizophrenia
Latent schizophrenic reaction
Schizophrenia:
- borderline
- incipient
- prepsychotic
- prodromal
- pseudoneurotic
- pseudopsychopathic

EXCLUDES schizoid personality (301.20-301.22)

√5ᵗʰ 295.6 Residual schizophrenia
Chronic undifferentiated schizophrenia
Restzustand (schizophrenic)
Schizophrenic residual state

√5ᵗʰ 295.7 Schizo-affective type
Cyclic schizophrenia
Mixed schizophrenic and affective psychosis
Schizo-affective psychosis
Schizophreniform psychosis, affective type

√5ᵗʰ 295.8 Other specified types of schizophrenia
Acute (undifferentiated) schizophrenia
Atypical schizophrenia
Cenesthopathic schizophrenia

EXCLUDES infantile autism (299.0)

√5ᵗʰ 295.9 Unspecified schizophrenia
Schizophrenia:
- NOS
- mixed NOS
- undifferentiated NOS

Schizophrenic reaction NOS
Schizophreniform psychosis NOS

√4ᵗʰ 296 Affective psychoses

INCLUDES episodic affective disorders
EXCLUDES neurotic depression (300.4)
reactive depressive psychosis (298.0)
reactive excitation (298.1)

The following fifth-digit subclassification is for use with categories 296.0-296.6:
- 0 unspecified
- 1 mild
- 2 moderate
- 3 severe, without mention of psychotic behavior
- 4 severe, specified as with psychotic behavior
- 5 in partial or unspecified remission
- 6 in full remission

√5ᵗʰ 296.0 Manic disorder, single episode
Hypomania (mild) NOS
Hypomanic psychosis
Mania (monopolar) NOS
Manic-depressive psychosis or reaction:
- hypomanic
- manic

} single episode or unspecified

EXCLUDES circular type, if there was a previous attack of depression (296.4)

DEF: Mood disorder identified by hyperactivity; may show extreme agitation or exaggerated excitability; speech and thought processes may be accelerated.

MENTAL DISORDERS

§ ✓5th 296.1 Manic disorder, recurrent episode
Any condition classifiable to 296.0, stated to be recurrent
EXCLUDES *circular type, if there was a previous attack of depression (296.4)*

§ ✓5th 296.2 Major depressive disorder, single episode
Depressive psychosis
Endogenous depression
Involutional melancholia
Manic-depressive psychosis
  or reaction,
  depressed type
Monopolar depression
Psychotic depression
} single episode or unspecified

EXCLUDES *circular type, if previous attack was of manic type (296.5)*
depression NOS (311)
reactive depression (neurotic) (300.4)
psychotic (298.0)

DEF: Mood disorder that produces depression; may exhibit as sadness, low self-esteem, or guilt feelings; other manifestations may be withdrawal from friends and family; interrupted normal sleep.

§ ✓5th 296.3 Major depressive disorder, recurrent episode
Any condition classifiable to 296.2, stated to be recurrent
EXCLUDES *circular type, if previous attack was of manic type (296.5)*
depression NOS (311)
reactive depression (neurotic) (300.4)
psychotic (298.0)

§ ✓5th 296.4 Bipolar affective disorder, manic
Bipolar disorder, now manic
Manic-depressive psychosis, circular type but currently manic
EXCLUDES *brief compensatory or rebound mood swings (296.99)*

§ ✓5th 296.5 Bipolar affective disorder, depressed
Bipolar disorder, now depressed
Manic-depressive psychosis, circular type but currently depressed
EXCLUDES *brief compensatory or rebound mood swings (296.99)*

§ ✓5th 296.6 Bipolar affective disorder, mixed
Manic-depressive psychosis, circular type, mixed

296.7 Bipolar affective disorder, unspecified
Atypical bipolar affective disorder NOS
Manic-depressive psychosis, circular type, current condition not specified as either manic or depressive

DEF: Manic-depressive disorder referred to as bipolar because of the mood range from manic to depressive.

✓5th 296.8 Manic-depressive psychosis, other and unspecified
  296.80 Manic-depressive psychosis, unspecified
    Manic-depressive: Manic-depressive:
      reaction NOS   syndrome NOS
  296.81 Atypical manic disorder
  296.82 Atypical depressive disorder
  296.89 Other
    Manic-depressive psychosis, mixed type

✓5th 296.9 Other and unspecified affective psychoses
EXCLUDES *psychogenic affective psychoses (298.0-298.8)*

§ Requires fifth-digit. See beginning of category 296 for codes and definitions.

MENTAL DISORDERS

296.90 Unspecified affective psychosis
Affective psychosis NOS
Melancholia NOS

296.99 Other specified affective psychoses
Mood swings:
 brief compensatory
 rebound

297 Paranoid states (Delusional disorders)
INCLUDES paranoid disorders
EXCLUDES acute paranoid reaction (298.3)
 alcoholic jealousy or paranoid state (291.5)
 paranoid schizophrenia (295.3)

297.0 Paranoid state, simple

297.1 Paranoia
Chronic paranoid psychosis
Sander's disease
Systematized delusions
EXCLUDES paranoid personality disorder (301.0)

297.2 Paraphrenia
Involutional paranoid state   Paraphrenia (involutional)
Late paraphrenia

DEF: Paranoid schizophrenic disorder that persists over a prolonged period but does not distort personality despite persistent delusions.

297.3 Shared paranoid disorder
Folie à deux   Induced psychosis or paranoid disorder

DEF: Mental disorder two people share; first person with the delusional disorder convinces second person because of a close relationship and shared experiences to accept the delusions.

297.8 Other specified paranoid states
Paranoia querulans
Sensitiver Beziehungswahn
EXCLUDES acute paranoid reaction or state (298.3)
 senile paranoid state (290.20)

297.9 Unspecified paranoid state
Paranoid: Paranoid:
 disorder NOS   reaction NOS
 psychosis NOS   state NOS

298 Other nonorganic psychoses
INCLUDES psychotic conditions due to or provoked by:
 emotional stress
 environmental factors as major part of etiology

298.0 Depressive type psychosis
Psychogenic depressive psychosis
Psychotic reactive depression
Reactive depressive psychosis
EXCLUDES manic-depressive psychosis, depressed type (296.2-296.3)
 neurotic depression (300.4)
 reactive depression NOS (300.4)

298.1 Excitative type psychosis
Acute hysterical psychosis   Reactive excitation
Psychogenic excitation
EXCLUDES manic-depressive psychosis, manic type (296.0-296.1)

DEF: Affective disorder similar to manic-depressive psychosis, in the manic phase, seemingly brought on by stress.

  Additional Digit Required
MSP Medicare Secondary Payer   ▶◀ Revised Text   ● New Code   ▲ Revised Code Title
Unspecified Code   Other Specified Code   Manifestation Code

298.2 Reactive confusion
Psychogenic confusion
Psychogenic twilight state
EXCLUDES acute confusional state (293.0)

DEF: Confusion, disorientation, cloudiness in consciousness; brought on by severe emotional upheaval.

298.3 Acute paranoid reaction
Acute psychogenic paranoid psychosis
Bouffée délirante
EXCLUDES paranoid states (297.0-297.9)

298.4 Psychogenic paranoid psychosis
Protracted reactive paranoid psychosis

298.8 Other and unspecified reactive psychosis
Brief reactive psychosis NOS
Hysterical psychosis
Psychogenic psychosis NOS
Psychogenic stupor
EXCLUDES acute hysterical psychosis (298.1)

298.9 Unspecified psychosis
Atypical psychosis
Psychosis NOS

√4th 299 Psychoses with origin specific to childhood
INCLUDES pervasive developmental disorders
EXCLUDES adult type psychoses occurring in childhood, as:
 affective disorders (296.0-296.9)
 manic-depressive disorders (296.0-296.9)
 schizophrenia (295.0-295.9)

The following fifth-digit subclassification is for use with category 299:
 0 current or active state
 1 residual state

√5th 299.0 Infantile autism
Childhood autism   Kanner's syndrome
Infantile psychosis
EXCLUDES disintegrative psychosis (299.1)
 Heller's syndrome (299.1)
 schizophrenic syndrome of childhood (299.9)

DEF: Severe mental disorder of children, results in impaired social behavior; abnormal development of communicative skills, appears to be unaware of the need for emotional support and offers little emotional response to family members.

√5th 299.1 Disintegrative psychosis
Heller's syndrome
Use additional code to identify any associated neurological disorder
EXCLUDES infantile autism (299.0)
 schizophrenic syndrome of childhood (299.9)

DEF: Mental disease of children identified by impaired development of reciprocal social skills, verbal and nonverbal communication skills, imaginative play.

√5th 299.8 Other specified early childhood psychoses
Atypical childhood psychosis
Borderline psychosis of childhood
EXCLUDES simple stereotypes without psychotic disturbance (307.3)

MENTAL DISORDERS

✓5ᵗʰ **299.9 Unspecified**
　　Child psychosis NOS
　　Schizophrenia, childhood type NOS
　　Schizophrenic syndrome of childhood NOS
　　　EXCLUDES *schizophrenia of adult type occurring in childhood (295.0-295.9)*

NEUROTIC DISORDERS, PERSONALITY DISORDERS, AND OTHER NONPSYCHOTIC MENTAL DISORDERS (300-316)

✓4ᵗʰ **300 Neurotic disorders**

✓5ᵗʰ **300.0 Anxiety states**
　　　EXCLUDES *anxiety in:*
　　　　　acute stress reaction (308.0)
　　　　　transient adjustment reaction (309.24)
　　　　neurasthenia (300.5)
　　　　psychophysiological disorders (306.0-306.9)
　　　　separation anxiety (309.21)

DEF: Mental disorder characterized by anxiety and avoidance behavior not particularly related to any specific situation or stimulus; symptoms include emotional instability, apprehension, fatigue.

300.00 Anxiety state, unspecified
　　Anxiety:　　　　Anxiety:
　　　neurosis　　　　state (neurotic)
　　　reaction　　　Atypical anxiety disorder

300.01 Panic disorder
　　Panic:
　　　attack
　　　state

DEF: Neurotic disorder characterized by recurrent panic or anxiety, apprehension, fear or terror; symptoms include shortness of breath, palpitations, dizziness, faintness or shakiness; fear of dying may persist or fear of other morbid consequences.

300.02 Generalized anxiety disorder

300.09 Other

✓5ᵗʰ **300.1 Hysteria**
　　　EXCLUDES *adjustment reaction (309.0-309.9)*
　　　　anorexia nervosa (307.1)
　　　　gross stress reaction (308.0-308.9)
　　　　hysterical personality (301.50-301.59)
　　　　psychophysiologic disorders (306.0-306.9)

300.10 Hysteria, unspecified

300.11 Conversion disorder
　　Astasia-abasia, hysterical
　　Conversion hysteria or reaction
　　Hysterical
　　　blindness
　　　deafness
　　　paralysis

DEF: Mental disorder that impairs physical functions with no physiological basis; sensory motor symptoms include seizures, paralysis, temporary blindness; increase in stress or avoidance of unpleasant responsibilities may precipitate.

300.12 Psychogenic amnesia
　　Hysterical amnesia

✓4ᵗʰ
✓5ᵗʰ Additional Digit Required　　　Unspecified Code　　　Other Specified Code　　　Manifestation Code

 Medicare Secondary Payer　　▶◀ Revised Text　　● New Code　　▲ Revised Code Title

2002 Ingenix, Inc.

MENTAL DISORDERS

300.13 Psychogenic fugue
Hysterical fugue
DEF: Dissociative hysteria; identified by loss of memory, flight from familiar surroundings; conscious activity is not associated with perception of surroundings, no later memory of episode.

300.14 Multiple personality
Dissociative identity disorder

300.15 Dissociative disorder or reaction, unspecified
DEF: Hysterical neurotic episode; sudden but temporary changes in perceived identity, memory, consciousness, segregated memory patterns exist separate from dominant personality.

300.16 Factitious illness with psychological symptoms
Compensation neurosis
Ganser's syndrome, hysterical
DEF: A disorder characterized by the purposeful assumption of mental illness symptoms; the symptoms are not real, possibly representing what the patient imagines mental illness to be like, and are acted out more often when another person is present.

300.19 Other and unspecified factitious illness
Factitious illness (with physical symptoms) NOS
EXCLUDES multiple operations or hospital addiction syndrome (301.51)

✓5th **300.2 Phobic disorders**
EXCLUDES anxiety state not associated with a specific situation or object (300.00-300.09)
obsessional phobias (300.3)

300.20 Phobia, unspecified
Anxiety-hysteria NOS
Phobia NOS

300.21 Agoraphobia with panic attacks
Fear of:
  open spaces ⎫
  streets   ⎬ with panic attacks
  travel   ⎭

300.22 Agoraphobia without mention of panic attacks
Any condition classifiable to 300.21 without mention of panic attacks

300.23 Social phobia
Fear of: Fear of:
  eating in public   washing in public
  public speaking

300.29 Other isolated or simple phobias
Acrophobia   Claustrophobia
Animal phobias   Fear of crowds

300.3 Obsessive-compulsive disorders
Anancastic neurosis   Obsessional phobia [any]
Compulsive neurosis
EXCLUDES obsessive-compulsive symptoms occurring in:
  endogenous depression (296.2-296.3)
  organic states (eg., encephalitis)
  schizophrenia (295.0-295.9)

MENTAL DISORDERS

300.4 Neurotic depression
Anxiety depression
Depression with anxiety
Depressive reaction
Dysthymic disorder
Neurotic depressive state
Reactive depression

> **EXCLUDES** adjustment reaction with depressive symptoms (309.0-309.1)
> depression NOS (311)
> manic-depressive psychosis, depressed type (296.2-296.3)
> reactive depressive psychosis (298.0)

DEF: Depression without psychosis; less severe depression related to personal change or unexpected circumstances; also referred to as "reactional depression."

300.5 Neurasthenia
Fatigue neurosis
Nervous debility
Psychogenic:
   asthenia
   general fatigue
Use additional code to identify any associated physical disorder

> **EXCLUDES** anxiety state (300.00-300.09)
> neurotic depression (300.4)
> psychophysiological disorders (306.0-306.9)
> specific nonpsychotic mental disorders following organic brain damage (310.0-310.9)

DEF: Physical and mental symptoms caused primarily by what is known as mental exhaustion; symptoms include chronic weakness, fatigue.

300.6 Depersonalization syndrome
Depersonalization disorder
Derealization (neurotic)
Neurotic state with depersonalization episode

> **EXCLUDES** depersonalization associated with:
> anxiety (300.00-300.09)
> depression (300.4)
> manic-depressive disorder or psychosis (296.0-296.9)
> schizophrenia (295.0-295.9)

DEF: Dissociative disorder characterized by feelings of strangeness about self or body image; symptoms include dizziness, anxiety, fear of insanity, loss of reality of surroundings.

300.7 Hypochondriasis
Body dysmorphic disorder

> **EXCLUDES** hypochondriasis in:
> hysteria (300.10-300.19)
> manic-depressive psychosis, depressed type (296.2-296.3)
> neurasthenia (300.5)
> obsessional disorder (300.3)
> schizophrenia (295.0-295.9)

√5ᵗʰ **300.8 Other neurotic disorders**

300.81 Somatization disorder
Briquet's disorder
Severe somatoform disorder

300.82 Undifferentiated somatoform disorder
Atypical somatoform disorder
Somatoform disorder NOS

DEF: Disorders in which patients have symptoms that suggest an organic disease but no evidence of physical disorder after repeated testing.

Additional Digit Required
Unspecified Code
Other Specified Code
Manifestation Code
MSP Medicare Secondary Payer
▶◀ Revised Text
● New Code
▲ Revised Code Title

300.89 Other
  Occupational neurosis, including writers' cramp
  Psychasthenia
  Psychasthenic neurosis

300.9 Unspecified neurotic disorder
  Neurosis NOS
  Psychoneurosis NOS

✓4th **301 Personality disorders**
  INCLUDES   character neurosis
  Use additional code to identify any associated neurosis or psychosis, or physical condition
  EXCLUDES   nonpsychotic personality disorder associated with organic brain syndromes (310.0-310.9)

301.0 Paranoid personality disorder
  Fanatic personality
  Paranoid personality (disorder)
  Paranoid traits
  EXCLUDES   acute paranoid reaction (298.3)
            alcoholic paranoia (291.5)
            paranoid schizophrenia (295.3)
            paranoid states (297.0-297.9)

✓5th **301.1 Affective personality disorder**
  EXCLUDES   affective psychotic disorders (296.0-296.9)
            neurasthenia (300.5)
            neurotic depression (300.4)

  301.10 Affective personality disorder, unspecified
  301.11 Chronic hypomanic personality disorder
    Chronic hypomanic disorder
    Hypomanic personality
  301.12 Chronic depressive personality disorder
    Chronic depressive disorder
    Depressive character or personality
  301.13 Cyclothymic disorder
    Cycloid personality
    Cyclothymia
    Cyclothymic personality

✓5th **301.2 Schizoid personality disorder**
  EXCLUDES   schizophrenia (295.0-295.9)

  301.20 Schizoid personality disorder, unspecified
  301.21 Introverted personality
  301.22 Schizotypal personality

301.3 Explosive personality disorder
  Aggressive: Emotional instability
    personality   (excessive)
    reaction   Pathological emotionality
  Aggressiveness   Quarrelsomeness
  EXCLUDES   dyssocial personality (301.7)
            hysterical neurosis (300.10-300.19)

301.4 Compulsive personality disorder
  Anancastic personality
  Obsessional personality
  EXCLUDES   obsessive-compulsive disorder (300.3)
            phobic state (300.20-300.29)

✓5th **301.5 Histrionic personality disorder**
  EXCLUDES   hysterical neurosis (300.10-300.19)
  DEF: Extreme emotional behavior, often theatrical; often concerned about own appeal; may demand attention, exhibit seductive behavior.

MENTAL DISORDERS

301.50 Histrionic personality disorder, unspecified
Hysterical personality NOS

301.51 Chronic factitious illness with physical symptoms
Hospital addiction syndrome
Multiple operations syndrome
Munchausen syndrome

301.59 Other histrionic personality disorder
Personality:
    emotionally unstable
    labile
Personality:
    psychoinfantile

301.6 Dependent personality disorder
Asthenic personality   Passive personality
Inadequate personality
> **EXCLUDES**   neurasthenia (300.5)
>   passive-aggressive personality (301.84)

DEF: Overwhelming feeling of helplessness; fears of abandonment may persist; difficulty in making personal decisions without confirmation by others; low self-esteem due to irrational sensitivity to criticism.

301.7 Antisocial personality disorder
Amoral personality
Asocial personality
Dyssocial personality
Personality disorder with predominantly sociopathic or asocial manifestation
> **EXCLUDES**   disturbance of conduct without specifiable personality disorder (312.0-312.9)
>   explosive personality (301.3)

DEF: Continuous antisocial behavior that violates rights of others; social traits include extreme aggression, total disregard for traditional social rules.

✓5th 301.8 Other personality disorders

  301.81 Narcissistic personality
    DEF: Grandiose fantasy or behavior, lack of social empathy, hypersensitive to the lack of others' judgment, exploits others; also sense of entitlement to have expectations met, need for continual admiration.

  301.82 Avoidant personality
    DEF: Personality disorder marked by feelings of social inferiority; sensitivity to criticism, emotionally restrained due to fear of rejection.

  301.83 Borderline personality
    DEF: Personality disorder characterized by unstable moods, self-image, and interpersonal relationships; uncontrolled anger, impulsive and self-destructive acts, fears of abandonment, feelings of emptiness and boredom, recurrent suicide threats or self-mutilation.

  301.84 Passive-aggressive personality
    DEF: Pattern of procrastination and refusal to meet standards; introduce own obstacles to success and exploit failure.

  301.89 Other
    Personality:
      eccentric
      "haltlose" type
      immature
    Personality:
      masochistic
      psychoneurotic
> **EXCLUDES**   psychoinfantile personality (301.59)

MENTAL DISORDERS

301.9 Unspecified personality disorder
    Pathological personality NOS
    Personality disorder NOS
    Psychopathic:
        constitutional state
        personality (disorder)

√4th **302 Sexual deviations and disorders**
    EXCLUDES   sexual disorder manifest in:
        organic brain syndrome (290.0-294.9, 310.0-310.9)
        psychosis (295.0-298.9)

302.0 Ego-dystonic homosexuality
    Ego-dystonic lesbianism
    Homosexual conflict disorder
    EXCLUDES   homosexual pedophilia (302.2)

302.1 Zoophilia
    Bestiality
DEF: A sociodeviant disorder marked by engaging in sexual intercourse with animals.

302.2 Pedophilia
DEF: A sociodeviant condition of adults characterized by sexual activity with children.

302.3 Transvestism
    EXCLUDES   trans-sexualism (302.5)
DEF: The desire to dress in clothing of opposite sex.

302.4 Exhibitionism
DEF: Sexual deviant behavior; exposure of genitals to strangers; behavior prompted by intense sexual urges and fantasies.

√5th **302.5 Trans-sexualism**
    EXCLUDES   transvestism (302.3)
DEF: Gender identity disturbance; overwhelming desire to change anatomic sex, due to belief that individual is a member of the opposite sex.

302.50 With unspecified sexual history
302.51 With asexual history
302.52 With homosexual history
302.53 With heterosexual history

302.6 Disorders of psychosexual identity
    Feminism in boys
    Gender identity disorder of childhood
    EXCLUDES   gender identity disorder in adult (302.85)
        homosexuality (302.0)
        trans-sexualism (302.50-302.53)
        transvestism (302.3)

√5th **302.7 Psychosexual dysfunction**
    EXCLUDES   impotence of organic origin (607.84)
        normal transient symptoms from ruptured hymen
        transient or occasional failures of erection due to fatigue,
            anxiety, alcohol, or drugs

302.70 Psychosexual dysfunction, unspecified
302.71 With inhibited sexual desire
302.72 With inhibited sexual excitement
    Frigidity   Impotence
302.73 With inhibited female orgasm ♀
302.74 With inhibited male orgasm ♂
302.75 With premature ejaculation ♂

MENTAL DISORDERS 302.76–303.9

302.76 With functional dyspareunia ♀
   Dyspareunia, psychogenic
   DEF: Difficult or painful sex due to psychosomatic state.

302.79 With other specified psychosexual dysfunctions

√5ᵗʰ **302.8 Other specified psychosexual disorders**

302.81 Fetishism
   DEF: Psychosexual disorder noted for intense sexual urges and arousal precipitated by fantasies; use of inanimate objects, such as clothing, to stimulate sexual arousal, orgasm.

302.82 Voyeurism
   DEF: Psychosexual disorder characterized by uncontrollable impulse to observe others, without their knowledge, who are nude or engaged in sexual activity.

302.83 Sexual masochism
   DEF: Psychosexual disorder noted for need to achieve sexual gratification through humiliating or hurtful acts inflicted on self.

302.84 Sexual sadism
   DEF: Psychosexual disorder noted for need to achieve sexual gratification through humiliating or hurtful acts inflicted on someone else.

302.85 Gender identity disorder of adolescent or adult life

302.89 Other
   Nymphomania   Satyriasis

302.9 Unspecified psychosexual disorder
   Pathologic sexuality NOS
   Sexual deviation NOS

√4ᵗʰ **303 Alcohol dependence syndrome**
   Use additional code to identify any associated condition, as:
      alcoholic psychoses (291.0-291.9)
      drug dependence (304.0-304.9)
      physical complications of alcohol, such as:
         cerebral degeneration (331.7)
         cirrhosis of liver (571.2)
         epilepsy (345.0-345.9)
         gastritis (535.3)
         hepatitis (571.1)
         liver damage NOS (571.3)
   EXCLUDES drunkenness NOS (305.0)

   The following fifth-digit subclassification is for use with category 303:
      0 **unspecified**
      1 continuous
      2 episodic
      3 in remission

√5ᵗʰ **303.0 Acute alcoholic intoxication**
   Acute drunkenness in alcoholism

√5ᵗʰ **303.9 Other and unspecified alcohol dependence**
   Chronic alcoholism
   Dipsomania

√4ᵗʰ Additional Digit Required   Unspecified Code   Other Specified Code   Manifestation Code
√5ᵗʰ
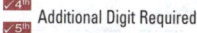 Medicare Secondary Payer   ▶◀ Revised Text   ● New Code   ▲ Revised Code Title

304 Drug dependence

EXCLUDES nondependent abuse of drugs (305.1-305.9)

The following fifth-digit subclassification is for use with category 304:
- 0 unspecified
- 1 continuous
- 2 episodic
- 3 in remission

304.0 Opioid type dependence
- Heroin
- Meperidine
- Methadone
- Morphine
- Opium
- Opium alkaloids and their derivatives
- Synthetics with morphine-like effects

304.1 Barbiturate and similarly acting sedative or hypnotic dependence
- Barbiturates
- Nonbarbiturate sedatives and tranquilizers with a similar effect:
  - chlordiazepoxide
  - diazepam
  - glutethimide
  - meprobamate
  - methaqualone

304.2 Cocaine dependence
- Coca leaves and derivatives

304.3 Cannabis dependence
- Hashish
- Hemp
- Marihuana

304.4 Amphetamine and other psychostimulant dependence
- Methylphenidate
- Phenmetrazine

304.5 Hallucinogen dependence
- Dimethyltryptamine [DMT]
- Lysergic acid diethylamide [LSD] and derivatives
- Mescaline
- Psilocybin

304.6 Other specified drug dependence
- Absinthe addiction
- Glue sniffing

EXCLUDES tobacco dependence (305.1)

304.7 Combinations of opioid type drug with any other

304.8 Combinations of drug dependence excluding opioid type drug

304.9 Unspecified drug dependence
- Drug addiction NOS
- Drug dependence NOS

305 Nondependent abuse of drugs

Note: Includes cases where a person, for whom no other diagnosis is possible, has come under medical care because of the maladaptive effect of a drug on which he is not dependent and that he has taken on his own initiative to the detriment of his health or social functioning.

EXCLUDES alcohol dependence syndrome (303.0-303.9)
drug dependence (304.0-304.9)
drug withdrawal syndrome (292.0)
poisoning by drugs or medicinal substances (960.0-979.9)

The following fifth-digit subclassification is for use with codes 305.0, 305.2-305.9:
- 0 unspecified
- 1 continuous
- 2 episodic
- 3 in remission

MENTAL DISORDERS

305.0 Alcohol abuse
√5th
Drunkenness NOS
Excessive drinking of alcohol NOS
"Hangover" (alcohol)
Inebriety NOS
> **EXCLUDES** acute alcohol intoxication in alcoholism (303.0)
> alcoholic psychoses (291.0-291.9)

305.1 Tobacco use disorder
Tobacco dependence
> **EXCLUDES** history of tobacco use (V15.82)

305.2 Cannabis abuse
√5th

305.3 Hallucinogen abuse
√5th
Acute intoxication from hallucinogens ["bad trips"]
LSD reaction

305.4 Barbiturate and similarly acting sedative or hypnotic abuse
√5th

305.5 Opioid abuse
√5th

305.6 Cocaine abuse
√5th

305.7 Amphetamine or related acting sympathomimetic abuse
√5th

305.8 Antidepressant type abuse
√5th

305.9 Other, mixed, or unspecified drug abuse
√5th
"Laxative habit"
Misuse of drugs NOS
Nonprescribed use of drugs or patent medicinals

306 Physiological malfunction arising from mental factors
√4th
> **INCLUDES** psychogenic:
> physical symptoms } not involving
> physiological   tissue
> manifestations   damage

> **EXCLUDES** hysteria (300.11-300.19)
> physical symptoms secondary to a psychiatric disorder classified elsewhere
> psychic factors associated with physical conditions involving tissue damage classified elsewhere (316)
> specific nonpsychotic mental disorders following organic brain damage (310.0-310.9)

DEF: Functional disturbances or interruptions due to mental or psychological causes; no tissue damage sustained in these conditions.

306.0 Musculoskeletal
Psychogenic paralysis   Psychogenic torticollis
> **EXCLUDES** Gilles de la Tourette's syndrome (307.23)
> paralysis as hysterical or conversion reaction (300.11)
> tics (307.20-307.22)

306.1 Respiratory
Psychogenic: Psychogenic:
  air hunger   hyperventilation
  cough   yawning
  hiccough
> **EXCLUDES** psychogenic asthma (316 and 493.9)

MENTAL DISORDERS

306.2 Cardiovascular
Cardiac neurosis
Cardiovascular neurosis
Neurocirculatory asthenia
Psychogenic cardiovascular disorder
> **EXCLUDES** psychogenic paroxysmal tachycardia (316 and 427.2)

DEF: Neurocirculatory asthenia: functional nervous and circulatory irregularities with palpitations, dyspnea, fatigue, rapid pulse, precordial pain, fear of effort, discomfort during exercise, anxiety; also called DaCosta's syndrome, Effort syndrome, Irritable or Soldier's Heart.

306.3 Skin
Psychogenic pruritus
> **EXCLUDES** psychogenic:
> alopecia (316 and 704.00)
> dermatitis (316 and 692.9)
> eczema (316 and 691.8 or 692.9)
> urticaria (316 and 708.0-708.9)

306.4 Gastrointestinal
Aerophagy
Cyclical vomiting, psychogenic
Diarrhea, psychogenic
Nervous gastritis
Psychogenic dyspepsia
> **EXCLUDES** cyclical vomiting NOS (536.2)
> globus hystericus (300.11)
> mucous colitis (316 and 564.9)
> psychogenic:
> cardiospasm (316 and 530.0)
> duodenal ulcer (316 and 532.0-532.9)
> gastric ulcer (316 and 531.0-531.9)
> peptic ulcer NOS (316 and 533.0-533.9)
> vomiting NOS (307.54)

DEF: Aerophagy: excess swallowing of air, usually unconscious; related to anxiety; results in distended abdomen or belching, often interpreted by the patient as a physical disorder.

√5th 306.5 Genitourinary
> **EXCLUDES** enuresis, psychogenic (307.6)
> frigidity (302.72)
> impotence (302.72)
> psychogenic dyspareunia (302.76)

306.50 Psychogenic genitourinary malfunction, unspecified

306.51 Psychogenic vaginismus ♀
Functional vaginismus
DEF: Psychogenic response resulting in painful contractions of vaginal canal muscles; can be severe enough to prevent sexual intercourse.

306.52 Psychogenic dysmenorrhea ♀
306.53 Psychogenic dysuria
306.59 Other

306.6 Endocrine

306.7 Organs of special sense
> **EXCLUDES** hysterical blindness or deafness (300.11)
> psychophysical visual disturbances (368.16)

306.8 Other specified psychophysiological malfunction
Bruxism
Teeth grinding

306.9 Unspecified psychophysiological malfunction
Psychophysiologic disorder NOS
Psychosomatic disorder NOS

MENTAL DISORDERS

✓4th 307 Special symptoms or syndromes, not elsewhere classified

Note: This category is intended for use if the psychopathology is manifested by a single specific symptom or group of symptoms which is not part of an organic illness or other mental disorder classifiable elsewhere.

EXCLUDES   those due to mental disorders classified elsewhere
those of organic origin

307.0 Stammering and stuttering

EXCLUDES   dysphasia (784.5)
lisping or lalling (307.9)
retarded development of speech (315.31-315.39)

307.1 Anorexia nervosa

EXCLUDES   eating disturbance NOS (307.50)
feeding problem (783.3)
   of nonorganic origin (307.59)
loss of appetite (783.0)
   of nonorganic origin (307.59)

✓5th 307.2 Tics

EXCLUDES   nail-biting or thumb-sucking (307.9)
stereotypes occurring in isolation (307.3)
tics of organic origin (333.3)

DEF: Involuntary muscle response usually confined to the face, shoulders.

307.20 Tic disorder, unspecified
307.21 Transient tic disorder of childhood
307.22 Chronic motor tic disorder
307.23 Gilles de la Tourette's disorder
Motor-verbal tic disorder

DEF: Syndrome of facial and vocal tics in childhood; progresses to spontaneous or involuntary jerking, obscene utterances, other uncontrollable actions considered inappropriate.

307.3 Stereotyped repetitive movements
Body-rocking   Spasmus nutans
Head banging   Stereotypes NOS

EXCLUDES   tics (307.20-307.23)
of organic origin (333.3)

✓5th 307.4 Specific disorders of sleep of nonorganic origin

EXCLUDES   narcolepsy (347)
those of unspecified cause (780.50-780.59)

307.40 Nonorganic sleep disorder, unspecified
307.41 Transient disorder of initiating or maintaining sleep

Hyposomnia   } associated with
Insomnia   intermittent
Sleeplessness   emotional reactions
                 or conflicts

307.42 Persistent disorder of initiating or maintaining sleep
Hyposomnia, insomnia, or sleeplessness associated with:
   anxiety
   conditioned arousal
   depression (major) (minor)
   psychosis

307.43 Transient disorder of initiating or maintaining wakefulness
Hypersomnia associated with acute or intermittent emotional reactions or conflicts

---

✓4th
✓5th   Additional Digit Required   Unspecified Code   Other Specified Code   Manifestation Code
 Medicare Secondary Payer   ▶◀ Revised Text   ● New Code   ▲ Revised Code Title

2002 Ingenix, Inc.

307.44 Persistent disorder of initiating or maintaining wakefulness
Hypersomnia associated with depression (major) (minor)

307.45 Phase-shift disruption of 24-hour sleep-wake cycle
Irregular sleep-wake rhythm, nonorganic origin
Jet lag syndrome
Rapid time-zone change
Shifting sleep-work schedule

307.46 Somnambulism or night terrors
DEF: Sleepwalking marked by extreme terror, panic, screaming, confusion; no recall of event upon arousal; term may refer to simply the act of sleepwalking.

307.47 Other dysfunctions of sleep stages or arousal from sleep
Nightmares: Sleep drunkenness
  NOS
  REM-sleep type

307.48 Repetitive intrusions of sleep
Repetitive intrusion of sleep with:
  atypical polysomnographic features
  environmental disturbances
  repeated REM-sleep interruptions

307.49 Other
"Short-sleeper"
Subjective insomnia complaint

√5ᵗʰ **307.5 Other and unspecified disorders of eating**
EXCLUDES   anorexia:
             nervosa (307-1)
             of unspecified cause (783.0)
           overeating, of unspecified cause (783.6)
           vomiting:
             NOS (787.0)
             cyclical (536.2)
             psychogenic (306.4)

307.50 Eating disorder, unspecified

307.51 Bulimia
Overeating of nonorganic origin
DEF: Mental disorder commonly characterized by binge eating followed by self-induced vomiting; perceptions of being fat; and fear the inability to stop eating voluntarily.

307.52 Pica
Perverted appetite of nonorganic origin
DEF: Compulsive eating disorder characterized by craving for substances, other than food; such as paint chips or dirt.

307.53 Psychogenic rumination
Regurgitation, of nonorganic origin, of food with reswallowing
EXCLUDES   obsessional rumination (300.3)

307.54 Psychogenic vomiting

307.59 Other
Infantile feeding
  disturbances   } of nonorganic
Loss of appetite   origin

307.6 Enuresis
Enuresis (primary) (secondary) of nonorganic origin
EXCLUDES   enuresis of unspecified cause (788.3)
DEF: Involuntary urination past age of normal control; also called bedwetting; no trace to biological problem; focus on psychological issues.

MENTAL DISORDERS

307.7 Encopresis
Encopresis (continuous) (discontinuous) of nonorganic origin
EXCLUDES encopresis of unspecified cause (787.6)

DEF: Inability to control bowel movements; cause traced to psychological, not biological, problems.

√5th 307.8 Psychalgia
307.80 Psychogenic pain, site unspecified
307.81 Tension headache
EXCLUDES headache:
NOS (784.0)
migraine (346.0-346.9)

307.89 Other
Psychogenic backache
EXCLUDES pains not specifically attributable to a psychological cause (in):
back (724.5)
joint (719.4)
limb (729.5)
lumbago (724.2)
rheumatic (729.0)

307.9 Other and unspecified special symptoms or syndromes, not elsewhere classified
Hair plucking   Masturbation
Lalling   Nail-biting
Lisping   Thumb-sucking

√4th 308 Acute reaction to stress
INCLUDES catastrophic stress
combat fatigue
gross stress reaction (acute)
transient disorders in response to exceptional physical or mental stress which usually subside within hours or days
EXCLUDES adjustment reaction or disorder (309.0-309.9)
chronic stress reaction (309.1-309.9)

308.0 Predominant disturbance of emotions
Anxiety
Emotional crisis   } as acute reaction to exceptional [gross] stress
Panic state

308.1 Predominant disturbance of consciousness
Fugues as acute reaction to exceptional [gross] stress

308.2 Predominant psychomotor disturbance
Agitation states } as acute reaction to
Stupor   exceptional [gross] stress

308.3 Other acute reactions to stress
Acute situational disturbance
Brief or acute posttraumatic stress disorder
EXCLUDES prolonged posttraumatic emotional disturbance (309.81)

308.4 Mixed disorders as reaction to stress
308.9 Unspecified acute reaction to stress

√4th 309 Adjustment reaction
INCLUDES adjustment disorders
reaction (adjustment) to chronic stress
EXCLUDES acute reaction to major stress (308.0-308.9)
neurotic disorders (300.0-300.9)

√4th √5th Additional Digit Required
MSP Medicare Secondary Payer
▶◀ Revised Text
Unspecified Code
● New Code
Other Specified Code
▲ Revised Code Title
Manifestation Code

2002 Ingenix, Inc.

Volume 1 — 155

MENTAL DISORDERS

309.0 Brief depressive reaction
Adjustment disorder with depressed mood
Grief reaction
> EXCLUDES affective psychoses (296.0-296.9)
> neurotic depression (300.4)
> prolonged depressive reaction (309.1)
> psychogenic depressive psychosis (298.0)

309.1 Prolonged depressive reaction
> EXCLUDES affective psychoses (296.0-296.9)
> brief depressive reaction (309.0)
> neurotic depression (300.4)
> psychogenic depressive psychosis (298.0)

309.2 With predominant disturbance of other emotions

309.21 Separation anxiety disorder
DEF: Abnormal apprehension by a child when physically separated from support environment; byproduct of abnormal symbiotic child-parent relationship.

309.22 Emancipation disorder of adolescence and early adult life
DEF: Adjustment reaction of late adolescence; conflict over independence from parental supervision; symptoms include difficulty in making decisions, increased reliance on parental advice, deliberate adoption of values in opposition of parents.

309.23 Specific academic or work inhibition

309.24 Adjustment reaction with anxious mood

309.28 Adjustment reaction with mixed emotional features
Adjustment reaction with anxiety and depression

309.29 Other
Culture shock

309.3 With predominant disturbance of conduct
Conduct disturbance } as adjustment reaction
Destructiveness
> EXCLUDES destructiveness in child (312.9)
> disturbance of conduct NOS (312.9)
> dyssocial behavior without manifest psychiatric disorder (V71.01-V71.02)
> personality disorder with predominantly sociopathic or asocial manifestations (301.7)

309.4 With mixed disturbance of emotions and conduct

309.8 Other specified adjustment reactions

309.81 Prolonged posttraumatic stress disorder
Chronic posttraumatic stress disorder
Concentration camp syndrome
> EXCLUDES posttraumatic brain syndrome:
> nonpsychotic (310.2)
> psychotic (293.0-293.9)

DEF: Preoccupation with traumatic events beyond normal experience; events such as rape, personal assault, combat, natural disasters, accidents, torture precipitate disorder; also recurring flashbacks of trauma; symptoms include difficulty remembering, sleeping, or concentrating, and guilt feelings for surviving.

309.82 Adjustment reaction with physical symptoms

309.83 Adjustment reaction with withdrawal
Elective mutism as adjustment reaction
Hospitalism (in children) NOS

309.89 Other

309.9 Unspecified adjustment reaction
Adaptation reaction NOS
Adjustment reaction NOS

MENTAL DISORDERS

✓4th 310 Specific nonpsychotic mental disorders due to organic brain damage

EXCLUDES *neuroses, personality disorders, or other nonpsychotic conditions occurring in a form similar to that seen with functional disorders but in association with a physical condition (300.0-300.9, 301.0-301.9)*

310.0 Frontal lobe syndrome
Lobotomy syndrome
Postleucotomy syndrome [state]

EXCLUDES *postcontusion syndrome (310.2)*

310.1 Organic personality syndrome
Cognitive or personality change of other type, of nonpsychotic severity
Mild memory disturbance
Organic psychosyndrome of nonpsychotic severity
Presbyophrenia NOS
Senility with mental changes of nonpsychotic severity

DEF: Personality disorder caused by organic factors, such as brain lesions, head trauma, or cerebrovascular accident (CVA).

310.2 Postconcussion syndrome
Postcontusion syndrome or encephalopathy
Posttraumatic brain syndrome, nonpsychotic
Status postcommotio cerebri

EXCLUDES *frontal lobe syndrome (310.0)*
postencephalitic syndrome (310.8)
any organic psychotic conditions following head injury (293.0-294.0)

DEF: Nonpsychotic disorder due to brain trauma, causes symptoms unrelated to any disease process; symptoms include amnesia, serial headaches, rapid heartbeat, fatigue, disrupted sleep patterns, inability to concentrate.

310.8 Other specified nonpsychotic mental disorders following organic brain damage
Postencephalitic syndrome
Other focal (partial) organic psychosyndromes

310.9 Unspecified nonpsychotic mental disorder following organic brain damage

311 Depressive disorder, not elsewhere classified
Depressive disorder NOS
Depressive state NOS
Depression NOS

EXCLUDES *acute reaction to major stress with depressive symptoms (308.0)*
affective personality disorder (301.10-301.13)
affective psychoses (296.0-296.9)
brief depressive reaction (309.0)
depressive states associated with stressful events (309.0-309.1)
disturbance of emotions specific to childhood and adolescence, with misery and unhappiness (313.1)
mixed adjustment reaction with depressive symptoms (309.4)
neurotic depression (300.4)
prolonged depressive adjustment reaction (309.1)
psychogenic depressive psychosis (298.0)

MENTAL DISORDERS

✓4ᵗʰ **312 Disturbance of conduct, not elsewhere classified**

> **EXCLUDES** adjustment reaction with disturbance of conduct (309.3)
> drug dependence (304.0-304.9)
> dyssocial behavior without manifest psychiatric disorder (V71.01-V71.02)
> personality disorder with predominantly sociopathic or asocial manifestations (301.7)
> sexual deviations (302.0-302.9)

The following fifth-digit subclassification is for use with categories 312.0-312.2:
- 0 unspecified
- 1 mild
- 2 moderate
- 3 severe

✓5ᵗʰ **312.0 Undersocialized conduct disorder, aggressive type**
Aggressive outburst   Unsocialized aggressive
Anger reaction   disorder

DEF: Mental condition identified by behaviors disrespectful of others' rights and of age-appropriate social norms or rules; symptoms include bullying, vandalism, verbal and physical abusiveness, lying, stealing, defiance.

✓5ᵗʰ **312.1 Undersocialized conduct disorder, unaggressive type**
Childhood truancy, unsocialized
Solitary stealing
Tantrums

✓5ᵗʰ **312.2 Socialized conduct disorder**
Childhood truancy, socialized   Group delinquency

> **EXCLUDES** gang activity without manifest psychiatric disorder (V71.01)

✓5ᵗʰ **312.3 Disorders of impulse control, not elsewhere classified**
- 312.30 Impulse control disorder, unspecified
- 312.31 Pathological gambling
- 312.32 Kleptomania
- 312.33 Pyromania
- 312.34 Intermittent explosive disorder
- 312.35 Isolated explosive disorder
- 312.39 Other

312.4 Mixed disturbance of conduct and emotions
Neurotic delinquency

> **EXCLUDES** compulsive conduct disorder (312.3)

✓5ᵗʰ **312.8 Other specified disturbances of conduct, not elsewhere classified**
- 312.81 Conduct disorder, childhood onset type
- 312.82 Conduct disorder, adolescent onset type
- 312.89 Other conduct disorder

312.9 Unspecified disturbance of conduct
Delinquency (juvenile)

✓4ᵗʰ **313 Disturbance of emotions specific to childhood and adolescence**

> **EXCLUDES** adjustment reaction (309.0-309.9)
> emotional disorder of neurotic type (300.0-300.9)
> masturbation, nail-biting, thumbsucking, and other isolated symptoms (307.0-307.9)

313.0 Overanxious disorder
Anxiety and fearfulness } of childhood and
Overanxious disorder   } adolescence

> **EXCLUDES** abnormal separation anxiety (309.21)
> anxiety states (300.00-300.09)
> hospitalism in children (309.83)
> phobic state (300.20-300.29)

MENTAL DISORDERS

313.1 **Misery and unhappiness disorder**
  EXCLUDES *depressive neurosis (300.4)*

√5ᵗʰ **313.2** **Sensitivity, shyness, and social withdrawal disorder**
  EXCLUDES *infantile autism (299.0)*
         schizoid personality (301.20-301.22)
         schizophrenia (295.0-295.9)

  313.21 Shyness disorder of childhood
    Sensitivity reaction of childhood or adolescence

  313.22 Introverted disorder of childhood
    Social withdrawal ⎫
    Withdrawal   ⎬ of childhood or adolescence
    reaction   ⎭

  313.23 Elective mutism
    EXCLUDES *elective mutism as adjustment reaction (309.83)*

313.3 **Relationship problems**
  Sibling jealousy
  EXCLUDES *relationship problems associated with aggression, destruction, or other forms of conduct disturbance (312.0-312.9)*

√5ᵗʰ **313.8** **Other or mixed emotional disturbances of childhood or adolescence**

  313.81 Oppositional disorder
    DEF: Mental disorder of children noted for pervasive opposition, defiance of authority.

  313.82 Identity disorder
    DEF: Distress of adolescents caused by inability to form acceptable self-identity; uncertainty about career choice, sexual orientation, moral values.

  313.83 Academic underachievement disorder

  313.89 Other   P

313.9 **Unspecified emotional disturbance of childhood or adolescence**   P

√4ᵗʰ **314** **Hyperkinetic syndrome of childhood**
  EXCLUDES *hyperkinesis as symptom of underlying disorder—code the underlying disorder*

  DEF: A behavioral disorder usually diagnosed at an early age; characterized by the inability to focus attention for a normal period of time.

√5ᵗʰ **314.0** **Attention deficit disorder**
    Adult   Child

  314.00 Without mention of hyperactivity
    Predominantly inattentive type

  314.01 With hyperactivity
    Combined type
    Overactivity NOS
    Predominantly hyperactive/impulsive type
    Simple disturbance of attention with overactivity

314.1 **Hyperkinesis with developmental delay**
  Developmental disorder of hyperkinesis
  Use additional code to identify any associated neurological disorder

314.2 **Hyperkinetic conduct disorder**
  Hyperkinetic conduct disorder without developmental delay
  EXCLUDES *hyperkinesis with significant delays in specific skills (314.1)*

314.8 **Other specified manifestations of hyperkinetic syndrome**

314.9 **Unspecified hyperkinetic syndrome**
  Hyperkinetic reaction of childhood or adolescence NOS
  Hyperkinetic syndrome NOS

MENTAL DISORDERS

✓4th 315 Specific delays in development
   EXCLUDES *that due to a neurological disorder (320.0-389.9)*

   ✓5th 315.0 Specific reading disorder
      315.00 Reading disorder, unspecified
      315.01 Alexia
         DEF: Lack of ability to understand written language; manifestation of aphasia.
      315.02 Developmental dyslexia
         DEF: Serious impairment of reading skills unexplained in relation to general intelligence and teaching processes; it can be inherited or congenital.
      315.09 Other
         Specific spelling difficulty

   315.1 Specific arithmetical disorder
      Dyscalculia

   315.2 Other specific learning difficulties
      EXCLUDES *specific arithmetical disorder (315.1)*
      specific reading disorder (315.00-315.09)

   ✓5th 315.3 Developmental speech or language disorder
      315.31 Developmental language disorder
         Developmental aphasia
         Expressive language disorder
         Word deafness
         EXCLUDES *acquired aphasia (784.3)*
         elective mutism (309.83, 313.0, 313.23)
      315.32 Receptive language disorder (mixed)
         Receptive expressive language disorder
      315.39 Other
         Developmental articulation disorder
         Dyslalia
         EXCLUDES *lisping and lalling (307.9)*
         stammering and stuttering (307.0)

   315.4 Coordination disorder
      Clumsiness syndrome
      Dyspraxia syndrome
      Specific motor development disorder

   315.5 Mixed development disorder

   315.8 Other specified delays in development

   315.9 Unspecified delay in development
      Developmental disorder NOS

316 Psychic factors associated with diseases classified elsewhere
   Psychologic factors in physical conditions classified elsewhere
   Use additional code to identify the associated physical condition, as:
   psychogenic:
      asthma (493.9)
      dermatitis (692.9)
      duodenal ulcer (532.0-532.9)
      eczema (691.8, 692.9)
      gastric ulcer (531.0-531.9)
      mucous colitis (564.9)
      paroxysmal tachycardia (427.2)
      ulcerative colitis (556)
      urticaria (708.0-708.9)
   psychosocial dwarfism (259.4)
      EXCLUDES *physical symptoms and physiological malfunctions, not involving tissue damage, of mental origin (306.0-306.9)*

NERVOUS SYSTEM AND SENSE ORGANS 317–320.81

MENTAL RETARDATION (317-319)

Use additional code(s) to identify any associated psychiatric or physical condition(s)

317 Mild mental retardation
High-grade defect
IQ 50-70
Mild mental subnormality

✓4th **318 Other specified mental retardation**

318.0 Moderate mental retardation
IQ 35-49   Moderate mental subnormality

318.1 Severe mental retardation
IQ 20-34   Severe mental subnormality

318.2 Profound mental retardation
IQ under 20   Profound mental subnormality

319 Unspecified mental retardation
Mental deficiency NOS
Mental subnormality NOS

6. NERVOUS SYSTEM AND SENSE ORGANS (320-389)

INFLAMMATORY DISEASES OF THE CENTRAL NERVOUS SYSTEM (320-326)

✓4th **320 Bacterial meningitis**

INCLUDES:
arachnoiditis
leptomeningitis
meningitis   } bacterial
meningoencephalitis
meningomyelitis
pachymeningitis

DEF: Bacterial infection causing inflammation of the lining of the brain and/or spinal cord.

320.0 Hemophilus meningitis
Meningitis due to Hemophilus influenzae [H. influenzae]

320.1 Pneumococcal meningitis

320.2 Streptococcal meningitis

320.3 Staphylococcal meningitis

320.7 Meningitis in other bacterial diseases classified elsewhere
Code first underlying disease, as:
actinomycosis (039.8)
listeriosis (027.0)
typhoid fever (002.0)
whooping cough (033.0-033.9)

EXCLUDES:
meningitis (in):
epidemic (036.0)
gonococcal (098.82)
meningococcal (036.0)
salmonellosis (003.21)
syphilis:
NOS (094.2)
congenital (090.42)
meningovascular (094.2)
secondary (091.81)
tuberculous (013.0)

✓5th **320.8 Meningitis due to other specified bacteria**

320.81 Anaerobic meningitis
Bacteroides (fragilis)
Gram-negative anaerobes

✓4th / ✓5th Additional Digit Required   Unspecified Code   Other Specified Code   Manifestation Code

MSP Medicare Secondary Payer   ▶◀ Revised Text   ● New Code   ▲ Revised Code Title

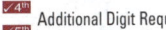2002 Ingenix, Inc.   Volume 1 — 161

320.82 Meningitis due to gram-negative bacteria, not elsewhere classified
- Aerobacter aerogenes
- Escherichia coli [E. coli]
- Friedländer bacillus
- Klebsiella pneumoniae
- Proteus morganii
- Pseudomonas

EXCLUDES gram-negative anaerobes (320.81)

320.89 Meningitis due to other specified bacteria
- Bacillus pyocyaneus

320.9 Meningitis due to unspecified bacterium
Meningitis:
- bacterial NOS
- purulent NOS
- pyogenic NOS
- suppurative NOS

✓4th **321 Meningitis due to other organisms**

INCLUDES arachnoiditis, leptomeningitis, meningitis, pachymeningitis } due to organisms other than bacteria

DEF: Infection causing inflammation of the lining of the brain and/or spinal cord, due to organisms other than bacteria.

321.0 Cryptococcal meningitis
Code first underlying disease (117.5)

321.1 Meningitis in other fungal diseases
Code first underlying disease (110.0-118)
EXCLUDES meningitis in:
- candidiasis (112.83)
- coccidioidomycosis (114.2)
- histoplasmosis (115.01, 115.11, 115.91)

321.2 Meningitis due to viruses not elsewhere classified
Code first underlying disease, as:
meningitis due to arbovirus (060.0-066.9)
EXCLUDES meningitis (due to):
- abacterial (047.0-047.9)
- adenovirus (049.1)
- aseptic NOS (047.9)
- Coxsackie (virus)(047.0)
- ECHO virus (047.1)
- enterovirus (047.0-047.9)
- herpes simplex virus (054.72)
- herpes zoster virus (053.0)
- lymphocytic choriomeningitis virus (049.0)
- mumps (072.1)
- viral NOS (047.9)
- meningo-eruptive syndrome (047.1)

321.3 Meningitis due to trypanosomiasis
Code first underlying disease (086.0-086.9)

321.4 Meningitis in sarcoidosis
Code first underlying disease (135)

321.8 Meningitis due to other nonbacterial organisms classified elsewhere
Code first underlying disease
EXCLUDES leptospiral meningitis (100.81)

NERVOUS SYSTEM AND SENSE ORGANS   322–323.2

√4th 322 Meningitis of unspecified cause

INCLUDES: arachnoiditis
leptomeningitis
meningitis
pachymeningitis
} with no organism specified as cause

DEF: Infection causing inflammation of the lining of the brain and/or spinal cord, due to unspecified cause.

322.0 Nonpyogenic meningitis
Meningitis with clear cerebrospinal fluid

322.1 Eosinophilic meningitis

322.2 Chronic meningitis

322.9 Meningitis, unspecified

√4th 323 Encephalitis, myelitis, and encephalomyelitis

INCLUDES: acute disseminated encephalomyelitis
meningoencephalitis, except bacterial
meningomyelitis, except bacterial
myelitis (acute):
   ascending
   transverse

EXCLUDES: bacterial:
   meningoencephalitis (320.0-320.9)
   meningomyelitis (320.0-320.9)

DEF: Encephalitis: inflammation of brain tissues.

DEF: Myelitis: inflammation of the spinal cord.

DEF: Encephalomyelitis: inflammation of brain and spinal cord.

323.0 Encephalitis in viral diseases classified elsewhere
Code first underlying disease, as:
   cat-scratch disease (078.3)
   infectious mononucleosis (075)
   ornithosis (073.7)

EXCLUDES: encephalitis (in):
   arthropod-borne viral (062.0-064)
   herpes simplex (054.3)
   mumps (072.2)
   other viral diseases of central nervous system (049.8-049.9)
   poliomyelitis (045.0-045.9)
   rubella (056.01)
   slow virus infections of central nervous system (046.0-046.9)
   viral NOS (049.9)

323.1 Encephalitis in rickettsial diseases classified elsewhere
Code first underlying disease (080-083.9)

DEF: Inflammation of the brain caused by rickettsial disease carried by louse, tick, or mite.

323.2 Encephalitis in protozoal diseases classified elsewhere
Code first underlying disease, as:
   malaria (084.0-084.9)
   trypanosomiasis (086.0-086.9)

DEF: Inflammation of the brain caused by protozoal disease carried by mosquitoes and flies.

323.4 Other encephalitis due to infection classified elsewhere
Code first underlying disease
EXCLUDES encephalitis (in):
meningococcal (036.1)
syphilis:
NOS (094.81)
congenital (090.41)
toxoplasmosis (130.0)
tuberculosis (013.6)
meningoencephalitis due to free-living ameba [Naegleria] (136.2)

323.5 Encephalitis following immunization procedures
Encephalitis ⎫ postimmunization or
Encephalomyelitis ⎭ postvaccinal
Use additional E code to identify vaccine

323.6 Postinfectious encephalitis
Code first underlying disease
EXCLUDES encephalitis:
postchickenpox (052.0)
postmeasles (055.0)
DEF: Infection, inflammation of brain several weeks following the outbreak of a systemic infection.

323.7 Toxic encephalitis
Code first underlying cause, as:
carbon tetrachloride (982.1)
hydroxyquinoline derivatives (961.3)
lead (984.0-984.9)
mercury (985.0)
thallium (985.8)

323.8 Other causes of encephalitis

323.9 Unspecified cause of encephalitis

4th 324 Intracranial and intraspinal abscess

324.0 Intracranial abscess
Abscess (embolic):   Abscess (embolic) of brain
  cerebellar   [any part]:
  cerebral   epidural
                              extradural
                              otogenic
                              subdural
EXCLUDES tuberculous (013.3)

324.1 Intraspinal abscess
Abscess (embolic) of spinal cord [any part]:
epidural
extradural
subdural
EXCLUDES tuberculous (013.5)

324.9 Of unspecified site
Extradural or subdural abscess NOS

NERVOUS SYSTEM AND SENSE ORGANS

325 Phlebitis and thrombophlebitis of intracranial venous sinuses

Embolism
Endophlebitis
Phlebitis, septic or suppurative
Thrombophlebitis
Thrombosis
} of cavernous, lateral, or other intracranial or unspecified intracranial venous sinus

EXCLUDES that specified as:
complicating pregnancy, childbirth, or the puerperium (671.5)
of nonpyogenic origin (437.6)

DEF: Inflammation and formation of blood clot in a vein within the brain or its lining.

326 Late effects of intracranial abscess or pyogenic infection

Note: This category is to be used to indicate conditions whose primary classification is to 320-325 [excluding 320.7, 321.0-321.8, 323.0-323.4, 323.6-323.7] as the cause of late effects, themselves classifiable elsewhere. The "late effects" include conditions specified as such, or as sequelae, which may occur at any time after the resolution of the causal condition.

Use additional code to identify condition, as:
hydrocephalus (331.4)
paralysis (342.0-342.9, 344.0-344.9)

HEREDITARY AND DEGENERATIVE DISEASES OF THE CENTRAL NERVOUS SYSTEM (330-337)

EXCLUDES hepatolenticular degeneration (275.1)
multiple sclerosis (340)
other demyelinating diseases of central nervous system (341.0-341.9)

√4th 330 Cerebral degenerations usually manifest in childhood

Use additional code to identify associated mental retardation

330.0 Leukodystrophy

Krabbe's disease
Leukodystrophy
  NOS
  globoid cell
  metachromatic
  sudanophilic
Pelizaeus-Merzbacher disease
Sulfatide lipidosis

DEF: Hereditary disease of arylsulfatase or cerebroside sulfatase; characterized by a diffuse loss of myelin in CNS; infantile form causes blindness, motor disturbances, rigidity, mental deterioration and, occasionally, convulsions.

330.1 Cerebral lipidoses

Amaurotic (familial) idiocy
Disease:
  Batten
  Jansky-Bielschowsky
  Kufs'
Disease:
  Spielmeyer-Vogt
  Tay-Sachs
Gangliosidosis

DEF: Genetic disorder causing abnormal lipid accumulation in the reticuloendothelial cells of the brain.

330.2 ▲ Cerebral degeneration in generalized lipidoses

Code first underlying disease, as:
Fabry's disease (272.7)
Gaucher's disease (272.7)
Niemann-Pick disease (272.7)
sphingolipidosis (272.7)

NERVOUS SYSTEM AND SENSE ORGANS

330.3 Cerebral degeneration of childhood in other diseases classified elsewhere
Code first underlying disease, as:
Hunter's disease (277.5)
mucopolysaccharidosis (277.5)

330.8 Other specified cerebral degenerations in childhood
Alpers' disease or gray-matter degeneration
Infantile necrotizing encephalomyelopathy
Leigh's disease
Subacute necrotizing encephalopathy or encephalomyelopathy

330.9 Unspecified cerebral degeneration in childhood

√4th **331 Other cerebral degenerations**

331.0 Alzheimer's disease
DEF: Diffuse atrophy of cerebral cortex; causing a progressive decline in intellectual and physical functions, including memory loss, personality changes and profound dementia.

331.1 Pick's disease
DEF: Rare, progressive degenerative brain disease, similar to Alzheimer's; cortical atrophy affects the frontal and temporal lobes.

331.2 Senile degeneration of brain
EXCLUDES   senility NOS (797)

331.3 Communicating hydrocephalus
EXCLUDES   congenital hydrocephalus (741.0, 742.3)
DEF: Subarachnoid hemorrhage and meningitis causing excess buildup of cerebrospinal fluid in cavities due to nonabsorption of fluid back through fluid pathways.

331.4 Obstructive hydrocephalus
Acquired hydrocephalus NOS
EXCLUDES   congenital hydrocephalus (741.0, 742.3)
DEF: Obstruction of cerebrospinal fluid passage from brain into spinal canal.

331.7 Cerebral degeneration in diseases classified elsewhere
Code first underlying disease, as:
alcoholism (303.0-303.9)
beriberi (265.0)
cerebrovascular disease (430-438)
congenital hydrocephalus (741.0, 742.3)
neoplastic disease (140.0-239.9)
myxedema (244.0-244.9)
vitamin B_{12} deficiency (266.2)
EXCLUDES   cerebral degeneration in:
Jakob-Creutzfeldt disease (046.1)
progressive multifocal leukoencephalopathy (046.3)
subacute spongiform encephalopathy (046.1)

√5th **331.8 Other cerebral degeneration**

331.81 Reye's syndrome
DEF: Rare childhood illness, often developed after a bout of viral upper respiratory infection; characterized by vomiting, elevated serum transaminase, changes in liver and other viscera; symptoms may be followed by an encephalopathic phase with brain swelling, distur-bances of consciousness and seizures; can be fatal.

331.89 Other
Cerebral ataxia

331.9 Cerebral degeneration, unspecified

NERVOUS SYSTEM AND SENSE ORGANS

✓4th 332 Parkinson's disease

332.0 Paralysis agitans
Parkinsonism or Parkinson's disease:
  NOS
  idiopathic
  primary

DEF: Form of parkinsonism; progressive, occurs in senior years; characterized by masklike facial expression; condition affects ability to stand erect, walk smoothly; weakened muscles, also tremble and involuntarily movement.

332.1 Secondary Parkinsonism
Parkinsonism due to drugs
Use additional E code to identify drug, if drug-induced
  EXCLUDES Parkinsonism (in):
    Huntington's disease (333.4)
    progressive supranuclear palsy (333.0)
    Shy-Drager syndrome (333.0)
    syphilitic (094.82)

✓4th 333 Other extrapyramidal disease and abnormal movement disorders
  INCLUDES other forms of extrapyramidal, basal ganglia, or striatopallidal disease
  EXCLUDES abnormal movements of head NOS (781.0)

333.0 Other degenerative diseases of the basal ganglia
Atrophy or degeneration:
  olivopontocerebellar [Déjérine-Thomas syndrome]
  pigmentary pallidal [Hallervorden-Spatz disease]
  striatonigral
Parkinsonian syndrome associated with:
  idiopathic orthostatic hypotension
  symptomatic orthostatic hypotension
Progressive supranuclear ophthalmoplegia
Shy-Drager syndrome

333.1 Essential and other specified forms of tremor
Benign essential tremor
Familial tremor
Use additional E code to identify drug, if drug-induced
  EXCLUDES tremor NOS (781.0)

333.2 Myoclonus
Familial essential myoclonus
Progressive myoclonic epilepsy
Unverricht-Lundborg disease
Use additional E code to identify drug, if drug-induced

DEF: Spontaneous movements or contractions of muscles.

333.3 Tics of organic origin
Use additional E code to identify drug, if drug-induced
  EXCLUDES Gilles de la Tourette's syndrome (307.23)
    habit spasm (307.22)
    tic NOS (307.20)

333.4 Huntington's chorea

DEF: Genetic disease; characterized by chronic progressive mental deterioration; dementia and death within 15 years of onset.

333.5 Other choreas
Hemiballism(us)
Paroxysmal choreo-athetosis
Use additional E code to identify drug, if drug-induced
  EXCLUDES Sydenham's or rheumatic chorea (392.0-392.9)

333.6 Idiopathic torsion dystonia
Dystonia:
   deformans progressiva
   musculorum deformans
(Schwalbe-) Ziehen-Oppenheim disease
DEF: Sustained muscular contractions, causing twisting and repetitive movements that result in abnormal postures of trunk and limbs; etiology unknown.

333.7 Symptomatic torsion dystonia
Athetoid cerebral palsy [Vogt's disease]
Double athetosis (syndrome)
Use additional E code to identify drug, if drug-induced

√5th **333.8 Fragments of torsion dystonia**
Use additional E code to identify drug, if drug-induced

333.81 Blepharospasm
DEF: Uncontrolled winking or blinking due to orbicularis oculi muscle spasm.

333.82 Orofacial dyskinesia
DEF: Uncontrolled movement of mouth or facial muscles.

333.83 Spasmodic torticollis
EXCLUDES   torticollis:
   NOS (723.5)
   hysterical (300.11)
   psychogenic (306.0)
DEF: Uncontrolled movement of head due to spasms of neck muscle.

333.84 Organic writers' cramp
EXCLUDES   pychogenic (300.89)

333.89 Other

√5th **333.9 Other and unspecified extrapyramidal diseases and abnormal movement disorders**

333.90 Unspecified extrapyramidal disease and abnormal movement disorder

333.91 Stiff-man syndrome

333.92 Neuroleptic malignant syndrome
Use additional E code to identify drug

333.93 Benign shuddering attacks

333.99 Other
Restless legs

√4th **334 Spinocerebellar disease**
EXCLUDES   olivopontocerebellar degeneration (333.0)
peroneal muscular atrophy (356.1)

334.0 Friedreich's ataxia
DEF: Genetic recessive disease of children; sclerosis of dorsal, lateral spinal cord columns; characterized by ataxia, speech impairment, swaying and irregular movements, with muscle paralysis, especially of lower limbs.

334.1 Hereditary spastic paraplegia

334.2 Primary cerebellar degeneration
Cerebellar ataxia: Primary cerebellar
   Marie's   degeneration:
   Sanger-Brown   NOS
   Dyssynergia cerebellaris   hereditary
      myoclonica   sporadic

334.3 Other cerebellar ataxia
Cerebellar ataxia NOS
Use additional E code to identify drug, if drug-induced

NERVOUS SYSTEM AND SENSE ORGANS

334.4 *Cerebellar ataxia in diseases classified elsewhere*
  Code first underlying disease, as:
    alcoholism (303.0-303.9)
    myxedema (244.0-244.9)
    neoplastic disease (140.0-239.9)

334.8 **Other spinocerebellar diseases**
  Ataxia-telangiectasia [Louis-Bar syndrome]
  Corticostriatal-spinal degeneration

334.9 Spinocerebellar disease, unspecified

√4th **335 Anterior horn cell disease**

  335.0 **Werdnig-Hoffmann disease**
    Infantile spinal muscular atrophy
    Progressive muscular atrophy of infancy

  DEF: Spinal muscle atrophy manifested in prenatal period or shortly after birth; symptoms include hypotonia, atrophy of skeletal muscle; death occurs in infancy.

  √5th **335.1** **Spinal muscular atrophy**
    335.10 Spinal muscular atrophy, unspecified
    335.11 **Kugelberg-Welander disease**
      Spinal muscular atrophy:
        familial
        juvenile

  DEF: Hereditary; juvenile muscle atrophy; appears during first two decades of life; due to lesions of anterior horns of spinal cord; includes wasting, diminution of lower body muscles and twitching.

    335.19 Other
      Adult spinal muscular atrophy

  √5th **335.2** **Motor neuron disease**
    335.20 **Amyotrophic lateral sclerosis**
      Motor neuron disease (bulbar) (mixed type)
    335.21 **Progressive muscular atrophy**
      Duchenne-Aran muscular atrophy
      Progressive muscular atrophy (pure)
    335.22 **Progressive bulbar palsy**
    335.23 **Pseudobulbar palsy**
    335.24 **Primary lateral sclerosis**
    335.29 Other

  335.8 **Other anterior horn cell diseases**
  335.9 Anterior horn cell disease, unspecified

√4th **336 Other diseases of spinal cord**

  336.0 **Syringomyelia and syringobulbia**
  336.1 **Vascular myelopathies**
    Acute infarction of spinal cord (embolic) (nonembolic)
    Arterial thrombosis of spinal cord
    Edema of spinal cord
    Hematomyelia
    Subacute necrotic myelopathy

  336.2 *Subacute combined degeneration of spinal cord in diseases classified elsewhere*
    Code first underlying disease, as:
      pernicious anemia (281.0)
      other vitamin B_{12} deficiency anemia (281.1)
      vitamin B_{12} deficiency (266.2)

 Additional Digit Required   Unspecified Code 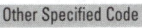 Other Specified Code Manifestation Code

MSP Medicare Secondary Payer   ▶◀ Revised Text   ● New Code   ▲ Revised Code Title

NERVOUS SYSTEM AND SENSE ORGANS

336.3 **Myelopathy in other diseases classified elsewhere**
Code first underlying disease, as:
myelopathy in neoplastic disease (140.0-239.9)
EXCLUDES   myelopathy in:
intervertebral disc disorder (722.70-722.73)
spondylosis (721.1, 721.41-721.42, 721.91)

336.8 **Other myelopathy**
Myelopathy: Myelopathy:
  drug-induced   radiation-induced
Use additonal E code to identify cause

336.9 **Unspecified disease of spinal cord**
Cord compression NOS   Myelopathy NOS
EXCLUDES   myelitis (323.0-323.9)
spinal (canal) stenosis (723.0, 724.00-724.09)

√4th **337 Disorders of the autonomic nervous system**
INCLUDES   disorders of peripheral autonomic, sympathetic, parasympathetic, or vegetative system
EXCLUDES   familial dysautonomia [Riley-Day syndrome] (742.8)

337.0 **Idiopathic peripheral autonomic neuropathy**
Carotid sinus syncope or syndrome
Cervical sympathetic dystrophy or paralysis

337.1 **Peripheral autonomic neuropathy in disorders classified elsewhere**
Code first underlying disease, as:
amyloidosis (277.3)
diabetes (250.6)

√5th **337.2** **Reflex sympathetic dystrophy**
DEF: Disturbance of the sympathetic nervous system evidenced by sweating, pain, pallor and edema following injury to nerves or blood vessels.

337.20 **Reflex sympathetic dystrophy, unspecified**
337.21 Reflex sympathetic dystrophy of the upper limb
337.22 Reflex sympathetic dystrophy of the lower limb
337.29 **Reflex sympathetic dystrophy of other specified site**

337.3 Autonomic dysreflexia
Use additional code to identify the cause, such as:
decubitus ulcer (707.0)
fecal impaction (560.39)
urinary tract infection (599.0)

DEF: Noxious stimuli evokes paroxysmal hypertension, bradycardia, excess sweating, headache, pilomotor responses, facial flushing, and nasal congestion due to uncontrolled parasympathetic nerve response; usually occurs in patients with spinal cord injury above major sympathetic outflow tract (T_6).

337.9 **Unspecified disorder of autonomic nervous system**

OTHER DISORDERS OF THE CENTRAL NERVOUS SYSTEM (340-349)

340 Multiple sclerosis   A
Disseminated or multiple sclerosis:
NOS
brain stem
cord
generalized

√4th **341 Other demyelinating diseases of central nervous system**
341.0 Neuromyelitis optica

NERVOUS SYSTEM AND SENSE ORGANS 341.1–343.3

341.1 Schilder's disease
Baló's concentric sclerosis
Encephalitis periaxialis:
  concentrica [Baló's]
  diffusa [Schilder's]

DEF: Chronic leukoencephalopathy of children and adolescents; symptoms include blindness, deafness, bilateral spasticity and progressive mental deterioration.

341.8 Other demyelinating diseases of central nervous system
Central demyelination of corpus callosum
Central pontine myelinosis
Marchiafava (-Bignami) disease

341.9 Demyelinating disease of central nervous system, unspecified

√4th **342 Hemiplegia and hemiparesis**

Note: This category is to be used when hemiplegia (complete) (incomplete) is reported without further specification, or is stated to be old or long-standing but of unspecified cause. The category is also for use in multiple coding to identify these types of hemiplegia resulting from any cause.

> EXCLUDES   congenital (343.1)
>   hemiplegia due to late effect of cerebrovascular accident (438.20-438.22)
>   infantile NOS (343.4)

The following fifth-digits are for use with codes 342.0-342.9:
  0 affecting unspecified side
  1 affecting dominant side
  2 affecting nondominant side

√5th **342.0 Flaccid hemiplegia**
√5th **342.1 Spastic hemiplegia**
√5th **342.8 Other specified hemiplegia**
√5th **342.9 Hemiplegia, unspecified**

√4th **343 Infantile cerebral palsy**

> INCLUDES   cerebral:
>   palsy NOS
>   spastic infantile paralysis
>   congenital spastic paralysis (cerebral)
>   Little's disease
>   paralysis (spastic) due to birth injury:
>   intracranial
>   spinal

> EXCLUDES   hereditary cerebral paralysis, such as:
>   hereditary spastic paraplegia (334.1)
>   Vogt's disease (333.7)
>   spastic paralysis specified as noncongenital or noninfantile (344.0-344.9)

343.0 Diplegic
Congenital diplegia   Congenital paraplegia
DEF: Paralysis affecting both sides of the body simultaneously.

343.1 Hemiplegic
Congenital hemiplegia
> EXCLUDES   infantile hemiplegia NOS (343.4)

343.2 Quadriplegic
Tetraplegic

343.3 Monoplegic

343.4 **Infantile hemiplegia**
Infantile hemiplegia (postnatal) NOS

343.8 Other specified infantile cerebral palsy

343.9 Infantile cerebral palsy, unspecified
Cerebral palsy NOS

√4th **344 Other paralytic syndromes**

Note: This category is to be used when the listed conditions are reported without further specification or are stated to be old or long-standing but of unspecified cause. The category is also for use in multiple coding to identify these conditions resulting from any cause.

INCLUDES   paralysis (complete) (incomplete), except as classifiable to 342 and 343

EXCLUDES   congenital or infantile cerebral palsy (343.0-343.9)
hemiplegia (342.0-342.9)
congenital or infantile (343.1, 343.4)

√5th **344.0 Quadriplegia and quadriparesis**

344.00 Quadriplegia unspecified

344.01 C_1-C_4 complete

344.02 C_1-C_4 incomplete

344.03 C_5-C_7 complete

344.04 C_5-C_7 incomplete

344.09 Other

344.1 Paraplegia
Paralysis of both lower limbs
Paraplegia (lower)

344.2 Diplegia of upper limbs
Diplegia (upper)
Paralysis of both upper limbs

√5th **344.3 Monoplegia of lower limb**
Paralysis of lower limb

EXCLUDES   monoplegia of lower limb due to late effect of cerebrovascular accident (438.40-438.42)

344.30 Affecting unspecified side

344.31 Affecting dominant side

344.32 Affecting nondominant side

√5th **344.4 Monoplegia of upper limb**
Paralysis of upper limb

EXCLUDES   monoplegia of upper limb due to late effect of cerebrovascular accident (438.30-438.32)

344.40 Affecting unspecified side

344.41 Affecting dominant side

344.42 Affecting nondominant side

344.5 Unspecified monoplegia

√5th **344.6 Cauda equina syndrome**

DEF: Dull pain and paresthesias in sacrum, perineum and bladder due to compression of spinal nerve roots; pain radiates down buttocks, back of thigh, calf of leg and into foot with prickling, burning sensations.

344.60 Without mention of neurogenic bladder

344.61 With neurogenic bladder
Acontractile bladder
Autonomic hyperreflexia of bladder
Cord bladder
Detrusor hyperreflexia

NERVOUS SYSTEM AND SENSE ORGANS   344.8–345.4

√5ᵗʰ 344.8 Other specified paralytic syndromes

344.81 Locked-in state

DEF: State of consciousness where patients are paralyzed and unable to respond to environmental stimuli; patients have eye movements, and stimuli can enter the brain but patients cannot respond to stimuli.

344.89 Other specified paralytic syndrome

344.9 Paralysis, unspecified

√4ᵗʰ 345 Epilepsy

EXCLUDES   progressive myoclonic epilepsy (333.2)

DEF: Brain disorder characterized by electrical-like disturbances; may include occasional impairment or loss of consciousness, abnormal motor phenomena and psychic or sensory disturbances.

The following fifth-digit subclassification is for use with categories 345.0, .1, .4–.9:
- 0 without mention of intractable epilepsy
- 1 with intractable epilepsy, so stated

√5ᵗʰ 345.0 Generalized nonconvulsive epilepsy
Absences:
  atonic
  typical
Minor epilepsy
Petit mal
Pykno-epilepsy
Seizures:
  akinetic
  atonic

√5ᵗʰ 345.1 Generalized convulsive epilepsy
Epileptic seizures:
  clonic
  myoclonic
  tonic
Epileptic seizures:
  tonic-clonic
  Grand mal
  Major epilepsy

EXCLUDES   convulsions:
  NOS (780.3)
  infantile (780.3)
  newborn (779.0)
infantile spasms (345.6)

DEF: Convulsive seizures with tension of limbs (tonic) or rhythmic contractions (clonic).

345.2 Petit mal status
Epileptic absence status

DEF: Minor myoclonic spasms and sudden momentary loss of consciousness in epilepsy.

345.3 Grand mal status
Status epilepticus NOS

EXCLUDES   epilepsia partialis continua (345.7)
status:
  psychomotor (345.7)
  temporal lobe (345.7)

DEF: Sudden loss of consciousness followed by generalized convulsions in epilepsy.

√5ᵗʰ 345.4 Partial epilepsy, with impairment of consciousness
Epilepsy:
  limbic system
  partial:
    secondarily generalized
    with memory and ideational disturbances
  psychomotor
  psychosensory
  temporal lobe
Epileptic automatism

345.5 Partial epilepsy, without mention of impairment of consciousness
Epilepsy:
    Bravais-Jacksonian NOS
    focal (motor) NOS
    Jacksonian NOS
    motor partial
    partial NOS
Epilepsy:
    sensory-induced
    somatomotor
    somatosensory
    visceral
    visual

345.6 Infantile spasms
Hypsarrhythmia   Salaam attacks
Lightning spasms
EXCLUDES salaam tic (781.0)

345.7 Epilepsia partialis continua
Kojevnikov's epilepsy
DEF: Continuous muscle contractions and relaxation; result of abnormal neural discharge.

345.8 Other forms of epilepsy
Epilepsy: Epilepsy:
    cursive [running]   gelastic

345.9 Epilepsy, unspecified
Epileptic convulsions, fits, or seizures NOS
EXCLUDES convulsive seizure or fit NOS (780.3)

346 Migraine
DEF: Benign vascular headache of extreme pain; commonly associated with irritability, nausea, vomiting and often photophobia; premonitory visual hallucination of a crescent in the visual field (scotoma).

The following fifth-digit subclassification is for use with category 346:
    0 without mention of intractable migraine
    1 with intractable migraine, so stated

346.0 Classical migraine
Migraine preceded or accompanied by transient focal neurological phenomena
Migraine with aura

346.1 Common migraine
Atypical migraine   Sick headache

346.2 Variants of migraine
Cluster headache
Histamine cephalgia
Horton's neuralgia
Migraine:
    abdominal
    basilar
Migraine:
    lower half
    retinal
Neuralgia:
    ciliary
    migrainous

346.8 Other forms of migraine
Migraine: Migraine:
    hemiplegic   ophthalmoplegic

346.9 Migraine, unspecified

347 Cataplexy and narcolepsy
DEF: Cataplexy: sudden onset of muscle weakness with loss of tone and strength; caused by aggressive or spontaneous emotions.

DEF: Narcolepsy: brief, recurrent, uncontrollable episodes of sound sleep.

348 Other conditions of brain

348.0 Cerebral cysts
Arachnoid cyst   Porencephaly, acquired
Porencephalic cyst   Pseudoporencephaly
EXCLUDES porencephaly (congenital) (742.4)

NERVOUS SYSTEM AND SENSE ORGANS

NERVOUS SYSTEM AND SENSE ORGANS

348.1 Anoxic brain damage
> **EXCLUDES** that occurring in:
> abortion (634-638 with .7, 639.8)
> ectopic or molar pregnancy (639.8)
> labor or delivery (668.2, 669.4)
> that of newborn (767.0, 768.0-768.9, 772.1-772.2)

Use additional E code to identify cause
DEF: Brain injury due to lack of oxygen, other than birth trauma.

348.2 Benign intracranial hypertension
Pseudotumor cerebri
> **EXCLUDES** hypertensive encephalopathy (437.2)

DEF: Elevated pressure in brain due to fluid retention in brain cavities.

348.3 Encephalopathy, unspecified

348.4 Compression of brain
Compression ⎫
Herniation ⎬ brain (stem)

Posterior fossa compression syndrome
DEF: Elevated pressure in brain due to blood clot, tumor, fracture, abscess, other condition.

348.5 Cerebral edema
DEF: Elevated pressure in the brain due to fluid retention in brain tissues.

348.8 Other conditions of brain
Cerebral: Cerebral:
  calcification   fungus

348.9 Unspecified condition of brain

√4th **349 Other and unspecified disorders of the nervous system**

349.0 Reaction to spinal or lumbar puncture
Headache following lumbar puncture

349.1 Nervous system complications from surgically implanted device
> **EXCLUDES** immediate postoperative complications (997.00-997.09)
> mechanical complications of nervous system device (996.2)

349.2 Disorders of meninges, not elsewhere classified
Adhesions, meningeal (cerebral) (spinal)
Cyst, spinal meninges
Meningocele, acquired
Pseudomeningocele, acquired

√5th **349.8 Other specified disorders of nervous system**

349.81 Cerebrospinal fluid rhinorrhea
> **EXCLUDES** cerebrospinal fluid otorrhea (388.61)

DEF: Cerebrospinal fluid discharging from the nose; caused by fracture of frontal bone with tearing of dura mater and arachnoid.

349.82 Toxic encephalopathy
Use additional E code, if desired, to identify cause
DEF: Brain tissue degeneration due to toxic substance.

349.89 Other

349.9 Unspecified disorders of nervous system
Disorder of nervous system (central) NOS

NERVOUS SYSTEM AND SENSE ORGANS 350–352.0

DISORDERS OF THE PERIPHERAL NERVOUS SYSTEM (350-359)

EXCLUDES diseases of:
acoustic [8th] nerve (388.5)
oculomotor [3rd, 4th, 6th] nerves (378.0-378.9)
optic [2nd] nerve (377.0-377.9)
peripheral autonomic nerves (337.0-337.9)
neuralgia
neuritis } NOS or "rheumatic" (729.2)
radiculitis

peripheral neuritis in pregnancy (646.4)

✓4th **350 Trigeminal nerve disorders**
  INCLUDES disorders of 5th cranial nerve

  350.1 Trigeminal neuralgia
  Tic douloureux   Trigeminal neuralgia NOS
  Trifacial neuralgia
  EXCLUDES postherpetic (053.12)

  350.2 Atypical face pain
  350.8 Other specified trigeminal nerve disorders
  350.9 Trigeminal nerve disorder, unspecified

✓4th **351 Facial nerve disorders**
  INCLUDES disorders of 7th cranial nerve
  EXCLUDES that in newborn (767.5)

  351.0 Bell's palsy
  Facial palsy
  DEF: Unilateral paralysis of face due to lesion on facial nerve; produces facial distortion.

  351.1 Geniculate ganglionitis
  Geniculate ganglionitis NOS
  EXCLUDES herpetic (053.11)
  DEF: Inflammation of tissue at bend in facial nerve.

  351.8 Other facial nerve disorders
  Facial myokymia   Melkersson's syndrome
  351.9 Facial nerve disorder, unspecified

✓4th **352 Disorders of other cranial nerves**
  352.0 Disorders of olfactory [1st] nerve

✓4th
✓5th Additional Digit Required   Unspecified Code   Other Specified Code   Manifestation Code
 Medicare Secondary Payer   ▶◀ Revised Text   ● New Code   ▲ Revised Code Title

2002 Ingenix, Inc.   Volume 1 — 177

NERVOUS SYSTEM AND SENSE ORGANS

Cranial Nerves

- Olfactory bulb (I)
- Optic nerve (II)
- Oculomotor nerve (III)
- Trochlear nerve (IV)
- Trigeminal nerve (V)
- Abducens nerve (VI)
- Facial nerve (VII)
- Vestibulocochlear nerve (VIII)
- Glossopharyngeal nerve (IX)
- Vagus nerve (X)
- Accessory nerve (XI)
- Hypoglossal nerve (XII)

Pons

352.1 Glossopharyngeal neuralgia
DEF: Pain between throat and ear along petrosal and jugular ganglia.

352.2 Other disorders of glossopharyngeal [9th] nerve

352.3 Disorders of pneumogastric [10th] nerve
Disorders of vagal nerve
EXCLUDES *paralysis of vocal cords or larynx (478.30-478.34)*
DEF: Nerve disorder affecting ear, tongue, pharynx, larynx, esophagus, viscera and thorax.

352.4 Disorders of accessory [11th] nerve
DEF: Nerve disorder affecting palate, pharynx, larynx, thoracic viscera, sternocleidomastoid and trapezius muscles.

352.5 Disorders of hypoglossal [12th] nerve
DEF: Nerve disorder affecting tongue muscles.

352.6 Multiple cranial nerve palsies
Collet-Sicard syndrome   Polyneuritis cranialis

352.9 Unspecified disorder of cranial nerves

√4th **353 Nerve root and plexus disorders**
EXCLUDES conditions due to:
intervertebral disc disorders (722.0-722.9)
spondylosis (720.0-721.9)
vertebrogenic disorders (723.0-724.9)

353.0 Brachial plexus lesions
Cervical rib syndrome
Costoclavicular syndrome
Scalenus anticus syndrome
Thoracic outlet syndrome
EXCLUDES *brachial neuritis or radiculitis NOS (723.4)*
that in newborn (767.6)
DEF: Acquired disorder in tissue along nerves in shoulder; causes corresponding motor and sensory dysfunction.

353.1 Lumbosacral plexus lesions
DEF: Acquired disorder in tissue along nerves in lower back; causes corresponding motor and sensory dysfunction.

353.2 Cervical root lesions, not elsewhere classified
353.3 Thoracic root lesions, not elsewhere classified
353.4 Lumbosacral root lesions, not elsewhere classified
353.5 Neuralgic amyotrophy
Parsonage-Aldren-Turner syndrome

NERVOUS SYSTEM AND SENSE ORGANS

353.6 **Phantom limb (syndrome)**
DEF: Abnormal tingling or a burning sensation, transient aches, and intermittent or continuous pain perceived as originating in the absent limb.

353.8 Other nerve root and plexus disorders
353.9 Unspecified nerve root and plexus disorder

354 Mononeuritis of upper limb and mononeuritis multiplex
DEF: Inflammation of a single nerve; known as mononeuritis multiplex when several nerves in unrelated body areas are affected.

354.0 **Carpal tunnel syndrome**
Median nerve entrapment   Partial thenar atrophy
DEF: Compression of median nerve by tendons; causes pain, tingling, numbness and burning sensation in hand.

354.1 Other lesion of median nerve
Median nerve neuritis

354.2 **Lesion of ulnar nerve**
Cubital tunnel syndrome
Tardy ulnar nerve palsy

354.3 **Lesion of radial nerve**
Acute radial nerve palsy

354.4 **Causalgia of upper limb**
EXCLUDES causalgia:
NOS (355.9)
lower limb (355.71)
DEF: Peripheral nerve damage, upper limb; usually due to injury; causes burning sensation and trophic skin changes.

354.5 **Mononeuritis multiplex**
Combinations of single conditions classifiable to 354 or 355

354.8 Other mononeuritis of upper limb
354.9 Mononeuritis of upper limb, unspecified

355 Mononeuritis of lower limb

355.0 **Lesion of sciatic nerve**
EXCLUDES sciatica NOS (724.3)
DEF: Acquired disorder of sciatic nerve; causes motor and sensory dysfunction in back, buttock and leg.

355.1 **Meralgia paresthetica**
Lateral cutaneous femoral nerve of thigh compression or syndrome
DEF: Inguinal ligament entraps lateral femoral cutaneous nerve; causes tingling, pain and numbness along outer thigh.

355.2 Other lesion of femoral nerve
355.3 **Lesion of lateral popliteal nerve**
Lesion of common peroneal nerve
355.4 **Lesion of medial popliteal nerve**
355.5 **Tarsal tunnel syndrome**
DEF: Compressed, entrapped posterior tibial nerve; causes tingling, pain and numbness in sole of foot.

355.6 **Lesion of plantar nerve**
Morton's metatarsalgia, neuralgia, or neuroma

NERVOUS SYSTEM AND SENSE ORGANS

√5ᵗʰ 355.7　Other mononeuritis of lower limb

　　355.71　Causalgia of lower limb
　　　　　　EXCLUDES　causalgia:
　　　　　　　　　　　　　NOS (355.9)
　　　　　　　　　　　　　upper limb (354.4)
　　　　　　DEF: Dysfunction of lower limb peripheral nerve, usually due to injury; causes burning pain and trophic skin changes.

　　355.79　Other mononeuritis of lower limb

355.8　Mononeuritis of lower limb, unspecified

355.9　Mononeuritis of unspecified site
　　　　Causalgia NOS
　　　　EXCLUDES　causalgia:
　　　　　　　　　　　lower limb (355.71)
　　　　　　　　　　　upper limb (354.4)

√4ᵗʰ 356　Hereditary and idiopathic peripheral neuropathy

356.0　Hereditary peripheral neuropathy
　　　　Déjérine-Sottas disease

356.1　Peroneal muscular atrophy
　　　　Charcôt-Marie-Tooth disease　　Neuropathic muscular atrophy
　　　　DEF: Genetic disorder, in muscles innervated by peroneal nerves; symptoms include muscle wasting in lower limbs and locomotor difficulties.

356.2　Hereditary sensory neuropathy
　　　　DEF: Inherited disorder in dorsal root ganglia, optic nerve, and cerebellum, causing sensory losses, shooting pains, and foot ulcers.

356.3　Refsum's disease
　　　　Heredopathia atactica polyneuritiformis
　　　　DEF: Genetic disorder of lipid metabolism; causes persistent, painful inflammation of nerves and retinitis pigmentosa.

356.4　Idiopathic progressive polyneuropathy

356.8　Other specified idiopathic peripheral neuropathy
　　　　Supranuclear paralysis

356.9　Unspecified

√4ᵗʰ 357　Inflammatory and toxic neuropathy

357.0　Acute infective polyneuritis
　　　　Guillain-Barré syndrome　　Postinfectious polyneuritis
　　　　DEF: Guillain-Barré syndrome: acute demyelinatry polyneuropathy preceded by viral illness (i.e., herpes, cytomegalovirus [CMV], Epstein-Barr virus [EBV]) or a bacterial illness; areflexic motor paralysis with mild sensory disturbance and acellular rise in spinal fluid protein.

357.1　Polyneuropathy in collagen vascular disease
　　　　Code first underlying disease, as:
　　　　　　disseminated lupus erythematosus (710.0)
　　　　　　polyarteritis nodosa (446.0)
　　　　　　rheumatoid arthritis (714.0)

357.2　Polyneuropathy in diabetes
　　　　Code first underlying disease (250.6)

357.3　Polyneuropathy in malignant disease
　　　　Code first underlying disease (140.0-208.9)

NERVOUS SYSTEM AND SENSE ORGANS

357.4 Polyneuropathy in other diseases classified elsewhere
Code first underlying disease, as:
amyloidosis (277.3)
beriberi (265.0)
deficiency of B vitamins (266.0-266.9)
diphtheria (032.0-032.9)
hypoglycemia (251.2)
pellagra (265.2)
porphyria (277.1)
sarcoidosis (135)
uremia (585)
> EXCLUDES polyneuropathy in: polyneuropathy in:
>   herpes zoster (053.13)   mumps (072.72)

357.5 Alcoholic polyneuropathy

357.6 Polyneuropathy due to drugs
Use additional E code to identify drug

357.7 Polyneuropathy due to other toxic agents
Use additional E code to identify toxic agent

√5th **357.8 Other**

357.81 Chronic inflammatory demyelinating polyneuritis
DEF: Inflammation of peripheral nerves resulting in destruction of myelin sheath; associated with diabetes mellitus, dysproteinemias, renal failure and malnutrition; symptoms include tingling, numbness, burning pain, diminished tendon reflexes, weakness, and atrophy in lower extremities.

357.82 Critical illness polyneuropathy
Acute motor neuropathy

357.89 Other inflammatory and toxic neuropathy

357.9 Unspecified

√4th **358 Myoneural disorders**

358.0 Myasthenia gravis
DEF: Autoimmune disorder of acetylcholine at neuromuscular junction; causing fatigue of voluntary muscles.

358.1 Myasthenic syndromes in diseases classified elsewhere
Amyotrophy
Eaton-Lambert syndrome } from stated cause classified elsewhere

Code first underlying disease, as:
botulism (005.1)
diabetes mellitus (250.6)
hypothyroidism (244.0-244.9)
malignant neoplasm (140.0-208.9)
pernicious anemia (281.0)
thyrotoxicosis (242.0-242.9)

358.2 Toxic myoneural disorders
Use additional E code to identify toxic agent

358.8 Other specified myoneural disorders

358.9 Myoneural disorders, unspecified

√4th **359 Muscular dystrophies and other myopathies**
> EXCLUDES idiopathic polymyositis (710.4)

NERVOUS SYSTEM AND SENSE ORGANS

359.0 Congenital hereditary muscular dystrophy
Benign congenital myopathy
Central core disease
Centronuclear myopathy
Myotubular myopathy
Nemaline body disease

EXCLUDES arthrogryposis multiplex congenita (754.89)

DEF: Genetic disorder; causing progressive or nonprogressive muscle weakness.

359.1 Hereditary progressive muscular dystrophy
Muscular dystrophy: Muscular dystrophy:
  NOS   Gower's
  distal   Landouzy-Déjérine
  Duchenne   limb-girdle
  Erb's   ocular
  fascioscapulohumeral   oculopharyngeal

DEF: Genetic degenerative, muscle disease; causes progressive weakness, wasting of muscle with no nerve involvement.

359.2 Myotonic disorders
Dystrophia myotonica   Paramyotonia congenita
Eulenburg's disease   Steinert's disease
Myotonia congenita   Thomsen's disease

DEF: Impaired movement due to spasmatic, rigid muscles.

359.3 Familial periodic paralysis
Hypokalemic familial periodic paralysis

DEF: Genetic disorder; characterized by rapidly progressive flaccid paralysis; attacks often occur after exercise or exposure to cold or dietary changes.

359.4 Toxic myopathy
Use additional E code to identify toxic agent

DEF: Muscle disorder caused by toxic agent.

359.5 Myopathy in endocrine diseases classified elsewhere
Code first underlying disease, as:
   Addison's disease (255.4)
   Cushing's syndrome (255.0)
   hypopituitarism (253.2)
   myxedema (244.0-244.9)
   thyrotoxicosis (242.0-242.9)

DEF: Muscle disorder secondary to dysfunction in hormone secretion.

359.6 Symptomatic inflammatory myopathy in diseases classified elsewhere
Code first underlying disease, as:
   amyloidosis (277.3)
   disseminated lupus erythematosus (710.0)
   malignant neoplasm (140.0-208.9)
   polyarteritis nodosa (446.0)
   rheumatoid arthritis (714.0)
   sarcoidosis (135)
   scleroderma (710.1)
   Sjögren's disease (710.2)

√5th 359.8 Other myopathies
  359.81 Critical illness myopathy
     Acute necrotizing myopathy
     Acute quadriplegic myopathy
     Intensive care (ICU) myopathy
     Myopathy of critical illness
  359.89 Other myopathies

359.9 Myopathy, unspecified

NERVOUS SYSTEM AND SENSE ORGANS 360–360.14

DISORDERS OF THE EYE AND ADNEXA (360-379)

360 Disorders of the globe
  INCLUDES: disorders affecting multiple structures of eye

360.0 Purulent endophthalmitis
  360.00 Purulent endophthalmitis, unspecified
  360.01 Acute endophthalmitis
  360.02 Panophthalmitis
  360.03 Chronic endophthalmitis
  360.04 Vitreous abscess

360.1 Other endophthalmitis
  360.11 Sympathetic uveitis
    DEF: Inflammation of vascular layer of uninjured eye; follows injury to other eye.

  360.12 Panuveitis
    DEF: Inflammation of entire vascular layer of eye, including choroid, iris and ciliary body.

  360.13 Parasitic endophthalmitis NOS
    DEF: Parasitic infection causing inflammation of the entire eye.

  360.14 Ophthalmia nodosa
    DEF: Conjunctival inflammation caused by embedded hairs.

360.19 Other
   Phacoanaphylactic endophthalmitis

√5th 360.2 Degenerative disorders of globe

360.20 Degenerative disorder of globe, unspecified

360.21 Progressive high (degenerative) myopia
   Malignant myopia
   DEF: Severe, progressive nearsightedness in adults, complicated by serious disease of the choroid; leads to retinal detachment and blindness.

360.23 Siderosis
   DEF: Iron pigment deposits within tissue of eyeball; caused by high iron content of blood.

360.24 Other metallosis
   Chalcosis
   DEF: Metal deposits, other than iron, within eyeball tissues.

360.29 Other
   EXCLUDES   xerophthalmia (264.7)

√5th 360.3 Hypotony of eye

360.30 Hypotony, unspecified
   DEF: Low osmotic pressure causing lack of tone, tension and strength.

360.31 Primary hypotony

360.32 Ocular fistula causing hypotony
   DEF: Low intraocular pressure due to leak through abnormal passage.

360.33 Hypotony associated with other ocular disorders

360.34 Flat anterior chamber
   DEF: Low pressure behind cornea, causing compression.

√5th 360.4 Degenerated conditions of globe

360.40 Degenerated globe or eye, unspecified

360.41 Blind hypotensive eye
   Atrophy of globe
   Phthisis bulbi
   DEF: Vision loss due to extremely low intraocular pressure.

360.42 Blind hypertensive eye
   Absolute glaucoma
   DEF: Vision loss due to painful, high intraocular pressure.

360.43 Hemophthalmos, except current injury
   EXCLUDES   traumatic (871.0-871.9, 921.0-921.9)
   DEF: Pool of blood within eyeball, not from current injury.

360.44 Leucocoria
   DEF: Whitish mass or reflex in the pupil behind lens; also called cat's eye reflex; often indicative of retinoblastoma.

√5th 360.5 Retained (old) intraocular foreign body, magnetic
   EXCLUDES   current penetrating injury with magnetic foreign body (871.5)
              retained (old) foreign body of orbit (376.6)

360.50 Foreign body, magnetic, intraocular, unspecified

360.51 Foreign body, magnetic, in anterior chamber

360.52 Foreign body, magnetic, in iris or ciliary body

360.53 Foreign body, magnetic, in lens

360.54 Foreign body, magnetic, in vitreous

360.55 Foreign body, magnetic, in posterior wall

360.59 Foreign body, magnetic, in other or multiple sites

NERVOUS SYSTEM AND SENSE ORGANS 360.6–361.19

√5th 360.6 Retained (old) intraocular foreign body, nonmagnetic
Retained (old) foreign body:
NOS
nonmagnetic

> **EXCLUDES** current penetrating injury with (nonmagnetic) foreign body (871.6)
> retained (old) foreign body in orbit (376.6)

- 360.60 **Foreign body, intraocular, unspecified**
- 360.61 Foreign body in anterior chamber
- 360.62 Foreign body in iris or ciliary body
- 360.63 Foreign body in lens
- 360.64 Foreign body in vitreous
- 360.65 Foreign body in posterior wall
- 360.69 Foreign body in other or multiple sites

√5th 360.8 Other disorders of globe
- 360.81 Luxation of globe
  DEF: Displacement of eyeball.
- 360.89 Other

360.9 Unspecified disorder of globe

√4th 361 Retinal detachments and defects
DEF: Light-sensitive layer at back of eye, separates from blood supply; disrupting vision.

√5th 361.0 Retinal detachment with retinal defect
Rhegmatogenous retinal detachment

> **EXCLUDES** detachment of retinal pigment epithelium (362.42-362.43)
> retinal detachment (serous) (without defect) (361.2)

- 361.00 **Retinal detachment with retinal defect, unspecified**
- 361.01 Recent detachment, partial, with single defect
- 361.02 Recent detachment, partial, with multiple defects
- 361.03 Recent detachment, partial, with giant tear
- 361.04 Recent detachment, partial, with retinal dialysis
  Dialysis (juvenile) of retina (with detachment)
- 361.05 Recent detachment, total or subtotal
- 361.06 Old detachment, partial
  Delimited old retinal detachment
- 361.07 Old detachment, total or subtotal

√5th 361.1 Retinoschisis and retinal cysts

> **EXCLUDES** juvenile retinoschisis (362.73)
> microcystoid degeneration of retina (362.62)
> parasitic cyst of retina (360.13)

- 361.10 **Retinoschisis, unspecified**
  DEF: Separation of retina due to degenerative process of aging; should not be confused with acute retinal detachment.
- 361.11 Flat retinoschisis
  DEF: Slow, progressive split of retinal sensory layers.
- 361.12 Bullous retinoschisis
  DEF: Fluid retention between split retinal sensory layers.
- 361.13 Primary retinal cysts
- 361.14 Secondary retinal cysts
- 361.19 Other
  Pseudocyst of retina

√4th / √5th Additional Digit Required   Unspecified Code   Other Specified Code   Manifestation Code
 Medicare Secondary Payer   ▶◀ Revised Text   ● New Code   ▲ Revised Code Title

2002 Ingenix, Inc.   Volume 1 — 185

361.2 Serous retinal detachment
Retinal detachment without retinal defect
> EXCLUDES central serous retinopathy (362.41)
> retinal pigment epithelium detachment (362.42-362.43)

√5th **361.3 Retinal defects without detachment**
> EXCLUDES chorioretinal scars after surgery for detachment (363.30-363.35)
> peripheral retinal degeneration without defect (362.60-362.66)

361.30 Retinal defect, unspecified
Retinal break(s) NOS

361.31 Round hole of retina without detachment

361.32 Horseshoe tear of retina without detachment
Operculum of retina without mention of detachment

361.33 Multiple defects of retina without detachment

√5th **361.8 Other forms of retinal detachment**

361.81 Traction detachment of retina
Traction detachment with vitreoretinal organization

361.89 Other

361.9 Unspecified retinal detachment

√4th **362 Other retinal disorders**
> EXCLUDES chorioretinal scars (363.30-363.35)
> chorioretinitis (363.0-363.2)

√5th **362.0 Diabetic retinopathy**
Code first diabetes (250.5)
DEF: Retinal changes in diabetes of long duration; causes hemorrhages, microaneurysms, waxy deposits and proliferative noninflammatory degenerative disease of retina.

362.01 *Background diabetic retinopathy*
Diabetic macular edema
Diabetic retinal edema
Diabetic retinal microaneurysms
Diabetic retinopathy NOS

362.02 *Proliferative diabetic retinopathy*

√5th **362.1 Other background retinopathy and retinal vascular changes**

362.10 Background retinopathy, unspecified

362.11 Hypertensive retinopathy
DEF: Retinal irregularities caused by systemic hypertension.

362.12 Exudative retinopathy
Coats' syndrome

362.13 Changes in vascular appearance
Vascular sheathing of retina
Use additional code for any associated atherosclerosis (440.8)

362.14 Retinal microaneurysms NOS
DEF: Microscopic dilation of retinal vessels in nondiabetic.

362.15 Retinal telangiectasia
DEF: Dilation of blood vessels of the retina.

362.16 Retinal neovascularization NOS
Neovascularization:
choroidal
subretinal
DEF: New and abnormal vascular growth in the retina.

362.17 Other intraretinal microvascular abnormalities
Retinal varices

NERVOUS SYSTEM AND SENSE ORGANS 362.18–362.52

362.18 Retinal vasculitis
Eales' disease
Retinal:
  arteritis
  endarteritis
Retinal:
  perivasculitis
  phlebitis
DEF: Inflammation of retinal blood vessels.

√5th **362.2 Other proliferative retinopathy**
  362.21 Retrolental fibroplasia
    DEF: Fibrous tissue in vitreous, from retina to lens, causing blindness; associated with premature infants requiring high amounts of oxygen.

  362.29 Other nondiabetic proliferative retinopathy

√5th **362.3 Retinal vascular occlusion**
DEF: Obstructed blood flow to and from retina.

  362.30 Retinal vascular occlusion, unspecified
  362.31 Central retinal artery occlusion
  362.32 Arterial branch occlusion
  362.33 Partial arterial occlusion
    Hollenhorst plaque   Retinal microembolism
  362.34 Transient arterial occlusion
    Amaurosis fugax
  362.35 Central retinal vein occlusion
  362.36 Venous tributary (branch) occlusion
  362.37 Venous engorgement
    Occlusion:
      incipient } of retinal vein
      partial

√5th **362.4 Separation of retinal layers**
  EXCLUDES retinal detachment (serous) (361.2)
                rhegmatogenous (361.00-361.07)

  362.40 Retinal layer separation, unspecified
  362.41 Central serous retinopathy
    DEF: Serous-filled blister causing detachment of retina from pigment epithelium.

  362.42 Serous detachment of retinal pigment epithelium
    Exudative detachment of retinal pigment epithelium
    DEF: Blister of fatty fluid causing detachment of retina from pigment epithelium.

  362.43 Hemorrhagic detachment of retinal pigment epithelium
    DEF: Blood-filled blister causing detachment of retina from pigment epithelium.

√5th **362.5 Degeneration of macula and posterior pole**
  EXCLUDES degeneration of optic disc (377.21-377.24)
                hereditary retinal degeneration [dystrophy] (362.70-362.77)

  362.50 Macular degeneration (senile), unspecified
  362.51 Nonexudative senile macular degeneration
    Senile macular degeneration:
      atrophic
      dry
  362.52 Exudative senile macular degeneration
    Kuhnt-Junius degeneration
    Senile macular degeneration:
      disciform
      wet
    DEF: Leakage in macular blood vessels with loss of visual acuity.

 Additional Digit Required   Unspecified Code   Other Specified Code   Manifestation Code
MSP Medicare Secondary Payer   ▶◀ Revised Text   ● New Code   ▲ Revised Code Title

NERVOUS SYSTEM AND SENSE ORGANS

- **362.53 Cystoid macular degeneration**
  Cystoid macular edema
  DEF: Retinal swelling and cyst formation in macula.
- **362.54 Macular cyst, hole, or pseudohole**
- **362.55 Toxic maculopathy**
  Use additional E code to identify drug, if drug induced
- **362.56 Macular puckering**
  Preretinal fibrosis
- **362.57 Drusen (degenerative)**
  DEF: White, hyaline deposits on Bruch's membrane (lamina basalis choroideae).

√5th **362.6 Peripheral retinal degenerations**
  EXCLUDES hereditary retinal degeneration [dystrophy] (362.70-362.77)
  retinal degeneration with retinal defect (361.00-361.07)

- **362.60 Peripheral retinal degeneration, unspecified**
- **362.61 Paving stone degeneration**
  DEF: Degeneration of peripheral retina; causes thinning through which choroid is visible.
- **362.62 Microcystoid degeneration**
  Blessig's cysts   Iwanoff's cysts
- **362.63 Lattice degeneration**
  Palisade degeneration of retina
  DEF: Degeneration of retina; often bilateral, usually benign; characterized by lines intersecting at irregular intervals in peripheral retina; retinal thinning and retinal holes may occur.
- **362.64 Senile reticular degeneration**
  DEF: Net-like appearance of retina; sign of degeneration.
- **362.65 Secondary pigmentary degeneration**
  Pseudoretinitis pigmentosa
- **362.66 Secondary vitreoretinal degenerations**

√5th **362.7 Hereditary retinal dystrophies**
DEF: Genetically induced progressive changes in retina.

- **362.70 Hereditary retinal dystrophy, unspecified**
- **362.71 *Retinal dystrophy in systemic or cerebroretinal lipidoses***
  Code first underlying disease, as:
  cerebroretinal lipidoses (330.1)
  systemic lipidoses (272.7)
- **362.72 *Retinal dystrophy in other systemic disorders and syndromes***
  Code first underlying disease, as:
  Bassen-Kornzweig syndrome (272.5)
  Refsum's disease (356.3)
- **362.73 Vitreoretinal dystrophies**
  Juvenile retinoschisis
- **362.74 Pigmentary retinal dystrophy**
  Retinal dystrophy, albipunctate
  Retinitis pigmentosa
- **362.75 Other dystrophies primarily involving the sensory retina**
  Progressive cone(-rod) dystrophy
  Stargardt's disease
- **362.76 Dystrophies primarily involving the retinal pigment epithelium**
  Fundus flavimaculatus
  Vitelliform dystrophy

NERVOUS SYSTEM AND SENSE ORGANS 362.77–363.12

362.77 Dystrophies primarily involving Bruch's membrane
Dystrophy:
hyaline
pseudoinflammatory foveal
Hereditary drusen

√5ᵗʰ **362.8 Other retinal disorders**
> EXCLUDES chorioretinal inflammations (363.0-363.2)
> chorioretinal scars (363.30-363.35)

362.81 Retinal hemorrhage
Hemorrhage:
preretinal
retinal (deep) (superficial)
subretinal

362.82 Retinal exudates and deposits

362.83 Retinal edema
Retinal: Retinal:
cotton wool spots   edema (localized) (macular) (peripheral)
DEF: Retinal swelling due to fluid accumulation.

362.84 Retinal ischemia
DEF: Reduced retinal blood supply.

362.85 Retinal nerve fiber bundle defects

362.89 Other retinal disorders

362.9 Unspecified retinal disorder

√4ᵗʰ **363 Chorioretinal inflammations, scars, and other disorders of choroid**

√5ᵗʰ **363.0 Focal chorioretinitis and focal retinochoroiditis**
> EXCLUDES focal chorioretinitis or retinochoroiditis in:
> histoplasmosis (115.02, 115.12, 115.92)
> toxoplasmosis (130.2)
> congenital infection (771.2)

363.00 Focal chorioretinitis, unspecified
Focal:
choroiditis or chorioretinitis NOS
retinitis or retinochoroiditis NOS

363.01 Focal choroiditis and chorioretinitis, juxtapapillary

363.03 Focal choroiditis and chorioretinitis of other posterior pole

363.04 Focal choroiditis and chorioretinitis, peripheral

363.05 Focal retinitis and retinochoroiditis, juxtapapillary
Neuroretinitis

363.06 Focal retinitis and retinochoroiditis, macular or paramacular

363.07 Focal retinitis and retinochoroiditis of other posterior pole

363.08 Focal retinitis and retinochoroiditis, peripheral

√5ᵗʰ **363.1 Disseminated chorioretinitis and disseminated retinochoroiditis**
> EXCLUDES disseminated choroiditis or chorioretinitis in secondary syphilis (091.51)
> neurosyphilitic disseminated retinitis or retinochoroiditis (094.83)
> retinal (peri)vasculitis (362.18)

363.10 Disseminated chorioretinitis, unspecified
Disseminated:
choroiditis or chorioretinitis NOS
retinitis or retinochoroiditis NOS

363.11 Disseminated choroiditis and chorioretinitis, posterior pole

363.12 Disseminated choroiditis and chorioretinitis, peripheral

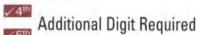

| √4ᵗʰ √5ᵗʰ Additional Digit Required | Unspecified Code | Other Specified Code | ▲ Manifestation Code |
| MSP Medicare Secondary Payer | ▶◀ Revised Text | ● New Code | ▲ Revised Code Title |

2002 Ingenix, Inc.   Volume 1 — 189

363.13 Disseminated choroiditis and chorioretinitis, generalized
  Code first any underlying disease, as:
    tuberculosis (017.0)
363.14 Disseminated retinitis and retinochoroiditis, metastatic
363.15 Disseminated retinitis and retinochoroiditis, pigment epitheliopathy
  Acute posterior multifocal placoid pigment epitheliopathy
  DEF: Widespread inflammation of retina and choroid; characterized by pigmented epithelium involvement.

√5th **363.2 Other and unspecified forms of chorioretinitis and retinochoroiditis**
  EXCLUDES panophthalmitis (360.02)
            sympathetic uveitis (360.11)
            uveitis NOS (364.3)

363.20 Chorioretinitis, unspecified
  Choroiditis NOS   Uveitis, posterior NOS
  Retinitis NOS

363.21 Pars planitis
  Posterior cyclitis
  DEF: Inflammation of peripheral retina and ciliary body; characterized by bands of white cells.

363.22 Harada's disease
  DEF: Retinal detachment and bilateral widespread exudative choroiditis; symptoms include headache, vomiting, increased lymphocytes in cerebrospinal fluid; and temporary or permanent deafness may occur.

√5th **363.3 Chorioretinal scars**
  Scar (postinflammatory) (postsurgical) (posttraumatic):
    choroid
    retina

363.30 Chorioretinal scar, unspecified
363.31 Solar retinopathy
  DEF: Retinal scarring caused by solar radiation.
363.32 Other macular scars
363.33 Other scars of posterior pole
363.34 Peripheral scars
363.35 Disseminated scars

√5th **363.4 Choroidal degenerations**
363.40 Choroidal degeneration, unspecified
  Choroidal sclerosis NOS
363.41 Senile atrophy of choroid
  DEF: Wasting away of choroid; due to aging.
363.42 Diffuse secondary atrophy of choroid
  DEF: Wasting away of choroid in systemic disease.
363.43 Angioid streaks of choroid
  DEF: Degeneration of choroid; characterized by dark brown steaks radiating from optic disk; occurs with pseudoxanthoma, elasticum or Paget's disease.

√5th **363.5 Hereditary choroidal dystrophies**
  Hereditary choroidal atrophy:
    partial [choriocapillaris]
    total [all vessels]

363.50 Hereditary choroidal dystrophy or atrophy, unspecified
363.51 Circumpapillary dystrophy of choroid, partial
363.52 Circumpapillary dystrophy of choroid, total
  Helicoid dystrophy of choroid

363.53 Central dystrophy of choroid, partial
Dystrophy, choroidal:
central areolar
circinate

363.54 Central choroidal atrophy, total
Dystrophy, choroidal:
central gyrate
serpiginous

363.55 Choroideremia
DEF: Hereditary choroid degeneration, occurs in first decade; characterized by constricted visual field and ultimately blindness in males; less debilitating in females.

363.56 Other diffuse or generalized dystrophy, partial
Diffuse choroidal sclerosis

363.57 Other diffuse or generalized dystrophy, total
Generalized gyrate atrophy, choroid

√5th **363.6 Choroidal hemorrhage and rupture**
363.61 Choroidal hemorrhage, unspecified
363.62 Expulsive choroidal hemorrhage
363.63 Choroidal rupture

√5th **363.7 Choroidal detachment**
363.70 Choroidal detachment, unspecified
363.71 Serous choroidal detachment
DEF: Detachment of choroid from sclera; due to blister of serous fluid.

363.72 Hemorrhagic choroidal detachment
DEF: Detachment of choroid from sclera; due to blood-filled blister.

363.8 Other disorders of choroid
363.9 Unspecified disorder of choroid

√4th **364 Disorders of iris and ciliary body**

√5th **364.0 Acute and subacute iridocyclitis**
Anterior uveitis ⎫
Cyclitis   ⎬ acute
Iridocyclitis   ⎭ subacute
Iritis

EXCLUDES   gonococcal (098.41)
           herpes simplex (054.44)
           herpes zoster (053.22)

364.00 Acute and subacute iridocyclitis, unspecified
364.01 Primary iridocyclitis
364.02 Recurrent iridocyclitis
364.03 Secondary iridocyclitis, infectious
364.04 Secondary iridocyclitis, noninfectious
Aqueous:
cells
fibrin
flare

364.05 Hypopyon
DEF: Accumulation of white blood cells between cornea and lens.

√5th **364.1 Chronic iridocyclitis**
EXCLUDES   posterior cyclitis (363.21)
364.10 Chronic iridocyclitis, unspecified

364.11 Chronic iridocyclitis in diseases classified elsewhere
Code first underlying disease, as:
sarcoidosis (135)
tuberculosis (017.3)
> **EXCLUDES** syphilitic iridocyclitis (091.52)

DEF: Persistent inflammation of iris and ciliary body; due to underlying disease or condition.

√5th **364.2 Certain types of iridocyclitis**
> **EXCLUDES** posterior cyclitis (363.21)
> sympathetic uveitis (360.11)

364.21 Fuchs' heterochromic cyclitis
DEF: Chronic cyclitis characterized by differences in the color of the two irises; the lighter iris appears in the inflamed eye.

364.22 Glaucomatocyclitic crises
DEF: One-sided form of secondary open angle glaucoma; recurrent, uncommon and of short duration; causes high intraocular pressure, rarely damage.

364.23 Lens-induced iridocyclitis
DEF: Inflammation of iris; due to immune reaction to proteins in lens following trauma or other lens abnormality.

364.24 Vogt-Koyanagi syndrome
DEF: Uveomeningitis with exudative iridocyclitis and choroiditis; causes depigmentation of hair and skin, detached retina; tinnitus and loss of hearing may occur.

364.3 Unspecified iridocyclitis
Uveitis NOS

√5th **364.4 Vascular disorders of iris and ciliary body**
364.41 Hyphema
Hemorrhage of iris or ciliary body
DEF: Hemorrhage in anterior chamber; also called hyphemia or "blood shot" eyes.

364.42 Rubeosis iridis
Neovascularization of iris or ciliary body
DEF: Blood vessel and connective tissue formation on surface of iris; symptomatic of diabetic retinopathy, central retinal vein occlusion and retinal detachment.

√5th **364.5 Degenerations of iris and ciliary body**
364.51 Essential or progressive iris atrophy
364.52 Iridoschisis
DEF: Splitting of iris into two layers.

364.53 Pigmentary iris degeneration
Acquired heterochromia ⎫
Pigment dispersion ⎬ of iris
  syndrome ⎪
Translucency ⎭

364.54 Degeneration of pupillary margin
Atrophy of sphincter ⎫
Ectropion of pigment ⎬ of iris
  epithelium ⎭

364.55 Miotic cysts of pupillary margin
DEF: Serous-filled sacs in pupillary margin of iris.

364.56 Degenerative changes of chamber angle
364.57 Degenerative changes of ciliary body

NERVOUS SYSTEM AND SENSE ORGANS

364.59 Other iris atrophy
Iris atrophy (generalized) (sector shaped)

√5th **364.6 Cysts of iris, ciliary body, and anterior chamber**
EXCLUDES miotic pupillary cyst (364.55)
parasitic cyst (360.13)

364.60 Idiopathic cysts
DEF: Fluid-filled sacs in iris or ciliary body; unknown etiology.

364.61 Implantation cysts
Epithelial down-growth, anterior chamber
Implantation cysts (surgical) (traumatic)

364.62 Exudative cysts of iris or anterior chamber

364.63 Primary cyst of pars plana
DEF: Fluid-filled sacs of outermost ciliary ring.

364.64 Exudative cyst of pars plana
DEF: Protein, fatty-filled sacs of outermost ciliary ring; due to fluid lead from blood vessels.

√5th **364.7 Adhesions and disruptions of iris and ciliary body**
EXCLUDES flat anterior chamber (360.34)

364.70 Adhesions of iris, unspecified
Synechiae (iris) NOS

364.71 Posterior synechiae
DEF: Adhesion binding iris to lens.

364.72 Anterior synechiae
DEF: Adhesion binding the iris to cornea.

364.73 Goniosynechiae
Peripheral anterior synechiae
DEF: Adhesion binding the iris to cornea at the angle of the anterior chamber.

364.74 Pupillary membranes
Iris bombé   Pupillary:
Pupillary: seclusion
  occlusion
DEF: Membrane traversing the pupil and blocking vision.

364.75 Pupillary abnormalities
Deformed pupil   Rupture of sphincter, pupil
Ectopic pupil

364.76 Iridodialysis
DEF: Separation of the iris from the ciliary body base; due to trauma or surgical accident.

364.77 Recession of chamber angle
DEF: Receding of anterior chamber angle of the eye; restricts vision.

364.8 Other disorders of iris and ciliary body
Prolapse of iris NOS
EXCLUDES prolapse of iris in recent wound (871.1)

364.9 Unspecified disorder of iris and ciliary body

√4th **365 Glaucoma**
EXCLUDES blind hypertensive eye [absolute glaucoma] (360.42)
congenital glaucoma (743.20-743.22)
DEF: Rise in intraocular pressure which restricts blood flow; multiple causes.

√4th Additional Digit Required
√5th
 Medicare Secondary Payer

Unspecified Code

Other Specified Code

Manifestation Code

▶◀ Revised Text

● New Code

▲ Revised Code Title

√5th **365.0 Borderline glaucoma [glaucoma suspect]**
365.00 Preglaucoma, unspecified
365.01 Open angle with borderline findings
Open angle with:
borderline intraocular pressure
cupping of optic discs
DEF: Minor block of aqueous outflow from eye.

365.02 Anatomical narrow angle
365.03 Steroid responders
365.04 Ocular hypertension
DEF: High fluid pressure within eye; no apparent cause.

√5th **365.1 Open-angle glaucoma**
365.10 Open-angle glaucoma, unspecified
Wide-angle glaucoma NOS
365.11 Primary open angle glaucoma
Chronic simple glaucoma
DEF: High intraocular pressure, despite free flow of aqueous.

365.12 Low tension glaucoma
365.13 Pigmentary glaucoma
DEF: High intraocular pressure; due to iris pigment granules blocking aqueous flow.

365.14 Glaucoma of childhood
Infantile or juvenile glaucoma
365.15 Residual stage of open angle glaucoma

√5th **365.2 Primary angle-closure glaucoma**
365.20 Primary angle-closure glaucoma, unspecified
365.21 Intermittent angle-closure glaucoma
Angle-closure glaucoma:
interval
subacute
DEF: Recurring attacks of high intraocular pressure; due to blocked aqueous flow.

365.22 Acute angle-closure glaucoma
DEF: Sudden, severe rise in intraocular pressure due to blockage in aqueous drainage.

365.23 Chronic angle-closure glaucoma
365.24 Residual stage of angle-closure glaucoma

√5th **365.3 Corticosteroid-induced glaucoma**
DEF: Elevated intraocular pressure; due to long-term corticosteroid therapy.

365.31 Glaucomatous stage
365.32 Residual stage

√5th **365.4 Glaucoma associated with congenital anomalies, dystrophies, and systemic syndromes**
365.41 *Glaucoma associated with chamber angle anomalies*
Code first associated disorder, as:
Axenfeld's anomaly (743.44)
Rieger's anomaly or syndrome (743.44)
365.42 *Glaucoma associated with anomalies of iris*
Code first associated disorder, as:
aniridia (743.45)
essential iris atrophy (364.51)
365.43 *Glaucoma associated with other anterior segment anomalies*
Code first associated disorder, as:
microcornea (743.41)

NERVOUS SYSTEM AND SENSE ORGANS 365.44–366.00

- **365.44 Glaucoma associated with systemic syndromes**
  Code first associated disease, as
    neurofibromatosis (237.7)
    Sturge-Weber (-Dimitri) syndrome (759.6)

√5ᵗʰ **365.5 Glaucoma associated with disorders of the lens**
- **365.51 Phacolytic glaucoma**
  Use additional code for associated hypermature cataract (366.18)
  DEF: Elevated intraocular pressure; due to lens protein blocking aqueous flow.

- **365.52 Pseudoexfoliation glaucoma**
  Use additional code for associated pseudoexfoliation of capsule (366.11)
  DEF: Glaucoma characterized by small grayish particles deposited on the lens.

- **365.59 Glaucoma associated with other lens disorders**
  Use additional code for associated disorder, as:
    dislocation of lens (379.33-379.34)
    spherophakia (743.36)

√5ᵗʰ **365.6 Glaucoma associated with other ocular disorders**
- **365.60 Glaucoma associated with unspecified ocular disorder**
- **365.61 Glaucoma associated with pupillary block**
  Use additional code for associated disorder, as:
    seclusion of pupil [iris bombé] (364.74)
  DEF: Acute, open-angle glaucoma caused by mature cataract; aqueous flow is blocked by lens material and macrophages.

- **365.62 Glaucoma associated with ocular inflammations**
  Use additional code for associated disorder, as:
    glaucomatocyclitic crises (364.22)
    iridocyclitis (364.0-364.3)

- **365.63 Glaucoma associated with vascular disorders**
  Use additional code for associated disorder, as:
    central retinal vein occlusion (362.35)
    hyphema (364.41)

- **365.64 Glaucoma associated with tumors or cysts**
  Use additional code for associated disorder, as:
    benign neoplasm (224.0-224.9)
    epithelial down-growth (364.61)
    malignant neoplasm (190.0-190.9)

- **365.65 Glaucoma associated with ocular trauma**
  Use additional code for associated condition, as:
    contusion of globe (921.3)
    recession of chamber angle (364.77)

√5ᵗʰ **365.8 Other specified forms of glaucoma**
- **365.81 Hypersecretion glaucoma**
- **365.82 Glaucoma with increased episcleral venous pressure**
- **365.83 Aqueous misdirection**
  Malignant glaucoma
- **365.89 Other specified glaucoma**

365.9 Unspecified glaucoma

√4ᵗʰ **366 Cataract**
  EXCLUDES congenital cataract (743.30-743.34)
  DEF: A variety of conditions that create a cloudy, or calcified lens that obstructs vision.

√5ᵗʰ **366.0 Infantile, juvenile, and presenile cataract**
- **366.00 Nonsenile cataract, unspecified**

√4ᵗʰ / √5ᵗʰ Additional Digit Required   Unspecified Code   Other Specified Code   Manifestation Code
MSP Medicare Secondary Payer   ▶◀ Revised Text   ● New Code   ▲ Revised Code Title

2002 Ingenix, Inc.

366.01 Anterior subcapsular polar cataract
DEF: Defect within the front, center lens surface.

366.02 Posterior subcapsular polar cataract
DEF: Defect within the rear, center lens surface.

366.03 Cortical, lamellar, or zonular cataract
DEF: Opacities radiating from center to edge of lens; appear as thin, concentric layers of lens.

366.04 Nuclear cataract

366.09 Other and combined forms of nonsenile cataract

√5th **366.1** Senile cataract

366.10 Senile cataract, unspecified   A

366.11 Pseudoexfoliation of lens capsule   A

366.12 Incipient cataract   A
    Cataract: Cataract:
      coronary   punctate
      immature NOS Water clefts
DEF: Minor disorders of lens not affecting vision; due to aging.

366.13 Anterior subcapsular polar senile cataract   A

366.14 Posterior subcapsular polar senile cataract   A

366.15 Cortical senile cataract   A

366.16 Nuclear sclerosis   A
    Cataracta brunescens
    Nuclear cataract

366.17 Total or mature cataract   A

366.18 Hypermature cataract   A
    Morgagni cataract

366.19 Other and combined forms of senile cataract   A

√5th **366.2** Traumatic cataract

366.20 Traumatic cataract, unspecified

366.21 Localized traumatic opacities
    Vossius' ring

366.22 Total traumatic cataract

366.23 Partially resolved traumatic cataract

√5th **366.3** Cataract secondary to ocular disorders

366.30 Cataracta complicata, unspecified

366.31 *Glaucomatous flecks (subcapsular)*
    Code first underlying glaucoma (365.0-365.9)

366.32 *Cataract in inflammatory disorders*
    Code first underlying condition, as:
      chronic choroiditis (363.0-363.2)

366.33 *Cataract with neovascularization*
    Code first underlying condition, as:
      chronic iridocyclitis (364.10)

366.34 *Cataract in degenerative disorders*
    Sunflower cataract
    Code first underlying condition, as:
      chalcosis (360.24)
      degenerative myopia (360.21)
      pigmentary retinal dystrophy (362.74)

√5th **366.4** Cataract associated with other disorders

366.41 *Diabetic cataract*
    Code first diabetes (250.5)

N Newborn Age: 0   **P** Pediatric Age: 0-17   **M** Maternity Age: 12-55   **A** Adult Age: 15-124

NERVOUS SYSTEM AND SENSE ORGANS 366.42–367.1

Cataract

366.42 Tetanic cataract
　　Code first underlying disease, as:
　　　calcinosis (275.4)
　　　hypoparathyroidism (252.1)

366.43 Myotonic cataract
　　Code first underlying disorder (359.2)

366.44 Cataract associated with other syndromes
　　Code first underlying condition, as:
　　　craniofacial dysostosis (756.0)
　　　galactosemia (271.1)

366.45 Toxic cataract
　　Drug-induced cataract
　　Use additional E code to identify drug or other toxic substance

366.46 Cataract associated with radiation and other physical influences
　　Use additional E code to identify cause

√5ᵗʰ **366.5 After-cataract**

366.50 After-cataract, unspecified
　　Secondary cataract NOS

366.51 Soemmering's ring
　　DEF: A donut-shaped lens remnant and a capsule behind the pupil as a result of cataract surgery or trauma.

366.52 Other after-cataract, not obscuring vision

366.53 After-cataract, obscuring vision

366.8 Other cataract
　　Calcification of lens

366.9 Unspecified cataract

√4ᵗʰ **367 Disorders of refraction and accommodation**

367.0 Hypermetropia
　　Far-sightedness
　　Hyperopia
　　DEF: Refraction error, called also hyperopia, focal point is posterior to retina; abnormally short anteroposterior diameter or subnormal refractive power; causes farsightedness.

367.1 Myopia
　　Near-sightedness
　　DEF: Refraction error, focal point is anterior to retina; causes near-sightedness.

NERVOUS SYSTEM AND SENSE ORGANS

√5th **367.2 Astigmatism**
 367.20 Astiginatism, unspecified
 367.21 Regular astigmatism
 367.22 Irregular astiginatism

√5th **367.3 Anisometropia and aniseikonia**
 367.31 Anisometropia
  DEF: Eyes with refractive powers that differ by at least one diopter.

 367.32 Aniseikonia
  DEF: Eyes with unequal retinal imaging; usually due to refractive error.

367.4 Presbyopia
 DEF: Loss of crystalline lens elasticity; causes errors of accommodation; due to aging.

√5th **367.5 Disorders of accommodation**
 367.51 Paresis of accommodation
  Cycloplegia
  DEF: Partial paralysis of ciliary muscle; causing focus problems.

 367.52 Total or complete internal ophthalmoplegia
  DEF: Total paralysis of ciliary muscle; large pupil incapable of focus.

 367.53 Spasm of accommodation
  DEF: Abnormal contraction of ciliary muscle; causes focus problems.

√5th **367.8 Other disorders of refraction and accommodation**
 367.81 Transient refractive change
 367.89 Other
  Drug-induced } disorders of refraction
  Toxic   & accommodation

367.9 Unspecified disorder of refraction and accommodation

√4th **368 Visual disturbances**
 EXCLUDES electrophysiological disturbances (794.11-794.14)

√5th **368.0 Amblyopia ex anopsia**
 DEF: Vision impaired due to disuse; esotropia often cause.

 368.00 Amblyopia, unspecified
 368.01 Strabismic amblyopia
  Suppression amblyopia
 368.02 Deprivation amblyopia
  DEF: Decreased vision associated with suppressed retinal image of one eye.
 368.03 Refractive amblyopia

√5th **368.1 Subjective visual disturbances**
 368.10 Subjective visual disturbance, unspecified
 368.11 Sudden visual loss
 368.12 Transient visual loss
  Concentric fading   Scintillating scotoma
 368.13 Visual discomfort
  Asthenopia   Photophobia
  Eye strain
 368.14 Visual distortions of shape and size
  Macropsia   Micropsia
  Metamorphopsia
 368.15 Other visual distortions and entoptic phenomena
  Photopsia   Refractive:
  Refractive: polyopia
   diplopia   Visual halos

NERVOUS SYSTEM AND SENSE ORGANS 368.16–368.51

368.16 Psychophysical visual disturbances
Visual:
 agnosia
 disorientation syndrome
 hallucinations

368.2 Diplopia
Double vision

√5th **368.3 Other disorders of binocular vision**

368.30 Binocular vision disorder, unspecified

368.31 Suppression of binocular vision

368.32 Simultaneous visual perception without fusion

368.33 Fusion with defective stereopsis
DEF: Faulty depth perception though normal ability to focus.

368.34 Abnormal retinal correspondence

√5th **368.4 Visual field defects**

368.40 Visual field defect, unspecified

368.41 Scotoma involving central area
Scotoma: Scotoma:
 central   paracentral
 centrocecal
DEF: Vision loss (blind spot) in central five degrees of visual field.

368.42 Scotoma of blind spot area
Enlarged: Paracecal scotoma
 angioscotoma
 blind spot

368.43 Sector or arcuate defects
Scotoma: Scotoma:
 arcuate   Seidel
 Bjerrum
DEF: Arc-shaped blind spot caused by retinal nerve damage.

368.44 Other localized visual field defect
Scotoma: Visual field defect:
 NOS   nasal step
 ring   peripheral

368.45 Generalized contraction or constriction

368.46 Homonymous bilateral field defects
Hemianopsia (altitudinal) (homonymous)
Quadrant anopia
DEF: Disorders found in the corresponding vertical halves of the visual fields of both eyes.

368.47 Heteronymous bilateral field defects
Hemianopsia:
 binasal
 bitemporal
DEF: Disorders in the opposite halves of the visual fields of both eyes.

√5th **368.5 Color vision deficiencies**
Color blindness

368.51 Protan defect
Protanomaly
Protanopia
DEF: Mild difficulty distinguishing green and red hues with shortened spectrum; sex-linked affecting one percent of males.

√4th
√5th Additional Digit Required   Unspecified Code   Other Specified Code   Manifestation Code
 Medicare Secondary Payer   ▶◀ Revised Text   ● New Code   ▲ Revised Code Title

2002 Ingenix, Inc.   Volume 1 — 199

368.52 Deutan defect
 Deuteranomaly
 Deuteranopia
 DEF: Male-only disorder; difficulty in distinguishing green and red, no shortened spectrum.

368.53 Tritan defect
 Tritanomaly
 Tritanopia
 DEF: Difficulty in distinguishing blue and yellow; occurs often due to drugs, retinal detachment and central nervous system diseases.

368.54 Achromatopsia
 Monochromatism (cone) (rod)
 DEF: Complete color blindness; caused by disease, injury to retina, optic nerve or pathway.

368.55 Acquired color vision deficiencies

368.59 Other color vision deficiencies

√5th **368.6 Night blindness**
 Nyctalopia
 DEF: Nyctalopia: disorder of vision in dim light or night blindness.

368.60 Night blindness, unspecified

368.61 Congenital night blindness
 Hereditary night blindness
 Oguchi's disease

368.62 Acquired night blindness
 EXCLUDES that due to vitamin A deficiency (264.5)

368.63 Abnormal dark adaptation curve
 Abnormal threshold } of cones or rods
 Delayed adaptation

368.69 Other night blindness

368.8 Other specified visual disturbances
 Blurred vision NOS

368.9 Unspecified visual disturbance

√4th **369 Blindness and low vision**

Note: Visual impairment refers to a functional limitation of the eye (e.g., limited visual acuity or visual field). It should be distinguished from visual disability, indicating a limitation of the abilities of the individual (e.g., limited reading skills, vocational skills), and from visual handicap, indicating a limitation of personal and socioeconomic independence (e.g., limited mobility, limited employability).

The levels of impairment defined in the table on page 201 are based on the recommendations of the WHO Study Group on Prevention of Blindness (Geneva, November 6–10, 1972; WHO Technical Report Series 518), and of the International Council of Ophthalmology (1976).

Note that definitions of blindness vary in different settings.

For international reporting WHO defines blindness as profound impairment. This definition can be applied to blindness of one eye (369.1, 369.6) and to blindness of the individual (369.0).

For determination of benefits in the U.S.A., the definition of legal blindness as severe impairment is often used. This definition applies to blindness of the individual only.

EXCLUDES correctable impaired vision due to refractive errors (367.0-367.9)

NERVOUS SYSTEM AND SENSE ORGANS 369.0–369.07

Classification		LEVELS OF VISUAL IMPAIRMENT	Additional descriptors which may be encountered
"legal"	WHO	Visual acuity and/or visual field limitation (whichever is worse)	
LEGAL BLINDNESS (U.S.A.) both eyes	(NEAR-) NORMAL VISION	RANGE OF NORMAL VISION 20/10 20/13 20/16 20/20 20/25 2.0 1.6 1.25 1.0 0.8	
		NEAR-NORMAL VISION 20/30 20/40 20/50 20/60 0.7 0.6 0.5 0.4 0.3	
	LOW VISION	MODERATE VISUAL IMPAIRMENT 20/70 20/80 20/100 20/125 20/160 0.25 0.20 0.16 0.12	Moderate low vision
		SEVERE VISUAL IMPAIRMENT 20/200 20/250 20/320 20/400 0.10 0.08 0.06 0.05 Visual field: 20 degrees or less	Severe low vision, "Legal" blindness
	BLINDNESS (WHO) one or both eyes	PROFOUND VISUAL IMPAIRMENT 20/500 20/630 20/800 20/1000 0.04 0.03 0.025 0.02 Count fingers at: less than 3m (10 ft.) Visual field: 10 degrees or less	Profound low vision, Moderate blindness
		NEAR-TOTAL VISUAL IMPAIRMENT Visual acuity: less than 0.02 (20/1000) Count fingers at: 1m (3 ft.) or less Hand movements: 5m (15 ft.) or less Light projection, light perception Visual field: 5 degrees or less	Severe blindness, Near-total blindness
		TOTAL VISUAL IMPAIRMENT No light perception (NLP)	Total blindness

Visual acuity refers to best achievable acuity with correction.
Non-listed Snellen fractions may be classified by converting to the nearest decimal equivalent, e.g. 10/200 = 0.05, 6/30 = 0.20.
CF (count fingers) without designation of distance, may be classified to profound impairment.
HM (hand motion) without designation of distance, may be classified to near-total impairment.
Visual field measurements refer to the largest field diameter for a 1/100 white test object.

√5th **369.0 Profound impairment, both eyes**

369.00 Impairment level not further specified
   Blindness:
      NOS according to WHO definition
      both eyes

369.01 Better eye: total impairment; lesser eye: total impairment

369.02 Better eye: near-total impairment; lesser eye: not further specified

369.03 Better eye: near-total impairment; lesser eye: total impairment

369.04 Better eye: near-total impairment; lesser eye: near-total impairment

369.05 Better eye: profound impairment; lesser eye: not further specified

369.06 Better eye: profound impairment; lesser eye: total impairment

369.07 Better eye: profound impairment; lesser eye: near-total impairment

---

√4th √5th Additional Digit Required   Unspecified Code   Other Specified Code   Manifestation Code
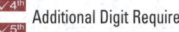 Medicare Secondary Payer   ▶◀ Revised Text   ● New Code   ▲ Revised Code Title

2002 Ingenix, Inc.   Volume 1 — 201

369.08 Better eye: profound impairment; lesser eye: profound impairment

√5th **369.1** Moderate or severe impairment, better eye, profound impairment lesser eye

369.10 Impairment level not further specified
Blindness, one eye, low vision other eye

369.11 Better eye: severe impairment; lesser eye: blind, not further specified

369.12 Better eye: severe impairment; lesser eye: total impairment

369.13 Better eye: severe impairment; lesser eye: near-total impairment

369.14 Better eye: severe impairment; lesser eye: profound impairment

369.15 Better eye: moderate impairment; lesser eye: blind, not further specified

369.16 Better eye: moderate impairment; lesser eye: total impairment

369.17 Better eye: moderate impairment; lesser eye: near-total impairment

369.18 Better eye: moderate impairment; lesser eye: profound impairment

√5th **369.2** Moderate or severe impairment, both eyes

369.20 Impairment level not further specified
Low vision, both eyes NOS

369.21 Better eye: severe impairment; lesser eye: not further specified

369.22 Better eye: severe impairment; lesser eye: severe impairment

369.23 Better eye: moderate impairment; lesser eye: not further specified

369.24 Better eye: moderate impairment; lesser eye: severe impairment

369.25 Better eye: moderate impairment; lesser eye: moderate impairment

369.3 Unqualified visual loss, both eyes
> **EXCLUDES** blindness NOS:
> legal [U.S.A. definition] (369.4)
> WHO definition (369.00)

369.4 Legal blindness, as defined in U.S.A.
Blindness NOS according to U.S.A. definition
> **EXCLUDES** legal blindness with specification of impairment level (369.01-369.08, 369.11-369.14, 369.21-369.22)

√5th **369.6** Profound impairment, one eye

369.60 Impairment level not further specified
Blindness, one eye

369.61 One eye: total impairment; other eye; not specified

369.62 One eye: total impairment; other eye: near-normal vision

369.63 One eye: total impairment; other eye: normal vision

369.64 One eye: near-total impairment; other eye: not specified

369.65 One eye: near-total impairment; other eye: near-normal vision

369.66 One eye: near-total impairment; other eye: normal vision

369.67 One eye: profound impairment; other eye: not specified

369.68 One eye: profound impairment; other eye: near-normal vision

369.69 One eye: profound impairment; other eye: normal vision

√5th **369.7** Moderate or severe impairment, one eye

369.70 Impairment level not further specified
Low vision, one eye

369.71 One eye: severe impairment; other eye: not specified

369.72 One eye: severe impairment; other eye: near-normal vision

369.73 One eye: severe impairment; other eye: normal vision

NERVOUS SYSTEM AND SENSE ORGANS

- **369.74** One eye: moderate impairment; other eye: not specified
- **369.75** One eye: moderate impairment; other eye: near-normal vision
- **369.76** One eye: moderate impairment; other eye: normal vision
- **369.8** Unqualified visual loss, one eye
- **369.9** Unspecified visual loss

✓4th 370 Keratitis

✓5th 370.0 Corneal ulcer
> **EXCLUDES** that due to vitamin A deficiency (264.3)

- **370.00** Corneal ulcer, unspecified
- **370.01** Marginal corneal ulcer
- **370.02** Ring corneal ulcer
- **370.03** Central corneal ulcer
- **370.04** Hypopyon ulcer
  Serpiginous ulcer
  DEF: Corneal ulcer with an accumulation of pus in the eye's anterior chamber.
- **370.05** Mycotic corneal ulcer
  DEF: Fungal infection causing corneal tissue loss.
- **370.06** Perforated corneal ulcer
  DEF: Tissue loss through all layers of cornea.
- **370.07** Mooren's ulcer
  DEF: Tissue loss, with chronic inflammation, at junction of cornea and sclera; seen in elderly.

✓5th 370.2 Superficial keratitis without conjunctivitis
> **EXCLUDES** dendritic [herpes simplex] keratitis (054.42)

- **370.20** Superficial keratitis, unspecified
- **370.21** Punctate keratitis
  Thygeson's superficial punctate keratitis
  DEF: Formation of cellular and fibrinous deposits (keratic precipitates) on posterior surface; deposits develop after injury or iridocyclitis.
- **370.22** Macular keratitis
  Keratitis: Keratitis:
    areolar   stellate
    nummular   striate
- **370.23** Filamentary keratitis
  DEF: Keratitis characterized by twisted filaments of mucoid material on the cornea's surface.
- **370.24** Photokeratitis
  Snow blindness
  Welders' keratitis
  DEF: Painful, inflamed cornea; due to extended exposure to ultraviolet light.

✓5th 370.3 Certain types of keratoconjunctivitis
- **370.31** Phlyctenular keratoconjunctivitis
  Phlyctenulosis
  Use additional code for any associated tuberculosis (017.3)
  DEF: Miniature blister on conjunctiva or cornea; associated with tuberculosis and malnutrition disorders.
- **370.32** Limbar and corneal involvement in vernal conjunctivitis
  Use additional code for vernal conjunctivitis (372.13)
  DEF: Corneal itching and inflammation in conjunctivitis; often limited to lining of eyelids.

370.33 Keratoconjunctivitis sicca, not specified as Sjögren's
　　EXCLUDES　Sjögren's syndrome (710.2)
　　DEF: Inflammation of conjunctiva and cornea; characterized by "horny" looking tissue and excess blood in these areas; decreased flow of lacrimal (tear) is a contributing factor.

370.34 Exposure keratoconjunctivitis
　　DEF: Incomplete closure of eyelid causing dry, inflamed eye.

370.35 Neurotrophic keratoconjunctivitis

√5th **370.4 Other and unspecified keratoconjunctivitis**

370.40 Keratoconjunctivitis, unspecified
　　Superficial keratitis with conjunctivitis NOS

370.44 Keratitis or keratoconjunctivitis in exanthema
　　Code first underlying condition (050.0-052.9)
　　EXCLUDES　herpes simplex (054.43)
　　　　　　　herpes zoster (053.21)
　　　　　　　measles (055.71)

370.49 Other
　　EXCLUDES　epidemic keratoconjunctivitis (077.1)

√5th **370.5 Interstitial and deep keratitis**

370.50 Interstitial keratitis, unspecified

370.52 Diffuse interstitial keratitis
　　Cogan's syndrome
　　DEF: Inflammation of cornea; with deposits in middle corneal layers; may obscure vision.

370.54 Sclerosing keratitis
　　DEF: Chronic corneal inflammation leading to opaque scarring.

370.55 Corneal abscess
　　DEF: Pocket of pus and inflammation on the cornea.

370.59 Other
　　EXCLUDES　disciform herpes simplex keratitis (054.43)
　　　　　　　syphilitic keratitis (090.3)

√5th **370.6 Corneal neovascularization**

370.60 Corneal neovascularization, unspecified

370.61 Localized vascularization of cornea
　　DEF: Limited infiltration of cornea by new blood vessels.

370.62 Pannus (corneal)
　　DEF: Buildup of superficial vascularization and granulated tissue under epithelium of cornea.

370.63 Deep vascularization of cornea
　　DEF: Deep infiltration of cornea by new blood vessels.

370.64 Ghost vessels (corneal)

370.8 Other forms of keratitis

370.9 Unspecified keratitis

√4th **371 Corneal opacity and other disorders of cornea**

√5th **371.0 Corneal scars and opacities**
　　EXCLUDES　that due to vitamin A deficiency (264.6)

371.00 Corneal opacity, unspecified
　　Corneal scar NOS

371.01 Minor opacity of cornea
　　Corneal nebula

371.02 Peripheral opacity of cornea
　　Corneal macula not interfering with central vision

NERVOUS SYSTEM AND SENSE ORGANS — 371.03–371.44

371.03 Central opacity of cornea
Corneal:
leucoma ⎫ interfering with central
macula ⎬ vision

371.04 Adherent leucoma
DEF: Dense, opaque corneal growth adhering to the iris; also spelled as leukoma.

371.05 Phthisical cornea
Code first underlying tuberculosis (017.3)

√5th **371.1 Corneal pigmentations and deposits**
371.10 Corneal deposit, unspecified
371.11 Anterior pigmentations
Stähli's lines
371.12 Stromal pigmentations
Hematocornea
371.13 Posterior pigmentations
Krukenberg spindle
371.14 Kayser-Fleischer ring
DEF: Copper deposits forming ring at outer edge of cornea; seen in Wilson's disease and other liver disorders.
371.15 Other deposits associated with metabolic disorders
371.16 Argentous deposits
DEF: Silver deposits in cornea.

√5th **371.2 Corneal edema**
371.20 Corneal edema, unspecified
371.21 Idiopathic corneal edema
DEF: Corneal swelling and fluid retention of unknown cause.
371.22 Secondary corneal edema
DEF: Corneal swelling and fluid retention caused by an underlying disease, injury, or condition.
371.23 Bullous keratopathy
DEF: Corneal degeneration; characterized by recurring, rupturing epithelial "blisters;" ruptured blebs expose corneal nerves, cause great pain; occurs in glaucoma, iridocyclitis and Fuchs' epithelial dystrophy.
371.24 Corneal edema due to wearing of contact lenses

√5th **371.3 Changes of corneal membranes**
371.30 Corneal membrane change, unspecified
371.31 Folds and rupture of Bowman's membrane
371.32 Folds in Descemet's membrane
371.33 Rupture in Descemet's membrane

√5th **371.4 Corneal degenerations**
371.40 Corneal degeneration, unspecified
371.41 Senile corneal changes
Arcus senilis   Hassall-Henle bodies
371.42 Recurrent erosion of cornea
EXCLUDES Mooren's ulcer (370.07)
371.43 Band-shaped keratopathy
DEF: Horizontal bands of superficial corneal calcium deposits.
371.44 Other calcerous degenerations of cornea

√4th / √5th Additional Digit Required
MSP Medicare Secondary Payer
▶◀ Revised Text
Unspecified Code
● New Code
Other Specified Code
▲ Revised Code Title
Manifestation Code

2002 Ingenix, Inc.   Volume 1 — 205

371.45 Keratomalacia NOS
> **EXCLUDES** that due to vitamin A deficiency (264.4)

DEF: Destruction of the cornea by keratinization of the epithelium with ulceration and perforation of the cornea; seen in cases of vitamin A deficiency.

371.46 Nodular degeneration of cornea
Salzmann's nodular dystrophy

371.48 Peripheral degenerations of cornea
Marginal degeneration of cornea [Terrien's]

371.49 Other
Discrete colliquative keratopathy

√5th **371.5 Hereditary corneal dystrophies**
DEF: Genetic disorder; leads to opacities, edema or lesions of cornea.

371.50 Corneal dystrophy, unspecified
371.51 Juvenile epithelial corneal dystrophy
371.52 Other anterior corneal dystrophies
Corneal dystrophy:
  microscopic cystic
  ring-like

371.53 Granular corneal dystrophy
371.54 Lattice corneal dystrophy
371.55 Macular corneal dystrophy
371.56 Other stromal corneal dystrophies
Crystalline corneal dystrophy

371.57 Endothelial corneal dystrophy
Combined corneal dystrophy
Cornea guttata
Fuchs' endothelial dystrophy

371.58 Other posterior corneal dystrophies
Polymorphous corneal dystrophy

√5th **371.6 Keratoconus**
DEF: Bilateral bulging protrusion of anterior cornea; often due to noninflammatory thinning.

371.60 Keratoconus, unspecified
371.61 Keratoconus, stable condition
371.62 Keratoconus, acute hydrops

√5th **371.7 Other corneal deformities**
371.70 Corneal deformity, unspecified
371.71 Corneal ectasia
DEF: Bulging protrusion of thinned, scarred cornea.

371.72 Descemetocele
DEF: Protrusion of Descemet's membrane into cornea.

371.73 Corneal staphyloma
DEF: Protrusion of cornea into adjacent tissue.

√5th **371.8 Other corneal disorders**
371.81 Corneal anesthesia and hypoesthesia
DEF: Decreased or absent sensitivity of cornea.

371.82 Corneal disorder due to contact lens
> **EXCLUDES** corneal edema due to contact lens (371.24)

DEF: Contact lens wear causing cornea disorder, excluding swelling.

371.89 Other
371.9 Unspecified corneal disorder

NERVOUS SYSTEM AND SENSE ORGANS   372–372.30

✓4ʰ 372 Disorders of conjunctiva
> **EXCLUDES** keratoconjunctivitis (370.3-370.4)

✓5ʰ 372.0 Acute conjunctivitis

372.00 Acute conjunctivitis, unspecified

372.01 Serous conjunctivitis, except viral
> **EXCLUDES** viral conjunctivitis NOS (077.9)

372.02 Acute follicular conjunctivitis
Conjunctival folliculosis NOS
> **EXCLUDES** conjunctivitis:
> adenoviral (acute follicular) (077.3)
> epidemic hemorrhagic (077.4)
> inclusion (077.0)
> Newcastle (077.8)
> epidemic keratoconjunctivitis (077.1)
> pharyngoconjunctival fever (077.2)

DEF: Severe conjunctival inflammation with dense infiltrations of lymphoid tissues of inner eyelids; may be traced to a viral or chlamydial etiology.

372.03 Other mucopurulent conjunctivitis
Catarrhal conjunctivitis
> **EXCLUDES** blennorrhea neonatorum (gonococcal) (098.40)
> neonatal conjunctivitis(771.6)
> ophthalmia neonatorum NOS (771.6)

372.04 Pseudomembranous conjunctivitis
Membranous conjunctivitis
> **EXCLUDES** diphtheritic conjunctivitis (032.81)

DEF: Severe inflammation of conjunctiva; false membrane develops on inner surface of eyelid; membrane can be removed without harming epithelium, due to bacterial infections, toxic and allergic factors, and viral infections.

372.05 Acute atopic conjunctivitis
DEF: Sudden, severe conjunctivitis due to allergens.

✓5ʰ 372.1 Chronic conjunctivitis

372.10 Chronic conjunctivitis, unspecified
372.11 Simple chronic conjunctivitis
372.12 Chronic follicular conjunctivitis
DEF: Persistent inflammation of conjunctiva; with infiltration of lymphoid tissue of inner eyelids.

372.13 Vernal conjunctivitis
372.14 Other chronic allergic conjunctivitis
372.15 *Parasitic conjunctivitis*
Code first underlying disease, as:
filariasis (125.0-125.9)
mucocutaneous leishmaniasis (085.5)

✓5ʰ 372.2 Blepharoconjunctivitis

372.20 Blepharoconjunctivitis, unspecified
372.21 Angular blepharoconjunctivitis
DEF: Inflammation at junction of upper and lower eyelids; may block lacrimal secretions.

372.22 Contact blepharoconjunctivitis

✓5ʰ 372.3 Other and unspecified conjunctivitis

372.30 Conjunctivitis, unspecified

  Additional Digit Required   Unspecified Code   Other Specified Code   Manifestation Code
MSP Medicare Secondary Payer   ▶◀ Revised Text   ● New Code   ▲ Revised Code Title

2002 Ingenix, Inc.   Volume 1 — 207

372.31 Rosacea conjunctivitis
Code first underlying rosacea dermatitis (695.3)

372.33 Conjunctivitis in mucocutaneous disease
Code first underlying disease, as:
erythema multiforme (695.1)
Reiter's disease (099.3)
EXCLUDES ocular pemphigoid (694.61)

372.39 **Other**

√5th **372.4 Pterygium**
EXCLUDES pseudopterygium (372.52)
DEF: Wedge-shaped, conjunctival thickening that advances from the inner corner of the eye toward the cornea.

372.40 **Pterygium, unspecified**
372.41 Peripheral pterygium, stationary
372.42 Peripheral pterygium, progressive
372.43 Central pterygium
372.44 Double pterygium
372.45 Recurrent pterygium

√5th **372.5 Conjunctival degenerations and deposits**
372.50 **Conjunctival degeneration, unspecified**
372.51 Pinguecula
DEF: Proliferative spot on the bulbar conjunctiva located near the sclerocorneal junction, usually on the nasal side; it is seen in elderly people.

372.52 Pseudopterygium
DEF: Conjunctival scar joined to the cornea; it looks like a pterygium but is not attached to the tissue.

372.53 Conjunctival xerosis
EXCLUDES conjunctival xerosis due to vitamin A deficiency (264.0, 264.1, 264.7)
DEF: Dry conjunctiva due to vitamin A deficiency; related to Bitot's spots; may develop into xerophthalmia and keratomalacia.

372.54 Conjunctival concretions
DEF: Calculus or deposit on conjunctiva.

372.55 Conjunctival pigmentations
Conjunctival argyrosis
DEF: Color deposits in conjunctiva.

372.56 Conjunctival deposits

√5th **372.6 Conjunctival scars**
372.61 Granuloma of conjunctiva
372.62 Localized adhesions and strands of conjunctiva
DEF: Abnormal fibrous connections in conjunctiva.

372.63 Symblepharon
Extensive adhesions of conjunctiva
DEF: Adhesion of the eyelids to the eyeball.

372.64 Scarring of conjunctiva
Contraction of eye socket (after enucleation)

√5th **372.7 Conjunctival vascular disorders and cysts**
372.71 Hyperemia of conjunctiva
DEF: Conjunctival blood vessel congestion causing eye redness.

NERVOUS SYSTEM AND SENSE ORGANS

- **372.72 Conjunctival hemorrhage**
  - Hyposphagma
  - Subconjunctival hemorrhage
- **372.73 Conjunctival edema**
  - Chemosis of conjunctiva
  - Subconjunctival edema
  - DEF: Fluid retention and swelling in conjunctival tissue.
- **372.74 Vascular abnormalities of conjunctiva**
  - Aneurysm(ata) of conjunctiva
- **372.75 Conjunctival cysts**
  - DEF: Abnormal sacs of fluid in conjunctiva.

√5th **372.8 Other disorders of conjunctiva**
- **372.81 Conjunctivochalasis**
  - DEF: Bilateral condition of redundant conjunctival tissue between globe and lower eyelid margin; may cover lower punctum, interferring with normal tearing.
- **372.89 Other disorders of conjunctiva**

372.9 Unspecified disorder of conjunctiva

√4th **373 Inflammation of eyelids**

√5th **373.0 Blepharitis**
- EXCLUDES blepharoconjunctivitis (372.20-372.22)
- **373.00 Blepharitis, unspecified**
- **373.01 Ulcerative blepharitis**
- **373.02 Squamous blepharitis**

√5th **373.1 Hordeolum and other deep inflammation of eyelid**
- DEF: Purulent, localized, staphylococcal infection in sebaceous glands of eyelids.
- **373.11 Hordeolum externum**
  - Hordeolum NOS   Stye
  - DEF: Infection of oil gland in eyelash follicles.
- **373.12 Hordeolum internum**
  - Infection of meibomian gland
  - DEF: Infection of oil gland of eyelid margin.
- **373.13 Abscess of eyelid**
  - Furuncle of eyelid
  - DEF: Inflamed pocket of pus on eyelid.

373.2 Chalazion
- Meibomian (gland) cyst
- EXCLUDES infected meibomian gland (373.12)
- DEF: Chronic inflammation of the meibomian gland, causing an eyelid mass.

√5th **373.3 Noninfectious dermatoses of eyelid**
- **373.31 Eczematous dermatitis of eyelid**
- **373.32 Contact and allergic dermatitis of eyelid**
- **373.33 Xeroderma of eyelid**
- **373.34 Discoid lupus erythematosus of eyelid**

373.4 Infective dermatitis of eyelid of types resulting in deformity
- Code first underlying disease, as:
  - leprosy (030.0-030.9)
  - lupus vulgaris (tuberculous) (017.0)
  - yaws (102.0-102.9)

√4th / √5th Additional Digit Required   Unspecified Code   Other Specified Code   Manifestation Code

  Medicare Secondary Payer   ▶◀ Revised Text   ● New Code   ▲ Revised Code Title

Entropion and Ectropion

Normal eyelashes

Entropion — Lower eyelashes curve toward eye tissue, irritating the conjunctiva and cornea

Ectropion — Lower eyelid droops, causing excessive dryness and irritation

373.5 Other infective dermatitis of eyelid
Code first underlying disease, as:
actinomycosis (039.3)
impetigo (684)
mycotic dermatitis (110.0-111.9)
vaccinia (051.0)
postvaccination (999.0)
EXCLUDES herpes:
simplex (054.41)
zoster (053.20)

373.6 Parasitic infestation of eyelid
Code first underlying disease, as:
leishmaniasis (085.0-085.9)
loiasis (125.2)
onchocerciasis (125.3)
pediculosis (132.0)

373.8 Other inflammations of eyelids

373.9 Unspecified inflammation of eyelid

√4th **374 Other disorders of eyelids**

√5th **374.0 Entropion and trichiasis of eyelid**
DEF: Entropion: turning inward of eyelid edge toward eyeball.
DEF: Trichiasis: ingrowing eyelashes marked by irritation with possible distortion of sight.

374.00 Entropion, unspecified
374.01 Senile entropion
374.02 Mechanical entropion
374.03 Spastic entropion
374.04 Cicatricial entropion
374.05 Trichiasis without entropion

√5th **374.1 Ectropion**
DEF: Turning outward (eversion) of eyelid edge; exposes palpebral conjunctiva; dryness, irritation result.

374.10 Ectropion, unspecified
374.11 Senile ectropion
374.12 Mechanical ectropion
374.13 Spastic ectropion
374.14 Cicatricial ectropion

NERVOUS SYSTEM AND SENSE ORGANS 374.2–374.54

√5ᵗʰ **374.2 Lagophthalmos**
DEF: Incomplete closure of eyes; causes dry eye and other complications.

- 374.20 Lagophthalmos, unspecified
- 374.21 Paralytic lagophthalmos
- 374.22 Mechanical lagophthalmos
- 374.23 Cicatricial lagophthalmos

√5ᵗʰ **374.3 Ptosis of eyelid**

- 374.30 Ptosis of eyelid, unspecified
- 374.31 Paralytic ptosis
  DEF: Drooping of upper eyelid due to nerve disorder.
- 374.32 Myogenic ptosis
  DEF: Drooping of upper eyelid due to muscle disorder.
- 374.33 Mechanical ptosis
  DEF: Outside force causes drooping of upper eyelid.
- 374.34 Blepharochalasis
  Pseudoptosis
  DEF: Loss of elasticity causing skin to hang over eyelid margin; due to intercellular tissue atrophy.

√5ᵗʰ **374.4 Other disorders affecting eyelid function**

EXCLUDES   blepharoclonus (333.81)
blepharospasm (333.81)
facial nerve palsy (351.0)
third nerve palsy or paralysis (378.51-378.52)
tic (psychogenic) (307.20-307.23)
organic (333.3)

- 374.41 Lid retraction or lag
- 374.43 Abnormal innervation syndrome
  Jaw-blinking   Paradoxical facial movements
- 374.44 Sensory disorders
- 374.45 Other sensorimotor disorders
  Deficient blink reflex
- 374.46 Blepharophimosis
  Ankyloblepharon
  DEF: Narrowing of palpebral fissure horizontally; caused by laterally displaced inner canthi; either acquired or congenital.

√5ᵗʰ **374.5 Degenerative disorders of eyelid and periocular area**

- 374.50 Degenerative disorder of eyelid, unspecified
- 374.51 Xanthelasma
  Xanthoma (planum) (tuberosum) of eyelid
  Code first underlying condition (272.0-272.9)
  DEF: Fatty tumors of eyelid linked to high fat content of blood.
- 374.52 Hyperpigmentation of eyelid
  Chloasma   Dyspigmentation
  DEF: Excess pigment of eyelid.
- 374.53 Hypopigmentation of eyelid
  Vitiligo of eyelid
  DEF: Lack of color pigment of the eyelid.
- 374.54 Hypertrichosis of eyelid
  DEF: Excess eyelash growth.

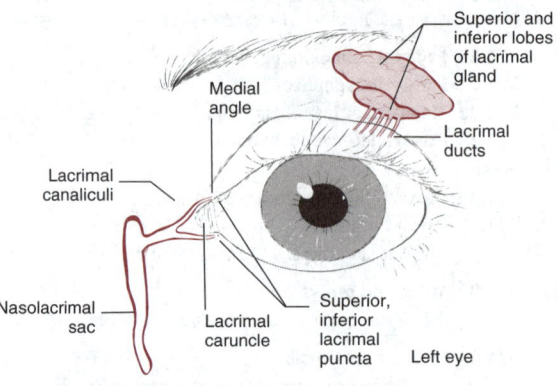

Lacrimal System

- 374.55 **Hypotrichosis of eyelid**
  Madarosis of eyelid
  DEF: Less than normal, or absent, eyelashes.
- 374.56 Other degenerative disorders of skin affecting eyelid
- 374.8 Other disorders of eyelid
  - 374.81 **Hemorrhage of eyelid**
    EXCLUDES black eye (921.0)
  - 374.82 **Edema of eyelid**
    Hyperemia of eyelid
    DEF: Swelling and fluid retention in eyelid.
  - 374.83 **Elephantiasis of eyelid**
    DEF: Filarial disease causing dermatitis and enlarged eyelid.
  - 374.84 **Cysts of eyelids**
    Sebaceous cyst of eyelid
  - 374.85 **Vascular anomalies of eyelid**
  - 374.86 **Retained foreign body of eyelid**
  - 374.87 **Dermatochalasis**
    DEF: Loss of elasticity causing skin under eye to sag.
  - 374.89 Other disorders of eyelid
- 374.9 Unspecified disorder of eyelid
- 375 Disorders of lacrimal system
  - 375.0 Dacryoadenitis
    - 375.00 Dacryoadenitis, unspecified
    - 375.01 **Acute dacryoadenitis**
      DEF: Severe, sudden inflammation of lacrimal gland.
    - 375.02 **Chronic dacryoadenitis**
      DEF: Persistent inflammation of lacrimal gland.
    - 375.03 **Chronic enlargement of lacrimal gland**
  - 375.1 Other disorders of lacrimal gland
    - 375.11 **Dacryops**
      DEF: Overproduction and constant flow of tears; may cause distended lacrimal duct.
    - 375.12 Other lacrimal cysts and cystic degeneration
    - 375.13 **Primary lacrimal atrophy**
    - 375.14 **Secondary lacrimal atrophy**
      DEF: Wasting away of lacrimal gland due to another disease.

375.15 **Tear film insufficiency, unspecified**
Dry eye syndrome
DEF: Eye dryness and irritation due to insufficient tear production.

375.16 Dislocation of lacrimal gland

✓5th 375.2 Epiphora
DEF: Abnormal development of tears due to stricture of lacrimal passages.

375.20 **Epiphora, unspecified as to cause**
375.21 Epiphora due to excess lacrimation
DEF: Tear overflow due to overproduction.

375.22 Epiphora due to insufficient drainage
DEF: Tear overflow due to blocked drainage.

✓5th 375.3 Acute and unspecified inflammation of lacrimal passages
EXCLUDES neonatal dacryocystitis (771.6)

375.30 **Dacryocystitis, unspecified**
375.31 Acute canaliculitis, lacrimal
375.32 Acute dacryocystitis
Acute peridacryocystitis
375.33 Phlegmonous dacryocystitis
DEF: Infection of tear sac with pockets of pus.

✓5th 375.4 Chronic inflammation of lacrimal passages
375.41 Chronic canaliculitis
375.42 Chronic dacryocystitis
375.43 Lacrimal mucocele

✓5th 375.5 Stenosis and insufficiency of lacrimal passages
375.51 Eversion of lacrimal punctum
DEF: Abnormal turning outward of tear duct.

375.52 Stenosis of lacrimal punctum
DEF: Abnormal narrowing of tear duct.

375.53 Stenosis of lacrimal canaliculi
375.54 Stenosis of lacrimal sac
DEF: Abnormal narrowing of tear sac.

375.55 Obstruction of nasolacrimal duct, neonatal
EXCLUDES congenital anomaly of nasolacrimal duct (743.65)
DEF: Acquired, abnormal obstruction of lacrimal system, from eye to nose; in an infant.

375.56 Stenosis of nasolacrimal duct, acquired
375.57 Dacryolith
DEF: Concretion or stone in lacrimal system.

✓5th 375.6 Other changes of lacrimal passages
375.61 Lacrimal fistula
DEF: Abnormal communication from lacrimal system.

375.69 **Other**

✓5th 375.8 Other disorders of lacrimal system
375.81 Granuloma of lacrimal passages
DEF: Abnormal nodules within lacrimal system.

375.89 **Other**

✓4th
✓5th   Additional Digit Required
MSP   Medicare Secondary Payer

Unspecified Code
▶◀ Revised Text

Other Specified Code
● New Code

Manifestation Code
▲ Revised Code Title

2002 Ingenix, Inc.

NERVOUS SYSTEM AND SENSE ORGANS

- **375.9** Unspecified disorder of lacrimal system
- √4th **376** Disorders of the orbit
  - √5th **376.0** Acute inflammation of orbit
    - **376.00** Acute inflammation of orbit, unspecified
    - **376.01** Orbital cellulitis
      - Abscess of orbit
      - DEF: Infection of tissue between orbital bone and eyeball.
    - **376.02** Orbital periostitis
      - DEF: Inflammation of connective tissue covering orbital bone.
    - **376.03** Orbital osteomyelitis
      - DEF: Inflammation of orbital bone.
    - **376.04** Tenonitis
  - √5th **376.1** Chronic inflammatory disorders of orbit
    - **376.10** Chronic inflammation of orbit, unspecified
    - **376.11** Orbital granuloma
      - Pseudotumor (inflammatory) of orbit
      - DEF: Abnormal nodule between orbital bone and eyeball.
    - **376.12** Orbital myositis
      - DEF: Painful inflammation of eye muscles.
    - **376.13** Parasitic infestation of orbit
      - Code first underlying disease, as:
        - hydatid infestation of orbit (122.3, 122.6, 122.9)
        - myiasis of orbit (134.0)
  - √5th **376.2** Endocrine exophthalmos
    - Code first underlying thyroid disorder (242.0-242.9)
    - **376.21** Thyrotoxic exophthalmos
      - DEF: Bulging eyes due to hyperthyroidism.
    - **376.22** Exophthalmic ophthalmoplegia
      - DEF: Inability to rotate eye due to bulging eyes.
  - √5th **376.3** Other exophthalmic conditions
    - **376.30** Exophthalmos, unspecified
      - DEF: Abnormal protrusion of eyeball.
    - **376.31** Constant exophthalmos
      - DEF: Continuous, abnormal protrusion or bulging of eyeball.
    - **376.32** Orbital hemorrhage
      - DEF: Bleeding behind the eyeball, causing forward bulge.
    - **376.33** Orbital edema or congestion
      - DEF: Fluid retention behind eyeball, causing forward bulge.
    - **376.34** Intermittent exophthalmos
    - **376.35** Pulsating exophthalmos
      - DEF: Bulge or protrusion; associated with a carotid-cavernous fistula.
    - **376.36** Lateral displacement of globe
      - DEF: Abnormal displacement of the eyeball away from nose, toward temple.
  - √5th **376.4** Deformity of orbit
    - **376.40** Deformity of orbit, unspecified
    - **376.41** Hypertelorism of orbit
      - DEF: Abnormal increase in interorbital distance; associated with congenital facial deformities; may be accompanied by mental deficiency.

N Newborn Age: 0   P Pediatric Age: 0-17   M Maternity Age: 12-55   A Adult Age: 15-124

NERVOUS SYSTEM AND SENSE ORGANS 376.42–377.16

- **376.42 Exostosis of orbit**
  DEF: Abnormal bony growth of orbit.
- **376.43 Local deformities due to bone disease**
  DEF: Acquired abnormalities of orbit; due to bone disease.
- **376.44 Orbital deformities associated with craniofacial deformities**
- **376.45 Atrophy of orbit**
  DEF: Wasting away of bone tissue of orbit.
- **376.46 Enlargement of orbit**
- **376.47 Deformity due to trauma or surgery**

√5th **376.5 Enophthalmos**
DEF: Recession of eyeball deep into eye socket.
- **376.50 Enophthalmos, unspecified as to cause**
- **376.51 Enophthalmos due to atrophy of orbital tissue**
- **376.52 Enophthalmos due to trauma or surgery**

376.6 Retained (old) foreign body following penetrating wound of orbit
Retrobulbar foreign body

√5th **376.8 Other orbital disorders**
- **376.81 Orbital cysts**
  Encephalocele of orbit
- **376.82 Myopathy of extraocular muscles**
  DEF: Disease in the muscles that control eyeball movement.
- **376.89 Other**

376.9 Unspecified disorder of orbit

√4th **377 Disorders of optic nerve and visual pathways**

√5th **377.0 Papilledema**
- **377.00 Papilledema, unspecified**
- **377.01 Papilledema associated with increased intracranial pressure**
- **377.02 Papilledema associated with decreased ocular pressure**
- **377.03 Papilledema associated with retinal disorder**
- **377.04 Foster-Kennedy syndrome**
  DEF: Retrobulbar optic neuritis, central scotoma and optic atrophy; caused by tumors in frontal lobe of brain that press downward.

√5th **377.1 Optic atrophy**
- **377.10 Optic atrophy, unspecified**
- **377.11 Primary optic atrophy**
  EXCLUDES neurosyphilitic optic atrophy (094.84)
- **377.12 Postinflammatory optic atrophy**
  DEF: Adverse effect of inflammation causing wasting away of eye.
- **377.13 Optic atrophy associated with retinal dystrophies**
  DEF: Progressive changes in retinal tissue due to metabolic disorder causing wasting away of eye.
- **377.14 Glaucomatous atrophy [cupping] of optic disc**
- **377.15 Partial optic atrophy**
  Temporal pallor of optic disc
- **377.16 Hereditary optic atrophy**
  Optic atrophy:
      dominant hereditary
      Leber's

√4th Additional Digit Required
√5th
 Medicare Secondary Payer   ▶◀ Revised Text   ● New Code   ▲ Revised Code Title

Unspecified Code   Other Specified Code   Manifestation Code

2002 Ingenix, Inc.   Volume 1 — 215

377.2 Other disorders of optic disc
- **377.21** Drusen of optic disc
- **377.22** Crater-like holes of optic disc
- **377.23** Coloboma of optic disc
  DEF: Ocular malformation caused by the failure of fetal fissure of optic stalk to close.
- **377.24** Pseudopapilledema

377.3 Optic neuritis
EXCLUDES meningococcal optic neuritis (036.81)
- **377.30** Optic neuritis, unspecified
- **377.31** Optic papillitis
  DEF: Swelling and inflammation of optic disc.
- **377.32** Retrobulbar neuritis (acute)
  EXCLUDES syphilitic retrobulbar neuritis (094.85)
  DEF: Inflammation of optic nerve immediately behind the eyeball.
- **377.33** Nutritional optic neuropathy
  DEF: Malnutrition causing optic nerve disorder.
- **377.34** Toxic optic neuropathy
  Toxic amblyopia
  DEF: Toxic substance causing optic nerve disorder.
- **377.39** Other
  EXCLUDES ischemic optic neuropathy (377.41)

377.4 Other disorders of optic nerve
- **377.41** Ischemic optic neuropathy
  DEF: Decreased blood flow affecting optic nerve.
- **377.42** Hemorrhage in optic nerve sheaths
  DEF: Bleeding in meningeal lining of optic nerve.
- **377.49** Other
  Compression of optic nerve

377.5 Disorders of optic chiasm
- **377.51** Associated with pituitary neoplasms and disorders
  DEF: Abnormal pituitary growth causing disruption in nerve chain from retina to brain.
- **377.52** Associated with other neoplasms
  DEF: Abnormal growth, other than pituitary, causing disruption in nerve chain from retina to brain.
- **377.53** Associated with vascular disorders
  DEF: Vascular disorder causing disruption in nerve chain from retina to brain.
- **377.54** Associated with inflammatory disorders
  DEF: Inflammatory disease causing disruption in nerve chain from retina to brain.

377.6 Disorders of other visual pathways
- **377.61** Associated with neoplasms
- **377.62** Associated with vascular disorders
- **377.63** Associated with inflammatory disorders

377.7 Disorders of visual cortex
EXCLUDES visual:
  agnosia (368.16)
  hallucinations (368.16)
  halos (368.15)

NERVOUS SYSTEM AND SENSE ORGANS 377.71–378.13

Eye Musculature

Superior rectus · Superior oblique · Lateral rectus · Medial rectus · Inferior oblique · Inferior rectus

Muscles and actions (right eye)

R. L. Monocular (one eye only) esotropia (inward)

Monocular exotropia (outward)

Monocular hypertropia (upward)

377.71 Associated with neoplasms
377.72 Associated with vascular disorders
377.73 Associated with inflammatory disorders
377.75 Cortical blindness
DEF: Blindness due to brain disorder, rather than eye disorder.

377.9 Unspecified disorder of optic nerve and visual pathways

√4th **378 Strabismus and other disorders of binocular eye movements**
EXCLUDES nystagmus and other irregular eye movements (379.50-379.59)
DEF: Misalignment of the eyes due to imbalance in extraocular muscles.

√5th **378.0 Esotropia**
Convergent concomitant strabismus
EXCLUDES intermittent esotropia (378.20-378.22)
DEF: Visual axis deviation created by one eye fixing upon an image and the other eye deviating inward.

378.00 Esotropia, unspecified
378.01 Monocular esotropia
378.02 Monocular esotropia with A pattern
378.03 Monocular esotropia with V pattern
378.04 Monocular esotropia with other noncomitancies
  Monocular esotropia with X or Y pattern
378.05 Alternating esotropia
378.06 Alternating esotropia with A pattern
378.07 Alternating esotropia with V pattern
378.08 Alternating esotropia with other noncomitancies
  Alternating esotropia with X or Y pattern

√5th **378.1 Exotropia**
Divergent concomitant strabismus
EXCLUDES intermittent exotropia (378.20, 378.23-378.24)
DEF: Visual axis deviation created by one eye fixing upon an image and the other eye deviating outward.

378.10 Exotropia, unspecified
378.11 Monocular exotropia
378.12 Monocular exotropia with A pattern
378.13 Monocular exotropia with V pattern

- **378.14 Monocular exotropia with other noncomitancies**
  Monocular exotropia with X or Y pattern
- **378.15** Alternating exotropia
- **378.16** Alternating exotropia with A pattern
- **378.17** Alternating exotropia with V pattern
- **378.18 Alternating exotropia with other noncomitancies**
  Alternating exotropia with X or Y pattern

√5ᵗʰ **378.2** Intermittent heterotropia
   EXCLUDES *vertical heterotropia (intermittent) (378.31)*
   DEF: Deviation of eyes seen only at intervals; it is also called strabismus.

- **378.20 Intermittent heterotropia, unspecified**
  Intermittent:
    esotropia NOS
    exotropia NOS
- **378.21** Intermittent esotropia, monocular
- **378.22** Intermittent esotropia, alternating
- **378.23** Intermittent exotropia, monocular
- **378.24** Intermittent exotropia, alternating

√5ᵗʰ **378.3** Other and unspecified heterotropia
- **378.30 Heterotropia, unspecified**
- **378.31** Hypertropia
  Vertical heterotropia (constant) (intermittent)
- **378.32** Hypotropia
- **378.33** Cyclotropia
- **378.34** Monofixation syndrome
  Microtropia
- **378.35** Accommodative component in esotropia

√5ᵗʰ **378.4** Heterophoria
   DEF: Deviation occurring only when the other eye is covered.

- **378.40 Heterophoria, unspecified**
- **378.41** Esophoria
- **378.42** Exophoria
- **378.43** Vertical heterophoria
- **378.44** Cyclophoria
- **378.45** Alternating hyperphoria

√5ᵗʰ **378.5** Paralytic strabismus
   DEF: Deviation of the eye due to nerve paralysis affecting muscle.

- **378.50 Paralytic strabismus, unspecified**
- **378.51** Third or oculomotor nerve palsy, partial
- **378.52** Third or oculomotor nerve palsy, total
- **378.53** Fourth or trochlear nerve palsy
- **378.54** Sixth or abducens nerve palsy
- **378.55** External ophthalmoplegia
- **378.56** Total ophthalmoplegia

√5ᵗʰ **378.6** Mechanical strabismus
   DEF: Deviation of the eye due to an outside force on extraocular muscle.

- **378.60 Mechanical strabismus, unspecified**
- **378.61** Brown's (tendon) sheath syndrome
  DEF: Congenital or acquired shortening of the anterior sheath of the superior oblique muscle; the eye is unable to move upward and inward; it is usually unilateral.
- **378.62 Mechanical strabismus from other musculofascial disorders**
- **378.63** Limited duction associated with other conditions

NERVOUS SYSTEM AND SENSE ORGANS

√5ᵗʰ 378.7 Other specified strabismus
    378.71 Duane's syndrome
        DEF: Congenital, affects one eye; due to abnormal fibrous bands attached to rectus muscle; inability to abduct affected eye with retraction of globe.

    378.72 Progressive external ophthalmoplegia
        DEF: Paralysis progressing from one eye muscle to another.

    378.73 Strabismus in other neuromuscular disorders

√5ᵗʰ 378.8 Other disorders of binocular eye movements
    EXCLUDES   nystagmus (379.50-379.56)

    378.81 Palsy of conjugate gaze
        DEF: Muscle dysfunction impairing parallel movement of the eye.

    378.82 Spasm of conjugate gaze
        DEF: Muscle contractions impairing parallel movement of eye.

    378.83 Convergence insufficiency or palsy
    378.84 Convergence excess or spasm
    378.85 Anomalies of divergence
    378.86 Internuclear ophthalmoplegia
        DEF: Eye movement anomaly due to brainstem lesion.

    378.87 Other dissociated deviation of eye movements
        Skew deviation

378.9 Unspecified disorder of eye movements
    Ophthalmoplegia NOS   Strabismus NOS

√4ᵗʰ 379 Other disorders of eye

√5ᵗʰ 379.0 Scleritis and episcleritis
    EXCLUDES   syphilitic episcleritis (095.0)

    379.00 Scleritis, unspecified
        Episcleritis NOS

    379.01 Episcleritis periodica fugax
        DEF: Hyperemia (engorgement) of the sclera and overlying conjunctiva characterized by a sudden onset and short duration.

    379.02 Nodular episcleritis
        DEF: Inflammation of the outermost layer of the sclera, with formation of nodules.

    379.03 Anterior scleritis
    379.04 Scleromalacia perforans
        DEF: Scleral thinning, softening and degeneration; seen with rheumatoid arthritis.

    379.05 Scleritis with corneal involvement
        Scleroperikeratitis

    379.06 Brawny scleritis
        DEF: Severe inflammation of the sclera; with thickened corneal margins.

    379.07 Posterior scleritis
        Sclerotenonitis

    379.09 Other
        Scleral abscess

√5ᵗʰ 379.1 Other disorders of sclera
    EXCLUDES   blue sclera (743.47)

    379.11 Scleral ectasia
        Scleral staphyloma NOS
        DEF: Protrusion of the contents of the eyeball where the sclera has thinned.

 Additional Digit Required   Unspecified Code   Other Specified Code   Manifestation Code

MSP Medicare Secondary Payer   ▶◀ Revised Text   ● New Code   ▲ Revised Code Title

2002 Ingenix, Inc.   Volume 1 — 219

379.12 Staphyloma posticum
DEF: Ring-shaped protrusion or bulging of sclera and uveal tissue at posterior pole of eye.

379.13 Equatorial staphyloma
DEF: Ring-shaped protrusion or bulging of sclera and uveal tissue midway between front and back of eye.

379.14 Anterior staphyloma, localized
379.15 Ring staphyloma
379.16 Other degenerative disorders of sclera
379.19 Other

√5th 379.2 Disorders of vitreous body
DEF: Disorder of clear gel that fills space between retina and lens.

379.21 Vitreous degeneration
Vitreous: Vitreous:
cavitation liquefaction
detachment

379.22 Crystalline deposits in vitreous
Asteroid hyalitis Synchysis scintillans

379.23 Vitreous hemorrhage
379.24 Other vitreous opacities
Vitreous floaters

379.25 Vitreous membranes and strands
379.26 Vitreous prolapse
DEF: Slipping of vitreous from normal position.

379.29 Other disorders of vitreous
EXCLUDES vitreous abscess (360.04)

√5th 379.3 Aphakia and other disorders of lens
EXCLUDES after-cataract (366.50-366.53)

379.31 Aphakia
EXCLUDES cataract extraction status (V45.61)
DEF: Absence of eye's crystalline lens.

379.32 Subluxation of lens
379.33 Anterior dislocation of lens
DEF: Lens displaced toward iris.

379.34 Posterior dislocation of lens
DEF: Lens displaced backward toward vitreous.

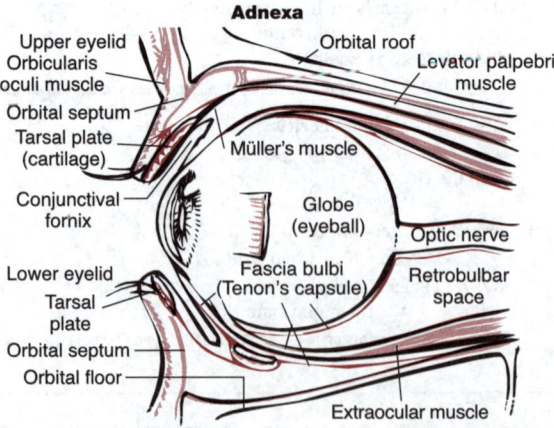

Adnexa

NERVOUS SYSTEM AND SENSE ORGANS

379.39 Other disorders of lens

√5th **379.4** Anomalies of pupillary function

379.40 Abnormal pupillary function, unspecified

379.41 Anisocoria
DEF: Unequal pupil diameter.

379.42 Miosis (persistent), not due to miotics
DEF: Abnormal contraction of pupil less than 2 millimeters.

379.43 Mydriasis (persistent), not due to mydriatics
DEF: Morbid dilation of pupil.

379.45 Argyll Robertson pupil, atypical
Argyll Robertson phenomenon or pupil, nonsyphilitic
EXCLUDES Argyll Robertson pupil (syphilitic) (094.89)
DEF: Failure of pupil to respond to light; affects both eyes; may be caused by diseases such as syphilis of the central nervous system or miosis.

379.46 Tonic pupillary reaction
Adie's pupil or syndrome

379.49 Other
Hippus   Pupillary paralysis

√5th **379.5** Nystagmus and other irregular eye movements

379.50 Nystagmus, unspecified
DEF: Involuntary, rapid, rhythmic movement of eyeball; vertical, horizontal, rotatory or mixed; cause may be congenital, acquired, physiological, neurological, myopathic, or due to ocular diseases.

379.51 Congenital nystagmus

379.52 Latent nystagmus

379.53 Visual deprivation nystagmus

379.54 Nystagmus associated with disorders of the vestibular system

379.55 Dissociated nystagmus

379.56 Other forms of nystagmus

379.57 Deficiencies of saccadic eye movements
Abnormal optokinetic response
DEF: Saccadic eye movements; small, rapid, involuntary movements by both eyes simultaneously, due to changing point of fixation on visualized object.

379.58 Deficiencies of smooth pursuit movements

379.59 Other irregularities of eye movements
Opsoclonus

Ear and Mastoid Process

Helix, Antihelix, Concha, Mastoid process, External auditory meatus, Tragus, Antitragus

NERVOUS SYSTEM AND SENSE ORGANS

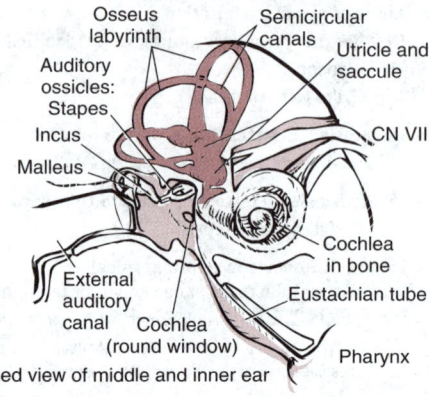

Middle and Inner Ear
Exposed view of middle and inner ear

379.8 Other specified disorders of eye and adnexa

√5th **379.9 Unspecified disorder of eye and adnexa**
- 379.90 Disorder of eye, unspecified
- 379.91 Pain in or around eye
- 379.92 Swelling or mass of eye
- 379.93 Redness or discharge of eye
- 379.99 Other ill-defined disorders of eye
  - EXCLUDES blurred vision NOS (368.8)

DISEASES OF THE EAR AND MASTOID PROCESS (380-389)

√4th **380 Disorders of external ear**

√5th **380.0 Perichondritis of pinna**
Perichondritis of auricle
- 380.00 Perichondritis of pinna, unspecified
- 380.01 Acute perichondritis of pinna
- 380.02 Chronic perichondritis of pinna

√5th **380.1 Infective otitis externa**
- 380.10 Infective otitis externa, unspecified
  - Otitis externa (acute): NOS, circumscribed, diffuse
  - Otitis externa (acute): hemorrhagica, infective NOS
- 380.11 Acute infection of pinna
  - EXCLUDES furuncular otitis externa (680.0)
- 380.12 Acute swimmers' ear
  - Beach ear   Tank ear
  - DEF: Otitis externa due to swimming.
- 380.13 Other acute infections of external ear
  - Code first underlying disease, as:
    - erysipelas (035)
    - impetigo (684)
    - seborrheic dermatitis (690.10-690.18)
  - EXCLUDES herpes simplex (054.73)
  - herpes zoster (053.71)
- 380.14 Malignant otitis externa
  - DEF: Severe necrotic otitis externa; due to bacteria.

NERVOUS SYSTEM AND SENSE ORGANS

380.15 Chronic mycotic otitis externa
Code first underlying disease, as:
aspergillosis (117.3)
otomycosis NOS (111.9)
EXCLUDES candidal otitis externa (112.82)

380.16 Other chronic infective otitis externa
Chronic infective otitis externa NOS

√5ᵗʰ **380.2 Other otitis externa**

380.21 Cholesteatoma of external ear
Keratosis obturans of external ear (canal)
EXCLUDES cholesteatoma NOS (385.30-385.35)
postmastoidectomy (383.32)
DEF: Cystlike mass filled with debris, including cholesterol; rare, congenital condition.

380.22 Other acute otitis externa
Acute otitis externa: Acute otitis externa:
actinic   eczematoid
chemical   reactive
contact

380.23 Other chronic otitis externa
Chronic otitis externa NOS

√5ᵗʰ **380.3 Noninfectious disorders of pinna**

380.30 Disorder of pinna, unspecified

380.31 Hematoma of auricle or pinna

380.32 Acquired deformities of auricle or pinna
EXCLUDES cauliflower ear (738.7)

380.39 Other
EXCLUDES gouty tophi of ear (274.81)

380.4 Impacted cerumen
Wax in ear

√5ᵗʰ **380.5 Acquired stenosis of external ear canal**
Collapse of external ear canal

380.50 Acquired stenosis of external ear canal, unspecified as to cause

380.51 Secondary to trauma
DEF: Narrowing of external ear canal; due to trauma.

380.52 Secondary to surgery
DEF: Postsurgical narrowing of external ear canal.

380.53 Secondary to inflammation
DEF: Narrowing, external ear canal; due to chronic inflammation.

√5ᵗʰ **380.8 Other disorders of external ear**

380.81 Exostosis of external ear canal

380.89 Other

380.9 Unspecified disorder of external ear

√4ᵗʰ / √5ᵗʰ Additional Digit Required   ▶◀ Revised Text   ● New Code   ▲ Revised Code Title
MSP Medicare Secondary Payer   Unspecified Code   Other Specified Code   Manifestation Code

NERVOUS SYSTEM AND SENSE ORGANS

√4ᵗʰ **381 Nonsuppurative otitis media and Eustachian tube disorders**

√5ᵗʰ **381.0 Acute nonsuppurative otitis media**
Acute tubotympanic catarrh
Otitis media, acute or subacute:
  catarrhal
  exudative
  transudative
  with effusion
  EXCLUDES *otitic barotrauma (993.0)*

381.00 Acute nonsuppurative otitis media, unspecified

381.01 Acute serous otitis media
Acute or subacute secretory otitis media
DEF: Sudden, severe infection of middle ear.

381.02 Acute mucoid otitis media
Acute or subacute seromucinous otitis media
Blue drum syndrome
DEF: Sudden, severe infection of middle ear, with mucous.

381.03 Acute sanguinous otitis media
DEF: Sudden, severe infection of middle ear, with blood.

381.04 Acute allergic serous otitis media
381.05 Acute allergic mucoid otitis media
381.06 Acute allergic sanguinous otitis media

√5ᵗʰ **381.1 Chronic serous otitis media**
Chronic tubotympanic catarrh

381.10 Chronic serous otitis media, simple or unspecified
DEF: Persistent infection of middle ear, without pus.

381.19 Other
Serosanguinous chronic otitis media

√5ᵗʰ **381.2 Chronic mucoid otitis media**
Glue ear
EXCLUDES *adhesive middle ear disease (385.10-385.19)*
DEF: Chronic condition; characterized by viscous fluid in middle ear; due to obstructed Eustachian tube.

381.20 Chronic mucoid otitis media, simple or unspecified
381.29 Other
Mucosanguinous chronic otitis media

381.3 Other and unspecified chronic nonsuppurative otitis media
Otitis media, chronic: Otitis media, chronic:
  allergic   seromucinous
  exudative   transudative
  secretory   with effusion

381.4 Nonsuppurative otitis media, not specified as acute or chronic
Otitis media: Otitis media:
  allergic   seromucinous
  catarrhal   serous
  exudative   transudative
  mucoid   with effusion
  secretory

√5ᵗʰ **381.5 Eustachian salpingitis**

381.50 Eustachian salpingitis, unspecified
381.51 Acute Eustachian salpingitis
DEF: Sudden, severe inflammation of Eustachian tube.

381.52 Chronic Eustachian salpingitis
DEF: Persistent inflammation of Eustachian tube.

NERVOUS SYSTEM AND SENSE ORGANS 381.6–382.3

√5th 381.6 **Obstruction of Eustachian tube**
Stenosis } of Eustachian tube
Stricture

   381.60 <mark>Obstruction of Eustachian tube, unspecified</mark>
   381.61 **Osseous obstruction of Eustachian tube**
     Obstruction of Eustachian tube from cholesteatoma, polyp, or other osseous lesion
   381.62 **Intrinsic cartilagenous obstruction of Eustachian tube**
     DEF: Blockage of Eustachian tube; due to cartilage overgrowth.
   381.63 **Extrinsic cartilagenous obstruction of Eustachian tube**
     Compression of Eustachian tube

  381.7 **Patulous Eustachian tube**
   DEF: Distended, oversized Eustachian tube.

√5th 381.8 **Other disorders of Eustachian tube**
   381.81 **Dysfunction of Eustachian tube**
   381.89 Other

  381.9 <mark>Unspecified Eustachian tube disorder</mark>

√4th **382 Suppurative and unspecified otitis media**

√5th 382.0 **Acute suppurative otitis media**
   Otitis media, acute: Otitis media, acute:
    necrotizing NOS purulent

   382.00 **Acute suppurative otitis media without spontaneous rupture of ear drum**
     DEF: Sudden, severe inflammation of middle ear, with pus.
   382.01 **Acute suppurative otitis media with spontaneous rupture of ear drum**
     DEF: Sudden, severe inflammation of middle ear, with pressure tearing ear drum tissue.
   382.02 *Acute suppurative otitis media in diseases classified elsewhere*
     Code first underlying disease, as:
      influenza (487.8)
      scarlet fever (034.1)
     EXCLUDES postmeasles otitis (055.2)

  382.1 **Chronic tubotympanic suppurative otitis media**
   Benign chronic
    suppurative otitis } (with anterior
    media   perforation of ear
   Chronic tubotympanic drum)
    disease
   DEF: Inflammation of tympanic cavity and auditory tube; with pus formation.

  382.2 **Chronic atticoantral suppurative otitis media**
   Chronic atticoantral
    disease   } (with posterior or superior
   Persistent mucosal marginal perforation
    disease   of ear drum)
   DEF: Inflammation of upper tympanic membrane and mastoid antrum; with pus formation.

  382.3 <mark>Unspecified chronic suppurative otitis media</mark>
   Chronic purulent otitis media
    EXCLUDES tuberculous otitis media (017.4)

382.4 Unspecified suppurative otitis media
Purulent otitis media NOS

382.9 Unspecified otitis media
Otitis media:
  NOS
  acute NOS
Otitis media:
  chronic NOS

√4th **383 Mastoiditis and related conditions**

√5th **383.0 Acute mastoiditis**
Abscess of mastoid   Empyema of mastoid

383.00 Acute mastoiditis without complications
DEF: Sudden, severe inflammation of mastoid air cells.

383.01 Subperiosteal abscess of mastoid
DEF: Pocket of pus within mastoid bone.

383.02 Acute mastoiditis with other complications
Gradenigo's syndrome

383.1 Chronic mastoiditis
Caries of mastoid
Fistula of mastoid
EXCLUDES   tuberculous mastoiditis (015.6)
DEF: Persistent inflammation of mastoid air cells.

√5th **383.2 Petrositis**
Coalescing osteitis
Inflammation   } of petrous bone
Osteomyelitis

383.20 Petrositis, unspecified

383.21 Acute petrositis
DEF: Sudden, severe inflammation of dense bone behind ear.

383.22 Chronic petrositis
DEF: Persistent inflammation of dense bone behind ear.

√5th **383.3 Complications following mastoidectomy**

383.30 Postmastoidectomy complication, unspecified

383.31 Mucosal cyst of postmastoidectomy cavity
DEF: Mucous-lined cyst cavity following removal of mastoid bone.

383.32 Recurrent cholesteatoma of postmastoidectomy cavity
DEF: Cystlike mass of cell debris in cavity following removal of mastoid bone.

383.33 Granulations of postmastoidectomy cavity
Chronic inflammation of postmastoidectomy cavity
DEF: Granular tissue in cavity following removal of mastoid bone.

√5th **383.8 Other disorders of mastoid**

383.81 Postauricular fistula
DEF: Abnormal passage behind mastoid cavity.

383.89 Other

383.9 Unspecified mastoiditis

√4th **384 Other disorders of tympanic membrane**

√5th **384.0 Acute myringitis without mention of otitis media**

384.00 Acute myringitis, unspecified
Acute tympanitis NOS
DEF: Sudden, severe inflammation of ear drum.

384.01 Bullous myringitis
Myringitis bullosa hemorrhagica
DEF: Type of viral otitis media characterized by the appearance of serous or hemorrhagic blebs on the tympanic membrane.

384.09 Other

384.1 Chronic myringitis without mention of otitis media
Chronic tympanitis
DEF: Persistent inflammation of ear drum; with no evidence of middle ear infection.

384.2 Perforation of tympanic membrane
Perforation of ear drum: NOS, persistent posttraumatic
Perforation of ear drum: postinflammatory
EXCLUDES otitis media with perforation of tympanic membrane (382.00-382.9)
traumatic perforation [current injury] (872.61)

- 384.20 Perforation of tympanic membrane, unspecified
- 384.21 Central perforation of tympanic membrane
- 384.22 Attic perforation of tympanic membrane
  Pars flaccida
- 384.23 Other marginal perforation of tympanic membrane
- 384.24 Multiple perforations of tympanic membrane
- 384.25 Total perforation of tympanic membrane

384.8 Other specified disorders of tympanic membrane
- 384.81 Atrophic flaccid tympanic membrane
  Healed perforation of ear drum
- 384.82 Atrophic nonflaccid tympanic membrane

384.9 Unspecified disorder of tympanic membrane

385 Other disorders of middle ear and mastoid
EXCLUDES mastoiditis (383.0-383.9)

385.0 Tympanosclerosis
- 385.00 Tympanosclerosis, unspecified as to involvement
- 385.01 Tympanosclerosis involving tympanic membrane only
  DEF: Tough, fibrous tissue impeding functions of ear drum.
- 385.02 Tympanosclerosis involving tympanic membrane and ear ossicles
  DEF: Tough, fibrous tissue impeding functions of middle ear bones (stapes, malleus, incus).

Cholesteatoma
Middle ear chamber
Cholesteatoma sac
Ear drum

NERVOUS SYSTEM AND SENSE ORGANS

385.03 Tympanosclerosis involving tympanic membrane, ear ossicles, and middle ear
DEF: Tough, fibrous tissue impeding functions of ear drum, middle ear bones and middle ear canal.

385.09 Tympanosclerosis involving other combination of structures

√5th **385.1 Adhesive middle ear disease**
Adhesive otitis
Otitis media: chronic adhesive
Otitis media: fibrotic
EXCLUDES glue ear (381.20-381.29)
DEF: Adhesions of middle ear structures.

385.10 Adhesive middle ear disease, unspecified as to involvement
385.11 Adhesions of drum head to incus
385.12 Adhesions of drum head to stapes
385.13 Adhesions of drum head to promontorium
385.19 Other adhesions and combinations

√5th **385.2 Other acquired abnormality of ear ossicles**
385.21 Impaired mobility of malleus
Ankylosis of malleus
385.22 Impaired mobility of other ear ossicles
Ankylosis of ear ossicles, except malleus
385.23 Discontinuity or dislocation of ear ossicles
DEF: Disruption in auditory chain; created by malleus, incus and stapes.
385.24 Partial loss or necrosis of ear ossicles
DEF: Tissue loss in malleus, incus and stapes.

√5th **385.3 Cholesteatoma of middle ear and mastoid**
Cholesterosis
Epidermosis   } of (middle) ear
Keratosis
Polyp
EXCLUDES cholesteatoma:
external ear canal (380.21)
recurrent of postmastoidectomy cavity (383.32)
DEF: Cystlike mass of middle ear and mastoid antrum filled with debris, including cholesterol.

385.30 Cholesteatoma, unspecified
385.31 Cholesteatoma of attic
385.32 Cholesteatoma of middle ear
385.33 Cholesteatoma of middle ear and mastoid
DEF: Cystlike mass of cell debris in middle ear and mastoid air cells behind ear.
385.35 Diffuse cholesteatosis

√5th **385.8 Other disorders of middle ear and mastoid**
385.82 Cholesterin granuloma
DEF: Granuloma formed of fibrotic tissue; contains cholesterol crystals surrounded by foreign-body cells; found in the middle ear and mastoid area.
385.83 Retained foreign body of middle ear
385.89 Other

385.9 Unspecified disorder of middle ear and mastoid

√4th **386 Vertiginous syndromes and other disorders of vestibular system**
EXCLUDES vertigo NOS (780.4)

NERVOUS SYSTEM AND SENSE ORGANS 386.0–386.50

√5ᵗʰ **386.0 Ménière's disease**
Endolymphatic hydrops
Lermoyez's syndrome
Ménière's syndrome or vertigo

DEF: Distended membranous labyrinth of middle ear from endolymphatic hydrops; causes ischemia, failure of nerve function; hearing and balance dysfunction; symptoms include fluctuating deafness, ringing in ears and dizziness.

386.00 Ménière's disease, unspecified
Ménière's disease (active)

386.01 Active Ménière's disease, cochleovestibular

386.02 Active Ménière's disease, cochlear

386.03 Active Ménière's disease, vestibular

386.04 Inactive Ménière's disease
Ménière's disease in remission

√5ᵗʰ **386.1 Other and unspecified peripheral vertigo**
EXCLUDES epidemic vertigo (078.81)

386.10 Peripheral vertigo, unspecified

386.11 Benign paroxysmal positional vertigo
Benign paroxysmal positional nystagmus

386.12 Vestibular neuronitis
Acute (and recurrent) peripheral vestibulopathy

DEF: Transient benign vertigo, unknown cause; characterized by response to caloric stimulation on one side, nystagmus with rhythmic movement of eyes; normal auditory function present; occurs in young adults.

386.19 Other
Aural vertigo
Otogenic vertigo

386.2 Vertigo of central origin
Central positional nystagmus
Malignant positional vertigo

√5ᵗʰ **386.3 Labyrinthitis**

386.30 Labyrinthitis, unspecified

386.31 Serous labyrinthitis
Diffuse labyrinthitis

DEF: Inflammation of labyrinth; with fluid buildup.

386.32 Circumscribed labyrinthitis
Focal labyrinthitis

386.33 Suppurative labyrinthitis
Purulent labyrinthitis

DEF: Inflammation of labyrinth; with pus.

386.34 Toxic labyrinthitis

DEF: Inflammation of labyrinth; due to toxic reaction.

386.35 Viral labyrinthitis

√5ᵗʰ **386.4 Labyrinthine fistula**

386.40 Labyrinthine fistula, unspecified

386.41 Round window fistula

386.42 Oval window fistula

386.43 Semicircular canal fistula

386.48 Labyrinthine fistula of combined sites

√5ᵗʰ **386.5 Labyrinthine dysfunction**

386.50 Labyrinthine dysfunction, unspecified

√4ᵗʰ / √5ᵗʰ Additional Digit Required   Unspecified Code   Other Specified Code   Manifestation Code

 Medicare Secondary Payer   ▶◀ Revised Text   ● New Code   ▲ Revised Code Title

386.51 **Hyperactive labyrinth, unilateral**
  DEF: Oversensitivity of labyrinth to auditory signals; affecting one ear.

386.52 **Hyperactive labyrinth, bilateral**
  DEF: Oversensitivity of labyrinth to auditory signals; affecting both ears.

386.53 **Hypoactive labyrinth, unilateral**
  DEF: Reduced sensitivity of labyrinth to auditory signals; affecting one ear.

386.54 **Hypoactive labyrinth, bilateral**
  DEF: Reduced sensitivity of labyrinth to auditory signals; affecting both ears.

386.55 **Loss of labyrinthine reactivity, unilateral**
  DEF: Reduced reaction of labyrinth to auditory signals, affecting one ear.

386.56 **Loss of labyrinthine reactivity, bilateral**
  DEF: Reduced reaction of labyrinth to auditory signals; affecting both ears.

386.58 **Other forms and combinations**

386.8 **Other disorders of labyrinth**

386.9 **Unspecified vertiginous syndromes and labyrinthine disorders**

√4th **387 Otosclerosis**
  INCLUDES   otospongiosis
  DEF: Synonym for otospongiosis, spongy bone formation in the labyrinth bones of the ear; it causes progressive hearing impairment.

387.0 **Otosclerosis involving oval window, nonobliterative**
  DEF: Tough, fibrous tissue impeding functions of oval window.

387.1 **Otosclerosis involving oval window, obliterative**
  DEF: Tough, fibrous tissue blocking oval window.

387.2 **Cochlear otosclerosis**
  Otosclerosis involving: Otosclerosis involving:
    otic capsule   round window
  DEF: Tough, fibrous tissue impeding functions of cochlea.

387.8 **Other otosclerosis**

387.9 **Otosclerosis, unspecified**

√4th **388 Other disorders of ear**

  √5th **388.0** **Degenerative and vascular disorders of ear**

  388.00 **Degenerative and vascular disorders, unspecified**

  388.01 **Presbyacusis**
    DEF: Progressive, bilateral perceptive hearing loss caused by advancing age; it is also known as presbycusis.

  388.02 **Transient ischemic deafness**
    DEF: Restricted blood flow to auditory organs causing temporary hearing loss.

  √5th **388.1** **Noise effects on inner ear**

  388.10 **Noise effects on inner ear, unspecified**

  388.11 **Acoustic trauma (explosive) to ear**
    Otitic blast injury

  388.12 **Noise-induced hearing loss**

  388.2 **Sudden hearing loss, unspecified**

  √5th **388.3** **Tinnitus**
    DEF: Abnormal noises in ear; may be heard by others beside the affected individual; noises include ringing, clicking, roaring and buzzing.

  388.30 **Tinnitus, unspecified**
  388.31 Subjective tinnitus
  388.32 Objective tinnitus

NERVOUS SYSTEM AND SENSE ORGANS

√5ᵗʰ **388.4 Other abnormal auditory perception**
 388.40 Abnormal auditory perception, unspecified
 388.41 Diplacusis
  DEF: Perception of a single auditory sound as two sounds at two different levels of intensity.

 388.42 Hyperacusis
  DEF: Exceptionally acute sense of hearing caused by such conditions as Bell's palsy; this term may also refer to painful sensitivity to sounds.

 388.43 Impairment of auditory discrimination
  DEF: Impaired ability to distinguish tone of sound.

 388.44 Recruitment
  DEF: Perception of abnormally increased loudness caused by a slight increase in sound intensity; it is a term used in audiology.

388.5 Disorders of acoustic nerve
 Acoustic neuritis
 Degeneration ⎫
 Disorder ⎭ of acoustic or eighth nerve

 EXCLUDES acoustic neuroma (225.1)
  syphilitic acoustic neuritis (094.86)

√5ᵗʰ **388.6 Otorrhea**
 388.60 Otorrhea, unspecified
  Discharging ear NOS
 388.61 Cerebrospinal fluid otorrhea
  EXCLUDES cerebrospinal fluid rhinorrhea (349.81)
  DEF: Spinal fluid leakage from ear.

 388.69 Other
  Otorrhagia

√5ᵗʰ **388.7 Otalgia**
 388.70 Otalgia, unspecified
  Earache NOS
 388.71 Otogenic pain
 388.72 Referred pain

388.8 Other disorders of ear
388.9 Unspecified disorder of ear

√4ᵗʰ **389 Hearing loss**
√5ᵗʰ **389.0 Conductive hearing loss**
 Conductive deafness
 DEF: Dysfunction in sound-conducting structures of external or middle ear causing hearing loss.

 389.00 Conductive hearing loss, unspecified
 389.01 Conductive hearing loss, external ear
 389.02 Conductive hearing loss, tympanic membrane
 389.03 Conductive hearing loss, middle ear
 389.04 Conductive hearing loss, inner ear
 389.08 Conductive hearing loss of combined types

√4ᵗʰ/√5ᵗʰ Additional Digit Required   Unspecified Code   Other Specified Code   Manifestation Code
MSP Medicare Secondary Payer   ▶◀ Revised Text   ● New Code   ▲ Revised Code Title

2002 Ingenix, Inc.

389.1–391.2 CIRCULATORY SYSTEM

√5ᵗʰ **389.1 Sensorineural hearing loss**
Perceptive hearing loss or deafness
EXCLUDES abnormal auditory perception (388.40-388.44)
psychogenic deafness (306.7)
DEF: Nerve conduction causing hearing loss.

389.10 Sensorineural hearing loss, unspecified
389.11 Sensory hearing loss
389.12 Neural hearing loss
389.14 Central hearing loss
389.18 Sensorineural hearing loss of combined types

389.2 Mixed conductive and sensorineural hearing loss
Deafness or hearing loss of type classifiable to 389.0 with type classifiable to 389.1

389.7 Deaf mutism, not elsewhere classifiable
Deaf, nonspeaking

389.8 Other specified forms of hearing loss

389.9 Unspecified hearing loss
Deafness NOS

7. DISEASES OF THE CIRCULATORY SYSTEM (390-459)

ACUTE RHEUMATIC FEVER (390-392)

DEF: Febrile disease occurs mainly in children or young adults following throat infection by group A streptococci; symptoms include fever, joint pain, lesions of heart, blood vessels and joint connective tissue, abdominal pain, skin changes, and chorea.

390 Rheumatic fever without mention of heart involvement
Arthritis, rheumatic, acute or subacute
Rheumatic fever (active) (acute)
Rheumatism, articular, acute or subacute
EXCLUDES that with heart involvement (391.0-391.9)

√4ᵗʰ **391 Rheumatic fever with heart involvement**
EXCLUDES chronic heart diseases of rheumatic origin (393.0-398.9) unless rheumatic fever is also present or there is evidence of recrudescence or activity of the rheumatic process

391.0 Acute rheumatic pericarditis
Rheumatic:
fever (active) (acute) with pericarditis
pericarditis (acute)
Any condition classifiable to 390 with pericarditis
EXCLUDES that not specified as rheumatic (420.0-420.9)
DEF: Sudden, severe inflammation of heart lining due to rheumatic fever.

391.1 Acute rheumatic endocarditis
Rheumatic:
endocarditis, acute
fever (active) (acute) with endocarditis or valvulitis
valvulitis acute
Any condition classifiable to 390 with endocarditis or valvulitis
DEF: Sudden, severe inflammation of heart cavities due to rheumatic fever.

391.2 Acute rheumatic myocarditis
Rheumatic fever (active) (acute) with myocarditis
Any condition classifiable to 390 with myocarditis
DEF: Sudden, severe inflammation of heart muscles due to rheumatic fever.

CIRCULATORY SYSTEM

391.8 Other acute rheumatic heart disease
Rheumatic:
fever (active) (acute) with other or multiple types of heart involvement
pancarditis, acute
Any condition classifiable to 390 with other or multiple types of heart involvement

391.9 Acute rheumatic heart disease, unspecified
Rheumatic:
carditis, acute
fever (active) (acute) with unspecified type of heart involvement
heart disease, active or acute
Any condition classifiable to 390 with unspecified type of heart involvement

392 Rheumatic chorea
INCLUDES   Sydenham's chorea
EXCLUDES   chorea:
NOS (333.5)
Huntington's (333.4)

DEF: Childhood disease linked with rheumatic fever and streptococcal infections; symptoms include spasmodic, involuntary movements of limbs or facial muscles, psychic symptoms, and irritability.

392.0 With heart involvement
Rheumatic chorea with heart involvement of any type classifiable to 391

392.9 Without mention of heart involvement

CHRONIC RHEUMATIC HEART DISEASE (393-398)

393 Chronic rheumatic pericarditis
Adherent pericardium, rheumatic
Chronic rheumatic:
mediastinopericarditis
myopericarditis
EXCLUDES   pericarditis NOS or not specified as rheumatic (423.0-423.9)

DEF: Persistent inflammation of heart lining due to rheumatic heart disease.

394 Diseases of mitral valve
EXCLUDES   that with aortic valve involvement (396.0-396.9)

394.0 Mitral stenosis
Mitral (valve):   Mitral (valve):
  obstruction (rheumatic)   stenosis NOS

DEF: Narrowing, of mitral valve between left atrium and left ventricle due to rheumatic heart disease.

394.1 Rheumatic mitral insufficiency
Rheumatic mitral: Rheumatic mitral:
  incompetence   regurgitation
EXCLUDES   that not specified as rheumatic (424.0)

DEF: Malfunction of mitral valve between left atrium and left ventricle due to rheumatic heart disease.

394.2 Mitral stenosis with insufficiency
Mitral stenosis with incompetence or regurgitation

DEF: A narrowing or stricture of the mitral valve situated between the left atrium and left ventricle. The stenosis interferes with blood flow from the atrium into the ventricle. If the valve does not completely close, it becomes insufficient (inadequate) and cannot prevent regurgitation (abnormal backward flow) into the atrium when the left ventricle contracts. This abnormal function is also called incompetence.

CIRCULATORY SYSTEM

394.9 **Other and unspecified mitral valve diseases**
Mitral (valve):   Mitral (valve):
   disease (chronic)   failure

✓4th **395 Diseases of aortic valve**
> **EXCLUDES**   that not specified as rheumatic (424.1)
> that with mitral valve involvement (396.0-396.9)

395.0 **Rheumatic aortic stenosis**
Rheumatic aortic (valve) obstruction
DEF: Narrowing of the aortic valve; results in backflow into ventricle due to rheumatic heart disease.

395.1 **Rheumatic aortic insufficiency**
Rheumatic aortic: Rheumatic aortic:
   incompetence   regurgitation
DEF: Malfunction of the aortic valve; results in backflow into left ventricle due to rheumatic heart disease.

395.2 **Rheumatic aortic stenosis with insufficiency**
Rheumatic aortic stenosis with incompetence or regurgitation
DEF: Malfunction and narrowing, of the aortic valve; results in backflow into left ventricle due to rheumatic heart disease.

395.9 **Other and unspecified rheumatic aortic diseases**
Rheumatic aortic (valve) disease

✓4th **396 Diseases of mitral and aortic valves**
> **INCLUDES**   involvement of both mitral and aortic valves, whether specified as rheumatic or not

396.0 **Mitral valve stenosis and aortic valve stenosis**
Atypical aortic (valve) stenosis
Mitral and aortic (valve) obstruction (rheumatic)

396.1 **Mitral valve stenosis and aortic valve insufficiency**

396.2 **Mitral valve insufficiency and aortic valve stenosis**

396.3 **Mitral valve insufficiency and aortic valve insufficiency**
Mitral and aortic (valve):   Mitral and aortic (valve):
   incompetence   regurgitation

396.8 **Multiple involvement of mitral and aortic valves**
Stenosis and insufficiency of mitral or aortic valve with stenosis or insufficiency, or both, of the other valve

396.9 **Mitral and aortic valve diseases, unspecified**

✓4th **397 Diseases of other endocardial structures**

397.0 **Diseases of tricuspid valve**
Tricuspid (valve) (rheumatic):   Tricuspid (valve) (rheumatic):
   disease   regurgitation
   insufficiency   stenosis
   obstruction
DEF: Malfunction of the valve between right atrium and right ventricle due to rheumatic heart disease.

397.1 **Rheumatic diseases of pulmonary valve**
> **EXCLUDES**   that not specified as rheumatic (424.3)

397.9 **Rheumatic diseases of endocardium, valve unspecified**
Rheumatic:
   endocarditis (chronic)
   valvulitis (chronic)
> **EXCLUDES**   that not specified as rheumatic (424.90-424.99)

CIRCULATORY SYSTEM

√4ᵗʰ **398 Other rheumatic heart disease**

398.0 Rheumatic myocarditis
Rheumatic degeneration of myocardium
EXCLUDES   myocarditis not specified as rheumatic (429.0)
DEF: Chronic inflammation of heart muscle due to rheumatic heart disease.

√5ᵗʰ **398.9 Other and unspecified rheumatic heart diseases**

398.90 Rheumatic heart disease, unspecified
Rheumatic: Rheumatic:
  carditis   heart disease NOS
EXCLUDES   carditis not specified as rheumatic (429.89)
heart disease NOS not specified as rheumatic (429.9)

398.91 Rheumatic heart failure (congestive)
Rheumatic left ventricular failure
DEF: Decreased cardiac output, edema and hypertension due to rheumatic heart disease.

398.99 Other

HYPERTENSIVE DISEASE (401-405)

EXCLUDES   that complicating pregnancy, childbirth, or the puerperium (642.0-642.9)
that involving coronary vessels (410.00-414.9)

√4ᵗʰ **401 Essential hypertension**
INCLUDES   high blood pressure
hyperpiesia
hyperpiesis
hypertension (arterial) (essential) (primary) (systemic)
hypertensive vascular:
  degeneration
  disease
EXCLUDES   elevated blood pressure without diagnosis of hypertension (796.2)
pulmonary hypertension (416.0-416.9)
that involving vessels of:
  brain (430-438)
  eye (362.11)
DEF: Hypertension that occurs without apparent organic cause; idiopathic.

401.0 Malignant
DEF: Severe high arterial blood pressure; results in necrosis in kidney, retina, etc.; hemorrhages occur and death commonly due to uremia or rupture of cerebral vessel.

401.1 Benign
DEF: Mildly elevated arterial blood pressure.

401.9 Unspecified

√4ᵗʰ **402 Hypertensive heart disease**
▶Use additional code to specify type of heart failure (428.0, 428.20-428.23, 428.30-428.33, 428.40-428.43)◀
INCLUDES   hypertensive:
  cardiomegaly
  cardiopathy
  cardiovascular disease
  heart (disease) (failure)
  any condition classifiable to 428, 429.0-429.3, 429.8, 429.9 due to hypertension

CIRCULATORY SYSTEM

- √5th **402.0 Malignant**
  - ▲ **402.00** Without heart failure
  - ▲ **402.01** With heart failure
- √5th **402.1 Benign**
  - ▲ **402.10** Without heart failure
  - ▲ **402.11** With heart failure
- √5th **402.9 Unspecified**
  - ▲ **402.90** Without heart failure
  - ▲ **402.91** With heart failure

√4th **403 Hypertensive renal disease**

INCLUDES
- arteriolar nephritis
- arteriosclerosis of:
  - kidney
  - renal arterioles
- arteriosclerotic nephritis (chronic) (interstitial)
- hypertensive:
  - nephropathy
  - renal failure
  - uremia (chronic)
- nephrosclerosis
- renal sclerosis with hypertension
- any condition classifiable to 585, 586, or 587 with any condition classifiable to 401

EXCLUDES
- acute renal failure (584.5-584.9)
- renal disease stated as not due to hypertension
- renovascular hypertension (405.0-405.9 with fifth-digit 1)

The following fifth-digit subclassification is for use with category 403:
- 0 without mention of renal failure
- 1 with renal failure

- √5th **403.0 Malignant**
- √5th **403.1 Benign**
- √5th **403.9 Unspecified**

√4th **404 Hypertensive heart and renal disease**

▶Use additional code to specify type of heart failure (428.0, 428.20-428.23, 428.30-428.33, 428.40-428.43)◀

INCLUDES disease:
- cardiorenal
- cardiovascular renal
- any condition classifiable to 402 with any condition classifiable to 403

The following fifth-digit subclassification is for use with category 404:
- ▲ 0 without mention of heart failure or renal failure
- ▲ 1 with heart failure
- 2 with renal failure
- ▲ 3 with heart failure and renal failure

- √5th **404.0 Malignant**
- √5th **404.1 Benign**
- √5th **404.9 Unspecified**

√4th **405 Secondary hypertension**

DEF: High arterial blood pressure due to or with a variety of primary diseases, such as renal disorders, CNS disorders, endocrine, and vascular diseases.

- √5th **405.0 Malignant**
  - **405.01** Renovascular
  - **405.09** Other

CIRCULATORY SYSTEM

Sections of Heart Muscle

✓5th **405.1 Benign**
  405.11 Renovascular
  405.19 Other

✓5th **405.9 Unspecified**
  405.91 Renovascular
  405.99 Other

ISCHEMIC HEART DISEASE (410-414)

INCLUDES that with mention of hypertension
Use additional code to identify presence of hypertension (401.0-405.9)

✓4th **410 Acute myocardial infarction**
  INCLUDES cardiac infarction
      coronary (artery):
        embolism
        occlusion
        rupture
        thrombosis
      infarction of heart, myocardium, or ventricle
      rupture of heart, myocardium, or ventricle
      any condition classifiable to 414.1-414.9 specified as acute or with a stated duration of 8 weeks or less

DEF: A sudden insufficiency of blood supply to an area of the heart muscle; usually due to a coronary artery occlusion.

The following fifth-digit subclassification is for use with category 410:
  0 episode of care unspecified
    Use when the source document does not contain sufficient information for the assignment of fifth digit 1 or 2.
  1 initial episode of care
    Use fifth-digit 1 to designate the first episode of care (regardless of facility site) for a newly diagnosed myocardial infarction. The fifth-digit 1 is assigned regardless of the number of times a patient may be transferred during the initial episode of care.
  2 subsequent episode of care
    Use fifth-digit 2 to designate an episode of care following the initial episode when the patient is admitted for further observation, evaluation or treatment for a myocardial infarction that has received initial treatment, but is still less than 8 weeks old.

| ✓4th ✓5th Additional Digit Required | Unspecified Code | Other Specified Code | Manifestation Code |
| MSP Medicare Secondary Payer | ▶◀ Revised Text | ● New Code | ▲ Revised Code Title |

2002 Ingenix, Inc.

CIRCULATORY SYSTEM 410.0–411.0

Acute Myocardial Infarction
Anatomic Sites
- Anterolateral 410.0
- Other lateral 410.5
- Posterobasal 410.6
- Posterolateral 410.5
- Anteroseptal 410.1
- Inferoposterior 410.3
- Atrium only 410.8
- Septum only
- Papillary muscle
- Apical 410.1
- Other and septum 410.4

§ √5th **410.0 Of anterolateral wall** A

§ √5th **410.1 Of other anterior wall** A
Infarction:
anterior (wall)
NOS   (with contiguous portion of
anteroapical   intraventricular septum)
anteroseptal

§ √5th **410.2 Of inferolateral wall** A

§ √5th **410.3 Of inferoposterior wall** A

§ √5th **410.4 Of other inferior wall** A
Infarction:
diaphragmatic   (with contiguous portion
wall NOS   of intraventricular
inferior (wall) NOS   septum)

§ √5th **410.5 Of other lateral wall** A
Infarction: Infarction:
apical-lateral   high lateral
basal-lateral   posterolateral

§ √5th **410.6 True posterior wall infarction** A
Infarction: Infarction:
posterobasal   strictly posterior

§ √5th **410.7 Subendocardial infarction** A
Nontransmural infarction

§ √5th **410.8 Of other specified sites** A
Infarction of: Infarction of:
atrium   septum alone
papillary muscle

§ √5th **410.9 Unspecified site** A
Acute myocardial infarction NOS
Coronary occlusion NOS

√4th **411 Other acute and subacute forms of ischemic heart disease**

411.0 Postmyocardial infarction syndrome A
Dressler's syndrome
DEF: Complication developing several days/weeks after myocardial infarction; symptoms include fever, leukocytosis, chest pain, evidence of pericarditis, pleurisy, and pneumonitis; tendency to recur.

§ Requires fifth-digit. See beginning of category 410 for codes and definitions.

N Newborn Age: 0   P Pediatric Age: 0-17   M Maternity Age: 12-55   A Adult Age: 15-124

CIRCULATORY SYSTEM   411.1–413.1

411.1 Intermediate coronary syndrome   ▲
    Impending infarction   Preinfarction syndrome
    Preinfarction angina   Unstable angina
    EXCLUDES   angina (pectoris) (413.9)
                    decubitus (413.0)
    DEF: A condition representing an intermediate stage between angina of effort and acute myocardial infarction. It is often documented by the physician as "unstable angina."

√5ᵗʰ **411.8 Other**

  411.81 Acute coronary occlusion without myocardial infarction   ▲
    Acute coronary (artery):
        embolism   ⎫ without or not
        obstruction   ⎬ resulting in
        occlusion   ⎪ myocardial
        thrombosis   ⎭ infarction
        EXCLUDES   obstruction without infarction due to atherosclerosis
                        ▶(414.00-414.06)◀
                        occlusion without infarction due to atherosclerosis
                        ▶(414.00-414.06)◀
    DEF: Interrupted blood flow to a portion of the heart; without tissue death.

  411.89 Other   ▲
    Coronary insufficiency (acute)
    Subendocardial ischemia

412 Old myocardial infarction   ▲
    Healed myocardial infarction
    Past myocardial infarction diagnosed on ECG [EKG] or other special investigation, but currently presenting no symptoms

√4ᵗʰ **413 Angina pectoris**
    DEF: Severe constricting pain in the chest, often radiating from the precordium to the left shoulder and down the arm, due to ischemia of the heart muscle; usually caused by coronary disease; pain is often precipitated by effort or excitement.

  413.0 Angina decubitus   ▲
    Nocturnal angina
    DEF: Angina occurring only in the recumbent position.

  413.1 Prinzmetal angina   ▲
    Variant angina pectoris
    DEF: Angina occurring when patient is recumbent; associated with ST-segment elevations.

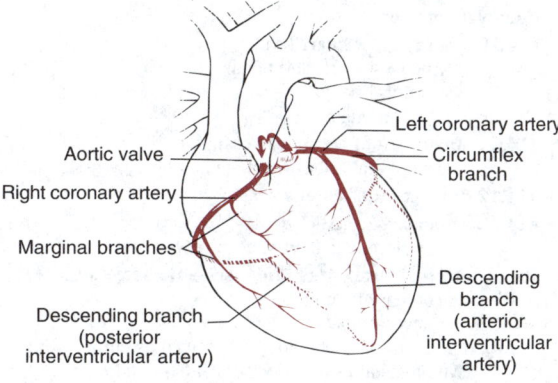

Arteries of the Heart

√4ᵗʰ/√5ᵗʰ Additional Digit Required   **Unspecified Code**   ● Other Specified Code   ▲ Manifestation Code
MSP Medicare Secondary Payer   ▶◀ Revised Text   ● New Code   ▲ Revised Code Title

2002 Ingenix, Inc.   October 2002 • Volume 1 — 239

413.9 Other and unspecified angina pectoris
    Angina:
        NOS
        cardiac
        of effort
    Anginal syndrome
    Status anginosus
    Stenocardia
    Syncope anginosa
    EXCLUDES preinfarction angina (411.1)

√4th **414 Other forms of chronic ischemic heart disease**
    EXCLUDES arteriosclerotic cardiovascular disease [ASCVD] (429.2)
        cardiovascular:
            arteriosclerosis or sclerosis (429.2)
            degeneration or disease (429.2)

√5th **414.0 Coronary atherosclerosis**
    Arteriosclerotic heart disease [ASHD]
    Atherosclerotic heart disease
    Coronary (artery):
        arteriosclerosis
        arteritis or endarteritis
        atheroma
        sclerosis
        stricture
    EXCLUDES embolism of graft (996.72)
        occlusion NOS of graft (996.72)
        thrombus of graft (996.72)
    DEF: A chronic condition marked by thickening and loss of elasticity of the coronary artery; caused by deposits of plaque containing cholesterol, lipoid material and lipophages.

    414.00 Of unspecified type of vessel, native or graft
    414.01 Of native coronary artery
        DEF: Plaque deposits in natural heart vessels.
    414.02 Of autologous vein bypass graft
        DEF: Plaque deposit in grafted vein originating within patient.
    414.03 Of nonautologous biological bypass graft
        DEF: Plaque deposits in grafted vessel originating outside patient.
    414.04 Of artery bypass graft
        Internal mammary artery
        DEF: Plaque deposits in grafted artery originating within patient.
    414.05 Of unspecified type of bypass graft
        Bypass graft NOS
    414.06 Of coronary artery of transplanted heart

√5th **414.1 Aneurysm of heart**
    414.10 Aneurysm of heart (wall)
        Aneurysm (arteriovenous):
            mural
            ventricular
    414.11 Aneurysm of coronary vessels
        Aneurysm (arteriovenous) of coronary vessels
    414.12 Dissection of coronary artery
    414.19 Other aneurysm of heart
        Arteriovenous fistula, acquired, of heart

414.8 Other specified forms of chronic ischemic heart disease
    Chronic coronary insufficiency
    Ischemia, myocardial (chronic)
    Any condition classifiable to 410 specified as chronic, or presenting with symptoms after 8 weeks from date of infarction
    EXCLUDES coronary insufficiency (acute) (411.89)

CIRCULATORY SYSTEM

414.9 Chronic ischemic heart disease, unspecified
Ischemic heart disease NOS

DISEASES OF PULMONARY CIRCULATION (415-417)

√4ᵗʰ **415** Acute pulmonary heart disease

415.0 Acute cor pulmonale
EXCLUDES cor pulmonale NOS (416.9)
DEF: A heart-lung disease marked by dilation and failure of the right side of heart; due to pulmonary embolism; ventilatory function is impaired and pulmonary hypertension results within hours.

√5ᵗʰ **415.1** Pulmonary embolism and infarction
Pulmonary (artery) (vein):
  apoplexy
  embolism
  infarction (hemorrhagic)
  thrombosis
EXCLUDES that complicating:
  abortion (634-638 with .6, 639.6)
  ectopic or molar pregnancy (639.6)
  pregnancy, childbirth, or the puerperium (673.0-673.8)

DEF: Embolism: closure of the pulmonary artery or branch; due to thrombosis (blood clot).

DEF: Infarction: necrosis of lung tissue; due to obstructed arterial blood supply, most often by pulmonary embolism.

415.11 Iatrogenic pulmonary embolism and infarction
415.19 Other

√4ᵗʰ **416** Chronic pulmonary heart disease

416.0 Primary pulmonary hypertension
Idiopathic pulmonary arteriosclerosis
Pulmonary hypertension (essential) (idiopathic) (primary)
DEF: A rare increase in pulmonary circulation, often resulting in right ventricular failure or fatal syncope.

416.1 Kyphoscoliotic heart disease
DEF: High blood pressure within the lungs as a result of curvature of the spine.

416.8 Other chronic pulmonary heart diseases
Pulmonary hypertension, secondary

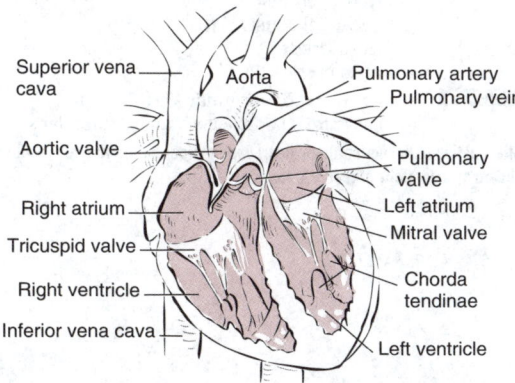

Heart Anatomy

√4ᵗʰ √5ᵗʰ Additional Digit Required
MSP Medicare Secondary Payer
 Unspecified Code
▶◀ Revised Text
 Other Specified Code
● New Code
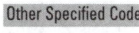 Manifestation Code
▲ Revised Code Title

2002 Ingenix, Inc.

Blood Flow

416.9 Chronic pulmonary heart disease, unspecified
Chronic cardiopulmonary disease
Cor pulmonale (chronic) NOS

√4th **417** Other diseases of pulmonary circulation

417.0 Arteriovenous fistula of pulmonary vessels
EXCLUDES congenital arteriovenous fistula (747.3)
DEF: Abnormal communication between blood vessels within lung.

417.1 Aneurysm of pulmonary artery
EXCLUDES congenital aneurysm (747.3)

417.8 Other specified diseases of pulmonary circulation
Pulmonary:
  arteritis
  endarteritis
  Rupture } of pulmonary vessel
  Stricture

417.9 Unspecified disease of pulmonary circulation

OTHER FORMS OF HEART DISEASE (420-429)

√4th **420** Acute pericarditis
INCLUDES acute:
  mediastinopericarditis
  myopericarditis
  pericardial effusion
  pleuropericarditis
  pneumopericarditis
EXCLUDES acute rheumatic pericarditis (391.0)
  postmyocardial infarction syndrome [Dressler's] (411.0)
DEF: Inflammation of the pericardium (heart sac); pericardial friction rub results from this inflammation and is heard as a scratchy or leathery sound.

CIRCULATORY SYSTEM

420.0 Acute pericarditis in diseases classified elsewhere
  Code first underlying disease, as:
    actinomycosis (039.8)
    amebiasis (006.8)
    nocardiosis (039.8)
    tuberculosis (017.9)
    uremia (585)
  EXCLUDES pericarditis (acute) (in):
    Coxsackie (virus) (074.21)
    gonococcal (098.83)
    histoplasmosis (115.0-115.9 with fifth-digit 3)
    meningococcal infection (036.41)
    syphilitic (093.81)

√5th **420.9 Other and unspecified acute pericarditis**

  420.90 Acute pericarditis, unspecified
    Pericarditis (acute):
      NOS
      infective NOS
      sicca

  420.91 Acute idiopathic pericarditis
    Pericarditis, acute:
      benign
      nonspecific
      viral

  420.99 Other
    Pericarditis (acute):
      pneumococcal
      purulent
      staphylococcal
      streptococcal
      suppurative
    Pneumopyopericardium
    Pyopericardium
      EXCLUDES pericarditis in diseases classified elsewhere (420.0)

√4th **421 Acute and subacute endocarditis**
  DEF: Bacterial inflammation of the endocardium (intracardiac area); major symptoms include fever, fatigue, heart murmurs, splenomegaly, embolic episodes and areas of infarction.

  421.0 Acute and subacute bacterial endocarditis
    Endocarditis (acute)   Endocarditis (acute)
      (chronic) (subacute):   (chronic) (subacute):
      bacterial   ulcerative
      infective NOS   vegetative
      lenta   Infective aneurysm
      malignant   Subacute bacterial
      purulent   endocarditis [SBE]
      septic
    Use additional code to identify infectious organism [e.g., Streptococcus 041.0, Staphylococcus 041.1]

421.1 Acute and subacute infective endocarditis in diseases classified elsewhere

Code first underlying disease, as:
blastomycosis (116.0)
Q fever (083.0)
typhoid (fever) (002.0)

EXCLUDES endocarditis (in):
Coxsackie (virus) (074.22)
gonococcal (098.84)
histoplasmosis (115.0-115.9 with fifth-digit 4)
meningococcal infection (036.42)
monilial (112.81)

421.9 Acute endocarditis, unspecified

Endocarditis ⎫
Myoendocarditis ⎬ acute or subacute
Periendocarditis ⎭

EXCLUDES acute rheumatic endocarditis (391.1)

✓4th 422 Acute myocarditis

EXCLUDES acute rheumatic myocarditis (391.2)

DEF: Acute inflammation of the muscular walls of the heart (myocardium).

422.0 Acute myocarditis in diseases classified elsewhere

Code first underlying disease, as:
myocarditis (acute):
influenzal (487.8)
tuberculous (017.9)

EXCLUDES myocarditis (acute) (due to):
aseptic, of newborn (074.23)
Coxsackie (virus) (074.23)
diphtheritic (032.82)
meningococcal infection (036.43)
syphilitic (093.82)
toxoplasmosis (130.3)

✓5th 422.9 Other and unspecified acute myocarditis

422.90 Acute myocarditis, unspecified
Acute or subacute (interstitial) myocarditis

422.91 Idiopathic myocarditis
Myocarditis (acute or subacute):
Fiedler's
giant cell
isolated (diffuse) (granulomatous)
nonspecific granulomatous

422.92 Septic myocarditis
Myocarditis, acute or subacute:
pneumococcal
staphylococcal
Use additional code to identify infectious organism [e.g., Staphylococcus 041.1]

EXCLUDES myocarditis, acute or subacute:
in bacterial diseases classified elsewhere (422.0)
streptococcal (391.2)

422.93 Toxic myocarditis
DEF: Inflammation of the heart muscle due to an adverse reaction to certain drugs or chemicals reaching the heart through the bloodstream.

422.99 Other

CIRCULATORY SYSTEM

✓4th **423 Other diseases of pericardium**
    EXCLUDES that specified as rheumatic (393)

  423.0 Hemopericardium
    DEF: Blood in the pericardial sac (pericardium).

  423.1 Adhesive pericarditis
    Adherent pericardium
    Fibrosis of pericardium
    Milk spots
    Pericarditis:
      adhesive
      obliterative
    Soldiers' patches
    DEF: Two layers of serous pericardium adhere to each other by fibrous adhesions.

  423.2 Constrictive pericarditis
    Concato's disease
    Pick's disease of heart (and liver)
    DEF: Inflammation identified by a rigid, thickened and sometimes calcified pericardium; ventricles of the heart cannot be adequately filled and congestive heart failure may result.

  423.8 Other specified diseases of pericardium
    Calcification }
    Fistula } of pericardium

  423.9 Unspecified disease of pericardium

✓4th **424 Other diseases of endocardium**
    EXCLUDES bacterial endocarditis (421.0-421.9)
        rheumatic endocarditis (391.1, 394.0-397.9)
        syphilitic endocarditis (093.20-093.24)

  424.0 Mitral valve disorders
    Mitral (valve):
      incompetence }
      insufficiency } NOS of specified cause, except rheumatic
      regurgitation }

    EXCLUDES mitral (valve):
        disease (394.9)
        failure (394.9)
        stenosis (394.0)
      the listed conditions:
        specified as rheumatic (394.1)
        unspecified as to cause but with mention of:
          diseases of aortic valve (396.0-396.9)
          mitral stenosis or obstruction (394.2)

  424.1 Aortic valve disorders
    Aortic (valve):
      incompetence }
      insufficiency } NOS of specified cause, except rheumatic
      regurgitation }
      stenosis }

    EXCLUDES hypertrophic subaortic stenosis (425.1)
      that specified as rheumatic (395.0-395.9)
      that of unspecified cause but with mention of diseases of mitral valve (396.0-396.9)

Normal Heart Valve Function

Heart Valve Disorders

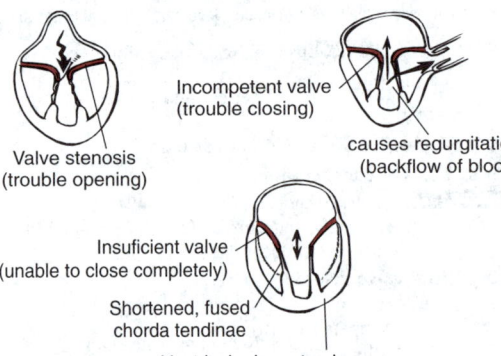

- 424.2 **Tricuspid valve disorders, specified as nonrheumatic**
  Tricuspid valve:
  incompetence
  insufficiency   } of specified cause,
  regurgitation   except
  stenosis   rheumatic

  EXCLUDES rheumatic or of unspecified cause (397.0)

- 424.3 **Pulmonary valve disorders**
  Pulmonic: Pulmonic:
  incompetence NOS   regurgitation NOS
  insufficiency NOS   stenosis NOS

  EXCLUDES that specified as rheumatic (397.1)

- √5th 424.9 **Endocarditis, valve unspecified**
  - 424.90 **Endocarditis, valve unspecified, unspecified cause**
    Endocarditis (chronic):
      NOS
      nonbacterial thrombotic
    Valvular:
      incompetence
      insufficiency   } of unspecified valve,
      regurgitation   unspecified cause
      stenosis
    Valvulitis (chronic)

CIRCULATORY SYSTEM 424.91–425.5

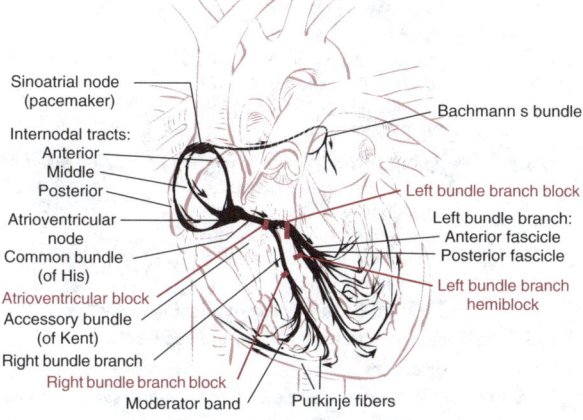

Nerve Conduction of the Heart

424.91 Endocarditis in diseases classified elsewhere
Code first underlying disease as:
atypical verrucous endocarditis [Libman-Sacks] (710.0)
disseminated lupus erythematosus (710.0)
tuberculosis (017.9)
EXCLUDES syphilitic (093.20-093.24)

424.99 Other
Any condition classifiable to 424.90 with specified cause, except rheumatic
EXCLUDES endocardial fibroelastosis (425.3)
that specified as rheumatic (397.9)

✓4th 425 Cardiomyopathy
INCLUDES myocardiopathy

425.0 Endomyocardial fibrosis

425.1 Hypertrophic obstructive cardiomyopathy
Hypertrophic subaortic stenosis (idiopathic)
DEF: Cardiomyopathy marked by left ventricle hypertrophy, enlarged septum; results in obstructed blood flow.

425.2 Obscure cardiomyopathy of Africa
Becker's disease
Idiopathic mural endomyocardial disease

425.3 Endocardial fibroelastosis
Elastomyofibrosis
DEF: A condition marked by left ventricle hypertrophy and conversion of the endocardium into a thick fibroelastic coat; capacity of the ventricle may be reduced, but is often increased.

425.4 Other primary cardiomyopathies
Cardiomyopathy:
  NOS
  congestive
  constrictive
  familial
  hypertrophic
Cardiomyopathy:
  idiopathic
  nonobstructive
  obstructive
  restrictive
Cardiovascular collagenosis

425.5 Alcoholic cardiomyopathy
DEF: Heart disease as result of excess alcohol consumption.

425.7 Nutritional and metabolic cardiomyopathy
Code first underlying disease, as:
amyloidosis (277.3)
beriberi (265.0)
cardiac glycogenosis (271.0)
mucopolysaccharidosis (277.5)
thyrotoxicosis (242.0-242.9)

EXCLUDES gouty tophi of heart (274.82)

425.8 Cardiomyopathy in other diseases classified elsewhere
Code first underlying disease, as:
Friedreich's ataxia (334.0)
myotonia atrophica (359.2)
progressive muscular dystrophy (359.1)
sarcoidosis (135)

EXCLUDES cardiomyopathy in Chagas' disease (086.0)

425.9 Secondary cardiomyopathy, unspecified

✓4th 426 Conduction disorders
DEF: Disruption or disturbance in the electrical impulses that regulate heartbeats.

426.0 Atrioventricular block, complete
Third degree atrioventricular block

✓5th 426.1 Atrioventricular block, other and unspecified

426.10 Atrioventricular block, unspecified
Atrioventricular [AV] block (incomplete) (partial)

426.11 First degree atrioventricular block
Incomplete atrioventricular block, first degree
Prolonged P-R interval NOS

426.12 Mobitz (type) II atrioventricular block
Incomplete atrioventricular block:
Mobitz (type) II
second degree, Mobitz (type) II

DEF: Impaired conduction of excitatory impulse from cardiac atrium to ventricle through AV node.

426.13 Other second degree atrioventricular block
Incomplete atrioventricular block:
Mobitz (type) I [Wenckebach's]
second degree:
NOS
Mobitz (type) I
with 2:1 atrioventricular response [block]
Wenckebach's phenomenon

DEF: Wenckebach's phenomenon: impulses generated at constant rate to sinus node, P-R interval lengthens; results in cycle of ventricular inadequacy and shortened P-R interval; second-degree A-V block commonly called "Mobitz type 1."

426.2 Left bundle branch hemiblock
Block:
left anterior fascicular
left posterior fascicular

426.3 Other left bundle branch block
Left bundle branch block:
NOS
anterior fascicular with posterior fascicular
complete
main stem

426.4 Right bundle branch block

CIRCULATORY SYSTEM

√5th **426.5 Bundle branch block, other and unspecified**
  426.50 Bundle branch block, unspecified
  426.51 Right bundle branch block and left posterior fascicular block
  426.52 Right bundle branch block and left anterior fascicular block
  426.53 Other bilateral bundle branch block
    Bifascicular block NOS
    Bilateral bundle branch block NOS
    Right bundle branch with left bundle branch block (incomplete) (main stem)
  426.54 Trifascicular block

426.6 Other heart block
  Intraventricular block: Sinoatrial block
    NOS Sinoauricular block
    diffuse
    myofibrillar

426.7 Anomalous atrioventricular excitation
  Atrioventricular conduction:
    accelerated
    accessory
    pre-excitation
  Ventricular pre-excitation
  Wolff-Parkinson-White syndrome
  DEF: Wolff-Parkinson-White: normal conduction pathway is bypassed; results in short P-R interval on EKG; tendency to supraventricular tachycardia.

√5th **426.8 Other specified conduction disorders**
  426.81 Lown-Ganong-Levine syndrome
    Syndrome of short P-R interval, normal QRS complexes, and supraventricular tachycardias
  426.89 Other
    Dissociation:
      atrioventricular [AV]
      interference
      isorhythmic
    Nonparoxysmal AV nodal tachycardia

426.9 Conduction disorder, unspecified
  Heart block NOS
  Stokes-Adams syndrome

√4th **427 Cardiac dysrhythmias**
  EXCLUDES that complicating:
    abortion (634-638 with .7, 639.8)
    ectopic or molar pregnancy (639.8)
    labor or delivery (668.1, 669.4)
  DEF: Disruption or disturbance in the rhythm of heartbeats.

  427.0 Paroxysmal supraventricular tachycardia
    Paroxysmal tachycardia: Paroxysmal tachycardia:
      atrial [PAT] junctional
      atrioventricular [AV] nodal
    DEF: Rapid atrial rhythm.

  427.1 Paroxysmal ventricular tachycardia
    Ventricular tachycardia (paroxysmal)
    DEF: Rapid ventricular rhythm.

427.2 Paroxysmal tachycardia, unspecified
Bouveret-Hoffmann syndrome
Paroxysmal tachycardia:
   NOS
   essential

√5th **427.3 Atrial fibrillation and flutter**
   427.31 Atrial fibrillation
      DEF: Irregular, rapid atrial contractions.

   427.32 Atrial flutter
      DEF: Regular, rapid atrial contractions.

√5th **427.4 Ventricular fibrillation and flutter**
   427.41 Ventricular fibrillation
      DEF: Irregular, rapid ventricular contractions.

   427.42 Ventricular flutter
      DEF: Regular, rapid, ventricular contractions.

427.5 Cardiac arrest
   Cardiorespiratory arrest

√5th **427.6 Premature beats**
   427.60 Premature beats, unspecified
      Ectopic beats   Premature contractions
      Extrasystoles   or systoles NOS
      Extrasystolic arrhythmia

   427.61 Supraventricular premature beats
      Atrial premature beats, contractions, or systoles

   427.69 Other
      Ventricular premature beats, contractions, or systoles

√5th **427.8 Other specified cardiac dysrhythmias**
   427.81 Sinoatrial node dysfunction
      Sinus bradycardia: Syndrome:
         persistent   sick sinus
         severe   tachycardia-bradycardia
      EXCLUDES sinus bradycardia NOS (427.89)
      DEF: Complex cardiac arrhythmia; appears as severe sinus bradycardia, sinus bradycardia with tachycardia, or sinus bradycardia with atrioventricular block.

   427.89 Other
      Rhythm disorder: Rhythm disorder:
         coronary sinus   nodal
         ectopic   Wandering (atrial) pacemaker
      EXCLUDES carotid sinus syncope (337.0)
                ▶neonatal bradycardia (779.81)◀
                ▶neonatal tachycardia (779.82)◀
                reflex bradycardia (337.0)
                tachycardia NOS (785.0)

427.9 Cardiac dysrhythmia, unspecified
   Arrhythmia (cardiac) NOS

√4th **428 Heart failure**
   ▶Code, if applicable, heart failure due to hypertension first (402.0-402.9, with fifth-digit 1 or 404.0-404.9 with fifth-digit 1 or 3)◀
   EXCLUDES following cardiac surgery (429.4)
             rheumatic (398.91)
             that complicating:
                abortion (634-638 with .7, 639.8)
                ectopic or molar pregnancy (639.8)
                labor or delivery (668.1, 669.4)

CIRCULATORY SYSTEM 428.0–429.0

▲ **428.0 Congestive heart failure, unspecified**
Congestive heart disease
Right heart failure (secondary to left heart failure)
EXCLUDES ▶*fluid overload NOS (276.6)*◀
DEF: Mechanical inadequacy; caused by inability of heart to pump and circulate blood; results in fluid collection in lungs, hypertension, congestion and edema of tissue.

428.1 Left heart failure
Acute edema of lung } with heart disease NOS
Acute pulmonary edema } or heart failure
Cardiac asthma
Left ventricular failure
DEF: Mechanical inadequacy of left ventricle; causing fluid in lungs.

√5th **428.2 Systolic heart failure**
EXCLUDES combined systolic and diastolic heart failure (428.40-428.43)
• 428.20 Unspecified
• 428.21 Acute
• 428.22 Chronic
• 428.23 Acute on chronic

√5th **428.3 Diastolic heart failure**
EXCLUDES combined systolic and diastolic heart failure (428.40-428.43)
• 428.30 Unspecified
• 428.31 Acute
• 428.32 Chronic
• 428.33 Acute on chronic

√5th **428.4 Combined systolic and diastolic heart failure**
• 428.40 Unspecified
• 428.41 Acute
• 428.42 Chronic
• 428.43 Acute on chronic

428.9 Heart failure, unspecified
Cardiac failure NOS   Myocardial failure NOS
Heart failure NOS   Weak heart

√4th **429 Ill-defined descriptions and complications of heart disease**

429.0 Myocarditis, unspecified
Myocarditis:
 NOS
 chronic (interstitial) } (with mention of
 fibroid   arteriosclerosis)
 senile
Use additional code to identify presence of arteriosclerosis
EXCLUDES acute or subacute (422.0-422.9)
rheumatic (398.0)
 acute (391.2)
that due to hypertension (402.0-402.9)

CIRCULATORY SYSTEM

429.1 Myocardial degeneration
Degeneration of heart or myocardium:
    fatty
    mural
    muscular   (with mention of arteriosclerosis)
Myocardial:
    degeneration
    disease

Use additional code to identify presence of arteriosclerosis
EXCLUDES *that due to hypertension (402.0-402.9)*

429.2 Cardiovascular disease, unspecified
Arteriosclerotic cardiovascular disease [ASCVD]
Cardiovascular arteriosclerosis
Cardiovascular:
    degeneration
    disease   (with mention of arteriosclerosis)
    sclerosis

Use additional code to identify presence of arteriosclerosis
EXCLUDES *that due to hypertension (402.0-402.9)*

429.3 Cardiomegaly
Cardiac:
    dilatation
    hypertrophy
Ventricular dilatation
EXCLUDES *that due to hypertension (402.0-402.9)*

429.4 Functional disturbances following cardiac surgery
Cardiac insufficiency   following cardiac surgery
Heart failure   or due to prosthesis

Postcardiotomy syndrome
Postvalvulotomy syndrome
EXCLUDES *cardiac failure in the immediate postoperative period (997.1)*

429.5 Rupture of chordae tendineae
DEF: Torn tissue, between heart valves and papillary muscles.

429.6 Rupture of papillary muscle
DEF: Torn muscle, between chordae tendineae and heart wall.

Berry Aneurysm

CIRCULATORY SYSTEM

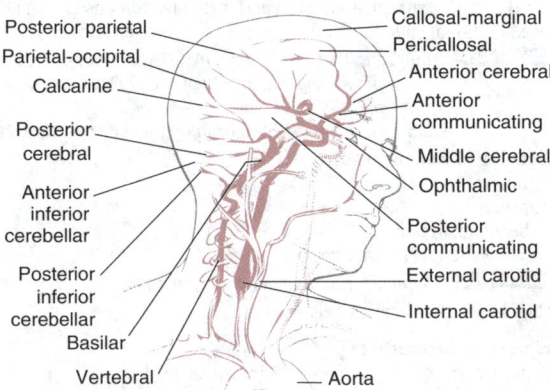

Cerebrovascular Arteries

429.7 Certain sequelae of myocardial infarction, not elsewhere classified
Use additional code to identify the associated myocardial infarction:
with onset of 8 weeks or less (410.00-410.92)
with onset of more than 8 weeks (414.8)

EXCLUDES congenital defects of heart (745, 746)
coronary aneurysm (414.11)
disorders of papillary muscle (429.6, 429.81)
postmyocardial infarction syndrome (411.0)
rupture of chordae tendineae (429.5)

429.71 Acquired cardiac septal defect
EXCLUDES acute septal infarction (410.00-410.92)

DEF: Abnormal communication, between opposite heart chambers; due to defect of septum; not present at birth.

429.79 Other
Mural thrombus (atrial) (ventricular), acquired, following myocardial infarction

429.8 Other ill-defined heart diseases

429.81 Other disorders of papillary muscle
Papillary muscle: Papillary muscle:
  atrophy   incompetence
  degeneration   incoordination
  dysfunction   scarring

429.82 Hyperkinetic heart disease
DEF: Condition of unknown origin in young adults; marked by increased cardiac output at rest, increased rate of ventricular ejection; may lead to heart failure.

429.89 Other
Carditis
EXCLUDES that due to hypertension (402.0-402.9)

429.9 Heart disease, unspecified
Heart disease (organic) NOS
Morbus cordis NOS
EXCLUDES that due to hypertension (402.0-402.9)

Additional Digit Required | Unspecified Code | Other Specified Code | Manifestation Code
MSP Medicare Secondary Payer | ▶◀ Revised Text | ● New Code | ▲ Revised Code Title

2002 Ingenix, Inc.

CEREBROVASCULAR DISEASE (430-438)

INCLUDES with mention of hypertension (conditions classifiable to 401-405)
Use additional code to identify presence of hypertension

EXCLUDES any condition classifiable to 430-434, 436, 437 occurring during pregnancy, childbirth, or the puerperium, or specified as puerperal (674.0)

▶iatrogenic cerebrovascular infarction or hemorrhage (997.02)◀

430 Subarachnoid hemorrhage
Meningeal hemorrhage
Ruptured:
    berry aneurysm
    (congenital) cerebral aneurysm NOS

EXCLUDES syphilitic ruptured cerebral aneurysm (094.87)

DEF: Bleeding in space between brain and lining.

431 Intracerebral hemorrhage
Hemorrhage (of):
  basilar
  bulbar
  cerebellar
  cerebral
  cerebromeningeal
  cortical

Hemorrhage (of):
  internal capsule
  intrapontine
  pontine
  subcortical
  ventricular
Rupture of blood vessel in brain

DEF: Bleeding within the brain.

✓4th 432 Other and unspecified intracranial hemorrhage

432.0 Nontraumatic extradural hemorrhage
Nontraumatic epidural hemorrhage
DEF: Bleeding, nontraumatic, between skull and brain lining.

432.1 Subdural hemorrhage
Subdural hematoma, nontraumatic
DEF: Bleeding, between outermost and other layers of brain lining.

432.9 Unspecified intracranial hemorrhage
Intracranial hemorrhage NOS

✓4th 433 Occlusion and stenosis of precerebral arteries

INCLUDES
  embolism
  narrowing
  obstruction
  thrombosis
of basilar, carotid, and vertebral arteries

EXCLUDES insufficiency NOS of precerebral arteries (435.0-435.9)

DEF: Blockage, stricture, arteries branching into brain.

The following fifth-digit subclassification is for use with category 433:
  0 without mention of cerebral infarction
  1 with cerebral infarction

- ✓5th **433.0** Basilar artery
- ✓5th **433.1** Carotid artery
- ✓5th **433.2** Vertebral artery
- ✓5th **433.3** Multiple and bilateral
- ✓5th **433.8** Other specified precerebral artery
- ✓5th **433.9** Unspecified precerebral artery
    Precerebral artery NOS

CIRCULATORY SYSTEM

✓4th 434 Occlusion of cerebral arteries

The following fifth-digit subclassification is for use with category 434:
 0 without mention of cerebral infarction
 1 with cerebral infarction

- ✓5th **434.0 Cerebral thrombosis**
  Thrombosis of cerebral arteries
- ✓5th **434.1 Cerebral embolism**
- ✓5th **434.9 Cerebral artery occlusion, unspecified**

✓4th 435 Transient cerebral ischemia

INCLUDES cerebrovascular insufficiency (acute) with transient focal neurological signs and symptoms
insufficiency of basilar, carotid, and vertebral arteries
spasm of cerebral arteries

EXCLUDES *acute cerebrovascular insufficiency NOS (437.1)*
that due to any condition classifiable to 433 (433.0-433.9)

DEF: Temporary restriction of blood flow, to arteries branching into brain.

435.0 Basilar artery syndrome
435.1 Vertebral artery syndrome
435.2 Subclavian steal syndrome
  DEF: Cerebrovascular insufficiency, due to occluded subclavian artery; symptoms include pain in mastoid and posterior head regions, flaccid paralysis of arm and diminished or absent radical pulse on affected side.

435.3 Vertebrobasilar artery syndrome
  DEF: Transient ischemic attack; due to brainstem dysfunction; symptoms include confusion, vertigo, binocular blindness, diplopia, unilateral or bilateral weakness and paresthesis of extremities.

435.8 Other specified transient cerebral ischemias
435.9 Unspecified transient cerebral ischemia
  Impending cerebrovascular accident
  Intermittent cerebral ischemia
  Transient ischemic attack [TIA]

436 Acute, but ill-defined, cerebrovascular disease

Apoplexy, apoplectic: Cerebral seizure
 NOS   Cerebrovascular accident
 attack   [CVA] NOS
 cerebral   Stroke
 seizure

EXCLUDES *any condition classifiable to categories 430-435*
▶*postoperative cerebrovascular accident (997.02)*◀

✓4th 437 Other and ill-defined cerebrovascular disease

437.0 Cerebral atherosclerosis
  Atheroma of cerebral arteries
  Cerebral arteriosclerosis

437.1 Other generalized ischemic cerebrovascular disease
  Acute cerebrovascular insufficiency NOS
  Cerebral ischemia (chronic)

437.2 Hypertensive encephalopathy
  DEF: Cerebral manifestations (such as visual disturbances and headache) due to high blood pressure.

 Unspecified Code   Other Specified Code   ▲ Manifestation Code
MSP Medicare Secondary Payer   ▶◀ Revised Text   ● New Code   ▲ Revised Code Title

CIRCULATORY SYSTEM

437.3 Cerebral aneurysm, nonruptured
Internal carotid artery, intracranial portion
Internal carotid artery NOS
EXCLUDES congenital cerebral aneurysm, nonruptured (747.81)
internal carotid artery, extracranial portion (442.81)

437.4 Cerebral arteritis
DEF: Inflammation of a cerebral artery or arteries.

437.5 Moyamoya disease
DEF: Cerebrovascular ischemia; vessels occlude and rupture causing tiny hemorrhages at base of brain; predominantly affects Japanese.

437.6 Nonpyogenic thrombosis of intracranial venous sinus
EXCLUDES pyogenic (325)

437.7 Transient global amnesia
DEF: Episode of short-term memory loss, not often recurrent; pathogenesis unknown; with no signs or symptoms of neurological disorder.

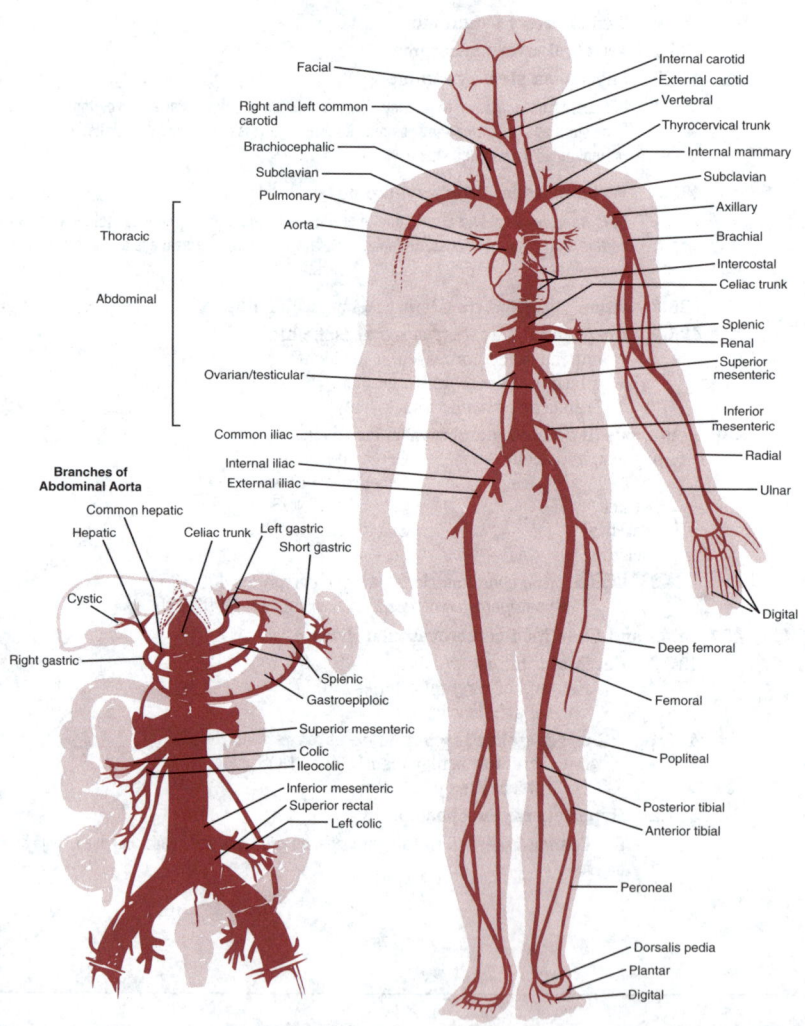

Map of Major Arteries

CIRCULATORY SYSTEM

437.8 Other
437.9 Unspecified
   Cerebrovascular disease or lesion NOS

✓4th **438 Late effects of cerebrovascular disease**
   Note: This category is to be used to indicate conditions in 430-437 as the cause of late effects. The "late effects" include conditions specified as such, as sequelae, which may occur at any time after the onset of the causal condition.

   438.0 Cognitive deficits

✓5th **438.1** Speech and language deficits
   438.10 Speech and language deficit, unspecified
   438.11 Aphasia
      DEF: Impairment or absence of the ability to communicate by speech, writing or signs or to comprehend the spoken or written language due to disease or injury to the brain. Total aphasia is the loss of function of both sensory and motor areas of the brain.
   438.12 Dysphasia
      DEF: Impaired speech; marked by inability to sequence language.
   438.19 Other speech and language deficits

✓5th **438.2** Hemiplegia/hemiparesis
   DEF: Paralysis of one side of the body.
   438.20 Hemiplegia affecting unspecified side
   438.21 Hemiplegia affecting dominant side
   438.22 Hemiplegia affecting nondominant side

✓5th **438.3** Monoplegia of upper limb
   DEF: Paralysis of one limb or one muscle group.
   438.30 Monoplegia of upper limb affecting unspecified side
   438.31 Monoplegia of upper limb affecting dominant side
   438.32 Monoplegia of upper limb affecing nondominant side

✓5th **438.4** Monoplegia of lower limb
   438.40 Monoplegia of lower limb affecting unspecified side
   438.41 Monoplegia of lower limb affecting dominant side
   438.42 Monoplegia of lower limb affecting nondominant side

✓5th **438.5** Other paralytic syndrome
      Use additional code to identify type of paralytic syndrome, such as:
         locked-in state (344.81)
         quadriplegia (344.00-344.09)
      EXCLUDES late effects of cerebrovascular accident with:
         hemiplegia/hemiparesis (438.20-438.22)
         monoplegia of lower limb (438.40-438.42)
         monoplegia of upper limb (438.30-438.32)
   438.50 Other paralytic syndrome affecting unspecified side
   438.51 Other paralytic syndrome affecting dominant side
   438.52 Other paralytic syndrome affecting nondominant side
   438.53 Other paralytic syndrome, bilateral

● **438.6** Alterations of sensations
      Use additional code to identify the altered sensation

● **438.7** Disturbances of vision
      Use additional code to identify the visual disturbance

CIRCULATORY SYSTEM

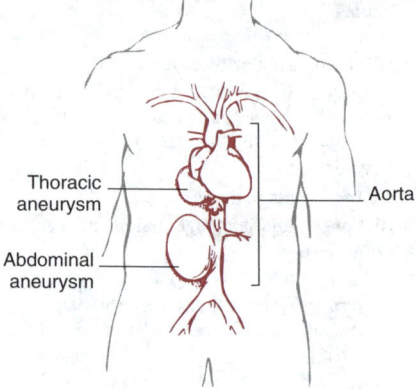

Thoracic, Abdominal and Aortic Aneurysm

√5th **438.8 Other late effects of cerebrovascular disease**

438.81 Apraxia
DEF: Inability to activate learned movements; no known sensory or motor impairment.

438.82 Dysphagia
DEF: Inability or difficulty in swallowing.

438.83 Facial weakness
Facial droop

438.84 Ataxia

438.85 Vertigo

438.89 Other late effects of cerebrovascular disease
Use additional code to identify the late effect

438.9 Unspecified late effects of cerebrovascular disease

DISEASES OF ARTERIES, ARTERIOLES, AND CAPILLARIES (440-448)

√4th **440 Atherosclerosis**
INCLUDES   arteriolosclerosis
arteriosclerosis (obliterans) (senile)
arteriosclerotic vascular disease
atheroma
degeneration:
    arterial
    arteriovascular
    vascular
endarteritis deformans or obliterans
senile:
    arteritis
    endarteritis
EXCLUDES ▶atheroembolism (445.01-445.89)◀
atherosclerosis of bypass graft of the extremities (403.30-403.32)
DEF: Stricture and reduced elasticity of an artery; due to plaque deposits.

440.0 Of aorta   A

440.1 Of renal artery   A
EXCLUDES   atherosclerosis of renal arterioles (403.00-403.91)

√5th **440.2 Of native arteries of the extremities**
EXCLUDES   atherosclerosis of bypass graft of the extremities (440.30-440.32)

440.20 Atherosclerosis of the extremities, unspecified   A

CIRCULATORY SYSTEM 440.21–440.9

440.21 Atherosclerosis of the extremities with intermittent claudication   A
DEF: Atherosclerosis; marked by pain, tension and weakness after walking; no symptoms while at rest.

440.22 Atherosclerosis of the extremities with rest pain   A
INCLUDES   any condition classifiable to 440.21
DEF: Atherosclerosis, marked by pain, tension and weakness while at rest.

440.23 Atherosclerosis of the extremities with ulceration   A
Use additional code for any associated ulceration (707.10-707.9)
INCLUDES   any condition classifiable to 440.21 and 440.22

440.24 Atherosclerosis of the extremities with gangrene   A
INCLUDES   any condition classifiable to 440.21, 440.22, and 440.23 with ischemic gangrene 785.4
EXCLUDES   gas gangrene (040.0)

440.29 Other   A

√5th **440.3 Of bypass graft of extremities**
EXCLUDES   atherosclerosis of native arteries of the extremities (440.21-440.24)
embolism [occlusion NOS] [thrombus] of graft (996.74)

440.30 Of unspecified graft   A
440.31 Of autologous vein bypass graft   A
440.32 Of nonautologous biological bypass graft   A

440.8 Of other specified arteries   A
EXCLUDES   basilar (433.0)
carotid (433.1)
cerebral (437.0)
coronary ▶(414.00-414.06)◀
mesenteric (557.1)
precerebral (433.0-433.9)
pulmonary (416.0)
vertebral (433.2)

440.9 Generalized and unspecified atherosclerosis   A
Arteriosclerotic vascular disease NOS
EXCLUDES   arteriosclerotic cardiovascular disease [ASCVD] (429.2)

Arterial Diseases and Disorders

2002 Ingenix, Inc.

CIRCULATORY SYSTEM

441 Aortic aneurysm and dissection
EXCLUDES syphilitic aortic aneurysm (093.0)
traumatic aortic aneurysm (901.0, 902.0)

441.0 Dissection of aorta
DEF: Dissection or splitting of wall of the aorta; due to blood entering through intimal tear or interstitial hemorrhage.

- 441.00 Unspecified site
- 441.01 Thoracic
- 441.02 Abdominal
- 441.03 Thoracoabdominal

441.1 Thoracic aneurysm, ruptured
441.2 Thoracic aneurysm without mention of rupture
441.3 Abdominal aneurysm, ruptured
441.4 Abdominal aneurysm without mention of rupture
441.5 Aortic aneurysm of unspecified site, ruptured
Rupture of aorta NOS
441.6 Thoracoabdominal aneurysm, ruptured
441.7 Thoracoabdominal aneurysm, without mention of rupture
441.9 Aortic aneurysm of unspecified site without mention of rupture
Aneurysm
Dilatation } of aorta
Hyaline necrosis

442 Other aneurysm
INCLUDES aneurysm (ruptured) (cirsoid) (false) (varicose)
aneurysmal varix

EXCLUDES arteriovenous aneurysm or fistula:
acquired (447.0)
congenital (747.60-747.69)
traumatic (900.0-904.9)

DEF: Dissection or splitting of arterial wall; due to blood entering through intimal tear or interstitial hemorrhage.

442.0 Of artery of upper extremity
442.1 Of renal artery
442.2 Of iliac artery
442.3 Of artery of lower extremity
Aneurysm:
femoral   } artery
popliteal

442.8 Of other specified artery

442.81 Artery of neck
Aneurysm of carotid artery (common) (external) (internal, extracranial portion)
EXCLUDES internal carotid artery, intracranial portion (437.3)

442.82 Subclavian artery
442.83 Splenic artery
442.84 Other visceral artery
Aneurysm:
celiac
gastroduodenal
gastroepiploic   } artery
hepatic
pancreaticoduodenal
superior mesenteric

CIRCULATORY SYSTEM

442.89 Other
Aneurysm:
mediastinal ⎫
spinal   ⎬ artery

> EXCLUDES: cerebral (nonruptured) (437.3)
> congenital (747.81)
> ruptured (430)
> coronary (414.11)
> heart (414.10)
> pulmonary (417.1)

442.9 Of unspecified site

443 Other peripheral vascular disease

443.0 Raynaud's syndrome
Raynaud's:
  disease
  phenomenon (secondary)
Use additional code to identify gangrene (785.4)

DEF: Constriction of the arteries, due to cold or stress; bilateral ischemic attacks of fingers, toes, nose or ears; symptoms include pallor, paresthesia and pain; more common in females.

443.1 Thromboangiitis obliterans [Buerger's disease]
Presenile gangrene

DEF: Inflammatory disease of extremity blood vessels, mainly the lower; occurs primarily in young men and leads to tissue ischemia and gangrene.

443.2 Other arterial dissection
> EXCLUDES: dissection of aorta (441.00-441.03)
> dissection of coronary arteries (414.12)

443.21 Dissection of carotid artery
443.22 Dissection of iliac artery
443.23 Dissection of renal artery
443.24 Dissection of vertebral artery
443.29 Dissection of other artery

443.8 Other specified peripheral vascular diseases

443.81 Peripheral angiopathy in diseases classified elsewhere
Code first underlying disease, as:
  diabetes mellitus (250.7)

443.89 Other
Acrocyanosis   Erythrocyanosis
Acroparesthesia: Erythromelalgia
  simple [Schultze's type]
  vasomotor [Nothnagel's type]
> EXCLUDES: chilblains (991.5)
> frostbite (991.0-991.3)
> immersion foot (991.4)

443.9 Peripheral vascular disease, unspecified
Intermittent claudication NOS
Peripheral:
  angiopathy NOS
  vascular disease NOS
Spasm of artery
> EXCLUDES: atherosclerosis of the arteries of the extremities (440.20-440.22)
> spasm of cerebral artery (435.0-435.9)

CIRCULATORY SYSTEM

✓4ᵗʰ 444 Arterial embolism and thrombosis
　　INCLUDES　infarction:
　　　　　　　　　embolic
　　　　　　　　　thrombotic
　　　　　　　　occlusion
　　EXCLUDES　▶atheroembolism (445.01-445.89)◀
　　　　　　　that complicating:
　　　　　　　　abortion (634-638 with .6, 639.6)
　　　　　　　　ectopic or molar pregnancy (639.6)
　　　　　　　　pregnancy, childbirth, or the pueperium (673.0-673.8)

　444.0 Of abdominal aorta
　　　Aortic bifurcation syndrome　　Leriche's syndrome
　　　Aortoiliac obstruction　　　　　Saddle embolus

　444.1 Of thoracic aorta
　　　Embolism or thrombosis of aorta (thoracic)

✓5ᵗʰ 444.2 Of arteries of the extremities
　444.21 Upper extremity
　444.22 Lower extremity
　　　Arterial embolism or thrombosis:
　　　　femoral
　　　　peripheral NOS
　　　　popliteal
　　　　EXCLUDES　iliofemoral (444.81)

✓5ᵗʰ 444.8 Of other specified artery
　444.81 Iliac artery
　444.89 Other
　　　EXCLUDES
　　　　basilar (433.0)
　　　　carotid (433.1)
　　　　cerebral (434.0-434.9)
　　　　coronary (410.00-410.92)
　　　　mesenteric (557.0)
　　　　ophthalmic (362.30-362.34)
　　　　precerebral (433.0-433.9)
　　　　pulmonary (415.19)
　　　　renal (593.81)
　　　　retinal (362.30-362.34)
　　　　vertebral (433.2)

　444.9 Of unspecified artery

✓4ᵗʰ 445 Atheroembolism
　　INCLUDES　atherothrombotic microembolism
　　　　　　　cholesterol embolism

✓5ᵗʰ 445.0 Of extremities
　445.01 Upper extremity
　445.02 Lower extremity

✓5ᵗʰ 445.8 Of other sites
　445.81 Kidney
　　　Use additional code for any associated kidney failure (584, 585)
　445.89 Other site

✓4ᵗʰ 446 Polyarteritis nodosa and allied conditions
　446.0 Polyarteritis nodosa
　　　Disseminated necrotizing periarteritis
　　　Necrotizing angiitis
　　　Panarteritis (nodosa)
　　　Periarteritis (nodosa)

　　DEF: Inflammation of small and mid-size arteries; symptoms related to involved arteries in kidneys, muscles, gastrointestinal tract and heart; results in tissue death.

CIRCULATORY SYSTEM

446.1   Acute febrile mucocutaneous lymph node syndrome [MCLS]
Kawasaki disease

DEF: Acute febrile disease of children; marked by erythema of conjunctiva and mucous membranes of upper respiratory tract, skin eruptions and edema.

✓5ᵗʰ   446.2   Hypersensitivity angiitis

> EXCLUDES   antiglomerular basement membrane disease without pulmonary hemorrhage (583.89)

446.20   Hypersensitivity angiitis, unspecified

446.21   Goodpasture's syndrome
Antiglomerular basement membrane antibody-mediated nephritis with pulmonary hemorrhage
Use additional code to identify renal disease (583.81)

DEF: Glomerulonephritis associated with hematuria, progresses rapidly; results in death from renal failure.

446.29   Other specified hypersensitivity angiitis

446.3   Lethal midline granuloma
Malignant granuloma of face

DEF: Granulomatous lesion; in nose or paranasal sinuses; often fatal; occurs chiefly in males.

446.4   Wegener's granulomatosis
Necrotizing respiratory granulomatosis
Wegener's syndrome

DEF: A disease occurring mainly in men; marked by necrotizing granulomas and ulceration of the upper respiratory tract; underlying condition is a vasculitis affecting small vessels and is possibly due to an immune disorder.

446.5   Giant cell arteritis
Cranial arteritis   Temporal arteritis
Horton's disease

DEF: Inflammation of arteries; due to giant cells affecting carotid artery branches, resulting in occlusion; symptoms include fever, headache and neurological problems; occurs in elderly.

446.6   Thrombotic microangiopathy
Moschcowitz's syndrome
Thrombotic thrombocytopenic purpura

DEF: Blockage of small blood vessels; due to hyaline deposits; symptoms include purpura, CNS disorders; results in protracted disease or rapid death.

446.7   Takayasu's disease
Aortic arch arteritis
Pulseless disease

DEF: Progressive obliterative arteritis of brachiocephalic trunk, left subclavian, and left common carotid arteries above aortic arch; results in ischemia in brain, heart and arm; pulses impalpable in head, neck and arms; more common in young adult females.

✓4ᵗʰ   447   Other disorders of arteries and arterioles

447.0   Arteriovenous fistula, acquired
Arteriovenous aneurysm, acquired

> EXCLUDES   cerebrovascular (437.3)
> coronary (414.19)
> pulmonary (417.0)
> surgically created arteriovenous shunt or fistula:
>   complication (996.1, 996.61-996.62)
>   status or presence (V45.1)
> traumatic (900.0-904.9)

DEF: Communication between an artery and vein caused by error in healing.

CIRCULATORY SYSTEM

Map of Major Veins

447.1 **Stricture of artery**

447.2 **Rupture of artery**
Erosion
Fistula, except arteriovenous } of artery
Ulcer

EXCLUDES *traumatic rupture of artery (900.0-904.9)*

447.3 **Hyperplasia of renal artery**
Fibromuscular hyperplasia of renal artery
DEF: Overgrowth of cells in muscular lining of renal artery.

447.4 Celiac artery compression syndrome
Celiac axis syndrome
Marable's syndrome

447.5 Necrosis of artery

447.6 Arteritis, unspecified
Aortitis NOS   Endarteritis NOS
EXCLUDES arteritis, endarteritis:
   aortic arch (446.7)
   cerebral (437.4)
   coronary ▶(414.00-414.06)◀
   deformans (440.0-440.9)
   obliterans (440.0-440.9)
   pulmonary (417.8)
   senile (440.0-440.9)
polyarteritis NOS (446.0)
syphilitic aortitis (093.1)

447.8 Other specified disorders of arteries and arterioles
Fibromuscular hyperplasia of arteries, except renal

447.9 Unspecified disorders of arteries and arterioles

√4th **448 Disease of capillaries**

448.0 Hereditary hemorrhagic telangiectasia
Rendu-Osler-Weber disease

DEF: Genetic disease with onset after puberty; results in multiple telangiectases, dilated venules on skin and mucous membranes; recurrent bleeding may occur.

448.1 Nevus, non-neoplastic
Nevus:
   araneus
   senile
   spider
   stellar
EXCLUDES neoplastic (216.0-216.9)
   port wine (757.32)
   strawberry (757.32)

DEF: Enlarged or malformed blood vessels of skin; results in reddish swelling, skin patch, or birthmark.

448.9 Other and unspecified capillary diseases
Capillary:
   hemorrhage
   hyperpermeability
   thrombosis
EXCLUDES capillary fragility (hereditary) (287.8)

DISEASES OF VEINS AND LYMPHATICS, AND OTHER DISEASES OF CIRCULATORY SYSTEM (451-459)

√4th **451 Phlebitis and thrombophlebitis**
- INCLUDES: endophlebitis
  inflammation, vein
  periphlebitis
  suppurative phlebitis

Use additional E code to identify drug, if drug-induced

EXCLUDES: that complicating:
  abortion (634-638 with .7, 639.8)
  ectopic or molar pregnancy (639.8)
  pregnancy, childbirth, or the puerperium (671.0-671.9)
  that due to or following:
  implant or catheter device (996.61-996.62)
  infusion, perfusion, or transfusion (999.2)

DEF: Inflammation of a vein (phlebitis) with formation of a thrombus (thrombophlebitis).

- **451.0 Of superficial vessels of lower extremities**
  Saphenous vein (greater) (lesser)
- √5th **451.1 Of deep vessels of lower extremities**
  - **451.11 Femoral vein (deep) (superficial)**
  - **451.19 Other**
    Femoropopliteal vein   Tibial vein
    Popliteal vein
- **451.2 Of lower extremities, unspecified**
- √5th **451.8 Of other sites**

  EXCLUDES: intracranial venous sinus (325)
    nonpyogenic (437.6)
    portal (vein) (572.1)

  - **451.81 Iliac vein**
  - **451.82 Of superficial veins of upper extremities**
    Antecubital vein   Cephalic vein
    Basilic vein
  - **451.83 Of deep veins of upper extremities**
    Brachial vein   Ulnar vein
    Radial vein
  - **451.84 Of upper extremities, unspecified**
  - **451.89 Other**
    Axillary vein   Thrombophlebitis of
    Jugular vein   breast (Mondor's
    Subclavian vein   disease)
- **451.9 Of unspecified site**

452 Portal vein thrombosis
Portal (vein) obstruction

EXCLUDES: hepatic vein thrombosis (453.0)
  phlebitis of portal vein (572.1)

DEF: Formation of a blood clot in main vein of liver.

√4th **453 Other venous embolism and thrombosis**

EXCLUDES: that complicating:
  abortion (634-638 with .7, 639.8)
  ectopic or molar pregnancy (639.8)
  pregnancy, childbirth, or the puerperium (671.0-671.9)
  that with inflammation, phlebitis, and thrombophlebitis (451.0-451.9)

CIRCULATORY SYSTEM

453.0 **Budd-Chiari syndrome**
Hepatic vein thrombosis
DEF: Thrombosis or other obstruction of hepatic vein; symptoms include enlarged liver, extensive collateral vessels, intractable ascites and severe portal hypertension.

453.1 **Thrombophlebitis migrans**
DEF: Slow, advancing thrombophlebitis; appearing first in one vein then another.

453.2 **Of vena cava**

453.3 **Of renal vein**

453.8 **Of other specified veins**
EXCLUDES: cerebral (434.0-434.9)
coronary (410.00-410.92)
intracranial venous sinus (325)
  nonpyogenic (437.6)
mesenteric (557.0)
portal (452)
precerebral (433.0-433.9)
pulmonary (415.19)

453.9 **Of unspecified site**
Embolism of vein   Thrombosis (vein)

454 **Varicose veins of lower extremities**
EXCLUDES: that complicating pregnancy, childbirth, or the puerperium (671.0)
DEF: Dilated leg veins; due to incompetent vein valves that allow reversed blood flow and cause tissue erosion or weakness of wall; may be painful.

454.0 **With ulcer**
Varicose ulcer (lower extremity, any part)
Varicose veins with ulcer of lower extremity [any part] or of unspecified site
Any condition classifiable to 454.9 with ulcer or specified as ulcerated

454.1 **With inflammation**
Stasis dermatitis
Varicose veins with inflammation of lower extremity [any part] or of unspecified site
Any condition classifiable to 454.9 with inflammation or specified as inflamed

454.2 **With ulcer and inflammation**
Varicose veins with ulcer and inflammation of lower extremity [any part] or of unspecified site
Any condition classifiable to 454.9 with ulcer and inflammation

454.8 **With other complications**
Edema
Pain
Swelling

454.9 **Asymptomatic varicose veins**
Phlebectasia
Varicose veins } of lower extremity [any part] or of unspecified site
Varix
▶Varicose veins NOS◀

455 **Hemorrhoids**
INCLUDES: hemorrhoids (anus) (rectum)
piles
varicose veins, anus or rectum
EXCLUDES: that complicating pregnancy, childbirth, or the puerperium (671.8)
DEF: Varicose condition of external hemorrhoidal veins causing painful swellings at the anus.

CIRCULATORY SYSTEM

- **455.0** Internal hemorrhoids without mention of complication
- **455.1** Internal thrombosed hemorrhoids
- **455.2** Internal hemorrhoids with other complication
  - Internal hemorrhoids:
    - bleeding
    - prolapsed
  - Internal hemorrhoids:
    - strangulated
    - ulcerated
- **455.3** External hemorrhoids without mention of complication
- **455.4** External thrombosed hemorrhoids
- **455.5** External hemorrhoids with other complication
  - External hemorrhoids:
    - bleeding
    - prolapsed
  - External hemorrhoids:
    - strangulated
    - ulcerated
- **455.6** Unspecified hemorrhoids without mention of complication
  - Hemorrhoids NOS
- **455.7** Unspecified thrombosed hemorrhoids
  - Thrombosed hemorrhoids, unspecified whether internal or external
- **455.8** Unspecified hemorrhoids with other complication
  - Hemorrhoids, unspecified whether internal or external:
    - bleeding
    - prolapsed
    - strangulated
    - ulcerated
- **455.9** Residual hemorrhoidal skin tags
  - Skin tags, anus or rectum

√4ᵗʰ **456 Varicose veins of other sites**

- **456.0** Esophageal varices with bleeding
  - DEF: Distended, tortuous, veins of lower esophagus, usually due to portal hypertension.
- **456.1** Esophageal varices without mention of bleeding

√5ᵗʰ **456.2** Esophageal varices in diseases classified elsewhere
  - Code first underlying disease, as:
    - cirrhosis of liver (571.0-571.9)
    - portal hypertension (572.3)
  - **456.20** *With bleeding*
  - **456.21** *Without mention of bleeding*
- **456.3** Sublingual varices
  - DEF: Distended, tortuous veins beneath tongue.
- **456.4** Scrotal varices ♂
  - Varicocele
- **456.5** Pelvic varices
  - Varices of broad ligament
- **456.6** Vulval varices ♀
  - Varices of perineum
  - **EXCLUDES** that complicating pregnancy, childbirth, or the puerperium (671.1)
- **456.8** Varices of other sites
  - Varicose veins of nasal septum (with ulcer)
  - **EXCLUDES** placental varices (656.7)
    - retinal varices (362.17)
    - varicose ulcer of unspecified site (454.0)
    - varicose veins of unspecified site (454.9)

CIRCULATORY SYSTEM

✓4th 457 Noninfectious disorders of lymphatic channels

457.0 Postmastectomy lymphedema syndrome

Elephantiasis
Obliteration of lymphatic vessel } due to mastectomy

DEF: Reduced lymphatic circulation following mastectomy; symptoms include swelling of the arm on the operative side.

457.1 Other lymphedema

Elephantiasis
  (nonfilarial) NOS
Lymphangiectasis
Lymphedema:
  acquired (chronic)

Lymphedema:
  praecox
  secondary
Obliteration, lymphatic vessel

EXCLUDES elephantiasis (nonfilarial):
    congenital (757.0)
    eyelid (374.83)
    vulva (624.8)

DEF: Fluid retention due to reduced lymphatic circulation; due to other than mastectomy.

457.2 Lymphangitis

Lymphangitis:
  NOS
  chronic

Lymphangitis:
  subacute

EXCLUDES acute lymphangitis (682.0-682.9)

457.8 Other noninfectious disorders of lymphatic channels

Chylocele (nonfilarial)
Chylous:
  ascites
  cyst

Lymph node or vessel:
  fistula
  infarction
  rupture

EXCLUDES chylocele:
    filarial (125.0-125.9)
    tunica vaginalis (nonfilarial) (608.84)

457.9 Unspecified noninfectious disorder of lymphatic channels

✓4th 458 Hypotension

INCLUDES hypopiesis
EXCLUDES cardiovascular collapse (785.50)
    maternal hypotension syndrome (669.2)
    shock (785.50-785.59)
    Shy-Drager syndrome (333.0)

458.0 Orthostatic hypotension

Hypotension:
  orthostatic (chronic)
  postural

DEF: Low blood pressure; occurs when standing.

458.1 Chronic hypotension

Permanent idiopathic hypotension

DEF: Persistent low blood pressure.

458.2 Iatrogenic hypotension

Postoperative hypotension

DEF: Abnormally low blood pressure; due to medical treatment.

458.8 Other specified hypotension

458.9 Hypotension, unspecified

Hypotension (arterial) NOS

2002 Ingenix, Inc.

CIRCULATORY SYSTEM

✓4th 459 Other disorders of circulatory system

459.0 Hemorrhage, unspecified
Rupture of blood vessel NOS
Spontaneous hemorrhage NEC
EXCLUDES hemorrhage:
  gastrointestinal NOS (578.9)
  in newborn NOS (772.9)
  secondary or recurrent following trauma (958.2)
  traumatic rupture of blood vessel (900.0-904.9)

✓5th 459.1 Postphlebitic syndrome
▶Chronic venous hypertension due to deep vein thrombosis◀
EXCLUDES ▶chronic venous hypertension without deep vein thrombosis (459.30-459.39)◀
DEF: Various conditions following deep vein thrombosis; including edema, pain, stasis dermatitis, cellulitis, varicose veins and ulceration of the lower leg.

- **459.10 Postphlebitic syndrome without complications**
  Asymptomatic postphlebitic syndrome
  Postphlebitic syndrome NOS
- **459.11 Postphlebitic syndrome with ulcer**
- **459.12 Postphlebitic syndrome with inflammation**
- **459.13 Postphlebitic syndrome with ulcer and inflammation**
- **459.19 Postphlebitic syndrome with other complication**

459.2 Compression of vein
Stricture of vein
Vena cava syndrome (inferior) (superior)

✓5th 459.3 Chronic venous hypertension (idiopathic)
Stasis edema
EXCLUDES chronic venous hypertension due to deep vein thrombosis (459.10-459.19)
varicose veins (454.0-454.9)

- **459.30 Chronic venous hypertension without complications**
  Asymptomatic chronic venous hypertension
  Chronic venous hypertension NOS
- **459.31 Chronic venous hypertension with ulcer**
- **459.32 Chronic venous hypertension with inflammation**
- **459.33 Chronic venous hypertension with ulcer and inflammation**
- **459.39 Chronic venous hypertension with other complication**

✓5th 459.8 Other specified disorders of circulatory system

459.81 Venous (peripheral) insufficiency, unspecified
Chronic venous insufficiency NOS
Use additional code for any associated ulceration (707.10-707.9)
DEF: Insufficient drainage, venous blood, any part of body, results in edema or dermatosis.

459.89 Other
Collateral circulation (venous), any site
Phlebosclerosis
Venofibrosis

459.9 Unspecified circulatory system disorder

8. DISEASES OF THE RESPIRATORY SYSTEM (460-519)

Use additional code to identify infectious organism

ACUTE RESPIRATORY INFECTIONS (460-466)

EXCLUDES pneumonia and influenza (480.0-487.8)

460 Acute nasopharyngitis [common cold]

Coryza (acute)
Nasal catarrh, acute
Nasopharyngitis:
  NOS
  acute
Nasopharyngitis:
  infective NOS
Rhinitis:
  acute
  infective

EXCLUDES nasopharyngitis, chronic (472.2)
pharyngitis:
  acute or unspecified (462)
  chronic (472.1)
rhinitis:
  allergic (477.0-477.9)
  chronic or unspecified (472.0)
sore throat:
  acute or unspecified (462)
  chronic (472.1)

DEF: Acute inflammation of mucous membranes; extends from nares to pharynx.

√4ᵗʰ 461 Acute sinusitis

INCLUDES
abscess
empyema
infection
inflammation
suppuration
} acute, of sinus (accessory) (nasal)

EXCLUDES chronic or unspecified sinusitis (473.0-473.9)

- **461.0 Maxillary**
  Acute antritis
- **461.1 Frontal**
- **461.2 Ethmoidal**
- **461.3 Sphenoidal**
- **461.8 Other acute sinusitis**
  Acute pansinusitis
- **461.9 Acute sinusitis, unspecified**
  Acute sinusitis NOS

462 Acute pharyngitis

Acute sore throat NOS
Pharyngitis (acute):
    NOS
    gangrenous
    infective
    phlegmonous
    pneumococcal
Pharyngitis (acute):
    staphylococcal
    suppurative
    ulcerative
Sore throat (viral) NOS
Viral pharyngitis

EXCLUDES   abscess:
    peritonsillar [quinsy] (475)
    pharyngeal NOS (478.29)
    retropharyngeal (478.24)
chronic pharyngitis (472.1)
infectious mononucleosis (075)
that specified as (due to):
    Coxsackie (virus) (074.0)
    gonococcus (098.6)
    herpes simplex (054.79)
    influenza (487.1)
    septic (034.0)
    streptococcal (034.0)

463 Acute tonsillitis

Tonsillitis (acute):
    NOS
    follicular
    gangrenous
    infective
    pneumococcal
Tonsillitis (acute):
    septic
    staphylococcal
    suppurative
    ulcerative
    viral

EXCLUDES   chronic tonsillitis (474.0)
hypertrophy of tonsils (474.1)
peritonsillar abscess [quinsy] (475)
sore throat:
    acute or NOS (462)
    septic (034.0)
streptococcal tonsillitis (034.0)

✓4th 464 Acute laryngitis and tracheitis

EXCLUDES   that associated with influenza (487.1)
that due to Streptococcus (034.0)

✓5th 464.0 Acute laryngitis

Laryngitis (acute):
    NOS
    edematous
    Hemophilus influenzae [H. influenzae]
    pneumococcal
    septic
    suppurative
    ulcerative

EXCLUDES   chronic laryngitis (476.0-476.1)
influenzal laryngitis (487.1)

464.00 Without mention of obstruction
464.01 With obstruction

✓5th 464.1 Acute tracheitis

Tracheitis (acute):
    NOS
    catarrhal
Tracheitis (acute):
    viral

EXCLUDES   chronic tracheitis (491.8)

RESPIRATORY SYSTEM

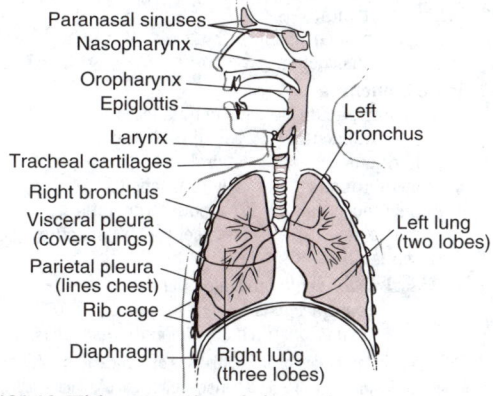

Respiratory System

464.10 Without mention of obstruction
464.11 With obstruction

✓5th **464.2 Acute laryngotracheitis**
  Laryngotracheitis (acute)
  Tracheitis (acute) with laryngitis (acute)
  EXCLUDES chronic laryngotracheitis (476.1)

464.20 Without mention of obstruction
464.21 With obstruction

✓5th **464.3 Acute epiglottitis**
  Viral epiglottitis
  EXCLUDES epiglottitis, chronic (476.1)

464.30 Without mention of obstruction
464.31 With obstruction

464.4 Croup
  Croup syndrome
  DEF: Acute laryngeal obstruction due to allergy, foreign body or infection; symptoms include barking cough, hoarseness and harsh, persistent high-pitched respiratory sound.

✓5th **464.5 Supraglottitis, unspecified**
  DEF: A rapidly advancing generalized upper respiratory infection of the lingual tonsillar area, epiglottic folds, false vocal cords, and the epiglottis; seen most commonly in children, but can affect people of any age.

464.50 Without mention of obstruction
464.51 With obstruction

✓4th **465 Acute upper respiratory infections of multiple or unspecified sites**
  EXCLUDES upper respiratory infection due to:
    influenza (487.1)
    Streptococcus (034.0)

465.0 Acute laryngopharyngitis
  DEF: Acute infection of the vocal cords and pharynx.

465.8 Other multiple sites
  Multiple URI

465.9 Unspecified site
  Acute URI NOS
  Upper respiratory infection (acute)

✓4th ✓5th Additional Digit Required | Unspecified Code | Other Specified Code | Manifestation Code
MSP Medicare Secondary Payer | ▶◀ Revised Text | ● New Code | ▲ Revised Code Title

2002 Ingenix, Inc.

Volume 1 — 273

466 Acute bronchitis and bronchiolitis
INCLUDES that with:
    bronchospasm
    obstruction

466.0 Acute bronchitis
Bronchitis, acute or subacute:
  fibrinous
  membranous
  pneumococcal
  purulent
  septic

Bronchitis, acute or subacute:
  viral
  with tracheitis
Croupous bronchitis
Tracheobronchitis, acute

EXCLUDES acute bronchitis with:
  bronchiectasis (494.1)
  chronic obstructive pulmonary disease (491.21)

DEF: Acute inflammation of main branches of bronchial tree due to infectious or irritant agents; symptoms include cough with a varied production of sputum, fever, substernal soreness, and lung rales.

466.1 Acute bronchiolitis
Bronchiolitis (acute)   Capillary pneumonia

DEF: Acute inflammation of finer subdivisions of bronchial tree due to infectious or irritant agents; symptoms include cough with a varied production of sputum, fever, substernal soreness, and lung rales.

- **466.11** Acute bronchiolitis due to respiratory syncytial virus (RSV)
- **466.19** Acute bronchiolitis due to other infectious organisms
    Use additional code to identify organism

OTHER DISEASES OF THE UPPER RESPIRATORY TRACT (470-478)

470 Deviated nasal septum
Deflected septum (nasal) (acquired)
EXCLUDES congenital (754.0)

471 Nasal polyps
EXCLUDES adenomatous polyps (212.0)

- **471.0 Polyp of nasal cavity**
  Polyp: Polyp:
    choanal   nasopharyngeal
- **471.1 Polypoid sinus degeneration**
  Woakes' syndrome or ethmoiditis
- **471.8 Other polyp of sinus**
  Polyp of sinus: Polyp of sinus:
    accessory   maxillary
    ethmoidal   sphenoidal
- **471.9 Unspecified nasal polyp**
  Nasal polyp NOS

472 Chronic pharyngitis and nasopharyngitis

- **472.0 Chronic rhinitis**
  Ozena   Rhinitis:
  Rhinitis: hypertrophic
    NOS   obstructive
    atrophic   purulent
    granulomatous ulcerative
  EXCLUDES allergic rhinitis (477.0-477.9)

DEF: Persistent inflammation of mucous membranes of nose.

RESPIRATORY SYSTEM

472.1 Chronic pharyngitis
  Chronic sore throat
  Pharyngitis:
    atrophic
  Pharyngitis:
    granular (chronic)
    hypertrophic

472.2 Chronic nasopharyngitis
  EXCLUDES acute or unspecified nasopharyngitis (460)
  DEF: Persistent inflammation of mucous membranes extending from nares to pharynx.

√4th **473 Chronic sinusitis**
  INCLUDES
    abscess
    empyema   (chronic) of sinus
    infection   (accessory) (nasal)
    suppuration
  EXCLUDES acute sinusitis (461.0-461.9)

  473.0 Maxillary
    Antritis (chronic)
  473.1 Frontal
  473.2 Ethmoidal
    EXCLUDES Woakes' ethmoiditis (471.1)
  473.3 Sphenoidal
  473.8 Other chronic sinusitis
    Pansinusitis (chronic)
  473.9 Unspecified sinusitis (chronic)
    Sinusitis (chronic) NOS

√4th **474 Chronic disease of tonsils and adenoids**
  √5th **474.0 Chronic tonsillitis and adenoiditis**
    EXCLUDES acute or unspecified tonsillitis (463)
    474.00 Chronic tonsillitis
    474.01 Chronic adenoiditis
    474.02 Chronic tonsillitis and adenoiditis

Upper Respiratory System

√4th / √5th Additional Digit Required   Unspecified Code   Other Specified Code   Manifestation Code
MSP Medicare Secondary Payer   ▶◀ Revised Text   ● New Code   ▲ Revised Code Title

2002 Ingenix, Inc.

Paranasal Sinuses

√5th **474.1 Hypertrophy of tonsils and adenoids**
Enlargement }
Hyperplasia } of tonsils or adenoids
Hypertrophy }

EXCLUDES that with:
adenoiditis (474.01)
adenoiditis and tonsillitis (474.02)
tonsillitis (474.00)

474.10 Tonsils with adenoids
474.11 Tonsils alone
474.12 Adenoids alone

474.2 Adenoid vegetations
DEF: Fungus-like growth of lymph tissue between the nares and pharynx.

474.8 Other chronic disease of tonsils and adenoids
Amygdalolith   Tonsillar tag
Calculus, tonsil   Ulcer, tonsil
Cicatrix of tonsil (and adenoid)

474.9 Unspecified chronic disease of tonsils and adenoids
Disease (chronic) of tonsils (and adenoids)

475 Peritonsillar abscess
Abscess of tonsil   Quinsy
Peritonsillar cellulitis
EXCLUDES tonsillitis:
acute or NOS (463)
chronic (474.0)

√4th **476 Chronic laryngitis and laryngotracheitis**
476.0 Chronic laryngitis
Laryngitis: Laryngitis:
catarrhal   sicca
hypertrophic

476.1 Chronic laryngotracheitis
Laryngitis, chronic, with tracheitis (chronic)
Tracheitis, chronic, with laryngitis
EXCLUDES chronic tracheitis (491.8)
laryngitis and tracheitis, acute or unspecified (464.00-464.51)

RESPIRATORY SYSTEM

✓4ᵗʰ 477 Allergic rhinitis
  INCLUDES allergic rhinitis (nonseasonal) (seasonal)
  hay fever
  spasmodic rhinorrhea
  EXCLUDES allergic rhinitis with asthma (bronchial) (493.0)

DEF: True immunoglobulin E (IgE)-mediated allergic reaction of nasal mucosa; seasonal (typical hay fever) or perennial (year-round allergens: dust, food, dander).

- **477.0 Due to pollen**
  Pollinosis
- **477.1 Due to food**
- **477.8 Due to other allergen**
- **477.9 Cause unspecified**

✓4ᵗʰ 478 Other diseases of upper respiratory tract

- **478.0 Hypertrophy of nasal turbinates**
  DEF: Overgrowth, enlargement of shell-shaped bones, in nasal cavity.

- **478.1 Other diseases of nasal cavity and sinuses**
  Abscess ⎫
  Necrosis ⎬ of nose (septum)
  Ulcer ⎭
  Cyst or mucocele of sinus (nasal)
  Rhinolith
  EXCLUDES varicose ulcer of nasal septum (456.8)

✓5ᵗʰ 478.2 Other diseases of pharynx, not elsewhere classified
  - **478.20 Unspecified disease of pharynx**
  - **478.21 Cellulitis of pharynx or nasopharynx**
  - **478.22 Parapharyngeal abscess**
  - **478.24 Retropharyngeal abscess**
    DEF: Purulent infection, behind pharynx and front of precerebral fascia.
  - **478.25 Edema of pharynx or nasopharynx**
  - **478.26 Cyst of pharynx or nasopharynx**
  - **478.29 Other**
    Abscess of pharynx or nasopharynx
    EXCLUDES ulcerative pharyngitis (462)

✓5ᵗʰ 478.3 Paralysis of vocal cords or larynx
  DEF: Loss of motor ability of vocal cords or larynx; due to nerve or muscle damage.
  - **478.30 Paralysis, unspecified**
    Laryngoplegia   Paralysis of glottis
  - **478.31 Unilateral, partial**
  - **478.32 Unilateral, complete**
  - **478.33 Bilateral, partial**
  - **478.34 Bilateral, complete**

- **478.4 Polyp of vocal cord or larynx**
  EXCLUDES adenomatous polyps (212.1)

- **478.5 Other diseases of vocal cords**
  Abscess ⎫
  Cellulitis ⎬ of vocal cords
  Granuloma ⎪
  Leukoplakia ⎭
  Chorditis (fibrinous) (nodosa) (tuberosa)
  Singers' nodes

✓4ᵗʰ / ✓5ᵗʰ Additional Digit Required
MSP Medicare Secondary Payer
▶◀ Revised Text
Unspecified Code
● New Code
Other Specified Code
▲ Revised Code Title
Manifestation Code

2002 Ingenix, Inc.

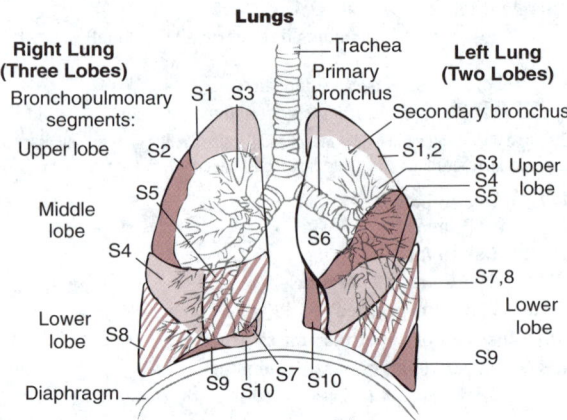

478.6 **Edema of larynx**
Edema (of):
glottis
subglottic
supraglottic

√5th 478.7 **Other diseases of larynx, not elsewhere classified**

478.70 Unspecified disease of larynx

478.71 Cellulitis and perichondritis of larynx
DEF: Inflammation of deep soft tissues or lining of bone of the larynx.

478.74 Stenosis of larynx

478.75 Laryngeal spasm
Laryngismus (stridulus)
DEF: Involuntary muscle contraction of the larynx.

478.79 Other
Abscess
Necrosis
Obstruction } of larynx
Pachyderma
Ulcer

EXCLUDES ulcerative laryngitis (464.00-464.01)

478.8 **Upper respiratory tract hypersensitivity reaction, site unspecified**
EXCLUDES hypersensitivity reaction of lower respiratory tract, as:
extrinsic allergic alveolitis (495.0-495.9)
pneumoconiosis (500-505)

478.9 **Other and unspecified diseases of upper respiratory tract**
Abscess
Cicatrix } of trachea

RESPIRATORY SYSTEM

PNEUMONIA AND INFLUENZA (480-487)

EXCLUDES pneumonia:
- allergic or eosinophilic (518.3)
- aspiration:
  - NOS (507.0)
  - newborn (770.1)
  - solids and liquids (507.0-507.8)
- congenital (770.0)
- lipoid (507.1)
- passive (514)
- rheumatic (390)

√4th **480 Viral pneumonia**
- 480.0 Pneumonia due to adenovirus
- 480.1 Pneumonia due to respiratory syncytial virus
- 480.2 Pneumonia due to parainfluenza virus
- 480.8 Pneumonia due to other virus not elsewhere classified
  - **EXCLUDES** congenital rubella pneumonitis (771.0)
    - influenza with pneumonia, any form (487.0)
    - pneumonia complicating viral diseases classified elsewhere (484.1-484.8)
- 480.9 Viral pneumonia, unspecified

481 Pneumococcal pneumonia [Streptococcus pneumoniae pneumonia]
- Lobar pneumonia, organism unspecified

√4th **482 Other bacterial pneumonia**
- 482.0 Pneumonia due to Klebsiella pneumoniae
- 482.1 Pneumonia due to Pseudomonas
- 482.2 Pneumonia due to Hemophilus influenzae [H. influenzae]
- √5th 482.3 Pneumonia due to Streptococcus
  - **EXCLUDES** Streptococcus pneumoniae (481)
  - 482.30 Streptococcus, unspecified
  - 482.31 Group A
  - 482.32 Group B
  - 482.39 Other Streptococcus
- √5th 482.4 Pneumonia due to Staphylococcus
  - 482.40 Pneumonia due to Staphylococcus, unspecified
  - 482.41 Pneumonia due to Staphylococcus aureus
  - 482.49 Other Staphylococcus pneumonia
- √5th 482.8 Pneumonia due to other specified bacteria
  - **EXCLUDES** pneumonia, complicating infectious disease classified elsewhere (484.1-484.8)
  - 482.81 Anaerobes
    - Bacteroides (melaninogenicus)
    - Gram-negative anaerobes
  - 482.82 Escherichia coli [E. coli]
  - 482.83 Other gram-negative bacteria
    - Gram-negative pneumonia NOS
    - Proteus
    - Serratia marcescens
    - **EXCLUDES** gram-negative anaerobes (482.81)
      - Legionnaires' disease (482.84)

√4th Additional Digit Required
√5th
 Medicare Secondary Payer
▶◀ Revised Text
Unspecified Code
● New Code
Other Specified Code
▲ Revised Code Title
Manifestation Code

482.84 Legionnaires' disease
DEF: Severe and often fatal infection by *Legionella pneumophilia*; symptoms include high fever, gastrointestinal pain, headache, myalgia, dry cough, and pneumonia; transmitted airborne via air conditioning systems, humidifiers, water faucets, shower heads; not person-to-person contact.

482.89 Other specified bacteria

482.9 Bacterial pneumonia unspecified

✓4th **483 Pneumonia due to other specified organism**

483.0 Mycoplasma pneumoniae
Eaton's agent   Pleuropneumonia-like organism [PPLO]

483.1 Chlamydia

483.8 Other specified organism

✓4th **484 Pneumonia in infectious diseases classified elsewhere**
EXCLUDES influenza with pneumonia, any form (487.0)

484.1 Pneumonia in cytomegalic inclusion disease
Code first underlying disease, as (078.5)

484.3 Pneumonia in whooping cough
Code first underlying disease, as (033.0-033.9)

484.5 Pneumonia in anthrax
Code first underlying disease (022.1)

484.6 Pneumonia in aspergillosis
Code first underlying disease (117.3)

484.7 Pneumonia in other systemic mycoses
Code first underlying disease
EXCLUDES pneumonia in:
candidiasis (112.4)
coccidioidomycosis (114.0)
histoplasmosis (115.0-115.9 with fifth-digit 5)

484.8 Pneumonia in other infectious diseases classified elsewhere
Code first underlying disease, as:
Q fever (083.0)
typhoid fever (002.0)
EXCLUDES pneumonia in:
actinomycosis (039.1)
measles (055.1)
nocardiosis (039.1)
ornithosis (073.0)
Pneumocystis carinii (136.3)
salmonellosis (003.22)
toxoplasmosis (130.4)
tuberculosis (011.6)
tularemia (021.2)
varicella (052.1)

485 Bronchopneumonia, organism unspecified
Bronchopneumonia: Pneumonia:
  hemorrhagic   lobular
  terminal   segmental
Pleurobronchopneumonia
EXCLUDES bronchiolitis (acute) (466.11-466.19)
chronic (491.8)
lipoid pneumonia (507.1)

486 Pneumonia, organism unspecified
EXCLUDES hypostatic or passive pneumonia (514)
influenza with pneumonia, any form (487.0)
inhalation or aspiration pneumonia due to foreign materials (507.0-507.8)
pneumonitis due to fumes and vapors (506.0)

RESPIRATORY SYSTEM 487–491.0

√4th 487 Influenza

> **EXCLUDES** Hemophilus influenzae [H. influenzae]:
> infection NOS (041.5)
> laryngitis (464.00-464.01)
> meningitis (320.0)
> pneumonia (482.2)

487.0 With pneumonia
Influenza with pneumonia, any form
Influenzal:
bronchopneumonia
pneumonia

487.1 With other respiratory manifestations
Influenza NOS
Influenzal:
laryngitis
pharyngitis
respiratory infection (upper) (acute)

487.8 With other manifestations
Encephalopathy due to influenza
Influenza with involvement of gastrointestinal tract
> **EXCLUDES** "intestinal flu" [viral gastroenteritis] (008.8)

CHRONIC OBSTRUCTIVE PULMONARY DISEASE AND ALLIED CONDITIONS (490-496)

490 Bronchitis, not specified as acute or chronic
Bronchitis NOS:
catarrhal
with tracheitis NOS
Tracheobronchitis NOS
> **EXCLUDES** bronchitis:
> allergic NOS (493.9)
> asthmatic NOS (493.9)
> due to fumes and vapors (506.0)

√4th 491 Chronic bronchitis
> **EXCLUDES** chronic obstructive asthma (493.2)

491.0 Simple chronic bronchitis
Catarrhal bronchitis, chronic
Smokers' cough

Bronchioli and Alveoli

  Additional Digit Required | Unspecified Code | ● Other Specified Code | ▲ Manifestation Code
MSP Medicare Secondary Payer ▶◀ Revised Text ● New Code ▲ Revised Code Title

2002 Ingenix, Inc.

491.1 Mucopurulent chronic bronchitis
Bronchitis (chronic) (recurrent):
fetid
mucopurulent
purulent

DEF: Chronic bronchial infection characterized by both mucus and pus secretions in the bronchial tree; recurs after asymptomatic periods; signs are coughing, expectoration and secondary changes in the lung.

√5th **491.2 Obstructive chronic bronchitis**
Bronchitis:
  emphysematous
  obstructive (chronic) (diffuse)
Bronchitis with:
  chronic airway obstruction
  emphysema

EXCLUDES asthmatic bronchitis (acute) NOS (493.9)
chronic obstructive asthma (493.2)

491.20 Without mention of acute exacerbation
Emphysema with chronic bronchitis

491.21 With acute exacerbation
Acute bronchitis with chronic obstructive pulmonary disease [COPD]
Acute and chronic obstructive bronchitis
Acute exacerbation of chronic obstructive pulmonary disease [COPD]
Emphysema with both acute and chronic bronchitis

EXCLUDES chronic obstructive asthma with acute exacerbation (493.22)

491.8 Other chronic bronchitis
Chronic:
  tracheitis
  tracheobronchitis

491.9 Unspecified chronic bronchitis

√4th **492 Emphysema**

492.0 Emphysematous bleb
Giant bullous emphysema
Ruptured emphysematous bleb
Tension pneumatocele
Vanishing lung

DEF: Formation of vesicle or bulla in emphysematous lung, more than one millimeter; contains serum or blood.

492.8 Other emphysema
Emphysema (lung or pulmonary):
  NOS
  centriacinar
  centrilobular
  obstructive
  panacinar
  panlobular
Emphysema (lung or pulmonary):
  unilateral
  vesicular
MacLeod's syndrome
Swyer-James syndrome
Unilateral hyperlucent lung

EXCLUDES emphysema:
with both acute and chronic bronchitis (491.21)
with chronic bronchitis (491.2)
compensatory (518.2)
due to fumes and vapors (506.4)
interstitial (518.1)
  newborn (770.2)
mediastinal (518.1)
surgical (subcutaneous) (998.81)
traumatic (958.7)

RESPIRATORY SYSTEM

✓4th 493 Asthma
> **EXCLUDES** *wheezing NOS (786.07)*
>
> The following fifth-digit subclassification is for use with category 493:
> - 0 without mention of status asthmaticus or acute exacerbation or unspecified
> - 1 with status asthmaticus
> - 2 with acute exacerbation
>
> DEF: Status asthmaticus: Severe, intractable episode of asthma unresponsive to normal therapeutic measures.

✓5th 493.0 Extrinsic asthma
> Asthma: Asthma:
>   allergic with   hay
>   stated cause   platinum
>   atopic Hay fever with asthma
>   childhood
>
> **EXCLUDES** *asthma:*
>   *allergic NOS (493.9)*
>   *detergent (507.8)*
>   *miners' (500)*
>   *wood (495.8)*
>
> DEF: Transient stricture of airway diameters of bronchi; due to environmental factor; also called allergic (bronchial) asthma.

✓5th 493.1 Intrinsic asthma
> Late-onset asthma
>
> DEF: Transient stricture, of airway diameters of bronchi; due to pathophysiological disturbances.

✓5th 493.2 Chronic obstructive asthma
> Asthma with chronic obstructive pulmonary disease [COPD]
> ▶Chronic asthmatic bronchitis◀
>
> **EXCLUDES** *acute bronchitis (466.0)*
>   *chronic obstructive bronchitis (491.2)*
>
> DEF: Persistent narrowing of airway diameters in the bronchial tree, restricting airflow and causing constant labored breathing.

✓5th 493.9 Asthma, unspecified
> Asthma (bronchial) (allergic NOS)
> Bronchitis:
>   allergic
>   asthmatic

✓4th 494 Bronchiectasis
> Bronchiectasis (fusiform) (postinfectious) (recurrent)
> Bronchiolectasis
>
> **EXCLUDES** *congenital (748.61)*
>   *tuberculous bronchiectasis (current disease) (011.5)*
>
> DEF: Dilation of bronchi; due to infection or chronic conditions; causes decreased lung capacity and recurrent infections of lungs.

  494.0 Bronchiectasis without acute exacerbation
  494.1 Bronchiectasis with acute exacerbation
> Acute bronchitis with bronchiectasis

✓4th / ✓5th Additional Digit Required   Unspecified Code   Other Specified Code   Manifestation Code
MSP Medicare Secondary Payer   ▶◀ Revised Text   ● New Code   ▲ Revised Code Title

2002 Ingenix, Inc.

RESPIRATORY SYSTEM

✓4th 495 Extrinsic allergic alveolitis
  INCLUDES allergic alveolitis and pneumonitis due to inhaled organic dust particles of fungal, thermophilic actinomycete, or other origin
  DEF: Pneumonitis due to particles inhaled into lung, often at workplace; symptoms include cough, chills, fever, increased heart and respiratory rates; develops within hours of exposure.

- **495.0 Farmers' lung**
- **495.1 Bagassosis**
- **495.2 Bird-fanciers' lung**
  Budgerigar-fanciers' disease or lung
  Pigeon-fanciers' disease or lung
- **495.3 Suberosis**
  Cork-handlers' disease or lung
- **495.4 Malt workers' lung**
  Alveolitis due to Aspergillus clavatus
- **495.5 Mushroom workers' lung**
- **495.6 Maple bark-strippers' lung**
  Alveolitis due to Cryptostroma corticale
- **495.7 "Ventilation" pneumonitis**
  Allergic alveolitis due to fungal, thermophilic actinomycete, and other organisms growing in ventilation [air conditioning] systems
- **495.8 Other specified allergic alveolitis and pneumonitis**
  Cheese-washers' lung
  Coffee workers' lung
  Fish-meal workers' lung
  Furriers' lung
  Grain-handlers' disease or lung
  Pituitary snuff-takers' disease
  Sequoiosis or red-cedar asthma
  Wood asthma
- **495.9 Unspecified allergic alveolitis and pneumonitis**
  Alveolitis, allergic (extrinsic)
  Hypersensitivity pneumonitis

496 Chronic airway obstruction, not elsewhere classified 🅰
  Note: This code is not to be used with any code from categories 491-493
  Chronic:
    nonspecific lung disease
    obstructive lung disease
    obstructive pulmonary disease [COPD] NOS
  EXCLUDES chronic obstructive lung disease [COPD] specified (as) (with):
    allergic alveolitis (495.0-495.9)
    asthma (493.2)
    bronchiectasis (494.0-494.1)
    bronchitis (491.20-491.21)
      with emphysema (491.20-491.21)
    emphysema (492.0-492.8)

PNEUMOCONIOSES AND OTHER LUNG DISEASES DUE TO EXTERNAL AGENTS (500-508)
DEF: Permanent deposits of particulate matter, within lungs; due to occupational or environmental exposure; results in chronic induration and fibrosis. (See specific listings in 500-508 code range)

500 Coal workers' pneumoconiosis 🅰
  Anthracosilicosis   Coal workers' lung
  Anthracosis   Miner's asthma
  Black lung disease

501 Asbestosis 🅰

RESPIRATORY SYSTEM

502 Pneumoconiosis due to other silica or silicates
    Pneumoconiosis due to talc
    Silicotic fibrosis (massive) of lung
    Silicosis (simple) (complicated)

503 Pneumoconiosis due to other inorganic dust
    Aluminosis (of lung)   Graphite fibrosis (of lung)
    Bauxite fibrosis (of lung)   Siderosis
    Berylliosis   Stannosis

504 Pneumonopathy due to inhalation of other dust
    Byssinosis   Flax-dressers' disease
    Cannabinosis
    EXCLUDES allergic alveolitis (495.0-495.9)
            asbestosis (501)
            bagassosis (495.1)
            farmers' lung (495.0)

505 Pneumoconiosis, unspecified

✓4th **506 Respiratory conditions due to chemical fumes and vapors**
    Use additional E code to identify cause

    506.0 Bronchitis and pneumonitis due to fumes and vapors
        Chemical bronchitis (acute)

    506.1 Acute pulmonary edema due to fumes and vapors
        Chemical pulmonary edema (acute)
        EXCLUDES acute pulmonary edema NOS (518.4)
                chronic or unspecified pulmonary edema (514)

    506.2 Upper respiratory inflammation due to fumes and vapors

    506.3 Other acute and subacute respiratory conditions due to fumes and vapors

    506.4 Chronic respiratory conditions due to fumes and vapors
        Emphysema (diffuse) (chronic)
        Obliterative bronchiolitis (chronic) (subacute)   } due to inhalation of chemical fumes and vapors
        Pulmonary fibrosis (chronic)

    506.9 Unspecified respiratory conditions due to fumes and vapors
        Silo-fillers' disease

✓4th **507 Pneumonitis due to solids and liquids**
    EXCLUDES fetal aspiration pneumonitis (770.1)

    507.0 Due to inhalation of food or vomitus
        Aspiration pneumonia (due to):   Aspiration pneumonia (due to):
        NOS   milk
        food (regurgitated)   saliva
        gastric secretions   vomitus

    507.1 Due to inhalation of oils and essences
        Lipoid pneumonia (exogenous)
        EXCLUDES endogenous lipoid pneumonia (516.8)

    507.8 Due to other solids and liquids
        Detergent asthma

✓4th **508 Respiratory conditions due to other and unspecified external agents**
    Use additional E code to identify cause

    508.0 Acute pulmonary manifestations due to radiation
        Radiation pneumonitis

    508.1 Chronic and other pulmonary manifestations due to radiation
        Fibrosis of lung following radiation

✓4th / ✓5th Additional Digit Required   Unspecified Code   Other Specified Code   Manifestation Code
 Medicare Secondary Payer   ▶◀ Revised Text   ● New Code   ▲ Revised Code Title

2002 Ingenix, Inc.

508.8 Respiratory conditions due to other specified external agents
508.9 Respiratory conditions due to unspecified external agent

OTHER DISEASES OF RESPIRATORY SYSTEM (510-519)

4th 510 Empyema
Use additional code to identify infectious organism (041.0-041.9)
> **EXCLUDES** abscess of lung (513.0)

DEF: Purulent infection, within pleural space.

510.0 With fistula
Fistula:
    bronchocutaneous
    bronchopleural
    hepatopleural
Fistula:
    mediastinal
    pleural
    thoracic
Any condition classifiable to 510.9 with fistula

DEF: Purulent infection of respiratory cavity; with communication from cavity to another structure.

510.9 Without mention of fistula
Abscess:
    pleura
    thorax
Empyema (chest) (lung)
    (pleura)
Fibrinopurulent pleurisy
Pleurisy:
    purulent
Pleurisy:
    septic
    seropurulent
    suppurative
Pyopneumothorax
Pyothorax

4th 511 Pleurisy
> **EXCLUDES** malignant pleural effusion (197.2)
> pleurisy with mention of tuberculosis, current disease (012.0)

DEF: Inflammation of serous membrane of lungs and lining of thoracic cavity; causes exudation in cavity or membrane surface.

511.0 Without mention of effusion or current tuberculosis
Adhesion, lung or pleura
Calcification of pleura
Pleurisy (acute) (sterile):
    diaphragmatic
    fibrinous
    interlobar
Pleurisy:
    NOS
    pneumococcal
    staphylococcal
    streptococcal
Thickening of pleura

511.1 With effusion, with mention of a bacterial cause other than tuberculosis
Pleurisy with effusion (exudative) (serous):
    pneumococcal
    staphylococcal
    streptococcal
    other specified nontuberculous bacterial cause

511.8 Other specified forms of effusion, except tuberculous
Encysted pleurisy
Hemopneumothorax
Hemothorax
Hydropneumothorax
Hydrothorax
> **EXCLUDES** traumatic (860.2-860.5, 862.29, 862.39)

511.9 Unspecified pleural effusion
Pleural effusion NOS
Pleurisy:
    exudative
    serofibrinous
Pleurisy:
    serous
    with effusion NOS

RESPIRATORY SYSTEM

✓4ᵗʰ 512 Pneumothorax
DEF: Collapsed lung; due to gas or air in pleural space.

512.0 Spontaneous tension pneumothorax
DEF: Leaking air from lung into lining causing collapse.

512.1 Iatrogenic pneumothorax
Postoperative pneumothorax
DEF: Air trapped in the lining of the lung following surgery.

512.8 Other spontaneous pneumothorax
Pneumothorax:
 NOS
 acute
Pneumothorax:
 chronic

EXCLUDES pneumothorax:
 congenital (770.2)
 traumatic (860.0-860.1, 860.4-860.5)
 tuberculous, current disease (011.7)

✓4ᵗʰ 513 Abscess of lung and mediastinum

513.0 Abscess of lung
Abscess (multiple) of lung
Gangrenous or necrotic pneumonia
Pulmonary gangrene or necrosis

513.1 Abscess of mediastinum

514 Pulmonary congestion and hypostasis
Hypostatic:
 bronchopneumonia
 pneumonia
Passive pneumonia
Pulmonary congestion (chronic) (passive)
Pulmonary edema:
 NOS
 chronic

EXCLUDES acute pulmonary edema:
 NOS (518.4)
 with mention of heart disease or failure (428.1)

DEF: Excessive retention of interstitial fluid in the lungs and pulmonary vessels; due to poor circulation.

515 Postinflammatory pulmonary fibrosis
Cirrhosis of lung
Fibrosis of lung (atrophic)
 (confluent) (massive)
 (perialveolar)
 (peribronchial)
Induration of lung
} chronic or unspecified

DEF: Fibrosis and scarring of the lungs due to inflammatory reaction.

✓4ᵗʰ 516 Other alveolar and parietoalveolar pneumonopathy

516.0 Pulmonary alveolar proteinosis
DEF: Reduced ventilation; due to proteinaceous deposits on alveoli; symptoms include dyspnea, cough, chest pain, weakness, weight loss, and hemoptysis.

516.1 Idiopathic pulmonary hemosiderosis
Essential brown induration of lung
Code first underlying disease (275.0)
DEF: Fibrosis of alveolar walls; marked by abnormal amounts hemosiderin in lungs; primarily affects children; symptoms include anemia, fluid in lungs, and blood in sputum; etiology unknown.

516.2 Pulmonary alveolar microlithiasis
DEF: Small calculi in pulmonary alveoli resembling sand-like particles on x-ray.

RESPIRATORY SYSTEM

516.3 Idiopathic fibrosing alveolitis
Alveolar capillary block
Diffuse (idiopathic) (interstitial) pulmonary fibrosis
Hamman-Rich syndrome

516.8 Other specified alveolar and parietoalveolar pneumonopathies
Endogenous lipoid pneumonia
Interstitial pneumonia (desquamative) (lymphoid)
> EXCLUDES lipoid pneumonia, exogenous or unspecified (507.1)

516.9 Unspecified alveolar and parietoalveolar pneumonopathy

✓4th 517 Lung involvement in conditions classified elsewhere
> EXCLUDES rheumatoid lung (714.81)

517.1 Rheumatic pneumonia
Code first underlying disease (390)

517.2 Lung involvement in systemic sclerosis
Code first underlying disease (710.1)

517.8 Lung involvement in other diseases classified elsewhere
Code first underlying disease, as:
 amyloidosis (277.3)
 polymyositis (710.4)
 sarcoidosis (135)
 Sjögren's disease (710.2)
 systemic lupus erythematosus (710.0)
> EXCLUDES syphilis (095.1)

✓4th 518 Other diseases of lung

518.0 Pulmonary collapse
Atelectasis   Middle lobe syndrome
Collapse of lung
> EXCLUDES atelectasis:
> congenital (partial) (770.5)
>   primary (770.4)
> tuberculous, current disease (011.8)

518.1 Interstitial emphysema
Mediastinal emphysema
> EXCLUDES surgical (subcutaneous) emphysema (998.81)
> that in fetus or newborn (770.2)
> traumatic emphysema (958.7)

DEF: Escaped air from the alveoli trapped in the interstices of the lung; trauma or cough may cause the disease.

518.2 Compensatory emphysema

DEF: Distention of all or part of the lung caused by disease processes or surgical intervention that decreased volume in another part of the lung; overcompensation reaction to the loss of capacity in another part of the lung.

518.3 Pulmonary eosinophilia
Eosinophilic asthma   Pneumonia:
Löffler's syndrome   eosinophilic
Pneumonia: Tropical eosinophilia
 allergic

DEF: Infiltration, into pulmonary parenchyma of eosinophilia; results in cough, fever, and dyspnea.

518.4 Acute edema of lung, unspecified
Acute pulmonary edema NOS   Pulmonary edema, postoperative
> EXCLUDES pulmonary edema:
> acute, with mention of heart disease or failure (428.1)
> chronic or unspecified (514)
> due to external agents (506.0-508.9)

DEF: Severe, sudden fluid retention within lung tissues.

N Newborn Age: 0   P Pediatric Age: 0-17   M Maternity Age: 12-55   A Adult Age: 15-124

RESPIRATORY SYSTEM

518.5 Pulmonary insufficiency following trauma and surgery
Adult respiratory distress syndrome
Pulmonary insufficiency following:
  shock
  surgery
  trauma
Shock lung
> EXCLUDES   adult respiratory distress syndrome associated with other conditions (518.82)
> pneumonia:
>   aspiration (507.0)
>   hypostatic (514)
> respiratory failure in other conditions (518.81, 518.83-518.84)

518.6 Allergic bronchopulmonary aspegillosis
DEF: Noninvasive hypersensitive reaction; due to allergic reaction to *Aspergillus fumigatus* (mold).

518.8 Other diseases of lung

518.81 Acute respiratory failure
Respiratory failure NOS
> EXCLUDES   acute and chronic respiratory failure (518.84)
> acute respiratory distress (518.82)
> chronic respiratory failure (518.83)
> respiratory arrest (799.1)
> respiratory failure, newborn ▶(770.84)◀

518.82 Other pulmonary insufficiency, not elsewhere classified
Acute respiratory distress
Acute respiratory insufficiency
Adult respiratory distress syndrome NEC
> EXCLUDES   adult respiratory distress syndrome associated with trauma and surgery (518.5)
> pulmonary insufficiency following trauma and surgery (518.5)
> respiratory distress:
>   NOS (786.09)
>   newborn ▶(770.89)◀
>   syndrome, newborn (769)
> shock lung (518.5)

518.83 Chronic respiratory failure

518.84 Acute and chronic respiratory failure
Acute on chronic respiratory failure

518.89 Other diseases of lung, not elsewhere classified
Broncholithiasis   Lung disease NOS
Calcification of lung   Pulmolithiasis
DEF: Broncholithiasis: calculi in lumen of transbronchial tree.
DEF: Pulmolithiasis: calculi in lung.

519 Other diseases of respiratory system

519.0 Tracheostomy complications

519.00 Tracheostomy complication, unspecified

519.01 Infection of tracheostomy
Use additional code to identify type of infection, such as:
  abscess or cellulitis of neck (682.1)
  septicemia (038.0-038.9)
Use additional code to identify organism (041.00-041.9)

519.02 **Mechanical complication of tracheostomy**
Tracheal stenosis due to tracheostomy

519.09 **Other tracheostomy complications**
Hemorrhage due to tracheostomy
Tracheoesophageal fistula due to tracheostomy

519.1 **Other diseases of trachea and bronchus, not elsewhere classified**

Calcification
Stenosis   } of bronchus or trachea
Ulcer

519.2 **Mediastinitis**
DEF: Inflammation of tissue between organs behind sternum.

519.3 **Other diseases of mediastinum, not elsewhere classified**

Fibrosis
Hernia   } of mediastinum
Retraction

519.4 **Disorders of diaphragm**
Diaphragmitis   Relaxation of diaphragm
Paralysis of diaphragm
> **EXCLUDES** congenital defect of diaphragm (756.6)
> diaphragmatic hernia (551-553 with .3)
> congenital (756.6)

519.8 **Other diseases of respiratory system, not elsewhere classified**

519.9 **Unspecified disease of respiratory system**
Respiratory disease (chronic) NOS

9. DISEASES OF THE DIGESTIVE SYSTEM (520-579)

DISEASES OF ORAL CAVITY, SALIVARY GLANDS, AND JAWS (520-529)

✓4th **520 Disorders of tooth development and eruption**

520.0 **Anodontia**
Absence of teeth (complete) (congenital) (partial)
Hypodontia
Oligodontia
> **EXCLUDES** acquired absence of teeth (525.10-525.19)

520.1 **Supernumerary teeth**
Distomolar
Fourth molar
Mesiodens
Paramolar
Supplemental teeth
> **EXCLUDES** supernumerary roots (520.2)

520.2 **Abnormalities of size and form**

Concrescence
Fusion   } of teeth
Gemination

Dens evaginatus   Microdontia
Dens in dente   Peg-shaped [conical] teeth
Dens invaginatus   Supernumerary roots
Enamel pearls   Taurodontism
Macrodontia   Tuberculum paramolare
> **EXCLUDES** that due to congenital syphilis (090.5)
> tuberculum Carabelli, which is regarded as a normal variation

DIGESTIVE SYSTEM

Digestive System

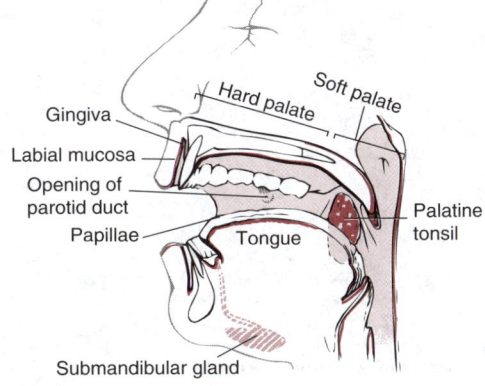

The Oral Cavity

520.3 Mottled teeth
Dental fluorosis
Mottling of enamel
Nonfluoride enamel opacities

520.4 Disturbances of tooth formation
Aplasia and hypoplasia of cementum
Dilaceration of tooth
Enamel hypoplasia (neonatal) (postnatal) (prenatal)
Horner's teeth
Hypocalcification of teeth
Regional odontodysplasia
Turner's tooth
> **EXCLUDES** Hutchinson's teeth and mulberry molars in congenital syphilis (090.5)
> mottled teeth (520.3)

520.5 Hereditary disturbances in tooth structure, not elsewhere classified
Amelogenesis ⎫
Dentinogenesis ⎬ imperfecta
Odontogenesis ⎭

Dentinal dysplasia   Shell teeth

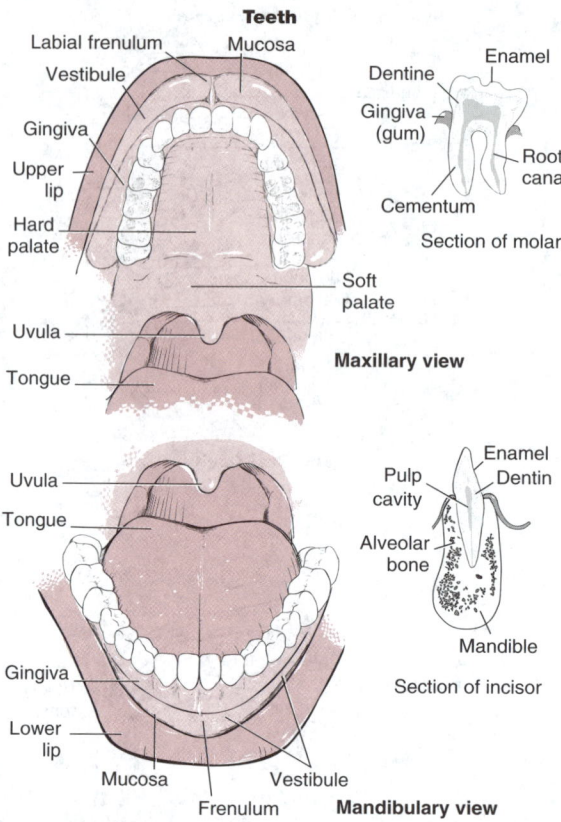

520.6 Disturbances in tooth eruption

Teeth:
  embedded
  impacted
  natal
  neonatal
  primary [deciduous]:
    persistent
    shedding, premature

Tooth eruption:
  late
  obstructed
  premature

EXCLUDES exfoliation of teeth (attributable to disease of surrounding tissues) (525.0-525.19)
impacted or embedded teeth with abnormal position of such teeth or adjacent teeth (524.3)

520.7 Teething syndrome

520.8 Other specified disorders of tooth development and eruption
Color changes during tooth formation
Pre-eruptive color changes
EXCLUDES posteruptive color changes (521.7)

520.9 Unspecified disorder of tooth development and eruption

DIGESTIVE SYSTEM

✓4ᵗʰ **521 Diseases of hard tissues of teeth**

✓5ᵗʰ **521.0 Dental caries**

521.00 Dental caries, unspecified

521.01 Dental caries limited to enamel
Initial caries   White spot lesion

521.02 Dental caries extending into dentine

521.03 Dental caries extending into pulp

521.04 Arrested dental caries

521.05 Odontoclasia
Infantile melanodontia   Melanodontoclasia
> EXCLUDES internal and external resorption of teeth (521.4)

DEF: A pathological dental condition described as stained areas, loss of tooth substance, and hypoplasia linked to nutritional deficiencies during tooth development and to cariogenic oral conditions; synonyms are melanodontoclasia and infantile melanodontia.

521.09 Other dental caries

521.1 Excessive attrition
Approximal wear
Occlusal wear

521.2 Abrasion
Abrasion:
  dentifrice
  habitual
  occupational   } of teeth
  ritual
  traditional
Wedge defect NOS

521.3 Erosion
Erosion of teeth:
  NOS
  due to:
    medicine
    persistent vomiting
  idiopathic
  occupational

521.4 Pathological resorption
Internal granuloma of pulp
Resorption of tooth or root (external) (internal)
DEF: Loss of dentin and cementum due to disease process.

521.5 Hypercementosis
Cementation hyperplasia
DEF: Excess deposits of cementum, on tooth root.

521.6 Ankylosis of teeth
DEF: Adhesion of tooth to surrounding bone.

521.7 Posteruptive color changes
Staining [discoloration] of teeth:
  NOS
  due to:
    drugs
    metals
    pulpal bleeding
> EXCLUDES accretions [deposits] on teeth (523.6)
> pre-eruptive color changes (520.8)

✓4ᵗʰ / ✓5ᵗʰ Additional Digit Required   Unspecified Code   ● Other Specified Code   ▲ Manifestation Code

MSP Medicare Secondary Payer   ▶◀ Revised Text   ● New Code   ▲ Revised Code Title

DIGESTIVE SYSTEM

521.8 **Other specified diseases of hard tissues of teeth**
Irradiated enamel
Sensitive dentin

521.9 **Unspecified disease of hard tissues of teeth**

√4ᵗʰ **522 Diseases of pulp and periapical tissues**

522.0 **Pulpitis**
Pulpal:
  abscess
  polyp
Pulpitis:
  acute
  chronic (hyperplastic) (ulcerative)
  suppurative

522.1 **Necrosis of the pulp**
Pulp gangrene
DEF: Death of pulp tissue.

522.2 **Pulp degeneration**
Denticles
Pulp calcifications
Pulp stones

522.3 **Abnormal hard tissue formation in pulp**
Secondary or irregular dentin

522.4 **Acute apical periodontitis of pulpal origin**
DEF: Severe inflammation of periodontal ligament due to pulpal inflammation or necrosis.

522.5 **Periapical abscess without sinus**
Abscess: Abscess:
  dental   dentoalveolar
EXCLUDES *periapical abscess with sinus (522.7).*

522.6 **Chronic apical periodontitis**
Apical or periapical granuloma
Apical periodontitis NOS

522.7 **Periapical abscess with sinus**
Fistula: Fistula:
  alveolar process   dental

522.8 **Radicular cyst**
Cyst: Cyst:
  apical (periodontal)   radiculodental
  periapical   residual radicular
EXCLUDES *lateral developmental or lateral periodontal cyst (526.0)*
DEF: Cyst in tissue around tooth apex due to chronic infection of granuloma around root.

522.9 **Other and unspecified diseases of pulp and periapical tissues**

√4ᵗʰ **523 Gingival and periodontal diseases**

523.0 **Acute gingivitis**
EXCLUDES *acute necrotizing ulcerative gingivitis (101)*
herpetic gingivostomatitis (054.2)

523.1 **Chronic gingivitis**
Gingivitis (chronic):   Gingivitis (chronic):
  NOS   simple marginal
  desquamative   ulcerative
  hyperplastic   Gingivostomatitis
EXCLUDES *herpetic gingivostomatitis (054.2)*

523.2 **Gingival recession**
Gingival recession (generalized) (localized) (postinfective) (postoperative)

DIGESTIVE SYSTEM

523.3 Acute periodontitis
    Acute: Paradontal abscess
       pericementitis   Periodontal abscess
       pericoronitis
    EXCLUDES   *acute apical periodontitis (522.4)*
                           periapical abscess (522.5, 522.7)
    DEF: Severe inflammation, of tissues supporting teeth.

523.4 Chronic periodontitis
    Alveolar pyorrhea   Periodontitis:
    Chronic pericoronitis   NOS
    Pericementitis (chronic)   complex
                             simplex
    EXCLUDES   *chronic apical periodontitis (522.6)*

523.5 Periodontosis

523.6 Accretions on teeth
    Dental calculus: Deposits on teeth:
       subgingival   materia alba
       supragingival   soft
    Deposits on teeth: tartar
       betel   tobacco
    DEF: Foreign material on tooth surface, usually plaque or calculus.

523.8 Other specified periodontal diseases
    Giant cell:
       epulis
       peripheral granuloma
    Gingival:
       cysts
       enlargement NOS
       fibromatosis
    Gingival polyp
    Periodontal lesions due to traumatic occlusion
    Peripheral giant cell granuloma
    EXCLUDES   *leukoplakia of gingiva (528.6)*

523.9 Unspecified gingival and periodontal disease

✓4ᵗʰ 524 Dentofacial anomalies, including malocclusion

    ✓5ᵗʰ 524.0 Major anomalies of jaw size
        EXCLUDES   *hemifacial atrophy or hypertrophy (754.0)*
                         unilateral condylar hyperplasia or hypoplasia of mandible (526.89)

       524.00 Unspecified anomaly
           DEF: Unspecified deformity of jaw size.

       524.01 Maxillary hyperplasia
           DEF: Overgrowth or overdevelopment of upper jaw bone.

       524.02 Mandibular hyperplasia
           DEF: Overgrowth or overdevelopment of lower jaw bone.

       524.03 Maxillary hypoplasia
           DEF: Incomplete or underdeveloped, upper jaw bone.

       524.04 Mandibular hypoplasia
           DEF: Incomplete or underdeveloped, lower jaw bone.

       524.05 Macrogenia
           DEF: Enlarged, jaw, especially chin; affects bone, soft tissue, or both.

✓4ᵗʰ ✓5ᵗʰ Additional Digit Required   Unspecified Code   Other Specified Code   Manifestation Code

 Medicare Secondary Payer   ▶◀ Revised Text   ● New Code   ▲ Revised Code Title

2002 Ingenix, Inc.

524.06 Microgenia
DEF: Underdeveloped mandible, characterized by an extremely small chin.

524.09 Other specified anomaly

√5ᵗʰ **524.1 Anomalies of relationship of jaw to cranial base**

524.10 Unspecified anomaly
Prognathism   Retrognathism
DEF: Prognathism: protrusion of lower jaw.

DEF: Retrognathism: jaw is located posteriorly to a normally positioned jaw; backward position of mandible.

524.11 Maxillary asymmetry
DEF: Absence of symmetry of maxilla.

524.12 Other jaw asymmetry

524.19 Other specified anomaly

524.2 Anomalies of dental arch relationship
Crossbite (anterior) (posterior)
Disto-occlusion
Mesio-occlusion
Midline deviation
Open bite (anterior) (posterior)
Overbite (excessive):
   deep
   horizontal
   vertical
Overjet
Posterior lingual occlusion of mandibular teeth
Soft tissue impingement

> **EXCLUDES** hemifacial atrophy or hypertrophy (754.0)
> unilateral condylar hyperplasia or hypoplasia of mandible (526.89)

524.3 Anomalies of tooth position
Crowding
Diastema
Displacement } of tooth, teeth
Rotation
Spacing, abnormal
Transposition

Impacted or embedded teeth with abnormal position of such teeth or adjacent teeth

524.4 Malocclusion, unspecified
DEF: Malposition of top and bottom teeth; interferes with chewing.

524.5 Dentofacial functional abnormalities
Abnormal jaw closure
Malocclusion due to:
   abnormal swallowing
   mouth breathing
   tongue, lip, or finger habits

√5ᵗʰ **524.6 Temporomandibular joint disorders**

> **EXCLUDES** current temporomandibular joint:
> dislocation (830.0-830.1)
> strain (848.1)

524.60 Temporomandibular joint disorders, unspecified
Temporomandibular joint-pain-dysfunction syndrome [TMJ]

524.61 Adhesions and ankylosis (bony or fibrous)
DEF: Stiffening or union of temporomandibular joint due to bony or fibrous union across joint.

DIGESTIVE SYSTEM 524.62–526.1

- **524.62 Arthralgia of temporomandibular joint**
  DEF: Pain in temporomandibular joint; not inflammatory in nature.
- **524.63 Articular disc disorder (reducing or non-reducing)**
- **524.69 Other specified temporomandibular joint disorders**

√5ᵗʰ **524.7 Dental alveolar anomalies**
- **524.70 Unspecified alveolar anomaly**
- **524.71 Alveolar maxillary hyperplasia**
  DEF: Excessive tissue formation in the dental alveoli of upper jaw.
- **524.72 Alveolar mandibular hyperplasia**
  DEF: Excessive tissue formation in the dental alveoli of lower jaw.
- **524.73 Alveolar maxillary hypoplasia**
  DEF: Incomplete or underdeveloped, alveolar tissue of upper jaw.
- **524.74 Alveolar mandibular hypoplasia**
  DEF: Incomplete or underdeveloped, alveolar tissue of lower jaw.
- **524.79 Other specified alveolar anomaly**

524.8 Other specified dentofacial anomalies
524.9 Unspecified dentofacial anomalies

√4ᵗʰ **525 Other diseases and conditions of the teeth and supporting structures**
- **525.0 Exfoliation of teeth due to systemic causes**
  DEF: Deterioration of teeth and surrounding structures due to systemic disease.

√5ᵗʰ **525.1 Loss of teeth due to trauma, extraction, or periodontal disease**
- **525.10 Acquired absence of teeth, unspecified**
  Edentulism   Tooth extraction status, NOS
- **525.11 Loss of teeth due to trauma**
- **525.12 Loss of teeth due to periodontal disease**
- **525.13 Loss of teeth due to caries**
- **525.19 Other loss of teeth**

525.2 Atrophy of edentulous alveolar ridge
525.3 Retained dental root
525.8 Other specified disorders of the teeth and supporting structures
  Enlargement of alveolar ridge NOS
  Irregular alveolar process
525.9 Unspecified disorder of the teeth and supporting structures

√4ᵗʰ **526 Diseases of the jaws**
- **526.0 Developmental odontogenic cysts**
  Cyst: Cyst:
    dentigerous   lateral periodontal
    eruption   primordial
    follicular   Keratocyst
    lateral developmental
  EXCLUDES   radicular cyst (522.8)
- **526.1 Fissural cysts of jaw**
  Cyst: Cyst:
    globulomaxillary   median palatal
    incisor canal   nasopalatine
    median anterior maxillary   palatine of papilla
  EXCLUDES   cysts of oral soft tissues (528.4)

√4ᵗʰ
√5ᵗʰ Additional Digit Required   Unspecified Code   Other Specified Code   Manifestation Code
 Medicare Secondary Payer   ▶◀ Revised Text   ● New Code   ▲ Revised Code Title

2002 Ingenix, Inc.   Volume 1 — 297

526.2 Other cysts of jaws
    Cyst of jaw: Cyst of jaw:
      NOS   hemorrhagic
      aneurysmal   traumatic

526.3 Central giant cell (reparative) granuloma
    EXCLUDES *peripheral giant cell granuloma (523.8)*

526.4 Inflammatory conditions
    Abscess
    Osteitis
    Osteomyelitis   } of jaw (acute) (chronic) (suppurative)
      (neonatal)
    Periostitis

    Sequestrum of jaw bone
    EXCLUDES *alveolar osteitis (526.5)*

526.5 Alveolitis of jaw
    Alveolar osteitis
    Dry socket
    DEF: Inflammation, of alveoli or tooth socket.

√5th **526.8 Other specified diseases of the jaws**
    526.81 Exostosis of jaw
        Torus mandibularis
        Torus palatinus
        DEF: Spur or bony outgrowth on the jaw.

    526.89 Other
        Cherubism
        Fibrous dysplasia
        Latent bone cyst   } of jaw(s)
        Osteoradionecrosis

        Unilateral condylar hyperplasia or hypoplasia of mandible

526.9 Unspecified disease of the jaws

√4th **527 Diseases of the salivary glands**

527.0 Atrophy
    DEF: Wasting away, necrosis of salivary gland tissue.

527.1 Hypertrophy
    DEF: Overgrowth or overdeveloped salivary gland tissue.

527.2 Sialoadenitis
    Parotitis: Sialoangitis
      NOS   Sialodochitis
      allergic
      toxic
    EXCLUDES *epidemic or infectious parotitis (072.0-072.9)*
                      uveoparotid fever (135)
    DEF: Inflammation of salivary gland.

527.3 Abscess

527.4 Fistula
    EXCLUDES *congenital fistula of salivary gland (750.24)*

527.5 Sialolithiasis
    Calculus   } of salivary gland or duct
    Stone
    Sialodocholithiasis

DIGESTIVE SYSTEM

527.6 Mucocele
Mucous:
extravasation cyst of salivary gland
retention cyst of salivary gland
Ranula
DEF: Dilated salivary gland cavity filled with mucous.

527.7 Disturbance of salivary secretion
Hyposecretion   Sialorrhea
Ptyalism   Xerostomia

527.8 Other specified diseases of the salivary glands
Benign lymphoepithelial lesion of salivary gland
Sialectasia
Sialosis
Stenosis } of salivary duct
Stricture

527.9 Unspecified disease of the salivary glands

√4th **528 Diseases of the oral soft tissues, excluding lesions specific for gingiva and tongue**

528.0 Stomatitis
Stomatitis: Vesicular stomatitis
  NOS
  ulcerative
EXCLUDES stomatitis:
  acute necrotizing ulcerative (101)
  aphthous (528.2)
  gangrenous (528.1)
  herpetic (054.2)
  Vincent's (101)
DEF: Inflammation of oral mucosa; labial and buccal mucosa, tongue, plate, floor of the mouth, and gingivae.

528.1 Cancrum oris
Gangrenous stomatitis   Noma
DEF: A severely gangrenous lesion of mouth due to fusospirochetal infection; destroys buccal, labial and facial tissues; can be fatal; found primarily in debilitated and malnourished children.

528.2 Oral aphthae
Aphthous stomatitis
Canker sore
Periadenitis mucosa necrotica recurrens
Recurrent aphthous ulcer
Stomatitis herpetiformis
EXCLUDES herpetic stomatitis (054.2)
DEF: Small oval or round ulcers of the mouth marked by a grayish exudate and a red halo effect.

528.3 Cellulitis and abscess
Cellulitis of mouth (floor)   Oral fistula
Ludwig's angina
EXCLUDES abscess of tongue (529.0)
cellulitis or abscess of lip (528.5)
fistula (of):
  dental (522.7)
  lip (528.5)
gingivitis (523.0-523.1)

528.4 Cysts
- Dermoid cyst
- Epidermoid cyst
- Epstein's pearl
- Lymphoepithelial cyst
- Nasoalveolar cyst
- Nasolabial cyst

} of mouth

EXCLUDES cyst:
- gingiva (523.8)
- tongue (529.8)

528.5 Diseases of lips
- Abscess
- Cellulitis
- Fistula
- Hypertrophy

} of lip(s)

Cheilitis: Cheilodynia
- NOS   Cheilosis
- angular

EXCLUDES
- actinic cheilitis (692.79)
- congenital fistula of lip (750.25)
- leukoplakia of lips (528.6)

528.6 Leukoplakia of oral mucosa, including tongue
- Leukokeratosis of oral mucosa
- Leukoplakia of: gingiva
- Leukoplakia of: lips
- Leukoplakia of: tongue

EXCLUDES
- carcinoma in situ (230.0, 232.0)
- leukokeratosis nicotina palati (528.7)

DEF: Thickened white patches of epithelium on mucous membranes of mouth.

528.7 Other disturbances of oral epithelium, including tongue
- Erythroplakia
- Focal epithelial hyperplasia
- Leukoedema

} of mouth or tongue

Leukokeratosis nicotina palati

EXCLUDES
- carcinoma in situ (230.0, 232.0)
- leukokeratosis NOS (702)

528.8 Oral submucosal fibrosis, including of tongue

528.9 Other and unspecified diseases of the oral soft tissues
- Cheek and lip biting   Melanoplakia
- Denture sore mouth   Papillary hyperplasia of palate
- Denture stomatitis

- Eosinophilic granuloma
- Irritative hyperplasia
- Pyogenic granuloma
- Ulcer (traumatic)

} of oral mucosa

✓4th 529 Diseases and other conditions of the tongue

529.0 Glossitis
- Abscess
- Ulceration (traumatic)

} of tongue

EXCLUDES glossitis:
- benign migratory (529.1)
- Hunter's (529.4)
- median rhomboid (529.2)
- Moeller's (529.4)

DIGESTIVE SYSTEM

529.1 **Geographic tongue**
Benign migratory glossitis
Glossitis areata exfoliativa

DEF: Chronic glossitis; marked by filiform papillae atrophy and inflammation; no known etiology.

529.2 **Median rhomboid glossitis**

DEF: A noninflammatory, congenital disease characterized by rhomboid-like lesions at the middle third of the tongue's dorsal surface.

529.3 **Hypertrophy of tongue papillae**
Black hairy tongue   Hypertrophy of foliate papillae
Coated tongue   Lingua villosa nigra

529.4 **Atrophy of tongue papillae**
Bald tongue   Glossitis:
Glazed tongue   Moeller's
Glossitis: Glossodynia exfoliativa
  Hunter's   Smooth atrophic tongue

529.5 **Plicated tongue**
Fissured ⎫
Furrowed ⎬ tongue
Scrotal ⎭

EXCLUDES fissure of tongue, congenital (750.13)

DEF: Cracks, fissures or furrows, on dorsal surface of tongue.

529.6 **Glossodynia**
Glossopyrosis   Painful tongue
EXCLUDES glossodynia exfoliativa (529.4)

529.8 **Other specified conditions of the tongue**
Atrophy   ⎫
Crenated ⎬ (of) tongue
Enlargement ⎬
Hypertrophy ⎭

Glossocele
Glossoptosis

EXCLUDES
erythroplasia of tongue (528.7)
leukoplakia of tongue (528.6)
macroglossia (congenital) (750.15)
microglossia (congenital) (750.16)
oral submucosal fibrosis (528.8)

529.9 **Unspecified condition of the tongue**

DISEASES OF ESOPHAGUS, STOMACH, AND DUODENUM (530-537)

√4th 530 Diseases of esophagus
EXCLUDES esophageal varices (456.0-456.2)

530.0 **Achalasia and cardiospasm**
Achalasia (of cardia)   Megaesophagus
Aperistalsis of esophagus
EXCLUDES congenital cardiospasm (750.7)

DEF: Failure of smooth muscle fibers to relax, at gastrointestinal junctures; such as esophagogastric sphincter when swallowing.

530.1 Esophagitis

Abscess of esophagus
Esophagitis:
  NOS
  chemical
Esophagitis:
  peptic
  postoperative
  regurgitant

Use additional E code to identify cause, if induced by chemical
EXCLUDES   tuberculous esophagitis (017.8)

530.10 Esophagitis, unspecified

530.11 Reflux esophagitis
DEF: Inflammation of lower esophagus; due to regurgitated gastric acid from malfunctioning lower esophageal sphincter; causes heartburn and substernal pain.

530.12 Acute esophagitis
DEF: An acute inflammation of the mucous lining or submucosal coat of the esophagus.

530.19 Other esophagitis

530.2 Ulcer of esophagus
Ulcer of esophagus
  fungal
  peptic
Ulcer of esophagus due to ingestion of:
  aspirin
  chemicals
  medicines

Use additional E code to identify cause, if induced by chemical or drug

530.3 Stricture and stenosis of esophagus
Compression of esophagus
Obstruction of esophagus
EXCLUDES   congenital stricture of esophagus (750.3)

530.4 Perforation of esophagus
Rupture of esophagus
EXCLUDES   traumatic perforation of esophagus (862.22, 862.32, 874.4-874.5)

530.5 Dyskinesia of esophagus
Corkscrew esophagus   Esophagospasm
Curling esophagus   Spasm of esophagus
EXCLUDES   cardiospasm (530.0)

DEF: Difficulty performing voluntary esophageal movements.

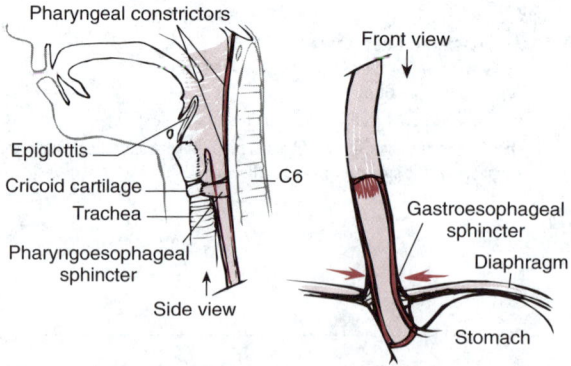

Esophagus

DIGESTIVE SYSTEM

530.6 **Diverticulum of esophagus, acquired**
Diverticulum, acquired:
  epiphrenic
  pharyngoesophageal
  pulsion
  subdiaphragmatic
  traction
  Zenker's (hypopharyngeal)
Esophageal pouch, acquired
Esophagocele, acquired
  EXCLUDES *congenital diverticulum of esophagus (750.4)*

530.7 **Gastroesophageal laceration-hemorrhage syndrome**
Mallory-Weiss syndrome
DEF: Laceration of distal esophagus and proximal stomach due to vomiting, hiccups or other sustained activity.

√5th **530.8** **Other specified disorders of esophagus**

530.81 Esophageal reflux
Gastroesophageal reflux
  EXCLUDES *reflux esophagitis (530.11)*
DEF: Regurgitation of the gastric contents into esophagus and possibly pharynx; where aspiration may occur between the vocal cords and down into the trachea.

530.82 Esophageal hemorrhage
  EXCLUDES *hemorrhage due to esophageal varices (456.0-456.2)*

530.83 Esophageal leukoplakia

530.84 Tracheoesophageal fistula
  EXCLUDES *congenital tracheoesophageal fistula (750.3)*

530.89 Other
  EXCLUDES *Paterson-Kelly syndrome (280.8)*

530.9 **Unspecified disorder of esophagus**

√4th **531 Gastric ulcer**
  INCLUDES ulcer (peptic):
    prepyloric
    pylorus
    stomach
Use additional E code to identify drug, if drug-induced
  EXCLUDES *peptic ulcer NOS (533.0-533.9)*

The following fifth-digit subclassification is for use with category 531:
  0 without mention of obstruction
  1 with obstruction

DEF: Destruction of tissue in lumen of stomach due to action of gastric acid and pepsin on gastric mucosa decreasing resistance to ulcers.

√5th **531.0** **Acute with hemorrhage**
√5th **531.1** **Acute with perforation**
√5th **531.2** **Acute with hemorrhage and perforation**
√5th **531.3** **Acute without mention of hemorrhage or perforation**
√5th **531.4** **Chronic or unspecified with hemorrhage**
√5th **531.5** **Chronic or unspecified with perforation**
√5th **531.6** **Chronic or unspecified with hemorrhage and perforation**
√5th **531.7** **Chronic without mention of hemorrhage or perforation**
√5th **531.9** **Unspecified as acute or chronic, without mention of hemorrhage or perforation**

DIGESTIVE SYSTEM

Stomach diagram with labels: Stomach, Esophagus, Diaphragm, Cardiac portion, Fundus, Pylorus, Greater curvature, Pancreas, Sphincter of Oddi, Pancreatic duct, Common bile duct, Proximal duodenum

✓4th **532 Duodenal ulcer**

[INCLUDES] erosion (acute) of duodenum
ulcer (peptic):
   duodenum
   postpyloric

Use additional E code to identify drug, if drug-induced

[EXCLUDES] *peptic ulcer NOS (533.0-533.9)*

The following fifth-digit subclassification is for use with category 532:
  0 without mention of obstruction
  1 with obstruction

DEF: Ulcers in duodenum due to action of gastric acid and pepsin on mucosa decreasing resistance to ulcers.

✓5th **532.0** Acute with hemorrhage
✓5th **532.1** Acute with perforation
✓5th **532.2** Acute with hemorrhage and perforation
✓5th **532.3** Acute without mention of hemorrhage or perforation
✓5th **532.4** Chronic or unspecified with hemorrhage
✓5th **532.5** Chronic or unspecified with perforation
✓5th **532.6** Chronic or unspecified with hemorrhage and perforation
✓5th **532.7** Chronic without mention of hemorrhage or perforation
✓5th **532.9** **Unspecified as acute or chronic, without mention of hemorrhage or perforation**

✓4th **533 Peptic ulcer, site unspecified**

[INCLUDES] gastroduodenal ulcer NOS
peptic ulcer NOS
stress ulcer NOS

Use additional E code to identify drug, if drug-induced

[EXCLUDES] *peptic ulcer:*
   duodenal (532.0-532.9)
   gastric (531.0-531.9)

The following fifth-digit subclassification is for use with category 533:
  0 without mention of obstruction
  1 with obstruction

✓5th **533.0** Acute with hemorrhage
✓5th **533.1** Acute with perforation

DIGESTIVE SYSTEM

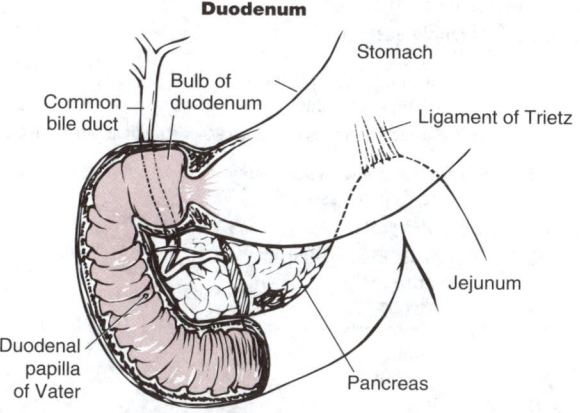

- √5th **533.2** Acute with hemorrhage and perforation
- √5th **533.3** Acute without mention of hemorrhage and perforation
- √5th **533.4** Chronic or unspecified with hemorrhage
- √5th **533.5** Chronic or unspecified with perforation
- √5th **533.6** Chronic or unspecified with hemorrhage and perforation
- √5th **533.7** Chronic without mention of hemorrhage or perforation
- √5th **533.9** Unspecified as acute or chronic, without mention of hemorrhage or perforation

√4th **534 Gastrojejunal ulcer**

INCLUDES ulcer (peptic) or erosion:
anastomotic
gastrocolic
gastrointestinal
gastrojejunal
jejunal
marginal
stomal

EXCLUDES primary ulcer of small intestine (569.82)

The following fifth-digit subclassification is for use with category 534:
0 without mention of obstruction
1 with obstruction

- √5th **534.0** Acute with hemorrhage
- √5th **534.1** Acute with perforation
- √5th **534.2** Acute with hemorrhage and perforation
- √5th **534.3** Acute without mention of hemorrhage or perforation
- √5th **534.4** Chronic or unspecified with hemorrhage
- √5th **534.5** Chronic or unspecified with perforation
- √5th **534.6** Chronic or unspecified with hemorrhage and perforation
- √5th **534.7** Chronic without mention of hemorrhage or perforation
- √5th **534.9** Unspecified as acute or chronic, without mention of hemorrhage or perforation

√4th **535 Gastritis and duodenitis**

The following fifth-digit subclassification is for use with category 535:
0 without mention of hemorrhage
1 with hemorrhage

DIGESTIVE SYSTEM

§ ✓5th **535.0 Acute gastritis**

§ ✓5th **535.1 Atrophic gastritis**
Gastritis:
   atrophic-hyperplastic
   chronic (atrophic)
DEF: Inflammation of stomach, with mucous membrane atrophy and peptic gland destruction.

§ ✓5th **535.2 Gastric mucosal hypertrophy**
Hypertrophic gastritis

§ ✓5th **535.3 Alcoholic gastritis**

§ ✓5th **535.4 Other specified gastritis**
Gastritis:
   allergic
   bile induced
   irritant
   superficial
   toxic

§ ✓5th **535.5 Unspecified gastritis and gastroduodenitis**

§ ✓5th **535.6 Duodenitis**
DEF: Inflammation of intestine, between pylorus and jejunum.

✓4th **536 Disorders of function of stomach**
   EXCLUDES *functional disorders of stomach specified as psychogenic (306.4)*

536.0 Achlorhydria
DEF: Absence of gastric acid due to gastric mucosa atrophy; unresponsive to histamines; also known as gastric anacidity.

536.1 Acute dilatation of stomach
Acute distention of stomach

536.2 Persistent vomiting
Habit vomiting
Persistent vomiting [not of pregnancy]
Uncontrollable vomiting
   EXCLUDES *excessive vomiting in pregnancy (643.0-643.9)*
   vomiting NOS (787.0)

536.3 Gastroparesis
DEF: Slight degree of paralysis within muscular coat of stomach.

✓5th **536.4 Gastrostomy complications**

   536.40 Gastrostomy complication, unspecified

   536.41 Infection of gastrostomy
      Use additional code to specify type of infection, such as:
         abscess or cellulitis of abdomen (682.2)
         septicemia (038.0-038.9)
      Use additional code to identify organism (041.00-041.9)

   536.42 Mechanical complication of gastrostomy

   536.49 Other gastrostomy complications

536.8 Dyspepsia and other specified disorders of function of stomach
Achylia gastrica   Hyperchlorhydria
Hourglass contraction   Hypochlorhydria
   of stomach   Indigestion
Hyperacidity
   EXCLUDES *achlorhydria (536.0)*
   heartburn (787.1)

§ Requires fifth-digit. See beginning of category 535 for codes and definitions.

DIGESTIVE SYSTEM

536.9 **Unspecified functional disorder of stomach**
Functional gastrointestinal:
  disorder
  disturbance
  irritation

✓4th **537 Other disorders of stomach and duodenum**

537.0 **Acquired hypertrophic pyloric stenosis**
Constriction ⎫
Obstruction ⎬ of pylorus, acquired or adult
Stricture ⎭

EXCLUDES congenital or infantile pyloric stenosis (750.5)

537.1 **Gastric diverticulum**
EXCLUDES congenital diverticulum of stomach (750.7)
DEF: Herniated sac or pouch, within stomach or duodenum.

537.2 **Chronic duodenal ileus**
DEF: Persistent obstruction between pylorus and jejunum.

537.3 **Other obstruction of duodenum**
Cicatrix ⎫
Stenosis ⎬
Stricture ⎬ of duodenum
Volvulus ⎭

EXCLUDES congenital obstruction of duodenum (751.1)

537.4 **Fistula of stomach or duodenum**
Gastrocolic fistula   Gastrojejunocolic fistula

537.5 **Gastroptosis**
DEF: Downward displacement of stomach.

537.6 **Hourglass stricture or stenosis of stomach**
Cascade stomach
EXCLUDES congenital hourglass stomach (750.7)
hourglass contraction of stomach (536.8)

✓5th **537.8** **Other specified disorders of stomach and duodenum**

537.81 Pylorospasm
EXCLUDES congenital pylorospasm (750.5)
DEF: Spasm of the pyloric sphincter.

537.82 Angiodysplasia of stomach and duodenum (without mention of hemorrhage)

537.83 Angiodysplasia of stomach and duodenum with hemorrhage
DEF: Bleeding of stomach and duodenum due to vascular abnormalities.

● **537.84** Dieulafoy lesion (hemorrhagic) of stomach and duodenum

537.89 Other
Gastric or duodenal:
  prolapse
  rupture
Intestinal metaplasia of gastric mucosa
Passive congestion of stomach
EXCLUDES diverticula of duodenum (562.00-562.01)
gastrointestinal hemorrhage (578.0-578.9)

537.9 **Unspecified disorder of stomach and duodenum**

DIGESTIVE SYSTEM

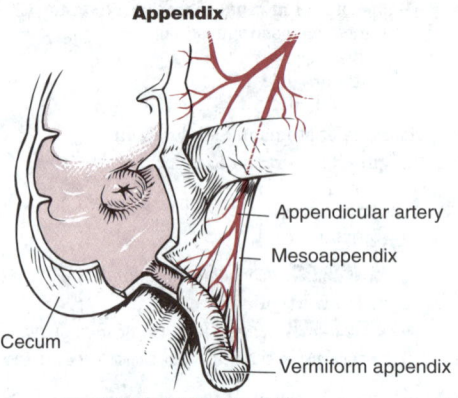

APPENDICITIS (540-543)

✓4th 540 Acute appendicitis
DEF: Inflammation of vermiform appendix due to fecal obstruction, neoplasm or foreign body of appendiceal lumen; causes infection, edema and infarction of appendiceal wall; may result in mural necrosis, and perforation.

540.0 With generalized peritonitis
Appendicitis (acute): with:
  fulminating   perforation
  gangrenous   peritonitis (generalized)
  obstructive   rupture
Cecitis (acute)

Rupture of appendix
EXCLUDES *acute appendicitis with peritoneal abscess (540.1)*

540.1 With peritoneal abscess
With generalized peritonitis
Abscess of appendix

540.9 Without mention of peritonitis
Acute:
  appendicitis:
    fulminating
    gangrenous   without mention of
    inflamed   perforation,
    obstructive   peritonitis, or rupture
    cecitis

541 Appendicitis, unqualified
542 Other appendicitis
Appendicitis: Appendicitis:
  chronic   relapsing
  recurrent   subacute
EXCLUDES *hyperplasia (lymphoid) of appendix (543.0)*

✓4th 543 Other diseases of appendix
543.0 Hyperplasia of appendix (lymphoid)
DEF: Proliferation of cells in appendix tissue.

DIGESTIVE SYSTEM

543.9 **Other and unspecified diseases of appendix**
Appendicular or appendiceal:
  colic
  concretion
  fistula
Diverticulum
Fecalith
Intussusception } of appendix
Mucocele
Stercolith

HERNIA OF ABDOMINAL CAVITY (550-553)

INCLUDES hernia:
  acquired
  congenital, except diaphragmatic or hiatal

√4th **550 Inguinal hernia**
  INCLUDES bubonocele
  inguinal hernia (direct) (double) (indirect) (oblique) (sliding)
  scrotal hernia

The following fifth-digit subclassification is for use with category 550:
  0 **unilateral or unspecified (not specified as recurrent)**
    Unilateral NOS
  1 **unilateral or unspecified, recurrent**
  2 **bilateral (not specified as recurrent)**
    Bilateral NOS
  3 **bilateral, recurrent**

DEF: Hernia: protrusion of an abdominal organ or tissue through inguinal canal.

DEF: Indirect inguinal hernia: (external or oblique) leaves abdomen through deep inguinal ring, passes through inguinal canal lateral to the inferior epigastric artery.

DEF: Direct inguinal hernia: (internal) emerges between inferior epigastric artery and rectus muscle edge.

√5th **550.0 Inguinal hernia, with gangrene**
  Inguinal hernia with gangrene (and obstruction)

√5th **550.1 Inguinal hernia, with obstruction, without mention of gangrene**
  Inguinal hernia with mention of incarceration, irreducibility, or strangulation

√5th **550.9 Inguinal hernia, without mention of obstruction or gangrene**
  Inguinal hernia NOS

√4th **551 Other hernia of abdominal cavity, with gangrene**
  INCLUDES that with gangrene (and obstruction)

√5th **551.0 Femoral hernia with gangrene**
  551.00 Unilateral or unspecified (not specified as recurrent)
    Femoral hernia NOS with gangrene
  551.01 Unilateral or unspecified, recurrent
  551.02 Bilateral (not specified as recurrent)
  551.03 Bilateral, recurrent

551.1 Umbilical hernia with gangrene
  Parumbilical hernia specified as gangrenous

√5th **551.2 Ventral hernia with gangrene**
  551.20 Ventral, unspecified, with gangrene

Inguinal Hernia

551.21 Incisional, with gangrene
Hernia:
postoperative } specified as
recurrent, ventral } gangrenous

551.29 Other
Epigastric hernia specified as gangrenous

551.3 Diaphragmatic hernia with gangrene
Hernia:
hiatal (esophageal)
(sliding) } specified as
paraesophageal } gangrenous
Thoracic stomach

EXCLUDES congenital diaphragmatic hernia (756.6)

551.8 Hernia of other specified sites, with gangrene
Any condition classifiable to 553.8 if specified as gangrenous

551.9 Hernia of unspecified site, with gangrene
Any condition classifiable to 553.9 if specified as gangrenous

√4th **552 Other hernia of abdominal cavity, with obstruction, but without mention of gangrene**

EXCLUDES that with mention of gangrene (551.0-551.9)

√5th **552.0 Femoral hernia with obstruction**
Femoral hernia specified as incarcerated, irreducible, strangulated, or causing obstruction

552.00 Unilateral or unspecified (not specified as recurrent)
552.01 Unilateral or unspecified, recurrent
552.02 Bilateral (not specified as recurrent)
552.03 Bilateral, recurrent

DIGESTIVE SYSTEM

Femoral Hernia

552.1 Umbilical hernia with obstruction
Parumbilical hernia specified as incarcerated, irreducible, strangulated, or causing obstruction

✓5ᵗʰ **552.2 Ventral hernia with obstruction**
Ventral hernia specified as incarcerated, irreducible, strangulated, or causing obstruction

552.20 Ventral, unspecified, with obstruction

552.21 Incisional, with obstruction
Hernia:
postoperative ⎤
recurrent,   ⎬ specified as incarcerated, irreducible, strangulated, or causing obstruction
ventral   ⎦

552.29 Other
Epigastric hernia specified as incarcerated, irreducible, strangulated, or causing obstruction

552.3 Diaphragmatic hernia with obstruction
Hernia:
hiatal (esophageal) ⎤
 (sliding)   ⎬ specified as incarcerated, irreducible, strangulated, or causing obstruction
paraesophageal   ⎥
Thoracic stomach   ⎦

> **EXCLUDES** congenital diaphragmatic hernia (756.6)

552.8 Hernia of other specified sites, with obstruction
Any condition classifiable to 553.8 if specified as incarcerated, irreducible, strangulated, or causing obstruction

552.9 Hernia of unspecified site, with obstruction
Any condition classifiable to 553.9 if specified as incarcerated, irreducible, strangulated, or causing obstruction

✓4ᵗʰ **553 Other hernia of abdominal cavity without mention of obstruction or gangrene**

> **EXCLUDES** the listed conditions with mention of:
> gangrene (and obstruction) (551.0-551.9)
> obstruction (552.0-552.9)

✓5ᵗʰ **553.0 Femoral hernia**

553.00 Unilateral or unspecified (not specified as recurrent)
Femoral hernia NOS

553.01 Unilateral or unspecified, recurrent

553.02 Bilateral (not specified as recurrent)

553.03 Bilateral, recurrent

DIGESTIVE SYSTEM

Hernia of Abdominal Cavity

- Hiatal hernia
- Diaphragm
- Epigastric hernia
- Incisional hernia
- Umbilical hernia
- Inguinal hernia

553.1 Umbilical hernia
Parumbilical hernia

✓5th **553.2 Ventral hernia**
    553.20 Ventral, unspecified
    553.21 Incisional
        Hernia:
            postoperative
            recurrent, ventral
    553.29 Other
        Hernia:
            epigastric
            spigelian

553.3 Diaphragmatic hernia
    Hernia:
        hiatal (esophageal) (sliding)
        paraesophageal
    Thoracic stomach
        EXCLUDES congenital:
            diaphragmatic hernia (756.6)
            hiatal hernia (750.6)
            esophagocele (530.6)

DIGESTIVE SYSTEM

553.8 Hernia of other specified sites
Hernia:
 ischiatic
 ischiorectal
 lumbar
 obturator
Hernia:
 pudendal
 retroperitoneal
 sciatic
Other abdominal hernia of specified site
> **EXCLUDES** vaginal enterocele (618.6)

553.9 Hernia of unspecified site
Enterocele
Epiplocele
Hernia:
 NOS
 interstitial
Hernia:
 intestinal
 intra-abdominal
Rupture (nontraumatic)
Sarcoepiplocele

NONINFECTIOUS ENTERITIS AND COLITIS (555-558)

✓4th 555 Regional enteritis
> **INCLUDES** Crohn's disease
> Granulomatous enteritis
> **EXCLUDES** ulcerative colitis (556)

DEF: Inflammation of intestine; classified to site.

555.0 Small intestine
Ileitis:
 regional
 segmental
 terminal
Regional enteritis or Crohn's disease of:
 duodenum
 ileum
 jejunum

555.1 Large intestine
Colitis:
 granulmatous
 regional
 transmural
Regional enteritis or Crohn's disease of:
 colon
 large bowel
 rectum

555.2 Small intestine with large intestine
Regional ileocolitis

555.9 Unspecified site
Crohn's disease NOS
Regional enteritis NOS

✓4th 556 Ulcerative colitis
DEF: Chronic inflammation of mucosal lining of intestinal tract; may be single area or entire colon.

556.0 Ulcerative (chronic) enterocolitis
556.1 Ulcerative (chronic) ileocolitis
556.2 Ulcerative (chronic) proctitis
556.3 Ulcerative (chronic) proctosigmoiditis
556.4 Pseudopolyposis of colon
556.5 Left-sided ulcerative (chronic) colitis
556.6 Universal ulcerative (chronic) colitis
Pancolitis
556.8 Other ulcerative colitis
556.9 Ulcerative colitis, unspecified
Ulcerative enteritis NOS

DIGESTIVE SYSTEM

✓4th 557 Vascular insufficiency of intestine
    EXCLUDES *necrotizing enterocolitis of the newborn (777.5)*
DEF: Inadequacy of intestinal vessels.

- **557.0 Acute vascular insufficiency of intestine**
  Acute:
    hemorrhagic enterocolitis
    ischemic colitis, enteritis, or enterocolitis
    massive necrosis of intestine
  Bowel infarction
  Embolism of mesenteric artery
  Fulminant enterocolitis
  Hemorrhagic necrosis of intestine
  Infarction of appendices epiploicae
  Intestinal gangrene
  Intestinal infarction (acute) (agnogenic) (hemorrhagic) (nonocclusive)
  Mesenteric infarction (embolic) (thrombotic)
  Necrosis of intestine
  Terminal hemorrhagic enteropathy
  Thrombosis of mesenteric artery

- **557.1 Chronic vascular insufficiency of intestine**
  Angina, abdominal
  Chronic ischemic colitis, enteritis, or enterocolitis
  Ischemic stricture of intestine
  Mesenteric:
    angina
    artery syndrome (superior)
    vascular insufficiency

- **557.9 Unspecified vascular insufficiency of intestine**
  Alimentary pain due to vascular insufficiency
  Ischemic colitis, enteritis, or enterocolitis NOS

✓4th 558 Other and unspecified noninfectious gastroenteritis and colitis
    EXCLUDES *infectious:*
        colitis, enteritis, or gastroenteritis (009.0-009.1)
        diarrhea (009.2-009.3)

- **558.1 Gastroenteritis and colitis due to radiation**
  Radiation enterocolitis

- **558.2 Toxic gastroenteritis and colitis**
  Use additional E code, if desired, to identify cause

- **558.3 Allergic gastroenteritis and colitis**
  DEF: True immunoglobulin E (IgE)-mediated allergic reaction of the lining of the stomach, intestines, or colon to food proteins; causes nausea, vomiting, diarrhea, and abdominal cramping.

- **558.9 Other and unspecified noninfectious gastroenteritis and colitis**
  Colitis
  Enteritis
  Gastroenteritis   } NOS, dietetic, or
  Ileitis   noninfectious
  Jejunitis
  Sigmoiditis

DIGESTIVE SYSTEM 560–560.39

OTHER DISEASES OF INTESTINES AND PERITONEUM (560-569)

✓4th 560 Intestinal obstruction without mention of hernia

> **EXCLUDES** duodenum (537.2-537.3)
> inguinal hernia with obstruction (550.1)
> intestinal obstruction complicating hernia (552.0-552.9)
> mesenteric:
>   embolism (557.0)
>   infarction (557.0)
>   thrombosis (557.0)
> neonatal intestinal obstruction (277.01, 777.1-777.2, 777.4)

560.0 Intussusception
Intussusception (colon) (intestine) (rectum)
Invagination of intestine or colon

> **EXCLUDES** intussusception of appendix (543.9)

DEF: Prolapse of a bowel section into adjacent section; occurs primarily in children; symptoms include paroxysmal pain, vomiting, presence of lower abdominal tumor and blood, and mucous passage from rectum.

560.1 Paralytic ileus
Adynamic ileus
Ileus (of intestine) (of bowel) (of colon)
Paralysis of intestine or colon

> **EXCLUDES** gallstone ileus (560.31)

DEF: Obstruction of ileus due to inhibited bowel motility.

560.2 Volvulus
Knotting
Strangulation   } of intestine, bowel, or
Torsion   colon
Twist

DEF: Entanglement of bowel; causes obstruction; may compromise bowel circulation.

✓5th 560.3 Impaction of intestine

560.30 Impaction of intestine, unspecified
Impaction of colon

560.31 Gallstone ileus
Obstruction of intestine by gallstone

560.39 Other
Concretion of intestine   Fecal impaction
Enterolith

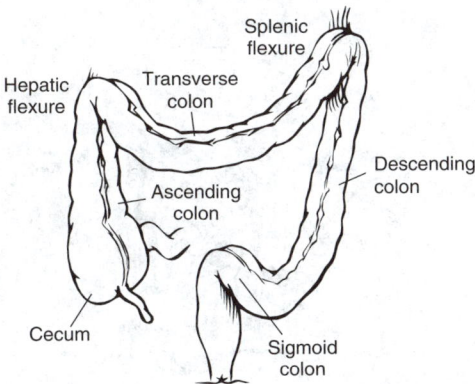

Large Intestine

✓4th Additional Digit Required   Unspecified Code   Other Specified Code   Manifestation Code
✓5th
MSP Medicare Secondary Payer   ▶◀ Revised Text   ● New Code   ▲ Revised Code Title

2002 Ingenix, Inc.   Volume 1 — 315

DIGESTIVE SYSTEM

√5th **560.8 Other specified intestinal obstruction**

560.81 Intestinal or peritoneal adhesions with obstruction (postoperative) (postinfection)
- EXCLUDES: adhesions without obstruction (568.0)
- DEF: Obstruction of peritoneum or intestine due to abnormal union of tissues.

560.89 Other
- Mural thickening causing obstruction
- EXCLUDES: ischemic stricture of intestine (557.1)

560.9 Unspecified intestinal obstruction
- Enterostenosis
- Obstruction
- Occlusion
- Stenosis
- Stricture

  } of intestine or colon

- EXCLUDES: congenital stricture or stenosis of intestine (751.1-751.2)

√4th **562 Diverticula of intestine**

Use additional code to identify any associated:
peritonitis (567.0-567.9)

EXCLUDES:
- congenital diverticulum of colon (751.5)
- diverticulum of appendix (543.9)
- Meckel's diverticulum (751.0)

√5th **562.0 Small intestine**

562.00 Diverticulosis of small intestine (without mention of hemorrhage)
Diverticulosis:
- duodenum
- ileum
- jejunum

} without mention of diverticulitis

DEF: Saclike herniations of mucous lining of small intestine.

562.01 Diverticulitis of small intestine (without mention of hemorrhage)
Diverticulitis (with diverticulosis):
- duodenum
- ileum
- jejunum
- small intestine

DEF: Inflamed saclike herniations of mucous lining of small intestine.

Volvulus, Diverticulitis

- Knotted intestine (volvulus)
- Diverticulum

DIGESTIVE SYSTEM

- **562.02** Diverticulosis of small intestine with hemorrhage
- **562.03** Diverticulitis of small intestine with hemorrhage

√5th **562.1** Colon

- **562.10** Diverticulosis of colon (without mention of hemorrhage)

  Diverticulosis:
  NOS
  intestine (large)
  Diverticular disease (colon)
  } without mention of diverticulitis

  DEF: Saclike herniations of mucous lining of large intestine

- **562.11** Diverticulitis of colon (without mention of hemorrhage)

  Diverticulitis (with diverticulosis):
  NOS
  colon
  intestine (large)

  DEF: Inflamed saclike herniations of mucosal lining of large intestine.

- **562.12** Diverticulosis of colon with hemorrhage
- **562.13** Diverticulitis of colon with hemorrhage

√4th **564** Functional digestive disorders, not elsewhere classified

  EXCLUDES functional disorders of stomach (536.0-536.9)
  those specified as psychogenic (306.4)

√5th **564.0** Constipation

- **564.00** Constipation, unspecified
- **564.01** Slow transit constipation

  DEF: Delay in the transit of fecal material through the colon secondary to smooth muscle dysfunction or decreased peristaltic contractions along the colon: also called colonic inertia or delayed transit.

- **564.02** Outlet dysfunction constipation

  DEF: Failure to relax the paradoxical contractions of the striated pelvic floor muscles during the attempted defecation.

- **564.09** Other constipation

564.1 Irritable bowel syndrome

  Irritable colon   Spastic colon

  DEF: Functional gastrointestinal disorder (FGID); symptoms following meals include diarrhea, constipation, abdominal pain; other symptoms include bloating, gas, distended abdomen, nausea, vomiting, appetite loss, emotional distress, and depression.

564.2 Postgastric surgery syndromes

  Dumping syndrome   Postgastrectomy syndrome
  Jejunal syndrome   Postvagotomy syndrome

  EXCLUDES malnutrition following gastrointestinal surgery (579.3)
  postgastrojejunostomy ulcer (534.0-534.9)

564.3 Vomiting following gastrointestinal surgery

  Vomiting (bilious) following gastrointestinal surgery

564.4 Other postoperative functional disorders

  Diarrhea following gastrointestinal surgery

  EXCLUDES colostomy and enterostomy complications (569.60-569.69)

564.5 Functional diarrhea

  EXCLUDES diarrhea:
  NOS (787.91)
  psychogenic (306.4)

  DEF: Diarrhea with no detectable organic cause.

564.6 Anal spasm

  Proctalgia fugax

√4th/√5th Additional Digit Required   Unspecified Code   Other Specified Code   Manifestation Code

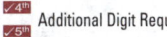 Medicare Secondary Payer   ►◄ Revised Text   ● New Code   ▲ Revised Code Title

2002 Ingenix, Inc.

564.7 Megacolon, other than Hirschsprung's
Dilatation of colon

EXCLUDES megacolon:
congenital [Hirschsprung's] (751.3)
toxic (556)

DEF: Enlarged colon; congenital or acquired; can occur acutely or become chronic.

✓5th 564.8 Other specified functional disorders of intestine
EXCLUDES malabsorption (579.0-579.9)

564.81 Neurogenic bowel
DEF: Disorder of bowel due to spinal cord lesion above conus medullaris; symptoms include precipitous micturition, nocturia, catheter intolerance, headache, sweating, nasal obstruction and spastic contractions.

564.89 Other functional disorders of intestine
Atony of colon

DEF: Absence of normal bowel tone or strength.

564.9 Unspecified functional disorder of intestine

✓4th 565 Anal fissure and fistula

565.0 Anal fissure
Tear of anus, nontraumatic

EXCLUDES traumatic (863.89, 863.99)

DEF: Ulceration of cleft at anal mucosa; causes pain, itching, bleeding, infection, and sphincter spasm; may occur with hemorrhoids.

565.1 Anal fistula
Fistula:
  anorectal
  rectal
  rectum to skin

EXCLUDES fistula of rectum to internal organs—see Alphabetic Index
ischiorectal fistula (566)
rectovaginal fistula (619.1)

DEF: Abnormal opening on cutaneous surface near anus; may lack connection with rectum.

566 Abscess of anal and rectal regions
Abscess:
  ischiorectal
  perianal
  perirectal
Cellulitis:
  anal

Cellulitis:
  perirectal
  rectal
Ischiorectal fistula

✓4th 567 Peritonitis
EXCLUDES peritonitis:
benign paroxysmal (277.3)
pelvic, female (614.5, 614.7)
periodic familial (277.3)
puerperal (670)
with or following:
  abortion (634-638 with .0, 639.0)
  appendicitis (540.0-540.1)
  ectopic or molar pregnancy (639.0)

DEF: Inflammation of the peritoneal cavity.

567.0 Peritonitis in infectious diseases classified elsewhere
Code first underlying disease

EXCLUDES peritonitis:
gonococcal (098.86)
syphilitic (095.2)
tuberculous (014.0)

DIGESTIVE SYSTEM

567.1 Pneumococcal peritonitis
567.2 **Other suppurative peritonitis**
    Abscess (of):
        abdominopelvic
        mesenteric
        omentum
        peritoneum
        retrocecal
        retroperitoneal
        subdiaphragmatic
    Abscess (of):
        subhepatic
        subphrenic
    Peritonitis (acute):
        general
        pelvic, male
        subphrenic
        suppurative

567.8 **Other specified peritonitis**
    Chronic proliferative peritonitis
    Fat necrosis of peritoneum
    Mesenteric saponification
    Peritonitis due to:
        bile
        urine

567.9 **Unspecified peritonitis**
    Peritonitis:
        NOS
    Peritonitis:
        of unspecified cause

√4th **568 Other disorders of peritoneum**

    568.0 Peritoneal adhesions (postoperative) (postinfection)
        Adhesions (of):
            abdominal (wall)
            diaphragm
            intestine
            male pelvis
        Adhesions (of):
            mesenteric
            omentum
            stomach
        Adhesive bands

        EXCLUDES adhesions:
            pelvic, female (614.6)
            with obstruction:
                duodenum (537.3)
                intestine (560.81)

    DEF: Abnormal union of tissues in peritoneum.

√5th **568.8 Other specified disorders of peritoneum**
    568.81 Hemoperitoneum (nontraumatic)
    568.82 Peritoneal effusion (chronic)
        EXCLUDES ascites NOS (789.5)
    DEF: Persistent leakage of fluid within peritoneal cavity.

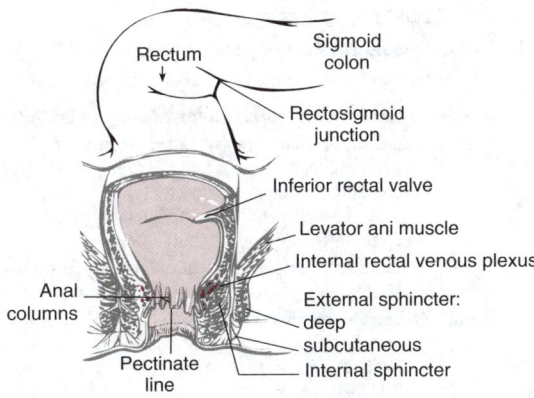

Rectum and Anus

568.89 Other
  Peritoneal:
    cyst
    granuloma

568.9 Unspecified disorder of peritoneum

√4ᵗʰ **569 Other disorders of intestine**

569.0 Anal and rectal polyp
  Anal and rectal polyp NOS
  EXCLUDES adenomatous anal and rectal polyp (211.4)

569.1 Rectal prolapse
  Procidentia:
    anus (sphincter)
    rectum (sphincter)
  Proctoptosis
  Prolapse:
    anal canal
    rectal mucosa
  EXCLUDES prolapsed hemorrhoids (455.2, 455.5)

569.2 Stenosis of rectum and anus
  Stricture of anus (sphincter)

569.3 Hemorrhage of rectum and anus
  EXCLUDES gastrointestinal bleeding NOS (578.9)
    melena (578.1)

√5ᵗʰ **569.4 Other specified disorders of rectum and anus**

  569.41 Ulcer of anus and rectum
    Solitary ulcer ⎫ of anus (sphincter) or
    Stercoral ulcer ⎭ rectum (sphincter)

  569.42 Anal or rectal pain

  569.49 Other
    Granuloma ⎫ of rectum (sphincter)
    Rupture   ⎭
    Hypertrophy of anal papillae
    Proctitis NOS
    EXCLUDES fistula of rectum to:
      internal organs—see Alphabetic Index
      skin (565.1)
      hemorrhoids (455.0-455.9)
      incontinence of sphincter ani (787.6)

569.5 Abscess of intestine
  EXCLUDES appendiceal abscess (540.1)

√5ᵗʰ **569.6 Colostomy and enterostomy complications**
  DEF: Complication in a surgically created opening, from intestine to surface skin.

  569.60 Colostomy and enterostomy complication, unspecified

  569.61 Infection of colostomy or enterostomy
    Use additional code to identify organism (041.00-041.9)
    Use additional code to specify type of infection, such as:
      abscess or cellulitis of abdomen (682.2)
      septicemia (038.0-038.9)

  569.62 Mechanical complication of colostomy and enterostomy
    Malfunction of colostomy and enterostomy

  569.69 Other complication
    Fistula
    Hernia
    Prolapse

DIGESTIVE SYSTEM

✓5th 569.8 Other specified disorder of intestine

    569.81 Fistula of intestine, excluding rectum and anus
        Fistula: Fistula:
        abdominal wall   enteroenteric
        enterocolic   ileorectal

        EXCLUDES *fistula of intestine to internal organs—see Alphabetic Index*
            persistent postoperative fistula (998.6)

    569.82 Ulceration of intestine
        Primary ulcer of intestine
        Ulceration of colon
        EXCLUDES *that with perforation (569.83)*

    569.83 Perforation of intestine

    569.84 Angiodysplasia of intestine (without mention of hemorrhage)
        DEF: Small vascular abnormalities of the intestinal tract without bleeding problems.

    569.85 Angiodysplasia of intestine with hemorrhage
        DEF: Small vascular abnormalities of the intestinal tract with bleeding problems.

•   **569.86 Dieulafoy lesion (hemorrhagic) of intestine**

    569.89 Other
        Enteroptosis
        Granuloma   } of intestine
        Prolapse

        Pericolitis
        Perisigmoiditis
        Visceroptosis
        EXCLUDES *gangrene of intestine, mesentery, or omentum (557.0)*
            hemorrhage of intestine NOS (578.9)
            obstruction of intestine (560.0-560.9)

569.9 Unspecified disorder of intestine

OTHER DISEASES OF DIGESTIVE SYSTEM (570-579)

570 Acute and subacute necrosis of liver
    Acute hepatic failure
    Acute or subacute hepatitis, not specified as infective
    Necrosis of liver (acute) (diffuse) (massive) (subacute)
    Parenchymatous degeneration of liver
    Yellow atrophy (liver) (acute) (subacute)
    EXCLUDES *icterus gravis of newborn (773.0-773.2)*
        serum hepatitis (070.2-070.3)
        that with:
            abortion (634-638 with .7, 639.8)
            ectopic or molar pregnancy (639.8)
            pregnancy, childbirth, or the puerperium (646.7)
        viral hepatitis (070.0-070.9)

✓4th 571 Chronic liver disease and cirrhosis

    571.0 Alcoholic fatty liver   ▲

    571.1 Acute alcoholic hepatitis   ▲
        Acute alcoholic liver disease

    571.2 Alcoholic cirrhosis of liver   ▲
        Florid cirrhosis
        Laennec's cirrhosis (alcoholic)
    DEF: Fibrosis and dysfunction, of liver; due to alcoholic liver disease.

    571.3 Alcoholic liver damage, unspecified   ▲

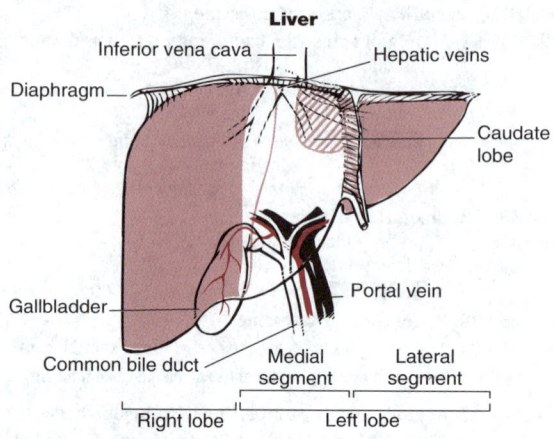

- ✓5th **571.4 Chronic hepatitis**

  EXCLUDES viral hepatitis (acute) (chronic) (070.0-070.9)

  571.40 Chronic hepatitis, unspecified
  571.41 Chronic persistent hepatitis
  571.49 Other
  Chronic hepatitis:
  active
  aggressive
  Recurrent hepatitis

- **571.5 Cirrhosis of liver without mention of alcohol**
  Cirrhosis of liver: Cirrhosis of liver:
  NOS   postnecrotic
  cryptogenic   Healed yellow atrophy
  macronodular   (liver)
  micronodular   Portal cirrhosis
  posthepatitic

  DEF: Fibrosis and dysfunction of liver; not alcohol related.

- **571.6 Biliary cirrhosis**
  Chronic nonsuppurative destructive cholangitis
  Cirrhosis:
    cholangitic
    cholestatic

- **571.8 Other chronic nonalcoholic liver disease**
  Chronic yellow atrophy (liver)
  Fatty liver, without mention of alcohol

- **571.9 Unspecified chronic liver disease without mention of alcohol**

✓4th **572 Liver abscess and sequelae of chronic liver disease**

  572.0 Abscess of liver

  EXCLUDES amebic liver abscess (006.3)

  572.1 Portal pyemia
  Phlebitis of portal vein   Pylephlebitis
  Portal thrombophlebitis   Pylethrombophlebitis

  DEF: Inflammation of portal vein or branches; may be due to intestinal disease; symptoms include fever, chills, jaundice, sweating, and abscess in various body parts.

  572.2 Hepatic coma
  Hepatic encephalopathy
  Hepatocerebral intoxication
  Portal-systemic encephalopathy

DIGESTIVE SYSTEM

572.3 Portal hypertension
DEF: Abnormally high blood pressure in the portal vein.

572.4 Hepatorenal syndrome
> EXCLUDES that following delivery (674.8)

DEF: Hepatic and renal failure characterized by cirrhosis with ascites or obstructive jaundice, oliguria, and low sodium concentration.

572.8 Other sequelae of chronic liver disease

✓4th 573 Other disorders of liver
> EXCLUDES amyloid or lardaceous degeneration of liver (277.3)
> congenital cystic disease of liver (751.62)
> glycogen infiltration of liver (271.0)
> hepatomegaly NOS (789.1)
> portal vein obstruction (452)

573.0 Chronic passive congestion of liver
DEF: Blood accumulation in liver tissue.

573.1 Hepatitis in viral diseases classified elsewhere
Code first underlying disease as:
  Coxsackie virus disease (074.8)
  cytomegalic inclusion virus disease (078.5)
  infectious mononucleosis (075)
> EXCLUDES hepatitis (in):
> mumps (072.71)
> viral (070.0-070.9)
> yellow fever (060.0-060.9)

573.2 Hepatitis in other infectious diseases classified elsewhere
Code first underlying disease, as:
  malaria (084.9)
> EXCLUDES hepatitis in:
> late syphilis (095.3)
> secondary syphilis (091.62)
> toxoplasmosis (130.5)

573.3 Hepatitis, unspecified
Toxic (noninfectious) hepatitis
Use additional E code to identify cause

573.4 Hepatic infarction

573.8 Other specified disorders of liver
Hepatoptosis

573.9 Unspecified disorder of liver

✓4th 574 Cholelithiasis
The following fifth-digit subclassification is for use with category 574:
  0 without mention of obstruction
  1 with obstruction

✓5th 574.0 Calculus of gallbladder with acute cholecystitis   ▲
Biliary calculus
Calculus of cystic duct } with acute cholecystitis
Cholelithiasis

Any condition classifiable to 574.2 with acute cholecystitis

✓4th / ✓5th Additional Digit Required   Unspecified Code   Other Specified Code   Manifestation Code
MSP Medicare Secondary Payer   ▶◀ Revised Text   ● New Code   ▲ Revised Code Title

2002 Ingenix, Inc.

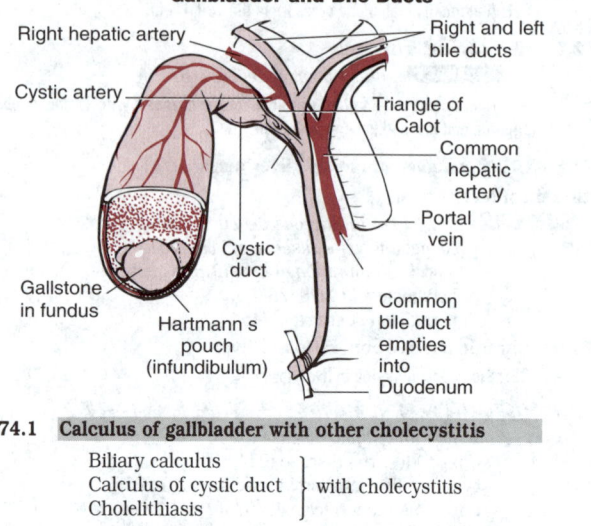

Gallbladder and Bile Ducts

§ √5th **574.1 Calculus of gallbladder with other cholecystitis**
  Biliary calculus
  Calculus of cystic duct } with cholecystitis
  Cholelithiasis

  Cholecystitis with cholelithiasis NOS
  Any condition classifiable to 574.2 with cholecystitis (chronic)

§ √5th **574.2 Calculus of gallbladder without mention of cholecystitis**
  Biliary: Cholelithiasis NOS
    calculus NOS   Colic (recurrent) of
    colic NOS   gallbladder
  Calculus of cystic duct Gallstone (impacted)

§ √5th **574.3 Calculus of bile duct with acute cholecystitis**
  Calculus of bile
    duct [any]   } with acute cholecystitis
  Choledocholithiasis

  Any condition classifiable to 574.5 with acute cholecystitis

§ √5th **574.4 Calculus of bile duct with other cholecystitis**
  Calculus of bile duct [any]
  Choledocholithiasis } with cholecystitis (chronic)

  Any condition classifiable to 574.5 with cholecystitis (chronic)

§ √5th **574.5 Calculus of bile duct without mention of cholecystitis**
  Calculus of: Choledocholithiasis
    bile duct [any]   Hepatic:
    common duct   colic (recurrent)
    hepatic duct   lithiasis

§ √5th **574.6 Calculus of gallbladder and bile duct with acute cholecystitis**
  Any condition classifiable to 574.0 and 574.3

§ √5th **574.7 Calculus of gallbladder and bile duct with other cholecystitis**
  Any condition classifiable to 574.1 and 574.4

§ √5th **574.8 Calculus of gallbladder and bile duct with acute and chronic cholecystitis**
  Any condition classifiable to 574.6 and 574.7

§ √5th **574.9 Calculus of gallbladder and bile duct without cholecystitis**
  Any condition classifiable to 574.2 and 574.5

§ Requires fifth-digit. See beginning of category 574 for codes and definitions.

DIGESTIVE SYSTEM

✓4ᵗʰ 575 Other disorders of gallbladder

575.0 Acute cholecystitis
Abscess of gallbladder
Angiocholecystitis
Cholecystitis:
  emphysematous (acute) ⎫
  gangrenous   ⎬ without mention
  suppurative   ⎭ of calculus
Empyema of gallbladder
Gangrene of gallbladder

> **EXCLUDES** that with:
> acute and chronic cholecystitis (575.12)
> choledocholithiasis (574.3)
> choledocholithiasis and cholelithiasis (574.6)
> cholelithiasis (574.0)

✓5ᵗʰ 575.1 Other cholecystitis
Cholecystitis:
  NOS   ⎫ without mention of calculus
  chronic ⎭

> **EXCLUDES** that with:
> choledocholithiasis (574.4)
> choledocholithiasis and cholelithiasis (574.8)
> cholelithiasis (574.1)

575.10 Cholecystitis, unspecified
Cholecystitis NOS

575.11 Chronic cholecystitis

575.12 Acute and chronic cholecystitis

575.2 Obstruction of gallbladder
Occlusion ⎫
Stenosis   ⎬ of cystic duct or gallbladder without
Stricture ⎭   mention of calculus

> **EXCLUDES** that with calculus (574.0-574.2 with fifth-digit 1)

575.3 Hydrops of gallbladder
Mucocele of gallbladder
DEF: Serous fluid accumulation in bladder.

575.4 Perforation of gallbladder
Rupture of cystic duct or gallbladder

575.5 Fistula of gallbladder
Fistula:
  cholecystoduodenal
  cholecystoenteric

575.6 Cholesterolosis of gallbladder
Strawberry gallbladder
DEF: Cholesterol deposits in gallbladder tissue.

575.8 Other specified disorders of gallbladder

Adhesions
Atrophy
Cyst   } (of) cystic duct or gallbladder
Hypertrophy
Nonfunctioning
Ulcer

Biliary dyskinesia
> **EXCLUDES** Hartmann's pouch of intestine (V44.3)
> nonvisualization of gallbladder (793.3)

575.9 Unspecified disorder of gallbladder

√4ᵗʰ **576 Other disorders of biliary tract**
> **EXCLUDES** that involving the:
> cystic duct (575.0-575.9)
> gallbladder (575.0-575.9)

576.0 Postcholecystectomy syndrome   **A**
DEF: Jaundice or abdominal pain following cholecystectomy.

576.1 Cholangitis

Cholangitis:	Cholangitis:
NOS	recurrent
acute	sclerosing
ascending	secondary
chronic	stenosing
primary	suppurative

576.2 Obstruction of bile duct

Occlusion } of bile duct, except cystic
Stenosis   } duct, without mention
Stricture } of calculus

> **EXCLUDES** congenital (751.61)
> that with calculus (574.3-574.5 with fifth-digit 1)

576.3 Perforation of bile duct
Rupture of bile duct, except cystic duct

576.4 Fistula of bile duct
Choledochoduodenal fistula

576.5 Spasm of sphincter of Oddi

DIGESTIVE SYSTEM

576.8 Other specified disorders of biliary tract
- Adhesions ⎫
- Atrophy ⎪
- Cyst ⎬ of bile duct [any]
- Hypertrophy ⎪
- Stasis ⎪
- Ulcer ⎭

EXCLUDES congenital choledochal cyst (751.69)

576.9 Unspecified disorder of biliary tract

577 Diseases of pancreas

577.0 Acute pancreatitis
- Abscess of pancreas
- Necrosis of pancreas:
  - acute
  - infective
- Pancreatitis:
  - NOS
  - acute (recurrent)
  - apoplectic
  - hemorrhagic
  - subacute
  - suppurative

EXCLUDES mumps pancreatitis (072.3)

577.1 Chronic pancreatitis
- Chronic pancreatitis:
  - NOS
  - infectious
  - interstitial
- Pancreatitis:
  - painless
  - recurrent
  - relapsing

577.2 Cyst and pseudocyst of pancreas

577.8 Other specified diseases of pancreas
- Atrophy ⎫
- Calculus ⎪
- Cirrhosis ⎬ of pancreas
- Fibrosis ⎭

Pancreatic: Pancreatic:
  infantilism   necrosis:
  necrosis: fat
    NOS   Pancreatolithiasis
    aseptic

EXCLUDES fibrocystic disease of pancreas ►(277.00-277.09)◄
islet cell tumor of pancreas (211.7)
pancreatic steatorrhea (579.4)

577.9 Unspecified disease of pancreas

DIGESTIVE SYSTEM

✓4th 578 Gastrointestinal hemorrhage
EXCLUDES that with mention of:
> angiodysplasia of stomach and duodenum (537.83)
> angiodysplasia of intestine (569.85)
> diverticulitis, intestine:
>> large (562.13)
>> small (562.03)
>
> diverticulosis, intestine:
>> large (562.12)
>> small (562.02)
>
> gastritis and duodenitis (535.0-535.6)
> ulcer:
>> duodenal, gastric, gastrojejuunal or peptic (531.00-534.91)

578.0 Hematemesis
> Vomiting of blood

578.1 Blood in stool
> Melena
> **EXCLUDES** melena of the newborn (772.4, 777.3)
> occult blood (792.1)

578.9 Hemorrhage of gastrointestinal tract, unspecified
> Gastric hemorrhage
> Intestinal hemorrhage

✓4th 579 Intestinal malabsorption

579.0 Celiac disease
> Celiac:
>> crisis
>> infantilism
>> rickets
>
> Gee (-Herter) disease
> Gluten enteropathy
> Idiopathic steatorrhea
> Nontropical sprue
>
> **DEF:** Malabsorption syndrome due to gluten consumption; symptoms include fetid, bulky, frothy, oily stools; distended abdomen, gas, weight loss, asthenia, electrolyte depletion and vitamin B, D and K deficiency.

579.1 Tropical sprue
> Sprue:
>> NOS
>> tropical
>
> Tropical steatorrhea
>
> **DEF:** Diarrhea, occurs in tropics; may be due to enteric infection and malnutrition.

579.2 Blind loop syndrome
> Postoperative blind loop syndrome
>
> **DEF:** Obstruction or impaired passage in small intestine due to alterations, from strictures or surgery; causes stasis, abnormal bacterial flora, diarrhea, weight loss, multiple vitamin deficiency, and megaloblastic anemia.

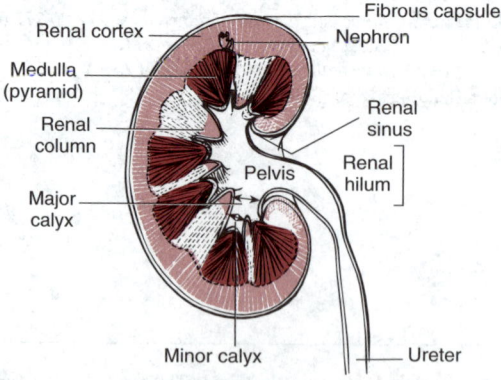

Kidney

GENITOURINARY SYSTEM

579.3 Other and unspecified postsurgical nonabsorption
   Hypoglycemia ⎱ following gastrointestinal
   Malnutrition ⎰ surgery

579.4 Pancreatic steatorrhea
   DEF: Excess fat in feces due to absence of pancreatic juice in intestine.

579.8 Other specified intestinal malabsorption
   Enteropathy: Steatorrhea (chronic)
      exudative
      protein-losing

579.9 Unspecified intestinal malabsorption
   Malabsorption syndrome NOS

10. DISEASES OF THE GENITOURINARY SYSTEM (580-629)

NEPHRITIS, NEPHROTIC SYNDROME, AND NEPHROSIS (580-589)
   EXCLUDES *hypertensive renal disease (403.00-403.91)*

✓4th **580 Acute glomerulonephritis**
   INCLUDES acute nephritis
   DEF: Acute, severe inflammation in tuft of capillaries that filter the kidneys.

   580.0 With lesion of proliferative glomerulonephritis
      Acute (diffuse) proliferative glomerulonephritis
      Acute poststreptococcal glomerulonephritis

   580.4 With lesion of rapidly progressive glomerulonephritis
      Acute nephritis with lesion of necrotizing glomerulitis
      DEF: Acute glomerulonephritis; progresses to ESRD with diffuse epithelial proliferation.

✓5th **580.8 With other specified pathological lesion in kidney**

   580.81 Acute glomerulonephritis in diseases classified elsewhere
      Code first underlying disease, as:
         infectious hepatitis (070.0-070.9)
         mumps (072.79)
         subacute bacterial endocarditis (421.0)
         typhoid fever (002.0)

   580.89 Other
      Glomerulonephritis, acute, with lesion of:
         exudative nephritis
         interstitial (diffuse) (focal) nephritis

   580.9 Acute glomerulonephritis with unspecified pathological lesion in kidney
      Glomerulonephritis: ⎫
         NOS   ⎪
         hemorrhagic   ⎬ specified as acute
      Nephritis   ⎪
      Nephropathy   ⎭

✓4th **581 Nephrotic syndrome**
   DEF: Disease process marked by symptoms such as; extensive edema, notable proteinuria, hypoalbuminemia, and susceptibility to intercurrent infections.

   581.0 With lesion of proliferative glomerulonephritis

581.1 With lesion of membranous glomerulonephritis
Epimembranous nephritis
Idiopathic membranous glomerular disease
Nephrotic syndrome with lesion of:
   focal glomerulosclerosis
   sclerosing membranous glomerulonephritis
   segmental hyalinosis

581.2 With lesion of membranoproliferative glomerulonephritis
Nephrotic syndrome with lesion (of):
   endothelial
   hypocomplementemic persistent
   lobular
   mesangiocapillary   } glomerulonephritis
   mixed membranous and proliferative

DEF: Glomerulonephritis combined with clinical features of nephrotic syndrome; characterized by uneven thickening of glomerular capillary walls and mesangial cell increase; slowly progresses to ESRD.

581.3 With lesion of minimal change glomerulonephritis
Foot process disease   Minimal change:
Lipoid nephrosis   glomerulitis
Minimal change: nephrotic syndrome
   glomerular disease

√5ᵗʰ **581.8 With other specified pathological lesion in kidney**

581.81 Nephrotic syndrome in diseases classified elsewhere
Code first underlying disease, as:
   amyloidosis (277.3)
   diabetes mellitus (250.4)
   malaria (084.9)
   polyarteritis (446.0)
   systemic lupus erythematosus (710.0)
   EXCLUDES nephrosis in epidemic hemorrhagic fever (078.6)

581.89 Other
Glomerulonephritis with edema and lesion of:
   exudative nephritis
   interstitial (diffuse) (focal) nephritis

GENITOURINARY SYSTEM

581.9 Nephrotic syndrome with unspecified pathological lesion in kidney
Glomerulonephritis with edema NOS
Nephritis:
nephrotic NOS
with edema NOS
Nephrosis NOS
Renal disease with edema NOS

√4th **582 Chronic glomerulonephritis**
INCLUDES chronic nephritis

DEF: Slow progressive type of nephritis characterized by inflammation of the capillary loops in the glomeruli of the kidney, which leads to renal failure.

582.0 With lesion of proliferative glomerulonephritis
Chronic (diffuse) proliferative glomerulonephritis

582.1 With lesion of membranous glomerulonephritis
Chronic glomerulonephritis:
membranous
sclerosing
Focal glomerulosclerosis
Segmental hyalinosis

582.2 With lesion of membranoproliferative glomerulonephritis
Chronic glomerulonephritis:
endothelial
hypocomplementemic persistent
lobular
membranoproliferative
mesangiocapillary
mixed membranous and proliferative

DEF: Chronic glomerulonephritis with mesangial cell proliferation.

582.4 With lesion of rapidly progressive glomerulonephritis
Chronic nephritis with lesion of necrotizing glomerulitis

DEF: Chronic glomerulonephritisrapidly progresses to ESRD; marked by diffuse epithelial proliferation.

√5th **582.8 With other specified pathological lesion in kidney**

582.81 Chronic glomerulonephritis in diseases classified elsewhere
Code first underlying disease, as:
amyloidosis (277.3)
systemic lupus erythematosus (710.0)

582.89 Other
Chronic glomerulonephritis with lesion of:
exudative nephritis
interstitial (diffuse) (focal) nephritis

582.9 Chronic glomerulonephritis with unspecified pathological lesion in kidney
Glomerulonephritis:
  NOS
  hemorrhagic   ⎫
Nephritis   ⎬ specified as chronic
Nephropathy   ⎭

Additional Digit Required
MSP Medicare Secondary Payer   ◀ Revised Text   ● New Code   ▲ Revised Code Title

2002 Ingenix, Inc.

√4th **583 Nephritis and nephropathy, not specified as acute or chronic**
INCLUDES "renal disease" so stated, not specified as acute or chronic but with stated pathology or cause

583.0 With lesion of proliferative glomerulonephritis
Proliferative:
  glomerulonephritis (diffuse) NOS
Proliferative
  nephritis NOS
  nephropathy NOS

583.1 With lesion of membranous glomerulonephritis
Membranous:
  glomerulonephritis NOS
  nephritis NOS
Membranous nephropathy:
  NOS

DEF: Kidney inflammation or dysfunction with deposits on glomerular capillary basement membranes.

583.2 With lesion of membranoproliferative glomerulonephritis
Membranoproliferative:
  glomerulonephritis NOS
  nephritis NOS
  nephropathy NOS
Nephritis NOS, with lesion of:
  hypocomplementemic persistent
  lobular
  mesangiocapillary
  mixed membranous and proliferative
} glomerulonephritis

DEF: Kidney inflammation or dysfunction with mesangial cell proliferation.

583.4 With lesion of rapidly progressive glomerulonephritis
Necrotizing or rapidly progressive:
  glomerulitis NOS
  glomerulonephritis NOS
  nephritis NOS
  nephropathy NOS
Nephritis, unspecified, with lesion of necrotizing glomerulitis

DEF: Kidney inflammation or dysfunction; rapidly progresses to ESRD marked by diffuse epithelial proliferation.

583.6 With lesion of renal cortical necrosis
Nephritis NOS } with (renal) cortical
Nephropathy NOS } necrosis

Renal cortical necrosis NOS

583.7 With lesion of renal medullary necrosis
Nephritis NOS } with (renal) medullary
Nephropathy NOS } [papillary] necrosis

GENITOURINARY SYSTEM

√5ᵗʰ 583.8 With other specified pathological lesion in kidney

583.81 Nephritis and nephropathy, not specified as acute or chronic, in diseases classified elsewhere
Code first underlying disease, as:
amyloidosis (277.3)
diabetes mellitus (250.4)
gonococcal infection (098.19)
Goodpasture's syndrome (446.21)
systemic lupus erythematosus (710.0)
tuberculosis (016.0)
EXCLUDES gouty nephropathy (274.10)
syphilitic nephritis (095.4)

583.89 Other
Glomerulitis   with lesion of:
Glomerulonephritis   exudative
Nephritis   nephritis
Nephropathy   interstitial
Renal disease   nephritis

583.9 With unspecified pathological lesion in kidney
Glomerulitis NOS   Nephritis NOS
Glomerulonephritis NOS Nephropathy NOS
EXCLUDES nephropathy complicating pregnancy, labor, or the puerperium (642.0-642.9, 646.2)
renal disease NOS with no stated cause (593.9)

√4ᵗʰ 584 Acute renal failure
EXCLUDES following labor and delivery (669.3)
posttraumatic (958.5)
that complicating:
abortion (634-638 with .3, 639.3)
ectopic or molar pregnancy (639.3)

DEF: State resulting from increasing urea and related substances from the blood (azotemia), often with urine output of less than 500 ml per day.

584.5 With lesion of tubular necrosis
Lower nephron nephrosis
Renal failure with (acute) tubular necrosis
Tubular necrosis:
NOS
acute
DEF: Acute decline in kidney efficiency with destruction of tubules.

584.6 With lesion of renal cortical necrosis
DEF: Acute decline in kidney efficiency with destruction of renal tissues that filter blood.

584.7 With lesion of renal medullary [papillary] necrosis
Necrotizing renal papillitis
DEF: Acute decline in kidney efficiency with destruction of renal tissues that collect urine.

584.8 With other specified pathological lesion in kidney
584.9 Acute renal failure, unspecified

GENITOURINARY SYSTEM

585 Chronic renal failure
   Chronic uremia
   Use additional code to identify manifestation as:
      uremic:
         neuropathy (357.4)
         pericarditis (420.0)
   EXCLUDES *that with any condition classifiable to 401 (403.0-403.9 with fifth-digit 1)*

586 Renal failure, unspecified
   Uremia NOS
   EXCLUDES *following labor and delivery (669.3)*
      posttraumatic renal failure (958.5)
      that complicating:
         abortion (634-638 with .3, 639.3)
         ectopic or molar pregnancy (639.3)
      uremia:
         extrarenal (788.9)
         prerenal (788.9)
      with any condition classifiable to 401 (403.0-403.9 with fifth-digit 1)

DEF: Renal failure: kidney functions cease; malfunction may be due to inability to excrete metabolized substances or retain level of electrolytes.

DEF: Uremia: excess urea, creatinine and other nitrogenous products of protein and amino acid metabolism in blood due to reduced excretory function in bilateral kidney disease; also called azotemia.

587 Renal sclerosis, unspecified
   Atrophy of kidney
   Contracted kidney
   Renal:
      cirrhosis
      fibrosis
   EXCLUDES *nephrosclerosis (arteriolar) (arteriosclerotic) (403.00-403.92)*
      with hypertension (403.00-403.91)

Genitourinary System

GENITOURINARY SYSTEM

√4th 588 Disorders resulting from impaired renal function

588.0 Renal osteodystrophy
Azotemic osteodystrophy
Phosphate-losing tubular disorders
Renal:
  dwarfism
  infantilism
  rickets

DEF: Bone disorder that results in various bone diseases such as osteomalacia, osteoporosis or osteosclerosis; caused by impaired renal function, an abnormal level of phosphorus in the blood and impaired stimulation of the parathyroid.

588.1 Nephrogenic diabetes insipidus
  EXCLUDES *diabetes insipidus NOS (253.5)*

DEF: Type of diabetes due to renal tubules inability to reabsorb water; not responsive to vasopressin; may develop into chronic renal insufficiency.

588.8 Other specified disorders resulting from impaired renal function
Hypokalemic nephropathy
Secondary hyperparathyroidism (of renal origin)
  EXCLUDES *secondary hypertension (405.0-405.9)*

588.9 Unspecified disorder resulting from impaired renal function

√4th 589 Small kidney of unknown cause

589.0 Unilateral small kidney
589.1 Bilateral small kidneys
589.9 Small kidney, unspecified

OTHER DISEASES OF URINARY SYSTEM (590-599)

√4th 590 Infections of kidney
Use additional code to identify organism, such as Escherichia coli [E. coli] (041.4)

√5th 590.0 Chronic pyelonephritis
Chronic pyelitis
Chronic pyonephrosis
▶Code, if applicable, any causal condition first◀
590.00 Without lesion of renal medullary necrosis
590.01 With lesion of renal medullary necrosis

√5th 590.1 Acute pyelonephritis
Acute pyelitis   Acute pyonephrosis
590.10 Without lesion of renal medullary necrosis
590.11 With lesion of renal medullary necrosis

590.2 Renal and perinephric abscess
Abscess: Abscess:
  kidney   perirenal
  nephritic   Carbuncle of kidney

590.3 Pyeloureteritis cystica
Infection of renal pelvis and ureter
Ureteritis cystica

DEF: Inflammation and formation of submucosal cysts in the kidney, pelvis, and ureter.

√5th 590.8 Other pyelonephritis or pyonephrosis, not specified as acute or chronic
590.80 Pyelonephritis, unspecified
Pyelitis NOS
Pyelonephritis NOS

590.81 Pyelitis or pyelonephritis in diseases classified elsewhere
Code first underlying disease, as:
tuberculosis (016.0)

590.9 Infection of kidney, unspecified
EXCLUDES urinary tract infection NOS (599.0)

591 Hydronephrosis
Hydrocalycosis   Hydroureteronephrosis
Hydronephrosis
EXCLUDES congenital hydronephrosis (753.29)
hydroureter (593.5)

DEF: Distention of kidney and pelvis, with urine build-up due to ureteral obstruction; pyonephrosis may result.

✓4ᵗʰ 592 Calculus of kidney and ureter
EXCLUDES nephrocalcinosis (275.4)

592.0 Calculus of kidney
Nephrolithiasis NOS   Staghorn calculus
Renal calculus or stone   Stone in kidney
EXCLUDES uric acid nephrolithiasis (274.11)

592.1 Calculus of ureter
Ureteric stone   Ureterolithiasis

592.9 Urinary calculus, unspecified

✓4ᵗʰ 593 Other disorders of kidney and ureter

593.0 Nephroptosis
Floating kidney   Mobile kidney

593.1 Hypertrophy of kidney

593.2 Cyst of kidney, acquired
Cyst (multiple) (solitary) of kidney, not congenital
Peripelvic (lymphatic) cyst
EXCLUDES calyceal or pyelogenic cyst of kidney (591)
congenital cyst of kidney (753.1)
polycystic (disease of) kidney (753.1)

DEF: Abnormal, fluid-filled sac in the kidney, not present at birth.

593.3 Stricture or kinking of ureter
Angulation } of ureter (post-operative)
Constriction

Stricture of pelviureteric junction
DEF: Stricture or knot in tube connecting kidney to bladder.

593.4 Other ureteric obstruction
Idiopathic retroperitoneal fibrosis
Occlusion NOS of ureter
EXCLUDES that due to calculus (592.1)

593.5 Hydroureter
EXCLUDES congenital hydroureter (753.22)
hydroureteronephrosis (591)

593.6 Postural proteinuria
Benign postural proteinuria
Orthostatic proteinuria
EXCLUDES proteinuria NOS (791.0)

DEF: Excessive amounts of serum protein in the urine caused by the body position, e.g., orthostatic and lordotic.

✓5ᵗʰ 593.7 Vesicoureteral reflux
DEF: Backflow of urine, from bladder into ureter due to obstructed bladder neck.

GENITOURINARY SYSTEM

- **593.70** Unspecified or without reflux nephropathy
- **593.71** With reflux nephropathy, unilateral
- **593.72** With reflux nephropathy, bilateral
- **593.73** With reflux nephropathy NOS

✓5th **593.8** Other specified disorders of kidney and ureter

- **593.81** Vascular disorders of kidney
  - Renal (artery): embolism
  - Renal (artery): hemorrhage
  - Renal (artery): thrombosis
  - Renal infarction

- **593.82** Ureteral fistula
  - Intestinoureteral fistula
  - **EXCLUDES** fistula between ureter and female genital tract (619.0)
  - **DEF:** Abnormal communication, between tube connecting kidney to bladder and another structure.

- **593.89** Other
  - Adhesions, kidney or ureter
  - Periureteritis
  - Polyp of ureter
  - Pyelectasia
  - Ureterocele
  - **EXCLUDES** tuberculosis of ureter (016.2)
  - ureteritis cystica (590.3)

593.9 Unspecified disorder of kidney and ureter
- Renal disease NOS
- Salt-losing nephritis or syndrome
- **EXCLUDES** cystic kidney disease (753.1)
  - nephropathy, so stated (583.0-583.9)
  - renal disease:
    - acute (580.0-580.9)
    - arising in pregnancy or the puerperium (642.1-642.2, 642.4-642.7, 646.2)
    - chronic (582.0-582.9)
    - not specified as acute or chronic, but with stated pathology or cause (583.0-583.9)

✓4th **594 Calculus of lower urinary tract**

- **594.0** Calculus in diverticulum of bladder
  - **DEF:** Stone or mineral deposit in abnormal sac on the bladder wall.

- **594.1** Other calculus in bladder
  - Urinary bladder stone
  - **EXCLUDES** staghorn calculus (592.0)
  - **DEF:** Stone or mineral deposit in bladder.

- **594.2** Calculus in urethra
  - **DEF:** Stone or mineral deposit in tube that empties urine from bladder.

- **594.8** Other lower urinary tract calculus

- **594.9** Calculus of lower urinary tract, unspecified
  - **EXCLUDES** calculus of urinary tract NOS (592.9)

✓4th **595 Cystitis**
- **EXCLUDES** prostatocystitis (601.3)
- Use additional code to identify organism, such as Escherichia coli [E. coli] (041.4)

- **595.0** Acute cystitis
  - **EXCLUDES** trigonitis (595.3)
  - **DEF:** Acute inflammation of bladder.

- Additional Digit Required ✓4th ✓5th
- Unspecified Code
- Other Specified Code
- Manifestation Code
- **MSP** Medicare Secondary Payer
- ▶◀ Revised Text
- ● New Code
- ▲ Revised Code Title

Bladder Anterior View

Lateral View

595.1 Chronic interstitial cystitis
Hunner's ulcer   Submucous cystitis
Panmural fibrosis of bladder
DEF: Inflamed lesion affecting bladder wall; symptoms include urinary frequency, pain on bladder filling, nocturia, and distended bladder.

595.2 Other chronic cystitis
Chronic cystitis NOS   Subacute cystitis
EXCLUDES   trigonitis (595.3)
DEF: Persistent inflammation of bladder.

595.3 Trigonitis
Follicular cystitis   Urethrotrigonitis
Trigonitis (acute) (chronic)
DEF: Inflammation of the triangular area of the bladder called the trigonum vesicae.

595.4 Cystitis in diseases classified elsewhere
Code first underlying disease, as:
    actinomycosis (039.8)
    amebiasis (006.8)
    bilharziasis (120.0-120.9)
    Echinococcus infestation (122.3, 122.6)
EXCLUDES   cystitis:
        diphtheritic (032.84)
        gonococcal (098.11, 098.31)
        monilial (112.2)
        trichomonal (131.09)
        tuberculous (016.1)

GENITOURINARY SYSTEM

595.8 **Other specified types of cystitis**

    595.81 Cystitis cystica
        DEF: Inflammation of the bladder characterized by formation of multiple cysts.

    595.82 Irradiation cystitis
        Use additional E code to identify cause
        DEF: Inflammation of the bladder due to effects of radiation.

    595.89 Other
        Abscess of bladder
        Cystitis:
           bullous
        Cystitis:
           emphysematous
           glandularis

595.9 Cystitis, unspecified

596 Other disorders of bladder
Use additional code to identify urinary incontinence (625.6, 788.30-788.39)

    596.0 Bladder neck obstruction
        Contracture (acquired) ⎫
        Obstruction (acquired) ⎬ of bladder neck or vesicourethral orifice
        Stenosis (acquired) ⎭

        EXCLUDES congenital (753.6)

        DEF: Bladder outlet and vesicourethral obstruction; occurs more often in males as a consequence of benign prostatic hypertrophy or prostatic cancer; may also occur in either sex due to strictures, following radiation, cystoscopy, catheterization, injury, infection, blood clots, bladder cancer, impaction or disease compressing bladder neck.

    596.1 Intestinovesical fistula
        Fistula:
           enterovesical
           vesicocolic
        Fistula:
           vesicoenteric
           vesicorectal
        DEF: Abnormal communication, between intestine and bladder.

    596.2 Vesical fistula, not elsewhere classified
        Fistula:
           bladder NOS
           urethrovesical
        Fistula:
           vesicocutaneous
           vesicoperineal
        EXCLUDES *fistula between bladder and female genital tract (619.0)*
        DEF: Abnormal communication between bladder and another structure.

    596.3 Diverticulum of bladder
        Diverticulitis ⎫
        Diverticulum (acquired) (false) ⎬ of bladder

        EXCLUDES *that with calculus in diverticulum of bladder (594.0)*
        DEF: Abnormal pouch in bladder wall.

    596.4 Atony of bladder
        High compliance bladder
        Hypotonicity ⎫
        Inertia ⎬ of bladder

        EXCLUDES *neurogenic bladder (596.54)*
        DEF: Distended, bladder with loss of expulsive force; linked to CNS disease.

GENITOURINARY SYSTEM

√5th **596.5 Other functional disorders of bladder**
  EXCLUDES *cauda equina syndrome with neurogenic bladder (344.61)*

596.51 Hypertonicity of bladder
  Hyperactivity
  Overactive bladder
  DEF: Abnormal tension of muscular wall of bladder; may appear after surgery of voluntary nerve.

596.52 Low bladder compliance
  DEF: Low bladder capacity; causes increased pressure and frequent urination.

596.53 Paralysis of bladder
  DEF: Impaired bladder motor function due to nerve or muscle damage.

596.54 Neurogenic bladder NOS
  DEF: Unspecified dysfunctional bladder due to lesion of central, peripheral nervous system; may result in incontinence, residual urine retention, urinary infection, stones and renal failure.

596.55 Detrusor sphincter dyssynergia
  DEF: Instability of the urinary bladder sphincter muscle associated with urinary incontinence.

596.59 Other functional disorder of bladder
  Detrusor instability
  DEF: Detrusor instability: instability of bladder; marked by uninhibited contractions often leading to incontinence.

596.6 Rupture of bladder, nontraumatic

596.7 Hemorrhage into bladder wall
  Hyperemia of bladder
  EXCLUDES *acute hemorrhagic cystitis (595.0)*

596.8 Other specified disorders of bladder
  Bladder: Bladder:
    calcified   hemorrhage
    contracted   hypertrophy
  EXCLUDES *cystocele, female (618.0, 618.2-618.4)*
  hernia or prolapse of bladder, female (618.0, 618.2-618.4)

596.9 Unspecified disorder of bladder

√4th **597 Urethritis, not sexually transmitted, and urethral syndrome**
  EXCLUDES *nonspecific urethritis, so stated (099.4)*

597.0 Urethral abscess
  Abscess: Abscess of:
    periurethral   Cowper's gland
    urethral (gland)   Littré's gland
  Abscess of: Periurethral cellulitis
    bulbourethral gland
  EXCLUDES *urethral caruncle (599.3)*
  DEF: Pocket of pus in tube that empties urine from the bladder.

√5th **597.8 Other urethritis**
  597.80 Urethritis, unspecified
  597.81 Urethral syndrome NOS
  597.89 Other
    Adenitis, Skene's glands
    Cowperitis
    Meatitis, urethral
    Ulcer, urethra (meatus)
    Verumontanitis
    EXCLUDES *trichomonal (131.02)*

GENITOURINARY SYSTEM 598–599.7

✓4th 598 Urethral stricture
   Use additional code to identify urinary incontinence (625.6, 788.30-788.39)
   INCLUDES pinhole meatus
             stricture of urinary meatus
   EXCLUDES *congenital stricture of urethra and urinary meatus (753.6)*
   DEF: Narrowing of tube that empties urine from bladder.

   ✓5th 598.0 Urethral stricture due to infection
      598.00 Due to unspecified infection
      598.01 Due to infective diseases classified elsewhere
         Code first underlying disease, as:
            gonococcal infection (098.2)
            schistosomiasis (120.0-120.9)
            syphilis (095.8)
   598.1 Traumatic urethral stricture
      Stricture of urethra: Stricture of urethra:
        late effect of injury   postobstetric
      EXCLUDES *postoperative following surgery on genitourinary tract (598.2)*
   598.2 Postoperative urethral stricture
      Postcatheterization stricture of urethra
   598.8 Other specified causes of urethral stricture
   598.9 Urethral stricture, unspecified

✓4th 599 Other disorders of urethra and urinary tract
   599.0 Urinary tract infection, site not specified
      EXCLUDES *candidiasis of urinary tract (112.2)*
                ▶*urinary tract infection of newborn (771.82)*◀
      Use additional code to identify organism, such as Escherichia coli [E. coli] (041.4)
   599.1 Urethral fistula
      Fistula: Urinary fistula NOS
        urethroperineal
        urethrorectal
      EXCLUDES *fistula:*
                   urethroscrotal (608.89)
                   urethrovaginal (619.0)
                   urethrovesicovaginal (619.0)
   599.2 Urethral diverticulum
      DEF: Abnormal pouch in urethral wall.
   599.3 Urethral caruncle
      Polyp of urethra
   599.4 Urethral false passage
      DEF: Abnormal opening in urethra due to surgery, trauma or disease.
   599.5 Prolapsed urethral mucosa
      Prolapse of urethra   Urethrocele
      EXCLUDES *urethrocele, female (618.0, 618.2-618.4)*
   599.6 Urinary obstruction, unspecified
      Obstructive uropathy NOS
      Urinary (tract) obstruction NOS
      Use additional code to identify urinary incontinence (625.6, 788.30-788.39)
      EXCLUDES *obstructive nephropathy NOS (593.89)*
   599.7 Hematuria
      Hematuria (benign) (essential)
      EXCLUDES *hemoglobinuria (791.2)*
      DEF: Blood in urine.

Medicare Secondary Payer   ▶◀ Revised Text   ● New Code   ▲ Revised Code Title

✓4th Additional Digit Required   Unspecified Code   Other Specified Code   Manifestation Code

2002 Ingenix, Inc.   October 2002 • Volume 1 — 341

599.8–600.1 GENITOURINARY SYSTEM

✓5th 599.8 Other specified disorders of urethra and urinary tract
Use additional code to identify urinary incontinence (625.6, 788.30-788.39)
EXCLUDES symptoms and other conditions classifiable to 788.0-788.2, 788.4-788.9, 791.0-791.9

599.81 Urethral hypermobility
DEF: Hyperactive urethra.

599.82 Intrinsic (urethral) spincter deficiency [ISD]
DEF: Malfunctioning urethral sphincter.

599.83 Urethral instability
DEF: Inconsistent functioning of urethra.

599.84 Other specified disorders of urethra
Rupture of urethra (nontraumatic)
Urethral:
  cyst
  granuloma
DEF: Rupture of urethra; due to herniation or breaking down of tissue; not due to trauma.

DEF: Urethral cyst: abnormal sac in urethra; usually fluid filled.

DEF: Granuloma: inflammatory cells forming small nodules in urethra.

599.89 Other specified disorders of urinary tract

599.9 Unspecified disorder of urethra and urinary tract

DISEASES OF MALE GENITAL ORGANS (600-608)

✓4th 600 Hyperplasia of prostate
Use additional code to identify urinary incontinence (788.30-788.39)
DEF: Fibrostromal proliferation in periurethral glands, causes blood in urine; etiology unknown.

600.0 Hypertrophy (benign) of prostate A♂
Benign prostatic hypertrophy   Smooth enlarged prostate
Enlargement of prostate   Soft enlarged prostate

600.1 Nodular prostate A♂
Hard, firm prostate   Multinodular prostate
EXCLUDES malignant neoplasm of prostate (185)
DEF: Hard, firm nodule in prostate.

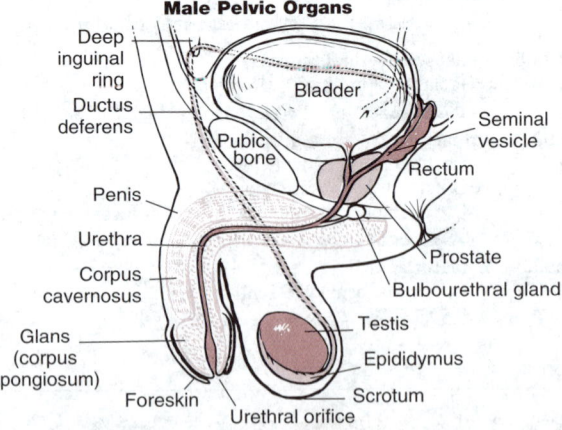

Male Pelvic Organs

342 — Volume 1

GENITOURINARY SYSTEM 600.2–601.4

Common Inguinal Canal Anomalies

600.2 Benign localized hyperplasia of prostate
Adenofibromatous hypertrophy of prostate
Adenoma of prostate
Fibroadenoma of prostate
Fibroma of prostate
Myoma of prostate
Polyp of prostate
> EXCLUDES benign neoplasms of prostate (222.2)
> hypertrophy of prostate (600.0)
> malignant neoplasm of prostate (185)

DEF: Benign localized hyperplasia is a clearly defined epithelial tumor. Other terms used for this condition are adenofibromatous hypertrophy of prostate, adenoma of prostate, fibroadenoma of prostate, fibroma of prostate, myoma of prostate, and polyp of prostate.

600.3 Cyst of prostate
DEF: Sacs of fluid, which differentiate this from either nodular or adenomatous tumors.

600.9 Hyperplasia of prostate, unspecified
Median bar
Prostatic obstruction NOS

√4th 601 Inflammatory diseases of prostate
Use additional code to identify organism, such as Staphylococcus (041.1), or Streptococcus (041.0)

601.0 Acute prostatitis

601.1 Chronic prostatitis

601.2 Abscess of prostate

601.3 Prostatocystitis

601.4 Prostatitis in diseases classified elsewhere
Code first underlying disease, as:
actinomycosis (039.8)
blastomycosis (116.0)
syphilis (095.8)
tuberculosis (016.5)
> EXCLUDES prostatitis:
> gonococcal (098.12, 098.32)
> monilial (112.2)
> trichomonal (131.03)

601.8 Other specified inflammatory diseases of prostate A ♂
    Prostatitis: Prostatitis:
      cavitary   granulomatous
      diverticular

601.9 Prostatitis, unspecified A ♂
    Prostatitis NOS

✓4ᵗʰ **602 Other disorders of prostate**

602.0 Calculus of prostate A ♂
    Prostatic stone
    DEF: Stone or mineral deposit in prostate.

602.1 Congestion or hemorrhage of prostate A ♂
    DEF: Bleeding or fluid collection in prostate.

602.2 Atrophy of prostate A ♂
602.3 Dysplasia of prostate A ♂
    Prostatic intraepithelial ▶neoplasia◀ I (PIN I)
    Prostatic intraepithelial ▶neoplasia◀ II (PIN II)
        EXCLUDES   prostatic intraepithelial ▶neoplasia◀ III (PIN III) (233.4)
    DEF: Abnormality of shape and size of the intraepithelial tissues of the prostate; pre-malignant condition characteristized by stalks and absence of a basilar cell layer; synonyms are intraductal dysplasia, large acinar atypical hyperplasia, atypical primary hyperplasia, hyperplasia with malignant changes, marked atypia, or duct-acinar dysplasia.

602.8 Other specified disorders of prostate A ♂
    Fistula ⎫
    Infarction ⎬ of prostate
    Stricture ⎭

    Periprostatic adhesions

602.9 Unspecified disorder of prostate A ♂

✓4ᵗʰ **603 Hydrocele**
    INCLUDES   hydrocele of spermatic cord, testis, or tunica vaginalis
    EXCLUDES   congenital (778.6)
    DEF: Circumscribed collection of fluid in tunica vaginalis, spermatic cord or testis.

603.0 Encysted hydrocele
603.1 Infected hydrocele
    Use additional code to identify organism
603.8 Other specified types of hydrocele
603.9 Hydrocele, unspecified

✓4ᵗʰ **604 Orchitis and epididymitis**
    Use additional code to identify organism, such as Escherichia coli [E. coli] (041.4), Staphylococcus (041.1), or Streptococcus (041.0)

604.0 Orchitis, epididymitis, and epididymo-orchitis, with abscess ♂
    Abscess of epididymis or testis

✓5ᵗʰ **604.9** Other orchitis, epididymitis, and epididymo-orchitis, without mention of abscess

    604.90 Orchitis and epididymitis, unspecified ♂

Torsion of Testes

Torsion of testis

Testes after correction showing bilateral fixation

- Spermatic cord

604.91 Orchitis and epididymitis in diseases classified elsewhere ♂
Code first underlying disease, as:
diphtheria (032.89)
filariasis (125.0-125.9)
syphilis (095.8)
EXCLUDES orchitis:
gonococcal (098.13, 098.33)
mumps (072.0)
tuberculous (016.5)
tuberculous epididymitis (016.4)

604.99 Other ♂

605 Redundant prepuce and phimosis ♂
Adherent prepuce   Phimosis (congenital)
Paraphimosis   Tight foreskin
DEF: Constriction of preputial orifice causing inability of the prepuce to be drawn back over the glans; it may be congenital or caused by infection.

✓4th 606 Infertility, male

606.0 Azoospermia A ♂
Absolute infertility
Infertility due to:
germinal (cell) aplasia
spermatogenic arrest (complete)
DEF: Absence of spermatozoa in the semen or inability to produce spermatozoa.

606.1 Oligospermia A ♂
Infertility due to:
germinal cell desquamation
hypospermatogenesis
incomplete spermatogenic arrest
DEF: Insufficient number of sperm in semen.

606.8 Infertility due to extratesticular causes A ♂
Infertility due to: Infertility due to:
drug therapy   radiation
infection   systemic disease
obstruction of efferent
ducts

606.9 Male infertility, unspecified A ♂

GENITOURINARY SYSTEM

607 Disorders of penis
EXCLUDES phimosis (605)

607.0 Leukoplakia of penis
Kraurosis of penis
EXCLUDES carcinoma in situ of penis (233.5)
erythroplasia of Queyrat (233.5)
DEF: White, thickened patches on glans penis.

607.1 Balanoposthitis
Balanitis
Use additional code to identify organism
DEF: Inflammation of glans penis and prepuce.

607.2 Other inflammatory disorders of penis
Abscess
Boil
Carbuncle
Cellulitis
} of corpus cavernosum or penis

Cavernitis (penis)
Use additional code to identify organism
EXCLUDES herpetic infection (054.13)

607.3 Priapism
Painful erection
DEF: Prolonged penile erection without sexual stimulation.

607.8 Other specified disorders of penis

607.81 Balanitis xerotica obliterans
Induratio penis plastica
DEF: Inflammation of the glans penis, caused by stricture of the opening of the prepuce.

607.82 Vascular disorders of penis
Embolism
Hematoma (nontraumatic)
Hemorrhage
Thrombosis
} of corpus cavernosum or penis

607.83 Edema of penis
DEF: Fluid retention within penile tissues.

607.84 Impotence of organic origin
EXCLUDES nonorganic or unspecified (302.72)
DEF: Physiological cause interfering with erection.

607.89 Other
Atrophy
Fibrosis
Hypertrophy
Ulcer (chronic)
} of corpus cavernosum or penis

607.9 Unspecified disorder of penis

608 Other disorders of male genital organs

608.0 Seminal vesiculitis
Abscess
Cellulitis
} of seminal vesicle

Vesiculitis (seminal)
Use additional code to identify organism
EXCLUDES gonococcal infection (098.14, 098.34)
DEF: Inflammation of seminal vesicle.

GENITOURINARY SYSTEM   608.1–608.9

608.1 Spermatocele ♂
DEF: Cystic enlargement of the epididymis or the testis; the cysts contain spermatozoa.

608.2 Torsion of testis ♂
Torsion of: Torsion of:
  epididymis   testicle
  spermatic cord
DEF: Twisted or rotated testis; may compromise blood flow.

608.3 Atrophy of testis ♂

608.4 Other inflammatory disorders of male genital organs ♂
Abscess ⎤
Boil   ⎬ of scrotum, spermatic cord, testis
Carbuncle⎮ [except abscess], tunica
Cellulitis⎦ vaginalis, or vas deferens

Vasitis
Use additional code to identify organism
EXCLUDES abscess of testis (604.0)

√5ᵗʰ **608.8 Other specified disorders of male genital organs**

  608.81 Disorders of male genital organs in diseases classified elsewhere ♂
    Code first underlying disease, as:
      filariasis (125.0-125.9)
      tuberculosis (016.5)

  608.82 Hematospermia ♂
    DEF: Presence of blood in the ejaculate; relatively common, affecting men of any age after puberty; cause is often difficult to determine since the semen originates in several organs, often the result of a viral bacterial infection and inflammation.

  608.83 Vascular disorders ♂
    Hematoma (non- ⎤ of seminal vesicle, spermatic
      traumatic)   ⎬ cord, testis, scrotum,
    Hemorrhage   ⎮ tunica vaginalis, or vas
    Thrombosis   ⎦ deferens

    Hematocele NOS, male

  608.84 Chylocele of tunica vaginalis ♂
    DEF: Chylous effusion into tunica vaginalis; due to infusion of lymphatic fluids.

  608.85 Stricture ♂
    Stricture of: Stricture of:
      spermatic cord   vas deferens
      tunica vaginalis

  608.86 Edema ♂

  608.87 Retrograde ejaculation ♂
    DEF: Condition where the semen travels to the bladder rather than out through the urethra due to damaged nerves causing the bladder neck to remain open during ejaculation.

  608.89 Other ♂
    Atrophy   ⎤
    Fibrosis   ⎬ of seminal vesicle, spermatic cord,
    Hypertrophy⎮ testis, scrotum, tunica
    Ulcer   ⎦ vaginalis, or vas deferens

    EXCLUDES atrophy of testis (608.3)

608.9 Unspecified disorder of male genital organs ♂

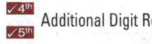 Additional Digit Required
MSP Medicare Secondary Payer   ▶◀ Revised Text

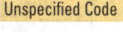 Unspecified Code   ● New Code

 Other Specified Code   Manifestation Code   ▲ Revised Code Title

2002 Ingenix, Inc.   Volume 1 — 347

DISORDERS OF BREAST (610-611)

✓4ᵗʰ **610 Benign mammary dysplasias**

- **610.0 Solitary cyst of breast**
  Cyst (solitary) of breast

- **610.1 Diffuse cystic mastopathy** [A]
  Chronic cystic mastitis   Fibrocystic disease of
  Cystic breast   breast
  DEF: Extensive formation of nodular cysts in breast tissue; symptoms include tenderness, change in size and hyperplasia of ductal epithelium.

- **610.2 Fibroadenosis of breast**
  Fibroadenosis of breast: Fibroadenosis of breast:
  NOS   diffuse
  chronic   periodic
  cystic   segmental
  DEF: Non-neoplastic nodular condition of breast.

- **610.3 Fibrosclerosis of breast**
  DEF: Fibrous tissue in breast.

- **610.4 Mammary duct ectasia**
  Comedomastitis   Mastitis:
  Duct ectasia   periductal
                    plasma cell
  DEF: Atrophy of duct epithelium; causes distended collecting ducts of mammary gland; drying up of breast secretion, intraductal inflammation and periductal and interstitial chronic inflammatory reaction.

- **610.8 Other specified benign mammary dysplasias**
  Mazoplasia   Sebaceous cyst of breast

- **610.9 Benign mammary dysplasia, unspecified**

✓4ᵗʰ **611 Other disorders of breast**

> **EXCLUDES** that associated with lactation or the puerperium (675.0-676.9)

- **611.0 Inflammatory disease of breast**
  Abscess (acute) (chronic)   Mastitis (acute) (subacute)
    (nonpuerperal) of: (nonpuerperal):
    areola   NOS
    breast   infective
    Mammillary fistula   retromammary
                                submammary

> **EXCLUDES** carbuncle of breast (680.2)
> chronic cystic mastitis (610.1)
> neonatal infective mastitis (771.5)
> thrombophlebitis of breast [Mondor's disease] (451.89)

- **611.1 Hypertrophy of breast**
  Gynecomastia   Hypertrophy of breast:
  Hypertrophy of breast: massive pubertal
  NOS

- **611.2 Fissure of nipple**

- **611.3 Fat necrosis of breast**
  Fat necrosis (segmental) of breast
  DEF: Splitting of neutral fats in adipose tissue cells as a result of trauma; a firm circumscribed mass is then formed in the breast.

- **611.4 Atrophy of breast**

- **611.5 Galactocele**
  DEF: Milk-filled cyst in breast; due to blocked duct.

- **611.6 Galactorrhea not associated with childbirth**
  DEF: Flow of milk not associated with childbirth or pregnancy.

[N] Newborn Age: 0   [P] Pediatric Age: 0-17   [M] Maternity Age: 12-55   [A] Adult Age: 15-124

GENITOURINARY SYSTEM

√5th 611.7 Signs and symptoms in breast
- **611.71 Mastodynia**
  - Pain in breast
- **611.72 Lump or mass in breast**
- **611.79 Other**
  - Induration of breast   Nipple discharge
  - Inversion of nipple   Retraction of nipple

611.8 Other specified disorders of breast
- Hematoma (nontraumatic) } of breast
- Infarction
- Occlusion of breast duct
- Subinvolution of breast (postlactational) (postpartum)

611.9 Unspecified breast disorder

INFLAMMATORY DISEASE OF FEMALE PELVIC ORGANS (614-616)
Use additional code to identify organism, such as Staphylococcus (041.1), or Streptococcus (041.0)

> **EXCLUDES** that associated with pregnancy, abortion, childbirth, or the puerperium (630-676.9)

√4th 614 Inflammatory disease of ovary, fallopian tube, pelvic cellular tissue, and peritoneum

> **EXCLUDES** endometritis (615.0-615.9)
> major infection following delivery (670)
> that complicating:
>   abortion (634-638 with .0, 639.0)
>   ectopic or molar pregnancy (639.0)
>   pregnancy or labor (646.6)

614.0 Acute salpingitis and oophoritis ♀
Any condition classifiable to 614.2, specified as acute or subacute
DEF: Acute inflammation, of ovary and fallopian tube.

614.1 Chronic salpingitis and oophoritis ♀
Hydrosalpinx
Salpingitis:
  follicularis
  isthmica nodosa
Any condition classifiable to 614.2, specified as chronic
DEF: Persistent inflammation of ovary and fallopian tube.

614.2 Salpingitis and oophoritis not specified as acute, subacute, or chronic ♀
Abscess (of):   Pyosalpinx
  fallopian tube   Perisalpingitis
  ovary   Salpingitis
  tubo-ovarian   Salpingo-oophoritis
Oophoritis   Tubo-ovarian inflammatory
Perioophoritis   disease

> **EXCLUDES** gonococcal infection (chronic) (098.37)
> acute (098.17)
> tuberculous (016.6)

614.3 Acute parametritis and pelvic cellulitis ♀
Acute inflammatory pelvic disease
Any condition classifiable to 614.4, specified as acute
DEF: Parametritis: inflammation of the parametrium; pelvic cellulitis is a synonym for parametritis.

√4th / √5th Additional Digit Required   Unspecified Code   Other Specified Code   Manifestation Code
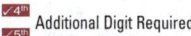 Medicare Secondary Payer   ▶◀ Revised Text   ● New Code   ▲ Revised Code Title

Female Genitourinary System

- **614.4 Chronic or unspecified parametritis and pelvic cellulitis** ♀
  Abscess (of):
  - broad ligament
  - parametrium
  - pelvis, female
  - pouch of Douglas
  } chronic or NOS

  Chronic inflammatory pelvic disease
  Pelvic cellulitis, female
  EXCLUDES tuberculous (016.7)

- **614.5 Acute or unspecified pelvic peritonitis, female** ♀
- **614.6 Pelvic peritoneal adhesions, female (postoperative) (postinfection)** ♀
  Adhesions:
  - peritubal
  - tubo-ovarian

  Use additional code to identify any associated infertility (628.2)

  DEF: Fibrous scarring abnormally joining structures within abdomen.

- **614.7 Other chronic pelvic peritonitis, female** ♀
  EXCLUDES tuberculous (016.7)
- **614.8 Other specified inflammatory disease of female pelvic organs and tissues** ♀
- **614.9 Unspecified inflammatory disease of female pelvic organs and tissues** ♀
  Pelvic infection or inflammation, female NOS
  Pelvic inflammatory disease [PID]

√4th **615 Inflammatory diseases of uterus, except cervix**
  EXCLUDES following delivery (670)
  hyperplastic endometritis (621.3)
  that complicating:
    abortion (634-638 with .0, 639.0)
    ectopic or molar pregnancy (639.0)
    pregnancy or labor (646.6)

- **615.0 Acute** ♀
  Any condition classifiable to 615.9, specified as acute or subacute
- **615.1 Chronic** ♀
  Any condition classifiable to 615.9, specified as chronic
- **615.9 Unspecified inflammatory disease of uterus** ♀
  - Endometritis
  - Endomyometritis
  - Metritis
  - Myometritis
  - Perimetritis
  - Pyometra
  - Uterine abscess

GENITOURINARY SYSTEM

√4th **616 Inflammatory disease of cervix, vagina, and vulva**
> **EXCLUDES** that complicating:
> abortion (634-638 with .0, 639.0)
> ectopic or molar pregnancy (639.0)
> pregnancy, childbirth, or the puerperium (646.6)

616.0 Cervicitis and endocervicitis ♀
Cervicitis ⎫ with or without mention of
Endocervicitis ⎭ erosion or ectropion

Nabothian (gland) cyst or follicle
> **EXCLUDES** erosion or ectropion without mention of cervicitis (622.0)

√5th **616.1 Vaginitis and vulvovaginitis**
DEF: Inflammation or infection of vagina or external female genitalia.

616.10 Vaginitis and vulvovaginitis, unspecified ♀
Vaginitis:
  NOS
  postirradiation
Vulvitis NOS
Vulvovaginitis NOS
Use additional code to identify organism, such as Escherichia coli [E. coli] (041.4), Staphylococcus (041.1), or Streptococcus (041.0)
> **EXCLUDES** noninfective leukorrhea (623.5)
> postmenopausal or senile vaginitis (627.3)

616.11 Vaginitis and vulvovaginitis in diseases classified elsewhere ♀
Code first underlying disease, as:
  pinworm vaginitis (127.4)
> **EXCLUDES** herpetic vulvovaginitis (054.11)
> monilial vulvotaginitis (112.1)
> trichomonal vaginitis or vulvovaginitis (131.01)

616.2 Cyst of Bartholin's gland ♀
Bartholin's duct cyst
DEF: Fluid-filled sac within gland of vaginal orifice.

616.3 Abscess of Bartholin's gland ♀
Vulvovaginal gland abscess

616.4 Other abscess of vulva ♀
Abscess ⎫
Carbuncle ⎬ of vulva
Furuncle ⎭

√5th **616.5 Ulceration of vulva**
616.50 Ulceration of vulva, unspecified ♀
Ulcer NOS of vulva

616.51 Ulceration of vulva in diseases classified elsewhere ♀
Code first underlying disease, as:
  Behçet's syndrome (136.1)
  tuberculosis (016.7)
> **EXCLUDES** vulvar ulcer (in):
> gonococcal (098.0)
> herpes simplex (054.12)
> syphilitic (091.0)

√4th √5th Additional Digit Required | **Unspecified Code** | Other Specified Code | ▲ Manifestation Code
MSP Medicare Secondary Payer | ▶◀ Revised Text | ● New Code | ▲ Revised Code Title

616.8 Other specified inflammatory diseases of cervix, vagina, and vulva ♀
Caruncle, vagina or labium
Ulcer, vagina

EXCLUDES noninflammatory disorders of:
cervix (622.0-622.9)
vagina (623.0-623.9)
vulva (624.0-624.9)

616.9 Unspecified inflammatory disease of cervix, vagina and vulva ♀

OTHER DISORDERS OF FEMALE GENITAL TRACT (617-629)

√4th **617 Endometriosis**
DEF: What resembles uterine mucosa (endometrial tissue) is found in the pelvic cavity.

617.0 Endometriosis of uterus ♀
Adenomyosis   Endometriosis:
Endometriosis: internal
  cervix   myometrium

EXCLUDES stromal endometriosis (236.0)

DEF: Aberrant uterine mucosal tissue; creating products of menses and inflamed uterine tissues.

617.1 Endometriosis of ovary ♀
Chocolate cyst of ovary
Endometrial cystoma of ovary

DEF: Aberrant uterine tissue; creating products of menses and inflamed ovarian tissues.

617.2 Endometriosis of fallopian tube ♀
DEF: Aberrant uterine tissue; creating products of menses and inflamed tissues of fallopian tubes.

617.3 Endometriosis of pelvic peritoneum ♀
Endometriosis: Endometriosis:
  broad ligament   parametrium
  cul-de-sac (Douglas')   round ligament

DEF: Aberrant uterine tissue; creating products of menses and inflamed peritoneum tissues.

617.4 Endometriosis of rectovaginal septum and vagina ♀
DEF: Aberrant uterine tissue; creating products of menses and inflamed tissues in and behind vagina.

Common Sites of Endometriosis

Common sites of endometriosis, in descending order of frequency:
(1) ovary
(2) cul de sac
(3) uterosacral ligaments
(4) broad ligaments
(5) fallopian tube
(6) uterovesical fold
(7) round ligament
(8) vermiform appendix
(9) vagina
(10) rectovaginal septum

GENITOURINARY SYSTEM

617.5 Endometriosis of intestine ♀
    Endometriosis: Endometriosis:
      appendix   rectum
      colon
    DEF: Aberrant uterine tissue; creating products of menses and inflamed intestinal tissues.

617.6 Endometriosis in scar of skin ♀
617.8 Endometriosis of other specified sites ♀
    Endometriosis: Endometriosis:
      bladder   umbilicus
      lung   vulva

617.9 Endometriosis, site unspecified ♀

√4ᵗʰ 618 Genital prolapse
    Use additional code to identify urinary incontinence (625.6, 788.31, 788.33-788.39)
    EXCLUDES *that complicating pregnancy, labor, or delivery (654.4)*

  618.0 Prolapse of vaginal walls without mention of uterine prolapse ♀
    Cystocele
    Cystourethrocele
    Proctocele, female
    Rectocele   } without mention of uterine
    Urethrocele, female   prolapse
    Vaginal prolapse
    EXCLUDES *that with uterine prolapse (618.2-618.4)*
              enterocele (618.6)
              vaginal vault prolapse following hysterectomy (618.5)

  618.1 Uterine prolapse without mention of vaginal wall prolapse ♀
    Descensus uteri   Uterine prolapse:
    Uterine prolapse: first degree
      NOS   second degree
      complete   third degree
    EXCLUDES *that with mention of cystocele, urethrocele, or rectocele (618.2-618.4)*

  618.2 Uterovaginal prolapse, incomplete ♀
    DEF: Downward displacement of uterus downward into vagina.

  618.3 Uterovaginal prolapse, complete ♀
    DEF: Downward displacement of uterus exposed within external genitalia.

  618.4 Uterovaginal prolapse, unspecified ♀
  618.5 Prolapse of vaginal vault after hysterectomy ♀
  618.6 Vaginal enterocele, congenital or acquired ♀
    Pelvic enterocele, congenital or acquired
    DEF: Vaginal vault hernia formed by the loop of the small intestine protruding into the rectal vaginal pouch; can also accompany uterine prolapse or follow hysterectomy.

  618.7 Old laceration of muscles of pelvic floor ♀
  618.8 Other specified genital prolapse ♀
    Incompetence or weakening of pelvic fundus
    Relaxation of vaginal outlet or pelvis

  618.9 Unspecified genital prolapse ♀

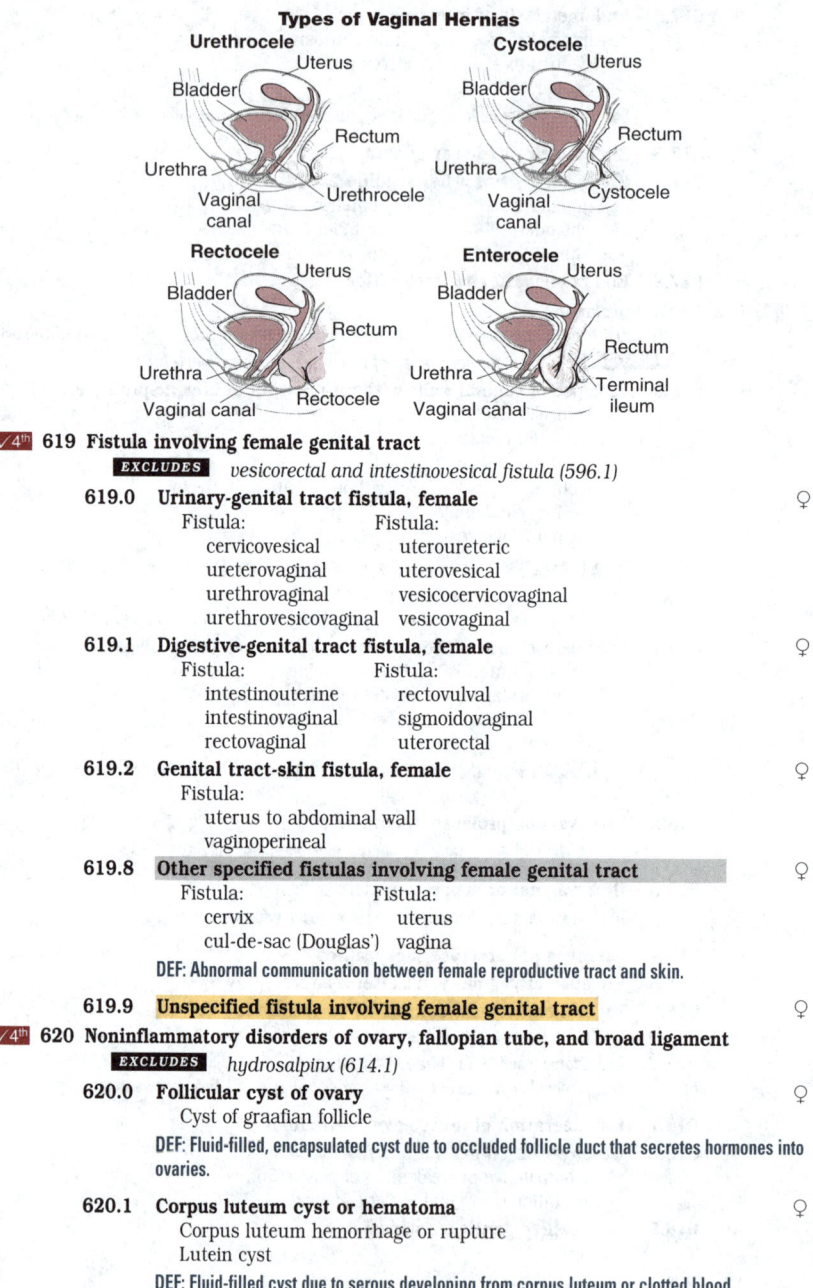

Types of Vaginal Hernias

619 Fistula involving female genital tract
   EXCLUDES: *vesicorectal and intestinovesical fistula (596.1)*

   619.0 Urinary-genital tract fistula, female ♀
      Fistula:
         cervicovesical
         ureterovaginal
         urethrovaginal
         urethrovesicovaginal
      Fistula:
         uteroureteric
         uterovesical
         vesicocervicovaginal
         vesicovaginal

   619.1 Digestive-genital tract fistula, female ♀
      Fistula:
         intestinouterine
         intestinovaginal
         rectovaginal
      Fistula:
         rectovulval
         sigmoidovaginal
         uterorectal

   619.2 Genital tract-skin fistula, female ♀
      Fistula:
         uterus to abdominal wall
         vaginoperineal

   619.8 Other specified fistulas involving female genital tract ♀
      Fistula:
         cervix
         cul-de-sac (Douglas')
      Fistula:
         uterus
         vagina
      DEF: Abnormal communication between female reproductive tract and skin.

   619.9 Unspecified fistula involving female genital tract ♀

620 Noninflammatory disorders of ovary, fallopian tube, and broad ligament
   EXCLUDES: *hydrosalpinx (614.1)*

   620.0 Follicular cyst of ovary ♀
      Cyst of graafian follicle
      DEF: Fluid-filled, encapsulated cyst due to occluded follicle duct that secretes hormones into ovaries.

   620.1 Corpus luteum cyst or hematoma ♀
      Corpus luteum hemorrhage or rupture
      Lutein cyst
      DEF: Fluid-filled cyst due to serous developing from corpus luteum or clotted blood.

GENITOURINARY SYSTEM   620.2–621.2

620.2 Other and unspecified ovarian cyst ♀
　　Cyst:
　　　NOS
　　　corpus albicans
　　　retention NOS　　} of ovary
　　　serous
　　　theca-lutein
　　Simple cystoma of ovary
　　EXCLUDES cystadenoma (benign) (serous) (220)
　　　　developmental cysts (752.0)
　　　　neoplastic cysts (220)
　　　　polycystic ovaries (256.4)
　　　　Stein-Leventhal syndrome (256.4)

620.3 Acquired atrophy of ovary and fallopian tube ♀
　　Senile involution of ovary

620.4 Prolapse or hernia of ovary and fallopian tube ♀
　　Displacement of ovary and fallopian tube
　　Salpingocele

620.5 Torsion of ovary, ovarian pedicle, or fallopian tube ♀
　　Torsion:　　　　　Torsion:
　　　accessory tube　　hydatid of Morgagni

620.6 Broad ligament laceration syndrome ♀
　　Masters-Allen syndrome

620.7 Hematoma of broad ligament ♀
　　Hematocele, broad ligament
　　DEF: Blood within peritoneal fold that supports uterus.

620.8 Other noninflammatory disorders of ovary, fallopian tube, and broad ligament ♀
　　Cyst　　} of broad ligament or fallopian tube
　　Polyp
　　
　　Infarction　} of ovary or fallopian tube
　　Rupture
　　
　　Hematosalpinx
　　EXCLUDES hematosalpinx in ectopic pregnancy (639.2)
　　　　peritubal adhesions (614.6)
　　　　torsion of ovary, ovarian pedicle, or fallopian tube (620.5)

620.9 Unspecified noninflammatory disorder of ovary, fallopian tube, and broad ligament ♀

✓4ᵗʰ **621 Disorders of uterus, not elsewhere classified**

621.0 Polyp of corpus uteri ♀
　　Polyp:　　　　Polyp:
　　　endometrium　　uterus NOS
　　EXCLUDES cervical polyp NOS (622.7)

621.1 Chronic subinvolution of uterus ♀
　　EXCLUDES puerperal (674.8)
　　DEF: Abnormal size of uterus after delivery; the uterus does not return to its normal size after the birth of a child.

621.2 Hypertrophy of uterus ♀
　　Bulky or enlarged uterus
　　EXCLUDES puerperal (674.8)

 Additional Digit Required   Unspecified Code   Other Specified Code   ▲ Manifestation Code
MSP Medicare Secondary Payer   ▶◀ Revised Text   ● New Code   ▲ Revised Code Title

621.3–622 GENITOURINARY SYSTEM

621.3 Endometrial cystic hyperplasia ♀
Hyperplasia (adenomatous) (cystic) (glandular) of endometrium
Hyperplastic endometritis
DEF: Abnormal cystic overgrowth of endometrial tissue.

621.4 Hematometra ♀
Hemometra
EXCLUDES that in congenital anomaly (752.2-752.3)
DEF: Accumulated blood in uterus.

621.5 Intrauterine synechiae ♀
Adhesions of uterus   Band(s) of uterus

621.6 Malposition of uterus ♀
Anteversion
Retroflexion } of uterus
Retroversion
EXCLUDES malposition complicating pregnancy, labor, or delivery (654.3-654.4)
prolapse of uterus (618.1-618.4)

621.7 Chronic inversion of uterus ♀
EXCLUDES current obstetrical trauma (665.2)
prolapse of uterus (618.1-618.4)

621.8 Other specified disorders of uterus, not elsewhere classified ♀
Atrophy, acquired
Cyst
Fibrosis NOS   } of uterus
Old laceration (postpartum)
Ulcer
EXCLUDES bilharzial fibrosis (120.0-120.9)
endometriosis (617.0)
fistulas (619.0-619.8)
inflammatory diseases (615.0-615.9)

621.9 Unspecified disorder of uterus ♀

√4th **622 Noninflammatory disorders of cervix**
EXCLUDES abnormality of cervix complicating pregnancy, labor, or delivery (654.5-654.6)
fistula (619.0-619.8)

Uterus and Ovaries

GENITOURINARY SYSTEM 622.0–622.9

622.0 Erosion and ectropion of cervix ♀
  Eversion ⎱ of cervix
  Ulcer ⎰
  EXCLUDES *that in chronic cervicitis (616.0)*
  DEF: Ulceration or turning outward of uterine cervix.

622.1 Dysplasia of cervix (uteri) ♀
  Anaplasia of cervix
  Cervical atypism
  ▶Cervical intraepithelial neoplasia I (CIN I)
  Cervical intraepithelial neoplasia II (CIN II)
  High grade squamous intraepithelial dysplasia (HGSIL)
  Low grade squamous intraepithelial dysplasia (LGSIL)◀
  EXCLUDES *carcinoma in situ of cervix (233.1)*
  cervical intraepithelial neoplasia III [CIN III] (233.1)

622.2 Leukoplakia of cervix (uteri) ♀
  DEF: Abnormal cell structures in portal between uterus and vagina.
  EXCLUDES *carcinoma in situ of cervix (233.1)*
  DEF: Thickened, white patches on portal between uterus and vagina.

622.3 Old laceration of cervix ♀
  Adhesions ⎫
  Band(s) ⎬ of cervix
  Cicatrix (postpartum) ⎭
  EXCLUDES *current obstetrical trauma (665.3)*
  DEF: Scarring or other evidence of old wound on cervix.

622.4 Stricture and stenosis of cervix ♀
  Atresia (acquired) ⎫
  Contracture ⎬ of cervix
  Occlusion ⎭

  Pinpoint os uteri
  EXCLUDES *congenital (752.49)*
  that complicating labor (654.6)

622.5 Incompetence of cervix ♀
  EXCLUDES *complicating pregnancy (654.5)*
  that affecting fetus or newborn (761.0)
  DEF: Inadequate functioning of cervix; marked by abnormal widening during pregnancy; causing miscarriage.

622.6 Hypertrophic elongation of cervix ♀
  DEF: Overgrowth of cervix tissues extending down into vagina.

622.7 Mucous polyp of cervix ♀
  Polyp NOS of cervix
  EXCLUDES *adenomatous polyp of cervix (219.0)*

622.8 Other specified noninflammatory disorders of cervix ♀
  Atrophy (senile) ⎫
  Cyst ⎬ of cervix
  Fibrosis ⎪
  Hemorrhage ⎭
  EXCLUDES *endometriosis (617.0)*
  fistula (619.0-619.8)
  inflammatory diseases (616.0)

622.9 Unspecified noninflammatory disorder of cervix ♀

GENITOURINARY SYSTEM

✓4ᵗʰ 623 Noninflammatory disorders of vagina
> **EXCLUDES** abnormality of vagina complicating pregnancy, labor, or delivery (654.7)
> congenital absence of vagina (752.49)
> congenital diaphragm or bands (752.49)
> fistulas involving vagina (619.0-619.8)

623.0 Dysplasia of vagina ♀
> **EXCLUDES** carcinoma in situ of vagina (233.3)

623.1 Leukoplakia of vagina ♀
DEF: Thickened white patches on vaginal canal.

623.2 Stricture or atresia of vagina ♀
Adhesions (postoperative) (postradiation) of vagina
Occlusion of vagina
Stenosis, vagina
Use additional E code to identify any external cause
> **EXCLUDES** congenital atresia or stricture (752.49)

623.3 Tight hymenal ring ♀
Rigid hymen
Tight hymenal ring } acquired or congenital
Tight introitus
> **EXCLUDES** imperforate hymen (752.42)

623.4 Old vaginal laceration ♀
> **EXCLUDES** old laceration involving muscles of pelvic floor (618.7)

DEF: Scarring or other evidence of old wound on vagina.

623.5 Leukorrhea, not specified as infective ♀
Leukorrhea NOS of vagina
Vaginal discharge NOS
> **EXCLUDES** trichomonal (131.00)

DEF: Viscid whitish discharge, from vagina.

623.6 Vaginal hematoma ♀
> **EXCLUDES** current obstetrical trauma (665.7)

623.7 Polyp of vagina ♀

623.8 Other specified noninflammatory disorders of vagina ♀
Cyst
Hemorrhage } of vagina

623.9 Unspecified noninflammatory disorder of vagina ♀

✓4ᵗʰ 624 Noninflammatory disorders of vulva and perineum
> **EXCLUDES** abnormality of vulva and perineum complicating pregnancy, labor, or delivery (654.8)
> condyloma acuminatum (078.1)
> fistulas involving:
>   perineum — see Alphabetic Index
>   vulva (619.0-619.8)
> vulval varices (456.6)
> vulvar involvement in skin conditions (690-709.9)

624.0 Dystrophy of vulva ♀
Kraurosis
Leukoplakia } of vulva
> **EXCLUDES** carcinoma in situ of vulva (233.3)

624.1 Atrophy of vulva ♀

624.2 Hypertrophy of clitoris ♀
> **EXCLUDES** that in endocrine disorders (255.2, 256.1)

GENITOURINARY SYSTEM

624.3 **Hypertrophy of labia** ♀
Hypertrophy of vulva NOS
DEF: Overgrowth of fleshy folds on either side of vagina.

624.4 **Old laceration or scarring of vulva** ♀
DEF: Scarring or other evidence of old wound on external female genitalia.

624.5 **Hematoma of vulva**
EXCLUDES that complicating delivery (664.5)
DEF: Blood in tissue of external genitalia.

624.6 **Polyp of labia and vulva** ♀

624.8 **Other specified noninflammatory disorders of vulva and perineum** ♀

Cyst
Edema } of vulva
Stricture

624.9 **Unspecified noninflammatory disorder of vulva and perineum** ♀

✓4ᵗʰ **625 Pain and other symptoms associated with female genital organs**

625.0 **Dyspareunia** ♀
EXCLUDES psychogenic dyspareunia (302.76)
DEF: Difficult or painful sexual intercourse.

625.1 **Vaginismus** ♀
Colpospasm   Vulvismus
EXCLUDES psychogenic vaginismus (306.51)
DEF: Vaginal spasms; due to involuntary contraction of musculature; prevents intercourse.

625.2 **Mittelschmerz** ♀
Intermenstrual pain   Ovulation pain
DEF: Pain occurring between menstrual periods.

625.3 **Dysmenorrhea** ♀
Painful menstruation
EXCLUDES psychogenic dysmenorrhea (306.52)

625.4 **Premenstrual tension syndromes** ♀
Menstrual:
  migraine
  molimen
Premenstual syndrome
Premenstrual tension NOS

625.5 **Pelvic congestion syndrome** ♀
Congestion-fibrosis syndrome   Taylor's syndrome
DEF: Excessive accumulated of blood in vessels of pelvis; may occur after orgasm; causes abnormal menstruation, lower back pain and vaginal discharge.

625.6 **Stress incontinence, female** ♀
EXCLUDES mixed incontinence (788.33)
stress incontinence, male (788.32)
DEF: Involuntary leakage of urine due to insufficient sphincter control; occurs upon sneezing, laughing, coughing, sudden movement or lifting.

625.8 **Other specified symptoms associated with female genital organs** ♀

625.9 **Unspecified symptom associated with female genital organs** ♀

GENITOURINARY SYSTEM

√4th **626 Disorders of menstruation and other abnormal bleeding from female genital tract**
  EXCLUDES menopausal and premenopausal bleeding (627.0)
  pain and other symptoms associated with menstrual cycle (625.2-625.4)
  postmenopausal bleeding (627.1)

626.0 Absence of menstruation ♀
  Amenorrhea (primary) (secondary)

626.1 Scanty or infrequent menstruation ♀
  Hypomenorrhea   Oligomenorrhea

626.2 Excessive or frequent menstruation ♀
  Heavy periods   Menorrhagia
  Menometrorrhagia   Plymenorrhea
  EXCLUDES premenopausal(627.0)
  that in puberty (626.3)

626.3 Puberty bleeding ♀
  Excessive bleeding associated with onset of menstrual periods
  Pubertal menorrhagia

626.4 Irregular menstrual cycle ♀
  Irregular: Irregular:
    bleeding NOS   periods
    menstruation

626.5 Ovulation bleeding ♀
  Regular intermenstrual bleeding

626.6 Metrorrhagia ♀
  Bleeding unrelated to menstrual cycle
  Irregular intermenstrual bleeding

626.7 Postcoital bleeding ♀
  DEF: Bleeding from vagina after sexual intercourse.

626.8 Other ♀
  Dysfunctional or functional uterine hemorrhage NOS
  Menstruation:
    retained
    suppression of

626.9 Unspecified ♀

√4th **627 Menopausal and postmenopausal disorders**
  EXCLUDES asymptomatic age-related (natural)
  postmenopausal status (V49.81)

627.0 Premenopausal menorrhagia ♀
  Excessive bleeding associated with onset of menopause
  Menorrhagia:
    climacteric
    menopausal
    preclimacteric

627.1 Postmenopausal bleeding ♀

▲ **627.2 Symptomatic menopausal or female climacteric states** ♀
  Symptoms, such as flushing, sleeplessness, headache, lack of concentration, associated with the menopause

627.3 Postmenopausal atrophic vaginitis ♀
  Senile (atrophic) vaginitis

▲ **627.4 Symptomatic states associated with artificial menopause** ♀
  Postartificial menopause syndromes
  Any condition classifiable to 627.1, 627.2, or 627.3 which follows induced menopause
  DEF: Conditions arising after hysterectomy.

N Newborn Age: 0   P Pediatric Age: 0-17   M Maternity Age: 12-55   A Adult Age: 15-124

GENITOURINARY SYSTEM

627.8 Other specified menopausal and postmenopausal disorders ♀
EXCLUDES: premature menopause NOS (256.31)

627.9 Unspecified menopausal and postmenopausal disorder ♀

✓4th **628 Infertility, female**
INCLUDES: primary and secondary sterility

DEF: Infertility: inability to conceive for at least one year with regular intercourse.

DEF: Primary infertility: occurring in patients who have never conceived.

DEF: Secondary infertility; occurring in patients who have previously conceived.

628.0 Associated with anovulation ♀
Anovulatory cycle
Use additional code for any associated Stein-Leventhal syndrome (256.4)

628.1 Of pituitary-hypothalamic origin ♀
Code first underlying cause, as:
adiposogenital dystrophy (253.8)
anterior pituitary disorder (253.0-253.4)

628.2 Of tubal origin ♀
Infertility associated with congenital anomaly of tube
Tubal:
block
occlusion
stenosis
Use additional code for any associated peritubal adhesions (614.6)

628.3 Of uterine origin ♀
Infertility associated with congenital anomaly of uterus
Nonimplantation
Use additional code for any associated tuberculous endometritis (016.7)

628.4 Of cervical or vaginal origin ♀
Infertility associated with:
anomaly of cervical mucus
congenital structural anomaly
dysmucorrhea

628.8 Of other specified origin ♀
628.9 Of unspecified origin ♀

✓4th **629 Other disorders of female genital organs**

629.0 Hematocele, female, not elsewhere classified ♀
EXCLUDES: hematocele or hematoma:
broad ligament (620.7)
fallopian tube (620.8)
that associated with ectopic pregnancy
▶(633.00-633.91)◀
uterus (621.4)
vagina (623.6)
vulva (624.5)

629.1 Hydrocele, canal of Nuck ♀
Cyst of canal of Nuck (acquired)
EXCLUDES: congenital (752.41)

629.8 Other specified disorders of female genital organs ♀
629.9 Unspecified disorder of female genital organs ♀
Habitual aborter without current pregnancy

11. COMPLICATIONS OF PREGNANCY, CHILDBIRTH, AND THE PUERPERIUM (630-677)

ECTOPIC AND MOLAR PREGNANCY (630-633)

Use additional code from category 639 to identify any complications

630 Hydatidiform mole
Trophoblastic disease NOS
Vesicular mole

> **EXCLUDES** *chorioadenoma (destruens) (236.1)*
> *chorionepithelioma (181)*
> *malignant hydatidiform mole (236.1)*

DEF: Abnormal product of pregnancy; marked by mass of cysts resembling bunch of grapes due to chorionic villi proliferation, and dissolution; must be surgically removed.

631 Other abnormal product of conception
Blighted ovum
Mole:
  NOS
  carneous
  fleshy
  stone

632 Missed abortion
Early fetal death before completion of 22 weeks' gestation with retention of dead fetus
Retained products of conception, not following spontaneous or induced abortion or delivery

> **EXCLUDES** *failed induced abortion (638.0-638.9)*
> *fetal death (intrauterine) (late) (656.4)*
> *missed delivery (656.4)*
> *that with abnormal product of conception (630, 631)*

√4th 633 Ectopic pregnancy

> **INCLUDES** ruptured ectopic pregnancy

DEF: Fertilized egg develops outside uterus.

√5th 633.0 Abdominal pregnancy
Intraperitoneal pregnancy
- **633.00 Abdominal pregnancy without intrauterine pregnancy**
- **633.01 Abdominal pregnancy with intrauterine pregnancy**

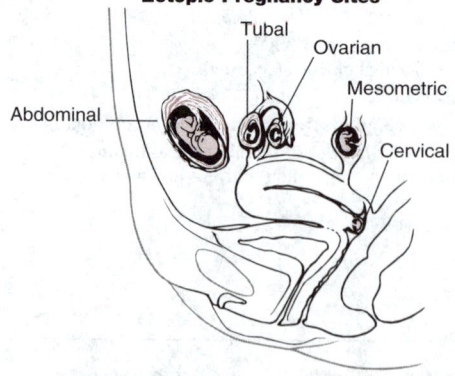

Ectopic Pregnancy Sites

COMPLICATIONS OF PREGNANCY, CHILDBIRTH, & PUERPERIUM

633.1 Tubal pregnancy
Fallopian pregnancy
Rupture of (fallopian) tube due to pregnancy
Tubal abortion

- 633.10 Tubal pregnancy without intrauterine pregnancy
- 633.11 Tubal pregnancy with intrauterine pregnancy

633.2 Ovarian pregnancy

- 633.20 Ovarian pregnancy without intrauterine pregnancy
- 633.21 Ovarian pregnancy with intrauterine pregnancy

633.8 Other ectopic pregnancy
Pregnancy:
  cervical
  combined
  cornual
Pregnancy:
  intraligamentous
  mesometric
  mural

- 633.80 Other ectopic pregnancy without intrauterine pregnancy
- 633.81 Other ectopic pregnancy with intrauterine pregnancy

633.9 Unspecified ectopic pregnancy

- 633.90 Unspecified ectopic pregnancy without intrauterine pregnancy
- 633.91 Unspecified ectopic pregnancy with intrauterine pregnancy

OTHER PREGNANCY WITH ABORTIVE OUTCOME (634-639)

The following fourth-digit subdivisions are for use with categories 634-638:

.0 Complicated by genital tract and pelvic infection
Endometritis
Salpingo-oophoritis
Sepsis NOS
Septicemia NOS
Any condition classifiable to 639.0, with condition classifiable to 634-638

> **EXCLUDES** urinary tract infection (634-638 with .7)

.1 Complicated by delayed or excessive hemorrhage
Afibrinogenemia
Defibrination syndrome
Intravascular hemolysis
Any condition classifiable to 639.1, with condition classifiable to 634-638

.2 Complicated by damage to pelvic organs and tissues
Laceration, perforation, or tear of:
  bladder
  uterus
Any condition classifiable to 639.2, with condition classifiable to 634-638

.3 Complicated by renal failure
Oliguria
Uremia
Any condition classifiable to 639.3, with condition classifiable to 634-638

.4 Complicated by metabolic disorder
Electrolyte imbalance with conditions classifiable to 634-638

.5 Complicated by shock
Circulatory collapse
Shock (postoperative) (septic)
Any condition classifiable to 639.5, with condition classifiable to 634-638

COMPLICATIONS OF PREGNANCY, CHILDBIRTH, & PUERPERIUM

.6 **Complicated by embolism**
Embolism:
NOS
amniotic fluid
pulmonary
Any condition classifiable to 639.6, with condition classifiable to 634-638

.7 **With other specified complications**
Cardiac arrest or failure
Urinary tract infection
Any condition classifiable to 639.8, with condition classifiable to 634-638

.8 **With unspecified complication**

.9 **Without mention of complication**

§ ✓4th **634 Spontaneous abortion**

INCLUDES   miscarriage
spontaneous abortion

Requires fifth-digit to identify stage:
0 unspecified
1 incomplete
2 complete

DEF: Spontaneous premature expulsion of the products of conception from the uterus.

- ✓5th 634.0 Complicated by genital tract and pelvic infection
- ✓5th 634.1 Complicated by delayed or excessive hemorrhage
- ✓5th 634.2 Complicated by damage to pelvic organs or tissues
- ✓5th 634.3 Complicated by renal failure
- ✓5th 634.4 Complicated by metabolic disorder
- ✓5th 634.5 Complicated by shock
- ✓5th 634.6 Complicated by embolism
- ✓5th 634.7 With other specified complications
- ✓5th 634.8 With unspecified complication
- ✓5th 634.9 Without mention of complication

§ ✓4th **635 Legally induced abortion**

INCLUDES   abortion or termination of pregnancy:
elective
legal
therapeutic

EXCLUDES   menstrual extraction or regulation (V25.3)

Requires fifth-digit to identify stage:
0 unspecified
1 incomplete
2 complete

DEF: Intentional expulsion of products of conception from uterus performed by medical professionals inside boundaries of law.

- ✓5th 635.0 Complicated by genital tract and pelvic infection
- ✓5th 635.1 Complicated by delayed or excessive hemorrhage
- ✓5th 635.2 Complicated by damage to pelvic organs or tissues
- ✓5th 635.3 Complicated by renal failure
- ✓5th 635.4 Complicated by metabolic disorder
- ✓5th 635.5 Complicated by shock

§ See beginning of section 634-639 for fourth-digit definitions.

COMPLICATIONS OF PREGNANCY, CHILDBIRTH, & PUERPERIUM 635.6–638

- √5th **635.6** Complicated by embolism
- √5th **635.7** With other specified complications
- √5th **635.8** With unspecified complication
- √5th **635.9** Without mention of complication

§ √4th **636 Illegally induced abortion**

INCLUDES abortion:
  criminal
  illegal
  self-induced

Requires fifth-digit to identify stage:
  0 unspecified
  1 incomplete
  2 complete

DEF: Intentional expulsion of products of conception from uterus; outside boundaries of law.

- √5th **636.0** Complicated by genital tract and pelvic infection
- √5th **636.1** Complicated by delayed or excessive hemorrhage
- √5th **636.2** Complicated by damage to pelvic organs or tissues
- √5th **636.3** Complicated by renal failure
- √5th **636.4** Complicated by metabolic disorder
- √5th **636.5** Complicated by shock
- √5th **636.6** Complicated by embolism
- √5th **636.7** With other specified complications
- √5th **636.8** With unspecified complication
- √5th **636.9** Without mention of complication

§ √4th **637 Unspecified abortion**

INCLUDES abortion NOS
  retained products of conception following abortion, not classifiable elsewhere

Requires fifth-digit to identify stage:
  0 unspecified
  1 incomplete
  2 complete

- √5th **637.0** Complicated by genital tract and pelvic infection
- √5th **637.1** Complicated by delayed or excessive hemorrhage
- √5th **637.2** Complicated by damage to pelvic organs or tissues
- √5th **637.3** Complicated by renal failure
- √5th **637.4** Complicated by metabolic disorder
- √5th **637.5** Complicated by shock
- √5th **637.6** Complicated by embolism
- √5th **637.7** With other specified complications
- √5th **637.8** With unspecified complication
- √5th **637.9** Without mention of complication

§ √4th **638 Failed attempted abortion**

INCLUDES failure of attempted induction of (legal) abortion
EXCLUDES incomplete abortion (634.0-637.9)

DEF: Continued pregnancy despite an attempted legal abortion.

§ See beginning of section 634-639 for fourth-digit definitions.

√4th/√5th Additional Digit Required   Unspecified Code   Other Specified Code   Manifestation Code
MSP Medicare Secondary Payer   ▶◀ Revised Text   ● New Code   ▲ Revised Code Title

638.0–639.4 COMPLICATIONS OF PREGNANCY, CHILDBIRTH, & PUERPERIUM

- **638.0** Complicated by genital tract and pelvic infection [M ♀]
- **638.1** Complicated by delayed or excessive hemorrhage [M ♀]
- **638.2** Complicated by damage to pelvic organs or tissues [M ♀]
- **638.3** Complicated by renal failure [M ♀]
- **638.4** Complicated by metabolic disorder [M ♀]
- **638.5** Complicated by shock [M ♀]
- **638.6** Complicated by embolism [M ♀]
- **638.7** With other specified complications [M ♀]
- **638.8** With unspecified complication [M ♀]
- **638.9** Without mention of complication [M ♀]

✓4th **639 Complications following abortion and ectopic and molar pregnancies**

> Note: This category is provided for use when it is required to classify separately the complications classifiable to the fourth-digit level in categories 634-638; for example:
>
> a) when the complication itself was responsible for an episode of medical care, the abortion, ectopic or molar pregnancy itself having been dealt with at a previous episode
>
> b) when these conditions are immediate complications of ectopic or molar pregnancies classifiable to 630-633 where they cannot be identified at fourth-digit level.

639.0 Genital tract and pelvic infection [M ♀]

Endometritis
Parametritis
Pelvic peritonitis
Salpingitis   } following conditions classifiable to 630-638
Salpingo-oophoritis
Sepsis NOS
Septicemia NOS

> **EXCLUDES** urinary tract infection (639.8)

639.1 Delayed or excessive hemorrhage [M ♀]

Afibrinogenemia
Defibrination syndrome   } following conditions classifiable to 630-638
Intravascular hemolysis

639.2 Damage to pelvic organs and tissues [M ♀]

Laceration, perforation,
  or tear of:
    bladder
    bowel
    broad ligament   } following conditions classifiable to 630-638
    cervix
    periurethral tissue
    uterus
    vagina

639.3 Renal failure [M ♀]

Oliguria
Renal:
    failure (acute)
    shutdown   } following conditions classifiable to 630-638
    tubular necrosis
Uremia

639.4 Metabolic disorders [M ♀]

Electrolyte imbalance following conditions classifiable to 630-638

COMPLICATIONS OF PREGNANCY, CHILDBIRTH, & PUERPERIUM 639.5–639.9

639.5 Shock MQ
    Circulatory collapse
    Shock (postoperative) (septic)
    } following conditions classifiable to 630-638

639.6 Embolism MQ
    Embolism:
      NOS
      air
      amniotic fluid
      blood-clot
      fat
      pulmonary
      pyemic
      septic
      soap
    } following conditions classifiable to 630-638

639.8 Other specified complications following abortion or ectopic and molar pregnancy MQ
    Acute yellow atrophy or necrosis of liver
    Cardiac arrest or failure
    Cerebral anoxia
    Urinary tract infection
    } following conditions classifiable to 630-638

639.9 Unspecified complication following abortion or ectopic and molar pregnancy MQ
    Complication(s) not further specified following conditions classifiable to 630-638

COMPLICATIONS MAINLY RELATED TO PREGNANCY (640-648)

INCLUDES the listed conditions even if they arose or were present during labor, delivery, or the puerperium

The following fifth-digit subclassification is for use with categories 640-648 to denote the current episode of care. Valid fifth-digits are in [brackets] under each code.

0 unspecified as to episode of care or not applicable

1 delivered, with or without mention of antepartum condition
    Antepartum condition with delivery
    Delivery NOS (with mention of antepartum complication during current episode of care)
    Intrapartum obstetric condition (with mention of antepartum complication during current episode of care)
    Pregnancy, delivered (with mention of antepartum complication during current episode of care)

2 delivered, with mention of postpartum complication
    Delivery with mention of puerperal complication during current episode of care

3 antepartum condition or complication
    Antepartum obstetric condition, not delivered during the current episode of care

4 postpartum condition or complication
    Postpartum or puerperal obstetric condition or complication following delivery that occurred:
      during previous episode of care
      outside hospital, with subsequent admission for observation or care

---

✓4th ✓5th Additional Digit Required   **Unspecified Code**   ● Other Specified Code   ▲ Manifestation Code
 Medicare Secondary Payer   ▶◀ Revised Text   ● New Code   ▲ Revised Code Title

2002 Ingenix, Inc.   Volume 1 — 367

COMPLICATIONS OF PREGNANCY, CHILDBIRTH, & PUERPERIUM

✓4th 640 Hemorrhage in early pregnancy
INCLUDES hemorrhage before completion of 22 weeks' gestation

§ ✓5th 640.0 Threatened abortion
[0,1,3] DEF: Bloody discharge during pregnancy; cervix may be dilated and pregnancy is threatened, but the pregnancy is not terminated.

§ ✓5th 640.8 Other specified hemorrhage in early pregnancy
[0,1,3]

§ ✓5th 640.9 Unspecified hemorrhage in early pregnancy
[0,1,3]

✓4th 641 Antepartum hemorrhage, abruptio placentae, and placenta previa

§ ✓5th 641.0 Placenta previa without hemorrhage
[0,1,3]
Low implantation of placenta
Placenta previa noted:
  during pregnancy
  before labor (and delivered by cesarean delivery)
} without hemorrhage

DEF: Placenta implanted in lower segment of uterus; commonly causes hemorrhage in the last trimester of pregnancy.

§ ✓5th 641.1 Hemorrhage from placenta previa
[0,1,3]
Low-lying placenta
Placenta previa:
  incomplete
  marginal
  partial
  total
} NOS or with hemorrhage (intrapartum)

EXCLUDES hemorrhage from vasa previa (663.5)

§ ✓5th 641.2 Premature separation of placenta
[0,1,3]
Ablatio placentae
Abruptio placentae
Accidental antepartum hemorrhage
Couvelaire uterus
Detachment of placenta (premature)
Premature separation of normally implanted placenta

DEF: Abruptio placentae: premature detachment of the placenta, characterized by shock, oliguria and decreased fibrinogen.

§ ✓5th 641.3 Antepartum hemorrhage associated with coagulation defects
[0,1,3]
Antepartum or intrapartum hemorrhage associated with:
  afibrinogenemia
  hyperfibrinolysis
  hypofibrinogenemia

DEF: Uterine hemorrhage prior to delivery.

§ ✓5th 641.8 Other antepartum hemorrhage
[0,1,3]
Antepartum or intrapartum hemorrhage associated with:
  trauma
  uterine leiomyoma

§ ✓5th 641.9 Unspecified antepartum hemorrhage
[0,1,3]
Hemorrhage: Hemorrhage:
  antepartum NOS   of pregnancy NOS
  intrapartum NOS

§ Requires fifth-digit. Valid digits are in [brackets] under each code. See beginning of section 640–648 for codes and definitions.

N Newborn Age: 0   **P** Pediatric Age: 0-17   **M** Maternity Age: 12-55   **A** Adult Age: 15-124

COMPLICATIONS OF PREGNANCY, CHILDBIRTH, & PUERPERIUM   642–642.4

Placenta Previa

Low (marginal) implantation   Partial placenta previa   Total placenta previa

√4ᵗʰ **642 Hypertension complicating pregnancy, childbirth, and the puerperium**

§ √5ᵗʰ **642.0 Benign essential hypertension complicating pregnancy, childbirth, and the puerperium**
[0-4]
    Hypertension:
      benign essential
      chronic NOS
      essential
      pre-existing NOS
    } specified as complicating, or as a reason for obstetric care during pregnancy, childbirth, or the puerperium

§ √5ᵗʰ **642.1 Hypertension secondary to renal disease, complicating pregnancy, childbirth, and the puerperium**
[0-4]
    Hypertension secondary to renal disease, specified as complicating, or as a reason for obstetric care during pregnancy, childbirth, or the puerperium

§ √5ᵗʰ **642.2 Other pre-existing hypertension complicating pregnancy, childbirth, and the puerperium**
[0-4]
    Hypertensive:
      heart and renal disease
      heart disease
      renal disease
    Malignant hypertension
    } specified as complicating, or as a reason for obstetric care during pregnancy, childbirth, or the puerperium

§ √5ᵗʰ **642.3 Transient hypertension of pregnancy**
[0-4]
    Gestational hypertension
    Transient hypertension, so described, in pregnancy, childbirth, or the puerperium

§ √5ᵗʰ **642.4 Mild or unspecified pre-eclampsia**
[0-4]
    Hypertension in pregnancy, childbirth, or the puerperium, not specified as pre-existing, with either albuminuria or edema, or both; mild or unspecified
    Pre-eclampsia: Toxemia (pre-eclamptic):
      NOS   NOS
      mild   mild

        EXCLUDES   albuminuria in pregnancy, without mention of hypertension (646.2)
                        edema in pregnancy, without mention of hypertension (646.1)

§ Requires fifth-digit. Valid digits are in [brackets] under each code. See beginning of section 640–648 for codes and definitions.

Abruptio Placentae
Partial separation (concealed bleeding) — Partial separation (apparent hemorrhage) — Complete separation (concealed hemorrhage)

§ ✓5th **642.5** **Severe pre-eclampsia**
[0-4]
  Hypertension in pregnancy, childbirth, or the puerperium, not specified as pre-existing, with either albuminuria or edema, or both; specified as severe
  Pre-eclampsia, severe
  Toxemia (pre-eclamptic), severe

§ ✓5th **642.6** **Eclampsia**
[0-4]
  Toxemia:
    eclamptic
    with convulsions

§ ✓5th **642.7** **Pre-eclampsia or eclampsia superimposed on pre existing hypertension**
[0-4]
  Conditions classifiable to 642.4-642.6, with conditions classifiable to 642.0-642.2

§ ✓5th **642.9** **Unspecified hypertension complicating pregnancy, childbirth, or the puerperium**
[0-4]
  Hypertension NOS, without mention of albuminuria or edema, complicating pregnancy, childbirth, or the puerperium

✓4th **643** **Excessive vomiting in pregnancy**
  INCLUDES   hyperemesis
             vomiting:
               persistent   } arising during pregnancy
               vicious
             hyperemesis gravidarum

§ ✓5th **643.0** **Mild hyperemesis gravidarum**
[0,1,3]
  Hyperemesis gravidarum, mild or unspecified, starting before the end of the 22nd week of gestation
  DEF: Detrimental vomiting and nausea.

§ ✓5th **643.1** **Hyperemesis gravidarum with metabolic disturbance**
[0,1,3]
  Hyperemesis gravidarum, starting before the end of the 22nd week of gestation, with metabolic disturbance, such as:
    carbohydrate depletion
    dehydration
    electrolyte imbalance

§ ✓5th **643.2** **Late vomiting of pregnancy**
[0,1,3]
  Excessive vomiting starting after 22 completed weeks of gestation

§ Requires fifth-digit. Valid digits are in [brackets] under each code. See beginning of section 640–648 for codes and definitions.

COMPLICATIONS OF PREGNANCY, CHILDBIRTH, & PUERPERIUM 643.8–646.3

§ ✓5th 643.8 Other vomiting complicating pregnancy M ♀
[0,1,3]   Vomiting due to organic disease or other cause, specified as complicating pregnancy, or as a reason for obstetric care during pregnancy
Use additional code to specify cause

§ ✓5th 643.9 Unspecified vomiting of pregnancy M ♀
[0,1,3]   Vomiting as a reason for care during pregnancy, length of gestation unspecified

✓4th 644 Early or threatened labor

§ ✓5th 644.0 Threatened premature labor M ♀
[0,3]   Premature labor after 22 weeks, but before 37 completed weeks of gestation without delivery
EXCLUDES *that occurring before 22 completed weeks of gestation (640.0)*

§ ✓5th 644.1 Other threatened labor M ♀
[0,3]   False labor:
NOS
after 37 completed weeks of gestation   } without delivery
Threatened labor NOS

§ ✓5th 644.2 Early onset of delivery M ♀
[0,1]   Onset (spontaneous) of delivery
Premature labor with onset of delivery   } before 37 completed weeks of gestation

✓4th 645 Late pregnancy

§ ✓5th 645.1 Post term pregnancy M ♀
[0,1,3]   Pregnancy over 40 completed weeks to 42 completed weeks gestation

§ ✓5th 645.2 Prolonged pregnancy M ♀
[0,1,3]   Pregnancy which has advanced beyond 42 completed weeks of gestation

✓4th 646 Other complications of pregnancy, not elsewhere classified
Use additional code(s) to further specify complication

§ ✓5th 646.0 Papyraceous fetus M ♀
[0,1,3]   DEF: Fetus retained in the uterus beyond natural term, exhibits parchment-like skin.

§ ✓5th 646.1 Edema or excessive weight gain in pregnancy, without mention of hypertension M ♀
[0-4]
Gestational edema   Maternal obesity syndrome
EXCLUDES *that with mention of hypertension (642.0-642.)*

§ ✓5th 646.2 Unspecified renal disease in pregnancy, without mention of hypertension M ♀
[0-4]
Albuminuria
Nephropathy NOS   } in pregnancy or the puerperium, without
Renal disease NOS   mention of hypertension
Uremia

Gestational proteinuria
EXCLUDES *that with mention of hypertension (642.0-642.9)*

§ ✓5th 646.3 Habitual aborter M ♀
[0,1,3]   EXCLUDES with current abortion (634.0-634.9)
without current pregnancy (629.9)
DEF: Three or more consecutive spontaneous abortions.

§ Requires fifth-digit. Valid digits are in [brackets] under each code. See beginning of section 640–648 for codes and definitions.

✓4th / ✓5th Additional Digit Required | Unspecified Code | Other Specified Code | Manifestation Code
MSP Medicare Secondary Payer | ▶◀ Revised Text | ● New Code | ▲ Revised Code Title

646.4–647.9 COMPLICATIONS OF PREGNANCY, CHILDBIRTH, & PUERPERIUM

§ ✓5ᵗʰ **646.4** Peripheral neuritis in pregnancy ⓂⒻ
[0-4]

§ ✓5ᵗʰ **646.5** Asymptomatic bacteriuria in pregnancy ⓂⒻ
[0-4]

§ ✓5ᵗʰ **646.6** Infections of genitourinary tract in pregnancy ⓂⒻ
[0-4]
Conditions classifiable to 590, 595, 597, 599.0, 616 complicating pregnancy, childbirth, or the puerperium
Conditions classifiable to ▶(614.0-614.5, 614.7-614.9, 615)◀ complicating pregnancy or labor
EXCLUDES major puerperal infection (670)

§ ✓5ᵗʰ **646.7** Liver disorders in pregnancy ⓂⒻ
[0,1,3]
Acute yellow atrophy of liver (obstetric) (true)
Icterus gravis } of pregnancy
Necrosis of liver

EXCLUDES hepatorenal syndrome following delivery (674.8)
viral hepatitis (647.6)

§ ✓5ᵗʰ **646.8** Other specified complications of pregnancy ⓂⒻ
[0-4]
Fatigue during pregnancy
Herpes gestationis
Insufficient weight gain of pregnancy
Uterine size-date discrepancy

§ ✓5ᵗʰ **646.9** Unspecified complication of pregnancy ⓂⒻ
[0,1,3]

✓4ᵗʰ **647** Infectious and parasitic conditions in the mother classifiable elsewhere, but complicating pregnancy, childbirth, or the puerperium
INCLUDES the listed conditions when complicating the pregnant state, aggravated by the pregnancy, or when a main reason for obstetric care
EXCLUDES those conditions in the mother known or suspected to have affected the fetus (655.0-655.9)
Use additional code(s) to further specify complication

§ ✓5ᵗʰ **647.0** Syphilis ⓂⒻ
[0-4] Conditions classifiable to 090-097

§ ✓5ᵗʰ **647.1** Gonorrhea ⓂⒻ
[0-4] Conditions classifiable to 098

§ ✓5ᵗʰ **647.2** Other venereal diseases ⓂⒻ
[0-4] Conditions classifiable to 099

§ ✓5ᵗʰ **647.3** Tuberculosis ⓂⒻ
[0-4] Conditions classifiable to 010-018

§ ✓5ᵗʰ **647.4** Malaria ⓂⒻ
[0-4] Conditions classifiable to 084

§ ✓5ᵗʰ **647.5** Rubella ⓂⒻ
[0-4] Conditions classifiable to 056

§ ✓5ᵗʰ **647.6** Other viral diseases ⓂⒻ
[0-4] Conditions classifiable to 042 and 050-079, except 056

§ ✓5ᵗʰ **647.8** Other specified infectious and parasitic diseases ⓂⒻ
[0-4]

§ ✓5ᵗʰ **647.9** Unspecified infection or infestation ⓂⒻ
[0-4]

§ Requires fifth-digit. Valid digits are in [brackets] under each code. See beginning of section 640–648 for codes and definitions.

Ⓝ Newborn Age: 0   Ⓟ Pediatric Age: 0-17   Ⓜ Maternity Age: 12-55   Ⓐ Adult Age: 15-124

COMPLICATIONS OF PREGNANCY, CHILDBIRTH, & PUERPERIUM 648–648.9

✓4th **648 Other current conditions in the mother classifiable elsewhere, but complicating pregnancy, childbirth, or the puerperium**

> INCLUDES the listed conditions when complicating the pregnant state, aggravated by the pregnancy, or when a main reason for obstetric care
>
> EXCLUDES those conditions in the mother known or suspected to have affected the fetus (655.0-665.9)
>
> Use additional code(s) to identify the condition

§ ✓5th **648.0 Diabetes mellitus** M ♀
[0-4] Conditions classifiable to 250
> EXCLUDES gestational diabetes (648.8)

§ ✓5th **648.1 Thyroid dysfunction** M ♀
[0-4] Conditions classifiable to 240-246

§ ✓5th **648.2 Anemia** M ♀
[0-4] Conditions classifiable to 280-285

§ ✓5th **648.3 Drug dependence** M ♀
[0-4] Conditions classifiable to 304

§ ✓5th **648.4 Mental disorders** M ♀
[0-4] Conditions classifiable to 290-303, 305-316, 317-319

§ ✓5th **648.5 Congenital cardiovascular disorders** M ♀
[0-4] Conditions classifiable to 745-747

§ ✓5th **648.6 Other cardiovascular diseases** M ♀
[0-4] Conditions classifiable to 390-398, 410-429
> EXCLUDES cerebrovascular disorders in the puerperium (674.0)
> venous complications (671.0-671.9)

§ ✓5th **648.7 Bone and joint disorders of back, pelvis, and lower limbs** M ♀
[0-4] Conditions classifiable to 720-724, and those classifiable to 711-719 or 725-738, specified as affecting the lower limbs

§ ✓5th **648.8 Abnormal glucose tolerance** M ♀
[0-4] Conditions classifiable to 790.2
Gestational diabetes
DEF: Glucose intolerance arising in pregnancy, resolving at end of pregnancy.

§ ✓5th **648.9 Other current conditions classifiable elsewhere** M ♀
[0-4] Conditions classifiable to 440-459
Nutritional deficiencies [conditions classifiable to 260-269]

NORMAL DELIVERY, AND OTHER INDICATIONS FOR CARE IN PREGNANCY, LABOR, AND DELIVERY (650-659)

The following fifth-digit subclassification is for use with categories 651-659 to denote the current episode of care. Valid fifth-digits are in [brackets] under each code.

0 **unspecified as to episode of care or not applicable**
1 delivered, with or without mention of antepartum condition
2 delivered, with mention of postpartum complication
3 antepartum condition or complication
4 postpartum condition or complication

§ Requires fifth-digit. Valid digits are in [brackets] under each code. See beginning of section 640-648 for codes and definitions.

✓4th Additional Digit Required
✓5th
MSP Medicare Secondary Payer

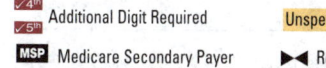

▶ Revised Text   ● New Code   ▲ Revised Code Title

2002 Ingenix, Inc.   Volume 1 — 373

650–652.4 COMPLICATIONS OF PREGNANCY, CHILDBIRTH, & PUERPERIUM

650 Normal delivery
Delivery requiring minimal or no assistance, with or without episiotomy, without fetal manipulation [e.g., rotation version] or instrumentation [forceps] of spontaneous, cephalic, vaginal, full-term, single, live-born infant. This code is for use as a single diagnosis code and is not to be used with any other code in the range 630-676.

> **EXCLUDES** breech delivery (assisted) (spontaneous) NOS (652.2)
> delivery by vacuum extractor, forceps, cesarean section, or breech extraction, without specified complication (669.5-669.7)

Use additional code to indicate outcome of delivery (V27.0)

✓4th **651 Multiple gestation**

§ ✓5th **651.0 Twin pregnancy**
[0,1,3]

§ ✓5th **651.1 Triplet pregnancy**
[0,1,3]

§ ✓5th **651.2 Quadruplet pregnancy**
[0,1,3]

§ ✓5th **651.3 Twin pregnancy with fetal loss and retention of one fetus**
[0,1,3]   Vanishing twin syndrome (651.33)

§ ✓5th **651.4 Triplet pregnancy with fetal loss and retention of one or more fetus(es)**
[0,1,3]

§ ✓5th **651.5 Quadruplet pregnancy with fetal loss and retentio of one or more fetus(es)**
[0,1,3]

§ ✓5th **651.6 Other multiple pregnancy with fetal loss and retention of one or more fetus(es)**
[0,1,3]

§ ✓5th **651.8 Other specified multiple gestation**
[0,1,3]

§ ✓5th **651.9 Unspecified multiple gestation**
[0,1,3]

✓4th **652 Malposition and malpresentation of fetus**
Code first any associated obstructed labor (660.0)

§ ✓5th **652.0 Unstable lie**
[0,1,3]   DEF: Changing fetal position.

§ ✓5th **652.1 Breech or other malpresentation successfully converted to cephalic presentation**
[0,1,3]   Cephalic version NOS

§ ✓5th **652.2 Breech presentation without mention of version**
[0,1,3]   Breech delivery (assisted) (spontaneous) NOS
Buttocks presentation
Complete breech
Frank breech

> **EXCLUDES** footling presentation (652.8)
> incomplete breech (652.8)

DEF: Fetal presentation of buttocks or feet at birth canal.

§ ✓5th **652.3 Transverse or oblique presentation**
[0,1,3]   Oblique lie   Transverse lie

> **EXCLUDES** transverse arrest of fetal head (660.3)

DEF: Delivery of fetus, shoulder first.

§ ✓5th **652.4 Face or brow presentation**
[0,1,3]   Mentum presentation

---

§ Requires fifth-digit. Valid digits are in [brackets] under each code. See beginning of section 640–648 for codes and definitions.

 Newborn Age: 0   Pediatric Age: 0-17   Maternity Age: 12-55   A Adult Age: 15-124

COMPLICATIONS OF PREGNANCY, CHILDBIRTH, & PUERPERIUM 652.5–653.6

§ ✓5ᵗʰ **652.5 High head at term** Ⓜ♀
  [0,1,3]   Failure of head to enter pelvic brim

§ ✓5ᵗʰ **652.6 Multiple gestation with malpresentation of one fetus or more** Ⓜ♀
  [0,1,3]

§ ✓5ᵗʰ **652.7 Prolapsed arm** Ⓜ♀
  [0,1,3]

§ ✓5ᵗʰ **652.8 Other specified malposition or malpresentation** Ⓜ♀
  [0,1,3]   Compound presentation

§ ✓5ᵗʰ **652.9 Unspecified malposition or malpresentation** Ⓜ♀
  [0,1,3]

✓4ᵗʰ **653 Disproportion**
  Code first any associated obstructed labor (660.1)

§ ✓5ᵗʰ **653.0 Major abnormality of bony pelvis, not further specified** Ⓜ♀
  [0,1,3]   Pelvic deformity NOS

§ ✓5ᵗʰ **653.1 Generally contracted pelvis** Ⓜ♀
  [0,1,3]   Contracted pelvis NOS

§ ✓5ᵗʰ **653.2 Inlet contraction of pelvis** Ⓜ♀
  [0,1,3]   Inlet contraction (pelvis)

§ ✓5ᵗʰ **653.3 Outlet contraction of pelvis** Ⓜ♀
  [0,1,3]   Outlet contraction (pelvis)

§ ✓5ᵗʰ **653.4 Fetopelvic disproportion** Ⓜ♀
  [0,1,3]   Cephalopelvic disproportion NOS
          Disproportion of mixed maternal and fetal origin, with normally formed fetus

§ ✓5ᵗʰ **653.5 Unusually large fetus causing disproportion** Ⓜ♀
  [0,1,3]   Disproportion of fetal origin with normally formed fetus
          Fetal disproportion NOS
          EXCLUDES *that when the reason for medical care was concern for the fetus (656.6).*

§ ✓5ᵗʰ **653.6 Hydrocephalic fetus causing disproportion** Ⓜ♀
  [0,1,3]   **EXCLUDES** *that when the reason for medical care was concern for the fetus (655.0).*

Malposition and Malpresentation

Breech
Shoulder (arm prolapse)
Mother's pelvis
Face (mentum)
Compound (extremity together with head)
Oblique

§ Requires fifth-digit. Valid digits are in [brackets] under each code. See beginning of section 640–648 for codes and definitions.

✓4ᵗʰ Additional Digit Required
✓5ᵗʰ
MSP Medicare Secondary Payer
▶◀ Revised Text
Unspecified Code
● New Code
Other Specified Code
▲ Revised Code Title
Manifestation Code

2002 Ingenix, Inc.
Volume 1 — 375

653.7–654.6 COMPLICATIONS OF PREGNANCY, CHILDBIRTH, & PUERPERIUM

§ ✓5th **653.7** Other fetal abnormality causing disproportion
[0,1,3]
Conjoined twins
Fetal:
 ascites
 hydrops
Fetal:
 myelomeningocele
 sacral teratoma
 tumor

§ ✓5th **653.8** Disproportion of other origin
[0,1,3]
EXCLUDES   shoulder (girdle) dystocia (660.4)

§ ✓5th **653.9** Unspecified disproportion
[0,1,3]

✓4th **654 Abnormality of organs and soft tissues of pelvis**
INCLUDES   the listed conditions during pregnancy, childbirth, or the puerperium
Code first any associated obstructed labor (660.2)

§ ✓5th **654.0** Congenital abnormalities of uterus
[0-4]
Double uterus   Uterus bicornis

§ ✓5th **654.1** Tumors of body of uterus
[0-4]
Uterine fibroids

§ ✓5th **654.2** Previous cesarean delivery
[0,1,3]
Uterine scar from previous cesarean delivery

§ ✓5th **654.3** Retroverted and incarcerated gravid uterus
[0-4]
DEF: Retroverted: tilted back uterus; no change in angle of longitudinal axis.
DEF: Incarcerated: immobile, fixed uterus.

§ ✓5th **654.4** Other abnormalities in shape or position of gravid uterus
[0-4]   and of neighboring structures
Cystocele   Prolapse of gravid uterus
Pelvic floor repair   Rectocele
Pendulous abdomen   Rigid pelvic floor

§ ✓5th **654.5** Cervical incompetence
[0-4]
Presence of Shirodkar suture with or without mention of cervical incompetence
DEF: Abnormal cervix; tendency to dilate in second trimester; causes premature fetal expulsion.
DEF: Shirodkar suture: purse-string suture used to artificially close incompetent cervix.

§ ✓5th **654.6** Other congenital or acquired abnormality of cervix
[0-4]
Cicatricial cervix   Rigid cervix (uteri)
Polyp of cervix   Stenosis or stricture of cervix
Previous surgery to cervix   Tumor of cervix

Cephalopelvic Disproportion

Pubic symphysis

Cephalopelvic disproportion due to: Contraction of pelvic inlet, or large fetus, or hydrocephalus

Ischial tuberosity

Contraction of pelvic outlet (from below)

Pubic symphysis

Pelvic inlet from above

§ Requires fifth-digit. Valid digits are in [brackets] under each code. See beginning of section 640–648 for codes and definitions.

 Newborn Age: 0   Pediatric Age: 0-17   Maternity Age: 12-55   Adult Age: 15-124

COMPLICATIONS OF PREGNANCY, CHILDBIRTH, & PUERPERIUM 654.7–656.0

§ ✓5th **654.7** Congenital or acquired abnormality of vagina [M]♀
[0-4]
Previous surgery to vagina   Stricture of vagina
Septate vagina   Tumor of vagina
Stenosis of vagina (acquired) (congenital)

§ ✓5th **654.8** Congenital or acquired abnormality of vulva [M]♀
[0-4]
Fibrosis of perineum   Rigid perineum
Persistent hymen   Tumor of vulva
Previous surgery to perineum or vulva
EXCLUDES *varicose veins of vulva (671.1)*

§ ✓5th **654.9** Other and unspecified [M]♀
[0-4]
Uterine scar NEC

✓4th **655** Known or suspected fetal abnormality affecting management of mother
INCLUDES the listed conditions in the fetus as a reason for observation or obstetrical care of the mother, or for termination of pregnancy

§ ✓5th **655.0** Central nervous system malformation in fetus [M]♀
[0,1,3]
Fetal or suspected fetal:
 anencephaly
 hydrocephalus
 spina bifida (with myelomeningocele)

§ ✓5th **655.1** Chromosomal abnormality in fetus [M]♀
[0,1,3]

§ ✓5th **655.2** Hereditary disease in family possibly affecting fetus [M]♀
[0,1,3]

§ ✓5th **655.3** Suspected damage to fetus from viral disease in the mother [M]♀
[0,1,3]
Suspected damage to fetus from maternal rubella

§ ✓5th **655.4** Suspected damage to fetus from other disease in the mother [M]♀
[0,1,3]
Suspected damage to fetus from maternal:
 alcohol addiction
 listeriosis
 toxoplasmosis

§ ✓5th **655.5** Suspected damage to fetus from drugs [M]♀
[0,1,3]

§ ✓5th **655.6** Suspected damage to fetus from radiation [M]♀
[0,1,3]

§ ✓5th **655.7** Decreased fetal movements [M]♀
[0,1,3]

§ ✓5th **655.8** Other known or suspected fetal abnormality, not elsewhere classified [M]♀
[0,1,3]
Suspected damage to fetus from:
 environmental toxins
 intrauterine contraceptive device

§ ✓5th **655.9** Unspecified [M]♀
[0,1,3]

✓4th **656** Other fetal and placental problems affecting management of mother

§ ✓5th **656.0** Fetal-maternal hemorrhage [M]♀
[0,1,3]
Leakage (microscopic) of fetal blood into maternal circulation

---

§ Requires fifth-digit. Valid digits are in [brackets] under each code. See beginning of section 640–648 for codes and definitions.

656.1–658.1 COMPLICATIONS OF PREGNANCY, CHILDBIRTH, & PUERPERIUM

§ ✓5th **656.1 Rhesus isoimmunization**
[0,1,3]
    Anti-D [Rh] antibodies   Rh incompatibility
DEF: Antibodies developing against Rh factor; mother with Rh negative develops antibodies against Rh positive fetus.

§ ✓5th **656.2 Isoimmunization from other and unspecified blood-group incompatibility**
[0,1,3]
    ABO isoimmunization

§ ✓5th **656.3 Fetal distress**
[0,1,3]
    Fetal metabolic acidemia
    EXCLUDES abnormal fetal acid-base balance (656.8)
        abnormality in fetal heart rate or rhythm (659.7)
        fetal bradycardia (659.7)
        fetal distress NOS (656.8)
        fetal tachycardia (659.7)
        meconium in liquor (656.8)
DEF: Life-threatening disorder; fetal anoxia, hemolytic disease and other miscellaneous diseases cause fetal distress.

§ ✓5th **656.4 Intrauterine death**
[0,1,3]
    Fetal death:
        NOS
        after completion of 22 weeks' gestation
        late
    Missed delivery
    EXCLUDES missed abortion (632)

§ ✓5th **656.5 Poor fetal growth**
[0,1,3]
    "Light-for-dates"   "Small-for-dates"
    "Placental insufficiency"

§ ✓5th **656.6 Excessive fetal growth**
[0,1,3]
    "Large-for-dates"

§ ✓5th **656.7 Other placental conditions**
[0,1,3]
    Abnormal placenta   Placental infarct
    EXCLUDES placental polyp (674.4)
        placentitis (658.4)

§ ✓5th **656.8 Other specified fetal and placental problems**
[0,1,3]
    Abnormal acid-base balance   Lithopedian
    Intrauterine acidosis   Meconium in liquor
DEF: Lithopedion: Calcified fetus; not expelled by mother.

§ ✓5th **656.9 Unspecified fetal and placental problem**
[0,1,3]

✓4th **657 Polyhydramnios**
[0,1,3]
  § ✓5th Use 0 as fourth-digit for this category
    Hydramnios
DEF: Excess amniotic fluid.

✓4th **658 Other problems associated with amniotic cavity and membranes**
    EXCLUDES amniotic fluid embolism (673.1)

§ ✓5th **658.0 Oligohydramnios**
[0,1,3]
    Oligohydramnios without mention of rupture of membranes
DEF: Deficient amount of amniotic fluid.

§ ✓5th **658.1 Premature rupture of membranes**
[0,1,3]
    Rupture of amniotic sac less than 24 hours prior to the onset of labor

§ Requires fifth-digit. Valid digits are in [brackets] under each code. See beginning of section 640–648 for codes and definitions.

N Newborn Age: 0   P Pediatric Age: 0-17   M Maternity Age: 12-55   A Adult Age: 15-124

COMPLICATIONS OF PREGNANCY, CHILDBIRTH, & PUERPERIUM 658.2–659.9

§ ✓5ᵗʰ 658.2 **Delayed delivery after spontaneous or unspecified rupture of membranes**
[0,1,3]
    Prolonged rupture of membranes NOS
    Rupture of amniotic sac 24 hours or more prior to the onset of labor

§ ✓5ᵗʰ 658.3 **Delayed delivery after artificial rupture of membranes**
[0,1,3]

§ ✓5ᵗʰ 658.4 **Infection of amniotic cavity**
[0,1,3]
    Amnionitis   Membranitis
    Chorioamnionitis   Placentitis

§ ✓5ᵗʰ 658.8 **Other**
[0,1,3]
    Amnion nodosum   Amniotic cyst

§ ✓5ᵗʰ 658.9 **Unspecified**
[0,1,3]

✓4ᵗʰ 659 **Other indications for care or intervention related to labor and delivery, not elsewhere classified**

§ ✓5ᵗʰ 659.0 **Failed mechanical induction**
[0,1,3]
    Failure of induction of labor by surgical or other instrumental methods

§ ✓5ᵗʰ 659.1 **Failed medical or unspecified induction**
[0,1,3]
    Failed induction NOS
    Failure of induction of labor by medical methods, such as oxytocic drugs

§ ✓5ᵗʰ 659.2 **Maternal pyrexia during labor, unspecified**
[0,1,3]
DEF: Fever during labor.

§ ✓5ᵗʰ 659.3 **Generalized infection during labor**
[0,1,3]
    Septicemia during labor

§ ✓5ᵗʰ 659.4 **Grand multiparity**
[0,1,3]
    EXCLUDES supervision only, in pregnancy (V23.3)
                    without current pregnancy (V61.5)
DEF: Having borne six or more children previously.

§ ✓5ᵗʰ 659.5 **Elderly primigravida**
[0,1,3]
    First pregnancy in a woman who will be 35 years of age or older at expected date of delivery
    EXCLUDES supervision only, in pregnancy (V23.81)

§ ✓5ᵗʰ 659.6 **Elderly multigravida**
[0,1,3]
    Second or more pregnancy in a woman who will be 35 years of age or older at expected date of delivery
    EXCLUDES elderly primigravida 659.5
                    supervision only, in pregnancy (V23.82)

§ ✓5ᵗʰ 659.7 **Abnormality in fetal heart rate or rhythm**
[0,1,3]
    Depressed fetal heart tones
    Fetal:
        bradycardia
        tachycardia
    Fetal heart rate decelerations
    Non-reassuring fetal heart rate or rhythm

§ ✓5ᵗʰ 659.8 **Other specified indications for care or intervention related to labor and delivery**
[0,1,3]
    Pregnancy in a female less than 16 years old at expected date of delivery
    Very young maternal age

§ ✓5ᵗʰ 659.9 **Unspecified indication for care or intervention related to labor and delivery**
[0,1,3]

§ Requires fifth-digit. Valid digits are in [brackets] under each code. See beginning of section 640–648 for codes and definitions.

COMPLICATIONS OF PREGNANCY, CHILDBIRTH, & PUERPERIUM

COMPLICATIONS OCCURRING MAINLY IN THE COURSE OF LABOR AND DELIVERY (660-669)

The following fifth-digit subclassification is for use with categories 660-669 to denote the current episode of care. Valid fifth-digits are in [brackets] under each code.

0 unspecified as to episode of care or not applicable
1 delivered, with or without mention of antepartum condition
2 delivered, with mention of postpartum complication
3 antepartum condition or complication
4 postpartum condition or complication

660 Obstructed labor

§ **660.0 Obstruction caused by malposition of fetus at onset of labor**
[0,1,3]
Any condition classifiable to 652, causing obstruction during labor
Use additional code from 652.0-652.9 to identify condition

§ **660.1 Obstruction by bony pelvis**
[0,1,3]
Any condition classifiable to 653, causing obstruction during labor
Use additional code from 653.0-653.9 to identify condition

§ **660.2 Obstruction by abnormal pelvic soft tissues**
[0,1,3]
Prolapse of anterior lip of cervix
Any condition classifiable to 654, causing obstruction during labor
Use additional code from 654.0-654.9 to identify condition

§ **660.3 Deep transverse arrest and persistent occipitoposterior position**
[0,1,3]

§ **660.4 Shoulder (girdle) dystocia**
[0,1,3]
Impacted shoulders
DEF: Obstructed labor due to impacted fetal shoulders.

§ **660.5 Locked twins**
[0,1,3]

§ **660.6 Failed trial of labor, unspecified**
[0,1,3]
Failed trial of labor, without mention of condition or suspected condition

§ **660.7 Failed forceps or vacuum extractor, unspecified**
[0,1,3]
Application of ventouse or forceps, without mention of condition

§ **660.8 Other causes of obstructed labor**
[0,1,3]

§ **660.9 Unspecified obstructed labor**
[0,1,3]
Dystocia: Dystocia:
  NOS   maternal NOS
  fetal NOS

661 Abnormality of forces of labor

§ **661.0 Primary uterine inertia**
[0,1,3]
Failure of cervical dilation
Hypotonic uterine dysfunction, primary
Prolonged latent phase of labor
DEF: Lack of efficient contractions during labor causing prolonged labor.

§ **661.1 Secondary uterine inertia**
[0,1,3]
Arrested active phase of labor
Hypotonic uterine dysfunction, secondary

§ Requires fifth-digit. Valid digits are in [brackets] under each code. See beginning of section 640-648 for codes and definitions.

COMPLICATIONS OF PREGNANCY, CHILDBIRTH, & PUERPERIUM — 661.2–663.8

§ √5th **661.2** **Other and unspecified uterine inertia** M ♀
[0,1,3]
  Desultory labor   Poor contractions
  Irregular labor   Slow slope active phase
                           of labor

§ √5th **661.3** **Precipitate labor** M ♀
[0,1,3] DEF: Rapid labor and delivery.

§ √5th **661.4** **Hypertonic, incoordinate, or prolonged uterine contractions** M ♀
[0,1,3]
  Cervical spasm
  Contraction ring (dystocia)
  Dyscoordinate labor
  Hourglass contraction of uterus
  Hypertonic uterine dysfunction
  Incoordinate uterine action
  Retraction ring (Bandl's) (pathological)
  Tetanic contractions
  Uterine dystocia NOS
  Uterine spasm

§ √5th **661.9** **Unspecified abnormality of labor** M ♀
[0,1,3]

√4th **662** **Long labor**

§ √5th **662.0** **Prolonged first stage** M ♀
[0,1,3]

§ √5th **662.1** **Prolonged labor, unspecified** M ♀
[0,1,3]

§ √5th **662.2** **Prolonged second stage** M ♀
[0,1,3]

§ √5th **662.3** **Delayed delivery of second twin, triplet, etc.** M ♀
[0,1,3]

√4th **663** **Umbilical cord complications**

§ √5th **663.0** **Prolapse of cord** M ♀
[0,1,3]
  Presentation of cord
  DEF: Abnormal presentation of fetus; marked by protruding umbilical cord during labor; can cause fetal death.

§ √5th **663.1** **Cord around neck, with compression** M ♀
[0,1,3]
  Cord tightly around neck

§ √5th **663.2** **Other and unspecified cord entanglement, with compression** M ♀
[0,1,3]
  Entanglement of cords of twins in mono-amniotic sac
  Knot in cord (with compression)

§ √5th **663.3** **Other and unspecified cord entanglement, without mention of compression** M ♀
[0,1,3]

§ √5th **663.4** **Short cord** M ♀
[0,1,3]

§ √5th **663.5** **Vasa previa** M ♀
[0,1,3] DEF: Abnormal presentation of fetus marked by blood vessels of umbilical cord in front of fetal head.

§ √5th **663.6** **Vascular lesions of cord** M ♀
[0,1,3]
  Bruising of cord   Thrombosis of vessels of
  Hematoma of cord   cord

§ √5th **663.8** **Other umbilical cord complications** M ♀
[0,1,3]
  Velamentous insertion of umbilical cord

§ Requires fifth-digit. Valid digits are in [brackets] under each code. See beginning of section 640–648 for codes and definitions.

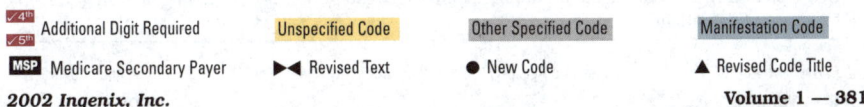

√4th/√5th Additional Digit Required   Unspecified Code   Other Specified Code   Manifestation Code
MSP Medicare Secondary Payer   ▶◀ Revised Text   ● New Code   ▲ Revised Code Title

COMPLICATIONS OF PREGNANCY, CHILDBIRTH, & PUERPERIUM

§ ✓5th **663.9** **Unspecified umbilical cord complication** M ♀
[0,1,3]

✓4th **664 Trauma to perineum and vulva during delivery**
   INCLUDES   damage from instruments
               that from extension of episiotomy

§ ✓5th **664.0** **First-degree perineal laceration** M ♀
[0,1,4]
Perineal laceration, rupture, or tear involving:
- fourchette
- skin
- hymen
- vagina
- labia
- vulva

§ ✓5th **664.1** **Second-degree perineal laceration** M ♀
[0,1,4]
Perineal laceration, rupture, or tear (following episiotomy) involving:
- pelvic floor
- perineal muscles
- vaginal muscles

   EXCLUDES   that involving anal sphincter (664.2)

§ ✓5th **664.2** **Third-degree perineal laceration** M ♀
[0,1,4]
Perineal laceration, rupture, or tear (following episiotomy) involving:
- anal sphincter
- rectovaginal septum
- sphincter NOS

   EXCLUDES   that with anal or rectal mucosal laceration (664.3)

§ ✓5th **664.3** **Fourth-degree perineal laceration** M ♀
[0,1,4]
Perineal laceration, rupture, or tear as classifiable to 664.2 and involving also:
- anal mucosa
- rectal mucosa

§ ✓5th **664.4** **Unspecified perineal laceration** M ♀
[0,1,4]
Central laceration

§ ✓5th **664.5** **Vulval and perineal hematoma** M ♀
[0,1,4]

§ ✓5th **664.8** **Other specified trauma to perineum and vulva** M ♀
[0,1,4]

§ ✓5th **664.9** **Unspecified trauma to perineum and vulva** M ♀
[0,1,4]

Perineal Lacerations

First degree
Anus
Second degree
Third degree
Fourth degree

§ Requires fifth-digit. Valid digits are in [brackets] under each code. See beginning of section 640–648 for codes and definitions.

N Newborn Age: 0   P Pediatric Age: 0-17   M Maternity Age: 12-55   A Adult Age: 15-124

COMPLICATIONS OF PREGNANCY, CHILDBIRTH, & PUERPERIUM 665–667

✓4ᵗʰ **665 Other obstetrical trauma**
  INCLUDES damage from instruments

§ ✓5ᵗʰ **665.0 Rupture of uterus before onset of labor** M♀
  [0,1,3]

§ ✓5ᵗʰ **665.1 Rupture of uterus during labor** M♀
  [0,1] Rupture of uterus NOS

§ ✓5ᵗʰ **665.2 Inversion of uterus** M♀
  [0,2,4]

§ ✓5ᵗʰ **665.3 Laceration of cervix** M♀
  [0,1,4]

§ ✓5ᵗʰ **665.4 High vaginal laceration** M♀
  [0,1,4] Laceration of vaginal wall or sulcus without mention of perineal laceration

§ ✓5ᵗʰ **665.5 Other injury to pelvic organs** M♀
  [0,1,4] Injury to:
      bladder
      urethra

§ ✓5ᵗʰ **665.6 Damage to pelvic joints and ligaments** M♀
  [0,1,4] Avulsion of inner symphyseal cartilage
      Damage to coccyx
      Separation of symphysis (pubis)

§ ✓5ᵗʰ **665.7 Pelvic hematoma** M♀
  [0,1,2,4] Hematoma of vagina

§ ✓5ᵗʰ **665.8 Other specified obstetrical trauma** M♀
  [0-4]

§ ✓5ᵗʰ **665.9 Unspecified obstetrical trauma** M♀
  [0-4]

✓4ᵗʰ **666 Postpartum hemorrhage**

§ ✓5ᵗʰ **666.0 Third-stage hemorrhage** M♀
  [0,2,4] Hemorrhage associated with retained, trapped, or adherent placenta
      Retained placenta NOS

§ ✓5ᵗʰ **666.1 Other immediate postpartum hemorrhage** M♀
  [0,2,4] Atony of uterus
      Hemorrhage within the first 24 hours following delivery of placenta
      Postpartum hemorrhage (atonic) NOS

§ ✓5ᵗʰ **666.2 Delayed and secondary postpartum hemorrhage** M♀
  [0,2,4] Hemorrhage:
        after the first 24 hours following delivery
        associated with retained portions of placenta or membranes
      Postpartum hemorrhage specified as delayed or secondary
      Retained products of conception NOS, following delivery

§ ✓5ᵗʰ **666.3 Postpartum coagulation defects** M♀
  [0,2,4] Postpartum: Postpartum:
      afibrinogenemia   fibrinolysis

✓4ᵗʰ **667 Retained placenta or membranes, without hemorrhage**
  Requires fifth-digit; valid digits are in [brackets] under each code. See beginning of section 660-669 for definitions.

  DEF: Postpartum condition resulting from failure to expel placental membrane tissues due to failed contractions of uterine wall.

§ Requires fifth-digit. Valid digits are in [brackets] under each code. See beginning of section 640–648 for codes and definitions.

✓4ᵗʰ / ✓5ᵗʰ Additional Digit Required   Unspecified Code   Other Specified Code   Manifestation Code
MSP Medicare Secondary Payer   ▶◀ Revised Text   ● New Code   ▲ Revised Code Title

2002 Ingenix, Inc.

667.0–669.5 COMPLICATIONS OF PREGNANCY, CHILDBIRTH, & PUERPERIUM

§ ✓5th **667.0 Retained placenta without hemorrhage** M♀
[0,2,4]
   Placenta accreta ⎫
   Retained placenta: ⎬ without hemorrhage
     NOS ⎪
     total ⎭

§ ✓5th **667.1 Retained portions of placenta or membranes, without hemorrhage** M♀
[0,2,4]   Retained products of conception following delivery, without hemorrhage

✓4th **668 Complications of the administration of anesthetic or other sedation in labor and delivery**

   INCLUDES complications arising from the administration of a general or local anesthetic, analgesic, or other sedation in labor and delivery

   EXCLUDES reaction to spinal or lumbar puncture (349.0)
            spinal headache (349.0)

   Use additional code(s) to further specify complication

§ ✓5th **668.0 Pulmonary complications** M♀
[0-4]
   Inhalation [aspiration] of ⎫
     stomach contents ⎪ following anesthesia
     or secretions ⎬ or other sedation in
   Mendelson's syndrome ⎪ labor or
   Pressure collapse of lung ⎭ delivery

§ ✓5th **668.1 Cardiac complications** M♀
[0-4]   Cardiac arrest or failure following anesthesia or other sedation in labor and delivery

§ ✓5th **668.2 Central nervous system complications** M♀
[0-4]   Cerebral anoxia following anesthesia or other sedation in labor and delivery

§ ✓5th **668.8 Other complications of anesthesia or other sedation in labor and delivery** M♀
[0-4]

§ ✓5th **668.9 Unspecified complication of anesthesia and other sedation** M♀
[0-4]

✓4th **669 Other complications of labor and delivery, not elsewhere classified**

§ ✓5th **669.0 Maternal distress** M♀
[0-4]   Metabolic disturbance in labor and delivery

§ ✓5th **669.1 Shock during or following labor and delivery** M♀
[0-4]   Obstetric shock

§ ✓5th **669.2 Maternal hypotension syndrome** M♀
[0-4]   DEF: Low arterial blood pressure, in mother, during labor and delivery.

§ ✓5th **669.3 Acute renal failure following labor and delivery** M♀
[0,2,4]

§ ✓5th **669.4 Other complications of obstetrical surgery and procedures** M♀
[0-4]
   Cardiac: ⎫
     arrest ⎬ following cesarean or other obstetrical surgery or
     failure ⎪ procedure, including delivery NOS
   Cerebral anoxia ⎭

   EXCLUDES complications of obstetrical surgical wounds (674.1-674.3)

§ ✓5th **669.5 Forceps or vacuum extractor delivery without mention of indication** M♀
[0,1]
   Delivery by ventouse, without mention of indication

---

§ Requires fifth-digit. Valid digits are in [brackets] under each code. See beginning of section 640–648 for codes and definitions.

N Newborn Age: 0   P Pediatric Age: 0-17   M Maternity Age: 12-55   A Adult Age: 15-124

COMPLICATIONS OF PREGNANCY, CHILDBIRTH, & PUERPERIUM 669.6–671.4

§ ✓5ᵗʰ **669.6** Breech extraction, without mention of indication M ♀
[0,1]   EXCLUDES   breech delivery NOS (652.2)

§ ✓5ᵗʰ **669.7** Cesarean delivery, without mention of indication M ♀
[0,1]

§ ✓5ᵗʰ **669.8** Other complications of labor and delivery M ♀
[0-4]

§ ✓5ᵗʰ **669.9** Unspecified complication of labor and delivery M ♀
[0-4]

COMPLICATIONS OF THE PUERPERIUM (670-677)

Note: Categories 671 and 673-676 include the listed conditions even if they occur during pregnancy or childbirth.

The following fifth-digit subclassification is for use with categories 670-676 to denote the current episode of care. Valid fifth-digits are in [brackets] under each code.

0 unspecified as to episode of care or not applicable
1 delivered, with or without mention of antepartum condition
2 delivered, with mention of postpartum complication
3 antepartum condition or complication
4 postpartum condition or complication

✓4ᵗʰ **670** Major puerperal infection
[0,2,4]

§ ✓5ᵗʰ Use 0 as fourth-digit for this category
Puerperal: Puerperal:
  endometritis   peritonitis
  fever (septic)   pyemia
  pelvic: salpingitis
    cellulitis   septicemia
    sepsis
   EXCLUDES   infection following abortion (639.0)
             minor genital tract infection following delivery (646.6)
             puerperal pyrexia NOS (672)
             puerperal fever NOS (672)
             puerperal pyrexia of unknown origin (672)
             urinary tract infection following delivery (646.6)
DEF: Infection and inflammation, following childbirth.

✓4ᵗʰ **671** Venous complications in pregnancy and the puerperium

§ ✓5ᵗʰ **671.0** Varicose veins of legs M ♀
[0-4]   Varicose veins NOS
           DEF: Distended, tortuous veins on legs associated with pregnancy.

§ ✓5ᵗʰ **671.1** Varicose veins of vulva and perineum M ♀
[0-4]   DEF: Distended, tortuous veins on external female genitalia associated with pregnancy.

§ ✓5ᵗʰ **671.2** Superficial thrombophlebitis M ♀
[0-4]   Thrombophlebitis (superficial)

§ ✓5ᵗʰ **671.3** Deep phlebothrombosis, antepartum M ♀
[0,1,3]   Deep-vein thrombosis, antepartum

§ ✓5ᵗʰ **671.4** Deep phlebothrombosis, postpartum M ♀
[0,2,4]   Deep-vein thrombosis, postpartum
           Pelvic thrombophlebitis, postpartum
           Phlegmasia alba dolens (puerperal)

§ Requires fifth-digit. Valid digits are in [brackets] under each code. See beginning of section 640–648 for codes and definitions.

✓4ᵗʰ/✓5ᵗʰ Additional Digit Required   Unspecified Code   Other Specified Code   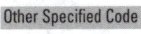 Manifestation Code
MSP Medicare Secondary Payer   ▶◀ Revised Text   ● New Code   ▲ Revised Code Title

2002 Ingenix, Inc.   Volume 1 — 385

671.5–674.3 COMPLICATIONS OF PREGNANCY, CHILDBIRTH, & PUERPERIUM

- § √5th **671.5 Other phlebitis and thrombosis**
  [0-4]
      Cerebral venous thrombosis
      Thrombosis of intracranial venous sinus
- § √5th **671.8 Other venous complications**
  [0-4]
      Hemorrhoids
- § √5th **671.9 Unspecified venous complication**
  [0-4]
      Phlebitis NOS   Thrombosis NOS

√4th **672 Pyrexia of unknown origin during the puerperium**
[0,2,4]
- § √5th
  Use 0 as fourth-digit for this category
  Postpartum fever NOS
  Puerperal fever NOS
  Puerperal pyrexia NOS

DEF: Fever of unknown origin experienced by the mother after childbirth.

√4th **673 Obstetrical pulmonary embolism**
Requires fifth-digit; valid digits are in [brackets] under each code. See beginning of section 670-676 for definitions.

INCLUDES   pulmonary emboli in pregnancy, childbirth, or the puerperium, or specified as puerperal

EXCLUDES   *embolism following abortion (639.6)*

- § √5th **673.0 Obstetrical air embolism**
  [0-4]
  DEF: Sudden blocking of pulmonary artery with air or nitrogen bubbles during puerperium..
- § √5th **673.1 Amniotic fluid embolism**
  [0-4]
  DEF: Sudden onset of pulmonary artery blockage from amniotic fluid entering the mother's circulation near the end of pregnancy due to strong uterine contractions.
- § √5th **673.2 Obstetrical blood-clot embolism**
  [0-4]
      Puerperal pulmonary embolism NOS
  DEF: Blood clot blocking artery in the lung; associated with pregnancy.
- § √5th **673.3 Obstetrical pyemic and septic embolism**
  [0-4]
- § √5th **673.8 Other pulmonary embolism**
  [0-4]
      Fat embolism

√4th **674 Other and unspecified complications of the puerperium, not elsewhere classified**
- § √5th **674.0 Cerebrovascular disorders in the puerperium**
  [0-4]
      Any condition classifiable to 430-434, 436-437 occurring during pregnancy, childbirth, or the puerperium, or specified as puerperal

  EXCLUDES   *intracranial venous sinus thrombosis (671.5)*
- § √5th **674.1 Disruption of cesarean wound**
  [0,2,4]
      Dehiscence or disruption of uterine wound

  EXCLUDES   ▶*uterine rupture before onset of labor (665.0)*
                  uterine rupture during labor (665.1)◀
- § √5th **674.2 Disruption of perineal wound**
  [0,2,4]
      Breakdown of perineum   Disruption of wound of:
      Disruption of wound of: perineal laceration
        episiotomy   Secondary perineal tear
- § √5th **674.3 Other complications of obstetrical surgical wounds**
  [0,2,4]
      Hematoma
      Hemorrhage } of cesarean section or perineal wound
      Infection

  EXCLUDES   *damage from instruments in delivery (664.0-665.9)*

§ Requires fifth-digit. Valid digits are in [brackets] under each code. See beginning of section 640–648 for codes and definitions.

COMPLICATIONS OF PREGNANCY, CHILDBIRTH, & PUERPERIUM 674.4–676.5

§ √5ᵗʰ **674.4** Placental polyp
  [0,2,4]

§ √5ᵗʰ **674.8** Other
  [0,2,4]
  Hepatorenal syndrome, following delivery
  Postpartum:
   cardiomyopathy
   subinvolution of uterus
   uterine hypertrophy

§ √5ᵗʰ **674.9** Unspecified
  [0,2,4]
  Sudden death of unknown cause during the puerperium

√4ᵗʰ **675** Infections of the breast and nipple associated with childbirth
  INCLUDES: the listed conditions during pregnancy, childbirth, or the puerperium

§ √5ᵗʰ **675.0** Infections of nipple
  [0-4]
  Abscess of nipple

§ √5ᵗʰ **675.1** Abscess of breast
  [0-4]
  Abscess:
   mammary
   subareolar
   submammary
  Mastitis:
   purulent
   retromammary
   submammary

§ √5ᵗʰ **675.2** Nonpurulent mastitis
  [0-4]
  Lymphangitis of breast
  Mastitis:
   NOS
   interstitial
   parenchymatous

§ √5ᵗʰ **675.8** Other specified infections of the breast and nipple
  [0-4]

§ √5ᵗʰ **675.9** Unspecified infection of the breast and nipple
  [0-4]

√4ᵗʰ **676** Other disorders of the breast associated with childbirth and disorders of lactation
  INCLUDES: the listed conditions during pregnancy, the puerperium, or lactation

§ √5ᵗʰ **676.0** Retracted nipple
  [0-4]

§ √5ᵗʰ **676.1** Cracked nipple
  [0-4]
  Fissure of nipple

§ √5ᵗʰ **676.2** Engorgement of breasts
  [0-4]
  DEF: Abnormal accumulation of milk in ducts of breast.

§ √5ᵗʰ **676.3** Other and unspecified disorder of breast
  [0-4]

§ √5ᵗʰ **676.4** Failure of lactation
  [0-4]
  Agalactia
  DEF: Abrupt ceasing of milk secretion by breast.

§ √5ᵗʰ **676.5** Suppressed lactation
  [0-4]

---

§ Requires fifth-digit. Valid digits are in [brackets] under each code. See beginning of section 640–648 for codes and definitions.

√4ᵗʰ / √5ᵗʰ Additional Digit Required   Unspecified Code   Other Specified Code   Manifestation Code
MSP Medicare Secondary Payer   ▶◀ Revised Text   ● New Code   ▲ Revised Code Title

676.6–680 SKIN AND SUBCUTANEOUS TISSUE

§ √5th **676.6** Galactorrhea M ♀
[0-4]   EXCLUDES *galactorrhea not associated with childbirth (611.6)*
DEF: Excessive or persistent milk secretion by breast; may be in absence of nursing.

§ √5th **676.8** **Other disorders of lactation** M ♀
[0-4]   Galactocele
DEF: Galactocele: obstructed mammary gland, creating retention cyst, results in milk-filled cysts enlarging mammary gland.

§ √5th **676.9** **Unspecified disorder of lactation** M ♀
[0-4]

677 Late effect of complication of pregnancy, childbirth, and the puerperium M ♀
Note: This category is to be used to indicate conditions in 632-648.9 and 651-676.9 as the cause of the late effect, themselves classifiable elsewhere. The "late effects" include conditions specified as such, or as sequelae, which may occur at any time after puerperium.
Code first any sequelae

12. DISEASES OF THE SKIN AND SUBCUTANEOUS TISSUE (680-709)

INFECTIONS OF SKIN AND SUBCUTANEOUS TISSUE (680-686)

EXCLUDES *certain infections of skin classified under "Infectious and Parasitic Diseases," such as:*
erysipelas (035)
erysipeloid of Rosenbach (027.1)
herpes:
simplex (054.0-054.9)
zoster (053.0-053.9)
molluscum contagiosum (078.0)
viral warts (078.1)

√4th **680** **Carbuncle and furuncle**
INCLUDES   boil
            furunculosis

DEF: Carbuncle: necrotic boils in skin and subcutaneous tissue of neck or back mainly due to staphylococcal infection.

DEF: Furuncle: Circumscribed inflammation of corium and subcutaneous tissue due to staphylococcal infection.

Skin and Subcutaneous Layer

Labels: Hair follicle, Epidermis, Dermis, Hypodermis (subcutaneous layer), Bulb, Sebaceous gland, Arrector pili muscle, Thick-skin epidermis, Hair shaft, Pacinian corpuscle, Hair matrix, Sweat (eccrine gland), Sensory nerve, Blood vessels

§ Requires fifth-digit. Valid digits are in [brackets] under each code. See beginning of section 640–648 for codes and definitions.

N Newborn Age: 0   P Pediatric Age: 0-17   M Maternity Age: 12-55   A Adult Age: 15-124

SKIN AND SUBCUTANEOUS TISSUE

680.0 Face
- Ear [any part]
- Face [any part, except eye]
- Nose (septum)
- Temple (region)

  EXCLUDES eyelid (373.13)
  lacrimal apparatus (375.31)
  orbit (376.01)

680.1 Neck

680.2 Trunk
- Abdominal wall
- Back [any part, except buttocks]
- Breast
- Chest wall
- Flank
- Groin
- Pectoral region
- Perineum
- Umbilicus

  EXCLUDES buttocks (680.5)
  external genital organs:
    female (616.4)
    male (607.2, 608.4)

680.3 Upper arm and forearm
- Arm [any part, except hand]
- Axilla
- Shoulder

680.4 Hand
- Finger [any]
- Thumb
- Wrist

680.5 Buttock
- Anus
- Gluteal region

680.6 Leg, except foot
- Ankle
- Hip
- Knee
- Thigh

680.7 Foot
- Heel
- Toe

680.8 Other specified sites
- Head [any part, except face]
- Scalp

  EXCLUDES external genital organs:
    female (616.4)
    male (607.2, 608.4)

680.9 Unspecified site
- Boil NOS
- Carbuncle NOS
- Furuncle NOS

√4th **681 Cellulitis and abscess of finger and toe**

  INCLUDES that with lymphangitis

  Use additional code to identify organism, such as Staphylococcus (041.1)

  DEF: Acute suppurative inflammation and edema in subcutaneous tissue or muscle of finger or toe.

√5th **681.0 Finger**

  681.00 Cellulitis and abscess, unspecified

681.01 Felon
- Pulp abscess
- Whitlow

EXCLUDES herpetic whitlow (054.6)

DEF: Painful abscess of fingertips caused by infection in the closed space of terminal phalanx.

681.02 Onychia and paronychia of finger
- Panaritium } of finger
- Perionychia

DEF: Onychia: inflammation of nail matrix; causes nail loss.

DEF: Paronychia: inflammation of tissue folds around nail.

√5th **681.1 Toe**

681.10 Cellulitis and abscess, unspecified

681.11 Onychia and paronychia of toe
- Panaritium } of toe
- Perionychia

681.9 Cellulitis and abscess of unspecified digit
Infection of nail NOS

√4th **682 Other cellulitis and abscess**

INCLUDES
- abscess (acute)
- cellulitis (diffuse) } (with lymphangitis)
- lymphangitis, acute   except of finger or toe

Use additional code to identify organism, such as Staphylococcus (041.1)

EXCLUDES lymphangitis (chronic) (subacute) (457.2)

DEF: Cellulitis: Acute suppurative inflammation of deep subcutaneous tissue and sometimes muscle due to infection of wound, burn or other lesion.

682.0 Face
- Cheek, external
- Chin
- Forehead
- Nose, external
- Submandibular
- Temple (region)

EXCLUDES
- ear [any part] (380.10-380.16)
- eyelid (373.13)
- lacrimal apparatus (375.31)
- lip (528.5)
- mouth (528.3)
- nose (internal) (478.1)
- orbit (376.01)

682.1 Neck

682.2 Trunk
- Abdominal wall
- Back [any part, except buttock]
- Chest wall
- Flank
- Groin
- Pectoral region
- Perineum
- Umbilicus, except newborn

EXCLUDES
- anal and rectal regions (566)
- breast:
  - NOS (611.0)
  - puerperal (675.1)
- external genital organs:
  - female (616.3-616.4)
  - male (604.0, 607.2, 608.4)
- umbilicus, newborn (771.4)

SKIN AND SUBCUTANEOUS TISSUE

682.3 **Upper arm and forearm**
　　Arm [any part, except hand]
　　Axilla
　　Shoulder
　　　EXCLUDES　hand (682.4)

682.4 **Hand, except fingers and thumb**
　　Wrist
　　　EXCLUDES　finger and thumb (681.00-681.02)

682.5 **Buttock**
　　Gluteal region
　　　EXCLUDES　anal and rectal regions (566)

682.6 **Leg, except foot**
　　Ankle
　　Hip
　　Knee
　　Thigh

682.7 **Foot, except toes**
　　Heel
　　　EXCLUDES　toe (681.10-681.11)

682.8 **Other specified sites**
　　Head [except face]
　　Scalp
　　　EXCLUDES　face (682.0)

682.9 **Unspecified site**
　　Abscess NOS　　　　Lymphangitis, acute NOS
　　Cellulitis NOS
　　　EXCLUDES　lymphangitis NOS (457.2)

683 Acute lymphadenitis
　　Abscess (acute)
　　Adenitis, acute　　　} lymph gland or node,
　　Lymphadenitis, acute　　　except mesenteric

　　Use additional code to identify organism, such as Staphylococcus (041.1)
　　　EXCLUDES　enlarged glands NOS (785.6)
　　　　lymphadenitis:
　　　　　chronic or subacute, except mesenteric (289.1)
　　　　　mesenteric (acute) (chronic) (subacute) (289.2)
　　　　　unspecified (289.3)

DEF: Acute inflammation of lymph nodes due to primary infection located elsewhere in the body.

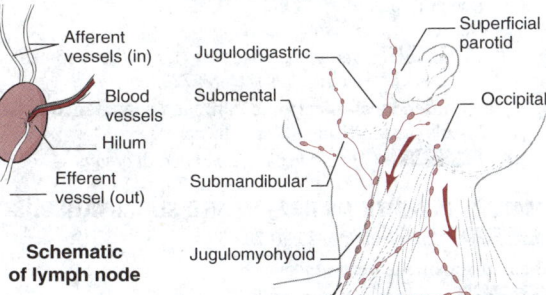

Schematic of lymph node

Lymphatic drainage of the head, neck, and face

SKIN AND SUBCUTANEOUS TISSUE

684 Impetigo
Impetiginization of other dermatoses
Impetigo (contagiosa) [any site] [any organism]:
- bullous
- circinate
- neonatorum
- simplex

Pemphigus neonatorum

EXCLUDES impetigo herpetiformis (694.3)

DEF: Infectious skin disease commonly occurring in children; caused by group A streptococci or *Staphylococcus aureus*; skin lesions usually appear on the face and consist of subcorneal vesicles and bullae that burst and form yellow crusts.

√4th 685 Pilonidal cyst

INCLUDES fistula } coccygeal or pilonidal
sinus

DEF: Hair-containing cyst or sinus in the tissues of the sacrococcygeal area; often drains through opening at the postanal dimple.

685.0 With abscess
685.1 Without mention of abscess

√4th 686 Other local infections of skin and subcutaneous tissue
Use additional code to identify any infectious organism (041.0-041.8)

√5th 686.0 Pyoderma
Dermatitis:
- purulent
- septic

Dermatitis:
- suppurative

DEF: Nonspecific purulent skin disease related most to furuncles, pustules, or possibly carbuncles.

686.00 Pyoderma, unspecified
686.01 Pyoderma gangrenosum
DEF: Persistent debilitating skin disease, characterized by irregular, boggy, blue-red ulcerations, with central healing and undermined edges.

686.09 Other pyoderma

686.1 Pyogenic granuloma
Granuloma:
- septic
- suppurative

Granuloma:
- telangiectaticum

EXCLUDES pyogenic granuloma of oral mucosa (528.9)

DEF: Solitary polypoid capillary hemangioma often asociated with local irritation, trauma, and superimposed inflammation; located on the skin and gingival or oral mucosa.

686.8 Other specified local infections of skin and subcutaneous tissue
- Bacterid (pustular)
- Dermatitis vegetans
- Ecthyma
- Perlèche

EXCLUDES dermatitis infectiosa eczematoides (690.8)
panniculitis (729.30-729.39)

686.9 Unspecified local infection of skin and subcutaneous tissue
Fistula of skin NOS   Skin infection NOS

EXCLUDES fistula to skin from internal organs — see Alphabetic Index

OTHER INFLAMMATORY CONDITIONS OF SKIN AND SUBCUTANEOUS TISSUE (690-698)

EXCLUDES panniculitis (729.30-729.39)

√4th 690 Erythematosquamous dermatosis

EXCLUDES
- eczematous dermatitis of eyelid (373.31)
- parakeratosis variegata (696.2)
- psoriasis (696.0-696.1)
- seborrheic keratosis (702.11-702.19)

DEF: Dry material desquamated from the scalp, associated with disease.

SKIN AND SUBCUTANEOUS TISSUE   690.1–691.8

Stages of Pilonidal Disease
- Normal follicle
- Stretched follicle
- Infected follicle
- Acute abscess
- Chronic abscess
- Epithelial tube

√5th **690.1 Seborrheic dermatitis**
- **690.10 Seborrheic dermatitis, unspecified**
  Seborrheic dermatitis NOS

√5th **690.1 Seborrheic dermatitis**
- **690.10 Seborrheic dermatitis, unspecified**
  Seborrheic dermatitis NOS
- **690.11 Seborrhea capitis**
  Cradle cap
- **690.12 Seborrheic infantile dermatitis**
- **690.18 Other seborrheic dermatitis**

690.8 Other erythematosquamous dermatosis

√4th **691 Atopic dermatitis and related conditions**

DEF: Atopic dermatitis: chronic, pruritic, inflammatory skin disorder found on the face and antecubital and popliteal fossae; noted in persons with a hereditary predisposition to pruritus, and often accompanied by allergic rhinitis, hay fever, asthma, and extreme itching; also called allergic dermatitis, allergic or atopic eczema, or disseminated neurodermatitis.

691.0 Diaper or napkin rash
  Ammonia dermatitis
  Diaper or napkin:
    dermatitis
    erythema
  Diaper or napkin:
    rash
  Psoriasiform napkin eruption

691.8 Other atopic dermatitis and related conditions
  Atopic dermatitis
  Besnier's prurigo
  Eczema:
    atopic
    flexural
    intrinsic (allergic)
  Neurodermatitis:
    atopic
    diffuse (of Brocq)

SKIN AND SUBCUTANEOUS TISSUE

✓4th 692 Contact dermatitis and other eczema
  - **INCLUDES** dermatitis:
    - NOS
    - contact
    - occupational
    - venenata
  - eczema (acute) (chronic):
    - NOS
    - allergic
    - erythematous
    - occupational
  - **EXCLUDES**
    - allergy NOS (995.3)
    - contact dermatitis of eyelids (373.32)
    - dermatitis due to substances taken internally (693.0-693.9)
    - eczema of external ear (380.22)
    - perioral dermatitis (695.3)
    - urticarial reactions (708.0-708.9, 995.1)

DEF: Contact dermatitis: acute or chronic dermatitis caused by initial irritant effect of a substance, or by prior sensitization to a substance coming once again in contact with skin.

692.0 Due to detergents

692.1 Due to oils and greases

692.2 Due to solvents
  Dermatitis due to solvents of:
  - chlorocompound ⎫
  - cyclohexane ⎬
  - ester ⎬ group
  - glycol ⎬
  - hydrocarbon ⎬
  - ketone ⎭

692.3 Due to drugs and medicines in contact with skin
  Dermatitis (allergic) (contact) due to:
  - arnica
  - fungicides
  - iodine
  - keratolytics
  - mercurials

  Dermatitis (allergic) (contact) due to:
  - neomycin
  - pediculocides
  - phenols
  - scabicides
  - any drug applied to skin

  Dermatitis medicamentosa due to drug applied to skin
  Use additional E code to identify drug
  - **EXCLUDES**
    - allergy NOS due to drugs (995.2)
    - dermatitis due to ingested drugs (693.0)
    - dermatitis medicamentosa NOS (693.0)

692.4 Due to other chemical products
  Dermatitis due to:
  - acids
  - adhesive plaster
  - alkalis
  - caustics
  - dichromate

  Dermatitis due to:
  - insecticide
  - nylon
  - plastic
  - rubber

SKIN AND SUBCUTANEOUS TISSUE — 692.5–692.73

692.5 Due to food in contact with skin
Dermatitis, contact, due to:
  cereals
  fish
  flour
Dermatitis, contact, due to:
  fruit
  meat
  milk

EXCLUDES dermatitis due to:
  dyes (692.89)
  ingested foods (693.1)
  preservatives (692.89)

692.6 Due to plants [except food]
Dermatitis due to:
  lacquer tree [Rhus verniciflua]
  poison:
    ivy [Rhus toxicodendron]
    oak [Rhus diversiloba]
    sumac [Rhus venenata]
    vine [Rhus radicans]
  primrose [Primula]
  ragweed [Senecio jacobae]
  other plants in contact with the skin

EXCLUDES allergy NOS due to pollen (477.0)
  nettle rash (708.8)

√5th 692.7 Due to solar radiation

EXCLUDES sunburn due to other ultraviolet radiation exposure (692.82)

692.70 Unspecified dermatitis due to sun

692.71 Sunburn
  First degree sunburn   Sunburn NOS

692.72 Acute dermatitis due to solar radiation
  Acute solar skin damage NOS
  Berlogue dermatitis
  Photoallergic response
  Phototoxic response
  Polymorphus light eruption

EXCLUDES sunburn (692.71, 692.76-692.77)
  Use additional E code to identify drug, if drug induced

DEF: Berloque dermatitis: phytophotodermatitis due to sun exposure after use of a product containing bergamot oil; causes red patches, which may turn brown.

DEF: Photoallergic response: dermatitis due to hypersensitivity to the sun; causes papulovesicular, eczematous or exudative eruptions.

DEF: Phototoxic response: chemically induced sensitivity to sun causes burn-like reaction, occasionally vesiculation and subsequent hyperpigmentation.

DEF: Polymorphous light eruption: inflammatory skin eruptions due to sunlight exposure; eruptions differ in size and shape.

DEF: Acute solar skin damage (NOS): rapid, unspecified injury to skin from sun.

692.73 Actinic reticuloid and actinic granuloma

DEF: Actinic reticuloid: dermatosis aggravated by light, causes chronic eczema-like eruption on exposed skin which extends to other unexposed surfaces; occurs in the eldery.

DEF: Actinic granuloma: inflammatory response of skin to sun causing small nodule of microphages.

692.74 Other chronic dermatitis due to solar radiation
　　Solar elastosis
　　Chronic solar skin damage NOS
　　　EXCLUDES　actinic [solar] keratosis (702.0)

DEF: Solar elastosis: premature aging of skin of light-skinned people; causes inelasticity, thinning or thickening, wrinkling, dryness, scaling and hyperpigmentation.

DEF: Chronic solar skin damage (NOS): chronic skin impairment due to exposure to the sun, not otherwise specified.

692.75 Disseminated superficial actinic porokeratosis (DSAP)
DEF: Autosomal dominant skin condition occurring in skin that has been overexposed to the sun. Primarily affects women over the age of 16; characterized by numerous superficial annular, keratotic, brownish-red spots or thickenings with depressed centers and sharp, ridged borders. High risk that condition will evolve into squamous cell carcinoma.

692.76 Sunburn of second degree
692.77 Sunburn of third degree
692.79 Other dermatitis due to solar radiation
　　Hydroa aestivale
　　Photodermatitis　　⎫
　　Photosensitiveness　⎬ (due to sun)
　　　　　　　　　　　⎭
　　Solar skin damage NOS

√5ᵗʰ **692.8 Due to other specified agents**
692.81 Dermatitis due to cosmetics
692.82 Dermatitis due to other radiation
　　Infrared rays　　Tanning bed
　　Light　　　　　 Ultraviolet rays
　　Radiation NOS　 X-rays
　　　EXCLUDES　solar radiation (692.70-692.79)

692.83 Dermatitis due to metals
　　Jewelry

692.89 Other
　　Dermatitis due to:
　　　cold weather
　　　dyes
　　　furs
　　　hot weather
　　　preservatives
　　　ultraviolet rays, except from sun
　　　EXCLUDES　allergy NOS due to animal hair, dander (animal), or
　　　　　　　　　　dust (477.8)
　　　　　　　　sunburn (692.71, 692.76-692.77)

692.9 Unspecified cause
　　Dermatitis:　　　　　Dermatitis:
　　　NOS　　　　　　　　venenata NOS
　　　contact NOS　　　　Eczema NOS

√4ᵗʰ **693 Dermatitis due to substances taken internally**
　　　EXCLUDES　adverse effect NOS of drugs and medicines (995.2)
　　　　　　　　allergy NOS (995.3)
　　　　　　　　contact dermatitis (692.0-692.9)
　　　　　　　　urticarial reactions (708.0-708.9, 995.1)

DEF: Inflammation of skin due to ingested substance.

SKIN AND SUBCUTANEOUS TISSUE 693.0–694.9

693.0 Due to drugs and medicines
Dermatitis medicamentosa NOS
Use additional E code to identify drug
EXCLUDES that due to drugs in contact with skin (692.3)

693.1 Due to food

693.8 Due to other specified substances taken internally

693.9 Due to unspecified substance taken internally
EXCLUDES dermatitis NOS (692.9)

✓4th **694 Bullous dermatoses**

694.0 Dermatitis herpetiformis
Dermatosis herpetiformis Hydroa herpetiformis
Duhring's disease
EXCLUDES herpes gestationis (646.8)
dermatitis herpetiformis:
juvenile (694.2)
senile (694.5)

DEF: Chronic, relapsing multisystem disease manifested most in the cutaneous system; seen as an extremely pruritic eruption of various combinations of lesions that frequently heal leaving hyperpigmentation or hypopigmentation and occasionally scarring; usually associated with an asymptomatic gluten-sensitive enteropathy, and immunogenic factors are believed to play a role in its origin.

694.1 Subcorneal pustular dermatosis
Sneddon-Wilkinson disease or syndrome

DEF: Chronic relapses of sterile pustular blebs beneath the horny skin layer of the trunk and skin folds; resembles dermatitis herpetiformis.

694.2 Juvenile dermatitis herpetiformis
Juvenile pemphigoid

694.3 Impetigo herpetiformis

DEF: Rare dermatosis associated with pregnancy; marked by itching pustules in third trimester, hypocalcemia, tetany, fever and lethargy; may result in maternal or fetal death.

694.4 Pemphigus
Pemphigus: Pemphigus:
  NOS   malignant
  erythematosus   vegetans
  foliaceus   vulgaris
EXCLUDES pemphigus neonatorum (684)

DEF: Chronic, relapsing, sometimes fatal skin diseases; causes vesicles, bullae; autoantibodies against intracellular connections cause acantholysis.

694.5 Pemphigoid
Benign pemphigus NOS
Bullous pemphigoid
Herpes circinatus bullosus
Senile dermatitis herpetiformis

✓5th **694.6 Benign mucous membrane pemphigoid**
Cicatricial pemphigoid
Mucosynechial atrophic bullous dermatitis

694.60 Without mention of ocular involvement

694.61 With ocular involvement
Ocular pemphigus

694.8 Other specified bullous dermatoses
EXCLUDES herpes gestationis (646.8)

694.9 Unspecified bullous dermatoses

✓4th
✓5th Additional Digit Required   Unspecified Code   Other Specified Code   Manifestation Code
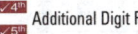 Medicare Secondary Payer   ▶◀ Revised Text   ● New Code   ▲ Revised Code Title

2002 Ingenix, Inc.   Volume 1 — 397

SKIN AND SUBCUTANEOUS TISSUE

✓4th **695 Erythematous conditions**

695.0 Toxic erythema
Erythema venenatum

695.1 Erythema multiforme
Erythema iris
Herpes iris
Lyell's syndrome
Scalded skin syndrome
Stevens-Johnson syndrome
Toxic epidermal necrolysis

DEF: Symptom complex with a varied skin eruption pattern of macular, bullous, papular, nodose, or vesicular lesions on the neck, face, and legs; gastritis and rheumatic pains are also noticeable, first-seen symptoms; complex is secondary to a number of factors, including infections, ingestants, physical agents, malignancy and pregnancy.

695.2 Erythema nodosum
EXCLUDES *tuberculous erythema nodosum (017.1)*

DEF: Panniculitis (an inflammatory reaction of the subcutaneous fat) of women, usually seen as a hypersensitivity reaction to various infections, drugs, sarcoidosis, and specific enteropathies; the acute stage is often associated with other symptoms, including fever, malaise, and arthralgia; the lesions are pink to blue in color, appear in crops as tender nodules and are found on the front of the legs below the knees.

695.3 Rosacea
Acne:
   erythematosa
   rosacea
Perioral dermatitis
Rhinophyma

DEF: Chronic skin disease, usually of the face, characterized by persistent erythema and sometimes by telangiectasis with acute episodes of edema, engorgement papules, and pustules.

695.4 Lupus erythematosus
Lupus:
   erythematodes (discoid)
   erythematosus (discoid), not disseminated
EXCLUDES *lupus (vulgaris) NOS (017.0)*
systemic [disseminated] lupus erythematosus (710.0)

DEF: Group of connective tissue disorders occurring as various cutaneous diseases of unknown origin; it primarily affects women between the ages of 20 and 40.

✓5th **695.8 Other specified erythematous conditions**

695.81 Ritter's disease
Dermatitis exfoliativa neonatorum

DEF: Infectious skin disease of infants and young children marked by eruptions ranging from a localized bullous type to widespread development of easily ruptured fine vesicles and bullae; results in exfoliation of large planes of skin and leaves raw areas; also called staphylococcal scalded skin syndrome.

695.89 Other
Erythema intertrigo
Intertrigo
Pityriasis rubra (Hebra)
EXCLUDES *mycotic intertrigo (111.0-111.9)*

695.9 Unspecified erythematous condition
Erythema NOS   Erythroderma (secondary)

✓4th **696 Psoriasis and similar disorders**

696.0 Psoriatic arthropathy
DEF: Psoriasis associated with inflammatory arthritis; often involves interphalangeal joints.

SKIN AND SUBCUTANEOUS TISSUE

696.1 Other psoriasis
  Acrodermatitis continua
  Dermatitis repens
  Psoriasis:
    NOS
    any type, except arthropathic
  EXCLUDES psoriatic arthropathy (696.0)

696.2 Parapsoriasis
  Parakeratosis variegata
  Parapsoriasis lichenoides chronica
  Pityriasis lichenoides et varioliformis
  DEF: Erythrodermas similar to lichen, planus and psoriasis; symptoms include redness and itching; resistant to treatment.

696.3 Pityriasis rosea
  Pityriasis circinata (et maculata)
  DEF: Common, self-limited rash of unknown etiology marked by a solitary erythematous, salmon or fawn-colored herald plaque on the trunk, arms or thighs; followed by development of papular or macular lesions that tend to peel and form a scaly collarette.

696.4 Pityriasis rubra pilaris
  Devergie's disease
  Lichen ruber acuminatus
  EXCLUDES pityriasis rubra (Hebra) (695.89)
  DEF: Inflammatory disease of hair follicles; marked by firm, red lesions topped by horny plugs; may form patches; occurs on fingers elbows, knees.

696.5 Other and unspecified pityriasis
  Pityriasis:
    NOS
    alba
    streptogenes
  EXCLUDES pityriasis:
    simplex (690.18)
    versicolor (111.0)

696.8 Other

4th 697 Lichen
  EXCLUDES lichen:
    obtusus corneus (698.3)
    pilaris (congenital) (757.39)
    ruber acuminatus (696.4)
    sclerosus et atrophicus (701.0)
    scrofulosus (017.0)
    simplex chronicus (698.3)
    spinulosus (congenital) (757.39)
    urticatus (698.2)

697.0 Lichen planus
  Lichen:
    planopilaris
    ruber planus
  DEF: Inflammatory, pruritic skin disease; marked by angular, flat-top, violet-colored papules; may be acute and widespread or chronic and localized.

697.1 Lichen nitidus
  Pinkus' disease
  DEF: Chronic, inflammatory, usually asymptomatic skin disorder, characterized by numerous glistening, flat-topped, discrete, smooth, skin-colored micropapules most often on penis, lower abdomen, inner thighs, wrists, forearms, breasts and buttocks.

697.8 Other lichen, not elsewhere classified
Lichen:
ruber moniliforme
striata

697.9 Lichen, unspecified

√4ᵗʰ **698 Pruritus and related conditions**
   EXCLUDES *pruritus specified as psychogenic (306.3)*

DEF: Pruritus: Intense, persistent itching due to irritation of sensory nerve endings from organic or psychogenic causes.

698.0 Pruritus ani
Perianal itch

698.1 Pruritus of genital organs

698.2 Prurigo
Lichen urticatus
Prurigo:
   NOS
   Hebra's
   mitis
   simplex
Urticaria papulosa (Hebra)
   EXCLUDES *prurigo nodularis (698.3)*

698.3 Lichenification and lichen simplex chronicus
Hyde's disease
Neurodermatitis (circumscripta) (local)
Prurigo nodularis
   EXCLUDES *neurodermatitis, diffuse (of Brocq) (691.8)*

DEF: Lichenification: thickening of skin due to prolonged rubbing or scratching.

DEF: Lichen simplex chronicus: eczematous dermatitis, of face, neck, extremities, scrotum, vulva, and perianal region due to repeated itching, rubbing and scratching; spontaneous or evolves with other dermatoses.

698.4 Dermatitis factitia [artefacta]
Dermatitis ficta
Neurotic excoriation
Use additional code to identify any associated mental disorder

DEF: Various types of self-inflicted skin lesions characterized in appearance as an erythema to a gangrene.

698.8 Other specified pruritic conditions
Pruritus:
   hiemalis
   senilis
Winter itch

698.9 Unspecified pruritic disorder
Itch NOS
Pruritus NOS

SKIN AND SUBCUTANEOUS TISSUE

OTHER DISEASES OF SKIN AND SUBCUTANEOUS TISSUE (700-709)

EXCLUDES   conditions confined to eyelids (373.0-374.9)
congenital conditions of skin, hair, and nails (757.0-757.9)

700 Corns and callosities
Callus
Clavus

DEF: Corns: conical or horny thickening of skin on toes, due to friction, pressure from shoes and hosiery; pain and inflammation may develop.

DEF: Callosities: localized overgrowth (hyperplasia) of the horny epidermal layer due to pressure or friction.

✓4ᵗʰ 701 Other hypertrophic and atrophic conditions of skin
EXCLUDES   dermatomyositis (710.3)
hereditary edema of legs (757.0)
scleroderma (generalized) (710.1)

701.0 Circumscribed scleroderma
Addison's keloid
Dermatosclerosis, localized
Lichen sclerosus et atrophicus
Morphea
Scleroderma, circumscribed or localized

DEF: Thickened, hardened, skin and subcutaneous tissue; may involve musculoskeletal system.

701.1 Keratoderma, acquired
Acquired:
    ichthyosis
    keratoderma palmaris et plantaris
Elastosis perforans serpiginosa
Hyperkeratosis:
    NOS
    follicularis in cutem penetrans
    palmoplantaris climacterica
Keratoderma:
    climactericum
    tylodes, progressive
Keratosis (blennorrhagica)

EXCLUDES   Darier's disease [keratosis follicularis] (congenital) (757.39)
keratosis:
    arsenical (692.4)
    gonococcal (098.81)

701.2 Acquired acanthosis nigricans
Keratosis nigricans

DEF: Diffuse velvety hyperplasia of the spinous skin layer of the axilla and other body folds marked by gray, brown, or black pigmentation; in adult form it is often associated with an internal carcinoma (malignant acanthosis nigricans) in a benign, nevoid form it is relatively generalized; benign juvenile form with obesity is sometimes caused by an endocrine disturbance.

701.3 Striae atrophicae
Atrophic spots of skin
Atrophoderma maculatum
Atrophy blanche (of Milian)
Degenerative colloid atrophy
Senile degenerative atrophy
Striae distensae

DEF: Bands of atrophic, depressed, wrinkled skin associated with stretching of skin from pregnancy, obesity, or rapid growth during puberty.

✓4ᵗʰ ✓5ᵗʰ Additional Digit Required   **Unspecified Code**   **Other Specified Code**   **Manifestation Code**
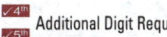 Medicare Secondary Payer   ▶◀ Revised Text   ● New Code   ▲ Revised Code Title

SKIN AND SUBCUTANEOUS TISSUE

701.4 Keloid scar
Cheloid
Hypertrophic scar
Keloid

DEF: Overgrowth of scar tissue due to excess amounts of collagen during connective tissue repair; occurs mainly on upper trunk, face.

701.5 Other abnormal granulation tissue
Excessive granulation

701.8 Other specified hypertrophic and atrophic conditions of skin
Acrodermatitis atrophicans chronica
Atrophia cutis senilis
Atrophoderma neuriticum
Confluent and reticulate papillomatosis
Cutis laxa senilis
Elastosis senilis
Folliculitis ulerythematosa reticulata
Gougerot-Carteaud syndrome or disease

701.9 Unspecified hypertrophic and atrophic conditions of skin
Atrophoderma

√4th **702 Other dermatoses**
EXCLUDES carcinoma in situ (232.0-232.9)

702.0 Actinic keratosis
DEF: Wart-like growth, red or skin-colored; may form a cutaneous horn.

√5th **702.1 Seborrheic keratosis**
DEF: Common, benign, lightly pigmented, warty growth composed of basaloid cells.

702.11 Inflamed seborrheic keratosis
702.19 Other seborrheic keratosis
Seborrheic keratosis NOS

702.8 Other specified dermatoses

√4th **703 Diseases of nail**
EXCLUDES congenital anomalies (757.5)
onychia and paronychia (681.02, 681.11)

703.0 Ingrowing nail
Ingrowing nail with infection
Unguis incarnatus
EXCLUDES infection, nail NOS (681.9)

703.8 Other specified diseases of nail
Dystrophia unguium   Onychauxis
Hypertrophy of nail   Onychogryposis
Koilonychia   Onycholysis
Leukonychia (punctata) (striata)

703.9 Unspecified disease of nail

√4th **704 Diseases of hair and hair follicles**
EXCLUDES congenital anomalies (757.4)

√5th **704.0 Alopecia**
EXCLUDES madarosis (374.55)
syphilitic alopecia (091.82)

DEF: Lack of hair, especially on scalp; often called baldness; may be partial or total; occurs at any age.

704.00 Alopecia, unspecified
Baldness
Loss of hair

SKIN AND SUBCUTANEOUS TISSUE

704.01 Alopecia areata
Ophiasis

DEF: Alopecia areata: usually reversible, inflammatory, patchy hair loss found in beard or scalp.

DEF: Ophiasis: alopecia areata of children; marked by band around temporal and occipital scalp margins.

704.02 Telogen effluvium

DEF: Shedding of hair from premature telogen development in follicles due to stress, including shock, childbirth, surgery, drugs or weight loss.

704.09 Other
Folliculitis decalvans
Hypotrichosis:
  NOS
  postinfectional NOS
Pseudopelade

704.1 Hirsutism
Hypertrichosis: Polytrichia
  NOS
  lanuginosa, acquired
  EXCLUDES hypertrichosis of eyelid (374.54)

DEF: Excess hair growth; often in unexpected places and amounts.

704.2 Abnormalities of the hair
Atrophic hair   Trichiasis:
Clastothrix   NOS
Fragilitas crinium   cicatrical
                    Trichorrhexis (nodosa)
  EXCLUDES trichiasis of eyelid (374.05)

704.3 Variations in hair color
Canities (premature)
Grayness, hair (premature)
Heterochromia of hair
Poliosis:
  NOS
  circumscripta, acquired

704.8 Other specified diseases of hair and hair follicles
Folliculitis: Sycosis:
  NOS   NOS
  abscedens et suffodiens   barbae [not parasitic]
  pustular   lupoid
Perifolliculitis: vulgaris
  NOS
  capitis abscedens et suffodiens
  scalp

704.9 Unspecified disease of hair and hair follicles

705 Disorders of sweat glands

705.0 Anhidrosis
Hypohidrosis   Oligohidrosis
DEF: Lack or deficiency of ability to sweat.

705.1 Prickly heat
Heat rash   Sudamina
Miliaria rubra (tropicalis)

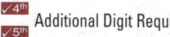 Additional Digit Required
Unspecified Code   Other Specified Code   Manifestation Code
MSP Medicare Secondary Payer   ▶◀ Revised Text   ● New Code   ▲ Revised Code Title

2002 Ingenix, Inc.   Volume 1 — 403

SKIN AND SUBCUTANEOUS TISSUE

√5th **705.8 Other specified disorders of sweat glands**

705.81 Dyshidrosis
Cheiropompholyx   Pompholyx
DEF: Vesicular eruption, on hands, feet causing itching and burning.

705.82 Fox-Fordyce disease
DEF: Chronic, usually pruritic disease chiefly of women evidenced by small follicular papular eruptions, especially in the axillary and pubic areas; develops from the closure and rupture of the affected apocrine glands' intraepidermal portion of the ducts.

705.83 Hidradenitis
Hidradenitis suppurativa
DEF: Inflamed sweat glands.

705.89 Other
Bromhidrosis   Granulosis rubra nasi
Chromhidrosis   Urhidrosis
EXCLUDES hidrocystoma (216.0-216.9)
hyperhidrosis (780.8)

DEF: Bromhidrosis: foul-smelling axillary sweat due to decomposed bacteria.

DEF: Chromhidrosis: secretion of colored sweat.

DEF: Granulosis ubra nasi: ideopathic condition of children; causes redness, sweating around nose, face and chin; tends to end by puberty.

DEF: Urhidrosis: urinous substance, such as uric acid, in sweat; occurs in uremia.

705.9 Unspecified disorder of sweat glands
Disorder of sweat glands NOS

√4th **706 Diseases of sebaceous glands**

706.0 Acne varioliformis
Acne: Acne:
  frontalis   necrotica

DEF: Rare form of acne characterized by persistent brown papulopustules usually on the brow and temporoparietal part of the scalp.

706.1 Other acne
Acne: Acne:
  NOS   vulgaris
  conglobata   Blackhead
  cystic   Comedo
  pustular
EXCLUDES acne rosacea (695.3)

706.2 Sebaceous cyst
Atheroma, skin   Wen
Keratin cyst
DEF: Benign epidermal cyst, contains sebum and keratin; presents as firm, circumscribed nodule.

706.3 Seborrhea
EXCLUDES seborrhea:
  capitis (690.11)
  sicca (690.18)
seborrheic:
  dermatitis (690.10)
  keratosis (702.11-702.19)

DEF: Seborrheic dermatitis marked by excessive secretion of sebum; the sebum forms an oily coating, crusts, or scales on the skin; it is also called hypersteatosis.

SKIN AND SUBCUTANEOUS TISSUE

706.8 **Other specified diseases of sebaceous glands**
Asteatosis (cutis)   Xerosis cutis

706.9 **Unspecified disease of sebaceous glands**

✓4th **707 Chronic ulcer of skin**

> INCLUDES   non-infected sinus of skin
> non-healing ulcer
>
> EXCLUDES   specific infections classified under "Infectious and Parasitic Diseases" (001.0-136.9)
> varicose ulcer (454.0, 454.2)

707.0 Decubitus ulcer
Bed sore   Plaster ulcer
Decubitus ulcer [any site]   Pressure ulcer

✓5th **707.1 Ulcer of lower limbs, except decubitus**
Ulcer, chronic:
  neurogenic ⎫
  trophic   ⎬ of lower limb

▶Code, if applicable, any casual condition first:◀
atherosclerosis of the extremities with ulceration (440.23)
▶chronic venous hypertension with ulcer (459.31)
chronic venous hypertension with ulcer and inflammation (459.33)◀
diabetes mellitus (250.80-250.83)
▶postphlebitic syndrome with ulcer (459.11)
postphlebitic syndrome with ulcer and inflammation (459.13)◀

707.10 Ulcer of lower limb, unspecified
707.11 Ulcer of thigh
707.12 Ulcer of calf
707.13 Ulcer of ankle
707.14 Ulcer of heel and midfoot
Plantar surface of midfoot
707.15 Ulcer of other part of foot
Toes
707.19 Ulcer of other part of lower limb

707.8 Chronic ulcer of other specified sites
Ulcer, chronic:
  neurogenic ⎫
  trophic   ⎬ of other specified sites

707.9 Chronic ulcer of unspecified site
Chronic ulcer NOS
Trophic ulcer NOS
Tropical ulcer NOS
Ulcer of skin NOS

✓4th **708 Urticaria**

> EXCLUDES   edema:
>   angioneurotic (995.1)
>   Quincke's (995.1)
> hereditary angioedema (277.6)
> urticaria:
>   giant (995.1)
>   papulosa (Hebra) (698.2)
>   pigmentosa (juvenile) (congenital) (757.33)

DEF: Skin disorder marked by raised edematous patches of skin or mucous membrane with intense itching; also called hives.

SKIN AND SUBCUTANEOUS TISSUE

Six Stages of Decubitus Ulcers

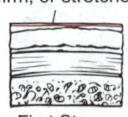
First Stage — Skin is warm, firm, or stretched

Second Stage — Bacteria enter

Third Stage — Fat layer exposed

Fourth Stage — Muscle necrosis

Fifth Stage — Advanced muscle necrosis

Sixth Stage — Bone necrosis

- **708.0 Allergic urticaria**
- **708.1 Idiopathic urticaria**
- **708.2 Urticaria due to cold and heat**
  Thermal urticaria
- **708.3 Dermatographic urticaria**
  Dermatographia   Factitial urticaria
- **708.4 Vibratory urticaria**
- **708.5 Cholinergic urticaria**
- **708.8 Other specified urticaria**
  Nettle rash   Urticaria:
  Urticaria: recurrent periodic
  chronic
- **708.9 Urticaria, unspecified**
  Hives NOS

√4th **709 Other disorders of skin and subcutaneous tissue**

√5th **709.0 Dyschromia**
  EXCLUDES albinism (270.2)
  pigmented nevus (216.0-216.9)
  that of eyelid (374.52-374.53)
  DEF: Pigment disorder of skin or hair.

- **709.00 Dyschromia, unspecified**
- **709.01 Vitiligo**
  DEF: Persistent, progressive development of nonpigmented white patches on otherwise normal skin.
- **709.09 Other**

709.1 Vascular disorders of skin
  Angioma serpiginosum
  Purpura (primary) annularis telangiectodes

709.2 Scar conditions and fibrosis of skin
  Adherent scar (skin)
  Cicatrix
  Disfigurement (due to scar)
  Fibrosis, skin NOS
  Scar NOS

SKIN AND SUBCUTANEOUS TISSUE

Cutaneous Lesions

Surface Lesions
Fissure — Polyp growth — Ulcer

Solid Lesions
Flat macule — Slightly elevated wheal — Solid papule

Sac Lesions
Cyst — Clear fluid vesicle — Pustule

709.3 Degenerative skin disorders
Calcinosis:
  circumscripta
  cutis
Colloid milium
Degeneration, skin
Deposits, skin
Senile dermatosis NOS
Subcutaneous calcification

709.4 Foreign body granuloma of skin and subcutaneous tissue
  EXCLUDES residual foreign body without granuloma of skin and subcutaneous tissue (729.6)
  that of muscle (728.82)

709.8 Other specified disorders of skin
Epithelial hyperplasia
Menstrual dermatosis
Vesicular eruption

DEF: Epithelial hyperplasia: increased number of epitheleal cells.

DEF: Vesicular eruption: liquid-filled structures appearing through skin.

709.9 Unspecified disorder of skin and subcutaneous tissue
Dermatosis NOS

MUSCULOSKELETAL SYSTEM

Joint Structures

13. DISEASES OF THE MUSCULOSKELETAL SYSTEM AND CONNECTIVE TISSUE (710-739)

The following fifth-digit subclassification is for use with categories 711-712, 715-716, 718-719, and 730:

0 **site unspecified**
1 **shoulder region**
    Acromioclavicular joint(s)   Scapula
    Clavicle   Sternoclavicular joint(s)
    Glenohumeral joint(s)
2 **upper arm**
    Elbow joint   Humerus
3 **forearm**
    Radius   Wrist joint
    Ulna
4 **hand**
    Carpus   Phalanges [fingers]
    Metacarpus
5 **pelvic region and thigh**
    Buttock   Hip (joint)
    Femur
6 **lower leg**
    Fibula   Patella
    Knee joint   Tibia
7 **ankle and foot**
    Ankle joint   Phalanges, foot
    Digits [toes]   Tarsus
    Metatarsus   Other joints in foot
8 **other specified sites**
    Head   Skull
    Neck   Trunk
    Ribs   Vertebral column
9 **multiple sites**

MUSCULOSKELETAL SYSTEM

ARTHROPATHIES AND RELATED DISORDERS (710-719)

EXCLUDES disorders of spine (720.0-724.9)

✓4th 710 Diffuse diseases of connective tissue

INCLUDES all collagen diseases whose effects are not mainly confined to a single system

EXCLUDES those affecting mainly the cardiovascular system, i.e., polyarteritis nodosa and allied conditions (446.0-446.7)

Use additional code to identify manifestation, as:
  lung involvement (517.8)
  myopathy (359.6)

710.0 Systemic lupus erythematosus
  Disseminated lupus erythematosus
  Libman-Sacks disease
  Use additional code to identify manifestation, as:
    endocarditis (424.91)
    nephritis (583.81)
      chronic (582.81)
    nephrotic syndrome (581.81)

  EXCLUDES lupus erythematosus (discoid) NOS (695.4)

  DEF: A chronic multisystemic inflammatory disease affecting connective tissue; marked by anemia, leukopenia, muscle and joint pains, fever, rash of a butterfly pattern around cheeks and forehead area; of unknown etiology.

710.1 Systemic sclerosis
  Acrosclerosis
  CRST syndrome
  Progressive systemic sclerosis
  Scleroderma
  ▶Use additional code to identify manifestation, as:
    lung involvement (517.8)
    myopathy (359.6)◀

  EXCLUDES circumscribed scleroderma (701.0)

  DEF: Systemic disease, involving excess fibrotic collagen build-up; symptoms include thickened skin; fibrotic degenerative changes in various organs; and vascular abnormalities; condition occurs more often in females.

710.2 Sicca syndrome
  Keratoconjunctivitis sicca
  Sjögren's disease

  DEF: Autoimmune disease; associated with keratoconjunctivitis, laryngopharyngitis, rhinitis, dry mouth, enlarged parotid gland, and chronic polyarthritis.

710.3 Dermatomyositis
  Poikilodermatomyositis
  Polymyositis with skin involvement

  DEF: Polymyositis associated with flat-top purple papules on knuckles; marked by upper eyelid rash, edema of eyelids and orbit area, red rash on forehead, neck, shoulders, trunk and arms; symptoms include fever, weight loss aching muscles; visceral cancer (in individuals older than 40).

710.4 Polymyositis

  DEF: Chronic, progressive, inflammatory skeletal muscle disease; causes weakness of limb girdles, neck, pharynx; may precede or follow scleroderma, Sjogren's disease, systemic lupus erythematosus, arthritis, or malignancy.

710.5 Eosinophilia myalgia syndrome
Toxic oil syndrome
Use additional E code to identify drug, if drug induced

DEF: Eosinophilia myalgia syndrome (EMS): inflammatory, multisystem fibrosis; associated with ingesting elemetary L-tryptophan; symptoms include myalgia, weak limbs and bulbar muscles, distal sensory loss, areflexia, arthralgia, cough, fever, fatigue, skin rashes, myopathy, and eosinophil counts greater than 1000/microliter.

DEF: Toxic oil syndrome: syndrome silimar to EMS due to ingesting contaminated cooking oil.

710.8 Other specified diffuse diseases of connective tissue
Multifocal fibrosclerosis (idiopathic) NEC
Systemic fibrosclerosing syndrome

710.9 Unspecified diffuse connective tissue disease
Collagen disease NOS

√4ᵗʰ 711 Arthropathy associated with infections

INCLUDES: arthritis, arthropathy, polyarthritis, polyarthropathy } associated with conditions classifiable below

EXCLUDES: rheumatic fever (390)

The following fifth-digit subclassification is for use with category 711; valid digits are in [brackets] under each code.

```
0  site unspecified
1  shoulder region
2  upper arm
3  forearm
4  hand
5  pelvic region and thigh
6  lower leg
7  ankle and foot
8  other specified sites
9  multiple sites
```

§ √5ᵗʰ 711.0 Pyogenic arthritis
[0-9]
Arthritis or polyarthritis (due to):
coliform [Escherichia coli]
Hemophilus influenzae [H. influenzae]
pneumococcal
Pseudomonas
staphylococcal
streptococcal
Pyarthrosis
Use additional code to identify infectious organism (041.0-041.8)

DEF: Infectious arthritis caused by various bacteria; marked by inflamed synovial membranes, and purulent effusion in joints.

§ √5ᵗʰ 711.1 Arthropathy associated with Reiter's disease and nonspecific urethritis
[0-9]
Code first underlying disease as:
nonspecific urethritis (099.4)
Reiter's disease (099.3)

DEF: Reiter's disease: joint disease marked by diarrhea, urethritis, conjunctivitis, keratosis and arthritis; of unknown etiology; affects young males.

DEF: Urethritis: inflamed urethra.

---

§ Requires fifth-digit. Valid digits are in [brackets] under each code. See beginning of section 710-719 for codes and definitions.

N Newborn Age: 0   **P** Pediatric Age: 0-17   **M** Maternity Age: 12-55   **A** Adult Age: 15-124

MUSCULOSKELETAL SYSTEM   711.2–712

§ ✓5th 711.2 Arthropathy in Behçet's syndrome
[0-9]   *Code first underlying disease (136.1)*
DEF: Behçet's syndrome: chronic inflammatory disorder, of unknown etiology; affects small blood vessels; causes ulcers of oral and pharyngeal mucous membranes and genitalia, skin lesions, retinal vasculitis, optic atrophy and severe uveitis.

§ ✓5th 711.3 Postdysenteric arthropathy
[0-9]   *Code first underlying disease as:*
       dysentery (009.0)
       enteritis, infectious (008.0-009.3)
       paratyphoid fever (002.1-002.9)
       typhoid fever (002.0)
   EXCLUDES   salmonella arthritis (003.23)

§ ✓5th 711.4 Arthropathy associated with other bacterial diseases
[0-9]   *Code first underlying disease as:*
       diseases classifiable to 010-040, 090-099, except as in 711.1, 711.3, and 713.5
       leprosy (030.0-030.9)
       tuberculosis (015.0-015.9)
   EXCLUDES   gonococcal arthritis (098.50)
                  meningococcal arthritis (036.82)

§ ✓5th 711.5 Arthropathy associated with other viral diseases
[0-9]   *Code first underlying disease as:*
       diseases classifiable to 045-049, 050-079, 480, 487
       O'nyong nyong (066.3)
   EXCLUDES   that due to rubella (056.71)

§ ✓5th 711.6 Arthropathy associated with mycoses
[0-9]   *Code first underlying disease (110.0-118)*

§ ✓5th 711.7 Arthropathy associated with helminthiasis
[0-9]   *Code first underlying disease as:*
       filariasis (125.0-125.9)

§ ✓5th 711.8 Arthropathy associated with other infectious and parasitic diseases
[0-9]   *Code first underlying disease as:*
       diseases classifiable to 080-088, 100-104, 130-136
   EXCLUDES   arthropathy associated with sarcoidosis (713.7)

§ ✓5th 711.9 Unspecified infective arthritis
[0-9]   Infective arthritis or polyarthritis (acute) (chronic) (subacute) NOS

✓4th 712 Crystal arthropathies
   INCLUDES   crystal-induced arthritis andsynovitis
   EXCLUDES   gouty arthropathy (274.0)
DEF: Joint disease due to urate crystal deposit in joints or synovial membranes.

The following fifth-digit subclassification is for use with category 712; valid digits are in [brackets] under each code. See definitions prior to category 710.
   0 site unspecified   5 pelvic region and thigh
   1 shoulder region   6 lower leg
   2 upper arm   7 ankle and foot
   3 forearm   8 other specified sites
   4 hand   9 multiple sites

§ Requires fifth-digit. Valid digits are in [brackets] under each code. See beginning of section 710-719 for codes and definitions.

✓4th / ✓5th Additional Digit Required   Unspecified Code   Other Specified Code   Manifestation Code
 Medicare Secondary Payer   ▶◀ Revised Text   ● New Code   ▲ Revised Code Title

2002 Ingenix, Inc.   Volume 1 — 411

MUSCULOSKELETAL SYSTEM

§ ✓5th **712.1 Chondrocalcinosis due to dicalcium phosphate crystals**
[0-9] Chondrocalcinosis due to dicalcium phosphate crystals (with other crystals)
Code first underlying disease (275.4)

§ ✓5th **712.2 Chondrocalcinosis due to pyrophosphate crystals**
[0-9] Code first underlying disease (275.4)

§ ✓5th **712.3 Chondrocalcinosis, unspecified**
[0-9] Code first underlying disease (275.4)

§ ✓5th **712.8 Other specified crystal arthropathies**
[0-9]

§ ✓5th **712.9 Unspecified crystal arthropathy**
[0-9]

✓4th **713 Arthropathy associated with other disorders classified elsewhere**

INCLUDES arthritis
arthropathy   } associated with conditions classifiable below
polyarthritis
polyarthropathy

713.0 Arthropathy associated with other endocrine and metabolic disorders
Code first underlying disease as:
acromegaly (253.0)
hemochromatosis (275.0)
hyperparathyroidism (252.0)
hypogammaglobulinemia (279.00-279.09)
hypothyroidism (243-244.9)
lipoid metabolism disorder (272.0-272.9)
ochronosis (270.2)
EXCLUDES arthropathy associated with:
amyloidosis (713.7)
crystal deposition disorders, except gout (712.1-712.9)
diabetic neuropathy (713.5)
gouty arthropathy (274.0)

713.1 Arthropathy associated with gastrointestinal conditions other than infections
Code first underlying disease as:
regional enteritis (555.0-555.9)
ulcerative colitis (556)

713.2 Arthropathy associated with hematological disorders
Code first underlying disease as:
hemoglobinopathy (282.4-282.7)
hemophilia (286.0-286.2)
leukemia (204.0-208.9)
malignant reticulosis (202.3)
multiple myelomatosis (203.0)
EXCLUDES arthropathy associated with Henoch-Schönlein purpura (713.6)

713.3 Arthropathy associated with dermatological disorders
Code first underlying disease as:
erythema multiforme (695.1)
erythema nodosum (695.2)
EXCLUDES psoriatic arthropathy (696.0)

713.4 Arthropathy associated with respiratory disorders
Code first underlying disease as:
diseases classifiable to 490-519
EXCLUDES arthropathy associated with respiratory infections (711.0, 711.4-711.8)

§ Requires fifth-digit. Valid digits are in [brackets] under each code. See beginning of section 710-719 for codes and definitions.

N Newborn Age: 0   P Pediatric Age: 0-17   M Maternity Age: 12-55   A Adult Age: 15-124

MUSCULOSKELETAL SYSTEM

713.5 Arthropathy associated with neurological disorders

Charcôt's arthropathy
Neuropathic arthritis
} associated with diseases classifiable elsewhere

Code first underlying disease as:
 neuropathic joint disease [Charcôt's joints]:
  NOS (094.0)
  diabetic (250.6)
  syringomyelic (336.0)
  tabetic [syphilitic] (094.0)

713.6 Arthropathy associated with hypersensitivity reaction
Code first underlying disease as:
 Henoch (-Schönlein) purpura (287.0)
 serum sickness (999.5)
 EXCLUDES allergic arthritis NOS (716.2)

713.7 Other general diseases with articular involvement
Code first underlying disease as:
 amyloidosis (277.3)
 familial Mediterranean fever (277.3)
 sarcoidosis (135)

713.8 Arthropathy associated with other conditions classifiable elsewhere
Code first underlying disease as:
 conditions classifiable elsewhere except as in 711.1-711.8, 712, and 713.0-713.7

✓4th **714 Rheumatoid arthritis and other inflammatory polyarthropathies**
EXCLUDES rheumatic fever (390)
 rheumatoid arthritis of spine NOS (720.0)

714.0 Rheumatoid arthritis
Arthritis or polyarthritis:
 atrophic
 rheumatic (chronic)
Use additional code to identify manifestation, as:
 myopathy (359.6)
 polyneuropathy (357.1)
 EXCLUDES juvenile rheumatoid arthritis NOS (714.30)
DEF: Chronic systemic disease principally of joints, manifested by inflammatory changes in articular structures and synovial membranes, atrophy, and loss in bone density.

714.1 Felty's syndrome
Rheumatoid arthritis with splenoadenomegaly and leukopenia
DEF: Syndrome marked by rheumatoid arthritis, splenomegaly, leukopenia, pigmented spots on lower extremity skin, anemia, and thrombocytopenia.

714.2 Other rheumatoid arthritis with visceral or systemic involvement
Rheumatoid carditis

✓5th **714.3 Juvenile chronic polyarthritis**
DEF: Rheumatoid arthritis of more than one joint; lasts longer than six weeks in age 17 or younger; symptoms include fever, erythematous rash, weight loss, lymphadenopathy, hepatosplenomegaly and pericarditis.

714.30 Polyarticular juvenile rheumatoid arthritis, chronic or unspecified
Juvenile rheumatoid arthritis NOS
Still's disease

714.31–715.3 MUSCULOSKELETAL SYSTEM

- **714.31** Polyarticular juvenile rheumatoid arthritis, acute
- **714.32** Pauciarticular juvenile rheumatoid arthritis
- **714.33** Monoarticular juvenile rheumatoid arthritis

714.4 Chronic postrheumatic arthropathy
Chronic rheumatoid nodular fibrositis
Jaccoud's syndrome
DEF: Persistent joint disorder; follows previous rheumatic infection.

✓5th **714.8 Other specified inflammatory polyarthropathies**
- **714.81 Rheumatoid lung**
  Caplan's syndrome
  Diffuse interstitial rheumatoid disease of lung
  Fibrosing alveolitis, rheumatoid
  DEF: Lung disorders associated with rheumatoid arthritis.
- **714.89 Other**

714.9 Unspecified inflammatory polyarthropathy
Inflammatory polyarthropathy or polyarthritis NOS
EXCLUDES polyarthropathy NOS (716.5)

✓4th **715 Osteoarthrosis and allied disorders**
Note: Localized, in the subcategories below, includes bilateral involvement of the same site.
INCLUDES arthritis or polyarthritis:
- degenerative
- hypertrophic
- degenerative joint disease
- osteoarthritis

EXCLUDES Marie-Strümpell spondylitis (720.0)
osteoarthrosis [osteoarthritis] of spine (721.0-721.9)

The following fifth-digit subclassification is for use with category 715; valid digits are in [brackets] under each code. See definitions prior to category 710.
- 0 site unspecified
- 1 shoulder region
- 2 upper arm
- 3 forearm
- 4 hand
- 5 pelvic region and thigh
- 6 lower leg
- 7 ankle and foot
- 8 other specified sites
- 9 multiple sites

§ ✓5th **715.0 Osteoarthrosis, generalized**
[0,4,9]
Degenerative joint disease, involving multiple joints
Primary generalized hypertrophic osteoarthrosis
DEF: Chronic noninflammatory arthritis; marked by degenerated articular cartilage and enlarged bone; symptoms include pain and stiffness with activity; occurs among elderly.

§ ✓5th **715.1 Osteoarthrosis, localized, primary**
[0-8]
Localized osteoarthropathy, idiopathic

§ ✓5th **715.2 Osteoarthrosis, localized, secondary**
[0-8]
Coxae malum senilis

§ ✓5th **715.3 Osteoarthrosis, localized, not specified whether primary or secondary**
[0-8]
Otto's pelvis

§ Requires fifth-digit. Valid digits are in [brackets] under each code. See beginning of section 710-719 for codes and definitions.

N Newborn Age: 0   P Pediatric Age: 0-17   M Maternity Age: 12-55   A Adult Age: 15-124

MUSCULOSKELETAL SYSTEM 715.8–716.4

§ ✓5ᵗʰ **715.8** Osteoarthrosis involving, or with mention of more
[0,9]   than one site, but not specified as generalized

§ ✓5ᵗʰ **715.9** Osteoarthrosis, unspecified whether generalized or localized
[0-8]

§ ✓4ᵗʰ **716 Other and unspecified arthropathies**
      EXCLUDES *cricoarytenoid arthropathy (478.79)*

The following fifth-digit subclassification is for use with category 716; valid digits are in [brackets] under each code. See definitions prior to category 710.

      0 site unspecified
      1 shoulder region
      2 upper arm
      3 forearm
      4 hand
      5 pelvic region and thigh
      6 lower leg
      7 ankle and foot
      8 other specified sites
      9 multiple sites

§ ✓5ᵗʰ **716.0** Kaschin-Beck disease
[0-9]   Endemic polyarthritis
      DEF: Chronic degenerative disease of spine and peripheral joints; occurs in eastern Siberian, northern Chinese, and Korean youth; may a mycotoxicosis caused by eating cereals infected with fungus.

§ ✓5ᵗʰ **716.1** Traumatic arthropathy
[0-9]

§ ✓5ᵗʰ **716.2** Allergic arthritis
[0-9]   **EXCLUDES** *arthritis associated with Henoch-Schönlein purpura or serum sickness (713.6)*

§ ✓5ᵗʰ **716.3** Climacteric arthritis   ♀
[0-9]   Menopausal arthritis
      DEF: Ovarian hormone deficiency; causes pain in small joints, shoulders, elbows or knees; affects females at menopause; also called arthropathia ovaripriva.

§ ✓5ᵗʰ **716.4** Transient arthropathy
[0-9]   **EXCLUDES** *palindromic rheumatism (719.3)*

Disruption and Tears of Meniscus

Bucket-handle   Flap-type   Peripheral

Horizontal cleavage   Vertical   Congenital discoid meniscus

§ Requires fifth-digit. Valid digits are in [brackets] under each code. See beginning of section 710-719 for codes and definitions.

✓4ᵗʰ/✓5ᵗʰ Additional Digit Required | Unspecified Code | Other Specified Code | Manifestation Code
MSP Medicare Secondary Payer | ▶◀ Revised Text | ● New Code | ▲ Revised Code Title

MUSCULOSKELETAL SYSTEM

Internal Derangements of Knee

§ ✓5ᵗʰ **716.5 Unspecified polyarthropathy or polyarthritis**
[0-9]

§ ✓5ᵗʰ **716.6 Unspecified monoarthritis**
[0-8]   Coxitis

§ ✓5ᵗʰ **716.8 Other specified arthropathy**
[0-9]

§ ✓5ᵗʰ **716.9 Arthropathy, unspecified**
[0-9]
Arthritis ⎫
Arthropathy ⎬ (acute) (chronic) (subacute)

Articular rheumatism (chronic)
Inflammation of joint NOS

✓4ᵗʰ **717 Internal derangement of knee**

INCLUDES degeneration ⎫
rupture, old ⎬ of articular cartilage or meniscus of knee
tear, old ⎭

EXCLUDES acute derangement of knee (836.0-836.6)
ankylosis (718.5)
contracture (718.4)
current injury (836.0-836.6)
deformity (736.4-736.6)
recurrent dislocation (718.3)

717.0 Old bucket handle tear of medial meniscus
Old bucket handle tear of unspecified cartilage

717.1 Derangement of anterior horn of medial meniscus

717.2 Derangement of posterior horn of medial meniscus

717.3 Other and unspecified derangement of medial meniscus
Degeneration of internal semilunar cartilage

✓5ᵗʰ **717.4 Derangement of lateral meniscus**

717.40 Derangement of lateral meniscus, unspecified

717.41 Bucket handle tear of lateral meniscus

717.42 Derangement of anterior horn of lateral meniscus

717.43 Derangement of posterior horn of lateral meniscus

717.49 Other

---

§ Requires fifth-digit. Valid digits are in [brackets] under each code. See beginning of section 710-719 for codes and definitions.

MUSCULOSKELETAL SYSTEM

717.5 Derangement of meniscus, not elsewhere classified
Congenital discoid meniscus
Cyst of semilunar cartilage
Derangement of semilunar cartilage NOS

717.6 Loose body in knee
Joint mice, knee
Rice bodies, knee (joint)
DEF: The presence in the joint synovial area of a small, frequently calcified, loose body created from synovial membrane, organized fibrin fragments of articular cartilage or arthritis osteophytes.

717.7 Chondromalacia of patella
Chondromalacia patellae
Degeneration [softening] of articular cartilage of patella
DEF: Softened patella cartilage.

√5th **717.8 Other internal derangement of knee**
  717.81 Old disruption of lateral collateral ligament
  717.82 Old disruption of medial collateral ligament
  717.83 Old disruption of anterior cruciate ligament
  717.84 Old disruption of posterior cruciate ligament
  717.85 Old disruption of other ligaments of knee
    Capsular ligament of knee
  717.89 Other
    Old disruption of ligaments of knee NOS

717.9 Unspecified internal derangement of knee
Derangement NOS of knee

√4th **718 Other derangement of joint**
  EXCLUDES current injury (830.0-848.9)
  jaw (524.6)

The following fifth-digit subclassification is for use with category 718; valid digits are in [brackets] under each code. See definitions prior to category 710.
  0 site unspecified
  1 shoulder region
  2 upper arm
  3 forearm
  4 hand
  5 pelvic region and thigh
  6 lower leg
  7 ankle and foot
  8 other specified sites
  9 multiple sites

§ √5th **718.0 Articular cartilage disorder**
[0-5,7-9]
  Meniscus: Meniscus:
    disorder   tear, old
    rupture, old   Old rupture of ligament(s) of
                            joint NOS
  EXCLUDES articular cartilage disorder:
    in ochronosis (270.2)
    knee (717.0-717.9)
    chondrocalcinosis (275.4)
    metastatic calcification (275.4)

---

§ Requires fifth-digit. Valid digits are in [brackets] under each code. See beginning of section 710-719 for codes and definitions.

MUSCULOSKELETAL SYSTEM

Joint Derangements and Disorders

- Loose body in joint
- Dislocation of joint
- Joint contracture
- Ankylosis of joint
- Synovial effusion (fluid)
- Hemarthrosis (blood)

§ ✓5th **718.1 Loose body in joint**
[0-5,7-9] Joint mice
EXCLUDES knee (717.6)
DEF: Calcified loose bodies in synovial fluid; due to arthritic osteophytes.

§ ✓5th **718.2 Pathological dislocation**
[0-9] Dislocation or displacement of joint, not recurrent and not current injury
Spontaneous dislocation (joint)

§ ✓5th **718.3 Recurrent dislocation of joint**
[0-9]

§ ✓5th **718.4 Contracture of joint**
[0-9]

§ ✓5th **718.5 Ankylosis of joint**
[0-9] Ankylosis of joint (fibrous) (osseous)
EXCLUDES spine (724.9)
stiffness of joint without mention of ankylosis (719.5)
DEF: Immobility and solidification, of joint; due to disease, injury or surgical procedure.

§ ✓5th **718.6 Unspecified intrapelvic protrusion of acetabulum**
[0,5] Protrusio acetabuli, unspecified
DEF: Sinking of the floor of acetabulum; causing femoral head to protrude, limits hip movement; of unknown etiology.

§ ✓5th **718.7 Developmental dislocation of joint**
[0-9] EXCLUDES ▶congenital dislocation of joint (754.0-755.8)
traumatic dislocation of joint (830-839)◀

§ ✓5th **718.8 Other joint derangement, not elsewhere classified**
[0-9] Flail joint (paralytic)
Instability of joint
EXCLUDES deformities classifiable to 736 (736.0-736.9)

§ ✓5th **718.9 Unspecified derangement of joint**
[0-5,7-9] EXCLUDES knee (717.9)

§ Requires fifth-digit. Valid digits are in [brackets] under each code. See beginning of section 710-719 for codes and definitions.

MUSCULOSKELETAL SYSTEM

✓4th 719 Other and unspecified disorders of joint

EXCLUDES jaw (524.6)

The following fifth-digit subclassification is for use with category 719; valid digits are in [brackets] under each code. See definitions prior to category 710.

0 site unspecified
1 shoulder region
2 upper arm
3 forearm
4 hand
5 pelvic region and thigh
6 lower leg
7 ankle and foot
8 other specified sites
9 multiple sites

§ ✓5th 719.0 Effusion of joint
[0-9]
Hydrarthrosis
Swelling of joint, with or without pain
EXCLUDES intermittent hydrarthrosis (719.3)

§ ✓5th 719.1 Hemarthrosis
[0-9]
EXCLUDES current injury (840.0-848.9)

§ ✓5th 719.2 Villonodular synovitis
[0-9]
DEF: Overgrowth of synovial tissue, especially at knee joint; due to macrophage infiltration of giant cells in synovial villi and fibrous nodules.

§ ✓5th 719.3 Palindromic rheumatism
[0-9]
Hench-Rosenberg syndrome
Intermittent hydrarthrosis

DEF: Recurrent episodes of afebrile arthritis and periarthritis marked by their complete disappearance after a few days or hours; causes swelling, redness, and disability usually affecting only one joint; no known cause; affects adults of either sex.

§ ✓5th 719.4 Pain in joint
[0-9]
Arthralgia

§ ✓5th 719.5 Stiffness of joint, not elsewhere classified
[0-9]

§ ✓5th 719.6 Other symptoms referable to joint
[0-9]
Joint crepitus   Snapping hip

§ ✓5th 719.7 Difficulty in walking
[0,5-9]
EXCLUDES abnormality of gait (781.2)

§ ✓5th 719.8 Other specified disorders of joint
[0-9]
Calcification of joint   Fistula of joint
EXCLUDES temporomandibular joint-pain-dysfunction syndrome [Costen's syndrome] (524.6)

§ ✓5th 719.9 Unspecified disorder of joint
[0-9]

---

§ Requires fifth-digit. Valid digits are in [brackets] under each code. See beginning of section 710-719 for codes and definitions.

Normal Anatomy of Vertebral Disc

DORSOPATHIES (720-724)

EXCLUDES curvature of spine (737.0-737.9)
osteochondrosis of spine (juvenile) (732.0)
adult (732.8)

√4th **720 Ankylosing spondylitis and other inflammatory spondylopathies**

720.0 Ankylosing spondylitis
Rheumatoid arthritis of spine NOS
Spondylitis:
  Marie-Strümpell
  rheumatoid

DEF: Rheumatoid arthritis of spine and sacroiliac joints; fusion and deformity in spine follows; affects mainly males; cause unknown.

720.1 Spinal enthesopathy
Disorder of peripheral ligamentous or muscular attachments of spine
Romanus lesion

DEF: Tendinous or muscular vertebral bone attachment abnormality.

720.2 Sacroiliitis, not elsewhere classified
Inflammation of sacroiliac joint NOS

DEF: Pain due to inflammation in joint, at juncture of sacrum and hip.

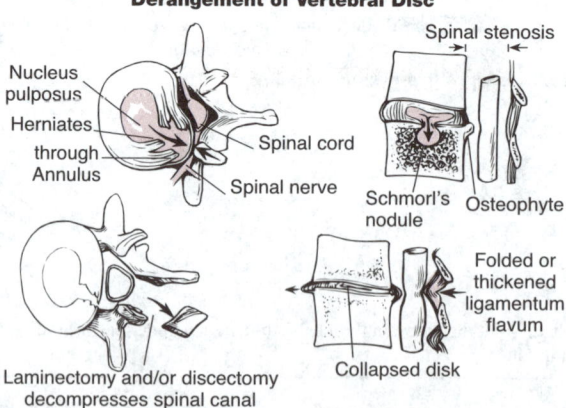

Derangement of Vertebral Disc

MUSCULOSKELETAL SYSTEM

720.8 Other inflammatory spondylopathies

720.81 *Inflammatory spondylopathies in diseases classified elsewhere*
Code first underlying disease as:
tuberculosis (015.0)

720.89 Other

720.9 Unspecified inflammatory spondylopathy
Spondylitis NOS

721 Spondylosis and allied disorders
DEF: Degenerative changes in spinal joint.

721.0 Cervical spondylosis without myelopathy
Cervical or cervicodorsal:
arthritis
osteoarthritis
spondylarthritis

721.1 Cervical spondylosis with myelopathy
Anterior spinal artery compression syndrome
Spondylogenic compression of cervical spinal cord
Vertebral artery compression syndrome

721.2 Thoracic spondylosis without myelopathy
Thoracic: Thoracic:
arthritis   spondylarthritis
osteoarthritis

721.3 Lumbosacral spondylosis without myelopathy
Lumbar or lumbosacral: Lumbar or lumbosacral:
arthritis   spondylarthritis
osteoarthritis

721.4 Thoracic or lumbar spondylosis with myelopathy

721.41 Thoracic region
Spondylogenic compression of thoracic spinal cord

721.42 Lumbar region
Spondylogenic compression of lumbar spinal cord

721.5 Kissing spine
Baastrup's syndrome
DEF: Compression of spinous processes of adjacent vertebrae; due to mutual contact.

721.6 Ankylosing vertebral hyperostosis

721.7 Traumatic spondylopathy
Kümmell's disease or spondylitis

Spinal Stenosis in Cervical Region

721.8 **Other allied disorders of spine**

√5th **721.9 Spondylosis of unspecified site**

721.90 Without mention of myelopathy
Spinal:
  arthritis (deformans) (degenerative) (hypertrophic)
  osteoarthritis NOS
Spondylarthrosis NOS

721.91 With myelopathy
Spondylogenic compression of spinal cord NOS

√4th **722 Intervertebral disc disorders**

722.0 Displacement of cervical intervertebral disc without myelopathy [A]
Neuritis (brachial) or radiculitis due to displacement or rupture of cervical intervertebral disc
Any condition classifiable to 722.2 of the cervical or cervicothoracic intervertebral disc

√5th **722.1 Displacement of thoracic or lumbar intervertebral disc without myelopathy**

722.10 Lumbar intervertebral disc without myelopathy [A]
Lumbago or sciatica due to displacement of intervertebral disc
Neuritis or radiculitis due to displacement or rupture of lumbar intervertebral disc
Any condition classifiable to 722.2 of the lumbar or lumbosacral intervertebral disc

722.11 Thoracic intervertebral disc without myelopathy [A]
Any condition classifiable to 722.2 of thoracic intervertebral disc

722.2 Displacement of intervertebral disc, site unspecified, without myelopathy [A]
Discogenic syndrome NOS
Herniation of nucleus pulposus NOS
Intervertebral disc NOS:
  extrusion
  prolapse
  protrusion
  rupture
Neuritis or radiculitis due to displacement or rupture of intervertebral disc

√5th **722.3 Schmorl's nodes**

DEF: Irregular bone defect in the margin of the vertebral body; causes herniation into end plate of vertebral body.

722.30 Unspecified region [A]
722.31 Thoracic region [A]
722.32 Lumbar region [A]
722.39 Other [A]

722.4 Degeneration of cervical intervertebral disc
Degeneration of cervicothoracic intervertebral disc

√5th **722.5 Degeneration of thoracic or lumbar intervertebral disc**
722.51 Thoracic or thoracolumbar intervertebral disc [A]
722.52 Lumbar or lumbosacral intervertebral disc [A]

722.6 Degeneration of intervertebral disc, site unspecified [A]
Degenerative disc disease NOS
Narrowing of intervertebral disc or space NOS

√5th **722.7 Intervertebral disc disorder with myelopathy**
722.70 Unspecified region [A]
722.71 Cervical region [A]
722.72 Thoracic region [A]
722.73 Lumbar region [A]

MUSCULOSKELETAL SYSTEM 722.8–723.8

√5ᵗʰ 722.8 Postlaminectomy syndrome
DEF: Spinal disorder due to spinal laminectomy surgery.

- 722.80 Unspecified region ▲
- 722.81 Cervical region ▲
- 722.82 Thoracic region ▲
- 722.83 Lumbar region ▲

√5ᵗʰ 722.9 Other and unspecified disc disorder
Calcification of intervertebral cartilage or disc
Discitis

- 722.90 Unspecified region ▲
- 722.91 Cervical region ▲
- 722.92 Thoracic region ▲
- 722.93 Lumbar region ▲

√4ᵗʰ 723 Other disorders of cervical region
> EXCLUDES conditions due to:
> intervertebral disc disorders (722.0-722.9)
> spondylosis (721.0-721.9)

723.0 Spinal stenosis in cervical region

723.1 Cervicalgia
Pain in neck
DEF: Pain in cervical spine or neck region.

723.2 Cervicocranial syndrome
Barré-Liéou syndrome
Posterior cervical sympathetic syndrome
DEF: Neurologic disorder of upper cervical spine and nerve roots.

723.3 Cervicobrachial syndrome (diffuse)
DEF: Complex of symptoms due to scalenus anterior muscle compressing the brachial plexus; pain radiates from shoulder to arm or back of neck.

723.4 Brachial neuritis or radiculitis NOS
Cervical radiculitis
Radicular syndrome of upper limbs

723.5 Torticollis, unspecified
Contracture of neck
> EXCLUDES congenital (754.1)
> due to birth injury (767.8)
> hysterical (300.11)
> ►ocular torticollis (781.93)◄
> psychogenic (306.0)
> spasmodic (333.83)
> traumatic, current (847.0)

DEF: Abnormally positioned neck relative to head; due to cervical muscle or fascia contractions; also called wryneck.

723.6 Panniculitis specified as affecting neck
DEF: Inflammation of the panniculus adiposus (subcutaneous fat) in the neck.

723.7 Ossification of posterior longitudinal ligament in cervical region

723.8 Other syndromes affecting cervical region
Cervical syndrome NEC
Klippel's disease
Occipital neuralgia

Bunion

- **723.9** Unspecified musculoskeletal disorders and symptoms referable to neck
  Cervical (region) disorder NOS

✓4th **724 Other and unspecified disorders of back**
  EXCLUDES: collapsed vertebra (code to cause, e.g., osteoporosis, 733.00-733.09)
  conditions due to:
    intervertebral disc disorders (722.0-722.9)
    spondylosis (721.0-721.9)

  ✓5th **724.0 Spinal stenosis, other than cervical**
    724.00 Spinal stenosis, unspecified region — A
    724.01 Thoracic region — A
    724.02 Lumbar region — A
    724.09 Other — A
  724.1 Pain in thoracic spine
  724.2 Lumbago
    Low back pain   Lumbalgia
    Low back syndrome
  724.3 Sciatica
    Neuralgia or neuritis of sciatic nerve
    EXCLUDES: specified lesion of sciatic nerve (355.0)
  724.4 Thoracic or lumbosacral neuritis or radiculitis, unspecified
    Radicular syndrome of lower limbs
  724.5 Backache, unspecified
    Vertebrogenic (pain) syndrome NOS
  724.6 Disorders of sacrum
    Ankylosis } lumbosacral or sacroiliac (joint)
    Instability
  ✓5th **724.7 Disorders of coccyx**
    724.70 Unspecified disorder of coccyx
    724.71 Hypermobility of coccyx
    724.79 Other
      Coccygodynia
  724.8 Other symptoms referable to back
    Ossification of posterior longitudinal ligament NOS
    Panniculitis specified as sacral or affecting back
  724.9 Other unspecified back disorders
    Ankylosis of spine NOS
    Compression of spinal nerve root NEC
    Spinal disorder NOS
    EXCLUDES: sacroiliitis (720.2)

MUSCULOSKELETAL SYSTEM 725–726.69

RHEUMATISM, EXCLUDING THE BACK (725-729)

INCLUDES: disorders of muscles and tendons and their attachments, and of other soft tissues

725 Polymyalgia rheumatica
DEF: Joint and muscle pain, pelvis, and shoulder girdle stiffness, high sedimentation rate and temporal arteritis; occurs in elderly.

√4ᵗʰ 726 Peripheral enthesopathies and allied syndromes
Note: Enthesopathies are disorders of peripheral ligamentous or muscular attachments.
EXCLUDES: spinal enthesopathy (720.1)

- **726.0** Adhesive capsulitis of shoulder
- **√5ᵗʰ 726.1** Rotator cuff syndrome of shoulder and allied disorders
  - **726.10** Disorders of bursae and tendons in shoulder region, unspecified
    - Rotator cuff syndrome NOS
    - Supraspinatus syndrome NOS
  - **726.11** Calcifying tendinitis of shoulder
  - **726.12** Bicipital tenosynovitis
  - **726.19** Other specified disorders
    - EXCLUDES: complete rupture of rotator cuff, nontraumatic (727.61)
- **726.2** Other affections of shoulder region, not elsewhere classified
  - Periarthritis of shoulder   Scapulohumeral fibrositis
- **√5ᵗʰ 726.3** Enthesopathy of elbow region
  - **726.30** Enthesopathy of elbow, unspecified
  - **726.31** Medial epicondylitis
  - **726.32** Lateral epicondylitis
    - Epicondylitis NOS   Tennis elbow
    - Golfers' elbow
  - **726.33** Olecranon bursitis
    - Bursitis of elbow
  - **726.39** Other
- **726.4** Enthesopathy of wrist and carpus
  - Bursitis of hand or wrist
  - Periarthritis of wrist
- **726.5** Enthesopathy of hip region
  - Bursitis of hip   Psoas tendinitis
  - Gluteal tendinitis   Trochanteric tendinitis
  - Iliac crest spur
- **√5ᵗʰ 726.6** Enthesopathy of knee
  - **726.60** Enthesopathy of knee, unspecified
    - Bursitis of knee NOS
  - **726.61** Pes anserinus tendinitis or bursitis
    - DEF: Inflamed tendons of sartorius, gracilis and semitendinosus muscles of medial aspect of knee.
  - **726.62** Tibial collateral ligament bursitis
    - Pellegrini-Stieda syndrome
  - **726.63** Fibular collateral ligament bursitis
  - **726.64** Patellar tendinitis
  - **726.65** Prepatellar bursitis
  - **726.69** Other
    - Bursitis:
      - infrapatellar
      - subpatellar

 Additional Digit Required   Unspecified Code   Other Specified Code   Manifestation Code

MSP Medicare Secondary Payer   ▶◀ Revised Text   ● New Code   ▲ Revised Code Title

2002 Ingenix, Inc.   Volume 1 — 425

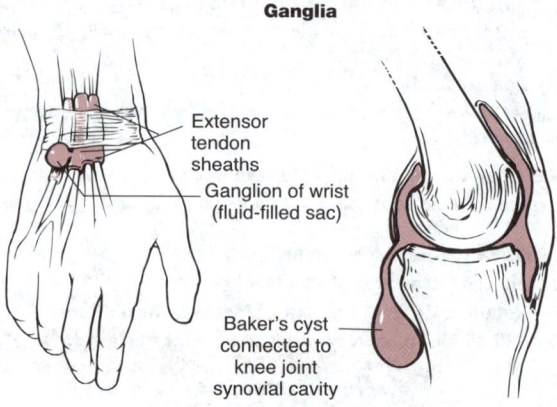

Ganglia

- ✓5th **726.7 Enthesopathy of ankle and tarsus**
  - **726.70 Enthesopathy of ankle and tarsus, unspecified**
    - Metatarsalgia NOS
    - EXCLUDES: Morton's metatarsalgia (355.6)
  - **726.71 Achilles bursitis or tendinitis**
  - **726.72 Tibialis tendinitis**
    - Tibialis (anterior) (posterior) tendinitis
  - **726.73 Calcaneal spur**
    - DEF: Overgrowth of calcaneous bone; causes pain on walking; due to chronic avulsion injury of plantar fascia from calcaneus.
  - **726.79 Other**
    - Peroneal tendinitis
- **726.8 Other peripheral enthesopathies**
- ✓5th **726.9 Unspecified enthesopathy**
  - **726.90 Enthesopathy of unspecified site**
    - Capsulitis NOS
    - Periarthritis NOS
    - Tendinitis NOS
  - **726.91 Exostosis of unspecified site**
    - Bone spur NOS

- ✓4th **727 Other disorders of synovium, tendon, and bursa**
  - ✓5th **727.0 Synovitis and tenosynovitis**
    - **727.00 Synovitis and tenosynovitis, unspecified**
      - Synovitis NOS
      - Tenosynovitis NOS
    - **727.01 Synovitis and tenosynovitis in diseases classified elsewhere**
      - Code first underlying disease as:
        - tuberculosis (015.0-015.9)
      - EXCLUDES:
        - crystal-induced (275.4)
        - gonococcal (098.51)
        - gouty (274.0)
        - syphilitic (095.7)
    - **727.02 Giant cell tumor of tendon sheath**
    - **727.03 Trigger finger (acquired)**
      - DEF: Stenosing tenosynovitis or nodule in flexor tendon; cessation of flexion or extension movement in finger, followed by snapping into place.
    - **727.04 Radial styloid tenosynovitis**
      - de Quervain's disease

MUSCULOSKELETAL SYSTEM 727.05–727.82

- **727.05** Other tenosynovitis of hand and wrist
- **727.06** Tenosynovitis of foot and ankle
- **727.09** Other

727.1 **Bunion**
DEF: Enlarged first metatarsal head due to inflamed bursa; results in laterally displaced great toe.

727.2 **Specific bursitides often of occupational origin**
Beat:
 elbow
 hand
 knee
Miners':
 elbow
 knee
Chronic crepitant synovitis of wrist

727.3 **Other bursitis**
Bursitis NOS
EXCLUDES bursitis:
 gonococcal (098.52)
 subacromial (726.19)
 subcoracoid (726.19)
 subdeltoid (726.19)
 syphilitic (095.7)
 "frozen shoulder" (726.0)

√5th **727.4** **Ganglion and cyst of synovium, tendon, and bursa**
- **727.40** Synovial cyst, unspecified
  EXCLUDES that of popliteal space (727.51)
- **727.41** Ganglion of joint
- **727.42** Ganglion of tendon sheath
- **727.43** Ganglion, unspecified
- **727.49** Other
  Cyst of bursa

√5th **727.5** **Rupture of synovium**
- **727.50** Rupture of synovium, unspecified
- **727.51** Synovial cyst of popliteal space
  Baker's cyst (knee)
- **727.59** Other

√5th **727.6** **Rupture of tendon, nontraumatic**
- **727.60** Nontraumatic rupture of unspecified tendon
- **727.61** Complete rupture of rotator cuff
- **727.62** Tendons of biceps (long head)
- **727.63** Extensor tendons of hand and wrist
- **727.64** Flexor tendons of hand and wrist
- **727.65** Quadriceps tendon
- **727.66** Patellar tendon
- **727.67** Achilles tendon
- **727.68** Other tendons of foot and ankle
- **727.69** Other

√5th **727.8** **Other disorders of synovium, tendon, and bursa**
- **727.81** Contracture of tendon (sheath)
  Short Achilles tendon (acquired)
- **727.82** Calcium deposits in tendon and bursa
  Calcification of tendon NOS
  Calcific tendinitis NOS
  EXCLUDES peripheral ligamentous or muscular attachments (726.0-726.9)

√4th Additional Digit Required
√5th
 Medicare Secondary Payer
 Unspecified Code
▶◀ Revised Text
Other Specified Code
● New Code
Manifestation Code
▲ Revised Code Title

2002 Ingenix, Inc.

727.83 Plica syndrome
Plica knee
DEF: A fold in the synovial tissue that begins to form before birth, creating a septum between two pockets of synovial tissue; two most common plicae are the medial patellar plica and the suprapatellar plica. Plica syndrome, or plica knee, refers to symptomatic plica. Experienced by females more commonly than males.

727.89 Other
Abscess of bursa or tendon
> EXCLUDES   xanthomatosis localized to tendons (272.7)

727.9 Unspecified disorder of synovium, tendon, and bursa

728 Disorders of muscle, ligament, and fascia
> EXCLUDES   enthesopathies (726.0-726.9)
> muscular dystrophies (359.0-359.1)
> myoneural disorders (358.0-358.9)
> myopathies (359.2-359.9)
> old disruption of ligaments of knee (717.81-717.89)

728.0 Infective myositis
Myositis:
  purulent
  suppurative
> EXCLUDES   myositis:
>   epidemic (074.1)
>   interstitial (728.81)
>   syphilitic (095.6)
>   tropical (040.81)

DEF: Inflamed connective septal tissue of muscle.

728.1 Muscular calcification and ossification

728.10 Calcification and ossification, unspecified
Massive calcification (paraplegic)

728.11 Progressive myositis ossificans
DEF: Progressive myositic disease; marked by bony tissue formed by voluntary muscle; occurs among very young.

728.12 Traumatic myositis ossificans
Myositis ossificans (circumscripta)

728.13 Postoperative heterotopic calcification
DEF: Abnormal formation of calcium deposits in muscular tissue after surgery, marked by a corresponding loss of muscle tone and tension.

728.19 Other
Polymyositis ossificans

728.2 Muscular wasting and disuse atrophy, not elsewhere classified
Amyotrophia NOS   Myofibrosis
> EXCLUDES   neuralgic amyotrophy (353.5)
>   progressive muscular atrophy (335.0-335.9)

728.3 Other specific muscle disorders
Arthrogryposis
Immobility syndrome (paraplegic)
> EXCLUDES   arthrogryposis multiplex congenita (754.89)
>   stiff-man syndrome (333.91)

728.4 Laxity of ligament

728.5 Hypermobility syndrome

728.6 Contracture of palmar fascia
Dupuytren's contracture

DEF: Dupuytren's contracture: flexion deformity of finger, due to shortened, thickened fibrosing of palmar fascia; cause unknown; associated with long-standing epilepsy; occurs more often in males.

MUSCULOSKELETAL SYSTEM 728.7–729.0

✓5ᵗʰ 728.7 Other fibromatoses

728.71 Plantar fascial fibromatosis
Contracture of plantar fascia
Plantar fasciitis (traumatic)
DEF: Plantar fascia fibromatosis; causes nodular swelling and pain; not associated with contractures.

728.79 Other
Garrod's or knuckle pads
Nodular fasciitis
Pseudosarcomatous fibromatosis (proliferative) (subcutaneous)
DEF: Knuckle pads: pea-size nodules on dorsal surface of interphalangeal joints; new growth of fibrous tissue with thickened dermis and epidermis.

✓5ᵗʰ 728.8 Other disorders of muscle, ligament, and fascia

728.81 Interstitial myositis
DEF: Inflammation of septal connective parts of muscle tissue.

728.82 Foreign body granuloma of muscle
Talc granuloma of muscle

728.83 Rupture of muscle, nontraumatic

728.84 Diastasis of muscle
Diastasis recti (abdomen)
> EXCLUDES diastasis recti complicating pregnancy, labor, and delivery (665.8)

DEF: Muscle separation, such as recti abdominis after repeated pregnancies.

728.85 Spasm of muscle

728.86 Necrotizing fasciitis
Use additional code to identify:
infectious organism (041.00-041.89)
gangrene (785.4), if applicable
DEF: Fulminating infection begins with extensive cellulitis, spreads to superficial and deep fascia; causes thrombosis of subcutaneous vessels, and gangrene of underlying tissue.

728.89 Other
Eosinophilic fasciitis
Use additional E code to identify drug, if drug induced
DEF: Eosinophilic fasciitis: inflammation of fascia of extremities associated with eosinophilia, edema, and swelling; occurs alone or as part of myalgia syndrome.

728.9 Unspecified disorder of muscle, ligament, and fascia

✓4ᵗʰ 729 Other disorders of soft tissues
> EXCLUDES acroparesthesia (443.89)
> carpal tunnel syndrome (354.0)
> disorders of the back (720.0-724.9)
> entrapment syndromes (354.0-355.9)
> palindromic rheumatism (719.3)
> periarthritis (726.0-726.9)
> psychogenic rheumatism (306.0)

729.0 Rheumatism, unspecified and fibrositis
DEF: General term describes diseases of muscle, tendon, nerve, joint, or bone; symptoms include pain and stiffness.

MUSCULOSKELETAL SYSTEM

729.1 **Myalgia and myositis, unspecified**
Fibromyositis NOS

DEF: Myalgia: muscle pain.

DEF: Myositis: inflamed voluntary muscle.

DEF: Fibromyositis: inflamed fibromuscular tissue.

729.2 **Neuralgia, neuritis, and radiculitis, unspecified**
EXCLUDES brachial radiculitis (723.4)
cervical radiculitis (723.4)
lumbosacral radiculitis (724.4)
mononeuritis (354.0-355.9)
radiculitis due to intervertebral disc involvement (722.0-722.2, 722.7)
sciatica (724.3)

DEF: Neuralgia: [aroxysmal pain along nerve symptoms include brief pain and tenderness at point nerve exits.

DEF: Neuritis: inflamed nerve, symptoms include paresthesia, paralysis and loss of reflexes at nerve site.

DEF: Radiculitis: inflamed nerve root.

√5th **729.3** **Panniculitis, unspecified**
DEF: Inflammatory reaction of subcutaneous fat; causes nodules; often develops in abdominal region.

729.30 **Panniculitis, unspecified site**
Weber-Christian disease

DEF: Febrile, nodular, nonsuppurative, relapsing inflammation of subcutaneous fat.

729.31 **Hypertrophy of fat pad, knee**
Hypertrophy of infrapatellar fat pad

729.39 **Other site**
EXCLUDES panniculitis specified as (affecting):
back (724.8)
neck (723.6)
sacral (724.8)

729.4 **Fasciitis, unspecified**
EXCLUDES necrotizing fasciitis (728.86)
nodular fasciitis (728.79)

729.5 **Pain in limb**

729.6 **Residual foreign body in soft tissue**
EXCLUDES foreign body granuloma:
muscle (728.82)
skin and subcutaneous tissue (709.4)

√5th **729.8** **Other musculoskeletal symptoms referable to limbs**
729.81 Swelling of limb
729.82 Cramp
729.89 **Other**
EXCLUDES abnormality of gait (781.2)
tetany (781.7)
transient paralysis of limb (781.4)

729.9 **Other and unspecified disorders of soft tissue**
Polyalgia

MUSCULOSKELETAL SYSTEM

OSTEOPATHIES, CHONDROPATHIES, AND ACQUIRED MUSCULOSKELETAL DEFORMITIES (730-739)

✓4th 730 Osteomyelitis, periostitis, and other infections involving bone

> **EXCLUDES** jaw (526.4-526.5)
> petrous bone (383.2)

Use additional code to identify organism, such as Staphylococcus (041.1)

DEF: Osteomyelitis: bacterial inflammation of bone tissue and marrow.

DEF: Periostitis: inflammation of specialized connective tissue; causes swelling of bone and aching pain.

The following fifth-digit subclassification is for use with category 730; valid digits are in [brackets] under each code. See definitions prior to category 710.

```
0  site unspecified
1  shoulder region
2  upper arm
3  forearm
4  hand
5  pelvic region and thigh
6  lower leg
7  ankle and foot
8  other specified sites
9  multiple sites
```

§ ✓5th 730.0 Acute osteomyelitis
[0-9]
Abscess of any bone except accessory sinus, jaw, or mastoid
Acute or subacute osteomyelitis, with or without mention of periostitis

§ ✓5th 730.1 Chronic osteomyelitis
[0-9]
Brodie's abscess
Chronic or old osteomyelitis, with or without mention of periostitis
Sclerosing osteomyelitis of Garré
Sequestrum of bone
> **EXCLUDES** aseptic necrosis of bone (733.40-733.49)

§ ✓5th 730.2 Unspecified osteomyelitis
[0-9]
Osteitis or osteomyelitis NOS, with or without mention of periostitis

§ ✓5th 730.3 Periostitis without mention of osteomyelitis
[0-9]
Abscess of periosteum } without mention of osteomyelitis
Periostosis
> **EXCLUDES** that in secondary syphilis (091.61)

§ ✓5th 730.7 Osteopathy resulting from poliomyelitis
[0-9]
Code first underlying disease (045.0-045.9)

§ ✓5th 730.8 Other infections involving bone in diseases classified elsewhere
[0-9]
Code first underlying disease as:
  tuberculosis (015.0-015.9)
  typhoid fever (002.0)
> **EXCLUDES** syphilis of bone NOS (095.5)

§ ✓5th 730.9 Unspecified infection of bone
[0-9]

---

§ Requires fifth-digit. Valid digits are in [brackets] under each code. See beginning of section 710-719 for codes and definitions.

| ✓4th / ✓5th Additional Digit Required | Unspecified Code | Other Specified Code | Manifestation Code |
| MSP Medicare Secondary Payer | ▶◀ Revised Text | ● New Code | ▲ Revised Code Title |

2002 Ingenix, Inc.   Volume 1 — 431

MUSCULOSKELETAL SYSTEM

✓4th **731 Osteitis deformans and osteopathies associated with other disorders classified elsewhere**
DEF: Osteitis deformans: Bone disease marked by episodes of increased bone loss, excessive repair attempts follow; causes weakened, deformed bones with increased mass, bowed long bones, deformed flat bones, pain and pathological fractures; may be fatal if associated with congestive heart failure, giant cell tumors or bone sarcoma; also called Paget's disease.

731.0 Osteitis deformans without mention of bone tumor
Paget's disease of bone

731.1 *Osteitis deformans in diseases classified elsewhere*
Code first underlying disease as:
malignant neoplasm of bone (170.0-170.9)

731.2 Hypertrophic pulmonary osteoarthropathy
Bamberger-Marie disease
DEF: Clubbing, of fingers and toes; related to enlarged ends of long bones; due to chronic lung and heart disease.

731.8 *Other bone involvement in diseases classified elsewhere*
Code first underlying disease as:
diabetes mellitus (250.8)
Use additional code to specify bone condition, such as:
acute osteomyelitis (730.00-730.09)

✓4th **732 Osteochondropathies**
DEF: Conditions related to both bone and cartilage, or conditions in which cartilage is converted to bone (enchondral ossification).

732.0 Juvenile osteochondrosis of spine
Juvenile osteochondrosis (of):
marginal or vertebral epiphysis (of Scheuermann)
spine NOS
Vertebral epiphysitis
> EXCLUDES adolescent postural kyphosis (737.0)

732.1 Juvenile osteochondrosis of hip and pelvis
Coxa plana
Ischiopubic synchondrosis (of van Neck)
Osteochondrosis (juvenile) of:
acetabulum
head of femur (of Legg-Calvé-Perthes)
iliac crest (of Buchanan)
symphysis pubis (of Pierson)
Pseudocoxalgia

732.2 Nontraumatic slipped upper femoral epiphysis
Slipped upper femoral epiphysis NOS

732.3 Juvenile osteochondrosis of upper extremity
Osteochondrosis (juvenile) of:
capitulum of humerus (of Panner)
carpal lunate (of Kienbock)
hand NOS
head of humerus (of Haas)
heads of metacarpals (of Mauclaire)
lower ulna (of Burns)
radial head (of Brailsford)
upper extremity NOS

MUSCULOSKELETAL SYSTEM

732.4 **Juvenile osteochondrosis of lower extremity, excluding foot**
Osteochondrosis (juvenile) of:
lower extremity NOS
primary patellar center (of Köhler)
proximal tibia (of Blount)
secondary patellar center (of Sinding-Larsen)
tibial tubercle (of Osgood-Schlatter)
Tibia vara

732.5 **Juvenile osteochondrosis of foot**
Calcaneal apophysitis
Epiphysitis, os calcis
Osteochondrosis (juvenile) of:
astragalus (of Diaz)
calcaneum (of Sever)
foot NOS
metatarsal:
second (of Freiberg)
fifth (of Iselin)
os tibiale externum (of Haglund)
tarsal navicular (of Köhler)

732.6 **Other juvenile osteochondrosis**
Apophysitis
Epiphysitis } specified as juvenile, of other site, or site NOS
Osteochondritis
Osteochondrosis

732.7 **Osteochondritis dissecans**

732.8 **Other specified forms of osteochondropathy**
Adult osteochondrosis of spine

732.9 **Unspecified osteochondropathy**
Apophysitis
Epiphysitis } NOS
Osteochondritis   not specified as adult or juvenile, of unspecified site
Osteochondrosis

√4th 733 **Other disorders of bone and cartilage**
EXCLUDES bone spur (726.91)
cartilage of, or loose body in, joint (717.0-717.9, 718.0-718.9)
giant cell granuloma of jaw (526.3)
osteitis fibrosa cystica generalisata (252.0)
osteomalacia (268.2)
polyostotic fibrous dysplasia of bone (756.54)
prognathism, retrognathism (524.1)
xanthomatosis localized to bone (272.7)

√5th 733.0 **Osteoporosis**
DEF: Bone mass reduction that ultimately results in fractures after minimal trauma; dorsal kyphosis or loss of height often occur.

733.00 **Osteoporosis, unspecified**
Wedging of vertebra NOS

733.01 **Senile osteoporosis**
Postmenopausal osteoporosis

733.02 **Idiopathic osteoporosis**

733.03 **Disuse osteoporosis**

733.09 **Other**
Drug-induced osteoporosis
Use additional E code to identify drug

733.1 Pathologic fracture
 Spontaneous fracture
 EXCLUDES stress fracture (733.93-733.95)
 traumatic fracture (800-829)
 DEF: Fracture due to bone structure weakening by pathological processes (e.g., osteoporosis, neoplasms and osteomalacia).

 733.10 Pathologic fracture, unspecified site
 733.11 Pathologic fracture of humerus
 733.12 Pathologic fracture of distal radius and ulna
  Wrist NOS
 733.13 Pathologic fracture of vertebrae
  Collapse of vertebra NOS
 733.14 Pathologic fracture of neck of femur
  Femur NOS   Hip NOS
 733.15 Pathologic fracture of other specified part of femur
 733.16 Pathologic fracture of tibia or fibula
  Ankle NOS
 733.19 Pathologic fracture of other specified site

733.2 Cyst of bone
 733.20 Cyst of bone (localized), unspecified
 733.21 Solitary bone cyst
  Unicameral bone cyst
 733.22 Aneurysmal bone cyst
 DEF: Solitary bone lesion, bulges into periosteum; marked by calcified rim.

 733.29 Other
  Fibrous dysplasia (monostotic)
  EXCLUDES cyst of jaw (526.0-526.2, 526.89)
   osteitis fibrosa cystica (252.0)
   polyostotic fibrousdyplasia of bone (756.54)

733.3 Hyperostosis of skull
 Hyperostosis interna frontalis
 Leontiasis ossium
 DEF: Abnormal bone growth on inner aspect of cranial bones.

733.4 Aseptic necrosis of bone
 EXCLUDES osteochondropathies (732.0-732.9)
 DEF: Infraction of bone tissue due to a nonfectious etiology, such as a fracture, ischemic disorder or administration of immunosuppressive drugs; leads to degenerative joint disease or nonunion of fractures.

 733.40 Aseptic necrosis of bone, site unspecified
 733.41 Head of humerus
 733.42 Head and neck of femur
  Femur NOS
  EXCLUDES Legg-Calvé-Perthes disease (732.1)
 733.43 Medial femoral condyle
 733.44 Talus
 733.49 Other

733.5 Osteitis condensans
 Piriform sclerosis of ilium
 DEF: Idiopathic condition marked by low back pain; associated with oval or triangular sclerotic, opaque bone next to sacroiliac joints in the ileum.

733.6 Tietze's disease
 Costochondral junction syndrome   Costochondritis
 DEF: Painful, idiopathic, nonsuppurative, swollen costal cartilage sometimes confused with cardiac symptoms because the anterior chest pain resembles that of coronary artery disease.

MUSCULOSKELETAL SYSTEM

Acquired Deformities of Toe

- Hallux valgus
- Hallux varus
- Hallux malleus (hammer of big toe)
- Hammertoe

733.7 Algoneurodystrophy
Disuse atrophy of bone   Sudeck's atrophy
DEF: Painful, idiopathic.

√5ᵗʰ 733.8 Malunion and nonunion of fracture
733.81 Malunion of fracture
733.82 Nonunion of fracture
Pseudoarthrosis (bone)

√5ᵗʰ 733.9 Other and unspecified disorders of bone and cartilage
733.90 Disorder of bone and cartilage, unspecified
733.91 Arrest of bone development or growth
Epiphyseal arrest
733.92 Chondromalacia
Chondromalacia:
  NOS
  localized, except patella
  systemic
  tibial plateau
  EXCLUDES chondromalacia of patella (717.7)
DEF: Articular cartilage softening..

733.93 Stress fracture of tibia or fibula
Stress reaction of tibia or fibula
733.94 Stress fracture of the metatarsals
Stress reaction of metatarsals
733.95 Stress fracture of other bone
Stress reaction of other bone
733.99 Other
Diaphysitis
Hypertrophy of bone
Relapsing polychondritis

734 Flat foot
Pes planus (acquired)
Talipes planus (acquired)
EXCLUDES congenital (754.61)
rigid flat foot (754.61)
spastic (everted) flat foot (754.61)

√4ᵗʰ / √5ᵗʰ Additional Digit Required   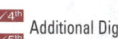 Unspecified Code   ● Other Specified Code   ▲ Manifestation Code
MSP Medicare Secondary Payer   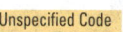 Revised Text   ● New Code   ▲ Revised Code Title

2002 Ingenix, Inc.   Volume 1 — 435

Acquired Deformities of Forearm

Cubitus valgus — Cubitus varus — Varus deformity of wrist — Valgus deformity of wrist — Claw hand — Wrist drop — Club hand

- ✓4th **735 Acquired deformities of toe**

  EXCLUDES congenital (754.60-754.69, 755.65-755.66)

  735.0 Hallux valgus (acquired)
  DEF: Angled displacement of the great toe, causing it to ride over or under other toes.

  735.1 Hallux varus (acquired)
  DEF: Angled displacement of the great toe toward the body midline, away from the other toes.

  735.2 Hallux rigidus
  DEF: Limited flexion movement at metatarsophalangeal joint of great toe; due to degenerative joint disease.

  735.3 Hallux malleus
  DEF: Extended proximal phalanx, flexed distal phalanges, of great toe; foot resembles claw or hammer.

  735.4 Other hammer toe (acquired)

  735.5 Claw toe (acquired)
  DEF: Hyperextended proximal phalanges, flexed middle and distal phalanges.

  735.8 Other acquired deformities of toe

  735.9 Unspecified acquired deformity of toe

- ✓4th **736 Other acquired deformities of limbs**

  EXCLUDES congenital (754.3-755.9)

  - ✓5th **736.0 Acquired deformities of forearm, excluding fingers**

    736.00 Unspecified deformity
    Deformity of elbow, forearm, hand, or wrist (acquired) NOS

    736.01 Cubitus valgus (acquired)
    DEF: Deviation of the elbow away from the body midline upon extension; it occurs when the palm is turning outward.

    736.02 Cubitus varus (acquired)
    DEF: Elbow joint displacement angled laterally; when the forearm is extended, it is deviated toward the midline of the body; also called "gun stock" deformity.

    736.03 Valgus deformity of wrist (acquired)
    DEF: Abnormal angulation away from the body midline.

    736.04 Varus deformity of wrist (acquired)
    DEF: Abnormal angulation toward the body midline.

MUSCULOSKELETAL SYSTEM

Acquired Deformities of Hip

Acquired Deformities of Lower Limb

- **736.05 Wrist drop (acquired)**
  DEF: Inability to extend the hand at the wrist due to extensor muscle paralysis.

- **736.06 Claw hand (acquired)**
  DEF: Flexion and atrophy of the hand and fingers; found in ulnar nerve lesions, syringomyelia, and leprosy.

- **736.07 Club hand, acquired**
  DEF: Twisting of the hand out of shape or position; caused by the congenital absence of the ulna or radius.

- **736.09 Other**

736.1 Mallet finger
DEF: Permanently flexed distal phalanx.

736.2 Other acquired deformities of finger

- **736.20 Unspecified deformity**
  Deformity of finger (acquired) NOS

- **736.21 Boutonniere deformity**
  DEF: A complete or partial protrusion of a joint finger through a defect in the extensor aponeurosis; also called buttonhole deformity.

- **736.22 Swan-neck deformity**
  DEF: Flexed distal and hyperextended proximal interphalangeal joint.

✓4ᵗʰ Additional Digit Required
✓5ᵗʰ
MSP Medicare Secondary Payer ▶◀ Revised Text   ● New Code   ▲ Revised Code Title

Unspecified Code   Other Specified Code   Manifestation Code

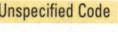

MUSCULOSKELETAL SYSTEM

736.29 Other
> EXCLUDES   *trigger finger (727.03)*

√5th **736.3 Acquired deformities of hip**

736.30 Unspecified deformity
Deformity of hip (acquired) NOS

736.31 Coxa valga (acquired)
DEF: Increase of at least 140 degrees in the angle formed by the axis of the head and the neck of the femur, and the axis of its shaft.

736.32 Coxa vara (acquired)
DEF: The bending downward of the neck of the femur; causing difficulty in movement; a right angle or less may be formed by the axis of the head and neck of the femur, and the axis of its shaft.

736.39 Other

√5th **736.4 Genu valgum or varum (acquired)**

736.41 Genu valgum (acquired)
DEF: Abnormally close together and an abnormally large space between the ankles; also called "knock-knees."

736.42 Genu varum (acquired)
DEF: Abnormally separated knees and the inward bowing of the legs; it is also called "bowlegs."

736.5 Genu recurvatum (acquired)
DEF: Hyperextended knees; also called "backknee."

736.6 Other acquired deformities of knee
Deformity of knee (acquired) NOS

√5th **736.7 Other acquired deformities of ankle and foot**
> EXCLUDES   *deformities of toe (acquired) (735.0-735.9)*
> *pes planus (acquired) (734)*

736.70 Unspecified deformity of ankle and foot, acquired

736.71 Acquired equinovarus deformity
Clubfoot, acquired
> EXCLUDES   *clubfoot not specified as acquired (754.5-754.7)*

736.72 Equinus deformity of foot, acquired
DEF: A plantar flexion deformity that forces people to walk on their toes.

736.73 Cavus deformity of foot
> EXCLUDES   *that with claw foot (736.74)*

DEF: Abnormally high longitudinal arch of the foot.

736.74 Claw foot, acquired
DEF: High foot arch with hyperextended toes at metatarsophalangeal joint and flexed toes at distal joints; also called "main en griffe."

736.75 Cavovarus deformity of foot, acquired
DEF: Inward turning of the heel from the midline of the leg and an abnormally high longitudinal arch.

736.76 Other calcaneus deformity

736.79 Other
Acquired:
  pes   } not elsewhere classified
  talipes

√5th **736.8 Acquired deformities of other parts of limbs**

736.81 Unequal leg length (acquired)

MUSCULOSKELETAL SYSTEM

Kyphosis and Lordosis

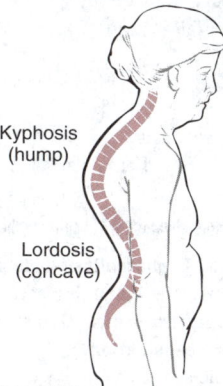

736.89 Other
    Deformity (acquired):
      arm or leg, not elsewhere classified
      shoulder

736.9 Acquired deformity of limb, site unspecified

737 Curvature of spine
    EXCLUDES congenital (754.2)

737.0 Adolescent postural kyphosis
    EXCLUDES osteochondrosis of spine (juvenile) (732.0)
        adult (732.8)

737.1 Kyphosis (acquired)
    737.10 Kyphosis (acquired) (postural)
    737.11 Kyphosis due to radiation
    737.12 Kyphosis, postlaminectomy
    737.19 Other
        EXCLUDES that associated with conditions classifiable elsewhere (737.41)

737.2 Lordosis (acquired)
    DEF: Swayback appearance created by an abnormally increased spinal curvature; it is also referred to as "hollow back" or "saddle back."

Scoliosis and Kyphoscoliosis

Scoliosis

Kyphoscoliosis

MUSCULOSKELETAL SYSTEM

- **737.20** Lordosis (acquired) (postural)
- **737.21** Lordosis, postlaminectomy
- **737.22** Other postsurgical lordosis
- **737.29** Other
  > EXCLUDES that associated with conditions classifiable elsewhere (737.42)

✓5ᵗʰ **737.3** Kyphoscoliosis and scoliosis

DEF: Kyphoscoliosis: backward and lateral curvature of the spinal column; it is found in vertebral osteochondrosis.

DEF: Scoliosis: an abnormal deviation of the spine to the left or right of the midline

- **737.30** Scoliosis [and kyphoscoliosis], idiopathic
- **737.31** Resolving infantile idiopathic scoliosis
- **737.32** Progressive infantile idiopathic scoliosis
- **737.33** Scoliosis due to radiation
- **737.34** Thoracogenic scoliosis
- **737.39** Other
  > EXCLUDES that associated with conditions classifiable elsewhere (737.43)
  > that in kyphoscoliotic heart disease (416.1)

✓5ᵗʰ **737.4** Curvature of spine associated with other conditions
  Code first associated condition as:
    Charcôt-Marie-Tooth disease (356.1)
    mucopolysaccharidosis (277.5)
    neurofibromatosis (237.7)
    osteitis deformans (731.0)
    osteitis fibrosa cystica (252.0)
    osteoporosis (733.00-733.09)
    poliomyelitis (138)
    tuberculosis [Pott's curvature] (015.0)

- **737.40** Curvature of spine, unspecified
- **737.41** Kyphosis
- **737.42** Lordosis
- **737.43** Scoliosis

737.8 Other curvatures of spine

737.9 Unspecified curvature of spine
  Curvature of spine (acquired) (idiopathic) NOS
  Hunchback, acquired
  > EXCLUDES deformity of spine NOS (738.5)

✓4ᵗʰ **738** Other acquired deformity
  > EXCLUDES congenital (754.0-756.9, 758.0-759.9)
  > dentofacial anomalies (524.0-524.9)

738.0 Acquired deformity of nose
  Deformity of nose (acquired)
  Overdevelopment of nasal bones
  > EXCLUDES deflected or deviated nasal septum (470)

✓5ᵗʰ **738.1** Other acquired deformity of head
- **738.10** Unspecified deformity
- **738.11** Zygomatic hyperplasia
  DEF: Abnormal enlargement of the zygoma (processus zygomaticus temporalis).
- **738.12** Zygomatic hypoplasia
  DEF: Underdevelopment of the zygoma (processus zygomaticus temporalis).
- **738.19** Other specified deformity

738.2 Acquired deformity of neck

MUSCULOSKELETAL SYSTEM

738.3 Acquired deformity of chest and rib
Deformity: Pectus:
  chest (acquired)   carinatum, acquired
  rib (acquired)   excavatum, acquired

738.4 Acquired spondylolisthesis
Degenerative spondylolisthesis
Spondylolysis, acquired
  EXCLUDES congenital (756.12)
DEF: Vertebra displaced forward over another; due to bilateral defect in vertebral arch, eroded articular surface of posterior facts and elongated pedicle between fifth lumbar vertebra and sacrum.

738.5 Other acquired deformity of back or spine
Deformity of spine NOS
  EXCLUDES curvature of spine (737.0-737.9)

738.6 Acquired deformity of pelvis
Pelvic obliquity
  EXCLUDES intrapelvic protrusion of acetabulum (718.6)
           that in relation to labor and delivery (653.0-653.4, 653.8-653.9)
DEF: Pelvic obliquity: slanting or inclination of the pelvis at an angle between 55 and 60 degrees between the plane of the pelvis and the horizontal plane.

738.7 Cauliflower ear
DEF: Abnormal external ear; due to injury, subsequent perichondritis.

738.8 Acquired deformity of other specified site
Deformity of clavicle

738.9 Acquired deformity of unspecified site

√4th 739 Nonallopathic lesions, not elsewhere classified
  INCLUDES segmental dysfunction
           somatic dysfunction
DEF: Disability, loss of function or abnormality of a body part that is neither classifiable to a particular system nor brought about therapeutically to counteract another disease.

739.0 Head region
Occipitocervical region

739.1 Cervical region
Cervicothoracic region

739.2 Thoracic region
Thoracolumbar region

739.3 Lumbar region
Lumbosacral region

739.4 Sacral region
Sacrococcygeal region   Sacroiliac region

739.5 Pelvic region
Hip region   Pubic region

739.6 Lower extremities

739.7 Upper extremities
Acromioclavicular region
Sternoclavicular region

739.8 Rib cage
Costochondral region   Sternochondral region
Costovertebral region

739.9 Abdomen and other

14. CONGENITAL ANOMALIES (740-759)

√4th **740 Anencephalus and similar anomalies**

740.0 Anencephalus
Acrania   Hemicephaly
Amyelencephalus   Hemianencephaly
DEF: Fetus without cerebrum, cerebellum and flat bones of skull.

740.1 Craniorachischisis
DEF: Congenital slit in cranium and vertebral column.

740.2 Iniencephaly
DEF: Spinal cord passes through enlarged occipital bone (foramen magnum); absent vertebral bone layer and spinal processes; resulting in both reduction in number and proper fusion of the vertebrae.

√4th **741 Spina bifida**

EXCLUDES spina bifida occulta (756.17)

DEF: Lack of closure of spinal cord's bony encasement; marked by cord protrusion into lumbosacral area; evident by elevated alpha-fetoprotein of amniotic fluid.

The following fifth-digit subclassification is for use with category 741:
  0 unspecified region
  1 cervical region
  2 dorsal [thoracic] region
  3 lumbar region

√5th **741.0 With hydrocephalus**
Arnold-Chiari syndrome, type II
Any condition classifiable to 741.9 with any condition classifiable to 742.3
Chiari malformation, type II

√5th **741.9 Without mention of hydrocephalus**
Hydromeningocele (spinal)   Myelocystocele
Hydromyelocele   Rachischisis
Meningocele (spinal)   Spina bifida (aperta)
Meningomyelocele   Syringomyelocele
Myelocele

√4th **742 Other congenital anomalies of nervous system**

742.0 Encephalocele
Encephalocystocele   Hydromeningocele, cranial
Encephalomyelocele   Meningocele, cerebral
Hydroencephalocele   Meningoencephalocele
DEF: Brain tissue protrudes through skull defect.

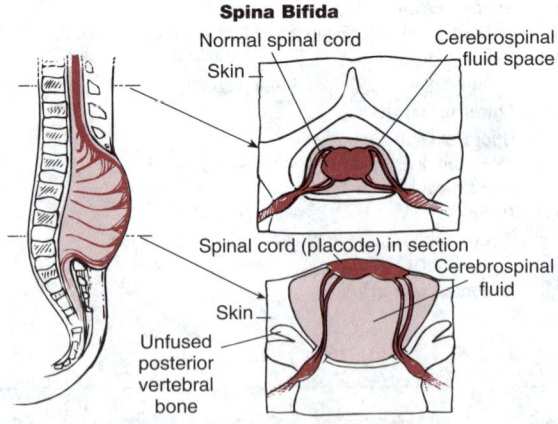

Spina Bifida

CONGENITAL ANOMALIES

742.1   Microcephalus
Hydromicrocephaly
Micrencephaly
DEF: Extremely small head or brain.

742.2   Reduction deformities of brain
Absence
Agenesis
Aplasia
Hypoplasia
} of part of brain

Agyria
Arhinencephaly
Holoprosencephaly
Microgyria

742.3   Congenital hydrocephalus
Aqueduct of Sylvius:
   anomaly
   obstruction, congenital
   stenosis
Atresia of foramina of Magendie and Luschka
Hydrocephalus in newborn

EXCLUDES hydrocephalus:
   acquired (331.3-331.4)
   due to congenital toxoplasmosis (771.2)
   with any condition classifiable to 741.9 (741.0)

DEF: Fluid accumulation within the skull; involves subarachnoid (external) or ventricular (internal) brain spaces.

Normal Ventricles and Hydrocephalus

CONGENITAL ANOMALIES

742.4 Other specified anomalies of brain
- Congenital cerebral cyst
- Macroencephaly
- Macrogyria
- Megalencephaly
- Multiple anomalies of brain NOS
- Porencephaly
- Ulegyria

√5th **742.5 Other specified anomalies of spinal cord**

742.51 Diastematomyelia
DEF: Congenital anomaly often associated with spina bifida; the spinal cord is separated into halves by a bony tissue resembling a "spike" (a spicule), each half surrounded by a dural sac.

742.53 Hydromyelia
- Hydrorhachis

DEF: Dilated central spinal cord canal; characterized by increased fluid accumulation.

742.59 Other
- Amyelia
- Atelomyelia
- Congenital anomaly of spinal meninges
- Defective development of cauda equina
- Hypoplasia of spinal cord
- Myelatelia
- Myelodysplasia

742.8 Other specified anomalies of nervous system
- Agenesis of nerve
- Displacement of brachial plexus
- Familial dysautonomia
- Jaw-winking syndrome
- Marcus-Gunn syndrome
- Riley-Day syndrome

EXCLUDES neurofibromatosis (237.7)

742.9 Unspecified anomaly of brain, spinal cord, and nervous system
- Anomaly
- Congenital:
  - disease
  - lesion
- Deformity

of:
- brain
- nervous system
- spinal cord

√4th **743 Congenital anomalies of eye**

√5th **743.0 Anophthalmos**
DEF: Complete absence of the eyes or the presence of vestigial eyes.

743.00 Clinical anophthalmos, unspecified
- Agenesis
- Congenital absence } of eye
- Anophthalmos NOS

743.03 Cystic eyeball, congenital

743.06 Cryptophthalmos
DEF: Eyelids continue over eyeball, results in apparent absence of eyelids.

√5th **743.1 Microphthalmos**
- Dysplasia
- Hypoplasia } of eye
- Rudimentary eye

DEF: Abnormally small eyeballs, may be opacities of cornea and lens, scarring of choroid and retina.

CONGENITAL ANOMALIES

743.10 Microphthalmos, unspecified
743.11 Simple microphthalmos
743.12 Microphthalmos associated with other anomalies of eye and adnexa

√5ᵗʰ **743.2** **Buphthalmos**
  Glaucoma: Hydrophthalmos
    congenital
    newborn
  EXCLUDES glaucoma of childhood (365.14)
                 traumatic glaucoma due to birth injury (767.8)
  DEF: Distended, enlarged fibrous coats of eye; due to intraocular pressure of congenital glaucoma.

743.20 Buphthalmos, unspecified
743.21 Simple buphthalmos
743.22 Buphthalmos associated with other ocular anomalies
    Keratoglobus, congenital ⎫ associated with
    Megalocornea   ⎭ buphthalmos

√5ᵗʰ **743.3** Congenital cataract and lens anomalies
  EXCLUDES infantile cataract (366.00-366.09)
  DEF: Opaque eye lens.

743.30 Congenital cataract, unspecified
743.31 Capsular and subcapsular cataract
743.32 Cortical and zonular cataract
743.33 Nuclear cataract
743.34 Total and subtotal cataract, congenital
743.35 Congenital aphakia
    Congenital absence of lens
743.36 Anomalies of lens shape
    Microphakia   Spherophakia
743.37 Congenital ectopic lens
743.39 Other

√5ᵗʰ **743.4** Coloboma and other anomalies of anterior segment
  DEF: Coloboma: ocular tissue defect associated with defect of ocular fetal intraocular fissure; may cause small pit on optic disk, major defects of iris, ciliary body, choroid, and retina.

743.41 Anomalies of corneal size and shape
    Microcornea
    EXCLUDES that associated with buphthalmos (743.22)
743.42 Corneal opacities, interfering with vision, congenital
743.43 Other corneal opacities, congenital
743.44 Specified anomalies of anterior chamber, chamber angle, and related structures
    Anomaly: Anomaly:
      Axenfeld's   Rieger's
      Peters'
743.45 Aniridia
  DEF: Incompletely formed or absent iris; affects both eyes; dominant trait; also called congenital hyperplasia of iris.
743.46 Other specified anomalies of iris and ciliary body
    Anisocoria, congenital   Coloboma of iris
    Atresia of pupil   Corectopia
743.47 Specified anomalies of sclera
743.48 Multiple and combined anomalies of anterior segment

√4ᵗʰ Additional Digit Required | Unspecified Code | Other Specified Code | Manifestation Code
√5ᵗʰ
MSP Medicare Secondary Payer | ▶◀ Revised Text | ● New Code | ▲ Revised Code Title

2002 Ingenix, Inc.   Volume 1 — 445

743.49 Other

√5th **743.5 Congenital anomalies of posterior segment**

743.51 Vitreous anomalies
Congenital vitreous opacity

743.52 Fundus coloboma
DEF: Absent retinal and choroidal tissue; occurs in lower fundus; a bright white ectatic zone of exposed sclera extends into and changes the optic disk.

743.53 Chorioretinal degeneration, congenital

743.54 Congenital folds and cysts of posterior segment

743.55 Congenital macular changes

743.56 Other retinal changes, congenital

743.57 Specified anomalies of optic disc
Coloboma of optic disc (congenital)

743.58 Vascular anomalies
Congenital retinal aneurysm

743.59 Other

√5th **743.6 Congenital anomalies of eyelids, lacrimal system, and orbit**

743.61 Congenital ptosis
DEF: Drooping of eyelid.

743.62 Congenital deformities of eyelids
Ablepharon　　　Congenital:
Absence of eyelid　　ectropion
Accessory eyelid　　entropion

743.63 Other specified congenital anomalies of eyelid
Absence, agenesis, of cilia

743.64 Specified congenital anomalies of lacrimal gland

743.65 Specified congenital anomalies of lacrimal passages
Absence, agenesis of:
　lacrimal apparatus
　punctum lacrimale
Accessory lacrimal canal

743.66 Specified congenital anomalies of orbit

743.69 Other
Accessory eye muscles

743.8 Other specified anomalies of eye
　EXCLUDES　congenital nystagmus (379.51)
　　　　　　ocular albinism (270.2)
　　　　　　retinitis pigmentosa (362.74)

743.9 Unspecified anomaly of eye
Congenital:
　anomaly NOS　}
　deformity NOS } of eye [any part]

√4th **744 Congenital anomalies of ear, face, and neck**
　EXCLUDES　anomaly of:
　　　　　　cervical spine (754.2, 756.10-756.19)
　　　　　　larynx (748.2-748.3)
　　　　　　nose (748.0-748.1)
　　　　　　parathyroid gland (759.2)
　　　　　　thyroid gland (759.2)
　　　　　　cleft lip (749.10-749.25)

√5th **744.0 Anomalies of ear causing impairment of hearing**
　EXCLUDES　congenital deafness without mention of cause (389.0-389.9)

744.00 Unspecified anomaly of ear with impairment of hearing

CONGENITAL ANOMALIES 744.01–744.47

744.01 Absence of external ear
Absence of:
auditory canal (external)
auricle (ear) (with stenosis or atresia of auditory canal)

744.02 Other anomalies of external ear with impairment of hearing
Atresia or stricture of auditory canal (external)

744.03 Anomaly of middle ear, except ossicles
Atresia or stricture of osseous meatus (ear)

744.04 Anomalies of ear ossicles
Fusion of ear ossicles

744.05 Anomalies of inner ear
Congenital anomaly of: Congenital anomaly of:
   membranous labyrinth   organ of Corti

744.09 Other
Absence of ear, congenital

744.1 Accessory auricle
Accessory tragus   Supernumerary:
Polyotia   ear
Preauricular appendage   lobule

DEF: Redundant tissue or structures of ear.

√5th 744.2 Other specified anomalies of ear
EXCLUDES that with impairment of hearing (744.00-744.09)

744.21 Absence of ear lobe, congenital

744.22 Macrotia
DEF: Abnormally large pinna of ear.

744.23 Microtia
DEF: Hypoplasia of pinna; associated with absent or closed auditory canal.

744.24 Specified anomalies of Eustachian tube
Absence of Eustachian tube

744.29 Other
Bat ear   Prominence of auricle
Darwin's tubercle   Ridge ear
Pointed ear
EXCLUDES preauricular sinus (744.46)

744.3 Unspecified anomaly of ear
Congenital:
   anomaly NOS } of ear, not elsewhere
   deformity NOS }   classified

√5th 744.4 Branchial cleft cyst or fistula; preauricular sinus
DEF: Coloboma: malclosure of the intraoccular fissure in embryo resulting in defects to optic disk, iris, ciliary body, choroid, or retina.

744.41 Branchial cleft sinus or fistula
Branchial:
   sinus (external) (internal)
   vestige
DEF: Cyst due to failed closure of embryonic branchial cleft.

744.42 Branchial cleft cyst

744.43 Cervical auricle

744.46 Preauricular sinus or fistula

744.47 Preauricular cyst

√4th / √5th Additional Digit Required   Unspecified Code   Other Specified Code   Manifestation Code
 Medicare Secondary Payer   ▶◀ Revised Text   ● New Code   ▲ Revised Code Title

2002 Ingenix, Inc.   Volume 1 — 447

744.49 Other
Fistula (of): auricle, congenital
Fistula (of): cervicoaural

744.5 Webbing of neck
Pterygium colli
DEF: Thick, triangular skinfold, stretches from lateral side of neck across shoulder; associated with Turner's and Noonan's syndromes.

✓5th **744.8 Other specified anomalies of face and neck**

744.81 Macrocheilia
Hypertrophy of lip, congenital
DEF: Abnormally large lips.

744.82 Microcheilia
DEF: Abnormally small lips.

744.83 Macrostomia
DEF: Bilateral or unilateral anomaly, of mouth due to malformed maxillary and mandibular processes; results in mouth extending toward ear.

744.84 Microstomia
DEF: Abnormally small mouth.

744.89 Other
EXCLUDES congenital fistula of lip (750.25)
musculoskeletal anomalies (754.0-754.1, 756.0)

744.9 Unspecified anomalies of face and neck
Congenital:
anomaly NOS } of face [any part] or
deformity NOS } neck [any part]

✓4th **745 Bulbus cordis anomalies and anomalies of cardiac septal closure**

745.0 Common truncus
Absent septum
Communication } between aorta and
(abnormal) } pulmonary artery

Aortic septal defect
Common aortopulmonary trunk
Persistent truncus arteriosus

✓5th **745.1 Transposition of great vessels**

745.10 Complete transposition of great vessels
Transposition of great vessels:
NOS
classical

745.11 Double outlet right ventricle
Dextratransposition of aorta
Incomplete transposition of great vessels
Origin of both great vessels from right ventricle
Taussig-Bing syndrome or defect

745.12 Corrected transposition of great vessels

745.19 Other

745.2 Tetralogy of Fallot
Fallot's pentalogy
Ventricular septal defect with pulmonary stenosis or atresia, dextraposition of aorta, and hypertrophy of right ventricle
EXCLUDES Fallot's triad (746.09)
DEF: Obstructed cardiac outflow causes pulmonary stenosis, interventricular septal defect and right ventricular hypertrophy.

CONGENITAL ANOMALIES 745.3–746.09

745.3 Common ventricle
Cor triloculare biatriatum   Single ventricle

745.4 Ventricular septal defect
Eisenmenger's defect or complex
Gerbo dedefect
Interventricular septal defect
Left ventricular-right atrial communication
Roger's disease
> EXCLUDES common atrioventricular canal type (745.69)
> single ventricle (745.3)

745.5 Ostium secundum type atrial septal defect
Defect: Patent or persistent:
  atrium secundum   foramen ovale
  fossa ovalis   ostium secundum
Lutembacher's syndrome
DEF: Opening in atrial septum due to failure of the septum secondum and the endocardial cushions to fuse; there is a rim of septum surrounding the defect.

√5th **745.6 Endocardial cushion defects**
DEF: Atrial and/or ventricular septa defects causing abnormal fusion of cushions in atrioventricular canal.

745.60 Endocardial cushion defect, unspecified type
DEF: Septal defect due to imperfect fusion of endocardial cushions.

745.61 Ostium primum defect
Persistent ostium primum
DEF: Opening in low, posterior septum primum; causes cleft in basal portion of atrial septum; associated with cleft mitral valve.

745.69 Other
Absence of atrial septum
Atrioventricular canal type ventricular septal defect
Common atrioventricular canal
Common atrium

745.7 Cor biloculare
Absence of atrial and ventricular septa
DEF: Atrial and ventricular septal defect; marked by heart with two cardiac chambers (one atrium, one ventricle), and one atrioventricular valve.

745.8 Other

745.9 Unspecified defect of septal closure
Septal defect NOS

√4th **746 Other congenital anomalies of heart**
> EXCLUDES endocardial fibroelastosis (425.3)

√5th **746.0 Anomalies of pulmonary valve**
> EXCLUDES infundibular or subvalvular pulmonic stenosis (746.83)
> tetralogy of Fallot (745.2)

746.00 Pulmonary valve anomaly, unspecified

746.01 Atresia, congenital
Congenital absence of pulmonary valve

746.02 Stenosis, congenital
DEF: Stenosis of opening between pulmonary artery and right ventricle; causes obstructed blood outflow from right ventricle.

746.09 Other
Congenital insufficiency of pulmonary valve
Fallot's triad or trilogy

  Additional Digit Required   Unspecified Code   Other Specified Code   Manifestation Code
MSP Medicare Secondary Payer   ▶◀ Revised Text   ● New Code   ▲ Revised Code Title
2002 Ingenix, Inc.

CONGENITAL ANOMALIES

Heart Defects

- Atrial septal defect
- Aortic stenosis
- Ventricular septal defect
- Patent ductus arteriosus
- Pulmonary stenosis
- Transposition of the great vessels
- Tetralogy of Fallot

746.1 Tricuspid atresia and stenosis, congenital
Absence of tricuspid valve

746.2 Ebstein's anomaly
DEF: Malformation of the tricuspid valve characterized by septal and posterior leaflets attaching to the wall of the right ventricle; causing the right ventricle to fuse with the atrium producing a large right atrium and a small ventricle; causes a malfunction of the right ventricle with accompanying complications such as heart failure and abnormal cardiac rhythm.

746.3 Congenital stenosis of aortic valve
Congenital aortic stenosis

> **EXCLUDES** congenital:
> subaortic stenosis (746.81)
> supravalvular aortic stenosis (747.22)

DEF: Stenosis of orifice of aortic valve; obstructs blood outflow from left ventricle.

746.4 Congenital insufficiency of aortic valve
Bicuspid aortic valve
Congenital aortic insufficiency

DEF: Impaired functioning of aortic valve due to incomplete closure; causes backflow (regurgitation) of blood from aorta to left ventricle.

746.5 Congenital mitral stenosis
Fused commissure
Parachute deformity   } of mitral valve
Supernumerary cusps

DEF: Stenosis of left atrioventricular orifice.

746.6 Congenital mitral insufficiency
DEF: Impaired functioning of mitral valve due to incomplete closure; causes backflow of blood from left ventricle to left atrium.

746.7 Hypoplastic left heart syndrome
Atresia, or marked hypoplasia, of aortic orifice or valve, with hypoplasia of ascending aorta and defective development of left ventricle (with mitral valve atresia)

√5th **746.8 Other specified anomalies of heart**

746.81 Subaortic stenosis
DEF: Stenosis, of left ventricular outflow tract due to fibrous tissue ring or septal hypertrophy below aortic valve.

746.82 Cor triatriatum
DEF: Transverse septum divides left atrium due to failed resorption of embryonic common pulmonary vein; results in three atrial chambers.

CONGENITAL ANOMALIES

746.83 Infundibular pulmonic stenosis
Subvalvular pulmonic stenosis
DEF: Stenosis of right ventricle outflow tract within infundibulum due to fibrous diaphragm below valve or long, narrow fibromuscular channel.

746.84 Obstructive anomalies of heart, not elsewhere classified
Uhl's disease

746.85 Coronary artery anomaly
Anomalous origin or communication of coronary artery
Arteriovenous malformation of coronary artery
Coronary artery:
  absence
  arising from aorta or pulmonary trunk
  single

746.86 Congenital heart block
Complete or incomplete atrioventricular [AV] block
DEF: Impaired conduction of electrical impulses; due to maldeveloped junctional tissue.

746.87 Malposition of heart and cardiac apex
Abdominal heart   Levocardia (isolated)
Dextrocardia   Mesocardia
Ectopia cordis
  EXCLUDES dextrocardia with complete transposition of viscera (759.3)

746.89 Other
Atresia } of cardiac vein
Hypoplasia
Congenital:
  cardiomegaly
  diverticulum, left ventricle
  pericardial defect

746.9 Unspecified anomaly of heart
Congenital:
  anomaly of heart NOS
  heart disease NOS

747 Other congenital anomalies of circulatory system

747.0 Patent ductus arteriosus
Patent ductus Botalli
Persistent ductus arteriosus
DEF: Open lumen in ductus arteriosus causes arterial blood recirculation in lungs; inhibits blood supply to aorta; symptoms such as shortness of breath more noticeable upon activity.

747.1 Coarctation of aorta
DEF: Localized deformity of aortic media seen as a severe constriction of the vessel lumen; major symptom is high blood pressure in the arms and low pressure in the legs; a CVA, rupture of the aorta, bacterial endocarditis or congestive heart failure can follow if left untreated.

747.10 Coarctation of aorta (preductal) (postductal)
Hypoplasia of aortic arch

747.11 Interruption of aortic arch

747.2 Other anomalies of aorta
747.20 Anomaly of aorta, unspecified

747.21 Anomalies of aortic arch
  Anomalous origin, right subclavian artery
  Dextraposition of aorta
  Double aortic arch
  Kommerell's diverticulum
  Overriding aorta
  Persistent:
    convolutions, aortic arch
    right aortic arch
  Vascular ring
  EXCLUDES hypoplasia of aortic arch (747.10)

747.22 Atresia and stenosis of aorta
  Absence ⎫
  Aplasia ⎬ of aorta
  Hypoplasia ⎪
  Stricture ⎭

  Supra (valvular)-aortic stenosis
  EXCLUDES congenital aortic (valvular) stenosis or stricture, so stated (746.3)
  hypoplasia of aorta in hypoplastic left heart syndrome (746.7)

747.29 Other
  Aneurysm of sinus of Valsalva
  Congenital:
    aneurysm ⎫
    dilation ⎬ of aorta

747.3 Anomalies of pulmonary artery
  Agenesis ⎫
  Anomaly ⎪
  Atresia ⎪
  Coarctation ⎬ of pulmonary artery
  Hypoplasia ⎪
  Stenosis ⎭

  Pulmonary arteriovenous aneurysm

✓5th **747.4 Anomalies of great veins**

747.40 Anomaly of great veins, unspecified
  Anomaly NOS of:
    pulmonary veins
    vena cava

747.41 Total anomalous pulmonary venous connection
  Total anomalous pulmonary venous return [TAPVR]:
    subdiaphragmatic
    supradiaphragmatic

747.42 Partial anomalous pulmonary venous connection
  Partial anomalous pulmonary venous return

747.49 Other anomalies of great veins
  Absence ⎫
  Congenital ⎬ of vena cava (inferior)
    stenosis ⎭ (superior)

  Persistent:
    left posterior cardinal vein
    left superior vena cava
  Scimitar syndrome
  Transposition of pulmonary veins NOS

CONGENITAL ANOMALIES 747.5–748.0

747.5 Absence or hypoplasia of umbilical artery
Single umbilical artery

747.6 Other anomalies of peripheral vascular system

Absence ⎫
Anomaly ⎬ of artery or vein, not elsewhere classified
Atresia ⎭

Arteriovenous aneurysm (peripheral)
Arteriovenous malformation of the peripheral vascular system
Congenital:
 aneurysm (peripheral)
Congenital:
 phlebectasia
 stricture, artery
 varix
Multiple renal arteries

EXCLUDES anomalies of:
 cerebral vessels (747.81)
 pulmonary artery (747.3)
 congenital retinal aneurysm (743.58)
 hemangioma (228.00-228.09)
 lymphangioma (228.1)

747.60 Anomaly of the peripheral vascular system, unspecified site

747.61 Gastrointestinal vessel anomaly

747.62 Renal vessel anomaly

747.63 Upper limb vessel anomaly

747.64 Lower limb vessel anomaly

747.69 Anomalies of other specified sites of peripheral vascular system

747.8 Other specified anomalies of circulatory system

747.81 Anomalies of cerebrovascular system
Arteriovenous malformation of brain
Cerebral arteriovenous aneurysm, congenital
Congenital anomalies of cerebral vessels
EXCLUDES ruptured cerebral (arteriovenous) aneurysm (430)

747.82 Spinal vessel anomaly
Arteriovenous malformation of spinal vessel

747.83 Persistent fetal circulation
Persistent pulmonary hypertension
Primary pulmonary hypertension of newborn

747.89 Other
Aneurysm, congenital, specified site not elsewhere classified
EXCLUDES congenital aneurysm:
 coronary (746.85)
 peripheral (747.6)
 pulmonary (747.3)
 retinal (743.58)

747.9 Unspecified anomaly of circulatory system

748 Congenital anomalies of respiratory system
EXCLUDES congenital defect of diaphragm (756.6)

748.0 Choanal atresia
Atresia ⎫ of nares (anterior)
Congenital stenosis ⎭ (posterior)

DEF: Occluded posterior nares (choana), bony or membranous due to failure of embryonic bucconasal membrane to rupture.

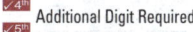
Medicare Secondary Payer

Additional Digit Required | Unspecified Code | Other Specified Code | Manifestation Code
▶◀ Revised Text | ● New Code | ▲ Revised Code Title

2002 Ingenix, Inc.

748.1 Other anomalies of nose
  Absent nose
  Accessory nose
  Cleft nose
  Congenital:
    deformity of nose
  Congenital:
    notching of tip of nose
    perforation of wall of
      nasal sinus
  Deformity of wall of nasal
    sinus
  > EXCLUDES congenital deviation of nasal septum (754.0)

748.2 Web of larynx
  Web of larynx:
    NOS
    glottic
  Web of larynx:
    subglottic
  DEF: Malformed larynx; marked by thin, translucent, or thick, fibrotic spread between vocal folds; affects speech.

748.3 Other anomalies of larynx, trachea, and bronchus
  Absence or agenesis of:
    bronchus
    larynx
    trachea
  Anomaly(of):
    cricoid cartilage
    epiglottis
    thyroid cartilage
    tracheal cartilage
  Atresia (of):
    epiglottis
    glottis
    larynx
    trachea
  Cleft thyroid, cartilage,
    congenital
  Congenital:
    dilation, trachea
    stenosis:
      larynx
      trachea
    tracheocele
  Diverticulum:
    bronchus
    trachea
  Fissure of epiglottis
  Laryngocele
  Posterior cleft of cricoid
    cartilage (congenital)
  Rudimentary tracheal
    bronchus
  Stridor, laryngeal,
    congenital

748.4 Congenital cystic lung
  Disease, lung:
    cystic, congenital
    polycystic, congenital
  Honeycomb lung, congenital
  > EXCLUDES acquired or unspecified cystic lung (518.89)
  DEF: Enlarged air spaces of lung parenchyma.

748.5 Agenesis, hypoplasia, and dysplasia of lung
  Absence of lung (fissures) (lobe)
  Aplasia of lung
  Hypoplasia of lung (lobe)
  Sequestration of lung

√5th **748.6 Other anomalies of lung**
  748.60 Anomaly of lung, unspecified
  748.61 Congenital bronchiectasis
  748.69 Other
    Accessory lung (lobe)
    Azygos lobe (fissure), lung

748.8 Other specified anomalies of respiratory system
  Abnormal communication between pericardial and pleural sacs
  Anomaly, pleural folds
  Atresia of nasopharynx
  Congenital cyst of mediastinum

748.9 Unspecified anomaly of respiratory system
  Anomaly of respiratory system NOS

CONGENITAL ANOMALIES

- ✓4th **749 Cleft palate and cleft lip**
  - ✓5th **749.0 Cleft palate**
    - 749.00 Cleft palate, unspecified
    - 749.01 Unilateral, complete
    - 749.02 Unilateral, incomplete
        Cleft uvula
    - 749.03 Bilateral, complete
    - 749.04 Bilateral, incomplete
  - ✓5th **749.1 Cleft lip**
        Cheiloschisis   Harelip
        Congenital fissure of lip   Labium leporinum
    - 749.10 Cleft lip, unspecified
    - 749.11 Unilateral, complete
    - 749.12 Unilateral, incomplete
    - 749.13 Bilateral, complete
    - 749.14 Bilateral, incomplete
  - ✓5th **749.2 Cleft palate with cleft lip**
        Cheilopalatoschisis
    - 749.20 Cleft palate with cleft lip, unspecified
    - 749.21 Unilateral, complete
    - 749.22 Unilateral, incomplete
    - 749.23 Bilateral, complete
    - 749.24 Bilateral, incomplete
    - 749.25 Other combinations

Cleft Lip and Palate

Unilateral cleft lip
No cleft palate

Cleft lip with cleft alveolar ridge
No cleft palate

Unilateral cleft lip and cleft palate
Alveolar ridge
Cleft palate

Prolabium
Bilateral cleft lip and cleft palate

Isolated cleft palate

CONGENITAL ANOMALIES

✓4th 750 Other congenital anomalies of upper alimentary tract
    EXCLUDES dentofacial anomalies (524.0-524.9)

750.0 Tongue tie
    Ankyloglossia
    DEF: Restricted tongue movement due to lingual frenum extending toward tip of tongue. Tongue may be fused to mouth floor affecting speech.

✓5th 750.1 Other anomalies of tongue
    750.10 Anomaly of tongue, unspecified
    750.11 Aglossia
        DEF: Absence of tongue.
    750.12 Congenital adhesions of tongue
    750.13 Fissure of tongue
        Bifid tongue   Double tongue
    750.15 Macroglossia
        Congenital hypertrophy of tongue
    750.16 Microglossia
        Hypoplasia of tongue
    750.19 Other

✓5th 750.2 Other specified anomalies of mouth and pharynx
    750.21 Absence of salivary gland
    750.22 Accessory salivary gland
    750.23 Atresia, salivary duct
        Imperforate salivary duct
    750.24 Congenital fistula of salivary gland
    750.25 Congenital fistula of lip
        Congenital (mucus) lip pits
    750.26 Other specified anomalies of mouth
        Absence of uvula
    750.27 Diverticulum of pharynx
        Pharyngeal pouch
    750.29 Other specified anomalies of pharynx
        Imperforate pharynx

750.3 Tracheoesophageal fistula, esophageal atresia and stenosis
    Absent esophagus   Congenital fistula:
    Atresia of esophagus   esophagobronchial
    Congenital: esophagotracheal
      esophageal ring   Imperforate esophagus
      stenosis of esophagus   Webbed esophagus
      stricture of esophagus

750.4 Other specified anomalies of esophagus
    Dilatation, congenital
    Displacement, congenital
    Diverticulum   } (of) esophagus
    Duplication
    Giant

    Esophageal pouch
    EXCLUDES congenital hiatus hernia (750.6)

750.5 Congenital hypertrophic pyloric stenosis
    Congenital or infantile:
      constriction
      hypertrophy
      spasm   } of pylorus
      stenosis
      stricture

    DEF: Obstructed pylorus due to overgrowth of pyloric muscle.

CONGENITAL ANOMALIES

750.6 Congenital hiatus hernia
Displacement of cardia through esophageal hiatus
> EXCLUDES congenital diaphragmatic hernia (756.6)

750.7 Other specified anomalies of stomach
Congenital:
  cardiospasm
  hourglass stomach
Displacement of stomach
Diverticulum of stomach, congenital
Duplication of stomach
Megalogastria
Microgastria
Transposition of stomach

750.8 Other specified anomalies of upper alimentary tract

750.9 Unspecified anomaly of upper alimentary tract
Congenital:
  anomaly NOS } of upper alimentary tract
  deformity NOS } [any part, except tongue]

√4th 751 Other congenital anomalies of digestive system

751.0 Meckel's diverticulum
Meckel's diverticulum (displaced) (hypertrophic)
Persistent:
  omphalomesenteric duct
  vitelline duct

DEF: Malformed sacs or appendages of ileum of small intestine; can cause strangulation, volvulus and intussusception.

751.1 Atresia and stenosis of small intestine
Atresia of: Atresia of:
  duodenum   intestine NOS
  ileum
Congenital:
  absence
  obstruction } of small intestine or
  stenosis   } intestine NOS
  stricture

Imperforate jejunum

751.2 Atresia and stenosis of large intestine, rectum, and anal canal
Absence:
  anus (congenital)
  appendix, congenital
  large intestine, congenital
  rectum
Atresia of:
  anus
  colon
  rectum
Congenital or infantile:
  obstruction of large intestine
  occlusion of anus
  stricture of anus
Imperforate:
  anus
  rectum
Stricture of rectum, congenital

Medicare Secondary Payer

751.3 Hirschsprung's disease and other congenital functional disorders of colon
　　Aganglionosis
　　Congenital dilation of colon
　　Congenital megacolon
　　Macrocolon

DEF: Hirschsprung's disease: enlarged or dilated colon (megacolon), with absence of ganglion cells in the narrowed wall distally; causes inability to defecate.

751.4 Anomalies of intestinal fixation
　　Congenital adhesions:　　　Rotation of cecum or colon:
　　　omental, anomalous　　　　failure of
　　　peritoneal　　　　　　　　incomplete
　　Jackson's membrane　　　　　insufficient
　　Malrotation of colon　　　　Universal mesentery

751.5 Other anomalies of intestine
　　Congenital diverticulum, colon
　　Dolichocolon
　　Duplication of:
　　　anus
　　　appendix
　　　cecum
　　　intestine
　　Ectopic anus
　　Megaloappendix
　　Megaloduodenum
　　Microcolon
　　Persistent cloaca
　　Transposition of:
　　　appendix
　　　colon
　　　intestine

√5th **751.6 Anomalies of gallbladder, bile ducts, and liver**

　　751.60 Unspecified anomaly of gallbladder, bile ducts, and liver

　　751.61 Biliary atresia
　　　　Congenital:
　　　　　absence　　　⎫
　　　　　hypoplasia　　⎬ of bile duct (common)
　　　　　obstruction　　⎪ or passage
　　　　　stricture　　　⎭

　　751.62 Congenital cystic disease of liver
　　　　Congenital polycystic disease of liver
　　　　Fibrocystic disease of liver

751.69 Other anomalies of gallbladder, bile ducts, and liver
Absence of:
gallbladder, congenital
liver (lobe)
Accessory:
hepatic ducts
liver
Congenital:
choledochal cyst
hepatomegaly
Duplication of:
biliary duct
cystic duct
gallbladder
liver
Floating:
gallbladder
liver
Intrahepatic gallbladder

751.7 Anomalies of pancreas
Absence
Accessory
Agenesis   } (of) pancreas
Annular
Hypoplasia

Ectopic pancreatic tissue
Pancreatic heterotopia
> **EXCLUDES** diabetes mellitus:
> congenital (250.0-250.9)
> neonatal (775.1)
> fibrocystic disease of pancreas ▶(277.00-277.09)◀

751.8 Other specified anomalies of digestive system
Absence (complete) (partial) of alimentary tract NOS
Duplication
Malposition, congenital } of digestive organs NOS

> **EXCLUDES** congenital diaphragmatic hernia (756.6)
> congenital hiatus hernia (750.6)

751.9 Unspecified anomaly of digestive system
Congenital:
anomaly NOS
deformity NOS } of digestive system NOS

√4th 752 Congenital anomalies of genital organs
> **EXCLUDES** syndromes associated with anomalies in the number and form of chromosomes (758.0-758.9)
> testicular feminization syndrome (257.8)

752.0 Anomalies of ovaries ♀
Absence, congenital
Accessory
Ectopic   } (of) ovary
Streak

√5th 752.1 Anomalies of fallopian tubes and broad ligaments
   752.10 Unspecified anomaly of fallopian tubes and broad ligaments ♀

CONGENITAL ANOMALIES

752.11 Embryonic cyst of fallopian tubes and broad ligaments ♀
    Cyst: Cyst:
      epoophoron   Gartner's duct
      fimbrial   parovarian

752.19 Other ♀
    Absence
    Accessory   } (of) fallopian tube or broad ligament
    Atresia

752.2 Doubling of uterus ♀
    Didelphic uterus
    Doubling of uterus [any degree] (associated with doubling of cervix and vagina)

752.3 Other anomalies of uterus ♀
    Absence, congenital
    Agenesis
    Aplasia   } (of) uterus
    Bicornuate

    Uterus unicornis
    Uterus with only one functioning horn

√5th **752.4 Anomalies of cervix, vagina, and external female genitalia**
  752.40 Unspecified anomaly of cervix, vagina, and external female genitalia ♀

  752.41 Embryonic cyst of cervix, vagina, and external female genitalia ♀
    Cyst of:
      canal of Nuck, congenital
      vagina, embryonal
      vulva, congenital
    DEF: Embryonic fluid-filled cysts, of cervix, vagina or external female genitalia.

  752.42 Imperforate hymen ♀
    DEF: Complete closure of membranous fold around external opening of vagina.

  752.49 Other anomalies of cervix, vagina, and external female genitalia ♀
    Absence   } of cervix, clitoris,
    Agenesis   vagina, or vulva

    Congenital stenosis or stricture of:
      cervical canal
      vagina
      EXCLUDES   *double vagina associated with total duplication (752.2)*

√5th **752.5 Undescended and retractile testicle**
  752.51 Undescended testis ♂
    Cryptorchism   Ectopic testis

  752.52 Retractile testis ♂

√5th **752.6 Hypospadias and epispadias and other penile anomalies**
  752.61 Hypospadias ♂
    DEF: Hypospadias: abnormal opening of urethra on the ventral surface of the penis or perineum; also a rare defect of vagina.

  752.62 Epispadias ♂
    Anaspadias
    DEF: Epispadias: urethra opening on dorsal surface of penis; in females appears as a slit in the upper wall of urethra.

CONGENITAL ANOMALIES 752.63–752.9

Hypospadias and Epispadias

Hypospadias (ventral view) — Glans penis, Glandular hypospadias, Penile hypospadias, Penile raphe, Scrotal hypospadias, Scrotum, Scrotal raphe

Epispadias (dorsal view) — Normal external urethral orifice, Glans penis, Foreskin (retracted), Epispadias

752.63 Congenital chordee ♂
DEF: Ventral bowing of penis due to fibrous band along corpus spongiosum; occurs with hypospadias.

752.64 Micropenis ♂
752.65 Hidden penis ♂
752.69 Other penile anomalies ♂

752.7 Indeterminate sex and pseudohermaphroditism
Gynandrism   Pseudohermaphroditism
Hermaphroditism   (male) (female)
Ovotestis   Pure gonadal dysgenesis
  EXCLUDES pseudohermaphroditism:
     female, with adrenocortical disorder (255.2)
     male, with gonadal disorder (257.8)
     with specified chromosomal anomaly (758.0-758.9)
     testicular feminization syndrome (257.8)

DEF: Pseudohermaphroditism: presence of gonads of one sex and external genitalia of other sex.

752.8 Other specified anomalies of genital organs
Absence of: Atresia of:
  prostate   ejaculatory duct
  spermatic cord   vas deferens
  vas deferens   Fusion of testes
Anorchism   Hypoplasia of testis
Aplasia (congenital) of: Monorchism
  prostate   Polyorchism
  round ligament
  testicle
  EXCLUDES congenital hydrocele (778.6)
     penile anomalies (752.61-752.69)
     phimosis or paraphimosis (605)

752.9 Unspecified anomaly of genital organs
Congenital:
  anomaly NOS } of genital organ, not
  deformity NOS }   elsewhere classified

CONGENITAL ANOMALIES

√4th 753 Congenital anomalies of urinary system

753.0 Renal agenesis and dysgenesis
Atrophy of kidney: Congenital absence of kidney(s)
  congenital   Hypoplasia of kidney(s)
  infantile

√5th 753.1 Cystic kidney disease
  EXCLUDES acquired cyst of kidney (593.2)

  753.10 Cystic kidney disease, unspecified
  753.11 Congenital single renal cyst
  753.12 Polycystic kidney, unspecified type
  753.13 Polycystic kidney, autosomal dominant
    DEF: Slow progressive disease characterized by bilateral cysts causing increased kidney size and impaired function.

  753.14 Polycystic kidney, autosomal recessive
    DEF: Rare disease characterized by multiple cysts involving kidneys and liver, producing renal and hepatic failure in childhood or adolescence.

  753.15 Renal dysplasia
  753.16 Medullary cystic kidney
    Nephronopthisis
    DEF: Diffuse kidney disease results in uremia onset prior to age 20.

  753.17 Medullary sponge kidney
    DEF: Dilated collecting tubules; usually asymptomatic but calcinosis in tubules may cause renal insufficiency.

  753.19 Other specified cystic kidney disease
    Multicystic kidney

√5th 753.2 Obstructive defects of renal pelvis and ureter

  753.20 Unspecified obstructive defect of renal pelvis and ureter
  753.21 Congenital obstruction of ureteropelvic junction
    DEF: Stricture at junction of ureter and renal pelvis.

  753.22 Congenital obstruction of ureterovesical junction
    Adynamic ureter
    Congenital hydroureter
    DEF: Stricture at junction of ureter and bladder.

  753.23 Congenital ureterocele
  753.29 Other

753.3 Other specified anomalies of kidney
  Accessory kidney   Fusion of kidneys
  Congenital: Giant kidney
    calculus of kidney   Horseshoe kidney
    displaced kidney   Hyperplasia of kidney
  Discoid kidney   Lobulation of kidney
  Double kidney with   Malrotation of kidney
    double pelvis   Trifid kidney (pelvis)
  Ectopic kidney

753.4 Other specified anomalies of ureter
  Absent ureter   Double ureter
  Accessory ureter   Ectopic ureter
  Deviation of ureter   Implantation, anomalous
  Displaced ureteric orifice   of ureter

753.5 Exstrophy of urinary bladder
  Ectopia vesicae
  Extroversion of bladder
  DEF: Absence of lower abdominal and anterior bladder walls with posterior bladder wall protrusion.

CONGENITAL ANOMALIES

753.6 Atresia and stenosis of urethra and bladder neck
  Congenital obstruction:
    bladder neck
    urethra
  Congenital stricture of:
    urethra (valvular)
    urinary meatus
    vesicourethral orifice
  Imperforate urinary meatus
  Impervious urethra
  Urethral valve formation

753.7 Anomalies of urachus
  Cyst   ⎫
  Fistula   ⎬ (of) urachussinus
  Patent   ⎭

  Persistent umbilical sinus

753.8 Other specified anomalies of bladder and urethra
  Absence, congenital of: Congenital urethrorectal
    bladder   fistula
    urethra   Congenital prolapse of:
  Accessory: bladder (mucosa)
    bladder   urethra
    urethra   Double:
  Congenital: urethra
    diverticulum of bladder   urinary meatus
    hernia of bladder

753.9 Unspecified anomaly of urinary system
  Congenital:
    anomaly NOS   ⎫ of urinary system [any part,
    deformity NOS ⎬   except urachus]

754 Certain congenital musculoskeletal deformities
  INCLUDES nonteratogenic deformities which are considered to be due to intrauterine malposition and pressure

754.0 Of skull, face, and jaw
  Asymmetry of face   Dolichocephaly
  Compression facies   Plagiocephaly
  Depressions in skull   Potter's facies
  Deviation of nasal   Squashed or bent nose,
    septum, congenital   congenital
  EXCLUDES   dentofacial anomalies (524.0-524.9)
             syphilitic saddle nose (090.5)

754.1 Of sternocleidomastoid muscle
  Congenital sternomastoid torticollis
  Congenital wryneck
  Contracture of sternocleidomastoid (muscle)
  Sternomastoid tumor

754.2 Of spine
  Congenital postural:
    lordosis
    scoliosis

754.3 Congenital dislocation of hip
  754.30 Congenital dislocation of hip, unilateral
    Congenital dislocation of hip NOS
  754.31 Congenital dislocation of hip, bilateral

754.32 Congenital subluxation of hip, unilateral
    Congenital flexion deformity, hip or thigh
    Predislocation status of hip at birth
    Preluxation of hip, congenital
754.33 Congenital subluxation of hip, bilateral
754.35 Congenital dislocation of one hip with subluxation of other hip

√5th **754.4** Congenital genu recurvatum and bowing of long bones of leg
754.40 Genu recurvatum
    DEF: Backward curving of knee joint.
754.41 Congenital dislocation of knee (with genu recurvatum)
    DEF: Elevated, outward rotation of heel; also called clubfoot.
754.42 Congenital bowing of femur
754.43 Congenital bowing of tibia and fibula
754.44 ==Congenital bowing of unspecified long bones of leg==

√5th **754.5** Varus deformities of feet
    EXCLUDES acquired (736.71, 736.75, 736.79)
754.50 Talipes varus
    Congenital varus deformity of foot, unspecified
    Pes varus
    DEF: Inverted foot marked by outer sole resting on ground.
754.51 Talipes equinovarus
    Equinovarus (congenital)
754.52 Metatarsus primus varus
    DEF: Malformed first metatarsal bone, with bone angled toward body.
754.53 Metatarsus varus
    DEF: Osseous adhesion of radius and ulna.
754.59 Other
    Talipes calcaneovarus

√5th **754.6** Valgus deformities of feet
    EXCLUDES valgus deformity of foot (acquired) (736.79)
754.60 Talipes valgus
    Congenital valgus deformity of foot, unspecified
754.61 Congenital pes planus
    Congenital rocker bottom flat foot
    Flat foot, congenital
        EXCLUDES pes planus (acquired) (734)
754.62 Talipes calcaneovalgus
754.69 Other
    Talipes: Talipes:
        equinovalgus   planovalgus

√5th **754.7** Other deformities of feet
    EXCLUDES acquired (736.70-736.79)
754.70 ==Talipes, unspecified==
    Congenital deformity of foot NOS
754.71 Talipes cavus
    Cavus foot (congenital)
754.79 Other
    Asymmetric talipes   Talipes:
    Talipes: equinus
        calcaneus

√5th **754.8** Other specified nonteratogenic anomalies
754.81 Pectus excavatum
    Congenital funnel chest

CONGENITAL ANOMALIES

754.82 Pectus carinatum
Congenital pigeon chest [breast]

754.89 Other
Club hand (congenital)
Congenital:
    deformity of chest wall
    dislocation of elbow
Generalized flexion contractures of lower limb joints, congenital
Spade-like hand (congenital)

√4th **755 Other congenital anomalies of limbs**
> EXCLUDES: those deformities classifiable to 754.0-754.8

√5th **755.0 Polydactyly**

755.00 Polydactyly, unspecified digits
Supernumerary digits

755.01 Of fingers
Accessory fingers

755.02 Of toes
Accessory toes

√5th **755.1 Syndactyly**
Symphalangy   Webbing of digits

755.10 Of multiple and unspecified sites

755.11 Of fingers without fusion of bone

755.12 Of fingers with fusion of bone

755.13 Of toes without fusion of bone

755.14 Of toes with fusion of bone

√5th **755.2 Reduction deformities of upper limb**

755.20 Unspecified reduction deformity of upper limb
Ectromelia NOS } of upper limb
Hemimelia NOS
Shortening of arm, congenital

755.21 Transverse deficiency of upper limb
Amelia of upper limb
Congenital absence of:
    fingers, all (complete or partial)
    forearm, including hand and fingers
    upper limb, complete
Congenital amputation of upper limb
Transverse hemimelia of upper limb

755.22 Longitudinal deficiency of upper limb, not elsewhere classified
Phocomelia NOS of upper limb
Rudimentary arm

755.23 Longitudinal deficiency, combined, involving humerus, radius, and ulna (complete or incomplete)
Congenital absence of arm and forearm (complete or incomplete) with or without metacarpal deficiency and/or phalangeal deficiency, incomplete
Phocomelia, complete, of upper limb

755.24 Longitudinal deficiency, humeral, complete or partial (with or without distal deficiencies, incomplete)
Congenital absence of humerus (with or without absence of some [but not all] distal elements)
Proximal phocomelia of upper limb

√4th Additional Digit Required
√5th
 Medicare Secondary Payer

Unspecified Code

▶◀ Revised Text

● New Code

Other Specified Code

Manifestation Code

▲ Revised Code Title

CONGENITAL ANOMALIES

755.25 Longitudinal deficiency, radioulnar, complete or partial (with or without distal deficiencies, incomplete)
Congenital absence of radius and ulna (with or without absence of some [but not all] distal elements)
Distal phocomelia of upper limb

755.26 Longitudinal deficiency, radial, complete or partial (with or without distal deficiencies, incomplete)
Agenesis of radius
Congenital absence of radius (with or without absence of some [but not all] distal elements)

755.27 Longitudinal deficiency, ulnar, complete or partial (with or without distal deficiencies, incomplete)
Agenesis of ulna
Congenital absence of ulna (with or without absence of some [but not all] distal elements)

755.28 Longitudinal deficiency, carpals or metacarpals, complete or partial (with or without incomplete phalangeal deficiency)

755.29 Longitudinal deficiency, phalanges, complete or partial
Absence of finger, congenital
Aphalangia of upper limb, terminal, complete or partial
> **EXCLUDES** terminal deficiency of all five digits (755.21)
> transverse deficiency of phalanges (755.21)

√5th 755.3 Reduction deformities of lower limb

755.30 Unspecified reduction deformity of lower limb
Ectromelia NOS } of lower limb
Hemimelia NOS
Shortening of leg, congenital

755.31 Transverse deficiency of lower limb
Amelia of lower limb
Congenital absence of:
  foot
  leg, including foot and toes
  lower limb, complete
  toes, all, complete
Transverse hemimelia of lower limb

755.32 Longitudinal deficiency of lower limb, not elsewhere classified
Phocomelia NOS of lower limb

755.33 Longitudinal deficiency, combined, involving femur, tibia, and fibula (complete or incomplete)
Congenital absence of thigh and (lower) leg (complete or incomplete) with or without metacarpal deficiency and/or phalangeal deficiency, incomplete
Phocomelia, complete, of lower limb

755.34 Longitudinal deficiency, femoral, complete or partial (with or without distal deficiencies, incomplete)
Congenital absence of femur (with or without absence of some [but not all] distal elements)
Proximal phocomelia of lower limb

755.35 Longitudinal deficiency, tibiofibular, complete or partial (with or without distal deficiencies, incomplete)
Congenital absence of tibia and fibula (with or without absence of some [but not all] distal elements)
Distal phocomelia of lower limb

755.36 Longitudinal deficiency, tibia, complete or partial (with or without distal deficiencies, incomplete)
Agenesis of tibia
Congenital absence of tibia (with or without absence of some [but not all] distal elements)

CONGENITAL ANOMALIES

755.37 Longitudinal deficiency, fibular, complete or partial (with or without distal deficiencies, incomplete)
Agenesis of fibula
Congenital absence of fibula (with or without absence of some [but not all] distal elements)

755.38 Longitudinal deficiency, tarsals or metatarsals, complete or partial (with or without incomplete phalangeal deficiency)

755.39 Longitudinal deficiency, phalanges, complete or partial
Absence of toe, congenital
Aphalangia of lower limb, terminal, complete or partial
> **EXCLUDES** terminal deficiency of all five digits (755.31)
> transverse deficiency of phalanges (755.31)

755.4 Reduction deformities, unspecified limb
Absence, congenital (complete or partial) of limb NOS
Amelia
Ectromelia
Hemimelia
Phocomelia } of unspecified limb

√5th 755.5 Other anomalies of upper limb, including shoulder girdle

755.50 Unspecified anomaly of upper limb

755.51 Congenital deformity of clavicle

755.52 Congenital elevation of scapula
Sprengel's deformity

755.53 Radioulnar synostosis

755.54 Madelung's deformity
DEF: Distal ulnar overgrowth or radial shortening; also called carpus curvus.

755.55 Acrocephalosyndactyly
Apert's syndrome
DEF: Premature cranial suture fusion (craniostenosis); marked by cone-shaped or pointed (acrocephaly) head and webbing of the fingers (syndactyly); it is very similar to craniofacial dysostosis.

755.56 Accessory carpal bones

755.57 Macrodactylia (fingers)
DEF: Abnormally large fingers, toes.

755.58 Cleft hand, congenital
Lobster-claw hand
DEF: Extended separation between fingers into metacarpus; also may refer to large fingers and absent middle fingers of hand.

755.59 Other
Cleidocranial dysostosis
Cubitus:
  valgus, congenital
  varus, congenital
> **EXCLUDES** club hand (congenital) (754.89)
> congenital dislocation of elbow (754.89)

√5th 755.6 Other anomalies of lower limb, including pelvic girdle

755.60 Unspecified anomaly of lower limb

755.61 Coxa valga, congenital
DEF: Abnormally wide angle between the neck and shaft of the femur.

755.62 Coxa vara, congenital
DEF: Diminished angle between neck and shaft of femur.

CONGENITAL ANOMALIES

755.63 Other congenital deformity of hip (joint)
Congenital anteversion of femur (neck)
EXCLUDES congenital dislocation of hip (754.30-754.35)

755.64 Congenital deformity of knee (joint)
Congenital:
  absence of patella
  genu valgum [knock-knee]
  genu varum [bowleg]
  Rudimentary patella

755.65 Macrodactylia of toes
DEF: Abnormally large toes.

755.66 Other anomalies of toes
Congenital: Congenital:
  hallux valgus   hammer toe
  hallux varus

755.67 Anomalies of foot, not elsewhere classified
Astragaloscaphoid synostosis
Calcaneonavicular bar
Coalition of calcaneus
Talonavicular synostosis
Tarsal coalitions

755.69 Other
Congenital:
  angulation of tibia
  deformity (of):
    ankle (joint)
    sacroiliac (joint)
  fusion of sacroiliac joint

755.8 Other specified anomalies of unspecified limb

755.9 Unspecified anomaly of unspecified limb
Congenital:
  anomaly NOS } of unspecified limb
  deformity NOS
EXCLUDES reduction deformity of unspecified limb (755.4)

✓4th 756 Other congenital musculoskeletal anomalies
EXCLUDES those deformities classifiable to 754.0-754.8

756.0 Anomalies of skull and face bones
Absence of skull bones   Imperfect fusion of skull
Acrocephaly   Oxycephaly
Congenital deformity   Platybasia
  of forehead   Premature closure of
Craniosynostosis   cranial sutures
Crouzon's disease   Tower skull
Hypertelorism   Trigonocephaly
EXCLUDES acrocephalosyndactyly [Apert's syndrome] (755.55)
dentofacial anomalies (524.0-524.9)
skull defects associated with brain anomalies, such as:
  anencephalus (740.0)
  encephalocele (742.0)
  hydrocephalus (742.3)
  microcephalus (742.1)

✓5th **756.1 Anomalies of spine**
756.10 Anomaly of spine, unspecified

756.11 Spondylolysis, lumbosacral region
Prespondylolisthesis (lumbosacral)
DEF: Bilateral or unilateral defect through the pars interarticularis of a vertebra causes spondylolisthesis.

756.12 Spondylolisthesis
DEF: Downward slipping of lumbar vertebra over next vertebra; usually related to pelvic deformity.

756.13 Absence of vertebra, congenital

756.14 Hemivertebra
DEF: Incomplete development of one side of a vertebra.

756.15 Fusion of spine [vertebra], congenital

756.16 Klippel-Feil syndrome
DEF: Short, wide neck; limits range of motion due to abnormal number of cervical vertebra or fused hemivertebrae.

756.17 Spina bifida occulta
> EXCLUDES spina bifida (aperta) (741.0-741.9)

DEF: Spina bifida marked by a bony spinal canal defect without a protrusion of the cord or meninges; it is diagnosed by radiography and has no symptoms.

756.19 Other
Platyspondylia
Supernumerary vertebra

756.2 Cervical rib
Supernumerary rib in the cervical region
DEF: Costa cervicalis: extra rib attached to cervical vertebra.

756.3 Other anomalies of ribs and sternum
Congenital absence of: Congenital:
  rib   fissure of sternum
  sternum   fusion of ribs
                                                    Sternum bifidum
> EXCLUDES nonteratogenic deformity of chest wall (754.81-754.89)

756.4 Chondrodystrophy
Achondroplasia   Enchondromatosis
Chondrodystrophia (fetalis) Ollier's disease
Dyschondroplasia
> EXCLUDES lipochondrodystrophy [Hurler's syndrome] (277.5)
>   Morquio's disease (277.5)

DEF: Abnormal development of cartilage.

√5th 756.5 Osteodystrophies

756.50 Osteodystrophy, unspecified

756.51 Osteogenesis imperfecta
Fragilitas ossium
Osteopsathyrosis
DEF: A collagen disorder commonly characterized by brittle, osteoporotic, easily fractured bones, hypermobility of joints, blue sclerae, and a tendency to hemorrhage.

756.52 Osteopetrosis
DEF: Abnormally dense bone, optic atrophy, hepatosplenomegaly, deafness; sclerosing depletes bone marrow and nerve foramina of skull; often fatal.

756.53 Osteopoikilosis
DEF: Multiple sclerotic foci on ends of long bones, stippling in round, flat bones; identified by x-ray.

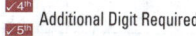 Additional Digit Required | Unspecified Code | Other Specified Code | Manifestation Code
MSP Medicare Secondary Payer ▶◀ Revised Text ● New Code ▲ Revised Code Title

756.54 Polyostotic fibrous dysplasia of bone
DEF: Fibrous tissue displaces bone results in segmented ragged-edge café-au-lait spots; occurs in girls of early puberty.

756.55 Chondroectodermal dysplasia
Ellis-van Creveld syndrome
DEF: Inadequate enchondral bone formation; impaired development of hair and teeth, polydactyly, and cardiac septum defects.

756.56 Multiple epiphyseal dysplasia

756.59 Other
Albright (-McCune)-Sternberg syndrome

756.6 Anomalies of diaphragm
Absence of diaphragm
Congenital hernia: diaphragmatic
Congenital hernia: foramen of Morgagni
Eventration of diaphragm

EXCLUDES congenital hiatus hernia (750.6)

✓5th 756.7 Anomalies of abdominal wall

756.70 Anomaly of abdominal wall, unspecified

756.71 Prune belly syndrome
Eagle-Barrett syndrome
Prolapse of bladder mucosa

DEF: Prune belly syndrome: absence of lower rectus abdominis muscle and lower and medial oblique muscles; results in dilated bladder and ureters, dysplastic kidneys and hydronephrosis; more common in male infants with undescended testicles.

756.79 Other congenital anomalies of abdominal wall
Exomphalos
Gastroschisis
Omphalocele

EXCLUDES umbilical hernia (551-553 with .1)

DEF: Exomphalos: umbilical hernia prominent navel.

DEF: Gastroschisis: fissure of abdominal wall, results in protruding small or large intestine.

DEF: Omphalocele: hernia of umbilicus due to impaired abdominal wall; results in membrane-covered intestine protruding through peritoneum and amnion.

✓5th 756.8 Other specified anomalies of muscle, tendon, fascia, and connective tissue

756.81 Absence of muscle and tendon
Absence of muscle (pectoral)

756.82 Accessory muscle

756.83 Ehlers-Danlos syndrome
DEF: Danlos syndrome: connective tissue disorder causes hyperextended skin and joints; results in fragile blood vessels with bleeding, poor wound healing and subcutaneous pseudotumors.

756.89 Other
Amyotrophia congenita
Congenital shortening of tendon

756.9 Other and unspecified anomalies of musculoskeletal system
Congenital:
anomaly NOS } of musculoskeletal system,
deformity NOS } not elsewhere classified

CONGENITAL ANOMALIES

√4th 757 Congenital anomalies of the integument
- INCLUDES: anomalies of skin, subcutaneous tissue, hair, nails, and breast
- EXCLUDES: hemangioma (228.00-228.09)
  pigmented nevus (216.0-216.9)

757.0 Hereditary edema of legs
Congenital lymphedema
Hereditary trophedema
Milroy's disease

757.1 Ichthyosis congenita
Congenital ichthyosis
Harlequin fetus
Ichthyosiform erythroderma
DEF: Overproduction of skin cells causes scaling of skin; may result in stillborn fetus or death soon after birth.

757.2 Dermatoglyphic anomalies
Abnormal palmar creases
DEF: Abnormal skin-line patterns of fingers, palms, toes and soles; initial finding of possible chromosomal abnormalities.

√5th 757.3 Other specified anomalies of skin

757.31 Congenital ectodermal dysplasia
DEF: Tissues and structures originate in embryonic ectoderm; includes anhidrotic and hidrotic ectodermal dysplasia and EEC syndrome.

757.32 Vascular hamartomas
Birthmarks   Strawberry nevus
Port-wine stain
DEF: Benign tumor of blood vessels; due to malformed angioblastic tissues.

757.33 Congenital pigmentary anomalies of skin
Congenital poikiloderma
Urticaria pigmentosa
Xeroderma pigmentosum
EXCLUDES: albinism (270.2)

757.39 Other
Accessory skin tags, congenital
Congenital scar
Epidermolysis bullosa
Keratoderma (congenital)
EXCLUDES: pilonidal cyst (685.0-685.1)

757.4 Specified anomalies of hair
Congenital: Congenital:
  alopecia   hypertrichosis
  atrichosis   monilethrix
  beaded hair   Persistent lanugo

757.5 Specified anomalies of nails
Anonychia   Congenital:
Congenital: leukonychia
  clubnail   onychauxis
  koilonychia   pachyonychia

757.6 Specified anomalies of breast
Absent   ⎫
Accessory   ⎬ breast or nipple
Supernumerary ⎭

Hypoplasia of breast
EXCLUDES: absence of pectoral muscle (756.81)

CONGENITAL ANOMALIES

757.8 **Other specified anomalies of the integument**

757.9 **Unspecified anomaly of the integument**
Congenital:
anomaly NOS } of integument
deformity NOS

✓4th **758 Chromosomal anomalies**
INCLUDES syndromes associated with anomalies in the number and form of chromosomes

758.0 **Down's syndrome**
Mongolism   Trisomy:
Translocation Down's   21 or 22
syndrome   G

758.1 **Patau's syndrome**
Trisomy: Trisomy:
13   D_1

DEF: Trisomy of 13th chromosome; characteristic failure to thrive, severe mental impairment, seizures, abnormal eyes, low-set ears and sloped forehead.

758.2 **Edwards' syndrome**
Trisomy: Trisomy:
18   E_3

DEF: Trisomy of 18th chromosome; characteristic mental and physical impairments; mainly affects females.

758.3 **Autosomal deletion syndromes**
Antimongolism syndrome   Cri-du-chat syndrome

DEF: Antimongolism syndrome: Deletions in 21st chromosome; characteristic oblique palpebral fissures, hypertonia, micrognathia, microcephaly, high-arched palate and impaired mental and physical growth.

DEF: Cri-du-chat syndrome: Abnormally large distance between two organs or parts, abnormally small brain and severe mental impairment; characteristic of abnormal 5th chromosome.

758.4 **Balanced autosomal translocation in normal individual**

758.5 **Other conditions due to autosomal anomalies**
Accessory autosomes NEC

758.6 **Gonadal dysgenesis**
Ovarian dysgenesis   XO syndrome
Turner's syndrome
EXCLUDES   *pure gonadal dysgenesis (752.7)*

DEF: Impaired embryonic development of seminiferous tubes; results in small testes, azoospermia, infertility and enlarged mammary glands.

758.7 **Klinefelter's syndrome**   ♂
XXY syndrome

✓5th **758.8** **Other conditions due to chromosome anomalies**
758.81 **Other conditions due to sex chromosome anomalies**
758.89 **Other**

758.9 **Conditions due to anomaly of unspecified chromosome**

✓4th **759 Other and unspecified congenital anomalies**

759.0 **Anomalies of spleen**
Aberrant
Absent   } spleen
Accessory

Congenital splenomegaly
Ectopic spleen
Lobulation of spleen

CONGENITAL ANOMALIES

759.1 Anomalies of adrenal gland
Aberrant
Absent } adrenal gland
Accessory

> EXCLUDES: adrenogenital disorders (255.2)
> congenital disorders of steroid metabolism (255.2)

759.2 Anomalies of other endocrine glands
Absent parathyroid gland
Accessory thyroid gland
Persistent thyroglossal or thyrolingual duct
Thyroglossal (duct) cyst

> EXCLUDES: congenital:
> goiter (246.1)
> hypothyroidism (243)

759.3 Situs inversus
Situs inversus or transversus:
 abdominalis
 thoracis
Transposition of viscera:
 abdominal
 thoracic

> EXCLUDES: dextrocardia without mention of complete transposition (746.87)

DEF: Laterally transposed thoracic and abdominal viscera.

759.4 Conjoined twins
Craniopagus   Thoracopagus
Dicephalus   Xiphopagus
Pygopagus

759.5 Tuberous sclerosis
Bourneville's disease   Epiloia

DEF: Hamartomas of brain, retina and viscera, impaired mental ability, seizures and adenoma sebaceum.

759.6 Other hamartoses, not elsewhere classified
Syndrome: Syndrome:
 Peutz-Jeghers   von Hippel-Lindau
 Sturge-Weber (-Dimitri)

> EXCLUDES: neurofibromatosis (237.7)

DEF: Peutz-Jeghers: hereditary syndrome characterized by hamartomas of small intestine

DEF: Sturge-Weber: congenital syndrome characterized by unilateral port-wine stain over trigeminal nerve, underlying meninges and cerebral cortex.

DEF: von Hipple-Lindau: hereditary syndrome of congenital angiomatosis of the retina and cerebellum.

759.7 Multiple congenital anomalies, so described
Congenital:
 anomaly, multiple NOS
 deformity, multiple NOS

√5th **759.8 Other specified anomalies**
759.81 Prader-Willi syndrome
759.82 Marfan syndrome
759.83 Fragile X syndrome

759.89 Other
Congenital malformation syndromes affecting multiple systems, not elsewhere classified
Laurence-Moon-Biedl syndrome

759.9 Congenital anomaly, unspecified

15. CERTAIN CONDITIONS ORIGINATING IN THE PERINATAL PERIOD (760-779)

INCLUDES conditions which have their origin in the perinatal period even though death or morbidity occurs later

Use additional code(s) to further specify condition

MATERNAL CAUSES OF PERINATAL MORBIDITY AND MORTALITY (760-763)

✓4th **760 Fetus or newborn affected by maternal conditions which may be unrelated to present pregnancy**

INCLUDES the listed maternal conditions only when specified as a cause of mortality or morbidity of the fetus or newborn

EXCLUDES maternal endocrine and metabolic disorders affecting fetus or newborn (775.0-775.9)

760.0 Maternal hypertensive disorders
Fetus or newborn affected by maternal conditions classifiable to 642

760.1 Maternal renal and urinary tract diseases
Fetus or newborn affected by maternal conditions classifiable to 580-599

760.2 Maternal infections
Fetus or newborn affected by maternal infectious disease classifiable to 001-136 and 487, but fetus or newborn not manifesting that disease
EXCLUDES congenital infectious diseases (771.0-771.8)
maternal genital tract and other localized infections (760.8)

760.3 Other chronic maternal circulatory and respiratory diseases
Fetus or newborn affected by chronic maternal conditions classifiable to 390-459, 490-519, 745-748

760.4 Maternal nutritional disorders
Fetus or newborn affected by:
maternal disorders classifiable to 260-269
maternal malnutrition NOS
EXCLUDES fetal malnutrition (764.10-764.29)

760.5 Maternal injury
Fetus or newborn affected by maternal conditions classifiable to 800-995

760.6 Surgical operation on mother
EXCLUDES cesarean section for present delivery (763.4)
damage to placenta from amniocentesis, cesarean section, or surgical induction (762.1)
previous surgery to uterus or pelvic organs (763.89)

✓5th **760.7 Noxious influences affecting fetus via placenta or breast milk**
Fetus or newborn affected by noxious substance transmitted via placenta or breast milk
EXCLUDES anesthetic and analgesic drugs administered during labor and delivery (763.5)
drug withdrawal syndrome in newborn (779.5)

760.70 Unspecified noxious substance
Fetus or newborn affected by:
Drug NEC

760.71 Alcohol
Fetal alcohol syndrome

760.72 Narcotics

760.73 Hallucinogenic agents

760.74 Anti-infectives
Antibiotics

760.75 Cocaine
760.76 Diethylstilbestrol [DES]
760.79 Other

Fetus or newborn affected by:
- immune sera ⎫
- medicinal agents ⎬ transmitted via placenta or breast milk
- NEC ⎪
- toxic substance NEC ⎭

760.8 Other specified maternal conditions affecting fetus or newborn

Maternal genital tract and other localized infection affecting fetus or newborn, but fetus or newborn not manifesting that disease

EXCLUDES maternal urinary tract infection affecting fetus or newborn (760.1)

760.9 Unspecified maternal condition affecting fetus or newborn

✓4th 761 Fetus or newborn affected by maternal complications of pregnancy

INCLUDES the listed maternal conditions only when specified as a cause of mortality or morbidity of the fetus or newborn

761.0 Incompetent cervix
DEF: Inadequate functioning of uterine cervix.

761.1 Premature rupture of membranes

761.2 Oligohydramnios
EXCLUDES that due to premature rupture of membranes (761.1)
DEF: Deficient amniotic fluid.

761.3 Polyhydramnios
Hydramnios (acute) (chronic)
DEF: Excess amniotic fluid.

761.4 Ectopic pregnancy
Pregnancy: Pregnancy:
  abdominal   tubal
  intraperitoneal

761.5 Multiple pregnancy
Triplet (pregnancy)   Twin (pregnancy)

761.6 Maternal death

761.7 Malpresentation before labor
Breech presentation ⎫
External version ⎪
Oblique lie ⎬ before labor
Transverse lie ⎪
Unstable lie ⎭

761.8 Other specified maternal complications of pregnancy affecting fetus or newborn
Spontaneous abortion, fetus

761.9 Unspecified maternal complication of pregnancy affecting fetus or newborn

✓4th 762 Fetus or newborn affected by complications of placenta, cord, and membranes

INCLUDES the listed maternal conditions only when specified as a cause of mortality or morbidity in the fetus or newborn

762.0 Placenta previa
DEF: Placenta developed in lower segment of uterus; causes hemorrhaging in last trimester.

762.1 Other forms of placental separation and hemorrhage [N]
    Abruptio placentae
    Antepartum hemorrhage
    Damage to placenta from amniocentesis, cesarean section, or surgical induction
    Maternal blood loss
    Premature separation of placenta
    Rupture of marginal sinus

762.2 Other and unspecified morphological and functional abnormalities of placenta [N]
    Placental: Placental:
      dysfunction   insufficiency
      infarction

762.3 Placental transfusion syndromes [N]
    Placental and cord abnormality resulting in twin-to-twin or other transplacental transfusion
    Use additional code to indicate resultant condition in fetus or newborn:
      fetal blood loss (772.0)
      polycythemia neonatorum (776.4)

762.4 Prolapsed cord [N]
    Cord presentation

762.5 Other compression of umbilical cord [N]
    Cord around neck   Knot in cord
    Entanglement of cord   Torsion of cord

762.6 Other and unspecified conditions of umbilical cord [N]
    Short cord
    Thrombosis
    Varices   } of umbilical cord
    Velamentous insertion

    Vasa previa
    EXCLUDES infection of umbilical cord (771.4)
        single umbilical artery (747.5)

762.7 Chorioamnionitis [N]
    Amnionitis   Placentitis
    Membranitis
    DEF: Inflamed fetal membrane.

762.8 Other specified abnormalities of chorion and amnion [N]

762.9 Unspecified abnormality of chorion and amnion [N]

✓4th **763 Fetus or newborn affected by other complications of labor and delivery**
    INCLUDES the listed conditions only when specified as a cause of mortality or morbidity in the fetus or newborn

763.0 Breech delivery and extraction [N]

763.1 Other malpresentation, malposition, and disproportion during labor and delivery [N]
    Fetus or newborn affected by:
      abnormality of bony pelvis
      contracted pelvis
      persistent occipitoposterior position
      shoulder presentation
      transverse lie
      conditions classifiable to 652, 653, and 660

763.2 Forceps delivery [N]
    Fetus or newborn affected by forceps extraction

763.3 Delivery by vacuum extractor [N]

763.4 Cesarean delivery [N]
    EXCLUDES placental separation or hemorrhage from cesarean section (762.1)

CONDITIONS IN THE PERINATAL PERIOD — 763.5–764.1

763.5 **Maternal anesthesia and analgesia**
Reactions and intoxications from maternal opiates and tranquilizers during labor and delivery
> **EXCLUDES** drug withdrawal syndrome in newborn (779.5)

763.6 **Precipitate delivery**
Rapid second stage

763.7 **Abnormal uterine contractions**
Fetus or newborn affected by:
contraction ring
hypertonic labor
hypotonic uterine dysfunction
uterine inertia or dysfunction
conditions classifiable to 661, except 661.3

√5th **763.8** **Other specified complications of labor and delivery affecting fetus or newborn**

763.81 Abnormality in fetal heart rate or rhythm before the onset of labor

763.82 Abnormality in fetal heart rate or rhythm during labor

763.83 Abnormality in fetal heart rate or rhythm, unspecified as to time of onset

763.89 Other specified complications of labor and delivery affecting fetus or newborn
Fetus or newborn affected by:
abnormality of maternal soft tissues
destructive operation on live fetus to facilitate delivery
induction of labor (medical)
previous surgery to uterus or pelvic organs
other conditions classifiable to 650-669
other procedures used in labor and delivery

763.9 Unspecified complication of labor and delivery affecting fetus or newborn

OTHER CONDITIONS ORIGINATING IN THE PERINATAL PERIOD (764-779)

The following fifth-digit subclassification is for use with ▶category 764 and codes 765.0 and 765.1◀ to denote birthweight:
0 unspecified [weight]
1 less than 500 grams
2 500-749 grams
3 750-999 grams
4 1,000-1,249 grams
5 1,250-1,499 grams
6 1,500-1,749 grams
7 1,750-1,999 grams
8 2,000-2,499 grams
9 2,500 grams and over

√4th **764** **Slow fetal growth and fetal malnutrition**

§ √5th **764.0** **"Light-for-dates" without mention of fetal malnutrition**
Infants underweight for gestational age
"Small-for-dates"

§ √5th **764.1** **"Light-for-dates" with signs of fetal malnutrition**
Infants "light-for-dates" classifiable to 764.0, who in addition show signs of fetal malnutrition, such as dry peeling skin and loss of subcutaneous tissue

§ Requires fifth-digit. See beginning of section 764–779, for codes and definitions.

CONDITIONS IN THE PERINATAL PERIOD

§ ✓5th **764.2 Fetal malnutrition without mention of "light-for-dates"** N
Infants, not underweight for gestational age, showing signs of fetal malnutrition, such as dry peeling skin and loss of subcutaneous tissue
Intrauterine malnutrition

§ ✓5th **764.9 Fetal growth retardation, unspecified** N
Intrauterine growth retardation

▲ ✓4th **765 Disorders relating to short gestation and low birthweight**
INCLUDES the listed conditions, without further specification, as causes of mortality, morbidity, or additional care, in fetus or newborn

§ ✓5th **765.0 Extreme immaturity** N
Note: Usually implies a birthweight of less than 1000 grams

§ ✓5th **765.1 Other preterm infants** N
Note: Usually implies a birthweight of 1000-2499 grams
Prematurity NOS
Prematurity or small size, not classifiable to 765.0 or as "light-for-dates" in 764
▶Use additional code for weeks of gestation (765.20-765.29)◀

✓5th **765.2 Weeks of gestation**
- **765.20** Unspecified weeks of gestation N
- **765.21** Less than 24 completed weeks of gestation N
- **765.22** 24 completed weeks of gestation N
- **765.23** 25-26 completed weeks of gestation N
- **765.24** 27-28 completed weeks of gestation N
- **765.25** 29-30 completed weeks of gestation N
- **765.26** 31-32 completed weeks of gestation N
- **765.27** 33-34 completed weeks of gestation N
- **765.28** 35-36 completed weeks of gestation N
- **765.29** 37 or more completed weeks of gestation N

✓4th **766 Disorders relating to long gestation and high birthweight**
INCLUDES the listed conditions, without further specification, as causes of mortality, morbidity, or additional care, in fetus or newborn

766.0 Exceptionally large baby N
Note: Usually implies a birthweight of 4500 grams or more.

766.1 Other "heavy-for-dates" infants N
Other fetus or infant "heavy-" or "large-for-dates" regardless of period of gestation

766.2 Post-term infant, not "heavy-for-dates" N
Fetus or infant with gestation period of 294 days or more [42 or more completed weeks], not "heavy-" or "large-for-dates"
Postmaturity NOS

✓4th **767 Birth trauma**

767.0 Subdural and cerebral hemorrhage N
Subdural and cerebral hemorrhage, whether described as due to birth trauma or to intrapartum anoxia or hypoxia
Subdural hematoma (localized)
Tentorial tear
Use additional code to identify cause
EXCLUDES intraventricular hemorrhage (772.10-772.14)
subarachnoid hemorrhage (772.2)

767.1 Injuries to scalp N
Caput succedaneum
Cephalhematoma
Chignon (from vacuum extraction)
Massive epicranial subaponeurotic hemorrhage

§ Requires fifth-digit. See beginning of section 764–779, for codes and definitions.

N Newborn Age: 0   P Pediatric Age: 0-17   M Maternity Age: 12-55   A Adult Age: 15-124

CONDITIONS IN THE PERINATAL PERIOD

767.2 Fracture of clavicle

767.3 **Other injuries to skeleton**
Fracture of: Fracture of:
   long bones   skull
EXCLUDES congenital dislocation of hip (754.30-754.35)
fracture of spine, congenital (767.4)

767.4 **Injury to spine and spinal cord**
Dislocation
Fracture   } of spine or spinal cord
Laceration   due to birth trauma
Rupture

767.5 **Facial nerve injury**
Facial palsy

767.6 **Injury to brachial plexus**
Palsy or paralysis: Palsy or paralysis:
   brachial   Klumpke (-Déjérine)
   Erb (-Duchenne)

767.7 **Other cranial and peripheral nerve injuries**
Phrenic nerve paralysis

767.8 **Other specified birth trauma**
Eye damage   Rupture of:
Hematoma of: liver
   liver (subcapsular)   spleen
   testes   Scalpel wound
   vulva   Traumatic glaucoma
EXCLUDES hemorrhage classifiable to 772.0-772.9

767.9 ==Birth trauma, unspecified==
Birth injury NOS

√4th 768 **Intrauterine hypoxia and birth asphyxia**
Use only when associated with newborn morbidity classifiable elsewhere
DEF: Oxygen intake insufficiency due to interrupted placental circulation or premature separation of placenta.

768.0 Fetal death from asphyxia or anoxia before onset of labor or at unspecified time

768.1 Fetal death from asphyxia or anoxia during labor

768.2 Fetal distress before onset of labor, in liveborn infant
Fetal metabolic acidemia before onset of labor, in liveborn infant

768.3 Fetal distress first noted during labor, in liveborn infant
Fetal metabolic acidemia first noted during labor, in liveborn infant

768.4 ==Fetal distress, unspecified as to time of onset, in liveborn infant==
Fetal metabolic acidemia unspecified as to time of onset, in liveborn infant

768.5 **Severe birth asphyxia**
Birth asphyxia with neurologic involvement

768.6 **Mild or moderate birth asphyxia**
Other specified birth asphyxia (without mention of neurologic involvement)

768.9 ==Unspecified birth asphyxia in liveborn infant==
Anoxia
Asphyxia   } NOS, in liveborn infant
Hypoxia

 Additional Digit Required   Revised Text   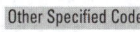 New Code

769 Respiratory distress syndrome
   Cardiorespiratory distress syndrome of newborn
   Hyaline membrane disease (pulmonary)
   Idiopathic respiratory distress syndrome [IRDS or RDS] of newborn
   Pulmonary hypoperfusion syndrome
   EXCLUDES transient tachypnea of newborn (770.6)

   DEF: Severe chest contractions upon air intake and expiratory grunting; infant appears blue due to oxygen deficiency and has rapid respiratory rate; formerly called hyaline membrane disease.

√4th **770 Other respiratory conditions of fetus and newborn**

   770.0 Congenital pneumonia
      Infective pneumonia acquired prenatally
      EXCLUDES pneumonia from infection acquired after birth (480.0-486)

   770.1 Meconium aspiration syndrome
      Aspiration of contents of birth canal NOS
      Meconium aspiration below vocal cords
      Pneumonitis:
         fetal aspiration
         meconium

      DEF: Aspiration of meconium by the newborn infant prior to delivery. Presence of meconium in the trachea or chest x-ray indicating patchy infiltrates in conjunction with chest hyperextension establishes this diagnosis.

   770.2 Interstitial emphysema and related conditions
      Pneumomediastinum ⎫
      Pneumopericardium ⎬ originating in the perinatal period
      Pneumothorax   ⎭

   770.3 Pulmonary hemorrhage
      Hemorrhage:
         alveolar (lung)   ⎫
         intra-alveolar (lung)   ⎬ originating in the perinatal period
         massive pulmonary   ⎭

   770.4 Primary atelectasis
      Pulmonary immaturity NOS
      DEF: Alveoli fail to expand causing insufficient air intake by newborn.

   770.5 Other and unspecified atelectasis
      Atelectasis: ⎫
         NOS   ⎪
         partial   ⎬ originating in the perinatal period
         secondary   ⎪
      Pulmonary collapse ⎭

   770.6 Transitory tachypnea of newborn
      Idiopathic tachypnea of newborn
      Wet lung syndrome
      EXCLUDES respiratory distress syndrome (769)
      DEF: Quick, shallow breathing of newborn; short-term problem.

   770.7 Chronic respiratory disease arising in the perinatal period
      Bronchopulmonary dysplasia
      Interstitial pulmonary fibrosis of prematurity
      Wilson-Mikity syndrome

√5th **770.8 Other respiratory problems after birth**
      770.81 Primary apnea of newborn
         Apneic spells of newborn NOS
         Essential apnea of newborn
         Sleep apnea of newborn

CONDITIONS IN THE PERINATAL PERIOD 770.82–771.89

- **770.82 Other apnea of newborn**
  Obstructive apnea of newborn
- **770.83 Cyanotic attacks of newborn**
- **770.84 Respiratory failure of newborn**
  EXCLUDES   respiratory distress syndrome (769)
- **770.89 Other respiratory problems after birth**

770.9 Unspecified respiratory condition of fetus and newborn

√4th **771 Infections specific to the perinatal period**
  INCLUDES   infections acquired before or during birth or via the umbilicus
  EXCLUDES   congenital pneumonia (770.0)
  congenital syphilis (090.0-090.9)
  maternal infectious disease as a cause of mortality or morbidity in fetus or newborn, but fetus or newborn not manifesting the disease (760.2)
  ophthalmia neonatorum due to gonococcus (098.40)
  other infections not specifically classified to this category

771.0 Congenital rubella
  Congenital rubella pneumonitis

771.1 Congenital cytomegalovirus infection
  Congenital cytomegalic inclusion disease

771.2 Other congenital infections
  Congenital: Congenital:
    herpes simplex   toxoplasmosis
    listeriosis   tuberculosis
    malaria

771.3 Tetanus neonatorum
  Tetanus omphalitis
  EXCLUDES   hypocalcemic tetany (775.4)
  DEF: Severe infection of central nervous system; due to exotoxin of tetanus bacillus from navel infection prompted by nonsterile technique during umbilical ligation.

771.4 Omphalitis of the newborn
  Infection:
    navel cord
    umbilical stump
  EXCLUDES   tetanus omphalitis (771.3)
  DEF: Inflamed umbilicus.

771.5 Neonatal infective mastitis
  EXCLUDES   noninfective neonatal mastitis (778.7)

771.6 Neonatal conjunctivitis and dacryocystitis
  Ophthalmia neonatorum NOS
  EXCLUDES   ophthalmia neonatorum due to gonococcus (098.40)

771.7 Neonatal Candida infection
  Neonatal moniliasis   Thrush in newborn

√5th **771.8 Other infection specific to the perinatal period**
  ▶Use additional code to identify organism◀
- **771.81 Septicemia [sepsis] of newborn**
- **771.82 Urinary tract infection of newborn**
- **771.83 Bacteremia of newborn**
- **771.89 Other infections specific to the perinatal period**
  Intra-amniotic infection of fetus NOS
  Infection of newborn NOS

CONDITIONS IN THE PERINATAL PERIOD

✓4ᵗʰ **772 Fetal and neonatal hemorrhage**
> **EXCLUDES** hematological disorders of fetus and newborn (776.0-776.9)

    772.0 Fetal blood loss [N]
        Fetal blood loss from:
            cut end of co-twin's cord
            placenta
            ruptured cord
            vasa previa
        Fetal exsanguination
        Fetal hemorrhage into:
            co-twin
            mother's circulation

✓5ᵗʰ   **772.1 Intraventricular hemorrhage** [N]
        Intraventricular hemorrhage from any perinatal cause
        772.10 Unspecified grade
        772.11 Grade I
            Bleeding into germinal matrix
        772.12 Grade II
            Bleeding into ventricle
        772.13 Grade III
            Bleeding with enlargement of ventricle
        772.14 Grade IV
            Bleeding into cerebral cortex

    772.2 Subarachnoid hemorrhage [N]
        Subarachnoid hemorrhage from any perinatal cause
> **EXCLUDES** subdural and cerebral hemorrhage (767.0)

    772.3 Umbilical hemorrhage after birth [N]
        Slipped umbilical ligature

    772.4 Gastrointestinal hemorrhage [N]
> **EXCLUDES** swallowed maternal blood (777.3)

    772.5 Adrenal hemorrhage [N]
    772.6 Cutaneous hemorrhage [N]
        Bruising ⎫
        Ecchymoses ⎬ in fetus or newborn
        Petechiae ⎪
        Superficial hematoma ⎭

    772.8 Other specified hemorrhage of fetus or newborn [N]
> **EXCLUDES** hemorrhagic disease of newborn (776.0)
>   pulmonary hemorrhage (770.3)

    772.9 Unspecified hemorrhage of newborn [N]

✓4ᵗʰ **773 Hemolytic disease of fetus or newborn, due to isoimmunization**
DEF: Hemolytic anemia of fetus or newborn due to maternal antibody formation against fetal erythrocytes; infant blood contains nonmaternal antigen.

    773.0 Hemolytic disease due to Rh isoimmunization [N]
        Anemia ⎫
        Erythroblastosis ⎪ due to RH:
            (fetalis) ⎬   antibodies
        Hemolytic disease ⎪   isoimmunization
            (fetus) (newborn) ⎪   maternal/fetal
        Jaundice ⎭   incompatibility

        Rh hemolytic disease
        Rh isoimmunization

CONDITIONS IN THE PERINATAL PERIOD   773.1–774.31

773.1   Hemolytic disease due to ABO isoimmunization
    ABO hemolytic disease
    ABO isoimmunization
    Anemia ⎫
    Erythroblastosis ⎬ due to ABO:
      (fetalis) ⎪   antibodies
    Hemolytic disease ⎬   isoimmunization
      (fetus) (newborn) ⎪   maternal/fetal
    Jaundice ⎭   incompatibility

DEF: Incompatible Rh fetal-maternal blood grouping; prematurely destroys red blood cells; detected by Coombs test.

773.2   Hemolytic disease due to other and unspecified isoimmunization
    Eythroblastosis (fetalis) (neonatorum) NOS
    Hemolytic disease (fetus) (newborn) NOS
    Jaundice or anemia due to other and unspecified blood-group incompatibility

773.3   Hydrops fetalis due to isoimmunization
    Use additional code to identify type of isoimmunization (773.0-773.2)

DEF: Massive edema of entire body and severe anemia; may result in fetal death or stillbirth.

773.4   Kernicterus due to isoimmunization
    Use additional code to identify type of isoimmunization (773.0-773.2)

DEF: Complication of erythroblastosis fetalis associated with severe neural symptoms, high blood bilirubin levels and nerve cell destruction; results in bilirubin-pigmented gray matter of central nervous system.

773.5   Late anemia due to isoimmunization

√4th **774   Other perinatal jaundice**

774.0   Perinatal jaundice from hereditary hemolytic anemias
    Code first underlying disease (282.0-282.9)

774.1   Perinatal jaundice from other excessive hemolysis
    Fetal or neonatal jaundice from:
      bruising
      drugs or toxins transmitted from mother
      infection
      polycythemia
      swallowed maternal blood
    Use additional code to identify cause
    EXCLUDES jaundice due to isoimmunization (773.0-773.2)

774.2   Neonatal jaundice associated with preterm delivery
    Hyperbilirubinemia of prematurity
    Jaundice due to delayed conjugation associated with preterm delivery

√5th **774.3   Neonatal jaundice due to delayed conjugation from other causes**

    774.30   Neonatal jaundice due to delayed conjugation, cause unspecified
    DEF: Jaundice of newborn with abnormal bilirubin metabolism; causes excess accumulated unconjugated bilirubin in blood.

    774.31   Neonatal jaundice due to delayed conjugation in diseases classified elsewhere
      Code first underlying diseases as:
        congenital hypothyroidism (243)
        Crigler-Najjar syndrome (277.4)
        Gilbert's syndrome (277.4)

 Additional Digit Required   Revised Text   ● New Code   ▲ Revised Code Title

Unspecified Code   Other Specified Code   Manifestation Code

MSP Medicare Secondary Payer

2002 Ingenix, Inc.   Volume 1 — 483

774.39 Other
     Jaundice due to delayed conjugation from causes, such as:
        breast milk inhibitors
        delayed development of conjugating system

774.4 Perinatal jaundice due to hepatocellular damage
     Fetal or neonatal hepatitis
     Giant cell hepatitis
     Inspissated bile syndrome

774.5 Perinatal jaundice from other causes
     Code first underlying cause as:
        congenital obstruction of bile duct (751.61)
        galactosemia (271.1)
        Mucoviscidosis ▶(277.00-277.09)◀

774.6 Unspecified fetal and neonatal jaundice
     Icterus neonatorum
     Neonatal hyperbilirubinemia (transient)
     Physiologic jaundice NOS in newborn
        EXCLUDES that in preterm infants (774.2)

774.7 Kernicterus not due to isoimmunization
     Bilirubin encephalopathy
     Kernicterus of newborn NOS
        EXCLUDES kernicterus due to isoimmunization (773.4)

✓4th 775 Endocrine and metabolic disturbances specific to the fetus and newborn
INCLUDES transitory endocrine and metabolic disturbances caused by the infant's response to maternal endocrine and metabolic factors, its removal from them, or its adjustment to extrauterine existence

775.0 Syndrome of "infant of a diabetic mother"
     Maternal diabetes mellitus affecting fetus or newborn (with hypoglycemia)

775.1 Neonatal diabetes mellitus
     Diabetes mellitus syndrome in newborn infant

775.2 Neonatal myasthenia gravis

775.3 Neonatal thyrotoxicosis
     Neonatal hyperthydroidism (transient)

775.4 Hypocalcemia and hypomagnesemia of newborn
     Cow's milk hypocalcemia
     Hypocalcemic tetany, neonatal
     Neonatal hypoparathyroidism
     Phosphate-loading hypocalcemia

775.5 Other transitory neonatal electrolyte disturbances
     Dehydration, neonatal

775.6 Neonatal hypoglycemia
        EXCLUDES infant of mother with diabetes mellitus (775.0)

775.7 Late metabolic acidosis of newborn

775.8 Other transitory neonatal endocrine and metabolic disturbances
     Amino-acid metabolic disorders described as transitory

775.9 Unspecified endocrine and metabolic disturbances specific to the fetus and newborn

✓4th 776 Hematological disorders of fetus and newborn
INCLUDES disorders specific to the fetus or newborn

776.0 Hemorrhagic disease of newborn
     Hemorrhagic diathesis of newborn
     Vitamin K deficiency of newborn
        EXCLUDES fetal or neonatal hemorrhage (772.0-772.9)

CONDITIONS IN THE PERINATAL PERIOD

776.1 Transient neonatal thrombocytopenia
Neonatal thrombocytopenia due to:
  exchange transfusion
  idiopathic maternal thrombocytopenia
  isoimmunization
DEF: Temporary decrease in blood platelets of newborn.

776.2 Disseminated intravascular coagulation in newborn
DEF: Disseminated intravascular coagulation of newborn: clotting disorder due to excess thromboplastic agents in blood as a result of disease or trauma; causes blood clotting within vessels and reduces available elements necessary for blood coagulation.

776.3 Other transient neonatal disorders of coagulation
Transient coagulation defect, newborn

776.4 Polycythemia neonatorum
Plethora of newborn   Polycythemia due to:
Polycythemia due to: maternal-fetal transfusion
  donor twin transfusion
DEF: Abnormal increase of total red blood cells of newborn.

776.5 Congenital anemia
Anemia following fetal blood loss
  EXCLUDES   anemia due to isoimmunization (773.0-773.2, 773.5)
              hereditary hemolytic anemias (282.0-282.9)

776.6 Anemia of prematurity

776.7 Transient neonatal neutropenia
Isoimmune neutropenia   Maternal transfer neutropenia
  EXCLUDES   congenital neutropenia (nontransient) (288.0)
DEF: Decreased neutrophilic leukocytes in blood of newborn.

776.8 Other specified transient hematological disorders

776.9 Unspecified hematological disorder specific to fetus or newborn

√4th 777 Perinatal disorders of digestive system
  INCLUDES   disorders specific to the fetus and newborn
  EXCLUDES   intestinal obstruction classifiable to 560.0-560.9

777.1 Meconium obstruction
Congenital fecaliths
Delayed passage of meconium
Meconium ileus NOS
Meconium plug syndrome
  EXCLUDES   meconium ileus in cystic fibrosis (277.01)
DEF: Meconium blocked digestive tract of newborn.

777.2 Intestinal obstruction due to inspissated milk

777.3 Hematemesis and melena due to swallowed maternal blood
Swallowed blood syndrome in newborn
  EXCLUDES   that not due to swallowed maternal blood (772.4)

777.4 Transitory ileus of newborn
  EXCLUDES   Hirschsprung's disease (751.3)

777.5 Necrotizing enterocolitis in fetus or newborn
Pseudomembranous enterocolitis in newborn
DEF: Acute inflammation of small intestine due to pseudomembranous plaque over ulceration; may be due to aggressive antibiotic therapy.

777.6 Perinatal intestinal perforation
Meconium peritonitis

777.8 Other specified perinatal disorders of digestive system

777.9 Unspecified perinatal disorder of digestive system

CONDITIONS IN THE PERINATAL PERIOD

✓4th **778 Conditions involving the integument and temperature regulation of fetus and newborn**

- **778.0 Hydrops fetalis not due to isoimmunization** [N]
  - Idiopathic hydrops
  - **EXCLUDES** hydrops fetalis due to isoimmunization (773.3)
  - DEF: Edema of entire body, unrelated to immune response.

- **778.1 Sclerema neonatorum** [N]
  - Subcutaneous fat necrosis
  - DEF: Diffuse, rapidly progressing white, waxy, nonpitting hardening of tissue, usually of legs and feet, life-threatening; found in preterm or debilitated infants; unknown etiology.

- **778.2 Cold injury syndrome of newborn** [N]
- **778.3 Other hypothermia of newborn** [N]
- **778.4 Other disturbances of temperature regulation of newborn** [N]
  - Dehydration fever in newborn
  - Environmentally-induced pyrexia
  - Hyperthermia in newborn
  - Transitory fever of newborn

- **778.5 Other and unspecified edema of newborn** [N]
  - Edema neonatorum

- **778.6 Congenital hydrocele** [N]
  - Congenital hydrocele of tunica vaginalis

- **778.7 Breast engorgement in newborn** [N]
  - Noninfective mastitis of newborn
  - **EXCLUDES** infective mastitis of newborn (771.5)

- **778.8 Other specified conditions involving the integument of fetus and newborn** [N]
  - Urticaria neonatorum
  - **EXCLUDES** impetigo neonatorum (684)
  - pemphigus neonatorum (684)

- **778.9 Unspecified condition involving the integument and temperature regulation of fetus and newborn** [N]

✓4th **779 Other and ill-defined conditions originating in the perinatal period**

- **779.0 Convulsions in newborn** [N]
  - Fits } in newborn
  - Seizures

- **779.1 Other and unspecified cerebral irritability in newborn** [N]
- **779.2 Cerebral depression, coma, and other abnormal cerebral signs** [N]
  - CNS dysfunction in newborn NOS

- **779.3 Feeding problems in newborn** [N]
  - Regurgitation of food
  - Slow feeding } in newborn
  - Vomiting

- **779.4 Drug reactions and intoxications specific tonewborn** [N]
  - Gray syndrome from chloramphenicol administration in newborn
  - **EXCLUDES** fetal alcohol syndrome (760.71)
  - reactions and intoxications from maternal opiates and tranquilizers (763.5)

- **779.5 Drug withdrawal syndrome in newborn** [N]
  - Drug withdrawal syndrome in infant of dependent mother
  - **EXCLUDES** fetal alcohol syndrome (760.71)

SYMPTOMS, SIGNS, AND ILL-DEFINED CONDITIONS 779.6–779.9

779.6 Termination of pregnancy (fetus)
Fetal death due to:
induced abortion
termination of pregnancy
EXCLUDES spontaneous abortion (fetus) (761.8)

779.7 Periventricular leukomalacia
DEF: Necrosis of white matter adjacent to lateral ventricles with the formation of cysts; cause of PVL has not been firmly established, but thought to be related to inadequate blood flow in certain areas of the brain.

√5th **779.8 Other specified conditions originating in the perinatal period**
- **779.81 Neonatal bradycardia**
  EXCLUDES abnormality in fetal heart rate or rhythm complicating labor and delivery (763.81-763.83)
  bradycardia due to birth asphyxia (768.5-768.9)
- **779.82 Neonatal tachycardia**
  EXCLUDES abnormality in fetal heart rate or rhythm complicating labor and delivery (763.81-763.83)
- **779.89 Other specified conditions originating in the perinatal period**

779.9 Unspecified condition originating in the perinatal period
Congenital debility NOS
Stillbirth NEC

16. SYMPTOMS, SIGNS, AND ILL-DEFINED CONDITIONS (780-799)

This section includes symptoms, signs, abnormal results of laboratory or other investigative procedures, and ill-defined conditions regarding which no diagnosis classifiable elsewhere is recorded.

Signs and symptoms that point rather definitely to a given diagnosis are assigned to some category in the preceding part of the classification. In general, categories 780-796 include the more ill-defined conditions and symptoms that point with perhaps equal suspicion to two or more diseases or to two or more systems of the body, and without the necessary study of the case to make a final diagnosis. Practically all categories in this group could be designated as "not otherwise specified," or as "unknown etiology," or as "transient." The Alphabetic Index should be consulted to determine which symptoms and signs are to be allocated here and which to more specific sections of the classification; the residual subcategories numbered .9 are provided for other relevant symptoms which cannot be allocated elsewhere in the classification.

The conditions and signs or symptoms included in categories 780-796 consist of: (a) cases for which no more specific diagnosis can be made even after all facts bearing on the case have been investigated; (b) signs or symptoms existing at the time of initial encounter that proved to be transient and whose causes could not be determined; (c) provisional diagnoses in a patient who failed to return for further investigation or care; (d) cases referred elsewhere for investigation or treatment before the diagnosis was made; (e) cases in which a more precise diagnosis was not available for any other reason; (f) certain symptoms which represent important problems in medical care and which it might be desired to classify in addition to a known cause.

SYMPTOMS, SIGNS, AND ILL-DEFINED CONDITIONS

SYMPTOMS (780-789)

√4th 780 General symptoms

√5th 780.0 Alteration of consciousness

EXCLUDES coma:
diabetic (250.2-250.3)
hepatic (572.2)
originating in the perinatal period (779.2)

780.01 Coma
DEF: State of unconsciousness from which the patient cannot be awakened.

780.02 Transient alteration of awareness
DEF: Temporary, recurring spells of reduced consciousness.

780.03 Persistent vegetative state
DEF: Persistent wakefulness without consciousness due to nonfunctioning cerebral cortex.

780.09 Other
Drowsiness   Stupor
Semicoma   Unconsciousness
Somnolence

780.1 Hallucinations
Hallucinations: Hallucinations:
  NOS   olfactory
  auditory   tactile
  gustatory

EXCLUDES those associated with mental disorders, as functional psychoses (295.0-298.9)
organic brain syndromes (290.0-294.9, 310.0-310.9)
visual hallucinations (368.16)

DEF: Perception of external stimulus in absence of stimulus; inability to distinguish between real and imagined.

780.2 Syncope and collapse
Blackout   (Near) (Pre) syncope
Fainting   Vasovagal attack

EXCLUDES carotid sinus syncope (337.0)
heat syncope (992.1)
neurocirculatory asthenia (306.2)
orthostatic hypotension (458.0)
shock NOS (785.50)

DEF: Sudden unconsciousness due to reduced blood flow to brain.

√5th 780.3 Convulsions

EXCLUDES convulsions:
epileptic (345.10-345.91)
in newborn (779.0)

DEF: Sudden, involuntary contractions of the muscles.

780.31 Febrile convulsions
Febrile seizure

780.39 Other convulsions
Convulsive disorder NOS
Fit NOS
Seizure NOS

780.4 Dizziness and giddiness
Light-headedness   Vertigo NOS

EXCLUDES Ménière's disease and other specified vertiginous syndromes (386.0-386.9)

DEF: Whirling sensations in head with feeling of falling.

SYMPTOMS, SIGNS, AND ILL-DEFINED CONDITIONS

√5ᵗʰ **780.5 Sleep disturbances**
> **EXCLUDES** that of nonorganic origin (307.40-307.49)

780.50 Sleep disturbance, unspecified

780.51 Insomnia with sleep apnea
DEF: Transient cessation of breathing disturbing sleep.

780.52 Other insomnia
Insomnia NOS
DEF: Inability to maintain adequate sleep cycle.

780.53 Hypersomnia with sleep apnea
DEF: Autonomic response inhibited during sleep; causes insufficient oxygen intake, acidosis and pulmonary hypertension.

780.54 Other hypersomnia
Hypersomnia NOS
DEF: Prolonged sleep cycle.

780.55 Disruptions of 24-hour sleep-wake cycle
Inversion of sleep rhythm
Irregular sleep-wake rhythm NOS
Non-24-hour sleep-wake rhythm

780.56 Dysfunctions associated with sleep stages or arousal from sleep

780.57 Other and unspecified sleep apnea

780.59 Other

780.6 Fever
Chills with fever
Fever NOS
Fever of unknown origin (FUO)
Hyperpyrexia NOS
Pyrexia
Pyrexia of unknown origin
> **EXCLUDES** pyrexia of unknown origin (during):
> in newborn (778.4)
> labor (659.2)
> the puerperium (672)

DEF: Elevated body temperature; no known cause.

√5ᵗʰ **780.7 Malaise and fatigue**
> **EXCLUDES** debility, unspecified (799.3)
> fatigue (during):
> combat (308.0-308.9)
> heat (992.6)
> pregnancy (646.8)
> neurasthenia (300.5)
> senile asthenia (797)

DEF: Indefinite feeling of debility or lack of good health.

780.71 Chronic fatigue syndrome
DEF: Persistent fatigue, symptoms include weak muscles, sore throat, lymphadenitis, headache, depression and mild fever; no known cause; also called chronic mononucleosis, benign myalgic encephalomyelitis, Iceland disease and neurasthenia.

SYMPTOMS, SIGNS, AND ILL-DEFINED CONDITIONS

780.79 Other malaise and fatigue
Asthenia NOS
Lethargy
Postviral (asthenic) syndrome
Tiredness

DEF: Asthenia: any weakness, lack of strength or loss of energy, especially neuromuscular.

DEF: Lethargy: listlessness, drowsiness, stupor and apathy.

DEF: Postviral (asthenia) syndrome: listlessness, drowsiness, stupor and apathy; follows acute viral infection.

DEF: Tiredness: general exhaustion or fatigue.

780.8 Hyperhidrosis
Diaphoresis
Excessive sweating

DEF: Excessive sweating, appears as droplets on skin; general or localized.

√5th **780.9 Other general symptoms**
  EXCLUDES hypothermia:
       NOS (accidental) (991.6)
       due to anesthesia (995.89)
       of newborn (778.2-778.3)
       memory disturbance as part of a pattern of mental disorder

• **780.91 Fussy infant (baby)**
• **780.92 Excessive crying of infant (baby)**
• **780.99 Other general symptoms**
Amnesia (retrograde)
Chill(s) NOS
Generalized pain
Hypothermia, not associated with low environmental temperature

√4th **781 Symptoms involving nervous and musculoskeletal systems**
  EXCLUDES depression NOS (311)
       disorders specifically relating to:
         back (724.0-724.9)
         hearing (388.0-389.9)
         joint (718.0-719.9)
         limb (729.0-729.9)
         neck (723.0-723.9)
         vision (368.0-369.9)
       pain in limb (729.5)

781.0 Abnormal involuntary movements
Abnormal head movements   Spasms NOS
Fasciculation   Tremor NOS
  EXCLUDES abnormal reflex (796.1)
       chorea NOS (333.5)
       infantile spasms (345.60-345.61)
       spastic paralysis (342.1, 343.0-344.9)
       specified movement disorders classifiable to 333 (333.0-333.9)
       that of nonorganic origin (307.2-307.3)

781.1 Disturbances of sensation of smell and taste
Anosmia   Parosmia
Parageusia

DEF: Anosmia: loss of sense of smell due to organic factors, including loss of olfactory nerve conductivity, cerebral disease, nasal fossae formation and peripheral olfactory nerve diseases; can also be psychological disorder.

DEF: Parageusia: distorted sense of taste, or bad taste in mouth.

DEF: Parosmia: distorted sense of smell.

SYMPTOMS, SIGNS, AND ILL-DEFINED CONDITIONS

781.2 Abnormality of gait
Gait:
  ataxic
  paralytic
  spastic
  staggering
  EXCLUDES ataxia:
    NOS (781.3)
    locomotor (progressive) (094.0)
    difficulty in walking (719.7)
DEF: Abnormal, asymmetric gait.

781.3 Lack of coordination
Ataxia NOS   Muscular incoordination
  EXCLUDES ataxic gait (781.2)
    cerebellar ataxia (334.0-334.9)
    difficulty in walking (719.7)
    vertigo NOS (780.4)

781.4 Transient paralysis of limb
Monoplegia, transient NOS
  EXCLUDES paralysis (342.0-344.9)

781.5 Clubbing of fingers
DEF: Enlarged soft tissue of distal fingers.

781.6 Meningismus
Dupré's syndrome   Meningism
DEF: Condition with signs and symptoms that resemble meningeal irritation; it is associated with febrile illness and dehydration with no evidence of infection.

781.7 Tetany
Carpopedal spasm
  EXCLUDES tetanus neonatorum (771.3)
    tetany:
      hysterical (300.11)
      newborn (hypocalcemic) (775.4)
      parathyroid (252.1)
      psychogenic (306.0)
DEF: Nerve and muscle hyperexcitability; symptoms include muscle spasms, twitching, cramps, laryngospasm with inspiratory stridor, hyperreflexia and choreiform movements.

781.8 Neurologic neglect syndrome
  Asomatognosia   Left-sided neglect
  Hemi-akinesia   Sensory extinction
  Hemi-inattention   Sensory neglect
  Hemispatial neglect   Visuospatial neglect

√5ᵗʰ 781.9 Other symptoms involving nervous and musculoskeletal systems

781.91 Loss of height
  EXCLUDES osteoporosis (733.00-733.09)

781.92 Abnormal posture

781.93 Ocular torticollis

781.99 Other symptoms involving nervous and musculoskeletal systems

SYMPTOMS, SIGNS, AND ILL-DEFINED CONDITIONS

√4th **782 Symptoms involving skin and other integumentary tissue**
  EXCLUDES symptoms relating to breast (611.71-611.79)

782.0 Disturbance of skin sensation
  Anesthesia of skin
  Burning or prickling sensation
  Hyperesthesia
  Hypoesthesia
  Numbness
  Paresthesia
  Tingling

782.1 Rash and other nonspecific skin eruption
  Exanthem
  EXCLUDES vesicular eruption (709.8)

782.2 Localized superficial swelling, mass, or lump
  Subcutaneous nodules
  EXCLUDES localized adiposity (278.1)

782.3 Edema
  Anasarca
  Dropsy
  Localized edema NOS
  EXCLUDES ascites (789.5)
  edema of:
    newborn NOS (778.5)
    pregnancy (642.0-642.9, 646.1)
  fluid retention (276.6)
  hydrops fetalis (773.3, 778.0)
  hydrothorax (511.8)
  nutritional edema (260, 262)

DEF: Edema: excess fluid in intercellular body tissue.

DEF: Anasarca: massive edema in all body tissues.

DEF: Dropsy: serous fluid accumulated in body cavity or cellular tissue.

DEF: Localized edema: edema in specific body areas.

782.4 Jaundice, unspecified, not of newborn
  Cholemia NOS   Icterus NOS
  EXCLUDES jaundice in newborn (774.0-774.7)
    due to isoimmunization (773.0-773.2, 773.4)

DEF: Bilirubin deposits of skin, causing yellow cast.

782.5 Cyanosis
  EXCLUDES newborn ▶(770.83)◀

DEF: Deficient oxygen of blood; causes blue cast to skin.

√5th **782.6 Pallor and flushing**
  782.61 Pallor
  782.62 Flushing
    Excessive blushing

782.7 Spontaneous ecchymoses
  Petechiae
  EXCLUDES ecchymosis in fetus or newborn (772.6)
    purpura (287.0-287.9)

DEF: Hemorrhagic spots of skin; resemble freckles.

782.8 Changes in skin texture
  Induration } of skin
  Thickening

782.9 Other symptoms involving skin and integumentary tissues

SYMPTOMS, SIGNS, AND ILL-DEFINED CONDITIONS

783 Symptoms concerning nutrition, metabolism, and development

783.0 Anorexia
Loss of appetite
EXCLUDES anorexia nervosa (307.1)
loss of appetite of nonorganic origin (307.59)

783.1 Abnormal weight gain
EXCLUDES excessive weight gain in pregnancy (646.1)
obesity (278.00)
morbid (278.01)

783.2 Abnormal loss of weight and underweight
783.21 Loss of weight
783.22 Underweight

783.3 Feeding difficulties and mismanagement
Feeding problem (elderly) (infant)
EXCLUDES feeding disturbance or problems:
in newborn (779.3)
of nonorganic origin (307.50-307.59)

783.4 Lack of expected normal physiological development in childhood
EXCLUDES delay in sexual development and puberty (259.0)
gonadal dysgenesis (758.6)
pituitary dwarfism (253.3)
slow fetal growth and fetal malnutrition (764.00-764.99)
specific delays in mental development (315.0-315.9)

783.40 Lack of normal physiological development, unspecified
Inadequate development
Lack of development

783.41 Failure to thrive
Failure to gain weight

DEF: Organic failure to thrive: acute or chronic illness that interferes with nutritional intake, absorption, metabolism excretion and energy requirements. Nonorganic FTT is symptom of neglect or abuse.

783.42 Delayed milestones
Late talker
Late walker

783.43 Short stature
Growth failure
Growth retardation
Lack of growth
Physical retardation

DEF: Constitutional short stature: stature inconsistent with chronological age. Genetic short stature is when skeletal maturation matches chronological age.

783.5 Polydipsia
Excessive thirst

783.6 Polyphagia
Excessive eating   Hyperalimentation NOS
EXCLUDES disorders of eating of nonorganic origin (307.50-307.59)

783.7 Adult failure to thrive

783.9 Other symptoms concerning nutrition, metabolism, and development
Hypometabolism
EXCLUDES abnormal basal metabolic rate (794.7)
dehydration (276.5)
other disorders of fluid, electrolyte, and acid-base balance (276.0-276.9)

Additional Digit Required | Unspecified Code | Other Specified Code | Manifestation Code
MSP Medicare Secondary Payer | ▶◀ Revised Text | ● New Code | ▲ Revised Code Title

2002 Ingenix, Inc.

SYMPTOMS, SIGNS, AND ILL-DEFINED CONDITIONS

√4th 784 Symptoms involving head and neck
    EXCLUDES encephalopathy NOS (348.3)
                     specific symptoms involving neck classifiable to 723 (723.0-723.9)

784.0 Headache
    Facial pain   Pain in head NOS
    EXCLUDES atypical face pain (350.2)
                migraine (346.0-346.9)
                tension headache (307.81)

784.1 Throat pain
    EXCLUDES dysphagia (787.2)
                neck pain (723.1)
                sore throat (462)
                     chronic (472.1)

784.2 Swelling, mass, or lump in head and neck
    Space-occupying lesion, intracranial NOS

784.3 Aphasia
    EXCLUDES developmental aphasia (315.31)
    DEF: Inability to communicate through speech, written word, or sign language.

√5th 784.4 Voice disturbance
    784.40 Voice disturbance, unspecified
    784.41 Aphonia
        Loss of voice
    784.49 Other
        Change in voice   Hypernasality
        Dysphonia   Hyponasality
        Hoarseness

784.5 Other speech disturbance
    Dysarthria   Slurred speech
    Dysphasia
    EXCLUDES stammering and stuttering (307.0)
                 that of nonorganic origin (307.0, 307.9)

√5th 784.6 Other symbolic dysfunction
    EXCLUDES developmental learning delays (315.0-315.9)
    784.60 Symbolic dysfunction, unspecified
    784.61 Alexia and dyslexia
        Alexia (with agraphia)
        DEF: Alexia: Inability to understand written word due to central brain lesion.

        DEF: Dyslexia: Ability to recognize letters but inability to read, spell, and write words; genetic.

    784.69 Other
        Acalculia   Agraphia NOS
        Agnosia   Apraxia

784.7 Epistaxis
    Hemorrhage from nose
    Nosebleed

784.8 Hemorrhage from throat
    EXCLUDES hemoptysis (786.3)

784.9 Other symptoms involving head and neck
    Choking sensation   Mouth breathing
    Halitosis   Sneezing

N Newborn Age: 0   **P** Pediatric Age: 0-17   **M** Maternity Age: 12-55   **A** Adult Age: 15-124

SYMPTOMS, SIGNS, AND ILL-DEFINED CONDITIONS   785–785.59

√4ᵗʰ **785 Symptoms involving cardiovascular system**
   EXCLUDES   heart failure NOS (428.9)

785.0 Tachycardia, unspecified
   Rapid heart beat
   EXCLUDES ▶neonatal tachycardia (779.82)◀
       paroxysmal tachycardia (427.0-427.2)
   DEF: Excessively rapid heart rate.

785.1 Palpitations
   Awareness of heart beat
   EXCLUDES   specified dysrhythmias (427.0-427.9)
   DEF: Shock syndrome: associated with myocardial infarction, cardiac tamponade and massive pulmonary embolism; symptoms include mental torpor, reduced blood pressure, tachycardia, pallor and cold, clammy skin.

785.2 Undiagnosed cardiac murmurs
   Heart murmurs NOS

785.3 Other abnormal heart sounds
   Cardiac dullness, increased or decreased
   Friction fremitus, cardiac
   Precordial friction

785.4 Gangrene
   Gangrene:
       NOS
       spreading cutaneous
   Gangrenous cellulitis
   Phagedena
   Code first any associated underlying condition
   EXCLUDES   gangrene of certain sites — see Alphabetic Index
       gangrene with atherosclerosis of the extremities (440.24)
       gas gangrene (040.0)
   DEF: Gangrene: necrosis of skin tissue due to bacterial infection, diabetes, embolus and vascular supply loss.

   DEF: Gangrenous cellulitis: group A streptococcal infection; begins with severe cellulitis, spreads to superficial and deep fascia; produces gangrene of underlying tissues.

√5ᵗʰ **785.5 Shock without mention of trauma**

   785.50 Shock, unspecified
       Failure of peripheral circulation

   785.51 Cardiogenic shock
       DEF: Peripheral circulatory failure due to heart insufficiencies.

   785.59 Other
       Shock: Shock:
           endotoxic   hypovolemic
           gram-negative   septic
       EXCLUDES   shock (due to):
           anesthetic (995.4)
           anaphylactic (995.0)
               due to serum (999.4)
           electric (994.8)
           following abortion (639.5)
           lightning (994.0)
           obstetrical (669.1)
           postoperative (998.0)
           traumatic (958.4)

√4ᵗʰ
√5ᵗʰ Additional Digit Required   **Unspecified Code**   Other Specified Code   ▲ Manifestation Code
 Medicare Secondary Payer   ▶◀ Revised Text   ● New Code   ▲ Revised Code Title

SYMPTOMS, SIGNS, AND ILL-DEFINED CONDITIONS

785.6 Enlargement of lymph nodes
Lymphadenopathy   "Swollen glands"
EXCLUDES   lymphadenitis (chronic) (289.1-289.3)
                acute (683)

785.9 Other symptoms involving cardiovascular system
Bruit (arterial)   Weak pulse

√4th **786 Symptoms involving respiratory system and other chest symptoms**

√5th **786.0 Dyspnea and respiratory abnormalities**

786.00 Respiratory abnormality, unspecified

786.01 Hyperventilation
EXCLUDES   hyperventilation, psychogenic (306.1)
DEF: Rapid breathing causes carbon dioxide loss from blood.

786.02 Orthopnea
DEF: Difficulty breathing except in upright position.

786.03 Apnea
EXCLUDES ▶apnea of newborn (770.81, 770.82)◀
               sleep apnea (780.51, 780.53, 780.57)
DEF: Cessation of breathing.

786.04 Cheyne-Stokes respiration
DEF: Rhythmic increase of depth and frequency of breathing with apnea; occurs in frontal lobe and diencephalic dysfunction.

786.05 Shortness of breath
DEF: Inability to take in sufficient oxygen.

786.06 Tachypnea
EXCLUDES   transitory tachypnea of newborn (770.6)
DEF: Abnormal rapid respiratory rate; called hyperventilation.

786.07 Wheezing
EXCLUDES   asthma (493.00-493.92)
DEF: Stenosis of respiratory passageway; causes whistling sound; due to asthma, coryza, croup, emphysema, hay fever, edema, and pleural effusion.

786.09 Other
EXCLUDES   respiratory distress:
                    following trauma and surgery (518.5)
                    newborn ▶(770.89)◀
                    syndrome (newborn) (769)
                    adult (518.5)
                respiratory failure (518.81, 518.83-518.84)
                    newborn ▶(770.84)◀

786.1 Stridor
EXCLUDES   congenital laryngeal stridor (748.3)
DEF: Obstructed airway causes harsh sound.

786.2 Cough
EXCLUDES   cough:
                    psychogenic (306.1)
                    smokers' (491.0)
                    with hemorrhage (786.3)

786.3 Hemoptysis
Cough with hemorrhage
Pulmonary hemorrhage NOS
EXCLUDES   pulmonary hemorrhage of newborn (770.3)
DEF: Coughing up blood or blood-stained sputum.

SYMPTOMS, SIGNS, AND ILL-DEFINED CONDITIONS 786.4–787.03

786.4 Abnormal sputum
Abnormal:
  amount
  color   } (of) sputum
  odor
  Excessive

✓5th **786.5 Chest pain**
  786.50 Chest pain, unspecified
  786.51 Precordial pain
    DEF: Chest pain over heart and lower thorax.
  786.52 Painful respiration
    Pain:
      anterior chest wall
      pleuritic
    Pleurodynia
    EXCLUDES epidemic pleurodynia (074.1)
  786.59 Other
    Discomfort
    Pressure   } in chest
    Tightness
    EXCLUDES pain in breast (611.71)

786.6 Swelling, mass, or lump in chest
  EXCLUDES lump in breast (611.72)

786.7 Abnormal chest sounds
  Abnormal percussion, chest
  Friction sounds, chest
  Rales
  Tympany, chest
  EXCLUDES wheezing (786.07)

786.8 Hiccough
  EXCLUDES psychogenic hiccough (306.1)

786.9 Other symptoms involving respiratory system and chest
  Breath-holding spell

✓4th **787 Symptoms involving digestive system**
  EXCLUDES constipation (564.00-564.09)
    pylorospasm (537.81)
      congenital (750.5)

✓5th **787.0 Nausea and vomiting**
  Emesis
  EXCLUDES hematemesis NOS (578.0)
    vomiting:
      bilious, following gastrointestinal surgery (564.3)
      cyclical (536.2)
        psychogenic (306.4)
      excessive, in pregnancy (643.0-643.9)
      habit (536.2)
      of newborn (779.3)
      psychogenic NOS (307.54)
  787.01 Nausea with vomiting
  787.02 Nausea alone
  787.03 Vomiting alone

 Additional Digit Required   Unspecified Code   Other Specified Code   Manifestation Code
MSP Medicare Secondary Payer   ▶◀ Revised Text   ● New Code   ▲ Revised Code Title

2002 Ingenix, Inc.   Volume 1 — 497

SYMPTOMS, SIGNS, AND ILL-DEFINED CONDITIONS

787.1 Heartburn
Pyrosis   Waterbrash
EXCLUDES dyspepsia or indigestion (536.8)

787.2 Dysphagia
Difficulty in swallowing

787.3 Flatulence, eructation, and gas pain
Abdominal distention (gaseous)
Bloating
Tympanites (abdominal) (intestinal)
EXCLUDES aerophagy (306.4)

DEF: Flatulence: excess air or gas in intestine or stomach.

DEF: Eructation: belching, expelling gas through mouth.

DEF: Gas pain: gaseous pressure affecting gastrointestinal system.

787.4 Visible peristalsis
Hyperperistalsis

DEF: Increase in involuntary movements of intestines.

787.5 Abnormal bowel sounds
Absent bowel sounds   Hyperactive bowel sounds

787.6 Incontinence of feces
Encopresis NOS
Incontinence of sphincter ani
EXCLUDES that of nonorganic origin (307.7)

787.7 Abnormal feces
Bulky stools
EXCLUDES abnormal stool content (792.1)
melena:
NOS (578.1)
newborn (772.4, 777.3)

√5th **787.9 Other symptoms involving digestive system**
EXCLUDES gastrointestinal hemorrhage (578.0-578.9)
intestinal obstruction (560.0-560.9)
specific functional digestive disorders:
esophagus (530.0-530.9)
stomach and duodenum (536.0-536.9)
those not elsewhere classified (564.00-564.9)

787.91 Diarrhea
Diarrhea NOS

787.99 Other
Change in bowel habits
Tenesmus (rectal)

DEF: Tenesmus: painful, ineffective straining at the rectum with limited passage of fecal matter.

√4th **788 Symptoms involving urinary system**
EXCLUDES hematuria (599.7)
nonspecific findings on examination of the urine (791.0-791.9)
small kidney of unknown cause (589.0-589.9)
uremia NOS (586)

788.0 Renal colic
Colic (recurrent) of: Colic (recurrent) of:
  kidney   ureter

DEF: Kidney pain.

788.1 Dysuria
Painful urination   Strangury

SYMPTOMS, SIGNS, AND ILL-DEFINED CONDITIONS

✓5th 788.2 Retention of urine
DEF: Inability to void.

788.20 Retention of urine, unspecified
788.21 Incomplete bladder emptying
788.29 Other specified retention of urine

✓5th 788.3 Incontinence of urine
▶Code, if applicable, any causal condition first, such as:◀
congenital ureterocele (753.23)
genital prolapse (618.0-618.9)
> **EXCLUDES** that of nonorganic origin (307.6)

788.30 Urinary incontinence, unspecified
Enuresis NOS

788.31 Urge incontinence
DEF: Inability to control urination, upon urge to urinate.

788.32 Stress incontinence, male ♂
> **EXCLUDES** stress incontinence, female (625.6)

DEF: Inability to control urination associated with weak sphincter in males.

788.33 Mixed incontinence, (male) (female)
Urge and stress

DEF: Urge, stress incontinence: involuntary discharge of urine due to anatomic displacement.

788.34 Incontinence without sensory awareness
DEF: Involuntary discharge of urine without sensory warning.

788.35 Post-void dribbling
DEF: Involuntary discharge of residual urine after voiding.

788.36 Nocturnal enuresis
DEF: Involuntary discharge of urine during the night.

788.37 Continuous leakage
DEF: Continuous, involuntary urine seepage.

788.39 Other urinary incontinence

✓5th 788.4 Frequency of urination and polyuria

788.41 Urinary frequency
Frequency of micturition

788.42 Polyuria
DEF: Excessive urination.

788.43 Nocturia
DEF: Urination affecting sleep patterns.

788.5 Oliguria and anuria
Deficient secretion of urine
Suppression of urinary secretion
> **EXCLUDES** that complicating:
> abortion (634-638 with .3, 639.3)
> ectopic or molar pregnancy (639.3)
> pregnancy, childbirth, or the puerperium (642.0-642.9, 646.2)

DEF: Oliguria: diminished urinary secretion related to fluid intake.

DEF: Anuria: lack of urinary secretion due to renal failure or obstructed urinary tract.

SYMPTOMS, SIGNS, AND ILL-DEFINED CONDITIONS

✓5ᵗʰ **788.6 Other abnormality of urination**

788.61 Splitting of urinary stream
Intermittent urinary stream

788.62 Slowing of urinary stream
Weak stream

788.69 Other

788.7 Urethral discharge
Penile discharge   Urethrorrhea

788.8 Extravasation of urine
DEF: Leaking or infiltration of urine into tissues.

788.9 Other symptoms involving urinary system
Extrarenal uremia   Vesical:
Vesical: tenesmus
  pain

✓4ᵗʰ **789 Other symptoms involving abdomen and pelvis**

EXCLUDES symptoms referable to genital organs:
  female (625.0-625.9)
  male (607.0-608.9)
  psychogenic (302.70-302.79)

The following fifth-digit subclassification is to be used for codes 789.0, 789.3, 789.4, 789.6:

  0 unspecified site
  1 right upper quadrant
  2 left upper quadrant
  3 right lower quadrant
  4 left lower quadrant
  5 periumbilic
  6 epigastric
  7 generalized
  9 other specified site
    Multiple sites

✓5ᵗʰ **789.0 Abdominal pain**
Colic:
  NOS
  infantile
Cramps, abdominal
EXCLUDES renal colic (788.0)

789.1 Hepatomegaly
Enlargement of liver

789.2 Splenomegaly
Enlargement of spleen

✓5ᵗʰ **789.3 Abdominal or pelvic swelling, mass, or lump**
Diffuse or generalized swelling or mass:
  abdominal NOS
  umbilical
EXCLUDES abdominal distention (gaseous) (787.3)
  ascites (789.5)

✓5ᵗʰ **789.4 Abdominal rigidity**

789.5 Ascites
Fluid in peritoneal cavity
DEF: Serous fluid effusion and accumulation in abdominal cavity.

✓5ᵗʰ **789.6 Abdominal tenderness**
Rebound tenderness

789.9 Other symptoms involving abdomen and pelvis
Umbilical: Umbilical:
  bleeding   discharge

SYMPTOMS, SIGNS, AND ILL-DEFINED CONDITIONS

NONSPECIFIC ABNORMAL FINDINGS (790-796)

√4th 790 Nonspecific findings on examination of blood
> **EXCLUDES** abnormality of:
>   platelets (287.0-287.9)
>   thrombocytes (287.0-287.9)
>   white blood cells (288.0-288.9)

√5th 790.0 Abnormality of red blood cells
> **EXCLUDES** anemia:
>   congenital (776.5)
>   newborn, due to isoimmunization (773.0-773.2, 773.5)
>   of premature infant (776.6)
>   other specified types (280.0-285.9)
> hemoglobin disorders (282.5-282.7)
> polycythemia:
>   familial (289.6)
>   neonatorum (776.4)
>   secondary (289.0)
>   vera (238.4)

790.01 Precipitous drop in hematocrit
Drop in hematocrit

790.09 Other abnormality of red blood cells
Abnormal red cell morphology NOS
Abnormal red cell volume NOS
Anisocytosis
Poikilocytosis

790.1 Elevated sedimentation rate

790.2 Abnormal glucose tolerance test
> **EXCLUDES** that complicating pregnancy, childbirth, or the puerperium (648.8)

790.3 Excessive blood level of alcohol
Elevated blood-alcohol

790.4 Nonspecific elevation of levels of transaminase or lactic acid dehydrogenase [LDH]

790.5 Other nonspecific abnormal serum enzyme levels
Abnormal serum level of:
  acid phosphatase
  alkaline phosphatase
  amylase
  lipase
> **EXCLUDES** deficiency of circulating enzymes (277.6)

790.6 Other abnormal blood chemistry
Abnormal blood level of: Abnormal blood level of:
  cobalt   magnesium
  copper   mineral
  iron   zinc
  lithium
> **EXCLUDES** abnormality of electrolyte or acid-base balance (276.0-276.9)
> hypoglycemia NOS (251.2)
> specific finding indicating abnormality of:
>   amino-acid transport and metabolism (270.0-270.9)
>   carbohydrate transport and metabolism (271.0-271.9)
>   lipid metabolism (272.0-272.9)
> uremia NOS (586)

√4th
√5th Additional Digit Required   Unspecified Code   Other Specified Code   Manifestation Code
MSP Medicare Secondary Payer   ▶◀ Revised Text   ● New Code   ▲ Revised Code Title

SYMPTOMS, SIGNS, AND ILL-DEFINED CONDITIONS

790.7 Bacteremia
  EXCLUDES ▶bacteremia of newborn (771.83)◀
  septicemia (038)
  Use additional code to identify organism (041)
  DEF: Bacterial infection of blood with no signs of infection.

790.8 Viremia, unspecified
  DEF: Presence of a virus in the blood stream.

✓5th **790.9 Other nonspecific findings on examination of blood**
  790.91 Abnormal arterial blood gases
  790.92 Abnormal coagulation profile
  Abnormal or prolonged:
  bleeding time
  coagulation time
  partial thromboplastin time [PTT]
  prothrombintime [PT]
  EXCLUDES coagulation (hemorrhagic) disorders (286.0-286.9)
  790.93 Elevated prostate specific antigen, (PSA) A ♂
  790.94 Euthyroid sick syndrome
  DEF: Transient alteration of thyroid hormone metabolism due to nonthyroid illness or stress.
  790.99 Other

✓4th **791 Nonspecific findings on examination of urine**
  EXCLUDES hematuria NOS (599.7)
  specific findings indicating abnormality of:
  amino-acid transport and metabolism (270.0-270.9)
  carbohydrate transport and metabolism (271.0-271.9)

  791.0 Proteinuria
  Albuminuria   Bence-Jones proteinuria
  EXCLUDES postural proteinuria (593.6)
  that arising during pregnancy or the puerperium (642.0-642.9, 646.2)
  DEF: Excess protein in urine.

  791.1 Chyluria
  EXCLUDES filarial (125.0-125.9)
  DEF: Excess chyle in urine.

  791.2 Hemoglobinuria
  DEF: Free hemoglobin in blood due to rapid hemolysis of red blood cells.

  791.3 Myoglobinuria
  DEF: Myoglobin (oxygen-transporting pigment) in urine.

  791.4 Biliuria
  DEF: Bile pigments in urine.

  791.5 Glycosuria
  EXCLUDES renal glycosuria (271.4)
  DEF: Sugar in urine.

  791.6 Acetonuria
  Ketonuria
  DEF: Excess acetone in urine.

  791.7 Other cells and casts in urine

SYMPTOMS, SIGNS, AND ILL-DEFINED CONDITIONS

791.9 Other nonspecific findings on examination of urine
Crystalluria
Elevated urine levels of:
  17-ketosteroids
  catecholamines
  indolacetic acid
Elevated urine levels of:
  vanillylmandelic acid [VMA]
Melanuria

✓4th **792 Nonspecific abnormal findings in other body substances**
EXCLUDES that in chromosomal analysis (795.2)

792.0 Cerebrospinal fluid

792.1 Stool contents
Abnormal stool color   Occult stool
Fat in stool   Pus in stool
Mucus in stool
EXCLUDES blood in stool [melena] (578.1)
          newborn (772.4, 777.3)

792.2 Semen ♂
Abnormal spermatozoa
EXCLUDES azoospermia (606.0)
          oligospermia (606.1)

792.3 Amniotic fluid M ♀
DEF: Nonspecific abnormal findings in amniotic fluid.

792.4 Saliva
EXCLUDES that in chromosomal analysis (795.2)

792.5 Cloudy (hemodialysis) (peritoneal) dialysis effluent

792.9 Other nonspecific abnormal findings in body substances
Peritoneal fluid   Synovial fluid
Pleural fluid   Vaginal fluids

✓4th **793 Nonspecific abnormal findings on radiological and other examination of body structure**
INCLUDES nonspecific abnormal findings of:
          thermography
          ultrasound examination [echogram]
          x-ray examination
EXCLUDES abnormal results of function studies and radioisotope scans (794.0-794.9)

793.0 Skull and head
EXCLUDES nonspecific abnormal echoencephalogram (794.01)

793.1 Lung field
Coin lesion } (of) lung
Shadow

DEF: Coin lesion of lung: coin-shaped, solitary pulmonary nodule; diagnosis includes tuberculoma, histoplasmoma, blastomycoma, coccidioidomycoma, primary carcinoma of the lung, metastatic carcinoma and benign pulmonary tumor.

793.2 Other intrathoracic organ
Abnormal: Abnormal:
  echocardiogram   ultrasound cardiogram
  heart shadow   Mediastinal shift

793.3 Biliary tract
Nonvisualization of gallbladder

793.4 Gastrointestinal tract

SYMPTOMS, SIGNS, AND ILL-DEFINED CONDITIONS

- **793.5 Genitourinary organs**
  - Filling defect:
    - bladder
    - kidney
  - Filling defect:
    - ureter
- **793.6 Abdominal area, including retroperitoneum**
- **793.7 Musculoskeletal system**
- ✓5th **793.8 Breast**
  - **793.80 Abnormal mammogram, unspecified**
  - **793.81 Mammographic microcalcification**
    - DEF: Calcium and cellular debris deposits in the breast that cannot be felt but can be detected on a mammogram; can be a sign of cancer, benign conditions, or changes in the breast tissue as a result of inflammation, injury, or obstructed duct.
  - **793.89 Other abnormal findings on radiological examination of breast**
- **793.9 Other**
  - Abnormal:
    - placental finding by x-ray or ultrasound method
    - radiological findings in skin and subcutaneous tissue
  - EXCLUDES abnormal finding by radioisotope localization of placenta (794.9)

- ✓4th **794 Nonspecific abnormal results of function studies**
  - INCLUDES radioisotope:
    - scans
    - uptake studies
    - scintiphotography
- ✓5th **794.0 Brain and central nervous system**
  - **794.00 Abnormal function study, unspecified**
  - **794.01 Abnormal echoencephalogram**
  - **794.02 Abnormal electroencephalogram [EEG]**
  - **794.09 Other**
    - Abnormal brain scan
- ✓5th **794.1 Peripheral nervous system and special senses**
  - **794.10 Abnormal response to nerve stimulation, unspecified**
  - **794.11 Abnormal retinal function studies**
    - Abnormal electroretinogram [ERG]
  - **794.12 Abnormal electro-oculogram [EOG]**
  - **794.13 Abnormal visually evoked potential**
  - **794.14 Abnormal oculomotor studies**
  - **794.15 Abnormal auditory function studies**
  - **794.16 Abnormal vestibular function studies**
  - **794.17 Abnormal electromyogram [EMG]**
    - EXCLUDES that of eye (794.14)
  - **794.19 Other**
- **794.2 Pulmonary**
  - Abnormal lung scan
  - Reduced:
    - ventilatory capacity
  - Reduced:
    - vital capacity
- ✓5th **794.3 Cardiovascular**
  - **794.30 Abnormal function study, unspecified**
  - **794.31 Abnormal electrocardiogram [ECG] [EKG]**
  - **794.39 Other**
    - Abnormal:
      - ballistocardiogram
      - phonocardiogram
    - Abnormal:
      - vectorcardiogram

SYMPTOMS, SIGNS, AND ILL-DEFINED CONDITIONS

794.4 Kidney
  Abnormal renal function test

794.5 Thyroid
  Abnormal thyroid: scan
  Abnormal thyroid: uptake

794.6 Other endocrine function study

794.7 Basal metabolism
  Abnormal basal metabolic rate [BMR]

794.8 Liver
  Abnormal liver scan

794.9 Other
  Bladder   Placenta
  Pancreas   Spleen

√4th **795 Nonspecific abnormal histological and immunological findings**
  EXCLUDES   *nonspecific abnormalities of red blood cells (790.01-790.09)*

√5th **795.0 Nonspecific abnormal Papanicolaou smear of cervix**
  EXCLUDES   ▶*carcinoma in-situ of cervix (233.1)*
  cervical intraepithelial neoplasia I (CIN I) (622.1)
  cervical intraepithelial neoplasia II (CIN II) (622.1)
  cervical intraepithelial neoplasia III (CIN III) (233.1)
  dyplasia of cervix (uteri) (622.1)
  high grade squamous intraepithelial dysplasia (HGSIL) (622.1)
  low grade squamous intraepithelial dysplasia (LGSIL) (622.1)◀

● **795.00 Nonspecific abnormal Papanicolaou smear of cervix, unspecified** ♀

● **795.01 Atypical squamous cell changes of undetermined significance favor benign (ASCUS favor benign)** ♀
  Atypical glandular cell changes of undetermined significance favor benign (AGCUS favor benign)

● **795.02 Atypical squamous cell changes of undetermined significance favor dysplasia (ASCUS favor dysplasia)** ♀
  Atypical glandular cell changes of undetermined significance favor dysplasia (AGCUS favor dysplasia)

● **795.09 Other nonspecific abnormal Papanicolaou smear of cervix** ♀
  Benign cellular changes
  Unsatisfactory smear

795.1 Nonspecific abnormal Papanicolaou smear of other site

795.2 Nonspecific abnormal findings on chromosomal analysis
  Abnormal karyotype

√5th **795.3 Nonspecific positive culture findings**
  Positive culture findings in:
    nose
    sputum
    throat
    wound
  EXCLUDES   *that of:*
    blood (790.7-790.8)
    urine (791.9)

● **795.31 Nonspecific positive findings for anthrax**
  Positive findings by nasal swab

● **795.39 Other nonspecific positive culture findings**

795.4 Other nonspecific abnormal histological findings

795.5–798.1 SYMPTOMS, SIGNS, AND ILL-DEFINED CONDITIONS

795.5 Nonspecific reaction to tuberculin skin test without active tuberculosis
Abnormal result of Mantoux test
PPD positive
Tuberculin (skin test):
  positive
  reactor

795.6 False positive serological test for syphilis
False positive Wassermann reaction

√5th **795.7 Other nonspecific immunological findings**
  EXCLUDES: *isoimmunization, in pregnancy (656.1-656.2)*
    affecting fetus or newborn (773.0-773.2)

  795.71 Nonspecific serologic evidence of human immunodeficiency virus [HIV]
    Inclusive human immunodeficiency [HIV] test (adult) (infant)
    Note: This code is ONLY to be used when a test finding is reported as nonspecific. Asymptomatic positive findings are coded to V08. If any HIV infection symptom or condition is present, see code 042. Negative findings are not coded.
    EXCLUDES: *acquired immunodeficiency syndrome [AIDS] (042)*
      asymptomatic human immunodeficiency virus, [HIV] infection status (V08)
      HIV infection, symptomatic (042)
      human immunodeficiency virus [HIV] disease (042)
      positive (status) NOS (V08)

  795.79 Other and unspecified nonspecific immunological findings
    Raised antibody titer
    Raised level of immunoglobulins

√4th **796 Other nonspecific abnormal findings**

  796.0 Nonspecific abnormal toxicological findings
    Abnormal levels of heavy metals or drugs in blood, urine, or other tissue
    EXCLUDES: *excessive blood level of alcohol (790.3)*

  796.1 Abnormal reflex

  796.2 Elevated blood pressure reading without diagnosis of hypertension
    Note: This category is to be used to record an episode of elevated blood pressure in a patient in whom no formal diagnosis of hypertension has been made, or as an incidental finding.

  796.3 Nonspecific low blood pressure reading

  796.4 Other abnormal clinical findings

  796.5 Abnormal finding on antenatal screening   M ♀

  796.9 Other

ILL-DEFINED AND UNKNOWN CAUSES OF MORBIDITY AND MORTALITY (797-799)

797 Senility without mention of psychosis
Old age   Senile:
Senescence   debility
Senile asthenia   exhaustion
  EXCLUDES: *senile psychoses (290.0-290.9)*

√4th **798 Sudden death, cause unknown**

  798.0 Sudden infant death syndrome   P
    Cot death   Sudden death of nonspecific
    Crib death   cause in infancy
    DEF: Sudden Infant Death Syndrome (SIDS): death of infant under age one due to nonspecific cause.

  798.1 Instantaneous death

Maternity Age: 12-55

SYMPTOMS, SIGNS, AND ILL-DEFINED CONDITIONS

798.2 **Death occurring in less than 24 hours from onset of symptoms, not otherwise explained**
Death known not to be violent or instantaneous, for which no cause could be discovered
Died without sign of disease

798.9 **Unattended death**
Death in circumstances where the body of the deceased was found and no cause could be discovered
Found dead

✓4th **799 Other ill-defined and unknown causes of morbidity and mortality**
DEF: Weakened organ functions due to complex chronic medical conditions.

799.0 **Asphyxia**
EXCLUDES asphyxia (due to):
  carbon monoxide (986)
  inhalation of food or foreign body (932-934.9)
  newborn (768.0-768.9)
  traumatic (994.7)
DEF: Lack of oxygen.

799.1 **Respiratory arrest**
Cardiorespiratory failure
EXCLUDES cardiac arrest (427.5)
  failure of peripheral circulation (785.50)
  respiratory distress:
    NOS (786.09)
    acute (518.82)
    following trauma and surgery (518.5)
    newborn ▶(770.89)◀
    syndrome (newborn) (769)
      adult (following trauma and surgery) (518.5)
    other (518.82)
  respiratory failure (518.81, 518.83-518.84)
    newborn ▶(770.84)◀
  respiratory insufficiency (786.09)
    acute (518.82)

799.2 **Nervousness**
"Nerves"

799.3 **Debility, unspecified**
EXCLUDES asthenia (780.79)
  nervous debility (300.5)
  neurasthenia (300.5)
  senile asthenia (797)

799.4 **Cachexia**
Wasting disease
EXCLUDES nutritional marasmus (261)

799.8 **Other ill-defined conditions**
DEF: General ill health and poor nutrition.

799.9 **Other unknown and unspecified cause**
Undiagnosed disease, not specified as to site or system involved
Unknown cause of morbidity or mortality

INJURY AND POISONING

17. INJURY AND POISONING (800-999)

Use E code(s) to identify the cause and intent of the injury or poisoning (E800-E999)

Note:

1. The principle of multiple coding of injuries should be followed wherever possible. Combination categories for multiple injuries are provided for use when there is insufficient detail as to the nature of the individual conditions, or for primary tabulation purposes when it is more convenient to record a single code; otherwise, the component injuries should be coded separately.

   Where multiple sites of injury are specified in the titles, the word "with" indicates involvement of both sites, and the word "and" indicates involvement of either or both sites. The word "finger" thumb.

2. Categories for "late effect" of injuries are to be found at 905-909.

FRACTURES (800-829)

EXCLUDES   malunion (733.81)
nonunion (733.82)
pathological or spontaneous fracture (733.10-733.19)
stress fracture (733.93-733.95)

The terms "condyle," "coronoid process," "ramus," and "symphysis" indicate the portion of the bone fractured, not the name of the bone involved.

The descriptions "closed" and "open" used in the fourth-digit subdivisions include the following terms:

   closed (with or without delayed healing):
      comminuted   impacted
      depressed   linear
      elevated   simple
      fissured   slipped epiphysis
      fracture NOS   spiral
      greenstick
   open (with or without delayed healing):
      compound   puncture
      infected   with foreign body
      missile

A fracture not indicated as closed or open should be classified as closed.

INJURY AND POISONING

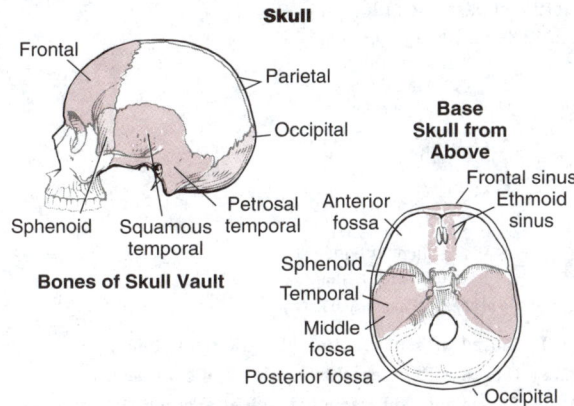

FRACTURE OF SKULL (800-804)

The following fifth-digit subclassification is for use with the appropriate codes in categories 800, 801, 803, and 804:

0 unspecified state of consciousness
1 with no loss of consciousness
2 with brief [less than one hour] loss of consciousness
3 with moderate [1-24 hours] loss of consciousness
4 with prolonged [more than 24 hours] loss of consciousness and return to pre-existing conscious level
5 with prolonged [more than 24 hours] loss of consciousness, without return to pre-existing conscious level
   Use fifth-digit 5 to designate when a patient is unconscious and dies before regaining consciousness, regardless of the duration of the loss of consciousness
6 with loss of consciousness of unspecified duration
9 with concussion, unspecified

✓4th **800 Fracture of vault of skull**
   INCLUDES: frontal bone
              parietal bone
   DEF: Fracture of bone that forms skull dome and protects brain.

§ ✓5th 800.0 Closed without mention of intracranial injury — MSP
§ ✓5th 800.1 Closed with cerebral laceration and contusion — MSP
§ ✓5th 800.2 Closed with subarachnoid, subdural, and extradural hemorrhage — MSP
§ ✓5th 800.3 Closed with other and unspecified intracranial hemorrhage — MSP
§ ✓5th 800.4 Closed with intracranial injury of other and unspecified nature — MSP
§ ✓5th 800.5 Open without mention of intracranial injury — MSP
§ ✓5th 800.6 Open with cerebral laceration and contusion — MSP
§ ✓5th 800.7 Open with subarachnoid, subdural, and extradural hemorrhage — MSP
§ ✓5th 800.8 Open with other and unspecified intracranial hemorrhage — MSP
§ ✓5th 800.9 Open with intracranial injury of other and unspecified nature — MSP

§ Requires fifth-digit. See beginning of section 800–804 for codes and definitions.

✓4th Additional Digit Required
✓5th
MSP Medicare Secondary Payer
▶◀ Revised Text
● New Code
Unspecified Code
Other Specified Code
▲ Revised Code Title
Manifestation Code

2002 Ingenix, Inc.

INJURY AND POISONING

√4ᵗʰ **801 Fracture of base of skull**

INCLUDES: fossa:
    anterior
    middle
    posterior
occiput bone
orbital roof
sinus:
    ethmoid
    frontal
sphenoid bone
temporal bone

DEF: Fracture of bone that forms skull floor.

§ √5ᵗʰ 801.0 Closed without mention of intracranial injury [MSP]
§ √5ᵗʰ 801.1 Closed with cerebral laceration and contusion [MSP]
§ √5ᵗʰ 801.2 Closed with subarachnoid, subdural, and extradural hemorrhage [MSP]
§ √5ᵗʰ 801.3 Closed with other and unspecified intracranial hemorrhage [MSP]
§ √5ᵗʰ 801.4 Closed with intracranial injury of other and unspecified nature [MSP]
§ √5ᵗʰ 801.5 Open without mention of intracranial injury [MSP]
§ √5ᵗʰ 801.6 Open with cerebral laceration and contusion [MSP]
§ √5ᵗʰ 801.7 Open with subarachnoid, subdural, and extradural hemorrhage [MSP]
§ √5ᵗʰ 801.8 Open with other and unspecified intracranial hemorrhage [MSP]
§ √5ᵗʰ 801.9 Open with intracranial injury of other and unspecified nature [MSP]

√4ᵗʰ **802 Fracture of face bones**

    802.0 Nasal bones, closed [MSP]
    802.1 Nasal bones, open [MSP]
√5ᵗʰ 802.2 Mandible, closed
        Inferior maxilla   Lower jaw (bone)
    802.20 Unspecified site [MSP]
    802.21 Condylar process [MSP]
    802.22 Subcondylar [MSP]
    802.23 Coronoid process [MSP]
    802.24 Ramus, unspecified [MSP]
    802.25 Angle of jaw [MSP]
    802.26 Symphysis of body [MSP]
    802.27 Alveolar border of body [MSP]

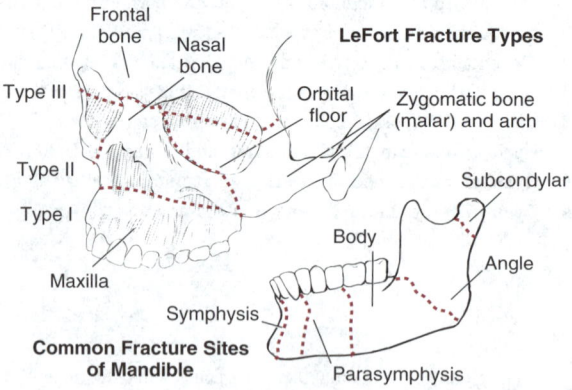

Facial Fractures

§ Requires fifth-digit. See beginning of section 800–804 for codes and definitions.

INJURY AND POISONING

802.28 Body, other and unspecified — MSP
802.29 Multiple sites — MSP

✓5th 802.3 Mandible, open
802.30 Unspecified site — MSP
802.31 Condylar process — MSP
802.32 Subcondylar — MSP
802.33 Coronoid process — MSP
802.34 Ramus, unspecified — MSP
802.35 Angle of jaw — MSP
802.36 Symphysis of body — MSP
802.37 Alveolar border of body — MSP
802.38 Body, other and unspecified — MSP
802.39 Multiple sites — MSP

802.4 Malar and maxillary bones, closed — MSP
  Superior maxilla   Zygoma
  Upper jaw (bone)   Zygomatic arch

802.5 Malar and maxillary bones, open — MSP
802.6 Orbital floor (blow-out), closed — MSP
802.7 Orbital floor (blow-out), open — MSP
802.8 Other facial bones, closed — MSP
  Alveolus
  Orbit:
    NOS
    part other than roof or floor
  Palate
  EXCLUDES orbital:
    floor (802.6)
    roof (801.0-801.9)

802.9 Other facial bones, open — MSP

✓4th 803 Other and unqualified skull fractures
  INCLUDES skull NOS
    skull multiple NOS

§ ✓5th 803.0 Closed without mention of intracranial injury — MSP
§ ✓5th 803.1 Closed with cerebral laceration and contusion — MSP
§ ✓5th 803.2 Closed with subarachnoid, subdural, and extradural hemorrhage — MSP
§ ✓5th 803.3 Closed with other and unspecified intracranial hemorrhage — MSP
§ ✓5th 803.4 Closed with intracranial injury of other and unspecified nature — MSP
§ ✓5th 803.5 Open without mention of intracranial injury — MSP
§ ✓5th 803.6 Open with cerebral laceration and contusion — MSP
§ ✓5th 803.7 Open with subarachnoid, subdural, and extradural hemorrhage — MSP
§ ✓5th 803.8 Open with other and unspecified intracranial hemorrhage — MSP
§ ✓5th 803.9 Open with intracranial injury of other and unspecified nature — MSP

✓4th 804 Multiple fractures involving skull or face with other bones
§ ✓5th 804.0 Closed without mention of intracranial injury — MSP
§ ✓5th 804.1 Closed with cerebral laceration and contusion — MSP
§ ✓5th 804.2 Closed with subarachnoid, subdural, and extradural hemorrhage — MSP
§ ✓5th 804.3 Closed with other and unspecified intracranial hemorrhage — MSP
§ ✓5th 804.4 Closed with intracranial injury of other and unspecified nature — MSP
§ ✓5th 804.5 Open without mention of intracranial injury — MSP
§ ✓5th 804.6 Open with cerebral laceration and contusion — MSP

§ Requires fifth-digit. See beginning of section 800–804 for codes and definitions.

✓4th / ✓5th Additional Digit Required
Unspecified Code
Other Specified Code
Manifestation Code
MSP Medicare Secondary Payer
▶◀ Revised Text
● New Code
▲ Revised Code Title

§ √5th	804.7	Open with subarachnoid, subdural, and extradural hemorrage	MSP
§ √5th	804.8	Open with other and unspecified intracranial hemorrhage	MSP
§ √5th	804.9	Open with intracranial injury of other and unspecified nature	MSP

FRACTURE OF NECK AND TRUNK (805-809)

√4th 805 Fracture of vertebral column without mention of spinal cord injury

INCLUDES   neural arch
spine
spinous process
transverse process
vertebra

The following fifth-digit subclassification is for use with codes 805.0-805.1:
0 cervical vertebra, unspecified level
1 first cervical vertebra
2 second cervical vertebra
3 third cervical vertebra
4 fourth cervical vertebra
5 fifth cervical vertebra
6 sixth cervical vertebra
7 seventh cervical vertebra
8 multiple cervical vertebrae

√5th 805.0 Cervical, closed   MSP
         Atlas   Axis
√5th 805.1 Cervical, open   MSP
      805.2 Dorsal [thoracic], closed   MSP

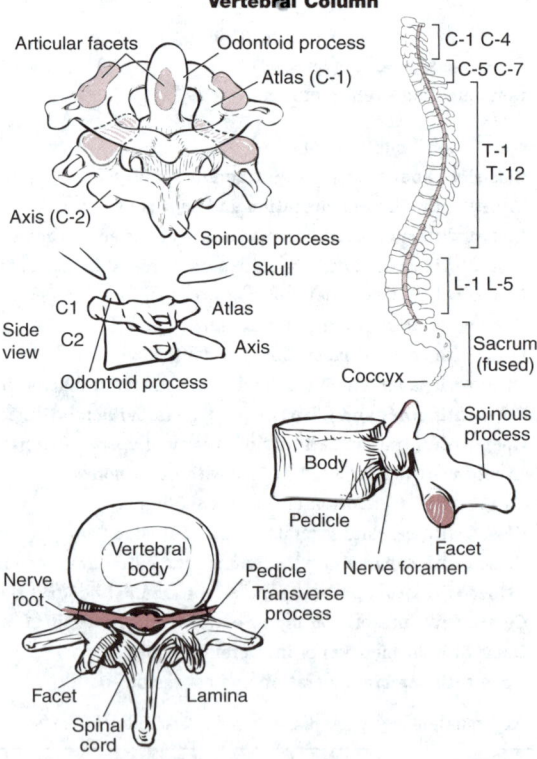

§ Requires fifth-digit. See beginning of section 800–804 for codes and definitions.

N Newborn Age: 0   P Pediatric Age: 0-17   M Maternity Age: 12-55   A Adult Age: 15-124

INJURY AND POISONING

805.3 Dorsal [thoracic], open — MSP
805.4 Lumbar, closed — MSP
805.5 Lumbar, open — MSP
805.6 Sacrum and coccyx, closed — MSP
805.7 Sacrum and coccyx, open — MSP
805.8 Unspecified, closed — MSP
805.9 Unspecified, open — MSP

√4th 806 **Fracture of vertebral column with spinal cord injury**
INCLUDES any condition classifiable to 805 with:
complete or incomplete transverse lesion (of cord)
hematomyelia
injury to:
cauda equina
nerve
paralysis
paraplegia
quadriplegia
spinal concussion

√5th 806.0 Cervical, closed
806.00 C_1-C_4 level with unspecified spinal cord injury — MSP
Cervical region NOS with spinal cord injury NOS
806.01 C_1-C_4 level with complete lesion of cord — MSP
806.02 C_1-C_4 level with anterior cord syndrome — MSP
806.03 C_1-C_4 level with central cord syndrome — MSP
806.04 C_1-C_4 level with other specified spinal cord injury — MSP
C_1-C_4 level with:
incomplete spinal cord lesion NOS
posterior cord syndrome
806.05 C_5-C_7 level with unspecified spinal cord injury — MSP
806.06 C_5-C_7 level with complete lesion of cord — MSP
806.07 C_5-C_7 level with anterior cord syndrome — MSP
806.08 C_5-C_7 level with central cord syndrome — MSP
806.09 C_5-C_7 level with other specified spinal cord injury — MSP
C_5-C_7 level with:
incomplete spinal cord lesion NOS
posterior cord syndrome

√5th 806.1 Cervical, open
806.10 C_1-C_4 level with unspecified spinal cord injury — MSP
806.11 C_1-C_4 level with complete lesion of cord — MSP
806.12 C_1-C_4 level with anterior cord syndrome — MSP
806.13 C_1-C_4 level with central cord syndrome — MSP
806.14 C_1-C_4 level with other specified spinal cord injury — MSP
C_1-C_4 level with:
incomplete spinal cord lesion NOS
posterior cord syndrome
806.15 C_5-C_7 level with unspecified spinal cord injury — MSP
806.16 C_5-C_7 level with complete lesion of cord — MSP
806.17 C_5-C_7 level with anterior cord syndrome — MSP
806.18 C_5-C_7 level with central cord syndrome — MSP
806.19 C_5-C_7 level with other specified spinal cord injury — MSP
C_5-C_7 level with:
incomplete spinal cord lesion NOS
posterior cord syndrome

√4th √5th Additional Digit Required | Unspecified Code | Other Specified Code | Manifestation Code
MSP Medicare Secondary Payer | Revised Text | 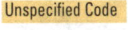 New Code | ▲ Revised Code Title

INJURY AND POISONING

√5th **806.2 Dorsal [thoracic], closed** [MSP]
- 806.20 T_1-T_6 level with unspecified spinal cord injury [MSP]
  Thoracic region NOS with spinal cord injury NOS
- 806.21 T_1-T_6 level with complete lesion of cord [MSP]
- 806.22 T_1-T_6 level with anterior cord syndrome [MSP]
- 806.23 T_1-T_6 level with central cord syndrome [MSP]
- 806.24 T_1-T_6 level with other specified spinal cord injury [MSP]
  T_1-T_6 level with:
    incomplete spinal cord lesion NOS
    posterior cord syndrome
- 806.25 T_7-T_{12} level with unspecified spinal cord injury [MSP]
- 806.26 T_7-T_{12} level with complete lesion of cord [MSP]
- 806.27 T_7-T_{12} level with anterior cord syndrome [MSP]
- 806.28 T_7-T_{12} level with central cord syndrome [MSP]
- 806.29 T_7-T_{12} level with other specified spinal cord injury [MSP]
  T_7-T_{12} level with:
    incomplete spinal cord lesion NOS
    posterior cord syndrome

√5th **806.3 Dorsal [thoracic], open**
- 806.30 T_1-T_6 level with unspecified spinal cord injury [MSP]
- 806.31 T_1-T_6 level with complete lesion of cord [MSP]
- 806.32 T_1-T_6 level with anterior cord syndrome [MSP]
- 806.33 T_1-T_6 level with central cord syndrome [MSP]
- 806.34 T_1-T_6 level with other specified spinal cord injury [MSP]
  T_1-T_6 level with:
    incomplete spinal cord lesion NOS
    posterior cord syndrome
- 806.35 T_7-T_{12} level with unspecified spinal cord injury [MSP]
- 806.36 T_7-T_{12} level with complete lesion of cord [MSP]
- 806.37 T_7-T_{12} level with anterior cord syndrome [MSP]
- 806.38 T_7-T_{12} level with central cord syndrome [MSP]
- 806.39 T_7-T_{12} level with other specified spinal cord injury [MSP]
  T_7-T_{12} level with:
    incomplete spinal cord lesion NOS
    posterior cord syndrome

806.4 Lumbar, closed [MSP]

806.5 Lumbar, open [MSP]

√5th **806.6 Sacrum and coccyx, closed**
- 806.60 With unspecified spinal cord injury [MSP]
- 806.61 With complete cauda equina lesion [MSP]
- 806.62 With other cauda equina injury [MSP]
- 806.69 With other spinal cord injury [MSP]

√5th **806.7 Sacrum and coccyx, open**
- 806.70 With unspecified spinal cord injury [MSP]
- 806.71 With complete cauda equina lesion [MSP]
- 806.72 With other cauda equina injury [MSP]
- 806.79 With other spinal cord injury [MSP]

806.8 Unspecified, closed [MSP]

806.9 Unspecified, open [MSP]

INJURY AND POISONING

✓4th **807 Fracture of rib(s), sternum, larynx, and trachea**

The following fifth-digit subclassification is for use with codes 807.0-807.1:

0 rib(s), unspecified
1 one rib
2 two ribs
3 three ribs
4 four ribs
5 five ribs
6 six ribs
7 seven ribs
8 eight or more ribs
9 multiple ribs, unspecified

- ✓5th 807.0 Rib(s), closed [MSP]
- ✓5th 807.1 Rib(s), open [MSP]
- 807.2 Sternum, closed [MSP]
  DEF: Break in flat bone (breast bone) in anterior thorax.
- 807.3 Sternum, open [MSP]
  DEF: Break, with open wound, in flat bone in mid anterior thorax.
- 807.4 Flail chest [MSP]
- 807.5 Larynx and trachea, closed [MSP]
  Hyoid bone   Trachea
  Thyroid cartilage
- 807.6 Larynx and trachea, open [MSP]

✓4th **808 Fracture of pelvis**

- 808.0 Acetabulum, closed
- 808.1 Acetabulum, open
- 808.2 Pubis, closed
- 808.3 Pubis, open
- ✓5th 808.4 Other specified part, closed
  - 808.41 Ilium
  - 808.42 Ischium
  - 808.43 Multiple pelvic fractures with disruption of pelvic circle
  - 808.49 Other
    Innominate bone
    Pelvic rim

Pelvis and Pelvic Fractures

✓4th
✓5th Additional Digit Required   Unspecified Code   Other Specified Code   Manifestation Code

 Medicare Secondary Payer   ▶◀ Revised Text   ● New Code   ▲ Revised Code Title

2002 Ingenix, Inc.   Volume 1 — 515

808.5–812.09 INJURY AND POISONING

√5th **808.5 Other specified part, open**
- 808.51 Ilium
- 808.52 Ischium
- 808.53 Multiple pelvic fractures with disruption of pelvic circle
- 808.59 Other

808.8 Unspecified, closed
808.9 Unspecified, open

√4th **809 Ill-defined fractures of bones of trunk**

INCLUDES: bones of trunk with other bones except those of skull and face
multiple bones of trunk

EXCLUDES: *multiple fractures of:*
pelvic bones alone (808.0-808.9)
ribs alone (807.0-807.1, 807.4)
ribs or sternum with limb bones (819.0-819.1, 828.0-828.1)
skull or face with other bones (804.0-804.9)

- 809.0 Fracture of bones of trunk, closed
- 809.1 Fracture of bones of trunk, open

FRACTURE OF UPPER LIMB (810-819)

√4th **810 Fracture of clavicle**

INCLUDES: collar bone
interligamentous part of clavicle

The following fifth-digit subclassification is for use with category 810:
- 0 **unspecified part**
  - Clavicle NOS
- 1 **sternal end of clavicle**
- 2 **shaft of clavicle**
- 3 **acromial end of clavicle**

√5th 810.0 Closed MSP
√5th 810.1 Open MSP

√4th **811 Fracture of scapula**

INCLUDES: shoulder blade

The following fifth-digit subclassification is for use with category 811:
- 0 **unspecified part**
- 1 **acromial process**
  - Acromion (process)
- 2 **coracoid process**
- 3 **glenoid cavity and neck of scapula**
- 9 **other**

√5th 811.0 Closed MSP
√5th 811.1 Open MSP

√4th **812 Fracture of humerus**
√5th **812.0 Upper end, closed**
- 812.00 **Upper end, unspecified part**
  - Proximal end   Shoulder
- 812.01 Surgical neck
  - Neck of humerus NOS
- 812.02 Anatomical neck
- 812.03 Greater tuberosity
- 812.09 **Other**
  - Head   Upper epiphysis

N Newborn Age: 0   P Pediatric Age: 0-17   M Maternity Age: 12-55   A Adult Age: 15-124

516 — Volume 1   2002 Ingenix, Inc.

INJURY AND POISONING 812.1–812.42

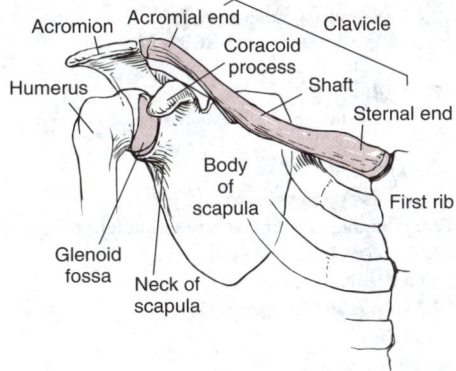

Right Clavicle and Scapula, Anterior View

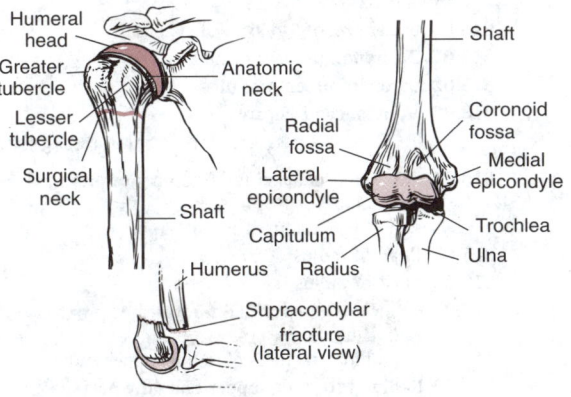

Right Humerus, Anterior View

√5th **812.1 Upper end, open**
812.10 Upper end, unspecified part
812.11 Surgical neck
812.12 Anatomical neck
812.13 Greater tuberosity
812.19 Other

√5th **812.2 Shaft or unspecified part, closed**
812.20 Unspecified part of humerus
  Humerus NOS Upper arm NOS
812.21 Shaft of humerus

√5th **812.3 Shaft or unspecified part, open**
812.30 Unspecified part of humerus
812.31 Shaft of humerus

√5th **812.4 Lower end, closed**
  Distal end of humerus
  Elbow
812.40 Lower end, unspecified part
812.41 Supracondylar fracture of humerus
812.42 Lateral condyle
  External condyle

√4th / √5th Additional Digit Required   Unspecified Code   Other Specified Code   Manifestation Code
MSP Medicare Secondary Payer   ◄► Revised Text   ● New Code   ▲ Revised Code Title

2002 Ingenix, Inc.   Volume 1 — 517

812.43–813.13 INJURY AND POISONING

- 812.43 Medial condyle
  - Internal epicondyle
- 812.44 Condyle(s), unspecified
  - Articular process NOS
  - Lower epiphysis NOS
- 812.49 Other
  - Multiple fractures of lower end
  - Trochlea

√5th 812.5 Lower end, open
- 812.50 Lower end, unspecified part
- 812.51 Supracondylar fracture of humerus
- 812.52 Lateral condyle
- 812.53 Medial condyle
- 812.54 Condyle(s), unspecified
- 812.59 Other

√4th 813 Fracture of radius and ulna

√5th 813.0 Upper end, closed
  - Proximal end
- 813.00 Upper end of forearm, unspecified
- 813.01 Olecranon process of ulna
- 813.02 Coronoid process of ulna
- 813.03 Monteggia's fracture
  - **DEF:** Fracture near the head of the ulnar shaft, causing dislocation of the radial head.
- 813.04 Other and unspecified fractures of proximal end of ulna (alone)
  - Multiple fractures of ulna, upper end
- 813.05 Head of radius
- 813.06 Neck of radius
- 813.07 Other and unspecified fractures of proximal end of radius (alone)
  - Multiple fractures of radius, upper end
- 813.08 Radius with ulna, upper end [any part]

√5th 813.1 Upper end, open
- 813.10 Upper end of forearm, unspecified
- 813.11 Olecranon process of ulna
- 813.12 Coronoid process of ulna
- 813.13 Monteggia's fracture

Right Radius and Ulna, Anterior View

INJURY AND POISONING

  813.14 **Other and unspecified fractures of proximal end of ulna (alone)**
  813.15 Head of radius
  813.16 Neck of radius
  813.17 **Other and unspecified fractures of proximal end of radius (alone)**
  813.18 Radius with ulna, upper end [any part]

✓5th 813.2 Shaft, closed
  813.20 **Shaft, unspecified**
  813.21 Radius (alone)
  813.22 Ulna (alone)
  813.23 Radius with ulna

✓5th 813.3 Shaft, open
  813.30 **Shaft, unspecified**
  813.31 Radius (alone)
  813.32 Ulna (alone)
  813.33 Radius with ulna

✓5th 813.4 Lower end, closed
   Distal end
  813.40 **Lower end of forearm, unspecified**
  813.41 Colles' fracture
   Smith's fracture
   DEF: Break of lower end of radius; associated with backward movement of the radius lower section.
  813.42 **Other fractures of distal end of radius (alone)**
   Dupuytren's fracture, radius
   Radius, lower end
   DEF: Dupuytren's fracture: fracture and dislocation of the forearm; the fracture is of the radius above the wrist, and the dislocation is of the ulna at the lower end.
  813.43 Distal end of ulna (alone)
   Ulna: Ulna:
    head   lower epiphysis
    lower end styloid process
  813.44 Radius with ulna, lower end
  813.45 Torus fracture of radius

✓5th 813.5 Lower end, open
  813.50 **Lower end of forearm, unspecified**
  813.51 Colles' fracture
  813.52 **Other fractures of distal end of radius (alone)**
  813.53 Distal end of ulna (alone)
  813.54 Radius with ulna, lower end

✓5th 813.8 Unspecified part, closed
  813.80 **Forearm, unspecified**
  813.81 **Radius (alone)**
  813.82 **Ulna (alone)**
  813.83 **Radius with ulna**

✓5th 813.9 Unspecified part, open
  813.90 **Forearm, unspecified**
  813.91 **Radius (alone)**
  813.92 **Ulna (alone)**
  813.93 **Radius with ulna**

✓4th / ✓5th Additional Digit Required **Unspecified Code** Other Specified Code Manifestation Code
MSP Medicare Secondary Payer ▶◀ Revised Text ● New Code ▲ Revised Code Title

814–816 INJURY AND POISONING

✓4th 814 Fracture of carpal bone(s)

The following fifth-digit subclassification is for use with category 814:
- 0 carpal bone, unspecified
  - Wrist NOS
- 1 navicular [scaphoid] of wrist
- 2 lunate [semilunar] bone of wrist
- 3 triquetral [cuneiform] bone of wrist
- 4 pisiform
- 5 trapezium bone [larger multangular]
- 6 trapezoid bone [smaller multangular]
- 7 capitate bone [os magnum]
- 8 hamate [unciform] bone
- 9 other

✓5th 814.0 Closed
✓5th 814.1 Open

✓4th 815 Fracture of metacarpal bone(s)

INCLUDES   hand [except finger]
           metacarpus

The following fifth-digit subclassification is for use with category 815:
- 0 metacarpal bone(s), site unspecified
- 1 base of thumb [first] metacarpal
  - Bennett's fracture
- 2 base of other metacarpal bone(s)
- 3 shaft of metacarpal bone(s)
- 4 neck of metacarpal bone(s)
- 9 multiple sites of metacarpus

✓5th 815.0 Closed
✓5th 815.1 Open

✓4th 816 Fracture of one or more phalanges of hand

INCLUDES   finger(s) thumb

The following fifth-digit subclassification is for use with category 816:
- 0 phalanx or phalanges, unspecified
- 1 middle or proximal phalanx or phalanges
- 2 distal phalanx or phalanges
- 3 multiple sites

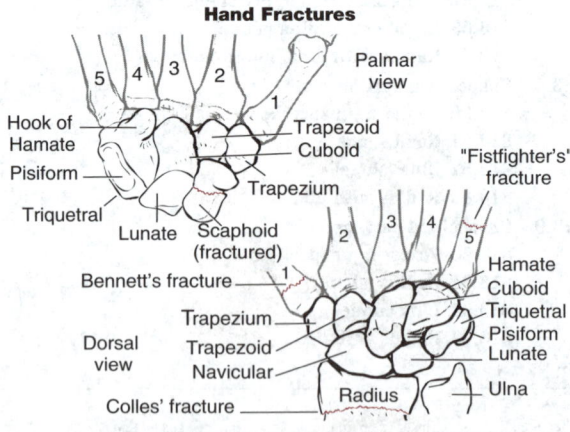

Hand Fractures

INJURY AND POISONING

    √5th 816.0 Closed
    √5th 816.1 Open

√4th **817** **Multiple fractures of hand bones**
        INCLUDES metacarpal bone(s) with phalanx or phalanges of same hand
    817.0 Closed
    817.1 Open

√4th **818** **Ill-defined fractures of upper limb**
        INCLUDES arm NOS
                      multiple bones of same upper limb
        EXCLUDES *multiple fractures of:*
                      metacarpal bone(s) with phalanx or phalanges (817.0-817.1)
                      phalanges of hand alone (816.0-816.1)
                      radius with ulna (813.0-813.9)
    818.0 Closed
    818.1 Open

√4th **819** **Multiple fractures involving both upper limbs, and upper limb with rib(s) and sternum**
        INCLUDES arm(s) with rib(s) or sternum
                      both arms [any bones]
    819.0 Closed
    819.1 Open

FRACTURE OF LOWER LIMB (820-829)

√4th **820** **Fracture of neck of femur**
    √5th 820.0 **Transcervical fracture, closed**
        820.00 Intracapsular section, unspecified
        820.01 Epiphysis (separation) (upper)
                  Transepiphyseal
        820.02 Midcervical section
                  Transcervical NOS
        820.03 Base of neck
                  Cervicotrochanteric section
        820.09 Other
                  Head of femur   Subcapital

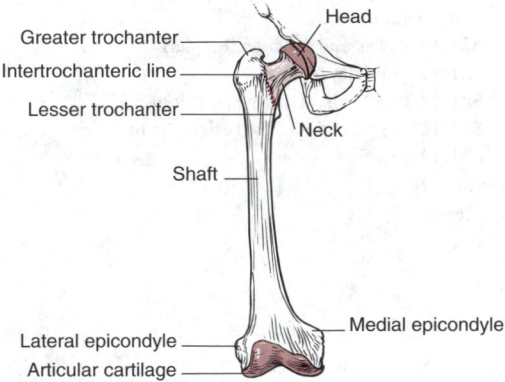

Right Femur, Anterior View

INJURY AND POISONING

- √5th **820.1** Transcervical fracture, open
  - 820.10 Intracapsular section, unspecified
  - 820.11 Epiphysis (separation) (upper)
  - 820.12 Midcervical section
  - 820.13 Base of neck
  - 820.19 Other
- √5th **820.2** Pertrochanteric fracture, closed
  - 820.20 Trochanteric section, unspecified
    - Trochanter: NOS
    - Trochanter: lesser
    - Trochanter: greater
  - 820.21 Intertrochanteric section
  - 820.22 Subtrochanteric section
- √5th **820.3** Pertrochanteric fracture, open
  - 820.30 Trochanteric section, unspecified
  - 820.31 Intertrochanteric section
  - 820.32 Subtrochanteric section
- **820.8** Unspecified part of neck of femur, closed
  - Hip NOS   Neck of femur NOS
- **820.9** Unspecified part of neck of femur, open

√4th **821** Fracture of other and unspecified parts of femur
- √5th **821.0** Shaft or unspecified part, closed
  - 821.00 Unspecified part of femur
    - Thigh   Upper leg
    - **EXCLUDES** hip NOS (820.8)
  - 821.01 Shaft
- √5th **821.1** Shaft or unspecified part, open
  - 821.10 Unspecified part of femur
  - 821.11 Shaft
- √5th **821.2** Lower end, closed
  - Distal end
  - 821.20 Lower end, unspecified part
  - 821.21 Condyle, femoral
  - 821.22 Epiphysis, lower (separation)
  - 821.23 Supracondylar fracture of femur
    - Multiple fractures of lower end
  - 821.29 Other
    - Multiple fractures of lower end
- √5th **821.3** Lower end, open
  - 821.30 Lower end, unspecified part
  - 821.31 Condyle, femoral
  - 821.32 Epiphysis, lower (separation)
  - 821.33 Supracondylar fracture of femur
  - 821.39 Other

√4th **822** Fracture of patella
- **822.0** Closed
- **822.1** Open

INJURY AND POISONING

Right Tibula and Fibula, Anterior View

√4th **823 Fracture of tibia and fibula**

> **EXCLUDES**   Dupuytren's fracture (824.4-824.5)
> ankle (824.4-824.5)
> radius (813.42, 813.52)
> Pott's fracture (824.4-824.5)
> that involving ankle (824.0-824.9)

The following fifth-digit subclassification is for use with category 823:
 0 tibia alone
 1 fibula alone
 2 fibula with tibia

√5th 823.0 **Upper end, closed**
  Head   Tibia:
  Proximal end   condyles
                      tuberosity

√5th 823.1 **Upper end, open**
√5th 823.2 **Shaft, closed**
√5th 823.3 **Shaft, open**
● √5th 823.4 **Torus fracture**
√5th 823.8 **Unspecified part, closed**
  Lower leg NOS
√5th 823.9 **Unspecified part, open**

√4th **824 Fracture of ankle**

824.0 **Medial malleolus, closed**
  Tibia involving: Tibia involving:
    ankle   malleolus
824.1 **Medial malleolus, open**
824.2 **Lateral malleolus, closed**
  Fibula involving: Fibula involving:
    ankle   malleolus
824.3 **Lateral malleolus, open**
824.4 **Bimalleolar, closed**
  Dupuytren's fracture, fibula   Pott's fracture

DEF: Bimalleolar, closed: Breaking of both nodules (malleoli) on either side of ankle joint, without an open wound.

DEF: Dupuytren's fracture (Pott's fracture): The breaking of the farthest end of the lower leg bone (fibula), with injury to the farthest end joint of the other lower leg bone (tibia).

824.5–826.1 — **INJURY AND POISONING**

- 824.5 **Bimalleolar, open**
- 824.6 **Trimalleolar, closed**
    Lateral and medial malleolus with anterior or posterior lip of tibia
- 824.7 **Trimalleolar, open**
- 824.8 **Unspecified, closed**
    Ankle NOS
- 824.9 **Unspecified, open**

✓4th **825 Fracture of one or more tarsal and metatarsal bones**
- 825.0 **Fracture of calcaneus, closed**
    Heel bone   Os calcis
- 825.1 **Fracture of calcaneus, open**

✓5th 825.2 **Fracture of other tarsal and metatarsal bones, closed**
- 825.20 **Unspecified bone(s) of foot [except toes]**
    Instep
- 825.21 **Astragalus**
    Talus
- 825.22 **Navicular [scaphoid], foot**
- 825.23 **Cuboid**
- 825.24 **Cuneiform, foot**
- 825.25 **Metatarsal bone(s)**
- 825.29 **Other**
    Tarsal with metatarsal bone(s) only
    EXCLUDES calcaneus (825.0)

✓5th 825.3 **Fracture of other tarsal and metatarsal bones, open**
- 825.30 **Unspecified bone(s) of foot [except toes]**
- 825.31 **Astragalus**
- 825.32 **Navicular [scaphoid], foot**
- 825.33 **Cuboid**
- 825.34 **Cuneiform, foot**
- 825.35 **Metatarsal bone(s)**
- 825.39 **Other**

✓4th **826 Fracture of one or more phalanges of foot**
    INCLUDES toe(s)
- 826.0 **Closed**
- 826.1 **Open**

Right Foot, Dorsal

N Newborn Age: 0   P Pediatric Age: 0–17   M Maternity Age: 12–55   A Adult Age: 15–124

2002 Ingenix, Inc.

INJURY AND POISONING

✓4th 827 Other, multiple, and ill-defined fractures of lower limb
- INCLUDES: leg NOS
  multiple bones of same lower limb
- EXCLUDES: multiple fractures of:
  - ankle bones alone (824.4-824.9)
  - phalanges of foot alone (826.0-826.1)
  - tarsal with metatarsal bones (825.29, 825.39)
  - tibia with fibula (823.0-823.9 with fifth-digit 2)

- 827.0 Closed
- 827.1 Open

✓4th 828 Multiple fractures involving both lower limbs, lower with upper limb, and lower limb(s) with rib(s) and sternum
- INCLUDES:
  - arm(s) with leg(s) [any bones]
  - both legs [any bones]
  - leg(s) with rib(s) or sternum

- 828.0 Closed MSP
- 828.1 Open MSP

✓4th 829 Fracture of unspecified bones
- 829.0 Unspecified bone, closed
- 829.1 Unspecified bone, open

DISLOCATION (830-839)

- INCLUDES:
  - displacement
  - subluxation
- EXCLUDES:
  - congenital dislocation (754.0-755.8)
  - pathological dislocation (718.2)
  - recurrent dislocation (718.3)

The descriptions "closed" and "open," used in the fourth-digit subdivisions, include the following terms:

closed:
- complete
- dislocation NOS
- partial
- simple
- uncomplicated

open:
- compound
- infected
- with foreign body

A dislocation not indicated as closed or open should be classified as closed.

✓4th 830 Dislocation of jaw
- INCLUDES:
  - jaw (cartilage) (meniscus)
  - mandible
  - maxilla (inferior)
  - temporomandibular (joint)

- 830.0 Closed dislocation
- 830.1 Open dislocation

INJURY AND POISONING

✓4th **831 Dislocation of shoulder**
> EXCLUDES: sternoclavicular joint (839.61, 839.71)
> sternum (839.61, 839.71)

The following fifth-digit subclassification is for use with category 831:
- 0 shoulder, unspecified
  Humerus NOS
- 1 anterior dislocation of humerus
- 2 posterior dislocation of humerus
- 3 inferior dislocation of humerus
- 4 acromioclavicular (joint)
  Clavicle
- 9 other
  Scapula

✓5th **831.0 Closed dislocation**
✓5th **831.1 Open dislocation**

✓4th **832 Dislocation of elbow**

The following fifth-digit subclassification is for use with category 832:
- 0 elbow unspecified
- 1 anterior dislocation of elbow
- 2 posterior dislocation of elbow
- 3 medial dislocation of elbow
- 4 lateral dislocation of elbow
- 9 other

✓5th **832.0 Closed dislocation**
✓5th **832.1 Open dislocation**

✓4th **833 Dislocation of wrist**

The following fifth-digit subclassification is for use with category 833:
- 0 wrist, unspecified part
  Carpal (bone)
  Radius, distal end
- 1 radioulnar (joint), distal
- 2 radiocarpal (joint)
- 3 midcarpal (joint)
- 4 carpometacarpal (joint)
- 5 metacarpal (bone), proximal end
- 9 other
  Ulna, distal end

✓5th **833.0 Closed dislocation**
✓5th **833.1 Open dislocation**

✓4th **834 Dislocation of finger**
> INCLUDES: finger(s)
> phalanx of hand
> thumb

The following fifth-digit subclassification is for use with category 834:
- 0 finger, unspecified part
- 1 metacarpophalangeal (joint)
  Metacarpal (bone), distal end
- 2 interphalangeal (joint), hand

✓5th **834.0 Closed dislocation**
✓5th **834.1 Open dislocation**

N Newborn Age: 0   P Pediatric Age: 0-17   M Maternity Age: 12-55   A Adult Age: 15-124

INJURY AND POISONING

✓4th 835 Dislocation of hip

The following fifth-digit subclassification is for use with category 835:
- 0 dislocation of hip, unspecified
- 1 posterior dislocation
- 2 obturator dislocation
- 3 other anterior dislocation

✓5th 835.0 Closed dislocation
✓5th 835.1 Open dislocation

✓4th 836 Dislocation of knee

EXCLUDES dislocation of knee:
old or pathological (718.2)
recurrent (718.3)
internal derangement of knee joint (717.0-717.5, 717.8-717.9)
old tear of cartilage or meniscus of knee (717.0-717.5, 717.8-717.9)

836.0 Tear of medial cartilage or meniscus of knee, current
Bucket handle tear:
 NOS
 medial meniscus } current injury

836.1 Tear of lateral cartilage or meniscus of knee, current

836.2 Other tear of cartilage or meniscus of knee, current
Tear of:
 cartilage
  (semilunar)
 meniscus } current injury, not specified as medial or lateral

836.3 Dislocation of patella, closed
836.4 Dislocation of patella, open

✓5th 836.5 Other dislocation of knee, closed
- 836.50 Dislocation of knee, unspecified
- 836.51 Anterior dislocation of tibia, proximal end
   Posterior dislocation of femur, distal end
- 836.52 Posterior dislocation of tibia, proximal end
   Anterior dislocation of femur, distal end
- 836.53 Medial dislocation of tibia, proximal end
- 836.54 Lateral dislocation of tibia, proximal end
- 836.59 Other

✓5th 836.6 Other dislocation of knee, open
- 836.60 Dislocation of knee, unspecified
- 836.61 Anterior dislocation of tibia, proximal end
- 836.62 Posterior dislocation of tibia, proximal end
- 836.63 Medial dislocation of tibia, proximal end
- 836.64 Lateral dislocation of tibia, proximal end
- 836.69 Other

✓4th 837 Dislocation of ankle

INCLUDES astragalus
fibula, distal end
navicular, foot
scaphoid, foot
tibia, distal end

837.0 Closed dislocation
837.1 Open dislocation

✓4th
✓5th Additional Digit Required | Unspecified Code | Other Specified Code | Manifestation Code
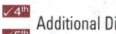 Medicare Secondary Payer | ▶◀ Revised Text | ● New Code | ▲ Revised Code Title

2002 Ingenix, Inc.

INJURY AND POISONING

✓4ᵗʰ 838 Dislocation of foot

The following fifth-digit subclassification is for use with category 838:
- 0 foot, unspecified
- 1 tarsal (bone), joint unspecified
- 2 midtarsal (joint)
- 3 tarsometatarsal (joint)
- 4 metatarsal (bone), joint unspecified
- 5 metatarsophalangeal (joint)
- 6 interphalangeal (joint), foot
- 9 other
   - Phalanx of foot
   - Toe(s)

✓5ᵗʰ **838.0** Closed dislocation
✓5ᵗʰ **838.1** Open dislocation

✓4ᵗʰ 839 Other, multiple, and ill-defined dislocations

✓5ᵗʰ **839.0** Cervical vertebra, closed
    Cervical spine   Neck
- 839.00 Cervical vertebra, unspecified — MSP
- 839.01 First cervical vertebra — MSP
- 839.02 Second cervical vertebra — MSP
- 839.03 Third cervical vertebra — MSP
- 839.04 Fourth cervical vertebra — MSP
- 839.05 Fifth cervical vertebra — MSP
- 839.06 Sixth cervical vertebra — MSP
- 839.07 Seventh cervical vertebra — MSP
- 839.08 Multiple cervical vertebrae — MSP

✓5ᵗʰ **839.1** Cervical vertebra, open
- 839.10 Cervical vertebra, unspecified — MSP
- 839.11 First cervical vertebra — MSP
- 839.12 Second cervical vertebra — MSP
- 839.13 Third cervical vertebra — MSP
- 839.14 Fourth cervical vertebra — MSP
- 839.15 Fifth cervical vertebra — MSP
- 839.16 Sixth cervical vertebra — MSP
- 839.17 Seventh cervical vertebra — MSP
- 839.18 Multiple cervical vertebrae — MSP

✓5ᵗʰ **839.2** Thoracic and lumbar vertebra, closed
- 839.20 Lumbar vertebra — MSP
- 839.21 Thoracic vertebra — MSP
   - Dorsal [thoracic] vertebra

✓5ᵗʰ **839.3** Thoracic and lumbar vertebra, open
- 839.30 Lumbar vertebra — MSP
- 839.31 Thoracic vertebra — MSP

✓5ᵗʰ **839.4** Other vertebra, closed
- 839.40 Vertebra, unspecified site
   - Spine NOS
- 839.41 Coccyx
- 839.42 Sacrum
   - Sacroiliac (joint)
- 839.49 Other

N Newborn Age: 0   **P** Pediatric Age: 0-17   **M** Maternity Age: 12-55   **A** Adult Age: 15-124

INJURY AND POISONING

√5ᵗʰ **839.5 Other vertebra, open**
    839.50 Vertebra, unspecified site
    839.51 Coccyx
    839.52 Sacrum
    839.59 Other

√5ᵗʰ **839.6 Other location, closed**
    839.61 Sternum
        Sternoclavicular joint
    839.69 Other
        Pelvis

√5ᵗʰ **839.7 Other location, open**
    839.71 Sternum   MSP
    839.79 Other   MSP

839.8 Multiple and ill-defined, closed   MSP
    Arm
    Back
    Hand
    Multiple locations, except fingers or toes alone
    Other ill-defined locations
    Unspecified location

839.9 Multiple and ill-defined, open   MSP

SPRAINS AND STRAINS OF JOINTS AND ADJACENT MUSCLES (840-848)

INCLUDES   avulsion
                hemarthrosis
                laceration   of:
                rupture   joint capsule
                sprain   ligament
                strain   muscle
                tear   tendon

EXCLUDES   *laceration of tendon in open wounds (880-884 and 890-894 with .2)*

√4ᵗʰ **840 Sprains and strains of shoulder and upper arm**
    840.0 Acromioclavicular (joint) (ligament)
    840.1 Coracoclavicular (ligament)
    840.2 Coracohumeral (ligament)
    840.3 Infraspinatus (muscle) (tendon)
    840.4 Rotator cuff (capsule)
        EXCLUDES   *complete rupture of rotator cuff, nontraumatic (727.61)*
    840.5 Subscapularis (muscle)
    840.6 Supraspinatus (muscle) (tendon)
    840.7 Superior glenoid labrum lesion
        SLAP lesion
        DEF: Detachment injury of the superior aspect of the glenoid labrum which is the ring of fibrocartilage attached to the rim of the glenoid cavity of the scapula.
    840.8 Other specified sites of shoulder and upper arm
    840.9 Unspecified site of shoulder and upper arm
        Arm NOS   Shoulder NOS

√4ᵗʰ **841 Sprains and strains of elbow and forearm**
    841.0 Radial collateral ligament
    841.1 Ulnar collateral ligament
    841.2 Radiohumeral (joint)
    841.3 Ulnohumeral (joint)

√4ᵗʰ / √5ᵗʰ Additional Digit Required   Unspecified Code   Other Specified Code   Manifestation Code
MSP Medicare Secondary Payer   ▶◀ Revised Text   ● New Code   ▲ Revised Code Title

841.8–846.2 INJURY AND POISONING

- 841.8 **Other specified sites of elbow and forearm**
- 841.9 **Unspecified site of elbow and forearm**
  Elbow NOS

✓4th 842 Sprains and strains of wrist and hand
 ✓5th 842.0 Wrist
  - 842.00 **Unspecified site**
  - 842.01 Carpal (joint)
  - 842.02 Radiocarpal (joint) (ligament)
  - 842.09 **Other**
    Radioulnar joint, distal
 ✓5th 842.1 Hand
  - 842.10 **Unspecified site**
  - 842.11 Carpometacarpal (joint)
  - 842.12 Metacarpophalangeal (joint)
  - 842.13 Interphalangeal (joint)
  - 842.19 **Other**
    Midcarpal (joint)

✓4th 843 Sprains and strains of hip and thigh
- 843.0 Iliofemoral (ligament)
- 843.1 Ischiocapsular (ligament)
- 843.8 **Other specified sites of hip and thigh**
- 843.9 **Unspecified site of hip and thigh**
  Hip NOS
  Thigh NOS

✓4th 844 Sprains and strains of knee and leg
- 844.0 Lateral collateral ligament of knee
- 844.1 Medial collateral ligament of knee
- 844.2 Cruciate ligament of knee
- 844.3 Tibiofibular (joint) (ligament), superior
- 844.8 **Other specified sites of knee and leg**
- 844.9 **Unspecified site of knee and leg**
  Knee NOS   Leg NOS

✓4th 845 Sprains and strains of ankle and foot
 ✓5th 845.0 Ankle
  - 845.00 **Unspecified site**
  - 845.01 Deltoid (ligament), ankle
    Internal collateral (ligament), ankle
  - 845.02 Calcaneofibular (ligament)
  - 845.03 Tibiofibular (ligament), distal
  - 845.09 **Other**
    Achilles tendon
 ✓5th 845.1 Foot
  - 845.10 **Unspecified site**
  - 845.11 Tarsometatarsal (joint) (ligament)
  - 845.12 Metatarsophalangeal (joint)
  - 845.13 Interphalangeal (joint), toe
  - 845.19 **Other**

✓4th 846 Sprains and strains of sacroiliac region
- 846.0 Lumbosacral (joint) (ligament)
- 846.1 Sacroiliac ligament
- 846.2 Sacrospinatus (ligament)

N Newborn Age: 0   P Pediatric Age: 0-17   M Maternity Age: 12-55   A Adult Age: 15-124

INJURY AND POISONING

846.3 **Sacrotuberous (ligament)**
846.8 Other specified sites of sacroiliac region
846.9 Unspecified site of sacroiliac region

✓4ᵗʰ **847 Sprains and strains of other and unspecified parts of back**
    EXCLUDES lumbosacral (846.0)

847.0 **Neck** [MSP]
    Anterior longitudinal (ligament), cervical
    Atlanto-axial (joints)
    Atlanto-occipital (joints)
    Whiplash injury
        EXCLUDES neck injury NOS (959.0)
            thyroid region (848.2)

847.1 **Thoracic**
847.2 **Lumbar**
847.3 **Sacrum**
    Sacrococcygeal (ligament)
847.4 **Coccyx**
847.9 Unspecified site of back
    Back NOS

✓4ᵗʰ **848 Other and ill-defined sprains and strains**
848.0 **Septal cartilage of nose**
848.1 **Jaw**
    Temporomandibular (joint) (ligament)
848.2 **Thyroid region**
    Cricoarytenoid (joint) (ligament)
    Cricothyroid (joint) (ligament)
    Thyroid cartilage
848.3 **Ribs**
    Chondrocostal (joint) } without mention of injury to sternum
    Costal cartilage

✓5ᵗʰ 848.4 **Sternum**
    848.40 Unspecified site
    848.41 **Sternoclavicular (joint) (ligament)**
    848.42 **Chondrosternal (joint)**
    848.49 Other
        Xiphoid cartilage
848.5 **Pelvis**
    Symphysis pubis
        EXCLUDES that in childbirth (665.6)
848.8 Other specified sites of sprains and strains
848.9 Unspecified site of sprain and strain

 Additional Digit Required   Unspecified Code   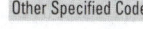 Other Specified Code   Manifestation Code
[MSP] Medicare Secondary Payer   ▶◀ Revised Text   ● New Code   ▲ Revised Code Title

850–851.5 INJURY AND POISONING

INTRACRANIAL INJURY, EXCLUDING THOSE WITH SKULL FRACTURE (850-854)

EXCLUDES intracranial injury with skull fracture (800-801 and 803-804, except .0 and .5)
open wound of head without intracranial injury (870.0-873.9)
skull fracture alone (800-801 and 803-804 with .0, .5)

The description "with open intracranial wound," used in the fourth-digit subdivisions, those specified as open or with mention of infection or foreign body.

The following fifth-digit subclassification is for use with categories 851-854:
- 0 **unspecified state of consciousness**
- 1 with no loss of consciousness
- 2 with brief [less than one hour] loss of consciousness
- 3 with moderate [1-24 hours] loss of consciousness
- 4 with prolonged [more than 24 hours] loss of consciousness and return to pre-existing conscious level
- 5 with prolonged [more than 24 hours] loss of consciousness, without return to pre-existing conscious level
  - Use fifth-digit 5 to designate when a patient is unconscious and dies before regaining consciousness, regardless of the duration of the loss of consciousness
- 6 **with loss of consciousness of unspecified duration**
- 9 **with concussion, unspecified**

✓4th **850 Concussion**
  - **INCLUDES** commotio cerebri
  - **EXCLUDES** concussion with:
    - cerebral laceration or contusion (851.0-851.9)
    - cerebral hemorrhage (852-853)
    - head injury NOS (959.01)

  - **850.0 With no loss of consciousness** [MSP]
    - Concussion with mental confusion or disorientation, without loss of consciousness
  - **850.1 With brief loss of consciousness** [MSP]
    - Loss of consciousness for less than one hour
  - **850.2 With moderate loss of consciousness** [MSP]
    - Loss of consciousness for 1-24 hours
  - **850.3 With prolonged loss of consciousness and return to pre-existing conscious level** [MSP]
    - Loss of consciousness for more than 24 hours with complete recovery
  - **850.4 With prolonged loss of consciousness, without return to pre-existing conscious level** [MSP]
  - **850.5 With loss of consciousness of unspecified duration** [MSP]
  - **850.9 Concussion, unspecified** [MSP]

✓4th **851 Cerebral laceration and contusion**
  - § ✓5th **851.0 Cortex (cerebral) contusion without mention of open intracranial wound** [MSP]
  - § ✓5th **851.1 Cortex (cerebral) contusion with open intracranial wound** [MSP]
  - § ✓5th **851.2 Cortex (cerebral) laceration without mention of open intracranial wound** [MSP]
  - § ✓5th **851.3 Cortex (cerebral) laceration with open intracranial wound** [MSP]
  - § ✓5th **851.4 Cerebellar or brain stem contusion without mention of open intracranial wound** [MSP]
  - § ✓5th **851.5 Cerebellar or brain stem contusion with open intracranial wound** [MSP]

§ Requires fifth-digit. See beginning of section 850–854 for codes and definitions.

[N] Newborn Age: 0   [P] Pediatric Age: 0-17   [M] Maternity Age: 12-55   [A] Adult Age: 15-124

INJURY AND POISONING 851.6–852.2

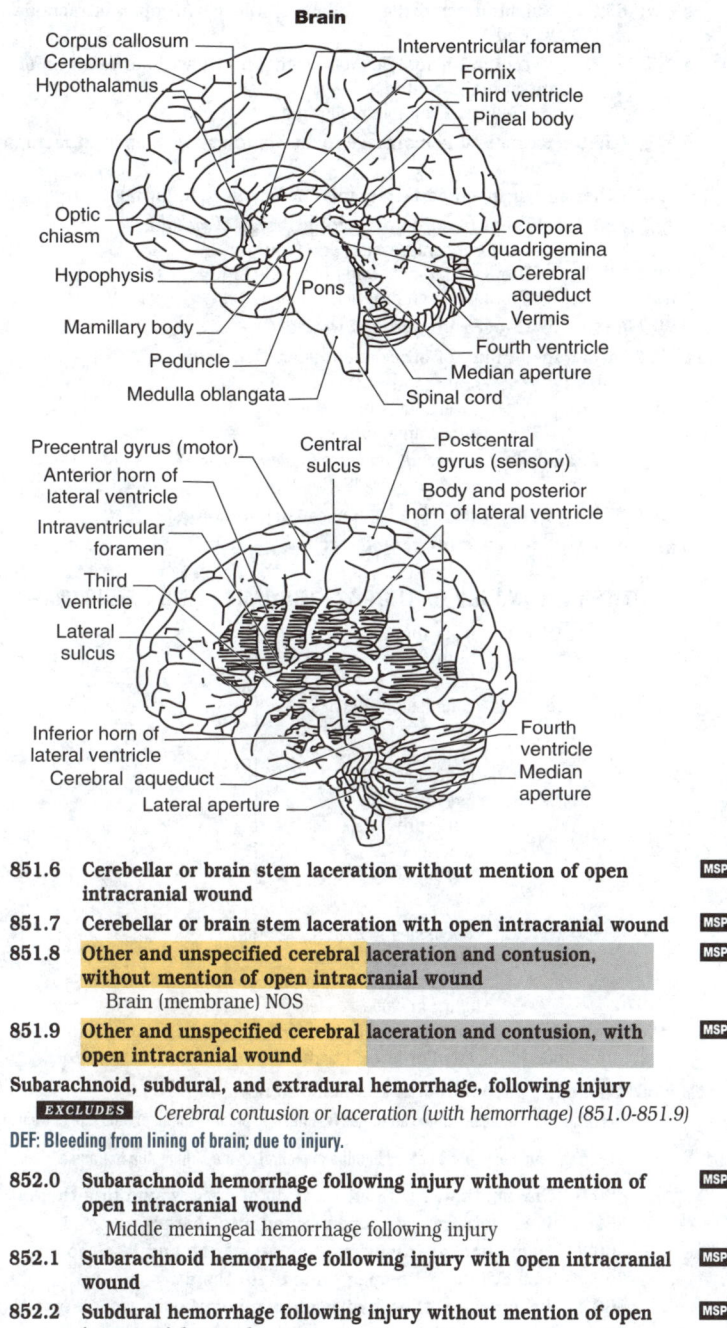

§ ✓5th	851.6	Cerebellar or brain stem laceration without mention of open intracranial wound	MSP
§ ✓5th	851.7	Cerebellar or brain stem laceration with open intracranial wound	MSP
§ ✓5th	851.8	Other and unspecified cerebral laceration and contusion, without mention of open intracranial wound Brain (membrane) NOS	MSP
§ ✓5th	851.9	Other and unspecified cerebral laceration and contusion, with open intracranial wound	MSP

✓4th **852 Subarachnoid, subdural, and extradural hemorrhage, following injury**

    EXCLUDES Cerebral contusion or laceration (with hemorrhage) (851.0-851.9)

    DEF: Bleeding from lining of brain; due to injury.

§ ✓5th	852.0	Subarachnoid hemorrhage following injury without mention of open intracranial wound Middle meningeal hemorrhage following injury	MSP
§ ✓5th	852.1	Subarachnoid hemorrhage following injury with open intracranial wound	MSP
§ ✓5th	852.2	Subdural hemorrhage following injury without mention of open intracranial wound	MSP

§ Requires fifth-digit. See beginning of section 850–854 for codes and definitions.

✓4th/✓5th Additional Digit Required   Unspecified Code   Other Specified Code   Manifestation Code

MSP Medicare Secondary Payer   ▶◀ Revised Text   ● New Code   ▲ Revised Code Title

2002 Ingenix, Inc.

INJURY AND POISONING

§ ✓5ᵗʰ **852.3** Subdural hemorrhage following injury with open intracranial wound [MSP]

§ ✓5ᵗʰ **852.4** Extradural hemorrhage following injury without mention of open intracranial wound [MSP]
    Epidural hematoma following injury

§ ✓5ᵗʰ **852.5** Extradural hemorrhage following injury with open intracranial wound [MSP]

✓4ᵗʰ **853 Other and unspecified intracranial hemorrhage following injury**

§ ✓5ᵗʰ **853.0** Without mention of open intracranial wound [MSP]
    Cerebral compression due to injury
    Intracranial hematoma following injury
    Traumatic cerebral hemorrhage

§ ✓5ᵗʰ **853.1** With open intracranial wound [MSP]

✓4ᵗʰ **854 Intracranial injury of other and unspecified nature**

    INCLUDES brain injury NOS
                  cavernous sinus
                  intracranial injury

    EXCLUDES any condition classifiable to 850-853
                 head injury NOS (959.01)

§ ✓5ᵗʰ **854.0** Without mention of open intracranial wound [MSP]

§ ✓5ᵗʰ **854.1** With open intracranial wound [MSP]

INTERNAL INJURY OF THORAX, ABDOMEN, AND PELVIS (860-869)

INCLUDES blast injuries
blunt trauma
bruise
concussion injuries (except cerebral)
crushing
hematoma   } of internal organs
laceration
puncture
tear
traumatic rupture

EXCLUDES concussion NOS (850.0-850.9)
flail chest (807.4)
foreign body entering through orifice (930.0-939.9)
injury to blood vessels (901.0-902.9)

The description "with open wound," used in the fourth-digit subdivisions, those with mention of infection or foreign body.

✓4ᵗʰ **860 Traumatic pneumothorax and hemothorax**

DEF: Traumatic pneumothorax: air or gas leaking into pleural space of lung due to trauma.

DEF: Traumatic hemothorax: blood buildup in pleural space of lung due to trauma.

860.0 Pneumothorax without mention of open wound into thorax [MSP]
860.1 Pneumothorax with open wound into thorax [MSP]
860.2 Hemothorax without mention of open wound into thorax [MSP]
860.3 Hemothorax with open wound into thorax [MSP]
860.4 Pneumohemothorax without mention of open wound into thorax [MSP]
860.5 Pneumohemothorax with open wound into thorax [MSP]

§ Requires fifth-digit. See beginning of section 850–854 for codes and definitions.

INJURY AND POISONING   861–863.0

✓4th 861 Injury to heart and lung
  EXCLUDES: *injury to blood vessels of thorax (901.0-901.9)*

  ✓5th 861.0 Heart, without mention of open wound into thorax
    861.00 Unspecified injury [MSP]
    861.01 Contusion [MSP]
       Cardiac contusion
       Myocardial contusion
       DEF: Bruising within the pericardium with no mention of open wound.

    861.02 Laceration without penetration of heart chambers [MSP]
       DEF: Tearing injury of heart tissue, without penetration of chambers; no open wound.

    861.03 Laceration with penetration of heart chambers [MSP]

  ✓5th 861.1 Heart, with open wound into thorax
    861.10 Unspecified injury [MSP]
    861.11 Contusion [MSP]
    861.12 Laceration without penetration of heart chambers [MSP]
    861.13 Laceration with penetration of heart chambers [MSP]

  ✓5th 861.2 Lung, without mention of open wound into thorax
    861.20 Unspecified injury [MSP]
    861.21 Contusion [MSP]
       DEF: Bruising of lung without mention of open wound.

    861.22 Laceration [MSP]

  ✓5th 861.3 Lung, with open wound into thorax
    861.30 Unspecified injury [MSP]
    861.31 Contusion [MSP]
    861.32 Laceration [MSP]

✓4th 862 Injury to other and unspecified intrathoracic organs
  EXCLUDES: *injury to blood vessels of thorax (901.0-901.9)*

  862.0 Diaphragm, without mention of open wound into cavity
  862.1 Diaphragm, with open wound into cavity

  ✓5th 862.2 Other specified intrathoracic organs, without mention of open wound into cavity
    862.21 Bronchus
    862.22 Esophagus
    862.29 Other
       Pleura   Thymus gland

  ✓5th 862.3 Other specified intrathoracic organs, with open wound into cavity
    862.31 Bronchus
    862.32 Esophagus
    862.39 Other

  862.8 Multiple and unspecified intrathoracic organs, without mention of open wound into cavity [MSP]
       Crushed chest
       Multiple intrathoracic organs

  862.9 Multiple and unspecified intrathoracic organs, with open wound into cavity

✓4th 863 Injury to gastrointestinal tract
  EXCLUDES: *anal sphincter laceration during delivery (664.2)*
           bile duct (868.0-868.1 with fifth-digit 2)
           gallbladder (868.0-868.1 with fifth-digit 2)

  863.0 Stomach, without mention of open wound into cavity [MSP]

✓4th / ✓5th Additional Digit Required | Unspecified Code | ● Other Specified Code | ▲ Manifestation Code
[MSP] Medicare Secondary Payer | Revised Text | ● New Code | ▲ Revised Code Title

2002 Ingenix, Inc.   Volume 1 — 535

INJURY AND POISONING

863.1 Stomach, with open wound into cavity [MSP]

√5th 863.2 Small intestine, without mention of open wound into cavity
    863.20 Small intestine, unspecified site [MSP]
    863.21 Duodenum [MSP]
    863.29 Other [MSP]

√5th 863.3 Small intestine, with open wound into cavity
    863.30 Small intestine, unspecified site [MSP]
    863.31 Duodenum [MSP]
    863.39 Other [MSP]

√5th 863.4 Colon or rectum, without mention of open wound into cavity
    863.40 Colon, unspecified site [MSP]
    863.41 Ascending [right] colon [MSP]
    863.42 Transverse colon [MSP]
    863.43 Descending [left] colon [MSP]
    863.44 Sigmoid colon [MSP]
    863.45 Rectum [MSP]
    863.46 Multiple sites in colon and rectum [MSP]
    863.49 Other [MSP]

√5th 863.5 Colon or rectum, with open wound into cavity
    863.50 Colon, unspecified site [MSP]
    863.51 Ascending [right] colon [MSP]
    863.52 Transverse colon [MSP]
    863.53 Descending [left] colon [MSP]
    863.54 Sigmoid colon [MSP]
    863.55 Rectum [MSP]
    863.56 Multiple sites in colon and rectum [MSP]
    863.59 Other [MSP]

√5th 863.8 Other and unspecified gastrointestinal sites, without mention of open wound into cavity [MSP]
    863.80 Gastrointestinal tract, unspecified site [MSP]
    863.81 Pancreas, head [MSP]
    863.82 Pancreas, body [MSP]
    863.83 Pancreas, tail [MSP]
    863.84 Pancreas, multiple and unspecified sites
    863.85 Appendix [MSP]
    863.89 Other [MSP]
        Intestine NOS

√5th 863.9 Other and unspecified gastrointestinal sites, with open wound into cavity
    863.90 Gastrointestinal tract, unspecified site [MSP]
    863.91 Pancreas, head [MSP]
    863.92 Pancreas, body [MSP]
    863.93 Pancreas, tail [MSP]
    863.94 Pancreas, multiple and unspecified sites [MSP]
    863.95 Appendix [MSP]
    863.99 Other [MSP]

INJURY AND POISONING

√4th 864 Injury to liver

The following fifth-digit subclassification is for use with category 864:
- 0 unspecified injury
- 1 hematoma and contusion
- 2 laceration, minor
  Laceration involving capsule only, or without significant involvement of hepatic parenchyma [i.e., less than 1 cm deep]
- 3 laceration, moderate
  Laceration involving parenchyma but without major disruption of parenchyma [i.e., less than 10 cm long and less than 3 cm deep]
- 4 laceration, major
  Laceration with significant disruption of hepatic parenchyma [i.e., 10 cm long and 3 cm deep]
  Multiple moderate lacerations, with or without hematoma
  Stellate lacerations of liver
- 5 laceration, unspecified
- 9 other

√5th 864.0 Without mention of open wound into cavity [MSP]
√5th 864.1 With open wound into cavity [MSP]

√4th 865 Injury to spleen

The following fifth-digit subclassification is for use with category 865:
- 0 unspecified injury
- 1 hematoma without rupture of capsule
- 2 capsular tears, without major disruption of parenchyma
- 3 laceration extending into parenchyma
- 4 massive parenchymal disruption
- 9 other

√5th 865.0 Without mention of open wound into cavity [MSP]
√5th 865.1 With open wound into cavity [MSP]

√4th 866 Injury to kidney

The following fifth-digit subclassification is for use with category 866:
- 0 unspecified injury
- 1 hematoma without rupture of capsule
- 2 laceration
- 3 complete disruption of kidney parenchyma

√5th 866.0 Without mention of open wound into cavity [MSP]
√5th 866.1 With open wound into cavity [MSP]

√4th 867 Injury to pelvic organs

EXCLUDES   injury during delivery (664.0-665.9)

867.0	Bladder and urethra, without mention of open wound into cavity	[MSP]
867.1	Bladder and urethra, with open wound into cavity	[MSP]
867.2	Ureter, without mention of open wound into cavity	[MSP]
867.3	Ureter, with open wound into cavity	[MSP]
867.4	Uterus, without mention of open wound into cavity	[MSP] ♀
867.5	Uterus, with open wound into cavity	[MSP] ♀
867.6	Other specified pelvic organs, without mention of open wound into cavity	[MSP]

Fallopian tube   Seminal vesicle
Ovary   Vas deferens
Prostate

√4th
√5th   Additional Digit Required
   Unspecified Code   Other Specified Code   Manifestation Code
MSP Medicare Secondary Payer   ▶◀ Revised Text   ● New Code   ▲ Revised Code Title

2002 Ingenix, Inc.

867.7	Other specified pelvic organs, with open wound into cavity	MSP
867.8	Unspecified pelvic organ, without mention of open wound into cavity	MSP
867.9	Unspecified pelvic organ, with open wound into cavity	MSP

√4th **868 Injury to other intra-abdominal organs**

The following fifth-digit subclassification is for use with category 868:
- 0 unspecified intra-abdominal organ
- 1 adrenal gland
- 2 bile duct and gallbladder
- 3 peritoneum
- 4 retroperitoneum
- 9 other and multiple intra-abdominal organs

√5th 868.0 Without mention of open wound into cavity   MSP
√5th 868.1 With open wound into cavity   MSP

√4th **869 Internal injury to unsupecified or ill-defined organs**

INCLUDES: internal injury NOS
multiple internal injury NOS

869.0 Without mention of open wound into cavity   MSP
869.1 With open wound into cavity   MSP

OPEN WOUND (870-897)

INCLUDES:
- animal bite
- avulsion
- cut
- laceration
- puncture wound
- traumatic amputation

EXCLUDES:
- burn (940.0-949.5)
- crushing (925-929.9)
- puncture of internal organs (860.0-869.1)
- superficial injury (910.0-919.9)
- that incidental to:
  - dislocation (830.0-839.9)
  - fracture (800.0-829.1)
  - internal injury (860.0-869.1)
  - intracranial injury (851.0-854.1)

The description "complicated" used in the fourth-digit subdivisions those with mention of delayed healing, delayed treatment, foreign body, or infection.

Use additional code to identify infection

OPEN WOUND OF HEAD, NECK, AND TRUNK (870-879)

√4th **870 Open wound of ocular adnexa**

- 870.0 Laceration of skin of eyelid and periocular area
- 870.1 Laceration of eyelid, full-thickness, not involving lacrimal passages
- 870.2 Laceration of eyelid involving lacrimal passages
- 870.3 Penetrating wound of orbit, without mention of foreign body
- 870.4 Penetrating wound of orbit with foreign body
  EXCLUDES: retained (old) foreign body in orbit (376.6)
- 870.8 Other specified open wounds of ocular adnexa
- 870.9 Unspecified open wound of ocular adnexa

INJURY AND POISONING 871–872.8

☑4th **871 Open wound of eyeball**
    EXCLUDES: 2nd cranial nerve [optic] injury (950.0-950.9)
                       3rd cranial nerve [oculomotor] injury (951.0)

    871.0 Ocular laceration without prolapse of intraocular tissue
        DEF: Tear in ocular tissue without displacing structures.

    871.1 Ocular laceration with prolapse or exposure of intraocular tissue

    871.2 Rupture of eye with partial loss of intraocular tissue
        DEF: Forcible tearing of eyeball, with tissue loss.

    871.3 Avulsion of eye
        Traumatic enucleation
        DEF: Traumatic extraction of eyeball from socket.

    871.4 Unspecified laceration of eye

    871.5 Penetration of eyeball with magnetic foreign body
        EXCLUDES: retained (old) magnetic foreign body in globe (360.50-360.59)

    871.6 Penetration of eyeball with (nonmagnetic) foreign body
        EXCLUDES: retained (old) (nonmagnetic) foreign body in globe (360.60-360.69)

    871.7 Unspecified ocular penetration

    871.9 Unspecified open wound of eyeball

☑4th **872 Open wound of ear**

  ☑5th **872.0 External ear, without mention of complication**
        872.00 External ear, unspecified site
        872.01 Auricle, ear
            Pinna
            DEF: Open wound of fleshy, outer ear.
        872.02 Auditory canal
            DEF: Open wound of passage from external ear to eardrum.

  ☑5th **872.1 External ear, complicated**
        872.10 External ear, unspecified site
        872.11 Auricle, ear
        872.12 Auditory canal

  ☑5th **872.6 Other specified parts of ear, without mention of complication**
        872.61 Ear drum
            Drumhead   Tympanic membrane
        872.62 Ossicles
        872.63 Eustachian tube
            DEF: Open wound of channel between nasopharynx and tympanic cavity.
        872.64 Cochlea
            DEF: Open wound of snail shell shaped tube of inner ear.
        872.69 Other and multiple sites

  ☑5th **872.7 Other specified parts of ear, complicated**
        872.71 Ear drum
        872.72 Ossicles
        872.73 Eustachian tube
        872.74 Cochlea
        872.79 Other and multiple sites

    872.8 Ear, part unspecified, without mention of complication
        Ear NOS

872.9–873.72 INJURY AND POISONING

    872.9 **Ear, part unspecified, complicated**
✓4th **873 Other open wound of head**
    873.0 Scalp, without mention of complication
    873.1 Scalp, complicated
✓5th 873.2 Nose, without mention of complication
        873.20 **Nose, unspecified site**
        873.21 Nasal septum
            DEF: Open wound between nasal passages.
        873.22 Nasal cavity
            DEF: Open wound of nostrils.
        873.23 Nasal sinus
            DEF: Open wound of mucous-lined respiratory cavities.
        873.29 Multiple sites
✓5th 873.3 Nose, complicated
        873.30 **Nose, unspecified site**
        873.31 Nasal septum
        873.32 Nasal cavity
        873.33 Nasal sinus
        873.39 Multiple sites
✓5th 873.4 Face, without mention of complication
        873.40 **Face, unspecified site**
        873.41 Cheek
        873.42 Forehead
            Eyebrow
        873.43 Lip
        873.44 Jaw
        873.49 **Other and multiple sites**
✓5th 873.5 Face, complicated
        873.50 **Face, unspecified site**
        873.51 Cheek
        873.52 Forehead
        873.53 Lip
        873.54 Jaw
        873.59 **Other and multiple sites**
✓5th 873.6 Internal structures of mouth, without mention of complication
        873.60 **Mouth, unspecified site**
        873.61 Buccal mucosa
            DEF: Open wound of inside of cheek.
        873.62 Gum (alveolar process)
        873.63 Tooth (broken)
        873.64 Tongue and floor of mouth
        873.65 Palate
            DEF: Open wound of roof of mouth.
        873.69 **Other and multiple sites**
✓5th 873.7 Internal structures of mouth, complicated
        873.70 **Mouth, unspecified site**
        873.71 Buccal mucosa
        873.72 Gum (alveolar process)

N Newborn Age: 0   **P** Pediatric Age: 0-17   **M** Maternity Age: 12-55   **A** Adult Age: 15-124

INJURY AND POISONING 873.73–878.5

- 873.73 Tooth (broken)
- 873.74 Tongue and floor of mouth
- 873.75 Palate
- 873.79 Other and multiple sites

873.8 **Other and unspecified open wound of head without mention of complication**
- Head NOS

873.9 **Other and unspecified open wound of head, complicated**

✓4th **874 Open wound of neck**

  ✓5th 874.0 Larynx and trachea, without mention of complication
- 874.00 Larynx with trachea
- 874.01 Larynx
- 874.02 Trachea

  ✓5th 874.1 Larynx and trachea, complicated
- 874.10 Larynx with trachea
- 874.11 Larynx
- 874.12 Trachea

- 874.2 Thyroid gland, without mention of complication
- 874.3 Thyroid gland, complicated
- 874.4 Pharynx, without mention of complication
  - Cervical esophagus
- 874.5 Pharynx, complicated
- 874.8 **Other and unspecified parts, without mention of complication**
  - Nape of neck   Throat NOS
  - Supraclavicular region
- 874.9 **Other and unspecified parts, complicated**

✓4th **875 Open wound of chest (wall)**
> EXCLUDES: open wound into thoracic cavity (860.0-862.9)
> traumatic pneumothorax and hemothorax (860.1, 860.3, 860.5)

- 875.0 Without mention of complication
- 875.1 Complicated

✓4th **876 Open wound of back**
> INCLUDES: loin
> lumbar region
>
> EXCLUDES: open wound into thoracic cavity (860.0-862.9)
> traumatic pneumothorax and hemothorax (860.1, 860.3, 860.5)

- 876.0 Without mention of complication
- 876.1 Complicated

✓4th **877 Open wound of buttock**
> INCLUDES: sacroiliac region

- 877.0 Without mention of complication
- 877.1 Complicated

✓4th **878 Open wound of genital organs (external), including traumatic amputation**
> EXCLUDES: injury during delivery (664.0-665.9)
> internal genital organs (867.0-867.9)

- 878.0 Penis, without mention of complication ♂
- 878.1 Penis, complicated ♂
- 878.2 Scrotum and testes, without mention of complication ♂
- 878.3 Scrotum and testes, complicated ♂
- 878.4 Vulva, without mention of complication ♀
  - Labium (majus) (minus)
- 878.5 Vulva, complicated ♀

✓4th/✓5th Additional Digit Required   **Unspecified Code**   Other Specified Code   Manifestation Code
MSP Medicare Secondary Payer   ▶◀ Revised Text   ● New Code   ▲ Revised Code Title

	878.6	Vagina, without mention of complication ♀
	878.7	Vagina, complicated ♀
	878.8	Other and unspecified parts, without mention of complication
	878.9	Other and unspecified parts, complicated

✓4th **879 Open wound of other and unspecified sites, except limbs**

- 879.0 Breast, without mention of complication
- 879.1 Breast, complicated
- 879.2 Abdominal wall, anterior, without mention of complication
  - Abdominal wall NOS
  - Epigastric region
  - Hypogastric region
  - Pubic region
  - Umbilical region
- 879.3 Abdominal wall, anterior, complicated
- 879.4 Abdominal wall, lateral, without mention of complication
  - Flank
  - Groin
  - Hypochondrium
  - Iliac (region)
  - Inguinal region
- 879.5 Abdominal wall, lateral, complicated
- 879.6 Other and unspecified parts of trunk, without mention of complication
  - Pelvic region
  - Perineum
  - Trunk NOS
- 879.7 Other and unspecified parts of trunk, complicated
- 879.8 Open wound(s) (multiple) of unspecified site(s) without mention of complication
  - Multiple open wounds NOS
  - Open wound NOS
- 879.9 Open wound(s) (multiple) of unspecified site(s), complicated

OPEN WOUND OF UPPER LIMB (880-887)

✓4th **880 Open wound of shoulder and upper arm**

The following fifth-digit subclassification is for use with category 880:
- 0 shoulder region
- 1 scapular region
- 2 axillary region
- 3 upper arm
- 9 multiple sites

- ✓5th 880.0 Without mention of complication
- ✓5th 880.1 Complicated
- ✓5th 880.2 With tendon involvement

✓4th **881 Open wound of elbow, forearm, and wrist**

The following fifth-digit subclassification is for use with category 881:
- 0 forearm
- 1 elbow
- 2 wrist

- ✓5th 881.0 Without mention of complication
- ✓5th 881.1 Complicated
- ✓5th 881.2 With tendon involvement

✓4th **882 Open wound of hand except finger(s) alone**

- 882.0 Without mention of complication
- 882.1 Complicated
- 882.2 With tendon involvement

INJURY AND POISONING

✓4ᵗʰ **883 Open wound of finger(s)**
  INCLUDES fingernail
            thumb (nail)
  883.0 Without mention of complication
  883.1 Complicated
  883.2 With tendon involvement

✓4ᵗʰ **884 Multiple and unspecified open wound of upper limb**
  INCLUDES arm NOS
            multiple sites of one upper limb
            upper limb NOS
  884.0 Without mention of complication
  884.1 Complicated
  884.2 With tendon involvement

✓4ᵗʰ **885 Traumatic amputation of thumb (complete) (partial)**
  INCLUDES thumb(s) (with finger(s) of either hand)
  885.0 Without mention of complication
  885.1 Complicated

✓4ᵗʰ **886 Traumatic amputation of other finger(s) (complete) (partial)**
  INCLUDES finger(s) of one or both hands, without mention of thumb(s)
  886.0 Without mention of complication
  886.1 Complicated

✓4ᵗʰ **887 Traumatic amputation of arm and hand (complete) (partial)**
  887.0 Unilateral, below elbow, without mention of complication [MSP]
  887.1 Unilateral, below elbow, complicated [MSP]
  887.2 Unilateral, at or above elbow, without mention of complication [MSP]
  887.3 Unilateral, at or above elbow, complicated [MSP]
  887.4 ==Unilateral, level not specified, without mention of complication== [MSP]
  887.5 ==Unilateral, level not specified, complicated== [MSP]
  887.6 Bilateral [any level], without mention of complication [MSP]
        One hand and other arm
  887.7 Bilateral [any level], complicated [MSP]

OPEN WOUND OF LOWER LIMB (890-897)

✓4ᵗʰ **890 Open wound of hip and thigh**
  890.0 Without mention of complication
  890.1 Complicated
  890.2 With tendon involvement

✓4ᵗʰ **891 Open wound of knee, leg [except thigh], and ankle**
  INCLUDES leg NOS
            multiple sites of leg, except thigh
  EXCLUDES *that of thigh (890.0-890.2)*
            with multiple sites of lower limb (894.0-894.2)
  891.0 Without mention of complication
  891.1 Complicated
  891.2 With tendon involvement

✓4ᵗʰ **892 Open wound of foot except toe(s) alone**
  INCLUDES heel
  892.0 Without mention of complication
  892.1 Complicated
  892.2 With tendon involvement

✓4ᵗʰ / ✓5ᵗʰ Additional Digit Required   Unspecified Code   ● Other Specified Code   ▲ Manifestation Code
 Medicare Secondary Payer   ◄► Revised Text   ● New Code   ▲ Revised Code Title

INJURY AND POISONING

✓4th 893 Open wound of toe(s)
   INCLUDES   toenail
- 893.0 Without mention of complication
- 893.1 Complicated
- 893.2 With tendon involvement

✓4th 894 Multiple and unspecified open wound of lower limb
   INCLUDES   lower limb NOS
   multiple sites of one lower limb, with thigh
- 894.0 Without mention of complication
- 894.1 Complicated
- 894.2 With tendon involvement

✓4th 895 Traumatic amputation of toe(s) (complete) (partial)
   INCLUDES   toe(s) of one or both feet
- 895.0 Without mention of complication
- 895.1 Complicated

✓4th 896 Traumatic amputation of foot (complete) (partial)
- 896.0 Unilateral, without mention of complication [MSP]
- 896.1 Unilateral, complicated [MSP]
- 896.2 Bilateral, without mention of complication [MSP]
   EXCLUDES   one foot and other leg (897.6-897.7)
- 896.3 Bilateral, complicated [MSP]

✓4th 897 Traumatic amputation of leg(s) (complete) (partial)
- 897.0 Unilateral, below knee, without mention of complication [MSP]
- 897.1 Unilateral, below knee, complicated [MSP]
- 897.2 Unilateral, at or above knee, without mention of complication [MSP]
- 897.3 Unilateral, at or above knee, complicated [MSP]
- 897.4 **Unilateral, level not specified, without mention of complication** [MSP]
- 897.5 **Unilateral, level not specified, complicated** [MSP]
- 897.6 Bilateral [any level], without mention of complication [MSP]
   One foot and other leg
- 897.7 Bilateral [any level], complicated [MSP]

INJURY TO BLOOD VESSELS (900-904)

INCLUDES   arterial hematoma
   avulsion
   cut
   laceration
   rupture
   traumatic aneurysm
      or fistula
         (arteriovenous)
} of blood vessel, secondary to other injuries e.g., fracture or open wound

EXCLUDES   accidental puncture or laceration during medical procedure (998.2)
   intracranial hemorrhage following injury (851.0-854.1)

✓4th 900 Injury to blood vessels of head and neck
- **✓5th 900.0 Carotid artery**
  - 900.00 **Carotid artery, unspecified** [MSP]
  - 900.01 Common carotid artery [MSP]
  - 900.02 External carotid artery [MSP]
  - 900.03 Internal carotid artery [MSP]

INJURY AND POISONING 900.1–902.39

- 900.1 Internal jugular vein [MSP]
- √5th 900.8 Other specified blood vessels of head and neck
  - 900.81 External jugular vein [MSP]
    - Jugular vein NOS
  - 900.82 Multiple blood vessels of head and neck [MSP]
  - 900.89 Other [MSP]
- 900.9 Unspecified blood vessel of head and neck [MSP]

√4th 901 Injury to blood vessels of thorax
  EXCLUDES   traumatic hemothorax (860.2-860.5)
- 901.0 Thoracic aorta
- 901.1 Innominate and subclavian arteries
- 901.2 Superior vena cava
- 901.3 Innominate and subclavian veins
- √5th 901.4 Pulmonary blood vessels
  - 901.40 Pulmonary vessel(s), unspecified
  - 901.41 Pulmonary artery
  - 901.42 Pulmonary vein
- √5th 901.8 Other specified blood vessels of thorax
  - 901.81 Intercostal artery or vein
  - 901.82 Internal mammary artery or vein
  - 901.83 Multiple blood vessels of thorax
  - 901.89 Other
    - Azygos vein
    - Hemiazygos vein
- 901.9 Unspecified blood vessel of thorax

√4th 902 Injury to blood vessels of abdomen and pelvis
- 902.0 Abdominal aorta
- √5th 902.1 Inferior vena cava
  - 902.10 Inferior vena cava, unspecified
  - 902.11 Hepatic veins
  - 902.19 Other
- √5th 902.2 Celiac and mesenteric arteries
  - 902.20 Celiac and mesenteric arteries, unspecified
  - 902.21 Gastric artery
  - 902.22 Hepatic artery
  - 902.23 Splenic artery
  - 902.24 Other specified branches of celiac axis
  - 902.25 Superior mesenteric artery (trunk)
  - 902.26 Primary branches of superior mesenteric artery
    - Ileocolic artery
  - 902.27 Inferior mesenteric artery
  - 902.29 Other
- √5th 902.3 Portal and splenic veins
  - 902.31 Superior mesenteric vein and primary subdivisions
    - Ileocolic vein
  - 902.32 Inferior mesenteric vein
  - 902.33 Portal vein
  - 902.34 Splenic vein
  - 902.39 Other
    - Cystic vein   Gastric vein

√4th / √5th Additional Digit Required   Unspecified Code   Other Specified Code   Manifestation Code
[MSP] Medicare Secondary Payer   ▶◀ Revised Text   ● New Code   ▲ Revised Code Title

2002 Ingenix, Inc.

902.4–904.52 INJURY AND POISONING

- √5th **902.4 Renal blood vessels**
  - 902.40 Renal vessel(s), unspecified
  - 902.41 Renal artery
  - 902.42 Renal vein
  - 902.49 Other
    - Suprarenal arteries
- √5th **902.5 Iliac blood vessels**
  - 902.50 Iliac vessel(s), unspecified
  - 902.51 Hypogastric artery
  - 902.52 Hypogastric vein
  - 902.53 Iliac artery
  - 902.54 Iliac vein
  - 902.55 Uterine artery ♀
  - 902.56 Uterine vein ♀
  - 902.59 Other
- √5th **902.8 Other specified blood vessels of abdomen and pelvis**
  - 902.81 Ovarian artery ♀
  - 902.82 Ovarian vein ♀
  - 902.87 Multiple blood vessels of abdomen and pelvis
  - 902.89 Other
- **902.9 Unspecified blood vessel of abdomen and pelvis**
- √4th **903 Injury to blood vessels of upper extremity**
  - √5th **903.0 Axillary blood vessels**
    - 903.00 Axillary vessel(s), unspecified
    - 903.01 Axillary artery
    - 903.02 Axillary vein
  - 903.1 Brachial blood vessels
  - 903.2 Radial blood vessels
  - 903.3 Ulnar blood vessels
  - 903.4 Palmar artery
  - 903.5 Digital blood vessels
  - 903.8 Other specified blood vessels of upper extremity
    - Multiple blood vessels of upper extremity
  - 903.9 Unspecified blood vessel of upper extremity
- √4th **904 Injury to blood vessels of lower extremity and unspecified sites**
  - 904.0 Common femoral artery
    - Femoral artery above profunda origin
  - 904.1 Superficial femoral artery
  - 904.2 Femoral veins
  - 904.3 Saphenous veins
    - Saphenous vein (greater) (lesser)
  - √5th **904.4 Popliteal blood vessels**
    - 904.40 Popliteal vessel(s), unspecified
    - 904.41 Popliteal artery
    - 904.42 Popliteal vein
  - √5th **904.5 Tibial blood vessels**
    - 904.50 Tibial vessel(s), unspecified
    - 904.51 Anterior tibial artery
    - 904.52 Anterior tibial vein

INJURY AND POISONING

- 904.53 Posterior tibial artery
- 904.54 Posterior tibial vein
- **904.6** Deep plantar blood vessels
- **904.7** ==Other specified blood vessels of lower extremity==
    Multiple blood vessels of lower extremity
- **904.8** ==Unspecified blood vessel of lower extremity==
- **904.9** ==Unspecified site==
    Injury to blood vessel NOS

LATE EFFECTS OF INJURIES, POISONINGS, TOXIC EFFECTS, AND OTHER EXTERNAL CAUSES (905-909)

Note: These categories are to be used to indicate conditions classifiable to 800-999 as the cause of late effects, which are themselves classified elsewhere. The "late effects" include those specified as such, or as sequelae, which may occur at any time after the acute injury.

✓4th **905 Late effects of musculoskeletal and connective tissue injuries**
- **905.0** Late effect of fracture of skull and face bones
    Late effect of injury classifiable to 800-804
- **905.1** Late effect of fracture of spine and trunk without mention of spinal cord lesion
    Late effect of injury classifiable to 805, 807-809
- **905.2** Late effect of fracture of upper extremities
    Late effect of injury classifiable to 810-819
- **905.3** Late effect of fracture of neck of femur
    Late effect of injury classifiable to 820
- **905.4** Late effect of fracture of lower extremities
    Late effect of injury classifiable to 821-827
- **905.5** Late effect of fracture of multiple and unspecified bones
    Late effect of injury classifiable to 828-829
- **905.6** Late effect of dislocation
    Late effect of injury classifiable to 830-839
- **905.7** Late effect of sprain and strain without mention of tendon injury
    Late effect of injury classifiable to 840-848, except tendon injury
- **905.8** Late effect of tendon injury
    Late effect of tendon injury due to:
        open wound [injury classifiable to 880-884 with .2, 890-894 with .2]
        sprain and strain [injury classifiable to 840-848]
- **905.9** Late effect of traumatic amputation
    Late effect of injury classifiable to 885-887, 895-897
    EXCLUDES *late amputation stump complication (997.60-997.69)*

✓4th **906 Late effects of injuries to skin and subcutaneous tissues**
- **906.0** Late effect of open wound of head, neck, and trunk
    Late effect of injury classifiable to 870-879
- **906.1** Late effect of open wound of extremities without mention of tendon injury
    Late effect of injury classifiable to 880-884, 890-894 except .2
- **906.2** Late effect of superficial injury
    Late effect of injury classifiable to 910-919
- **906.3** Late effect of contusion
    Late effect of injury classifiable to 920-924
- **906.4** Late effect of crushing
    Late effect of injury classifiable to 925-929
- **906.5** Late effect of burn of eye, face, head, and neck
    Late effect of injury classifiable to 940-941

Additional Digit Required | ==Unspecified Code== | Other Specified Code | Manifestation Code
MSP Medicare Secondary Payer | ▶◀ Revised Text | ● New Code | ▲ Revised Code Title

906.6 Late effect of burn of wrist and hand
Late effect of injury classifiable to 944
906.7 Late effect of burn of other extremities
Late effect of injury classifiable to 943 or 945
906.8 Late effect of burns of other specified sites
Late effect of injury classifiable to 942, 946-947
906.9 Late effect of burn of unspecified site
Late effect of injury classifiable to 948-949

√4th **907 Late effects of injuries to the nervous system**
907.0 Late effect of intracranial injury without mention of skull fracture
Late effect of injury classifiable to 850-854
907.1 Late effect of injury to cranial nerve
Late effect of injury classifiable to 950-951
907.2 Late effect of spinal cord injury
Late effect of injury classifiable to 806, 952
907.3 Late effect of injury to nerve root(s), spinal plexus(es), and other nerves of trunk
Late effect of injury classifiable to 953-954
907.4 Late effect of injury to peripheral nerve of shoulder girdle and upper limb
Late effect of injury classifiable to 955
907.5 Late effect of injury to peripheral nerve of pelvic girdle and lower limb
Late effect of injury classifiable to 956
907.9 Late effect of injury to other and unspecified nerve
Late effect of injury classifiable to 957

√4th **908 Late effects of other and unspecified injuries**
908.0 Late effect of internal injury to chest
Late effect of injury classifiable to 860-862
908.1 Late effect of internal injury to intra-abdominal organs
Late effect of injury classifiable to 863-866, 868
908.2 Late effect of internal injury to other internal organs
Late effect of injury classifiable to 867 or 869
908.3 Late effect of injury to blood vessel of head, neck, and extremities
Late effect of injury classifiable to 900, 903-904
908.4 Late effect of injury to blood vessel of thorax, abdomen, and pelvis
Late effect of injury classifiable to 901-902
908.5 Late effect of foreign body in orifice
Late effect of injury classifiable to 930-939
908.6 Late effect of certain complications of trauma
Late effect of complications classifiable to 958
908.9 Late effect of unspecified injury
Late effect of injury classifiable to 959

√4th **909 Late effects of other and unspecified external causes**
909.0 Late effect of poisoning due to drug, medicinal or biological substance
Late effect of conditions classifiable to 960-979
EXCLUDES *late effect of adverse effect of drug, medicinal or biological substance (909.5)*
909.1 Late effect of toxic effects of nonmedical substances
Late effect of conditions classifiable to 980-989
909.2 Late effect of radiation
Late effect of conditions classifiable to 990
909.3 Late effect of complications of surgical and medical care
Late effect of conditions classifiable to 996-999
909.4 Late effect of certain other external causes
Late effect of conditions classifiable to 991-994

INJURY AND POISONING

909.5 Late effect of adverse effect of drug, medical or biological substance

> EXCLUDES late effect of poisoning due to drug, medical or biological substance (909.0)

909.9 Late effect of other and unspecified external causes

SUPERFICIAL INJURY (910-919)

> EXCLUDES burn (blisters) (940.0-949.5)
> contusion (920-924.9)
> foreign body:
>   granuloma (728.82)
>   inadvertently left in operative wound (998.4)
>   residual in soft tissue (729.6)
> insect bite, venomous (989.5)
> open wound with incidental foreign body (870.0-897.7)

910 Superficial injury of face, neck, and scalp except eye

> INCLUDES cheek
> ear
> gum
> lip
> nose
> throat

> EXCLUDES eye and adnexa (918.0-918.9)

- **910.0** Abrasion or friction burn without mention of infection
- **910.1** Abrasion or friction burn, infected
- **910.2** Blister without mention of infection
- **910.3** Blister, infected
- **910.4** Insect bite, nonvenomous, without mention of infection
- **910.5** Insect bite, nonvenomous, infected
- **910.6** Superficial foreign body (splinter) without major open wound and without mention of infection
- **910.7** Superficial foreign body (splinter) without major open wound, infected
- **910.8** Other and unspecified superficial injury of face, neck, and scalp without mention of infection
- **910.9** Other and unspecified superficial injury of face, neck, and scalp, infected

911 Superficial injury of trunk

> INCLUDES abdominal wall
> anus
> back
> breast
> buttock
> mchest wall
> flank
> groin
> interscapular region
> labium (majus) (minus)
> penis
> perineum
> scrotum
> testis
> vagina
> vulva

> EXCLUDES hip (916.0-916.9)
> scapular region (912.0-912.9)

 Additional Digit Required | Unspecified Code | Other Specified Code | Manifestation Code
MSP Medicare Secondary Payer | ▶◀ Revised Text | ● New Code | ▲ Revised Code Title

INJURY AND POISONING

	911.0	Abrasion or friction burn without mention of infection
	911.1	Abrasion or friction burn, infected
	911.2	Blister without mention of infection
	911.3	Blister, infected
	911.4	Insect bite, nonvenomous, without mention of infection
	911.5	Insect bite, nonvenomous, infected
	911.6	Superficial foreign body (splinter) without major open wound and without mention of infection
	911.7	Superficial foreign body (splinter) without major open wound, infected
	911.8	Other and unspecified superficial injury of trunk, without mention of infection
	911.9	Other and unspecified superficial injury of trunk, infected

✓4th **912 Superficial injury of shoulder and upper arm**

> INCLUDES axilla
> scapular region

	912.0	Abrasion or friction burn without mention of infection
	912.1	Abrasion or friction burn, infected
	912.2	Blister without mention of infection
	912.3	Blister, infected
	912.4	Insect bite, nonvenomous, without mention of infection
	912.5	Insect bite, nonvenomous, infected
	912.6	Superficial foreign body (splinter) without major open wound and without mention of infection
	912.7	Superficial foreign body (splinter) without major open wound, infected
	912.8	Other and unspecified superficial injury of shoulder and upper arm without mention of infection
	912.9	Other and unspecified superficial injury of shoulder and upper arm, infected

✓4th **913 Superficial injury of elbow, forearm, and wrist**

	913.0	Abrasion or friction burn without mention of infection
	913.1	Abrasion or friction burn, infected
	913.2	Blister without mention of infection
	913.3	Blister, infected
	913.4	Insect bite, nonvenomous, without mention of infection
	913.5	Insect bite, nonvenomous, infected
	913.6	Superficial foreign body (splinter) without major open wound and without mention of infection
	913.7	Superficial foreign body (splinter) without major open wound, infected
	913.8	Other and unspecified superficial injury of elbow, forearm, and wrist without mention of infection
	913.9	Other and unspecified superficial injury of elbow, forearm, and wrist, infected

✓4th **914 Superficial injury of hand(s) except finger(s) alone**

	914.0	Abrasion or friction burn without mention of infection
	914.1	Abrasion or friction burn, infected
	914.2	Blister without mention of infection
	914.3	Blister, infected
	914.4	Insect bite, nonvenomous, without mention of infection
	914.5	Insect bite, nonvenomous, infected
	914.6	Superficial foreign body (splinter) without major open wound and without mention of infection
	914.7	Superficial foreign body (splinter) without major open wound, infected

INJURY AND POISONING 914.8–917.9

- **914.8** Other and unspecified superficial injury of hand without mention of infection
- **914.9** Other and unspecified superficial injury of hand, infected

√4th **915 Superficial injury of finger(s)**
  INCLUDES   fingernail
             thumb (nail)
- **915.0** Abrasion or friction burn without mention of infection
- **915.1** Abrasion or friction burn, infected
- **915.2** Blister without mention of infection
- **915.3** Blister, infected
- **915.4** Insect bite, nonvenomous, without mention of infection
- **915.5** Insect bite, nonvenomous, infected
- **915.6** Superficial foreign body (splinter) without major open wound and without mention of infection
- **915.7** Superficial foreign body (splinter) without major open wound, infected
- **915.8** Other and unspecified superficial injury of fingers without mention of infection
- **915.9** Other and unspecified superficial injury of fingers, infected

√4th **916 Superficial injury of hip, thigh, leg, and ankle**
- **916.0** Abrasion or friction burn without mention of infection
- **916.1** Abrasion or friction burn, infected
- **916.2** Blister without mention of infection
- **916.3** Blister, infected
- **916.4** Insect bite, nonvenomous, without mention of infection
- **916.5** Insect bite, nonvenomous, infected
- **916.6** Superficial foreign body (splinter) without major open wound and without mention of infection
- **916.7** Superficial foreign body (splinter) without major open wound, infected
- **916.8** Other and unspecified superficial injury of hip, thigh, leg, and ankle without mention of infection
- **916.9** Other and unspecified superficial injury of hip, thigh, leg, and ankle, infected

√4th **917 Superficial injury of foot and toe(s)**
  INCLUDES   heel
             toenail
- **917.0** Abrasion or friction burn without mention of infection
- **917.1** Abrasion or friction burn, infected
- **917.2** Blister without mention of infection
- **917.3** Blister, infected
- **917.4** Insect bite, nonvenomous, without mention of infection
- **917.5** Insect bite, nonvenomous, infected
- **917.6** Superficial foreign body (splinter) without major open wound and without mention of infection
- **917.7** Superficial foreign body (splinter) without major open wound, infected
- **917.8** Other and unspecified superficial injury of foot and toes without mention of infection
- **917.9** Other and unspecified superficial injury of foot and toes, infected

INJURY AND POISONING

√4th 918 Superficial injury of eye and adnexa
   EXCLUDES burn (940.0-940.9)
   foreign body on external eye (930.0-930.9)

   918.0 Eyelids and periocular area
   Abrasion   Superficial foreign body
   Insect bite   (splinter)

   918.1 Cornea
   Corneal abrasion   Superficial laceration
   EXCLUDES corneal injury due to contact lens (371.82)

   918.2 Conjunctiva

   918.9 Other and unspecified superficial injuries of eye
   Eye (ball) NOS

√4th 919 Superficial injury of other, multiple, and unspecified sites
   EXCLUDES multiple sites classifiable to the same three-digit category (910.0-918.9)

   919.0 Abrasion or friction burn without mention of infection
   919.1 Abrasion or friction burn, infected
   919.2 Blister without mention of infection
   919.3 Blister, infected
   919.4 Insect bite, nonvenomous, without mention of infection
   919.5 Insect bite, nonvenomous, infected
   919.6 Superficial foreign body (splinter) without major open wound and without mention of infection
   919.7 Superficial foreign body (splinter) without major open wound, infected
   919.8 Other and unspecified superficial injury without mention of infection
   919.9 Other and unspecified superficial injury, infected

CONTUSION WITH INTACT SKIN SURFACE (920-924)

INCLUDES bruise   } without fracture or open
              hematoma   }   wound

EXCLUDES concussion (850.0-850.9)
   hemarthrosis (840.0-848.9)
   internal organs (860.0-869.1)
   that incidental to:
      crushing injury (925-929.9)
      dislocation (830.0-839.9)
      fracture (800.0-829.1)
      internal injury (860.0-869.1)
      intracranial injury (850.0-854.1)
      nerve injury (950.0-957.9)
      open wound (870.0-897.7)

920 Contusion of face, scalp, and neck except eye(s)
   Cheek   Mandibular joint area
   Ear (auricle)   Nose
   Gum   Throat
   Lip

√4th 921 Contusion of eye and adnexa
   921.0 Black eye, not otherwise specified
   921.1 Contusion of eyelids and periocular area
   921.2 Contusion of orbital tissues
   921.3 Contusion of eyeball

INJURY AND POISONING

921.9 **Unspecified contusion of eye**
Injury of eye NOS

√4th 922 **Contusion of trunk**
    922.0 **Breast**
    922.1 **Chest wall**
    922.2 **Abdominal wall**
        Flank   Groin
  √5th 922.3 **Back**
        922.31 **Back**
            EXCLUDES *interscapular region (922.33)*
        922.32 **Buttock**
        922.33 **Interscapular region**
    922.4 **Genital organs**
        Labium (majus) (minus)   Vulva
        Penis   Vagina
        Perineum   Testis
        Scrotum
    922.8 **Multiple sites of trunk**
    922.9 **Unspecified part**
        Trunk NOS

√4th 923 **Contusion of upper limb**
  √5th 923.0 **Shoulder and upper arm**
        923.00 **Shoulder region**
        923.01 **Scapular region**
        923.02 **Axillary region**
        923.03 **Upper arm**
        923.09 **Multiple sites**
  √5th 923.1 **Elbow and forearm**
        923.10 **Forearm**
        923.11 **Elbow**
  √5th 923.2 **Wrist and hand(s), except finger(s) alone**
        923.20 **Hand(s)**
        923.21 **Wrist**
    923.3 **Finger**
        Fingernail   Thumb (nail)
    923.8 **Multiple sites of upper limb**
    923.9 **Unspecified part of upper limb**
        Arm NOS

√4th 924 **Contusion of lower limb and of other and unspecified sites**
  √5th 924.0 **Hip and thigh**
        924.00 **Thigh**
        924.01 **Hip**
  √5th 924.1 **Knee and lower leg**
        924.10 **Lower leg**
        924.11 **Knee**
  √5th 924.2 **Ankle and foot, excluding toe(s)**
        924.20 **Foot**
            Heel
        924.21 **Ankle**
    924.3 **Toe**
        Toenail

√4th √5th **Additional Digit Required**   **Unspecified Code**   **Other Specified Code**   **Manifestation Code**

 Medicare Secondary Payer   ▶◀ Revised Text   ● New Code   ▲ Revised Code Title

2002 Ingenix, Inc.

924.4 Multiple sites of lower limb
924.5 **Unspecified part of lower limb**
  Leg NOS
924.8 Multiple sites, not elsewhere classified
924.9 **Unspecified site**

CRUSHING INJURY (925-929)

EXCLUDES concussion (850.0-850.9)
fractures (800-829)
internal organs (860.0-869.1)
that incidental to:
  internal injury (860.0-869.1)
  intracranial injury (850.0-854.1)

√4th **925 Crushing injury of face, scalp, and neck**
  Cheek   Pharynx
  Ear   Throat
  Larynx

  925.1 **Crushing injury of face and scalp** MSP
    Cheek   Ear
  925.2 **Crushing injury of neck** MSP
    Larynx   Throat
    Pharynx

√4th **926 Crushing injury of trunk**
  EXCLUDES crush injury of internal organs (860.0-869.1)

  926.0 **External genitalia**
    Labium (majus) (minus)   Testis
    Penis   Vulva
    Scrotum
  √5th 926.1 **Other specified sites**
    926.11 Back
    926.12 Buttock
    926.19 Other
      Breast
      EXCLUDES crushing of chest (860.0-862.9)
  926.8 **Multiple sites of trunk** MSP
  926.9 **Unspecified site**
    Trunk NOS

√4th **927 Crushing injury of upper limb**
  √5th 927.0 **Shoulder and upper arm**
    927.00 Shoulder region
    927.01 Scapular region
    927.02 Axillary region
    927.03 Upper arm
    927.09 Multiple sites
  √5th 927.1 **Elbow and forearm**
    927.10 Forearm
    927.11 Elbow
  √5th 927.2 **Wrist and hand(s), except finger(s) alone**
    927.20 Hand(s)
    927.21 Wrist
  927.3 **Finger(s)**
  927.8 **Multiple sites of upper limb**

INJURY AND POISONING 927.9–933.1

     927.9 Unspecified site
        Arm NOS

√4ᵗʰ **928 Crushing injury of lower limb**

  √5ᵗʰ **928.0 Hip and thigh**
      928.00 Thigh
      928.01 Hip

  √5ᵗʰ **928.1 Knee and lower leg**
      928.10 Lower leg
      928.11 Knee

  √5ᵗʰ **928.2 Ankle and foot, excluding toe(s) alone**
      928.20 Foot
        Heel
      928.21 Ankle

  928.3 Toe(s)
  928.8 Multiple sites of lower limb
  928.9 Unspecified site
     Leg NOS

√4ᵗʰ **929 Crushing injury of multiple and unspecified sites**
     EXCLUDES multiple internal injury NOS (869.0-869.1)

  929.0 Multiple sites, not elsewhere classified MSP
  929.9 Unspecified site MSP

EFFECTS OF FOREIGN BODY ENTERING THROUGH ORIFICE (930-939)

     EXCLUDES foreign body:
          granuloma (728.82)
          inadvertently left in operative wound (998.4, 998.7)
          in open wound (800-839, 851-897)
          residual in soft tissues (729.6)
          superficial without major open wound (910-919 with .6 or .7)

√4ᵗʰ **930 Foreign body on external eye**
     EXCLUDES foreign body in penetrating wound of:
          eyeball (871.5-871.6)
            retained (old) (360.5-360.6)
          ocular adnexa (870.4)
            retained (old) (376.6)

  930.0 Corneal foreign body
  930.1 Foreign body in conjunctival sac
  930.2 Foreign body in lacrimal punctum
  930.8 Other and combined sites
  930.9 Unspecified site
     External eye NOS

931 Foreign body in ear
    Auditory canal   Auricle

932 Foreign body in nose
    Nasal sinus   Nostril

√4ᵗʰ **933 Foreign body in pharynx and larynx**

  933.0 Pharynx
     Nasopharynx   Throat NOS

  933.1 Larynx
     Asphyxia due to foreign body
     Choking due to:
       food (regurgitated)
       phlegm

√4ᵗʰ
√5ᵗʰ Additional Digit Required   Unspecified Code   Other Specified Code   Manifestation Code

 Medicare Secondary Payer   ▶◀ Revised Text   ● New Code   ▲ Revised Code Title

INJURY AND POISONING

✓4th **934 Foreign body in trachea, bronchus, and lung**
- 934.0 Trachea
- 934.1 Main bronchus
- 934.8 Other specified parts
  - Bronchioles   Lung
- 934.9 Respiratory tree, unspecified
  - Inhalation of liquid or vomitus, lower respiratory tract NOS

✓4th **935 Foreign body in mouth, esophagus, and stomach**
- 935.0 Mouth
- 935.1 Esophagus
- 935.2 Stomach

936 Foreign body in intestine and colon

937 Foreign body in anus and rectum
  Rectosigmoid (junction)

938 Foreign body in digestive system, unspecified
  Alimentary tract NOS
  Swallowed foreign body

✓4th **939 Foreign body in genitourinary tract**
- 939.0 Bladder and urethra
- 939.1 Uterus, any part ♀
  - EXCLUDES *intrauterine contraceptive device:*
    complications from (996.32, 996.65)
    presence of (V45.51)
- 939.2 Vulva and vagina ♀
- 939.3 Penis ♂
- 939.9 Unspecified site

BURNS (940-949)

INCLUDES burns from:
  electrical heating appliance
  electricity
  flame
  hot object
  lightning
  radiation
  chemical burns (external) (internal)
  scalds

EXCLUDES *friction burns (910-919 with .0, .1)*
  sunburn (692.71, 692.76-692.779)

✓4th **940 Burn confined to eye and adnexa**
- 940.0 Chemical burn of eyelids and periocular area
- 940.1 Other burns of eyelids and periocular area
- 940.2 Alkaline chemical burn of cornea and conjunctival sac
- 940.3 Acid chemical burn of cornea and conjunctival sac
- 940.4 Other burn of cornea and conjunctival sac
- 940.5 Burn with resulting rupture and destruction of eyeball
- 940.9 Unspecified burn of eye and adnexa

INJURY AND POISONING 941–942.3

Burns

Degrees of Burns

First (redness)   Second (blistering)   Third (full thickness)   Deep Third (deep necrosis) — Eschar

√4ᵗʰ 941 Burn of face, head, and neck

> EXCLUDES mouth (947.0)

The following fifth-digit subclassification is for use with category 941:

- 0 face and head, unspecified site
- 1 ear [any part]
- 2 eye (with other parts of face, head, and neck)
- 3 lip(s)
- 4 chin
- 5 nose (septum)
- 6 scalp [any part]
   Temple (region)
- 7 forehead and cheek
- 8 neck
- 9 multiple sites [except with eye] of face, head, and neck

- √5ᵗʰ **941.0 Unspecified degree**
- √5ᵗʰ **941.1** Erythema [first degree]
- √5ᵗʰ **941.2** Blisters, epidermal loss [second degree]
- √5ᵗʰ **941.3** Full-thickness skin loss [third degree NOS]
- √5ᵗʰ **941.4** Deep necrosis of underlying tissues [deep third degree] without mention of loss of a body part
- √5ᵗʰ **941.5** Deep necrosis of underlying tissues [deep third degree] with loss of a body part

√4ᵗʰ 942 Burn of trunk

> EXCLUDES scapular region (943.0-943.5 with fifth-digit 6)

The following fifth-digit subclassification is for use with category 942:

- 0 trunk, unspecified site
- 1 breast
- 2 chest wall, excluding breast and nipple
- 3 abdominal wall
   Flank   Groin
- 4 back [any part]
   Buttock   Interscapular region
- 5 genitalia
   Labium (majus) (minus)   Scrotum
   Penis   Testis
   Perineum   Vulva
- 9 other and multiple sites of trunk

- √5ᵗʰ **942.0 Unspecified degree**
- √5ᵗʰ **942.1** Erythema [first degree]
- √5ᵗʰ **942.2** Blisters, epidermal loss [second degree]
- √5ᵗʰ **942.3** Full-thickness skin loss [third degree NOS]

√4ᵗʰ / √5ᵗʰ Additional Digit Required   **Unspecified Code**   Other Specified Code   **Manifestation Code**
MSP Medicare Secondary Payer   ▶◀ Revised Text   ● New Code   ▲ Revised Code Title

2002 Ingenix, Inc.   Volume 1 — 557

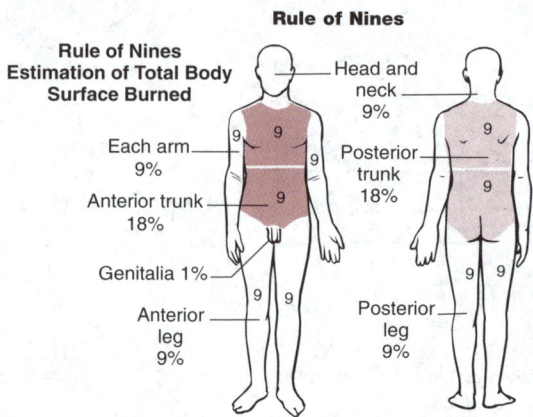

Rule of Nines

Rule of Nines Estimation of Total Body Surface Burned

- Head and neck 9%
- Each arm 9%
- Anterior trunk 18%
- Posterior trunk 18%
- Genitalia 1%
- Anterior leg 9%
- Posterior leg 9%

§ ✓5th **942.4** Deep necrosis of underlying tissues [deep third degree] without mention of loss of a body part

§ ✓5th **942.5** Deep necrosis of underlying tissues [deep third degree] with loss of a body part

✓4th **943** Burn of upper limb, except wrist and hand

The following fifth-digit subclassification is for use with category 943:
- 0 upper limb, unspecified site
- 1 forearm
- 2 elbow
- 3 upper arm
- 4 axilla
- 5 shoulder
- 6 scapular region
- 9 multiple sites of upper limb, except wrist and hand

✓5th **943.0** Unspecified degree
✓5th **943.1** Erythema [first degree]
✓5th **943.2** Blisters, epidermal loss [second degree]
✓5th **943.3** Full-thickness skin loss [third degree NOS]
✓5th **943.4** Deep necrosis of underlying tissues [deep third degree] without mention of loss of a body part
✓5th **943.5** Deep necrosis of underlying tissues [deep third degree] with loss of a body part

✓4th **944** Burn of wrist(s) and hand(s)

The following fifth-digit subclassification is for use with category 944:
- 0 hand, unspecified site
- 1 single digit [finger (nail)] other than thumb
- 2 thumb (nail)
- 3 two or more digits, not including thumb
- 4 two or more digits including thumb
- 5 palm
- 6 back of hand
- 7 wrist
- 8 multiple sites of wrist(s) and hand(s)

✓5th **944.0** Unspecified degree
✓5th **944.1** Erythema [first degree]

§ Requires fifth-digit. See beginning of category 942 for codes and definitions.

INJURY AND POISONING

- ✓5th **944.2** Blisters, epidermal loss [second degree]
- ✓5th **944.3** Full-thickness skin loss [third degree NOS]
- ✓5th **944.4** Deep necrosis of underlying tissues [deep third degree] without mention of loss of a body part
- ✓5th **944.5** Deep necrosis of underlying tissues [deep third degree] with loss of a body part

✓4th **945** Burn of lower limb(s)

The following fifth-digit subclassification is for use with category 945:
- 0 lower limb [leg], unspecified site
- 1 toe(s) (nail)
- 2 foot
- 3 ankle
- 4 lower leg
- 5 knee
- 6 thigh [any part]
- 9 multiple sites of lower limb(s)

- ✓5th **945.0** Unspecified degree
- ✓5th **945.1** Erythema [first degree]
- ✓5th **945.2** Blisters, epidermal loss [second degree]
- ✓5th **945.3** Full-thickness skin loss [third degree NOS]
- ✓5th **945.4** Deep necrosis of underlying tissues [deep third degree] without mention of loss of a body part
- ✓5th **945.5** Deep necrosis of underlying tissues [deep third degree] with loss of a body part

✓4th **946** Burns of multiple specified sites

INCLUDES   burns of sites classifiable to more than one three-digit category in 940-945

EXCLUDES   multiple burns NOS (949.0-949.5)

- **946.0** Unspecified degree
- **946.1** Erythema [first degree]
- **946.2** Blisters, epidermal loss [second degree]
- **946.3** Full-thickness skin loss [third degree NOS]
- **946.4** Deep necrosis of underlying tissues [deep third degree] without mention of loss of a body part
- **946.5** Deep necrosis of underlying tissues [deep third degree] with loss of a body part

✓4th **947** Burn of internal organs

INCLUDES   burns from chemical agents (ingested)

- **947.0** Mouth and pharynx
  - Gum
  - Tongue
- **947.1** Larynx, trachea, and lung
- **947.2** Esophagus
- **947.3** Gastrointestinal tract
  - Colon
  - Small intestine
  - Rectum
  - Stomach
- **947.4** Vagina and uterus ♀
- **947.8** Other specified sites
- **947.9** Unspecified site

INJURY AND POISONING

✓4th 948 Burns classified according to extent of body surface involved

Note: This category is to be used when the site of the burn is unspecified, or with categories 940-947 when the site is specified.

EXCLUDES   sunburn (692.71, 692.76-692.77)

The following fifth-digit subclassification is for use with category 948 to indicate the percent of body surface with third degree burn; valid digits are in [brackets] under each code:

- 0 less than 10 percent or unspecified
- 1 10-19%
- 2 20-29%
- 3 30-39%
- 4 40-49%
- 5 50-59%
- 6 60-69%
- 7 70-79%
- 8 80-89%
- 9 90% or more of body surface

✓5th **948.0** Burn [any degree] involving less than 10 percent of body surface
[0]

✓5th **948.1** 10-19 percent of body surface
[0-1]

✓5th **948.2** 20-29 percent of body surface
[0-2]

✓5th **948.3** 30-39 percent of body surface
[0-3]

✓5th **948.4** 40-49 percent of body surface
[0-4]

✓5th **948.5** 50-59 percent of body surface
[0-5]

✓5th **948.6** 60-69 percent of body surface
[0-6]

✓5th **948.7** 70-79 percent of body surface
[0-7]

✓5th **948.8** 80-89 percent of body surface
[0-8]

✓5th **948.9** 90 percent or more of body surface
[0-9]

✓4th 949 Burn, unspecified

INCLUDES   burn NOS multiple burns NOS

EXCLUDES   burn of unspecified site but with statement of the extent of body surface involved (948.0-948.9)

- 949.0 Unspecified degree
- 949.1 Erythema [first degree]
- 949.2 Blisters, epidermal loss [second degree]
- 949.3 Full-thickness skin loss [third degree NOS]
- 949.4 Deep necrosis of underlying tissues [deep third degree] without mention of loss of a body part
- 949.5 Deep necrosis of underlying tissues [deep third degree] with loss of a body part

INJURY AND POISONING

INJURY TO NERVES AND SPINAL CORD (950-957)

INCLUDES   division of nerve
lesion in continuity
traumatic neuroma } (with open wound)
traumatic transient
paralysis

EXCLUDES   accidental puncture or laceration during medical procedure (998.2)

✓4th **950 Injury to optic nerve and pathways**
- **950.0** Optic nerve injury
  Second cranial nerve
- **950.1** Injury to optic chiasm
- **950.2** Injury to optic pathways
- **950.3** Injury to visual cortex
- **950.9** Unspecified
  Traumatic blindness NOS

✓4th **951 Injury to other cranial nerve(s)**
- **951.0** Injury to oculomotor nerve
  Third cranial nerve
- **951.1** Injury to trochlear nerve
  Fourth cranial nerve
- **951.2** Injury to trigeminal nerve
  Fifth cranial nerve
- **951.3** Injury to abducens nerve
  Sixth cranial nerve
- **951.4** Injury to facial nerve
  Seventh cranial nerve
- **951.5** Injury to acoustic nerve
  Auditory nerve   Traumatic deafness NOS
  Eighth cranial nerve
- **951.6** Injury to accessory nerve
  Eleventh cranial nerve
- **951.7** Injury to hypoglossal nerve
  Twelfth cranial nerve
- **951.8** Injury to other specified cranial nerves
  Glossopharyngeal [9th cranial] nerve
  Olfactory [1st cranial] nerve
  Pneumogastric [10th cranial] nerve
  Traumatic anosmia NOS
  Vagus [10th cranial] nerve
- **951.9** Injury to unspecified cranial nerve

✓4th **952 Spinal cord injury without evidence of spinal bone injury**
- ✓5th **952.0** Cervical
  - **952.00** C_1-C_4 level with unspecified spinal cord injury
    Spinal cord injury, cervical region NOS
  - **952.01** C_1-C_4 level with complete lesion of spinal cord
  - **952.02** C_1-C_4 level with anterior cord syndrome
  - **952.03** C_1-C_4 level with central cord syndrome
  - **952.04** C_1-C_4 level with other specified spinal cord injury
    Incomplete spinal cord lesion at C_1-C_4 level:
    NOS
    with posterior cord syndrome
  - **952.05** C_5-C_7 level with unspecified spinal cord injury

---

✓4th Additional Digit Required
✓5th
 Medicare Secondary Payer   ▶◀ Revised Text   ● New Code
Unspecified Code   Other Specified Code   Manifestation Code
▲ Revised Code Title

2002 Ingenix, Inc.

- 952.06 C_5-C_7 level with complete lesion of spinal cord
- 952.07 C_5-C_7 level with anterior cord syndrome
- 952.08 C_5-C_7 level with central cord syndrome
- 952.09 C_5-C_7 level with other specified spinal cord injury
    Incomplete spinal cord lesion at C_5-C_7 level:
       NOS
       with posterior cord syndrome

√5th 952.1 Dorsal [thoracic]
- 952.10 T_1-T_6 level with unspecified spinal cord injury
    Spinal cord injury, thoracic region NOS
- 952.11 T_1-T_6 level with complete lesion of spinal cord
- 952.12 T_1-T_6 level with anterior cord syndrome
- 952.13 T_1-T_6 level with central cord syndrome
- 952.14 T_1-T_6 level with other specified spinal cord injury
    Incomplete spinal cord lesion at T_1-T_6 level:
       NOS
       with posterior cord syndrome
- 952.15 T_7-T_{12} level with unspecified spinal cord injury
- 952.16 T_7-T_{12} level with complete lesion of spinal cord
- 952.17 T_7-T_{12} level with anterior cord syndrome
- 952.18 T_7-T_{12} level with central cord syndrome
- 952.19 T_7-T_{12} level with other specified spinal cord injury
    Incomplete spinal cord lesion at T_7-T_{12} level:
       NOS
       with posterior cord syndrome

- 952.2 Lumbar
- 952.3 Sacral
- 952.4 Cauda equina
- 952.8 Multiple sites of spinal cord
- 952.9 Unspecified site of spinal cord

√4th 953 Injury to nerve roots and spinal plexus
- 953.0 Cervical root
- 953.1 Dorsal root
- 953.2 Lumbar root
- 953.3 Sacral root
- 953.4 Brachial plexus
- 953.5 Lumbosacral plexus
- 953.8 Multiple sites
- 953.9 Unspecified site

√4th 954 Injury to other nerve(s) of trunk, excluding shoulder and pelvic girdles
- 954.0 Cervical sympathetic
- 954.1 Other sympathetic
    Celiac ganglion or plexus   Splanchnic nerve(s)
    Inferior mesenteric plexus   Stellate ganglion
- 954.8 Other specified nerve(s) of trunk
- 954.9 Unspecified nerve of trunk

√4th 955 Injury to peripheral nerve(s) of shoulder girdle and upper limb
- 955.0 Axillary nerve
- 955.1 Median nerve
- 955.2 Ulnar nerve
- 955.3 Radial nerve
- 955.4 Musculocutaneous nerve

INJURY AND POISONING

- 955.5 Cutaneous sensory nerve, upper limb
- 955.6 Digital nerve
- 955.7 Other specified nerve(s) of shoulder girdle and upper limb
- 955.8 Multiple nerves of shoulder girdle and upper limb
- 955.9 Unspecified nerve of shoulder girdle and upper limb

√4ᵗʰ **956 Injury to peripheral nerve(s) of pelvic girdle and lower limb**
- 956.0 Sciatic nerve
- 956.1 Femoral nerve
- 956.2 Posterior tibial nerve
- 956.3 Peroneal nerve
- 956.4 Cutaneous sensory nerve, lower limb
- 956.5 Other specified nerve(s) of pelvic girdle and lower limb
- 956.8 Multiple nerves of pelvic girdle and lower limb
- 956.9 Unspecified nerve of pelvic girdle and lower limb

√4ᵗʰ **957 Injury to other and unspecified nerves**
- 957.0 Superficial nerves of head and neck
- 957.1 Other specified nerve(s)
- 957.8 Multiple nerves in several parts
    - Multiple nerve injury NOS
- 957.9 Unspecified site
    - Nerve injury NOS

CERTAIN TRAUMATIC COMPLICATIONS AND UNSPECIFIED INJURIES (958-959)

√4ᵗʰ **958 Certain early complications of trauma**

> **EXCLUDES** adult respiratory distress syndrome (518.5)
> flail chest (807.4)
> shock lung (518.5)
> that occurring during or following medical procedures (996.0-999.9)

- 958.0 **Air embolism**
    Pneumathemia

    > **EXCLUDES** that complicating:
    > abortion (634-638 with .6, 639.6)
    > ectopic or molar pregnancy (639.6)
    > pregnancy, childbirth, or the puerperium (673.0)

    DEF: Arterial obstruction due to introduction of air bubbles into the veins following surgery or trauma.

- 958.1 **Fat embolism**

    > **EXCLUDES** that complicating:
    > abortion (634-638 with .6, 639.6)
    > pregnancy, childbirth, or the puerperium (673.8)

    DEF: Arterial blockage due to the entrance of fat in circulatory system, after fracture of large bones or administration of corticosteroids.

- 958.2 Secondary and recurrent hemorrhage
- 958.3 Posttraumatic wound infection, not elsewhere classified

    > **EXCLUDES** infected open wounds — code to complicated open wound of site

INJURY AND POISONING

958.4 Traumatic shock [MSP]
Shock (immediate) (delayed) following injury
EXCLUDES shock:
anaphylactic (995.0)
due to serum (999.4)
anesthetic (995.4)
electric (994.8)
following abortion (639.5)
lightning (994.0)
nontraumatic NOS (785.50)
obstetric (669.1)
postoperative (998.0)
DEF: Shock, immediate or delayed following injury.

958.5 Traumatic anuria [MSP]
Crush syndrome
Renal failure following crushing
EXCLUDES that due to a medical procedure (997.5)
DEF: Complete suppression of urinary secretion by kidneys due to trauma.

958.6 Volkmann's ischemic contracture
Posttraumatic muscle contracture
DEF: Muscle deterioration due to loss of blood supply from injury or tourniquet; causes muscle contraction and results in inability to extend the muscles fully.

958.7 Traumatic subcutaneous emphysema
EXCLUDES subcutaneous emphysema resulting from a procedure (998.81)

958.8 Other early complications of trauma
DEF: Compartmental syndrome is abnormal pressure in confined anatomical space, as in swollen muscle restricted by fascia.

✓4th **959 Injury, other and unspecified**
INCLUDES injury NOS
EXCLUDES injury NOS of:
blood vessels (900.0-904.9)
eye (921.0-921.9)
internal organs (860.0-869.1)
intracranial sites (854.0-854.1)
nerves (950.0-951.9, 953.0-957.9)
spinal cord (952.0-952.9)

✓5th **959.0 Head, face and neck**

959.01 Head injury, unspecified [MSP]
EXCLUDES concussion (850.1-850.9)
with head injury NOS (850.0-850.9)
▶head injury NOS with loss of consciousness (850.1-850.5)◀
specified injuries (850.0-854.1)

959.09 Injury of face and neck [MSP]
Cheek   Mouth
Ear   Nose
Eyebrow   Throat
Lip

959.1 Trunk
Abdominal wall   External genital organs
Back   Flank
Breast   Groin
Buttock   Interscapular region
Chest wall   Perineum
EXCLUDES scapular region (959.2)

N Newborn Age: 0   P Pediatric Age: 0-17   M Maternity Age: 12-55   A Adult Age: 15-124

INJURY AND POISONING 959.2–960.4

959.2 Shoulder and upper arm
 Axilla   Scapular region

959.3 Elbow, forearm, and wrist

959.4 Hand, except finger

959.5 Finger
 Fingernail   Thumb (nail)

959.6 Hip and thigh
 Upper leg

959.7 Knee, leg, ankle, and foot

959.8 Other specified sites, including multiple
 EXCLUDES multiple sites classifiable to the same four-digit category (959.0-959.7)

959.9 Unspecified site

POISONING BY DRUGS, MEDICINAL AND BIOLOGICAL SUBSTANCES (960-979)

INCLUDES overdose of these substances
 wrong substance given or taken in error

EXCLUDES adverse effects ["hypersensitivity," "reaction," etc.] of correct substance properly administered. Such cases are to be classified according to the nature of the adverse effect, such as:
 adverse effect NOS (995.2)
 allergic lymphadenitis (289.3)
 aspirin gastritis (535.4)
 blood disorders (280.0-289.9)
 dermatitis:
  contact (692.0-692.9)
  due to ingestion (693.0-693.9)
 nephropathy (583.9)
 [The drug giving rise to the adverse effect may be identified by use of categories E930-E949.]
 drug dependence (304.0-304.9)
 drug reaction and poisoning affecting the newborn (760.0-779.9)
 nondependent abuse of drugs (305.0-305.9)
 pathological drug intoxication (292.2)
Use additional code to specify the effects of the poisoning

✓4th 960 Poisoning by antibiotics
EXCLUDES antibiotics:
 ear, nose, and throat (976.6)
 eye (976.5)
 local (976.0)

960.0 Penicillins
 Ampicillin   Cloxacillin
 Carbenicillin   Penicillin G

960.1 Antifungal antibiotics
 Amphotericin B   Nystatin
 Griseofulvin   Trichomycin
 EXCLUDES preparations intended for topical use (976.0-976.9)

960.2 Chloramphenicol group
 Chloramphenicol   Thiamphenicol

960.3 Erythromycin and other macrolides
 Oleandomycin   Spiramycin

960.4 Tetracycline group
 Doxycycline   Oxytetracycline
 Minocycline

INJURY AND POISONING

960.5 Cephalosporin group
Cephalexin   Cephaloridine
Cephaloglycin   Cephalothin

960.6 Antimycobacterial antibiotics
Cycloserine   Rifampin
Kanamycin   Streptomycin

960.7 Antineoplastic antibiotics
Actinomycin such as:
Bleomycin
Cactinomycin
Dactinomycin
Daunorubicin
Mitomycin

960.8 Other specified antibiotics

960.9 Unspecified antibiotic

√4th **961 Poisoning by other anti-infectives**
> EXCLUDES anti-infectives:
> ear, nose, and throat (976.6)
> eye (976.5)
> local (976.0)

961.0 Sulfonamides
Sulfadiazine   Sulfamethoxazole
Sulfafurazole

961.1 Arsenical anti-infectives

961.2 Heavy metal anti-infectives
Compounds of: Compounds of:
antimony   lead
bismuth   mercury
> EXCLUDES mercurial diuretics (974.0)

961.3 Quinoline and hydroxyquinoline derivatives
Chiniofon   Diiodohydroxyquin
> EXCLUDES antimalarial drugs (961.4)

961.4 Antimalarials and drugs acting on other blood protozoa
Chloroquine   Proguanil [chloroguanide]
Cycloguanil   Pyrimethamine
Primaquine   Quinine

961.5 Other antiprotozoal drugs
Emetine

961.6 Anthelmintics
Hexylresorcinol   Thiabendazole
Piperazine

961.7 Antiviral drugs
Methisazone
> EXCLUDES amantadine (966.4)
> cytarabine (963.1)
> idoxuridine (976.5)

961.8 Other antimycobacterial drugs
Ethambutol   Para-aminosalicylic acid
Ethionamide   derivatives
Isoniazid   Sulfones

961.9 Other and unspecified anti-infectives
Flucytosine   Nitrofuran derivatives

√4th **962 Poisoning by hormones and synthetic substitutes**
> EXCLUDES oxytocic hormones (975.0)

962.0 Adrenal cortical steroids
Cortisone derivatives
Desoxycorticosterone derivatives
Fluorinated corticosteroids

INJURY AND POISONING

962.1 **Androgens and anabolic congeners**
    Methandriol   Oxymetholone
    Nandrolone   Testosterone

962.2 **Ovarian hormones and synthetic substitutes**
    Contraceptives, oral
    Estrogens
    Estrogens and progestogens, combined
    Progestogens

962.3 **Insulins and antidiabetic agents**
    Acetohexamide
    Biguanide derivatives, oral
    Chlorpropamide
    Glucagon
    Insulin
    Phenformin
    Sulfonylurea derivatives, oral
    Tolbutamide

962.4 **Anterior pituitary hormones**
    Corticotropin   Somatotropin [growth
    Gonadotropin   hormone]

962.5 **Posterior pituitary hormones**
    Vasopressin
    EXCLUDES *oxytocic hormones (975.0)*

962.6 **Parathyroid and parathyroid derivatives**

962.7 **Thyroid and thyroid derivatives**
    Dextrothyroxin   Liothyronine
    Levothyroxine sodium   Thyroglobulin

962.8 **Antithyroid agents**
    Iodides   Thiourea
    Thiouracil

962.9 **Other and unspecified hormones and synthetic substitutes**

√4th **963 Poisoning by primarily systemic agents**

963.0 **Antiallergic and antiemetic drugs**
    Antihistamines   Diphenylpyraline
    Chlorpheniramine   Thonzylamine
    Diphenhydramine   Tripelennamine
    EXCLUDES *phenothiazine-based tranquilizers (969.1)*

963.1 **Antineoplastic and immunosuppressive drugs**
    Azathioprine   Cytarabine
    Busulfan   Fluorouracil
    Chlorambucil   Mercaptopurine
    Cyclophosphamide   thio-TEPA
    EXCLUDES *antineoplastic antibiotics (960.7)*

963.2 **Acidifying agents**

963.3 **Alkalizing agents**

963.4 **Enzymes, not elsewhere classified**
    Penicillinase

963.5 **Vitamins, not elsewhere classified**
    Vitamin A   Vitamin D
    EXCLUDES *nicotinic acid (972.2)*
                       vitamin K (964.3)

963.8 **Other specified systemic agents**
    Heavy metal antagonists

963.9 **Unspecified systemic agent**

 Additional Digit Required   Unspecified Code   Other Specified Code   Manifestation Code

MSP Medicare Secondary Payer   ▶◀ Revised Text   ● New Code   ▲ Revised Code Title

2002 Ingenix, Inc.

INJURY AND POISONING

✓4th 964 Poisoning by agents primarily affecting blood constituents

- **964.0 Iron and its compounds**
  - Ferric salts
  - Ferrous sulfate and other ferrous salts
- **964.1 Liver preparations and other antianemic agents**
  - Folic acid
- **964.2 Anticoagulants**
  - Coumarin
  - Heparin
  - Phenindione
  - Warfarin sodium
- **964.3 Vitamin K [phytonadione]**
- **964.4 Fibrinolysis-affecting drugs**
  - Aminocaproic acid
  - Streptodornase
  - Streptokinase
  - Urokinase
- **964.5 Anticoagulant antagonists and other coagulants**
  - Hexadimethrine
  - Protamine sulfate
- **964.6 Gamma globulin**
- **964.7 Natural blood and blood products**
  - Blood plasma
  - Human fibrinogen
  - Packed red cells
  - Whole blood
  - **EXCLUDES** transfusion reactions (999.4-999.8)
- **964.8 Other specified agents affecting blood constituents**
  - Macromolecular blood substitutes
  - Plasma expanders
- **964.9 Unspecified agent affecting blood constituents**

✓4th 965 Poisoning by analgesics, antipyretics, and antirheumatics

EXCLUDES drug dependence (304.0-304.9)
nondependent abuse (305.0-305.9)

- **✓5th 965.0 Opiates and related narcotics**
  - **965.00 Opium (alkaloids), unspecified**
  - **965.01 Heroin**
    - Diacetylmorphine
  - **965.02 Methadone**
  - **965.09 Other**
    - Codeine [methylmorphine]
    - Meperidine [pethidine]
    - Morphine
- **965.1 Salicylates**
  - Acetylsalicylic acid [aspirin]
  - Salicylic acid salts
- **965.4 Aromatic analgesics, not elsewhere classified**
  - Acetanilid
  - Paracetamol [acetaminophen]
  - Phenacetin [acetophenetidin]
- **965.5 Pyrazole derivatives**
  - Aminophenazone [aminopyrine]
  - Phenylbutazone
- **✓5th 965.6 Antirheumatics [antiphlogistics]**
  - **EXCLUDES** salicylates (965.1)
  - steroids (962.0-962.9)
  - **965.61 Propionic acid derivatives**
    - Fenoprofen
    - Flurbiprofen
    - Ibuprofen
    - Ketoprofen
    - Naproxen
    - Oxaprozin
  - **965.69 Other antirheumatics**
    - Gold salts
    - Indomethacin

INJURY AND POISONING 965.7–968.1

- **965.7 Other non-narcotic analgesics**
  - Pyrabital
- **965.8 Other specified analgesics and antipyretics**
  - Pentazocine
- **965.9 Unspecified analgesic and antipyretic**

✓4th 966 Poisoning by anticonvulsants and anti-Parkinsonism drugs

- **966.0 Oxazolidine derivatives**
  - Paramethadione   Trimethadione
- **966.1 Hydantoin derivatives**
  - Phenytoin
- **966.2 Succinimides**
  - Ethosuximide   Phensuximide
- **966.3 Other and unspecified anticonvulsants**
  - Primidone
  - EXCLUDES *barbiturates (967.0)*
  - *sulfonamides (961.0)*
- **966.4 Anti-Parkinsonism drugs**
  - Amantadine
  - Ethopropazine [profenamine]
  - Levodopa [L-dopa]

✓4th 967 Poisoning by sedatives and hypnotics

EXCLUDES *drug dependence (304.0-304.9)*
nondependent abuse (305.0-305.9)

- **967.0 Barbiturates**
  - Amobarbital [amylobarbitone]
  - Barbital [barbitone]
  - Butabarbital [butabarbitone]
  - Pentobarbital [pentobarbitone]
  - Phenobarbital [phenobarbitone]
  - Secobarbital [quinalbarbitone]
  - EXCLUDES *thiobarbiturate anesthetics (968.3)*
- **967.1 Chloral hydrate group**
- **967.2 Paraldehyde**
- **967.3 Bromine compounds**
  - Bromide   Carbromal (derivatives)
- **967.4 Methaqualone compounds**
- **967.5 Glutethimide group**
- **967.6 Mixed sedatives, not elsewhere classified**
- **967.8 Other sedatives and hypnotics**
- **967.9 Unspecified sedative or hypnotic**
  - Sleeping:
    - drug
    - pill   } NOS
    - tablet

✓4th 968 Poisoning by other central nervous system depressants and anesthetics

EXCLUDES *drug dependence (304.0-304.9)*
nondependent abuse (305.0-305.9)

- **968.0 Central nervous system muscle-tone depressants**
  - Chlorphenesin (carbamate)   Methocarbamol
  - Mephenesin
- **968.1 Halothane**

✓4th ✓5th Additional Digit Required   Unspecified Code   Other Specified Code   Manifestation Code
MSP Medicare Secondary Payer   ▶◀ Revised Text   ● New Code   ▲ Revised Code Title

2002 Ingenix, Inc.

968.2 Other gaseous anesthetics
  Ether
  Halogenated hydrocarbon derivatives, except halothane
  Nitrous oxide

968.3 Intravenous anesthetics
  Ketamine
  Methohexital [methohexitone]
  Thiobarbiturates, such as thiopental sodium

968.4 Other and unspecified general anesthetics

968.5 Surface [topical] and infiltration anesthetics
  Cocaine   Procaine
  Lidocaine [lignocaine] Tetracaine

968.6 Peripheral nerve- and plexus-blocking anesthetics

968.7 Spinal anesthetics

968.9 Other and unspecified local anesthetics

✓4th **969 Poisoning by psychotropic agents**
  EXCLUDES drug dependence (304.0-304.9)
            nondependent abuse (305.0-305.9)

969.0 Antidepressants
  Amitriptyline
  Imipramine
  Monoamine oxidase [MAO] inhibitors

969.1 Phenothiazine-based tranquilizers
  Chlorpromazine   Prochlorperazine
  Fluphenazine   Promazine

969.2 Butyrophenone-based tranquilizers
  Haloperidol   Trifluperidol
  Spiperone

969.3 Other antipsychotics, neuroleptics, and major tranquilizers

969.4 Benzodiazepine-based tranquilizers
  Chlordiazepoxide Lorazepam
  Diazepam   Medazepam
  Flurazepam   Nitrazepam

969.5 Other tranquilizers
  Hydroxyzine   Meprobamate

969.6 Psychodysleptics [hallucinogens]
  Cannabis (derivatives) Mescaline
  Lysergide [LSD]   Psilocin
  Marihuana (derivatives) Psilocybin

969.7 Psychostimulants
  Amphetamine   Caffeine
  EXCLUDES central appetite depressants (977.0)

969.8 Other specified psychotropic agents

969.9 Unspecified psychotropic agent

✓4th **970 Poisoning by central nervous system stimulants**

970.0 Analeptics
  Lobeline
  Nikethamide

970.1 Opiate antagonists
  Levallorphan
  Nalorphine
  Naloxone

970.8 Other specified central nervous system stimulants

970.9 Unspecified central nervous system stimulant

INJURY AND POISONING 971–973.2

✓4th **971 Poisoning by drugs primarily affecting the autonomic nervous system**

971.0 Parasympathomimetics [cholinergics]
Acetylcholine   Pilocarpine
Anticholinesterase:
  organophosphorus
  reversible

971.1 Parasympatholytics [anticholinergics and antimuscarinics] and spasmolytics
Atropine   Quaternary ammonium
Homatropine   derivatives
Hyoscine [scopolamine]
  EXCLUDES *papaverine (972.5)*

971.2 Sympathomimetics [adrenergics]
Epinephrine [adrenalin]   Levarterenol [noradrenalin]

971.3 Sympatholytics [antiadrenergics]
Phenoxybenzamine   Tolazolinehydrochloride

971.9 Unspecified drug primarily affecting autonomic nervous system

✓4th **972 Poisoning by agents primarily affecting the cardiovascular system**

972.0 Cardiac rhythm regulators
Practolol   Propranolol
Procainamide   Quinidine
  EXCLUDES *lidocaine (968.5)*

972.1 Cardiotonic glycosides and drugs of similar action
Digitalis glycosides   Strophanthins
Digoxin

972.2 Antilipemic and antiarteriosclerotic drugs
Clofibrate   Nicotinic acid derivatives

972.3 Ganglion-blocking agents
Pentamethonium bromide

972.4 Coronary vasodilators
Dipyridamole   Nitrites
Nitrates [nitroglycerin]

972.5 Other vasodilators
Cyclandelate   Papaverine
Diazoxide
  EXCLUDES *nicotinic acid (972.2)*

972.6 Other antihypertensive agents
Clonidine   Rauwolfia alkaloids
Guanethidine   Reserpine

972.7 Antivaricose drugs, including sclerosing agents
Sodium morrhuate   Zinc salts

972.8 Capillary-active drugs
Adrenochrome derivatives   Metaraminol

972.9 Other and unspecified agents primarily affecting the cardiovascular system

✓4th **973 Poisoning by agents primarily affecting the gastrointestinal system**

973.0 Antacids and antigastric secretion drugs
Aluminum hydroxide   Magnesium trisilicate

973.1 Irritant cathartics
Bisacodyl   Phenolphthalein
Castor oil

973.2 Emollient cathartics
Dioctyl sulfosuccinates

✓4th / ✓5th Additional Digit Required   Unspecified Code   Other Specified Code   Manifestation Code
 Medicare Secondary Payer   ▶◀ Revised Text   ● New Code   ▲ Revised Code Title

2002 Ingenix, Inc.   Volume 1 — 571

973.3 Other cathartics, including intestinal atonia drugs
  Magnesium sulfate

973.4 **Digestants**
  Pancreatin   Pepsin
  Papain

973.5 **Antidiarrheal drugs**
  Kaolin   Pectin
  EXCLUDES anti-infectives (960.0-961.9)

973.6 **Emetics**

973.8 Other specified agents primarily affecting the gastrointestinal system

973.9 Unspecified agent primarily affecting the gastrointestinal system

√4th **974 Poisoning by water, mineral, and uric acid metabolism drugs**

  974.0 **Mercurial diuretics**
    Chlormerodrin   Mersalyl
    Mercaptomerin

  974.1 **Purine derivative diuretics**
    Theobromine   Theophylline
    EXCLUDES aminophylline [theophylline ethylenediamine] (975.7)
    caffeine (969.7)

  974.2 **Carbonic acid anhydrase inhibitors**
    Acetazolamide

  974.3 **Saluretics**
    Benzothiadiazides   Chlorothiazide group

  974.4 Other diuretics
    Ethacrynic acid   Furosemide

  974.5 **Electrolytic, caloric, and water-balance agents**

  974.6 Other mineral salts, not elsewhere classified

  974.7 **Uric acid metabolism drugs**
    Allopurinol   Probenecid
    Colchicine

√4th **975 Poisoning by agents primarily acting on the smooth and skeletal muscles and respiratory system**

  975.0 **Oxytocic agents**
    Ergot alkaloids   Prostaglandins
    Oxytocin

  975.1 **Smooth muscle relaxants**
    Adiphenine   Metaproterenol [orciprenaline]
    EXCLUDES papaverine (972.5)

  975.2 **Skeletal muscle relaxants**

  975.3 Other and unspecified drugs acting on muscles

  975.4 **Antitussives**
    Dextromethorphan   Pipazethate

  975.5 **Expectorants**
    Acetylcysteine   Terpin hydrate
    Guaifenesin

  975.6 **Anti-common cold drugs**

  975.7 **Antiasthmatics**
    Aminophylline [theophylline ethylenediamine]

  975.8 Other and unspecified respiratory drugs

√4th **976 Poisoning by agents primarily affecting skin and mucous membrane, ophthalmological, otorhinolaryngological, and dental drugs**

  976.0 **Local anti-infectives and anti-inflammatory drugs**

  976.1 **Antipruritics**

  976.2 **Local astringents and local detergents**

INJURY AND POISONING

- 976.3 Emollients, demulcents, and protectants
- 976.4 Keratolytics, keratoplastics, other hair treatment drugs and preparations
- 976.5 Eye anti-infectives and other eye drugs
  Idoxuridine
- 976.6 Anti-infectives and other drugs and preparations for ear, nose, and throat
- 976.7 Dental drugs topically applied
  - EXCLUDES anti-infectives (976.0)
  local anesthetics (968.5)
- 976.8 Other agents primarily affecting skin and mucous membrane
  Spermicides [vaginal contraceptives]
- 976.9 Unspecified agent primarily affecting skin and mucous membrane

✓4th 977 Poisoning by other and unspecified drugs and medicinal substances
- 977.0 Dietetics
  Central appetite depressants
- 977.1 Lipotropic drugs
- 977.2 Antidotes and chelating agents, not elsewhere classified
- 977.3 Alcohol deterrents
- 977.4 Pharmaceutical excipients
  Pharmaceutical adjuncts
- 977.8 Other specified drugs and medicinal substances
  Contrast media used for diagnostic x-ray procedures
  Diagnostic agents and kits
- 977.9 Unspecified drug or medicinal substance

✓4th 978 Poisoning by bacterial vaccines
- 978.0 BCG
- 978.1 Typhoid and paratyphoid
- 978.2 Cholera
- 978.3 Plague
- 978.4 Tetanus
- 978.5 Diphtheria
- 978.6 Pertussis vaccine, including combinations with a pertussis component
- 978.8 Other and unspecified bacterial vaccines
- 978.9 Mixed bacterial vaccines, except combinations with a pertussis component

✓4th 979 Poisoning by other vaccines and biological substances
  - EXCLUDES gamma globulin (964.6)
- 979.0 Smallpox vaccine
- 979.1 Rabies vaccine
- 979.2 Typhus vaccine
- 979.3 Yellow fever vaccine
- 979.4 Measles vaccine
- 979.5 Poliomyelitis vaccine
- 979.6 Other and unspecified viral and rickettsial vaccines
  Mumps vaccine
- 979.7 Mixed viral-rickettsial and bacterial vaccines, except combinations with a pertussis component
  - EXCLUDES combinations with a pertussis component (978.6)
- 979.9 Other and unspecified vaccines and biological substances

980–984.0 INJURY AND POISONING

TOXIC EFFECTS OF SUBSTANCES CHIEFLY NONMEDICINAL AS TO SOURCE (980-989)

EXCLUDES burns from chemical agents (ingested) (947.0-947.9)
localized toxic effects indexed elsewhere (001.0-799.9)
respiratory conditions due to external agents (506.0-508.9)
Use additional code to specify the nature of the toxic effect

√4th **980 Toxic effect of alcohol**

980.0 Ethyl alcohol
Denatured alcohol   Grain alcohol
Ethanol
Use additional code to identify any associated:
acute alcohol intoxication (305.0)
in alcoholism (303.0)
drunkenness (simple) (305.0)
pathological (291.4)

980.1 Methyl alcohol
Methanol   Wood alcohol

980.2 Isopropyl alcohol
Dimethyl carbinol   Rubbing alcohol
Isopropanol

980.3 Fusel oil
Alcohol: Alcohol:
  amyl   propyl
  butyl

980.8 Other specified alcohols

980.9 Unspecified alcohol

981 Toxic effect of petroleum products
Benzine   Petroleum:
Gasoline   ether
Kerosene   naphtha
Paraffin wax   spirit

√4th **982 Toxic effect of solvents other than petroleum-based**

982.0 Benzene and homologues

982.1 Carbon tetrachloride

982.2 Carbon disulfide
Carbon bisulfide

982.3 Other chlorinated hydrocarbon solvents
Tetrachloroethylene   Trichloroethylene
EXCLUDES chlorinated hydrocarbon preparations other than solvents (989.2)

982.4 Nitroglycol

982.8 Other nonpetroleum-based solvents
Acetone

√4th **983 Toxic effect of corrosive aromatics, acids, and caustic alkalis**

983.0 Corrosive aromatics
Carbolic acid or phenol   Cresol

983.1 Acids
Acid: Acid:
  hydrochloric   sulfuric
  nitric

983.2 Caustic alkalis
Lye   Sodium hydroxide
Potassium hydroxide

983.9 Caustic, unspecified

√4th **984 Toxic effect of lead and its compounds (including fumes)**
INCLUDES that from all sources except medicinal substances

984.0 Inorganic lead compounds
Lead dioxide   Lead salts

INJURY AND POISONING

- **984.1** Organic lead compounds
  - Lead acetate
  - Tetraethyl lead
- **984.8** Other lead compounds
- **984.9** Unspecified lead compound

✓4th **985** Toxic effect of other metals
  - INCLUDES: that from all sources except medicinal substances
  - **985.0** Mercury and its compounds
    - Minamata disease
  - **985.1** Arsenic and its compounds
  - **985.2** Manganese and its compounds
  - **985.3** Beryllium and its compounds
  - **985.4** Antimony and its compounds
  - **985.5** Cadmium and its compounds
  - **985.6** Chromium
  - **985.8** Other specified metals
    - Brass fumes
    - Copper salts
    - Iron compounds
    - Nickel compounds
  - **985.9** Unspecified metal

986 Toxic effect of carbon monoxide
  - Carbon monoxide from any source

✓4th **987** Toxic effect of other gases, fumes, or vapors
  - **987.0** Liquefied petroleum gases
    - Butane
    - Propane
  - **987.1** Other hydrocarbon gas
  - **987.2** Nitrogen oxides
    - Nitrogen dioxide
    - Nitrous fumes
  - **987.3** Sulfur dioxide
  - **987.4** Freon
    - Dichloromonofluoromethane
  - **987.5** Lacrimogenic gas
    - Bromobenzyl cyanide
    - Ethyliodoacetate
    - Chloroacetophenone
  - **987.6** Chlorine gas
  - **987.7** Hydrocyanic acid gas
  - **987.8** Other specified gases, fumes, or vapors
    - Phosgene
    - Polyester fumes
  - **987.9** Unspecified gas, fume, or vapor

✓4th **988** Toxic effect of noxious substances eaten as food
  - EXCLUDES: allergic reaction to food, such as:
    - gastroenteritis (558.3)
    - rash (692.5, 693.1)
    - food poisoning (bacterial) (005.0-005.9)
    - toxic effects of food contaminants, such as:
      - aflatoxin and other mycotoxin (989.7)
      - mercury (985.0)
  - **988.0** Fish and shellfish
  - **988.1** Mushrooms
  - **988.2** Berries and other plants
  - **988.8** Other specified noxious substances eaten as food
  - **988.9** Unspecified noxious substance eaten as food

INJURY AND POISONING

✓4th **989 Toxic effect of other substances, chiefly nonmedicinal as to source**

989.0 Hydrocyanic acid and cyanides
Potassium cyanide   Sodium cyanide
EXCLUDES   gas and fumes (987.7)

989.1 Strychnine and salts

989.2 Chlorinated hydrocarbons
Aldrin   DDT
Chlordane   Dieldrin
EXCLUDES   chlorinated hydrocarbon solvents (982.0-982.3)

989.3 Organophosphate and carbamate
Carbaryl   Parathion
Dichlorvos   Phorate
Malathion   Phosdrin

989.4 Other pesticides, not elsewhere classified
Mixtures of insecticides

989.5 Venom
Bites of venomous snakes, lizards, and spiders
Tick paralysis

989.6 Soaps and detergents

989.7 Aflatoxin and other mycotoxin [food contaminants]

✓5th **989.8 Other substances, chiefly nonmedicinal as to source**

989.81 Asbestos
EXCLUDES   asbestosis (501)
exposure to asbestos (V15.84)

989.82 Latex

989.83 Silicone
EXCLUDES   silicone used in medical devices, implants and grafts (996.00-996.79)

989.84 Tobacco

989.89 Other

989.9 Unspecified substance, chiefly nonmedicinal as to source

OTHER AND UNSPECIFIED EFFECTS OF EXTERNAL CAUSES (990-995)

990 Effects of radiation, unspecified
Complication of: Radiation sickness
    phototherapy
    radiation therapy
EXCLUDES   specified adverse effects of radiation. Such conditions are to be classified according to the nature of the adverse effect, as:
    burns (940.0-949.5)
    dermatitis (692.7-692.8)
    leukemia (204.0-208.9)
    pneumonia (508.0)
    sunburn (692.71, 692.76-692.77)
[The type of radiation giving rise to the adverse effect may be identified by use of the E codes.]

✓4th **991 Effects of reduced temperature**

991.0 Frostbite of face

991.1 Frostbite of hand

991.2 Frostbite of foot

991.3 Frostbite of other and unspecified sites

991.4 Immersion foot
Trench foot
DEF: Paresthesia, edema, blotchy cyanosis of foot, the skin is soft (macerated), pale and wrinkled, and the sole is swollen with surface ridging and following sustained immersion in water.

INJURY AND POISONING

991.5 Chilblains
Erythema pernio   Perniosis
DEF: Red, swollen, itchy skin; follows damp cold exposure; also associated with pruritus and a burning feeling, in hands, feet, ears, and face in children, legs and toes in women, and hands and fingers in men.

991.6 Hypothermia
Hypothermia (accidental)
EXCLUDES: hypothermia following anesthesia (995.89)
hypothermia not associated with low environmental temperature ▶(780.99)◀
DEF: Reduced body temperature due to low environmental temperatures.

991.8 Other specified effects of reduced temperature

991.9 Unspecified effect of reduced temperature
Effects of freezing or excessive cold NOS

√4th 992 Effects of heat and light
EXCLUDES: burns (940.0-949.5)
diseases of sweat glands due to heat (705.0-705.9)
malignant hyperpyrexia following anesthesia (995.86)
sunburn (692.71, 692.76-692.77)

992.0 Heat stroke and sunstroke
Heat apoplexy   Siriasis
Heat pyrexia   Thermoplegia
Ictus solaris
DEF: Headache, vertigo, cramps and elevated body temperature due to high environmental temperatures.

992.1 Heat syncope
Heat collapse

992.2 Heat cramps

992.3 Heat exhaustion, anhydrotic
Heat prostration due to water depletion
EXCLUDES: that associated with salt depletion (992.4)

992.4 Heat exhaustion due to salt depletion
Heat prostration due to salt (and water) depletion

992.5 Heat exhaustion, unspecified
Heat prostration NOS

992.6 Heat fatigue, transient

992.7 Heat edema
DEF: Fluid retention due to high environmental temperatures.

992.8 Other specified heat effects

992.9 Unspecified

√4th 993 Effects of air pressure

993.0 Barotrauma, otitic
Aero-otitis media   Effects of high altitude on ears
DEF: Ringing ears, deafness, pain and vertigo due to air pressure changes.

993.1 Barotrauma, sinus
Aerosinusitis
Effects of high altitude on sinuses

993.2 Other and unspecified effects of high altitude
Alpine sickness   Hypobaropathy
Andes disease   Mountain sickness
Anoxia due to high altitude

 Additional Digit Required   Unspecified Code   Other Specified Code   Manifestation Code
MSP Medicare Secondary Payer   ▶◀ Revised Text   ● New Code   ▲ Revised Code Title

993.3 Caisson disease
Bends
Compressed-air disease
Decompression sickness
Divers' palsy or paralysis

DEF: Rapid reduction in air pressure while breathing compressed air; symptoms include skin lesions, joint pains, respiratory and neurological problems.

993.4 Effects of air pressure caused by explosion
993.8 Other specified effects of air pressure
993.9 Unspecified effect of air pressure

✓4th **994 Effects of other external causes**
    EXCLUDES *certain adverse effects not elsewhere classified (995.0-995.8)*

994.0 Effects of lightning
Shock from lightning   Struck by lightning NOS
    EXCLUDES *burns (940.0-949.5)*

994.1 Drowning and nonfatal submersion
Bathing cramp   Immersion

994.2 Effects of hunger
Deprivation of food   Starvation

994.3 Effects of thirst
Deprivation of water

994.4 Exhaustion due to exposure

994.5 Exhaustion due to excessive exertion
Overexertion

994.6 Motion sickness
Air sickness   Travel sickness
Seasickness

994.7 Asphyxiation and strangulation
Suffocation (by):
  bedclothes
  cave-in
  constriction
  mechanical
Suffocation (by):
  plastic bag
  pressure
  strangulation

    EXCLUDES *asphyxia from:*
        carbon monoxide (986)
        inhalation of food or foreign body (932-934.9)
        other gases, fumes, and vapors (987.0-987.9)

994.8 Electrocution and nonfatal effects of electric current
Shock from electric current
    EXCLUDES *electric burns (940.0-949.5)*

994.9 Other effects of external causes
Effects of:
  abnormal gravitational [G] forces or states
  weightlessness

INJURY AND POISONING

✓4th 995 Certain adverse effects not elsewhere classified
EXCLUDES complications of surgical and medical care (996.0-999.9)

995.0 Other anaphylactic shock

Allergic shock ⎫ NOS or due to adverse effect of
Anaphylactic ⎬ correct medicinal
   reaction ⎬ substance properly
Anaphylaxis ⎭ administered

Use additional E code to identify external cause, such as:
   adverse effects of correct medicinal substance properly administered [E930-E949]

EXCLUDES anaphylactic reaction to serum (999.4)
anaphylactic shock due to adverse food reaction (995.60-995.69)

DEF: Immediate sensitivity response after exposure to specific antigen; results in life-threatening respiratory distress; usually followed by vascular collapse, shock, urticaria, angioedema and pruritus.

995.1 Angioneurotic edema
Giant urticaria

EXCLUDES urticaria:
   due to serum (999.5)
   other specified (698.2, 708.0-708.9, 757.33)

DEF: Circulatory response of deep dermis, subcutaneous or submucosal tissues; causes localized edema and wheals.

995.2 Unspecified adverse effect of drug, medicinal and biological substance

Adverse effect ⎫
Allergic reaction ⎬ (due) to correct medicinal
Hypersensitivity ⎬ substance properly
Idiosyncrasy ⎭ administered

Drug: Drug:
   hypersensitivity NOS   reaction NOS

EXCLUDES pathological drug intoxication (292.2)

995.3 Allergy, unspecified
Allergic reaction NOS   Idiosyncrasy NOS
Hypersensitivity NOS

EXCLUDES allergic reaction NOS to correct medicinal substance properly administered (995.2)
specific types of allergic reaction, such as:
   allergic diarrhea (558.3)
   dermatitis (691.0-693.9)
   hayfever (477.0-477.9)

995.4 Shock due to anesthesia
Shock due to anesthesia in which the correct substance was properly administered

EXCLUDES complications of anesthesia in labor or delivery (668.0-668.9)
overdose or wrong substance given (968.0-969.9)
postoperative shock NOS (998.0)
specified adverse effects of anesthesia classified elsewhere, such as:
   anoxic brain damage (348.1)
   hepatitis (070.0-070.9), etc.
unspecified adverse effect of anesthesia (995.2)

995.5–995.82 INJURY AND POISONING

- ✓5th **995.5 Child maltreatment syndrome**
  Use additional code(s), if applicable, to identify any associated injuries
  Use additional E code to identify:
  nature of abuse (E960-E968)
  perpetrator (E967.0-E967.9)
  - **995.50 Child abuse, unspecified** [P]
  - 995.51 Child emotional/psychological abuse [P]
  - 995.52 Child neglect (nutritional) [P]
  - 995.53 Child sexual abuse [P]
  - 995.54 Child physical abuse [P]
    Battered baby or child syndrome
    EXCLUDES shaken infant syndrome (995.55)
  - 995.55 Shaken infant syndrome [P]
    Use additional code(s) to identify any associated injuries
  - **995.59 Other child abuse and neglect** [P]
    Multiple forms of abuse

- ✓5th **995.6 Anaphylactic shock due to adverse food reaction**
  Anaphylactic shock due to nonpoisonous foods
  - **995.60 Due to unspecified food**
  - 995.61 Due to peanuts
  - 995.62 Due to crustaceans
  - 995.63 Due to fruits and vegetables
  - 995.64 Due to tree nuts and seeds
  - 995.65 Due to fish
  - 995.66 Due to food additives
  - 995.67 Due to milk products
  - 995.68 Due to eggs
  - **995.69 Due to other specified food**

- **995.7 Other adverse food reactions, not elsewhere classified**
  Use additional code to identify the type of reaction, such as:
  hives (708.0)
  wheezing (786.07)
  EXCLUDES anaphylactic shock due to adverse food reaction (995.60-995.69)
  asthma (493.0, 493.9)
  dermatitis due to food (693.1)
  in contact with the skin (692.5)
  gastroenteritis and colitis due to food (558.3)
  rhinitis due to food (477.1)

- ✓5th **995.8 Other specified adverse effects, not elsewhere classified**
  - **995.80 Adult maltreatment, unspecified** [A]
    Abused person NOS
    Use additional code to identify:
    any associated injury
    perpetrator (E967.0-E967.9)
  - 995.81 Adult physical abuse [A]
    Battered:
    person syndrome NEC
    man
    spouse
    woman
    Use additional code to identify:
    any association injury
    nature of abuse (E960-E968)
    perpetrator (E967.0-E967.9)
  - 995.82 Adult emotional/psychological abuse [A]
    Use additional E code to identify perpetrator (E967.0-E967.9)

INJURY AND POISONING

995.83 Adult sexual abuse ▲
  Use additional code to identify:
    any associated injury
    perpetrator (E967.0-E967.9)

995.84 Adult neglect (nutritional) ▲
  Use addition code to identify:
    intent of neglect (E904.0, E968.4)
    perpetrator (E967.0-E967.9)

995.85 Other adult abuse and neglect ▲
  Multiple forms of abuse and neglect
  Use additional code to identify:
    any associated injury
    intent of neglect (E904.0, E968.4)
    nature of abuse (E960-E968)
    perpetrator (E967.0-E967.9)

995.86 Malignant hyperthermia
  Malignant hyperpyrexia due to anesthesia

995.89 Other
  Hypothermia due to anesthesia

√5th **995.9 Systemic inflammatory response syndrome (SIRS)**

  995.90 Systemic inflammatory response syndrome, unspecified
    SIRS NOS

  995.91 Systemic inflammatory response syndrome due to infectious process without organ dysfunction

  995.92 Systemic inflammatory response syndrome due to infectious process with organ dysfunction
    Severe sepsis
    Use additional code to specify organ dysfunction, such as:
      encephalopathy (348.3)
      heart failure (428.0-428.9)
      kidney failure (584.5-584.9, 585, 586)

  995.93 Systemic inflammatory response syndrome due to noninfectious process without organ dysfunction

  995.94 Systemic inflammatory response syndrome due to noninfectious process with organ dysfunction
    Use additional code to specify organ dysfunction, such as:
      encephalopathy (348.3)
      heart failure (428.0-428.9)
      kidney failure (584.5-584.9, 585, 586)

INJURY AND POISONING

COMPLICATIONS OF SURGICAL AND MEDICAL CARE, NOT ELSEWHERE CLASSIFIED (996-999)

> **EXCLUDES** adverse effects of medicinal agents (001.0-799.9, 995.0-995.8)
> burns from local applications and irradiation (940.0-949.5)
> complications of:
>   conditions for which the procedure was performed
>   surgical procedures during abortion, labor, and delivery (630-676.9)
> poisoning and toxic effects of drugs and chemicals (960.0-989.9)
> postoperative conditions in which no complications are present, such as:
>   artificial opening status (V44.0-V44.9)
>   closure of external stoma (V55.0-V55.9)
>   fitting of prosthetic device (V52.0-V52.9)
> specified complications classified elsewhere
>   anesthetic shock (995.4)
>   electrolyte imbalance (276.0-276.9)
>   postlaminectomy syndrome (722.80-722.83)
>   postmastectomy lymphedema syndrome (457.0)
>   postoperative psychosis (293.0-293.9)
>   any other condition classified elsewhere in the Alphabetic Index when described as due to a procedure

✓4th 996 Complications peculiar to certain specified procedures

> **INCLUDES** complications, not elsewhere classified, in the use of artificial substitutes [e.g., Dacron, metal, Silastic, Teflon] or natural sources [e.g., bone] involving:
>   anastomosis (internal)
>   graft (bypass) (patch)
>   implant
>   internal device:
>   catheter
>   electronic
>   fixation
>   prosthetic
>   reimplant
>   transplant

> **EXCLUDES** accidental puncture or laceration during procedure (998.2)
> complications of internal anastomosis of:
>   gastrointestinal tract (997.4)
>   urinary tract (997.5)
> other specified complications classified elsewhere, such as:
>   hemolytic anemia (283.1)
>   functional cardiac disturbances (429.4)
>   serum hepatitis (070.2-070.3)

✓5th 996.0 Mechanical complication of cardiac device, implant, and graft
Breakdown (mechanical)
Displacement
Leakage
Obstruction, mechanical
Perforation
Protrusion

- **996.00** Unspecified device, implant, and graft   MSP
- **996.01** Due to cardiac pacemaker (electrode)   MSP
- **996.02** Due to heart valve prosthesis   MSP
- **996.03** Due to coronary bypass graft   MSP
  > **EXCLUDES** atherosclerosis of graft (414.02, 414.03)
  > embolism [occlusion NOS] [thrombus] of graft (996.72)
- **996.04** Due to automatic implantable cardiac defibrillator
- **996.09** Other   MSP

INJURY AND POISONING

996.1 Mechanical complication of other vascular device, implant, and graft [MSP]
  femoral-popliteal bypass graft
  Mechanical complications involving:
    aortic (bifurcation) graft (replacement)
    arteriovenous:
      dialysis catheter ⎫
      fistula   ⎬ surgically created
      shunt   ⎭
    balloon (counterpulsation) device, intra-aortic
    carotid artery bypass graft
    umbrella device, vena cava
  EXCLUDES *atherosclerosis of biological graft (440.30-440.32)*
              embolism [occlusion NOS] [thrombus] of (biological) (synthetic) graft (996.74)
              peritoneal dialysis catheter (996.56)

996.2 Mechanical complication of nervous system device, implant, and graft [MSP]
  Mechanical complications involving:
    dorsal column stimulator
    electrodes implanted in brain [brain "pacemaker"]
    peripheral nerve graft
    ventricular (communicating) shunt

√5th 996.3 Mechanical complication of genitourinary device, implant, and graft
  996.30 Unspecified device, implant, and graft [MSP]
  996.31 Due to urethral [indwelling] catheter [MSP]
  996.32 Due to intrauterine contraceptive device [MSP ♀]
  996.39 Other [MSP]
    Cystostomy catheter
    Prosthetic reconstruction of vas deferens
    Repair (graft) of ureter without mention of resection
    EXCLUDES *complications due to:*
                external stoma of urinary tract (997.5)
                internal anastomosis of urinary tract (997.5)

996.4 Mechanical complication of internal orthopedic device, implant and graft [MSP]
  Mechanical complications involving:
    external (fixation) device utilizing internal screw(s), pin(s) or other methods of fixation
    grafts of bone, cartilage, muscle, or tendon
    internal (fixation) device such as nail, plate, rod, etc.
  EXCLUDES *complications of external orthopedic device, such as: pressure ulcer due to cast (707.0)*

√5th 996.5 Mechanical complications of other specified prosthetic device, implant, and graft
  Mechanical complications involving:
    prosthetic implant in: prosthetic implant in:
      bile duct   chin
      breast   orbit of eye
    nonabsorbable surgical material NOS
    other graft, implant, and internal device, not elsewhere classified
  996.51 Due to corneal graft

996.52 Due to graft of other tissue, not elsewhere classified
Skin graft failure or rejection
> **EXCLUDES** *failure of artificial skin graft (996.55)*
> *failure of decellularized allodermis (996.55)*
> *sloughing of temporary skin allografts or xenografts (pigskin)—omit code*

996.53 Due to ocular lens prosthesis
> **EXCLUDES** *contact lenses—code to condition*

996.54 Due to breast prosthesis
Breast capsule (prosthesis)
Mammary implant

996.55 Due to artificial skin graft and decellularized allodermis
Dislodgement
Displacement
Failure
Non-adherence
Poor incorporation
Shearing

996.56 Due to peritoneal dialysis catheter
> **EXCLUDES** *mechanical complication of arteriovenous dialysis catheter (996.1)*

996.59 Due to other implant and internal device, not elsewhere classified
Nonabsorbable surgical material NOS
Prosthetic implant in:
  bile duct
  chin
  orbit of eye

✓5th **996.6 Infection and inflammatory reaction due to internal prosthetic device, implant, and graft**

Infection (causing obstruction)
Inflammation
} due to (presence of) any device, implant, and graft classifiable to 996.0-996.5

Use additional code to identify specified infections

996.60 Due to unspecified device, implant, and graft

996.61 Due to cardiac device, implant, and graft
Cardiac pacemaker or defibrillator:
  electrode(s), lead(s)
  pulse generator
  subcutaneous pocket
Coronary artery bypass graft
Heart valve prosthesis

996.62 Due to other vascular device, implant, and graft
Arterial graft
Arteriovenous fistula or shunt
Infusion pump
Vascular catheter (arterial) (dialysis) (venous)

996.63 Due to nervous system device, implant, and graft
Electrodes implanted in brain
Peripheral nerve graft
Spinal canal catheter
Ventricular (communicating) shunt (catheter)

996.64 Due to indwelling urinary catheter
Use additional code to identify specified infections, such as:
  Cystitis (595.0-595.9)
  Sepsis (038.0-038.9)

996.65 Due to other genitourinary device, implant, and graft
   Intrauterine contraceptive device
996.66 Due to internal joint prosthesis
996.67 Due to other internal orthopedic device, implant, and graft
   Bone growth stimulator (electrode)
   Internal fixation device (pin) (rod) (screw)
996.68 Due to peritoneal dialysis catheter
   Exit-site infection or inflammation
996.69 Due to other internal prosthetic device, implant, and graft
   Breast prosthesis
   Ocular lens prosthesis
   Prosthetic orbital implant

√5th **996.7** Other complications of internal (biological) (synthetic) prosthetic device, implant, and graft

   Complication NOS
   occlusion NOS
   Embolism
   Fibrosis   } due to (presence of) any device, implant, and graft classifiable to 996.0-996.5
   Hemorrhage
   Pain
   Stenosis
   Thrombus

   EXCLUDES *transplant rejection (996.8)*

996.70 Due to unspecified device, implant, and graft
996.71 Due to heart valve prosthesis
996.72 Due to other cardiac device, implant, and graft
   Cardiac pacemaker or defibrillator:
      electrode(s), lead(s)
      subcutaneous pocket
   Coronary artery bypass (graft)
      EXCLUDES *occlusion due to atherosclerosis ▶(414.00-414.06)◀*
996.73 Due to renal dialysis device, implant, and graft
996.74 Due to other vascular device, implant, and graft
   EXCLUDES *occlusion of biological graft due to atherosclerosis (440.30-440.32)*
996.75 Due to nervous system device, implant, and graft
996.76 Due to genitourinary device, implant, and graft
996.77 Due to internal joint prosthesis
996.78 Due to other internal orthopedic device, implant, and graft
996.79 Due to other internal prosthetic device, implant, and graft

√5th **996.8** Complications of transplanted organ
   Transplant failure or rejection
   Use additional code to identify nature of complication, such as:
      Cytomegalovirus (CMV) infection (078.5)
996.80 Transplanted organ, unspecified
996.81 Kidney
996.82 Liver
996.83 Heart
996.84 Lung
996.85 Bone marrow
   Graft-versus-host disease (acute) (chronic)
996.86 Pancreas
996.87 Intestine

Medicare Secondary Payer

- **996.89** Other specified transplanted organ

√5th **996.9** Complications of reattached extremity or body part
- **996.90** Unspecified extremity
- **996.91** Forearm
- **996.92** Hand
- **996.93** Finger(s)
- **996.94** Upper extremity, other and unspecified
- **996.95** Foot and toe(s)
- **996.96** Lower extremity, other and unspecified
- **996.99** Other specified body part

√4th **997** **Complications affecting specified body system, not elsewhere classified**
Use additional code to identify complications
> EXCLUDES the listed conditions when specified as:
> causing shock (998.0)
> complications of:
> anesthesia:
> adverse effect (001.0-799.9, 995.0-995.8)
> in labor or delivery (668.0-668.9)
> poisoning (968.0-969.9)
> implanted device or graft (996.0-996.9)
> obstetrical procedures (669.0-669.4)
> reattached extremity (996.90-996.96)
> transplanted organ (996.80-996.89)

√5th **997.0** Nervous system complications
- **997.00** Nervous system complication, unspecified
- **997.01** Central nervous system complication
  Anoxic brain damage
  Cerebral hypoxia
  > EXCLUDES cerebrovascular hemorrhage or infarction (997.02)
- **997.02** Iatrogenic cerebrovascular infarction or hemorrhage
  Postoperative stroke
- **997.09** Other nervous system complications

997.1 Cardiac complications
Cardiac:
  arrest
  insufficiency   } during or resulting
Cardiorespiratory failure   from a
Heart failure   procedure
> EXCLUDES the listed conditions as long-term effects of cardiac surgery or due to the presence of cardiac prosthetic device (429.4)

997.2 Peripheral vascular complications
Phlebitis or thrombophlebitis during or resulting from a procedure
> EXCLUDES the listed conditions due to:
> implant or catheter device (996.62)
> infusion, perfusion, or transfusion (999.2)
> complications affecting blood vessels (997.71-997.79)

INJURY AND POISONING

997.3 Respiratory complications
  Mendelson's syndrome ⎫ resulting from a
  Pneumonia (aspiration) ⎭ procedure

  EXCLUDES iatrogenic [postoperative] pneumothorax (512.1)
  iatrogenic pulmonary embolism (415.11)
  Mendelson's syndrome in labor and delivery (668.0)
  specified complications classified elsewhere, such as:
    adult respiratory distress syndrome (518.5)
    pulmonary edema, postoperative (518.4)
    respiratory insufficiency, acute, postoperative (518.5)
    shock lung (518.5)
    tracheostomy complications (519.00-519.09)

  DEF: Mendelson's syndrome: acid pneumonitis due to aspiration of gastric acids, may occur after anesthesia or sedation.

997.4 Digestive system complications
  Complications of:
    intestinal (internal) anastomosis and bypass, not elsewhere classified, except that involving urinary tract
  Hepatic failure   ⎫
  Hepatorenal syndrome   ⎬ specified as due to a procedure
  Intestinal obstruction NOS ⎭

  EXCLUDES gastrostomy complications (536.40-536.49)
  specified gastrointestinal complications classified elsewhere, such as:
    blind loop syndrome (579.2)
    colostomy and enterostomy complications (569.60-569.69)
    gastrojejunal ulcer (534.0-534.9)
    infection of external stoma (569.61)
    pelvic peritoneal adhesions, female (614.6)
    peritoneal adhesions (568.0)
    peritoneal adhesions with obstruction (560.81)
    postcholecystectomy syndrome (576.0)
    postgastric surgery syndromes (564.2)

997.5 Urinary complications
  Complications of:
    external stoma of urinary tract
    internal anastomosis and bypass of urinary tract, including that involving intestinal tract
  Oliguria or anuria   ⎫
  Renal: ⎪
    failure (acute)   ⎬ specified as due to procedure
    insufficiency (acute)   ⎪
  Tubular necrosis (acute) ⎭

  EXCLUDES specified complications classified elsewhere, such as:
    postoperative stricture of:
      ureter (593.3)
      urethra (598.2)

√5th 997.6 Amputation stump complication
  EXCLUDES admission for treatment for a current traumatic amputation — code to complicated traumatic amputation
  phantom limb (syndrome) (353.6)

  997.60 Unspecified complication
  997.61 Neuroma of amputation stump
    DEF: Hyperplasia generated nerve cell mass following amputation.

997.62 Infection (chronic)
Use additional code to identify organism

997.69 Other

√5th **997.7 Vascular complications of other vessels**
EXCLUDES peripheral vascular complications (997.2)

997.71 Vascular complications of mesenteric artery

997.72 Vascular complications of renal artery

997.79 Vascular complications of other vessels

√5th **997.9 Complications affecting other specified body systems, not elsewhere classified**
EXCLUDES specified complications classified elsewhere, such as:
broad ligament laceration syndrome (620.6)
postartificial menopause syndrome (627.4)
postoperative stricture of vagina (623.2)

997.91 Hypertension
EXCLUDES essential hypertension (401.0-401.9)

997.99 Other
Vitreous touch syndrome
DEF: Vitreous protruding through pupil and attaches to corneal epithelium; causes aqueous fluid in vitreous body; marked by corneal edema, loss of lucidity; complication of cataract surgery.

√4th **998 Other complications of procedures, not elsewhere classified**

998.0 Postoperative shock
Collapse NOS
Shock (endotoxic)
(hypovolemic) (septic)
} during or resulting from a surgical procedure

EXCLUDES shock:
anaphylactic due to serum (999.4)
anesthetic (995.4)
electric (994.8)
following abortion (639.5)
obstetric (669.1)
traumatic (958.4)

√5th **998.1 Hemorrhage or hematoma or seroma complicating a procedure**
EXCLUDES hemorrhage, hematoma, or seroma:
complicating cesarean section or puerperal perineal wound (674.3)

998.11 Hemorrhage complicating a procedure

998.12 Hematoma complicating a procedure

998.13 Seroma complicating a procedure

998.2 Accidental puncture or laceration during a procedure
Accidental perforation by catheter or other instrument during a procedure on:
blood vessel
nerve
organ

EXCLUDES iatrogenic [postoperative] pneumothorax (512.1)
puncture or laceration caused by implanted device intentionally left in operation wound (996.0-996.5)
specified complications classified elsewhere, such as:
broad ligament laceration syndrome (620.6)
trauma from instruments during delivery (664.0-665.9)

INJURY AND POISONING

✓5ᵗʰ 998.3 Disruption of operation wound
    Dehiscence ⎫
    Rupture   ⎬ of operation wound

    EXCLUDES disruption of:
        cesarean wound (674.1)
        perineal wound, puerperal (674.2)

●   **998.31 Disruption of internal operation wound**
●   **998.32 Disruption of external operation wound**
    Disruption of operation wound NOS

998.4 Foreign body accidentally left during a procedure
    Adhesions   ⎫ due to foreign body accidentally
    Obstruction ⎬ left in operative wound or
    Perforation ⎭ body cavity during a procedure

    EXCLUDES obstruction or perforation caused by implanted device intentionally left in body (996.0-996.5)

✓5ᵗʰ 998.5 Postoperative infection
    EXCLUDES infection due to:
        implanted device (996.60-996.69)
        infusion, perfusion, or transfusion (999.3)
        postoperative obstetrical wound infection (674.3)

  998.51 Infected postoperative seroma
    Use additional code to identify organism
  998.59 Other postoperative infection
    Abscess:
      intra-abdominal ⎫
      stitch   ⎬
      subphrenic   ⎬ postoperative
      wound   ⎬
    Septicemia   ⎭

    Use additional code to identify infection

998.6 Persistent postoperative fistula

998.7 Acute reaction to foreign substance accidentally left during a procedure
    Peritonitis: Peritonitis:
      aseptic   chemical

✓5ᵗʰ 998.8 Other specified complications of procedures, not elsewhere classified
  998.81 Emphysema (subcutaneous) (surgical) resulting from a procedure
  998.82 Cataract fragments in eye following cataract surgery
  998.83 Non-healing surgical wound
  998.89 Other specified complications

998.9 Unspecified complication of procedure, not elsewhere classified
    Postoperative complication NOS
    EXCLUDES complication NOS of obstetrical, surgery or procedure (669.4)

999 Complications of medical care, not elsewhere classified

✓4th

INCLUDES complications, not elsewhere classified, of:
- dialysis (hemodialysis) (peritoneal) (renal)
- extracorporeal circulation
- hyperalimentation therapy
- immunization
- infusion
- inhalation therapy
- injection
- inoculation
- perfusion
- transfusion
- vaccination
- ventilation therapy

EXCLUDES specified complications classified elsewhere such as:
- complications of implanted device (996.0-996.9)
- contact dermatitis due to drugs (692.3)
- dementia dialysis (294.8)
  - transient (293.9)
- dialysis disequilibrium syndrome (276.0-276.9)
- poisoning and toxic effects of drugs and chemicals (960.0-989.9)
- postvaccinal encephalitis (323.5)
- water and electrolyte imbalance (276.0-276.9)

999.0 Generalized vaccinia

DEF: Skin eruption, self-limiting; follows vaccination; due to transient viremia with virus localized in skin.

999.1 Air embolism

Air embolism to any site following infusion, perfusion, or transfusion

EXCLUDES embolism specified as:
- complicating:
  - abortion (634-638 with .6, 639.6)
  - ectopic or molar pregnancy (639.6)
  - pregnancy, childbirth, or the puerperium (673.0)
- due to implanted device (996.7)
- traumatic (958.0)

999.2 Other vascular complications

Phlebitis
Thromboembolism
Thrombophlebitis
} following infusion, perfusion, or transfusion

EXCLUDES the listed conditions when specified as:
- due to implanted device (996.61-996.62, 996.72-996.74)
- postoperative NOS (997.2, 997.71-997.79)

999.3 Other infection

Infection
Sepsis
Septicemia
} following infusion, injection, transfusion, or vaccination

EXCLUDES the listed conditions when specified as:
- due to implanted device (996.60-996.69)
- postoperative NOS (998.51-998.59)

999.4 Anaphylactic shock due to serum

EXCLUDES shock:
- allergic NOS (995.0)
- anaphylactic:
  - NOS (995.0)
  - due to drugs and chemicals (995.0)

DEF: Life-threatening hypersensitivity to foreign serum; causes respiratory distress, vascular collapse, and shock.

INJURY AND POISONING

999.5 **Other serum reaction**
Intoxication by serum   Serum sickness
Protein sickness   Urticaria due to serum
Serum rash
EXCLUDES serum hepatitis (070.2-070.3)

DEF: Serum sickness: Hypersensitivity to foreign serum; causes fever, hives, swelling, and lymphadenopathy.

999.6 **ABO incompatibility reaction**
Incompatible blood transfusion
Reaction to blood group incompatibility in infusion or transfusion

999.7 **Rh incompatibility reaction**
Reactions due to Rh factor in infusion or transfusion

999.8 **Other transfusion reaction**
Septic shock due to transfusion
Transfusion reaction NOS
EXCLUDES postoperative shock (998.0)

999.9 **Other and unspecified complications of medical care, not elsewhere classified**
Complications, not elsewhere classified, of:
electroshock ⎫
inhalation   ⎬ therapy
ultrasound   ⎬
ventilation   ⎭

Unspecified misadventure of medical care
EXCLUDES unspecified complication of:
phototherapy (990)
radiation therapy (990)

SUPPLEMENTARY CLASSIFICATION OF FACTORS INFLUENCING HEALTH STATUS AND CONTACT WITH HEALTH SERVICES (V01-V83)

This classification is provided to deal with occasions when circumstances other than a disease or injury classifiable to categories 001-999 (the main part of ICD) are recorded as "diagnoses" or "problems." This can arise mainly in three ways:

a) When a person who is not currently sick encounters the health services for some specific purpose, such as to act as a donor of an organ or tissue, to receive prophylactic vaccination, or to discuss a problem which is in itself not a disease or injury. This will be a fairly rare occurrence among hospital inpatients, but will be relatively more common among hospital outpatients and patients of family practitioners, health clinics, etc.

b) When a person with a known disease or injury, whether it is current or resolving, encounters the health care system for a specific treatment of that disease or injury (e.g., dialysis for renal disease; chemotherapy for malignancy; cast change).

c) When some circumstance or problem is present which influences the person's health status but is not in itself a current illness or injury. Such factors may be elicited during population surveys, when the person may or may not be currently sick, or be recorded as an additional factor to be borne in mind when the person is receiving care for some current illness or injury classifiable to categories 001-999.

In the latter circumstances the V code should be used only as a supplementary code and should not be the one selected for use in primary, single cause tabulations. Examples of these circumstances are a personal history of certain diseases, or a person with an artificial heart valve in situ.

PERSONS WITH POTENTIAL HEALTH HAZARDS RELATED TO COMMUNICABLE DISEASES (V01-V06)

EXCLUDES *family history of infectious and parasitic diseases (V18.8)*
personal history of infectious and parasitic diseases (V12.0)

V01 Contact with or exposure to communicable diseases

- **V01.0 Cholera**
  Conditions classifiable to 001
- **V01.1 Tuberculosis**
  Conditions classifiable to 010-018
- **V01.2 Poliomyelitis**
  Conditions classifiable to 045
- **V01.3 Smallpox**
  Conditions classifiable to 050
- **V01.4 Rubella**
  Conditions classifiable to 056
- **V01.5 Rabies**
  Conditions classifiable to 071
- **V01.6 Venereal diseases**
  Conditions classifiable to 090-099
- **V01.7 Other viral diseases**
  Conditions classifiable to 042-078 and V08, except as above
- **V01.8 Other communicable diseases**
  Conditions classifiable to 001-136, except as above
  - V01.81 Anthrax
  - V01.89 Other communicable diseases
- **V01.9 Unspecified communicable disease**

V02 Carrier or suspected carrier of infectious diseases

- **V02.0 Cholera**
- **V02.1 Typhoid**
- **V02.2 Amebiasis**
- **V02.3 Other gastrointestinal pathogens**

V CODES

| | V02.4 | Diphtheria |
| ✓5th | V02.5 | Other specified bacterial diseases |

        V02.51 Group B streptococcus
        V02.52 Other streptococcus
        V02.59 Other specified bacterial disease
            Meningococcal
            Staphylococcal

✓5th V02.6 Viral hepatitis
        Hepatitis Australian-antigen [HAA] [SH] carrier
        Serum hepatitis carrier
        V02.60 Viral hepatitis carrier, unspecified
        V02.61 Hepatitis B carrier
        V02.62 Hepatitis C carrier
        V02.69 Other viral hepatitis carrier

V02.7 Gonorrhea
V02.8 Other venereal diseases
V02.9 Other specified infectious organism

✓4th **V03 Need for prophylactic vaccination and inoculation against bacterial diseases**
    EXCLUDES   *vaccination not carried out because of contraindication (V64.0)*
                             vaccines against combinations of diseases (V06.0-V06.9)

    V03.0 Cholera alone
    V03.1 Typhoid-paratyphoid alone [TAB]
    V03.2 Tuberculosis [BCG]
    V03.3 Plague
    V03.4 Tularemia
    V03.5 Diphtheria alone
    V03.6 Pertussis alone
    V03.7 Tetanus toxoid alone

✓5th V03.8 Other specified vaccinations against single bacterial diseases
        V03.81 Hemophilus influenza, type B [Hib]
        V03.82 Streptococcus pneumoniae [pneumococcus]
        V03.89 Other specified vaccination

    V03.9 Unspecified single bacterial disease

✓4th **V04 Need for prophylactic vaccination and inoculation against certain viral diseases**
    EXCLUDES   *vaccines against combinations of diseases (V06.0-V06.9)*

    V04.0 Poliomyelitis
    V04.1 Smallpox
    V04.2 Measles alone
    V04.3 Rubella alone
    V04.4 Yellow fever
    V04.5 Rabies
    V04.6 Mumps alone
    V04.7 Common cold
    V04.8 Influenza

✓4th **V05 Need for other prophylactic vaccination and inoculation against single diseases**
    EXCLUDES   *vaccines against combinations of diseases (V06.0-V06.9)*

    V05.0 Arthropod-borne viral encephalitis
    V05.1 Other arthropod-borne viral diseases
    V05.2 Leishmaniasis
    V05.3 Viral hepatitis

 Additional Digit Required   Unspecified Code   Other Specified Code   Manifestation Code

MSP Medicare Secondary Payer   ▶◀ Revised Text   ● New Code   ▲ Revised Code Title

V05.4–V09.0   V CODES

- **V05.4** Varicella
  Chickenpox
- **V05.8** Other specified disease
- **V05.9** Unspecified single disease

✓4th **V06 Need for prophylactic vaccination and inoculation against combinations of diseases**

    Note: Use additional single vaccination codes from categories V03-V05 to identify any vaccinations not included in a combination code.

- **V06.0** Cholera with typhoid-paratyphoid [cholera+TAB]
- **V06.1** Diphtheria-tetanus-pertussis, combined [DTP]
- **V06.2** Diphtheria-tetanus-pertussis with typhoid-paratyphoid [DTP+TAB]
- **V06.3** Diphtheria-tetanus-pertussis with poliomyelitis [DTP+polio]
- **V06.4** Measles-mumps-rubella [MMR]
- **V06.5** Tetanus-diphtheria [Td]
- **V06.6** Streptococcus pneumoniae [pneumococcus] and influenza
- **V06.8** Other combinations
  - EXCLUDES   *multiple single vaccination codes (V03.0-V05.9)*
- **V06.9** Unspecified combined vaccine

PERSONS WITH NEED FOR ISOLATION, OTHER POTENTIAL HEALTH HAZARDS AND PROPHYLACTIC MEASURES (V07-V09)

✓4th **V07 Need for isolation and other prophylactic measures**
  - EXCLUDES   *prophylactic organ removal (V50.41-V50.49)*

- **V07.0** Isolation
  Admission to protect the individual from his surroundings or for isolation of individual after contact with infectious diseases
- **V07.1** Desensitization to allergens
- **V07.2** Prophylactic immunotherapy
  Administration of:
      antivenin
      immune sera [gamma globulin]
      RhoGAM
      tetanus antitoxin

✓5th **V07.3** Other prophylactic chemotherapy
- **V07.31** Prophylactic fluoride administration
- **V07.39** Other prophylactic chemotherapy
  - EXCLUDES   *maintenance chemotherapy following disease (V58.1)*

- **V07.4** Postmenopausal hormone replacement therapy   ♀
- **V07.8** Other specified prophylactic measure
- **V07.9** Unspecified prophylactic measure

V08 Asymptomatic human immunodeficiency virus [HIV] infection status
  HIV positive NOS

    Note: This code is ONLY to be used when NO HIV infection symptoms or conditions are present. If any HIV infection symptoms or conditions are present, see code 042.

  - EXCLUDES   *AIDS (042)*
    human immunodeficiency virus [HIV] disease (042)
    exposure to HIV (V01.7)
    nonspecific serologic evidence of HIV (795.71)
    symptomatic human immunodeficiency virus [HIV] infection (042)

✓4th **V09 Infection with drug-resistant microorganisms**

    Note: This category is intended for use as an additional code for infectious conditions classified elsewhere to indicate the presence of drug-resistance of the infectious organism.

- **V09.0** Infection with microorganisms resistant to penicillins   SDx

V CODES

	V09.1	Infection with microorganisms resistant to cephalosporins and other B-lactam antibiotics	SDx
	V09.2	Infection with microorganisms resistant to macrolides	SDx
	V09.3	Infection with microorganisms resistant to tetracyclines	SDx
	V09.4	Infection with microorganisms resistant to aminoglycosides	SDx
√5th	V09.5	Infection with microorganisms resistant to quinolones and fluoroquinolones
	V09.50	Without mention of resistance to multiple quinolones and fluoroquinoles	SDx
	V09.51	With resistance to multiple quinolones and fluoroquinoles	SDx
	V09.6	Infection with microorganisms resistant to sulfonamides	SDx
√5th | V09.7 | Infection with microorganisms resistant to other specified antimycobacterial agents |

EXCLUDES Amikacin (V09.4)
Kanamycin (V09.4)
Streptomycin [SM] (V09.4)

| | V09.70 | Without mention of resistance to multiple antimycobacterial agents | SDx |
| | V09.71 | With resistance to multiple antimycobacterial agents | SDx |
√5th | V09.8 | Infection with microorganisms resistant to other specified drugs |
| | V09.80 | Without mention of resistance to multiple drugs | SDx |
| | V09.81 | With resistance to multiple drugs | SDx |
√5th | V09.9 | Infection with drug-resistant microorganisms, unspecified |
		Drug resistance, NOS
	V09.90	Without mention of multiple drug resistance	SDx
	V09.91	With multiple drug resistance	SDx
		Multiple drug resistance NOS

PERSONS WITH POTENTIAL HEALTH HAZARDS RELATED TO PERSONAL AND FAMILY HISTORY

EXCLUDES obstetric patients where the possibility that the fetus might be affected is the reason for observation or management during pregnancy (655.0-655.9)

√4th **V10 Personal history of malignant neoplasm**
√5th V10.0 Gastrointestinal tract
History of conditions classifiable to 140-159
V10.00 Gastrointestinal tract, unspecified
V10.01 Tongue
V10.02 Other and unspecified oral cavity and pharynx
V10.03 Esophagus
V10.04 Stomach
V10.05 Large intestine
V10.06 Rectum, rectosigmoid junction, and anus
V10.07 Liver
V10.09 Other
√5th V10.1 Trachea, bronchus, and lung
History of conditions classifiable to 162
V10.11 Bronchus and lung
V10.12 Trachea
√5th V10.2 Other respiratory and intrathoracic organs
History of conditions classifiable to 160, 161, 163-165
V10.20 Respiratory organ, unspecified

√4th Additional Digit Required
√5th
 Medicare Secondary Payer   ▶◀ Revised Text   ● New Code   ▲ Revised Code Title

Unspecified Code   Other Specified Code   Manifestation Code

2002 Ingenix, Inc.   Volume 1 — 595

V10.21–V10.89 V CODES

- **V10.21** Larynx
- **V10.22** Nasal cavities, middle ear, and accessory sinuses
- **V10.29** Other

V10.3 Breast
History of conditions classifiable to 174 and 175

√5ᵗʰ V10.4 Genital organs
History of conditions classifiable to 179-187
- **V10.40** Female genital organ, unspecified ♀
- **V10.41** Cervix uteri ♀
- **V10.42** Other parts of uterus ♀
- **V10.43** Ovary ♀
- **V10.44** Other female genital organs ♀
- **V10.45** Male genital organ, unspecified ♂
- **V10.46** Prostate ♂
- **V10.47** Testis ♂
- **V10.48** Epididymis ♂
- **V10.49** Other male genital organs ♂

√5ᵗʰ V10.5 Urinary organs
History of conditions classifiable to 188 and 189
- **V10.50** Urinary organ, unspecified
- **V10.51** Bladder
- **V10.52** Kidney
  - EXCLUDES renal pelvis (V10.53)
- **V10.53** Renal pelvis
- **V10.59** Other

√5ᵗʰ V10.6 Leukemia
Conditions classifiable to 204-208
  - EXCLUDES leukemia in remission (204-208)
- **V10.60** Leukemia, unspecified
- **V10.61** Lymphoid leukemia
- **V10.62** Myeloid leukemia
- **V10.63** Monocytic leukemia
- **V10.69** Other

√5ᵗʰ V10.7 Other lymphatic and hematopoietic neoplasms
Conditions classifiable to 200-203
  - EXCLUDES listed conditions in 200-203 in remission
- **V10.71** Lymphosarcoma and reticulosarcoma
- **V10.72** Hodgkin's disease
- **V10.79** Other

√5ᵗʰ V10.8 Personal history of malignant neoplasm of other sites
History of conditions classifiable to 170-173, 190-195
- **V10.81** Bone
- **V10.82** Malignant melanoma of skin
- **V10.83** Other malignant neoplasm of skin
- **V10.84** Eye
- **V10.85** Brain
- **V10.86** Other parts of nervous system
  - EXCLUDES peripheral sympathetic, and parasympathetic nerves (V10.89)
- **V10.87** Thyroid
- **V10.88** Other endocrine glands and related structures
- **V10.89** Other

V CODES

V10.9 **Unspecified personal history of malignant neoplasm**

✓4th **V11 Personal history of mental disorder**
- V11.0 Schizophrenia — SDx
  - EXCLUDES: that in remission (295.0-295.9 with fifth-digit 5)
- V11.1 Affective disorders — SDx
  - Personal history of manic-depressive psychosis
  - EXCLUDES: that in remission (296.0-296.6 with fifth-digit 5, 6)
- V11.2 Neurosis — SDx
- V11.3 Alcoholism — SDx
- V11.8 **Other mental disorders** — SDx
- V11.9 **Unspecified mental disorder** — SDx

✓4th **V12 Personal history of certain other diseases**
- ✓5th V12.0 Infectious and parasitic diseases
  - V12.00 **Unspecified infectious and parasitic disease** — SDx
  - V12.01 Tuberculosis — SDx
  - V12.02 Poliomyelitis — SDx
  - V12.03 Malaria — SDx
  - V12.09 **Other** — SDx
- V12.1 Nutritional deficiency — SDx
- V12.2 Endocrine, metabolic, and immunity disorders — SDx
  - EXCLUDES: history of allergy (V14.0-V14.9, V15.01-V15.09)
- V12.3 Diseases of blood and blood-forming organs — SDx
- ✓5th V12.4 Disorders of nervous system and sense organs
  - V12.40 **Unspecified disorder of nervous system and sense organs** — SDx
  - V12.41 Benign neoplasm of the brain — SDx
  - V12.49 **Other disorders of nervous system and sense organs** — SDx
- ✓5th V12.5 Diseases of circulatory system
  - EXCLUDES: old myocardial infarction (412)
    postmyocardial infarction syndrome (411.0)
  - V12.50 **Unspecified circulatory disease** — SDx
  - V12.51 Venous thrombosis and embolism — SDx
    - Pulmonary embolism
  - V12.52 Thrombophlebitis — SDx
  - V12.59 **Other** — SDx
- V12.6 Diseases of respiratory system — SDx
- ✓5th V12.7 Diseases of digestive system
  - V12.70 **Unspecified digestive disease** — SDx
  - V12.71 Peptic ulcer disease — SDx
  - V12.72 Colonic polyps — SDx
  - V12.79 **Other** — SDx

✓4th **V13 Personal history of other diseases**
- ✓5th V13.0 Disorders of urinary system
  - V13.00 **Unspecified urinary disorder** — SDx
  - V13.01 Urinary calculi — SDx
  - V13.09 **Other** — SDx
- V13.1 Trophoblastic disease — SDx ♀
  - EXCLUDES: supervision during a current pregnancy (V23.1)

Legend:
- ✓4th / ✓5th Additional Digit Required
- Unspecified Code
- Other Specified Code
- Manifestation Code
- MSP Medicare Secondary Payer
- ▶◀ Revised Text
- ● New Code
- ▲ Revised Code Title

2002 Ingenix, Inc.

V13.2–V15.09 V CODES

√5th **V13.2 Other genital system and obstetric disorders**
    EXCLUDES: *supervision during a current pregnancy of a woman with poor obstetric history (V23.0-V23.9)*
    habitual aborter (646.3)
    without current pregnancy (629.9)

- **V13.21 Personal history of pre-term labor** [SDx]
    EXCLUDES: *current pregnancy with history of pre-term labor (V23.41)*
- **V13.29 Other genital system and obstetric disorders** [SDx]

V13.3 Diseases of skin and subcutaneous tissue [SDx]
V13.4 Arthritis [SDx]
V13.5 Other musculoskeletal disorders [SDx]

√5th **V13.6 Congenital malformations**
    V13.61 Hypospadias [SDx] ♂
    V13.69 Other congenital malformations [SDx]

V13.7 Perinatal problems [SDx]
    EXCLUDES: *low birth weight status (V21.30-V21.35)*

V13.8 Other specified diseases [SDx]
V13.9 Unspecified disease [SDx]

√4th **V14 Personal history of allergy to medicinal agents**
    V14.0 Penicillin [SDx]
    V14.1 Other antibiotic agent [SDx]
    V14.2 Sulfonamides [SDx]
    V14.3 Other anti-infective agent [SDx]
    V14.4 Anesthetic agent [SDx]
    V14.5 Narcotic agent [SDx]
    V14.6 Analgesic agent [SDx]
    V14.7 Serum or vaccine [SDx]
    V14.8 Other specified medicinal agents [SDx]
    V14.9 Unspecified medicinal agent [SDx]

√4th **V15 Other personal history presenting hazards to health**

√5th **V15.0 Allergy, other than to medicinal agents**
    EXCLUDES: *allergy to food substance used as base for medicinal agent (V14.0-V14.9)*

    V15.01 Allergy to peanuts [SDx]
    V15.02 Allergy to milk products [SDx]
    EXCLUDES: *lactose intolerance (271.3)*
    V15.03 Allergy to eggs [SDx]
    V15.04 Allergy to seafood [SDx]
        Seafood (octopus) (squid) ink
        Shellfish
    V15.05 Allergy to other foods [SDx]
        Food additives
        Nuts other than peanuts
    V15.06 Allergy to insects [SDx]
        Bugs
        Insect bites and stings
        Spiders
    V15.07 Allergy to latex [SDx]
        Latex sensitivity
    V15.08 Allergy to radiographic dye [SDx]
        Contrast media used for diagnostic x-ray procedures
    V15.09 Other allergy, other than to medicinal agents [SDx]

[N] Newborn Age: 0   [P] Pediatric Age: 0-17   [M] Maternity Age: 12-55   [A] Adult Age: 15-124
[SDx] Secondary Diagnosis   [PDx] Primary Diagnosis

V CODES

V15.1 Surgery to heart and great vessels [SDx]
    EXCLUDES: *replacement by transplant or other means (V42.1-V42.2, V43.2-V43.4)*

V15.2 Surgery to other major organs [SDx]
    EXCLUDES: *replacement by transplant or other means (V42.0-V43.8)*

V15.3 Irradiation [SDx]
Previous exposure to therapeutic or other ionizing radiation

√5th **V15.4 Psychological trauma**
    EXCLUDES: *history of condition classifiable to 290-316 (V11.0-V11.9)*

    V15.41 History of physical abuse [SDx]
        Rape

    V15.42 History of emotional abuse [SDx]
        Neglect

    V15.49 Other [SDx]

V15.5 Injury [SDx]

V15.6 Poisoning [SDx]

V15.7 Contraception [SDx]
    EXCLUDES: *current contraceptive management (V25.0-V25.4)*
                    presence of intrauterine contraceptive device as incidental finding (V45.5)

√5th **V15.8 Other specified personal history presenting hazards to health**

    V15.81 Noncompliance with medical treatment [SDx]

    V15.82 History of tobacco use [SDx]
        EXCLUDES: *tobacco dependence (305.1)*

    V15.84 Exposure to asbestos [SDx]

    V15.85 Exposure to potentially hazardous body fluids [SDx]

    V15.86 Exposure to lead [SDx]

    V15.89 Other [SDx]

V15.9 Unspecified personal history presenting hazards to health [SDx]

√4th **V16 Family history of malignant neoplasm**

    V16.0 Gastrointestinal tract
        Family history of condition classifiable to 140-159

    V16.1 Trachea, bronchus, and lung
        Family history of condition classifiable to 162

    V16.2 Other respiratory and intrathoracic organs
        Family history of condition classifiable to 160-161, 163-165

    V16.3 Breast
        Family history of condition classifiable to 174

    √5th **V16.4 Genital organs**
        Family history of condition classifiable to 179-187

        V16.40 Genital organ, unspecified
        V16.41 Ovary
        V16.42 Prostate
        V16.43 Testis
        V16.49 Other

    √5th **V16.5 Urinary organs**
        Family history of condition classifiable to 189

        V16.51 Kidney
        V16.59 Other

    V16.6 Leukemia
        Family history of condition classifiable to 204-208

√4th √5th Additional Digit Required   Unspecified Code   Other Specified Code   Manifestation Code
MSP Medicare Secondary Payer   ▶◀ Revised Text   ● New Code   ▲ Revised Code Title

V CODES

V16.7 **Other lymphatic and hematopoietic neoplasms**
Family history of condition classifiable to 200-203
V16.8 **Other specified malignant neoplasm**
Family history of other condition classifiable to 140-199
V16.9 **Unspecified malignant neoplasm**

✓4th V17 Family history of certain chronic disabling diseases
V17.0 Psychiatric condition
EXCLUDES *family history of mental retardation (V18.4)*
V17.1 Stroke (cerebrovascular)
V17.2 **Other neurological diseases**
Epilepsy
Huntington's chorea
V17.3 Ischemic heart disease
V17.4 **Other cardiovascular diseases**
V17.5 Asthma
V17.6 **Other chronic respiratory conditions**
V17.7 Arthritis
V17.8 **Other musculoskeletal diseases**

✓4th V18 Family history of certain other specific conditions
V18.0 Diabetes mellitus
V18.1 **Other endocrine and metabolic diseases**
V18.2 Anemia
V18.3 **Other blood disorders**
V18.4 Mental retardation
V18.5 Digestive disorders
✓5th V18.6 Kidney diseases
V18.61 Polycystic kidney
V18.69 **Other kidney diseases**
V18.7 **Other genitourinary diseases**
V18.8 Infectious and parasitic diseases

✓4th V19 Family history of other conditions
V19.0 Blindness or visual loss
V19.1 **Other eye disorders**
V19.2 Deafness or hearing loss
V19.3 **Other ear disorders**
V19.4 Skin conditions
V19.5 Congenital anomalies
V19.6 Allergic disorders
V19.7 Consanguinity
V19.8 **Other condition**

PERSONS ENCOUNTERING HEALTH SERVICES IN CIRCUMSTANCES RELATED TO REPRODUCTION AND DEVELOPMENT (V20-V28)

✓4th V20 Health supervision of infant or child
V20.0 Foundling **PDx P**
V20.1 **Other healthy infant or child receiving care** **PDx P**
Medical or nursing care supervision of healthy infant in cases of:
maternal illness, physical or psychiatric
socioeconomic adverse condition at home
too many children at home preventing or interfering with normal care

---

N Newborn Age: 0 **P** Pediatric Age: 0-17 **M** Maternity Age: 12-55 **A** Adult Age: 15-124
600 — Volume 1 **SDx** Secondary Diagnosis **PDx** Primary Diagnosis *2002 Ingenix, Inc.*

V CODES

V20.2 Routine infant or child health check
 Developmental testing of infant or child
 Immunizations appropriate for age
 Routine vision and hearing testing
 Use additional code(s) to identify:
  special screening examination(s) performed (V73.0-V82.9)
   EXCLUDES special screening for developmental handicaps (V79.3)

V21 Constitutional states in development
 V21.0 Period of rapid growth in childhood
 V21.1 Puberty
 V21.2 Other adolescence
 V21.3 Low birth weight status
   EXCLUDES history of perinatal problems (V13.7)
  V21.30 Low birth weight status, unspecified
  V21.31 Low birth weight status, less than 500 grams
  V21.32 Low birth weight status, 500-999 grams
  V21.33 Low birth weight status, 1000-1499 grams
  V21.34 Low birth weight status, 1500-1999 grams
  V21.35 Low birth weight status, 2000-2500 grams
 V21.8 Other specified constitutional states in development
 V21.9 Unspecified constitutional state in development

V22 Normal pregnancy
  EXCLUDES pregnancy examination or test, pregnancy unconfirmed (V72.4)
 V22.0 Supervision of normal first pregnancy
 V22.1 Supervision of other normal pregnancy
 V22.2 Pregnant state, incidental
  Pregnant state NOS

V23 Supervision of high-risk pregnancy
 V23.0 Pregnancy with history of infertility
 V23.1 Pregnancy with history of trophoblastic disease
  Pregnancy with history of:
   hydatidiform mole
   vesicular mole
   EXCLUDES that without current pregnancy (V13.1)
 V23.2 Pregnancy with history of abortion
  Pregnancy with history of conditions classifiable to 634-638
   EXCLUDES habitual aborter:
     care during pregnancy (646.3)
     that without current pregnancy (629.9)
 V23.3 Grand multiparity
   EXCLUDES care in relation to labor and delivery (659.4)
    that without current pregnancy (V61.5)
 V23.4 Pregnancy with other poor obstetric history
  Pregnancy with history of other conditions classifiable to 630-676
  • **V23.41** Pregnancy with history of pre-term labor
  • **V23.49** Pregnancy with other poor obstetric history
 V23.5 Pregnancy with other poor reproductive history
  Pregnancy with history of stillbirth or neonatal death
 V23.7 Insufficient prenatal care
  History of little or no prenatal care

 Additional Digit Required
Unspecified Code
Other Specified Code
Manifestation Code
 Medicare Secondary Payer
▶◀ Revised Text
● New Code
▲ Revised Code Title

V23.8 Other high-risk pregnancy

V23.81 Elderly primigravida
First pregnancy in a woman who will be 35 years of age or older at expected date of delivery

EXCLUDES elderly primigravida complicating pregnancy (659.5)

V23.82 Elderly multigravida
Second or more pregnancy in a woman who will be 35 years of age or older at expected date of delivery

EXCLUDES elderly multigravida complicating pregnancy (659.6)

V23.83 Young primigravida
First pregnancy in a female less than 16 years old at expected date of delivery

EXCLUDES young primigravida complicating pregnancy (659.8)

V23.84 Young multigravida
Second or more pregnancy in a female less than 16 years old at expected date of delivery

EXCLUDES young multigravida complicating pregnancy (659.8)

V23.89 Other high-risk pregnancy

V23.9 Unspecified high-risk pregnancy

V24 Postpartum care and examination

V24.0 Immediately after delivery
Care and observation in uncomplicated cases

V24.1 Lactating mother
Supervision of lactation

V24.2 Routine postpartum follow-up

V25 Encounter for contraceptive management

V25.0 General counseling and advice

V25.01 Prescription of oral contraceptives

V25.02 Initiation of other contraceptive measures
Fitting of diaphragm
Prescription of foams, creams, or other agents

V25.09 Other
Family planning advice

V25.1 Insertion of intrauterine contraceptive device

V25.2 Sterilization
Admission for interruption of fallopian tubes or vas deferens

V25.3 Menstrual extraction
Menstrual regulation

V25.4 Surveillance of previously prescribed contraceptive methods
Checking, reinsertion, or removal of contraceptive device
Repeat prescription for contraceptive method
Routine examination in connection with contraceptive maintenance

EXCLUDES presence of intrauterine contraceptive device as incidental finding (V45.5)

V25.40 Contraceptive surveillance, unspecified
V25.41 Contraceptive pill
V25.42 Intrauterine contraceptive device
Checking, reinsertion, or removal of intrauterine device
V25.43 Implantable subdermal contraceptive
V25.49 Other contraceptive method

V25.5 Insertion of implantable subdermal contraceptive

V25.8 Other specified contraceptive management
Postvasectomy sperm count

EXCLUDES sperm count following sterilization reversal (V26.22)
sperm count for fertility testing (V26.21)

V CODES

- **V25.9** Unspecified contraceptive management
- ✓4th **V26** Procreative management
  - **V26.0** Tuboplasty or vasoplasty after previous sterilization
  - **V26.1** Artificial insemination ♀
  - ✓5th **V26.2** Investigation and testing
    - *EXCLUDES* postvasectomy sperm count (V25.8)
    - **V26.21** Fertility testing
      - Fallopian insufflation
      - Sperm count for fertility testing
      - *EXCLUDES* Genetic counseling and testing (V26.3)
    - **V26.22** Aftercare following sterilization reversal
      - Fallopian insufflation following sterilization reversal
      - Sperm count following sterilization reversal
    - **V26.29** Other investigation and testing
  - **V26.3** Genetic counseling and testing
    - *EXCLUDES* fertility testing (V26.21)
  - **V26.4** General counseling and advice
  - ✓5th **V26.5** Sterilization status
    - **V26.51** Tubal ligation status SDx ♀
      - *EXCLUDES* infertility not due to previous tubal ligation (628.0-628.9)
    - **V26.52** Vasectomy status SDx ♂
  - **V26.8** Other specified procreative management
  - **V26.9** Unspecified procreative management
- ✓4th **V27** Outcome of delivery
  - Note: This category is intended for the coding of the outcome of delivery on the mother's record.
  - **V27.0** Single liveborn M SDx ♀
  - **V27.1** Single stillborn M SDx ♀
  - **V27.2** Twins, both liveborn M SDx ♀
  - **V27.3** Twins, one liveborn and one stillborn M SDx ♀
  - **V27.4** Twins, both stillborn M SDx ♀
  - **V27.5** Other multiple birth, all liveborn M SDx ♀
  - **V27.6** Other multiple birth, some liveborn M SDx ♀
  - **V27.7** Other multiple birth, all stillborn M SDx ♀
  - **V27.9** Unspecified outcome of delivery M SDx ♀
    - Single birth } outcome to infant
    - Multiple birth } unspecified
- ✓4th **V28** Antenatal screening
  - *EXCLUDES* abnormal findings on screening — code to findings
    - routine prenatal care (V22.0-V23.9)
  - **V28.0** Screening for chromosomal anomalies by amniocentesis M ♀
  - **V28.1** Screening for raised alpha-fetoprotein levels in amniotic fluid M ♀
  - **V28.2** Other screening based on amniocentesis M ♀
  - **V28.3** Screening for malformation using ultrasonics
  - **V28.4** Screening for fetal growth retardation using ultrasonics
  - **V28.5** Screening for isoimmunization
  - **V28.6** Screening for Streptococcus B M ♀
  - **V28.8** Other specified antenatal screening
  - **V28.9** Unspecified antenatal screening

✓4th ✓5th Additional Digit Required | Unspecified Code | Other Specified Code | Manifestation Code
MSP Medicare Secondary Payer | ▶ Revised Text | ● New Code | ▲ Revised Code Title

V29–V41.6 V CODES

✓4ᵗʰ V29 Observation and evaluation of newborns and infants for suspected condition not found

Note: This category is to be used for newborns, within the neonatal period, (the first 28 days of life) who are suspected of having an abnormal condition resulting from exposure from the mother or the birth process, but without signs or symptoms, and, which after examination and observation, is found not to exist.

V29.0	Observation for suspected infectious condition	N PDx
V29.1	Observation for suspected neurological condition	N PDx
V29.2	Observation for suspected respiratory condition	N PDx
V29.3	Observation for suspected genetic or metabolic condition	N PDx
V29.8	Observation for other specified suspected condition	N PDx
V29.9	Observation for unspecified suspected condition	N PDx

LIVEBORN INFANTS ACCORDING TO TYPE OF BIRTH (V30-V39)

Note: These categories are intended for the coding of liveborn infants who are consuming health care [e.g., crib or bassinet occupancy].

The following fourth-digit subdivisions are for use with categories V30-V39:
- ✓5ᵗʰ 0 Born in hospital — N
- 1 Born before admission to hospital — N
- 2 Born outside hospital and not hospitalized

The following two fifth-digits are for use with the fourth-digit .0, Born in hospital:
- 0 delivered without mention of cesarean delivery
- 1 delivered by cesarean delivery

✓4ᵗʰ V30	Single liveborn	PDx
✓4ᵗʰ V31	Twin, mate liveborn	PDx
✓4ᵗʰ V32	Twin, mate stillborn	PDx
✓4ᵗʰ V33	Twin, unspecified	PDx
✓4ᵗʰ V34	Other multiple, mates all liveborn	PDx
✓4ᵗʰ V35	Other multiple, mates all stillborn	PDx
✓4ᵗʰ V36	Other multiple, mates live- and stillborn	PDx
✓4ᵗʰ V37	Other multiple, unspecified	PDx
✓4ᵗʰ V39	Unspecified	PDx

PERSONS WITH A CONDITION INFLUENCING THEIR HEALTH STATUS (V40-V49)

Note: These categories are intended for use when these conditions are recorded as "diagnoses" or "problems."

✓4ᵗʰ V40 Mental and behavioral problems

V40.0	Problems with learning	SDx
V40.1	Problems with communication [including speech]	SDx
V40.2	Other mental problems	SDx
V40.3	Other behavioral problems	SDx
V40.9	Unspecified mental or behavioral problem	SDx

✓4ᵗʰ V41 Problems with special senses and other special functions

V41.0	Problems with sight	SDx
V41.1	Other eye problems	SDx
V41.2	Problems with hearing	SDx
V41.3	Other ear problems	SDx
V41.4	Problems with voice production	SDx
V41.5	Problems with smell and taste	SDx
V41.6	Problems with swallowing and mastication	SDx

N Newborn Age: 0 P Pediatric Age: 0-17 M Maternity Age: 12-55 A Adult Age: 15-124
SDx Secondary Diagnosis PDx Primary Diagnosis

V CODES

V41.7 **Problems with sexual function** [SDx]
  EXCLUDES marital problems (V61.10)
         psychosexual disorders (302.0-302.9)
V41.8 Other problems with special functions [SDx]
V41.9 Unspecified problem with special functions [SDx]

✓4th V42 **Organ or tissue replaced by transplant**
  INCLUDES homologous or heterologous (animal) (human) transplant organ status
  V42.0 Kidney [SDx]
  V42.1 Heart [SDx]
  V42.2 Heart valve [SDx]
  V42.3 Skin [SDx]
  V42.4 Bone [SDx]
  V42.5 Cornea [SDx]
  V42.6 Lung [SDx]
  V42.7 Liver [SDx]
  ✓5th V42.8 Other specified organ or tissue
    V42.81 Bone marrow [SDx]
    V42.82 Peripheral stem cells [SDx]
    V42.83 Pancreas [SDx]
    V42.84 Intestines [SDx]
    V42.89 Other [SDx]
  V42.9 Unspecified organ or tissue [SDx]

✓4th V43 **Organ or tissue replaced by other means**
  INCLUDES replacement of organ by:
         artificial device
         mechanical device
         prosthesis
  EXCLUDES cardiac pacemaker in situ (V45.01)
         fitting and adjustment of prosthetic device (V52.0-V52.9)
         renal dialysis status (V45.1)
  V43.0 Eye globe [SDx]
  V43.1 Lens [SDx]
       Pseudophakos
  V43.2 Heart [SDx]
  V43.3 Heart valve [SDx]
  V43.4 Blood vessel [SDx]
  V43.5 Bladder [SDx]
  ✓5th V43.6 Joint
    V43.60 Unspecified joint [SDx]
    V43.61 Shoulder [SDx]
    V43.62 Elbow [SDx]
    V43.63 Wrist [SDx]
    V43.64 Hip [SDx]
    V43.65 Knee [SDx]
    V43.66 Ankle [SDx]
    V43.69 Other [SDx]
  V43.7 Limb
  ✓5th V43.8 Other organ or tissue
    V43.81 Larynx [SDx]
    V43.82 Breast [SDx]
    V43.83 Artificial skin [SDx]

✓4th
✓5th Additional Digit Required Unspecified Code Other Specified Code   Manifestation Code
MSP Medicare Secondary Payer   ▶◀ Revised Text   ● New Code   ▲ Revised Code Title

2002 Ingenix, Inc.   Volume 1 — 605

V43.89 Other — SDx

V44 Artificial opening status
EXCLUDES artificial openings requiring attention or management (V55.0-V55.9)

- **V44.0** Tracheostomy — SDx
- **V44.1** Gastrostomy — SDx
- **V44.2** Ileostomy — SDx
- **V44.3** Colostomy — SDx
- **V44.4** Other artificial opening of gastrointestinal tract
- **V44.5** Cystostomy
  - **V44.50** Cystostomy, unspecified — SDx
  - **V44.51** Cutaneous-vesicostomy — SDx
  - **V44.52** Appendico-vesicostomy — SDx
  - **V44.59** Other cystostomy — SDx
- **V44.6** Other artificial opening of urinary tract
  - Nephrostomy   Urethrostomy
  - Ureterostomy
- **V44.7** Artificial vagina — SDx
- **V44.8** Other artificial opening status — SDx
- **V44.9** Unspecified artificial opening status — SDx

V45 Other postsurgical states
EXCLUDES aftercare management (V51-V58.9)
malfunction or other complication — code to condition

- **V45.0** Cardiac device in situ
  - **V45.00** Unspecified cardiac device — SDx
  - **V45.01** Cardiac pacemaker — SDx
  - **V45.02** Automatic implantable cardiac defibrillator — SDx
  - **V45.09** Other specified cardiac device — SDx
    - Carotid sinus pacemaker in situ
- **V45.1** Renal dialysis status — SDx
  - Patient requiring intermittent renal dialysis
  - Presence of arterial-venous shunt (for dialysis)
  - **EXCLUDES** admission for dialysis treatment or session (V56.0)
- **V45.2** Presence of cerebrospinal fluid drainage device — SDx
  - Cerebral ventricle (communicating) shunt, valve, or device in situ
  - **EXCLUDES** malfunction (996.2)
- **V45.3** Intestinal bypass or anastomosis status — SDx
- **V45.4** Arthrodesis status — SDx
- **V45.5** Presence of contraceptive device
  - **EXCLUDES** checking, reinsertion, or removal of device (V25.42)
  - complication from device (996.32)
  - insertion of device (V25.1)
  - **V45.51** Intrauterine contraceptive device — SDx ♀
  - **V45.52** Subdermal contraceptive implant — SDx
  - **V45.59** Other — SDx
- **V45.6** States following surgery of eye and adnexa
  - Cataract extraction ⎫
  - Filtering bleb   ⎬ state following eye surgery
  - Surgical eyelid adhesion ⎭
  - **EXCLUDES** aphakia (379.31)
  - artificial eye globe (V43.0)
  - **V45.61** Cataract extraction status — SDx
    - Use additional code for associated artificial lens status (V43.1)
  - **V45.69** Other states following surgery of eye and adnexa — SDx

V CODES

√5th V45.7 Acquired absence of organ
    V45.71 Acquired absence of breast
    V45.72 Acquired absence of intestine (large) (small)
    V45.73 Acquired absence of kidney
    V45.74 **Other parts of urinary tract**
        Bladder
    V45.75 Stomach
    V45.76 Lung
    V45.77 Genital organs
    V45.78 Eye
    V45.79 **Other acquired absence of organ**

√5th V45.8 Other postsurgical status
    V45.81 Aortocoronary bypass status [SDx]
    V45.82 Percutaneous transluminal coronary angioplasty status [SDx]
    V45.83 Breast implant removal status [SDx]
    V45.84 Dental restoration status [SDx]
        Dental crowns status
        Dental filings status
    V45.89 Other [SDx]
        Presence of neuropacemaker or other electronic device
        EXCLUDES   *artificial heart valve in situ (V43.3)*
                          vascular prosthesis in situ (V43.4)

√4th V46 Other dependence on machines
    V46.0 Aspirator [SDx]
    V46.1 Respirator [SDx]
        Iron lung
  ● V46.2 Supplemental oxygen
        Long-term oxygen therapy
    V46.8 **Other enabling machines** [SDx]
        Hyperbaric chamber
        Possum [Patient-Operated-Selector-Mechanism]
        EXCLUDES   *cardiac pacemaker (V45.0)*
                          kidney dialysis machine (V45.1)
    V46.9 **Unspecified machine dependence** [SDx]

√4th V47 Other problems with internal organs [SDx]
    V47.0 Deficiencies of internal organs [SDx]
    V47.1 Mechanical and motor problems with internal organs [SDx]
    V47.2 **Other cardiorespiratory problems** [SDx]
        Cardiovascular exercise intolerance with pain (with):
            at rest
            less than ordinary activity
            ordinary activity
    V47.3 **Other digestive problems** [SDx]
    V47.4 **Other urinary problems** [SDx]
    V47.5 **Other genital problems** [SDx]
    V47.9 **Unspecified** [SDx]

√4th V48 Problems with head, neck, and trunk
    V48.0 Deficiencies of head [SDx]
        EXCLUDES   *deficiencies of ears, eyelids, and nose (V48.8)*
    V48.1 Deficiencies of neck and trunk [SDx]
    V48.2 Mechanical and motor problems with head [SDx]
    V48.3 Mechanical and motor problems with neck and trunk [SDx]

√4th / √5th   Additional Digit Required   **Unspecified Code**   Other Specified Code   **Manifestation Code**
MSP Medicare Secondary Payer   ►◄ Revised Text   ● New Code   ▲ Revised Code Title

V CODES

Code	Description	
V48.4	Sensory problem with head	SDx
V48.5	Sensory problem with neck and trunk	SDx
V48.6	Disfigurements of head	SDx
V48.7	Disfigurements of neck and trunk	SDx
V48.8	Other problems with head, neck, and trunk	SDx
V48.9	Unspecified problem with head, neck, or trunk	SDx

✓4th **V49 Other conditions influencing health status**

Code	Description	
V49.0	Deficiencies of limbs	SDx
V49.1	Mechanical problems with limbs	SDx
V49.2	Motor problems with limbs	SDx
V49.3	Sensory problems with limbs	SDx
V49.4	Disfigurements of limbs	SDx
V49.5	Other problems of limbs	SDx

✓5th **V49.6 Upper limb amputation status**

Code	Description	
V49.60	Unspecified level	SDx
V49.61	Thumb	SDx
V49.62	Other finger(s)	SDx
V49.63	Hand	SDx
V49.64	Wrist	SDx
	Disarticulation of wrist	
V49.65	Below elbow	SDx
V49.66	Above elbow	SDx
	Disarticulation of elbow	
V49.67	Shoulder	SDx
	Disarticulation of shoulder	

✓5th **V49.7 Lower limb amputation status**

Code	Description	
V49.70	Unspecified level	SDx
V49.71	Great toe	SDx
V49.72	Other toe(s)	SDx
V49.73	Foot	SDx
V49.74	Ankle	SDx
	Disarticulation of ankle	
V49.75	Below knee	SDx
V49.76	Above knee	SDx
	Disarticulation of knee	
V49.77	Hip	SDx
	Disarticulation of hip	

✓5th **V49.8 Other specified conditions influencing health status**

▲ V49.81 Asymptomatic postmenopausal status (age-related) (natural) A ♀

> EXCLUDES   menopausal and premenopausal disorders (627.0-627.9)
> postsurgical menopause (256.2)
> premature menopause (256.31)
> symptomatic menopause (627.0-627.9)

Code	Description	
V49.82	Dental sealant status	SDx
V49.89	Other specified conditions influencing health status	SDx
V49.9	Unspecified	SDx

N Newborn Age: 0   **P** Pediatric Age: 0-17   **M** Maternity Age: 12-55   **A** Adult Age: 15-124
SDx Secondary Diagnosis   **PDx** Primary Diagnosis

V CODES

PERSONS ENCOUNTERING HEALTH SERVICES FOR SPECIFIC PROCEDURES AND AFTERCARE (V50-V59)

Note: Categories V51-V58 are intended for use to indicate a reason for care in patients who may have already been treated for some disease or injury not now present, or who are receiving care to consolidate the treatment, to deal with residual states, or to prevent recurrence.

EXCLUDES follow-up examination for medical surveillance following treatment (V67.0-V67.9)

V50 Elective surgery for purposes other than remedying health states
- V50.0 Hair transplant
- V50.1 Other plastic surgery for unacceptable cosmetic appearance
  - Breast augmentation or reduction
  - Face-lift
  - **EXCLUDES** plastic surgery following healed injury or operation (V51)
- V50.2 Routine or ritual circumcision ♂
  - Circumcision in the absence of significant medical indication
- V50.3 Ear piercing
- V50.4 Prophylactic organ removal
  - **EXCLUDES** organ donations (V59.0-V59.9)
  - therapeutic organ removal — code to condition
  - V50.41 Breast
  - V50.42 Ovary ♀
  - V50.49 Other
- V50.8 Other
- V50.9 Unspecified

V51 Aftercare involving the use of plastic surgery SDx
- Plastic surgery following healed injury or operation
- **EXCLUDES** cosmetic plastic surgery (V50.1)
- plastic surgery as treatment for current injury — code to condition
- repair of scarred tissue — code to scar

V52 Fitting and adjustment of prosthetic device and implant
- **INCLUDES** removal of device
- **EXCLUDES** malfunction or complication of prosthetic device (996.0-996.7)
- status only, without need for care (V43.0-V43.8)
- V52.0 Artificial arm (complete) (partial)
- V52.1 Artificial leg (complete) (partial)
- V52.2 Artificial eye
- V52.3 Dental prosthetic device
- V52.4 Breast prosthesis and implant ♀
  - **EXCLUDES** admission for implant insertion (V50.1)
- V52.8 Other specified prosthetic device
- V52.9 Unspecified prosthetic device

V53 Fitting and adjustment of other device
- **INCLUDES** removal of device
- replacement of device
- **EXCLUDES** status only, without need for care (V45.0-V45.8)
- V53.0 Devices related to nervous system and special senses
  - V53.01 Fitting and adjustment of cerebral ventricular (communicating) shunt
  - V53.02 Neuropacemaker (brain) (peripheral nerve) (spinal cord)

Additional Digit Required | Unspecified Code | Other Specified Code | Manifestation Code
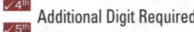 Medicare Secondary Payer | ▶◀ Revised Text | ● New Code | ▲ Revised Code Title

2002 Ingenix, Inc.

V53.09 Fitting and adjustment of other devices related to nervous system and special senses
  Auditory substitution device
  Visual substitution device

V53.1 Spectacles and contact lenses

V53.2 Hearing aid

√5th **V53.3** Cardiac device
  Reprogramming
  V53.31 Cardiac pacemaker
    EXCLUDES mechanical complication of cardiac pacemaker (996.01)
  V53.32 Automatic implantable cardiac defibrillator
  V53.39 Other cardiac device

V53.4 Orthodontic devices

V53.5 Other intestinal appliance
  EXCLUDES colostomy (V55.3)
    ileostomy (V55.2)
    other artificial opening of digestive tract (V55.4)

V53.6 Urinary devices
  Urinary catheter
  EXCLUDES cystostomy (V55.5)
    nephrostomy (V55.6)
    ureterostomy (V55.6)
    urethrostomy (V55.6)

V53.7 Orthopedic devices
  Orthopedic:
    brace
    cast
    corset
    shoes
  EXCLUDES other orthopedic aftercare (V54)

V53.8 Wheelchair

V53.9 Other and unspecified device

√4th **V54** Other orthopedic aftercare

V54.0 Aftercare involving removal of fracture plate or other internal fixation device
  Removal of:
    pins
    plates
    rods
    screws
  EXCLUDES malfunction of internal orthopedic device (996.4)
    other complication of nonmechanical nature (996.60-996.79)
    removal of external fixation device ▶(V54.89)◀

√5th **V54.1** Aftercare for healing traumatic fracture
  V54.10 Aftercare for healing traumatic fracture of arm, unspecified
  V54.11 Aftercare for healing traumatic fracture of upper arm
  V54.12 Aftercare for healing traumatic fracture of lower arm
  V54.13 Aftercare for healing traumatic fracture of hip
  V54.14 Aftercare for healing traumatic fracture of leg, unspecified
  V54.15 Aftercare for healing traumatic fracture of upper leg
    EXCLUDES aftercare for healing traumatic fracture of hip (V54.13)
  V54.16 Aftercare for healing traumatic fracture of lower leg
  V54.17 Aftercare for healing traumatic fracture of vertebrae
  V54.19 Aftercare for healing traumatic fracture of other bone

N Newborn Age: 0   P Pediatric Age: 0-17   M Maternity Age: 12-55   A Adult Age: 15-124
         Secondary Diagnosis   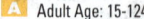 Primary Diagnosis

V CODES

√5th V54.2 Aftercare for healing pathologic fracture
- V54.20 Aftercare for healing pathologic fracture of arm, unspecified
- V54.21 Aftercare for healing pathologic fracture of upper arm
- V54.22 Aftercare for healing pathologic fracture of lower arm
- V54.23 Aftercare for healing pathologic fracture of hip
- V54.24 Aftercare for healing pathologic fracture of leg, unspecified
- V54.25 Aftercare for healing pathologic fracture of upper leg
  - EXCLUDES: aftercare for healing pathologic fracture of hip (V54.23)
- V54.26 Aftercare for healing pathologic fracture of lower leg
- V54.27 Aftercare for healing pathologic fracture of vertebrae
- V54.29 Aftercare for healing pathologic fracture of other bone

√5th V54.8 Other orthopedic aftercare
- V54.81 Aftercare following joint replacement
  - Use additional code to identify joint replacement site (V43.60-V43.69)
- V54.89 Other orthopedic aftercare
  - Aftercare for healing fracture NOS

V54.9 Unspecified orthopedic aftercare

√4th V55 Attention to artificial openings
- INCLUDES: adjustment or repositioning of catheter
  closure
  passage of sounds or bougies
  reforming
  removal or replacement of catheter
  toilet or cleansing
- EXCLUDES: complications of external stoma (519.00-519.09, 569.60-569.69, 997.4, 997.5)
  status only, without need for care (V44.0-V44.9)

- V55.0 Tracheostomy
- V55.1 Gastrostomy
- V55.2 Ileostomy
- V55.3 Colostomy
- V55.4 Other artificial opening of digestive tract
- V55.5 Cystostomy
- V55.6 Other artificial opening of urinary tract
  - Nephrostomy   Urethrostomy
  - Ureterostomy
- V55.7 Artificial vagina
- V55.8 Other specified artificial opening
- V55.9 Unspecified artificial opening

√4th V56 Encounter for dialysis and dialysis catheter care
- Use additional code to identify the associated condition
- EXCLUDES: dialysis preparation — code to condition
- V56.0 Extracorporeal dialysis
  - Dialysis (renal) NOS
  - EXCLUDES: dialysis status (V45.1)
- V56.1 Fitting and adjustment of extracorporeal dialysis catheter
  - Removal or replacement of catheter
  - Toilet or cleansing
  - Use additional code for any concurrent extracorporeal dialysis (V56.0)
- V56.2 Fitting and adjustment of peritoneal dialysis catheter
  - Use additional code for any concurrent peritoneal dialysis (V56.8)

V56.3–V58.5 V CODES

- ✓5th **V56.3 Encounter for adequacy testing for dialysis**
  - **V56.31** Encounter for adequacy testing for hemodialysis
  - **V56.32** Encounter for adequacy testing for peritoneal dialysis
    - Peritoneal equilibration test
- **V56.8 Other dialysis**
  - Peritoneal dialysis

- ✓4th **V57 Care involving use of rehabilitation procedures**
  - Use additional code to identify underlying condition
  - **V57.0** Breathing exercises
  - **V57.1 Other physical therapy**
    - Therapeutic and remedial exercises, except breathing
  - ✓5th **V57.2 Occupational therapy and vocational rehabilitation**
    - **V57.21** Encounter for occupational therapy
    - **V57.22** Encounter for vocational therapy
  - **V57.3** Speech therapy
  - **V57.4** Orthoptic training
  - ✓5th **V57.8 Other specified rehabilitation procedure**
    - **V57.81** Orthotic training
      - Gait training in the use of artificial limbs
    - **V57.89 Other**
      - Multiple training or therapy
  - **V57.9 Unspecified rehabilitation procedure**

- ✓4th **V58 Encounter for other and unspecified procedures and aftercare**
  - **EXCLUDES** convalescence and palliative care (V66)
  - **V58.0 Radiotherapy** `PDx`
    - Encounter or admission for radiotherapy
    - **EXCLUDES** encounter for radioactive implant — code to condition
      - radioactive iodine therapy — code to condition
  - **V58.1 Chemotherapy** `PDx`
    - Encounter or admission for chemotherapy
    - **EXCLUDES** prophylactic chemotherapy against disease which has never been present (V03.0-V07.9)
  - **V58.2 Blood transfusion, without reported diagnosis** `SDx`
  - **V58.3 Attention to surgical dressings and sutures** `PDx`
    - Change of dressings
    - Removal of sutures
  - ✓5th **V58.4 Other aftercare following surgery**
    - **EXCLUDES** aftercare following sterilization reversal surgery (V26.22)
      - attention to artificial openings (V55.0-V55.9)
      - orthopedic aftercare (V54.0-V54.9)
    - ▶Note: Codes from this subcategory should be used in conjunction with other aftercare codes to fully identify the reason for the aftercare encounter◀
    - **V58.41 Encounter for planned postoperative wound closure**
      - **EXCLUDES** disruption of operative wound (998.3)
    - • **V58.42 Aftercare following surgery for neoplasm**
      - Conditions classifiable to 140-239
    - • **V58.43 Aftercare following surgery for injury and trauma**
      - Conditions classifiable to 800-999
      - **EXCLUDES** aftercare for healing traumatic fracture (V54.10-V54.19)
    - **V58.49 Other specified aftercare following surgery**
  - **V58.5 Orthodontics** `PDx`
    - **EXCLUDES** fitting and adjustment of orthodontic device (V53.4)

`N` Newborn Age: 0   `P` Pediatric Age: 0-17   `M` Maternity Age: 12-55   `A` Adult Age: 15-124
`SDx` Secondary Diagnosis   `PDx` Primary Diagnosis

V CODES

V58.6–V58.9

✓5ᵗʰ **V58.6 Long-term (current) drug use**
    EXCLUDES   *drub abuse (305.00-305.93)*
                      drug dependence (304.00-304.93)

  V58.61 Long-term (current) use of anticoagulants
  V58.62 Long-term (current) use of antibiotics
  V58.69 Long-term (current) use of other medications
        High-risk medications

● ✓5ᵗʰ **V58.7 Aftercare following surgery to specified body systems, not elsewhere classified**

    Note: Codes from this subcategory should be used in conjunction with other aftercare codes to fully identify the reason for the aftercare encounter

●   **V58.71 Aftercare following surgery of the sense organs, NEC**
        Conditions classifiable to 360-379, 380-389

●   **V58.72 Aftercare following surgery of the nervous system, NEC**
        Conditions classifiable to 320-359
        EXCLUDES *aftercare following surgery of the sense organs, NEC (V58.71)*

●   **V58.73 Aftercare following surgery of the circulatory system, NEC**
        Conditions classifiable to 390-459

●   **V58.74 Aftercare following surgery of the respiratory system, NEC**
        Conditions classifiable to 460-519

●   **V58.75 Aftercare following surgery of the teeth, oral cavity and digestive system, NEC**
        Conditions classifiable to 520-579

●   **V58.76 Aftercare following surgery of the genitourinary system, NEC**
        Conditions classifiable to 580-629
        EXCLUDES *aftercare following sterilization reversal (V26.22)*

●   **V58.77 Aftercare following surgery of the skin and subcutaneous tissue, NEC**
        Conditions classifiable to 680-709

●   **V58.78 Aftercare following surgery of the musculoskeletal system, NEC**
        Conditions classifiable to 710-739

✓5ᵗʰ **V58.8 Other specified procedures and aftercare**

  V58.81 Fitting and adjustment of vascular catheter
        Removal or replacement of catheter
        Toilet or cleansing
        EXCLUDES *complication of renal dialysis (996.73)*
                      complication of vascular catheter (996.74)
                      dialysis preparation — code to condition
                      encounter for dialysis (V56.0-V56.8)
                      fitting and adjustment of dialysis catheter (V56.1)

  V58.82 Fitting and adjustment of nonvascular catheter, NEC
        Removal or replacement of catheter
        Toilet or cleansing
        EXCLUDES *fitting and adjustment of peritoneal dialysis catheter (V56.2)*
                      fitting and adjustment of urinary catheter (V53.6)

  V58.83 Encounter for therapeutic drug monitoring
        EXCLUDES *blood-drug testing for medicolegal reasons (V70.4)*
        ▶Use additional code for any associated long-term (current) drug use (V58.61-V58.69)◀

  V58.89 Other specified aftercare

V58.9 Unspecified aftercare   SDx

  Additional Digit Required   Unspecified Code   Other Specified Code   Manifestation Code
MSP Medicare Secondary Payer   ▶◀ Revised Text   ● New Code   ▲ Revised Code Title

V59 Donors

EXCLUDES examination of potential donor (V70.8)
self-donation of organ or tissue — code to condition

- **V59.0** Blood
  - V59.01 Whole blood `PDx`
  - V59.02 Stem cells `PDx`
  - V59.09 Other `PDx`
- **V59.1** Skin `PDx`
- **V59.2** Bone `PDx`
- **V59.3** Bone marrow `PDx`
- **V59.4** Kidney `PDx`
- **V59.5** Cornea `PDx`
- **V59.6** Liver `PDx`
- **V59.8** Other specified organ or tissue `PDx`
- **V59.9** Unspecified organ or tissue `PDx`

PERSONS ENCOUNTERING HEALTH SERVICES IN OTHER CIRCUMSTANCES (V60-V68)

V60 Housing, household, and economic circumstances

- **V60.0** Lack of housing `SDx`
  - Hobos
  - Social migrants
  - Tramps
  - Transients
  - Vagabonds
- **V60.1** Inadequate housing `SDx`
  - Lack of heating
  - Restriction of space
  - Technical defects in home preventing adequate care
- **V60.2** Inadequate material resources `SDx`
  - Economic problem
  - Poverty NOS
- **V60.3** Person living alone `SDx`
- **V60.4** No other household member able to render care `SDx`
  - Person requiring care (has) (is):
    - family member too handicapped, ill, or otherwise unsuited to render care
    - partner temporarily away from home
    - temporarily away from usual place of abode
  - **EXCLUDES** holiday relief care (V60.5)
- **V60.5** Holiday relief care `SDx`
  - Provision of health care facilities to a person normally cared for at home, to enable relatives to take a vacation
- **V60.6** Person living in residential institution `SDx`
  - Boarding school resident
- **V60.8** Other specified housing or economic circumstances `SDx`
- **V60.9** Unspecified housing or economic circumstance `SDx`

V61 Other family circumstances

INCLUDES when these circumstances or fear of them, affecting the person directly involved or others, are mentioned as the reason, justified or not, for seeking or receiving medical advice or care

- **V61.0** Family disruption
  - Divorce
  - Estrangement
- **V61.1** Counseling for marital and partner problems
  - **EXCLUDES** problems related to:
    - psychosexual disorders (302.0-302.9)
    - sexual function (V41.7)
  - **V61.10** Counseling for marital and partner problems, unspecified
    - Marital conflict   Partner conflict

V CODES

V61.11 Counseling for victim of spousal and partner abuse
  EXCLUDES encounter for treatment of current injuries due to abuse (995.80-995.85)

V61.12 Counseling for perpetrator of spousal and partner abuse

√5th **V61.2** Parent-child problems

V61.20 Counseling for parent-child problem, unspecified
  Concern about behavior of child
  Parent-child conflict

V61.21 Counseling for victim of child abuse
  Child battering   Child neglect
  EXCLUDES current injuries due to abuse (995.50-995.59)

V61.22 Counseling for perpetrator of parent child abuse
  EXCLUDES counseling for non-parental abuser (V62.83)

V61.29 Other
  Problem concerning adopted or foster child

V61.3 Problems with aged parents or in-laws

√5th **V61.4** Health problems within family

V61.41 Alcoholism in family

V61.49 Other
  Care of } sick or handicapped person in family
  Presence of } or household

V61.5 Multiparity

V61.6 Illegitimacy or illegitimate pregnancy M♀

V61.7 Other unwanted pregnancy M♀

V61.8 Other specified family circumstances
  Problems with family members NEC

V61.9 Unspecified family circumstance

√4th **V62** Other psychosocial circumstances
  INCLUDES those circumstances or fear of them, affecting the person directly involved or others, mentioned as the reason, justified or not, for seeking or receiving medical advice or care
  EXCLUDES previous psychological trauma (V15.41-V15.49)

V62.0 Unemployment SDx
  EXCLUDES circumstances when main problem is economic inadequacy or poverty (V60.2)

V62.1 Adverse effects of work environment SDx

V62.2 Other occupational circumstances or maladjustment SDx
  Career choice problem
  Dissatisfaction with employment

V62.3 Educational circumstances SDx
  Dissatisfaction with school environment
  Educational handicap

V62.4 Social maladjustment SDx
  Cultural deprivation
  Political, religious, or sex discrimination
  Social:
    isolation
    persecution

V62.5 Legal circumstances SDx
  Imprisonment
  Legal investigation
  Litigation
  Prosecution

√4th Additional Digit Required
√5th
 Medicare Secondary Payer
Unspecified Code
▶◀ Revised Text
Other Specified Code
● New Code
Manifestation Code
▲ Revised Code Title

V CODES

- **V62.6** Refusal of treatment for reasons of religion or conscience [SDx]
- ✓5th **V62.8** Other psychological or physical stress, not elsewhere classified
  - **V62.81** Interpersonal problems, not elsewhere classified [SDx]
  - **V62.82** Bereavement, uncomplicated [SDx]
    - EXCLUDES: bereavement as adjustment reaction (309.0)
  - **V62.83** Counseling for perpetrator of physical/sexual abuse [SDx]
    - EXCLUDES: counseling for perpetrator of parental child abuse (V61.22)
      counseling for perpetrator of spousal and partner abuse (V61.12)
  - **V62.89** Other [SDx]
    - Life circumstance problems
    - Phase of life problems
  - **V62.9** Unspecified psychosocial circumstance [SDx]
- ✓4th **V63** Unavailability of other medical facilities for care
  - **V63.0** Residence remote from hospital or other health care facility
  - **V63.1** Medical services in home not available
    - EXCLUDES: no other household member able to render care (V60.4)
  - **V63.2** Person awaiting admission to adequate facility elsewhere
  - **V63.8** Other specified reasons for unavailability of medical facilities
    - Person on waiting list undergoing social agency investigation
  - **V63.9** Unspecified reason for unavailability of medical facilities
- ✓4th **V64** Persons encountering health services for specific procedures, not carried out
  - **V64.0** Vaccination not carried out because of contraindication [SDx]
  - **V64.1** Surgical or other procedure not carried out because of contraindication [SDx]
  - **V64.2** Surgical or other procedure not carried out because of patient's decision
  - **V64.3** Procedure not carried out for other reasons [SDx]
  - **V64.4** Laparoscopic surgical procedure converted to open procedure [SDx]
- ✓4th **V65** Other persons seeking consultation without complaint or sickness
  - **V65.0** Healthy person accompanying sick person
    - Boarder
  - **V65.1** Person consulting on behalf of another person
    - Advice or treatment for nonattending third party
    - EXCLUDES: concern (normal) about sick person in family (V61.41-V61.49)
  - **V65.2** Person feigning illness
    - Malingerer
    - Peregrinating patient
  - **V65.3** Dietary surveillance and counseling
    - Dietary surveillance and counseling (in):
      - NOS
      - colitis
      - diabetes mellitus
      - food allergies or intolerance
      - gastritis
      - hypercholesterolemia
      - hypoglycemia
      - obesity

V CODES

√5th V65.4 Other counseling, not elsewhere classified
  Health:
    advice
    education
    instruction
  EXCLUDES counseling (for):
      contraception (V25.40-V25.49)
      genetic (V26.3)
      on behalf of third party (V65.1)
      procreative management (V26.4)

  V65.40 Counseling NOS
  V65.41 Exercise counseling
  V65.42 Counseling on substance use and abuse
  V65.43 Counseling on injury prevention
  V65.44 Human immunodeficiency virus [HIV] counseling
  V65.45 Counseling on other sexually transmitted diseases
  V65.49 Other specified counseling

  V65.5 Person with feared complaint in whom no diagnosis was made
      Feared condition not demonstrated
      Problem was normal state
      "Worried well"

  V65.8 Other reasons for seeking consultation
      EXCLUDES specified symptoms

  V65.9 Unspecified reason for consultation

√4th V66 Convalescence and palliative care
  V66.0 Following surgery `PDx`
  V66.1 Following radiotherapy `PDx`
  V66.2 Following chemotherapy `PDx`
  V66.3 Following psychotherapy and other treatment for mental disorder `PDx`
  V66.4 Following treatment of fracture `PDx`
  V66.5 Following other treatment `PDx`
  V66.6 Following combined treatment `PDx`
  V66.7 Encounter for palliative care `SDx`
      End-of-life care
      Hospice care
      Terminal care
      Code first underlying disease
  V66.9 Unspecified convalescence `PDx`

√4th V67 Follow-up examination
  INCLUDES surveillance only following completed treatment
  EXCLUDES surveillance of contraception (V25.40-V25.49)

  √5th V67.0 Following surgery
    V67.00 Following surgery, unspecified
    V67.01 Follow-up vaginal pap smear ♀
        Vaginal pap-smear, status-post hysterectomy for malignant condition
        Use additional code to identify:
          acquired absence of uterus (V45.77)
          personal history of malignant neoplasm (V10.40-V10.44)
        EXCLUDES vaginal pap smear status-post hysterectomy for non-malignant condition (V76.47)
    V67.09 Following other surgery
        EXCLUDES sperm count following sterilization reversal (V26.22)
          sperm count for fertility testing (V26.21)

Code	Description
V67.1	Following radiotherapy
V67.2	Following chemotherapy

Cancer chemotherapy follow-up

V67.3	Following psychotherapy and other treatment for mental disorder
V67.4	Following treatment of healed fracture

EXCLUDES current (healing) fracture aftercare (V54.0-V54.9)

√5th V67.5 Following other treatment

    V67.51 **Following completed treatment with high-risk medications, not elsewhere classified**

        EXCLUDES long-term (current) drug use (V58.61-V58.69)

    V67.59 Other

V67.6	Following combined treatment
V67.9	**Unspecified follow-up examination**

√4th V68 Encounters for administrative purposes

  V68.0 Issue of medical certificates   **PDx**

    Issue of medical certificate of: Issue of medical certificate of:
      cause of death   incapacity
      fitness

      EXCLUDES encounter for general medical examination (V70.0-V70.9)

  V68.1 Issue of repeat prescriptions   **PDx**

    Issue of repeat prescription for:
      appliance
      glasses
      medications

      EXCLUDES repeat prescription for contraceptives (V25.41-V25.49)

  V68.2 Request for expert evidence   **PDx**

√5th V68.8 Other specified administrative purpose

    V68.81 Referral of patient without examination or treatment   **PDx**

    V68.89 Other   **PDx**

  V68.9 **Unspecified administrative purpose**   **PDx**

√4th V69 Problems related to lifestyle

  V69.0 Lack of physical exercise

  V69.1 Inappropriate diet and eating habits

    EXCLUDES anorexia nervosa (307.1)
                 bulimia (783.6)
                 malnutrition and other nutritional deficiencies (260-269.9)
                 other and unspecified eating disorders (307.50-307.59)

  V69.2 High-risk sexual behavior

  V69.3 Gambling and betting

    EXCLUDES pathological gambling (312.31)

  V69.8 **Other problems related to lifestyle**

    Self-damaging behavior

  V69.9 **Problem related to lifestyle, unspecified**

PERSONS WITHOUT REPORTED DIAGNOSIS ENCOUNTERED DURING EXAMINATION AND INVESTIGATION OF INDIVIDUALS AND POPULATIONS (V70-V83)

Note: Nonspecific abnormal findings disclosed at the time of these examinations are classifiable to categories 790-796.

√4th V70 General medical examination

  Use additional code(s) to identify any special screening examination(s) performed (V73.0-V82.9)

  V70.0 Routine general medical examination at a health care facility   **PDx**

    Health checkup

    EXCLUDES health checkup of infant or child (V20.2)

V CODES

V70.1 General psychiatric examination, requested by the authority `PDx`
V70.2 General psychiatric examination, other and unspecified `PDx`
V70.3 Other medical examination for administrative purposes `PDx`
General medical examination for:
  admission to old age home
  adoption
  camp
  driving license
  immigration and naturalization
  insurance certification
  marriage
  prison
  school admission
  sports competition
  EXCLUDES attendance for issue of medical certificates (V68.0)
  pre-employment screening (V70.5)

V70.4 Examination for medicolegal reasons `PDx`
Blood-alcohol tests
Blood-drug tests
Paternity testing
  EXCLUDES examination and observation following:
  accidents (V71.3, V71.4)
  assault (V71.6)
  rape (V71.5)

V70.5 Health examination of defined subpopulations `PDx`
  Armed forces personnel   Prisoners
  Inhabitants of institutions Prostitutes
  Occupational health   Refugees
    examinations   School children
  Pre-employment screening   Students
  Preschool children

V70.6 Health examination in population surveys `PDx`
  EXCLUDES special screening (V73.0-V82.9)

V70.7 Examination of participant in clinical trial
Examination of participant or control in clinical research

V70.8 Other specified general medical examinations `PDx`
Examination of potential donor of organ or tissue

V70.9 Unspecified general medical examination `PDx`

√4th **V71 Observation and evaluation for suspected conditions not found**
  INCLUDES This category is to be used when persons without a diagnosis are suspected of having an abnormal condition, without signs or symptoms, which requires study, but after examination and observation, is found not to exist. This category is also for use for administrative and legal observation status.

√5th **V71.0 Observation for suspected mental condition**
  V71.01 Adult antisocial behavior `A` `PDx`
    Dyssocial behavior or gang activity in adult without manifest psychiatric disorder
  V71.02 Childhood or adolescent antisocial behavior `PDx`
    Dyssocial behavior or gang activity in child or adolescent without manifest psychiatric disorder
  V71.09 Other suspected mental condition `PDx`

V71.1 Observation for suspected malignant neoplasm `PDx`
V71.2 Observation for suspected tuberculosis `PDx`
V71.3 Observation following accident at work `PDx`

V CODES

	V71.4	**Observation following other accident**	PDx
		Examination of individual involved in motor vehicle traffic accident	
	V71.5	**Observation following alleged rape or seduction**	PDx
		Examination of victim or culprit	
	V71.6	**Observation following other inflicted injury**	PDx
		Examination of victim or culprit	
	V71.7	**Observation for suspected cardiovascular disease**	PDx
▲ ✓5th	**V71.8**	**Observation and evaluation for other specified suspected conditions**	
		V71.81 Abuse and neglect	PDx
		EXCLUDES adult abuse and neglect (995.80-995.85)	
		child abuse and neglect (995.50-995.59)	
●		V71.82 Observation and evaluation for suspected exposure to anthrax	
●		V71.83 Observation and evaluation for suspected exposure to other biological agent	
		V71.89 Other specified suspected conditions	PDx
	V71.9	**Observation for unspecified suspected condition**	PDx

✓4th **V72 Special investigations and examinations**

    INCLUDES   routine examination of specific system
    EXCLUDES   general medical examination (V70.0-V70.4)
                           general screening examination of defined population groups (V70.5, V70.6, V70.7)
                           routine examination of infant or child (V20.2)
Use additional code(s) to identify any special screening examination(s) performed (V73.0-V82.9)

	V72.0	**Examination of eyes and vision**	PDx
	V72.1	**Examination of ears and hearing**	PDx
	V72.2	**Dental examination**	PDx
	V72.3	**Gynecological examination**	PDx ♀
		Papanicolaou cervical smear as part of general gynecological examination	
		Pelvic examination (annual) (periodic)	
		Use additional code to identify routine vaginal Papanicolaou smear (V76.47)	
		EXCLUDES cervical Papanicolaou smear without general gynecological examination (V76.2)	
		routine examination in contraceptive management (V25.40-V25.49)	
	V72.4	**Pregnancy examination or test, pregnancy unconfirmed**	PDx ♀
		Possible pregnancy, not (yet) confirmed	
		EXCLUDES pregnancy examination with immediate confirmation (V22.0-V22.1)	
	V72.5	**Radiological examination, not elsewhere classified**	SDx
		Routine chest x-ray	
		EXCLUDES examination for suspected tuberculosis (V71.2)	
	V72.6	**Laboratory examination**	SDx
		EXCLUDES that for suspected disorder (V71.0-V71.9)	
	V72.7	**Diagnostic skin and sensitization tests**	PDx
		Allergy tests Skin tests for hypersensitivity	
		EXCLUDES diagnostic skin tests for bacterial diseases (V74.0-V74.9)	
✓5th	**V72.8**	**Other specified examinations**	
		V72.81 Pre-operative cardiovascular examination	PDx
		V72.82 Pre-operative respiratory examination	PDx
		V72.83 Other specified pre-operative examination	PDx
		V72.84 Pre-operative examination, unspecified	PDx
		V72.85 Other specified examination	PDx
	V72.9	**Unspecified examination**	PDx

N Newborn Age: 0   P Pediatric Age: 0-17   M Maternity Age: 12-55   A Adult Age: 15-124
SDx Secondary Diagnosis   PDx Primary Diagnosis

V CODES

✓4th **V73 Special screening examination for viral and chlamydial diseases**
- V73.0 Poliomyelitis
- V73.1 Smallpox
- V73.2 Measles
- V73.3 Rubella
- V73.4 Yellow fever
- V73.5 Other arthropod-borne viral diseases
  - Dengue fever
  - Hemorrhagic fever
  - Viral encephalitis:
    - mosquito-borne
    - tick-borne
- V73.6 Trachoma

✓5th V73.8 Other specified viral and chlamydial diseases
- V73.88 Other specified chlamydial diseases
- V73.89 Other specified viral diseases

✓5th V73.9 Unspecified viral and chlamydial disease
- V73.98 Unspecified chlamydial disease
- V73.99 Unspecified viral disease

✓4th **V74 Special screening examination for bacterial and spirochetal diseases**
INCLUDES diagnostic skin tests for these diseases
- V74.0 Cholera
- V74.1 Pulmonary tuberculosis
- V74.2 Leprosy [Hansen's disease]
- V74.3 Diphtheria
- V74.4 Bacterial conjunctivitis
- V74.5 Venereal disease
- V74.6 Yaws
- V74.8 Other specified bacterial and spirochetal diseases
  - Brucellosis
  - Leptospirosis
  - Plague
  - Tetanus
  - Whooping cough
- V74.9 Unspecified bacterial and spirochetal disease

✓4th **V75 Special screening examination for other infectious diseases**
- V75.0 Rickettsial diseases
- V75.1 Malaria
- V75.2 Leishmaniasis
- V75.3 Trypanosomiasis
  - Chagas' disease
  - Sleeping sickness
- V75.4 Mycotic infections
- V75.5 Schistosomiasis
- V75.6 Filariasis
- V75.7 Intestinal helminthiasis
- V75.8 Other specified parasitic infections
- V75.9 Unspecified infectious disease

✓4th **V76 Special screening for malignant neoplasms**
- V76.0 Respiratory organs
- ✓5th V76.1 Breast
  - V76.10 Breast screening, unspecified
  - V76.11 Screening mammogram for high-risk patient   ♀
  - V76.12 Other screening mammogram
  - V76.19 Other screening breast examination

✓4th / ✓5th Additional Digit Required | Unspecified Code | Other Specified Code | Manifestation Code
MSP Medicare Secondary Payer   ▶◀ Revised Text   ● New Code   ▲ Revised Code Title

V76.2–V78.9   V CODES

- **V76.2** Cervix ♀
  - Routine cervical Papanicolaou smear
  - EXCLUDES: *that as part of a general gynecological examination (V72.3)*
- **V76.3** Bladder
- ✓5th **V76.4** Other sites
  - **V76.41** Rectum
  - **V76.42** Oral cavity
  - **V76.43** Skin
  - **V76.44** Prostate ♂
  - **V76.45** Testis ♂
  - **V76.46** Ovary
  - **V76.47** Vagina
    - Vaginal pap smear status-post hysterectomy for non-malignant condition
    - Use additional code to identify acquired absence of uterus (V45.77)
    - EXCLUDES: *vaginal pap smear status-post hysterectomy for malignant condition (V67.01)*
  - **V76.49** Other sites
- ✓5th **V76.5** Intestine
  - **V76.50** Intestine, unspecified
  - **V76.51** Colon
    - EXCLUDES: *rectum (V76.41)*
  - **V76.52** Small intestine
- ✓5th **V76.8** Other neoplasm
  - **V76.81** Nervous system
  - **V76.89** Other neoplasm
- **V76.9** Unspecified

✓4th **V77** Special screening for endocrine, nutritional, metabolic, and immunity disorders
  - **V77.0** Thyroid disorders
  - **V77.1** Diabetes mellitus
  - **V77.2** Malnutrition
  - **V77.3** Phenylketonuria [PKU]
  - **V77.4** Galactosemia
  - **V77.5** Gout
  - **V77.6** Cystic fibrosis
    - Screening for mucoviscidosis
  - **V77.7** Other inborn errors of metabolism
  - **V77.8** Obesity
  - ✓5th **V77.9** Other and unspecified endocrine, nutritional, metabolic, and immunity disorders
    - **V77.91** Screening for lipoid disorders
      - Screening cholesterol level
      - Screening for hypercholesterolemia
      - Screening for hyperlipidemia
    - **V77.99** Other and unspecified endocrine, nutritional, metabolic, and immunity disorders

✓4th **V78** Special screening for disorders of blood and blood-forming organs
  - **V78.0** Iron deficiency anemia
  - **V78.1** Other and unspecified deficiency anemia
  - **V78.2** Sickle cell disease or trait
  - **V78.3** Other hemoglobinopathies
  - **V78.8** Other disorders of blood and blood-forming organs
  - **V78.9** Unspecified disorder of blood and blood-forming organs

---

N Newborn Age: 0   **P** Pediatric Age: 0-17   **M** Maternity Age: 12-55   **A** Adult Age: 15-124

 Secondary Diagnosis   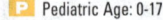 Primary Diagnosis

V CODES

✓4th V79 Special screening for mental disorders and developmental handicaps
    V79.0 Depression
    V79.1 Alcoholism
    V79.2 Mental retardation
    V79.3 Developmental handicaps in early childhood
    V79.8 Other specified mental disorders and developmental handicaps
    V79.9 Unspecified mental disorder and developmental handicap

✓4th V80 Special screening for neurological, eye, and ear diseases
    V80.0 Neurological conditions
    V80.1 Glaucoma
    V80.2 Other eye conditions
        Screening for:
            cataract
            congenital anomaly of eye
            senile macular lesions
        EXCLUDES   general vision examination (V72.0)
    V80.3 Ear diseases
        EXCLUDES   general hearing examination (V72.1)

✓4th V81 Special screening for cardiovascular, respiratory, and genitourinary diseases
    V81.0 Ischemic heart disease
    V81.1 Hypertension
    V81.2 Other and unspecified cardiovascular conditions
    V81.3 Chronic bronchitis and emphysema
    V81.4 Other and unspecified respiratory conditions
        EXCLUDES   screening for:
            lung neoplasm (V76.0)
            pulmonary tuberculosis (V74.1)
    V81.5 Nephropathy
        Screening for asymptomatic bacteriuria
    V81.6 Other and unspecified genitourinary conditions

✓4th V82 Special screening for other conditions
    V82.0 Skin conditions
    V82.1 Rheumatoid arthritis
    V82.2 Other rheumatic disorders
    V82.3 Congenital dislocation of hip
    V82.4 Maternal postnatal screening for chromosomal anomalies ♀
        EXCLUDES   antenatal screening by amniocentesis (V28.0)
    V82.5 Chemical poisoning and other contamination
        Screening for:
            heavy metal poisoning
            ingestion of radioactive substance
            poisoning from contaminated water supply
            radiation exposure
    V82.6 Multiphasic screening
    ✓5th V82.8 Other specified conditions
        V82.81 Osteoporosis
            Use additional code to identify:
                postmenopausal hormone replacement therapy status (V07.4)
                postmenopausal (natural) status (V49.81)
        V82.89 Other specified conditions
    V82.9 Unspecified condition

  Additional Digit Required   Unspecified Code   Other Specified Code   Manifestation Code
MSP Medicare Secondary Payer   ▶◀ Revised Text   ● New Code   ▲ Revised Code Title

V83–V83.89 V CODES

- ✓4th **V83 Genetic carrier status**
  - ✓5th **V83.0 Hemophilia A carrier**
    - V83.01 Asymptomatic hemophilia A carrier
    - V83.02 Symptomatic hemophilia A carrier
- ● ✓5th **V83.8 Other genetic carrier status**
- ●   V83.81 Cystic fibrosis gene carrier
- ●   V83.89 Other genetic carrier status

E CODES

SUPPLEMENTARY CLASSIFICATION OF EXTERNAL CAUSES OF INJURY AND POISONING (E800-E999)

This section is provided to permit the classification of environmental events, circumstances, and conditions as the cause of injury, poisoning, and other adverse effects. Where a code from this section is applicable, it is intended that it shall be used in addition to a code from one of the main chapters of ICD-9-CM, indicating the nature of the condition. Certain other conditions which may be stated to be due to external causes are classified in Chapters 1 to 16 of ICD-9-CM. For these, the "E" code classification should be used as an additional code for more detailed analysis.

Machinery accidents [other than those connected with transport] are classifiable to category E919, in which the fourth-digit allows a broad classification of the type of machinery involved. If a more detailed classification of type of machinery is required, it is suggested that the "Classification of Industrial Accidents according to Agency," prepared by the International Labor Office, be used in addition. This is reproduced in Appendix D for optional use.

Categories for "late effects" of accidents and other external causes are to be found at E929, E959, E969, E977, E989, and E999.

DEFINITIONS AND EXAMPLES RELATED TO TRANSPORT ACCIDENTS

(a) A transport accident (E800-E848) is any accident involving a device designed primarily for, or being used at the time primarily for, conveying persons or goods from one place to another.

> **INCLUDES** accidents involving:
> aircraft and spacecraft (E840-E845)
> watercraft (E830-E838)
> motor vehicle (E810-E825)
> railway (E800-E807)
> other road vehicles (E826-E829)

In classifying accidents which involve more than one kind of transport, the above order of precedence of transport accidents should be used.

Accidents involving agricultural and construction machines, such as tractors, cranes, and bulldozers, are regarded as transport accidents only when these vehicles are under their own power on a highway [otherwise the vehicles are regarded as machinery]. Vehicles which can travel on land or water, such as hovercraft and other amphibious vehicles, are regarded as watercraft when on the water, as motor vehicles when on the highway, and as off-road motor vehicles when on land, but off the highway.

> **EXCLUDES** accidents:
> in sports which involve the use of transport but where the transport vehicle itself was not involved in the accident
> involving vehicles which are part of industrial equipment used entirely on industrial premises
> occurring during transportation but unrelated to the hazards associated with the means of transportation [e.g., injuries received in a fight on board ship; transport vehicle involved in a cataclysm such as an earthquake]
> to persons engaged in the maintenance or repair of transport equipment or vehicle not in motion, unlesss injured by another vehicle in motion

(b) A railway accident is a transport accident involving a railway train or other railway vehicle operated on rails, whether in motion or not.

> **EXCLUDES** accidents:
> in repair shops
> in roundhouse or on turntable
> on railway premises but not involving a train or other railway vehicle

(c) A **railway train** or **railway vehicle** is any device with or without cars coupled to it, desiged for traffic on a railway.

> [INCLUDES] interurban:
> electric car ⎫ (operated chiefly on its own right-of-way, not
> streetcar ⎭ open to other traffic)
>
> railway train, any power [diesel] [electric] [steam]
>   funicular
>   monorail or two-rail
>   subterranean or elevated
> other vehicle designed to run on a railway track
>
> [EXCLUDES] *interurban electric cars [streetcars] specified to be operating on a right-of-way that forms part of the public street or highway [definition (n)]*

(d) A **railway** or **railroad** is a right-of-way designed for traffic on rails, which is used by carriages or wagons transporting passengers or freight, and by other rolling stock, and which is not open to other public vehicular traffic.

(e) A **motor vehicle** accident is a transport accident involving a motor vehicle. It is defined as a motor vehicle traffic accident or as a motor vehicle nontraffic accident according to whether the accident occurs on a public highway or elsewhere.

> [EXCLUDES] *injury or damage due to cataclysm*
> *injury or damage while a motor vehicle, not under its own power, is being loaded on, or unloaded from, another conveyance*

(f) A **motor vehicle traffic accident** is any motor vehicle accident occurring on a public highway [i.e., originating, terminating, or involving a vehicle partially on the highway]. A motor vehicle accident is assumed to have occurred on the highway unless another place is specified, except in the case of accidents involving only off-road motor vehicles which are classified as nontraffic accidents unless the contrary is stated.

(g) A **motor vehicle nontraffic accident** is any motor vehicle accident which occurs entirely in any place other than a public highway.

(h) A **public highway [trafficway]** or **street** is the entire width between property lines [or other boundary lines] of every way or place, of which any part is open to the use of the public for purposes of vehicular traffic as a matter of right or custom. A roadway is that part of the public highway designed, improved, and ordinarily used, for vehicular travel.

> [INCLUDES] approaches (public) to:
>   docks
>   public building
>   station
>
> [EXCLUDES] *driveway (private)*
> *parking lot*
> *ramp*
> *roads in:*
>   *airfield*
>   *farm*
>   *industrial premises*
>   *mine*
>   *private grounds*
>   *quarry*

E CODES

(i) A **motor vehicle** is any mechanically or electrically powered device, not operated on rails, upon which any person or property may be transported or drawn upon a highway. Any object such as a trailer, coaster, sled, or wagon being towed by a motor vehicle is considerd a part of the motor vehicle.

> INCLUDES
> automobile [any type]
> bus
> construction machinery, farm and industrial machinery, steam roller, tractor, army tank, highway grader, or similar vehicle on wheels or treads, while in transport under own power
> fire engine (motorized)
> motorcycle
> motorized bicycle [moped] or scooter
> trolley bus not operating on rails
> truck
> van

> EXCLUDES
> *devices used solely to move persons or materials within the confines of a building and its premises, such as:*
> *building elevator*
> *coal car in mine*
> *electric baggage or mail truck used solely within a railroad station*
> *electric truck used solely within an industrial plant*
> *moving overhead crane*

(j) A **motorcycle** is a two-wheeled motor vehicle having one or two riding saddles and sometimes having a third wheel for the support of a sidecar. The sidecar is considered part of the motorcycle.

> INCLUDES
> motorized:
>   bicycle [moped]
>   scooter
>   tricycle

(k) An **off-road motor vehicle** is a motor vehicle of special design, to enable it to negotiate rough or soft terrain or snow. Examples of special design are high construction, special wheels and tires, driven by treads, or support on a cushion of air.

> INCLUDES
> all terrain vehicle [ATV]
> army tank
> hovercraft, on land or swamp
> snowmobile

(l) A **driver** of a motor vehicle is the occupant of the motor vehicle operating it or intending to operate it. A **motorcyclist** is the driver of a motorcycle. Other authorized occupants of a motor vehicle are **passengers**.

(m) An **other road vehicle** is any device, except a motor vehicle, in, on, or by which any person or property may be transported on a highway.

> INCLUDES
> animal carrying a person or goods
> animal-drawn vehicles
> animal harnessed to conveyance
> bicycle [pedal cycle]
> streetcar
> tricycle (pedal)

> EXCLUDES
> *pedestrian conveyance [definition (q)]*

(n) A **streetcar** is a device designed and used primarily for transporting persons within a municipality, running on rails, usually subject to normal traffic control signals, and operated principally on a right-of-way that forms part of the traffic way. A trailer being towed by a streetcar is considered a part of the streetcar.

> INCLUDES
> interurban or intraurban electric or streetcar, when specified to be operating on a street or public highway
> tram (car)
> trolley (car)

(o) A **pedal cycle** is any road transport vehicle operated solely by pedals.

> INCLUDES bicycle
> pedal cycle
> tricycle
>
> EXCLUDES motorized bicycle [definition (i)]

(p) A **pedal cyclist** is any person riding on a pedal cycle or in a sidecar attached to such a vehicle.

(q) A **pedestrian conveyance** is any human powered device by which a pedestrian may move other than by walking or by which a walking person may move another pedestrian.

> INCLUDES baby carriage
> coaster wagon
> ice skates
> perambulator
> pushcart
> pushchair
> roller skates
> scooter
> skateboard
> skis
> sled
> wheelchair

(r) A **pedestrian** is any person involved in an accident who was not at the time of the accident riding in or on a motor vehicle, railroad train, streetcar, animal-drawn or other vehicle, or on a bicycle or animal.

> INCLUDES person:
> changing tire of vehicle
> in or operating a pedestrian conveyance
> making adjustment to motor of vehicle
> on foot

(s) A **watercraft** is any device for transporting passengers or goods on the water.

(t) A **small boat** is any watercraft propelled by paddle, oars, or small motor, with a passenger capacity of less than ten.

> INCLUDES boat NOS
> canoe
> coble
> dinghy
> punt
> raft
> rowboat
> rowing shell
> scull
> skiff
> small motorboat
>
> EXCLUDES barge
> lifeboat (used after abandoning ship)
> raft (anchored) being used as a diving platform
> yacht

(u) An **aircraft** is any device for transporting passengers or goods in the air.

> INCLUDES airplane [any type]
> balloon
> bomber
> dirigible
> glider (hang)
> military aircraft
> parachute

(v) A **commercial transport aircraft** is any device for collective passenger or freight transportation by air, whether run on commercial lines for profit or by government authorities, with the exception of military craft.

E CODES

RAILWAY ACCIDENTS (E800-E807)

Note: For definitions of railway accident and related terms see definitions (a) to (d).

EXCLUDES accidents involving railway train and:
- aircraft (E840.0-E845.9)
- motor vehicle (E810.0-E825.9)
- watercraft (E830.0-E838.9)

The following fourth-digit subdivisions are for use with categories E800-E807 to identify the injured person:

.0 Railway employee
Any person who by virtue of his employment in connection with a railway, whether by the railway company or not, is at increased risk of involvement in a railway accident, such as:
- catering staff of train
- driver
- guard
- porter
- postal staff on train
- railway fireman
- shunter
- sleeping car attendant

.1 Passenger on railway
Any authorized person traveling on a train, except a railway employee.

EXCLUDES
- intending passenger waiting at station (.8)
- unauthorized rider on railway vehicle (.8)

.2 Pedestrian
See definition (r)

.3 Pedal cyclist
See definition (p)

.8 Other specified person
- Intending passenger or bystander waiting at station
- Unauthorized rider on railway vehicle

.9 Unspecified person

§ ✓4ᵗʰ **E800 Railway accident involving collision with rolling stock**
INCLUDES
- collision between railway trains or railway vehicles, any kind
- collision NOS on railway
- derailment with antecedent collision with rolling stock or NOS

§ ✓4ᵗʰ **E801 Railway accident involving collision with other object**
INCLUDES collision of railway train with:
- buffers
- fallen tree on railway
- gates
- platform
- rock on railway
- streetcar
- other nonmotor vehicle
- other object

EXCLUDES collision with:
- aircraft (E840.0-E842.9)
- motor vehicle (E810.0-E810.9, E820.0-E822.9)

§ ✓4ᵗʰ **E802 Railway accident involving derailment without antecedent collision**

§ ✓4ᵗʰ **E803 Railway accident involving explosion, fire, or burning**
EXCLUDES
- explosion or fire, with antecedent derailment (E802.0-E802.9)
- explosion or fire, with mention of antecedent collision (E800.0-E801.9)

§ ✓4ᵗʰ **E804 Fall in, on, or from railway train**
INCLUDES fall while alighting from or boarding railway train
EXCLUDES fall related to collision, derailment, or explosion of railway train (E800.0-E803.9)

§ Requires fourth digit. See beginning of Section E800-E807 for options.

✓4ᵗʰ Fourth-digit Required ▶◀ Revised Text ● New Code ▲ Revised Code Title

§ ☑4ᵗʰ **E805 Hit by rolling stock**

　　INCLUDES:　crushed
　　　　　　　injured
　　　　　　　killed　　　　　} by railway train or part
　　　　　　　knocked down
　　　　　　　run over

　　EXCLUDES:　*pedestrian hit by object set in motion by railway train (E806.0-E806.9)*

§ ☑4ᵗʰ **E806 Other specified railway accident**

　　INCLUDES:　hit by object falling in railway train
　　　　　　　injured by door or window on railway train
　　　　　　　nonmotor road vehicle or pedestrian hit by object set in motion by railway train
　　　　　　　railway train hit by falling:
　　　　　　　　　earth NOS
　　　　　　　　　rock
　　　　　　　　　tree
　　　　　　　　　other object

　　EXCLUDES:　*railway accident due to cataclysm (E908-E909)*

§ ☑4ᵗʰ **E807 Railway accident of unspecified nature**

　　INCLUDES:　found dead　} on railway right-of-way
　　　　　　　injured　　　　 NOS
　　　　　　　railway accident NOS

MOTOR VEHICLE TRAFFIC ACCIDENTS (E810-E819)

Note: For definitions of motor vehicle traffic accident, and related terms, see definitions (e) to (k).

　　EXCLUDES:　*accidents involving motor vehicle and aircraft (E840.0-E845.9)*

The following fourth-digit subdivisions are for use with categories E810-E819 to identify the injured person:

.0 Driver of motor vehicle other than motorcycle
　　See definition (1)

.1 Passenger in motor vehicle other than motorcycle
　　See definition (1)

.2 Motorcyclist
　　See definition (1)

.3 Passenger on motorcycle
　　See definition (1)

.4 Occupant of streetcar

.5 Rider of animal; occupant of animal-drawn vehicle

.6 Pedal cyclist
　　See definition (p)

.7 Pedestrian
　　See definition (r)

.8 Other specified person
　　Occupant of vehicle other than above
　　Person in railway train involved in accident
　　Unauthorized rider of motor vehicle

.9 Unspecified person

§§ ☑4ᵗʰ **E810 Motor vehicle traffic accident involving collision with train**

　　EXCLUDES:　*motor vehicle collision with object set in motion by railway train (E815.0-E815.9)*
　　　　　　　　railway train hit by object set in motion by motor vehicle (E818.0-E818.9)

§ Requires fourth digit. See beginning of Section E800-E807 for options.
§§ Requires fourth digit. See beginning of Section E810-E819 for options.

§ ✓4ᵗʰ **E811 Motor vehicle traffic accident involving re-entrant collision with another motor vehicle**
>   INCLUDES collision between motor vehicle which accidentally leaves the roadway then re-enters the same roadway, or the opposite roadway on a divided highway, and another motor vehicle
>   EXCLUDES collision on the same roadway when none of the motor vehicles involved have left and re-entered the highway (E812.0-E812.9)

§ ✓4ᵗʰ **E812 Other motor vehicle traffic accident involving collision with motor vehicle**
>   INCLUDES collision with another motor vehicle parked, stopped, stalled, disabled, or abandoned on the highway
>   motor vehicle collision NOS
>   EXCLUDES collision with object set in motion by another motor vehicle (E815.0-E815.9)
>   re-entrant collision with another motor vehicle (E811.0-E811.9)

§ ✓4ᵗʰ **E813 Motor vehicle traffic accident involving collision with other vehicle**
>   INCLUDES collision between motor vehicle, any kind, and:
>   other road (nonmotor transport) vehicle, such as:
>   animal carrying a person
>   animal-drawn vehicle
>   pedal cycle
>   streetcar
>   EXCLUDES collision with:
>   object set in motion by nonmotor road vehicle (E815.0-E815.9)
>   pedestrian (E814.0-E814.9)
>   nonmotor road vehicle hit by object set in motion by motor vehicle (E818.0-E818.9)

§ ✓4ᵗʰ **E814 Motor vehicle traffic accident involving collision with pedestrian**
>   INCLUDES collision between motor vehicle, any kind, and pedestrian
>   pedestrian dragged, hit, or run over by motor vehicle, any kind
>   EXCLUDES pedestrian hit by object set in motion by motor vehicle (E818.0-E818.9)

§ ✓4ᵗʰ **E815 Other motor vehicle traffic accident involving collision on the highway**
>   INCLUDES collision (due to loss of control) (on highway) between motor vehicle, any kind, and:
>   abutment (bridge) (overpass)
>   animal (herded) (unattended)
>   fallen stone, traffic sign, tree, utility pole
>   guard rail or boundary fence
>   interhighway divider
>   landslide (not moving)
>   object set in motion by railway train or road vehicle (motor) (nonmotor)
>   object thrown in front of motor vehicle
>   other object, fixed, movable, or moving
>   safety island
>   temporary traffic sign or marker
>   wall of cut made for road
>   EXCLUDES collision with:
>   any object off the highway (resulting from loss of control) (E816.0-E816.9)
>   any object which normally would have been off the highway and is not stated to have been on it (E816.0-E816.9)
>   motor vehicle parked, stopped, stalled, disabled, or abandoned on highway (E812.0-E812.9)
>   moving landslide (E909)
>   motor vehicle hit by object:
>   set in motion by railway train or road vehicle (motor) (nonmotor) (E818.0-E818.9)
>   thrown into or on vehicle (E818.0-E818.9)

§ Requires fourth digit. See beginning of Section E810-E819 for options.

§ ✓4ᵗʰ **E816 Motor vehicle traffic accident due to loss of control, without collision on the highway**

INCLUDES motor vehicle:
- failing to make curve
- going out of control (due to):
  - blowout
  - burst tire
  - driver falling asleep
  - driver inattention
  - excessive speed
  - failure of mechanical part

and:
- coliding with object off the highway
- overturning
- stopping abruptly off the highway

EXCLUDES collision on highway following loss of control (E810.0-E815.9)
loss of control of motor vehicle following collision on the highway (E810.0-E815.9)

§ ✓4ᵗʰ **E817 Noncollision motor vehicle traffic accident while boarding or alighting**

INCLUDES
- fall down stairs of motor bus
- fall from car in street
- injured by moving part of the vehicle
- trapped by door of motor bus

while boarding or alighting

§ ✓4ᵗʰ **E818 Other noncollision motor vehicle traffic accident**

INCLUDES
- accidental poisoning from exhaust gas generated by
- breakage of any part of
- explosion of any part of
- fall, jump, or being accidentally pushed from
- fire starting in
- hit by object thrown into or on
- injured by being thrown against some part of, or object in
- injury from moving part of
- object falling in or on
- object thrown on

motor vehicle while in motion

- collision of railway train or road vehicle except motor vehicle, with object set in motion by motor vehicle
- motor vehicle hit by object set in motion by railway train or road vehicle (motor) (nonmotor)
- pedestrian, railway train, or road vehicle (motor) (nonmotor) hit by object set in motion by motor vehicle

EXCLUDES collision between motor vehicle and:
- object set in motion by railway train or road vehicle (motor) (nonmotor) (E815.0-E815.9)
- object thrown towards the motor vehicle (E815.0-E815.9)
- person overcome by carbon monoxide generated by stationary motor vehicle off the roadway with motor running (E868.2)

§ ✓4ᵗʰ **E819 Motor vehicle traffic accident of unspecified nature**

INCLUDES
- motor vehicle traffic accident NOS
- traffic accident NOS

§ Requires fourth digit. See beginning of Section E810-E819 for options.

E CODES

MOTOR VEHICLE NONTRAFFIC ACCIDENTS (E820-E825)

Note: For definitions of motor vehicle nontraffic accident and related terms see definition (a) to (k).

INCLUDES accidents involving motor vehicles being used in recreational or sporting activities off the highway
collision and noncollision motor vehicle accidents occurring entirely off the highway

EXCLUDES accidents involving motor vehicle and:
aircraft (E840.0-E845.9)
watercraft (E830.0-E838.9)
accidents, not on the public highway, involving agricultural and construction machinery but not involving another motor vehicle (E919.0, E919.2, E919.7)

The following fourth-digit subdivisions are for use with categories E820-E825 to identify the injured person:

.0 Driver of motor vehicle other than motorcycle
See definition (l)
.1 Passenger in motor vehicle other than motorcycle
See definition (l)
.2 Motorcyclist
See definition (l)
.3 Passenger on motorcycle
See definition (l)
.4 Occupant of streetcar
.5 Rider of animal; occupant of animal-drawn vehicle
.6 Pedal cyclist
See definition (p)
.7 Pedestrian
See definition (r)
.8 Other specified person
Occupant of vehicle other than above
Person on railway train involved in accident
Unauthorized rider of motor vehicle
.9 Unspecified person

§ ✓4ᵗʰ **E820 Nontraffic accident involving motor-driven snow vehicle**

INCLUDES breakage of part of
fall from
hit by   } motor-driven snow vehicle (not on
overturning of   public highway)
run over or dragged by

collision of motor-driven snow vehicle with:
animal (being ridden) (-drawn vehicle)
another off-road motor vehicle
other motor vehicle, not on public highway
railway train
other object, fixed or movable
injury caused by rough landing of motor-driven snow vehicle (after leaving ground on rough terrain)

EXCLUDES accident on the public highway involving motor driven snow vehicle (E810.0-E819.9)

§ Requires fourth digit. See beginning of Section E820-E825 for options.

✓4ᵗʰ Fourth-digit Required   ▶◀ Revised Text   ● New Code   ▲ Revised Code Title

§ ✓4ᵗʰ **E821 Nontraffic accident involving other off-road motor vehicle**

INCLUDES:
- breakage of part of
- fall from
- hit by
- overturning of
- run over or dragged by
- thrown against some part of or object in

} off-road motor vehicle, except snow vehicle (not on public highway)

collision with:
- animal (being ridden) (-drawn vehicle)
- another off-road motor vehicle, except snow vehicle
- other motor vehicle, not on public highway
- other object, fixed or movable

EXCLUDES:
- accident on public highway involving off-road motor vehicle (E810.0-E819.9)
- collision between motor driven snow vehicle and other off-road motor vehicle (E820.0-E820.9)
- hovercraft accident on water (E830.0-E838.9)

§ ✓4ᵗʰ **E822 Other motor vehicle nontraffic accident involving collision with moving object**

INCLUDES: collision, not on public highway, between motor vehicle, except off-road motor vehicle and:
- animal
- nonmotor vehicle
- other motor vehicle, except off-road motor vehicle
- pedestrian
- railway train
- other moving object

EXCLUDES: collision with:
- motor-driven snow vehicle (E820.0-E820.9)
- other off-road motor vehicle (E821.0-E821.9)

§ ✓4ᵗʰ **E823 Other motor vehicle nontraffic accident involving collision with stationary object**

INCLUDES: collision, not on public highway, between motor vehicle, except off-road motor vehicle, and any object, fixed or movable, but not in motion

§ ✓4ᵗʰ **E824 Other motor vehicle nontraffic accident while boarding and alighting**

INCLUDES:
- fall
- injury from moving part of motor vehicle
- trapped by door of motor vehicle

} while boarding or alighting from motor vehicle, except off-road motor vehicle, not on public highway

§ ✓4ᵗʰ **E825 Other motor vehicle nontraffic accident of other and unspecified nature**

INCLUDES:
- accidental poisoning from carbon monoxide generated by
- breakage of any part of
- explosion of any part of
- fall, jump, or being accidentally pushed from
- fire starting in
- hit by object thrown into, towards, or on
- injured by being thrown against some part of, or object in
- injury from moving part of
- object falling in or on

} motor vehicle while in motion, not on public highway

motor vehicle nontraffic accident NOS

EXCLUDES:
- fall from or in stationary motor vehicle (E884.9, E885.9)
- overcome by carbon monoxide or exhaust gas generated by stationary motor vehicle off the roadway with motor running (E868.2)
- struck by falling object from or in stationary motor vehicle (E916)

§ Requires fourth digit. See beginning of Section E820-E825 for options.

✓4ᵗʰ Fourth-digit Required ▶◀ Revised Text ● New Code ▲ Revised Code Title

E CODES

OTHER ROAD VEHICLE ACCIDENTS (E826-E829)

Note: Other road vehicle accidents are transport accidents involving road vehicles other than motor vehicles. For definitions of other road vehicle and related terms see definitions (m) to (o).

INCLUDES accidents involving other road vehicles being used in recreational or sporting activities

EXCLUDES collision of other road vehicle [any] with:
  aircraft (E840.0-E845.9)
  motor vehicle (E813.0-E813.9, E820.0-E822.9)
  railway train (E801.0-E801.9)

The following fourth-digit subdivisions are for use with categories E826-E829 to identify the injured person.

.0 **Pedestrian**
  See definition (r)
.1 **Pedal cyclist**
  See definition (p)
.2 **Rider of animal**
.3 **Occupant of animal-drawn vehicle**
.4 **Occupant of streetcar**
.8 **Other specified person**
.9 **Unspecified person**

§ ✓4ᵗʰ **E826 Pedal cycle accident**

[0-9] **INCLUDES** breakage of any part of pedal cycle
  collision between pedal cycle and:
    animal (being ridden) (herded) (unattended)
    another pedal cycle
    any pedestrian
    nonmotor road vehicle
    other object, fixed, movable, or moving, not set in motion by motor vehicle, railway train, or aircraft
  entanglement in wheel of pedal cycle
  fall from pedal cycle
  hit by object falling or thrown on the pedal cycle
  pedal cycle accident NOS
  pedal cycle overturned

§ ✓4ᵗʰ **E827 Animal-drawn vehicle accident**

[0,2-4,8,9] **INCLUDES** breakage of any part of vehicle
  collision between animal-drawn vehicle and:
    animal (being ridden) (herded) (unattended)
    nonmotor road vehicle, except pedal cycle
    pedestrian, pedestrian conveyance, or pedestrian vehicle
    other object, fixed, movable, or moving, not set in motion by motor vehicle, railway train, or aircraft
  fall from ⎫
  knocked down by ⎬ animal-drawn
  overturning of ⎬ vehicle
  run over by ⎬
  thrown from ⎭

EXCLUDES collision of animal-drawn vehicle with pedal cycle (E826.0-E826.9)

§ Requires fourth digit. See beginning of Section E826-E829 for options.

✓4ᵗʰ Fourth-digit Required   ▶◀ Revised Text   ● New Code   ▲ Revised Code Title

2002 Ingenix, Inc.   E Codes—11

E828–E829   E CODES

§ ✓4th **E828 Accident involving animal being ridden**
[0,2,4,8,9]

INCLUDES:
   collision between animal being ridden and:
      another animal
      nonmotor road vehicle, except pedal cycle, and animal-drawn vehicle
      pedestrian, pedestrian conveyance, or pedestrian vehicle
      other object, fixed, movable, or moving, not set in motion by motor vehicle, railway train, or aircraft
   fall from ⎫
   knocked down by ⎬ animal being ridden
   thrown from ⎪
   trampled by ⎭
   ridden animal stumbled and fell

EXCLUDES:
   collision of animal being ridden with:
      animal-drawn vehicle (E827.0-E827.9)
      pedal cycle (E826.0-E826.9)

§ ✓4th **E829 Other road vehicle accidents**
[0,4,8,9]

INCLUDES:
   accident while boarding or alighting from ⎫
   blow from object in ⎪ streetcar
   breakage of any part of ⎬ nonmotor road vehicle
   caught in door of- ⎪ not classifiable
   derailment of ⎪ to E826-E828
   fall in, on, or from ⎪
   fire in ⎭

   collision between streetcar or nonmotor road vehicle, except as in E826-E828, and:
      animal (not being ridden)
      another nonmotor road vehicle not classifiable to E826-E828
      pedestrian
      other object, fixed, movable, or moving, not set in motion by motor vehicle, railway train, or aircraft
   nonmotor road vehicle accident NOS
   streetcar accident NOS

EXCLUDES:
   collision with:
      animal being ridden (E828.0-E828.9)
      animal-drawn vehicle (E827.0-E827.9)
      pedal cycle (E826.0-E826.9)

§ Requires fourth digit. See beginning of Section E826-E829 for options.

✓4th Fourth-digit Required ▶◀ Revised Text ● New Code ▲ Revised Code Title

E CODES

WATER TRANSPORT ACCIDENTS (E830-E838)

Note: For definitions of water transport accident and related terms see definitions (a), (s), and (t).

INCLUDES watercraft accidents in the course of recreational activities

EXCLUDES accidents involving both aircraft, including objects set in motion by aircraft, and watercraft (E840.0-E845.9)

The following fourth-digit subdivisions are for use with categories E830-E838 to identify the injured person:

.0 Occupant of small boat, unpowered
.1 Occupant of small boat, powered
  See definition (t)
  EXCLUDES water skier (.4)
.2 Occupant of other watercraft — crew
  Persons:
    engaged in operation of watercraft
    providing passenger services [cabin attendants, ship's physician, catering personnel]
    working on ship during voyage in other capacity [musician in band, operators of shops and beauty parlors]
.3 Occupant of other watercraft — other than crew
  Passenger
  Occupant of lifeboat, other than crew, after abandoning ship
.4 Water skier
.5 Swimmer
.6 Dockers, stevedores
  Longshoreman employed on the dock in loading and unloading ships
.8 Other specified person
  Immigration and custom officials on board ship
  Person:
    accompanying passenger or member of crew visiting boat
  Pilot (guiding ship into port)
.9 Unspecified person

§ ✓4th **E830 Accident to watercraft causing submersion**

  INCLUDES submersion and drowning due to:
    boat overturning
    boat submerging
    falling or jumping from burning ship
    falling or jumping from crushed watercraft
    ship sinking
    other accident to watercraft

§ ✓4th **E831 Accident to watercraft causing other injury**

  INCLUDES any injury, except submersion and drowning, as a result of an accident to watercraft
    burned while ship on fire
    crushed between ships in collision
    crushed by lifeboat after abandoning ship
    fall due to collision or other accident to watercraft
    hit by falling object due to accident to watercraft
    injured in watercraft accident involving collision
    struck by boat or part thereof after fall or jump from damaged boat
  EXCLUDES burns from localized fire or explosion on board ship (E837.0-E837.9)

---

§ Requires fourth digit. See beginning of Section E830-E838 for options.

✓4th Fourth-digit Required   ▶◀ Revised Text   ● New Code   ▲ Revised Code Title

2002 Ingenix, Inc.   E Codes—13

§ ✓4th **E832 Other accidental submersion or drowning in water transport accident**

INCLUDES: submersion or drowning as a result of an accident other than accident to the watercraft, such as:
fall:
  from gangplank
  from ship
  overboard
thrown overboard by motion of ship
washed overboard

EXCLUDES: submersion or drowning of swimmer or diver who voluntarily jumps from boat not involved in an accident (E910.0-E910.9)

§ ✓4th **E833 Fall on stairs or ladders in water transport**

EXCLUDES: fall due to accident to watercraft (E831.0-E831.9)

§ ✓4th **E834 Other fall from one level to another in water transport**

EXCLUDES: fall due to accident to watercraft (E831.0-E831.9)

§ ✓4th **E835 Other and unspecified fall in water transport**

EXCLUDES: fall due to accident to watercraft (E831.0-E831.9)

§ ✓4th **E836 Machinery accident in water transport**

INCLUDES: injuries in water transport caused by:
  deck
  engine room
  galley   } machinery
  laundry
  loading

§ ✓4th **E837 Explosion, fire, or burning in watercraft**

INCLUDES: explosion of boiler on steamship
localized fire on ship

EXCLUDES: burning ship (due to collision or explosion) resulting in:
  submersion or drowning (E830.0-E830.9)
  other injury (E831.0-E831.9)

§ ✓4th **E838 Other and unspecified water transport accident**

INCLUDES: accidental poisoning by gases or fumes on ship
atomic power plant malfunction in watercraft
crushed between ship and stationary object [wharf]
crushed between ships without accident to watercraft
crushed by falling object on ship or while loading or unloading
hit by boat while water skiing
struck by boat or part thereof (after fall from boat)
watercraft accident NOS

AIR AND SPACE TRANSPORT ACCIDENTS (E840-E845)

Note: For definition of aircraft and related terms see definitions (u) and (v).

The following fourth-digit subdivisions are for use with categories E840-E845 to identify the injured person. Valid fourth digits are in [brackets] under codes E842-E845.

.0 Occupant of spacecraft
.1 Occupant of military aircraft, any
  Crew in military aircraft [air force] [army] [national guard] [navy]
  Passenger (civilian) (military) in military aircraft [air force] [army] [national guard] [navy]
  Troops in military aircraft [air force] [army] [national guard] [navy]

EXCLUDES: occupants of aircraft operated under jurisdiction of police departments (.5)
parachutist (.7)

.2 Crew of commercial aircraft (powered) in surface to surface transport

§ Requires fourth digit. See beginning of Section E830-E838 for options.

E CODES

.3 **Other occupant of commercial aircraft (powered) in surface to surface transport**
    Flight personnel:
        not part of crew
        on familiarization flight
    Passenger on aircraft (powered) NOS

.4 **Occupant of commercial aircraft (powered) in surface to air transport**
    Occupant [crew] [passenger] of aircraft (powered) engaged in activities, such as:
        aerial spraying (crops) (fire retardants)
        air drops of emergency supplies
        air drops of parachutists, except from military craft
        crop dusting
        lowering of construction material [bridge or telephone pole]
        sky writing

.5 **Occupant of other powered aircraft**
    Occupant [crew][passenger] of aircraft [powered] engaged in activities, such as:
        aerobatic flying
        aircraft racing
        rescue operation
        storm surveillance
        traffic surveillance
    Occupant of private plane NOS

.6 **Occupant of unpowered aircraft, except parachutist**
    Occupant of aircraft classifiable to E842

.7 **Parachutist (military) (other)**
    Person making voluntary descent
        EXCLUDES *person making descent after accident to aircraft (.1-.6)*

.8 **Ground crew, airline employee**
    Persons employed at airfields (civil) (military) or launching pads, not occupants of aircraft

.9 **Other person**

§ ✓4th **E840 Accident to powered aircraft at takeoff or landing**
    INCLUDES   collision of aircraft with any object, fixed, movable, or moving
                      crash
                      explosion on aircraft } while taking off or landing
                      fire on aircraft
                      forced landing

§ ✓4th **E841 Accident to powered aircraft, other and unspecified**
    INCLUDES   aircraft accident NOS
                      aircraft crash or wreck NOS
                      any accident to powered aircraft while in transit or when not specified whether in transit, taking off, or landing
                      collision of aircraft with another aircraft, bird, or any object, while in transit
                      explosion on aircraft while in transit
                      fire on aircraft while in transit

§ ✓4th **E842 Accident to unpowered aircraft**
    [6-9]   INCLUDES   any accident, except collision with powered aircraft, to:
                                balloon
                                glider
                                hang glider
                                kite carrying a person
                      hit by object falling from unpowered aircraft

§ Requires fourth digit. See beginning of Section E840-E845 for options.

✓4th Fourth-digit Required   ▶◀ Revised Text   ● New Code   ▲ Revised Code Title

§ ✓4ᵗʰ **E843 Fall in, on, or from aircraft**
[0-9] INCLUDES accident in boarding or alighting from aircraft, any kind
fall in, on, or from aircraft [any kind], while in transit, taking off, or landing, except when as a result of an accident to aircraft

§ ✓4ᵗʰ **E844 Other specified air transport accidents**
[0-9] INCLUDES hit by:
    aircraft
    object falling from aircraft
injury by or from:
    machinery on aircraft
    rotating propeller
    voluntary parachute descent
poisoning by carbon monoxide from aircraft while in transit
sucked into jet
} without accident to aircraft

any accident involving other transport vehicle (motor) (nonmotor) due to being hit by object set in motion by aircraft (powered)

EXCLUDES air sickness (E903)
effects of:
    high altitude (E902.0-E902.1)
    pressure change (E902.0-E902.1)
injury in parachute descent due to accident to aircraft (E840.0-E842.9)

§ ✓4ᵗʰ **E845 Accident involving spacecraft**
[0,8,9] INCLUDES launching pad accident
EXCLUDES effects of weightlessness in spacecraft (E928.0)

VEHICLE ACCIDENTS NOT ELSEWHERE CLASSIFIABLE (E846-E848)

E846 Accidents involving powered vehicles used solely within the buildings and premises of industrial or commercial establishment

Accident to, on, or involving:
    battery powered airport passenger vehicle
    battery powered trucks (baggage) (mail)
    coal car in mine
    logging car
    self propelled truck, industrial
    station baggage truck (powered)
    tram, truck, or tub (powered) in mine or quarry
Collision with:
    pedestrian
    other vehicle or object within premises
Explosion of
Fall from
Overturning of
Struck by
} powered vehicle, industrial or commercial

EXCLUDES accidental poisoning by exhaust gas from vehicle not elsewhere classifiable (E868.2)
injury by crane, lift (fork), or elevator (E919.2)

§ Requires fourth digit. See beginning of Section E840-E845 for options.

E CODES

E847 Accidents involving cable cars not running on rails
Accident to, on, or involving:
- cable car, not on rails
- ski chair-lift
- ski-lift with gondola
- téléférique

Breakage of cable
Caught or dragged by }
Fall or jump from } cable car, not on rails
Object thrown from or in }

E848 Accidents involving other vehicles, not elsewhere classifiable
Accident to, on, or involving:
- ice yacht
- land yacht
- nonmotor, nonroad vehicle NOS

✓4ᵗʰ E849 Place of occurrence
The following category is for use to denote the place where the injury or poisoning occurred.

E849.0 Home
- Apartment
- Boarding house
- Farm house
- Home premises
- House (residential)
- Noninstitutional place of residence
- Private:
  - driveway
- Private:
  - garage
  - garden
  - home
  - walk
- Swimming pool in private house or garden
- Yard of home

EXCLUDES home under construction but not yet occupied (E849.3)
institutional place of residence (E849.7)

E849.1 Farm
Farm:
- buildings
- land under cultivation

EXCLUDES farm house and home premises of farm (E849.0)

E849.2 Mine and quarry
- Gravel pit
- Sand pit
- Tunnel under construction

E849.3 Industrial place and premises
- Building under construction
- Dockyard
- Dry dock
- Factory
  - building
  - premises
- Garage (place of work)
- Industrial yard
- Loading platform (factory) (store)
- Plant, industrial
- Railway yard
- Shop (place of work)
- Warehouse
- Workhouse

E849.4 Place for recreation and sport

Amusement park	Public park
Baseball field	Racecourse
Basketball court	Resort NOS
Beach resort	Riding school
Cricket ground	Rifle range
Fives court	Seashore resort
Football field	Skating rink
Golf course	Sports palace
Gymnasium	Stadium
Hockey field	Swimming pool, public
Holiday camp	Tennis court
Ice palace	Vacation resort
Lake resort	
Mountain resort	
Playground, including school playground	

EXCLUDES that in private house or garden (E849.0)

E849.5 Street and highway

E849.6 Public building

Building (including adjacent grounds) used by the general public or by a particular group of the public, such as:

airport	music hall
bank	nightclub
café	office
casino	office building
church	opera house
cinema	post office
clubhouse	public hall
courthouse	radio broadcasting station
dance hall	restaurant
garage building (for car storage)	school (state) (public) (private)
hotel	shop, commercial
market (grocery or other commodity)	station (bus) (railway) store
movie house	theater

EXCLUDES home garage (E849.0)
industrial building or workplace (E849.3)

E849.7 Residential institution

Children's home	Old people's home
Dormitory	Orphanage
Hospital	Prison
Jail	Reform school

E849.8 Other specified places

Beach NOS	Pond or pool (natural)
Canal	Prairie
Caravan site NOS	Public place NOS
Derelict house	Railway line
Desert	Reservoir
Dock	River
Forest	Sea
Harbor	Seashore NOS
Hill	Stream
Lake NOS	Swamp
Mountain	Trailer court
Parking lot	Woods
Parking place	

E849.9 Unspecified place

E CODES

ACCIDENTAL POISONING BY DRUGS, MEDICINAL SUBSTANCES, AND BIOLOGICALS (E850-E858)

INCLUDES accidental overdose of drug, wrong drug given or taken in error, and drug taken inadvertently
accidents in the use of drugs and biologicals in medical and surgical procedures

EXCLUDES *administration with suicidal or homicidal intent or intent to harm, or in circumstances classifiable to E980-E989 (E950.0-E950.5, E962.0, E980.0-E980.5)*
correct drug properly administered in therapeutic or prophylactic dosage, as the cause of adverse effect (E930.0-E949.9)

See Alphabetic Index for more complete list of specific drugs to be classified under the fourth-digit subdivisions. The American Hospital Formulary numbers can be used to classify new drugs listed by the American Hospital Formulary Service (AHFS). See Appendix C.

✓4th E850 Accidental poisoning by analgesics, antipyretics, and antirheumatics

E850.0 Heroin
Diacetylmorphine

E850.1 Methadone

E850.2 Other opiates and related narcotics
Codeine [methylmorphine]   Morphine
Meperidine [pethidine]   Opium (alkaloids)

E850.3 Salicylates
Acetylsalicylic acid [aspirin]
Amino derivatives of salicylic acid
Salicylic acid salts

E850.4 Aromatic analgesics, not elsewhere classified
Acetanilid
Paracetamol [acetaminophen]
Phenacetin [acetophenetidin]

E850.5 Pyrazole derivatives
Aminophenazone [amidopyrine]
Phenylbutazone

E850.6 Antirheumatics [antiphlogistics]
Gold salts
Indomethacin
EXCLUDES *salicylates (E850.3)*
steroids (E858.0)

E850.7 Other non-narcotic analgesics
Pyrabital

E850.8 Other specified analgesics and antipyretics
Pentazocine

E850.9 Unspecified analgesic or antipyretic

E851 Accidental poisoning by barbiturates
Amobarbital [amylobarbitone]
Barbital [barbitone]
Butabarbital [butabarbitone]
Pentobarbital [pentobarbitone]
Phenobarbital [phenobarbitone]
Secobarbital [quinalbarbitone]
EXCLUDES *thiobarbiturates (E855.1)*

✓4th E852 Accidental poisoning by other sedatives and hypnotics

E852.0 Chloral hydrate group

E852.1 Paraldehyde

E852.2 Bromine compounds
Bromides
Carbromal (derivatives)

✓4th Fourth-digit Required ▶◀ Revised Text ● New Code ▲ Revised Code Title

E852.3 Methaqualone compounds
E852.4 Glutethimide group
E852.5 Mixed sedatives, not elsewhere classified
E852.8 Other specified sedatives and hypnotics
E852.9 Unspecified sedative or hypnotic
> Sleeping:
>   drug ⎫
>   pill   ⎬ NOS
>   tablet ⎭

✓4ᵗʰ **E853 Accidental poisoning by tranquilizers**

    E853.0 Phenothiazine-based tranquilizers
        Chlorpromazine   Prochlorperazine
        Fluphenazine   Promazine

    E853.1 Butyrophenone-based tranquilizers
        Haloperidol   Trifluperidol
        Spiperone

    E853.2 Benzodiazepine-based tranquilizers
        Chlordiazepoxide   Lorazepam
        Diazepam   Medazepam
        Flurazepam   Nitrazepam

    E853.8 Other specified tranquilizers
        Hydroxyzine   Meprobamate

    E853.9 Unspecified tranquilizer

✓4ᵗʰ **E854 Accidental poisoning by other psychotropic agents**

    E854.0 Antidepressants
        Amitriptyline
        Imipramine
        Monoamine oxidase [MAO] inhibitors

    E854.1 Psychodysleptics [hallucinogens]
        Cannabis derivatives   Mescaline
        Lysergide [LSD]   Psilocin
        Marihuana (derivatives) Psilocybin

    E854.2 Psychostimulants
        Amphetamine   Caffeine
             EXCLUDES *central appetite depressants (E858.8)*

    E854.3 Central nervous system stimulants
        Analeptics   Opiate antagonists

    E854.8 Other psychotropic agents

✓4ᵗʰ **E855 Accidental poisoning by other drugs acting on central and autonomic nervous system**

    E855.0 Anticonvulsant and anti-Parkinsonism drugs
        Amantadine
        Hydantoin derivatives
        Levodopa [L-dopa]
        Oxazolidine derivatives [paramethadione] [trimethadione]
        Succinimides

    E855.1 Other central nervous system depressants
        Ether
        Gaseous anesthetics
        Halogenated hydrocarbon derivatives
        Intravenous anesthetics
        Thiobarbiturates, such as thiopental sodium

    E855.2 Local anesthetics
        Cocaine   Procaine
        Lidocaine [lignocaine] Tetracaine

E CODES

- **E855.3 Parasympathomimetics [cholinergics]**
  - Acetylcholine
  - Pilocarpine
  - Anticholinesterase:
    - organophosphorus
    - reversible
- **E855.4 Parasympatholytics [anticholinergics and antimuscarinics] and spasmolytics**
  - Atropine
  - Homatropine
  - Hyoscine [scopolamine]
  - Quaternary ammonium derivatives
- **E855.5 Sympathomimetics [adrenergics]**
  - Epinephrine [adrenalin]
  - Levarterenol [noradrenalin]
- **E855.6 Sympatholytics [antiadrenergics]**
  - Phenoxybenzamine
  - Tolazoline hydrochloride
- **E855.8 Other specified drugs acting on central and autonomic nervous systems**
- **E855.9 Unspecified drug acting on central and autonomic nervous systems**

E856 Accidental poisoning by antibiotics

E857 Accidental poisoning by other anti-infectives

✓4th **E858 Accidental poisoning by other drugs**
- **E858.0 Hormones and synthetic substitutes**
- **E858.1 Primarily systemic agents**
- **E858.2 Agents primarily affecting blood constituents**
- **E858.3 Agents primarily affecting cardiovascular system**
- **E858.4 Agents primarily affecting gastrointestinal system**
- **E858.5 Water, mineral, and uric acid metabolism drugs**
- **E858.6 Agents primarily acting on the smooth and skeletal muscles and respiratory system**
- **E858.7 Agents primarily affecting skin and mucous membrane, ophthalmological, otorhinolaryngological, and dental drugs**
- **E858.8 Other specified drugs**
  - Central appetite depressants
- **E858.9 Unspecified drug**

ACCIDENTAL POISONING BY OTHER SOLID AND LIQUID SUBSTANCES, GASES, AND VAPORS (E860-E869)

Note: Categories in this section are intended primarily to indicate the external cause of poisoning states classifiable to 980-989. They may also be used to indicate external causes of localized effects classifiable to 001-799.

✓4th **E860 Accidental poisoning by alcohol, not elsewhere classified**
- **E860.0 Alcoholic beverages**
  - Alcohol in preparations intended for consumption
- **E860.1 Other and unspecified ethyl alcohol and its products**
  - Denatured alcohol
  - Ethanol NOS
  - Grain alcohol NOS
  - Methylated spirit
- **E860.2 Methyl alcohol**
  - Methanol
  - Wood alcohol
- **E860.3 Isopropyl alcohol**
  - Dimethyl carbinol
  - Isopropanol
  - Rubbing alcohol subsitute
  - Secondary propyl alcohol
- **E860.4 Fusel oil**
  - Alcohol:
    - amyl
    - butyl
  - Alcohol:
    - propyl
- **E860.8 Other specified alcohols**
- **E860.9 Unspecified alcohol**

☑4ᵗʰ **E861 Accidental poisoning by cleansing and polishing agents, disinfectants, paints, and varnishes**

E861.0 Synthetic detergents and shampoos

E861.1 Soap products

E861.2 Polishes

E861.3 Other cleansing and polishing agents
Scouring powders

E861.4 Disinfectants
Household and other disinfectants not ordinarily used on the person
EXCLUDES *carbolic acid or phenol (E864.0)*

E861.5 Lead paints

E861.6 Other paints and varnishes
Lacquers   Paints, other than lead
Oil colors   White washes

E861.9 Unspecified

☑4ᵗʰ **E862 Accidental poisoning by petroleum products, other solvents and their vapors, not elsewhere classified**

E862.0 Petroleum solvents
Petroleum: Petroleum:
  ether   naphtha
  benzine

E862.1 Petroleum fuels and cleaners
Antiknock additives to petroleum fuels
Gas oils
Gasoline or petrol
Kerosene
EXCLUDES *kerosene insecticides (E863.4)*

E862.2 Lubricating oils

E862.3 Petroleum solids
Paraffin wax

E862.4 Other specified solvents
Benzene

E862.9 Unspecified solvent

☑4ᵗʰ **E863 Accidental poisoning by agricultural and horticultural chemical and pharmaceutical preparations other than plant foods and fertilizers**
EXCLUDES *plant foods and fertilizers (E866.5)*

E863.0 Insecticides of organochlorine compounds
Benzene hexachloride   Dieldrin
Chlordane   Endrine
DDT   Toxaphene

E863.1 Insecticides of organophosphorus compounds
Demeton   Parathion
Diazinon   Phenylsulphthion
Dichlorvos   Phorate
Malathion   Phosdrin
Methyl parathion

E863.2 Carbamates
Aldicarb   Propoxur
Carbaryl

E863.3 Mixtures of insecticides

E863.4 Other and unspecified insecticides
Kerosene insecticides

E CODES

E863.5 Herbicides
  2, 4-Dichlorophenoxyacetic acid [2, 4-D]
  2, 4, 5-Trichlorophenoxyacetic acid [2, 4, 5-T]
  Chlorates
  Diquat
  Mixtures of plant foods and fertilizers with herbicides
  Paraquat

E863.6 Fungicides
  Organic mercurials (used in seed dressing)
  Pentachlorophenols

E863.7 Rodenticides
  Fluoroacetates   Warfarin
  Squill and derivatives   Zinc phosphide
  Thallium

E863.8 Fumigants
  Cyanides   Phosphine
  Methyl bromide

E863.9 Other and unspecified

✓4th **E864 Accidental poisoning by corrosives and caustics, not elsewhere classified**
  EXCLUDES those as components of disinfectants (E861.4)

E864.0 Corrosive aromatics
  Carbolic acid or phenol

E864.1 Acids
  Acid:
    hydrochloric
    nitric
    sulfuric

E864.2 Caustic alkalis
  Lye

E864.3 Other specified corrosives and caustics

E864.4 Unspecified corrosives and caustics

✓4th **E865 Accidental poisoning from poisonous foodstuffs and poisonous plants**
  INCLUDES any meat, fish, or shellfish
    plants, berries, and fungi eaten as, or in mistake for, food, or by a child
  EXCLUDES anaphylactic shock due to adverse food reaction (995.60-995.69)
    food poisoning (bacterial) (005.0-005.9)
    poisoning and toxic reactions to venomous plants (E905.6-E905.7)

E865.0 Meat

E865.1 Shellfish

E865.2 Other fish

E865.3 Berries and seeds

E865.4 Other specified plants

E865.5 Mushrooms and other fungi

E865.8 Other specified foods

E865.9 Unspecified foodstuff or poisonous plant

✓4th **E866 Accidental poisoning by other and unspecified solid and liquid substances**
  EXCLUDES these substances as a component of:
    medicines (E850.0-E858.9)
    paints (E861.5-E861.6)
    pesticides (E863.0-E863.9)
    petroleum fuels (E862.1)

E866.0 Lead and its compounds and fumes

E866.1 Mercury and its compounds and fumes

E866.2 Antimony and its compounds and fumes

E866.3 Arsenic and its compounds and fumes

E866.4 Other metals and their compounds and fumes
- Beryllium (compounds)
- Brass fumes
- Cadmium (compounds)
- Copper salts
- Iron (compounds)
- Manganese (compounds)
- Nickel (compounds)
- Thallium (compounds)

E866.5 Plant foods and fertilizers
> **EXCLUDES** mixtures with herbicides (E863.5)

E866.6 Glues and adhesives

E866.7 Cosmetics

E866.8 Other specified solid or liquid substances

E866.9 Unspecified solid or liquid substance

E867 Accidental poisoning by gas distributed by pipeline
- Carbon monoxide from incomplete combustion of piped gas
- Coal gas NOS
- Liquefied petroleum gas distributed through pipes (pure or mixed with air)
- Piped gas (natural) (manufactured)

✓4th E868 Accidental poisoning by other utility gas and other carbon monoxide

E868.0 Liquefied petroleum gas distributed in mobile containers
- Butane
- Liquefied hydrocarbon gas NOS
- Propane

} or carbon monoxide from incomplete combustion of these gases

E868.1 Other and unspecified utility gas
- Acetylene
- Gas NOS used for lighting, heating, or cooking
- Water gas

} or carbon monoxide from incomplete combustion of these gases

E868.2 Motor vehicle exhaust gas

Exhaust gas from:
- farm tractor, not in transit
- gas engine
- motor pump
- motor vehicle, not in transit
- any type of combustion engine not in watercraft

> **EXCLUDES** poisoning by carbon monoxide from:
> aircraft while in transit (E844.0-E844.9)
> motor vehicle while in transit (E818.0-E818.9)
> watercraft whether or not in transit (E838.0-E838.9)

E868.3 Carbon monoxide from incomplete combustion of other domestic fuels

Carbon monoxide from incomplete combustion of:
- coal
- coke
- kerosene
- wood

} in domestic stove or fireplace

> **EXCLUDES** carbon monoxide from smoke and fumes due to conflagration (E890.0-E893.9)

E868.8 Carbon monoxide from other sources

Carbon monoxide from:
- blast furnace gas
- incomplete combustion of fuels in industrial use
- kiln vapor

E868.9 Unspecified carbon monoxide

✓4th E869 Accidental poisoning by other gases and vapors

> **EXCLUDES** effects of gases used as anesthetics (E855.1, E938.2)
> fumes from heavy metals (E866.0-E866.4)
> smoke and fumes due to conflagration or explosion (E890.0-E899)

E869.0 Nitrogen oxides

E CODES

E869.1 **Sulfur dioxide**
E869.2 **Freon**
E869.3 **Lacrimogenic gas [tear gas]**
    Bromobenzyl cyanide   Ethyliodoacetate
    Chloroacetophenone
E869.4 **Second-hand tobacco smoke**
E869.8 **Other specified gases and vapors**
    Chlorine   Hydrocyanic acid gas
E869.9 **Unspecified gases and vapors**

MISADVENTURES TO PATIENTS DURING SURGICAL AND MEDICAL CARE (E870-E876)

> **EXCLUDES**   accidental overdose of drug and wrong drug given in error (E850.0-E858.9)
> surgical and medical procedures as the cause of abnormal reaction by the patient, without mention of misadventure at the time of procedure (E878.0-E879.9)

✓4ᵗʰ **E870 Accidental cut, puncture, perforation, or hemorrhage during medical care**
  E870.0 **Surgical operation**
  E870.1 **Infusion or transfusion**
  E870.2 **Kidney dialysis or other perfusion**
  E870.3 **Injection or vaccination**
  E870.4 **Endoscopic examination**
  E870.5 **Aspiration of fluid or tissue, puncture, and catheterization**
      Abdominal paracentesis   Lumbar puncture
      Aspirating needle biopsy Thoracentesis
      Blood sampling
> **EXCLUDES**   heart catheterization (E870.6)

  E870.6 **Heart catheterization**
  E870.7 **Administration of enema**
  E870.8 **Other specified medical care**
  E870.9 **Unspecified medical care**

✓4ᵗʰ **E871 Foreign object left in body during procedure**
  E871.0 **Surgical operation**
  E871.1 **Infusion or transfusion**
  E871.2 **Kidney dialysis or other perfusion**
  E871.3 **Injection or vaccination**
  E871.4 **Endoscopic examination**
  E871.5 **Aspiration of fluid or tissue, puncture, and catheterization**
      Abdominal paracentesis Lumbar puncture
      Aspiration needle biopsy Thoracentesis
      Blood sampling
> **EXCLUDES**   heart catheterization (E871.6)

  E871.6 **Heart catheterization**
  E871.7 **Removal of catheter or packing**
  E871.8 **Other specified procedures**
  E871.9 **Unspecified procedure**

✓4ᵗʰ **E872 Failure of sterile precautions during procedure**
  E872.0 **Surgical operation**
  E872.1 **Infusion or transfusion**
  E872.2 **Kidney dialysis and other perfusion**
  E872.3 **Injection or vaccination**
  E872.4 **Endoscopic examination**

✓4ᵗʰ Fourth-digit Required   ▶◀ Revised Text   ● New Code   ▲ Revised Code Title

E872.5 Aspiration of fluid or tissue, puncture, and catheterization
  Abdominal paracentesis   Lumbar puncture
  Aspiration needle biopsy   Thoracentesis
  Blood sampling
  EXCLUDES *heart catheterization (E872.6)*

E872.6 Heart catheterization
E872.8 Other specified procedures
E872.9 Unspecified procedure

✓4th **E873 Failure in dosage**
  EXCLUDES *accidental overdose of drug, medicinal or biological substance (E850.0-E858.9)*

E873.0 Excessive amount of blood or other fluid during transfusion or infusion
E873.1 Incorrect dilution of fluid during infusion
E873.2 Overdose of radiation in therapy
E873.3 Inadvertent exposure of patient to radiation during medical care
E873.4 Failure in dosage in electroshock or insulin-shock therapy
E873.5 Inappropriate [too hot or too cold] temperature in local application and packing
E873.6 Nonadministration of necessary drug or medicinal substance
E873.8 Other specified failure in dosage
E873.9 Unspecified failure in dosage

✓4th **E874 Mechanical failure of instrument or apparatus during procedure**
  E874.0 Surgical operation
  E874.1 Infusion and transfusion
    Air in system
  E874.2 Kidney dialysis and other perfusion
  E874.3 Endoscopic examination
  E874.4 Aspiration of fluid or tissue, puncture, and catheterization
    Abdominal paracentesis   Lumbar puncture
    Aspiration needle biopsy   Thoracentesis
    Blood sampling
    EXCLUDES *heart catheterization (E874.5)*
  E874.5 Heart catheterization
  E874.8 Other specified procedures
  E874.9 Unspecified procedure

✓4th **E875 Contaminated or infected blood, other fluid, drug, or biological substance**
  INCLUDES presence of:
    bacterial pyrogens
    endotoxin-producing bacteria
    serum hepatitis-producing agent

  E875.0 Contaminated substance transfused or infused
  E875.1 Contaminated substance injected or used for vaccination
  E875.2 Contaminated drug or biological substance administered by other means
  E875.8 Other
  E875.9 Unspecified

✓4th **E876 Other and unspecified misadventures during medical care**
  E876.0 Mismatched blood in transfusion
  E876.1 Wrong fluid in infusion
  E876.2 Failure in suture and ligature during surgical operation
  E876.3 Endotracheal tube wrongly placed during anesthetic procedure
  E876.4 Failure to introduce or to remove other tube or instrument
    EXCLUDES *foreign object left in body during procedure (E871.0-E871.9)*
  E876.5 Performance of inappropriate operation

E CODES

E876.8 Other specified misadventures during medical care
  Performance of inappropriate treatment NEC
E876.9 Unspecified misadventure during medical care

SURGICAL AND MEDICAL PROCEDURES AS THE CAUSE OF ABNORMAL REACTION OF PATIENT OR LATER COMPLICATION, WITHOUT MENTION OF MISADVENTURE AT THE TIME OF PROCEDURE (E878-E879)

INCLUDES procedures as the cause of abnormal reaction, such as:
  displacement or malfunction of prosthetic device
  hepatorenal failure, postoperative
  malfunction of external stoma
  postoperative intestinal obstruction
  rejection of transplanted organ

EXCLUDES *anesthetic management properly carried out as the cause of adverse effect (E937.0-E938.9)*
  infusion and transfusion, without mention of misadventure in the technique of procedure (E930.0-E949.9)

✓4th **E878 Surgical operation and other surgical procedures as the cause of abnormal reaction of patient, or of later complication, without mention of misadventure at the time of operation**

  E878.0 Surgical operation with transplant of whole organ
    Transplantation of: Transplantation of:
      heart   liver
      kidney

  E878.1 Surgical operation with implant of artificial internal device
    Cardiac pacemaker   Heart valve prosthesis
    Electrodes implanted in   Internal orthopedic
      brain   device

  E878.2 Surgical operation with anastomosis, bypass, or graft, with natural or artificial tissues used as implant
    Anastomosis: Graft of blood vessel,
      arteriovenous   tendon, or skin
      gastrojejunal
    EXCLUDES *external stoma (E878.3)*

  E878.3 Surgical operation with formation of external stoma
    Colostomy   Gastrostomy
    Cystostomy   Ureterostomy
    Duodenostomy

  E878.4 Other restorative surgery
  E878.5 Amputation of limb(s)
  E878.6 Removal of other organ (partial) (total)
  E878.8 Other specified surgical operations and procedures
  E878.9 Unspecified surgical operations and procedures

✓4th **E879 Other procedures, without mention of misadventure at the time of procedure, as the cause of abnormal reaction of patient, or of later complication**

  E879.0 Cardiac catheterization
  E879.1 Kidney dialysis
  E879.2 Radiological procedure and radiotherapy
    EXCLUDES *radio-opaque dyes for diagnostic x-ray procedures (E947.8)*
  E879.3 Shock therapy
    Electroshock therapy
    Insulin-shock therapy
  E879.4 Aspiration of fluid
    Lumbar puncture
    Thoracentesis
  E879.5 Insertion of gastric or duodenal sound
  E879.6 Urinary catheterization

E879.7 Blood sampling
E879.8 Other specified procedures
  Blood transfusion
E879.9 Unspecified procedure

ACCIDENTAL FALLS (E880-E888)

EXCLUDES *falls (in or from):*
  burning building (E890.8, E891.8)
  into fire (E890.0-E899)
  into water (with submersion or drowning) (E910.0-E910.9)
  machinery (in operation) (E919.0-E919.9)
  on edged, pointed, or sharp object (E920.0-E920.9)
  transport vehicle (E800.0-E845.9)
  vehicle not elsewhere classifiable (E846-E848)

✓4ᵗʰ **E880 Fall on or from stairs or steps**
  E880.0 Escalator
  E880.1 Fall on or from sidewalk curb
    EXCLUDES *fall from moving sidewalk (E885.9)*
  E880.9 Other stairs or steps

✓4ᵗʰ **E881 Fall on or from ladders or scaffolding**
  E881.0 Fall from ladder
  E881.1 Fall from scaffolding

E882 Fall from or out of building or other structure
  Fall from: Fall from:
    balcony   turret
    bridge   viaduct
    building   wall
    flagpole   window
    tower   Fall through roof
  EXCLUDES *collapse of a building or structure (E916)*
    fall or jump from burning building (E890.8, E891.8)

✓4ᵗʰ **E883 Fall into hole or other opening in surface**
  INCLUDES fall into: fall into:
                  cavity   shaft
                  dock   swimming pool
                  hole   tank
                  pit   well
                  quarry
  EXCLUDES *fall into water NOS (E910.9)*
    that resulting in drowning or submersion without mention of injury (E910.0-E910.9)

  E883.0 Accident from diving or jumping into water [swimming pool]
    Strike or hit:
      against bottom when jumping or diving into water
      wall or board of swimming pool
      water surface
    EXCLUDES *diving with insufficient air supply (E913.2)*
      effects of air pressure from diving (E902.2)
  E883.1 Accidental fall into well
  E883.2 Accidental fall into storm drain or manhole
  E883.9 Fall into other hole or other opening in surface

✓4ᵗʰ **E884 Other fall from one level to another**
  E884.0 Fall from playground equipment
    EXCLUDES *recreational machinery (E919.8)*
  E884.1 Fall from cliff
  E884.2 Fall from chair

E884.3 Fall from wheelchair
E884.4 Fall from bed
E884.5 Fall from other furniture
E884.6 Fall from commode
> Toilet

E884.9 Other fall from one level to another
> Fall from:
> > embankment
> > haystack
> > stationary vehicle
> > tree

✓4ᵗʰ **E885 Fall on same level from slipping, tripping, or stumbling**
- E885.0 Fall from (nonmotorized) scooter
- E885.1 Fall from roller skates
  > In-line skates
- E885.2 Fall from skateboard
- E885.3 Fall from skis
- E885.4 Fall from snowboard
- E885.9 Fall from other slipping, tripping, or stumbling
  > Fall on moving sidewalk

✓4ᵗʰ **E886 Fall on same level from collision, pushing, or shoving, by or with other person**
> **EXCLUDES** crushed or pushed by a crowd or human stampede (E917.1, E917.6)

E886.0 In sports
> Tackles in sports
> > **EXCLUDES** kicked, stepped on, struck by object, in sports (E917.0, E917.5)

E886.9 Other and unspecified
> Fall from collision of pedestrian (conveyance) with another pedestrian (conveyance)

E887 Fracture, cause unspecified

✓4ᵗʰ **E888 Other and unspecified fall**
> Accidental fall NOS
> Fall on same level NOS

E888.0 Fall resulting in striking against sharp object
> Use additional external cause code to identify object (E920)

E888.1 Fall resulting in striking against other object
E888.8 Other fall
E888.9 Unspecified fall
> Fall NOS

ACCIDENTS CAUSED BY FIRE AND FLAMES (E890-E899)

INCLUDES asphyxia or poisoning due to conflagration or ignition
burning by fire
secondary fires resulting from explosion

EXCLUDES arson (E968.0)
fire in or on:
> machinery (in operation) (E919.0-E919.9)
> transport vehicle other than stationary vehicle (E800.0-E845.9)
> vehicle not elsewhere classifiable (E846-E848)

E890 Conflagration in private dwelling

INCLUDES
conflagration in:
- apartment
- boarding house
- camping place
- caravan
- farmhouse
- house
- lodging house
- mobile home
- private garage
- rooming house
- tenement

conflagration originating from sources classifiable to E893-E898 in the above buildings

E890.0 Explosion caused by conflagration

E890.1 Fumes from combustion of polyvinylchloride [PVC] and similar material in conflagration

E890.2 Other smoke and fumes from conflagration

Carbon monoxide
Fumes NOS
Smoke NOS
} from conflagration in private building

E890.3 Burning caused by conflagration

E890.8 Other accident resulting from conflagration

Collapse of
Fall from
Hit by object falling from
Jump from
} burning private building

E890.9 Unspecified accident resulting from conflagration in private dwelling

E891 Conflagration in other and unspecified building or structure

Conflagration in:
- barn
- church
- convalescent and other residential home
- dormitory of educational institution
- factory
- farm outbuildings
- hospital
- hotel
- school
- store
- theater

Conflagration originating from sources classifiable to E893-E898, in the above buildings

E891.0 Explosion caused by conflagration

E891.1 Fumes from combustion of polyvinylchloride [PVC] and similar material in conflagration

E891.2 Other smoke and fumes from conflagration

Carbon monoxide
Fumes NOS
Smoke NOS
} from conflagration in building or structure

E891.3 Burning caused by conflagration

E891.8 Other accident resulting from conflagration

Collapse of
Fall from
Hit by object falling from
Jump from
} burning building or structure

E891.9 Unspecified accident resulting from conflagration of other and unspecified building or structure

E CODES

E892 Conflagration not in building or structure

Fire (uncontrolled) (in) (of):
- forest
- grass
- hay
- lumber
- mine

Fire (uncontrolled) (in) (of):
- prairie
- transport vehicle [any], except while in transit
- tunnel

✓4ᵗʰ E893 Accident caused by ignition of clothing

EXCLUDES ignition of clothing:
from highly inflammable material (E894)
with conflagration (E890.0-E892)

E893.0 From controlled fire in private dwelling
Ignition of clothing from:
normal fire (charcoal) (coal) (electric) (gas) (wood) in:
- brazier
- fireplace
- furnace
- stove

} in private dwelling (as listed in E890)

E893.1 From controlled fire in other building or structure
Ignition of clothing from:
normal fire (charcoal) (coal) (electric) (gas) (wood) in:
- brazier
- fireplace
- furnace
- stove

} in other building or structure (as listed in E891)

E893.2 From controlled fire not in building or structure
Ignition of clothing from:
- bonfire (controlled)
- brazier fire (controlled), not in building or structure
- trash fire (controlled)

EXCLUDES conflagration not in building (E892)
trash fire out of control (E892)

E893.8 From other specified sources
Ignition of clothing from:
- blowlamp
- blowtorch
- burning bedspread
- candle
- cigar
- cigarette
- lighter
- matches
- pipe
- welding torch

E893.9 Unspecified source
Ignition of clothing (from controlled fire NOS) (in building NOS) NOS

E894 Ignition of highly inflammable material

Ignition of:
- benzine
- gasoline
- fat
- kerosene
- paraffin
- petrol

} (with ignition of clothing)

EXCLUDES ignition of highly inflammable material with:
conflagration (E890.0-E892)
explosion (E923.0-E923.9)

E895 Accident caused by controlled fire in private dwelling
Burning by (flame of) normal fire (charcoal) (coal) (electric) (gas) (wood) in:
- brazier
- fireplace
- furnace
- stove

} in private dwelling (as listed in E890)

EXCLUDES   *burning by hot objects not producing fire or flames (E924.0-E924.9)*
ignition of clothing from these sources (E893.0)
poisoning by carbon monoxide from incomplete combustion of fuel (E867-E868.9)
that with conflagration (E890.0-E890.9)

E896 Accident caused by controlled fire in other and unspecified building or structure
Burning by (flame of) normal fire (charcoal) (coal) (electric) (gas) (wood) in:
- brazier
- fireplace
- furnace
- stove

} in other building or structure (as listed in E891)

EXCLUDES   *burning by hot objects not producing fire or flames (E924.0-E924.9)*
ignition of clothing from these sources (E893.1)
poisoning by carbon monoxide from incomplete combustion of fuel (E867-E868.9)
that with conflagration (E891.0-E891.9)

E897 Accident caused by controlled fire not in building or structure
Burns from flame of:
- bonfire
- brazier fire, not in building or structure
- trash fire

} controlled

EXCLUDES   *ignition of clothing from these sources (E893.2)*
trash fire out of control (E892)
that with conflagration (E892)

✓4ᵗʰ **E898 Accident caused by other specified fire and flames**
EXCLUDES   *conflagration (E890.0-E892)*
that with ignition of:
  clothing (E893.0-E893.9)
  highly inflammable material (E894)

E898.0 Burning bedclothes
Bed set on fire NOS

E898.1 Other

Burning by:
- blowlamp
- blowtorch
- candle
- cigar
- cigarette
- fire in room NOS

Burning by:
- lamp
- lighter
- matches
- pipe
- welding torch

E899 Accident caused by unspecified fire
Burning NOS

ACCIDENTS DUE TO NATURAL AND ENVIRONMENTAL FACTORS (E900-E909)

✓4ᵗʰ **E900 Excessive heat**

E900.0 Due to weather conditions
Excessive heat as the external cause of:
- ictus solaris
- siriasis
- sunstroke

E CODES

E900.1 Of man-made origin
    Heat (in):
        boiler room
        drying room
        factory
        furnace room
    Heat (in):
        generated in transport vehicle
        kitchen

E900.9 Of unspecified origin

✓4ᵗʰ E901 Excessive cold

E901.0 Due to weather conditions
    Excessive cold as the cause of:
        chilblains NOS
        immersion foot

E901.1 Of man-made origin
    Contact with or inhalation of:
        dry ice
        liquid air
        liquid hydrogen
        liquid nitrogen
    Prolonged exposure in:
        deep freeze unit
        refrigerator

E901.8 Other specified origin

E901.9 Of unspecified origin

✓4ᵗʰ E902 High and low air pressure and changes in air pressure

E902.0 Residence or prolonged visit at high altitude
    Residence or prolonged visit at high altitude as the cause of:
        Acosta syndrome
        Alpine sickness
        altitude sickness
        Andes disease
        anoxia, hypoxia
        barotitis, barodontalgia, barosinusitis, otitic barotrauma
        hypobarism, hypobaropathy
        mountain sickness
        range disease

E902.1 In aircraft
    Sudden change in air pressure in aircraft during ascent or descent as the cause of:
        aeroneurosis
        aviators' disease

E902.2 Due to diving
    High air pressure from rapid descent in water
    Reduction in atmospheric pressure while surfacing from deep water diving
    as the cause of:
        caisson disease
        divers' disease
        divers' palsy or paralysis

E902.8 Due to other specified causes
    Reduction in atmospheric pressure while surfacing from underground

E902.9 Unspecified cause

E903 Travel and motion

✓4ᵗʰ E904 Hunger, thirst, exposure, and neglect

    EXCLUDES any condition resulting from homicidal intent (E968.0-E968.9)
        hunger, thirst, and exposure resulting from accidents connected with transport (E800.0-E848)

E904.0 Abandonment or neglect of infants and helpless persons
Exposure to weather conditions ⎱ resulting from abandonment or
Hunger or thirst ⎰ neglect

Desertion of newborn
Inattention at or after birth
Lack of care (helpless person) (infant)
EXCLUDES *criminal [purposeful] neglect (E968.4)*

E904.1 Lack of food
Lack of food as the cause of:
  inanition   starvation
  insufficient nourishment
EXCLUDES *hunger resulting from abandonment or neglect (E904.0)*

E904.2 Lack of water
Lack of water as the cause of:
  dehydration   inanition
EXCLUDES *dehydration due to acute fluid loss (276.5)*

E904.3 Exposure (to weather conditions), not elsewhere classifiable
Exposure NOS
Humidity
Struck by hailstones
EXCLUDES *struck by lightning (E907)*

E904.9 Privation, unqualified
Destitution

√4ᵗʰ E905 Venomous animals and plants as the cause of poisoning and toxic reactions
INCLUDES chemical released by animal
insects
release of venom through fangs, hairs, spines, tentacles, and other venom apparatus
EXCLUDES *eating of poisonous animals or plants (E865.0-E865.9)*

E905.0 Venomous snakes and lizards
Cobra   Mamba
Copperhead snake   Rattlesnake
Coral snake   Sea snake
Fer de lance   Snake (venomous)
Gila monster   Viper
Krait   Water moccasin
EXCLUDES *bites of snakes and lizards known to be nonvenomous (E906.2)*

E905.1 Venomous spiders
Black widow spider   Tarantula (venomous)
Brown spider

E905.2 Scorpion

E905.3 Hornets, wasps, and bees
Yellow jacket

E905.4 Centipede and venomous millipede (tropical)

E905.5 Other venomous arthropods
Sting of:
  ant
  caterpillar

E CODES

E905.6 Venomous marine animals and plants
Puncture by sea urchin spine
Sting of:
  coral
  jelly fish
  nematocysts
  sea anemone
  sea cucumber
  other marine animal or plant
  > EXCLUDES   bites and other injuries caused by nonvenomous marine
  >   animal (E906.2-E906.8)
  >   bite of sea snake (venomous) (E905.0)

E905.7 Poisoning and toxic reactions caused by other plants
Injection of poisons or toxins into or through skin by plant thorns, spines, or other mechanisms
  > EXCLUDES   puncture wound NOS by plant thorns or spines (E920.8)

E905.8 Other specified

E905.9 Unspecified
Sting NOS   Venomous bite NOS

√4ᵗʰ **E906 Other injury caused by animals**
  > EXCLUDES   poisoning and toxic reactions caused by venomous animals and insects
  >   (E905.0-E905.9)
  >   road vehicle accident involving animals (E827.0-E828.9)
  >   tripping or falling over an animal (E885.9)

E906.0 Dog bite

E906.1 Rat bite

E906.2 Bite of nonvenomous snakes and lizards

E906.3 Bite of other animal except arthropod
Cats   Rodents, except rats
Moray eel   Shark

E906.4 Bite of nonvenomous arthropod
Insect bite NOS

E906.5 Bite by unspecified animal
Animal bite NOS

E906.8 Other specified injury caused by animal
Butted by animal
Fallen on by horse or other animal, not being ridden
Gored by animal
Implantation of quills of porcupine
Pecked by bird
Run over by animal, not being ridden
Stepped on by animal, not being ridden
  > EXCLUDES   injury by animal being ridden (E828.0-E828.9)

E906.9 Unspecified injury caused by animal

E907 Lightning
  > EXCLUDES   injury from:
  >   fall of tree or other object caused by lightning (E916)
  >   fire caused by lightning (E890.0-E892)

√4ᵗʰ **E908 Cataclysmic storms, and floods resulting from storms**
  > EXCLUDES   collapse of dam or man-made structure causing flood (E909.3)

E908.0 Hurricane
Storm surge
"Tidal wave" caused by storm action
Typhoon

E908.1 Tornado
  Cyclone
  Twisters

E908.2 Floods
  Torrential rainfall
  Flash flood
  > EXCLUDES: *collapse of dam or man-made structure causing flood (E909.3)*

E908.3 Blizzard (snow) (ice)

E908.4 Dust storm

E908.8 Other cataclysmic storms

E908.9 Unspecified cataclysmic storms, and floods resulting from storms
  Storm NOS

✓4th **E909 Cataclysmic earth surface movements and eruptions**

E909.0 Earthquakes

E909.1 Volcanic eruptions
  Burns from lava
  Ash inhalation

E909.2 Avalanche, landslide, or mudslide

E909.3 Collapse of dam or man-made structure

E909.4 Tidalwave caused by earthquake
  Tidalwave NOS
  Tsunami
  > EXCLUDES: *tidalwave caused by tropical storm (E908.0)*

E909.8 Other cataclysmic earth surface movements and eruptions

E909.9 Unspecified cataclysmic earth surface movements and eruptions

ACCIDENTS CAUSED BY SUBMERSION, SUFFOCATION, AND FOREIGN BODIES (E910-E915)

✓4th **E910 Accidental drowning and submersion**
  > INCLUDES: immersion
  > swimmers' cramp

  > EXCLUDES: *diving accident (NOS) (resulting in injury except drowning) (E883.0)*
  > *diving with insufficient air supply (E913.2)*
  > *drowning and submersion due to:*
  >   *cataclysm (E908-E909)*
  >   *machinery accident (E919.0-E919.9)*
  >   *transport accident (E800.0-E845.9)*
  > *effect of high and low air pressure (E902.2)*
  > *injury from striking against objects while in running water (E917.2)*

E910.0 While water-skiing
  Fall from water skis with submersion or drowning
  > EXCLUDES: *accident to water-skier involving a watercraft and resulting in submersion or other injury (E830.4, E831.4)*

E910.1 While engaged in other sport or recreational activity with diving equipment
  Scuba diving NOS   Underwater spear
  Skin diving NOS   fishing NOS

E910.2 While engaged in other sport or recreational activity without diving equipment
  Fishing or hunting, except from boat or with diving equipment
  Ice skating
  Playing in water
  Surfboarding
  Swimming NOS
  Voluntarily jumping from boat, not involved in accident, for swim NOS
  Wading in water
  > EXCLUDES: *jumping into water to rescue another person (E910.3)*

E CODES

E910.3 While swimming or diving for purposes other than recreation or sport
- Marine salvage
- Pearl diving
- Placement of fishing nets
- Rescue (attempt) of another person
- Underwater construction or repairs

} (with diving equipment)

E910.4 In bathtub

E910.8 Other accidental drowning or submersion
- Drowning in: quenching tank
- Drowning in: swimming pool

E910.9 Unspecified accidental drowning or submersion
- Accidental fall into water NOS
- Drowning NOS

E911 Inhalation and ingestion of food causing obstruction of respiratory tract or suffocation

Aspiration and inhalation of food [any] (into respiratory tract) NOS

- Asphyxia by
- Choked on
- Suffocation by

} food [including bone, seed in food, regurgitated food]

- Compression of trachea
- Interruption of respiration
- Obstruction of respiration

} by food lodged in esophagus

Obstruction of pharynx by food (bolus)

EXCLUDES injury, except asphyxia and obstruction of respiratory passage, caused by food (E915)

obstruction of esophagus by food without mention of asphyxia or obstruction of respiratory passage (E915)

E912 Inhalation and ingestion of other object causing obstruction of respiratory tract or suffocation

Aspiration and inhalation of foreign body except food (into respiratory tract) NOS
Foreign object [bean] [marble] in nose
Obstruction of pharynx by foreign body

- Compression
- Interruption of respiration
- Obstruction of respiration

} by foreign body in esophagus

EXCLUDES injury, except asphyxia and obstruction of respiratory passage, caused by foreign body (E915)

obstruction of esophagus by foreign body without mention of asphyxia or obstruction in respiratory passage (E915)

✓4th E913 Accidental mechanical suffocation

EXCLUDES mechanical suffocation from or by:
- accidental inhalation or ingestion of:
  - food (E911)
  - foreign object (E912)
- cataclysm (E908-E909)
- explosion (E921.0-E921.9, E923.0-E923.9)
- machinery accident (E919.0-E919.9)

E913.0 In bed or cradle

EXCLUDES suffocation by plastic bag (E913.1)

E913.1 By plastic bag

E913.2 Due to lack of air (in closed place)
- Accidentally closed up in refrigerator or other airtight enclosed space
- Diving with insufficient air supply

EXCLUDES suffocation by plastic bag (E913.1)

E913.3 By falling earth or other substance
Cave-in NOS
> EXCLUDES cave-in caused by cataclysmic earth surface movements and eruptions (E909)
> struck by cave-in without asphyxiation or suffocation (E916)

E913.8 Other specified means
Accidental hanging, except in bed or cradle

E913.9 Unspecified means
Asphyxia, mechanical NOS Suffocation NOS
Strangulation NOS

E914 Foreign body accidentally entering eye and adnexa
> EXCLUDES corrosive liquid (E924.1)

E915 Foreign body accidentally entering other orifice
> EXCLUDES aspiration and inhalation of foreign body, any, (into respiratory tract) NOS (E911-E912)

OTHER ACCIDENTS (E916-E928)

E916 Struck accidentally by falling object
Collapse of building, except on fire
Falling:
  rock
  snowslide NOS
  stone
  tree
Object falling from:
  machine, not in operation
  stationary vehicle
Code first:
  collapse of building on fire (E890.0-E891.9)
  falling object in:
    cataclysm (E908-E909)
    machinery accidents (E919.0-E919.9)
    transport accidents (E800.0-E845.9)
    vehicle accidents not elsewhere classifiable (E846-E848)
  object set in motion by:
    explosion (E921.0-E921.9, E923.0-E923.9)
    firearm (E922.0-E922.9)
    projected object (E917.0-E917.9)

✓4ᵗʰ **E917 Striking against or struck accidentally by objects or persons**
> INCLUDES
> bumping into or against
> colliding with
> kicking against   } object (moving) (projected) (stationary)
> stepping on   pedestrian conveyance
> struck by   person

> EXCLUDES fall from:
> collision with another person, except when caused by a crowd (E886.0-E886.9)
> stumbling over object (E885.9)
> fall resulting in striking against object (E888.0, E888.1)
> injury caused by:
>   assault (E960.0-E960.1, E967.0-E967.9)
>   cutting or piercing instrument (E920.0-E920.9)
>   explosion (E921.0-E921.9, E923.0-E923.9)
>   firearm (E922.0-E922.9)
>   machinery (E919.0-E919.9)
>   transport vehicle (E800.0-E845.9)
>   vehicle not elsewhere classifiable (E846-E848)

E CODES

E917.0 In sports without subsequent fall
    Kicked or stepped on during game (football) (rugby)
    Struck by hit or thrown ball
    Struck by hockey stick or puck

E917.1 Caused by a crowd, by collective fear or panic without subsequent fall
    Crushed ⎫
    Pushed ⎬ by crowd or human stampede
    Stepped on ⎭

E917.2 In running water without subsequent fall
    EXCLUDES   *drowning or submersion (E910.0-E910.9)*
                         that in sports (E917.0, E917.5)

E917.3 Furniture without subsequent fall
    EXCLUDES   *fall from furniture (E884.2, E884.4-E884.5)*

E917.4 Other stationary object without subsequent fall
    Bath tub   Lamp-post
    Fence

E917.5 Object in sports with subsequent fall
    Knocked down while boxing

E917.6 Caused by a crowd, by collective fear or panic with subsequent fall

E917.7 Furniture with subsequent fall
    EXCLUDES   *fall from furniture (E884.2, E884.4-E884.5)*

E917.8 Other stationary object with subsequent fall
    Bath tub
    Fence
    Lamp-post

E917.9 Other striking against with or without subsequent fall

E918 Caught accidentally in or between objects
    Caught, crushed, jammed, or pinched in or between moving or stationary objects, such as:
    escalator
    folding object
    hand tools, appliances, or implements
    sliding door and door frame
    under packing crate
    washing machine wringer
    EXCLUDES   *injury caused by:*
                         cutting or piercing instrument (E920.0-E920.9)
                         machinery (E919.0-E919.9)
                         transport vehicle (E800.0-E845.9)
                         vehicle not elsewhere classifiable (E846-E848)
                 struck accidentally by:
                         falling object (E916)
                         object (moving) (projected) (E917.0-E917.9)

E919 Accidents caused by machinery

INCLUDES
burned by
caught in (moving parts of)
collapse of
crushed by
cut or pierced by
drowning or submersion caused by
explosion of, on, in
fall from or into moving part of   } machinery (accident)
fire starting in or on
mechanical suffocation caused by
object falling from, on, in motion by
overturning of
pinned under
run over by
struck by
thrown from

caught between machinery and other object
machinery accident NOS

EXCLUDES
accidents involving machinery, not in operation (E884.9, E916-E918)
injury caused by:
    electric current in connection with machinery (E925.0-E925.9)
    escalator (E880.0, E918)
    explosion of pressure vessel in connection with machinery (E921.0-E921.9)
    moving sidewalk (E885.9)
    powered hand tools, appliances, and implements (E916-E918, E920.0-E921.9, E923.0-E926.9)
transport vehicle accidents involving machinery (E800.0-E848.9)
poisoning by carbon monoxide generated by machine (E868.8)

E919.0 Agricultural machines
Animal-powered agricultural machine
Combine
Derrick, hay
Farm machinery NOS
Farm tractor
Harvester
Hay mower or rake
Reaper
Thresher

EXCLUDES
that in transport under own power on the highway (E810.0-E819.9)
that being towed by another vehicle on the highway (E810.0-E819.9, E827.0-E827.9, E829.0-E829.9)
that involved in accident classifiable to E820-E829 (E820.0-E829.9)

E919.1 Mining and earth-drilling machinery
Bore or drill (land) (seabed)   Shaft lift
Shaft hoist   Under-cutter

EXCLUDES coal car, tram, truck, and tub in mine (E846)

E919.2 Lifting machines and appliances

Chain hoist
Crane
Derrick
Elevator (building) (grain)
Forklift truck
Lift
Pulley block
Winch

} except in agricultural or mining operations

EXCLUDES that being towed by another vehicle on the highway (E810.0-E819.9, E827.0-E827.9, E829.0-829.9)

that in transport under own power on the highway (E810.0-E819.9)

that involved in accident classifiable to E820-E829 (E820.0-E829.9)

E919.3 Metalworking machines

Abrasive wheel
Forging machine
Lathe
Mechanical shears

Metal:
  drilling machine
  milling machine
  power press
  rolling-mill
  sawing machine

E919.4 Woodworking and forming machines

Band saw
Bench saw
Circular saw
Molding machine

Overhead plane
Powered saw
Radial saw
Sander

EXCLUDES hand saw (E920.1)

E919.5 Prime movers, except electrical motors

Gas turbine
Internal combustion engine
Steam engine
Water driven turbine

EXCLUDES that being towed by other vehicle on the highway (E810.0-E819.9, E827.0-E827.9, E829.0-E829.9)

that in transport under own power on the highway (E810.0-E819.9)

E919.6 Transmission machinery

Transmission:
  belt
  cable
  chain
  gear

Transmission:
  pinion
  pulley
  shaft

E919.7 Earth moving, scraping, and other excavating machines

Bulldozer
Road scraper
Steam shovel

EXCLUDES that being towed by other vehicle on the highway (E810.0-E819.9, E827.0-E827.9, E829.0-E829.9)

that in transport under own power on the highway (E810.0-E819.9)

E919.8 Other specified machinery

Machines for manufacture of:
  clothing
  foodstuffs and beverages
  paper
Printing machine
Recreational machinery
Spinning, weaving, and textile machines

E919.9 Unspecified machinery

☑4ᵗʰ **E920 Accidents caused by cutting and piercing instruments or objects**

> INCLUDES   accidental injury (by) object:
> - edged
> - pointed
> - sharp

E920.0 Powered lawn mower

E920.1 Other powered hand tools
Any powered hand tool [compressed air] [electric] [explosive cartridge] [hydraulic power], such as:
- drill
- hand saw
- hedge clipper
- rivet gun
- snow blower
- staple gun

> EXCLUDES band saw (E919.4)
> bench saw (E919.4)

E920.2 Powered household appliances and implements
Blender
Electric:
- beater or mixer
- can opener
- fan
- knife
- sewing machine

Garbage disposal appliance

E920.3 Knives, swords, and daggers

E920.4 Other hand tools and implements

Axe	Paper cutter
Can opener NOS	Pitchfork
Chisel	Rake
Fork	Scissors
Hand saw	Screwdriver
Hoe	Sewing machine, not powered
Ice pick	Shovel
Needle (sewing)	

E920.5 Hypodermic needle
Contaminated needle
Needle stick

E920.8 Other specified cutting and piercing instruments or objects

Arrow	Nail
Broken glass	Plant thorn
Dart	Splinter
Edge of stiff paper	Tin can lid
Lathe turnings	

> EXCLUDES animal spines or quills (E906.8)
> flying glass due to explosion (E921.0-E923.9)

E920.9 Unspecified cutting and piercing instrument or object

☑4ᵗʰ **E921 Accident caused by explosion of pressure vessel**

> INCLUDES accidental explosion of pressure vessels, whether or not part of machinery

> EXCLUDES explosion of pressure vessel on transport vehicle (E800.0-E845.9)

E921.0 Boilers

E921.1 Gas cylinders
Air tank
Pressure gas tank

E CODES

E921.8 Other specified pressure vessels
    Aerosol can   Pressure cooker
    Automobile tire

E921.9 Unspecified pressure vessel

✓4ᵗʰ **E922 Accident caused by firearm, and air gun missile**

E922.0 Handgun
    Pistol   Revolver
    EXCLUDES Verey pistol (E922.8)

E922.1 Shotgun (automatic)

E922.2 Hunting rifle

E922.3 Military firearms
    Army rifle   Machine gun

E922.4 Air gun
    BB gun
    Pellet gun

• **E922.5 Paintball gun**

E922.8 Other specified firearm missile
    Verey pistol [flare]

E922.9 Unspecified firearm missile
    Gunshot wound NOS
    Shot NOS

✓4ᵗʰ **E923 Accident caused by explosive material**

  INCLUDES flash burns and other injuries resulting from explosion of explosive material
                ignition of highly explosive material with explosion

  EXCLUDES explosion:
                in or on machinery (E919.0-E919.9)
                on any transport vehicle, except stationary motor vehicle (E800.0-E848)
                with conflagration (E890.0, E891.0, E892)
                secondary fires resulting from explosion (E890.0-E899)

E923.0 Fireworks

E923.1 Blasting materials
    Blasting cap
    Detonator
    Dynamite
    Explosive [any] used in blasting operations

E923.2 Explosive gases
    Acetylene   Fire damp
    Butane   Gasoline fumes
    Coal gas   Methane
    Explosion in mine NOS   Propane

E923.8 Other explosive materials
    Bomb   Torpedo
    Explosive missile   Explosion in munitions:
    Grenade   dump
    Mine   factory
    Shell

E923.9 Unspecified explosive material
    Explosion NOS

✓4ᵗʰ **E924 Accident caused by hot substance or object, caustic or corrosive material, and steam**

  EXCLUDES burning NOS (E899)
                chemical burn resulting from swallowing a corrosive substance (E860.0-E864.4)
                fire caused by these substances and objects (E890.0-E894)
                radiation burns (E926.0-E926.9)
                therapeutic misadventures (E870.0-E876.9)

✓4ᵗʰ Fourth-digit Required   ▶◀ Revised Text   ● New Code   ▲ Revised Code Title

E924.0 Hot liquids and vapors, including steam
    Burning or scalding by:
        boiling water
        hot or boiling liquids not primarily caustic or corrosive
        liquid metal
        steam
        other hot vapor
    EXCLUDES   hot (boiling) tap water (E924.2)

E924.1 Caustic and corrosive substances
    Burning by: Burning by:
        acid [any kind]   corrosive substance
        ammonia   lye
        caustic oven cleaner   vitriol or other substance

E924.2 Hot (boiling) tap water

E924.8 Other
    Burning by:
        heat from electric heating appliance
        hot object NOS
        light bulb
        steam pipe

E924.9 Unspecified

✓4th **E925 Accident caused by electric current**
    INCLUDES   electric current from exposed wire, faulty appliance, high voltage
                cable, live rail, or open electric socket as the cause of:
                    burn
                    cardiac fibrillation
                    convulsion
                    electric shock
                    electrocution
                    puncture wound
                    respiratory paralysis
    EXCLUDES   burn by heat from electrical appliance (E924.8)
                lightning (E907)

E925.0 Domestic wiring and appliances

E925.1 Electric power generating plants, distribution stations, transmission lines
    Broken power line

E925.2 Industrial wiring, appliances, and electrical machinery
    Conductors
    Control apparatus
    Electrical equipment and machinery
    Transformers

E925.8 Other electric current
    Wiring and appliances in or on:
        farm [not farmhouse]
        outdoors
        public building
        residential institutions
        schools

E925.9 Unspecified electric current
    Burns or other injury from electric current NOS
    Electric shock NOS
    Electrocution NOS

E CODES

✓4th E926 Exposure to radiation

> **EXCLUDES** abnormal reaction to or complication of treatment without mention of misadventure (E879.2)
> atomic power plant malfunction in water transport (E838.0-E838.9)
> misadventure to patient in surgical and medical procedures (E873.2-E873.3)
> use of radiation in war operations (E996-E997.9)

E926.0 Radiofrequency radiation
Overexposure to:
  microwave radiation
  radar radiation
  radiofrequency
  radiofrequency radiation
  [any]
from:
  high-powered radio and television transmitters
  industrial radiofrequency induction heaters
  radar installations

E926.1 Infrared heaters and lamps
Exposure to infrared radiation from heaters and lamps as the cause of:
  blistering
  burning
  charring
  inflammatory change

> **EXCLUDES** physical contact with heater or lamp (E924.8)

E926.2 Visible and ultraviolet light sources
  Arc lamps
  Black light sources
  Electrical welding arc
  Oxygas welding torch
  Sun rays
  Tanning bed

> **EXCLUDES** excessive heat from these sources (E900.1-E900.9)

E926.3 X-rays and other electromagnetic ionizing radiation
  Gamma rays
  X-rays (hard) (soft)

E926.4 Lasers

E926.5 Radioactive isotopes
  Radiobiologicals
  Radiopharmaceuticals

E926.8 Other specified radiation
Artificially accelerated beams of ionized particles generated by:
  betatrons
  synchrotrons

E926.9 Unspecified radiation
  Radiation NOS

E927 Overexertion and strenuous movements
  Excessive physical exercise
  Overexertion (from):
    lifting
    pulling
    pushing
  Strenuous movements in:
    recreational activities
    other activities

✓4th E928 Other and unspecified environmental and accidental causes

E928.0 Prolonged stay in weightless environment
  Weightlessness in spacecraft (simulator)

E928.1 Exposure to noise
  Noise (pollution)
  Sound waves
  Supersonic waves

E928.2 Vibration

E928.3 Human bite

E928.8 Other

E928.9 Unspecified accident

Accident NOS
Blow NOS
Casualty (not due to war)
Decapitation
} stated as accidentally inflicted

Knocked down
Killed
Injury [any part of body, or unspecified]
Mangled
Wound
} stated as accidentally inflicted, but not otherwise specified

> **EXCLUDES** *fracture, cause unspecified (E887)*
> *injuries undetermined whether accidentally or purposely inflicted (E980.0-E989)*

LATE EFFECTS OF ACCIDENTAL INJURY (E929)

Note: This category is to be used to indicate accidental injury as the cause of death or disability from late effects, which are themselves classifiable elsewhere. The "late effects" include conditions reported as such, or as sequelae which may occur at any time after the attempted suicide or self-inflicted injury.

√4th E929 Late effects of accidental injury

> **EXCLUDES** *late effects of:*
> *surgical and medical procedures (E870.0-E879.9)*
> *therapeutic use of drugs and medicines (E930.0-E949.9)*

E929.0 Late effects of motor vehicle accident
Late effects of accidents classifiable to E810-E825

E929.1 Late effects of other transport accident
Late effects of accidents classifiable to E800-E807, E826-E838, E840-E848

E929.2 Late effects of accidental poisoning
Late effects of accidents classifiable to E850-E858, E860-E869

E929.3 Late effects of accidental fall
Late effects of accidents classifiable to E880-E888

E929.4 Late effects of accident caused by fire
Late effects of accidents classifiable to E890-E899

E929.5 Late effects of accident due to natural and environmental factors
Late effects of accidents classifiable to E900-E909

E929.8 Late effects of other accidents
Late effects of accidents classifiable to E910-E928.8

E929.9 Late effects of unspecified accident
Late effects of accidents classifiable to E928.9

DRUGS, MEDICINAL AND BIOLOGICAL SUBSTANCES CAUSING ADVERSE EFFECTS IN THERAPEUTIC USE (E930-E949)

> **INCLUDES** correct drug properly administered in therapeutic or prophylactic dosage, as the cause of any adverse effect including allergic or hypersensitivity reactions
>
> **EXCLUDES** *accidental overdose of drug and wrong drug given or taken in error (E850.0-E858.9)*
> *accidents in the technique of administration of drug or biological substance, such as accidental puncture during injection, or contamination of drug (E870.0-E876.9)*
> *administration with suicidal or homicidal intent or intent to harm, or in circumstances classifiable to E980-E989 (E950.0-E950.5, E962.0, E980.0-E980.5)*

See Alphabetic Index for more complete list of specific drugs to be classified under the fourth-digit subdivisions. The American Hospital Formulary numbers can be used to classify new drugs listed by the American Hospital Formulary Service (AHFS). See Appendix C.

E CODES

✓4th E930 Antibiotics

> EXCLUDES   that used as eye, ear, nose, and throat [ENT], and local anti-infectives (E946.0-E946.9)

E930.0 Penicillins
    Natural   Semisynthetic, such as:
    Synthetic   nafcillin
    Semisynthetic, such as: oxacillin
        ampicillin
        cloxacillin

E930.1 Antifungal antibiotics
    Amphotericin B   Hachimycin [trichomycin]
    Griseofulvin   Nystatin

E930.2 Chloramphenicol group
    Chloramphenicol   Thiamphenicol

E930.3 Erythromycin and other macrolides
    Oleandomycin   Spiramycin

E930.4 Tetracycline group
    Doxycycline   Oxytetracycline
    Minocycline

E930.5 Cephalosporin group
    Cephalexin   Cephaloridine
    Cephaloglycin   Cephalothin

E930.6 Antimycobacterial antibiotics
    Cycloserine   Rifampin
    Kanamycin   Streptomycin

E930.7 Antineoplastic antibiotics
    Actinomycins, such as: Actinomycins, such as:
        Bleomycin   Daunorubicin
        Cactinomycin   Mitomycin
        Dactinomycin

> EXCLUDES   other antineoplastic drugs (E933.1)

E930.8 Other specified antibiotics

E930.9 Unspecified antibiotic

✓4th E931 Other anti-infectives

> EXCLUDES   ENT, and local anti-infectives (E946.0-E946.9)

E931.0 Sulfonamides
    Sulfadiazine   Sulfamethoxazole
    Sulfafurazole

E931.1 Arsenical anti-infectives

E931.2 Heavy metal anti-infectives
    Compounds of: Compounds of:
        antimony   lead
        bismuth   mercury

> EXCLUDES   mercurial diuretics (E944.0)

E931.3 Quinoline and hydroxyquinoline derivatives
    Chiniofon   Diiodohydroxyquin

> EXCLUDES   antimalarial drugs (E931.4)

E931.4 Antimalarials and drugs acting on other blood protozoa
    Chloroquine phosphate   Proguanil [chloroguanide]
    Cycloguanil   Pyrimethamine
    Primaquine   Quinine (sulphate)

E931.5 Other antiprotozoal drugs
    Emetine

E931.6 Anthelmintics
    Hexylresorcinol   Piperazine
    Male fern oleoresin   Thiabendazole

E931.7 Antiviral drugs
    Methisazone
    EXCLUDES amantadine (E936.4)
                   cytarabine (E933.1)
                   idoxuridine (E946.5)

E931.8 Other antimycobacterial drugs
    Ethambutol   Para-aminosalicylic
    Ethionamide   acid derivatives
    Isoniazid   Sulfones

E931.9 Other and unspecified anti-infectives
    Flucytosine   Nitrofuranderivatives

✓4th E932 Hormones and synthetic substitutes

E932.0 Adrenal cortical steroids
    Cortisone derivatives
    Desoxycorticosterone derivatives
    Fluorinated corticosteroid

E932.1 Androgens and anabolic congeners
    Nandrolone phenpropionate
    Oxymetholone
    Testosterone and preparations

E932.2 Ovarian hormones and synthetic substitutes
    Contraceptives, oral
    Estrogens
    Estrogens and progestogens combined
    Progestogens

E932.3 Insulins and antidiabetic agents
    Acetohexamide   Phenformin
    Biguanide derivatives, oral Sulfonylurea
    Chlorpropamide   derivatives,
    Glucagon   oral
    Insulin   Tolbutamide
    EXCLUDES adverse effect of insulin administered for shock therapy (E879.3)

E932.4 Anterior pituitary hormones
    Corticotropin
    Gonadotropin
    Somatotropin [growth hormone]

E932.5 Posterior pituitary hormones
    Vasopressin
    EXCLUDES oxytocic agents (E945.0)

E932.6 Parathyroid and parathyroid derivatives

E932.7 Thyroid and thyroid derivatives
    Dextrothyroxine   Liothyronine
    Levothyroxine sodium Thyroglobulin

E932.8 Antithyroid agents
    Iodides   Thiourea
    Thiouracil

E932.9 Other and unspecified hormones and synthetic substitutes

✓4th E933 Primarily systemic agents

E933.0 Antiallergic and antiemetic drugs
    Antihistamines   Diphenylpyraline
    Chlorpheniramine Thonzylamine
    Diphenhydramine   Tripelennamine
    EXCLUDES phenothiazine-based tranquilizers (E939.1)

E CODES

E933.1 Antineoplastic and immunosuppressive drugs
- Azathioprine
- Busulfan
- Chlorambucil
- Cyclophosphamide
- Cytarabine
- Fluorouracil
- Mechlorethamine hydrochloride
- Mercaptopurine
- Triethylenethiophosphoramide [thio-TEPA]

  EXCLUDES *antineoplastic antibiotics (E930.7)*

E933.2 Acidifying agents

E933.3 Alkalizing agents

E933.4 Enzymes, not elsewhere classified
- Penicillinase

E933.5 Vitamins, not elsewhere classified
- Vitamin A
- Vitamin D

  EXCLUDES *nicotinic acid (E942.2)*
  vitamin K (E934.3)

E933.8 Other systemic agents, not elsewhere classified
- Heavy metal antagonists

E933.9 Unspecified systemic agent

✓4th E934 Agents primarily affecting blood constituents

E934.0 Iron and its compounds
- Ferric salts
- Ferrous sulphate and other ferrous salts

E934.1 Liver preparations and other antianemic agents
- Folic acid

E934.2 Anticoagulants
- Coumarin
- Heparin
- Phenindione
- Prothrombin synthesis inhibitor
- Warfarin sodium

E934.3 Vitamin K [phytonadione]

E934.4 Fibrinolysis-affecting drugs
- Aminocaproic acid
- Streptokinase
- Streptodornase
- Urokinase

E934.5 Anticoagulant antagonists and other coagulants
- Hexadimethrine bromide
- Protamine sulfate

E934.6 Gamma globulin

E934.7 Natural blood and blood products
- Blood plasma
- Packed red cells
- Human fibrinogen
- Whole blood

E934.8 Other agents affecting blood constituents
- Macromolecular blood substitutes

E934.9 Unspecified agent affecting blood constituents

✓4th E935 Analgesics, antipyretics, and antirheumatics

E935.0 Heroin
- Diacetylmorphine

E935.1 Methadone

E935.2 Other opiates and related narcotics
- Codeine [methylmorphine]
- Morphine
- Meperidine [pethidine]
- Opium (alkaloids)

E935.3 Salicylates
Acetylsalicylic acid [aspirin]
Amino derivatives of salicylic acid
Salicylic acid salts

E935.4 Aromatic analgesics, not elsewhere classified
Acetanilid
Paracetamol [acetaminophen]
Phenacetin [acetophenetidin]

E935.5 Pyrazole derivatives
Aminophenazone [aminopyrine]
Phenylbutazone

E935.6 Antirheumatics [antiphlogistics]
Gold salts   Indomethacin
> **EXCLUDES** salicylates (E935.3)
> steroids (E932.0)

E935.7 Other non-narcotic analgesics
Pyrabital

E935.8 Other specified analgesics and antipyretics
Pentazocine

E935.9 Unspecified analgesic and antipyretic

✓4ᵗʰ **E936 Anticonvulsants and anti-Parkinsonism drugs**

E936.0 Oxazolidine derivatives
Paramethadione
Trimethadione

E936.1 Hydantoin derivatives
Phenytoin

E936.2 Succinimides
Ethosuximide
Phensuximide

E936.3 Other and unspecified anticonvulsants
Beclamide
Primidone

E936.4 Anti-Parkinsonism drugs
Amantadine
Ethopropazine [profenamine]
Levodopa [L-dopa]

✓4ᵗʰ **E937 Sedatives and hypnotics**

E937.0 Barbiturates
Amobarbital [amylobarbitone]   Pentobarbital [pentobarbitone]
Barbital [barbitone]   Phenobarbital [phenobarbitone]
Butabarbital [butabarbitone]   Secobarbital [quinalbarbitone]
> **EXCLUDES** thiobarbiturates (E938.3)

E937.1 Chloral hydrate group

E937.2 Paraldehyde

E937.3 Bromine compounds
Bromide
Carbromal (derivatives)

E937.4 Methaqualone compounds

E937.5 Glutethimide group

E937.6 Mixed sedatives, not elsewhere classified

E937.8 Other sedatives and hypnotics

E937.9 Unspecified
Sleeping:
 drug
 pill   } NOS
 tablet

E CODES

✓4th E938 Other central nervous system depressants and anesthetics
- **E938.0 Central nervous system muscle-tone depressants**
  - Chlorphenesin (carbamate)
  - Mephenesin
  - Methocarbamol
- **E938.1 Halothane**
- **E938.2 Other gaseous anesthetics**
  - Ether
  - Halogenated hydrocarbon derivatives, except halothane
  - Nitrous oxide
- **E938.3 Intravenous anesthetics**
  - Ketamine
  - Methohexital [methohexitone]
  - Thiobarbiturates, such as thiopental sodium
- **E938.4 Other and unspecified general anesthetics**
- **E938.5 Surface and infiltration anesthetics**
  - Cocaine
  - Procaine
  - Lidocaine [lignocaine]
  - Tetracaine
- **E938.6 Peripheral nerve- and plexus-blocking anesthetics**
- **E938.7 Spinal anesthetics**
- **E938.9 Other and unspecified local anesthetics**

✓4th E939 Psychotropic agents
- **E939.0 Antidepressants**
  - Amitriptyline
  - Imipramine
  - Monoamine oxidase [MAO] inhibitors
- **E939.1 Phenothiazine-based tranquilizers**
  - Chlorpromazine
  - Prochlorperazine
  - Fluphenazine
  - Promazine
  - Phenothiazine
- **E939.2 Butyrophenone-based tranquilizers**
  - Haloperidol
  - Trifluperidol
  - Spiperone
- **E939.3 Other antipsychotics, neuroleptics, and major tranquilizers**
- **E939.4 Benzodiazepine-based tranquilizers**
  - Chlordiazepoxide
  - Lorazepam
  - Diazepam
  - Medazepam
  - Flurazepam
  - Nitrazepam
- **E939.5 Other tranquilizers**
  - Hydroxyzine
  - Meprobamate
- **E939.6 Psychodysleptics [hallucinogens]**
  - Cannabis (derivatives)
  - Mescaline
  - Lysergide [LSD]
  - Psilocin
  - Marihuana (derivatives)
  - Psilocybin
- **E939.7 Psychostimulants**
  - Amphetamine
  - Caffeine
  - **EXCLUDES** central appetite depressants (E947.0)
- **E939.8 Other psychotropic agents**
- **E939.9 Unspecified psychotropic agent**

✓4th E940 Central nervous system stimulants
- **E940.0 Analeptics**
  - Lobeline
  - Nikethamide
- **E940.1 Opiate antagonists**
  - Levallorphan
  - Naloxone
  - Nalorphine

E940.8 Other specified central nervous system stimulants
E940.9 Unspecified central nervous system stimulant

✓4th **E941 Drugs primarily affecting the autonomic nervous system**
  E941.0 Parasympathomimetics [cholinergics]
    Acetylcholine   Pilocarpine
    Anticholinesterase:
      organophosphorus
      reversible
  E941.1 Parasympatholytics [anticholinergics and antimuscarinics] and spasmolytics
    Atropine   Hyoscine [scopolamine]
    Homatropine   Quaternary ammonium derivatives
    EXCLUDES papaverine (E942.5)
  E941.2 Sympathomimetics [adrenergics]
    Epinephrine [adrenalin]   Levarterenol [noradrenalin]
  E941.3 Sympatholytics [antiadrenergics]
    Phenoxybenzamine   Tolazolinehydrochloride
  E941.9 Unspecified drug primarily affecting the autonomic nervous system

✓4th **E942 Agents primarily affecting the cardiovascular system**
  E942.0 Cardiac rhythm regulators
    Practolol   Propranolol
    Procainamide   Quinidine
  E942.1 Cardiotonic glycosides and drugs of similar action
    Digitalis glycosides   Strophanthins
    Digoxin
  E942.2 Antilipemic and antiarteriosclerotic drugs
    Cholestyramine   Nicotinic acid derivatives
    Clofibrate   Sitosterols
    EXCLUDES dextrothyroxine (E932.7)
  E942.3 Ganglion-blocking agents
    Pentamethonium bromide
  E942.4 Coronary vasodilators
    Dipyridamole   Nitrites
    Nitrates [nitroglycerin]   Prenylamine
  E942.5 Other vasodilators
    Cyclandelate   Hydralazine
    Diazoxide   Papaverine
  E942.6 Other antihypertensive agents
    Clonidine   Rauwolfia alkaloids
    Guanethidine   Reserpine
  E942.7 Antivaricose drugs, including sclerosing agents
    Monoethanolamine   Zinc salts
  E942.8 Capillary-active drugs
    Adrenochrome derivatives
    Bioflavonoids
    Metaraminol
  E942.9 Other and unspecified agents primarily affecting the cardiovascular system

✓4th **E943 Agents primarily affecting gastrointestinal system**
  E943.0 Antacids and antigastric secretion drugs
    Aluminum hydroxide   Magnesium trisilicate
  E943.1 Irritant cathartics
    Bisacodyl   Phenolphthalein
    Castor oil
  E943.2 Emollient cathartics
    Sodium dioctyl sulfosuccinate
  E943.3 Other cathartics, including intestinal atonia drugs
    Magnesium sulfate

E CODES

E943.4 Digestants
    Pancreatin   Pepsin
    Papain

E943.5 Antidiarrheal drugs
    Bismuth subcarbonate   Pectin
    Kaolin
    EXCLUDES anti-infectives (E930.0-E931.9)

E943.6 Emetics

E943.8 Other specified agents primarily affecting the gastrointestinal system

E943.9 Unspecified agent primarily affecting the gastrointestinal system

✓4th **E944 Water, mineral, and uric acid metabolism drugs**

E944.0 Mercurial diuretics
    Chlormerodrin   Mercurophylline
    Mercaptomerin   Mersalyl

E944.1 Purine derivative diuretics
    Theobromine   Theophylline
    EXCLUDES aminophylline [theophylline ethylenediamine] (E945.7)

E944.2 Carbonic acid anhydrase inhibitors
    Acetazolamide

E944.3 Saluretics
    Benzothiadiazides   Chlorothiazide group

E944.4 Other diuretics
    Ethacrynic acid   Furosemide

E944.5 Electrolytic, caloric, and water-balance agents

E944.6 Other mineral salts, not elsewhere classified

E944.7 Uric acid metabolism drugs
    Cinchophen and congeners   Phenoquin
    Colchicine   Probenecid

✓4th **E945 Agents primarily acting on the smooth and skeletal muscles and respiratory system**

E945.0 Oxytocic agents
    Ergot alkaloids   Prostaglandins

E945.1 Smooth muscle relaxants
    Adiphenine   Metaproterenol [orciprenaline]
    EXCLUDES papaverine (E942.5)

E945.2 Skeletal muscle relaxants
    Alcuronium chloride   Suxamethonium chloride

E945.3 Other and unspecified drugs acting on muscles

E945.4 Antitussives
    Dextromethorphan   Pipazethate hydrochloride

E945.5 Expectorants
    Acetylcysteine   Ipecacuanha
    Cocillana   Terpin hydrate
    Guaifenesin [glyceryl guaiacolate]

E945.6 Anti-common cold drugs

E945.7 Antiasthmatics
    Aminophylline [theophylline ethylenediamine]

E945.8 Other and unspecified respiratory drugs

✓4th **E946 Agents primarily affecting skin and mucous membrane, ophthalmological, otorhinolaryngological, and dental drugs**

E946.0 Local anti-infectives and anti-inflammatory drugs

E946.1 Antipruritics

E946.2 Local astringents and local detergents

E946.3 Emollients, demulcents, and protectants

E946.4 Keratolytics, kerstoplastics, other hair treatment drugs and preparations
E946.5 Eye anti-infectives and other eye drugs
   Idoxuridine
E946.6 Anti-infectives and other drugs and preparations for ear, nose, and throat
E946.7 Dental drugs topically applied
E946.8 Other agents primarily affecting skin and mucous membrane
   Spermicides
E946.9 Unspecified agent primarily affecting skin and mucous membrane

√4th **E947** Other and unspecified drugs and medicinal substances
   E947.0 Dietetics
   E947.1 Lipotropic drugs
   E947.2 Antidotes and chelating agents, not elsewhere classified
   E947.3 Alcohol deterrents
   E947.4 Pharmaceutical excipients
   E947.8 Other drugs and medicinal substances
      Contrast media used for diagnostic x-ray procedures
      Diagnostic agents and kits
   E947.9 Unspecified drug or medicinal substance

√4th **E948** Bacterial vaccines
   E948.0 BCG vaccine
   E948.1 Typhoid and paratyphoid
   E948.2 Cholera
   E948.3 Plague
   E948.4 Tetanus
   E948.5 Diphtheria
   E948.6 Pertussis vaccine, including combinations with a pertussis component
   E948.8 Other and unspecified bacterial vaccines
   E948.9 Mixed bacterial vaccines, except combinations with a pertussis component

√4th **E949** Other vaccines and biological substances
   EXCLUDES   *gamma globulin (E934.6)*
   E949.0 Smallpox vaccine
   E949.1 Rabies vaccine
   E949.2 Typhus vaccine
   E949.3 Yellow fever vaccine
   E949.4 Measles vaccine
   E949.5 Poliomyelitis vaccine
   E949.6 Other and unspecified viral and rickettsial vaccines
      Mumps vaccine
   E949.7 Mixed viral-rickettsial and bacterial vaccines, except combinations with a pertussis component
      EXCLUDES   *combinations with a pertussis component (E948.6)*
   E949.9 Other and unspecified vaccines and biological substances

SUICIDE AND SELF-INFLICTED INJURY (E950-E959)
   INCLUDES   injuries in suicide and attempted suicide
      self-inflicted injuries specified as intentional

√4th **E950** Suicide and self-inflicted poisoning by solid or liquid substances
   E950.0 Analgesics, antipyretics, and antirheumatics
   E950.1 Barbiturates
   E950.2 Other sedatives and hypnotics
   E950.3 Tranquilizers and other psychotropic agents
   E950.4 Other specified drugs and medicinal substances

E CODES

E950.5–E958.9

- E950.5 Unspecified drug or medicinal substance
- E950.6 Agricultural and horticultural chemical and pharmaceutical preparations other than plant foods and fertilizers
- E950.7 Corrosive and caustic substances
  - Suicide and self-inflicted poisoning by substances classifiable to E864
- E950.8 Arsenic and its compounds
- E950.9 Other and unspecified solid and liquid substances

✓4th **E951 Suicide and self-inflicted poisoning by gases in domestic use**
- E951.0 Gas distributed by pipeline
- E951.1 Liquefied petroleum gas distributed in mobile containers
- E951.8 Other utility gas

✓4th **E952 Suicide and self-inflicted poisoning by other gases and vapors**
- E952.0 Motor vehicle exhaust gas
- E952.1 Other carbon monoxide
- E952.8 Other specified gases and vapors
- E952.9 Unspecified gases and vapors

✓4th **E953 Suicide and self-inflicted injury by hanging, strangulation, and suffocation**
- E953.0 Hanging
- E953.1 Suffocation by plastic bag
- E953.8 Other specified means
- E953.9 Unspecified means

E954 Suicide and self-inflicted injury by submersion [drowning]

✓4th **E955 Suicide and self-inflicted injury by firearms, air guns and explosives**
- E955.0 Handgun
- E955.1 Shotgun
- E955.2 Hunting rifle
- E955.3 Military firearms
- E955.4 Other and unspecified firearm
  - Gunshot NOS   Shot NOS
- E955.5 Explosives
- E955.6 Air gun
  - BB gun
  - Pellet gun
- ● E955.7 Paintball gun
- E955.9 Unspecified

E956 Suicide and self-inflicted injury by cutting and piercing instrument

✓4th **E957 Suicide and self-inflicted injuries by jumping from high place**
- E957.0 Residential premises
- E957.1 Other man-made structures
- E957.2 Natural sites
- E957.9 Unspecified

✓4th **E958 Suicide and self-inflicted injury by other and unspecified means**
- E958.0 Jumping or lying before moving object
- E958.1 Burns, fire
- E958.2 Scald
- E958.3 Extremes of cold
- E958.4 Electrocution
- E958.5 Crashing of motor vehicle
- E958.6 Crashing of aircraft
- E958.7 Caustic substances, except poisoning
  - **EXCLUDES** poisoning by caustic substance (E950.7)
- E958.8 Other specified means
- E958.9 Unspecified means

✓4th Fourth-digit Required   ▶◀ Revised Text   ● New Code   ▲ Revised Code Title

E959 Late effects of self-inflicted injury

Note: This category is to be used to indicate circumstances classifiable to E950-E958 as the cause of death or disability from late effects, which are themselves classifiable elsewhere. The "late effects" include conditions reported as such, or as sequelae which may occur at any time after the attempted suicide or self-inflicted injury.

HOMICIDE AND INJURY PURPOSELY INFLICTED BY OTHER PERSONS (E960-E969)

INCLUDES injuries inflicted by another person with intent to injure or kill, by any means

EXCLUDES injuries due to:
  legal intervention (E970-E978)
  operations of war (E990-E999)
  ▶terrorism (979)◀

✓4th E960 Fight, brawl, rape

E960.0 Unarmed fight or brawl
  Beatings NOS
  Brawl or fight with hands, fists, feet
  Injured or killed in fight NOS
  EXCLUDES homicidal:
    injury by weapons (E965.0-E966, E969)
    strangulation (E963)
    submersion (E964)

E960.1 Rape

E961 Assault by corrosive or caustic substance, except poisoning

Injury or death purposely caused by corrosive or caustic substance, such as:
  acid [any]
  corrosive substance
  vitriol
EXCLUDES burns from hot liquid (E968.3)
  chemical burns from swallowing a corrosive substance (E962.0-E962.9)

✓4th E962 Assault by poisoning

E962.0 Drugs and medicinal substances
  Homicidal poisoning by any drug or medicinal substance

E962.1 Other solid and liquid substances

E962.2 Other gases and vapors

E962.9 Unspecified poisoning

E963 Assault by hanging and strangulation

Homicidal (attempt):   Homicidal (attempt):
  garrotting or ligature   strangulation
  hanging   suffocation

E964 Assault by submersion [drowning]

✓4th E965 Assault by firearms and explosives

E965.0 Handgun
  Pistol   Revolver

E965.1 Shotgun

E965.2 Hunting rifle

E965.3 Military firearms

E965.4 Other and unspecified firearm

E965.5 Antipersonnel bomb

E965.6 Gasoline bomb

E965.7 Letter bomb

E965.8 Other specified explosive
  Bomb NOS (placed in):   Dynamite
    car
    house

E CODES

E965.9 Unspecified explosive

E966 Assault by cutting and piercing instrument
    Assassination (attempt), homicide (attempt) by any instrument classifiable under E920

Homicidal:
    cut
    puncture   } any part of body
    stab
    Stabbed

✓4th **E967 Perpetrator of child and adult abuse**
    Note: Selection of the correct perpetrator code is based on the relationship between the perpetrator and the victim.

E967.0 By father, stepfather, or boyfriend
    Male partner of child's parent or guardian

E967.1 By other specified person

E967.2 By mother, stepmother, or girlfriend
    Female partner of child's parent or guardian

E967.3 By spouse or partner
    Abuse of spouse or partner by ex-spouse or ex-partner

E967.4 By child

E967.5 By sibling

E967.6 By grandparent

E967.7 By other relative

E967.8 By non-related caregiver

E967.9 By unspecified person

✓4th **E968 Assault by other and unspecified means**

E968.0 Fire
    Arson
    Homicidal burns NOS
    EXCLUDES *burns from hot liquid (E968.3)*

E968.1 Pushing from a high place

E968.2 Striking by blunt or thrown object

E968.3 Hot liquid
    Homicidal burns by scalding

E968.4 Criminal neglect
    Abandonment of child, infant, or other helpless person with intent to injure or kill

E968.5 Transport vehicle
    Being struck by other vehicle or run down with intent to injure
    Pushed in front of, thrown from, or dragged by moving vehicle with intent to injure

E968.6 Air gun
    BB gun   Pellet gun

E968.7 Human bite

E968.8 Other specified means

E968.9 Unspecified means
    Assassination (attempt) NOS
    Homicidal (attempt):
        injury NOS   wound NOS
    Manslaughter (nonaccidental)
    Murder (attempt) NOS
    Violence, non-accidental

E969 Late effects of injury purposely inflicted by other person

Note: This category is to be used to indicate circumstances classifiable to E960-E968 as the cause of death or disability from late effects, which are themselves classifiable elsewhere. The "late effects" include conditions reported as such, or as sequelae which may occur at any time after injury purposely inflicted by another person.

LEGAL INTERVENTION (E970-E978)

INCLUDES injuries inflicted by the police or other law-enforcing agents, including military on duty, in the course of arresting or attempting to arrest lawbreakers, suppressing disturbances, maintaining order, and other legal action

legal execution

EXCLUDES *injuries caused by civil insurrections (E990.0-E999)*

E970 Injury due to legal intervention by firearms
- Gunshot wound
- Injury by:
  - machine gun
  - revolver
- Injury by:
  - rifle pellet or rubber bullet
  - shot NOS

E971 Injury due to legal intervention by explosives
- Injury by:
  - dynamite
  - explosive shell
- Injury by:
  - grenade
  - mortar bomb

E972 Injury due to legal intervention by gas
- Asphyxiation by gas
- Injury by tear gas
- Poisoning by gas

E973 Injury due to legal intervention by blunt object
- Hit, struck by:
  - baton (nightstick)
  - blunt object
- Hit, struck by:
  - stave

E974 Injury due to legal intervention by cutting and piercing instrument
- Cut
- Incised wound
- Injured by bayonet
- Stab wound

E975 Injury due to legal intervention by other specified means
- Blow
- Manhandling

E976 Injury due to legal intervention by unspecified means

E977 Late effects of injuries due to legal intervention

Note: This category is to be used to indicate circumstances classifiable to E970-E976 as the cause of death or disability from late effects, which are themselves classifiable elsewhere. The "late effects" include conditions reported as such, or as sequelae, which may occur at any time after the injury due to legal intervention.

E978 Legal execution

All executions performed at the behest of the judiciary or ruling authority [whether permanent or temporary] as:
- asphyxiation by gas
- beheading, decapitation (by guillotine)
- capital punishment
- electrocution
- hanging
- poisoning
- shooting
- other specified means

E CODES

TERRORISM (E979)

- ✓4th **E979 Terrorism**
    Injuries resulting from the unlawful use of force or violence against persons or property to intimidate or coerce a Government, the civilian population, or any segment thereof, in furtherance of political or social objective

- **E979.0 Terrorism involving explosion of marine weapons**
    Depth-charge
    Marine mine
    Mine NOS, at sea or in harbour
    Sea-based artillery shell
    Torpedo
    Underwater blast

- **E979.1 Terrorism involving destruction of aircraft**
    Aircraft used as a weapon
    Aircraft:
        burned
        exploded
        shot down
    Crushed by falling aircraft

- **E979.2 Terrorism involving other explosions and fragments**
    Antipersonnel bomb (fragments)
    Blast NOS
    Explosion (of):
        artillery shell
        breech-block
        cannon block
        mortar bomb
        munitions being used in terrorism
        NOS
    Fragments from:
        artillery shell
        bomb
        grenade
        guided missile
        land-mine
        rocket
        shell
        shrapnel
    Mine NOS

- **E979.3 Terrorism involving fires, conflagraton and hot substances**
    Burning building or structure:
        collapse of
        fall from
        hit by falling object in
        jump from
    Conflagraton NOS
    Fire (causing):
        Asphyxia
        Burns
        NOS
        Other injury
    Melting of fittings and furniture in burning
    Petrol bomb
    Smouldering building or structure

✓4th Fourth-digit Required ▶◀ Revised Text ● New Code ▲ Revised Code Title

- **E979.4 Terrorism involving firearms**
    Bullet:
        carbine
        machine gun
        pistol
        rifle
        rubber (rifle)
    Pellets (shotgun)

- **E979.5 Terrorism involving nuclear weapons**
    Blast effects
    Exposure to ionizing radiation from nuclear weapon
    Fireball effects
    Heat from nuclear weapon
    Other direct and secondary effects of nuclear weapons

- **E979.6 Terrorism involving biological weapons**
    Anthrax
    Cholera
    Smallpox

- **E979.7 Terrorism involving chemical weapons**
    Gases, fumes, chemicals
    Hydrogen cyanide
    Phosgene
    Sarin

- **E979.8 Terrorism involving other means**
    Drowning and submersion
    Lasers
    Piercing or stabbing instruments
    Terrorism NOS

- **E979.9 Terrorism, secondary effects**
    Note: This code is for use to identify conditions occurring subsequent to a terrorist attack not those that are due to the initial terrorist act
    EXCLUDES late effect of terrorist attack (E999.1)

INJURY UNDETERMINED WHETHER ACCIDENTALLY OR PURPOSELY INFLICTED (E980-E989)

Note: Categories E980-E989 are for use when it is unspecified or it cannot be determined whether the injuries are accidental (unintentional), suicide (attempted), or assault.

√4th **E980 Poisoning by solid or liquid substances, undetermined whether accidentally or purposely inflicted**

E980.0 Analgesics, antipyretics, and antirheumatics

E980.1 Barbiturates

E980.2 Other sedatives and hypnotics

E980.3 Tranquilizers and other psychotropic agents

E980.4 Other specified drugs and medicinal substances

E980.5 Unspecified drug or medicinal substance

E980.6 Corrosive and caustic substances
    Poisoning, undetermined whether accidental or purposeful, by substances classifiable to E864

E980.7 Agricultural and horticultural chemical and pharmaceutical preparations other than plant foods and fertilizers

E980.8 Arsenic and its compounds

E980.9 Other and unspecified solid and liquid substances

√4th **E981 Poisoning by gases in domestic use, undetermined whether accidentally or purposely inflicted**

E CODES

      E981.0 Gas distributed by pipeline
      E981.1 Liquefied petroleum gas distributed in mobile containers
      E981.8 Other utility gas

✓4th **E982** Poisoning by other gases, undetermined whether accidentally or purposely inflicted
      E982.0 Motor vehicle exhaust gas
      E982.1 Other carbon monoxide
      E982.8 Other specified gases and vapors
      E982.9 Unspecified gases and vapors

✓4th **E983** Hanging, strangulation, or suffocation, undetermined whether accidentally or purposely inflicted
      E983.0 Hanging
      E983.1 Suffocation by plastic bag
      E983.8 Other specified means
      E983.9 Unspecified means

E984 Submersion [drowning], undetermined whether accidentally or purposely inflicted

✓4th **E985** Injury by firearms, air guns and explosives, undetermined whether accidentally or purposely inflicted
      E985.0 Handgun
      E985.1 Shotgun
      E985.2 Hunting rifle
      E985.3 Military firearms
      E985.4 Other and unspecified firearm
      E985.5 Explosives
      E985.6 Air gun
            BB gun
            Pellet gun
●   E985.7 Paintball gun

E986 Injury by cutting and piercing instruments, undetermined whether accidentally or purposely inflicted

✓4th **E987** Falling from high place, undetermined whether accidentally or purposely inflicted
      E987.0 Residential premises
      E987.1 Other man-made structures
      E987.2 Natural sites
      E987.9 Unspecified site

✓4th **E988** Injury by other and unspecified means, undetermined whether accidentally or purposely inflicted
      E988.0 Jumping or lying before moving object
      E988.1 Burns, fire
      E988.2 Scald
      E988.3 Extremes of cold
      E988.4 Electrocution
      E988.5 Crashing of motor vehicle
      E988.6 Crashing of aircraft
      E988.7 Caustic substances, except poisoning
      E988.8 Other specified means
      E988.9 Unspecified means

✓4th Fourth-digit Required   ▶◀ Revised Text   ● New Code   ▲ Revised Code Title

E989 Late effects of injury, undetermined whether accidentally or purposely inflicted

Note: This category is to be used to indicate circumstances classifiable to E980-E988 as the cause of death or disability from late effects, which are themselves classifiable elsewhere. The "late effects" include conditions reported as such, or as sequelae, which may occur at any time after injury, undetermined whether accidentally or purposely inflicted.

INJURY RESULTING FROM OPERATIONS OF WAR (E990-E999)

INCLUDES injuries to military personnel and civilians caused by war and civil insurrections and occurring during the time of war and insurrection

EXCLUDES accidents during training of military personnel manufacture of war material and transport, unless attributable to enemy action

✓4th E990 Injury due to war operations by fires and conflagrations

INCLUDES asphyxia, burns, or other injury originating from fire caused by a fire-producing device or indirectly by any conventional weapon

- **E990.0 From gasoline bomb**
- **E990.9 From other and unspecified source**

✓4th E991 Injury due to war operations by bullets and fragments

- **E991.0 Rubber bullets (rifle)**
- **E991.1 Pellets (rifle)**
- **E991.2 Other bullets**

    Bullet [any, except rubber bullets and pellets]
    - carbine
    - machine gun
    - pistol
    - rifle
    - shotgun

- **E991.3 Antipersonnel bomb (fragments)**
- **E991.9 Other and unspecified fragments**

    Fragments from:
    - artillery shell
    - bombs, except anti-personnel
    - grenade
    - guided missile

    Fragments from:
    - land mine
    - rockets
    - shell
    - Shrapnel

E992 Injury due to war operations by explosion of marine weapons

- Depth charge
- Marine mines
- Mine NOS, at sea or in harbor
- Sea-based artillery shell
- Torpedo
- Underwater blast

E993 Injury due to war operations by other explosion

- Accidental explosion of munitions being used in war
- Accidental explosion of own weapons
- Air blast NOS
- Blast NOS
- Explosion NOS
- Explosion of:
    - artillery shell
    - breech block
    - cannon block
    - mortar bomb
- Injury by weapon burst

E994 Injury due to war operations by destruction of aircraft

- Airplane:
    - burned
    - exploded
- Airplane:
    - shot down
- Crushed by falling airplane

E995 Injury due to war operations by other and unspecified forms of conventional warfare

- Battle wounds
- Bayonet injury
- Drowned in war operations

E CODES

E996 Injury due to war operations by nuclear weapons
    Blast effects
    Exposure to ionizing radiation from nuclear weapons
    Fireball effects
    Heat
    Other direct and secondary effects of nuclear weapons

✓4ᵗʰ **E997 Injury due to war operations by other forms of unconventional warfare**
    E997.0 Lasers
    E997.1 Biological warfare
    E997.2 Gases, fumes, and chemicals
    E997.8 Other specified forms of unconventional warfare
    E997.9 Unspecified form of unconventional warfare

E998 Injury due to war operations but occurring after cessation of hostilities
    Injuries due to operations of war but occurring after cessation of hostilities by any means classifiable under E990-E997
    Injuries by explosion of bombs or mines placed in the course of operations of war, if the explosion occurred after cessation of hostilities

E999 Late effect of injury due to war operations
    ▶Note: This category is to be used to indicate circumstances classifiable to E979, E990-E998 as the cause of death or disability from late effects, which are themselves classifiable elsewhere. The "late effects" include conditions reported as such, or as sequelae, which may occur at any time after the injury, resulting from operations of war or terrorism◀

- **E999.0 Late effect of injury due to war operations**
- **E999.1 Late effect of injury due to terrorism**

Notes

Official ICD•9•CM Government Appendixes

MORPHOLOGY OF NEOPLASMS

The World Health Organization has published an adaptation of the International Classification of Diseases for oncology (ICD-O). It contains a coded nomenclature for the morphology of neoplasms, which is reproduced here for those who wish to use it in conjunction with Chapter 2 of the International Classification of Diseases, 9th Revision, Clinical Modification.

The morphology code numbers consist of five digits; the first four identify the histological type of the neoplasm and the fifth indicates its behavior. The one-digit behavior code is as follows:

/0 Benign
/1 Uncertain whether benign or malignant
    Borderline malignancy
/2 Carcinoma in situ
    Intraepithelial
    Noninfiltrating
    Noninvasive
/3 Malignant, primary site
/6 Malignant, metastatic site
    Secondary site
/9 Malignant, uncertain whether primary or metastatic site

In the nomenclature below, the morphology code numbers include the behavior code appropriate to the histological type of neoplasm, but this behavior code should be changed if other reported information makes this necessary. For example, "chordoma (M9370/3)" is assumed to be malignant; the term "benign chordoma" should be coded M9370/0. Similarly, "superficial spreading adenocarcinoma (M8143/3)" described as "noninvasive" should be coded M8143/2 and "melanoma (M8720/3)" described as "secondary" should be coded M8720/6.

The following table shows the correspondence between the morphology code and the different sections of Chapter 2:

Morphology Code Histology/Behavior			ICD-9-CM Chapter 2
Any	0	210-229	Benign neoplasms
M8000-M8004	1	239	Neoplasms of unspecified nature
M8010+	1	235-238	Neoplasms of uncertain behavior
Any	2	230-234	Carcinoma in situ
Any	3	140-195 200-208	Malignant neoplasms, stated or presumed to be primary
Any	6	196-198	Malignant neoplasms, stated or presumed to be secondary

The ICD-O behavior digit /9 is inapplicable in an ICD context, since all malignant neoplasms are presumed to be primary (/3) or secondary (/6) according to other information on the medical record.

Only the first-listed term of the full ICD-O morphology nomenclature appears against each code number in the list below. The ICD-9-CM Alphabetical Index (Volume 2), however, includes all the ICD-O synonyms as well as a number of other morphological names still likely to be encountered on medical records but omitted from ICD-O as outdated or otherwise undesirable.

A coding difficulty sometimes arises where a morphological diagnosis contains two qualifying adjectives that have different code numbers. An example is "transitional cell epidermoid carcinoma." "Transitional cell carcinoma NOS" is M8120/3 and "epidermoid carcinoma NOS" is M8070/3. In such circumstances, the higher number (M8120/3 in this example) should be used, as it is usually more specific.

CODED NOMENCLATURE FOR MORPHOLOGY OF NEOPLASMS

M800 Neoplasms NOS
M8000/0 Neoplasm, benign
M8000/1 Neoplasm, uncertain whether benign or malignant
M8000/3 Neoplasm, malignant
M8000/6 Neoplasm, metastatic
M8000/9 Neoplasm, malignant, uncertain whether primary or metastatic
M8001/0 Tumor cells, benign
M8001/1 Tumor cells, uncertain whether benign or malignant
M8001/3 Tumor cells, malignant
M8002/3 Malignant tumor, small cell type
M8003/3 Malignant tumor, giant cell type
M8004/3 Malignant tumor, fusiform cell type

M801-M804 Epithelial neoplasms NOS
M8010/0 Epithelial tumor, benign
M8010/2 Carcinoma in situ NOS
M8010/3 Carcinoma NOS
M8010/6 Carcinoma, metastatic NOS
M8010/9 Carcinomatosis

2002 Ingenix, Inc.

Appendix A: Morphology of Neoplasms

APPENDIX A: MORPHOLOGY OF NEOPLASMS

M8011/0	Epithelioma, benign	**M812-M813**	**Transitional cell papillomas and carcinomas**
M8011/3	Epithelioma, malignant		
M8012/3	Large cell carcinoma NOS	M8120/0	Transitional cell papilloma NOS
M8020/3	Carcinoma, undifferentiated type NOS	M8120/1	Urothelial papilloma
M8021/3	Carcinoma, anaplastic type NOS	M8120/2	Transitional cell carcinoma in situ
M8022/3	Pleomorphic carcinoma	M8120/3	Transitional cell carcinoma NOS
M8030/3	Giant cell and spindle cell carcinoma	M8121/0	Schneiderian papilloma
M8031/3	Giant cell carcinoma	M8121/1	Transitional cell papilloma, inverted type
M8032/3	Spindle cell carcinoma		
M8033/3	Pseudosarcomatous carcinoma	M8121/3	Schneiderian carcinoma
M8034/3	Polygonal cell carcinoma	M8122/3	Transitional cell carcinoma, spindle cell type
M8035/3	Spheroidal cell carcinoma		
M8040/1	Tumorlet	M8123/3	Basaloid carcinoma
M8041/3	Small cell carcinoma NOS	M8124/3	Cloacogenic carcinoma
M8042/3	Oat cell carcinoma	M8130/3	Papillary transitional cell carcinoma
M8043/3	Small cell carcinoma, fusiform cell type	**M814-M838**	**Adenomas and adenocarcinomas**
M805-M808	**Papillary and squamous cell neoplasms**		
		M8140/0	Adenoma NOS
M8050/0	Papilloma NOS (except Papilloma of urinary bladder M8120/1)	M8140/1	Bronchial adenoma NOS
		M8140/2	Adenocarcinoma in situ
M8050/2	Papillary carcinoma in situ	M8140/3	Adenocarcinoma NOS
M8050/3	Papillary carcinoma NOS	M8140/6	Adenocarcinoma, metastatic NOS
M8051/0	Verrucous papilloma	M8141/3	Scirrhous adenocarcinoma
M8051/3	Verrucous carcinoma NOS	M8142/3	Linitis plastica
M8052/0	Squamous cell papilloma	M8143/3	Superficial spreading adenocarcinoma
M8052/3	Papillary squamous cell carcinoma	M8144/3	Adenocarcinoma, intestinal type
M8053/0	Inverted papilloma	M8145/3	Carcinoma, diffuse type
M8060/0	Papillomatosis NOS	M8146/0	Monomorphic adenoma
M8070/2	Squamous cell carcinoma in situ NOS	M8147/0	Basal cell adenoma
M8070/3	Squamous cell carcinoma NOS	M8150/0	Islet cell adenoma
M8070/6	Squamous cell carcinoma, metastatic NOS	M8150/3	Islet cell carcinoma
		M8151/0	Insulinoma NOS
M8071/3	Squamous cell carcinoma, keratinizing type NOS	M8151/3	Insulinoma, malignant
		M8152/0	Glucagonoma NOS
M8072/3	Squamous cell carcinoma, large cell, nonkeratinizing type	M8152/3	Glucagonoma, malignant
		M8153/1	Gastrinoma NOS
M8073/3	Squamous cell carcinoma, small cell, nonkeratinizing type	M8153/3	Gastrinoma, malignant
		M8154/3	Mixed islet cell and exocrine adenocarcinoma
M8074/3	Squamous cell carcinoma, spindle cell type		
		M8160/0	Bile duct adenoma
M8075/3	Adenoid squamous cell carcinoma	M8160/3	Cholangiocarcinoma
M8076/2	Squamous cell carcinoma in situ with questionable stromal invasion	M8161/0	Bile duct cystadenoma
		M8161/3	Bile duct cystadenocarcinoma
M8076/3	Squamous cell carcinoma, microinvasive	M8170/0	Liver cell adenoma
		M8170/3	Hepatocellular carcinoma NOS
M8080/2	Queyrat's erythroplasia	M8180/0	Hepatocholangioma, benign
M8081/2	Bowen's disease	M8180/3	Combined hepatocellular carcinoma and cholangiocarcinoma
M8082/3	Lymphoepithelial carcinoma		
M809-M811	**Basal cell neoplasms**	M8190/0	Trabecular adenoma
M8090/1	Basal cell tumor	M8190/3	Trabecular adenocarcinoma
M8090/3	Basal cell carcinoma NOS	M8191/0	Embryonal adenoma
M8091/3	Multicentric basal cell carcinoma	M8200/0	Eccrine dermal cylindroma
M8092/3	Basal cell carcinoma, morphea type	M8200/3	Adenoid cystic carcinoma
M8093/3	Basal cell carcinoma, fibroepithelial type	M8201/3	Cribriform carcinoma
		M8210/0	Adenomatous polyp NOS
M8094/3	Basosquamous carcinoma	M8210/3	Adenocarcinoma in adenomatous polyp
M8095/3	Metatypical carcinoma	M8211/0	Tubular adenoma NOS
M8096/0	Intraepidermal epithelioma of Jadassohn	M8211/3	Tubular adenocarcinoma
		M8220/0	Adenomatous polyposis coli
M8100/0	Trichoepithelioma	M8220/3	Adenocarcinoma in adenomatous polyposis coli
M8101/0	Trichofolliculoma		
M8102/0	Tricholemmoma	M8221/0	Multiple adenomatous polyps
M8110/0	Pilomatrixoma	M8230/3	Solid carcinoma NOS
		M8231/3	Carcinoma simplex

APPENDIX A: MORPHOLOGY OF NEOPLASMS

M8240/1	Carcinoid tumor NOS	M8375/0	Adrenal cortical adenoma, mixed cell type
M8240/3	Carcinoid tumor, malignant		
M8241/1	Carcinoid tumor, argentaffin NOS	M8380/0	Endometrioid adenoma NOS
M8241/3	Carcinoid tumor, argentaffin, malignant	M8380/1	Endometrioid adenoma, borderline malignancy
M8242/1	Carcinoid tumor, nonargentaffin NOS		
M8242/3	Carcinoid tumor, nonargentaffin, malignant	M8380/3	Endometrioid carcinoma
		M8381/0	Endometrioid adenofibroma NOS
M8243/3	Mucocarcinoid tumor, malignant	M8381/1	Endometrioid adenofibroma, borderline malignancy
M8244/3	Composite carcinoid		
M8250/1	Pulmonary adenomatosis	M8381/3	Endometrioid adenofibroma, malignant
M8250/3	Bronchiolo-alveolar adenocarcinoma	**M839-M842 Adnexal and skin appendage neoplasms**	
M8251/0	Alveolar adenoma		
M8251/3	Alveolar adenocarcinoma	M8390/0	Skin appendage adenoma
M8260/0	Papillary adenoma NOS	M8390/3	Skin appendage carcinoma
M8260/3	Papillary adenocarcinoma NOS	M8400/0	Sweat gland adenoma
M8261/1	Villous adenoma NOS	M8400/1	Sweat gland tumor NOS
M8261/3	Adenocarcinoma in villous adenoma	M8400/3	Sweat gland adenocarcinoma
M8262/3	Villous adenocarcinoma	M8401/0	Apocrine adenoma
M8263/0	Tubulovillous adenoma	M8401/3	Apocrine adenocarcinoma
M8270/0	Chromophobe adenoma	M8402/0	Eccrine acrospiroma
M8270/3	Chromophobe carcinoma	M8403/0	Eccrine spiradenoma
M8280/0	Acidophil adenoma	M8404/0	Hidrocystoma
M8280/3	Acidophil carcinoma	M8405/0	Papillary hydradenoma
M8281/0	Mixed acidophil-basophil adenoma	M8406/0	Papillary syringadenoma
M8281/3	Mixed acidophil-basophil carcinoma	M8407/0	Syringoma NOS
M8290/0	Oxyphilic adenoma	M8410/0	Sebaceous adenoma
M8290/3	Oxyphilic adenocarcinoma	M8410/3	Sebaceous adenocarcinoma
M8300/0	Basophil adenoma	M8420/0	Ceruminous adenoma
M8300/3	Basophil carcinoma	M8420/3	Ceruminous adenocarcinoma
M8310/0	Clear cell adenoma	**M843 Mucoepidermoid neoplasms**	
M8310/3	Clear cell adenocarcinoma NOS	M8430/1	Mucoepidermoid tumor
M8311/1	Hypernephroid tumor	M8430/3	Mucoepidermoid carcinoma
M8312/3	Renal cell carcinoma	**M844-M849 Cystic, mucinous, and serous neoplasms**	
M8313/0	Clear cell adenofibroma		
M8320/3	Granular cell carcinoma	M8440/0	Cystadenoma NOS
M8321/0	Chief cell adenoma	M8440/3	Cystadenocarcinoma NOS
M8322/0	Water-clear cell adenoma	M8441/0	Serous cystadenoma NOS
M8322/3	Water-clear cell adenocarcinoma	M8441/1	Serous cystadenoma, borderline malignancy
M8323/0	Mixed cell adenoma		
M8323/3	Mixed cell adenocarcinoma	M8441/3	Serous cystadenocarcinoma NOS
M8324/0	Lipoadenoma	M8450/0	Papillary cystadenoma NOS
M8330/0	Follicular adenoma	M8450/1	Papillary cystadenoma, borderline malignancy
M8330/3	Follicular adenocarcinoma NOS		
M8331/3	Follicular adenocarcinoma, well differentiated type	M8450/3	Papillary cystadenocarcinoma NOS
		M8460/0	Papillary serous cystadenoma NOS
M8332/3	Follicular adenocarcinoma, trabecular type	M8460/1	Papillary serous cystadenoma, borderline malignancy
		M8460/3	Papillary serous cystadenocarcinoma
M8333/0	Microfollicular adenoma		
M8334/0	Macrofollicular adenoma	M8461/0	Serous surface papilloma NOS
M8340/3	Papillary and follicular adenocarcinoma	M8461/1	Serous surface papilloma, borderline malignancy
M8350/3	Nonencapsulated sclerosing carcinoma	M8461/3	Serous surface papillary carcinoma
M8360/1	Multiple endocrine adenomas	M8470/0	Mucinous cystadenoma NOS
M8361/1	Juxtaglomerular tumor	M8470/1	Mucinous cystadenoma, borderline malignancy
M8370/0	Adrenal cortical adenoma NOS		
M8370/3	Adrenal cortical carcinoma	M8470/3	Mucinous cystadenocarcinoma NOS
M8371/0	Adrenal cortical adenoma, compact cell type	M8471/0	Papillary mucinous cystadenoma NOS
		M8471/1	Papillary mucinous cystadenoma, borderline malignancy
M8372/0	Adrenal cortical adenoma, heavily pigmented variant		
		M8471/3	Papillary mucinous cystadenocarcinoma
M8373/0	Adrenal cortical adenoma, clear cell type		
		M8480/0	Mucinous adenoma
M8374/0	Adrenal cortical adenoma, glomerulosa cell type	M8480/3	Mucinous adenocarcinoma
		M8480/6	Pseudomyxoma peritonei

APPENDIX A: MORPHOLOGY OF NEOPLASMS

M8481/3	Mucin-producing adenocarcinoma
M8490/3	Signet ring cell carcinoma
M8490/6	Metastatic signet ring cell carcinoma

M850-M854 Ductal, lobular, and medullary neoplasms

M8500/2	Intraductal carcinoma, noninfiltrating NOS
M8500/3	Infiltrating duct carcinoma
M8501/2	Comedocarcinoma, noninfiltrating
M8501/3	Comedocarcinoma NOS
M8502/3	Juvenile carcinoma of the breast
M8503/0	Intraductal papilloma
M8503/2	Noninfiltrating intraductal papillary adenocarcinoma
M8504/0	Intracystic papillary adenoma
M8504/2	Noninfiltrating intracystic carcinoma
M8505/0	Intraductal papillomatosis NOS
M8506/0	Subareolar duct papillomatosis
M8510/3	Medullary carcinoma NOS
M8511/3	Medullary carcinoma with amyloid stroma
M8512/3	Medullary carcinoma with lymphoid stroma
M8520/2	Lobular carcinoma in situ
M8520/3	Lobular carcinoma NOS
M8521/3	Infiltrating ductular carcinoma
M8530/3	Inflammatory carcinoma
M8540/3	Paget's disease, mammary
M8541/3	Paget's disease and infiltrating duct carcinoma of breast
M8542/3	Paget's disease, extramammary (except Paget's disease of bone)

M855 Acinar cell neoplasms

M8550/0	Acinar cell adenoma
M8550/1	Acinar cell tumor
M8550/3	Acinar cell carcinoma

M856-M858 Complex epithelial neoplasms

M8560/3	Adenosquamous carcinoma
M8561/0	Adenolymphoma
M8570/3	Adenocarcinoma with squamous metaplasia
M8571/3	Adenocarcinoma with cartilaginous and osseous metaplasia
M8572/3	Adenocarcinoma with spindle cell metaplasia
M8573/3	Adenocarcinoma with apocrine metaplasia
M8580/0	Thymoma, benign
M8580/3	Thymoma, malignant

M859-M867 Specialized gonadal neoplasms

M8590/1	Sex cord-stromal tumor
M8600/0	Thecoma NOS
M8600/3	Theca cell carcinoma
M8610/0	Luteoma NOS
M8620/1	Granulosa cell tumor NOS
M8620/3	Granulosa cell tumor, malignant
M8621/1	Granulosa cell-theca cell tumor
M8630/0	Androblastoma, benign
M8630/1	Androblastoma NOS
M8630/3	Androblastoma, malignant
M8631/0	Sertoli-Leydig cell tumor
M8632/1	Gynandroblastoma
M8640/0	Tubular androblastoma NOS
M8640/3	Sertoli cell carcinoma
M8641/0	Tubular androblastoma with lipid storage
M8650/0	Leydig cell tumor, benign
M8650/1	Leydig cell tumor NOS
M8650/3	Leydig cell tumor, malignant
M8660/0	Hilar cell tumor
M8670/0	Lipid cell tumor of ovary
M8671/0	Adrenal rest tumor

M868-M871 Paragangliomas and glomus tumors

M8680/1	Paraganglioma NOS
M8680/3	Paraganglioma, malignant
M8681/1	Sympathetic paraganglioma
M8682/1	Parasympathetic paraganglioma
M8690/1	Glomus jugulare tumor
M8691/1	Aortic body tumor
M8692/1	Carotid body tumor
M8693/1	Extra-adrenal paraganglioma NOS
M8693/3	Extra-adrenal paraganglioma, malignant
M8700/0	Pheochromocytoma NOS
M8700/3	Pheochromocytoma, malignant
M8710/3	Glomangiosarcoma
M8711/0	Glomus tumor
M8712/0	Glomangioma

M872-M879 Nevi and melanomas

M8720/0	Pigmented nevus NOS
M8720/3	Malignant melanoma NOS
M8721/3	Nodular melanoma
M8722/0	Balloon cell nevus
M8722/3	Balloon cell melanoma
M8723/0	Halo nevus
M8724/0	Fibrous papule of the nose
M8725/0	Neuronevus
M8726/0	Magnocellular nevus
M8730/0	Nonpigmented nevus
M8730/3	Amelanotic melanoma
M8740/0	Junctional nevus
M8740/3	Malignant melanoma in junctional nevus
M8741/2	Precancerous melanosis NOS
M8741/3	Malignant melanoma in precancerous melanosis
M8742/2	Hutchinson's melanotic freckle
M8742/3	Malignant melanoma in Hutchinson's melanotic freckle
M8743/3	Superficial spreading melanoma
M8750/0	Intradermal nevus
M8760/0	Compound nevus
M8761/1	Giant pigmented nevus
M8761/3	Malignant melanoma in giant pigmented nevus
M8770/0	Epithelioid and spindle cell nevus
M8771/3	Epithelioid cell melanoma
M8772/3	Spindle cell melanoma NOS
M8773/3	Spindle cell melanoma, type A
M8774/3	Spindle cell melanoma, type B
M8775/3	Mixed epithelioid and spindle cell melanoma
M8780/0	Blue nevus NOS
M8780/3	Blue nevus, malignant
M8790/0	Cellular blue nevus

APPENDIX A: MORPHOLOGY OF NEOPLASMS

M880 Soft tissue tumors and sarcomas NOS
M8800/0 Soft tissue tumor, benign
M8800/3 Sarcoma NOS
M8800/9 Sarcomatosis NOS
M8801/3 Spindle cell sarcoma
M8802/3 Giant cell sarcoma (except of bone M9250/3)
M8803/3 Small cell sarcoma
M8804/3 Epithelioid cell sarcoma

M881-M883 Fibromatous neoplasms
M8810/0 Fibroma NOS
M8810/3 Fibrosarcoma NOS
M8811/0 Fibromyxoma
M8811/3 Fibromyxosarcoma
M8812/0 Periosteal fibroma
M8812/3 Periosteal fibrosarcoma
M8813/0 Fascial fibroma
M8813/3 Fascial fibrosarcoma
M8814/3 Infantile fibrosarcoma
M8820/0 Elastofibroma
M8821/1 Aggressive fibromatosis
M8822/1 Abdominal fibromatosis
M8823/1 Desmoplastic fibroma
M8830/0 Fibrous histiocytoma NOS
M8830/1 Atypical fibrous histiocytoma
M8830/3 Fibrous histiocytoma, malignant
M8831/0 Fibroxanthoma NOS
M8831/1 Atypical fibroxanthoma
M8831/3 Fibroxanthoma, malignant
M8832/0 Dermatofibroma NOS
M8832/1 Dermatofibroma protuberans
M8832/3 Dermatofibrosarcoma NOS

M884 Myxomatous neoplasms
M8840/0 Myxoma NOS
M8840/3 Myxosarcoma

M885-M888 Lipomatous neoplasms
M8850/0 Lipoma NOS
M8850/3 Liposarcoma NOS
M8851/0 Fibrolipoma
M8851/3 Liposarcoma, well differentiated type
M8852/0 Fibromyxolipoma
M8852/3 Myxoid liposarcoma
M8853/3 Round cell liposarcoma
M8854/3 Pleomorphic liposarcoma
M8855/3 Mixed type liposarcoma
M8856/0 Intramuscular lipoma
M8857/0 Spindle cell lipoma
M8860/0 Angiomyolipoma
M8860/3 Angiomyoliposarcoma
M8861/0 Angiolipoma NOS
M8861/1 Angiolipoma, infiltrating
M8870/0 Myelolipoma
M8880/0 Hibernoma
M8881/0 Lipoblastomatosis

M889-M892 Myomatous neoplasms
M8890/0 Leiomyoma NOS
M8890/1 Intravascular leiomyomatosis
M8890/3 Leiomyosarcoma NOS
M8891/1 Epithelioid leiomyoma
M8891/3 Epithelioid leiomyosarcoma
M8892/1 Cellular leiomyoma
M8893/0 Bizarre leiomyoma
M8894/0 Angiomyoma

M8894/3 Angiomyosarcoma
M8895/0 Myoma
M8895/3 Myosarcoma
M8900/0 Rhabdomyoma NOS
M8900/3 Rhabdomyosarcoma NOS
M8901/3 Pleomorphic rhabdomyosarcoma
M8902/3 Mixed type rhabdomyosarcoma
M8903/0 Fetal rhabdomyoma
M8904/0 Adult rhabdomyoma
M8910/3 Embryonal rhabdomyosarcoma
M8920/3 Alveolar rhabdomyosarcoma

M893-M899 Complex mixed and stromal neoplasms
M8930/3 Endometrial stromal sarcoma
M8931/1 Endolymphatic stromal myosis
M8932/0 Adenomyoma
M8940/0 Pleomorphic adenoma
M8940/3 Mixed tumor, malignant NOS
M8950/3 Mullerian mixed tumor
M8951/3 Mesodermal mixed tumor
M8960/1 Mesoblastic nephroma
M8960/3 Nephroblastoma NOS
M8961/3 Epithelial nephroblastoma
M8962/3 Mesenchymal nephroblastoma
M8970/3 Hepatoblastoma
M8980/3 Carcinosarcoma NOS
M8981/3 Carcinosarcoma, embryonal type
M8982/0 Myoepithelioma
M8990/0 Mesenchymoma, benign
M8990/1 Mesenchymoma NOS
M8990/3 Mesenchymoma, malignant
M8991/3 Embryonal sarcoma

M900-M903 Fibroepithelial neoplasms
M9000/0 Brenner tumor NOS
M9000/1 Brenner tumor, borderline malignancy
M9000/3 Brenner tumor, malignant
M9010/0 Fibroadenoma NOS
M9011/0 Intracanalicular fibroadenoma NOS
M9012/0 Pericanalicular fibroadenoma
M9013/0 Adenofibroma NOS
M9014/0 Serous adenofibroma
M9015/0 Mucinous adenofibroma
M9020/0 Cellular intracanalicular fibroadenoma
M9020/1 Cystosarcoma phyllodes NOS
M9020/3 Cystosarcoma phyllodes, malignant
M9030/0 Juvenile fibroadenoma

M904 Synovial neoplasms
M9040/0 Synovioma, benign
M9040/3 Synovial sarcoma NOS
M9041/3 Synovial sarcoma, spindle cell type
M9042/3 Synovial sarcoma, epithelioid cell type
M9043/3 Synovial sarcoma, biphasic type
M9044/3 Clear cell sarcoma of tendons and aponeuroses

M905 Mesothelial neoplasms
M9050/0 Mesothelioma, benign
M9050/3 Mesothelioma, malignant
M9051/0 Fibrous mesothelioma, benign
M9051/3 Fibrous mesothelioma, malignant
M9052/0 Epithelioid mesothelioma, benign
M9052/3 Epithelioid mesothelioma, malignant
M9053/0 Mesothelioma, biphasic type, benign
M9053/3 Mesothelioma, biphasic type, malignant
M9054/0 Adenomatoid tumor NOS

APPENDIX A: MORPHOLOGY OF NEOPLASMS

M906-M909 Germ cell neoplasms
M9060/3	Dysgerminoma
M9061/3	Seminoma NOS
M9062/3	Seminoma, anaplastic type
M9063/3	Spermatocytic seminoma
M9064/3	Germinoma
M9070/3	Embryonal carcinoma NOS
M9071/3	Endodermal sinus tumor
M9072/3	Polyembryoma
M9073/1	Gonadoblastoma
M9080/0	Teratoma, benign
M9080/1	Teratoma NOS
M9080/3	Teratoma, malignant NOS
M9081/3	Teratocarcinoma
M9082/3	Malignant teratoma, undifferentiated type
M9083/3	Malignant teratoma, intermediate type
M9084/0	Dermoid cyst
M9084/3	Dermoid cyst with malignant transformation
M9090/0	Struma ovarii NOS
M9090/3	Struma ovarii, malignant
M9091/1	Strumal carcinoid

M910 Trophoblastic neoplasms
M9100/0	Hydatidiform mole NOS
M9100/1	Invasive hydatidiform mole
M9100/3	Choriocarcinoma
M9101/3	Choriocarcinoma combined with teratoma
M9102/3	Malignant teratoma, trophoblastic

M911 Mesonephromas
M9110/0	Mesonephroma, benign
M9110/1	Mesonephric tumor
M9110/3	Mesonephroma, malignant
M9111/1	Endosalpingioma

M912-M916 Blood vessel tumors
M9120/0	Hemangioma NOS
M9120/3	Hemangiosarcoma
M9121/0	Cavernous hemangioma
M9122/0	Venous hemangioma
M9123/0	Racemose hemangioma
M9124/3	Kupffer cell sarcoma
M9130/0	Hemangioendothelioma, benign
M9130/1	Hemangioendothelioma NOS
M9130/3	Hemangioendothelioma, malignant
M9131/0	Capillary hemangioma
M9132/0	Intramuscular hemangioma
M9140/3	Kaposi's sarcoma
M9141/0	Angiokeratoma
M9142/0	Verrucous keratotic hemangioma
M9150/0	Hemangiopericytoma, benign
M9150/1	Hemangiopericytoma NOS
M9150/3	Hemangiopericytoma, malignant
M9160/0	Angiofibroma NOS
M9161/1	Hemangioblastoma

M917 Lymphatic vessel tumors
M9170/0	Lymphangioma NOS
M9170/3	Lymphangiosarcoma
M9171/0	Capillary lymphangioma
M9172/0	Cavernous lymphangioma
M9173/0	Cystic lymphangioma
M9174/0	Lymphangiomyoma
M9174/1	Lymphangiomyomatosis
M9175/0	Hemolymphangioma

M918-M920 Osteomas and osteosarcomas
M9180/0	Osteoma NOS
M9180/3	Osteosarcoma NOS
M9181/3	Chondroblastic osteosarcoma
M9182/3	Fibroblastic osteosarcoma
M9183/3	Telangiectatic osteosarcoma
M9184/3	Osteosarcoma in Paget's disease of bone
M9190/3	Juxtacortical osteosarcoma
M9191/0	Osteoid osteoma NOS
M9200/0	Osteoblastoma

M921-M924 Chondromatous neoplasms
M9210/0	Osteochondroma
M9210/1	Osteochondromatosis NOS
M9220/0	Chondroma NOS
M9220/1	Chondromatosis NOS
M9220/3	Chondrosarcoma NOS
M9221/0	Juxtacortical chondroma
M9221/3	Juxtacortical chondrosarcoma
M9230/0	Chondroblastoma NOS
M9230/3	Chondroblastoma, malignant
M9240/3	Mesenchymal chondrosarcoma
M9241/0	Chondromyxoid fibroma

M925 Giant cell tumors
M9250/1	Giant cell tumor of bone NOS
M9250/3	Giant cell tumor of bone, malignant
M9251/1	Giant cell tumor of soft parts NOS
M9251/3	Malignant giant cell tumor of soft parts

M926 Miscellaneous bone tumors
M9260/3	Ewing's sarcoma
M9261/3	Adamantinoma of long bones
M9262/0	Ossifying fibroma

M927-M934 Odontogenic tumors
M9270/0	Odontogenic tumor, benign
M9270/1	Odontogenic tumor NOS
M9270/3	Odontogenic tumor, malignant
M9271/0	Dentinoma
M9272/0	Cementoma NOS
M9273/0	Cementoblastoma, benign
M9274/0	Cementifying fibroma
M9275/0	Gigantiform cementoma
M9280/0	Odontoma NOS
M9281/0	Compound odontoma
M9282/0	Complex odontoma
M9290/0	Ameloblastic fibro-odontoma
M9290/3	Ameloblastic odontosarcoma
M9300/0	Adenomatoid odontogenic tumor
M9301/0	Calcifying odontogenic cyst
M9310/0	Ameloblastoma NOS
M9310/3	Ameloblastoma, malignant
M9311/0	Odontoameloblastoma
M9312/0	Squamous odontogenic tumor
M9320/0	Odontogenic myxoma
M9321/0	Odontogenic fibroma NOS
M9330/0	Ameloblastic fibroma
M9330/3	Ameloblastic fibrosarcoma
M9340/0	Calcifying epithelial odontogenic tumor

M935-M937 Miscellaneous tumors
M9350/1	Craniopharyngioma
M9360/1	Pinealoma
M9361/1	Pineocytoma
M9362/3	Pineoblastoma
M9363/0	Melanotic neuroectodermal tumor
M9370/3	Chordoma

APPENDIX A: MORPHOLOGY OF NEOPLASMS

M938-M948 Gliomas
M9380/3 Glioma, malignant
M9381/3 Gliomatosis cerebri
M9382/3 Mixed glioma
M9383/1 Subependymal glioma
M9384/1 Subependymal giant cell astrocytoma
M9390/0 Choroid plexus papilloma NOS
M9390/3 Choroid plexus papilloma, malignant
M9391/3 Ependymoma NOS
M9392/3 Ependymoma, anaplastic type
M9393/1 Papillary ependymoma
M9394/1 Myxopapillary ependymoma
M9400/3 Astrocytoma NOS
M9401/3 Astrocytoma, anaplastic type
M9410/3 Protoplasmic astrocytoma
M9411/3 Gemistocytic astrocytoma
M9420/3 Fibrillary astrocytoma
M9421/3 Pilocytic astrocytoma
M9422/3 Spongioblastoma NOS
M9423/3 Spongioblastoma polare
M9430/3 Astroblastoma
M9440/3 Glioblastoma NOS
M9441/3 Giant cell glioblastoma
M9442/3 Glioblastoma with sarcomatous component
M9443/3 Primitive polar spongioblastoma
M9450/3 Oligodendroglioma NOS
M9451/3 Oligodendroglioma, anaplastic type
M9460/3 Oligodendroblastoma
M9470/3 Medulloblastoma NOS
M9471/3 Desmoplastic medulloblastoma
M9472/3 Medullomyoblastoma
M9480/3 Cerebellar sarcoma NOS
M9481/3 Monstrocellular sarcoma

M949-M952 Neuroepitheliomatous neoplasms
M9490/0 Ganglioneuroma
M9490/3 Ganglioneuroblastoma
M9491/0 Ganglioneuromatosis
M9500/3 Neuroblastoma NOS
M9501/3 Medulloepithelioma NOS
M9502/3 Teratoid medulloepithelioma
M9503/3 Neuroepithelioma NOS
M9504/3 Spongioneuroblastoma
M9505/1 Ganglioglioma
M9506/0 Neurocytoma
M9507/0 Pacinian tumor
M9510/3 Retinoblastoma NOS
M9511/3 Retinoblastoma, differentiated type
M9512/3 Retinoblastoma, undifferentiated type
M9520/3 Olfactory neurogenic tumor
M9521/3 Esthesioneurocytoma
M9522/3 Esthesioneuroblastoma
M9523/3 Esthesioneuroepithelioma

M953 Meningiomas
M9530/0 Meningioma NOS
M9530/1 Meningiomatosis NOS
M9530/3 Meningioma, malignant
M9531/0 Meningotheliomatous meningioma
M9532/0 Fibrous meningioma
M9533/0 Psammomatous meningioma
M9534/0 Angiomatous meningioma
M9535/0 Hemangioblastic meningioma
M9536/0 Hemangiopericytic meningioma
M9537/0 Transitional meningioma
M9538/1 Papillary meningioma
M9539/3 Meningeal sarcomatosis

M954-M957 Nerve sheath tumor
M9540/0 Neurofibroma NOS
M9540/1 Neurofibromatosis NOS
M9540/3 Neurofibrosarcoma
M9541/0 Melanotic neurofibroma
M9550/0 Plexiform neurofibroma
M9560/0 Neurilemmoma NOS
M9560/1 Neurinomatosis
M9560/3 Neurilemmoma, malignant
M9570/0 Neuroma NOS

M958 Granular cell tumors and alveolar soft part sarcoma
M9580/0 Granular cell tumor NOS
M9580/3 Granular cell tumor, malignant
M9581/3 Alveolar soft part sarcoma

M959-M963 Lymphomas, NOS or diffuse
M9590/0 Lymphomatous tumor, benign
M9590/3 Malignant lymphoma NOS
M9591/3 Malignant lymphoma, non Hodgkin's type
M9600/3 Malignant lymphoma, undifferentiated cell type NOS
M9601/3 Malignant lymphoma, stem cell type
M9602/3 Malignant lymphoma, convoluted cell type NOS
M9610/3 Lymphosarcoma NOS
M9611/3 Malignant lymphoma, lymphoplasmacytoid type
M9612/3 Malignant lymphoma, immunoblastic type
M9613/3 Malignant lymphoma, mixed lymphocytic-histiocytic NOS
M9614/3 Malignant lymphoma, centroblastic-centrocytic, diffuse
M9615/3 Malignant lymphoma, follicular center cell NOS
M9620/3 Malignant lymphoma, lymphocytic, well differentiated NOS
M9621/3 Malignant lymphoma, lymphocytic, intermediate differentiation NOS
M9622/3 Malignant lymphoma, centrocytic
M9623/3 Malignant lymphoma, follicular center cell, cleaved NOS
M9630/3 Malignant lymphoma, lymphocytic, poorly differentiated NOS
M9631/3 Prolymphocytic lymphosarcoma
M9632/3 Malignant lymphoma, centroblastic type NOS
M9633/3 Malignant lymphoma, follicular center cell, noncleaved NOS

M964 Reticulosarcomas
M9640/3 Reticulosarcoma NOS
M9641/3 Reticulosarcoma, pleomorphic cell type
M9642/3 Reticulosarcoma, nodular

M965-M966 Hodgkin's disease
M9650/3 Hodgkin's disease NOS
M9651/3 Hodgkin's disease, lymphocytic predominance
M9652/3 Hodgkin's disease, mixed cellularity
M9653/3 Hodgkin's disease, lymphocytic depletion NOS

APPENDIX A: MORPHOLOGY OF NEOPLASMS

M9654/3	Hodgkin's disease, lymphocytic depletion, diffuse fibrosis	M9802/3	Subacute leukemia NOS
		M9803/3	Chronic leukemia NOS
M9655/3	Hodgkin's disease, lymphocytic depletion, reticular type	M9804/3	Aleukemic leukemia NOS

M981 Compound leukemias

M9656/3 Hodgkin's disease, nodular sclerosis NOS
M9810/3 Compound leukemia

M982 Lymphoid leukemias

M9657/3 Hodgkin's disease, nodular sclerosis, cellular phase
M9820/3 Lymphoid leukemia NOS
M9821/3 Acute lymphoid leukemia
M9660/3 Hodgkin's paragranuloma
M9822/3 Subacute lymphoid leukemia
M9661/3 Hodgkin's granuloma
M9823/3 Chronic lymphoid leukemia
M9662/3 Hodgkin's sarcoma
M9824/3 Aleukemic lymphoid leukemia

M969 Lymphomas, nodular or follicular

M9825/3 Prolymphocytic leukemia
M9690/3 Malignant lymphoma, nodular NOS

M983 Plasma cell leukemias

M9691/3 Malignant lymphoma, mixed lymphocytic-histiocytic, nodular
M9830/3 Plasma cell leukemia

M984 Erythroleukemias

M9692/3 Malignant lymphoma, centroblastic-centrocytic, follicular
M9840/3 Erythroleukemia
M9841/3 Acute erythremia
M9842/3 Chronic erythremia
M9693/3 Malignant lymphoma, lymphocytic, well differentiated, nodular

M985 Lymphosarcoma cell leukemias

M9850/3 Lymphosarcoma cell leukemia
M9694/3 Malignant lymphoma, lymphocytic, intermediate differentiation, nodular

M986 Myeloid leukemias

M9860/3 Myeloid leukemia NOS
M9695/3 Malignant lymphoma, follicular center cell, cleaved, follicular
M9861/3 Acute myeloid leukemia
M9862/3 Subacute myeloid leukemia
M9696/3 Malignant lymphoma, lymphocytic, poorly differentiated, nodular
M9863/3 Chronic myeloid leukemia
M9864/3 Aleukemic myeloid leukemia
M9697/3 Malignant lymphoma, centroblastic type, follicular
M9865/3 Neutrophilic leukemia
M9866/3 Acute promyelocytic leukemia
M9698/3 Malignant lymphoma, follicular center cell, noncleaved, follicular

M987 Basophilic leukemias

M9870/3 Basophilic leukemia

M970 Mycosis fungoides

M988 Eosinophilic leukemias

M9700/3 Mycosis fungoides
M9880/3 Eosinophilic leukemia
M9701/3 Sezary's disease

M989 Monocytic leukemias

M971-M972 Miscellaneous reticuloendothelial neoplasms

M9890/3 Monocytic leukemia NOS
M9891/3 Acute monocytic leukemia
M9710/3 Microglioma
M9892/3 Subacute monocytic leukemia
M9720/3 Malignant histiocytosis
M9893/3 Chronic monocytic leukemia
M9721/3 Histiocytic medullary reticulosis
M9894/3 Aleukemic monocytic leukemia
M722/3 Letterer-Siwe's disease

M990-M994 Miscellaneous leukemias

M973 Plasma cell tumors

M9900/3 Mast cell leukemia
M9730/3 Plasma cell myeloma
M9910/3 Megakaryocytic leukemia
M9731/0 Plasma cell tumor, benign
M9920/3 Megakaryocytic myelosis
M9731/1 Plasmacytoma NOS
M9930/3 Myeloid sarcoma
M9731/3 Plasma cell tumor, malignant
M9940/3 Hairy cell leukemia

M974 Mast cell tumors

M995-M997 Miscellaneous myeloproliferative and lymphoproliferative disorders

M9740/1 Mastocytoma NOS
M9740/3 Mast cell sarcoma
M9741/3 Malignant mastocytosis
M9950/1 Polycythemia vera

M975 Burkitt's tumor

M9951/1 Acute panmyelosis
M9750/3 Burkitt's tumor
M9960/1 Chronic myeloproliferative disease

M980-M994 Leukemias

M9961/1 Myelosclerosis with myeloid metaplasia

M980 Leukemias NOS

M9962/1 Idiopathic thrombocythemia
M9800/3 Leukemia NOS
M9970/1 Chronic lymphoproliferative disease
M9801/3 Acute leukemia NOS

APPENDIX B: GLOSSARY OF MENTAL DISORDERS

Glossary of Mental Disorders

The psychiatric terms which appear in Chapter 5, "Mental Disorders," are listed here in alphabetic sequence. Many of the glossary descriptions originally appeared in the section on Mental Disorders in the *International Classification of Diseases, 9th Revision*,[1] and others are included to define the psychiatric conditions added to *ICD-9-CM*. The additional definitions are based on material furnished by the *American Psychiatric Association's Task Force on Nomenclature and Statistics*[2] and from *A Psychiatric Glossary*.[3] In a few instances definitions were obtained from *Dorland's Illustrated Medical Dictionary*[4] and from *Stedman's Medical Dictionary, Illustrated*.[5]

1. *Manual of the International Classification of Diseases, Injuries, and Causes of Death*, 9th Revision. World Health Organization, Geneva, Switzerland, 1975.
2. American Psychiatric Association, Task Force on Nomenclature and Statistics, Robert L. Spitzer, Chairman.
3. *A Psychiatric Glossary*, Fourth Edition, American Psychiatric Association, Washington, D.C., 1975.
4. *Dorland's Illustrated Medical Dictionary*, Twenty-fifth Edition, W.B. Saunders Company, Philadelphia, 1974.
5. *Stedman's Medical Dictionary*, Illustrated, Twenty-third Edition, the Williams and Wilkins Company, Baltimore, 1976.

Academic underachievement disorder – Failure to achieve in most school tasks despite adequate intellectual capacity, a supportive and encouraging social environment, and apparent effort. The failure occurs in the absence of a demonstrable specific learning disability and is caused by emotional conflict not clearly associated with any other mental disorder.[2]

Adaptation reaction — *see* Adjustment reaction

Adjustment reaction or disorder – Mild or transient disorders lasting longer than acute stress reactions which occur in individuals of any age without any apparent pre-existing mental disorder. Such disorders are often relatively circumscribed or situation-specific, are generally reversible, and usually last only a few months. They are usually closely related in time and content to stresses such as bereavement, migration, or other experiences. Reactions to major stress that last longer than a few days are also included. In children such disorders are associated with no significant distortion of development.[1]

conduct disturbance – Mild or transient disorders in which the main disturbance predominantly involves a disturbance of conduct (e.g., an adolescent grief reaction resulting in aggressive or antisocial disorder).[1]

depressive reaction – States of depression, not specifiable as manic-depressive, psychotic, or neurotic.[1]
- **brief** – Generally transient, in which the depressive symptoms are usually closely related in time and content to some stressful event.[1]
- **prolonged** – Generally long-lasting, usually developing in association with prolonged exposure to a stressful situation.[1]

emotional disturbance – An adjustment disorder in which the main symptoms are emotional in type (e.g., anxiety, fear, worry) but not specifically depressive.[1]

mixed conduct and emotional disturbance – An adjustment reaction in which both emotional disturbance and disturbance of conduct are prominent features.[1]

Affective psychoses – Mental disorders, usually recurrent, in which there is a severe disturbance of mood (mostly compounded of depression and anxiety but also manifested as elation, and excitement) which is accompanied by one or more of the following – delusions, perplexity, disturbed attitude to self, disorder of perception and behavior; these are all in keeping with the individual's prevailing mood (as are hallucinations when they occur). There is a strong tendency to suicide. For practical reasons, mild disorders of mood may also be included here if the symptoms match closely the descriptions given; this applies particularly to mild hypomania.[1]
- **bipolar** – A manic-depressive psychosis which has appeared in both the depressive and manic form, either alternating or separated by an interval of normality.[1]
  - **atypical** – An episode of affective psychosis with some, but not all, of the features of the one form of the disorder in individuals who have had a previous episode of the other form of the disorder.[2]
  - **depressed** – A manic-depressive psychosis, circular type, in which the depressive form is currently present.[1]
  - **manic** – A manic-depressive psychosis, circular type, in which the manic form is currently present.[1]

APPENDIX B: GLOSSARY OF MENTAL DISORDERS

    mixed – A manic-depressive psychosis, circular type, in which both manic and depressive symptoms are present at the same time.[1]

depressed type – A manic-depressive psychosis in which there is a widespread depressed mood of gloom and wretchedness with some degree of anxiety. There is often reduced activity but there may be restlessness and agitation. There is marked tendency to recurrence; in a few cases this may be at regular intervals.[1]

    atypical – An affective depressive disorder that cannot be classified as a manic-depressive psychosis, depressed type, or chronic depressive personality disorder, or as an adjustment disorder.[2]

manic type – A manic-depressive psychosis characterized by states of elation or excitement out of keeping with the individual's circumstances and varying from enhanced liveliness (hypomania) to violent, almost uncontrollable, excitement. Aggression and anger, flight of ideas, distractibility, impaired judgment, and grandiose ideas are common.[1]

mixed type – Manic-depressive psychosis syndromes corresponding to both the manic and depressed types, but which for other reasons cannot be classified more specifically.[1]

Aggressive personality — see Personality disorder, explosive type

Agoraphobia — see agoraphobia under Phobia

Alcohol dependence syndrome – A state, psychic and usually also physical, resulting from taking alcohol, characterized by behavioral and other responses that always include a compulsion to take alcohol on a continuous or periodic basis in order to experience its psychic effects, and sometimes to avoid the discomfort of its absence; tolerance may or may not be present. A person may be dependent on alcohol and other drugs; if so, also record the diagnosis of drug dependence to identify the agent. If alcohol dependence is associated with alcoholic psychosis or with physical complications, *both* diagnoses should be recorded.[1]

Alcohol intoxication

    acute – A psychic and physical state resulting from alcohol ingestion characterized by slurred speech, unsteady gait, poor coordination, flushed facies, nystagmus, sluggish reflexes, fetor alcoholica, loud speech, emotional instability (e.g., jollity followed by lugubriousness), excessive conviviality, loquacity, and poorly inhibited sexual and aggressive behavior.[2]

    idiosyncratic – Acute psychotic episodes induced by relatively small amounts of alcohol. These are regarded as individual idiosyncratic reactions to alcohol, not due to excessive consumption and without conspicuous neurological signs of intoxication.[1]

    pathological – see Alcohol intoxication, idiosyncratic

Alcoholic psychoses – Organic psychotic states due mainly to excessive consumption of alcohol; defects of nutrition are thought to play an important role.[1]

alcohol abstinence syndrome — see alcohol withdrawal syndrome below

alcohol amnestic syndrome – A syndrome of prominent and lasting reduction of memory span, including striking loss of recent memory, disordered time appreciation and confabulation, occurring in alcoholics as the sequel to an acute alcoholic psychosis (especially delirium tremens) or, more rarely, in the course of chronic alcoholism. It is usually accompanied by peripheral neuritis and may be associated with Wernicke's encephalopathy.[1]

alcohol withdrawal delirium [delirium tremens] – Acute or subacute organic psychotic states in alcoholics, characterized by clouded consciousness, disorientation, fear, illusions, delusions, hallucinations of any kind, notably visual and tactile, and restlessness, tremor and sometimes fever.[1]

alcohol withdrawal hallucinosis – A psychosis usually of less than six months' duration, with slight or no clouding of consciousness and much anxious restlessness in which auditory hallucinations, mostly of voices uttering insults and threats, predominate.[1]

alcohol withdrawal syndrome – Tremor of hands, tongue, and eyelids following cessation of prolonged heavy drinking of alcohol. Nausea and vomiting, dry mouth, headache, heavy perspiration, fitful sleep, acute anxiety attacks, mood depression, feelings of guilt and remorse, and irritability are associated features.[2]

alcohol delirium — see alcohol withdrawal delirium above

alcoholic dementia – Nonhallucinatory dementias occurring in association with alcoholism, but not characterized by the features of either alcohol withdrawal delirium [delirium tremens] or alcohol amnestic syndrome [Korsakoff's alcoholic psychosis].[1]

alcoholic hallucinosis — see alcohol withdrawal hallucinosis above

alcoholic jealousy – Chronic paranoid psychosis characterized by delusional jealousy and associated with alcoholism.[1]

alcoholic paranoia — see Alcoholic jealousy

APPENDIX B: GLOSSARY OF MENTAL DISORDERS

alcoholic polyneuritic psychosis — see alcohol amnestic syndrome above

Alcoholism
acute — see Alcohol intoxication, acute
chronic — see Alcohol dependence syndrome

Alexia - Loss of a previously possessed reading facility that cannot be explained by defective visual acuity.[3]

Amnesia, psychogenic - A form of dissociative hysteria in which there is a temporary disturbance in the ability to recall important personal information which has already been registered and stored in memory. The sudden onset of this disturbance in the absence of an underlying organic mental disorder, and the extent of the disturbance being too great to be explained by ordinary forgetfulness, are the essential features.[2]

Amnestic syndrome - A syndrome of prominent and lasting reduction of memory span, including striking loss of recent memory, disordered time appreciation, and confabulation. The commonest causes are chronic alcoholism [alcohol amnestic syndrome; Korsakoff's alcoholic psychosis], chronic barbiturate dependence, and malnutrition. An amnestic syndrome may be the predominating disturbance in the early states of presenile and senile dementia, arteriosclerotic dementia, and in encephalitis and other inflammatory and degenerative diseases in which there is particular bilateral involvement of the temporal lobes, and certain temporal lobe tumors.[2]
alcoholic — see alcohol amnestic syndrome under Alcoholic psychoses

Amoral personality — see Personality disorder, antisocial type

Anancastic [anankastic] neurosis — see Neurotic disorder, obsessive-compulsive

Anancastic [anankastic] personality — see Personality disorder, compulsive type

Anorexia nervosa - A disorder in which the main features are persistent active refusal to eat and marked loss of weight. The level of activity and alertness is characteristically high in relation to the degree of emaciation. Typically the disorder begins in teenage girls but it may sometimes begin before puberty and rarely it occurs in males. Amenorrhea is usual and there may be a variety of other physiological changes including slow pulse and respiration, low body temperature, and dependent edema. Unusual eating habits and attitudes toward food are typical and sometimes starvation follows or alternates with periods of overeating. The accompanying psychiatric symptoms are diverse.[1]

Anxiety hysteria — see phobia under Neurotic disorders

Anxiety state (neurotic) - Apprehension, tension, or uneasiness that stems from the anticipation of danger, the source of which is largely unknown or unrecognized.[3]
atypical - An anxiety disorder that does not fulfill the criteria of generalized or panic attack anxiety. An example might be an individual with a single morbid fear.[2]
generalized - A disorder of at least six months' duration in which the predominant feature is limited to diffuse and persistent anxiety without the specific symptoms that characterize phobic disorders, panic disorder, or obsessive-compulsive disorder.[2]
panic attack - An episodic and often chronic, recurrent disorder in which the predominant features are anxiety attacks and nervousness. The anxiety attacks are manifested by discrete periods of sudden onset of intense apprehension, fearfulness, or terror often associated with feelings of impending doom.[2]

Aphasia, developmental - A delay in the production of spoken language. Rarely, there is also a developmental delay in the comprehension of speech sounds.[1]

Arteriosclerotic dementia - Dementia attributable, because of physical signs (on examination of the central nervous system), to degenerative arterial disease of the brain. Symptoms suggesting a focal lesion in the brain are common. There may be a fluctuating or patchy intellectual defect with insight, and an intermittent course is common. Clinical differentiation from senile or presenile dementia, which may coexist with it, may be very difficult or impossible. The diagnosis of cerebral atherosclerosis should also be recorded.[1]

Asocial personality — see Personality disorder, antisocial type

Astasia-abasia, hysterical - A form of conversion hysteria in which the individual is unable to stand or walk although the legs are otherwise under control.[4]

Asthenia, psychogenic — see neurasthenia under Neurotic disorders

Asthenic personality — see Personality disorder, dependent type

Attention deficit disorder — see Attention deficit disorder under Hyperkinetic syndrome of childhood.

Autism, infantile - A syndrome present from birth or beginning almost invariably in the first 30 months. Responses to auditory and sometimes to visual stimuli are abnormal, and there are usually severe problems in the understanding of spoken language. Speech is delayed and,

APPENDIX B: GLOSSARY OF MENTAL DISORDERS

if it develops, is characterized by echolalia, the reversal of pronouns, immature grammatical structure, and inability to use abstract terms. There is generally an impairment in the social use of both verbal and gestural language. Problems in social relationships are most severe before the age of five years and include an impairment in the development of eye-to-eye gaze, social attachments, and cooperative play. Ritualistic behavior is usual and may include abnormal routines, resistance to change, attachment to odd objects, and stereotyped patterns of play. The capacity for abstract or symbolic thought and for imaginative play is diminished. Intelligence ranges from severely subnormal to normal or above. Performance is usually better on tasks involving rote memory or visuospatial skills than on those requiring symbolic or linguistic skills.[1]

Avoidant personality — see Personality disorder, avoidant type

"Bad trips" - Acute intoxication from hallucinogen abuse, manifested by hallucinatory states lasting only a few days or less.[1]

Barbiturate abuse - Cases where an individual has taken the drug to the detriment of his health or social functioning, in doses above or for periods beyond those normally regarded as therapeutic.[1]

Bestiality — see Zoophilia

Bipolar disorder — see Affective psychosis, bipolar

   atypical — see Affective psychosis, bipolar, atypical

Body-rocking — see Stereotyped repetitive movements

Borderline personality — see Personality disorder, borderline type

Borderline psychosis of childhood — see Psychosis, atypical childhood

Borderline schizophrenia — see Schizophrenia, latent

Bouffée délirante — see Paranoid reaction, acute

Briquet's disorder — see Somatization disorder under Neurotic disorders

Bulimia - An episodic pattern of overeating [binge eating] accompanied by an awareness of the disordered eating pattern with a fear of not being able to stop eating voluntarily. Depressive moods and self-deprecating thoughts follow the episodes of binge eating.[2]

Catalepsy schizophrenia — see Schizophrenia, catatonic type

Catastrophic stress — see Gross stress reaction

Catatonia (schizophrenic) — see Schizophrenia, catatonic type

Character neurosis — see Personality disorders

Childhood autism — see Autism, infantile

Childhood type schizophrenia — see Psychosis, child

Chronic alcoholic brain syndrome — see Alcoholic dementia under Alcoholic psychoses

Clay-eating — see Pica

Clumsiness syndrome — see Coordination disorder under Developmental delay disorders, specific

Combat fatigue — see Posttraumatic disorder, acute

Compensation neurosis — see Compensation neurosis under Neurotic disorders

Compulsive conduct disorder — see Impulse control disorders under Conduct disorders

Compulsive neurosis — see Neurotic disorder, obsessive-compulsive

Compulsive personality — see Personality disorder, compulsive type

Concentration camp syndrome — see Posttraumatic stress disorder, prolonged

Conduct disorders - Disorders mainly involving aggressive and destructive behavior and disorders involving delinquency. It should be used for abnormal behavior, in individuals of any age, which gives rise to social disapproval but which is not part of any other psychiatric condition. Minor emotional disturbances may also be present. To be included, the behavior, as judged by its frequency, severity, and type of associations with other symptoms, must be abnormal in its context. Disturbances of conduct are distinguished from an adjustment reaction by a longer duration and by a lack of close relationship in time and content to some stress. They differ from a personality disorder by the absence of deeply ingrained maladaptive patterns of behavior present from adolescence or earlier.[1]

   impulse control disorders - A failure to resist an impulse, drive, or temptation to perform some action which is harmful to the individual or to others. The impulse may or may not be consciously resisted, and the act may or may not be premeditated or planned. Prior to committing the act, there is an increasing sense of tension, and at the time of committing the act, there is an experience of either pleasure, gratification, or release. Immediately following the act, there may or may not be genuine regret, self-reproach, or guilt.[2] See also Intermittent explosive disorder, Isolated

APPENDIX B: GLOSSARY OF MENTAL DISORDERS

explosive disorder, Kleptomania, Pathological gambling, and Pyromania.

mixed disturbance of conduct and emotions – A disorder characterized by features of undersocialized and socialized disturbance of conduct, but in which there is also considerable emotional disturbance as shown, for example, by anxiety, misery, or obsessive manifestations.[1]

socialized conduct disorder – Conduct disorders in individuals who have acquired the values or behavior of a delinquent peer group to whom they are loyal and with whom they characteristically steal, play truant, and stay out late at night. There may also be sexual promiscuity.[1]

undersocialized conduct disturbance

    aggressive type – A disorder characterized by a persistent pattern of disrespect for the feelings and well-being of others (bullying, physical aggression, cruel behavior, hostility, verbal abusiveness, impudence, defiance, negativism), aggressive antisocial behavior (destructiveness, stealing, persistent lying, frequent truancy, and vandalism), and failure to develop close and stable relationships with others.[2]

    unaggressive type – A disorder in which there is a lack of concern for the rights and feelings of others to a degree which indicates a failure to establish a normal degree of affection, empathy, or bond with others. There are two patterns of behavior found. In one, the child is fearful and timid, lacking self-assertiveness, resorts to self-protective and manipulative lying, indulges in whining demandingness and temper tantrums, feels rejected and unfairly treated, and is mistrustful of others. In the other pattern of the disorder, the child approaches others strictly for his own gains and acts exclusively because of exploitative and extractive goals. The child lies brazenly and steals, appearing to feel no guilt, and forms no social bonds to other individuals.[2]

Confusion, psychogenic — *see* Psychosis, reactive confusion

Confusion, reactive — *see* Psychosis, reactive confusion

Confusional state
    acute — *see* Delirium, acute
    epileptic — *see* Delirium, acute
    subacute — *see* Delirium, subacute

Conversion hysteria — *see* Hysteria, conversion type under Neurotic disorders

Coordination disorder — *see* Coordination disorder under Developmental delay disorders, specific

Culture shock – A form of stress reaction associated with an individual's assimilation into a new culture which is vastly different from that in which he was raised.[5]

Cyclic schizophrenia — *see* Schizophrenia, schizo-affective type

Cyclothymic personality or disorder — *see* Personality disorder, cyclothymic type

Delirium – Transient organic psychotic conditions with a short course in which there is a rapidly developing onset of disorganization of higher mental processes manifested by some degree of impairment of information processing, impaired or abnormal attention, perception, memory, and thinking. Clouded consciousness, confusion, disorientation, delusions, illusions, and often vivid hallucinations predominate in the clinical picture.[1,2]

    acute – short-lived states, lasting hours or days, of the above type.[1]

    subacute – states of the above type in which the symptoms, usually less florid, last for several weeks or longer, during which they may show marked fluctuations in intensity.[1]

Delirium tremens — *see* Alcohol withdrawal delirium under Alcoholic psychoses

Delusions, systematized — *see* Paranoia

Dementia – A decrement in intellectual functioning of sufficient severity to interfere with occupational or social performance, or both. There is impairment of memory and abstract thinking, the ability to learn new skills, problem solving, and judgment. There is often also personality change or impairment in impulse control. Dementia in organic psychoses may be of a chronic or progressive nature, which if untreated are usually irreversible and terminal.[1,2]

    alcoholic — *see* Alcoholic dementia under Alcoholic psychoses

    arteriosclerotic — *see* Arteriosclerotic dementia

    multi-infarct — *see* Arteriosclerotic dementia

    presenile — *see* Presenile dementia

    repeated infarct — *see* Arteriosclerotic dementia

    senile — *see* Senile dementia

Depersonalization syndrome — *see* Depersonalization syndrome under Neurotic disorders

APPENDIX B: GLOSSARY OF MENTAL DISORDERS

Depression – States of depression, usually of moderate but occasionally of marked intensity, which have no specifically manic-depressive or other psychotic depressive features, and which do not appear to be associated with stressful events or other features specified under neurotic depression.[1]

anxiety — *see* Depression under Neurotic disorders

endogenous — *see* Affective psychosis, depressed type

monopolar — *see* Affective psychosis, depressed type

neurotic — *see* Depression under Neurotic disorders

psychotic — *see* Affective psychosis, depressed type

psychotic reactive — *see* Psychosis, depressive

reactive — *see* Depression under Neurotic disorders

reactive psychotic — *see* Psychosis, depressive

Depressive personality or character — *see* Personality disorder, chronic depressive type

Depressive reaction — *see* Depressive reaction under Adjustment reaction

Depressive psychosis — *see* Affective psychosis, depressed type

Derealization (neurotic) — *see* Depersonalization syndrome under Neurotic disorders

Developmental delay disorders, specific – A group of disorders in which a specific delay in development is the main feature. For many the delay is not explicable in terms of general intellectual retardation or of inadequate schooling. In each case development is related to biological maturation, but it is also influenced by nonbiological factors. A diagnosis of a specific developmental delay carries no etiological implications. A diagnosis of specific delay in development should not be made if it is due to a known neurological disorder.[1]

arithmetical disorder – Disorders in which the main feature is a serious impairment in the development of arithmetical skills.[1]

articulation disorder – A delay in the development of normal word-sound production resulting in defects of articulation. Omissions or substitutions of consonants are most frequent.[1]

coordination disorder – Disorders in which the main feature is a serious impairment in the development of motor coordination which is not explicable in terms of general intellectual retardation. The clumsiness is commonly associated with perceptual difficulties.[1]

mixed development disorder – A delay in the development of one specific skill (e.g., reading, arithmetic, speech, or coordination) is frequently associated with lesser delays in other skills. When this occurs, the diagnosis should be made according to the skill most seriously impaired. The mixed category should be used only where the mixture of delayed skills is such that no one skill is preponderantly affected.[1]

motor retardation — *see* Coordination disorder above

reading disorder or retardation – Disorders in which the main feature is a serious impairment in the development of reading or spelling skills which is not explicable in terms of general intellectual retardation or of inadequate schooling. Speech or language difficulties, impaired right-left differentiation, perceptuo-motor problems, and coding difficulties are frequently associated. Similar problems are often present in other members of the family. Adverse psychosocial factors may be present.[1]

speech or language disorder – Disorders in which the main feature is a serious impairment in the development of speech or language (syntax or semantic) which is not explicable in terms of general intellectual retardation. Most commonly there is a delay in the development of normal word-sound production resulting in defects of articulation. Omissions or substitutions of consonants are most frequent. There may also be a delay in the production of spoken language. Rarely, there is also a developmental delay in the comprehension of sounds. Includes cases in which delay is largely due to environmental privation.[1]

Dipsomania — *see* Alcohol dependence syndrome

Disorganized schizophrenia — *see* Schizophrenia, disorganized type

Dissociative hysteria — *see* Hysteria, dissociative type under Neurotic disorders

Drug abuse – Includes cases where an individual, for whom no other diagnosis is possible, has come under medical care because of the maladaptive effect of a drug on which he is not dependent (*see* Drug dependence) and that he has taken on his own initiative to the detriment of his health or social functioning. When drug abuse is secondary to a psychiatric disorder, record the disorder as an additional diagnosis.[1]

Drug dependence – A state, psychic and sometimes also physical dependence, resulting from taking a drug, characterized by behavioral and other responses that always include a compulsion to take a drug on a continuous or periodic basis in order to experience its psychic effects, and

APPENDIX B: GLOSSARY OF MENTAL DISORDERS

sometimes to avoid the discomfort of its absence. Tolerance may or may not be present. A person may be dependent on more than one drug.[1]

Drug psychoses – Organic mental syndromes which are due to consumption of drugs (notably amphetamines, barbiturates, and opiate and LSD groups) and solvents. Some of the syndromes in this group are not as severe as most conditions labeled "psychotic," but they are included here for practical reasons. The drug should be identified, and also a diagnosis of drug dependence should be recorded, if present.[1]

drug-induced hallucinosis – Hallucinatory states of more than a few days, but not more than a few months' duration, associated with large or prolonged intake of drugs, notably of the amphetamine and LSD groups. Auditory hallucinations usually predominate and there may be anxiety or restlessness. States following LSD or other hallucinogens lasting only a few days or less ["bad trips"] are not included.[1]

drug-induced organic delusional syndrome – Paranoid states of more than a few days, but not more than a few months' duration, associated with large or prolonged intake of drugs, notably of the amphetamine and LSD groups.[1]

drug withdrawal syndrome – States associated with drug withdrawal ranging from severe, as specified for alcohol withdrawal delirium [delirium tremens], to less severe states characterized by one or more symptoms such as convulsions, tremor, anxiety, restlessness, gastrointestinal and muscular complaints, and mild disorientation and memory disturbance.[1]

Drunkenness
acute — *see* Alcohol intoxication, acute
pathologic — *see* Alcohol intoxication, idiosyncratic
simple – A state of inebriation due to alcohol consumption without conspicuous neurological signs of intoxication.[2]
sleep – An inability to fully arouse from the sleep state characterized by failure to attain full consciousness after arousal.[2]

Dyscalculia — *see* Arithmetical disorder under Developmental delay disorders, specific

Dyslalia — *see* Articulation disorder under Developmental delay disorders, specific

Dyslexia, developmental – A disorder in which the main feature is a serious impairment of reading skills which is not explicable in terms of general intellectual retardation or of inadequate schooling. Word-blindness and strephosymbolia (tendency to reverse letters and words in reading) are included.[1,3]

Dysmenorrhea, psychogenic – Painful menstruation due to disturbance of psychic control.[4]

Dyspareunia, functional — *see* Functional dyspareunia under Psychosexual dysfunctions

Dyspraxia syndrome — *see* Coordination disorder under Developmental delay disorders, specific

Dyssocial personality — *see* Personality disorder, antisocial type

Dysuria, psychogenic – Difficulty in passing urine due to psychic factors.[4]

Eating disorders – A group of disorders characterized by a conspicuous disturbance in eating behavior.[2] *See also* Bulimia, Pica, and Rumination, psychogenic.

Eccentric personality — *see* Personality disorder, eccentric type

Elective mutism – A pervasive and persistent refusal to speak in situations not attributable to a mental disorder. In some cases the behavior may manifest a form of withdrawal reaction to a specific stressful situation, or as a predominant feature in children exhibiting shyness or social withdrawal disorders.[2]

Emancipation disorder – An adjustment reaction in adolescents or young adults in which there is symptomatic expression (e.g., difficulty in making independent decisions, increased dependence on parental advice, adoption of values deliberately oppositional to parents) of a conflict over independence following the recent assumption of a status in which the individual is more independent of parental control or supervision.[2]

Emotional disturbances specific to childhood and adolescence – Less well-differentiated emotional disorders characteristic of the childhood period. When the emotional disorder takes the form of a neurosis, the appropriate diagnosis should be made. These disorders differ from adjustment reactions in terms of longer duration and by the lack of close relationship in time and content to some stress.[1] *See also* Academic underachievement disorder, Elective mutism, Identity disorder, Introverted disorder of childhood, Misery and unhappiness disorder, Oppositional disorder, Overanxious disorder, and Shyness disorder of childhood.

Encopresis – A disorder in which the main manifestation is the persistent voluntary or involuntary passage of formed stools of normal or near-normal consistency into places not intended for that purpose in the individual's own sociocultural setting. Sometimes the child has failed to gain bowel control, and sometimes he has

APPENDIX B: GLOSSARY OF MENTAL DISORDERS

gained control but then later again became encopretic. There may be a variety of associated psychiatric symptoms and there may be smearing of feces. The condition would not usually be diagnosed under the age of four years.[1]

Endogenous depression — see Affective psychosis, depressed type

Enuresis - A disorder in which the main manifestation is a persistent involuntary voiding of urine by day or night which is considered abnormal for the age of the individual. Sometimes the child will have failed to gain bladder control and in other cases he will have gained control and then lost it. Episodic or fluctuating enuresis should be included. The disorder would not usually be diagnosed under the age of four years.[1]

Epileptic confusional or twilight state — see Delirium, acute

Excitation
   catatonic — see Schizophrenia, catatonic type
   psychogenic — see Psychosis, excitative type
   reactive — see Psychosis, excitative type

Exhaustion delirium — see Stress reaction, acute

Exhibitionism - Sexual deviation in which the main sexual pleasure and gratification is derived from exposure of the genitals to a person of the opposite sex.[1]

Explosive personality disorder — see Personality disorder, explosive type

Factitious illness - A form of hysterical neurosis in which there are physical or psychological symptoms that are not real, genuine, or natural, which are produced by the individual and are under his voluntary control.[2]
   physical symptom type - The presentation of physical symptoms that may be total fabrication, self-inflicted, an exaggeration or exacerbation of a pre-existing physical condition, or any combination or variation of these.[2]
   psychological symptom type - The voluntary production of symptoms suggestive of a mental disorder. Behavior may mimic psychosis or, rather, the individual's idea of psychosis.[2]

Fanatic personality — see Personality disorder, paranoid type

Fatigue neurosis — see Neurasthenia under Neurotic disorders

Feeble-minded — see Mental retardation, mild

Fetishism - A sexual deviation in which nonliving objects are utilized as a preferred or exclusive method of stimulating erotic arousal.[2]

Finger-flicking — see Stereotyped repetitive movements

Folie à deux — see Shared paranoid disorder

Frigidity - A psychosexual dysfunction in which there is partial or complete failure to attain or maintain the lubrication-swelling response of sexual excitement until completion of the sexual act.[2]

Frontal lobe syndrome — Changes in behavior following damage to the frontal areas of the brain or following interference with the connections of those areas. There is a general diminution of self-control, foresight, creativity, and spontaneity, which may be manifest as increased irritability, selfishness, restlessness, and lack of concern for others. Conscientiousness and powers of concentration are often diminished, but measurable deterioration of intellect or memory is not necessarily present. The overall picture is often one of emotional dullness, lack of drive, and slowness; but, particularly in persons previously with energetic, restless, or aggressive characteristics, there may be a change towards impulsiveness, boastfulness, temper outbursts, silly fatuous humor, and the development of unrealistic ambitions; the direction of change usually depends upon the previous personality. A considerable degree of recovery is possible and may continue over the course of several years.[1]

Fugue, psychogenic - A form of dissociative hysteria characterized by an episode of wandering with inability to recall one's prior identity. Both onset and recovery are rapid. Following recovery there is no recollection of events which took place during the fugue state.[2]

Ganser's syndrome (hysterical) - A form of factitious illness in which the patient voluntarily produces symptoms suggestive of a mental disorder.[2]

Gender identity disorder — see Gender identity disorder under Psychosexual identity disorders

Gilles de la Tourette's disorder or syndrome — see Gilles de la Tourette's disorder under Tics

Grief reaction — see Depressive reaction, brief under Adjustment reaction

Gross stress reaction — see Stress reaction, acute

Group delinquency — see Socialized conduct disorder under Conduct disorders

Habit spasm — see Chronic motor tic disorder under Tics

Hangover (alcohol) — see Drunkenness, simple

Head-banging — see Stereotyped repetitive movements

APPENDIX B: GLOSSARY OF MENTAL DISORDERS

Hebephrenia — *see* Schizophrenia, disorganized type

Heller's syndrome — *see* Psychosis, disintegrative

High grade defect — *see* Mental retardation, mild

Homosexuality – Exclusive or predominant sexual attraction for persons of the same sex with or without physical relationship. Record homosexuality as a diagnosis whether or not it is considered as a mental disorder.[1]

Hospital addiction syndrome — *see* Munchausen syndrome

Hospital hoboes — *see* Munchausen syndrome

Hospitalism – A mild or transient adjustment reaction characterized by withdrawal seen in hospitalized patients. In young children this may be manifested by elective mutism.[1]

Hyperkinetic syndrome of childhood – Disorders in which the essential features are short attention span and distractibility. In early childhood the most striking symptom is disinhibited, poorly organized and poorly regulated extreme overactivity but in adolescence this may be replaced by underactivity. Impulsiveness, marked mood fluctuations, and aggression are also common symptoms. Delays in the development of specific skills are often present and disturbed, poor relationships are common. If the hyperkinesis is symptomatic of an underlying disorder, the diagnosis of the underlying disorder is recorded instead.[1]

    attention deficit disorder – Cases of hyperkinetic syndrome in which short attention span, distractibility, and overactivity are the main manifestations without significant disturbance of conduct or delay in specific skills.[1]

    hyperkinesis with developmental delay – Cases in which the hyperkinetic syndrome is associated with speech delay, clumsiness, reading difficulties, or other delays of specific skills.[1]

    hyperkinetic conduct disorder – Cases in which the hyperkinetic syndrome is associated with marked conduct disturbance but not developmental delay.[1]

Hypersomnia – A disorder of initiating arousal from sleep or maintaining wakefulness.[2]

    persistent – Chronic difficulty in initiating arousal from sleep or maintaining wakefulness associated with major or minor depressive mental disorders.[2]

    transient – Episodes of difficulty in arousal from sleep or maintaining wakefulness associated with acute or intermittent emotional reactions or conflicts.[2]

Hypochondriasis — *see* Hypochondriasis under Neurotic disorders

Hypomania — *see* Affective psychosis, manic type

Hypomanic personality — *see* Personality disorder, chronic hypomanic type

Hyposomnia — *see* Insomnia

Hysteria — *see* Hysteria under Neurotic disorders

    anxiety — *see* Phobia under Neurotic disorders

    psychosis — *see* Psychosis, reactive

        acute — *see* Psychosis, excitative type

Hysterical personality — *see* Personality disorder, histrionic type

Identity disorder – An emotional disorder caused by distress over the inability to reconcile aspects of the self into a relatively coherent and acceptable sense of self, not secondary to another mental disorder. The disturbance is manifested by intense subjective distress regarding uncertainty about a variety of issues relating to identity, including long-term goals, career choice, friendship patterns, values, and loyalties.[2]

Idiocy — *see* Mental retardation, profound

Imbecile — *see* Mental retardation, moderate

Impotence – A psychosexual dysfunction in which there is partial or complete failure to attain or maintain erection until completion of the sexual act.[2]

Impulse control disorder — *see* Impulse control disorders under Conduct disorders

Inadequate personality — *see* Personality disorder, dependent type

Induced paranoid disorder — *see* Shared paranoid disorder

Inebriety — *see* Drunkenness, simple

Infantile autism — *see* Autism, infantile

Insomnia – A disorder of initiating or maintaining sleep.[2]

    persistent – A chronic state of sleeplessness associated with chronic anxiety, major or minor depressive disorders, or psychoses.[2]

    transient – Episodes of sleeplessness associated with acute or intermittent emotional reactions or conflicts.[2]

Intermittent explosive disorder – Recurrent episodes of sudden and significant loss of control of aggressive impulses, not accounted for by any other mental disorder, which results in serious assault or destruction of property. The magnitude of the behavior during an episode is grossly out of proportion to any psychosocial stressors which may have played a role in eliciting the episode of lack of control. Following each episode there is genuine regret or self-reproach at the consequences of the action and the

APPENDIX B: GLOSSARY OF MENTAL DISORDERS

inability to control the aggressive impulse.[2]

Introverted disorder of childhood – An emotional disturbance in children chiefly manifested by a lack of interest in social relationships and indifference to social praise or criticism.[2]

Introverted personality — see Personality disorder, introverted type

Involutional melancholia — see Affective psychosis, depressed type

Involutional paranoid state — see Paraphrenia

Isolated explosive disorder – A disorder of impulse control in which there is a single discrete episode characterized by failure to resist an impulse which leads to a single, violent externally-directed act, which has a catastrophic impact on others, and for which the available information does not justify the diagnosis of another mental disorder.[2]

Isolated phobia — see Simple phobia under Phobia

Jet lag syndrome – A phase-shift disruption of the 24-hour sleep-wake cycle due to rapid time-zone changes experienced in long-distance travel.[2]

Kanner's syndrome — see Autism, infantile

Kleptomania – A disorder of impulse control characterized by a recurrent failure to resist impulses to steal objects not for immediate use or their monetary value. An increasing sense of tension is experienced prior to committing the act, with an intense experience of gratification at the time of committing the theft.[2]

Korsakoff's psychosis
  alcoholic — see Alcohol amnestic syndrome under Alcoholic psychoses
  nonalcoholic — see Amnestic syndrome

Latent schizophrenia — see Schizophrenia, latent

Lesbianism — see Homosexuality

Lobotomy syndrome — see Frontal lobe syndrome

LSD reaction – Acute intoxication from hallucinogen abuse, manifested by hallucinatory states lasting only a few days or less.[1]

Major depressive disorder — see Affective psychosis, depressed type

Malingering – A clinical picture in which the predominant feature is the presentation of fake or grossly exaggerated physical or psychiatric illness apparently under voluntary control. In contrast to factitious illness, the symptoms produced in malingering are in pursuit of a goal which, when known, is recognizable and obviously understandable in light of knowledge of the individual's circumstances. Examples of understandable goals include, but are not limited to, becoming a "patient" in order to avoid conscription or military duty, avoid work, obtain financial compensation, evade criminal prosecution, and obtain drugs.[2]

Mania (monopolar) — see Affective psychosis, manic type

Manic-depressive psychosis
  circular type — see Affective psychosis, bipolar
  depressed type — see Affective psychosis, depressed type
  manic type — see Affective psychosis, manic type
  mixed type — see Affective psychosis, mixed type

Manic disorder — see Affective psychosis, manic type
  atypical — see Affective psychosis, manic type, atypical

Masochistic personality — see Personality disorder, masochistic type

Melancholia — see Affective psychoses
  involutional — see Affective psychosis, depressed type

Mental retardation – A condition of arrested or incomplete development of mind which is especially characterized by subnormality of intelligence. The coding should be made on the individual's current level of functioning *without regard to its nature* or causation, such as psychosis, cultural deprivation, Down's syndrome, etc. Where there is a specific cognitive handicap — such as in speech — the diagnosis of mental retardation should be based on assessments of cognition *outside the area of specific handicap*. The assessment of intellectual level should be based on whatever information is available, including clinical evidence, adaptive behavior, and psychometric findings. The IQ levels given are based on a test with a mean of 100 and a standard deviation of 15, such as the Wechsler scales. They are provided only as a guide and should not be applied rigidly. Mental retardation often involves psychiatric disturbances and may often develop as a result of some physical disease or injury. In these cases, an additional diagnosis should be recorded to identify any associated condition, psychiatric or physical.[1]

  mild mental retardation – IQ criteria 50–70. Individuals with this level of retardation are usually educable. During the preschool period they can develop social and communication skills, have minimal retardation in sensorimotor areas, and often are not distinguished from normal children until a later age. During the school age period they can learn academic skills up to approximately the sixth-grade level. During the

APPENDIX B: GLOSSARY OF MENTAL DISORDERS

adult years, they can usually achieve social and vocational skills adequate for minimum self-support, but may need guidance and assistance when under social or economic stress.[1]

moderate mental retardation – IQ criteria 35–49. Individuals with this level of retardation are usually trainable. During the preschool period they can talk or learn to communicate. They have poor social awareness and fair motor development. During the school age period they can profit from training in social and occupational skills, but they are unlikely to progress beyond the second-grade level in academic subjects. During their adult years they may achieve self-maintenance in unskilled or semi-skilled work under sheltered conditions. They need supervision and guidance when under mild social or economic stress.[2]

severe mental retardation – IQ criteria 20–34. Individuals with this level of retardation evidence poor motor development, minimal speech, and are generally unable to profit from training and self-help during the preschool period. During the school age period they can talk or learn to communicate, can be trained in elementary health habits, and may profit from systematic habit training. During the adult years they may contribute partially to self-maintenance under complete supervision.[2]

profound mental retardation – IQ criteria under 20. Individuals with this level of retardation evidence minimal capacity for sensorimotor functioning and need nursing care during the preschool period. During the school age period some further motor development may occur, and they may respond to minimal or limited training in self-help. During the adult years some motor and speech development may occur, and they may achieve very limited self-care and need nursing care.[2]

Merycism — see Rumination, psychogenic

Minimal brain dysfunction [MBD] — see Hyperkinetic syndrome of childhood

Misery and unhappiness disorder – An emotional disorder characteristic of childhood in which the main symptoms involve misery and unhappiness. There may also be eating and sleep disturbances.

Mood swings (brief compensatory) (rebound) – Mild disorders of mood (depression and anxiety or elation and excitement, occurring alternatingly or episodically) seen in affective psychosis.[1]

Motor tic disorders — see Tics

Motor-verbal tic disorder — see Gilles de la Tourette's disorder under Tics

Multi-infarct dementia or psychosis — see Arteriosclerotic dementia

Multiple operations syndrome — see Munchausen syndrome

Multiple personality – A form of dissociative hysteria in which there is the domination of the individual at any one time by one of two or more distinct personalities. Each personality is a fully-integrated and complex unit with memories, behavior patterns, and social friendships which determine the nature of the individual's acts when uppermost in consciousness.[2]

Munchausen syndrome – A chronic form of factitious illness in which the individual demonstrates a plausible presentation of voluntarily produced physical symptomatology of such a degree that he is able to obtain and sustain multiple hospitalizations.[2]

Narcissistic personality — see Personality disorder, narcissistic type

Nervous debility — see Neurasthenia under Neurotic disorders

Neurasthenia — see Neurasthenia under Neurotic disorders

Neurotic delinquency — see Mixed disturbance of conduct and emotions under Conduct disorders

Neurotic disorders – Neurotic disorders are mental disorders without any demonstrable organic basis in which the individual may have considerable insight and has unimpaired reality testing, in that he usually does not confuse his morbid subjective experiences and fantasies with external reality. Behavior may be greatly affected although usually remaining within socially acceptable limits, but personality is not disorganized. The principal manifestations include excessive anxiety, hysterical symptoms, phobias, obsessional and compulsive symptoms, and depression.[1]

anxiety states – Various combinations of physical and mental manifestations of anxiety, not attributable to real danger and occurring either in attacks [see Anxiety state, panic attacks] or as a persisting state [see Anxiety state, generalized]. The anxiety is usually diffuse and may extend to panic. Other neurotic features such as obsessional or hysterical symptoms may be present but do not dominate the clinical picture.[1]

compensation neurosis – Certain unconscious neurotic reactions in which features of secondary gain, such as a situational or financial advantage, are prominent.[3]

depersonalization – A neurotic disorder with an unpleasant state of disturbed perception in which external objects or parts of one's own body are experienced as changed in their quality, unreal, remote, or automatized. The patient is aware of the subjec-

2002 Ingenix, Inc.   Resources—19

APPENDIX B: GLOSSARY OF MENTAL DISORDERS

tive nature of the change he experiences. If depersonalization occurs as a feature of anxiety, schizophrenia, or other mental disorder, the condition is classified according to the major psychiatric disorder.[1]

depression – A neurotic disorder characterized by disproportionate depression which has usually recognizably ensued on a distressing experience; it does not include among its features delusions or hallucinations, and there is often preoccupation with the psychic trauma which preceded the illness, e.g., loss of a cherished person or possession. Anxiety is also frequently present and mixed states of anxiety and depression should be included here. The distinction between depressive neurosis and psychosis should be made not only upon the degree of depression but also on the presence or absence of other neurotic and psychotic characteristics, and upon the degree of disturbance of the individual's behavior.[1]

hypochondriasis – A neurotic disorder in which the conspicuous features are excessive concern with one's health in general or the integrity and functioning of some part of one's body, or less frequently, one's mind. It is usually associated with anxiety and depression. It may occur as a feature of some other severe mental disorder (e.g., manic-depressive psychosis, depressed type, schizophrenia, hysteria) and in that case should be classified according to the corresponding major disorder.[1]

hysteria – A neurotic mental disorder in which motives, of which the patient seems unaware, produce either a restriction of the field of consciousness or disturbances of motor or sensory function which may seem to have psychological advantage or symbolic value.[1] There are three subtypes –

    conversion type – The chief or only symptoms of the hysterical neurosis consist of psychogenic disturbance of function in some part of the body, e.g., paralysis, tremor, blindness, deafness, seizures.[1]

    dissociative type – The most prominent feature of the hysterical neurosis is a narrowing of the field of consciousness which seems to serve an unconscious purpose and is commonly accompanied or followed by a selective amnesia. There may be dramatic but essentially superficial changes of personality [multiple personality], or sometimes the patient enters into a wandering state [fugue].[1]

factitious illness – Physical or psychological symptoms that are not real, genuine, or natural, which are produced by the individual and are under his voluntary control.[2]

neurasthenia – A neurotic disorder characterized by fatigue, irritability, headache, depression, insomnia, difficulty in concentration, and lack of capacity for enjoyment [anhedonia]. It may follow or accompany an infection or exhaustion, or arise from continued emotional stress. If neurasthenia is associated with a physical disorder, the latter should also be recorded as a diagnosis.[1]

obsessive-compulsive – States in which the outstanding symptom is a feeling of subjective compulsion, which must be resisted, to carry out some action, to dwell on an idea, to recall an experience, or to ruminate on an abstract topic. Unwanted thoughts which intrude, the insistency of words or ideas, ruminations or trains of thought are perceived by the individual to be inappropriate or nonsensical. The obsessional urge or idea is recognized as alien to the personality but as coming from within the self. Obsessional actions may be quasi-ritual performances designed to relieve anxiety, e.g., washing the hands to cope with contamination. Attempts to dispel the unwelcome thoughts or urges may lead to a severe inner struggle, with intense anxiety.[1]

occupational – A neurosis characterized by a functional disorder of a group of muscles used chiefly in one's occupation, marked by the occurrence of spasm, paresis, or incoordination on attempt to repeat the habitual movements (e.g., writer's cramp).[5]

phobic disorders – Neurotic states with abnormally intense dread of certain objects or specific situations which would not normally have that effect. If the anxiety tends to spread from a specified situation or object to a wider range of circumstances, it becomes akin to or identical with anxiety state and should be classified as such.[1] See also Phobia.

somatization disorder – A chronic, but fluctuating, neurotic disorder which begins early in life and is characterized by recurrent and multiple somatic complaints for which medical attention is sought but which are not apparently due to any physical illness. Complaints are presented in a dramatic, vague, or exaggerated way, or are part of a complicated medical history in which often many specific diagnoses have allegedly been made by other physicians. Complaints invariably refer to many organ systems (headache, fatigue, palpitations, fainting, nausea and vomiting, abdominal pains, bowel trouble, allergies, menstrual and sexual difficulties), and the individual

APPENDIX B: GLOSSARY OF MENTAL DISORDERS

frequently receives medical care from a number of physicians, sometimes simultaneously.[2]

Neurosis — *see* Neurotic disorders

Nightmares – Anxiety attacks occurring in dreams during REM sleep.[2]

Night terrors – A pathology of arousal from stage 4 sleep in which the individual experiences excessive terror and extreme panic (screaming, verbalizations), symptoms of autonomic activity, confusion, and poor recall for event.[2]

Nymphomania – Abnormal and excessive need or desire in the woman for sexual intercourse.[3]

Obsessional personality — *see* Personality disorder, compulsive type

Occupational neurosis — *see* Neurotic disorder, occupational

Oneirophrenia — *see* Schizophrenia, acute episode

Oppositional disorder of childhood or adolescence – A disorder characterized by pervasive opposition to all in authority regardless of self-interest, a continuous argumentativeness, and an unwillingness to respond to reasonable persuasion, not accounted for by a conduct disorder, adjustment disorder, or a psychosis of childhood. The oppositional behavior in this disorder is evoked by any demand, rule, suggestion, request, or admonishment placed on the individual.[2]

Organic affective syndrome – A clinical picture in which the predominating symptoms closely resemble those seen in either the depressive or manic affective disorders, occurring in the presence of evidence or history of a specific organic factor which is etiologically related to the disturbance, such as head trauma, endocranial tumors, and exocranial tumors secreting neurotoxic diatheses (e.g., pancreatic carcinoma). Excessive use of steroids, Cushing's syndrome, and other endocrine disorders may lead to an organic affective syndrome.[2]

Organic personality syndrome – Chronic, mild states of memory disturbance and intellectual deterioration, of nonpsychotic nature, often accompanied by increased irritability, querulousness, lassitude, and complaints of physical weakness. These states are often associated with old age, and may precede more severe states due to brain damage classifiable under senile or presenile dementia, dementia associated with other chronic organic psychotic brain syndromes, or delirium, delusions, hallucinosis, and depression in transient organic psychotic conditions.[1]

Organic psychosyndrome, focal (partial) – A nonpsychotic organic mental disorder resembling the postconcussion syndrome associated with localized diseases of the brain or surrounding tissues.[1]

Organic psychotic conditions – Syndromes in which there is impairment of orientation, memory, comprehension, calculation, learning capacity, and judgment. These are the essential features but there may also be shallowness or lability of affect, or a more persistent disturbance of mood, lowering of ethical standards and exaggeration or emergence of personality traits, and diminished capacity for independent decision.[1] *See also* Alcohol psychoses, Arteriosclerotic dementia, Drug psychoses, Presenile dementia, and Senile dementia.

mixed paranoid and affective – Organic psychosis in which depressive and paranoid symptoms are the main features.[1]

transient – States characterized by clouded consciousness, confusion, disorientation, illusions, and often vivid hallucinations. They are usually due to some intra- or extracerebral toxic, infectious, metabolic or other systemic disturbance and are generally reversible. Depressive and paranoid symptoms may also be present but are not the main feature. The diagnosis of the associated physical or neurological condition should also be recorded.[1]

> **acute delirium** – Short-lived states, lasting hours or days, of the above type.[1]
>
> **subacute delirium** – States of the above type in which the symptoms, usually less florid, last for several weeks or longer during which they may show marked fluctuations in intensity.[1]

Organic reaction — *see* Organic psychotic conditions, transient

Overanxious disorder – An ill-defined emotional disorder characteristic of childhood in which the main symptoms involve anxiety and fearfulness.[1]

Panic disorder — *see* Panic attack under Anxiety state

Paranoia – A rare chronic psychosis in which logically constructed systematized delusions have developed gradually without concomitant hallucinations or the schizophrenic type of disordered thinking. The delusions are mostly of grandeur (the paranoiac prophet or inventor), persecution, or somatic abnormality.[1]

alcoholic — *see* Alcoholic jealousy under Alcoholic psychoses

querulans – A paranoid state which, though in many ways akin to schizophrenic or

APPENDIX B: GLOSSARY OF MENTAL DISORDERS

affective states, differs from other paranoid states and psychogenic paranoid psychosis.[1]

senile — see Paraphrenia

Paranoid personality — see Personality disorder, paranoid type

Paranoid reaction, acute – Paranoid states apparently provoked by some emotional stress. The stress is often misconstrued as an attack or threat. Such states are particularly prone to occur in prisoners or as acute reactions to a strange and threatening environment, e.g., in immigrants.[1]

Paranoid schizophrenia — see Schizophrenia, paranoid type

Paranoid state

involutional — see Paraphrenia

senile — see Paraphrenia

simple – A psychosis, acute or chronic, not classifiable as schizophrenia or affective psychosis, in which delusions, especially of being influenced, persecuted, or treated in some special way, are the main symptoms. The delusions are of a fairly fixed, elaborate, and systematized kind.[1]

Paranoid traits — see Personality disorder, paranoid type

Paraphilia — see Sexual deviations

Paraphrenia – Paranoid psychosis in which there are conspicuous hallucinations, often in several modalities. Affective symptoms and disordered thinking, if present, do not dominate the clinical picture, and the personality is well preserved.[1]

Paraphrenic schizophrenia — see Schizophrenia, paranoid type

Passive-aggressive personality — see Personality disorder, passive-aggressive type

Passive personality — see Personality disorder, dependent type

Pathological

alcohol intoxication — see Alcohol intoxication, idiosyncratic

drug intoxication – Individual idiosyncratic reactions to comparatively small quantities of a drug, which take the form of acute, brief psychotic states of any type.[1]

drunkenness — see Alcohol intoxication, idiosyncratic

gambling – A disorder of impulse control characterized by a chronic and progressive preoccupation with gambling and urge to gamble, with subsequent gambling behavior that compromises, disrupts, or damages personal, family, and vocational pursuits.[2]

personality — see Personality disorder

Pedophilia – Sexual deviations in which an adult engages in sexual activity with a child of the same or opposite sex.[1]

Peregrinating patient — see Malingering

Personality disorders – Deeply ingrained maladaptive patterns of behavior generally recognizable by the time of adolescence or earlier and continuing throughout most of adult life, although often becoming less obvious in middle or old age. The personality is abnormal either in the balance of its components, their quality and expression, or in its total aspect. Because of this deviation or psychopathy the patient suffers or others have to suffer, and there is an adverse effect upon the individual or on society. It includes what is sometimes called psychopathic personality, but if this is determined primarily by malfunctioning of the brain, it should be classified as one of the nonpsychotic organic brain syndromes. When the patient exhibits an anomaly of personality directly related to his neurosis or psychosis, e.g., schizoid personality and schizophrenia or anancastic personality and obsessive compulsive neurosis, the relevant neurosis or psychosis which is in evidence should be diagnosed in addition.[1]

affective type – A chronic personality disorder characterized by lifelong predominance of a pronounced mood. The illness does not have a clear onset, and there may be intermittent periods of disturbed mood separated by periods of normal mood.[1]

anancastic [anankastic] type — see Personality disorder, compulsive type

antisocial type – A personality disorder characterized by disregard for social obligations, lack of feeling for others, and impetuous violence or callous unconcern. There is a gross disparity between behavior and the prevailing social norms. Behavior is not readily modifiable by experience, including punishment. People with this personality are often affectively cold, and may be abnormally aggressive or irresponsible. Their tolerance to frustration is low; they blame others or offer plausible rationalizations for the behavior which brings them into conflict with society.[1]

asthenic type — see Personality disorder, dependent type

avoidant type – Individuals with this disorder exhibit excessive social inhibitions and shyness, a tendency to withdraw from opportunities for developing close relationships, and a fearful expectation that they will be belittled and humiliated. Desires for affection and acceptance are strong, but they are unwilling to enter relationships unless given unusually strong guarantees that they will be uncritically accepted. Therefore, they have few close relationships and suffer from feelings of loneliness and isolation.[2]

borderline type – Individuals with this disorder are characterized by instability in a variety of areas, including interpersonal

APPENDIX B: GLOSSARY OF MENTAL DISORDERS

relationships, behavior, mood, and self image. Interpersonal relationships are often intense and unstable with marked shifts of attitude over time. Frequently there is impulsive and unpredictable behavior which is potentially physically self-damaging. There may be problems tolerating being alone, and chronic feelings of emptiness or boredom.[2]

chronic depressive type – An affective personality disorder characterized by lifelong predominance of a chronic nonpsychotic disturbance involving either intermittent or sustained periods of depressed mood (marked by worry, pessimism, low output of energy, and a sense of futility).[2]

chronic hypomanic type – An affective personality disorder characterized by lifelong predominance of a chronic nonpsychotic disturbance involving either intermittent or sustained periods of abnormally elevated mood (unshakable optimism and an enhanced zest for life and activity).[2]

compulsive type – A personality disorder characterized by feelings of personal insecurity, doubt, and incompleteness leading to excessive conscientiousness, checking, stubbornness, and caution. There may be insistent and unwelcome thoughts or impulses which do not attain the severity of an obsessional neurosis. There is perfectionism and meticulous accuracy and a need to check repeatedly in an attempt to ensure this. Rigidity and excessive doubt may be conspicuous.[1]

cyclothymic type – A chronic nonpsychotic disturbance involving depressed and elevated mood, lasting at least two years, separated by periods of normal mood.[2]

dependent type – A personality disorder characterized by passive compliance with the wishes of elders and others and a weak inadequate response to the demands of daily life. Lack of vigor may show itself in the intellectual or emotional spheres; there is little capacity for enjoyment.[1]

eccentric type – A personality disorder characterized by oddities of behavior which do not conform to the clinical syndromes of personality disorders described elsewhere.[2]

explosive type – A personality disorder characterized by instability of mood with liability to intemperate outbursts of anger, hate, violence, or affection. Aggression may be expressed in words or in physical violence. The outbursts cannot readily be controlled by the affected persons, who are not otherwise prone to antisocial behavior.[1]

histrionic type – A personality disorder characterized by shallow, labile affectivity, dependence on others, craving for appreciation and attention, suggestibility, and theatricality. There is often sexual immaturity, e.g., frigidity and over-responsiveness to stimuli. Under stress hysterical symptoms [neurosis] may develop.[1]

hysterical type — see Personality disorder, histrionic type

inadequate type — see Personality disorder, dependent type

introverted type – A form of schizoid personality in which the essential features are a profound defect in the ability to form social relationships and to respond to the usual forms of social reinforcements. Such patients are characteristically "loners" who do not appear distressed by their social distance and are not interested in greater social involvement.[2]

masochistic type – A personality disorder in which the individual appears to arrange life situations so as to be defeated and humiliated.[2]

narcissistic type – A personality disorder in which interpersonal difficulties are caused by an inflated sense of self-worth, and indifference to the welfare of others. Achievement deficits and social irresponsibilities are justified and sustained by a boastful arrogance, expansive fantasies, facile rationalization, and frank prevarication.[2]

paranoid type – A personality disorder in which there is excessive sensitiveness to setbacks or to what are taken to be humiliations and rebuffs, a tendency to distort experience by misconstruing the neutral or friendly actions of others as hostile or contemptuous, and a combative and tenacious sense of personal rights. There may be a proneness to jealousy or excessive self-importance. Such persons may feel helplessly humiliated and put upon; others, likewise excessively sensitive, are aggressive and insistent. In all cases there is excessive self-reference.[1]

passive-aggressive type – A personality disorder characterized by aggressive behavior manifested in passive ways, such as obstructionism, pouting, procrastination, intentional inefficiency, or stubbornness. The *aggression* often arises from resentment at failing to find gratification in a relationship with an individual or institution upon which the individual is overdependent.[3]

passive type — see Personality disorder, dependent type

schizoid type – A personality disorder in which there is withdrawal from affectional, social, and other contacts with autistic preference for fantasy and introspective reserve. Behavior may be slightly eccentric or indicate avoidance of competitive situations. Apparent coolness and detachment may mask an incapacity to express feeling.[1]

schizotypal type – A form of schizoid personality in which individuals with this disorder manifest various oddities of thinking, per-

APPENDIX B: GLOSSARY OF MENTAL DISORDERS

ception, communication, and behavior. The disturbance in thinking may be expressed as magical thinking, ideas of reference, or paranoid ideation. Perceptual disturbances may include recurrent illusions and derealization [depersonalization]. Frequently, but not invariably, the behavioral manifestations include social isolation and constricted or inappropriate affect which interferes with rapport in face-to-face interaction without any of the frank psychotic features which characterize schizophrenia.[2]

Phobia – Neurotic states with abnormally intense dread of certain objects or specific situations which would not normally have that effect. If the anxiety tends to spread from a specified situation or object to a wider range of circumstances, it becomes akin to or identical with anxiety state, and should be classified as such.[1]

acrophobia – Fear of heights[3]

agoraphobia – Fear of leaving the familiar setting of the home, and is almost always preceded by a phase during which there are recurrent panic attacks. Because of the anticipatory fear of helplessness when having a panic attack, the patient is reluctant or refuses to be alone, travel or walk alone, or to be in situations where there is no ready access to help, such as in crowds, closed or open spaces, or crowded stores.[2]

ailurophobia – Fear of cats[3]

algophobia – Fear of pain[3]

claustrophobia – Fear of closed spaces[3]

isolated phobia — see Simple phobia below

mysophobia – Fear of dirt or germs[3]

obsessional — see Neurotic disorder, obsessive-compulsive

panphobia – Fear of everything[3]

simple phobia – Fear of a discrete object or situation which is neither fear of leaving the familiar setting of the home [agoraphobia], or of being observed by others in certain situations [social phobia]. Examples of simple phobia are fear of animals, acrophobia, and claustrophobia.[2]

social phobia – Fear of situations in which the subject is exposed to possible scrutiny by others, and the possibility exists that he may act in a fashion that will be considered shameful. The most common social phobias are fears of public speaking, blushing, eating in public, writing in front of others, or using public lavatories.[2]

xenophobia – Fear of strangers[3]

Pica – Perverted appetite of nonorganic origin in which there is persistent eating of non-nutritional substances. Typically, infants ingest paint, plaster, string, hair, or cloth. Older children may have access to animal droppings, sand, bugs, leaves, or pebbles. In the adult, eating of starch or clay-earth has been observed.[2]

Postconcussion syndrome – States occurring after generalized contusion of the brain, in which the symptom picture may resemble that of the frontal lobe syndrome or that of any of the neurotic disorders, but in which in addition, headache, giddiness, fatigue, insomnia, and a subjective feeling of impaired intellectual ability are usually prominent. Mood may fluctuate, and quite ordinary stress may produce exaggerated fear and apprehension. There may be marked intolerance of mental and physical exertion, undue sensitivity to noise, and hypochondriacal preoccupation. The symptoms are more common in persons who have previously suffered from neurotic or personality disorders, or when there is a possibility of compensation. This syndrome is particularly associated with the closed type of head injury when signs of localized brain damage are slight or absent, but it may also occur in other conditions.[1]

Postcontusion syndrome or encephalopathy — see Postconcussion syndrome

Postencephalitic syndrome – A nonpsychotic organic mental disorder resembling the postconcussion syndrome associated with central nervous system infections.[1]

Postleucotomy syndrome — see Frontal lobe syndrome

Posttraumatic brain syndrome, nonpsychotic — see Postconcussion syndrome

Posttraumatic organic psychosis — see Organic psychotic conditions, transient

Posttraumatic stress disorder – The development of characteristic symptoms (re-experiencing the traumatic event, numbing of responsiveness to or involvement with the external world, and a variety of other autonomic, dysphoric, or cognitive symptoms) after experiencing a psychologically traumatic event or events outside the normal range of human experience (e.g., rape or assault, military combat, natural catastrophes such as flood or earthquake, or other disaster, such as airplane crash, fires, bombings).[2]

acute – Brief, episodic, or recurrent disorders lasting less than six months' duration after the onset of trauma.[2]

prolonged – Chronic disorders of the above type lasting six months or more following the trauma.[2]

Premature ejaculation — see Premature ejaculation under Psychosexual dysfunctions

Prepsychotic schizophrenia — see Schizophrenia, latent

APPENDIX B: GLOSSARY OF MENTAL DISORDERS

Presbyophrenia — *see* Organic personality syndrome

Presenile dementia – Dementia occurring usually before the age of 65 in patients with the relatively rare forms of diffuse or lobar cerebral atrophy. The associated neurological condition (e.g., Alzheimer's disease, Pick's disease, Jakob-Creutzfeldt disease) should also be recorded as a diagnosis.[1]

Prodromal schizophrenia — *see* Schizophrenia, latent

Pseudoneurotic schizophrenia — *see* Schizophrenia, latent

Psychalgia – Pains of mental origin, e.g., headache or backache, for which a more precise medical or psychiatric diagnosis cannot be made.[1]

Psychasthenia – A functioning neurosis marked by stages of pathological fear or anxiety, obsessions, fixed ideas, tics, feelings of inadequacy, self-accusation, and pecular feelings of strangeness, unreality, and depersonalization.[4]

Psychic shock – A sudden disturbance of mental equilibrium produced by strong emotion in response to physical or mental stress.[4]

Psychic factors associated with physical diseases – Mental disturbances or psychic factors of any type thought to have played a major part in the etiology of physical conditions, usually involving tissue damage, classified elsewhere. The mental disturbance is usually mild and nonspecific, and the psychic factors (worry, fear, conflict, etc.) may be present without any overt psychiatric disorder. Examples of these conditions are asthma, dermatitis, eczema, duodenal ulcer, ulcerative colitis, and urticaria, specified as due to psychogenic factors. Use an additional diagnosis to identify the physical condition. In the rare instance that an overt psychiatric disorder is thought to have caused the physical condition, the psychiatric diagnosis should be recorded in addition.[1]

Psychoneurosis — *see* Neurotic disorders

Psycho-organic syndrome — *see* Organic psychotic conditions, transient

Psychopathic constitutional state — *see* Personality disorders

Psychopathic personality — *see* Personality disorders

Psychophysiological disorders – A variety of physical symptoms or types of physiological malfunctions of mental origin, not involving tissue damage, and usually mediated through the autonomic nervous system. The disorders are classified according to the body system involved. If the physical symptom is secondary to a psychiatric disorder classifiable elsewhere, the physical symptom is not classified as a psychophysiological disorder. If tissue damage is involved, then the diagnosis is classified as a *Psychic factor associated with diseases classified elsewhere.*[1]

Psychosexual dysfunctions – A group of disorders in which there is recurrent and persistent dysfunction encountered during sexual activity. The dysfunction may be lifelong or acquired, generalized or situational, and total or partial.[2]

   functional dyspareunia – Recurrent and persistent genital pain associated with coitus.[2]

   functional vaginismus – A history of recurrent and persistent involuntary spasm of the musculature of the outer one-third of the vagina that interferes with sexual activity.[2]

   inhibited female orgasm – Recurrent and persistent inhibition of the female orgasm as manifested by a delay or absence of orgasm following a normal sexual excitement phase during sexual activity.[2]

   inhibited male orgasm – Recurrent and persistent inhibition of the male orgasm as manifested by a delay or absence of either the emission or ejaculation phases, or more usually, both following an adequate phase of sexual excitement.[2]

   inhibited sexual desire – Persistent inhibition of desire for engaging in a particular form of sexual activity.[2]

   inhibited sexual excitement – Recurrent and persistent inhibition of sexual excitement during sexual activity, manifested either by partial or complete failure to attain or maintain erection until completion of the sexual act [impotence], or partial or complete failure to attain or maintain the lubrication-swelling response of sexual excitement until completion of the sexual act [frigidity].[2]

   premature ejaculation – Ejaculation occurs before the individual wishes it, because of recurrent and persistent absence of reasonable voluntary control of ejaculation and orgasm during sexual activity.[2]

Psychosexual gender identity disorders – Behavior occurring in preadolescents of immature psychosexuality, or in adults, in which there is an incongruence between the individual's anatomic sex and gender identity.[2]

   gender identity disorder – In children or in adults a condition in which the individual would prefer to be of the other sex, and strongly prefers the clothes, toys, activities, and companionship of the other sex. Cross-dressing is intermittent, although it may be frequent. In children the commonest form is feminism in boys.[2]

   trans-sexualism – A psychosexual identity disorder centered around fixed beliefs that

APPENDIX B: GLOSSARY OF MENTAL DISORDERS

the overt bodily sex is wrong. The resulting behavior is directed towards either changing the sexual organs by operation, or completely concealing the bodily sex by adopting both the dress and behavior of the opposite sex.[1]

Psychosomatic disorders — see Psychophysiological disorders

Psychosis – Mental disorders in which impairment of mental function has developed to a degree that interferes grossly with insight, ability to meet some ordinary demands of life or to maintain adequate contact with reality. It is not an exact or well defined term. Mental retardation is excluded.[1]

affective — see Affective psychoses

alcoholic — see Alcoholic psychoses

atypical childhood – A variety of atypical infantile psychoses which may show some, but not all, of the features of infantile autism. Symptoms may include stereotyped repetitive movements, hyperkinesis, self-injury, retarded speech development, echolalia, and impaired social relationships. Such disorders may occur in children of any level of intelligence but are particularly common in those with mental retardation.[1]

borderline, of childhood — see Psychosis, atypical childhood

child – A group of disorders in children, characterized by distortions in the timing, rate, and sequence of many psychological functions involving language development and social relations in which the severe qualitative abnormalities are not normal for any stage of development.[2] See also Autism, infantile, Psychosis, disintegrative, Psychosis, atypical childhood.

depressive — see Affective psychosis, depressed type

depressive type – A depressive psychosis which can be similar in its symptoms to manic-depressive psychosis, depressed type but is apparently provoked by saddening stress such as a bereavement, or a severe disappointment or frustration. There may be less diurnal variation of symptoms than in manic-depressive psychosis, depressed type, and the delusions are more often understandable in the context of the life experiences. There is usually a serious disturbance of behavior, e.g., major suicidal attempt.[1]

disintegrative – A disorder in which normal or near-normal development for the first few years is followed by a loss of social skills and of speech, together with a severe disorder of emotions, behavior, and relationships. Usually this loss of speech and of social competence takes place over a period of a few months and is accompanied by the emergence of overactivity and of stereotypies. In most cases there is intellectual impairment, but this is not a necessary part of the disorder. The condition may follow overt brain disease, such as measles encephalitis, but it may also occur in the absence of any known organic brain disease or damage. Any associated neurological disorder should also be recorded.[1]

epileptic – An organic psychotic condition associated with epilepsy.[1]

excitative type – An affective psychosis similar in its symptoms to manic-depressive psychosis, manic type, but apparently provoked by emotional stress.[1]

hypomanic — see Affective psychosis, manic type

hysterical — see Psychosis, reactive

    acute — see Psychosis, excitative type

induced — see Shared paranoid disorder

infantile — see Autism, infantile

infective — see Organic psychotic conditions, transient

Korsakoff's

    alcoholic — see alcohol amnestic syndrome under Alcoholic psychoses

    nonalcoholic — see Amnestic syndrome

manic-depressive — see Affective psychoses

multi-infarct — see Arteriosclerotic dementia

paranoid

    chronic — see Paranoia

    protracted reactive — see Psychosis, paranoid, psychogenic

    psychogenic – Psychogenic or reactive paranoid psychosis of any type which is more protracted than the reactions described under Paranoid reaction, acute.[1]

    acute — see Paranoid reaction, acute

postpartum — see Psychosis, puerperal

psychogenic — see Psychosis, reactive

    depressive — see Psychosis, depressive type

puerperal – Any psychosis occurring within a fixed period (approximately 90 days) after childbirth.[3] The diagnosis should be classified according to the predominant symptoms or characteristics, such as schizophrenia, affective psychosis, paranoid states, or other specified psychosis.

reactive – A psychotic condition which is largely or entirely attributable to a recent life experience. This diagnosis is not used for the wider range of psychoses in which environmental factors play some, but not the *major*, part in etiology.[1]

    brief – A florid psychosis of at least a few hours' duration but lasting no more than two weeks, with sudden onset

APPENDIX B: GLOSSARY OF MENTAL DISORDERS

immediately following a severe environmental stress and eventually terminating in complete recovery to the pre-psychotic state.[2]

confusion – Mental disorders with clouded consciousness, disorientation (though less marked than in organic confusion), and diminished accessibility often accompanied by excessive activity and apparently provoked by emotional stress.[1]

depressive — *see* Psychosis, depressive type

schizo-affective — *see* Schizophrenia, schizo-affective type

schizophrenic — *see* Schizophrenia

schizophreniform — *see* Schizophrenia

affective type — *see* Schizophrenia, schizo-affective type

confusional type — *see* Schizophrenia, acute episode

senile — *see* Senile dementia, delusional type

Pyromania – A disorder of impulse control characterized by a recurrent failure to resist impulses to set fires without regard for the consequences, or with deliberate destructive intent. Invariably there is intense fascination with the setting of fires, seeing fires burn, and a satisfaction with the resultant destruction.[2]

Relationship problems of childhood – Emotional disorders characteristic of childhood in which the main symptoms involve relationship problems.[1]

Repeated infarct dementia — *see* Arteriosclerotic dementia

Residual schizophrenia — *see* Schizophrenia, residual type

Restzustand (schizophrenia) — *see* Schizophrenia, residual type

Rumination

obsessional – The constant preoccupation with certain thoughts, with inability to dismiss them from the mind.[4] *See* Neurotic disorder, obsessive-compulsive.

psychogenic – In children the regurgitation of food, with failure to thrive or weight loss developing after a period of normal functioning. Food is brought up without nausea, retching, or disgust. The food is then ejected from the mouth, or chewed and reswallowed.[2]

Sander's disease — *see* Paranoia

Satyriasis – Pathologic or exaggerated sexual desire or excitement in the man.[3]

Schizoid personality disorder — *see* Personality disorder, schizoid type

Schizophrenia – A group of psychoses in which there is a fundamental disturbance of personality, a characteristic distortion of thinking, often a sense of being controlled by alien forces, delusions which may be bizarre, disturbed perception, abnormal affect out of keeping with the real situation, and autism. Nevertheless, clear consciousness and intellectual capacity are usually maintained. The disturbance of personality involves its most basic functions which give the normal person his feeling of individuality, uniqueness, and self-direction. The most intimate thoughts, feelings, and acts are often felt to be known to or shared by others and explanatory delusions may develop, to the effect that natural or supernatural forces are at work to influence the schizophrenic person's thoughts and actions in ways that are often bizarre. He may see himself as the pivot of all that happens. Hallucinations, especially of hearing, are common and may comment on the patient or address him. Perception is frequently disturbed in other ways; there may be perplexity, irrelevant features may become all-important and accompanied by passivity feelings, may lead the patient to believe that everyday objects and situations possess a special, usually sinister, meaning intended for him. In the characteristic schizophrenic disturbance of thinking, peripheral and irrelevant features of a total concept, which are inhibited in normal directed mental activity, are brought to the forefront and utilized in place of the elements relevant and appropriate to the situation. Thus, thinking becomes vague, elliptical and obscure, and its expression in speech sometimes incomprehensible. Breaks and interpolations in the flow of consecutive thought are frequent, and the patient may be convinced that his thoughts are being withdrawn by some outside agency. Mood may be shallow, capricious, or incongruous. Ambivalence and disturbance of volition may appear as inertia, negativism, or stupor. Catatonia may be present. The diagnosis "schizophrenia" should not be made unless there is, or has been evident during the same illness, characteristic disturbance of thought, perception, mood, conduct, or personality — preferably in at least two of these areas. The diagnosis should not be restricted to conditions running a protracted, deteriorating, or chronic course. In addition to making the diagnosis on the criteria just given, effort should be made to specify one of the following subtypes of schizophrenia, according to the predominant symptoms.[1]

APPENDIX B: GLOSSARY OF MENTAL DISORDERS

acute (undifferentiated) - Schizophrenia of florid nature which cannot be classified as simple, catatonic, hebephrenic, paranoid, or any other types.[1]

acute episode - Schizophrenic disorders, other than simple, hebephrenic, catatonic, and paranoid, in which there is a dream-like state with slight clouding of consciousness and perplexity. External things, people, and events may become charged with personal significance for the patient. There may be ideas of reference and emotional turmoil. In many such cases remission occurs within a few weeks or months, even without treatment.[1]

atypical — see Schizophrenia, acute (undifferentiated)

borderline — see Schizophrenia, latent

catatonic type - Includes as an essential feature prominent psychomotor disturbances often alternating between extremes such as hyperkinesis and stupor, or automatic obedience and negativism. Constrained attitudes may be maintained for long periods - if the patient's limbs are put in some unnatural position, they may be held there for some time after the external force has been removed. Severe excitement may be a striking feature of the condition. Depressive or hypomanic concomitants may be present.[1]

cenesthopathic — see Schizophrenia, acute (undifferentiated)

childhood type — see Psychosis, child

chronic undifferentiated — see Schizophrenia, residual

cyclic — see Schizophrenia, schizo-affective type

disorganized type - A form of schizophrenia in which affective changes are prominent, delusions and hallucinations fleeting and fragmentary, behavior irresponsible and unpredictable, and mannerisms common. The mood is shallow and inappropriate, accompanied by giggling or self-satisfied, self-absorbed smiling, or by a lofty manner, grimaces, mannerisms, pranks, hypochondriacal complaints, and reiterated phrases. Thought is disorganized. There is a tendency to remain solitary, and behavior seems empty of purpose and feeling. This form of schizophrenia usually starts between the ages of 15 and 25 years.[1]

hebephrenic type — see Schizophrenia, disorganized type

latent - It has not been possible to produce a generally acceptable description for this condition. It is not recommended for general use, but a description is provided for those who believe it to be useful - a condition of eccentric or inconsequent behavior and anomalies of affect which give the impression of schizophrenia though no definite and characteristic schizophrenic anomalies, present or past, have been manifest.[1]

paranoid type - The form of schizophrenia in which relatively stable delusions, which may be accompanied by hallucinations, dominate the clinical picture. The delusions are frequently of persecution, but may take other forms (for example, of jealousy, exalted birth, Messianic mission, or bodily change). Hallucinations and erratic behavior may occur; in some cases conduct is seriously disturbed from the outset, thought disorder may be gross, and affective flattening with fragmentary delusions and hallucinations may develop.[1]

prepsychotic — see Schizophrenia, latent

prodromal — see Schizophrenia, latent

pseudoneurotic — see Schizophrenia, latent

pseudopsychopathic — see Schizophrenia, latent

residual - A chronic form of schizophrenia in which the symptoms that persist from the acute phase have mostly lost their sharpness. Emotional response is blunted and thought disorder, even when gross, does not prevent the accomplishment of routine work.[1]

schizo-affective type - A psychosis in which pronounced manic or depressive features are intermingled with schizophrenic features and which tends towards remission without permanent defect, but which is prone to recur. The diagnosis should be made only when both the affective and schizophrenic symptoms are pronounced.[1]

simple type - A psychosis in which there is insidious development of oddities of conduct, inability to meet the demands of society, and decline in total performance. Delusions and hallucinations are not in evidence and the condition is less obviously psychotic than are the hebephrenic, catatonic, and paranoid types of schizophrenia. With increasing social impoverishment vagrancy may ensue and the patient becomes self-absorbed, idle, and aimless. Because the schizophrenic symptoms are not clear-cut, diagnosis of this form should be made sparingly, if at all.[1]

simplex — see Schizophrenia, simple type

Schizophrenic syndrome of childhood — see Psychosis, child

Schizophreniform
    attack — see Schizophrenia, acute episode
    disorder — see Schizophrenia, acute episode
    psychosis — see Schizophrenia
        affective type — see Schizophrenia, schizo-affective type
        confusional type — see Schizophrenia, acute episode

Schizotypal personality — see Personality disorder, schizotypal type

Senile dementia - Dementia occurring usually after the age of 65 in which any cerebral pathology other than that of

APPENDIX B: GLOSSARY OF MENTAL DISORDERS

senile atrophic change can be reasonably excluded.[1]

delirium – Senile dementia with a superimposed reversible episode of acute confusional state.[1]

delusional type – A type of senile dementia characterized by development in advanced old age, progressive in nature, in which delusions, varying from simple poorly formed paranoid delusions to highly formed paranoid delusional states, and hallucinations are also present.[1, 2]

depressed type – A type of senile dementia characterized by development in advanced old age, progressive in nature, in which depressive features, ranging from mild to severe forms of manic-depressive affective psychosis, are also present. Disturbance of the sleep-waking cycle and preoccupation with dead people are often particularly prominent.[1, 2]

paranoid type — see Senile dementia, delusional type

simple type — see Senile dementia

Sensitiver Beziehungswahn – A paranoid state which, though in many ways akin to schizophrenic or affective states, differs from paranoia, simple paranoid state, shared paranoid disorder, or psychogenic psychosis.[1]

Sensitivity reaction of childhood or adolescence — see Shyness disorder of childhood

Separation anxiety disorder – A clinical disorder in children in which the predominant disturbance is exaggerated distress at separation from parents, home, or other familial surroundings. When separation is instituted, the child may experience anxiety to the point of panic. In adults a similar disorder is seen in agoraphobic reactions.[2]

Sexual deviations – Abnormal sexual inclinations or behavior which are part of a referral problem. The limits and features of normal sexual behavior have not been stated absolutely in different societies and cultures, but are broadly such as serve approved social and biological purposes. The sexual activity of affected persons is directed primarily either towards people not of the opposite sex, or towards sexual acts not associated with coitus normally, or towards coitus performed under abnormal circumstances. If the anomalous behavior becomes manifest only during psychosis or other mental illness the condition should be classified under the major illness. It is common for more than one anomaly to occur together in the same individual; in that case the predominant deviation is classified. It is preferable not to diagnose sexual deviation in individuals who perform deviant sexual acts when normal sexual outlets are not available to them.[1] *See also* Exhibitionism, Fetishism, Homosexuality, Nymphomania, Pedophilia, Satyriasis, Sexual masochism, Sexual sadism, Transvestism, Voyeurism, and Zoophilia. Gender identity disorder and transsexualism are considered to be psychosexual gender identity disorders and are not included here.

Sexual masochism – A sexual deviation in which sexual arousal and pleasure is produced in an individual by his own physical or psychological suffering, and in which there are insistent and persistent fantasies wherein sexual excitement is produced as a result of suffering.[2]

Sexual sadism – A sexual deviation in which physical or psychological suffering inflicted on another person is utilized as a method of stimulating erotic excitement and orgasm, and in which there are insistent and persistent fantasies wherein sexual excitement is produced as a result of suffering inflicted on the partner.[2]

Shared paranoid disorder – Mainly delusional psychosis, usually chronic and often without florid features, which appears to have developed as a result of a close, if not dependent, relationship with another person who already has an established similar psychosis. The delusions are at least partly shared. The rare cases in which several persons are affected should also be included here.[1]

Shifting sleep-work schedule – A sleep disorder in which the phase-shift disruption of the 24-hour sleep-wake cycle occurs due to rapid changes in the individual's work schedule.[2]

Short sleeper – Individuals who typically need only 4–6 hours of sleep within the 24-hour cycle.[2]

Shyness disorder of childhood – A persistent and excessive shrinking from familiarity or contact with all strangers of sufficient severity as to interfere with peer functioning, yet there are warm and satisfying relationships with family members. A critical feature of this disorder is that the avoidant behavior with strangers persists even after prolonged exposure or contact.[2]

Sibling jealousy or rivalry – An emotional disorder related to competition between siblings for the love of a parent or for other recognition or gain.[3]

Simple phobia — see Simple phobia under Phobia

Situational disturbance, acute — see Stress reaction, acute

APPENDIX B: GLOSSARY OF MENTAL DISORDERS

Social phobia — *see* Social phobia under Phobia

Social withdrawal of childhood — *see* Introverted disorder of childhood

Socialized conduct disorder — *see* Socialized conduct disorder under Conduct disorders

Somatization disorder — *see* Somatization disorder under Neurotic disorders

Somatoform disorder, atypical — *see* Hypochondriasis under Neurotic disorders

Spasmus nutans — *see* Stereotyped repetitive movements

Specific academic or work inhibition – An adjustment reaction in which a specific academic or work inhibition occurs in an individual whose intellectual capacity, skills, and previous academic or work performance have been at least adequate, and in which the inhibition occurs despite apparent effort and is not due to any other mental disorder.[2]

Stammering — *see* Stuttering

Starch-eating — *see* Pica

Status postcommotio cerebri — *see* Postconcussion syndrome

Stereotyped repetitive movements – Disorders in which voluntary repetitive stereotyped movements, which are not due to any psychiatric or neurological condition, constitute the main feature. Includes head-banging, spasmus nutans, rocking, twirling, finger-flicking mannerisms, and eye poking. Such movements are particularly common in cases of mental retardation with sensory impairment or with environmental monotony.[1]

Stereotypies — *see* Stereotyped repetitive movements

Stress reaction
  acute – Acute transient disorders of any severity and nature of emotions, consciousness, and psychomotor states (singly or in combination) which occur in individuals, without any apparent pre-existing mental disorder, in response to exceptional physical or mental stress, such as natural catastrophe or battle, and which usually subside within hours or days.[1]
  chronic — *see* Adjustment reaction

Stupor
  catatonic — *see* Schizophrenia, catatonic type
  psychogenic — *see* Psychosis, reactive

Stuttering – Disorders in the rhythm of speech, in which the individual knows precisely what he wishes to say, but at the time is unable to say it because of an involuntary, repetitive prolongation or cessation of a sound.[1]

Subjective insomnia complaint – A complaint of insomnia made by the individual, which has not been investigated or proven.[2]

Tension headache – Headache of mental origin for which a more precise medical or psychiatric diagnosis cannot be made.[1]

Systematized delusions — *see* Paranoia

Tics – Disorders of no known organic origin in which the outstanding feature consists of quick, involuntary, apparently purposeless, and frequently repeated movements which are not due to any neurological condition. Any part of the body may be involved but the face is most frequently affected. Only one form of tic may be present, or there may be a combination of tics which are carried out simultaneously, alternatively, or consecutively.[1]

  chronic motor tic disorder – A tic disorder starting in childhood and persisting into adult life. The tic is limited to no more than three motor areas, and rarely has a verbal component.[2]

  Gilles de la Tourette's disorder [motor-verbal tic disorder] – A rare disorder occurring in individuals of any level of intelligence in which facial tics and tic-like throat noises become more marked and more generalized, and in which later whole words or short sentences (often with obscene content) are ejaculated spasmodically and involuntarily. There is some overlap with other varieties of tic.[1]

  transient tic disorder of childhood – Facial or other tics beginning in childhood, but limited to one year in duration.[2]

Tobacco use disorder – Cases in which tobacco is used to the detriment of a person's health or social functioning or in which there is tobacco dependence. Dependence is included here rather than under drug dependence because tobacco differs from other drugs of dependence in its psychotoxic effects.[1]

Tranquilizer abuse – Cases where an individual has taken the drug to the detriment of his health or social functioning, in doses above or for periods beyond those normally regarded as therapeutic.[1]

Transient organic psychotic condition — *see* Organic psychotic conditions, transient

Trans-sexualism — *see* Trans-sexualism under Psychosexual identity disorders

Transvestism – Sexual deviation in which there is recurrent and persistent dressing in clothes of the opposite sex, and initially in the early stage of the illness, for the purpose of sexual arousal.[2]

Twilight state
  confusional — *see* Delirium, acute
  psychogenic — *see* Psychosis, reactive confusion

APPENDIX B: GLOSSARY OF MENTAL DISORDERS

Undersocialized conduct disorder — see Undersocialized conduct disorder under Conduct disorders

Unsocialized aggressive disorder — see Undersocialized conduct disorder, aggressive type under Conduct disorders

Vaginismus, functional — see Functional vaginismus under Psychosexual dysfunctions

Vorbeireden – The symptom of the approximate answer or talking past the point, seen in the Ganser syndrome, a form of factitious illness.[2]

Voyeurism – A sexual deviation in which the individual repetitively seeks out situations in which he engages in looking at unsuspecting women who are either naked, in the act of disrobing, or engaging in sexual activity. The act of looking is accompanied by sexual excitement, frequently with orgasm. In its severe form, the act of peeping constitutes the preferred to exclusive sexual activity of the individual.[2]

Wernicke-Korsakoff syndrome — see Alcohol amnestic syndrome under Alcoholic psychoses

Withdrawal reaction of childhood or adolescence — see Introverted disorder of childhood

Word-deafness – A developmental delay in the comprehension of speech sounds.[1]

Zoophilia – Sexual or anal intercourse with animals.[1]

APPENDIX C: CLASSIFICATION OF DRUGS BY AHFS LIST

CLASSIFICATION OF DRUGS BY AMERICAN HOSPITAL FORMULARY SERVICE LIST NUMBER AND THEIR ICD-9-CM EQUIVALENTS

The coding of adverse effects of drugs is keyed to the continually revised Hospital Formulary of the American Hospital Formulary Service (AHFS) published under the direction of the American Society of Hospital Pharmacists.

The following section gives the ICD-9-CM diagnosis code for each AHFS list.

AHFS* List		ICD-9-CM Diagnosis Code
4:00	ANTIHISTAMINE DRUGS	963.0
8:00	ANTI-INFECTIVE AGENTS	
8:04	Amebacides	961.5
	hydroxyquinoline derivatives	961.3
	arsenical anti-infectives	961.1
8:08	Anthelmintics	961.6
	quinoline derivatives	961.3
8:12.04	Antifungal Antibiotics	960.1
	nonantibiotics	961.9
8:12.06	Cephalosporins	960.5
8:12.08	Chloramphenicol	960.2
8:12.12	The Erythromycins	960.3
8:12.16	The Penicillins	960.0
8:12.20	The Streptomycins	960.6
8:12.24	The Tetracyclines	960.4
8:12.28	Other Antibiotics	960.8
	antimycobacterial antibiotics	960.6
	macrolides	960.3
8:16	Antituberculars	961.8
	antibiotics	960.6
8:18	Antivirals	961.7
8:20	Plasmodicides (antimalarials)	961.4
8:24	Sulfonamides	961.0
8:26	The Sulfones	961.8
8:28	Treponemicides	961.2
8:32	Trichomonacides	961.5
	hydroxyquinoline derivatives	961.3
	nitrofuran derivatives	961.9
8:36	Urinary Germicides	961.9
	quinoline derivatives	961.3
8:40	Other Anti-Infectives	961.9
10:00	ANTINEOPLASTIC AGENTS	963.1
	antibiotics	960.7
	progestogens	962.2
12:00	AUTONOMIC DRUGS	
12:04	Parasympathomimetic (Cholinergic) Agents	971.0
12:08	Parasympatholytic (Cholinergic Blocking) Agents	971.1
12:12	Sympathomimetic (Adrenergic) Agents	971.2
12:16	Sympatholytic (Adrenergic Blocking) Agents	971.3
12:20	Skeletal Muscle Relaxants	975.2
	central nervous system muscle-tone depressants	968.0
16:00	BLOOD DERIVATIVES	964.7

AHFS* List		ICD-9-CM Diagnosis Code
20:00	BLOOD FORMATION AND COAGULATION	
20:04	Antianemia Drugs	964.1
20:04.04	Iron Preparations	964.0
20:04.08	Liver and Stomach Preparations	964.1
20:12.04	Anticoagulants	964.2
20:12.08	Antiheparin Agents	964.5
20:12.12	Coagulants	964.5
20.12.16	Hemostatics	964.5
	capillary-active drugs	972.8
	fibrinolysis-affecting agents	964.4
	natural products	964.7
24:00	CARDIOVASCULAR DRUGS	
24:04	Cardiac Drugs	972.9
	cardiotonic agents	972.1
	rhythm regulators	972.0
24:06	Antilipemic Agents	972.2
	thyroid derivatives	962.7
24:08	Hypotensive Agents	972.6
	adrenergic blocking agents	971.3
	ganglion-blocking agents	972.3
	vasodilators	972.5
24:12	Vasodilating Agents	972.5
	coronary	972.4
	nicotinic acid derivatives	972.2
24:16	Sclerosing Agents	972.7
28:00	CENTRAL NERVOUS SYSTEM DRUGS	
28:04	General Anesthetics	968.4
	gaseous anesthetics	968.2
	halothane	968.1
	intravenous anesthetics	968.3
28:08	Analgesics and Antipyretics	965.9
	antirheumatics	965.6
	aromatic analgesics	965.4
	non-narcotics NEC	965.7
	opium alkaloids	965.00
	heroin	965.01
	methadone	965.02
	specified type NEC	965.09
	pyrazole derivatives	965.5
	salicylates	965.1
	specified type NEC	965.8
28:10	Narcotic Antagonists	970.1
28:12	Anticonvulsants	966.3
	barbiturates	967.0
	benzodiazepine-based tranquilizers	969.4
	bromides	967.3
	hydantoin derivatives	966.1
	oxazolidine derivative	966.0
	succinimides	966.2
28:16.04	Antidepressants	969.0
28:16.08	Tranquilizers	969.5
	benzodiazepine-based	969.4
	butyrophenone-based	969.2
	major NEC	969.3
	phenothiazine-based	969.1
28:16.12	Other Psychotherapeutic Agents	969.8

APPENDIX C: CLASSIFICATION OF DRUGS BY AHFS LIST

AHFS* List		ICD-9-CM Diagnosis Code	AHFS* List		ICD-9-CM Diagnosis Code
28:20	Respiratory and Cerebral Stimulants	970.9	52:04.08	Sulfonamides ENT	976.6
	analeptics	970.0		ophthalmic	976.5
	anorexigenic agents	977.0	52:04.12	Miscellaneous Anti-Infectives	
	psychostimulants	969.7		ENT	976.6
	specified type NEC	970.8		ophthalmic	976.5
28:24	Sedatives and Hypnotics	967.9	52:08	Anti-Inflammatory Agents	
	barbiturates	967.0		ENT	976.6
	benzodiazepine-based tranquilizers	969.4		ophthalmic	976.5
			52:10	Carbonic Anhydrase Inhibitors	974.2
	chloral hydrate group	967.1	52:12	Contact Lens Solutions	976.5
	glutethamide group	967.5	52:16	Local Anesthetics	968.5
	intravenous anesthetics	968.3	52:20	Miotics	971.0
	methaqualone	967.4	52:24	Mydriatics	
	paraldehyde	967.2		adrenergics	971.2
	phenothiazine-based tranquilizers	969.1		anticholinergics	971.1
				antimuscarinics	971.1
	specified type NEC	967.8		parasympatholytics	971.1
	thiobarbiturates	968.3		spasmolytics	971.1
	tranquilizer NEC	969.5		sympathomimetics	971.2
36:00	DIAGNOSTIC AGENTS	977.8	52:28	Mouth Washes and Gargles	976.6
40:00	ELECTROLYTE, CALORIC, AND WATER BALANCE AGENTS NEC	974.5	52:32	Vasoconstrictors	971.2
			52:36	Unclassified Agents	
				ENT	976.6
40:04	Acidifying Agents	963.2		ophthalmic	976.5
40:08	Alkalinizing Agents	963.3	56:00	GASTROINTESTINAL DRUGS	
40:10	Ammonia Detoxicants	974.5	56:04	Antacids and Absorbents	973.0
40:12	Replacement Solutions NEC	974.5	56:08	Anti-Diarrhea Agents	973.5
	plasma volume expanders	964.8	56:10	Antiflatulents	973.8
40:16	Sodium-Removing Resins	974.5	56:12	Cathartics NEC	973.3
40:18	Potassium-Removing Resins	974.5		emollients	973.2
40:20	Caloric Agents	974.5		irritants	973.1
40:24	Salt and Sugar Substitutes	974.5	56:16	Digestants	973.4
40:28	Diuretics NEC	974.4	56:20	Emetics and Antiemetics	
	carbonic acid anhydrase inhibitors	974.2		antiemetics	963.0
				emetics	973.6
	mercurials	974.0	56:24	Lipotropic Agents	977.1
	purine derivatives	974.1	60:00	GOLD COMPOUNDS	965.6
	saluretics	974.3	64:00	HEAVY METAL ANTAGONISTS	963.8
40:36	Irrigating Solutions	974.5	68:00	HORMONES AND SYNTHETIC SUBSTITUTES	
40:40	Uricosuric Agents	974.7			
44:00	ENZYMES NEC	963.4	68:04	Adrenals	962.0
	fibrinolysis-affecting agents	964.4	68:08	Androgens	962.1
	gastric agents	973.4	68:12	Contraceptives	962.2
48:00	EXPECTORANTS AND COUGH PREPARATIONS		68:16	Estrogens	962.2
			68:18	Gonadotropins	962.4
	antihistamine agents	963.0	68:20	Insulins and Antidiabetic Agents	962.3
	antitussives	975.4			
	codeine derivatives	965.09	68:20.08	Insulins	962.3
	expectorants	975.5	68:24	Parathyroid	962.6
	narcotic agents NEC	965.09	68:28	Pituitary	
52:00	EYE, EAR, NOSE, AND THROAT PREPARATIONS			anterior	962.4
				posterior	962.5
52:04	Anti-Infectives		68:32	Progestogens	962.2
	ENT	976.6	68:34	Other Corpus Luteum Hormones	962.2
	ophthalmic	976.5	68:36	Thyroid and Antithyroid	
52:04.04	Antibiotics			antithyroid	962.8
	ENT	976.6		thyroid	962.7
	ophthalmic	976.5			
52:04.06	Antivirals				
	ENT	976.6			
	ophthalmic	976.5			

APPENDIX C: CLASSIFICATION OF DRUGS BY AHFS LIST

	AHFS* List	ICD-9-CM Diagnosis Code		AHFS* List	ICD-9-CM Diagnosis Code
72:00	LOCAL ANESTHETICS NEC	968.9	84:00	SKIN AND MUCOUS MEMBRANE PREPARATIONS	
	topical (surface) agents	968.5			
	infiltrating agents		84:04	Anti-Infectives	976.0
	(intradermal)		84:04.04	Antibiotics	976.0
	(subcutaneous)		84:04.08	Fungicides	976.0
	(submucosal)	968.5	84:04.12	Scabicides and Pediculicides	976.0
	nerve blocking agents		84:04.16	Miscellaneous Local	
	(peripheral)(plexus)			Anti-Infectives	976.0
	(regional)	968.6	84:06	Anti-Inflammatory Agents	976.0
	spinal	968.7	84:08	Antipruritics and Local	
76:00	OXYTOCICS	975.0		Anesthetics	
78:00	RADIOACTIVE AGENTS	990		antipruritics	976.1
80:00	SERUMS, TOXOIDS, AND			local anesthetics	968.5
	VACCINES		84:12	Astringents	976.2
80:04	Serums	979.9	84:16	Cell Stimulants and Proliferants	976.8
	immune globulin (gamma)		84:20	Detergents	976.2
	(human)	964.6	84:24	Emollients, Demulcents, and	
80:08	Toxoids NEC	978.8		Protectants	976.3
	diphtheria	978.5	84:28	Keratolytic Agents	976.4
	and tetanus	978.9	84:32	Keratoplastic Agents	976.4
	with pertussis		84:36	Miscellaneous Agents	976.8
	component	978.6	86:00	SPASMOLYTIC AGENTS	975.1
	tetanus	978.4		antiasthmatics	975.7
	and diphtheria	978.9		papaverine	972.5
	with pertussis			theophyllin	974.1
	component	978.6	88:00	VITAMINS	
80:12	Vaccines NEC	979.9	88:04	Vitamin A	963.5
	bacterial NEC	978.8	88:08	Vitamin B Complex	963.5
	with			hematopoietic vitamin	964.1
	other bacterial			nicotinic acid derivatives	972.2
	component	978.9	88:12	Vitamin C	963.5
	pertussis component	978.6	88:16	Vitamin D	963.5
	viral and rickettsial		88:20	Vitamin E	963.5
	component	979.7	88:24	Vitamin K Activity	964.3
	rickettsial NEC	979.6	88:28	Multivitamin Preparations	963.5
	with		92:00	UNCLASSIFIED THERAPEUTIC	
	bacterial component	979.7		AGENTS	977.8
	pertussis component	978.6			
	viral component	979.7			
	viral NEC	979.6			
	with				
	bacterial component	979.7			
	pertussis component	978.6			
	rickettsial component	979.7	* American Hospital Formulary Service		

APPENDIX D: INDUSTRIAL ACCIDENTS ACCORDING TO AGENCY

CLASSIFICATION OF INDUSTRIAL ACCIDENTS ACCORDING TO AGENCY

Annex B to the Resolution concerning Statistics of Employment Injuries adopted by the Tenth International Conference of Labor Statisticians on 12 October 1962

1 MACHINES

11	**Prime-Movers, except Electrical Motors**
111	*Steam engines*
112	*Internal combustion engines*
119	*Others*
12	**Transmission Machinery**
121	*Transmission shafts*
122	*Transmission belts, cables, pulleys, pinions, chains, gears*
129	*Others*
13	**Metalworking Machines**
131	*Power presses*
132	*Lathes*
133	*Milling machines*
134	*Abrasive wheels*
135	*Mechanical shears*
136	*Forging machines*
137	*Rolling-mills*
139	*Others*
14	**Wood and Assimilated Machines**
141	*Circular saws*
142	*Other saws*
143	*Molding machines*
144	*Overhand planes*
149	*Others*
15	**Agricultural Machines**
151	*Reapers (including combine reapers)*
152	*Threshers*
159	*Others*
16	**Mining Machinery**
161	*Under-cutters*
169	*Others*
19	**Other Machines Not Elsewhere Classified**
191	*Earth-moving machines, excavating and scraping machines, except means of transport*
192	*Spinning, weaving and other textile machines*
193	*Machines for the manufacture of foodstuffs and beverages*
194	*Machines for the manufacture of paper*
195	*Printing machines*
199	*Others*

2 MEANS OF TRANSPORT AND LIFTING EQUIPMENT

21	**Lifting Machines and Appliances**
211	*Cranes*
212	*Lifts and elevators*
213	*Winches*
214	*Pulley blocks*
219	*Others*
22	**Means of Rail Transport**
221	*Inter-urban railways*
222	*Rail transport in mines, tunnels, quarries, industrial establishments, docks, etc.*
229	*Others*
23	**Other Wheeled Means of Transport, Excluding Rail Transport**
231	*Tractors*
232	*Lorries*
233	*Trucks*
234	*Motor vehicles, not elsewhere classified*
235	*Animal-drawn vehicles*
236	*Hand-drawn vehicles*
239	*Others*
24	**Means of Air Transport**
25	**Means of Water Transport**
251	*Motorized means of water transport*
252	*Non-motorized means of water transport*
26	**Other Means of Transport**
261	*Cable-cars*
262	*Mechanical conveyors, except cable-cars*
269	*Others*

3 OTHER EQUIPMENT

31	**Pressure Vessels**
311	*Boilers*
312	*Pressurized containers*
313	*Pressurized piping and accessories*
314	*Gas cylinders*
315	*Caissons, diving equipment*
319	*Others*
32	**Furnaces, Ovens, Kilns**
321	*Blast furnaces*
322	*Refining furnaces*
323	*Other furnaces*
324	*Kilns*
325	*Ovens*
33	**Refrigerating Plants**
34	**Electrical Installations, Including Electric Motors, but Excluding Electric Hand Tools**
341	*Rotating machines*
342	*Conductors*
343	*Transformers*
344	*Control apparatus*
349	*Others*
35	**Electric Hand Tools**
36	**Tools, Implements, and Appliances, Except Electric Hand Tools**
361	*Power-driven hand tools, except electric hand tools*
362	*Hand tools, not power-driven*
369	*Others*
37	**Ladders, Mobile Ramps**
38	**Scaffolding**
39	**Other Equipment, Not Elsewhere Classified**

APPENDIX D: INDUSTRIAL ACCIDENTS ACCORDING TO AGENCY

4	MATERIALS, SUBSTANCES AND RADIATIONS	524	*Other traffic and working surfaces*
41	**Explosives**	525	*Floor openings and wall openings*
42	**Dusts, Gases, Liquids and Chemicals, Excluding Explosives**	526	*Environmental factors (lighting, ventilation, temperature, noise, etc.)*
421	*Dusts*	529	*Others*
422	*Gases, vapors, fumes*	**53**	**Underground**
423	*Liquids, not elsewhere classified*	531	*Roofs and faces of mine roads and tunnels, etc.*
424	*Chemicals, not elsewhere classified*	532	*Floors of mine roads and tunnels, etc.*
43	**Flying Fragments**	533	*Working-faces of mines, tunnels, etc.*
44	**Radiations**	534	*Mine shafts*
441	*Ionizing radiations*	535	*Fire*
449	*Others*	536	*Water*
49	**Other Materials and Substances Not Elsewhere Classified**	539	*Others*

5	WORKING ENVIRONMENT	6	OTHER AGENCIES, NOT ELSEWHERE CLASSIFIED
51	**Outdoor**	**61**	**Animals**
511	*Weather*	611	*Live animals*
512	*Traffic and working surfaces*	612	*Animal products*
513	*Water*	**69**	**Other Agencies, Not Elsewhere Classified**
519	*Others*		
52	**Indoor**	7	AGENCIES NOT CLASSIFIED
521	*Floors*		
522	*Confined quarters*		
523	*Stairs*		

APPENDIX E: LIST OF THREE-DIGIT CATEGORIES

LIST OF THREE-DIGIT CATEGORIES

1. INFECTIOUS AND PARASITIC DISEASES

Intestinal infectious diseases (001-009)
- 001 Cholera
- 002 Typhoid and paratyphoid fevers
- 003 Other salmonella infections
- 004 Shigellosis
- 005 Other food poisoning (bacterial)
- 006 Amebiasis
- 007 Other protozoal intestinal diseases
- 008 Intestinal infections due to other organisms
- 009 Ill-defined intestinal infections

Tuberculosis (010-018)
- 010 Primary tuberculous infection
- 011 Pulmonary tuberculosis
- 012 Other respiratory tuberculosis
- 013 Tuberculosis of meninges and central nervous system
- 014 Tuberculosis of intestines, peritoneum, and mesenteric glands
- 015 Tuberculosis of bones and joints
- 016 Tuberculosis of genitourinary system
- 017 Tuberculosis of other organs
- 018 Miliary tuberculosis

Zoonotic bacterial diseases (020-027)
- 020 Plague
- 021 Tularemia
- 022 Anthrax
- 023 Brucellosis
- 024 Glanders
- 025 Melioidosis
- 026 Rat-bite fever
- 027 Other zoonotic bacterial diseases

Other bacterial diseases (030-042)
- 030 Leprosy
- 031 Diseases due to other mycobacteria
- 032 Diphtheria
- 033 Whooping cough
- 034 Streptococcal sore throat and scarlatina
- 035 Erysipelas
- 036 Meningococcal infection
- 037 Tetanus
- 038 Septicemia
- 039 Actinomycotic infections
- 040 Other bacterial diseases
- 041 Bacterial infection in conditions classified elsewhere and of unspecified site

Human immunodeficiency virus (042)
- 042 Human immunodeficiency virus [HIV] disease

Poliomyelitis and other non-arthropod-borne viral diseases of central nervous system (045-049)
- 045 Acute poliomyelitis
- 046 Slow virus infection of central nervous system
- 047 Meningitis due to enterovirus
- 048 Other enterovirus diseases of central nervous system
- 049 Other non-arthropod-borne viral diseases of central nervous system

Viral diseases accompanied by exanthem (050-057)
- 050 Smallpox
- 051 Cowpox and paravaccinia
- 052 Chickenpox
- 053 Herpes zoster
- 054 Herpes simplex
- 055 Measles
- 056 Rubella
- 057 Other viral exanthemata

Arthropod-borne viral diseases (060-066)
- 060 Yellow fever
- 061 Dengue
- 062 Mosquito-borne viral encephalitis
- 063 Tick-borne viral encephalitis
- 064 Viral encephalitis transmitted by other and unspecified arthropods
- 065 Arthropod-borne hemorrhagic fever
- 066 Other arthropod-borne viral diseases

Other diseases due to viruses and Chlamydiae (070-079)
- 070 Viral hepatitis
- 071 Rabies
- 072 Mumps
- 073 Ornithosis
- 074 Specific diseases due to Coxsackievirus
- 075 Infectious mononucleosis
- 076 Trachoma
- 077 Other diseases of conjunctiva due to viruses and Chlamydiae
- 078 Other diseases due to viruses and Chlamydiae
- 079 Viral infection in conditions classified elsewhere and of unspecified site

Rickettsioses and other arthropod-borne diseases (080-088)
- 080 Louse-borne [epidemic] typhus
- 081 Other typhus
- 082 Tick-borne rickettsioses
- 083 Other rickettsioses
- 084 Malaria
- 085 Leishmaniasis
- 086 Trypanosomiasis
- 087 Relapsing fever
- 088 Other arthropod-borne diseases

Syphilis and other venereal diseases (090-099)
- 090 Congenital syphilis
- 091 Early syphilis, symptomatic
- 092 Early syphilis, latent
- 093 Cardiovascular syphilis
- 094 Neurosyphilis
- 095 Other forms of late syphilis, with symptoms
- 096 Late syphilis, latent

APPENDIX E: LIST OF THREE-DIGIT CATEGORIES

097	Other and unspecified syphilis
098	Gonococcal infections
099	Other venereal diseases

Other spirochetal diseases (100-104)
100	Leptospirosis
101	Vincent's angina
102	Yaws
103	Pinta
104	Other spirochetal infection

Mycoses (110-118)
110	Dermatophytosis
111	Dermatomycosis, other and unspecified
112	Candidiasis
114	Coccidioidomycosis
115	Histoplasmosis
116	Blastomycotic infection
117	Other mycoses
118	Opportunistic mycoses

Helminthiases (120-129)
120	Schistosomiasis [bilharziasis]
121	Other trematode infections
122	Echinococcosis
123	Other cestode infection
124	Trichinosis
125	Filarial infection and dracontiasis
126	Ancylostomiasis and necatoriasis
127	Other intestinal helminthiases
128	Other and unspecified helminthiases
129	Intestinal parasitism, unspecified

Other infectious and parasitic diseases (130-136)
130	Toxoplasmosis
131	Trichomoniasis
132	Pediculosis and phthirus infestation
133	Acariasis
134	Other infestation
135	Sarcoidosis
136	Other and unspecified infectious and parasitic diseases

Late effects of infectious and parasitic diseases (137-139)
137	Late effects of tuberculosis
138	Late effects of acute poliomyelitis
139	Late effects of other infectious and parasitic diseases

2. NEOPLASMS

Malignant neoplasm of lip, oral cavity, and pharynx (140-149)
140	Malignant neoplasm of lip
141	Malignant neoplasm of tongue
142	Malignant neoplasm of major salivary glands
143	Malignant neoplasm of gum
144	Malignant neoplasm of floor of mouth
145	Malignant neoplasm of other and unspecified parts of mouth
146	Malignant neoplasm of oropharynx
147	Malignant neoplasm of nasopharynx
148	Malignant neoplasm of hypopharynx
149	Malignant neoplasm of other and ill-defined sites within the lip, oral cavity, and pharynx

Malignant neoplasm of digestive organs and peritoneum (150-159)
150	Malignant neoplasm of esophagus
151	Malignant neoplasm of stomach
152	Malignant neoplasm of small intestine, including duodenum
153	Malignant neoplasm of colon
154	Malignant neoplasm of rectum, rectosigmoid junction, and anus
155	Malignant neoplasm of liver and intrahepatic bile ducts
156	Malignant neoplasm of gallbladder and extrahepatic bile ducts
157	Malignant neoplasm of pancreas
158	Malignant neoplasm of retroperitoneum and peritoneum
159	Malignant neoplasm of other and ill-defined sites within the digestive organs and peritoneum

Malignant neoplasm of respiratory and intrathoracic organs (160-165)
160	Malignant neoplasm of nasal cavities, middle ear, and accessory sinuses
161	Malignant neoplasm of larynx
162	Malignant neoplasm of trachea, bronchus, and lung
163	Malignant neoplasm of pleura
164	Malignant neoplasm of thymus, heart, and mediastinum
165	Malignant neoplasm of other and ill-defined sites within the respiratory system and intrathoracic organs

Malignant neoplasm of bone, connective tissue, skin, and breast (170-176)
170	Malignant neoplasm of bone and articular cartilage
171	Malignant neoplasm of connective and other soft tissue
172	Malignant melanoma of skin
173	Other malignant neoplasm of skin
174	Malignant neoplasm of female breast
175	Malignant neoplasm of male breast

Kaposi's sarcoma (176)
176	Kaposi's sarcoma

Malignant neoplasm of genitourinary organs (179-189)
179	Malignant neoplasm of uterus, part unspecified
180	Malignant neoplasm of cervix uteri
181	Malignant neoplasm of placenta
182	Malignant neoplasm of body of uterus
183	Malignant neoplasm of ovary and other uterine adnexa
184	Malignant neoplasm of other and unspecified female genital organs
185	Malignant neoplasm of prostate

APPENDIX E: LIST OF THREE-DIGIT CATEGORIES

186	Malignant neoplasm of testis
187	Malignant neoplasm of penis and other male genital organs
188	Malignant neoplasm of bladder
189	Malignant neoplasm of kidney and other unspecified urinary organs

Malignant neoplasm of other and unspecified sites (190-199)

190	Malignant neoplasm of eye
191	Malignant neoplasm of brain
192	Malignant neoplasm of other and unspecified parts of nervous system
193	Malignant neoplasm of thyroid gland
194	Malignant neoplasm of other endocrine glands and related structures
195	Malignant neoplasm of other and ill-defined sites
196	Secondary and unspecified malignant neoplasm of lymph nodes
197	Secondary malignant neoplasm of respiratory and digestive systems
198	Secondary malignant neoplasm of other specified sites
199	Malignant neoplasm without specification of site

Malignant neoplasm of lymphatic and hematopoietic tissue (200-208)

200	Lymphosarcoma and reticulosarcoma
201	Hodgkin's disease
202	Other malignant neoplasm of lymphoid and histiocytic tissue
203	Multiple myeloma and immunoproliferative neoplasms
204	Lymphoid leukemia
205	Myeloid leukemia
206	Monocytic leukemia
207	Other specified leukemia
208	Leukemia of unspecified cell type

Benign neoplasms (210-229)

210	Benign neoplasm of lip, oral cavity, and pharynx
211	Benign neoplasm of other parts of digestive system
212	Benign neoplasm of respiratory and intrathoracic organs
213	Benign neoplasm of bone and articular cartilage
214	Lipoma
215	Other benign neoplasm of connective and other soft tissue
216	Benign neoplasm of skin
217	Benign neoplasm of breast
218	Uterine leiomyoma
219	Other benign neoplasm of uterus
220	Benign neoplasm of ovary
221	Benign neoplasm of other female genital organs
222	Benign neoplasm of male genital organs
223	Benign neoplasm of kidney and other urinary organs
224	Benign neoplasm of eye
225	Benign neoplasm of brain and other parts of nervous system
226	Benign neoplasm of thyroid gland
227	Benign neoplasm of other endocrine glands and related structures
228	Hemangioma and lymphangioma, any site
229	Benign neoplasm of other and unspecified sites

Carcinoma in situ (230-234)

230	Carcinoma in situ of digestive organs
231	Carcinoma in situ of respiratory system
232	Carcinoma in situ of skin
233	Carcinoma in situ of breast and genitourinary system
234	Carcinoma in situ of other and unspecified sites

Neoplasms of uncertain behavior (235-238)

235	Neoplasm of uncertain behavior of digestive and respiratory systems
236	Neoplasm of uncertain behavior of genitourinary organs
237	Neoplasm of uncertain behavior of endocrine glands and nervous system
238	Neoplasm of uncertain behavior of other and unspecified sites and tissues

Neoplasms of unspecified nature (239)

239	Neoplasm of unspecified nature

3. ENDOCRINE, NUTRITIONAL AND METABOLIC DISEASES, AND IMMUNITY DISORDERS

Disorders of thyroid gland (240-246)

240	Simple and unspecified goiter
241	Nontoxic nodular goiter
242	Thyrotoxicosis with or without goiter
243	Congenital hypothyroidism
244	Acquired hypothyroidism
245	Thyroiditis
246	Other disorders of thyroid

Diseases of other endocrine glands (250-259)

250	Diabetes mellitus
251	Other disorders of pancreatic internal secretion
252	Disorders of parathyroid gland
253	Disorders of the pituitary gland and its hypothalamic control
254	Diseases of thymus gland
255	Disorders of adrenal glands
256	Ovarian dysfunction
257	Testicular dysfunction
258	Polyglandular dysfunction and related disorders
259	Other endocrine disorders

APPENDIX E: LIST OF THREE-DIGIT CATEGORIES

Nutritional deficiencies (260-269)
260 Kwashiorkor
261 Nutritional marasmus
262 Other severe protein-calorie malnutrition
263 Other and unspecified protein-calorie malnutrition
264 Vitamin A deficiency
265 Thiamine and niacin deficiency states
266 Deficiency of B-complex components
267 Ascorbic acid deficiency
268 Vitamin D deficiency
269 Other nutritional deficiencies

Other metabolic disorders and immunity disorders (270-279)
270 Disorders of amino-acid transport and metabolism
271 Disorders of carbohydrate transport and metabolism
272 Disorders of lipoid metabolism
273 Disorders of plasma protein metabolism
274 Gout
275 Disorders of mineral metabolism
276 Disorders of fluid, electrolyte, and acid-base balance
277 Other and unspecified disorders of metabolism
278 Obesity and other hyperalimentation
279 Disorders involving the immune mechanism

Diseases of blood and blood-forming organs (280-289)
280 Iron deficiency anemias
281 Other deficiency anemias
282 Hereditary hemolytic anemias
283 Acquired hemolytic anemias
284 Aplastic anemia
285 Other and unspecified anemias
286 Coagulation defects
287 Purpura and other hemorrhagic conditions
288 Diseases of white blood cells
289 Other diseases of blood and blood-forming organs

5. MENTAL DISORDERS

Organic psychotic conditions (290-294)
290 Senile and presenile organic psychotic conditions
291 Alcoholic psychoses
292 Drug psychoses
293 Transient organic psychotic conditions
294 Other organic psychotic conditions (chronic)

Other psychoses (295-299)
295 Schizophrenic psychoses
296 Affective psychoses
297 Paranoid states
298 Other nonorganic psychoses
299 Psychoses with origin specific to childhood

Neurotic disorders, personality disorders, and other nonpsychotic mental disorders (300-316)
300 Neurotic disorders
301 Personality disorders
302 Sexual deviations and disorders
303 Alcohol dependence syndrome
304 Drug dependence
305 Nondependent abuse of drugs
306 Physiological malfunction arising from mental factors
307 Special symptoms or syndromes, not elsewhere classified
308 Acute reaction to stress
309 Adjustment reaction
310 Specific nonpsychotic mental disorders following organic brain damage
311 Depressive disorder, not elsewhere classified
312 Disturbance of conduct, not elsewhere classified
313 Disturbance of emotions specific to childhood and adolescence
314 Hyperkinetic syndrome of childhood
315 Specific delays in development
316 Psychic factors associated with diseases classified elsewhere

Mental retardation (317-319)
317 Mild mental retardation
318 Other specified mental retardation
319 Unspecified mental retardation

6. DISEASES OF THE NERVOUS SYSTEM AND SENSE ORGANS

Inflammatory diseases of the central nervous system (320-326)
320 Bacterial meningitis
321 Meningitis due to other organisms
322 Meningitis of unspecified cause
323 Encephalitis, myelitis, and encephalomyelitis
324 Intracranial and intraspinal abscess
325 Phlebitis and thrombophlebitis of intracranial venous sinuses
326 Late effects of intracranial abscess or pyogenic infection

Hereditary and degenerative diseases of the central nervous system (330-337)
330 Cerebral degenerations usually manifest in childhood
331 Other cerebral degenerations
332 Parkinson's disease
333 Other extrapyramidal diseases and abnormal movement disorders
334 Spinocerebellar disease
335 Anterior horn cell disease
336 Other diseases of spinal cord
337 Disorders of the autonomic nervous system

APPENDIX E: LIST OF THREE-DIGIT CATEGORIES

Other disorders of the central nervous system (340-349)
340 Multiple sclerosis
341 Other demyelinating diseases of central nervous system
342 Hemiplegia and hemiparesis
343 Infantile cerebral palsy
344 Other paralytic syndromes
345 Epilepsy
346 Migraine
347 Cataplexy and narcolepsy
348 Other conditions of brain
349 Other and unspecified disorders of the nervous system

Disorders of the peripheral nervous system (350-359)
350 Trigeminal nerve disorders
351 Facial nerve disorders
352 Disorders of other cranial nerves
353 Nerve root and plexus disorders
354 Mononeuritis of upper limb and mononeuritis multiplex
355 Mononeuritis of lower limb
356 Hereditary and idiopathic peripheral neuropathy
357 Inflammatory and toxic neuropathy
358 Myoneural disorders
359 Muscular dystrophies and other myopathies

Disorders of the eye and adnexa (360-379)
360 Disorders of the globe
361 Retinal detachments and defects
362 Other retinal disorders
363 Chorioretinal inflammations and scars and other disorders of choroid
364 Disorders of iris and ciliary body
365 Glaucoma
366 Cataract
367 Disorders of refraction and accommodation
368 Visual disturbances
369 Blindness and low vision
370 Keratitis
371 Corneal opacity and other disorders of cornea
372 Disorders of conjunctiva
373 Inflammation of eyelids
374 Other disorders of eyelids
375 Disorders of lacrimal system
376 Disorders of the orbit
377 Disorders of optic nerve and visual pathways
378 Strabismus and other disorders of binocular eye movements
379 Other disorders of eye

Diseases of the ear and mastoid process (380-389)
380 Disorders of external ear
381 Nonsuppurative otitis media and Eustachian tube disorders
382 Suppurative and unspecified otitis media
383 Mastoiditis and related conditions
384 Other disorders of tympanic membrane
385 Other disorders of middle ear and mastoid
386 Vertiginous syndromes and other disorders of vestibular system
387 Otosclerosis
388 Other disorders of ear
389 Hearing loss

7. DISEASES OF THE CIRCULATORY SYSTEM

Acute rheumatic fever (390-392)
390 Rheumatic fever without mention of heart involvement
391 Rheumatic fever with heart involvement
392 Rheumatic chorea

Chronic rheumatic heart disease (393-398)
393 Chronic rheumatic pericarditis
394 Diseases of mitral valve
395 Diseases of aortic valve
396 Diseases of mitral and aortic valves
397 Diseases of other endocardial structures
398 Other rheumatic heart disease

Hypertensive disease (401-405)
401 Essential hypertension
402 Hypertensive heart disease
403 Hypertensive renal disease
404 Hypertensive heart and renal disease
405 Secondary hypertension

Ischemic heart disease (410-414)
410 Acute myocardial infarction
411 Other acute and subacute form of ischemic heart disease
412 Old myocardial infarction
413 Angina pectoris
414 Other forms of chronic ischemic heart disease

Diseases of pulmonary circulation (415-417)
415 Acute pulmonary heart disease
416 Chronic pulmonary heart disease
417 Other diseases of pulmonary circulation

Other forms of heart disease (420-429)
420 Acute pericarditis
421 Acute and subacute endocarditis
422 Acute myocarditis
423 Other diseases of pericardium
424 Other diseases of endocardium
425 Cardiomyopathy
426 Conduction disorders
427 Cardiac dysrhythmias
428 Heart failure
429 Ill-defined descriptions and complications of heart disease

APPENDIX E: LIST OF THREE-DIGIT CATEGORIES

Cerebrovascular disease (430-438)
430 Subarachnoid hemorrhage
431 Intracerebral hemorrhage
432 Other and unspecified intracranial hemorrhage
433 Occlusion and stenosis of precerebral arteries
434 Occlusion of cerebral arteries
435 Transient cerebral ischemia
436 Acute but ill-defined cerebrovascular disease
437 Other and ill-defined cerebrovascular disease
438 Late effects of cerebrovascular disease

Diseases of arteries, arterioles, and capillaries (440-448)
440 Atherosclerosis
441 Aortic aneurysm and dissection
442 Other aneurysm
443 Other peripheral vascular disease
444 Arterial embolism and thrombosis
445 Atheroembolism
446 Polyarteritis nodosa and allied conditions
447 Other disorders of arteries and arterioles
448 Diseases of capillaries

Diseases of veins and lymphatics, and other diseases of circulatory system (451-459)
451 Phlebitis and thrombophlebitis
452 Portal vein thrombosis
453 Other venous embolism and thrombosis
454 Varicose veins of lower extremities
455 Hemorrhoids
456 Varicose veins of other sites
457 Noninfective disorders of lymphatic channels
458 Hypotension
459 Other disorders of circulatory system

8. DISEASES OF THE RESPIRATORY SYSTEM

Acute respiratory infections (460-466)
460 Acute nasopharyngitis [common cold]
461 Acute sinusitis
462 Acute pharyngitis
463 Acute tonsillitis
464 Acute laryngitis and tracheitis
465 Acute upper respiratory infections of multiple or unspecified sites
466 Acute bronchitis and bronchiolitis

Other diseases of upper respiratory tract (470-478)
470 Deviated nasal septum
471 Nasal polyps
472 Chronic pharyngitis and nasopharyngitis
473 Chronic sinusitis
474 Chronic disease of tonsils and adenoids
475 Peritonsillar abscess
476 Chronic laryngitis and laryngotracheitis
477 Allergic rhinitis
478 Other diseases of upper respiratory tract

Pneumonia and influenza (480-487)
480 Viral pneumonia
481 Pneumococcal pneumonia [Streptococcus pneumoniae pneumonia]
482 Other bacterial pneumonia
483 Pneumonia due to other specified organism
484 Pneumonia in infectious diseases classified elsewhere
485 Bronchopneumonia, organism unspecified
486 Pneumonia, organism unspecified
487 Influenza

Chronic obstructive pulmonary disease and allied conditions (490-496)
490 Bronchitis, not specified as acute or chronic
491 Chronic bronchitis
492 Emphysema
493 Asthma
494 Bronchiectasis
495 Extrinsic allergic alveolitis
496 Chronic airways obstruction, not elsewhere classified

Pneumoconioses and other lung diseases due to external agents (500-508)
500 Coal workers' pneumoconiosis
501 Asbestosis
502 Pneumoconiosis due to other silica or silicates
503 Pneumoconiosis due to other inorganic dust
504 Pneumopathy due to inhalation of other dust
505 Pneumoconiosis, unspecified
506 Respiratory conditions due to chemical fumes and vapors
507 Pneumonitis due to solids and liquids
508 Respiratory conditions due to other and unspecified external agents

Other diseases of respiratory system (510-519)
510 Empyema
511 Pleurisy
512 Pneumothorax
513 Abscess of lung and mediastinum
514 Pulmonary congestion and hypostasis
515 Postinflammatory pulmonary fibrosis
516 Other alveolar and parietoalveolar pneumopathy

APPENDIX E: LIST OF THREE-DIGIT CATEGORIES

517 Lung involvement in conditions classified elsewhere
518 Other diseases of lung
519 Other diseases of respiratory system

9. DISEASES OF THE DIGESTIVE SYSTEM

Diseases of oral cavity, salivary glands, and jaws (520-529)
520 Disorders of tooth development and eruption
521 Diseases of hard tissues of teeth
522 Diseases of pulp and periapical tissues
523 Gingival and periodontal diseases
524 Dentofacial anomalies, including malocclusion
525 Other diseases and conditions of the teeth and supporting structures
526 Diseases of the jaws
527 Diseases of the salivary glands
528 Diseases of the oral soft tissues, excluding lesions specific for gingiva and tongue
529 Diseases and other conditions of the tongue

Diseases of esophagus, stomach, and duodenum (530-537)
530 Diseases of esophagus
531 Gastric ulcer
532 Duodenal ulcer
533 Peptic ulcer, site unspecified
534 Gastrojejunal ulcer
535 Gastritis and duodenitis
536 Disorders of function of stomach
537 Other disorders of stomach and duodenum

Appendicitis (540-543)
540 Acute appendicitis
541 Appendicitis, unqualified
542 Other appendicitis
543 Other diseases of appendix

Hernia of abdominal cavity (550-553)
550 Inguinal hernia
551 Other hernia of abdominal cavity, with gangrene
552 Other hernia of abdominal cavity, with obstruction, but without mention of gangrene
553 Other hernia of abdominal cavity without mention of obstruction or gangrene

Noninfective enteritis and colitis (555-558)
555 Regional enteritis
556 Ulcerative colitis
557 Vascular insufficiency of intestine
558 Other noninfective gastroenteritis and colitis

Other diseases of intestines and peritoneum (560-569)
560 Intestinal obstruction without mention of hernia
562 Diverticula of intestine
564 Functional digestive disorders, not elsewhere classified
565 Anal fissure and fistula
566 Abscess of anal and rectal regions
567 Peritonitis
568 Other disorders of peritoneum
569 Other disorders of intestine

Other diseases of digestive system (570-579)
570 Acute and subacute necrosis of liver
571 Chronic liver disease and cirrhosis
572 Liver abscess and sequelae of chronic liver disease
573 Other disorders of liver
574 Cholelithiasis
575 Other disorders of gallbladder
576 Other disorders of biliary tract
577 Diseases of pancreas
578 Gastrointestinal hemorrhage
579 Intestinal malabsorption

10. DISEASES OF THE GENITOURINARY SYSTEM

Nephritis, nephrotic syndrome, and nephrosis (580-589)
580 Acute glomerulonephritis
581 Nephrotic syndrome
582 Chronic glomerulonephritis
583 Nephritis and nephropathy, not specified as acute or chronic
584 Acute renal failure
585 Chronic renal failure
586 Renal failure, unspecified
587 Renal sclerosis, unspecified
588 Disorders resulting from impaired renal function
589 Small kidney of unknown cause

Other diseases of urinary system (590-599)
590 Infections of kidney
591 Hydronephrosis
592 Calculus of kidney and ureter
593 Other disorders of kidney and ureter
594 Calculus of lower urinary tract
595 Cystitis
596 Other disorders of bladder
597 Urethritis, not sexually transmitted, and urethral syndrome
598 Urethral stricture
599 Other disorders of urethra and urinary tract

Diseases of male genital organs (600-608)
600 Hyperplasia of prostate
601 Inflammatory diseases of prostate
602 Other disorders of prostate
603 Hydrocele
604 Orchitis and epididymitis
605 Redundant prepuce and phimosis

APPENDIX E: LIST OF THREE-DIGIT CATEGORIES

606	Infertility, male
607	Disorders of penis
608	Other disorders of male genital organs

Disorders of breast (610-611)

610	Benign mammary dysplasias
611	Other disorders of breast

Inflammatory disease of female pelvic organs (614-616)

614	Inflammatory disease of ovary, fallopian tube, pelvic cellular tissue, and peritoneum
615	Inflammatory diseases of uterus, except cervix
616	Inflammatory disease of cervix, vagina, and vulva

Other disorders of female genital tract (617-629)

617	Endometriosis
618	Genital prolapse
619	Fistula involving female genital tract
620	Noninflammatory disorders of ovary, fallopian tube, and broad ligament
621	Disorders of uterus, not elsewhere classified
622	Noninflammatory disorders of cervix
623	Noninflammatory disorders of vagina
624	Noninflammatory disorders of vulva and perineum
625	Pain and other symptoms associated with female genital organs
626	Disorders of menstruation and other abnormal bleeding from female genital tract
627	Menopausal and postmenopausal disorders
628	Infertility, female
629	Other disorders of female genital organs

11. COMPLICATIONS OF PREGNANCY, CHILDBIRTH AND THE PUERPERIUM

Ectopic and molar pregnancy and other pregnancy with abortive outcome (630-639)

630	Hydatidiform mole
631	Other abnormal product of conception
632	Missed abortion
633	Ectopic pregnancy
634	Spontaneous abortion
635	Legally induced abortion
636	Illegally induced abortion
637	Unspecified abortion
638	Failed attempted abortion
639	Complications following abortion and ectopic and molar pregnancies

Complications mainly related to pregnancy (640-648)

640	Hemorrhage in early pregnancy
641	Antepartum hemorrhage, abruptio placentae, and placenta previa
642	Hypertension complicating pregnancy, childbirth, and the puerperium
643	Excessive vomiting in pregnancy
644	Early or threatened labor
645	Prolonged pregnancy
646	Other complications of pregnancy, not elsewhere classified
647	Infective and parasitic conditions in the mother classifiable elsewhere but complicating pregnancy, childbirth, and the puerperium
648	Other current conditions in the mother classifiable elsewhere but complicating pregnancy, childbirth, and the puerperium

Normal delivery, and other indications for care in pregnancy, labor, and delivery (650-659)

650	Normal delivery
651	Multiple gestation
652	Malposition and malpresentation of fetus
653	Disproportion
654	Abnormality of organs and soft tissues of pelvis
655	Known or suspected fetal abnormality affecting management of mother
656	Other fetal and placental problems affecting management of mother
657	Polyhydramnios
658	Other problems associated with amniotic cavity and membranes
659	Other indications for care or intervention related to labor and delivery and not elsewhere classified

Complications occurring mainly in the course of labor and delivery (660-669)

660	Obstructed labor
661	Abnormality of forces of labor
662	Long labor
663	Umbilical cord complications
664	Trauma to perineum and vulva during delivery
665	Other obstetrical trauma
666	Postpartum hemorrhage
667	Retained placenta or membranes, without hemorrhage
668	Complications of the administration of anesthetic or other sedation in labor and delivery
669	Other complications of labor and delivery, not elsewhere classified

Complications of the puerperium (670-677)

670	Major puerperal infection
671	Venous complications in pregnancy and the puerperium
672	Pyrexia of unknown origin during the puerperium
673	Obstetrical pulmonary embolism

APPENDIX E: LIST OF THREE-DIGIT CATEGORIES

674 Other and unspecified complications of the puerperium, not elsewhere classified
675 Infections of the breast and nipple associated with childbirth
676 Other disorders of the breast associated with childbirth, and disorders of lactation
677 Late effect of complication of pregnancy, childbirth, and the puerperium

12. DISEASES OF THE SKIN AND SUBCUTANEOUS TISSUE

Infections of skin and subcutaneous tissue (680-686)
680 Carbuncle and furuncle
681 Cellulitis and abscess of finger and toe
682 Other cellulitis and abscess
683 Acute lymphadenitis
684 Impetigo
685 Pilonidal cyst
686 Other local infections of skin and subcutaneous tissue

Other inflammatory conditions of skin and subcutaneous tissue (690-698)
690 Erythematosquamous dermatosis
691 Atopic dermatitis and related conditions
692 Contact dermatitis and other eczema
693 Dermatitis due to substances taken internally
694 Bullous dermatoses
695 Erythematous conditions
696 Psoriasis and similar disorders
697 Lichen
698 Pruritus and related conditions

Other diseases of skin and subcutaneous tissue (700-709)
700 Corns and callosities
701 Other hypertrophic and atrophic conditions of skin
702 Other dermatoses
703 Diseases of nail
704 Diseases of hair and hair follicles
705 Disorders of sweat glands
706 Diseases of sebaceous glands
707 Chronic ulcer of skin
708 Urticaria
709 Other disorders of skin and subcutaneous tissue

13. DISEASES OF THE MUSCULOSKELETAL SYSTEM AND CONNECTIVE TISSUE

Arthropathies and related disorders (710-719)
710 Diffuse diseases of connective tissue
711 Arthropathy associated with infections
712 Crystal arthropathies
713 Arthropathy associated with other disorders classified elsewhere
714 Rheumatoid arthritis and other inflammatory polyarthropathies
715 Osteoarthrosis and allied disorders
716 Other and unspecified arthropathies
717 Internal derangement of knee
718 Other derangement of joint
719 Other and unspecified disorder of joint

Dorsopathies (720-724)
720 Ankylosing spondylitis and other inflammatory spondylopathies
721 Spondylosis and allied disorders
722 Intervertebral disc disorders
723 Other disorders of cervical region
724 Other and unspecified disorders of back

Rheumatism, excluding the back (725-729)
725 Polymyalgia rheumatica
726 Peripheral enthesopathies and allied syndromes
727 Other disorders of synovium, tendon, and bursa
728 Disorders of muscle, ligament, and fascia
729 Other disorders of soft tissues

Osteopathies, chondropathies, and acquired musculoskeletal deformities (730-739)
730 Osteomyelitis, periostitis, and other infections involving bone
731 Osteitis deformans and osteopathies associated with other disorders classified elsewhere
732 Osteochondropathies
733 Other disorders of bone and cartilage
734 Flat foot
735 Acquired deformities of toe
736 Other acquired deformities of limbs
737 Curvature of spine
738 Other acquired deformity
739 Nonallopathic lesions, not elsewhere classified

14. CONGENITAL ANOMALIES

740 Anencephalus and similar anomalies
741 Spina bifida
742 Other congenital anomalies of nervous system
743 Congenital anomalies of eye
744 Congenital anomalies of ear, face, and neck
745 Bulbus cordis anomalies and anomalies of cardiac septal closure
746 Other congenital anomalies of heart
747 Other congenital anomalies of circulatory system
748 Congenital anomalies of respiratory system
749 Cleft palate and cleft lip

APPENDIX E: LIST OF THREE-DIGIT CATEGORIES

750	Other congenital anomalies of upper alimentary tract	779	Other and ill-defined conditions originating in the perinatal period
751	Other congenital anomalies of digestive system		

16. SYMPTOMS, SIGNS, AND ILL-DEFINED CONDITIONS

752	Congenital anomalies of genital organs		**Symptoms (780-789)**
753	Congenital anomalies of urinary system	780	General symptoms
		781	Symptoms involving nervous and musculoskeletal systems
754	Certain congenital musculoskeletal deformities	782	Symptoms involving skin and other integumentary tissue
755	Other congenital anomalies of limbs		
756	Other congenital musculoskeletal anomalies	783	Symptoms concerning nutrition, metabolism, and development
757	Congenital anomalies of the integument	784	Symptoms involving head and neck
		785	Symptoms involving cardiovascular system
758	Chromosomal anomalies		
759	Other and unspecified congenital anomalies	786	Symptoms involving respiratory system and other chest symptoms
		787	Symptoms involving digestive system
	15. CERTAIN CONDITIONS ORIGINATING IN THE PERINATAL PERIOD	788	Symptoms involving urinary system
		789	Other symptoms involving abdomen and pelvis

Maternal causes of perinatal morbidity and mortality (760-763)

Nonspecific abnormal findings (790-796)

760	Fetus or newborn affected by maternal conditions which may be unrelated to present pregnancy	790	Nonspecific findings on examination of blood
		791	Nonspecific findings on examination of urine
761	Fetus or newborn affected by maternal complications of pregnancy	792	Nonspecific abnormal findings in other body substances
762	Fetus or newborn affected by complications of placenta, cord, and membranes	793	Nonspecific abnormal findings on radiological and other examination of body structure
763	Fetus or newborn affected by other complications of labor and delivery	794	Nonspecific abnormal results of function studies
		795	Nonspecific abnormal histological and immunological findings

Other conditions originating in the perinatal period (764-779)

764	Slow fetal growth and fetal malnutrition	796	Other nonspecific abnormal findings

Ill-defined and unknown causes of morbidity and mortality (797-799)

765	Disorders relating to short gestation and unspecified low birthweight	797	Senility without mention of psychosis
766	Disorders relating to long gestation and high birthweight	798	Sudden death, cause unknown
767	Birth trauma	799	Other ill-defined and unknown causes of morbidity and mortality
768	Intrauterine hypoxia and birth asphyxia		

17. INJURY AND POISONING

Fracture of skull (800-804)

769	Respiratory distress syndrome	800	Fracture of vault of skull
770	Other respiratory conditions of fetus and newborn	801	Fracture of base of skull
		802	Fracture of face bones
771	Infections specific to the perinatal period	803	Other and unqualified skull fractures
772	Fetal and neonatal hemorrhage	804	Multiple fractures involving skull or face with other bones
773	Hemolytic disease of fetus or newborn, due to isoimmunization		
774	Other perinatal jaundice		**Fracture of spine and trunk (805-809)**
775	Endocrine and metabolic disturbances specific to the fetus and newborn	805	Fracture of vertebral column without mention of spinal cord lesion
776	Hematological disorders of fetus and newborn	806	Fracture of vertebral column with spinal cord lesion
777	Perinatal disorders of digestive system	807	Fracture of rib(s), sternum, larynx, and trachea
778	Conditions involving the integument and temperature regulation of fetus and newborn	808	Fracture of pelvis

APPENDIX E: LIST OF THREE-DIGIT CATEGORIES

809	Ill-defined fractures of bones of trunk

Fracture of upper limb (810-819)
810	Fracture of clavicle
811	Fracture of scapula
812	Fracture of humerus
813	Fracture of radius and ulna
814	Fracture of carpal bone(s)
815	Fracture of metacarpal bone(s)
816	Fracture of one or more phalanges of hand
817	Multiple fractures of hand bones
818	Ill-defined fractures of upper limb
819	Multiple fractures involving both upper limbs, and upper limb with rib(s) and sternum

Fracture of lower limb (820-829)
820	Fracture of neck of femur
821	Fracture of other and unspecified parts of femur
822	Fracture of patella
823	Fracture of tibia and fibula
824	Fracture of ankle
825	Fracture of one or more tarsal and metatarsal bones
826	Fracture of one or more phalanges of foot
827	Other, multiple, and ill-defined fractures of lower limb
828	Multiple fractures involving both lower limbs, lower with upper limb, and lower limb(s) with rib(s) and sternum
829	Fracture of unspecified bones

Dislocation (830-839)
830	Dislocation of jaw
831	Dislocation of shoulder
832	Dislocation of elbow
833	Dislocation of wrist
834	Dislocation of finger
835	Dislocation of hip
836	Dislocation of knee
837	Dislocation of ankle
838	Dislocation of foot
839	Other, multiple, and ill-defined dislocations

Sprains and strains of joints and adjacent muscles (840-848)
840	Sprains and strains of shoulder and upper arm
841	Sprains and strains of elbow and forearm
842	Sprains and strains of wrist and hand
843	Sprains and strains of hip and thigh
844	Sprains and strains of knee and leg
845	Sprains and strains of ankle and foot
846	Sprains and strains of sacroiliac region
847	Sprains and strains of other and unspecified parts of back
848	Other and ill-defined sprains and strains

Intracranial injury, excluding those with skull fracture (850-854)
850	Concussion
851	Cerebral laceration and contusion
852	Subarachnoid, subdural, and extradural hemorrhage, following injury
853	Other and unspecified intracranial hemorrhage following injury
854	Intracranial injury of other and unspecified nature

Internal injury of chest, abdomen, and pelvis (860-869)
860	Traumatic pneumothorax and hemothorax
861	Injury to heart and lung
862	Injury to other and unspecified intrathoracic organs
863	Injury to gastrointestinal tract
864	Injury to liver
865	Injury to spleen
866	Injury to kidney
867	Injury to pelvic organs
868	Injury to other intra-abdominal organs
869	Internal injury to unspecified or ill-defined organs

Open wound of head, neck, and trunk (870-879)
870	Open wound of ocular adnexa
871	Open wound of eyeball
872	Open wound of ear
873	Other open wound of head
874	Open wound of neck
875	Open wound of chest (wall)
876	Open wound of back
877	Open wound of buttock
878	Open wound of genital organs (external), including traumatic amputation
879	Open wound of other and unspecified sites, except limbs

Open wound of upper limb (880-887)
880	Open wound of shoulder and upper arm
881	Open wound of elbow, forearm, and wrist
882	Open wound of hand except finger(s) alone
883	Open wound of finger(s)
884	Multiple and unspecified open wound of upper limb
885	Traumatic amputation of thumb (complete) (partial)
886	Traumatic amputation of other finger(s) (complete) (partial)
887	Traumatic amputation of arm and hand (complete) (partial)

APPENDIX E: LIST OF THREE-DIGIT CATEGORIES

Open wound of lower limb (890-897)
890 Open wound of hip and thigh
891 Open wound of knee, leg [except thigh], and ankle
892 Open wound of foot except toe(s) alone
893 Open wound of toe(s)
894 Multiple and unspecified open wound of lower limb
895 Traumatic amputation of toe(s) (complete) (partial)
896 Traumatic amputation of foot (complete) (partial)
897 Traumatic amputation of leg(s) (complete) (partial)

Injury to blood vessels (900-904)
900 Injury to blood vessels of head and neck
901 Injury to blood vessels of thorax
902 Injury to blood vessels of abdomen and pelvis
903 Injury to blood vessels of upper extremity
904 Injury to blood vessels of lower extremity and unspecified sites

Late effects of injuries, poisonings, toxic effects, and other external causes (905-909)
905 Late effects of musculoskeletal and connective tissue injuries
906 Late effects of injuries to skin and subcutaneous tissues
907 Late effects of injuries to the nervous system
908 Late effects of other and unspecified injuries
909 Late effects of other and unspecified external causes

Superficial injury (910-919)
910 Superficial injury of face, neck, and scalp except eye
911 Superficial injury of trunk
912 Superficial injury of shoulder and upper arm
913 Superficial injury of elbow, forearm, and wrist
914 Superficial injury of hand(s) except finger(s) alone
915 Superficial injury of finger(s)
916 Superficial injury of hip, thigh, leg, and ankle
917 Superficial injury of foot and toe(s)
918 Superficial injury of eye and adnexa
919 Superficial injury of other, multiple, and unspecified sites

Contusion with intact skin surface (920-924)
920 Contusion of face, scalp, and neck except eye(s)
921 Contusion of eye and adnexa
922 Contusion of trunk
923 Contusion of upper limb
924 Contusion of lower limb and of other and unspecified sites

Crushing injury (925-929)
925 Crushing injury of face, scalp, and neck
926 Crushing injury of trunk
927 Crushing injury of upper limb
928 Crushing injury of lower limb
929 Crushing injury of multiple and unspecified sites

Effects of foreign body entering through orifice (930-939)
930 Foreign body on external eye
931 Foreign body in ear
932 Foreign body in nose
933 Foreign body in pharynx and larynx
934 Foreign body in trachea, bronchus, and lung
935 Foreign body in mouth, esophagus, and stomach
936 Foreign body in intestine and colon
937 Foreign body in anus and rectum
938 Foreign body in digestive system, unspecified
939 Foreign body in genitourinary tract

Burns (940-949)
940 Burn confined to eye and adnexa
941 Burn of face, head, and neck
942 Burn of trunk
943 Burn of upper limb, except wrist and hand
944 Burn of wrist(s) and hand(s)
945 Burn of lower limb(s)
946 Burns of multiple specified sites
947 Burn of internal organs
948 Burns classified according to extent of body surface involved
949 Burn, unspecified

Injury to nerves and spinal cord (950-957)
950 Injury to optic nerve and pathways
951 Injury to other cranial nerve(s)
952 Spinal cord injury without evidence of spinal bone injury
953 Injury to nerve roots and spinal plexus
954 Injury to other nerve(s) of trunk excluding shoulder and pelvic girdles
955 Injury to peripheral nerve(s) of shoulder girdle and upper limb
956 Injury to peripheral nerve(s) of pelvic girdle and lower limb
957 Injury to other and unspecified nerves

Certain traumatic complications and unspecified injuries (958-959)
958 Certain early complications of trauma
959 Injury, other and unspecified

APPENDIX E: LIST OF THREE-DIGIT CATEGORIES

Poisoning by drugs, medicinals and biological substances (960-979)

960 Poisoning by antibiotics
961 Poisoning by other anti-infectives
962 Poisoning by hormones and synthetic substitutes
963 Poisoning by primarily systemic agents
964 Poisoning by agents primarily affecting blood constituents
965 Poisoning by analgesics, antipyretics, and antirheumatics
966 Poisoning by anticonvulsants and anti-Parkinsonism drugs
967 Poisoning by sedatives and hypnotics
968 Poisoning by other central nervous system depressants and anesthetics
969 Poisoning by psychotropic agents
970 Poisoning by central nervous system stimulants
971 Poisoning by drugs primarily affecting the autonomic nervous system
972 Poisoning by agents primarily affecting the cardiovascular system
973 Poisoning by agents primarily affecting the gastrointestinal system
974 Poisoning by water, mineral, and uric acid metabolism drugs
975 Poisoning by agents primarily acting on the smooth and skeletal muscles and respiratory system
976 Poisoning by agents primarily affecting skin and mucous membrane, ophthalmological, otorhinolaryngological, and dental drugs
977 Poisoning by other and unspecified drugs and medicinals
978 Poisoning by bacterial vaccines
979 Poisoning by other vaccines and biological substances

Toxic effects of substances chiefly nonmedicinal as to source (980-989)

980 Toxic effect of alcohol
981 Toxic effect of petroleum products
982 Toxic effect of solvents other than petroleum-based
983 Toxic effect of corrosive aromatics, acids, and caustic alkalis
984 Toxic effect of lead and its compounds (including fumes)
985 Toxic effect of other metals
986 Toxic effect of carbon monoxide
987 Toxic effect of other gases, fumes, or vapors
988 Toxic effect of noxious substances eaten as food
989 Toxic effect of other substances, chiefly nonmedicinal as to source

Other and unspecified effects of external causes (990-995)

990 Effects of radiation, unspecified
991 Effects of reduced temperature
992 Effects of heat and light
993 Effects of air pressure
994 Effects of other external causes
995 Certain adverse effects, not elsewhere classified

Complications of surgical and medical care, not elsewhere classified (996-999)

996 Complications peculiar to certain specified procedures
997 Complications affecting specified body systems, not elsewhere classified
998 Other complications of procedures, not elsewhere classified
999 Complications of medical care, not elsewhere classified

SUPPLEMENTARY CLASSIFICATION OF FACTORS INFLUENCING HEALTH STATUS AND CONTACT WITH HEALTH SERVICES

Persons with potential health hazards related to communicable diseases (V01-V09)

V01 Contact with or exposure to communicable diseases
V02 Carrier or suspected carrier of infectious diseases
V03 Need for prophylactic vaccination and inoculation against bacterial diseases
V04 Need for prophylactic vaccination and inoculation against certain viral diseases
V05 Need for other prophylactic vaccination and inoculation against single diseases
V06 Need for prophylactic vaccination and inoculation against combinations of diseases
V07 Need for isolation and other prophylactic measures
V08 Asymptomatic human immunodeficiency virus [HIV] infection status
V09 Infection with drug-resistant microorganisms

Persons with potential health hazards related to personal and family history (V10-V19)

V10 Personal history of malignant neoplasm
V11 Personal history of mental disorder
V12 Personal history of certain other diseases
V13 Personal history of other diseases
V14 Personal history of allergy to medicinal agents

APPENDIX E: LIST OF THREE-DIGIT CATEGORIES

V15	Other personal history presenting hazards to health	V53	Fitting and adjustment of other device
V16	Family history of malignant neoplasm	V54	Other orthopedic aftercare
		V55	Attention to artificial openings
V17	Family history of certain chronic disabling diseases	V56	Encounter for dialysis and dialysis catheter care
V18	Family history of certain other specific conditions	V57	Care involving use of rehabilitation procedures
V19	Family history of other conditions	V58	Encounter for other and unspecified procedures and aftercare

Persons encountering health services in circumstances related to reproduction and development (V20-V29)

V20	Health supervision of infant or child
V21	Constitutional states in development
V22	Normal pregnancy
V23	Supervision of high-risk pregnancy
V24	Postpartum care and examination
V25	Encounter for contraceptive management
V26	Procreative management
V27	Outcome of delivery
V28	Antenatal screening
V29	Observation and evaluation of newborns and infants for suspected condition not found

V59 Donors

Persons encountering health services in other circumstances (V60-V69)

V60	Housing, household, and economic circumstances
V61	Other family circumstances
V62	Other psychosocial circumstances
V63	Unavailability of other medical facilities for care
V64	Persons encountering health services for specific procedures, not carried out
V65	Other persons seeking consultation without complaint or sickness
V66	Convalescence and palliative care
V67	Follow-up examination
V68	Encounters for administrative purposes
V69	Problems related to lifestyle

Liveborn infants according to type of birth (V30-V39)

V30	Single liveborn
V31	Twin, mate liveborn
V32	Twin, mate stillborn
V33	Twin, unspecified
V34	Other multiple, mates all liveborn
V35	Other multiple, mates all stillborn
V36	Other multiple, mates live- and stillborn
V37	Other multiple, unspecified
V39	Unspecified

Persons with a condition influencing their health status (V40-V49)

V40	Mental and behavioral problems
V41	Problems with special senses and other special functions
V42	Organ or tissue replaced by transplant
V43	Organ or tissue replaced by other means
V44	Artificial opening status
V45	Other postsurgical states
V46	Other dependence on machines
V47	Other problems with internal organs
V48	Problems with head, neck, and trunk
V49	Problems with limbs and other problems

Persons encountering health services for specific procedures and aftercare (V50-V59)

V50	Elective surgery for purposes other than remedying health states
V51	Aftercare involving the use of plastic surgery
V52	Fitting and adjustment of prosthetic device

Persons without reported diagnosis encountered during examination and investigation of individuals and populations (V70-V83)

V70	General medical examination
V71	Observation and evaluation for suspected conditions not found
V72	Special investigations and examinations
V73	Special screening examination for viral and chlamydial diseases
V74	Special screening examination for bacterial and spirochetal diseases
V75	Special screening examination for other infectious diseases
V76	Special screening for malignant neoplasms
V77	Special screening for endocrine, nutritional, metabolic, and immunity disorders
V78	Special screening for disorders of blood and blood-forming organs
V79	Special screening for mental disorders and developmental handicaps
V80	Special screening for neurological, eye, and ear diseases
V81	Special screening for cardiovascular, respiratory, and genitourinary diseases
V82	Special screening for other conditions
V83	Genetic carrier status

APPENDIX E: LIST OF THREE-DIGIT CATEGORIES

SUPPLEMENTARY CLASSIFICATION OF EXTERNAL CAUSES OF INJURY AND POISONING

Railway accidents (E800-E807)
- E800 Railway accident involving collision with rolling stock
- E801 Railway accident involving collision with other object
- E802 Railway accident involving derailment without antecedent collision
- E803 Railway accident involving explosion, fire, or burning
- E804 Fall in, on, or from railway train
- E805 Hit by rolling stock
- E806 Other specified railway accident
- E807 Railway accident of unspecified nature

Motor vehicle traffic accidents (E810-E819)
- E810 Motor vehicle traffic accident involving collision with train
- E811 Motor vehicle traffic accident involving re-entrant collision with another motor vehicle
- E812 Other motor vehicle traffic accident involving collision with another motor vehicle
- E813 Motor vehicle traffic accident involving collision with other vehicle
- E814 Motor vehicle traffic accident involving collision with pedestrian
- E815 Other motor vehicle traffic accident involving collision on the highway
- E816 Motor vehicle traffic accident due to loss of control, without collision on the highway
- E817 Noncollision motor vehicle traffic accident while boarding or alighting
- E818 Other noncollision motor vehicle traffic accident
- E819 Motor vehicle traffic accident of unspecified nature

Motor vehicle nontraffic accidents (E820-E825)
- E820 Nontraffic accident involving motor-driven snow vehicle
- E821 Nontraffic accident involving other off-road motor vehicle
- E822 Other motor vehicle nontraffic accident involving collision with moving object
- E823 Other motor vehicle nontraffic accident involving collision with stationary object
- E824 Other motor vehicle nontraffic accident while boarding and alighting
- E825 Other motor vehicle nontraffic accident of other and unspecified nature

Other road vehicle accidents (E826-E829)
- E826 Pedal cycle accident
- E827 Animal-drawn vehicle accident
- E828 Accident involving animal being ridden
- E829 Other road vehicle accidents

Water transport accidents (E830-E838)
- E830 Accident to watercraft causing submersion
- E831 Accident to watercraft causing other injury
- E832 Other accidental submersion or drowning in water transport accident
- E833 Fall on stairs or ladders in water transport
- E834 Other fall from one level to another in water transport
- E835 Other and unspecified fall in water transport
- E836 Machinery accident in water transport
- E837 Explosion, fire, or burning in watercraft
- E838 Other and unspecified water transport accident

Air and space transport accidents (E840-E845)
- E840 Accident to powered aircraft at takeoff or landing
- E841 Accident to powered aircraft, other and unspecified
- E842 Accident to unpowered aircraft
- E843 Fall in, on, or from aircraft
- E844 Other specified air transport accidents
- E845 Accident involving spacecraft

Vehicle accidents, not elsewhere classifiable (E846-E849)
- E846 Accidents involving powered vehicles used solely within the buildings and premises of an industrial or commercial establishment
- E847 Accidents involving cable cars not running on rails
- E848 Accidents involving other vehicles, not elsewhere classifiable
- E849 Place of occurrence

Accidental poisoning by drugs, medicinal substances, and biologicals (E850-E858)
- E850 Accidental poisoning by analgesics, antipyretics, and antirheumatics
- E851 Accidental poisoning by barbiturates
- E852 Accidental poisoning by other sedatives and hypnotics
- E853 Accidental poisoning by tranquilizers
- E854 Accidental poisoning by other psychotropic agents
- E855 Accidental poisoning by other drugs acting on central and autonomic nervous systems
- E856 Accidental poisoning by antibiotics

APPENDIX E: LIST OF THREE-DIGIT CATEGORIES

E857 Accidental poisoning by anti-infectives
E858 Accidental poisoning by other drugs

Accidental poisoning by other solid and liquid substances, gases, and vapors (E860-E869)
E860 Accidental poisoning by alcohol, not elsewhere classified
E861 Accidental poisoning by cleansing and polishing agents, disinfectants, paints, and varnishes
E862 Accidental poisoning by petroleum products, other solvents and their vapors, not elsewhere classified
E863 Accidental poisoning by agricultural and horticultural chemical and pharmaceutical preparations other than plant foods and fertilizers
E864 Accidental poisoning by corrosives and caustics, not elsewhere classified
E865 Accidental poisoning from poisonous foodstuffs and poisonous plants
E866 Accidental poisoning by other and unspecified solid and liquid substances
E867 Accidental poisoning by gas distributed by pipeline
E868 Accidental poisoning by other utility gas and other carbon monoxide
E869 Accidental poisoning by other gases and vapors

Misadventures to patients during surgical and medical care (E870-E876)
E870 Accidental cut, puncture, perforation, or hemorrhage during medical care
E871 Foreign object left in body during procedure
E872 Failure of sterile precautions during procedure
E873 Failure in dosage
E874 Mechanical failure of instrument or apparatus during procedure
E875 Contaminated or infected blood, other fluid, drug, or biological substance
E876 Other and unspecified misadventures during medical care

Surgical and medical procedures as the cause of abnormal reaction of patient or later complication, without mention of misadventure at the time of procedure (E878-E879)
E878 Surgical operation and other surgical procedures as the cause of abnormal reaction of patient, or of later complication, without mention of misadventure at the time of operation
E879 Other procedures, without mention of misadventure at the time of procedure, as the cause of abnormal reaction of patient, or of later complication

Accidental falls (E880-E888)
E880 Fall on or from stairs or steps
E881 Fall on or from ladders or scaffolding
E882 Fall from or out of building or other structure
E883 Fall into hole or other opening in surface
E884 Other fall from one level to another
E885 Fall on same level from slipping, tripping, or stumbling
E886 Fall on same level from collision, pushing or shoving, by or with other person
E887 Fracture, cause unspecified
E888 Other and unspecified fall

Accidents caused by fire and flames (E890-E899)
E890 Conflagration in private dwelling
E891 Conflagration in other and unspecified building or structure
E892 Conflagration not in building or structure
E893 Accident caused by ignition of clothing
E894 Ignition of highly inflammable material
E895 Accident caused by controlled fire in private dwelling
E896 Accident caused by controlled fire in other and unspecified building or structure
E897 Accident caused by controlled fire not in building or structure
E898 Accident caused by other specified fire and flames
E899 Accident caused by unspecified fire

Accidents due to natural and environmental factors (E900-E909)
E900 Excessive heat
E901 Excessive cold
E902 High and low air pressure and changes in air pressure
E903 Travel and motion
E904 Hunger, thirst, exposure, and neglect
E905 Venomous animals and plants as the cause of poisoning and toxic reactions
E906 Other injury caused by animals
E907 Lightning
E908 Cataclysmic storms, and floods resulting from storms
E909 Cataclysmic earth surface movements and eruptions

APPENDIX E: LIST OF THREE-DIGIT CATEGORIES

Accidents caused by submersion, suffocation, and foreign bodies (E910-E915)
E910   Accidental drowning and submersion
E911   Inhalation and ingestion of food causing obstruction of respiratory tract or suffocation
E912   Inhalation and ingestion of other object causing obstruction of respiratory tract or suffocation
E913   Accidental mechanical suffocation
E914   Foreign body accidentally entering eye and adnexa
E915   Foreign body accidentally entering other orifice

Other accidents (E916-E928)
E916   Struck accidentally by falling object
E917   Striking against or struck accidentally by objects or persons
E918   Caught accidentally in or between objects
E919   Accidents caused by machinery
E920   Accidents caused by cutting and piercing instruments or objects
E921   Accident caused by explosion of pressure vessel
E922   Accident caused by firearm missile
E923   Accident caused by explosive material
E924   Accident caused by hot substance or object, caustic or corrosive material, and steam
E925   Accident caused by electric current
E926   Exposure to radiation
E927   Overexertion and strenuous movements
E928   Other and unspecified environmental and accidental causes

Late effects of accidental injury (E929)
E929   Late effects of accidental injury

Drugs, medicinal and biological substances causing adverse effects in therapeutic use (E930-E949)
E930   Antibiotics
E931   Other anti-infectives
E932   Hormones and synthetic substitutes
E933   Primarily systemic agents
E934   Agents primarily affecting blood constituents
E935   Analgesics, antipyretics, and antirheumatics
E936   Anticonvulsants and anti-Parkinsonism drugs
E937   Sedatives and hypnotics
E938   Other central nervous system depressants and anesthetics
E939   Psychotropic agents
E940   Central nervous system stimulants
E941   Drugs primarily affecting the autonomic nervous system
E942   Agents primarily affecting the cardiovascular system
E943   Agents primarily affecting gastrointestinal system
E944   Water, mineral, and uric acid metabolism drugs
E945   Agents primarily acting on the smooth and skeletal muscles and respiratory system
E946   Agents primarily affecting skin and mucous membrane, ophthalmological, otorhinolaryngological, and dental drugs
E947   Other and unspecified drugs and medicinal substances
E948   Bacterial vaccines
E949   Other vaccines and biological substances

Suicide and self-inflicted injury (E950-E959)
E950   Suicide and self-inflicted poisoning by solid or liquid substances
E951   Suicide and self-inflicted poisoning by gases in domestic use
E952   Suicide and self-inflicted poisoning by other gases and vapors
E953   Suicide and self-inflicted injury by hanging, strangulation, and suffocation
E954   Suicide and self-inflicted injury by submersion [drowning]
E955   Suicide and self-inflicted injury by firearms and explosives
E956   Suicide and self-inflicted injury by cutting and piercing instruments
E957   Suicide and self-inflicted injuries by jumping from high place
E958   Suicide and self-inflicted injury by other and unspecified means
E959   Late effects of self-inflicted injury

Homicide and injury purposely inflicted by other persons (E960-E969)
E960   Fight, brawl, and rape
E961   Assault by corrosive or caustic substance, except poisoning
E962   Assault by poisoning
E963   Assault by hanging and strangulation
E964   Assault by submersion [drowning]
E965   Assault by firearms and explosives
E966   Assault by cutting and piercing instrument
E967   Child and adult battering and other maltreatment
E968   Assault by other and unspecified means
E969   Late effects of injury purposely inflicted by other person

Legal intervention (E970-E978)
E970   Injury due to legal intervention by firearms

APPENDIX E: LIST OF THREE-DIGIT CATEGORIES

E971 Injury due to legal intervention by explosives
E972 Injury due to legal intervention by gas
E973 Injury due to legal intervention by blunt object
E974 Injury due to legal intervention by cutting and piercing instruments
E975 Injury due to legal intervention by other specified means
E976 Injury due to legal intervention by unspecified means
E977 Late effects of injuries due to legal intervention
E978 Legal execution

Terrorism (E979)
E979 Terrorism

Injury undetermined whether accidentally or purposely inflicted (E980-E989)
E980 Poisoning by solid or liquid substances, undetermined whether accidentally or purposely inflicted
E981 Poisoning by gases in domestic use, undetermined whether accidentally or purposely inflicted
E982 Poisoning by other gases, undetermined whether accidentally or purposely inflicted
E983 Hanging, strangulation, or suffocation, undetermined whether accidentally or purposely inflicted
E984 Submersion [drowning], undetermined whether accidentally or purposely inflicted
E985 Injury by firearms and explosives, undetermined whether accidentally or purposely inflicted
E986 Injury by cutting and piercing instruments, undetermined whether accidentally or purposely inflicted
E987 Falling from high place, undetermined whether accidentally or purposely inflicted
E988 Injury by other and unspecified means, undetermined whether accidentally or purposely inflicted
E989 Late effects of injury, undetermined whether accidentally or purposely inflicted

Injury resulting from operations of war (E990-E999)
E990 Injury due to war operations by fires and conflagrations
E991 Injury due to war operations by bullets and fragments
E992 Injury due to war operations by explosion of marine weapons
E993 Injury due to war operations by other explosion
E994 Injury due to war operations by destruction of aircraft
E995 Injury due to war operations by other and unspecified forms of conventional warfare
E996 Injury due to war operations by nuclear weapons
E997 Injury due to war operations by other forms of unconventional warfare
E998 Injury due to war operations but occurring after cessation of hostilities
E999 Late effects of injury due to war operations